SAVILL'S SYSTEM OF CLINICAL MEDICINE

SAVILL'S SYSTEM OF CLINICAL MEDICINE

DEALING WITH THE

DIAGNOSIS, PROGNOSIS, AND TREATMENT OF DISEASE

FOR

STUDENTS AND PRACTITIONERS

EDITED BY

E. C. WARNER, M.D., F.R.C.P.

FOURTEENTH EDITION

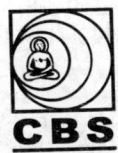

CBS Publishers & Distributors Pvt. Ltd.

New Delhi • Bengaluru • Chennai • Kochi • Kolkata • Mumbai
Hyderabad • Nagpur • Patna • Pune • Vijayawada

ISBN: 81-239-0911-X

First Indian Edition: 1980
Reprint: 1998, 2003, 2005

Copyright © E.C. Warner, 1964

First published in England by Edward Arnold (Publishers) Ltd.
41, Bedford Square, London, WCIB 3 DP.

Published by **Satish Kumar Jain** and produced by **Varun Jain** for
CBS Publishers & Distributors Pvt. Ltd.,
4819/XI Prahlad Street, 24 Ansari Road, Daryaganj, New Delhi - 110002
delhi@cbspd.com, cbspubs@airtelmail.in • www.cbspd.com
Ph.: 23289259, 23266861, 23266867 • Fax: 011-23243014

Corporate Office: 204 FIE, Industrial Area, Patparganj, Delhi - 110 092
Ph: 49344934 • Fax: 011-49344935
E-mail: publishing@cbspd.com • publicity@cbspd.com

Branches:
• *Bengaluru:* 2975, 17th Cross, K.R. Road, Bansankari 2nd Stage,
  Bengaluru - 70 • Ph: +91-80-26771678/79 • Fax: +91-80-26771680
  E-mail: csbng@gmail.com, bangalore@cbspd.com
• *Chennai:* No. 7, Subbaraya Street, Shenoy Nagar, Chennai - 600030
  Ph: +91-44-26681266, 26680620 • Fax: +91-44-42032115
  E-mail: chennai@cbspd.com
• *Kochi:* Ashana House, 39/1904, A.M. Thomas Road, Valanjambalam,
  Ernakulum, Kochi • Ph: +91-484-4059061-65
  Fax: +91-484-4059065 • E-mail: cochin@cbspd.com
• *Kolkata:* 6-B, Ground Floor, Rameshwar Shaw Road, Kolkata - 700014
  Ph: +91-33-22891126/7/8 • E-mail: kolkata@cbspd.com
• *Mumbai:* 83-C, Dr. E. Moses Road, Worli, Mumbai - 400018
  Ph: +91-9833017933, 022-24902340/41 • E-mail: mumbai@cbspd.com

Representatives:

• Hyderabad: 0-9885175004	• Nagpur: 0-9021734563
• Patna: 0-9334159340	• Pune: 0-9623451994
• Jharkhand: 0-9811541605	• Uttarakhand: 0-9716462459

Printed at:
India Binding House, Noida, UP (India)

PREFACE TO THE FOURTEENTH EDITION

MOST text-books of Medicine start by assuming the diagnosis of the various diseases, and then set out the symptoms which should be found. Over fifty years ago, Dr. T. D. Savill realised that this is not the way any practising physician goes to work in his consulting-room or at the bedside: what he does is to listen to the patient's history, select the principal (or cardinal) symptoms, and by a process of integration with the other clinical features, arrives at a tentative diagnosis. He then proceeds to consider the probable cause of the condition and any alternative diagnosis, he weighs up the prognosis and then undertakes the treatment of his patient. Dr. Savill therefore constructed a text-book of medicine on these lines—and the success of this Savill System is demonstrated once more by the ever increasing popularity of this book which has now reached its fourteenth edition.

It is no small task to combine the features of a system of this kind with the ever-increasing advances of medical knowledge and medical science: particularly have I attempted to show that there is still an art as well as a science in Medicine: correct diagnosis, the essential preliminary of correct treatment, is not a matter of studying the results of X-ray and other investigations. Medical practice at its best will always demand of the physician that he should first give time to assess the mental and physical symptoms of his patient before effecting a physical examination in an effort to arrive at a diagnosis; only a proportion of patients will then need X-rays and other ancillary methods to confirm or refute the diagnosis. For this art of diagnosis a long period of training as a physician, combined with a sympathy for the human problems created by disease and a knowledge of the pathological effects produced, are all necessary. This Art of Medicine, developed over the years by trained and observant medical men and women, is beyond the understanding of unskilled and untrained political planners.

This new edition is some 300 pages longer than its immediate predecessor; and it now contains 66 tables, 274 figures and 23 plates. A much more liberal use has been made of colours for 9 plates are thus presented, and in the neurological chapter two colours have often been used to outline the main tracts of the brain and spinal cord. I am fully conscious of the disadvantages of increasing the size of the book, but the advances in Medicine have made this inevitable; I am very grateful to the various contributors for allowing me such liberty in pruning their text in order to avoid repetition and to limit the size of this volume. Within the present compass the aim has been to add a description of most of the recently described diseases and of the techniques in common use. At the end of the book a new feature is the various tables which should be useful for quick reference: these give the average weights of normal men and women of different statures, the normal ranges of blood counts and the normal values obtained in the examination of the blood and other tissue fluids.

v

Chapter I, which describes the rules for clinical investigation as written by Dr. T. D. Savill, has been little altered over the years; no great change has been made in this new edition. In the chapters which follow, the Savill System as described in Chapter I has been kept to throughout. To bring the text up to date no page has escaped alteration in one way or another, and some chapters have been almost entirely rewritten. Chapter VI on the Lungs and Pleuræ has previously been the responsibility of Dr. Maurice Davidson. This time I have not had the help of his polished writing and so I have rewritten most of the chapter myself, and in so doing have borne in mind the great advances in X-ray techniques and in treatment of the pulmonary diseases due to chemotherapy and the antibiotics. To rewrite Chapter XIV dealing with Diseases of the Female Reproductive System I have been fortunate enough to enlis: the help of Dr. Josephine Barnes. In Chapter XVIII which deals with Diseases of the Skin, Dr. Arthur Rook has followed the outline plan used by Dr. Agnes Savill in so many previous editions, but he has rewritten the entire chapter in accordance with modern dermatological teaching and has added a section on disease of the nails. The long neurological chapter (Chapter XIX) has always been a credit to the book in the able hands of Dr. Redvers Ironside; in this edition he has found it necessary to rewrite almost the whole chapter and in doing so has lost none of his clarity of presentation. This time we agreed to separate the Diseases of the Special Senses from this chapter for they now merit a short chapter on their own (Chapter XX); it behoves every physician to have a good working knowledge of the various diseases affecting the Eyes and the Ears—especially when the former so often give fundamental information as to disease elsewhere and now that antibiotics have so greatly lessened the need for surgical interference in the ears. Happily Mr. Norman Fleming has been able to continue to give of his expert help in this extended version of Diseases of the Eyes and Mr. A. P. Ardouin has helped me write the section on Diseases of the Ears. I also welcome to this new edition Dr. P. B. S. Fowler who has been responsible for Chapter V dealing with the Pulse and Arteries, Dr. David Erskine who has revised the sections dealing with Ver°real Diseases, Dr. Twining McMath who has brought up to date the Infective Diseases (Chapter XV). Dr. E. Neumark has supplied the expert knowledge necessary to revise the description of the Diseases of the Blood in Chapter XVI. Other new contributors are Dr. F. D. Schofield who follows Dr. F. Murgatroyd in describing Tropical Diseases and Professor R. A. Shooter who has dealt with the problems of Preventive Methods and Immunity and with Chapter XXII on the Examination of Pathological Material. Professor Paul Polani has written and illustrated a new section which describes the ever-widening field of chromosomal abnormalities in relation to disease conditions.

It is sad to have to mention that two contributors died shortly after completing their sections. Dr. S. W. Patterson revised the Chapters dealing with Diseases of the Digestive System—I spent many profitable hours with him revising these, and recasting the Diseases of the Liver, Gall-bladder, Pancreas and Spleen which are now described under separate headings. Unfortunately Dr. Thomas Tennent has not lived to see in print the results of his labours in Chapter XXI relating to the Psychological Disorders.

I have again been fortunate in having the help of a team of experts who helped with previous editions. My best thanks are due to Dr. Geoffrey Bourne who revised the Cardiological Chapter (Chapter III), to Mr. L. R. Broster who helped with the Abdomen (Chapter IX), to Mr. W. A. Mill for parts of the Diseases of the Nose, Throat, Larynx and Œsophagus, to Mr. Arthur Gray who has again written the section on Sterility and to Dr. F. S. Warner who has revised Diseases of the Mouth.

It is impossible to draw up a list of all the new subjects which find a place in this System for the first time and only a few examples must suffice. Such are carcinoid tumours, the carpal tunnel syndrome, cryoglobulinæmia, erythræmic myelosis, hiatus hernia, kwashiorkor, the malabsorption syndrome and steatorrhœa, pleural biopsy, chronic œsophagitis, temporal arteritis and the Wolff-Parkinson-White syndrome. New tables include one on the newer antidiabetic drugs and insulins (Table XXV) and of necessity an entire revision of those dealing with the effects of the chemotherapeutic and antibiotic drugs on various organisms (Tables XXXV and XXXVI).

To these main contributors and to many others I must add my grateful thanks for such unstinting help. The latter include Dr. H. Post, Dr. Charles MacLean, Dr. Seymour Reynolds and Dr. David Sutton, who have lent X-ray films for reproduction; Dr. John Swale who has drawn up the tables of biochemical analyses and helped with his specialised knowledge on such subjects as paper chromatography and electrophoresis; Dr. D. O'Connell who helped to write the section on the effect of Ionising Radiations; and Dr. W. F. Dunham who has rewritten the section dealing with the Electrical Examination of Muscles and Nerves. Miss P. M. Turnbull has greatly assisted with a number of beautiful photographic reproductions which make a text-book of this kind so much more enjoyable. My especial thanks go to my secretary, Miss C. G. Sharvelle, who has spent so many hours and days typing the new material, to Dr. J. N. Mickerson who helped with the proof reading, and to Mr. Brian Armitage who is in charge in the Charing Cross Hospital Medical School library—he has undertaken the arduous and responsible task of preparing the index. I already see imperfections in the text but hope these are few and do not detract from a useful new Edition of this well-known text-book; particularly must I take responsibility for defects in Chapters II, IV, VI, VII, VIII, XIII, XVI and XVII which have been largely, or almost entirely rewritten by me. Throughout it has been my earnest endeavour to present the reader with a text which is written and presented in as clear a form as possible.

E. C. WARNER.

London, N.W.1

LIST OF CONTRIBUTORS

JOSEPHINE BARNES, M.A., D.M.(Oxon.), M.R.C.P.(Lond.), F.R.C.S.(Eng.), F.R.C.O.G., Consultant Obstetrician and Gynæcologist, Charing Cross Hospital and The Elizabeth Garrett Anderson Hospital.

GEOFFREY BOURNE, M.D., F.R.C.P., Consulting Physician and Consulting Cardiologist, St. Batholomew's Hospital.

L. R. BROSTER, O.B.E., M.A.(Oxon.), D.M., F.R.C.S.(Eng.), Consulting Surgeon, Charing Cross Hospital; Honorary Fellow of the American Surgical Association.

W. F. DUNHAM, B.A., B.M., B.Ch.(Oxon.), D.Phys.Med.(Eng.), Physician, Departments of Physical Medicine, Charing Cross Hospital and Wembley Hospital.

DAVID ERSKINE, M.D., D.P.H., Consultant Venereologist, Seamen's Group of Hospitals.

NORMAN FLEMING, M.B., Ch.B., D.O.M.S., Consulting Ophthalmic Surgeon, Prince of Wales's General Hospital, Tottenham.

P. B. S. FOWLER, D.M.(Oxon.), F.R.C.P.(Lond.), Consultant Physician, Charing Cross Hospital and Harrow Hospital.

ARTHUR GRAY, M.D., F.R.C.S.(Eng.), F.R.C.O.G., Consulting Obstetric and Gynæcological Surgeon, Charing Cross Hospital, The Hampstead General Hospital and The Miller General Hospital.

REDVERS IRONSIDE, M.B.(Aberdeen), F.R.C.P.(Lond.), Consultant Physician, Charing Cross Hospital; Senior Physician, Maida Vale Hospital for Nervous Diseases; Consulting Physician for Neurological Diseases, West London Hospital.

W. F. TWINING MCMATH, M.D., M.R.C.P.(Lond.), D.P.H., Physician-Superintendent, Neasden Hospital, London; Consultant Physician, West Hendon Hospital, and Spittlesea Infectious Diseases Hospital, Luton; Lecturer in Infectious Diseases, Charing Cross Hospital Medical School.

W. A. MILL, M.S., F.R.C.S., Consulting Surgeon, Ear, Nose and Throat Department, St. Thomas's Hospital, Royal Marsden Hospital and Royal Masonic Hospital.

E. NEUMARK, M.D.(Lond.), Lecturer in Pathology, St. Mary's Hospital Medical School; Medical Adviser to the Hæmophilia Society.

S. W. PATTERSON, M.D., D.Sc., F.R.C.P.(Lond.), late Senior Physician, Ruthin Castle Clinic.

PAUL E. POLANI, M.D.(Pisa), F.R.C.P.(Lond.), D.C.H.(Eng.), Prince Philip Professor of Pædiatric Research, Guy's Hospital Medical School.

ARTHUR ROOK, M.A., M.D.(Cantab.), F.R.C.P.(Lond.), Consultant Dermatologist, Addenbrooke's Hospital, Cambridge.

F. D. SCHOFIELD, M.D.(Cantab.), M.R.C.P.(Lond.), D.T.M. and H.(Eng.), recently Senior Lecturer, Dept. of Clinical Tropical Medicine, London School of Hygiene and Tropical Medicine; Asst. Director of Medical Services (Medical Research), Dept. of Health, Territory of Papua and New Guinea.

R. A. SHOOTER, M.A., M.D.(Cantab.), M.R.C.P.(Lond.), Professor of Bacteriology, University of London; Consultant Bacteriologist to St. Bartholomew's Hospital.

THOMAS TENNENT, M.D., F.R.C.P., D.P.H., D.P.M., late Medical Superintendent, St. Andrew's Hospital, Northampton; late Physician in Psychological Medicine, Northampton General Hospital.

E. C. WARNER, M.D., B.Sc., F.R.C.P.(Lond.), Physician, Charing Cross Hospital; recently Dean, Charing Cross Hospital Medical School; Senior Physician, Putney Hospital.

F. S. WARNER, F.D.S.R.C.S., L.R.C.P., M.R.C.S., Consultant Dental and Oral Surgeon, Guy's Hospital; Dean of Dental Studies, Guy's Hospital Dental School.

CONTENTS

LIST OF PLATES

LIST OF COLOUR PLATES

ILLUSTRATIONS IN THE TEXT

xii

LIST OF TABLES

INTRODUCTION

EVOLUTION

THOSE who ponder on general principles and methods will have observed that a considerable change has gradually taken place during the last half-century in the methods of studying the science and art of medicine. Formerly, men were content to observe the symptoms or effects of disease at the bedside and in the dead-house, and to speculate on the etiological connection of these two series of phenomena. Wherever the association of such phenomena during life and after death was sufficiently constant, they were spoken of collectively as a " disease " ; when a group of symptoms without anatomical lesion constantly recurred, it received a name and place among the list of " disorders." Then each disease or disorder was taken as a separate entity, its anatomy, symptoms, diagnosis and treatment were described, and its various possible etiological factors discussed ; and the result was known as " Descriptive " or " Systematic Medicine." The guiding principle of this descriptive process was the tracing from an assumed *cause* to a known *effect*.

In recent years great advances have been achieved, almost synchronously, in two very different directions. On the one hand great improvements have been made in the methods of observing and investigating the symptoms or effects of disease during life, and thus Clinical Medicine came into separate existence. On the other hand, with the rapid growth of chemical, biological and bacteriological sciences, and the elaboration of experimental methods in the investigation of disease processes, there has been the pathological approach, whose methods have been based upon experiment, and whose leading principle is the artificial production of a definite *cause* and the observing of its *effects*. The extraordinary advances made by these means, and the new light thus shed upon the science of medicine during the last few decades, have formed at once the wonder and delight of the civilised world.

As the result of these movements, treatises on Systematic Medicine, which attempt to deal at all fully with both the clinical and the pathological aspects of disease, have come to assume very considerable dimensions. In many of them there seems to be a tendency to become more and more pathological in their arrangement, and to treat diseases as separate entities, so that students of clinical medicine and busy practitioners, whose daily work consists of an endeavour to trace from *effect* to *cause*, have been heard to complain that they do not always find in them the clinical aid they seek.

ORIGIN

Immediately after embarking on medical practice I realised the importance for diagnostic purposes of reviewing the various diseases or pathological conditions which might give rise to a patient's leading symptom or symptoms, and being unable to find precisely the information desired in any of the current text-books, I proceeded to keep a brief record of all the cases I met arranged under the heading of their leading symptom. This book is based upon those records, which extend over many years, combined with the valuable knowledge imparted to me at the bedside by my teachers—more especially Dr. Charles Murchison, Dr. J. S. Bristowe, Professor J. M. Charcot and Sir William Broadbent. Hospital cliniques, at first of a general and later of a more special kind, have always been at my command; but it was at the Paddington Workhouse and Infirmary that the idea of this work was conceived, its foundations laid, and the chief part of its " skeleton " constructed. Here there has been a vast and almost unexplored field of every possible variety of disease, which can be studied from day to day from the beginning *to the end* of its course.

PLAN

In this work, the subject is approached from the standpoint of symptomatology. The principle throughout will be to trace from effect (symptoms) to cause (the morbid cause in operation). The order of sequence will be that which should be adopted in the examination of a patient. Thus, the first chapter will give a general scheme for the examination of a case, and will deal with certain general principles underlying methods of observation, diagnosis, prognosis and treatment. In the second chapter the physiognomy of disease will be discussed. The succeeding chapters will deal seriatim with the symptoms and signs referable to the several organs or anatomical regions of the body, and the disease which may cause those symptoms.

Each chapter is divided into three unequal parts. Part A. treats the *symptoms* which may indicate disease of the organ or region under discussion, the fallacies incidental to their detection, and a brief differential account of the various causes which may give rise to those symptoms. Part B. treats the *physical signs* of disease in that region, and the various methods used to elicit them. Part C., which constitutes the major portion of each chapter, is prefaced by a *clinical classification* of the various maladies affecting that region, and a summary of the routine procedure to be adopted; and this is followed by a series of sections dealing with the several *diseases*, arranged according to their clinical relationships. For example, in Chapter III., on The Heart—Part A. describes and differentiates the various causes of breathlessness, dropsy, palpitation, precordial pain and the other symptoms which may be indicative of heart disease; Part B. describes percussion, auscultation and the other methods of examining the heart; and Part C. deals seriatim with the various cardiac disorders, classified and arranged on a clinical basis.

SPECIAL FEATURES

Apart from this general plan, there are two features special to this work. The first part of each chapter, dealing with symptoms and their causes, forms a feature on which great labour has been expended. To make each list of causes complete without redundance, and to check the various data again and again in the light of experience, has involved an expenditure of time quite out of proportion to the space occupied. These lists will, I trust, be as useful to others as they have been to me in obtaining a clue to diagnosis.

Another feature consists of the italicised paragraphs in Part C. standing at the head of each section, which deal with each separate disease. These emphasise the salient features by which a disease may be recognised and differentiated from others belonging to the same clinical group. They are, in fact, brief clinical definitions, and form, metaphorically speaking, " sign-posts " or guides in the process of diagnosis. If, after carefully studying the lists of symptoms and their causes in Part A., and examining his patient (Part B.), the reader turns to these italicised paragraphs in Part C., the work will, it is hoped, serve as a " clinical index of diseases "; for by following the plan laid down he will shortly find himself reading a description of the diagnosis, prognosis, and treatment of the malady from which his patient is probably suffering; while adjacent to this are the disorders which clinically, and very often pathologically, resemble it, and for which in practice it is apt to be mistaken.

Such an arrangement as this must inevitably lead to some repetition, but this difficulty has been obviated to some extent by cross-references. I would also ask the reader to remember that nothing fixes things so well in our minds, or aids us so much in tracing those analogies to which I shall shortly refer, as constantly looking at the same facts from a different point of view.

An attempt has been made to present the various diseases in some kind of perspective by placing them as far as possible in order of importance and using different sized types. The relative importance of different subjects in medicine is largely a matter of opinion, and I cannot expect to escape criticism in this respect.

It is a standing accusation against medical writers that they are care-less in respect of literary style. I have striven to be intelligible rather than academic; and in general I must plead guilty to having endeavoured to follow the Duchess's advice to Alice in Wonderland, to " take care of the sense and the sounds will take care of themselves." When so large an area has to be covered, a certain amount of abbreviation is indispensable, and in order to condense my material, it has been my practice to adopt a numerical method of description. Some may take exception to this, though the student will find it to his advantage in the acquisition of knowledge.

ADVANTAGES

I may perhaps be pardoned for adverting to certain advantages which appear to me to be associated with the method that I have adopted of approaching clinical medicine. And first let me remark that this method of diagnosis is not what has been called a " process of exclusion." It is a positive rather than a negative process, for by carefully considering the various causal diseases which may be in operation and balancing the evidence for and against each, the physician is guided, not to the least improbable, but to the most probable diagnosis.

The advantages of passing in rapid review all the possible diseases which may give rise to a patient's leading symptom are very obvious to those actively engaged in clinical work. It is now often the method used in bedside teaching. Yet I am not aware that any work has yet been published which adopts precisely this plan of approaching clinical medicine.

This plan gives a truer view of nature's facts than one which deals with diseases as so many separate entities. We see a case in all its clinical and practical bearings. We not only learn that the diagnosis of a patient's illness can at best be only a question of the greatest probability, but with almost mathematical precision we can also assess the probability or improbability of each of the other possible causes in operation. We learn further that all diagnoses can only be provisional, and that the degree of probability of each possible cause changes from day to day, like the coloured pattern of the kaleidoscope, as the course of the disease unfolds itself before us.

The recognition of a clinical likeness between diseases has often led to the erection of a " working hypothesis " which by subsequent research has been found to be correct. Many of our greatest discoveries have been initiated in this way. It was, for instance, a process of this kind which led to the discovery that a large number of pyrexial disorders are of microbic origin. There are still a number, notably measles, small-pox and scarlatina, in which such a working hypothesis, based on clinical resemblances, forms at present the full extent of our knowledge; but so precise are these foundations that the microbic nature of these diseases is never doubted. Hypotheses framed in this way should always be tested and confirmed in the laboratory and dead-house, whenever the morbid conditions can be produced experimentally, or when they are attended by fatal results. But there are still a great many diseases, such, for instance, as the two great groups of clinical conditions we call hysteria and neurasthenia (conditions which form a considerable portion of the practitioner's daily work), which cannot, except in the most isolated instances, be observed in the dead-house, and which have not yet been reproduced in animals. In these cases the method of analogy or comparison to which I have just referred is not only a valuable means of investigation, it forms almost the only means we have.

Only few are able to devote the necessary time to laboratory research; but all can study their cases at the bedside in the way indicated, and many a valuable and often unrecorded idea as to treatment will occur to the practitioner who thinks out and traces analogies between diseases.

There is yet another advantage which has always appeared to me to accrue, especially to the young observer, by this process of balancing evidence and comparing diseases. It not only impresses important facts upon his memory, but it constitutes one of the best possible means of training him to habits of accurate and complete observation, and of systematic and productive thought. The scope of his horizon is widened, his faculty of systematising his knowledge becomes by practice wonderfully increased, and his reasoning powers strengthened and corrected. He finds intuitively that without accuracy in respect to the most minute details he may be led astray in the more important ones, that without system in the arrangement of his facts he will never be able to attach the proper significance and importance to each; and finally, that without judgment in attaching due weight to each item of evidence, his conclusions may be erroneous although his premises and facts are correct.

RESPONSIBILITIES

I have now described the scheme of this work, its purposes and scope—in a word, the ideal which I hope to compass; and I believe no one could approach a task of this kind without realising the responsibilities and difficulties involved in its execution. Amidst the bewildering records of medicine there are many excellent treatises both on systematic medicine and on one or other of the several departments of clinical medicine. These deal with their respective subjects in a manner which I cannot hope to rival, but they have afforded me no exact precedent or guide along the path I wished to travel. The contemplation of the wide range of knowledge and experience required, of the immense advances which have recently been made both in the theory and practice of medicine, of the supreme importance of the subjects here dealt with, involving as they do questions of life and death, has filled my mind with a painful sense of the obligation imposed upon me to sift my facts, and to cull my knowledge from all sources, but, before all, to obtain my material as far as possible by careful observation and patient thought from the book of nature which lay open before me from day to day at the bedside in infirmary, hospital and private practice.

In these circumstances I have gladly availed myself of the help and advice of many friends. It is especially difficult for me to express in measured terms my indebtedness to my wife, who has assisted me in the elaboration of this work during the greater part of four years. Her skill and knowledge have helped to give it such completeness as it may possess; her patient industry has afforded me not only assistance, but example; and her companionship and encouragement have made many rough places smooth, and have often transformed what at times seemed to be a laborious and interminable task into a pastime.

T. D. SAVILL

1909

A SYSTEM OF CLINICAL MEDICINE

CHAPTER I

CLINICAL METHODS

Preliminary Definitions—Case-Taking—Methods of Diagnosis, Prognosis and Treatment—Rules for Clinical Investigation.

§ 1. Definitions.—Disease is a departure from health, and is manifested in an individual during life by symptoms. These are of two kinds—" *subjective symptoms*," which are recognisable only by the patient, and present no external indication, such as pain, itching, or a feeling of chilliness; and " *objective symptoms*," [1] which can be detected by the observer—*e.g.*, abdominal enlargement or dullness on percussion. The word " symptom " is used in two senses. Sometimes it is used in a general sense to indicate all the subjective and objective evidence of a disease; but more usually it is employed in a narrower sense, as synonymous with subjective symptoms. Objective symptoms are usually spoken of as *signs*; and those objective symptoms which are made out by physical examination are known as *physical signs*.

Just as the value and significance of physical signs depend on the skill and experience of the physician who observes them, so the significance of subjective symptoms has to be weighed and considered in relation to the character and constitution of the patient who complains of them. Thus a certain symptom may appear trivial and unimportant to a patient of strong character not addicted to introspection, although serious disease may be present; whereas in women with a susceptible nervous system every subjective symptom, however slight, may cause great anxiety, exaggeration, and even real suffering. Submammary pain, for instance, in the first might indicate aneurysm; in the second, hysteria.

General (or constitutional) symptoms are those which relate to the whole body, such as debility or pyrexia.

A *latent disease* is one which is unattended by any very obvious symptoms. Thus, we speak of latent pulmonary tuberculosis when a patient suffering from tuberculosis of the lung has none of the more usual symptoms of that disorder. Physical signs are not necessarily absent in latent disease, but they are often difficult to detect. Some writers speak of a malady as being latent when pain, which is usually a prominent feature of the disease, is absent. Thus, pericarditis is ordinarily attended by a

---

[1] These words " subjective " and " objective " are borrowed from philosophy. Subjective reality is reality which exists in the mind only, whereas objective reality is that which can be demonstrated by means of tangible, visible or outward signs.

good deal of pain, but pain is absent in the latent form of pericarditis which so frequently complicates rheumatic fever, and in the latent peritonitis which complicates typhoid fever.

A *paroxysmal disorder* is one which comes on in the form of attacks separated by intervals of comparative health. Each attack or paroxysm consists of a stage of onset (usually more or less sudden), leading to an acme, and followed by a sudden or gradual decline in the severity of the symptoms. As instances of paroxysmal disorders may be mentioned Paroxysmal Tachycardia, Angina Pectoris, Epilepsy, Nervous Faints and Flush Storms and Paroxysmal Hæmoglobinuria.

§ 2. **Case-Taking.**—In clinical investigation, or case-taking, our object is, *first*, to elicit all the data of the case; and, *secondly*, by reasoning based on those data to arrive at its Diagnosis, Prognosis and Treatment. It will be found in actual practice that everything turns on the diagnosis; this is our first and principal object; the prognosis and treatment follow from this.

The investigation of a case consists of three parts: (A) The Interrogation of the Patient, (B) the Physical Examination, and (C) the further Investigation by Special Ancillary Methods (*e.g.*, Radiology, Clinical Pathology), where necessary. Students should always accustom themselves to learn all that is possible by interrogation before proceeding to the physical examination.

A. By **Interrogation of the Patient** we learn—

(*a*) What is his *chief* or cardinal symptom;
(*b*) The facts concerning the *present illness*;
(*c*) The patient's *previous history*;
(*d*) The patient's *personal history*; and
(*e*) His *family history*.

Throughout the interrogation of the patient it is well to follow THREE GENERAL RULES:

(1) *Avoid putting what barristers call " leading questions "*—*i.e.*, questions which suggest their own answer—*e.g.*, " Have you had a pain in the back ? " suggests an obvious answer to the patient. It might be put thus: " Have you had any pain, and if so, where ? " The patient should be encouraged to tell his own story, without interruption. Moreover, the very words he uses should be recorded between inverted commas, and on no account should his words be translated into scientific terms. Some say that leading questions are permissible when the patient is very ignorant and stupid, but these are the very cases in which leading questions should be specially avoided. The only legitimate way of putting a leading question is in an alternative form—*e.g.*, " Have you suffered from diarrhœa or constipation ? " Time, patience and tact are necessary to elicit the true facts of the case, without irrelevant detail. Our object is to learn what the patient *feels* and knows, not what he *thinks* of his disease; and our patience is often sorely tried by a long story of his own or his previous doctors' views on his case. Our record should be comprehensive, including all important data, negative as well as positive, yet concise—*i.e.*, excluding

irrelevant facts. Only experience and a knowledge of medicine can teach us what is or is not relevant. The beginner should strive after completeness rather than conciseness.

(2) *A chronological order* should always be adopted, both in eliciting and in recording the facts. Nothing is more wearisome than to wade through a mass of verbiage which mixes up dates. Dates should be recorded always in the same terms. It is very common, for instance, to read in students' reports that " breathlessness began in the year 1952," " palpitation started when the patient was aged forty," " œdema came on two years ago."

(3) Always adopt a kindly and *sympathetic manner*. Not only is it our bounden duty to be considerate and patient with those who suffer, but by entering into the spirit of the patient's sufferings we can often get at more important facts, and a truer narration of them, than can one whose harsh or abrupt manner causes the patient to shrink up like an oyster into its shell. Put your questions in as simple and non-technical a form as possible, and be sure that the patient attaches the same meaning to the words as you do. Much will depend on the tact of the physician, and two very good rules may here be added—viz., Never enquire concerning a family history of a lethal illness such as cancer before a patient whose illness is likely to be of that nature; Never put questions bearing on venereal disease before the husband or wife of the patient.

(*a*) THE CHIEF OR CARDINAL SYMPTOM.—The first question to ask a patient should always be the same " What do you complain of ? " Special attention should be paid to the main symptom for which the patient seeks advice or is admitted to hospital, because it is this symptom which guides most of our subsequent inquiries. It should always, as far as possible, be recorded in the patient's own words. *This book is based upon the patient's cardinal symptom;* and in the following chapters we shall, after each cardinal symptom, allude to the principal conditions for which it may be mistaken. The best way to avoid error is to verify your observations by repeating your examination.

(*b*) THE HISTORY OF THE PRESENT ILLNESS must be taken and recorded with care. It cannot too strongly be emphasised that in many diseases a full and accurate history of the illness may be the only method of arriving at a diagnosis, for physical signs may be absent or in abeyance (*e.g.*, in angina pectoris). Taking an average, it is fair to compute that of the information on which a diagnosis is ultimately founded, at least 50 per cent. comes from an accurate history, and rather less than 50 per cent. from the physical examination and subsequent special investigations. First ascertain *when* the illness started, by a question such as " When did you first notice or complain of this trouble ? " and this being answered: " Did you ever have this symptom before ? " Then elicit *where* the symptom is felt. The history should then reveal (i.) the mode of onset, whether sudden or gradual, (ii.) what the patient was doing at the time, and whether he attributed the onset to any cause. In many cases it is necessary to enquire into (iii.) whether the symptom is localised or widespread, (iv.) does it radiate to other areas; also (v.) the duration of the symptom, (vi.) whether it ended suddenly or gradually, (vii.) its severity, (viii) whether it has occurred since, and if so, how many times, and is it getting more or less severe; (ix.) what intervals of freedom have occurred, when the patient has been entirely free of the symptom; (x.) have other symptoms occurred in association with this chief symptom, and if so, what are they; (xi.) what does the patient do during the time of the symptom to relieve it; (xii.) has the patient found any measures of avail to ward off attacks, *e.g.*, drugs, diet, etc. In many cases, *e.g.*, in juvenile and unconscious persons, the history has to be elicited from near relatives or friends. It is useful also to know whether the patient has recently been, or is now, under medical care, not only because the symptoms may have been modified by treatment, but also because one of the most important ethical principles of the medical profession may be involved.[1] In all these enquiries the three general rules given above apply (p. 2).

(*c*) THE PREVIOUS HISTORY of the patient bears largely on the etiology, or *causation*, of his illness, and deals with any *illnesses* the patient may have had. Note in chronological order all ailments from which the patient has suffered prior to the present one, with the dates of their occurrence and their duration—*e.g.*, contagious diseases of childhood; and especially previous operations or serious illnesses. If the illnesses have been at all obscure, it is desirable to add a few of the leading symptoms to prove the nature of the alleged attacks, and in such instances inverted commas should be freely used. For instance " rheumatism " is a vague term which may mean any disease attended by pains in the limbs, such as are due to alcoholism, syphilis, tabes dorsalis or neurasthenia. The subject of syphilis should always be approached with delicacy in the case of women. Indirect information may often be gained by enquiring for prolonged sore throat, followed by loss of hair, enlarged glands, skin rashes, etc. In married women, a *series* of still-births, or children born with eruptions or snuffles, may have the same significance.

(*d*) THE PERSONAL HISTORY must be enquired into: such as (i.) present and previous occupations; (ii.) previous residence abroad; (iii.) the home conditions; (iv.) habits as to alcohol and tobacco and whether alcohol (*e.g.*, wine, beer or spirits) is taken between or with meals, because more harm is done by alcohol before meals (especially cocktails) than many times the same quantity taken with meals; (v.) the appetite; (vi.) the state of the digestion and the bowels; (vii.) the weight, and whether this is constant, being gained or lost; (viii.) the general state of the nervous system, *e.g.*, depression, excitability, nervousness; (ix.) the orientation of

---

[1] By-law CLVIX of the Royal College of Physicians of London runs as follows: " No Fellow, Member, or Licentiate of the College shall officiously. or under colour of a benevolent purpose, offer medical aid to, or prescribe for, any patient whom he knows to be under the care of another legally qualified Medical Practitioner." This is perhaps the most important guiding principle in the ethics and etiquette of the medical profession. On the other hand, this law gives us no proprietary right in a patient because we have once prescribed for him or his family. He ceases to be our patient directly he ceases our treatment for that particular ailment.

the patient to his (or her) work and to home life, and whether there are any special anxieties attached to these; (x.) the amount and quality of sleep. (xi.) In women, the previous state of the catamenia, and the number of pregnancies, miscarriages or still-births, should be noted.

(e) THE FAMILY HISTORY may, like the previous history, have a casual relationship to the patient's illness. The age and state of health if living, age and cause of death if dead, of near relations, should always be noted —i.e., father and mother, brothers and sisters, sons and daughters, also of husband or wife. Enquiry should also be made as to whether any members of the family (parents, grandparents, brothers, sisters, uncles, aunts or cousins) have suffered from tuberculosis, cancer, acute rheumatism, gout, nervous disease, asthma, heart disease, apoplexy, and especially those diseases to which the patient himself seems liable.

B. The Physical Examination (i.e., the State on Admission, or the Present Condition) may with advantage be prefaced by a few general remarks on how and what to observe.

(1) Here, again, having learned by interrogation our patient's chief complaint, we should ask ourselves, IS THERE ANY STRIKING OR PRE-DOMINANT SIGN OR APPEARANCE (Latin facies)? The importance of INSPECTING our patient cannot be overestimated. In these days of scientific instruments we are too apt to forget to use our faculties. By simply using our eyes many important data may be learned besides the colour of the skin, the condition of the teeth and gums, the general nutrition, the attitude or decubitus, and the facial expression. For instance, the manner in which a patient answers questions is often the first clue to anxiety, and a peculiar mode of speech is one of the pathognomonic signs of general paralysis of the insane, disseminated sclerosis and other diseases. Moreover, with experience we can by this means form a conclusion as to the kind of patient we have to deal with. Again, never be in a hurry; only by taking time can we fully appreciate all the points presented to us. This habit of " observing " the patient is only developed by long practice; it will never be developed if the young physician allows himself to be infected by the hurry of modern times.

(2) It is important always to commence our examination with that ORGAN TO WHICH THE SYMPTOMS ARE MAINLY REFERABLE. Some teachers direct their pupils to examine and report on the physiological systems always in the same order (first the heart, then the lungs, then the digestive system and so forth), whatever may be the illness. But such a course has three objections (i.) The student goes about his work in a mechanical fashion; (ii.) if the patient suffers from some serious disorder, such as peritonitis, he may be exhausted by a complete investigation of the chest and other parts during the acute illness; and (iii.) often it is a waste of time to examine all the organs with equal thoroughness. The same educational advantages and experience can be obtained by the other method, and in that way we come to the most important facts first.

(3) In all cases EVERY ORGAN IN THE BODY SHOULD BE CAREFULLY

EXAMINED; for although we may find in one physiological system sufficient mischief to account for the patient's symptoms, the other organs may reveal changes which considerably modify our treatment, our prognosis, and even our diagnosis. Whatever order is adopted, the student should not wander from organ to organ, but examine each physiological system thoroughly before proceeding to the next. It is well to get into the habit of adopting some such order of physical examination as the following: *First*, note the general condition; *secondly*, examine the organ chiefly affected; *thirdly*, the other organs in the following order: Thorax (heart and lungs), Abdomen (alimentary canal, liver, spleen and genito-urinary system), Head and Limbs (nervous and motor systems).

The examination should always be carried out *gently*, and *without undue exposure*. In serious cases, especially when the heart or lungs are involved, it is often well to postpone a thorough examination of some organs, so as not to risk harming the patient by exposing or fatiguing him. On the other hand, the young physician should never allow modesty to prevent his making a thorough examination. This rule is especially necessary in more sensitive patients, but a little firmness, tact, and a courteous demeanour will generally enable him to perform what is a duty both to his patient and to himself.

SCHEME OF CASE-TAKING

A. INTERROGATION OF PATIENT

(a) The patient's chief or **Cardinal Symptom**.
(b) Data concerning the **Present Illness**.
(c) The patient's **Previous History**.
(d) The **Personal History**.
(e) The **Family History**.

B. PHYSICAL EXAMINATION (i.e., Present Condition—Give Date) [1]

(a) **The general condition** may be summarised mainly under three headings: (i.) The Physiognomy or expression, especially in acute disease (Chapter II): (ii.) The Decubitus, Attitude, or Gait, especially in chronic disorders (Chapter II); (iii.) The Nutrition, General Conformation, and any Eruption on the skin (Chapter XVI). The temperature, pulse, respiration and weight should be noted.

(b) **Chest.**

　I. CARDIO-VASCULAR SYSTEM.　　　　　(Chapters III to V.)

　Symptoms.—Breathlessness, cardiac pain, palpitation.

---

[1] This scheme gives only the *chief points* which should be noted about the different physiological systems, with the object of excluding disease. For an exhaustive examination, such as must be made of the organ to which the patient's symptoms are mainly referable, the student should refer to the chapter dealing with the diseases of that organ.

Physical Signs.—Pulse: rate, rhythm, volume, tension, arterial wall. Heart: palpation, apex beat, percussion area, auscultation, œdema.

II. RESPIRATORY SYSTEM.   (Chapters VI and VII.)

Symptoms.—Cough, expectoration, dyspnœa, pain in chest.

Physical Signs.—Rate of respiration, inspection, palpation, percussion, auscultation. Examine throat and nose.

(c) **Abdomen.**

III. ALIMENTARY CANAL.   (Chapters VIII, IX, X, and XI.)

Symptoms.—Appetite, discomfort after food, nausea, pain, state of the bowels, colour of stools.

Physical Signs.—Examine mouth and tongue, gums, teeth and tonsils. Physical condition of abdomen as regards distension, and presence of fluid or tumour (inspection, palpation and percussion). Rectal examination.

IV. LIVER AND GALL-BLADDER.   (Chapter XII.)

Symptoms.—Pain, jaundice.

Physical Signs.—Size of liver (palpation and percussion), surface (if accessible), tenderness.

V. SPLEEN.   (Chapter XII.)

Any enlargement (palpation and percussion) or local pain.

VI. RENAL SYSTEM.   (Chapter XIII.)

Symptoms.—Any undue frequency of, or difficulty in, micturition. Any pain or œdema.

Physical Signs—(in a catheter specimen when necessary).

   (i.) *Urine:* quantity, colour, reaction, specific gravity, albumen, blood, sugar, bile, urobilin, acetone, aceto-acetic acid, deposit (microscopical examination).

   (ii.) *Kidney.*—Any enlargement, mobility or tenderness.

VII. GENERATIVE SYSTEM.   (Chapter XIV.)

Menstruation, frequency, duration, quantity, pain, intermenstrual discharge.

(d) **Head and Limbs.**

VIII. NERVOUS SYSTEM.   (Chapter XIX.)

Symptoms.—Headache, sleeplessness, neuralgia, etc.

Physical Signs.—Weakness or inco-ordination, muscular wasting, involuntary movements, gait. Reflexes, deep and superficial.

Sensation for touch, pain, temperature, vibration sense.

Cranial Nerves.—Vision, fundi, pupils, movements of the eyes. Movements of the face, masseters, palate and tongue, sternomastoids. Hearing. Smell. Taste.

Sympathetic System.—Flush storms, trophic lesions, vasomotor system, perspiration.

(e) **Blood.**

In anæmic and some other cases examine the blood (Chapter XVI).

Progress of Case.—Notes (daily of acute or febrile cases, twice a week of subacute, and once a week of chronic cases) should be made of the progress of the case; and much care is required here to avoid redundancy on the one hand, and on the other to record completely all important changes, or any fresh symptoms, and the results of special investigations. In acute febrile cases there ought to be a daily note, and the pulse, respiration and temperature should be charted every four hours. In chronic cases it will be sufficient to note, once a week, the persistence of the prominent symptoms or any change in the symptoms. In all cases any *sudden* change in the patient's symptoms or general condition should be recorded at once. Each note should have special reference to the previous one; and before taking a fresh note, the previous one should be read over. The treatment and its effects should always be incorporated.

History Sheets, Charts, Diagrams, etc.—A history sheet for recording the history of a patient should be ruled with one vertical line down the page one-third from the left-hand margin, so as to give space for information learned subsequently. It should have printed headings and spaces at the top, thus:

Diagnosis. (Space here for primary and secondary disease, filled in by physician afterwards.)

Name..............Age.........Sex...........Occupation ....

Address...........................Date of admission ....

Date of discharge (or death) ....

Chief symptom on admission ....

Temperature charts are of the greatest use to record the temperature and other features of diurnal variation. Outline diagrams or rubber stamps of the various regions of the body can be purchased, and are very useful.

A kind of shorthand code for physical signs is advocated by some authors, and, once learned, may be useful in saving time and space.

§ 3. Examination of Children and Infants.—Here the same general rules apply as to interrogation and physical examination, and we should first endeavour to ascertain the child's leading symptom, either from the patient or the relatives. There are, however, certain additional rules upon the adoption of which much of our success with children will depend.

1. First endeavour to establish friendly relations with your little patient. Often this is done by appearing not to notice the child at first; after a while he may make advances and investigate your watch-chain and be given a toy. A child dislikes being stared at. Time should always be given for the child to become accustomed to your presence, and anything like abruptness will defeat your aim.

2. The questions put to the child should always be of the simplest character—*e.g.*, " Where does it hurt you ? " Interrogation of the mother is essential to learn the age up to when the child remained healthy, the symptoms of the present and previous illnesses. In the case of an infant, enquire whether he was a full-time child, if born with instrumental aid, whether he was born healthy, his weight at birth and subsequently, and details about the methods of feeding. If the child is past early infancy, the same questions may still be put, and in addition enquire when he began to walk and talk, and when dentition commenced. Carefully record his present and past diet, his appetite and the state of the bowels. Ask also how long he sleeps, bearing

in mind that children require much more sleep than adults. Then ask for any recent illness in other members of the family.

PHYSICAL EXAMINATION.—Valuable as *attentive observation* may be with adults, it becomes quite indispensable with children, who cannot accurately describe their sensations. Much may be learned while you sit and allow the child to get accustomed to your presence. Notice his expression, the brightness of his eyes, his attitude, the colour of his skin, any rash present, the state of nutrition, his size as compared with age, his movements, the condition of his lips (moist or dry), the character of the breathing, the sound of his voice. If he cries, enquiry should be made whether this is constant or only periodic. If the child be asleep when first you enter, do not wake him, but notice all the above before he is disturbed. When awake, the limbs of a healthy child should be constantly on the move; drowsiness, dullness and listlessness are signs of pyrexia, and especially that of the contagious fevers. The hands are instinctively moved towards a seat of pain—*e.g.*, the head in meningitis. The state of the temper is altered in the prodromal stage of most diseases; but it is markedly peevish in the prodromal stage of meningitis. For other facial alterations, see **Facies** (§ 11). When the child is undressed for examination, the back of the chest should be examined first, while the child looks over the mother's shoulder at someone who attracts his attention with a bright object or a bunch of keys. Percussion should be delayed until the end of the examination.

§ 4. Methods of Diagnosis, Prognosis and Treatment.—Diagnosis, prognosis and treatment are the objects we had in view in eliciting all the facts concerning the patient by the process of " Case-taking." Of these three, **Diagnosis**—which, as the Greek word (διάγνωσις) implies, means the distinguishing or discernment of the disease—is by far the most important. Everything hinges on this, for without recognition of the disease, rational prognosis and treatment are impossible. It is well, therefore, to consider how the data we have elicited may be utilised in order to arrive at a diagnosis. Several different methods are employed:—

The method usually adopted, which is the outcome of the student's studies in systematic medicine, is to erect a *hypothetical diagnosis*, and to see whether the patient's symptoms tally with the description of the disease. When a child, for instance, with disorderly movements comes before us, the diagnosis of chorea at once occurs to our minds. The age of the patient, the character of the movements and all the obvious features of the case appear to correspond with that disorder. It does not seem necessary to consider any other suggestion. This method works well enough in straightforward, well-marked, typical cases; but in cases presenting anything unusual or atypical considerable difficulty may be experienced.

Another method of making a diagnosis is by a *process of exclusion*; that is, after studying the diseases which might possibly be in operation, we arrive at our diagnosis by excluding those which the disease least resembles. In such diseases as typhoid fever, where symptoms are few in number, this may be the only method possible. The patient, for instance, is suffering from a moderate degree of pyrexia, the illness came on gradually; that is all we may know about the case. There are many possible causes of such a condition, but we arrive at the conclusion that it is probably typhoid fever, because all the other possible diseases are rendered improbable for one reason or another.

The third method consists of *noting the cardinal symptoms* and *balancing the evidence* for and against all the possible causes which might give rise to them. In this method, after having elicited all the facts of the case, we return to the patient's *cardinal symptom*, enumerate in our own minds the various causes which might give rise to that symptom, and balance the evidence adduced by the other facts of the case for and against each one in turn. It may strike some as being a little tedious, but it is not so when we have got into the habit of employing it. It is certainly the one best adapted for the elucidation of obscure or atypical cases; and under all circumstances it presents a truer picture to our mind, because diagnosis can never be a matter of absolute certainty. At most a diagnosis is only a strong probability, and this method enables us to ascertain the exact amount of probability in each disease. Even in the simplest and most typical cases it is a good mental exercise for us to keep in mind the other lesions which might produce the same symptoms, and then we are always on the look-out for possible errors, and ready at any moment to review the diagnosis—a correct mental attitude when in the presence of Nature's phenomena. The chapters which follow are based on this method.

C. SPECIAL INVESTIGATIONS

Having arrived at a tentative diagnosis, it is advisable to confirm this by the use of X-rays, electrical tracings, pathological tests and other special methods of investigation. These should only be used in confirmation of a clinical diagnosis and *should never replace the Interrogation and the Physical Examination of the patient in the search for a diagnosis.* Remember that many diseases (*e.g.*, migraine, angina pectoris) do not produce changes which can be recognised by instrumental methods. Furthermore these investigations are by no means infallible: thus an X-ray film gives a pictorial representation of a number of shadows in a plane of one dimension and may not show a pathological shadow in a different plane. On the other hand confirmation of a clinical diagnosis can often be rendered much more certain by the use of such special methods.

EXAMPLE.—Let us suppose that the patient, a pale young woman, aged twenty-three, comes to us complaining of **vomiting blood** (*i.e.*, hæmatemesis).

First, we ascertain and verify this, the leading symptom, and find that she has really vomited a considerable quantity of blood.

Secondly, we INTERROGATE her as to the history of her present illness, her previous and family histories, and we find that she has suffered for several years from symptoms pointing to dyspepsia, and that latterly there has been severe pain in the epigastrium. There are always four features we have to investigate about every pain—its position, character, degree and constancy; and we find that this epigastric pain is a sharp pain, not constant, but coming on shortly after taking food, and that it is followed *and relieved* by vomiting. The other details of the case we will omit for the sake of brevity.

Thirdly, we proceed to the PHYSICAL EXAMINATION, first of the abdominal organs, but this reveals nothing abnormal. Then we go through the other physiological systems in order, observing (*a*) her General Condition (noting, for example, how pale and thin she is, and how weak she seems); (*b*) examining the Chest (Cardio-vascular and Respiratory systems); (c) the Head and Limbs (Nervous system); (d) the Blood must also be examined, because anæmia may be inferred from the pallor of her skin and mucous membranes.

Having elicited all the data by interrogation and physical examination, we return to the *cardinal symptom*—hæmatemesis [1]—and consider its various causes (see the section on Hæmatemesis) *seriatim*, taking the most probable cause first.

(a) SIMPLE ULCER OF THE STOMACH.

For: (i.) The profuseness of the hæmatemesis; (ii.) the character of the pain (brought on by food, relieved by vomiting); (iii.) the history of dyspepsia; (iv.) the age and sex of the patient.

Against: (i.) No tenderness in the epigastrium.

(b) CANCER OF THE STOMACH.

For: (i.) The vomiting of blood; (ii.) pain in the stomach; (iii.) pallor and emaciation; and so on.

Against: (i.) The blood vomited was too profuse, and had not the character special to cancer (coffee grounds); (ii.) the pain was only produced by food, and entirely disappeared after vomiting; (iii.) age of patient much too young.

(c) PORTAL OBSTRUCTION.

For: The profuseness of the hæmatemesis.

Against: (i.) Absence of abnormal signs in the liver; (ii.) absence of ascites, piles, and other symptoms of portal obstruction.

(d) OTHER AND LESS PROBABLE DIAGNOSES can be discussed in like manner, though each of these may be more summarily dismissed thus: *Vicarious menstruation* would not account for the dyspepsia, acute epigastric pain and other symptoms. *Leukæmia, Scurvy* and *other blood conditions,* if present, would present the other symptoms of those disorders.

It follows, therefore, that the balance of evidence is in favour of (a) SIMPLE ULCER OF THE STOMACH, partly because of the weighty arguments in its favour, and partly because the only argument against it is not vital, for tenderness may be absent when the ulcer is situated on the posterior wall of the stomach. Indeed, if a numerical value were given to each of the " reasons " for and against, it would be possible to express the precise degree of probability of each disease in the form of a mathematical ratio. This method may at first sight seem tedious, but after a little practice it becomes automatic and extremely simple; and it takes much less time than is here implied. Later, X-ray examination may confirm the diagnosis.

Prognosis (from the G.eek word προγνωσις) is a " foreknowledge " of the events which will happen—*i.e.,* of the probable course the disease will run. Nothing but wide experience, combined with careful and minute observation, will enable a physician to prophesy with any approach to accuracy. It will, however, be useful to bear in mind that the prognosis of a case depends upon four circumstances—viz., (1) the *usual course,*

[1] Here there was no difficulty about identifying or selecting which was the chief or most important symptom; but in another case the anæmia (or the vomiting or epigastric pain) might be the more serious or prominent symptom, the hæmatemesis consisting, perhaps, of a few streaks of blood. Then we should deal with the anæmia in the same way as hæmatemesis is here dealt with. Sometimes a good deal depends upon our choice of which is the "leading symptom," for it is not always the most prominent which is the most serious and important; and by an error in this respect we may be led far afield from the true disease. At times, however, it is useful to change the point of view we take of the case, by regarding it from another standpoint or leading symptom.

duration and event of the disease in operation (phthisis, for instance, runs a prolonged course, and until lately the event was almost invariably fatal); (2) the presence or absence of *untoward symptoms* (*e.g.*, profuse hæmoptysis in phthisis); (3) the presence or absence of *complications* (which are sometimes more fatal than the disease itself—*e.g.*, typhoid and many other fevers are fatal chiefly by their complications); and (4) the *causes* which are in operation, including among the predisposing causes such data as age and sex (gastro-enteritis, for example, in middle life is not a serious affection, but in infancy and old age it is often fatal).

As practical hints to the young physician, I would advise him—(1) Never to commit himself to a prognosis unasked, or before awaiting the result of treatment. More reputations are wrecked on the rock " Prognosis " than on any other. (2) Avoid giving a prognosis before all the facts of the case are to hand (including the results of X-ray and other special examinations). (3) It is also well to impress upon the friends that a " physician " cannot hope to be also a " prophet "; and that prognosis may depend on many factors in the case which are not yet revealed. (4) When the physician considers that the prognosis is grave, it is usually unwise even to hint this fact to the patient; however, it is essential to inform a responsible relative.

Treatment is what the patient comes to us for; and it may be of three kinds: (1) In *Specific* (*or Radical*) treatment our object is to cure the patient of his disease by the removal of the cause. This is the only truly scientific treatment, and it is based mainly upon a knowledge of the pathology of the disease. · (2) *Symptomatic* treatment is directed only to the relief of the symptoms. In some incurable maladies symptomatic treatment is the only kind possible, and all that we can do is to give physical and mental comfort to the patient and to ensure the co-operation of his relatives and friends. But in the practice of busy practitioners, the trouble and time needed for thorough investigation often lead to the use of symptomatic treatment at times when a more radical treatment is still possible. We should constantly guard against an unfortunate tendency to fall into a routine of symptomatic treatment. Both Specific and Symptomatic treatment may be either internal or external on the one hand, and either medicinal or dietetic and hygienic on the other. (3) *Preventive* treatment has within the last quarter of a century developed almost into a separate science, the science of Hygiene or Social Medicine.

§ 5. General Rules in Clinical Investigation.—There are certain habits which the student should strive to cultivate when he comes to the practical aspect of his profession; and he should remember Thackeray's saying: " Sow an act and you reap a habit; sow a habit and you reap a character; sow a character and you reap a destiny." Clinical medicine depends more than anything else on accurate, complete and well-directed observation, and there are six hints I would give to the student in this connection.

1. *Avoid superficiality* in your observations. Do not try to see many

cases in one day, but rather one or two cases *continuously from day to day*, so that you may follow a given disease throughout its entire course. It is of more value to follow up one case in this way than to see a dozen on one occasion only. Practical knowledge must be acquired gradually. The thought will often occur to the student how slowly he progresses with his clinical knowledge. This is partly apparent, partly real. It is partly apparent because a student does not realise at the time the value he derives from listening, for example, to the same cardiac murmur over and over again. It is partly real because it is only by patiently devoting the necessary time to the study of the same case from day to day that he will learn to make his observations adequate, thorough and precise. That is why many a brilliant intellect falls behind, and many a plodder comes to the front in our profession. It is vain to attempt to substitute genius for patient industry in this arena. You must learn for yourself the effects of this or that line of treatment; learn to correct and control the observations you make one day by your observations of the morrow; and above all, try to learn what is the sequel or termination of the case, especially in such instances as may lead you to the post-mortem room. There, more than anywhere else, the most brilliant diagnosticians learn from their own errors more than from a multitude of successful cases.

2. *Do not strive after what is rare and curious.* It follows as a matter of course that, other things being equal, a fact is more important in proportion as it is more common. Moreover, by studying *only* the exceptions to a rule, our minds will have a distorted view of clinical phenomena. Do not therefore be led astray by those pedants who seek after the singular and uncommon. It is well to see rare cases when the opportunity offers, but be careful that you mentally register them as rare.

3. *Do not study only acute and severe cases.* It is true that in acute diseases there is often more to be done, more heroic and decisive effects to be produced, or apparently produced, and therefore more credit and renown to be obtained. But we shall find in actual practice not one-tenth, perhaps not one-hundredth of our patients will be suffering from these complaints. Our success, therefore, in practice, whether measured by that laudable satisfaction at having done one's duty, or by the pecuniary reward of which every earnest labourer is worthy, will depend very much on our experience of, and our ability to treat, chronic and what we are too apt to call trivial complaints. For one case of Graves' or Addison's disease, the family doctor will have at least a hundred cases of dyspepsia, chronic rheumatism or chronic bronchitis. In the treatment of such complaints the greatest judgment and thoroughness are sometimes needed. No sudden or startling effects can be produced. Chronic diseases need persistent treatment, and it is only by experience that one can learn to produce those gradual effects which lead to a successful issue.

4. *Be accurate in your observations.* State facts precisely as you find them, no matter whether they accord with your hypothesis or not; and

state only what you find and know to be the truth. The study of clinical medicine, like the study of any other of Nature's phenomena, should inculcate in the mind of the student a love of truth. It is impossible to have any dealings with Nature without learning that truth is the key to the discovery of her secrets. Accuracy is one form of truth, and it is only by repeatedly going over your observations, and sifting the patient's statements, that you can ensure accuracy.

5. *Be complete in your examination of your patient.* It may not be possible or advisable to make a complete examination when you see your patient for the first time, or with a new illness. Many mistakes in diagnosis would be avoided if this rule were adhered to.

6. *Be systematic in the arrangement of your data,* for only by a systematic arrangement can you attach the proper importance to each observation, and get a firm grasp of the whole case. Nothing, for instance, is more liable to confuse and to prevent you from coming to a correct conclusion than wandering from one date to another without regard to the chronological sequence in the history of an illness. And again, in physical examination, nothing is so likely to lead you astray as wandering from organ to organ without first completing the examination of each.

§ 6. Classification of Diseases—Method of Procedure.—It has been customary, and the practice is convenient, to classify diseases into two great groups—Local and Constitutional. LOCAL diseases are those in which the principal, and perhaps the only, lesion is localised in one organ or situation, *e.g.,* facial neuralgia, ringworm. CONSTITUTIONAL diseases are those in which the disease has manifestations of general distribution, *e.g.,* acute rheumatism, typhoid fever and pyæmia.

It is convenient for clinical purposes to preserve this division, but the rapid advance of pathology has gradually transferred disorders from the "local" to the "constitutional" group. A large number of diseases formerly believed to be lesions of local origin (such, for instance, as pneumonia, endocarditis and peritonitis) are now known to be due to some general pathological process which, on reaching the blood, is carried all over the body and causes a special local manifestation in one situation.

From a pathological standpoint diseases are sometimes divided into two groups—Organic, those in which some anatomical change is found after death; and Functional, those in which we can, *in the present state of our knowledge,* find no structural alteration by modern methods. The anatomical or structural change is spoken of as the "lesion." The word "functional" must not be regarded as synonymous with "hysterical."

Now it so happens that local disorders are very often met with as complications or effects of constitutional or general conditions; and since in clinical work we are engaged in **tracing from effect to cause,** we shall, in the following chapters, take the local diseases which are manifested by a lesion *localised* in some particular organ first, and the *constitutional* conditions afterwards.

When a patient comes to us, and if, as the result of our inquiries, we find he is suffering from a symptom localised to some organ (*e.g.,* pain in the liver), turn to the chapters relating to the diseases of that organ (one of the Chapters III to XIV).

If, on the other hand, he has no localised symptom, but complains of malaise, feverishness or a sense of " bodily illness," turn to the chapters on constitutional diseases (Chapters XV to XXI).

CHAPTER II

THE FACIES, OR EXTERNAL APPEARANCE OF DISEASE [1]

In our scheme of case-taking it will be remembered that the first step in physical examination was to observe the patient's general condition; and it will also be remembered how great was the importance of an adequate inspection of the patient while he was telling us the story of his illness.

Some diseases can be identified almost at a glance, before the patient opens his lips, such, for instance, as Graves' Disease, Cretinism, Myxœdema, Facial Paralysis, Hydrocephalus, Chronic Alcoholism and some manifestations of Hereditary Syphilis, when these conditions have passed beyond the incipient stage. The existence of others can be very strongly suspected, such as Rickets, Post-nasal Adenoids (mouth-breathing children), Asthma, and Chronic Bronchitis with Dilated Right Heart.

But, apart from these, much may be learned from the first glance at a patient—from his *decubitus* (the way he lies), from his *attitude* or *gait*, from the expression of his *face*, the colour of his *skin*, and from the *general conformation* of his body—without the employment of any special methods or apparatus for diagnosis. It is to be feared that as scientific methods become more and more perfect, these means, which constitute one of the most useful and important aids to diagnosis and prognosis to the experienced busy practitioner, are apt to be neglected. But on the other hand, students and young practitioners had better not attempt "lightning diagnoses," or they will certainly fall into the most serious errors. Some men, it is true, seem to be especially gifted in this way; but it is only by long experience and the possession of special faculties that they can accomplish such feats.

It is a fundamental rule that your patient should face the light at all medical interviews. Similarly your own chair should be in the shade, lest the patient should read too readily what is passing through your mind. It is surprising what important clues can be obtained by an intelligent inspection of your patient, both as to his character and his disease.

The facies of a disease may be summarised under three headings: (A) THE PHYSIOGNOMY IN DISEASE. (B) THE DECUBITUS, ATTITUDE OR GAIT. (C) ALTERATIONS IN THE GENERAL CONFORMATION OF THE BODY.

Hints to be derived from an inspection of the hands are given under Diseases of the Extremities (Chapter XVII). The various diseases will be only mentioned here. The description and differentiation of the several affections referred to will be entered into more fully in the chapters which follow.

[1] The Latin word *facies* signifies an appearance, form or shape.

16

(A) THE PHYSIOGNOMY IN DISEASE

An observant physician can obtain important clues to diagnosis by the physiognomy—*i.e.*, the aspect and expression of the patient's face —even apart from the insight which can be gained by this means into his character.

§ 7. In **Acute Diseases** more can be learned from the position in which the patient lies (*i.e.*, his Decubitus, § 14) than from the physiognomy or expression of his face. But it is worth remembering that the face assumes an *anxious expression*, which is very characteristic in pericarditis, peritonitis, severe pneumonia, and during attacks of angina pectoris. The supervention of *acute pericarditis* in the course of rheumatic fever is often unsuspected, as there may be no local symptoms; but it may be recognised by this anxious expression, the dilated nostrils, and the flush upon the cheeks, which were (probably) at our last visit so pale. Again, in acute *lobar pneumonia*, the appearance is very distinctive. The flushed face, hot dry skin, widely dilating nostrils, the eruption of herpes near the mouth, and the profound disturbance of the pulse-respiration ratio (2 : 1 instead of 4 : 1, which is the normal), form a picture which greatly aids the recognition of the disease. The *Facies Hippocratica*—a facies or appearance, of which the description has been handed down from Hippocrates —is the forerunner of death from exhaustion, dehydration and wasting diseases, as in the final stages of acute peritonitis, cholera or malignant disease. The temples are hollow, the eyes sunken, the eyelids slightly parted, the eyes glazed, the lower jaw droops and the teeth are covered with sordes. The *Risus Sardonicus* is a fixed grin, met typically in tetanus. The corners of the mouth, which twitch at intervals, are drawn upwards as in laughter, and the features assume a fixed sarcastic expression.

§ 8. A few **Chronic Diseases** may be ^numerated in which the physiognomy is characteristic.

(i.) The aspect of a *phthisical* or *tuberculous* patient in the advanced stages often presents an appearance that enables the physician to hazard a diagnosis almost without further investigation. Especially in the young adult, the pale, emaciated face with sunken eyes, the circular crimson flush of hectic fever on the cheeks, the wasted body bathed from time to time in sweat, the hoarse voice and easily-provoked dyspnœa, collectively form a picture which is very characteristic.

(ii.) *Chronic bronchitis with dilated right heart* is a condition of extremely common occurrence in the practitioner's daily practice. These patients present a very characteristic picture with florid " healthy " looking cheeks, distended jugular veins in a person over forty.

(iii.) In *chronic alcoholism* there is a puffiness of the face and a congested watery look about the eyes (" a blear-eyed look "). The eyelids are puffy, so that the person is described by sailors as having " an eye like a poached egg." The cheeks and nose are often red and dotted with stellate venous capillaries. The abdomen is corpulent; and on holding out the hands and spreading the fingers, these show a fine rhythmical tremor. The whole picture is unmistakable, though the eyes alone will often tell the tale.

In various **diseases of the nervous system** the *face* presents a pathognomonic expression. The face is *distorted* in Bell's or facial paralysis, and in that rare condition facial hemiatrophy. In tabes dorsalis the unequal pupils, drooping eyelids and wrinkled forehead are diagnostic (§ 1022). Paralysis of the cervical sympathetic (Horner's syndrome) causes on the affected side a drooping upper eyelid with a narrowed palpebral fissure, and a constricted pupil. The expression is *vacant* in idiocy and in some hysterical subjects. A smooth, *expressionless* appearance (differing from the preceding in that there is a lack of mobility) is characteristic of paralysis agitans, and among rarer conditions, of double facial paralysis, the myopathies affecting the face muscles, and scleroderma. Very characteristic is the *spastic* smile, with open mouth, met in lenticular degeneration. Bulbar paralysis gives a characteristic, *mournful* or *sullen* appearance to the face; the orbicularis oris is paralysed, and allows the lower lip to pout; while the weakness of the zygomatici results in a drooping of the corners of the mouth, such as we usually associate with sorrow or sullenness of temper. In a more advanced stage the saliva dribbles out of the mouth. Certain *spasms* and *tremors* are recognised at a glance (§ 919 *et seq.*).

§ 9. Swelling of the Face and neck. (i.) If this is associated with œdema of the limbs and trunk, it is part of a generalised œdema. In the œdema of *renal disease*, the swelling is most obvious in the loose cellular tissues

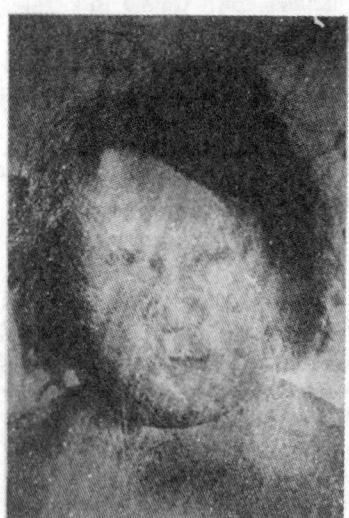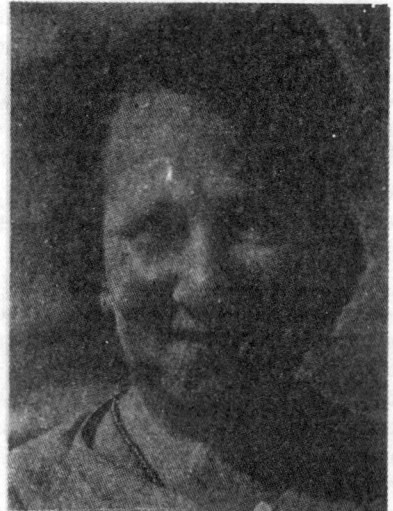

MYXŒDEMA. (FIG. 1) Before treatment. (FIG. 2.) After treatment with thyroid by mouth.

around the eyelids (Fig. 133). The puffiness of the eyelids due to renal disease is, however, greater in the morning than in the evening, and in this way may be distinguished from a similar condition due to arsenical poisoning or whooping-cough. The œdema of cardiac disease is more noticeable in the dependent parts of the body. In severe anæmia the pallor of the skin may be associated with some œdema.

Myxœdema is often recognised by a glance at the patient's face and hands (Fig. 1). There is a solid œdema and puffiness of the face—the body and limbs being also affected—but it does not *pit on pressure*. The vacant, stolid look, flushed cheeks, yellowish skin, scanty, coarse, dry hair, supra-clavicular pads and slow speech are equally typical of this disorder. The hands are flat, coarse and swollen (see ' § 575).

(ii.) Swelling which is confined to the face, accompanied sometimes by flushing after meals, is a symptom for which dyspeptic patients often seek advice (acne rosacea). It is also seen in urticaria. A *firm swelling* of the face occurs with scleroderma and scleredema. *Bilateral swelling* may be due to mumps and *unilateral swelling* to an infected tooth or antrum.

Chronic œdema around the eyelids must not be mistaken for myxœdema. It may be due to recurrent eczema, blepharitis, erysipelas or ethmoiditis. Transient exacerbations occur with fatigue and liver derangement. Œdema confined to the *head and neck* is found in those rare cases where there is pressure on the veins within the thorax, especially the superior vena cava, as in cases of mediastinal tumour.

In *acromegaly* the lower jaw, supra-orbital ridges, lips, cheeks and end of the nose are thickened and enlarged (Fig. 7 and § 615).

Various forms of parotitis, acute and chronic, cause swelling. Acute forms may appear in connection with specific fevers such as mumps (§ 495) or in the terminal stages of a long illness. In *Mikulicz' disease* there is a chronic bilateral painless swelling of the lachrymal and salivary glands, or of the latter only. The cause is unknown. The affected glands are densely infiltrated with lymphocytes, and do not recur if removed. In *Mikulicz' syndrome* swelling of the same glands occurs in lymphosarcoma, leukæmia, syphilis, tuberculosis, lymphadenoma, hepatic cirrhosis or lead poisoning, conditions to be eliminated before undertaking any operation. The *uveo-parotid syndrome* occurs occasionally with sarcoidosis (§§ 141 and 710). After an initial period of malaise, fever develops and iridocyclitis, bilateral facial palsy (§ 1081), bilateral parotid and lachrymal gland enlargements, occasionally polyneuritis and skin rashes occur.

§ 10. The **Complexion** and colour of the face will repay careful inspection, for thereby the trained observer will acquire useful information. Thus, the *pallor* of anæmic and toxæmic conditions is often very striking. So also is the dead white or *waxen puffy* appearance of parenchymatous nephritis; the *greyish pallor* of chronic interstitial nephritis and of hepatic cirrhosis; the *lemon* colour of pernicious anæmia; the *deeper yellow* colour of regular mepacrine dosage;[1] the *deep yellow* to *greenish-yellow* colour of jaundice; a *faint yellow tinge* with pallor occurs with old age, early jaundice, cholæmia and severe anæmia. A *muddy* sallow complexion may be associated with chronic constipation or other colonic disorders and with chronic nephritis. The *dull earthy* look occurs with malarial cachexia, cancer and chronic abdominal disease. The *purple* (or cyanotic) appearance of the cheeks and lips in congestive heart failure and congenital heart disease, and the congested appearance of polycythæmia, chronic bronchitis and chronic alcoholism, are distinctive; so also are the *grey* or *violet* complexion of

[1] It is only by long experience that one can distinguish these refinements of shade.

sulphhæmoglobinæmia and methæmoglobinæmia. *Dark rings* around the eyelids appear in states of fatigue; they often indicate want of sleep, intestinal disorder, a toxic state, and may be so pronounced in malaria as to resemble the ecchymosis of a bruise. *Bronzing* is seen with Addison's disease, arsenical poisoning, hæmochromatosis, Gaucher's disease, neurofibromatosis, occasionally in hyperthyroidism and in half-castes. *Greasiness of the face* occurs with acne vulgaris and seborrhœa oleosa.

§ 11. The **Face in Detail** merits a closer study, and, first, that most eloquent portion of it, the eyes.

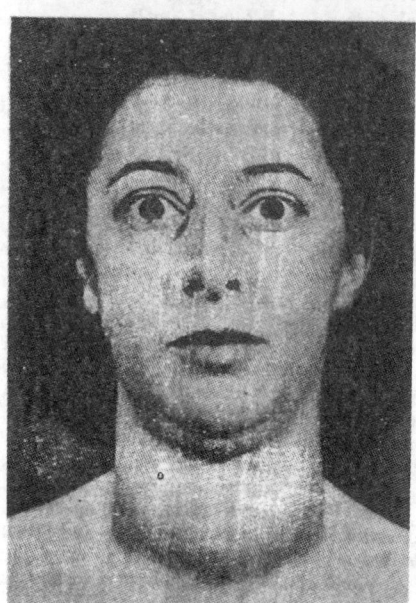

FIG. 3.—EXOPHTHALMIC GOITRE.

(i.) The *eyes may protrude* (Proptosis, Exophthalmos). They may give a deceptive appearance of protrusion when there is marked loss of intraorbital fat or severe dehydration. *Mild proptosis* is most commonly due to myopia and some degree is met as a family trait. *Marked proptosis* is usually due to Graves' disease (exophthalmic goitre) in association with an enlarged thyroid gland (Fig. 3). Other causes of unilateral or bilateral proptosis are retro-orbital or intra-ocular tumour, mucocœle of the ethmoid sinuses, chloroma, thrombosis of the cavernous sinus, irritation of the cervical sympathetic or advanced cerebral tumour. In children it is met with in oxycephaly and in the Hand-Schüller-Christian syndrome. *Malignant* or *progressive exophthalmos* may at first be unilateral: it is thought to be due to over-secretion of the thyrotropic hormone of the pituitary and may follow thyroidectomy.

The *eyeballs* may *recede* in paralysis of the cervical sympathetic, in wasting diseases, and in conditions of dehydration. The conjunctivæ show the pallor of anæmia; and in the sclerotic, or white of the eye, the tinge of *jaundice* can often be detected when the yellow colour of the skin is so slight as to escape notice. The sclerotic may also be yellow in severe anæmia and in old people; it may be bluish in congenital heart disease, in liver disease and in association with fragilitas ossium. The " *arcus senilis* " is a white ring of opacity in the cornea, just within its peripheral margin. It was once believed to indicate senile degeneration of the arteries and of other tissues, but this is erroneous. In adults who are subjects of hereditary syphilis, the corneæ may present *striæ* or the appearance of ground glass, due to interstitial keratitis, which may be confused with scars of corneal ulceration. Brownish-yellow, triangular pigmentation of the sclerotics, confined to the area uncovered by the lids, is seen in the Gaucher type of splenomegaly. Alterations of the *pupil* are dealt with in § 1059.

(ii.) The *lips* may show the pallor of anæmia on the one hand or the congestion or cyanosis of cardiac disease on the other. The mouth is held open when nasal obstruction is present, in idiocy, cretinism and certain paralyses. Fissures may be due to perlèche or, when indurated, to syphilis. Stellate scars around the lips are a record of previous or hereditary syphilis. Dryness of the lips occurs with fever, gastric disturbances and persistent mouth breathing. The position and movements of the mouth are characteristic in facial and bulbar paralysis, in the Landouzy-Déjérine type of myopathy, and in the tremors of general paralysis of the insane.

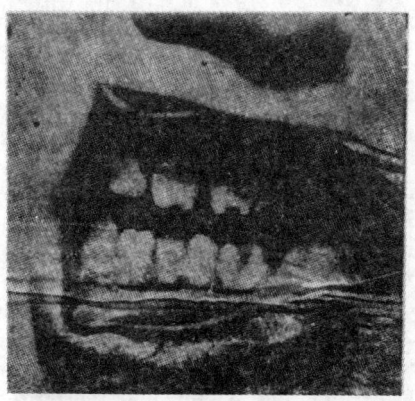

FIG. 4.—Hutchinson's Teeth.

(iii.) The *teeth and gums* may present evidence of pyorrhœa or of hereditary syphilis, in which disease the permanent incisors (erupting at the age of 7–8 years) are characteristically " pegged "—*i.e.*, narrow at the cutting edge, and notched (see also Hutchinson's teeth, § 204). Ridged teeth usually denote stomatitis in infancy.

(iv.) Depression of the bridge of the *nose*, if marked, is due to chronic rhinitis in childhood (usually of syphilitic origin), or to hyperteleorism. In such cases the nose is characteristically broad and flat, or small and " snub," like a button, the opera-glass nose of Fournier. The end of the nose is enlarged in acromegaly, myxœdema and rhinophyma.

(v.) The *ears* may reveal diagnostic evidence of lupus erythematosus, circulatory disturbances and the tophi of gout.

(vi.) Defective development may be recognised by " stigmata," such as epicanthic folds, hare-lip, cleft palate, accessory auricles and dermoid cysts.

(vii.) The *tongue* is considered in § 212 *et seq.*

§ 12. The **Physiognomy of Childhood** requires considerable experience to appreciate it fully; then it lends us invaluable aid.

(i.) *Infantile atrophy* or *marasmus* gives to an infant a very characteristic pinched or " senile " face. The complexion is greyish white, the face is sunken and livid, and the skin hangs in folds. The eyes lie deeply in their sockets from which the fat has disappeared, and thus give to the infant the appearance of a little wizened old man.

(ii.) When an infant is experiencing *pain* the face will sometimes give a clue to its situation. Thus, a wrinkling of the forehead or frown is indicative of pain in the head; a drawing-up of the mouth at the corners, producing marked naso-labial folds, points to severe abdominal pain; a dilatation of the nostrils and elevation of the eyebrows may suggest intra-thoracic discomfort; and in tabes mesenterica and other chronic wasting diseases the face gradually assumes a fixed or contracted condition, in which the angles of the mouth are depressed.

(iii.) Nothing is more characteristic than the *listless* and apathetic facies of children suffering from the early stages of fever.

(iv.) *Mouth-breathing children* (often due to post-nasal adenoids) have a very characteristic expression. The broad bridge of the nose and open mouth give a vacant, stupid appearance, which sometimes belies their intelligence, though sometimes they are, in fact, mentally backward.

(v.) The *fontanelles* afford useful information. A *depressed* fontanelle is due to dehydration and is an untoward sign in all acute illnesses of infancy—*e.g.*, diarrhœa and vomiting. The fontanelles *bulge* in inflammation of the meninges, and this is a useful diagnostic feature between true meningitis on the one hand, and fevers, *e.g.*, broncho-pneumonia and other diseases with cerebral symptoms, on the other. The fontanelles are bulging and tense in all diseases causing increased intracranial pressure—*e.g.*, cerebral tumour. Normally, the anterior fontanelle should close by the age of one and a half, and the posterior fontanelle at birth. In rickets and hydrocephalus the anterior fontanelle is late in closing.

(vi.) For *Cretinism* and *Mongolism* see § 19.

§ 13. Variations in the Form of the Skull are met in several complaints, and chiefly in children, because cases of marked deformity of the head seldom reach adult life, except in an institution for the mentally defective. The following are noteworthy:—

(i.) *Asymmetry* may be congenital, due to a difficult labour, or acquired in early life from the continual nursing of the infant on one arm. The head is flattened on the side on which it rests. Nursing on the other arm readily corrects the deformity.

(ii.) In *hydrocephalus* (§ 1037) the head is large out of all proportion to the face, and the forehead overhangs the face.

(iii.) In *rickets* the skull is large and square, but the forehead rises straight up and does not overhang. There are often bosses in the frontal and parietal regions.

(iv.) In *hereditary syphilis* the bones around the anterior fontanelle are thickened, and there are irregular areas of thickening and thinning (cranio-tabes), especially behind the ears. The condition resembles that found in rickets, with which it may co-exist.

(v.) In *microcephaly* the forehead is receding and the cranium very small. The children are mentally defective. In *scaphocephaly* the head is elongated and its lateral diameter diminished. *Brachycephaly* indicates that the head is shortened from before backwards: an extreme variety occurs in *oxycephaly* in which the head is very tall ("steeple-shaped"), with exophthalmos and slanting eyes. Defective mental development may co-exist with other "stigmata of degeneration," such as high arched palate, accessory auricles, etc.

(vi.) In *adults* signs of infantile malformations may be found. Localised thickenings may also be seen in osteitis deformans, leontiasis ossea and after injury.

(vii.) In *acromegaly* (§ 615) the lower jaw and often the nose are enlarged. The face is ovoid with the longer transverse diameter below. (See Fig. 7.)

(viii.) In *osteitis deformans* (Paget's disease) the face is ovoid but with the longer transverse diameter above.

(B) DECUBITUS (IN ACUTE CONDITIONS) AND ATTITUDE (IN CHRONIC DISEASES) [1]

§ 14. **Decubitus** signifies the position which a patient tends most constantly to assume, and it often gives a valuable clue to the disease, more especially in the diagnosis of **Acute Diseases,** and sometimes as to their probable issue as well. For example:

(i.) *Sitting up in bed,* propped up with pillows, on account of inability to bre᷍᷍᷍ᵤₑ in other positions (orthopnœɛ). ᷍᷍ characteristic of the extreme breathlessness which occurs in advanced cardiac, pulmonary or renal disease; and sometimes also in acute disease, such as pneumonia.

(ii.) *Lying on one side* is characteristic of considerable pleural effusion, pericarditis, or pneumonia on that side, as in this position free play is given to the healthy lung. When a patient with a chronic cough always lies on one side, suspect a cavity, bronchiectasis or empyema of that side. A patient curls up on one side in colic and in certain forms of meningitis.

(iii.) The *dorsal decubitus*—i.e., lying on the back—is seen in grave illnesses attended by marked prostration. (*a*) In the " typhoid state " the limbs are stretched out and completely relaxed. The typhoid state, so called from its occurrence in typhus and typhoid fevers, is a condition of profound prostration, attended by unconsciousness or muttering delirium, sordes on the teeth, and a dry, cracked tongue.

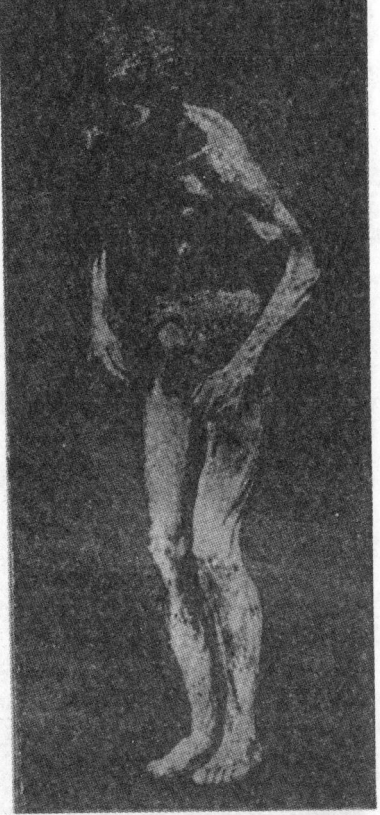

FIG. 5.—The attitude typical of PARALYSIS AGITANS; from a plaster cast by M. Paul Richer.

(*b*) If the prostration be due to peritonitis, the legs are drawn up, so as to relax the abdominal muscles; and for the same reason the breathing is thoracic and the abdomen is quite still. The greater flexion of one leg may give a clue as to the side on which the trouble exists.

(iv.) *Opisthotonos* is an arching of the back which occurs in some

[1] The various characteristic gaits are described in § 843.

convulsive and spasmodic disorders. It may be so great that only the head and heels touch the bed, especially in tetanus, hystero-epilepsy, strychnine poisoning and the cerebro-spinal meningitis of infants.

(v.) *Retraction of the head* is characteristic in cerebro-spinal and posterior basic meningitis. It is ; also met in the meningism of infants with digestive disorders, otitis media, or febrile states (§ 881), in dyspnœa—due to laryngeal obstruction and in rare cases of cervical caries.

(vi.) *Restlessness* occurs in many disorders, acute and chronic, and is generally a grave sign in the former—*e.g.*, in acute pericarditis. Sometimes, as in children, it is an indication of severe pain. *Carphology (καρφος,* the clothes; *λέγειν,* to pluck) is the picking at the bedclothes so characteristic of the " typhoid state." The hands seek after imaginary objects.

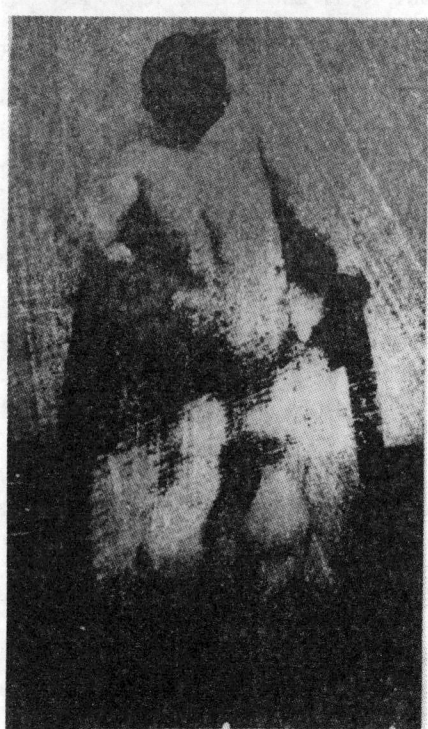

Subsultus tendinum is the muscular twitching or tremor which occurs in the same state. Both of these imply extreme cerebral depression. They are met in the malignant forms of the acute specific fevers, and are of the gravest possible import.

§ 15. The **Attitude** which is involuntarily assumed by a patient suffering from certain chronic diseases, if he be able to leave his bed, is very characteristic. Thus :

(i.) In *paralysis agitans* the head, neck and thorax are bent forwards, the arms are flexed at the elbows, the body moves stiffly, as if a statue, and the patient has the characteristic "festinating gait " (Fig. 5). The disease is recognisable at sight by the smooth, expressionless face, fixity of gaze (always

FIG. 6.—PSEUDO-HYPERTROPHIC PARALYSIS. [From Taylor, *Practice of Medicine,* J. & A. Churchill.]

looking forwards), the forward bending of the body, tremor of the hands, and the short steps which the patient takes as he shuffles along. (ii.) The attitude assumed by children suffering from *postdiphtheritic paralysis* is somewhat similar to the preceding, and is so characteristic that one can often detect the disease as the patient enters the room. The head hangs forward from weakness of the neck muscles, and the " flabbiness " of all the movements is peculiar. (iii.) The *rigidity of the spine* in spondylitis deformans, osteo-arthritis and spinal caries, gives a stiffness and awkward-ness to all the movements which is very noticeable.

(iv.) Duchenne's *pseudo-hypertrophic paralysis* (Fig. 6) is a comparatively rare condition, but the arching forwards of the back, prominence of the buttocks, scapulæ, and calves, and inability to rise from a recumbent posture without the aid of the hands are pathognomonic.

(C) The General Conformation

§ 16. Under this heading we note (*a*) whether the patient exhibits any loss of flesh (EMACIATION, *infra*); (*b*) whether he presents any increase in volume (GENERAL ENLARGEMENT, §§ 17 and 18); or (*c*) whether he presents any DEFORMITY or DWARFISM (§ 19).

Here we meet with several important diseases affecting the skeleton and general growth of the individual. The various causes of such altera-tions will only be mentioned here. They will be described and differentiated under the Diseases of Extremities, and elsewhere.

VARIATIONS IN HEALTH.—The terms "emaciation" and "General Enlargement of the Body" are only relative. The healthy man should have an elastic skin, firm muscles and small amount of subcutaneous fat; but *individual variations* are so great that no definite standard can be set up as normal. Health in the wiry, nervous man is consistent with a spare-ness that would indicate disease in his stouter and more phlegmatic brother. The same holds true with regard to *age*. A child has an amount of fatty covering that would be abnormal in adolescence; an old man has atrophy of the soft parts and prominence of the bones which in the middle-aged man could only accompany serious disease. The question of build is very largely one of *heredity*: stout parents usually have children who tend to become stout, and *vice versa*.

Emaciation is necessarily attended by more or less weakness, and the subject is dealt with under General Debility (Chapter XVI).

The chief causes of debility with emaciation are: Malignant disease, digestive disorders and privation, diabetes, tuberculosis, various nervous disorders, hyperthyroidism, pituitary cachexia (Simmonds' disease), sub-acute and chronic infections and toxæmias chronic nephritis, syphilis and pancreatic diseases; and in children, defective feeding, diarrhœa and chronic infections including tuberculosis and hereditary syphilis.

In *advanced life* the first cause which occurs to our minds, if the patient has lost flesh, is cancer; in *middle age*, diabetes; and in *young adults*, hyperthyroidism or tuberculosis. In tuberculosis of the lungs or else-where, loss of weight may occur before any physical signs can be detected; indeed, this symptom together with an intermitting pyrexia generally means latent tuberculosis. In *infancy* the two most common causes of acute or *rapid* wasting are defective feeding and acute gastro-enteritis. The most common causes of slow, progressive, or *chronic* wasting in infants are defective feeding and environment, cœliac disease and tuberculosis.

Emaciation of the face and upper part of the body, with enlargement below the waist, is seen in *lipodystrophia progressiva*, a rare disease probably of endocrine origin.

§ 17. General Enlargement of the body is usually due to *Obesity*. It is also seen with *Generalised Œdema* (see §§ 9, 18 and 29), *Myxœdema* (Fig. 1, § 9, and § 575), *Acromegaly* and in *Eunuchs*. Overactivity of the anterior lobe of the pituitary gland, when in a child, leads to gigantism;

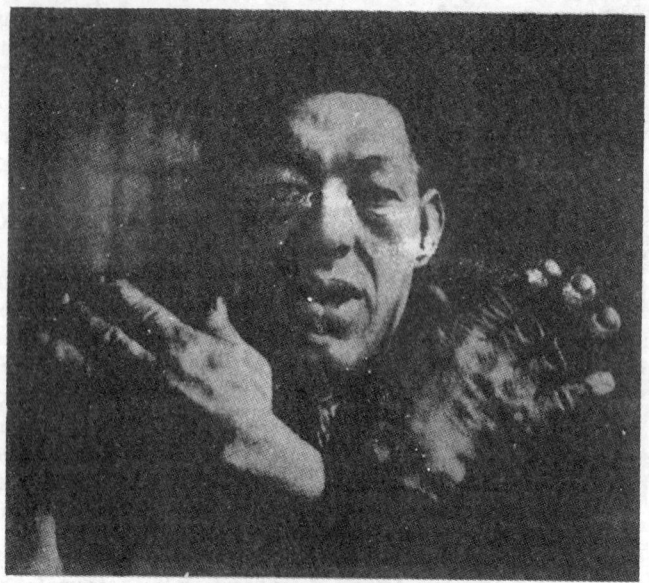

FIG. 7.—ACROMEGALY.

when occurring in the adult, it causes acromegaly. Enlargement of the body, with sexual precocity, may occur with tumours of the pineal gland. Obesity sometimes follows lesions of the nervous system, such as growths in the region of the hypothalamus.

§ 18. Obesity, the excessive accumulation of fat in the subcutaneous and deep tissues, is due to excessive intake as compared with output of calories. An individual is considered to be overweight when he or she is 10 per cent. or more above the ideal weight for the sex, age and height (Table at end of book).

Symptoms.—In modern civilised society, obesity is the cause of a greater amount of ill-health than any other single factor. It usually commences about middle age and often after childbirth. The ill effects of obesity are (i.) to cause general lack of energy (asthenia) for physical exertion and to

a less extent for mental work; (ii.) to contribute to cardio-vascular disease including atherosclerosis, coronary disease, myocardial degeneration and hypertension. (iii.) Orthopædic troubles which arise or are aggravated are postural strain of the lower back, osteo-arthritis of the lumbar spine, the hip or knee joints and also pes planus. (iv.) Varicose veins are more troublesome. (v.) Metabolic diseases and especially diabetes mellitus are a direct result of obesity as are (vi.) dyspepsia, gall-stone formation and hæmorrhoids. (vii.) Herniæ—especially of the umbilicus. (viii.) Respiratory symptoms include shortness of breath, chronic bronchitis and emphysema. (ix.) Sterility is not unusual in women. (x.) Obesity not only increases post-operative complications but makes abdominal operations technically more difficult. Taking exercise has little effect on obesity, for although exercise uses up calories it stimulates the appetite. On the other hand, most of the symptoms outlined above cause the obese patient to be relatively immobilised: this immobility together with an undiminished appetite produces a vicious circle and further gain in weight.

Etiology.—Some families show a hereditary tendency to obesity. Excessive appetite is largely a habit, associated with large meals and often double helpings of food. Another cause is eating between meals, particularly such foods as chocolates, cakes and pastries. These habits may be the result of emotional instability. Excessive consumption of alcohol and especially beer with its high calorie value, is another cause. It is well known that many start to gain weight after giving up cigarette smoking. Although the greater part of the gain in weight is due to the deposition of fat, there is also salt and water retention in the tissues—fat people often show a ridge of œdema above the shoes at the end of the day, independent of cardio-renal disease.

Varieties.—Two groups of cases are recognised: (a) the exogenous group where the chief factor is excessive appetite and overfeeding; (b) the endogenous group where endocrine factors are important.

(a) *Exogenous obesity.* In health the weight of an individual keeps remarkably steady: a temporary increase in calorie intake is compensated by an increased output. Comparable with the temperature-regulating mechanism there appears to be a weight-regulating mechanism in the hypothalamus, destruction of which causes obesity to develop. This mechanism prevents many people of slight build from gaining weight in spite of a large appetite. In others, this mechanism functions inefficiently and a large appetite causes the excessive intake of carbohydrate and fatty foods to be deposited as fat in the tissues: excess protein causes this much less often, partly on account of its stimulant effect on metabolism (specific dynamic action).

(b) *Endogenous obesity* occurs in certain endocrine diseases.

(i.) In *eunuchs, after* operative *removal of the ovaries* and at *menopause*, there is a considerable tendency to deposit fat on the trunk, breasts and around the shoulder and pelvic girdles: the forearms, hands, the lower legs and the feet remain slim. Since the gonads depress the function of the anterior lobe of the pituitary, their absence allows the pituitary to overact. This group is closely allied to the next.

(ii.) *Cushing's syndrome* arises when there is a basophil adenoma or a diffuse increase of these cells in the anterior lobe of the pituitary, or much more commonly when there is cortical hyperplasia (or even a cortical carcinoma) of the suprarenal (§ 263). Obesity chiefly affects the face, neck and trunk. There is also polycythæmia with a dusky skin, purple striæ distensæ on the abdomen, a considerable rise of blood pressure, hypertrichosis, impotence and amenorrhœa. Accompanying these are varying degrees of general weakness, glycosuria, osteoporosis and kyphosis.

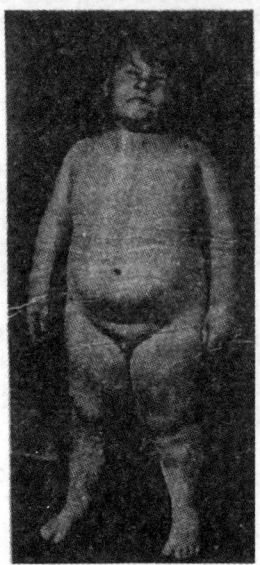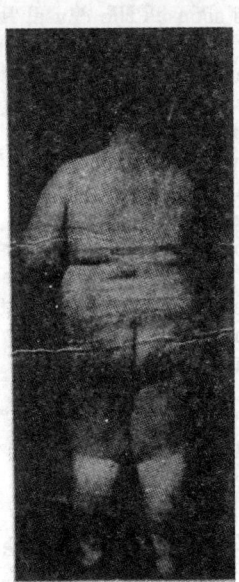

FIG. 8.
(Photographs taken by Mr. G. J. Potts.)
FRÖBLICH'S SYNDROME. Boy aged 5; weight 5 st. 4 lb.; has genital aplasia.

(iii.) *Adiposis Dolorosa* (Dercum's disease) is rare and occurs in women near the menopause. It is characterised by local subcutaneous and symmetrical deposition of a material probably mucoid in character, but the masses resemble lipomata. They are found chiefly over the deltoids or the triceps, and on the upper part of the body; and may occasionally spread downwards. In another form there is diffuse lipomatosis, only the hands and feet escaping. Pain is a constant symptom, due probably to pressure on the subcutaneous nerves. Small doses of thyroid, massage, and plenty of open-air exercise have given good results, but treatment has often been disappointing. The disease is probably due to overaction of the pituitary. The condition described by Bowlby as *diffuse lipoma*, which occurs in alcoholic men, may be mistaken for Dercum's disease.

(iv.) *Fröhlich's syndrome* is rare. It is characterised by dwarfism and a pituitary type of obesity in children, in whom sexual development never occurs. As in Frohlich's original case the hypothalamus may be destroyed by a cranio-pharyngioma,

or there may be a chromophobe adenoma of the anterior pituitary: in many cases no discoverable cause may be found.

(v.) *The Lawrence-Moon-Biedl syndrome* shows the characteristics of Fröhlich's syndrome, together with retinitis pigmentosa, mental retardation and polydactylism. It is familial but not hereditary.

(vi.) *Pineal tumours* with obesity have been recorded.

Prognosis.—In approximate figures, over the age of 30, the statistics of insurance companies show that the expectation of life is reduced by 1 per cent. for every 1 per cent. of weight in excess of the normal. In those affected by obesity it is always possible to reduce the weight but relapse occurs as soon as the causal factors reassert themselves. Loss of weight not only increases the sense of well-being: it often restores the sugar-tolerance of elderly persons to normal and causes hypertensive blood pressures to fall markedly.

Treatment.—(i.) *Diet.* The first essential is to reduce the calorie intake well below the output and to continue this until the requisite weight is lost. Particularly in elderly persons it is usually unwise to reduce to the ideal weight or to effect too rapid a weight reduction. In refractory cases it is better to commence treatment with a few days in bed, preferably in hospital. It is usually sufficient to give a diet which eliminates foods which are not essential and which are of high calorie value (*e.g.*, sugar, cream, ice-cream, pastries, thick soups), to limit foods such as bread and milk (§ 296), and to give bulk to the diet by allowing liberal amounts of salads, fruit and vegetables. If this scheme is not successful a diet consisting of protein, fruit and vegetables is usually effective (§ 296): alternatively a diet of 1,000 calories may be prescribed (§ 296). In all cases alcohol should be restricted and added salt forbidden at meal times to help decrease the appetite as well as to prevent sodium chloride and water retention. (ii.) *Drugs.* It is never wise to prescribe thyroid unless the patient shows signs of myxœdema: some who have used thyroid in large doses have been rendered diabetic. Dextro-amphetamine (5–10 mg.) given half an hour before breakfast and before lunch reduces the appetite and stimulates metabolism—if given later in the day it causes insomnia: particularly in those in whom *d*-amphetamine induces side effects, it may be prescribed with amylobarbitone (as in Drinamyl). A few doses of inject. mersalyl (intramuscularly) encourage loss of the retained salt and water. Di-nitrophenol is now considered too dangerous to use; and Preludin causes addiction, psychosis and other toxic effects. (iii.) Moderate exercise must be encouraged. (iv.) When emotional factors are responsible, psycho-therapy may be helpful. (v.) In endogenous obesity, appropriate endocrine preparations should be prescribed.

§ 19. **Dwarfism** means diminished stature, and does not imply mental or sexual retardation. It may arise from any cause which affects the growth or the adult structure of the bones of the trunk or limbs, whether local or constitutional. The common causes of a stunted condition of the body are :

(i.) *Curvature of the Spine*, which may take three forms: (i.) *kyphosis* (*i.e.*, the convexity projecting backwards) in the young is usually due to postural defects, tuberculosis or other disease of the vertebræ, or to lax ligaments, as in rickets. The latter disappears when the child is held up by the shoulders. Some degree of kyphosis and loss of stature occurs in most elderly persons: this is the result of muscular weakness and the diminution in thickness of the intervertebral discs. In some it becomes more severe as the result of senile osteoporosis and collapse of the vertebral bodies. Angular kyphosis is serious, as indicating organic disease of the bodies of the vertebræ. (ii.) *Lordosis* (*i.e.*, a forward projection), usually compensatory, or the result of muscular weakness; and (iii.) *scoliosis* (a lateral curve). A certain amount of scoliosis is normal to nearly everyone.

(ii.) *Rickets.*—In this disease there is curving of the long bones, together with altered epiphyseal growth. This results in " bandy legs," " knock-knee," and other familiar deformities (§ 608). Varieties occur in the form of *renal* and *cœliac rickets*.

(iii.) *Achondroplasia.*—A rare condition somewhat resembling, and formerly con-

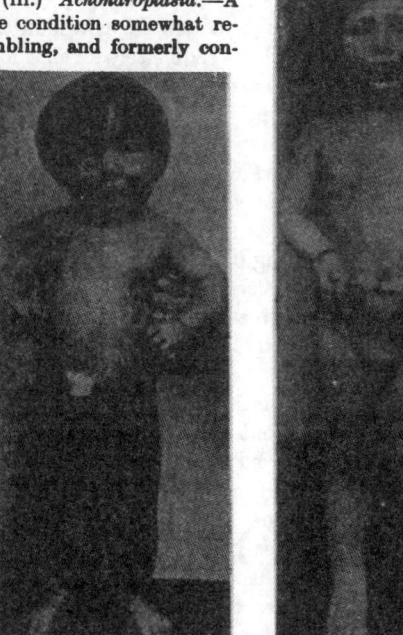
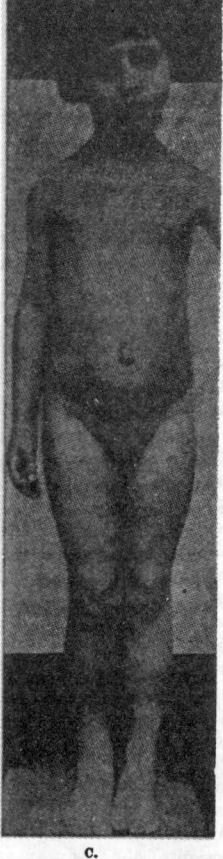

A.   B.   C.

FIG. 9.—Case of cretinism. A, aged 18 months. B and C after treatment, aged 38 and 66 months.

fused with, rickets (§ 616). The arms and legs are more shorte..ed than the body.

(iv.) *Congenital conditions or diseases acquired in early life*, especially tuberculosis, syphilis, malaria and cœliac disease. Also disease of the pancreas and poisoning by lead, mercury or morphia.

(v.) Although *Mongolism* and *Microcephaly* (§§ 13, 1194c) fall into this group on account of the lack of mental and physical growth and the sexual retardation, the changes produced make the subjects so unlike normal children that they are better described separately. In *Mongolism* (Down's Syndrome) defective development is met chiefly in the children of older parents. It is differentiated from cretinism by the fine hair, clear complexion, liveliness of manner, and broad head without an appreciable occipital prominence, and absence of constipation. The name is derived from the resemblance to the Mongolian races. The eyes are oval and slant upwards at the outer angle, the little finger tends to curve inwards; there is often a squint, with various " stigmata of degeneration " and often a congenital heart.

(vi.) *Cretinism* (§ 192) is a peculiar stunting of the growth which is either sporadic or is endemic among children in certain districts. The appearance is so distinctive that typical cases can be recognised at a distance (Fig. 9A). The face is broad and flat, and joined almost without a neck to the body. The skin and hair are coarse, the hands broad and stumpy, the stature stunted, for even when twenty years of age a cretin may be only 3 feet high. It is due to a diminished action of the thyroid gland; recovery usually results and is maintained while thyroid extract is being given (Fig. 9B and c), but for the best results it must be started as early in life as possible.

(vii.) *Pituitary deficiency*, especially of the growth-hormone-secreting cells of the anterior pituitary gland.

(viii.) In addition to the foregoing there are certain rare conditions, of which the celebrated Tom Thumb and his wife, and the race of pygmies of Africa met with by Sir H. M. Stanley and others are examples, in which the skeleton and the organs are diminished in size, but their proportions maintained. Such cases, however, seem to be functionally normal in every respect.

§ 20. **Infantilism** is a condition of dwarfism, combined with a developmental failure of the normal sexual and physical changes of puberty: the patient retains the stature, features, voice and often the mental proclivities of a child. Although the term infantilism is often applied to conditions in which there is dwarfism and in which sexual development never occurs, in many cases no hard and fast line can be drawn between pure dwarfism and infantilism as sexual changes may occur at an unusually late age. The principal cause of infantilism is a deficiency of the anterior pituitary involving the eosinophilic (growth-hormone-secreting) and the basophilic (gonado-trophic-hormone-secreting) cells. Such deficiency may follow an acute specific fever or be due to destruction of the cells of the anterior pituitary by a chromophobe adenoma or a craniopharyngioma—producing a condition closely resembling Simmonds' disease of childhood. In these cases union of the epiphyses is often delayed and so growth can proceed at a much later age than normal. *Ateliosis* may be of the same origin. It is hereditary; in the asexual form, there is delayed development of the whole body, but especially of the sexual organs; in another form improvement occurs at puberty, but the individual remains tiny. Under the name *progeria*, Hastings Gilford described a condition in which infantilism is associated with premature decay, the appearance, attitude and state of nutrition of the dwarf becoming senile, and degenerative changes occur in the vessels and viscera (§ 570). Primary thyroid deficiency gives rise to cretinism.

Treatment will depend on the primary cause, which should be sought. When there is evidence of a defect in the secretion of the growth-hormone or of the gonadotrophic hormone of the anterior pituitary, potent hormonal extracts should be injected. Thyroid medication is of major importance in the endocrine group, and injection of gonadotrophic and other hormones of the anterior lobe of the pituitary produce good results in experimental animals, and may benefit human beings. Even in the forms caused by toxaemia, thyroid should be given a trial.

Turner's syndrome is largely confined to females, the result of gonadal aplasia. There is retarded growth and formation of the epiphyses (possibly of pituitary origin), almost complete lack of development of the sex organs so that amenorrhœa is accompanied by great decrease in the size of the breasts, the external genitalia, the uterus and cervix with greatly diminished or absent pubic and axillary hair. A webbed neck is usual. Urine analysis shows deficient 17-ketosteroid secretion but a marked increase in follicle-stimulating hormone. The condition is rare in the male, and is due to an abnormal chromosomal pattern (45 instead of the normal 46 chromosomes, § 1315). *Treatment* in the female is with œstrogen therapy.

CHAPTER III

DISEASES OF THE HEART AND PERICARDIUM

§ 25. Physiology and Anatomy of the Heart.—Before considering systematically cardio-vascular disease, it is advisable to review the more important points regarding the physiological anatomy of the heart. The heart is developed as a tube of muscle which becomes bent on itself and develops diverticula, forming the chambers, auricular and ventricular, of the adult heart. This tube in the course of development becomes modified, but remains can be distinguished in the fully formed heart, and are of importance as they form the specialised tissues whose functions are the initiation and conduction of the normal cardiac impulse. This specialised system is made up of: (1) Sino-auricular node (Pacemaker), which is situated between the auricular openings of the superior and inferior venæ cavæ, and with which the extrinsic nerves are closely associated—(2) auriculo-ventricular node. Passing down from the auriculo-ventricular node is a neuro-muscular strand—(3) The Bundle of His, which has a special nerve and blood supply, and forms the main connecting link between auricles and ventricles. It lies just under the endocardium, under cover of the septal cusp of the tricuspid valve. The Bundle of His divides into—(4) A main right and left branch. The right branch, passing along the right side of the septum under the endocardium, runs along the moderator band and curves backwards to terminate chiefly in the base of the right ventricle and papillary muscles. The left branch passes along the left side of the septum, finally terminating in the wall of the left ventricle in close association with the cells of Purkinje. The different parts of this system are shown in Fig. 45.

The heart has a considerable reserve capacity; the maximum output during exertion is about six times that produced by the resting heart. The increase in the work done is frequently so sudden that the organ is subjected to strain as the result of sudden mechanical efforts or violent emotion. Injury is prevented by a series of protective mechanisms: the more important of which may be summarised as follows: (1) NERVOUS MECHANISMS.—*The Vagus* has two main sets of fibres in relation to the heart: (a) efferent fibres with the power of slowing, weakening or even stopping the beat; (b) afferent fibres (depressor nerve), which run from the arch of the aorta to the vaso-motor centre in the medulla and convey stimuli which lower the systemic blood pressure and so relieve the left heart. Overaction of the vagal mechanism may produce fainting attacks. The *carotid sinus*, situated at the bifurcation of the common carotid artery, is the focal point of vagal cardiac inhibition. A rise of blood pressure stretches the arterial wall and stimulates the rich network of nerve fibres arising in it: nerve impulses are conveyed by the sinus nerve to the glossopharyngeal nerve and thus to the vagal and vaso-motor centres in the medulla. Direct pressure on the sinus reflexly slows the heart rate and produces peripheral vaso-dilatation to such an extent that it can cause syncope. Such pressure may be digital, or from a stiff collar or other external object. More usually the stimulus is psychological, or the result of physical pain. Vaso-vagal attacks may be abrupt, or of more gradual onset. In the former case they must be distinguished from epilepsy, and in the latter from syncope caused by cerebral anæmia associated with vaso-motor failure. Bradycardia and very low blood pressure are the signs of a vaso-vagal attack. *Sympathetic* stimulation produces tachycardia.

(2) PAIN MECHANISM.—In most organs of the body a pain mechanism exists, the primary object of which is protection. In the case of the normal heart, the pain mechanism is one of the last called into play. *Afferent impulses* conduct painful sensations from the heart through sympathetic fibres. These leave the heart, and pass to the cervical and upper dorsal sympathetic ganglia of the left side, whence the

grey *rami communicantes* of the five upper dorsal segments pass the stimuli on to the spinal cord.

Heart sensations rarely become painful unless there is ventricular anoxæmia or pericarditis. Exercise cannot produce it in a healthy adult. The pain mechanism will be referred to again in connection with angina (§ 51).

(3) MYOCARDIAL MECHANISMS.—(a) In the absence of anoxæmia or toxæmia the myocardium maintains its tone. Excessive exertion produces no dilatation when such exertion has finished. In the diseased heart, however, dilatation occurs. It is probable that under certain conditions the tricuspid and mitral rings may relax so that the valves may be rendered for the time being incompetent and the pressure in the ventricles relieved. (b) The Moderator Band is a special band of muscle which crosses the cavity of the right ventricle and is reputed to prevent over-dilatation of this cavity; it contains the right branch of the Bundle of His.

(4) PERICARDIAL MECHANISMS.—The pericardium is a tough fibrous bag, the main function of which is to prevent over-distension of the auricles.

PART A. SYMPTOMATOLOGY

The GENERAL SYMPTOMS of cardiac disease, as distinct from the local signs referable to the heart, should be studied very carefully, inasmuch as the gravity of any given case depends not so much on the local signs present as on the general condition of the patient.

In the investigation of a case of cardiac disease the various methods have roughly the following relative values: history 40%, physical examination 25%, electrocardiography 20%, radiography 10%, and pathological and other special methods of diagnosis 5%. It is thus clear that the importance of an accurate evaluation of symptoms is very great.

The CARDINAL SYMPTOM of cardiac dysfunction is **Breathlessness.** When there is marked failure, **Œdema, Venous Engorgement** and **Cyanosis** are also present. **Pain, Palpitation** and **Cough** are found in certain cases. **Fainting Attacks,** although in the lay mind invariably attributed to the heart, have in practice only rarely a cardiac cause. **Lassitude** may be due to organic cardiac disease. **Sleeplessness** and **delirium** occur in cases of failure. **Fever** and its concomitant symptoms occur in acute affections. **Sudden** or **Unexpected Death** may terminate cardiac disease.

§ 26. **Breathlessness,** or Dyspnœa. Breathlessness may be present without cardiac disease; but it may be affirmed that no serious affection of the CARDIAC MUSCLE can exist without breathlessness. Dyspnœa is a physiological result of muscular exertion. It becomes pathological when evoked in excessive degree by an amount of exercise which previously had no such result. Two points to be elucidated are: (1) the amount of exercise now noticed to cause dyspnœa, and (2) the rapidity of development of the symptom. The severity of the myocardial failure and the progress of myocardial damage can, for example, be estimated clinically by assessing the effect of exertion upon the patient's breathing. When dyspnœa is severe the accessory muscles of respiration (*e.g.*, the scaleni and sterno-mastoid muscles) can be observed to come into action on inspiration.

Severe disease of the VALVES of the heart may exist for many years

—provided the disability so caused is adequately compensated by muscular hypertrophy—without the patient having any noteworthy symptoms, or even being aware of its existence. When the heart muscle fails to compensate for the valvular defect, breathlessness appears. When the patient is unable to breathe comfortably on lying down, or if the night is passed sitting upright in a chair, or propped up with pillows in bed, *orthopnœa* is present. It indicates pulmonary congestion from left-sided failure. It is absent in pure right-sided failure. This upright position relieves the embarrassed lung from the weight of the engorged liver, lowers the pressure in the venæ cavæ, assists the accessory muscles of respiration, and so reduces pulmonary congestion as far as possible. Towards the end in many cases of heart failure *Cheyne-Stokes' respiration* may be observed.

Sighing is frequently regarded as being due to organic heart disease, but this is not the case. It is suggestive of a cardio-vascular neurosis. It is frequently associated with vaso-motor instability, with a labile heart rate and blood pressure, or may result from great nervous or bodily fatigue. The sighing is often long-drawn and occurs at frequent intervals.

CAUSES OF BREATHLESSNESS (DYSPNŒA).—Difficult breathing may arise in five different groups of disorders.

1. **Myocardial Disease.**—The dyspnœa of heart disease has no intrinsic features which distinguish it from that due to other causes, but it is often associated with cyanosis. There is also usually a history, or evidence, of some of the other symptoms of cardiac disorder. Enlargement of the heart is nearly always present. If in a dyspnœic patient there is no enlargement, the dyspnœa is due to a cause other than heart disease.

2. **Mechanical Embarrassment of the Heart** by, for example, a peri-cardial or a pleural effusion, mediastinal tumours, a large aortic aneurysm, ascites, a dilated stomach. Obesity may be a subsidiary cause of dyspnœa.

3. **Pulmonary Disease,** of which chronic bronchitis with emphysema is the most common. *Acute pneumothorax* may also give rise to dyspnœa of sudden onset, generally with pain in the side (§ 126).

4. **Laryngeal or Tracheal Obstruction.**

5. **Blood Conditions.** Patients with a severe degree of anæmia are often markedly dyspnœic; in addition they often have palpitation, hæmic murmurs and œdema of the feet. Anæmic patients with dyspnœa prefer to lie flat, since there is no pulmonary congestion; cardiac patients with dyspnœa nearly always have congested lungs and therefore prefer to be propped up. *Acidæmia* due to diabetic ketosis or to urærnia, may cause dyspnœa, but this is present both at rest and on exercise.

§ 27. **Paroxysmal Dyspnœa** occurs in sudden attacks, chiefly at night. Cardiac causes are:—

(i.) mitral stenosis with severe pulmonary hypertension,
(ii.) chronic myocardial degeneration from coronary disease,
(iii.) hypertensive heart disease, which can be due to chronic nephritis (" renal asthma ").

In each case the cause is sudden left heart failure. The attacks are

clinically severe and similar to those of acute spasmodic asthma. The
patient is pale, sweating, distressed and orthopnœic. He frequently has
to grasp on to the back of a chair or to lean against the mantelpiece for
support. The attacks seem to arise as a direct result, possibly reflex, of
the pulmonary congestion. They usually persist from ten to thirty
minutes but may last longer. Multiple fine expiratory rhonchi are heard
all over the chest, cough is often present and the attacks may be associated
with acute pulmonary œdema, frothy yellow or pink sputum being coughed
up in considerable amount. Paroxysmal cardiac dyspnœa can be
differentiated from the paroxysmal attacks of acute asthma in that there
is no history of attacks in previous years, and examination reveals cardiac
enlargement (often with hypertension), with clinical and electrocardiographic evidence of chronic disease of the heart muscle.

Treatment of these attacks is by the injection of morphia gr. ¼ (intramusc. or intravenously) and by the inhalation of oxygen. Aminophylline
B.P. intravenously (0·24 G.) or intramuscularly (0·48 G.) is a useful
emergency measure. The development of attacks can be minimised or
prevented by the regular use of diuretics, by courses of aminophylline
(0·48 G.) intramusc. or as a suppository at bedtime on seven successive
days and in some cases by digitalis therapy.

OTHER CAUSES OF PAROXYSMAL DYSPNŒA are
1. ASTHMA, laryngismus stridulus and whooping-cough, the attacks of breathlessness are typically paroxysmal.
2. ACUTE PULMONARY ŒDEMA (§ 118).
3. INTRATHORACIC TUMOURS, such as carcinoma of the bronchus, thyroid enlargement (§§ 77–80).
4. NEUROTIC DYSPNŒA. Some neurotic patients are liable to attacks of rapid
respiration. These usually cease when the patient converses or thinks that he is
not being observed, or during sleep. If prolonged, tingling in the fingers and other
evidences of tetany are present (§ 1030). The heart rate may be rapid in these attacks.
5. THE LARYNGEAL CRISES of tabes dorsalis may take the form of paroxysmal
dyspnœa with a sense of suffocation, spasms of coughing, stridor and cyanosis.
6. FOREIGN BODIES in the trachea and retropharyngeal abscess in children, and
polypi or papillomata of the larynx, give rise to paroxysms of dyspnœa.

§ 28. Cheyne-Stokes' Respiration (so called after its first observers) consists, in its
typical form, of a series of eight or ten rapid inspirations gradually increasing in depth
and rapidity, and then dying gradually away, each series being separated by a pause
of some seconds (the stage of apnœa), in which there is little or no respiratory movement. It is due to slight dysfunction of the respiratory centre. The hyperpnœic
stage may produce such exaggerated movements as to wake the patient and cause
a sensation of acute discomfort.

In a modified form, without the apnœic pause, Cheyne-Stokes' breathing is not
infrequent. It is usually a serious symptom, and appears in cardiac patients towards
the end of life. It has less significance at the extremes of life, for it may be observed
during sleep in normal infants, and is occasionally compatible with a hale old age.

Its principal causes are as follows:
1. CEREBRAL ARTERIOSCLEROSIS; 2. CARDIAC DISEASE due to coronary atheroma;
3. URÆMIA; 4. Rapidly increased INTRACRANIAL PRESSURE such as occurs with
apoplexy, tuberculous meningitis, and in some cases of cerebral tumour; 5. ACUTE
HEPATIC NECROSIS in its advanced stages; 6. SUNSTROKE.

Treatment is by oxygen administration or in some cases the use of morphia, gr. ¼ by injection.   A course of daily intramuscular injections of aminophylline is useful, in doses of 0·48 G. in 2 ml. for 7–10 days.

§ 29. Œdema (Syn. dropsy) is the chronic effusion of fluid into the skin and subcutaneous tissues or into a serous cavity (as in hydrothorax, hydropericardium, ascites).   Anasarca is a form of GENERALISED ŒDEMA and is a very constant feature of some forms of cardiac disease.   Anasarca has to be differentiated from myxœdema, in which the swelling is harder, and does not pit on pressure.   It is best to apply the pressure over a bone, such as the lower end of the tibia on its inner aspect.

Causes.—The causes of localised œdema are given in Diseases of the Extremities (§ 580).   There are *three varieties of anasarca*, which differ from each other both pathologically in their origin, and clinically in the course they pursue.

1. **Cardiac Œdema** is primarily due to a diminished cardiac output giving rise to a fall in the filtration pressure in the renal glomeruli.   This results in the retention in the body of sodium ions and, by osmosis, of water also.   (1) It *starts* and, throughout the case predominates, in the *most dependent parts*, that is to say, in the legs if the patient has been walking about, or in the lower part of the back if he has been lying in bed.   On inquiry, the patient may complain that the ankles swell towards evening around the top of the boot.   (2) Other signs and symptoms of cardiac failure are present.   (3) In the history of the case dyspnœa will have preceded the dropsy.   Œdema does not occur with equal frequency in all forms of cardiac disease.   The œdema which complicates the rare cases of pure right heart failure are accompanied by much less dyspnœa and orthopnœa, because pulmonary congestion is absent.   Heart failure with manifest œdema is called *congestive heart failure*.   Œdema, in the absence of dyspnœa or of cardiac enlargement, is not due to heart disease; some other cause, such as phlebitis or obstruction to the vena cava, must be sought.   Œdema is often present in renal disease without dyspnœa; it then forms part of a general œdema.

2. **Hepatic Œdema** (1) usually begins and predominates *in the abdomen* (ascites), although the legs may swell subsequently.   (2) There may be also enlargement or other signs of the liver affection which has given rise to the condition; and if these be absent some other cause of obstruction to the portal vein should be sought (§ 260).   (3) The dyspnœa will have *followed* the abdominal enlargement.

3. **Renal Œdema** is (1) *general in its distribution* from the beginning, occurring in the legs and eyelids at the same time; though it is probable that the œdema around the eyes on rising in the morning first attracts the attention of the patient or his friends.   (2) Examination of the urine reveals the features of renal disease, but it should be remembered that some degree of albuminuria is common in heart failure.   The presence of many casts is strong evidence of a renal origin.   (3) The patient presents a characteristic pale or waxy appearance.   In some cases of anasarca associated with albuminuria the question arises whether the œdema is

renal or cardiac. This may sometimes be answered by finding the liver enlarged and the neck veins engorged for these are a natural accompaniment of congestive heart failure, though not of renal disease.

Prognosis.—Dropsy usually indicates a severe degree and a late stage of heart disease. The outlook varies greatly, according to the cause.

Treatment.—The principles are as follows: Absolute rest in bed; keep the patient warm; reduce the fluid intake to 30 to 40 oz. daily; give a small, dry, palatable, non-fermenting diet with a reduced sodium chloride content; also give digitalis and a mercurial diuretic—such as mersalyl ½–2 ml. intramuscularly, preceded for one day and accompanied by the administration of ammonium chloride 1 G. t.d.s., p.c. (in capsules).

Chlorothiazide (Saluric) 0·5–1·0 G., hydrochlorothiazide (Hydrosaluric) 25–100 mg., bendrofluazide (Aprinox, Neo-Naclex) 2·5–5·0 mg., hydroflumethazide (Naclex, Hydrenox) 25–50 mg., cyclopenthiazide (Navidrex) 0·25–0·50 mg., given once or twice daily for 2–3 days a week, are good diuretics which inhibit sodium and chloride reabsorption from the renal tubules; when large doses are used potass. chloride should be given to correct excessive potassium loss. They are less powerful than the mercurial diuretics but potentiate their effects. Tab. chlorthalidone (Hygroton) 100–200 mg. with a maintenance dose of 100 mg. each 2–4 days is a long-acting diuretic which is often very effective. Acetazolamide B.P. (Diamox) and theophyllin and sodium salicylate (diuretin) are now seldom used. If the œdema in the limbs is extensive, wrap them in cyanide gauze or some other dressing, as they are liable to eczema, erythema, cellulitis or exfoliative dermatitis. Should the above methods fail, multiple small punctures with needles or with small incisions through penicillin cream, or the insertion of Southey's tubes with aseptic precautions, may be practised; the patient's legs should have been dependent for several days to allow the fluid to accumulate. The abdomen or pleural cavity may require tapping. A pleural effusion constitutes a serious embarrassment to the heart and should be removed.

OBSCURE CAUSES OF GENERAL ŒDEMA (ANASARCA).—If, in a patient who complains of œdema, no marked evidences of cardiac, renal, or hepatic disease are discoverable, the following causes may be *suspected.*

1. In women with **poor muscular tone,** but who are otherwise normal, œdema of the legs and feet is found. It is common in multiparæ and the left leg is often the more severely affected, especially after a preceding phlebitis. It often accompanies varicose veins. Such patients generally have the symptom for many years, especially in hot weather; no marked dyspnœa and no cardiac enlargement are found.

2. **Anæmia** is not infrequently attended by some swelling of the ankles at the end of the day. Swelling of the feet and ankles may be present in the last stages of many diseases, such as phthisis, in septic and anæmic conditions and in cases of insufficient nutrition and old age.

3. Among other causes of œdema are Beri-Beri (§ 981) and **Epidemic Dropsy.** EPIDEMIC DROPSY occurs especially in India, but has been seen in South Africa and Mauritius. The cause is an unidentified toxic substance contained in the seeds of the Mexican Poppy (*Argemone Mexicana*), which become mixed with wheat or mustard crops.

Symptoms.—(i.) Anorexia, nausea, vomiting and diarrhœa are followed by (ii.) œdema of the legs. This may spread to other areas. (iii.) Severe dyspnœa is due to toxic myocardial damage with cardiac dilatation, a rapid weak pulse and a low blood pressure. (iv.) At an early stage the skin vessels become dilated, giving an irregular mottled appearance. (v.) Eye complications include glaucoma due to vascular dilatation of the ciliary body, and optic atrophy.

Treatment necessitates cessation of the contaminated food or mustard oil, rest in bed, digitalis, a low salt diet and inject. mersalyl (B.P.), tab. chlorothiazide or tab. chlorthalidone B.P. (Hygroton).

Famine Œdema is due to severe protein deficiency and arises from a lowered plasma albumin. It was common during the later years of World War II.

4. MILROY first described a **hereditary œdema** in which a solid œdema of the legs existed in many members of a family (§ 580).

5. **Congenital general œdema** (hydrops fœtalis, § 567 IV), a manifestation of erythroblastosis fœtalis, is usually fatal.

6. **Kwashiorkor** (Synonyms: Infantile Pellagra, Malignant Malnutrition, Fatty Liver Disease) is a syndrome found chiefly in children under 4 years of age in many parts of the world where poverty and ignorance are rife. The disease occurs after breast feeding is stopped when the child is put on to a high-carbohydrate, low-protein diet.

Symptoms.—There is always muscle wasting, though it is masked by an œdema which pits and responds to gravity. The child shows lack of progress and growth, becomes apathetic and difficult to feed. There is anæmia, sometimes macrocytic, and a reversed albumin/globulin ratio with a low total plasma protein. Other more variable features are diarrhœa, pellagrinous skin changes and a change in the hair, which becomes straight, soft and brown or reddish. If not treated the child will often die. Fibrotic changes in the liver, so common in the tropics, may possibly be a sequela in survivors.

Etiology.—The liver shows fatty infiltration, chiefly peri-portal. There is atrophy of the secretory cells of the pancreas, salivary glands and small intestine.

Treatment.—Very ill children may need intravenous plasma. Skimmed milk powder 4 oz. daily must be given, or at least one pint of ordinary milk daily if this is tolerated. The diet must otherwise be rich in protein with a low residue. Extra vitamins, if added to the diet early, are harmful; they should not be given until recovery is obvious. If malaria is found it should be treated at once, but helminth infections must wait till later. Every effort must be made to improve the child's home diet, to prevent relapses and permanent liver damage.

Venous Engorgement. In an advanced stage of heart failure the veins are continuously distended. This is visible chiefly in the veins of the neck and is increased during systole. The level below which the neck veins remain distended in a normal individual is the lower border of the manubrium sterni. In heart failure the veins remain swollen to a higher level according to the amount of increase in the pressure. If the neck veins are in a state of distension and there is no dyspnœa nor cardiac enlargement, the cause is to be sought in some lesion producing intra-thoracic venous obstruction, such as mediastinal tumour, aneurysm or constrictive pericarditis.

§ 30. Cyanosis, or bluish discoloration of the body surface, is due to an abnormal amount of reduced hæmoglobin in the peripheral capillary blood. *General cyanosis* which also affects the mucous membranes may be the result of (1) slowing of the general circulation, (2) insufficient aeration of the blood in the lungs, (3) admixture of venous with arterial blood in congenital heart disease, (4) polycythæmia (§ 31), (5) sulphæmoglobinæmia and methæmoglobinæmia (§ 32). When the blood stream is slowed, more oxygen is taken from the blood by the tissues. *Local cyanosis*, as in Raynaud's disease, is due to slowing of the peripheral circulation. It may be differentiated from general cyanosis, as in heart failure, by immersing the patient's hand in hot water for 10 minutes; in the former case the skin colour becomes pink, in the latter it remains blue.

Cardiac cyanosis is most pronounced in heart failure secondary to chronic pulmonary disease, or to mitral stenosis. It is found in congenital heart disease with pulmonary stenosis, or with gross auricular or ventricular septal defect. **Respiratory** causes of cyanosis are emphysema, bronchitis, asthma, pulmonary œdema, pneumonia and miliary tuberculosis.

Local cyanosis may be unilateral, as for example when an intrathoracic tumour is pressing upon the venous return of one arm. A venous thrombosis produces a similar effect. And see § 585.

Treatment of cyanosis.—The treatment of cyanosis of pulmonary origin depends on the cause. Oxygen, given by a B.L.B. or other type of mask, intra-nasal catheter, or oxygen tent or chamber, is most effective in emphysema, bronchitis, asthma, pulmonary œdema and pneumonia. Five per cent. CO_2 should be used with the oxygen when the breathing is shallow or when there is pulmonary collapse. Oxygen given by funnel is useless in every type of disease. Paracentesis of a pleural effusion always helps cardiac anoxæmia and cyanosis. In the absence of pulmonary œdema or bronchitis, oxygen is not of much use in heart failure, for the slowed circulation rate allows more, not less, time for the pulmonary capillary blood to be fully oxygenated. Heart failure with cyanosis is often benefited by rapid venesection and removal of 10 to 20 fl. oz. of blood, the particular indication for this being distension of the veins in the neck.

§ 31. Polycythæmia Rubra Vera (Synonyms: Erythræmia, Splenomegalic polycythæmia, Osler-Vaquez disease) is characterised by hyperplasia of the red-cell forming portion of the bone marrow, and to a lesser extent also of the white-cell and platelet producing portions. (i.) The patients are usually middle-aged and complain of headache, vertigo and visual disturbances, pains in the limbs and dyspnœa. (ii.) Their complexion is dusky red, deepening to cyanosis, particularly in cold weather. The superficial vessels in the skin are dilated. (iii.) The spleen is enlarged to a variable extent. (iv.) The liver is enlarged, either by engorgement with blood or occasionally by cirrhosis. (v.) The blood shows a marked increase in the number of red cells, white cells and platelets. The red cells may number up to 13 million per c.mm., and the hæmoglobin may rise to 120–160 per cent. (about 18 to 23 G. per 100 ml. of blood) with a colour index of about 0·7–0·9. The red cells may show polychromasia and occasional normoblasts. With the increase in the number of white cells myelocytes are present. Owing to the increase of red cells in the blood, its viscosity and the blood volume are raised and there is an increased tendency to thrombosis. (vi.) Hæmorrhages may occur from the distended vessels at any site. (vii.) Occasionally myeloid leukæmia develops terminally. When polycythæmia is accompanied by high blood pressure and arteriosclerosis, but no enlargement of the spleen, the condition is called *polycythæmia hypertonica* or **Gaisbock's disease**. This runs a chronic course; sometimes after many years death occurs from heart failure, cerebral hæmorrhage or thrombosis.

Erythrocytosis or secondary polycythæmia is a condition with an increase of the number of red cells without changes in white cells or platelets. It occurs most commonly with congenital cardiac abnormalities or with chronic pulmonary disease. When it is due to congenital stenosis or obliterative endarteritis of the pulmonary artery, this condition is known as **Ayerza's disease.** There is extreme dyspnœa, the blood pressure is normal or lowered, the spleen is not enlarged; the dilated conus of the pulmonary artery can be shown radiologically.

Treatment must be controlled by frequent blood counts. Drugs should not be used in polycythæmia secondary to pulmonary or cardiac conditions. It is therefore necessary to establish the correct diagnosis. Treatment may consist of (a) removing excess blood by repeated venesections; (b) inducing hæmolysis by drugs such as acetylphenylhydrazine gr. ¼ t.d.s. for 7–10 days, followed by a rest, or (c) depressing the bone marrow by irradiation or by the use of radiophosphorus, 3–8 millicuries intravenously at first followed by 1–5 millicuries every 3–6 months as long as the red cells number more than 6 million per c.mm.

§ 32. Rare causes of cyanosis are: **Sulph-hæmoglobinæmia** and **Methæmoglobinæmia.** The most prominent symptoms are (1) cyanosis of a peculiar greyish leaden colour; (2) marked weakness, vague pains and collapse; (3) constipation, sometimes alternating with offensive diarrhœa and most marked in sulph-hæmoglobinæmia; (4) periods of relative freedom followed by exacerbations. Two factors appear to be necessary for the formation of these compounds: (i.) some activating substance in the blood, and (ii.) absorption of sulphur or reducing substances from the bowel. It has been shown that sulphonamide compounds, metadinitrobenzene, trional, sulphonal, pamaquin, potassium chlorate, acetanilide, phenacetin and related compounds and certain aniline dyes, can act as such sensitising agents, and a history of taking these drugs can usually be obtained. Certain nitroso-bacilli, which have the power of reducing nitrogen compounds, have been isolated from the saliva and bowel, and are probably causal in those cases without a drug history (*enterogenous cyanosis*). Magnesium sulphate and other saline cathartics predispose by increasing the fluid content of the bowel, and hence bacterial fermentation. The *diagnosis* is based on the history and cyanosis without a cardiac or respiratory cause; it can be verified by spectroscopic examination of a sample of the blood. *Prognosis.*—This condition is not fatal, but may prove very resistant. In *treatment*, any possible sensitising drug must be excluded, and it is advisable to restrict sulphur in the diet; the constipation must be relieved by liquid paraffin or enemata. In severe cases, inhalations 2–3 times a day of 5 per cent. carbon dioxide in oxygen may be given. In cases due to nitroso-bacilli a vaccine of these organisms may be of value. The cyanosis of methæmoglobinæmia usually disappears within 48 hours of ceasing to take the drug, whilst that of sulph-hæmoglobinæmia may persist for very much longer. Methylene blue helps to relieve cyanosis: it is given in doses of gr. 1–2 t.d.s. by mouth, or 1–2 mg. per kilo intravenously. Ascorbic acid is effective in cases of familial methæmoglobinæmia.

A **Sallow Hue** of the skin is common in infective endocarditis. This sallowness is distinguished from jaundice by the absence of the yellow colour from the eyeballs and the absence of bile in the urine. Slight jaundice, however, does arise in cardiac disease, as a result of the hepatic congestion of severe cardiac failure.

Clubbing of the Fingers (§ 578) is found in heart disease in the following conditions. (1) The cyanotic forms of congenital heart disease. (2) Subacute bacterial endocarditis. (3) Rarely, slight clubbing is found in cases of chronic rheumatic carditis. (4) An aneurysm pressing on or affecting the flow in one subclavian artery may produce clubbing of the affected side (and see § 578).

§ 33. **Pain in the Chest** is absent in most forms of heart disease. It is present in coronary disease, less frequently in aortic insufficiency, and occasionally in mitral stenosis. Pain due to heart disease is usually proportional to the amount of exercise the patient is taking: it is generally substernal, sometimes præcordial in position and affects the upper rather than the lower part of the chest. It may radiate to either arm or to both, or to the neck or jaw (§ 51). Many cases of neuro-circulatory asthenia (effort syndrome) suffer from pain which is often submammary; hyperæsthesia of the precordium suggests a functional rather than an organic lesion.

The causes of præcordial pain are:

(a) Arising from **Organic affections outside the heart and pericardium.** Pectoral or intercostal fibrositis or " rheumatism "; neuritis which precedes or follows herpes zoster; carcinoma of the breast, bronchus or cardiac end of the stomach; hiatus hernia of the stomach; pleurisy and pneumothorax (§ 103); " cough fracture " of the ribs; spinal caries and carcinoma of the vertebræ, and tumours eroding the bones; the crises of tabes dorsalis; aneurysm. Muscular thoracic pain is increased by coughing or other muscular effort, and abolished by injection of a local anæsthetic; pleuritic pain is worse on breathing; herpetic pain is constant, and the pain of neoplasm is often worse at night.

(b) The pain may be of **Cardiac origin,** in which case it is usually called Angina (§ 51). It is the result of coronary ischæmia and occurs in three separate clinical conditions: (1) CORONARY THROMBOSIS (§ 52) produces an anginal pain, often of great severity. The onset is rapid, and the pain persists, with or without remission, for hours or even several days, during which time its intensity slowly subsides. (2) ANGINA OF EFFORT is characterised by an anginal pain which comes on during exertion, disappearing again when exertion ceases; its intensity is directly proportional to the amount of exercise taken. (3) SPASMODIC ANGINA leads to paroxysmal attacks of severe anginal pain lasting for some minutes, induced by exercise, emotion or cold, and relieved by nitrites; the pain is not proportional to exercise, and does not begin to subside directly exercise is stopped; angina of effort nearly always co-exists. These three forms of pain are due to an interference of blood flow through the coronary circulation. The interference in coronary thrombosis never completely disappears; that in angina of effort is temporary and only occurs when the heart activity is increased by exercise. The mechanism of an attack of spasmodic angina is not yet understood (see § 51).

(c) Pain of a cardiac type is also found in **neuro-circulatory asthenia,** effort syndrome, or disordered action of the heart (§§ 34, 53). The pain may be little more than a dull ache, when the term left submammary pain is often used, but it is sometimes acute and radiates to the left arm, thus simulating angina of effort or spasmodic angina. In such cases a careful history will reveal that it is not quantitative to exertion, is left-sided rather than central, and is closely related to fatigue or to emotion; and examination may reveal left submammary tenderness. The term angina innocens (§ 53) is a useful stimulus to correct diagnosis. In some cases intercostal or subscapular fibrositis seems to be a causative factor, but heart consciousness or fear are often the reasons for localisation of the pain to the præcordium. Sharp sudden stabs of pain sometimes occur in these cases, and accentuate the dull left-sided ache: syncopal attacks may follow these sharp stabs of pain. Organic heart disease is never indicated by pain of this type.

In cases of unexplained pain in the chest, and in the absence of cardiac signs, a *bronchial carcinoma, mediastinal tumour* or *aneurysm of the aorta*, either of the arch or of the descending aorta, should always be suspected, and an X-ray examination made (§§ 79-81).

Disease of the heart may also be an indirect cause of pain elsewhere than in the chest. For instance, with the engorged tender liver which is commonly associated with failure of the right side of the heart, the muscles and skin of the abdominal wall are often also tender. In coronary thrombosis and in acute pericarditis the pain may be referred entirely to the upper abdomen. A simple cause of epigastric tenderness which must never be forgotten in cases of heart and lung disease is muscular strain of the upper rectus muscle or diaphragm from the exertion of constant cough.

In the *treatment* of præcordial pain an endeavour should be made to ascertain and relieve the cause.

§ 34. Palpitation is consciousness of the heart's action. It arises under two sets of conditions, non-cardiac and cardiac. The essential symptomatic difference between the two types of palpitation is that in the *cardiac* group the onset is felt to be absolutely abrupt, as also in many cases is the termination of the paroxysm. The *non-cardiac* group is the larger and less serious; it includes:—

1. **Anæmia** where palpitation is a frequent and often a distressing feature.

2. **Dyspepsia.** Palpitation often comes on at night, especially after a heavy meal. It may, in these circumstances, be accompanied by nightmares, "night starts" and left chest pain.

3. Certain **Local Conditions,** such as thoracic or abdominal tumour, or dilated stomach, which hamper the heart's action, may produce palpitation, although the heart be healthy.

4. **Graves' Disease** (exophthalmic goitre). Palpitation and increased rate of the heart are prominent features. In quite a number of cases this and the other nervous symptoms of the disorder exist for months before the two diagnostic features—thyroid enlargement and exophthalmos— become obvious. Graves' disease should always be suspected in cases of persistent tachycardia (§ 186). In the type of thyrotoxicosis known as toxic adenoma cardiac disease with congestive failure and auricular fibrillation may exist without exophthalmos, and the true cause may thus escape notice (§ 191).

5. Early stages of **pulmonary tuberculosis** (§ 131).

6. **Nervous** conditions, such as fright, fear, or other emotion, especially after an exhausting illness. It also occurs in hysteria and anxiety neurosis.

7. **Effort syndrome,** neurocirculatory asthenia, Da Costa's syndrome,

cardiac neurosis, are all terms descriptive of a condition seen frequently in civilian life, but rising into prominence in times of war. The symptoms are largely cardio-vascular—extreme lassitude and fatigue, dyspnœa on slight exertion, palpitation, præcordial discomfort, submammary ache and angina innocens are the commonest cardiac manifestations. In addition, vaso-motor and psychological abnormalities are often present. Local sweating, especially of the axillæ and hands, tachycardia and lowered blood pressure on standing upright, fainting attacks and postural dizziness, are common. Psychologically there may be anxiety or hysteria, but far more frequently there is an idiosyncrasy of character rather than a neurosis, the individual being of the shy, hypersensitive, introspective type, who has avoided as far as possible situations in childhood or in adult life involving friction and physical or mental exposure and stress.

Treatment consists first in the thorough exclusion of all physical abnormalities. This is followed by explanation to the patient of the causes of his condition, and then by progressive exercises and interesting occupations, often while resident in a special treatment centre.

8. The excessive use of certain **Drugs** or **Articles of Diet**, notably tobacco, tea, coffee, and alcohol.

Cardiac causes of palpitation include: (1) gross cardiac lesions; (2) auricular flutter; (3) auricular fibrillation; and (4) paroxysmal tachycardia. These conditions are dealt with in Section C (§§ 63 *et seq.*).

Cough is a symptom which belongs chiefly to diseases of the lungs (§ 101), but it is met with in diseases of the cardio-vascular system in two circumstances. (*a*) Firstly, the lungs are always involved in left-sided failure; mitral stenosis produces a chronic pulmonary congestion, and coronary disease with left ventricular failure causes an acute or a chronic pulmonary congestion or œdema. The acute form is known as acute pulmonary œdema; this produces a sudden attack of severe cough, with copious, frothy, albuminous sputum, which may be pink (§§ 27, 118). (*b*) Secondly, from pressure. When an aortic aneurysm presses on the trachea or stretches the recurrent laryngeal nerve, a peculiar dry, brassy cough is present. Pericarditis or an enlarged left auricle in mitral stenosis may produce cough. Cough after effort may indicate heart failure.

§ 35. In **Syncope** there is transient loss of consciousness, due to anæmia of the brain. It is often preceded by giddiness, nausea, and a feeling of faintness. The face is ashen pale and the pulse and respiration feeble. Its advent is usually sudden, but recovery, after the attack has lasted some seconds, is gradual. Syncope is rarely caused by organic heart disease. With rare exceptions *patients with heart disease do not faint.*

Diagnosis.—Syncope has to be distinguished from *epilepsy* (§ 860). (1) Epilepsy is sometimes preceded by an aura, though this is evident to the patient only. Its advent is more sudden than syncope, the duration of the attack is shorter, and the return to consciousness almost as sudden and complete. (2) Syncope is rare without some definite determining cause, although it may be of a trivial nature—such as a heated room, or the sight of blood. *Aural vertigo* may be mistaken for syncope; for differential features, see § 826 *et seq.*

Causes.—(1) Deficiency of blood, *e.g.*, hæmorrhage. (2) Vaso-motor instability is seen in the common form of faint in which the abdominal vessels suddenly lose their " tone," dilate, and retain blood which is needed elsewhere. (3) Fainting is often due to vaso-vagal attacks (Lewis), in which as a result of disturbance of the carotid sinus or of the depressor nerve, vagal slowing of the heart is produced, which must not be confused with psychic (temporal-lobe) attacks (§ 864). The onset possibly follows a fright or other emotional disturbance. It is usually gradual, sometimes sudden. The patient sweats, loses consciousness, the heart rate is slowed and the blood pressure falls. The heart is not diseased, and the prognosis is good. (4) Senile syncope gives rise to attacks, preceded by giddiness, in old people who are the subjects of arterial degeneration (see § 833).

The **Vaso-motor** group is the largest. The " faints " occur chiefly in the upright position and in young, anæmic and nervous females and in boys at puberty; who, when exposed to grief, bereavement or any sudden emotion, or to overheated rooms, develop the familiar " fainting attack." (See also postural hypotension, § 89.)

Predisposing causes are:—(1) Anæmia, debility, hunger or starvation; (2) diminished resistance in the peripheral and splanchnic arteries, such as occurs with excessive heat, as in hot rooms or Turkish baths; (3) sudden assumption of the erect posture, as in jumping from bed, may produce syncope; (4) sometimes, in addition to the preceding, the splanchnic veins are suddenly dilated when the intra-abdominal pressure is rapidly lowered, as by emptying the bladder or by rapid paracentesis, and this leads to anæmia of the brain and syncope.

Cardiac causes are: certain cases of aortic incompetence or stenosis, Stokes-Adams' attacks in heart block, rare cases of auricular flutter or paroxysmal tachycardia or auricular fibrillation. In aortic stenosis there may be a direct relationship between exercise and fainting,

Prognosis.—Syncope in the young is usually not organic in origin, whereas in the aged it may be associated with cerebral arterio-sclerosis.

Treatment.—Place the patient immediately in a horizontal position with the head low. This may be most readily done on the floor, but if there is little space, instruct the patient to bend forward and lower the head between the knees. Apply sal volatile to the nostrils, throw cold water on the face. If recovery does not promptly take place, and the pulse be feeble, a hypodermic injection of leptazol or nikethamide B.P. (Coramine) may be given. For further treatment, see Collapse (§ 239). The underlying cause must be carefully sought and treated when the patient has recovered from the urgent syncopal condition.

Lassitude is the outstanding symptom of non-organic or functional heart disease. As an isolated symptom it is, however, a common forerunner of myocardial infarction.

Sleeplessness is a distressing symptom of severe heart failure, and is due to cerebral anoxæmia. Morphia has no deleterious effect upon the heart, but it should only be used for short periods of time owing to the danger of habit formation; it must not be given where there is much bronchitis. Paraldehyde in full doses, chloral hydrate alone or with nepenthe, soluble barbitone B.P. (Medinal), pentobarbitone B.P. (Nembutal) and phenobarbitone are useful. A hot drink of brandy or whisky at bedtime ("hot toddy") is a valuable but mild sedative. Oxygen inhalation is helpful when pulmonary œdema co-exists.

Delirium, generally worse at night, is a more severe result of the same cerebral anoxæmia. Should the remedies above mentioned fail, pethidine hydrochlor. 100 mg. by subcutaneous injection may be necessary, and can be repeated after 4 hours. Barbiturates may aggravate delirium in elderly patients.

Pyrexia and its concomitant symptoms (see Chapter XV) are present in many *acute disorders* of the heart and pericardium. The temperature in subacute bacterial endocarditis is usually of an intermittent or remittent type, with an irregular range, as in other forms of bacteræmia.

§ 36. Sudden or Unexpected Death due to heart disease is becoming increasingly common with the increased frequency of acute myocardial infarction. All the other cardiac causes are rare.

1. *Acute myocardial infarction* is common in middle-aged or elderly men, or in women who have passed middle age. Thrombosis of one of the larger coronary arteries causes instantaneous death, in those who are apparently in good health or in those who have had previous mild coronary episodes.

2. In *aortic valve disease*, stenosis much more often than regurgitation, death may suddenly supervene during apparently good health.

3. In *myocardial degeneration* and in *syphilitic aortitis* involving the coronary orifices, unexpected death may happen, the mechanism here being the onset of ventricular fibrillation, which condition is incompatible with life.

4. *Left ventricular failure* and sudden *heart block* are causes in elderly patients whereas *diphtheritic* myocarditis is now a rare cause in young people.

5. *Asthma, pulmonary embolism* from previous phlebitis, *fat embolism* from skeletal trauma and *air embolism* from thoracic paracentesis, may cause sudden death.

6. Neurological diseases which in their progress involve the *medulla* terminate suddenly; and thus, among the rarer causes, atlanto-axoid disease and syringomyelia may be mentioned.

7. *Cerebral hæmorrhage* especially involving the *pons* or *medulla* may also cause this.

8. *Poisons.*—Hydrocyanic acid acts very rapidly; others acting less quickly are cocaine, carbolic, volatile and non-volatile narcotics and anæsthetics.

9. Sudden rupture of a large cyst, an internal organ, acute disease of the suprarenals, or other cause of *Surgical shock* (§ 239).

10. Foreign bodies in the trachea, or other causes of *sudden asphyxia*, *e.g.*, reflex apnœa from irritation of the pleura (pleural shock).

11. During the *intravenous injection of drugs* to which the patient is hypersensitive.

§ 37. Status Lymphaticus (*Lymphatism*). In the past, sudden and unexpected death in children and adolescents used to be explained by a condition termed status lymphaticus. In this the patient was described as being pale and flabby, with an overgrowth of the thymus gland and of the lymphatic tissue throughout the body— but with no other symptoms. However, a report of a Committee of the Pathological Society (1931) revealed that no firm basis exists for this diagnosis. Even so anæsthetists recognise that such children are serious risks when given an anæsthetic or when exposed to anaphylactic or mental shocks.

PART B.—PHYSICAL EXAMINATION

§ 38. Landmarks of the Chest.—There is a *ridge* (Ludwig's angle) on the sternum between the manubrium and the body of the sternum; it can always be felt opposite the second costal cartilage; and the other ribs can be counted from the second one. The *nipple* is usually situated just external to the fourth costal cartilage, near its junction with the rib, At the back, the *lower angle* of the scapula just covers the seventh rib; and the *scapular line* is a vertical line drawn through the inferior angle of the scapula. The position and relations of the heart can be studied in Fig. 11.

Inspection.—First inspect the patient from the foot of the bed. In a cardiac case the bed-ridden patient is almost invariably propped up. The appearance is often characteristic: The throbbing neck vessels of aortic regurgitation; the malar flush of mitral stenosis; the undergrown body and reddish-blue appearance of congenital cyanotic heart lesions; the pinched patchy face, with the tortuous temporal arteries, and the often wasted body typical of arteriosclerosis; the sallow toxic, anxious face of infective endocarditis; the large white face of renal disease; the apprehensive look of the patient with angina, or the pale, puffy face of pericardial effusion are all characteristic.

Other points to look for are the respiratory rate, depth and rhythm: cyanosis: engorgement and pulsation of the jugular veins: presence or absence of carotid pulsation: epigastric pulsation: thyroid enlargement: clubbing of the fingers and, if present, whether the fingers are blue (congenital heart disease) or white (infective endocarditis). Œdema around the ankles should be noted.

The abdomen should be examined for distension. The presence of engorged veins, diminished respiratory movement, and the presence of ascites should all be observed.

Should the patient be confined to bed, attention should be directed to the position in which he lies or which he assumes. When the chest has been exposed, its shape and movements should be noted; also the cardiac impulse, its position and character, special attention being directed towards whether it is heaving (the true sign of cardiac hypertrophy) or slapping and diffuse in character. Systolic recession, indicative of adherent pericardium, should be looked for, not only in the region round the apex, but in the region of the epigastrium and also in the back (Broadbent's sign).

§ 39. Palpation and the Localisation of the Apex (see Figs. 11 and 12).— The apex beat is the point farthest downwards and to the left at which the cardiac impulse is distinctly felt in an intercostal space. After inspection it should be first palpated by the flat of the hand, and then localised with the finger tips. In an adult male it is normally situated in the fifth interspace ½ inch to the inner side of the mid-clavicular line, at a distance of about 3 inches from the mid-sternal line. *These and other cardiac measurements vary with the age* [1] *and proportions of the patient*—a fact which is apt to be forgotten. The *most external* portion of the apex beat should be marked by a dot with an aniline pencil. At the level of the apex, measure and note the distance from the mid-line to the apex; measure also the distance from the middle of the neck to the middle of the left clavicle. In health these measurements should be the same, or at least the apex should not lie to the left of the mid-clavicular line. Thus at the first examination the position of the apex can be accurately defined, in terms of the mid-clavicular line. Further measurements need only be made from the mid-line, provided the patient does not grow. The principal features to observe about the apex are—its POSITION, CHARACTER and FREQUENCY. The beat of the left ventricle is felt as a forward thrust, if the myocardium is healthy; that of the right is less well defined. It is important to bear in mind that the apex beat is considerably modified if the apex happens (as is not infrequent) to pulsate precisely behind a rib. Only when the apex beats in an intercostal space can the three above features be satisfactorily noted. The apex can sometimes be felt more distinctly when the patient leans forward. In dextrocardia the apex is on the right side of the chest.

Broadly speaking, two abnormal types of apex beat can be recognised: (1) heaving; (2) tapping. A *heaving* apex beat can be recognised by the forcible lift which the fingers experience at each systole when pressed over the apex. It is *the* sign of left ventricular hypertrophy and is typically met in cases of aortic regurgitation, hypertension, and, with modifications, in adherent pericardium. The *tapping* apex beat means a poorly contracting left ventricle, and this occurs in three conditions: (1) When the ventricle is badly filled, badly stretched and therefore badly stimulated, and consequently contracts badly; *e.g.*, mitral stenosis. (2) When the muscle has degenerated from coronary arterio-sclerosis. (3) When the muscle is poisoned as in diphtheria or other toxic states.

In *hypertrophy* of the left ventricle the apex beat is displaced chiefly

[1] In the child the heart normally differs a good deal from that of the adult. The apex is outside the nipple line until 6 years of age; it is, moreover, often in the fourth space. The right cardiac dullness extends slightly beyond the right margin of the sternum, while on auscultation the first sound at the apex is short (not long, dull and booming); at the base the pulmonary second sound is louder than the aortic second; finally, the rhythm is irregular owing to the heart speeding up during inspiration—sinus arrhythmia (§ 65).

downwards, and the cardiac impulse is forcible and heaving. In hypertrophy of the right ventricle there is pulsation in the epigastrium and in the lower interspaces, but the apex is in its normal site. With *dilatation* the impulse is diffuse and weak and the apex beat is moved to the left. The apex is *displaced* by collapse or fibrosis of the lung, as well as by empyema or pleurisy with effusion; if the latter be on the left side, the apex may even be displaced beyond the right border of the sternum (see Fig. 55). The apex is displaced to the *left* by severe depression of the lower sternum and by gross dorsal scoliosis. The apex beat is *obscured* by muscular or adipose chest walls or by emphysema. It is *feeble* with myocardial and pericardial disease, and with ventricular dilatation. With pericardial adhesions there is a *systolic retraction* of one or more interspaces; with hypertrophy of the heart a similar condition may be seen near the apex.

The apex rate should be counted and compared with the pulse. Where the beats are regular in force, the apex and pulse rates coincide, but where the rhythm and force are irregular, as in auricular fibrillation or with premature beats, apex and pulse rates may vary. The difference between the two is known as the pulse deficit.

THRILLS.—A thrill is a palpable " purring " sensation corresponding to the murmur of an organic lesion. If present, thrills should be timed with the carotid and their exact position noted; observe also whether they are constant or intermittent.

Thrills occurring during ventricular diastole. Two types of thrill are found in mitral stenosis, both being due to the flow of blood from left auricle to left ventricle. (*a*) The first, the *presystolic* or as it is sometimes called the auriculo-systolic thrill, is due to the blood flow produced by auricular systole. When the auricles fibrillate and no longer contract effectively, this thrill disappears. (*b*) The second is the *diastolic* thrill; it is due to the flow of blood from the left auricle to the ventricle through the stenosed valve during diastole, and is best felt early in diastole when the difference in the pressure in the two chambers is greatest. It may be found together with the presystolic thrill when the auricles are contracting or alone when they are fibrillating.

Thrills occurring during ventricular systole. A *systolic* thrill may be present at the apex in mitral regurgitation; at the pulmonary base in pulmonary stenosis; at the aortic base in aortic stenosis and aneurysm. Pericardial friction may produce a thrill. Systolic thrills are also common in congenital heart disease, especially in pulmonary stenosis and with interauricular and interventricular patency.

Any abnormal pulsation should be noted and investigated. Special attention should be directed towards the liver; and the spleen should also be palpated.

PALPATION OF THE ARTERIES. Note whether the brachial arteries are visible, tortuous, thickened; if the latter, note whether the thickening is uniform or otherwise, bearing in mind that if patchy in character, this usually indicates involvement of the muscle coat as well as of the intima.

The locomotor artery generally signifies two conditions, viz., a rigid vessel and a hypertrophied heart. Decreased pulsation in the femoral arteries, in a young person with hypertension, should suggest coarctation of the thoracic aorta.

In any routine examination of the cardio-vascular system, ophthalmoscopic inspection of the retinæ and of the retinal arteries furnishes valuable information as to the condition of the smaller arteries (§§ 92, 1126).

§ 40. **Percussion.**—By percussion one is able to make out the position and the approximate size of the heart. Cardiac dullness is elicited by percussion and gives more or less accurately the actual size of the heart. In a normal heart the right margin extends slightly beyond the right margin of the sternum; the left margin is slightly external to the apex, and just internal to the nipple line, while the upper border is approximately level with the third intercostal space (Fig. 11). The upper limit of the cardiac dullness is extended when there is dilatation of the pulmonary conus.

Method.—The student should lose no opportunity of PERCUSSING THE NORMAL HEART and of attending to the following points: (i.) *Having first localised the apex beat*, begin outside the cardiac area in a perfectly resonant area. The middle finger of the left hand should be held vertically and placed flat and *firmly* upon the chest wall in an interspace; then moved ¼ inch at a time towards the centre of the heart. (ii.) Use only one finger—the second of the right hand—as a hammer, making a short sharp tap with the finger *tip*. The percussing finger should rebound immediately—"staccato," as pianists say. The movement should be made from the *wrist*, or from the knuckle (metacarpo-phalangeal joint), as in playing the piano, and the tap should be a light one. (iii.) By listening attentively to the sound elicited, it will be noticed that it is dull and flat over the heart, like that produced by striking any solid object; but louder and more resonant outside the area, like the sound produced by striking an empty barrel. It is only possible to define in this way the right, the upper, and the left limits of the dull area, because at the lower limit the cardiac dullness is continuous with that of the liver.

FALLACIES.—Cardiac enlargement may be *obscured* by the hyper-resonance of emphysematous lungs, and in these circumstances enlargement of the heart or pericardium is very difficult to make out. We have then to rely upon other means than percussion. On the other hand, cardiac enlargement may be *simulated* by a fibrous retraction of the left lung, the heart, nevertheless, remaining of normal size; or thirdly, the heart may be *displaced* by an aneurysm or other mediastinal tumour pushing forward, and making the præcordial area appear larger. One or other border of the area of dullness may be *obscured* by pleural effusion. Ascites, pleural effusion or abdominal distension may actually *displace* the heart.

§ 41. **The Pulse.**—At this stage, one may well investigate the arterial pulse. The radial is the one commonly selected. The usual method of palpating the pulse is to place three fingers of the right hand on it, when the following points can be systematically investigated: (*a*) *Rate*. Whether abnormally fast or abnormally slow. (*b*) *Rhythm*. Whether regular or irregular; if the latter, the nature of the irregularity should be investigated. Irregular pulses can be classified in two groups: (1) regularly irregular or (2) irregularly irregular.   (c) The *Force* (estimated by the impact against the finger) depends upon the rapidity of the filling and emptying of the artery, *e.g.*, in aortic regurgitation, hyperthyroidism, anæmia and in certain febrile conditions, the force is considerable.   (d) The *Volume*, estimated by the lift and duration of the wave, gives one the output of the heart, *e.g.*, in athletes and hyperpiesis.   (e) The *Tension* is estimated by the obliterative force and indicates systolic blood pressure.   (f) The condition of the *Vessel Wall*.

The most common *regular irregularities* are: (1) Sinus arrhythmia (where the pulse speeds up during inspiration, and slows down during expiration), the slowing is vagal, and the irregularity is physiological (§ 65); (2) pulsus bigeminus or pulsus trigeminus (where the pulse beats in twos or threes followed by a pause), the result of regularly occurring premature beats; and (3) pulsus alternans (where big beats and little beats alternate at regular intervals), indicative of left ventricular failure (§ 73): this is of grave prognostic significance.   It is difficult to determine by palpating the pulse, but can invariably be detected by·the sphygmomanometer, the alternate beats coming through at a slightly lower systolic pressure.

The commonest *irregular irregularities* are: (1) The consistently irregular pulse due to auricular fibrillation.   Here the beats not only follow one another at irregular intervals, but are of unequal strength and volume. In addition the pulse rate may differ from the apex rate.   The great clinical test of the presence of auricular fibrillation is that the irregularity is increased by exercise (§ 69).   (2) The irregularity due to irregularly occurring premature beats or extrasystoles (§ 64).   This indicates myocardial hyper-irritability, resulting from fatigue, inflammation or degeneration. This irregularity is in most cases abolished when the rate is increased by exercise.

§ 42. **Auscultation.**—For auscultation much practice is required, and the student should never miss an opportunity of listening to the sounds of the heart, *particularly of the normal heart*.

The normal heart sounds are three in number—the *First*, or systolic sound, is long, dull and booming in character, and of lower pitch than the second sound.   It is best heard over the region of the apex beat, *i.e.*, left fifth intercostal space just internal to the mid-clavicular line.   It is the result of: (1) the contraction of the ventricular muscle, (2) the vibrations caused by the closure of the auriculo-ventricular valves.   The *Second* or diastolic sound is short, sharp, slapping, and higher pitched, and is heard at the apex and at the base on a level with the second costal cartilage. It has two components, being produced by the closure of the aortic and pulmonary semilunar valves.   The *Third* sound is mid-diastolic in time, is occasionally audible by the ordinary stethoscope, and can be easily detected by means of the cardio-phonograph.   Its origin is doubtful.   In diseased or damaged conditions of the heart not only are the normal heart sounds modified in various ways, to be described below, but adventitious sounds, murmurs or bruits, are liable to be produced either at the valve orifices or on the surface of the heart. When auscultating the heart, therefore, one should pay attention to (a) the characters of the normal heart sounds, and (b) the presence and character of any abnormal sounds (murmurs).

ALTERATIONS OF THE HEART SOUNDS AND THEIR SIGNIFICANCE.—AT THE APEX. From what has been said about the origin of the first sound,

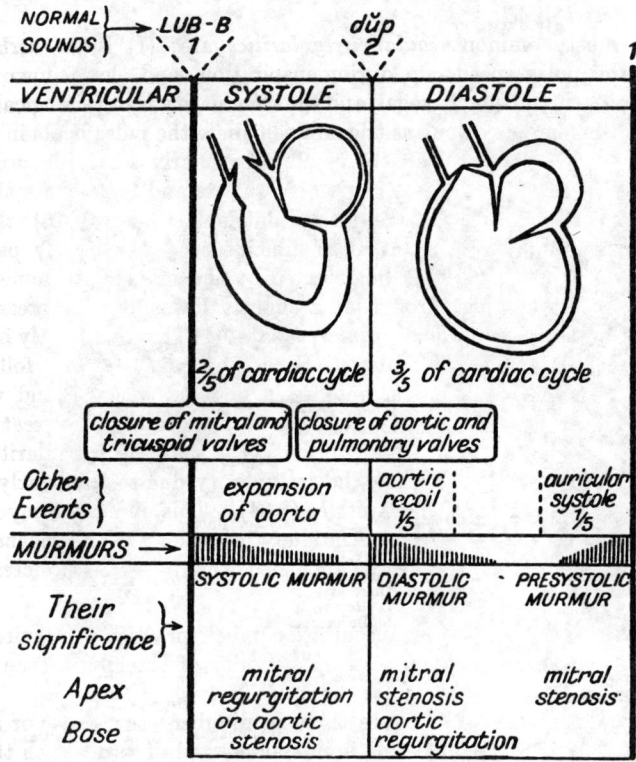

FIG. 10.—Diagram of a Cardiac Cycle, showing various events and their duration, how the different murmurs are produced, and their clinical significance. The student should study this and Fig. 11 very closely.

it is clear that its character will be modified by any condition which interferes with the contractility of the muscle or the closure of the auriculo-ventricular valves. This modification may be: (1) change in pitch, when the first sound becomes somewhat similar to the second sound, i.e., short and sharp in nature. This indicates a poorly contracting ventricle, due to inflammation, degeneration, toxæmia or non-stretching, e.g., mitral stenosis. It is also found in shock, or after severe hæmorrhage when the blood pressure is low. (2) Splitting due to a non-synchronising

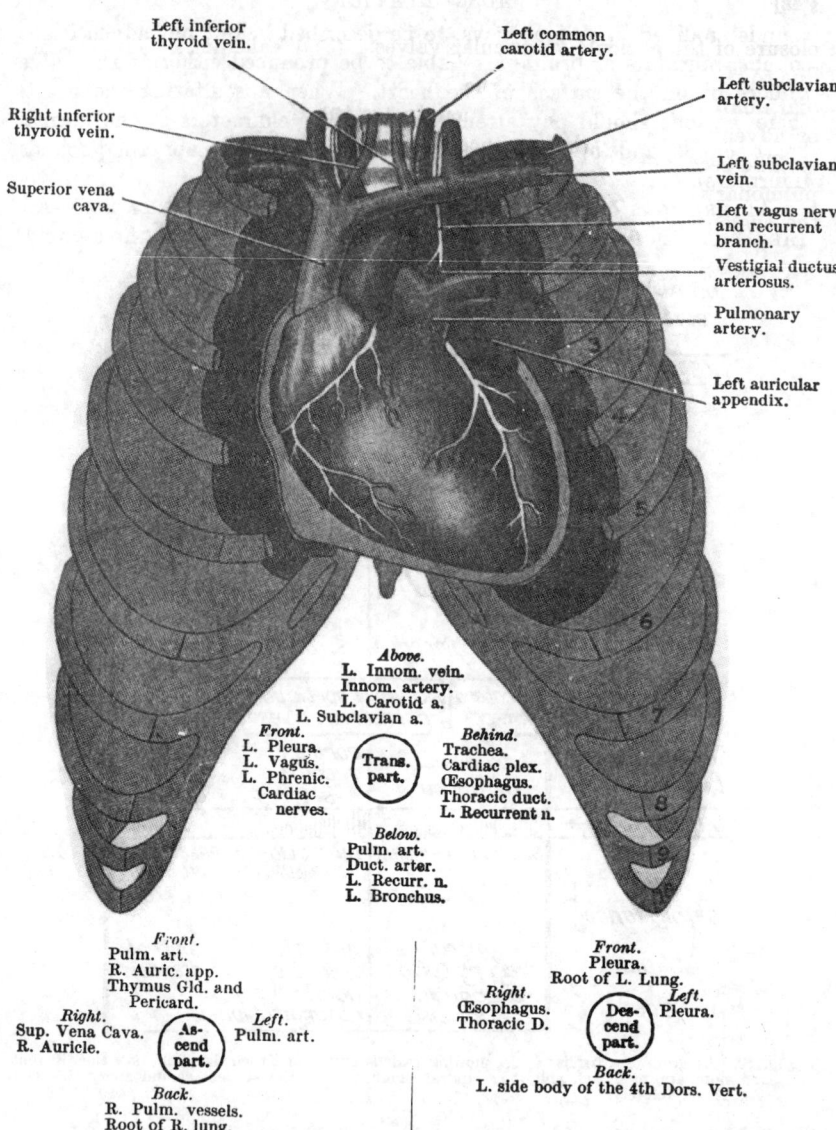

Left inferior thyroid vein.

Left common carotid artery.

Left subclavian artery.

Right inferior thyroid vein.

Left subclavian vein.

Superior vena cava.

Left vagus nerve and recurrent branch.

Vestigial ductus arteriosus.

Pulmonary artery.

Left auricular appendix.

Above.
L. Innom. vein.
Innom. artery.
L. Carotid a.
L. Subclavian a.

Front.
L. Pleura.
L. Vagus.
L. Phrenic.
Cardiac nerves.

Trans. part.

Behind.
Trachea.
Cardiac plex.
Œsophagus.
Thoracic duct.
L. Recurrent n.

Below.
Pulm. art.
Duct. arter.
L. Recurr. n.
L. Bronchus.

Front.
Pulm. art.
R. Auric. app.
Thymus Gld. and Pericard.

Right.
Sup. Vena Cava.
R. Auricle.

Ascend part.

Left.
Pulm. art.

Back.
R. Pulm. vessels.
Root of R. lung.

Front.
Pleura.
Root of L. Lung.

Right.
Œsophagus.
Thoracic D.

Descend part.

Left.
Pleura.

Back.
L. side body of the 4th Dors. Vert.

FIG. 11.—**The Heart and Great Vessels in Situ,** with lungs turned back. The right ventricle forms the greater part of the anterior surface of the heart. Above and to right of this is the right auricle, into which the superior vena cava opens, which collects the blood from the two innominate veins. Passing out from and above the right ventricle is the pulmonary artery, above which again is the remains of the ductus arteriosus, connecting it with the arch of the aorta. Just to the left of the pulmonary artery the left auricular appendix peeps round the corner. The arch of the aorta is seen coming forward from the left ventricle (which is at the back, and therefore only seen at the left margin of the heart), and from its upper convexity arise in order the innominate, left carotid and left subclavian arteries. The trachea is seen behind the vessels, and the vagus nerves are seen at the sides, that on the left passing down in front of the aorta but behind the root of the left lung. The relations of the ascending, descending, and transverse portions of the aorta are given diagrammatically above.

closure of the auriculo-ventricular valves. (3) Weakening or suppression due to pericardial effusion, emphysema, myocardial degeneration, myocardial infarction, etc.; or (4) partial or complete replacement by a murmur or adventitious sound.

The second sound at the apex, due to the closure of the aortic and pulmonary semilunar valves, may be (1) distinct; or (2) accentuated when the systemic or pulmonary tension is abnormally high.

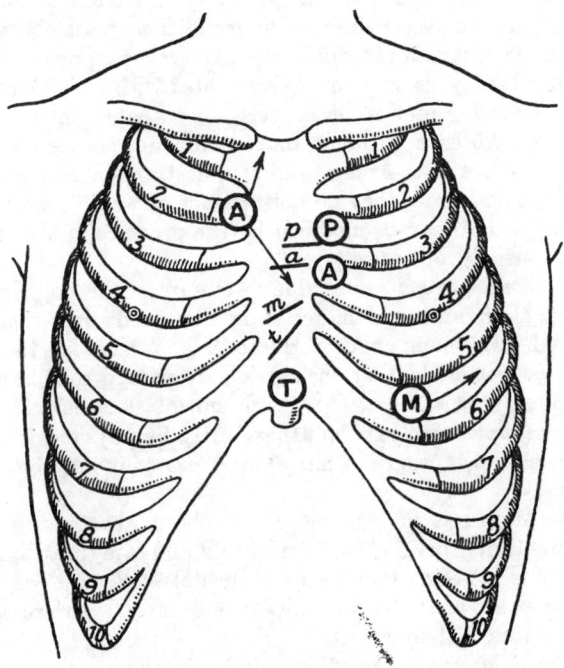

FIG. 12.—DIAGRAM SHOWING THE situation OF THE Cardiac Valves AND THE position IN WHICH THE SEVERAL murmurs ARE HEARD LOUDEST.

p = Pulmonary orifice, at level of upper border of third left costal cartilage.
a = Aortic orifice at level of lower border of third left costal cartilage.
m = Mitral orifice at level of lower border of fourth left costal cartilage.
t = Tricuspid orifice at level of fourth interspace, lying obliquely behind the sternum.
The positions where the sounds produced at the various orifices are best heard are indicated by the letters enclosed in circles. The arrows mark the direction in which murmurs produced at the corresponding orifices are conducted.
M, Mitral murmurs are best heard at the mitral area—*i.e.*, the apex.
A, Aortic murmurs are best heard at the aortic area—*i.e.*, second right costal cartilage; or along the left sternal border.
P, Pulmonary murmurs are best heard at the pulmonary area—*i.e.*, second left intercostal space.
T, Tricuspid murmurs are best heard at the tricuspid area—*i.e.*, at lower end of sternum.

A *canter, gallop* or *triple rhythm* is a condition in which there are three distinct sounds at or internal to the apex. The third sound may be heard, and often distinguished on palpation, at the apex (*a*) just before the normal first sound, probably due to an audible auricular systole; or (*b*) immediately after the normal second sound. The third sound may therefore be presystolic or proto-diastolic; in either case it is of low pitch and usually indicates left ventricular failure. It is frequent (i.) in large hearts with hypertension; (ii.) when coronary disease has caused failure with much dilatation; and (iii.) may be heard when conduction is defective in one or other branches of the Bundle of His (and see § 55).

AT THE BASE, the *Aortic second* sound, normally short, sharp and slapping, due to the closure of the aortic semilunar valves, may be (1) accentuated—indicative of a high peripheral resistance and a high blood pressure; (2) ringing, indicative of atheroma and often dilatation of the aorta and rigidity of the valves. This condition, most characteristic to those who are familiar with it, differs from an accentuation and has another significance. It may, or may not, be associated with a high blood pressure. The aortic second sound is often very accentuated in cases of aortic aneurysm. (3) Absence of the aortic second sound means either that the aortic valves do not close owing to injury, destruction or absence, or that they close so quietly that they do not produce an audible sound. (4) The aortic second sound may be modified by the presence of a murmur which replaces it partially or entirely.

The Pulmonary second sound, due to closure of the pulmonary valves, is also short, sharp and sudden, and in adults less distinct than the aortic second sound. In young children the reverse is the case—the pulmonary second sound being louder than the aortic. It, in turn, may be accentuated (high pulmonary tension), as occurs in mitral stenosis and acute lung conditions; reduplication or "splitting" may be physiological, especially in children, and also occurs in mitral stenosis; or it may be modified by a murmur.

CARDIAC MURMURS may be either systolic or diastolic in time. The latter are frequently divided into early, mid and late (presystolic) according to the time at which they occur in diastole. Further, murmurs may be produced either at the valve orifices—endocardial murmurs, or outside the heart—exocardial murmurs.

Endocardial Murmurs are of two kinds: (a) those indicating structural damage to the valves (organic), and (b) those indicating softening or loss of tone in the auriculo-ventricular rings (atonic or functional murmurs). Endocardial murmurs may generally be differentiated from exocardial murmurs by the following points: (1) *Endocardial* murmurs are best heard in defined areas corresponding to the normal valve sounds, (2) are conducted or propagated in a definite direction, (3) are harsh or blowing in character. *Exocardial* murmurs are: (1) superficial and often appear to be heard just under the stethoscope, (2) are usually not heard only over the valve area, (3) are not propagated in the same definite directions, (4) are not completely systolic or diastolic in time, (5) are often modified by pressure by the stethoscope, and are accentuated, diminished or removed by full inspiration or expiration. A single murmur of presystolic or diastolic time is usually an indication of organic disease at one of the cardiac orifices, but may be exocardial—*e.g.*, pericardial.

Functional Murmurs, which may be heard over either apex or base,

are usually soft and blowing in character. When present at the apex,
a functional murmur may be local or conducted to the axilla. They are
characterised by their variability under different conditions. Thus they
are often present when the patient is lying and disappear when he stands;
they may be heard during inspiration and not during expiration; they
may appear only after exercise and disappear during rest—or they may only
be audible when these conditions are reversed.

Hæmic Murmurs are frequently heard in anæmia and in some other
blood conditions (see Chapter XVI).[1] They are also common in thin-
chested adolescents, and in patients with Graves' disease. They are
usually systolic in time, are rarely double, are usually heard loudest in
the pulmonary area, and are heard best when the patient is lying down.

§ 43. **Estimation of Myocardial Efficiency.**—The measure of a heart's
efficiency is its capacity for work; this is true of all hearts, whether healthy
or diseased. Furthermore, it must be clearly borne in mind that many
hearts work perfectly, exhibiting no defects at all, when the patients are
at rest, but show serious derangements and definite evidence of myocardial
impairment when called upon to do extra work. *The fundamental symptom
of myocardial insufficiency is dyspnœa.* If dyspnœa is absent, the heart
muscle is not failing. The amount of dyspnœa is proportional to the
degree of myocardial failure. Dyspnœa is complained of by the patient;
it can also be observed objectively by the physician. When taking the
history an exact idea should be formed as to how far and how fast a patient
can walk, and whether hills or stairs cause shortness of breath. The
best test of cardiac function is the amount of work or exercise a patient
can take in the course of daily life. A patient who is made short of breath
by the exertion of undressing is unsafe for an exercise test and has a severe
degree of cardiac failure.

EFFECTS OF EXERCISE UPON THE HEART.—(*a*) *The Rate.*—The normal heart
responds to exercise by a gradual increase in rate. The increase is more or less uniform, the rate climbing up as exercise is increased. The normal heart rarely speeds
up to over 150 for any length of time. It rapidly returns to normal on ceasing the
exercise. A poisoned heart responds to exercise by undue acceleration, and only
slowly settles down to its normal rate; while in certain diseased conditions of the heart
one gets impaired acceleration, the rate scarcely altering at all. This may occur
in very fast hearts (*e.g.*, auricular flutter), or in very slow hearts (*e.g.*, heart-block).
Lastly, in a well-trained physiological heart, such as one meets with in young highly-
trained athletes, the rate does not climb on exercise but suddenly doubles (*e.g.*, at
the commencement of the exercise, the rate may be 42, and on exercise suddenly
becomes 84)—the so-called athletes' reaction.

(*b*) *Rhythm.*—The rhythm of the heart may be profoundly modified by exercise.
(1) An irregularity may be produced, and any heart that becomes irregular on exercise
is likely to be diseased. The most common irregularities revealed, or increased, by
exercise are auricular fibrillation, alternation (indicative of left ventricular failure),
a sign of grave significance, and in some cases, premature beats. (2) An existing
irregularity may be abolished. Practically speaking, the only irregularities abolished
by exercise are those caused by sinus arrhythmia and premature beats.

(*c*) *Sounds.*—Under the influence of exercise, normal heart sounds may be split

---

[1] These so-called hæmic murmurs are not due to anæmia *per se.*

or modified by the production of adventitious sounds or murmurs.   In mitral stenosis, exercise brings out the signs of the lesion.

(d) *Thrills.*—Thrills may be revealed.   This occurs in early mitral stenosis, when increased filling of the auricle results in increased stretching and increased contraction, and so produces a thrill, presystolic in time.   An existing thrill is increased by exercise or abolished by exhaustion or by tachycardia.

§ 44. Special Methods of Investigation.

1. **The Electrocardiograph** is an instrument for recording the minute electrical currents which are formed by the contraction of heart muscle.   The two principles usually employed in the instrument are those of the string galvanometer, and the cathode-ray oscillograph.   The electrical changes are recorded on a moving strip of sensitive film or paper, and the record is called an *Electrocardiogram*.   Records are usually taken by two different methods: (i.) Three standard limb leads have been in use for the last forty years.   With lead 1 the two electrodes are applied respectively to the right arm and the left arm; lead 2 to the right arm and the left leg; lead 3 to the left arm and the left leg. (ii.) Præcordial leads have recently been introduced.   With the unipolar electrode a succession of records are obtained from localised areas around the heart.   The præcordial (or exploring) electrode is moved to different areas of the chest wall, the indifferent electrode being composed of the attachments of all three limbs: this spreads the electrical effect to the "indifferent" half of the circuit and largely cancels it out.   Furthermore, resistances are introduced into the connections to the right arm, left arm and left leg which damp down still further the possible influences of the electrical currents obtained through the indifferent electrodes, thus increasing the influence of the currents obtained through the precordial or exploring electrode.

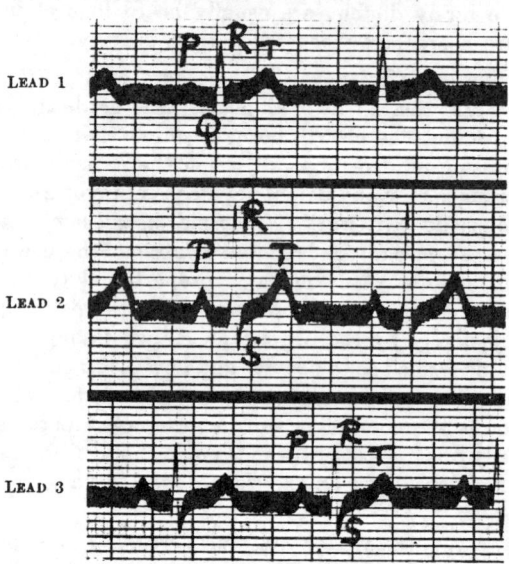

FIG. 13.—A normal tracing showing leads 1, 2 3.   (Thick lines indicate 0·2 of a second and thin lines 0·04 of a second.)

The usual præcordial unipolar leads are leads V1, V2, V3, V4, V5, V6 and .V7. V1 is obtained by placing the exploring electrode in the fourth space just to the right of the sternum.   V2 position is in the corresponding fourth space just to the left of the sternum.   V4 is in the fifth space in the mid-clavicular line, and V3 lies half-way between leads V2 and V4.   V5 is level with V4 in the anterior axillary line.   V6 is at the same level in the mid-axillary line, and V7 also at the same level in the posterior axillary line.   The information obtained by these præcordial leads is further discussed under coronary thrombosis (§ 52).   Unipolar electrocardiograms can also be taken from the right arm (a VR), the left arm (a VL) and the left leg (a VF).   Here the normal electrode limb attachments become the exploring electrodes and the indifferent electrodes are diffused as in the case of the unipolar præcordial leads.

When reading an electrocardiogram the following routine is advisable.   First observe if the whole of the tracing is slightly blurred by very fine oscillations: these are due to fine muscular tremors with failure of the patient to relax, and are common in nervous subjects and in Graves' disease. Next examine the " P " waves in all leads. These are produced by the auricles and for each lead should be uniform in shape and upright: occasionally in lead 3 they are diphasic or inverted in adipose patients with an abnormally elevated diaphragm. The amplitude of the " P " wave is increased if the auricles are hypertrophied, as in early mitral stenosis: while if the auricular muscle is diseased the wave is notched (*e.g.*, mitral stenosis). The " P " wave may be absent, and in its place there may or may not be irregularly occurring fine fibrillary waves (the ventricular waves being totally irregular): then auricular fibrillation is present (Fig. 14). Isolated " P " waves may be inverted, indicating that the auricles are here contracting from some ectopic pacemaker and not from the sino-auricular stimulus: these auricular premature beats may arise in any part of the auricular muscle, but the nearer they are to the sino-auricular node, the more closely does their shape approximate to normal (Fig. 15). If a series of these inverted or abnormal " P " waves occurs regularly at a rate higher than normal (between 120–200 per minute) and the ventricle contracts with each auricular beat, paroxysmal tachycardia (Fig. 40) is present. If no normal " P " waves are found, but instead there is visible a series of regular coarse undulations at a rate of between 200–300 per minute and best seen in leads 2 and 3, auricular flutter (Fig. 42) is present. Here the " QRST " follows either each second, third or fourth auricular undulation, giving an auriculo-ventricular ratio of 2 : 1, 3 : 1, or 4 : 1.

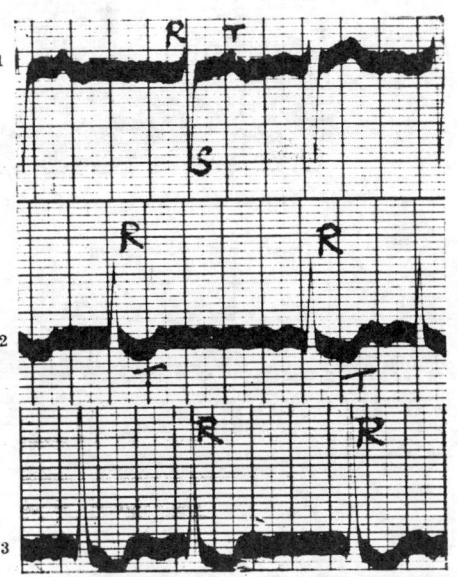

FIG. 14.—Auricular fibrillation. There is no " P " wave. Between the ventricular beats are seen fine fibrillary movements of the auricle. The ventricular rhythm is completely irregular. Note also the right axis deviation due to the fact that the tracing is from a case of advanced mitral stenosis.

Next measure the P–R interval. This represents the interval between the commencement of auricular and ventricular contractions, and is chiefly occupied by the time taken for the impulse to traverse the bundle of His. It should measure 0·12–0·20 sec. Heart-block is present in a minor degree if the P–R interval is prolonged beyond 0·20 sec. (Fig. 16), and in a greater degree if a ventricular beat drops out (Fig. 17): if a " P " wave is not followed by a QRS complex, but two, three or four " P " waves intervene between each QRS complex, then 2 : 1, 3 : 1 or 4 : 1 heart-block is present. If the interval between QRS and the nearest " P " wave varies continually, complete heart-block is present (Fig. 18). Occasionally the P–R interval is shortened. This is due to nodal rhythm with an abnormal pacemaker situated between the sino-auricular and auriculo-ventricular nodes (Fig. 19).

Next study the QRST portions representing ventricular action. The QRS portion should not exceed 0·10 sec.; this is increased when conduction is impaired in one branch of the bundle of His. Normally, the " R " wave is tallest in lead 2: left axis deviation (Fig. 20) is shown when the " R " wave is tallest in lead 1, and the " S " wave deepest in lead 3. Conversely, with right axis deviation (Fig. 14) the " S " wave is deepest in

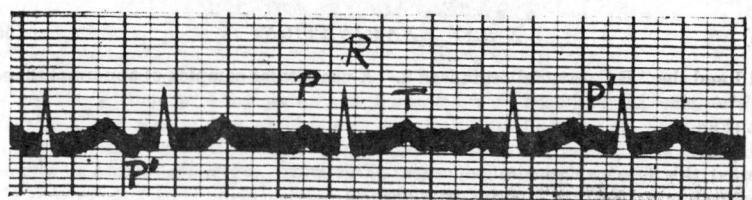

FIG. 15.—Two auricular premature beats (P') are shown, each arising from a different focus. The first ectopic " P " wave is inverted, showing its abnormal position of origin, and is also premature.

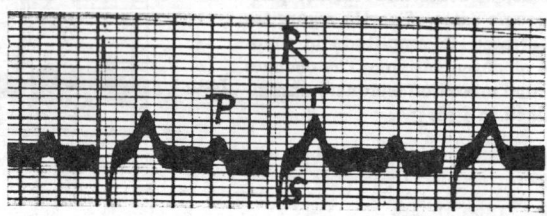

FIG. 16.—First stage of heart-block. " P-R " interval measures 0·3 of a second.

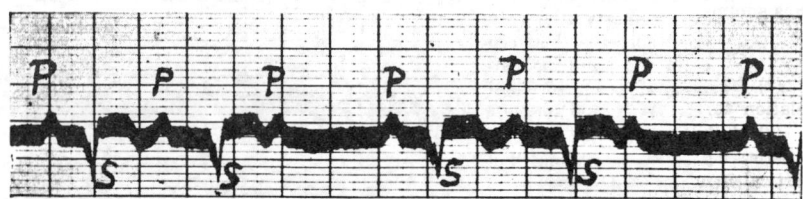

FIG. 17.—Heart-block. Stage of dropped beats. The " P-R " interval at first measures 0·20 of a second, then 0·25 of a second, and the third " P " wave fails to excite a ventricular contraction.

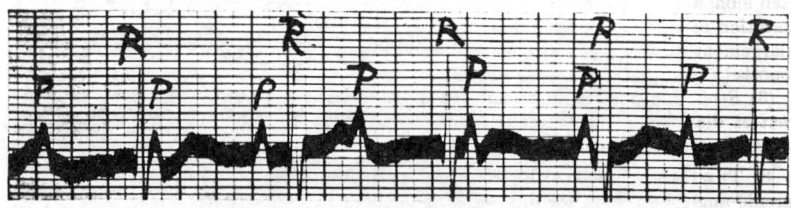

FIG. 18.—Complete heart-block. There is no relationship between the auricular and ventricular contractions.

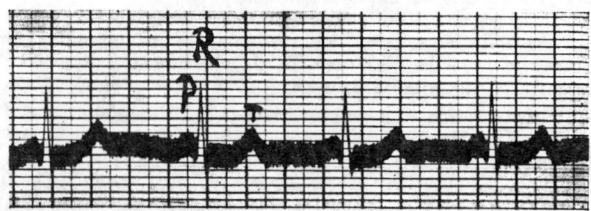

FIG. 19.—Tracing showing shortening of the " P-R " interval. This is due to nodal rhythm, in which the pacemaker is situated at the auriculo-ventricular node. In this instance the impulse reaches the auricles slightly before it reaches the ventricles.

lead 1 and the " R " wave tallest in lead 3. A ventricular complex of abnormal shape and size, placed between others which are normal, indicates a premature ventricular beat (Fig. 38). The start of the ST interval should be isoelectric and the " T " wave well formed and upright in all three leads, although if the " T " wave in lead 3 (T_3) is inverted this has no special significance. This wave, especially in lead 2, is well developed in proportion to the physiological state of the ventricular muscle. It is inverted in leads 1 and 2 by full doses of digitalis, in myocardial disease, in acute and chronic pericarditis, and in some cases of aortic regurgitation, and is decreased in amplitude in myocardial toxæmia or degeneration. The changes found in myocardial infarction (coronary thrombosis) are described in § 52.

2. **X-Ray investigation** is essential in the presence of cardio-vascular disease (Figs. 21 to 26). The technical details must be obtained from a special textbook; the main points to which attention should be directed may be thus summarised:—

A. THE HEART:—

(1) *Its position* in the mediastinum—its relation to the lungs and diaphragm.

(2) *Outline and form:* This is often characteristic, *e.g.*, in young healthy hearts it is vertical, in normal elderly people it is often more horizontal. With enlargement of the left ventricle it is boot-shaped with the long axis horizontal, while in pulmonary tuberculosis it is often elongated and tubular. Hypertrophy or dilatation of the left and right ventricles, and enlargement of the left auricle as in mitral stenosis (Figs. 22–25), are some of the chief points to be demonstrated by radiography.

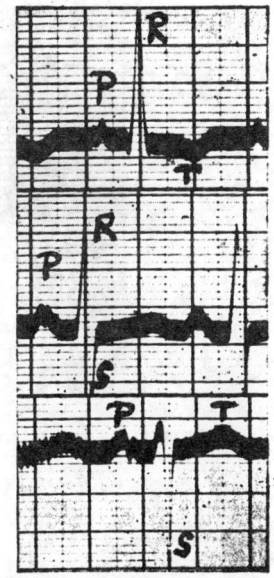

FIG. 20.—Left axis deviation, from a case of aortic regurgitation: " R " is tallest in lead 1, and " S " is deepest in lead 3.

(3) *Size:* The maximum transverse diameter of the heart is less than half the greatest diameter of the thorax. Thus a cardio-thoracic ratio of more than 0·50 is evidence of enlargement.

B. THE GREAT VESSELS: Examine especially in oblique positions; note the cardiophrenic angle; also look for dilatation or aneurysm; mediastinitis, growth or foreign body.

C. THE PERICARDIUM: Observe signs of adhesions or fluid.

3. **The Orthodiagraph** is an instrument whereby outline diagrams can be made, of the actual size of the heart itself, so that accurate measurements can be obtained not only of the heart but also of the great vessels, etc. An outline of the cardiac shadow, resulting from parallel rays, is traced on an X-ray screen. A six-foot X-ray film (*Teleradiogram*) is often substituted for this.

4. **Cardiac Catheterisation and Angiocardiography.** Cardiac catheterisation involves passing a long fine flexible catheter from the anticubital fossa via the superior vena cava into the right auricle, right ventricle, and pulmonary artery and its branches, and if there is a patency between the right and left sides of the heart, through such a patency. The information obtainable is (i.) the oxygen tension of the blood in these various positions; (ii.) the blood pressure; and (iii.) the visual appearance of the end of the catheter under the X-ray screen. Practical examples of the use of this method would be the discovery that the oxygen tension was measurably higher in the pulmonary artery than in the right auricle and ventricle. This would strongly suggest

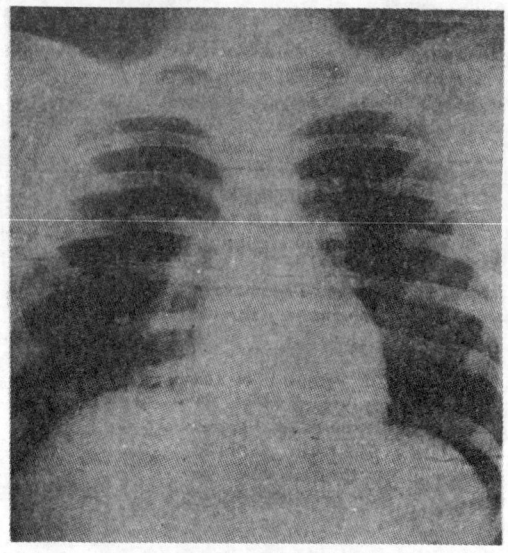

FIG. 21.—X-ray appearances of the heart and hilar shadows in a normal man.

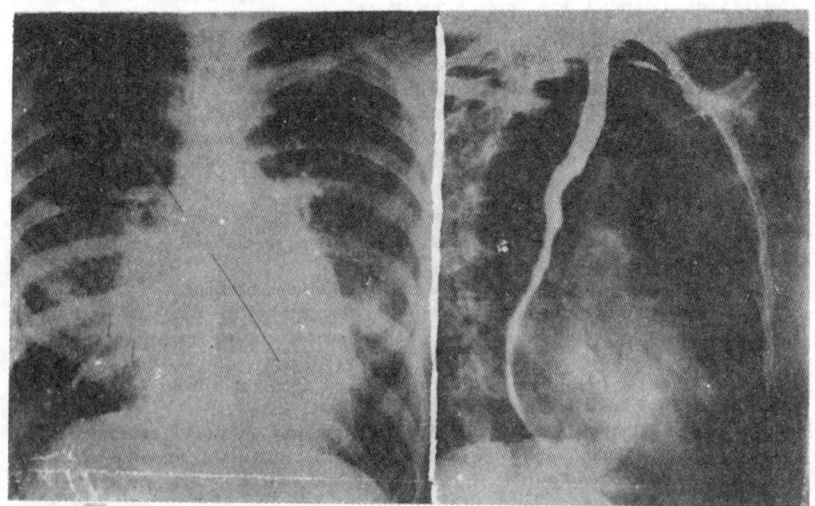

FIG. 22   FIG. 23

FIGS. 22 and 23.—X-ray appearances of the heart and lungs in a patient with mitral stenosis. In the antero-posterior view note the enlarged shadow of the pulmonary artery and left auricle; and also the marked congestion of the hilar shadows of the lungs. In the lateral view the enlarged left auricle is seen to compress and displace the lower end of the œsophagus.

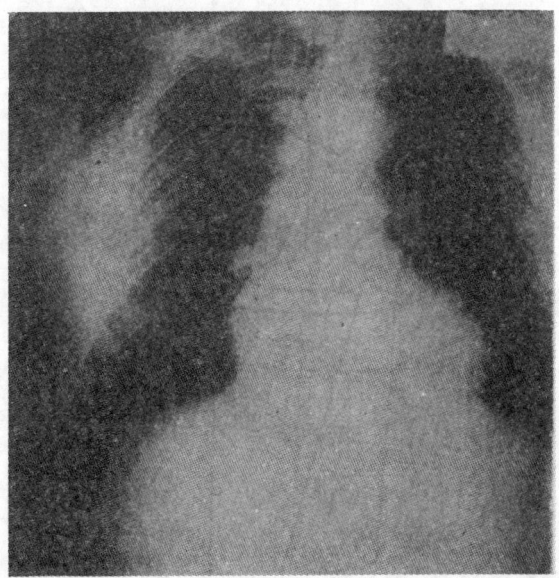

FIG. 24.—X-ray of the heart in a patient with hypertension, showing hypertrophy of the left ventricle.

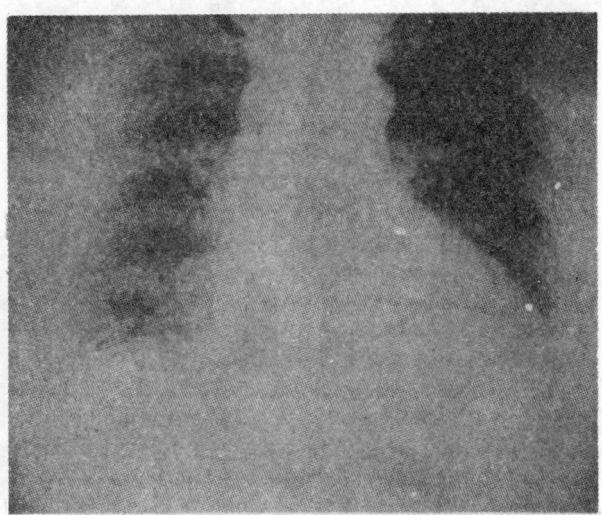

FIG. 25.—Chest X-ray showing hypertensive heart disease and left ventricular failure. Note the very large left ventricle and the pulmonary congestion.

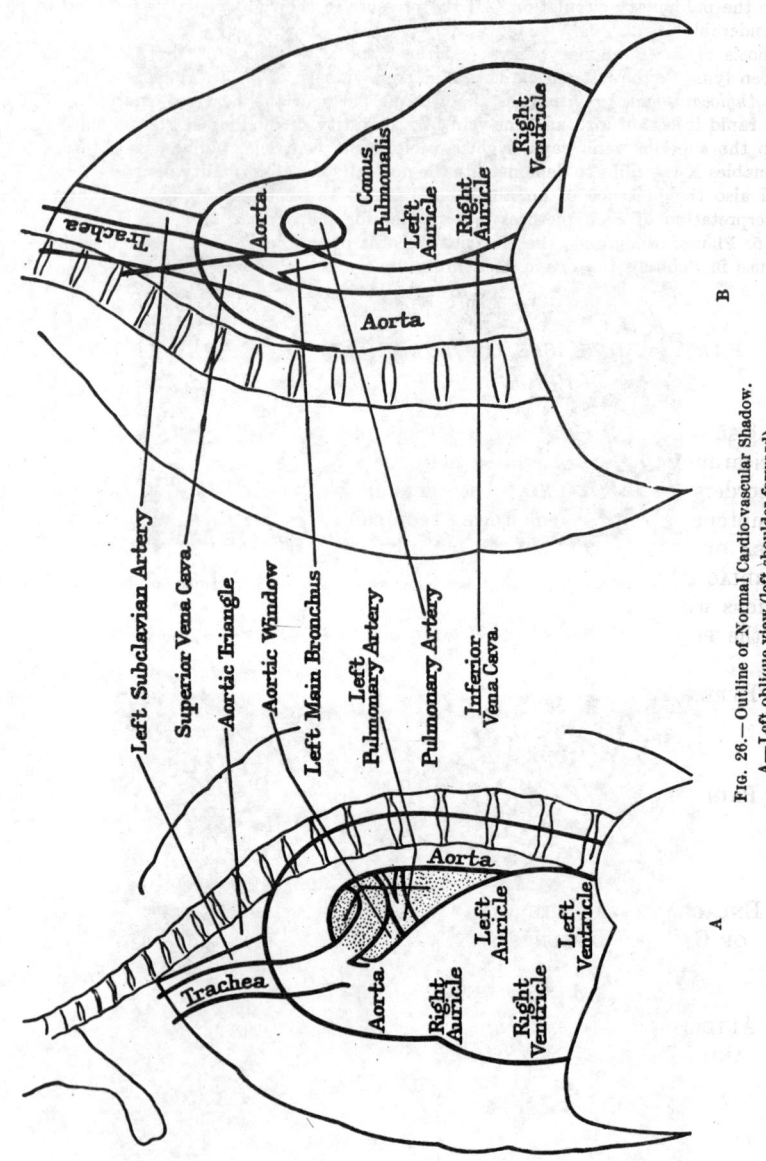

Fig. 26.—Outline of Normal Cardio-vascular Shadow.
A.—Left oblique view (left shoulder forward).
B.—Right oblique view (right shoulder forward).

the presence of a shunt of arterial blood, possibly from a patent ductus arteriosus, into the pulmonary circulation. If the pressure in the right ventricle is found to be considerably higher than that in the pulmonary artery there is clear evidence of stenosis of the pulmonary valve. If the catheter is visualised through the X-ray screen lying in the left auricle this is strong evidence of an atrial septal defect.

Angiocardiography visualises the various parts of the heart, in succession after the rapid injection into an arm vein of a quantity of diodone B.P. As this passes into the superior vena cava, right auricle, right ventricle, pulmonary artery, etc., it enables X-ray films to demonstrate the normality or abnormality of these chambers, and also the presence of an abnormal passage-way connection with any of them. Interpretation of such pictures is a matter for the expert.

5. **Phonocardiograms,** the electrical records of the heart sounds, are occasionally of use in defining the origin of a murmur.

PART C. DISEASES OF THE HEART AND PERICARDIUM: THEIR DIAGNOSIS, PROGNOSIS, AND TREATMENT

§ 45. **Classification.**—For practical purposes diseases of the heart and pericardium may be classified under five prominent differential features: Disorders WITH PYREXIA; Disorders in which PAIN is a characteristic symptom; Disorders which are accompanied by an ENLARGEMENT of the AREA OF CARDIAC DULLNESS; Disorders in which an ALTERATION of the CARDIAC SOUNDS, or a MURMUR, forms the diagnostic feature; and Conditions which are recognised by an ALTERATION of the RHYTHM or RATE of the PULSE.

A. PYREXIA .   .   .   .
  I. Pericarditis.
  II. Acute Endocarditis.

B. PAIN   .   .   .   .
  I. Angina of Effort.
  II. Spasmodic Angina.
  III. Coronary Thrombosis.
  IV. Angina Innocens (Pseudo-Angina).
  V. Pericarditis.

C. ENLARGEMENT OF THE AREA OF CARDIAC DULLNESS .
  I. Cardiac Hypertrophy.
  II. Cardiac Dilatation.
  III. Chronic Pericardial Effusion.
  IV. Adherent Pericardium.

D. ALTERED HEART SOUNDS AND MURMURS   .   .
  I. Myocardial Degeneration.
  II. Endocarditis.
  III. Congenital Heart Disease.
  IV. Pericarditis.

E. ALTERATION OF RHYTHM OR RATE OF PULSE   .
  I. Sinus Arrhythmia.
  II. Premature Beats (Extrasystoles).
  III. Paroxysmal Tachycardia.
  IV. Auricular Flutter.
  V. Auricular Fibrillation.
  VI. Bradycardia.
  VIII. Heart-Block.

The **Routine procedure** in the investigation of a cardio-vascular problem may be considered under the following headings—(1) The origin of the present symptoms, *e.g.*, whether they supervened on any definite illness, acute or chronic.

(2) The personal history, especially as regards (*a*) previous diseases such as rheumatic fever, growing pains, chorea, scarlet fever, tonsillitis, influenza, diphtheria, syphilis, etc.; (*b*) habits of life, especially as regards exercise, excessive weight, alcohol and tobacco.

(3) Family history. Certain diseases, *e.g.*, rheumatic fever, arterio-sclerosis, etc., tend to run in families and predispose to heart disease.

(4) Symptoms. The commonest symptoms associated with heart disease are dyspnœa, orthopnœa, lassitude, sleeplessness and pain. These are dealt with in Part A.

(5) Physical examination of the patient (Part B). Inasmuch as many hearts, when only slightly damaged, function normally when the patient is at rest and their " load " is light, but develop obvious defects of action under " load," it is essential to examine the patient three times—standing, lying, and after exercise. Further, it is convenient to divide the examination into: (*a*) Ordinary routine clinical examination, under which heading one would include the results of inspection (§ 38), palpation (§ 39), percussion (§ 40), the pulse (§ 41) and auscultation (§ 42); (*b*) cardiac efficiency tests (§ 43) used for ascertaining the reserve energy of the heart; (*c*) special instrumental methods of examinations (§ 44).

GROUP A. If the cardiac symptoms of which the patient complains are unattended by Pyrexia, turn to § 51. If the disease is **attended by Pyrexia,** it may be ACUTE PERICARDITIS or ACUTE ENDOCARDITIS, either rheumatic or infective in origin, or CORONARY THROMBOSIS. It must be remembered that cardiac patients are often subject to other febrile illnesses.

I. THE TEMPERATURE IS RAISED, *the patient is in evident distress, and the præcordial area of* DULLNESS IS INCREASED, *the shape of the dullness being* PYRAMIDAL, *with the point upwards.* A PERICARDIAL FRICTION SOUND *is audible. The disease is* ACUTE PERICARDITIS.

§ 46. Acute Pericarditis is an acute inflammation of the pericardial sac. It is not infrequently met as a primary affection. It supervenes during the course of many different diseases, and the symptoms of these may mask its onset. Rheumatic fever is its most common cause, and it should be remembered that it may be the first manifestation of this disease. We should always examine the heart daily in patients with rheumatic fever or the later stages of uræmia, because in these acute pericarditis may come on insidiously, without pain or tenderness. Its advent in rheumatic fever is marked by high fever, tachycardia, pallor and vomiting (especially in children) or by the occurrence of delirium.

Symptoms.—([1]) The patient wears an anxious, troubled look, and the cheeks are generally pallid; a distinct puffiness of the face, not amounting to obvious œdema, is often present; there are fever and a rapid pulse; the breathing is rapid, and he may complain of pain in the left chest (occasionally referred to the abdomen), increased by pressure, movement, or respiration; a short irritative unproductive cough is common. Abdominal rigidity may occur. (2) *Physical Signs.*—The præcordial dullness is increased in all directions. A friction sound is heard on auscultation. It is harsh, somewhat creaking in character, generally double, frequently triple, and occasionally systolic only. This may be distinguished from a murmur produced *within* the heart by (i.) usually being double, *i.e.*, accompanying the movements of the heart, and rarely exactly synchronous with the first and second sounds; (ii.) the second part of the rub is occasionally continuous with the first, without any diastolic pause; (iii.) it is often loudest at the root of the great vessels, over the third left costal cartilage; (iv.) it varies in its character from time to time, and is increased by firm pressure with the stethoscope; (v.) pressure will also elicit another character—viz., that the disease is usually accompanied by tenderness, as well as pain. The differentiation between peri- and endocardial murmurs is so important that it is also given in a tabular form below (Table I, p. 69). To distinguish pericardial from pleural friction is very easy, because the latter ceases if the patient holds his breath. Note that as the effusion occurs the murmur may become less distinct, but it rarely disappears entirely. It is again intensified as the effusion clears up. In many cases of acute pericarditis, with or without effusion, physical signs are to be found over the left lower lobe behind. These signs are those of collapse of the lung, and first occur, and are last to disappear, at the apex of the lobe; they may involve the whole lower lobe.

Second Stage, or stage of pericardial effusion. The inflammation may subside, but occasionally, in the course of a day or two, effusion of fluid occurs, and the pain and tenderness diminish. Effusion of more than half a pint is very rare in rheumatic pericarditis. When a LARGE EFFUSION does occur, the rub becomes less audible, though it may still be heard at the base of the heart. The breathlessness and other symptoms continue; cough becomes more troublesome; dysphagia and vomiting rarely occur. The neck veins are distended: pulsus paradoxus may be present. *The increased area of dullness*, due to pericardial effusion, may be greater than the enlargement from any other cause. (i.) It is of *triangular shape*, with apex upwards, reaching to the third, or even second, costal cartilage. (ii.) There is often actual or apparent *raising of the position of the apex beat.* (iii.) The *dullness extends to the left* of the apex beat. There is progressive weakening of the heart sounds at this time, from the associated myocarditis.

Etiology.—The causes may be classified under five headings: (1) acute infections, *e.g.*, rheumatism, scarlet fever, pneumonia, pyæmia, etc.; (2) extension from adjacent structures, *e.g.*, malignant disease and tuberculosis; (3) chronic nephritis; (4) coronary disease or infarction; (5) injury.

Course and Prognosis.—The duration of acute pericarditis varies widely, according to the cause, but it averages about fifteen to twenty-five days. It may undergo resolution with or without the formation of adhesions (Adherent Pericardium, § 56); or result in chronic pericardial effusion

(§ 56); or become purulent (Pyopericardium, § 47 below). Pericarditis with effusion is always a serious condition, but the prognosis depends on the underlying cause, the amount of distension of the pericardial sac, and the evidences of interference with the cardiac action—dyspnœa and cyanosis with feebleness, rapidity, and irregularity of the pulse. Pericarditis complicating rheumatism, like the other complications of that disease, tends to recover, but the myocardium is frequently damaged, and leads to cardiac dilatation (enlargement). In renal disease it is a serious though often latent affection; and in pyæmia, when it is generally purulent, is often fatal. In infancy and in debilitated patients it is also grave.

Diagnosis.—The diagnosis from acute endocarditis has been considered above, and in Table I, § 49. It is distinguished from enlargement of the

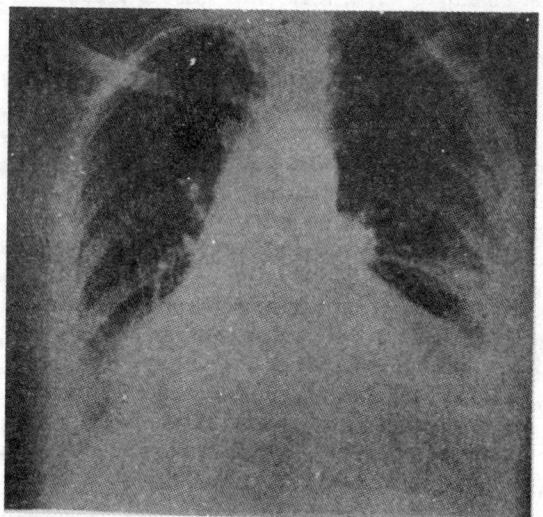

FIG. 27.—Chest X-ray showing the appearances in pericardial effusion.

heart by the following points: the left border of the dullness in pericardial effusion extends beyond the apex beat, and the apex beat may be displaced upwards; the right border of dullness has a convex outline and the cardio-hepatic angle at the right fifth intercostal space is obtuse; lack of movement of the epigastrium with respiration is another valuable sign. Both conditions may be present at the same time. X-Ray examination will usually enable one to verify the diagnosis when fluid is present. It should be remembered that inflammatory conditions of the *left lung* and *pleura* not infrequently give rise to a to-and-fro friction sound along the left border of the heart; this is produced by pleural and not by pericardial inflammation (pleuropericardial friction). The intensity of this friction often varies with respiration. The signs of consolidation of the left lower lobe described above may occasionally suggest a diagnosis of *lobar pneumonia.*

Treatment.—In the inflammatory stage the patient must be kept lying comfortably in bed. A fluid diet is advisable. A poultice or warm fomentation applied to the præcordium usually gives more relief than the ice-bag, though this undoubtedly relieves the symptoms, controls the restlessness of a young patient, and possibly also reduces the heart rate. If the pain is great, relief is often obtained from the application of four or five leeches over the præcordium. Blisters are occasionally used. If cyanosis, orthopnœa and venous distension are present, indicating considerable cardiac embarrassment, bleeding (15 to 20 oz.) is a prompt and efficacious measure. Opium by mouth, or morphia hypodermically, is of great value for the pain and distress, much smaller doses being given to children. The bowels should be regulated. Stimulants, such as nikethamide B.P. (Coramine), can be given when the blood pressure falls. Mersalyl is often useful in the more chronic forms of pericardial effusion. For hyperpyrexia and delirium tepid or cool sponging is a useful means of lowering the temperature, and will often induce sleep.

Treatment of the cause of the pericarditis should be combined with the foregoing—*e.g.*, sodium salicylate combined with alkalis for acute rheumatism. If the effusion becomes chronic, mersalyl is useful, but it must be used with care in nephritis.

PARACENTESIS PERICARDII.—When the amount of effusion becomes considerable, as shown by increasing dyspnœa, cyanosis, distension of the neck veins, tachycardia and lowered blood pressure, paracentesis pericardii should be performed. The site chosen for this procedure may be in the fifth left intercostal space just inside the mid-clavicular line, or one inch from the margin of the sternum in the same space; or in the angle between the xiphoid process and the left costal margin, near the lower end of the body of the sternum and passing upwards and inwards behind it into the pericardial sac. A trocar and cannula or an aspirating needle or a Potain aspirator may be employed. Eight or twelve or even forty ounces (in a chronic case) of fluid may be slowly removed; after mixing with a small amount of sodium citrate it should be examined pathologically. This operation is rarely required; it is never necessary in the rheumatic pericarditis of childhood.

§ 47. Pyopericarditis.—Sometimes in debilitated children and in the course of pyæmia, in phthisis and empyema, and in some other conditions, the fluid in the pericardium takes on a purulent or sero-purulent character. This is sometimes revealed (as is a collection of pus in other parts of the body) by (1) shivering attacks, (2) profuse perspirations, and (3) a temperature with wide variations in the course of a few hours, in addition to the clinical features of acute pericarditis above described. But it is difficult to diagnose, because the *friction sound is usually transient.* It is often fatal.

Pyopericarditis is the form which pericarditis frequently assumes in infancy, and is often not diagnosed. Progressive weakness, fever, anæmia, leucocytosis and X-ray examination may suggest the presence of pus.

Treatment.—A large sterilised (No. 10) needle should be very carefully introduced whenever the existence of pyopericardium is suspected. If the fluid withdrawn be of a purulent nature, paracentesis, followed by a local injection of penicillin, or free drainage, should be effected. Pyæmia or septicæmia should be treated by large doses of the antibiotic to which the organism is sensitive. Such treatment should

be continued for two weeks after the fever has entirely gone.   Tuberculous pericarditis
should be treated like tuberculous pleural effusion (1) by streptomycin, *para*-amino-
salicylic   acid   and   isoniazid,   (2)   by   paracentesis,   if   evidence   of   circulatory
embarrassment appears.

Pneumopericardium is a very rare condition in which air reaches the pericardial
sac from the lungs or stomach.

Hæmopericardium is rare.   Rupture of the heart following acute coronary occlusion,
aneurysm of the first part of the aorta or of the cardiac wall, wounds of the heart,
scurvy and some blood diseases, may lead to sudden death owing to the sudden
influx of blood into the pericardium.   A small amount of bleeding may be seen in
the pericarditis due to nephritis, malignant growths, acute rheumatism and tubercle.

§ **48. Latent Pericarditis**—*i.e.*, pericarditis without *symptoms* (though not necessarily without physical signs).   In most patients in whom we find a pericardial
effusion a history of acute pericarditis is obtainable; but it is not sufficiently recognised
that pericarditis may come on insidiously, without acute symptoms.   The effusion
may be discovered during routine examination of the heart, or perhaps not until
autopsy.   Moreover, at post-mortem a totally adherent pericardium is sometimes
found in a patient in whom careful inquiry has failed to reveal any symptoms pointing
to the heart during life.   In ACUTE RHEUMATISM *its advent may be indicated only
by delirium or vomiting.*

We now pass to the other acute disorder with pyrexia.—II. ACUTE
E..DOCARDITIS.

II. THE TEMPERATURE IS ELEVATED.   *The præcordial area of dullness
is not necessarily increased, and on auscultating the chest a* MITRAL *or* AORTIC
MURMUR *is added to the heart sounds—the disease is probably* ACUTE ENDO-
CARDITIS.   *It is not always easy to distinguish an endocardial from a pericardial murmur.*

§ **49. Acute Endocarditis** (Syn. Acute valvulitis) is acute inflammation of
the valves or of the mural endocardium of the heart.   It is usually attended
by enlargement of the præcordial dullness, because some degree of myocarditis and dilatation is associated with it.   In a large proportion of
cases it complicates some other disease; and, like pericarditis, it is most
frequently associated with acute rheumatism; it may even be the first
evidence of that disease.

There are two varieties of endocarditis with fever: RHEUMATIC Endocarditis, and INFECTIVE or MALIGNANT Endocarditis.

In RHEUMATIC ENDOCARDITIS: (1) *a murmur develops* at the apex or
base of the heart, corresponding to the mitral or aortic valves (see Fig. 12).
The mitral valve is most frequently involved in acute rheumatism, but
the mitral and aortic valves may be affected together, or rarely the aortic
valve alone.   The murmur is usually soft and heard over a limited area,
and only occasionally is it harsh soon after its appearance.   (2) There is
often some myocarditis sometimes causing cardiac dilatation, with a
weakened diffuse apical impulse and weak cardiac sounds.   (3) *Constitutional symptoms* may be marked when there are the general symptoms and
signs of rheumatic fever (§ 592); but in children these may be slight or
even absent.   The onset of endocarditis may then be suspected when
pallor supervenes, with loss of physical vigour, accompanied by an evening

rise in temperature and increase in pulse rate. Præcordial pain and distress are rarely found. The erythrocyte sedimentation rate is always raised when active endocarditis is present. The presence of rheumatic nodules (§ 592) around the elbows, wrists, knees and ankles usually indicates a severe form of active carditis.

Causes of Rheumatic Endocarditis.—It must be remembered that acute rheumatic endocarditis may complicate, not only rheumatic fever proper, but tonsillitis, chorea and scarlet fever. The patient is generally young, usually a child: the disease may be common in some families.

The *Diagnosis* of acute rheumatic endocarditis is sometimes difficult. The murmur will be found over the mitral or aortic valve, will immediately

TABLE I.—DIAGNOSIS OF ENDOCARDIAL FROM PERICARDIAL MURMURS

Endocardial Murmurs.	Pericardial Murmurs.
1. May accompany first or second sound only, or both.	Usually double—always superficial and are as loud in diastole as in systole; not quite synchronous with the heart sounds.
2. Often loudest at one of the valvular areas.	Usually loudest over third left costal cartilage (root of great vessels).
3. May be conducted into the axilla, or along the aorta and carotids.	Mostly confined to the præcordium.
4. Usually no pain or tenderness.	Often accompanied by pain.

follow a valve sound, will be localised and if conducted will follow the direction of the murmur of cardiac valvular disease (Fig. 12); it will not be materially affected by change of posture or by deep breathing. Care must be taken to avoid confusion with exocardial murmurs (§ 59). The distinction from pericardial murmurs is set out in Table I. In view of the great tendency to recurrence of acute rheumatism and of rheumatic endocarditis, a careful history of previous attacks should be taken: a mitral stenotic murmur is evidence of an attack of acute rheumatism at least six months previously. Therefore, if signs of an acute endocarditis are also present, the acute attack now suffered from cannot be the first. Pyrexia, tachycardia, an increase in the size of the heart and in the intensity of the murmur and a raised erythrocyte sedimentation rate indicate active inflammation of the valve or valves. *Subacute infective endocarditis* differs clinically (1) in the greater severity of the constitutional symptoms, with often a wide range of the diurnal temperature, and even rigors; (2) in the occurrence of systemic emboli; (3) the presence of splenomegaly, clubbing of the fingers and a positive blood culture. Subacute infective endocarditis often supervenes on a valve previously damaged by rheumatism, and the diagnosis may become difficult: persistent absence of

embolism and a persistently negative blood culture suggest an active
rheumatic lesion. Malignant endocarditis rarely supervenes upon a
recently active rheumatic lesion. The endocardial murmurs of syphilis
or of arteriosclerosis are not associated with pyrexia.

The *Prognosis* of rheumatic endocarditis, though the malady may last
for many weeks, or even months, is favourable as regards life, but the
damage to the cardiac valves is generally permanent, and then the prognosis turns on many important considerations (§ 61). A tendency to recur
is one of the most striking features of the disease.

Treatment should be directed primarily to the rheumatic fever: sodium
salicylate is usually thought to have no control over the cardiac lesion.
Digitalis is occasionally of use in cases of acute rheumatism with persistent
(regular) tachycardia or congestive failure. Iron is useful as ferri et
ammon. cit. 15 gr. t.d.s. for the anæmia which is so often present.
Penicillin is of no value in this condition. *Perfect rest*—hardly allowing
the patient to turn in bed—is absolutely essential. The patient should be
confined to bed until the temperature has been normal for at least 6 weeks,
the sedimentation rate has been normal for 2 weeks, the pulse rate has
remained normal for 3 weeks, anæmia has vanished, and the patient has
begun to put on weight. Careful treatment of the condition may require
prolonged rest in bed for 6 to 9 months (and see § 592). The erythrocyte
sedimentation rate is of great value in assessing the arrest of the active
process (§ 1210).

§ 50. **Infective, Bacterial, Malignant or Septic Endocarditis** is an acute
infection which attacks the heart valves or the endocardium already
damaged by previous disease. It is characterised by the presence of the
large vegetations, by local destruction of the valves, fever, bacteræmia
and multiple embolism. The disease probably never attacks a healthy
endocardium.

There are two clinical types. I. Subacute, which is fairly common ;
II. Acute, which is rarely seen.

I. *The patient, who may have been known to have* PREVIOUS CARDIAC
DISEASE, *runs a* TEMPERATURE *for some weeks and develops signs of* EM-
BOLISM. THE BLOOD CULTURE *is likely to grow* STREPTOCOCCUS VIRIDANS.
The disease is SUBACUTE BACTERIAL ENDOCARDITIS.

§ 50a. **Subacute Bacterial Endocarditis** (Syn. Subacute Infective Endocarditis).—Certain conditions predispose to the occurrence of the infection.
These are a heart valve previously damaged by rheumatism, rarely by
syphilis or atheroma, or a congenital heart lesion (especially a patent
ductus arteriosus, interventricular septal defect or a bicuspid aortic
valve). In 80–85 per cent. of cases, the infection is due to the *Streptococcus
viridans*, and it may follow extraction of infected teeth. Less commonly
the *H. influenzæ* is causal.

Symptoms.—The four cardinal findings are fever, a cardiac lesion, signs
of embolism and a positive blood culture. (i.) The fever may continue for

months (Fig. 173), the only complaints being general weakness, anorexia, headache, marked night sweating and transient pains in the joints or limbs. (ii.) Sooner or later a definite mitral or aortic valvular lesion is found: alternatively a congenital heart lesion is present. Sudden changes in the characters of the murmur may occur, and the heart undergoes enlargement. (iii.) Emboli may be gross or minute. Gross embolism affects most commonly the spleen, producing pain in the left hypochondrium and a palpable spleen; the kidney, producing macroscopic or microscopic hæmaturia and sometimes lumbar pain; the retinal artery, producing blindness; the cerebral vessels, producing hemiplegia or meningeal symptoms; and the arteries of the extremities, producing sudden pain in an arm, leg, finger or toe, pulsation then being absent distal to the block. More rarely mesenteric embolism may occur. Minute emboli produce a petechial rash, subconjunctival and retinal hæmorrhages and splinter hæmorrhages under the nails. Small red nodules on the fingers or toes (Osler's nodes) are diagnostic. As the disease progresses, rigors may occur, anæmia and progressive clubbing of the fingers develop and the skin may show a café au lait colour.

Diagnosis is confirmed by finding a positive blood culture, but this may remain persistently negative in 25 per cent. of cases. Even so the combination of symptoms and signs of the disease should suggest the diagnosis. The blood sedimentation rate is almost invariably high. Fever and a cardiac lesion occur in *acute* or *subacute rheumatism*, and pains in the joints are common, but a positive blood culture is never obtained. The joint lesions of acute rheumatism are brought to an end by full doses of salicylate, those of subacute bacterial endocarditis are unaffected. A cardiac lesion and systemic embolism occur in advanced mitral stenosis, but here the patient is afebrile, and auricular fibrillation is generally present; this irregularity is very rare in subacute bacterial endocarditis. Continued fever, possibly with a systolic cardiac murmur, may be present in other causes of severe *anæmia*, sometimes with splenic enlargement and petechiæ, but the blood count and response to treatment are generally diagnostic. *Hodgkin's disease, acute tuberculosis, E. coli pyelitis,* and other forms of *local sepsis* must in some cases be excluded.

Prognosis.—Without treatment by antibiotics, death is almost invariable. Early treatment results in a recovery rate of 75 per cent. Over a period of years, a relapse may occur in 20 per cent. of cases. Complications include myocardial dilatation and heart failure, the formation of mycotic aneurysms, temporary or permanent glomerulo-nephritis and embolism.

Treatment.—Whenever possible the invading organism should be isolated by blood culture and its sensitivity to penicillin and to the other antibiotics determined. When penicillin sensitive, 1–5 million units or more are given daily. If the organism is penicillin resistant or the patient sensitive to penicillin, other antibiotics (such as streptomycin or the tetracyclines) are given, alone or in combination, for a period of 6–8 weeks.

The anticoagulants are no longer considered necessary. If a transfusion is given for anæmia it must be given slowly. Rest in bed and attention to the general health are necessary until the patient is clearly convalescent, and preferably until the blood sedimentation rate is normal. To prevent recurrence, all dental extractions and endoscopies should be carried out under the cover of antibiotics. When the primary cause is an infection of a patent ductus arteriosus, this should usually be tied once the infection has been dealt with.

II. *The patient who has had a* RECENT SEVERE INFECTION *becomes more* SEVERELY ILL *with repeated* RIGORS *and a* POSITIVE BLOOD CULTURE. *The disease is likely to be* ACUTE INFECTIVE ENDOCARDITIS.

§ 50b. Acute Infective Endocarditis (Syn. Acute Bacterial or Septic Endocarditis) is relatively rare in comparison with Subacute Bacterial Endocarditis. The illness usually follows the infection which precedes it, especially in those with a poor resistance (*e.g.*, in diabetes). It is seen immediately after pneumonia, septic wounds, osteomyelitis, typhoid fever and other diseases which have failed to respond to appropriate antibiotic therapy.

Symptoms.—There is an exacerbation of the previously existing fever. The patient becomes more severely ill, perspires freely, with a high swinging temperature and usually repeated rigors. If the patient survives long enough signs of embolism and a positive blood culture as described in § 50*a* are found.

Etiology.—The organisms most commonly concerned are *Strep. hæmolyticus, pneumococcus, staphylococcus, gonococcus and E. typhosus.*

The *Treatment* is as for Subacute Bacterial Endocarditis, using still larger doses of the appropriate antibiotics.

GROUP B. We now turn to those cardiac disorders in which **Pain** is the leading feature. The other cardiac condition giving rise to pain is PERICARDITIS.

In PERICARDITIS the degree of pain is very variable; and it is recognised by the other symptoms and signs fully described in § 46.

The patient, probably a male, at or past middle life, is attacked by CONSTRICTION *and* PAIN IN THE CHEST—*the condition is* ANGINA PECTORIS.

§ 51. Angina Pectoris. There are four types of angina—I. Angina of Effort; II. Spasmodic Angina; III. Coronary Thrombosis (Status Anginosus); IV. Angina Innocens (Pseudo-angina). More than one of the varieties may be present in the same patient.

I. **Angina of Effort.** *Symptoms.*—The pain is usually dull and constricting, retrosternal and often radiating to the arms and to the neck. It is not present at rest and is proportional to the amount of exercise taken. It may or may not be accompanied by dyspnœa. It is often more marked if exercise is taken after a meal (and is thus sometimes mistaken for dyspepsia) and on exposure to cold. Hyperæsthesia is absent. The pain is relieved by nitrites.

Diagnosis.—An electrocardiographic record may show no signs of cardiac ischæmia; but when this is repeated immediately after exercise ischæmic changes occur, with depression of the ST interval and flattening or inversion of the T waves in some of the precordial or limb leads. These changes disappear after resting for five to ten minutes.

Etiology.—The pain is due to an inadequate coronary flow during exertion. It is caused by atheroma or by syphilitic aortitis. Even in cases with no sign of cardio-vascular disease a Wassermann reaction should still be done. Post mortem, one of three conditions may be found: (1) The heart itself may be unhealthy, as the result usually of changes in the coronary vessels; (2) the heart may be apparently healthy, but disease of the aorta may be present; (3) the heart and the vessels may both be diseased. The *immediate cause of the attack* is anoxia (lack of oxygen) of the heart muscle, due to increasing work thrown on the heart by physical effort, mental stress or mechanical embarrassment, such as is produced by cold (vaso-constriction of skin vessels), or distension of the stomach by food or flatulence.

Prognosis.—The two points to be clear about are (1) the sensitivity of the patient's nervous system; (2) other evidence of myocardial disease. The more anxious the patient the slighter will be the lesion which will cause pain, and the better is the outlook. A bad prognosis is suggested by considerable cardiac enlargement, high blood pressure, pulsus alternans, cardiac asthma, and marked dyspnœa. In the syphilitic cases, if treatment is sufficiently thorough, recovery may occur or the lesion may be arrested; the presence of aortic regurgitation makes the outlook more serious. Relatives should be told that the condition is serious, and that an exact prognosis is not possible. The condition of the cardiac muscle is the best guide to the probable course of a case (§§ 57 and 61).

Treatment.—The patient should be reassured. Undue apprehension and nervousness are apt to accentuate the symptoms. The term angina should not be mentioned to the patient. For the pain one or two tablets of glyceryl trinitrate B.P. should be crushed in the mouth or held under the tongue for a few minutes before being swallowed. Prophylactically, attention should be directed to lightening the cardiac burden, by adjustment of the mental and physical activities, treatment of adiposit and of dyspepsia. A glyceryl trinitrate tablet should be taken just before undertaking exertion which is likely to produce an attack of pain. Hurry and nervous tension must be avoided. Rest should be insisted on after every meal. Diet the patient strictly according to these principles: four meals daily (the object of four meals being that comparatively little food is introduced into the stomach at once); no fluid to be taken until some time after a meal, so as to avoid diluting the gastric juices and delaying digestion. Avoid bulky food which takes a long time to digest. If there is marked flatulence, in addition to the above regime, the following mixture can be given immediately after food: Spir. ammon. aromat., spir. ætheris nitrosi, spir. cajuputi, in equal parts, 60 min. to be taken in a little water.

Useful drugs are the long-acting nitrates such as pentaerythritol tetranitrate (Mycardol or Peritrate) t.d.s.; phenobarbitone gr. ½ t.d.s., p.c., or tab. phenobarb. et theobrom. (B.P.C.). Propyl thiouracil, to depress thyroid activity, is sometimes helpful in doses of 100 mg. t.d.s., p.c. Cervical sympathectomy is useful in selected cases. Continuous anticoagulant therapy is on trial.

II. **Spasmodic Angina.** The attack of pain is sudden, not proportional to exertion, severe, and often associated with a feeling of impending death. It is probably due to coronary spasm, accentuated by cold or emotion. Patients are usually of the male sex, and over 50 years of age. The disease also appears to affect by preference hypersensitive individuals.

These *Symptoms* may be superimposed on those of angina of effort; rarely they are present alone. The attack of spasmodic angina comes on quite suddenly, often after exertion, especially after a meal or in the cold. It consists of (1) acute pain in the chest, which radiates down the arms, especially the left: the site of the pain, as Mackenzie pointed out, is over the distribution of the four upper dorsal nerves, across the chest; the skin over this area may be hyperalgesic. The face is expressive of the pain which the patient suffers. Pallor and sweating are present. The patient usually keeps quite still, being afraid to move for fear of increasing the agony. The sense of suffocation, of bodily discomfort, constriction of the chest, and of impending dissolution is extreme. The attack lasts for a few seconds to a few minutes, and is liable to be aggravated if the patient ventures to move. (2) During an attack the heart's action is sometimes found to be unaltered, though palpitation may be complained of. The heart usually shows some enlargement, and the aortic valve may be diseased (see Etiology below). The blood pressure is raised: the pulse rate is in some cases increased. Electrocardiographic examination often shows some irregularity due to premature beats, and changes due to ischæmia which are especially marked after exercise (see angina of effort). (3) The mind remains clear throughout. Many attacks are accompanied or succeeded by a profuse flow of urine; others by profuse perspiration. The limbs and other parts which were the seat of pain may afterwards feel " numbed."

Etiology.—There is often a familial tendency. Coronary atheroma, severe aortic regurgitation and aortic syphilis are the commonest causes.

Prognosis.—The same considerations enter into the prognosis in spasmodic angina as in angina of effort, and death from coronary thrombosis is common.

Treatment.—The pain is relieved by amyl nitrite or nitroglycerin. Hot whisky and water is sometimes useful, especially at night. Attention should be paid to keeping the rooms and the bed well warmed, as many attacks are produced by passing from a warm room to a cold passage, and by getting into a cold bed at night. Good nights must be ensured by the use of barbiturates, chloral, or even morphia when necessary. If the cause of the condition is an inadequate oxygen supply, the object of treatment is twofold, namely: (1) to reduce the work of the heart, and (2) to increase the oxygen supply, *i.e.*, the blood supply to the muscle. Between attacks, the treatment is identical with that described for angina of effort.

There are two methods in use for blocking the stimuli in anginal pain, sympathectomy of the middle and lower cervical ganglia, and alcohol injection of the five upper dorsal sympathetic *rami communicantes*. The choice of appropriate cases is a matter for expert opinion, but it can be stated briefly that the chief indications for mechanical interference are: (1) The pain has a coronary origin; (2) syphilis has been excluded; (3) the cardiac function of the patient is otherwise good; (4) gross disease is absent.

§ 52. III. **Myocardial Infarction** (Syn. Coronary Thrombosis), is a condition in which a lesion of the coronary artery causes rapid ischæmia of an area of the ventricular heart muscle. It is much more common after the age of 40: up to the age of 60 it is more frequent in men than in women, but after this age it is equally common in the two sexes. Coronary thrombosis has now become the commonest cardiac cause of death.

Symptoms.—The cardinal symptom is pain in the chest which rapidly and progressively increases in severity. At first it may be mistaken for severe indigestion. Often commencing at night or when the patient is at rest, the pain is usually situated centrally beneath the upper, the middle, or the lower part of the sternum. It may radiate to either side of the sternum (more frequently to the left), into the arms, to the neck, to between the scapulæ or to the epigastrium. The pain lasts longer than in angina of effort and is not relieved by resting. The severity of the pain varies considerably. In a mild attack the pain may last for an hour, but in a severe attack the pain may persist for several successive days: it is uninfluenced by nitrites and usually needs morphia to relieve it. *Signs.* (1) Shock varies in intensity: in severe cases it may be profound, the patient being pale, frightened, restless, vomiting, sweating profusely and with a rapid fall in blood pressure. (2) Signs of heart failure may be observed, with dyspnœa even at rest. Right ventricular failure may produce cyanosis, distension of the neck veins and engorgement of the liver: left ventricular failure is accompanied by a poor pulse, weak heart sounds and triple rhythm at the apex and (3) Tachycardia is more common than bradycardia but abnormalities of rhythm and even heart block may occur (§ 71). (4), A pericardial rub may be heard for a day or two. (5) A few hours after the onset a raised sedimentation rate, a temperature of 100–101° and a leucocytosis are usual. (6) The serum glutamic oxaloacetic transaminase test of the serum demonstrates the presence in the blood of an enzyme released from the injured heart muscle. The normal value of 8–40 Sigma units begins to rise 12 hours after acute coronary occlusion to a peak value at 48 hours (even to over 200 units) and falls to normal by the fifth day. (7) The electrocardiographic changes are discussed on page 80.

The main differences between an attack of angina of effort and coronary thrombosis can be summarised as follows:

TABLE II

ANGINA OF EFFORT.	CORONARY THROMBOSIS.
I. Attack comes on during exercise, with cold or emotion. Especially after meals.	Attack comes on at any time, by day or night.
II. Patient is brought to a standstill by the pain, which then soon goes.	Patient is restless, collapsed, sweating and often slightly cyanosed or flushed.
III. Attacks last a few minutes.	Attacks may last some hours or days and are more agonising.
IV. Pain relieved by vaso-dilators.	Pain unaffected by vaso-dilators.
V. Arterial B.P. usually rises.	Arterial B.P. falls markedly. Venous pressure may be raised.
VI. No fever or leucocytosis.	Slight fever and leucocytosis within 24 hours.
VII. Erythrocyte sedimentation rate normal.	Erythrocyte sedimentation rate raised.
VIII. Friction sounds absent.	Pericardial friction often present after about the fourth day.
IX. Electrocardiogram. The tracing at rest is usually unchanged in shape.	Electrocardiogram always shows a changing QRST (Figs. 28–30).
X. Heart sounds clearly audible.	Heart sounds weak.
XI. Transaminase test negative.	Transaminase test positive.

Diagnosis.—Any sudden and persistent pain in the chest after the age of 40 should be viewed with suspicion and may require investigation with an electrocardiogram. Conditions simulating myocardial infarction are intercostal fibrositis, gall stone colic, pulmonary embolism, pneumothorax, perforated peptic ulcer and dissecting aneurysm. The pain of fibrositis is associated with local tenderness: both pain and tenderness disappear after injection of a local anæsthetic. In gall stone colic distension of the neck veins is not present: there may be a tinge of jaundice. The heart is normal clinically and electrocardiographically. In pulmonary embolism shortness of breath is present, pain is less severe or absent, the neck veins may be distended, hæmoptysis may occur and physical signs suggesting pulmonary œdema and pulmonary collapse may be present over the area of lung involved. It must be remembered that in pulmonary embolism the T wave over the right ventricular chest leads of the electrocardiogram is often inverted.

Etiology.—The primary disease is nearly always due to coronary atheroma. The acute lesion is frequently a thrombus and the myocardial lesion is an infarct. The relationship between the thrombosis and the infarction varies. In some patients the deficient blood supply to the area of heart muscle alone will induce the formation of a sudden infarct, the changes in the infarcted area being somewhat analogous to those of coagulation necrosis. Here the infarct occurs without the presence of clot in the vessel. But in some individuals a clot may occur in a coronary branch without infarction of the area supplied by such a vessel: this is because a sufficient collateral arterial supply has been already stimulated by the slow progressive narrowing of the branch in which the clot subsequently forms. Nevertheless, in most cases there is both a coronary clot and subsequent infarction.

The inflammation accompanying the infarct may involve the pericardium causing pericarditis, or the endocardium causing deposition of a mural clot inside the ventricular chamber. These clots may become detached and give rise to systemic embolism.

The underlying lesion of coronary atheroma is generally most prominent within an inch or so of the mouth of the coronary vessel. In some cases it would appear that a more acute coronary lesion, such as subintimal hæmorrhage, may be the precipitating cause of the coronary thrombosis. A raised blood cholesterol is present in many cases but this is probably only one of several causative factors, since a myocardial infarction does not necessarily develop in such individuals. Syphilis, subacute bacterial endocarditis and polyarteritis nodosa are exceedingly rare causes of myocardial infarction. In the U.S.A., some figures show those who smoke have twice the mortality of non-smokers.

The anterior descending branch of the left coronary artery is the vessel most frequently affected. The infarcted area is discoloured and in the acute stage is surrounded by an area in which hæmorrhage has occurred. Subsequent changes in the infarct vary according to the extent to which the blood supply has been cut off from the infarcted area. In a slight case little central fibrosis or scarring occurs, and revascularisation and recovery are considerable. This is either by reabsorption of the clot in the affected vessel, or by increase in the size and efficiency of collateral coronary branches. In a very severe case the infarct softens and rupture of the heart occurs. In a moderately severe case considerable fibrous tissue is laid down at the centre of the lesion and normal revascularisation and healing occur at the periphery of it. When recovery is reasonably good compensatory hypertrophy occurs in the adjacent ventricular muscle.

Prognosis.—Following coronary thrombosis sudden death may occur, particularly within the first three days. A bad prognosis is suggested by acute and prolonged pain, by severe initial shock, or the occurrence of a marked degree of right or left ventricular failure: those with hypertension and diabetes mellitus carry a worse prognosis. After a coronary thrombosis it is improbable that the heart will be as efficient as before, but in certain cases where the myocardium is otherwise healthy full functional recovery occurs. Points suggesting a favourable prognosis are absence of cardiac enlargement, of shortness of breath and of angina of effort in the convalescent period, and those with a normal blood pressure. A second thrombosis occurs in 25 per cent. of cases. The most serious complications are congestive heart failure, embolism from intraventricular clot (especially in the brain), rupture of the heart, cardiac irregularities due to paroxysmal tachycardia and deep vein thrombo-phlebitis in the legs causing pulmonary embolism.

Treatment.—Pain requires full doses of morphia which may have to be repeated two or even three times. Shock associated with great lowering of the systolic blood pressure to less than 100 mm. of mercury may call for the administration of nor-adrenalin in an intravenous drip of 5 per cent. glucose with half-normal saline at a rate of 10–20 drips a minute; start with 4 mg. per litre and increase to 8 mg., 16 mg., 24 mg., or even 32 mg. per litre if necessary, to maintain the systolic blood pressure at 100–110 mm. of mercury. Mephenteramine (Mephine) and metaraminol (Aramine) added to a slow intravenous drip or intramusc. are also valuable in raising the blood pressure. Anticoagulants have added to the efficiency of treatment. They prevent an extension of the original clot, the formation of intraventricular clot producing embolism and the deposition of silent thrombi in the femoral veins, which may cause serious pulmonary embolism. Mild cases have as good a prognosis, with or without anticoagulant therapy, but in severe cases statistics show that the prognosis is better when anticoagulants are used. Should the patient need to be under the influence of anticoagulants quickly, heparin must be given intravenously at once (15,000 units) and followed by ℮ similar quantity intramuscularly at eight-hour intervals for the first two days. Phenindione B.P. (Dindevan) is the other drug of choice. On successive days 200 mg., 100 mg., and 50 mg. are usually given, starting at the same time as the heparin. Subsequent dosage is determined by the prothrombin activity of the patient's blood; it is usually 50–100 mg. a day. At first daily prothrombin estimations (§ 1215) must be done, but later estimations may be spread to every second or third day as soon as the maintenance dose has been adequately determined. The prothrombin time of a fully treated patient should be 2 to 3 times that of the control blood. For example, if the prothrombin time of the control is 12 seconds that of the patient should be 30 seconds. The prothrombin index is then $\dfrac{12 \times 100}{30} = 40$ per cent. A dark coloured urine during anticoagulant therapy is of no importance, but the appearance of large numbers of red cells is an indication for caution. This anticoagulant treatment should be continued for three weeks in most cases. Anticoagulants must be given with caution to patients with recurrent epistaxis, peptic ulcer, hiatus hernia or other potential sources of bleeding. Bleeding from the nose, the kidneys, the gastro-intestinal tract, into the skin as purpura, or into the eye, may result from the use of phenindione in too high a dosage. *External Cardiac Massage* is now frequently used for sudden cardiac arrest, especially in acute myocardial infarction. To perform this the patient must be lying on a firm surface; and whenever possible the operator should kneel beside the patient. The heart is compressed between the ribs and sternum in front and the vertebræ behind, 20 to 30 times a minute; to do this considerable force must be suddenly applied to the precordium with the two hands placed one on top of the other. When it is thought that ventricular fibrillation may coexist, an electrical defibrillator must be used at the same time.

After the acute attack the patient should be kept in bed for three to six weeks depending on its severity. Old people should not be confined to bed for as long as this. During convalescence gradually increasing mobility

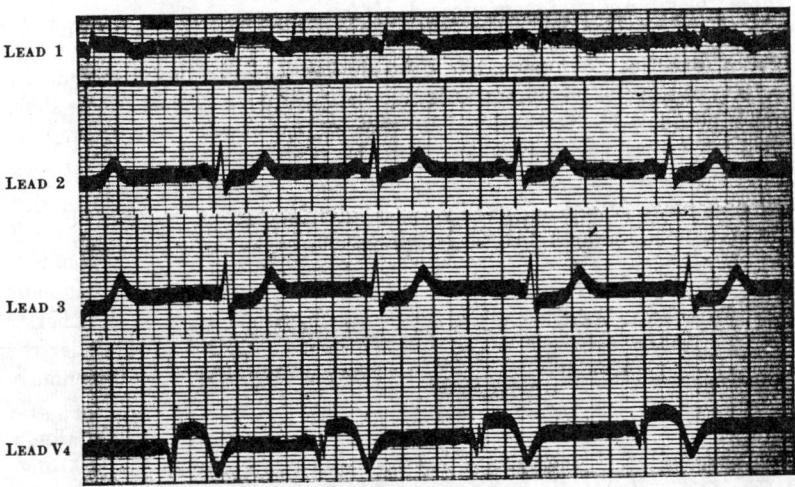

FIG. 28.—ELECTROCARDIOGRAM three days after an acute ANTERIOR CORONARY THROMBOSIS. Note S-T elevation in leads 1 and V_4, showing a positive Pardee sign in recent anterior myocardial infarction.

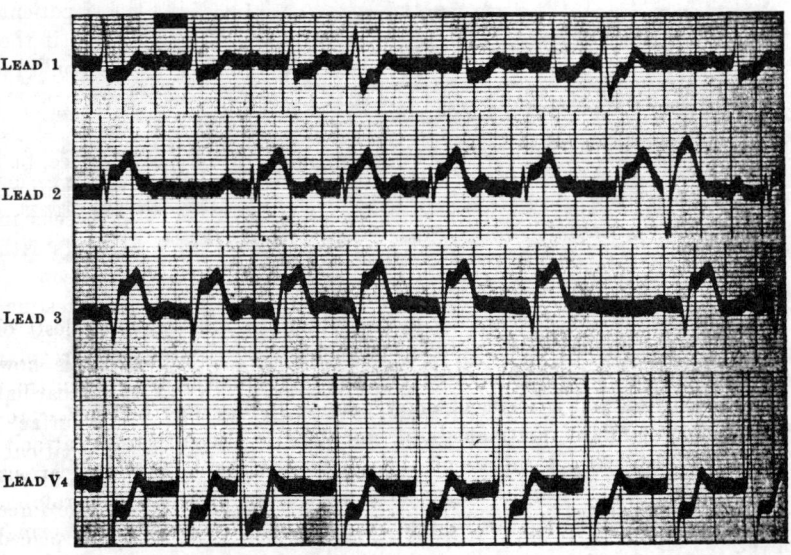

FIG. 29.—ELECTROCARDIOGRAM two days after an acute POSTERIOR CORONARY THROMBOSIS. Note the S-T elevation in leads 2 and 3, and the corresponding S-T depression in leads 1 and V_4: the characteristic Pardee sign in recent posterior myocardial infarction.

should be advised and even pressed.   *After-treatment.*—The patient should be encouraged gradually to increase his activities up to his previous normal level, provided that he remains free from shortness of breath and anginal pain.   It is of the greatest importance that the psychological effects should be kept in mind.   The fear induced by such an attack must be gradually dispelled by reassurance and by the knowledge that many patients recover a normal heart function after an attack of myocardial infarction.   On the other hand, physical and mental overwork and fatigue must be avoided. Weight should be reduced dietetically when necessary.   A low animal fat

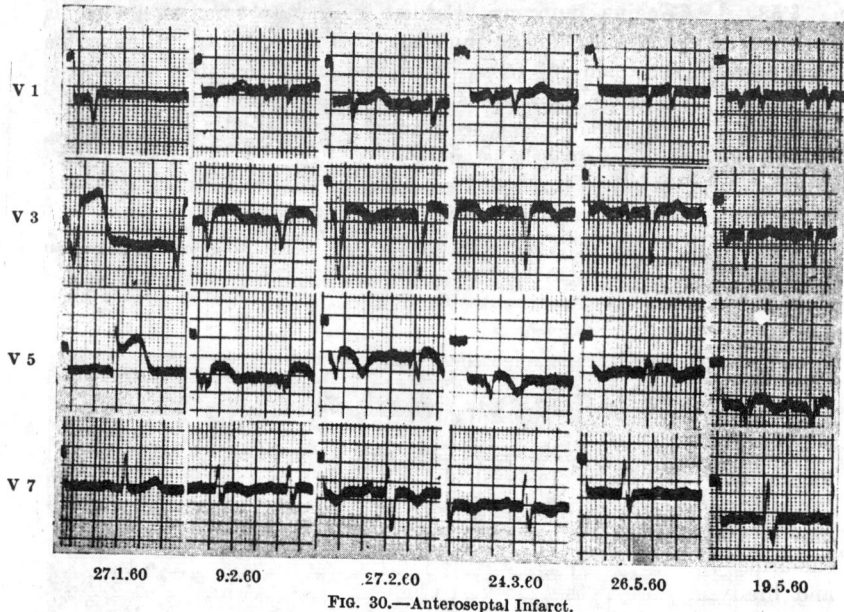

V 1

V 3

V 5

V 7

27.1.60   9:2.60   .27.2.60   24.3.60   26.5.60   19.5.60

FIG. 30.—Anteroseptal Infarct.

diet is a sensible measure in view of the sometimes high blood cholesterol figure.   Smoking should be abolished or much reduced, and regular examinations at intervals of three, six or twelve months are helpful from a psychological and a physical point of view.   The question as to prolonged anticoagulant treatment by phenindione to prevent further attacks is as yet undecided.   In a patient who is liable to thrombotic complications this may be wise.   If so it is essential to control the patient's prothrombin time at a figure less than the therapeutic one, namely at twice the normal level.

The *Electrocardiographic changes* in myocardial infarction (see Figs. 28 and 29) can be anatomically mapped out by the unipolar electrodes (§ 44).   They will show abnormalities of three distinct types.   Soon after the onset of myocardial infarction (Fig. 30) there is an S–T elevation (27–1–60) or depression, the so-called Pardee sign, which is due to a constant and uniform current of injury set up in the affected area of heart muscle.

The second type of change is that caused by ischæmia, or deficiency in the oxygen supply, to the myocardium, and which is shown by inversion of the T waves (27–2–60). The third type of injury is shown by the presence of Q waves and the absence of R waves: this indicates destruction of heart muscle tissue. The current of injury is transient, but the other two changes may be permanent. In Fig. 30 the S–T elevation due to a current of injury is well shown in the first three strips, but this has disappeared in the fourth strip. This is gradually replaced by inversion of the T waves. This change disappears as healing goes on, for instance lead V7 where the T wave is seen to be upright again in the last strip. In lead V3 there is no R wave in strips 1, 2, 3 and 4. There appears to be a slight R wave in the sixth strip as healing progresses.

§ 53. IV. **Angina Innocens.** Cardiac pain of a functional type is common and is labelled angina innocens or *pseudo-angina*. It must be distinguished from pain due to an organic lesion. The safest criterion is the relation to exercise. If there is never pain at rest, if it is strictly proportional to exercise and only occurs during exertion, it is of organic origin. Other evidences in favour of true angina are: the presence of dyspnœa, of cardiac enlargement, hypertension or aortic disease, and the absence of præcordial tenderness. Evidences in favour of angina innocens are: an increase of pain after exertion—not during it, the presence of palpitation, giddiness and fainting attacks, the presence of præcordial hyperæsthesia, evidence of an unstable nervous system or a history of nervous breakdown. In angina innocens there is no cardiac enlargement, and no evidence of cardiac disease clinically, electrocardiographically, or by X-ray. However, there is an exception to this rule in cases of mitral stenosis with pain; these patients have pain of the angina innocens type.

There is a second type of pain occasionally found in patients with angina innocens. It is almost identical with that described by Gowers (Vaso-vagal attacks of Gowers). These attacks have a sudden onset, there may be a sense of impending death; severe præcordial pain may radiate to the arms, or tingling in the arms may be complained of. Marked pallor and bradycardia are the most striking signs. The patient generally faints.

Prognosis. In angina innocens, though the symptoms may persist for years, there is no danger to life and recovery always occurs in time. The vaso-vagal attacks have no bad prognostic significance.

Treatment of angina innocens consists in reassuring the patient, in removing obvious physical abnormalities such as marked dental or tonsillar sepsis, in attempting to adjust any psychological stresses, and in allowing a gradual increase of exercise taken by the patient. Treatment in a special psycho-therapeutic centre is often advantageous. The best drugs are phenobarbitone and bromides.

GROUP C. We now consider those conditions in which examination reveals **Enlargement** of the **Area of Præcordial Dullness.**

a. If there is a history of acute onset, and there is PYREXIA, the condition is due to ACUTE PERICARDITIS, which is fully described in Group I, § 46, or to DILATATION secondary to a febrile process.

b. If there is no Pyrexia, the enlargement may be due to

    I. Cardiac Hypertrophy.

    II. Cardiac Dilatation.

    III. Chronic Pericardial Effusion.

    IV. Adherent Pericardium.

    V. Congenital heart disease (rare).

VI. Aortic Aneurysm and Mediastinal Tumours must be remembered, because their existence is often revealed by finding enlargement of the præcordial dullness, or dullness above, merging into that of the heart.

Chronic conditions which may be, but are NOT NECESSARILY, attended by ENLARGEMENT of the area of præcordial dullness should be borne in mind; their diagnosis may depend mainly on auscultation, and hence they are described under Groups D and E.

Method of Procedure.—It will be remembered that the routine examination of the heart consisted of (1) inspection; (2) palpation; (3) percussion of the præcordial dullness; (4) auscultation; and (5) in any patient in whom cardio-vascular disease is suspected, radiography and electrocardiography can give valuable help. The student should bear in mind the various *fallacies* which may give a false impression of cardiac enlargement, and also those conditions, such as emphysema, which obscure an enlarged heart (§ 40).

I. *The* APEX BEAT *is* BELOW *its normal position; the impulse is* FORCIBLE *and heaving; on auscultation, the first sound is* DULL *and prolonged. There is* HYPERTROPHY OF THE HEART.

§ 54. Hypertrophy of the Heart, and the dilatation which not infrequently accompanies or follows it, are certainly the commonest conditions which produce an increased area of præcordial dullness.

Cardiac Hypertrophy is an increase of the muscular substance of the heart, and its weight, which is normally about 250 G. in women and 300 G. in men, may be increased to 400–500 G., and on rare occasions to 600 G. Its *signs* are as follows: (1) The increase in the præcordial dullness is downwards and outwards if the left ventricle be hypertrophied, outwards only if the right ventricle; (2) the apex beats below and outside its normal position; (3) the impulse is unduly forcible, heaving or thrusting, the thrust of the hypertrophied right ventricle being generally felt in the epigastric notch; (4) on auscultation, the first sound is loud and prolonged. The pulse is firm, strong and bounding. (5) The electrocardiogram of ventricular hypertrophy shows a tall R wave and inversion of the T wave. In left ventricular hypertrophy these changes are seen in leads 1, VL, V5, V6 and V7, and in right ventricular hypertrophy exactly similar changes are seen in V1, V2, and sometimes V3, these unipolar leads being placed over the right ventricle.

Symptoms may be altogether absent if the hypertrophy accurately compensates for the obstruction in the circulation which has caused the hypertrophy. The patient may, indeed, be unaware of any cardiac disorder.

Etiology.—Hypertrophy is caused by an increase in the work to be performed. The part of the heart which undergoes hypertrophy is that immediately behind the lesion: the signs of such a lesion will be additional to those caused by hypertrophy. Thus, there will be three sets of signs: (*a*) Signs of hypertrophy of the heart as a whole; (*b*) signs of enlargement of the chamber specially involved; and (*c*) signs and symptoms of the cause. The following causes will be more readily understood by consulting Fig. 33 (p. 93), and it must be remembered that the enlargement is rarely in actual practice strictly limited to one chamber of the heart.

(*a*) HYPERTROPHY OF THE LEFT VENTRICLE is indicated by displacement of the apex beat *below* and to the left of its normal position. The apical impulse is strong, sustained and heaving in character. There is also enlargement of the area of cardiac dullness to the left. The pulse is strong unless modified by the presence of a valvular lesion, and the carotids may be seen to pulsate.

Etiology.—Hypertrophy is always secondary, and is proportional to the extent of the causative lesion, provided that compensation has occurred. It is an illustration of the physiological law that increased use leads to increased growth. Hypertrophy of the left ventricle is due to one of the following causes:—hypertension (§ 96), aortic regurgitation or stenosis, mitral regurgitation, healed chronic myocarditis and adherent pericardium. The largest of all hearts are those in which chronic pericarditis with adhesions is present (§ 56, IV). The writer has seen one such case where the heart weighed more than the liver. The commonest cause of marked enlargement is aortic regurgitation. Aortic stenosis produces only a slight degree of enlargement, the whole of which is due to hypertrophy. *Aneurysm of the aortic arch*, if unattended by valvular disease or by renal or arterial disease, does not *per se* cause cardiac hypertrophy; if enlargement is present, it is due to associated aortic regurgitation or hypertension. *Excessive muscular exercise*, whether athletic or laborious, may produce hypertrophy, and therefore the normal increase with age is more noticeable in men than in women.

(*b*) HYPERTROPHY OF THE RIGHT VENTRICLE is indicated by a heaving or thrusting impulse in the left parasternal area. It is the result of resistance to the emptying of the ventricle into the pulmonary vessels. This may occur in:

(i.) *Pulmonary diseases* attended by obstruction in the pulmonary circulation, of which *bronchitis with emphysema* is certainly the most frequent. This condition, a very common one, is identified by a history or evidence of lung disease (§ 143).

(ii.) *Mitral stenosis* is also a common cause, and should be borne in mind even in the absence of a presystolic murmur (§ 60).

(iii.) *Mitral regurgitation* (§ 58).

(iv.) Raised pulmonary pressure from pulmonary arterio-sclerosis, Ayerza's disease (see § 31).

(v.) Congenital pulmonary stenosis.

(*c*) HYPERTROPHY OF THE LEFT OR RIGHT AURICLE is always attended by dilatation. It cannot be recognised by physical signs but is shown by enlargement of the P waves in the electrocardiogram. Dilatation can be verified by X-ray examination (Figs. 22, 23).

Enlargement of the left auricle occurs in *mitral* regurgitation, but its chief cause is *mitral stenosis,* where it may be enormous. In the latter condition the physical signs are those of the valvular lesion: palpation generally reveals a thrill over the apex and careful auscultation may detect a presystolic or mid-diastolic murmur (§ 60).

Prognosis and Treatment.—Cardiac Hypertrophy is essentially a compensatory process for some condition which causes obstruction in the circulation. It is Nature's method of compensating for the increased work.

1. *If the cause be removable,* the prognosis is favourable. Treatment in such cases should therefore be directed to the removal of the cause—*e.g.,* high blood pressure.

2. *If the cause be not removable,* the prognosis of the case depends on the avoidance of myocardial failure, which will show itself symptomatically by dyspnœa and physically by dilatation. To accomplish the first, the general health should be improved by general hygienic measures. The patient should be encouraged to continue those physical activities which are possible and comfortable, and slowly to increase them.

3. The *existence of cardiac hypertrophy* usually indicates an added strain upon the heart muscle, either from valvular disease or from hypertension. If the muscle remains healthy it can support such a strain without failing.

II. *The* AREA OF DULLNESS IS INCREASED; *the position of the* APEX BEAT IS INDEFINITE; *the impulse is diffuse, wavy and slapping; on auscultation, the first sound is short and sharp. The condition is* CARDIAC DILATATION.

§ 55. Cardiac Dilatation (an important indication of " Myocardial failure ") suggests that the heart is " failing " to keep pace with the demand made upon it, that the reserve power of the muscle wall is becoming spent. Slight dilatation is the immediate physiological response of the heart to increased work. If increased work continues, hypertrophy normally follows. Physiological dilatation is limited by the pericardium. Severe or persistent dilatation, and the symptoms and signs of failure, are due to a common cause, the underlying myocardial failure—which is usually due to toxæmia or to anoxæmia.

As already stated (§ 26) cardiac dyspnœa is almost always accompanied by cardiac enlargement. The heart muscle usually fails because it is affected by one of the following conditions:

(i.) Subacute or chronic Rheumatic Disease, usually with involvement of the mitral or aortic valve.

(ii.) Coronary Atherosclerosis interfering with the oxygen supply to the heart muscle.

(iii.) Hypertensive Heart Disease when the coronary arterioles become narrowed and insufficient.

(iv.) Syphilis of the Aorta which interferes with the blood flow through the mouths of the coronary arteries as these leave the aorta.

(v.) Chronic Pulmonary Disease, particularly Emphysema.

Myocardial failure, nearly always accompanied by dilatation, generally involves both left and right ventricles. Usually the left side is first affected and its failure later causes the right ventricle to fail also. In rare cases the right ventricle fails alone: orthopnœa is absent in pure right ventricular failure. Heart failure with clinical œdema is called congestive heart failure.

(I) DILATATION OF THE LEFT VENTRICLE indicates some degree of **left ventricular failure.**

Physical Signs.—In the early stages we find: (1) the cardiac impulse by palpation is wavy and diffuse, and is displaced outwards rather than downwards: it may be so feeble as to be hardly perceptible. (2) There is increase in the area of cardiac dullness in a transverse direction to the left. (3) On auscultation the first sound is often reduced in volume and may be reduplicated. Both first and second sounds are often faint and the period of systolic output shortened. (4) Murmurs may be present from co-existing valvular disease, but a systolic murmur—the " murmur of dilatation "—may be heard apart from actual valvular disease, because the dilated auriculo-ventricular orifice allows a reflux of blood (§ 58, IIa). (5) The pulse may be feeble and rapid. *In the later stages,* when left ventricular failure is more severe, there may appear (1) pulmonary congestion and œdema. *Cardiac asthma* may follow. This is most noticeable in the night: it is revealed by orthopnœa, dyspnœa, cough, expectoration of mucus sometimes tinged with blood, or actual hæmoptysis. The physical signs are abundant rales and, sometimes, scattered patches of dullness at one or both bases. (2) In auricular fibrillation or *delirium cordis* the heart is so rapid and irregular that it becomes difficult to make out the relations of sounds and murmurs. (3) In *gallop rhythm* there is usually rapidity of action, together with a distinctly reduplicated first or second sound.

Gallop rhythm is a condition in which three heart sounds, instead of two, are heard in each cardiac cycle. *Pathological* causes are (i.) a Bundle-branch lesion (Figs. 46, 47). Owing to the fact that conduction is unequal down each branch of the bundle of His, the contraction of the two ventricles is slightly asynchronous. The first heart sound at the apex is thus reduplicated. (ii.) A reduplicated first sound may be present with left ventricular dilatation, generally in association with a failing heart in a patient with hypertension. (iii.) A third heart sound may be produced in the early stage of mitral stenosis by the discharge of blood from the left auricle through the mitral valve in mid-diastole. *Apart from disease,* three heart sounds may occur in two conditions: (i.) A physiological third heart sound heard at the apex as a very faint sound in the middle of diastole. (ii.) When the ventricular systole, by mechanical means, produces a sound outside the heart. This exocardial sound generally disappears either during full inspiration or during full expiration.

(II) DILATATION OF THE RIGHT VENTRICLE follows left-sided heart failure or is due to obstruction of the blood flow through the lungs. It causes enlargement of the area of cardiac dulness to the right, and often marked epigastric pulsation. Sooner or later the symptoms and signs of **right-sided heart failure occur :**

(i.) A *bruit* over the tricuspid orifice may be heard (see p. 96).

TABLE IIA.—DIAGNOSIS OF TYPICAL CARDIAC HYPERTROPHY FROM
TYPICAL DILATATION

	Apex-beat and Impulse.	Percussion.	Auscultation.
Hypertrophy	Left ventricle: forcible, heaving, thrusting apex; displaced downwards. Right ventricle: left parasternal thrust.	L. chambers: Area increased transversely to the l. and down. R. chambers: Area increased transversely to the l. and r.	Sounds muffled, prolonged and forcible.
Dilatation	Left ventricle: feeble, undulatory, diffuse apex; displaced to the left. Right ventricle-pulsation of liver in the epigastrium.	L. chambers: Area increased transversely to the l. R. chambers: Area increased transversely to the r. and l.	Sounds sharp and faint.

(ii.) *Fulness and pulsation* in the neck veins, due to tricuspid regurgitation.

(iii.) *Œdema,* which indicates congestion of the whole venous system. Cardiac œdema *starts and predominates in the legs* or *the back,* whichever may happen to have been in the most dependent position. The skin is tense, and is very liable to be attacked by erythematous, erysipelatous, and inflammatory conditions (cellulitis, ulcer, etc.). *Ascites* is generally present in the later stages. *Generalised cyanosis* is a consequence of the same venous stasis. A case of mitral disease, therefore, presents a marked contrast to one of aortic disease, where the countenance is often pale.

(iv.) *Engorgement of the liver* is evidenced by pain and tenderness in that region, and later jaundice of the skin. The liver is enlarged, and it may extend to the umbilicus: sometimes it pulsates, as may be shown by placing one hand on the right hypochondrium, and pressing the other beneath the back in the right lumbar region. In cases of *œdema with albuminuria,* when in doubt whether the œdema is of renal or cardiac origin, hepatic enlargement is a valuable diagnostic aid; its presence is usual in cardiac cases.

(v.) *Indigestion,* lack of appetite, a sense of discomfort in the stomach after meals, nausea or actual vomiting, with streaks of blood, indicate congestion of that organ.

(vi.) *Albuminuria,* with high-coloured scanty urine of high specific gravity (and possibly casts and some blood in long-standing cases), point to congestion of the kidney.

The *Causes of Cardiac Dilatation* are of extreme importance as bearing on the prognosis and treatment of cardiac valvular disease and other circulatory disorders. The *clinical conditions* which produce dilatation are practically identical with those which produce cardiac hypertrophy (§ 54), when they are persistent and *are associated with some condition which impairs the nutrition of the heart* (see Etiology). Undoubtedly the commonest causes of cardiac hypertrophy with dilatation are CARDIAC VALVULAR DISEASE, HYPERTENSION WITH MYOCARDIAL DEGENERATION (producing left-sided dilatation), and CHRONIC BRONCHITIS WITH EMPHYSEMA (producing right-sided dilatation). These are the possibilities which should first suggest themselves to the mind in a case where dilatation is evident.

Etiology.—Pathologically speaking, Dilatation falls under two heads:—Compensatory Dilatation and Dilatation due to failure.

Examples of *compensatory dilatation* are found in aortic and mitral regurgitation. In each case the left ventricle has to accommodate first the normal amount required for each normal systole, and secondly the quantity which will regurgitate through the damaged valves. *Dilatation due to failure* occurs whenever the heart muscle is sufficiently poisoned, or becomes anoxæmic. The commonest causes of this myocardial failure are: (*a*) Infections such as acute rheumatism, diphtheria, typhoid fever, septicæmia, pneumonia, influenza, malaria and possibly syphilis. (*b*) Poisons such as arsenic and alcohol. (*c*) Metabolic states such as hyper- and hypo-thyroidism, beri-beri, scurvy. (*d*) Cardiac *anoxia* is commonly due to: (i.) Severe anæmia of all kinds; (ii.) Coronary artery disease.

Any *sudden strain on an apparently normal heart* may produce acute dilatation. But no normal heart will dilate under strain. When such dilatation occurs, some mild infection or other lesion is present. Thus severe muscular exertion in athletes or soldiers who have not had any previous training may seem to cause the heart to fail. Instances are met with in hill-climbers who are "out of form," and others who take sudden and unaccustomed exercise. Breathlessness and heart consciousness may be caused in this way. Rest and gentle exercise are indicated. Prolonged fatigue may similarly overtax the heart muscle if it is already diseased.

The *Prognosis* and *Treatment* of Cardiac Dilatation are fully dealt with under Cardiac Valvular Disease (§§ 61 and 62).

III. *The area of dullness is* INCREASED UPWARDS, *and its shape is pyramidal, with the point upwards; the apex beat is raised, and the impulse is weak and undulatory; on auscultation, the sounds are feeble. The signs are of long standing. The disease is* CHRONIC PERICARDIAL EFFUSION.

§ 56. In **Chronic pericardial effusion** (Syn. Hydropericardium), the *Symptoms* are due to increasing intrapericardial pressure; there is increasing respiratory distress. *Signs:* (1) There is congestion of the neck veins. (2) The shape of the dullness is very characteristic, being pyramidal, with the narrow end upwards. (3) The apex of the heart is *raised*, and *to the right* of its normal position, because the roof of the pericardium is raised by the fluid, and takes the heart with it. (4) For the same reason, the left margin of præcordial dullness extends *beyond* the apex beat. (5) On auscultation, the heart sounds are distant and muffled. There may be irregularity and rapidity of the pulse, and difficulty of breathing from the impeded action of the heart and lungs. (6) Pulsus paradoxus may be present; this is an inspiratory diminution in pulse volume. (7) The physical signs at the base of the left lung are identical with those described with acute pericarditis (§ 46). (8) The X-ray shows a smooth, globular, rather pear-shaped cardiac outline.

Etiology.—Chronic effusion into the pericardium may originate in one of three ways. (1) As the result of Acute Pericarditis (§ 46), of which a history is generally obtainable, but by no means always (see Latent Pericarditis, § 48). (2) True hydropericardium seldom occurs excepting as part of a general œdema due to renal or cardiac disease, and therefore the urine should be carefully examined. In these circumstances dyspnœa is the most obvious symptom complained of and an X-ray examination should always be made if there is any doubt as to the existence of fluid. (3) When hydropericardium is not preceded by pericarditis, or is not part of a general œdema, new growth or tubercle should always be suspected.

The *Diagnosis* from Cardiac Dilatation is made by the shape of the dullness, which is square instead of pyramidal in dilatation; and by the heart sounds, which are clear and sharp in dilatation, muffled in effusion. X-ray examination shows a characteristic outline (see Fig. 27). Pleural effusion is attended by pulmonary symptoms and signs.

The *Prognosis* of hydropericardium depends on its causation, being favourable in Cause 1, adding only a little to the gravity of the primary disease in 2, and being necessarily fatal in malignancy: tuberculosis cases often recover.

Treatment.—The treatment of inflammatory effusion is dealt with in § 46. If part of a general œdema, our efforts must be directed to this. Counter-irritants are sometimes useful. Paracentesis should not be considered unless the cardiac embarrassment is urgent.

IV. **Adherent Pericardium.** The presence of adhesions between the parietal layer of the pericardium and the surrounding mediastinal structures is not now regarded as of clinical importance. The symptoms and signs previously attributed to this condition are to be regarded as the results of the chronic valvular disease or the disease of the myocardium. The only form of chronic pericarditis causing symptoms is constrictive pericarditis.

In CHRONIC CONSTRICTIVE PERICARDITIS (PICK'S DISEASE) there is adherence of the visceral and parietal layers with great thickening of the whole pericardium. The condition, which is usually regarded as of tuberculous origin, causes the heart to be constricted rather than enlarged. The condition may be *latent* when the pericardial thickening does not obstruct the auricular filling or the ventricular capacity during diastole. *Symptoms* arise when the auricles and the ventricles cannot fill adequately. At first this causes (i.) great distension of the neck veins without symptoms of heart failure; (ii.) inspiratory diminution of pulse volume or inspiratory lowering of systolic blood pressure (pulsus paradoxus). Later (iii.) dyspnœa and cyanosis develop; (iv.) there is gross ascites with a disproportionately smaller amount of peripheral œdema; (v.) the heart sounds are soft in character; (vi.) the electrocardiogram frequently shows low amplitude waves throughout, and in elderly persons auricular fibrillation. (vii.) Pericardial calcification is often visible on X-ray examination. In other cases, usually of rheumatic origin, there may be great cardiac enlargement and systolic recession along the attachments of the diaphragm in the ninth and tenth spaces behind (Broadbent's sign). The *Prognosis* in untreated cases of constrictive pericarditis is uniformly poor. *Treatment* is by pericardectomy—a measure of great value. Adhesions *per se* need no treatment.

V. In CONGENITAL HEART DISEASE the enlarged area of præcordial dullness varies with the lesion. There are usually characteristic murmurs. For the differential signs of this condition, see § 59.

VI. In ANEURYSM of the first part of the aortic arch, the upper part of the dull area is increased transversely, and there is dullness over the sternum. Auscultation may reveal a systolic or diastolic murmur and a loud, sharp, ringing aortic second sound (see § 80).

GROUP D. We now turn to those *conditions in which there is found an* **alteration of the heart sounds, or a murmur,** It is well to bear in mind several fallacies referred to on pp. 49, 54, 94, 95, 96 and 101.

In the absence of these, if *the heart sounds are* FAINT, the disease is MYOCARDIAL DEGENERATION, unless a thick chest wall or marked emphysema is present.

The second sound is ACCENTUATED *or* DOUBLE.   This may be due to (i.) High blood pressure; (ii.) aortic aneurysm; (iii.) pulmonary hypertension in mitral disease.

The first sound at the apex is unduly LOUD.   This may be due to: (i.) Nervousness of the patient; (ii.) mitral stenosis; (iii.) a thin chest wall; (iv.) hypertrophy of the ventricle.

The first sound is unduly SHORT.   This may be due to: (i.) Dilatation of the ventricles due to myocardial degeneration or toxæmia; (ii.) rapidity of the pulse; (iii.) incomplete filling of the left ventricle (mitral stenosis), resulting in an unduly hurried emptying.

I. *On auscultation the* HEART SOUNDS ARE VERY FEEBLE; *the impulse is weak and slapping.   No murmur is heard.*   MYOCARDIAL DEGENERATION *may be suspected.*

§ 57. **Myocardial Degeneration.**—The changes in the heart muscle may cause: (1) reduced tonicity, causing dilatation; (2) failure of contractility, causing circulatory inadequacy; (3) changes in the primitive musculature, causing irregularities of rhythm (see § 63).   The disease should be suspected when cardiac symptoms arise in a patient with cardiac enlargement, and when other diseases (such as of the valves, or hypertension) can be excluded.

Symptoms and Signs.—The heart is enlarged and there is often evidence of arterial disease elsewhere.   On exertion there is: (i.) undue dyspnœa; (ii.) marked lassitude; (iii.) palpitation; or (iv.) angina of effort.   (v.) Cardiac irregularities (§ 63) such as premature beats may be present at rest, and are often exaggerated by exercise.   Auricular fibrillation and occasionally auricular flutter occur.   When the disease is more advanced (vi.) dyspnœa may be present at night ("cardiac asthma"); (vii.) the cardiac impulse is feeble, the heart sounds poor and the radial pulse weak; (viii.) congestive failure may occur.   Myocardial degeneration usually affects both left and right ventricles in fairly equal degree.   When failure particularly affects the left ventricle, pulmonary congestion and œdema are prominent.   When emphysema is a causative factor, the failure chiefly involves the right ventricle.

The degree of degeneration is difficult to estimate clinically.   Guidance on this point may be obtained from (1) Estimation of the amount of exercise which can be carried out without distress, such as dyspnœa, pain, palpitation.   (2) The cardiac enlargement is always detectable radiologically, or clinically.   (3) The character of the heart sounds: especially shortening of the first sound.   (4) The systolic, and to a much less extent the diastolic, blood pressures fall from ventricular weakness; this produces a diminution in pulse pressure.   (5) Electrocardiographic changes, such as flattening or inversion of the " T " waves in leads 1 and 2, or the presence of a bundle-branch lesion, or the changes characteristic of coronary disease, are common.

Etiology.—Myocardial degeneration is a consequence of interference with the nutrition of the heart wall. In the majority of cases this is the result of coronary disease associated with a progressive interstitial fibrosis and fatty degeneration.

The Prognosis is uncertain. The earlier stages are insidious, so that by the time pronounced symptoms appear the damage may be irreparable. Some patients survive for years; those with marked Cheyne-Stokes' respiration or pulsus alternans die sooner. In the early stages of cardiac degeneration plenty of fresh air, exercise and good sleep are essential for increasing the reserve power of the unaffected muscle fibres, and if the patient responds to this treatment he may live for many years (Mackenzie). Prognosis and *Treatment* are discussed more fully in §§ 61, 62.

While auscultating the heart three questions should be in the physician's mind: (1) What is the character of the first sound ? (2) What is the character of the second sound ? (3) Is a murmur present ?

GROUP D. II. *A* **Murmur** *is present.* Its source may be:

(1) Endocardial—Endocarditis of valve or wall; narrowing or dilatation of orifice of valves; congenital abnormalities.

(2) Atonicity murmur due to muscular stretching of a valve ring.

(3) Cardio-pulmonary, Cardio-respiratory (§ 59).

(4) Pericardial—friction of Pericarditis (see §§ 46, 49).

(5) Functional and Hæmic murmurs (§§ 42 and 545).

The chief points to be considered in diagnosing the *source of a murmur* are given in § 42 and § 49 (Table I).

§ 58. Chronic Endocarditis Cardiac Valvular Disease—Cardiac murmurs.

—Disease of the valves of the heart is revealed on auscultation by the presence of a bruit or murmur, which is added to, or replaces, a normal heart sound.

Method of Procedure. Five features must be carefully investigated in any murmur: TIME OF OCCURRENCE. Whether it REPLACES or merely ACCOMPANIES the first or second sound; POSITION of maximum intensity; direction in which it is CONDUCTED; and CHARACTER. In order to be quite sure of the timing of a bruit, it is wise to place the thumb on the carotid artery while auscultating the chest.

The characters of PERICARDIAL MURMURS have already been given (§ 46); also their diagnosis from endocardial murmurs (Table I, p. 69).

Valvular disease is most commonly due in early life to endocarditis (acute or chronic), and in older persons, to chronic degenerative change. The effect is a thickening or puckering of the valves and ring, which results in one or both of two conditions: (a) Stenosis—i.e., a narrowing (στενόω, to contract) of the orifice, which prevents the blood flowing freely through it; or (b) Regurgitation, in which the valves are incompetent and allow a reflux of the blood to take place from imperfect meeting and

closure of the cusps.   The remote effect of these two conditions is similar
—viz., a retardation of the circulation of blood through that orifice.

It simplifies diagnosis very much that cardio-valvular disease arising
after birth is practically *confined to the left side of the heart—i.e.*, to the
mitral and aortic orifices.   Thus it happens that there are four principal
valvular lesions—MITRAL REGURGITATION, MITRAL STENOSIS, AORTIC
REGURGITATION and AORTIC STENOSIS.

TABLE III.—DIFFERENTIATION OF CARDIAC VALVULAR DISEASES

		Ausculta-tion.	Pulse.	Other Symptoms special to the Disease.
Mitral (apical murmurs).	*Regurgi-tation.*	*Systolic* murmur conducted into axilla.	Usually regular.	
	Stenosis.	*Presystolic and rumbling diastolic murmurs,* both localised to the apex beat area.	Small, mod-erately firm; very irregular with onset of auricular fibrillation.	Œdema, enlarged liver and ascites, etc., Hæmopty-sis; emboli, — with signs of congestion of organs.
Aortic (basal murmurs).	*Regurgi-tation.*	*Diastolic* murmur conducted down sternum.	" Water-hammer," rapid and compressible.	Throbbing of arteries of neck, — with symp-toms of cerebral anæmia and anginal attacks.
	Stenosis.[1]	*Systolic* murmur conducted into vessels of the neck.	Slow, regular, small and hard.	Syncopal attacks especially during exertion.

The student should study Fig. 10, p. 51, so as thoroughly to comprehend
the various events which occur during one complete cardiac cycle.   He
should also bear in mind that the left side of the heart is behind the right,
and that the left ventricle comes nearest to the surface only at the apex,
immediately behind or just below the fifth rib (Figs. 11 and 12, pp. 52
and 53).   He should also remember that a cardiac murmur is not produced *in* a diseased orifice, but by the eddies in the blood-stream beyond,
and is conducted in the direction of the stream of blood which is causing
the murmur.   For these reasons a murmur is not usually heard loudest
directly over the orifice diseased.   The student should also consult the
diagram of the circulation (Fig. 33).

Diagnosis of Cardiac Murmurs.—The first thing is to determine whether
a given murmur is related to the first or second sound of the heart—*i.e.*,
whether its time is systolic or diastolic.   (Note that the term systole is
used by clinicians to designate ventricular, not auricular, contraction.)
This will form a convenient basis of classification of cardiac murmurs.

[1] Real aortic stenosis is somewhat rare, but atheromatous roughening is common.

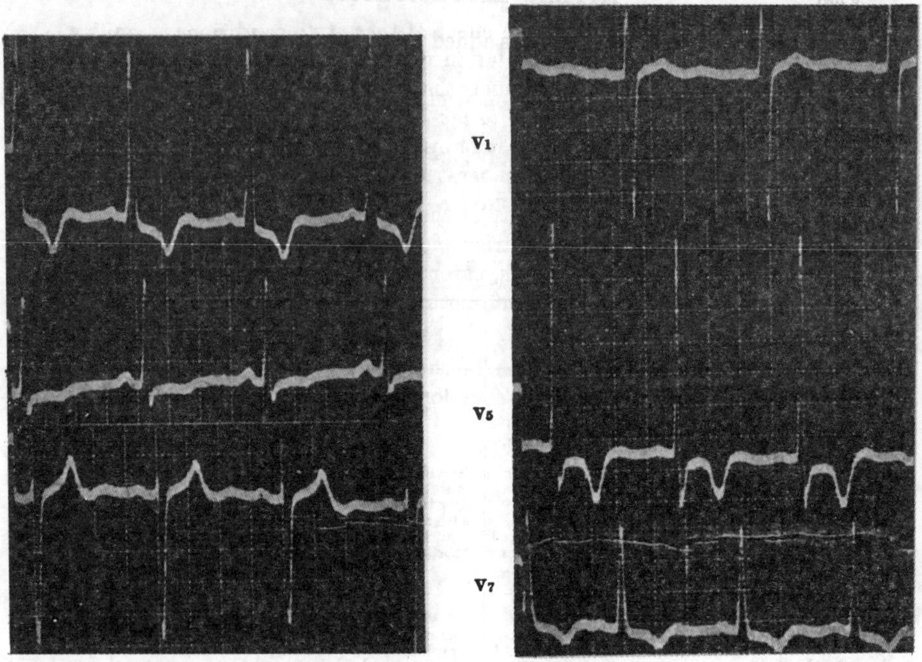

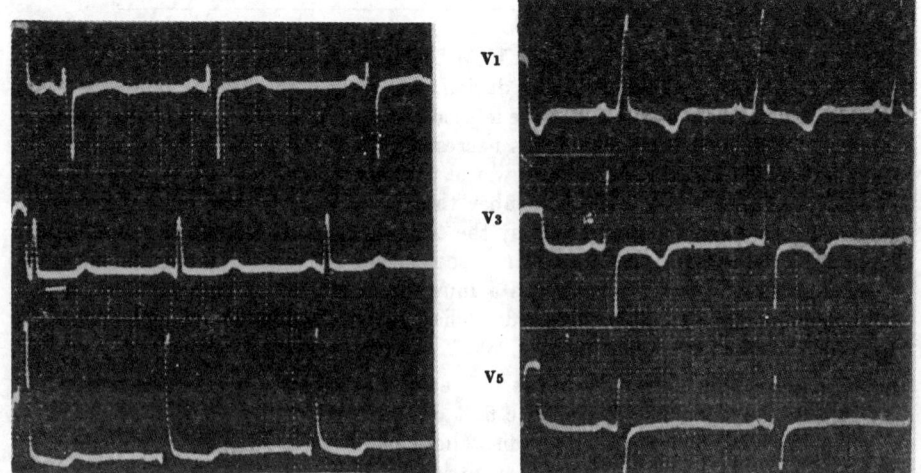

V1

V5

V7

FIG. 31.—Left Ventricular Hypertrophy.

V1

V3

V5

FIG. 32.—Right Ventricular Hypertrophy.

A. **Systolic Murmurs** are bruits added to or replacing the first sound and may be produced by the following causes, which are mentioned more or less in order of frequency: atheromatous degeneration, mitral regurgitation, hæmic and functional conditions (see § 42, and Anæmia, § 545), aortic stenosis, dilatation or aneurysm of the first part of the aorta, congenital lesions and tricuspid regurgitation: pulmonary stenosis, patent interventricular septum and patent ductus arteriosus.

I. **Atheromatous Degeneration** of the mitral or aortic valves is very common in the aged. It produces a harsh systolic murmur over the corresponding areas of the heart, but no symptoms result from this.

II. In **Mitral Regurgitation** the systolic murmur is characterised by (i.) being loudest at the apex; (ii.) being conducted to the axilla, and often audible behind, at the angle of the scapula. When regurgitation is marked, the apex is displaced downwards and outwards owing to the hypertrophy and dilatation of the left ventricle. There is accentuation of the second sound in the pulmonary area, due to hypertension in the pulmonary circulation. The pulse is soft; heart failure occurs late.

The ultimate mechanical effect of Mitral Regurgitation upon the heart and lungs is as follows: (1) owing to the reflux of blood from the ventricle during ventricular systole the auricle becomes dilated. (2) In order to drive on the increased volume of its contents the auricle hypertrophies. (3) Simultaneously the left ventricle dilates, and hypertrophies. It has to accommodate and to expel, not only its normal quota of blood, but also

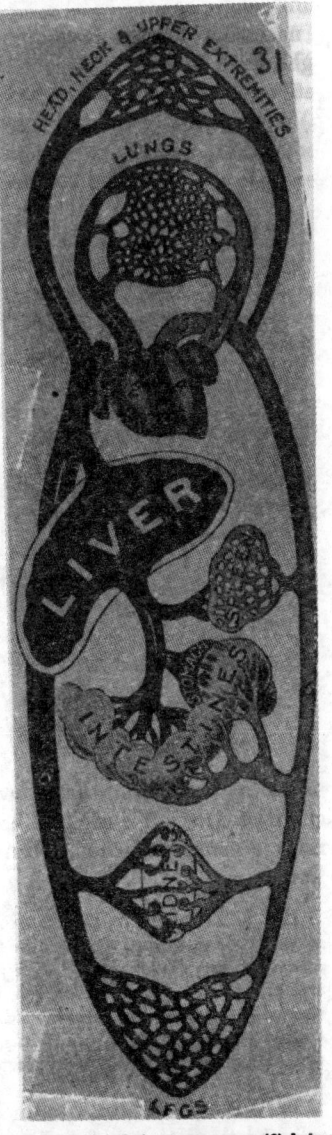

FIG. 33.—Scheme of the Circulation of the Blood.—The superior and inferior venæ cavæ (6) bring the blood back from the organs and tissues into the right auricle (1). Thence it passes into the right ventricle (2), through the pulmonary artery (7) into the lungs. Returning from the lungs by the pulmonary veins (9), it passes through the left auricle (3) and left ventricle (4), and is distributed by means of the aorta (5, 5) and the carotids (8) to the organs and tissues of the body. Notice that the blood from the stomach and intestines passes through the liver before joining the general circulation. (From Huxley's " Physiology," modified.)

the amount which regurgitates back into the left auricle. (4) When the left heart begins to fail it is unable to empty itself properly, and there is difficulty in the free passage of blood from the pulmonary veins. Thus pulmonary blood stasis tends to occur. (5) To overcome this stasis it is necessary for the right ventricle to hypertrophy. In cases of failure, right-sided dilatation supervenes, often with the onset of tricuspid incompetence. (6) So that in cases of Mitral Regurgitation there may occur: (a) dilatation and hypertrophy of left auricle and ventricle; (b) pulmonary congestion; and (c) dilatation and hypertrophy of the right auricle and ventricle. These changes are less marked and develop more slowly in

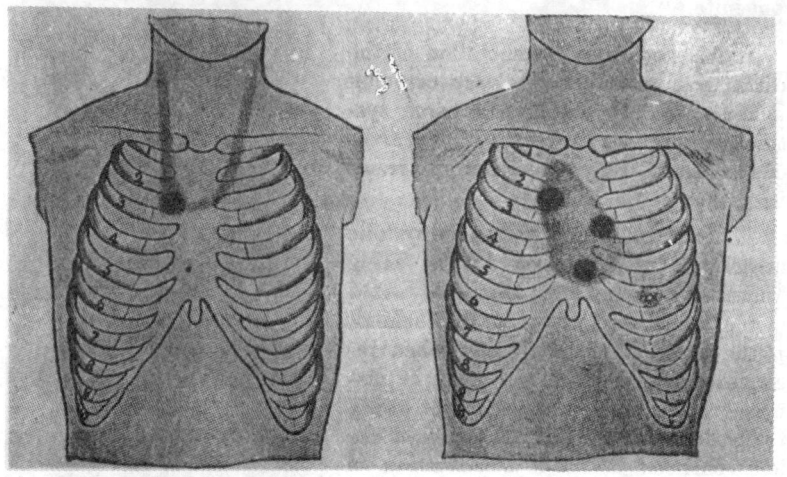

FIG. 34.—The systolic murmur of aortic stenosis. Depth of shading indicates intensity of murmur.

FIG. 35.—The diastolic murmur of aortic regurgitation. Depth of shading indicates intensity of murmur.

mitral regurgitation than they do in mitral stenosis, for in the latter condition the left auricle is less able to empty, and is kept in a state of more persistent tension. In mitral regurgitation the outlook is relatively good.

IIa. A MURMUR OF DILATATION (Atonicity M.), systolic in time, having all the above characters, and, like it, due to mitral regurgitation, may occur without definite disease of the valve, when the *left ventricle becomes dilated*, and the muscular ring around the valve *fails to complete* the closure of the mitral valve. This condition is especially apt to occur (i.) when dilatation of the left ventricle supervenes on hypertrophy, (ii.) in anæmia, and (iii.) in acute myocardial disease, *e.g.*, diphtheria and acute rheumatism, (iv.) in hypertensive heart disease.

III. **Aortic Stenosis** produces a mid-systolic bruit which must be distinguished from those of endocarditis and atheroma of the aortic orifice.

True narrowing of the aortic ring should not be diagnosed unless five signs are present: (i.) a loud mid-systolic bruit in the aortic area, conducted into the carotids. It is harsh, sometimes musical, and may be audible at the apex.   (ii.) There is usually a systolic thrill in the aortic area, second R. interspace, often best felt when the patient sits forward and at the end of expiration; (iii.) marked hypertrophy of the left ventricle; (iv.) a slow-rising, well-sustained, small pulse, often anacrotic in character; and (v.) a weak second sound with a low pulse pressure.   The calcified aortic valve may be visible on X-ray screening or on tomograms.

General Symptoms are almost wanting in aortic stenosis—other than anginal pain, due to coronary atheroma, pallor or sallowness of the face, and sudden attacks of giddiness or of fainting (syncope) on exertion.

Etiology.—The lesion is sometimes of rheumatic and sometimes of congenital origin; in many cases the cause is unknown.

IV. In DILATATION and in ANEURYSM OF THE COMMENCEMENT OF THE AORTA a systolic murmur is usually present.   The condition is a " relative stenosis," *i.e.*, though the aortic ring is normal in diameter it is small as compared with the diameter of the enlarged aorta.   A peculiar ringing character of the aortic second sound is the most constant cardiac physical sign (§ 80).

§ 59. V. Congenital Heart Disease is comparatively rare.

There are two groups—the cases without cyanosis and those with cyanosis.   Those *without cyanosis* include bicuspid aortic valve defect, imperfect ventricular septum, uncomplicated pulmonary stenosis and patent ductus arteriosus.   Those *with cyanosis* that survive generally have multiple defects which usually include pulmonary stenosis, or other abnormality in the size or position of the pulmonary artery.   Patency of the inter-auricular septum (atrial septum defect) does not usually cause cyanosis, but does so when the left ventricle fails later in life.

(1) Bicuspid aortic valve is not possible to diagnose during life, but should be suspected when aortic infective endocarditis develops in a patient whose heart previously was free from murmurs.

(2) Imperfect ventricular septum is characterised by a loud systolic murmur close to the sternum in the third and fourth left intercostal spaces.   The murmur is usually accompanied by a thrill.   There is usually no marked limitation of the cardiac function.

(3) In atrial septal defect there is a shunt from the left to the right auricle.   The whole heart is enlarged, especially the pulmonary conus, and the pulmonary arteries are enormous and are readily visible in the X-ray picture.   A systolic murmur and sometimes a thrill are present over the pulmonary area.   Cyanosis is absent at rest, but may appear during exertion: it may become permanent when heart failure sets in.

(4) Patent ductus arteriosus is characterised by slight ventricular hypertrophy, a loud continuous murmur throughout systole and diastole, loudest in systole, and present in the second left interspace near the sternal border.   A thrill usually co-exists.   The diastolic pressure is often lowered.   The X-ray shows a typical enlarged pulmonary conus.   If infective endocarditis supervenes, chemotherapy is effective and cure is possible by ligature of the ductus (§ 50*a*).

(5) Congenital pulmonary stenosis is characterised by a loud systolic murmur and thrill over the pulmonary base.   It is due to stenosis or hypoplasia of the pulmonary artery or of the pulmonary conus; the right ventricle hypertrophies proportionately.   When the lesion is present without a patent foramen ovale there is no cyanosis until the stenosis becomes so severe that the right ventricle begins to fail.   Other cases exist with a patent foramen ovale and cyanosis develops earlier, when the pressure in the right auricle rises above that in the left auricle.   The commonest lesion is known as *Fallot's tetralogy*—a combination of pulmonary stenosis, interventricular septal defect, an aorta which lies astride the interventricular septum and communicates with both ventricles, and great hypertrophy of the right ventricle (Fig. 36).

Fallot's tetralogy accounts for three-quarters of the cases of congenital heart disease with clubbing of the fingers and cyanosis, in adult life. Polycythæmia is usually present. Surgical anastomosis of the subclavian to the pulmonary artery (Blalock's operation) greatly benefits some cases.

Prognosis.—A congenital lesion may remain latent for years, though few cases survive to middle age. The acyanotic cases often die of a superadded infective endocarditis; the cyanotic group tend to develop pneumonia or tuberculosis. The prognosis is best if there is no sign of pulmonary stenosis, no clubbing of the fingers but only secondary polycythæmia. In childhood fatal bronchitis and broncho-pneumonia are common. The prognosis is serious in proportion to the degree of dyspnœa and cyanosis, pointing to deficient aëration of the blood, and in proportion to the other symptoms of " cardiac failure " (§ 61).

For *Treatment* see § 62.

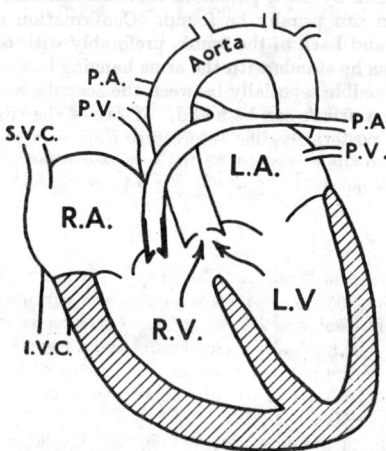

FIG 36.—Diagrammatic representation of Fallot's Tetralogy. Note the stenosed pulmonary valve (or infundibulum) and the over-riding aorta into which blood flows from both sides of the heart through a high interventricular septal defect. There is also a hypertrophied right ventricle.

VI.—**Tricuspid Regurgitation** takes place when that orifice is diseased or DILATED. Some maintain that if the valve be healthy, though dilated, no bruit can be heard, but in some cases of recurrent bronchitis a murmur is often present which comes and goes under treatment, and which is not found to be attended with any marked changes in the tricuspid valve after death. The murmur is characterised by being heard best at the tricuspid area—*i.e.*, on the left side of the lower part of the sternum. The best evidence of tricuspid regurgitation is an expansile systolic pulsation in the jugular veins: similar pulsation may be palpable in the enlarged liver.

VII. **Cardio-pulmonary or Cardio-respiratory Murmurs** are fairly common, and are probably produced by the expulsion of air from the adjacent lung tissue by the movements of the heart. They do not indicate a cardiac lesion and the lung is usually healthy. They are heard in various parts of the antero-lateral region of the chest. These murmurs have a blowing, whiffing, or " sipping " character, are usually systolic in time, and in rare cases double, though the systolic element is always loudest. Often they are not loudest at the apex, and come between the two sounds rather than with the first sound. A common variety is audible at the apex, getting louder as it is conducted into the axilla, and is only heard during inspiration. Sometimes they disappear when the patient alters his position or stands up. When he stops breathing, they may be weakened, abolished, or unaltered. These murmurs have no pathological significance.

VIII. The **Exocardial Murmur** is possibly due to a localised thickening of the visceral pericardium. Usually it is unattended by symptoms, but it may be of importance clinically, for it is apt to be mistaken for valvular disease. It is nearly always systolic and is not localised or conducted in the manner characteristic of any murmur of organic disease. In such cases the heart is normal clinically, radiologically and by the electrocardiograph.

IX. **Coarctation of the Aorta** is a rare condition due to congenital narrowing of the vessel, usually at the level of attachment of the remains of the ductus arteriosus to the aorta. It produces a systolic murmur over the back or the front of the chest. The narrowing may be annular and local or it may spread to the opening of the left subclavian artery. There is some dilatation of the ascending and transverse aorta and great narrowing at the coarctation: a collateral arterial supply reaches the lower half of the body via greatly enlarged and freely anastomosing internal mammary, scapular and intercostal arteries. *Symptoms* may be absent for many years and the condition revealed by the accidental discovery of a high blood pressure and left ventricular hypertrophy in a child or young person. Due to interference with the blood supply to the lower half of the body, there may be cramp, intermittent claudication and coldness of the legs and feet. *Signs.*—There is hypertension in the arm vessels and a low blood pressure in the legs—the blood pressure levels are more accurately compared on a sphygmomanometer by using palpation than auscultation: dorsal pedal and posterior tibial pulsation can usually be found. Confirmation is obtained by carefully inspecting the front and back of the trunk, preferably with an oblique light: if the patient slowly rotates as he stands with the arms hanging loosely forward, the pulsating arteries are usually visible especially between the scapulæ and the spine, and over these a distant systolic murmur can be heard. X-ray of the ribs may reveal notching of their lower borders posteriorly, due to pressure from enlarged collateral vessels. If the patient survives to the age of 40–50 the symptoms become those of hypertension and hypertensive heart disease. *Treatment* is with surgery, preferably in later childhood and before the age of 25: this is successful and devoid of undue risk.

X. **Endomyocardial Fibrosis** is probably the cause of much obscure cardiac disease in Africa; it is very rare in Great Britain. Mitral or tricuspid incompetence is due to large areas of fibrous tissue developing on the endocardial surface of the ventricles, involving the mitral and tricuspid valves. Heart failure occurs sooner or later. The *cause* is unknown.

§ 60. B. **Murmurs** heard in the **diastolic interval** may occupy either (*a*) the first half of that interval, replacing, accompanying, or following the second heart sound (*Diastolic* murmurs); or (*b*) they may occupy the second half of the interval, preceding and leading up to the first heart sound (*Presystolic* murmurs; see Fig. 37). The latter can be accurately defined and described as auriculo-systolic.

TABLE IV

Early Diastolic Murmurs	Late Diastolic Murmurs (Auriculo-systolic)
Aortic Regurgitation	
Mitral Stenosis	Mitral Stenosis
Dilatation of the Aortic Ring (Aneurysm)	Austin Flint Murmur.
Pulmonary regurgitation (rare)	Tricuspid Stenosis (very rare)

I. In **Aortic Regurgitation** the murmur is *diastolic* (Ventricular Diastolic). (i.) The diastolic murmur at the aortic valve (Fig. 35) must be listened for: (*a*) over the lower part and to the left of the sternum. It may be audible as far as the apex and indeed over the whole heart. This murmur may or may not be accompanied by a systolic murmur and is found typically in those cases of aortic regurgitation where the valve is the site of endocarditis or of aortic valve dilatation. (*b*) Over the junction of the second right costal cartilage with the sternum. Here the murmur may be loud, and just beneath the stethoscope. (*c*) Over the third left costal junction. Here the murmur is soft, blowing but distant, never harsh in character. This murmur should be carefully listened for in any case of mitral stenosis where the left ventricle is large. The diastolic aortic murmur of rheumatic valvulitis is best heard along the left sternal margin, that of the syphilitic lesion at the aortic base. (ii.) Owing to the amount of dilatation and hypertrophy of the left ventricle, the apex is displaced downwards and outwards more than in any other form of valvular disease. The increase in the size of the left ventricle is proportional to the amount of blood regurgitating. (iii.) The carotids visibly pulsate. Capillary pulsation is generally present, and is detected by drawing a line across the forehead, or by lightly pressing on the fingernail or on the lips with a glass slide; the alternate blush and pallor due to the pulsation in the capillaries is thus well brought out. The retinal arteries may also show visible pulsation. (iv.) In aortic regurgitation the pulse and the blood-pressure changes are of great diagnostic importance. The pulse wave is very forcible but is ill sustained, and this gives a marked pulsation in the carotids and the vessels of the limbs: it may be sufficiently marked to cause the head to nod to and fro with each heart-beat. It is best felt by clasping the flexor aspect of the patient's wrist with the flat of the hand and the fingers: pulsation is then felt in both radial and ulnar arteries and is increased by raising the forearm above the patient's head. Owing to the leakage back through the aortic valves during diastole, the volume of blood suddenly expelled into the aorta at the commencement of systole is markedly increased, with a forcible systolic wave in the whole arterial system, and a high systolic pressure: this is ill sustained, as during diastole blood leaves the arteries not only distally through dilated vessels, but also by leaking back through the aortic valves, with a correspondingly low diastolic pressure. The pulse therefore becomes " collapsing " or " water-hammer " (" Corrigan's pulse "): the pulse pressure is raised much above normal, and the diastolic pressure is lowered in close relation to the diastolic leak. A falling systolic pressure in aortic regurgitation usually means a failing myocardium. There is (v.) a pistol-shot sound over the arteries when the diastolic pressure is very low, and (vi.) a diastolic murmur (Durozier's murmur) over the large arteries.

The *appearance* of a patient with aortic regurgitation is often characteristic. (1) The rheumatic type occurs in children and young adults. There is marked pulsation in the neck, while the whole chest may be seen to pulsate with the heart-beat. The brachial arteries stand out prominently and seem to be definitely hypertrophied. (2) The syphilitic aortic case is usually middle-aged, and often presents signs of premature old age; the apex beat is less heaving in character, and more diffuse; angina and dyspnoea are frequently present, and often there are signs of arterial degeneration. (3) In the arteriosclerotic type the lesion is due to the associated atheroma.

As regards the *general symptoms*, pallor is generally stated to be characteristic but in fact this is not true (Lewis). Faintness and giddiness may occur, usually brought on by change of position; frontal headache and consciousness of the heart's action may be complained of, especially on first lying down at night. Pain may be present in the chest on exertion, but until failure sets in, beyond the consciousness of a forcibly acting heart, the patient is usually fit and able to do a large amount of physical work.

II. **Mitral Stenosis** is characterised by narrowing of the mitral orifice with obstruction to the free passage of blood from the left auricle to the left ventricle. It is always caused by a rheumatic infection.

The *appearance* of the mitral stenotic patient is often characteristic. It is most frequently met in women. The face shows a marked malar flush and, otherwise, a combination of cyanosis and pallor. The jugular veins may be engorged. The extremities are cold and pale in proportion to the systemic ischæmia. The pale Mitral Stenotic should always be regarded with suspicion as, generally speaking, one of the following conditions is present: (a) recrudescence of the rheumatic infection; (b) supervening malignant endocarditis; (c) some independent condition such as associated renal disease or anæmia.

Physical Examination.—(1) The *pulse* in Mitral Stenosis may be characteristic, and gives a guide to the condition of the systemic circulation and left side of the heart. The *volume* is small, due to the diminished output. The *rhythm* may be regular or irregular; in the latter case the irregularity is due either to ectopic beats or to auricular fibrillation. The *rate* is often rapid (round about 90). (2) The blood pressure is usually low, owing to diminished output and force of the left ventricle. It is sometimes reduced in volume after auricular fibrillation has set in. In older patients the blood pressure may be raised in proportion to the amount of associated arteriosclerosis. Should mitral stenosis become complicated by aortic regurgitation, the blood pressure tends to rise and the pulse volume and force increase. (3) *Cardiac Signs.*—*Inspection:* Pulsation is often visible to the left of the lower sternum owing to the dilatation and hypertrophy of the right ventricle; the apex beat itself can often be seen inside the nipple line somewhat diffuse in character. *Palpation:* The apex beat is slapping in character and well inside the nipple line. Typically, a presystolic thrill, and later a diastolic thrill, is felt at the apex (§ 39). The presystolic thrill may be intermittent and only brought out by exercise, deep breathing, or lying on the left side. Pulmonary conus pulsation may be increased over the pulmonary area. The pulmonary valve closes so forcibly that it can usually be felt. *Percussion:* The cardiac dullness is increased slightly, if at all. The right cardiac dullness measured from the mid-sternal line is increased. On the left, the cardiac dullness does not extend out to the nipple line unless there is some other associated condition such as mitral or aortic regurgitation, pericarditis, etc. *Auscultation:* In the early stages a faint diastolic murmur is audible, which after exercise, or in the left lateral position, may be accompanid by a typical crescendo presystolic murmur.[1]   Later, both murmurs appear at rest: then the first

---

[1] It may be difficult to differentiate early mitral stenosis from the overacting heart common in excited or neurotic young people and in thyrotoxicosis. At this

sound at the apex is sharp, split or markedly accentuated. This pre-systolic murmur, typical of mitral stenosis, is heard only over a limited area, and is not conducted outwards. Both presystolic and diastolic murmurs are accentuated *if the patient lies on the left side* (Fig. 37). The second sound at the apex is inaudible in a well-established mitral stenosis, while at the base the pulmonary second sound is markedly accentuated and split. The so-called opening snap, suggesting a split second sound, may be heard at the left sternal border opposite the third, fourth and fifth interspaces.

General Symptoms.—The commonest symptoms associated with mitral stenosis are: (1) Dyspnœa, at first only on strenuous exertion after meals, later after ordinary exertion (*e.g.*, stairs). It then becomes continuous and progressive, so that the patient is unable to lie down at nights (orthopnœa).

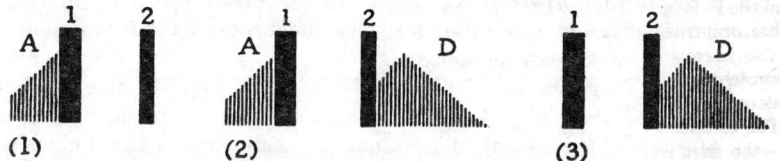

FIG. 37.—In mitral stenosis there are two murmurs, which occupy different parts of the diastolic interval—the presystolic or auriculo-systolic (A), and the diastolic (D) murmurs. The presystolic is present when the auricle is contracting; the diastolic is due to passive blood flow. The presystolic disappears when the auricles fibrillate. The figure shows:—(1) the presystolic murmur; (2) both murmurs; (3) the early diastolic alone as in fibrillation, the presystolic having disappeared. The splitting of the 2nd sound is omitted for clearness.

(2) Palpitation is at first intermittent, occurring after exertion, and is simply of the nature of a physiological tachycardia. Later on it becomes more or less continuous, occurring independently of effort. (3) Cough is a common symptom. The cause is probably pulmonary congestion, induced by exercise or change of position. It may be associated with marked cyanosis or with hæmoptysis. The underlying cause is congestion of the lungs. A severe type of cough is sometimes met with in embolism or infarction. Later developments are: (4) auricular fibrillation, flutter or premature beats; (5) hæmoptysis, embolism, right-sided failure with liver engorgement and ascites are common (§ 55). Embolism, generally cerebral producing hemiplegia, sometimes renal producing hæmaturia, may occur from the despatch into the blood stream of clots formed in the appendix of the dilated left auricle.

In order to understand the progressive variations of the physical signs and symptoms met with in Mitral Stenosis, it is necessary to say a few words about the anatomical changes which develop in this lesion. Broadly speaking, narrowing of the mitral orifice results in: (*a*) a tendency to dam up the blood in the left auricle, pulmonary and venous circulation in this order, so that the pressure tends to rise;

_____

stage the X-ray or electrocardiogram may give no help, and the best guide is the character of the first sound. In the excitable heart, although loud and roughened, the first sound is low-pitched; in mitral stenosis the pitch is higher and approximates to that of the second heart sound.

(b) there is a reduction in the left ventricular filling, with a reduced size of the left ventricle, a low tension pulse and a slapping first sound. The output and force are thus reduced and the systemic blood volume reduced. The damming of the blood in the pulmonary circulation is responsible for the physical signs met with in the chest, e.g., accentuated pulmonary second sound, basal crepitations, etc., and subsequently it produces right-sided heart failure with engorgement of the jugular veins, enlargement of the liver, peripheral œdema and other manifestations of congestive failure.

The progressive changes which occur in the myocardium in Mitral Stenosis and its actual condition at any phase of the disease can be followed by observing the changes in the electrocardiogram. The first result of Mitral Stenosis is increased auricular work and contraction, and this is reflected in the electrocardiogram by increase in the amplitude of the P or auricular waves, which still however retain their normal form. As the condition progresses, the two auricles become slightly divorced in their action, so that the P waves become flattened, widened and partly divided. Sometimes by the time this has occurred rheumatic fibrosis has involved the Bundle of His, with impairment of its conductivity, as is shown by an increase in the P–R interval (Fig. 16). Usually also, by now right ventricular " compensation " has occurred, so that the electrocardiogram suggests right ventricular hypertrophy. The narrowed mitral orifice results in imperfect filling and therefore incomplete stretching of the left ventricle, which consequently contracts poorly (hence the slapping character of the apex beat). The cause of the opening snap is unknown. The condition continues to progress, the muscle fails, the rhythm becomes irregular —the first irregularity noticed usually being due to premature beats of auricular origin (Fig. 15). This indicates myocardial hyper-irritability of the auricle, and is often succeeded by a complete irregularity due to auricular fibrillation (Fig. 14) which may rarely be preceded by a state of flutter (Fig. 42). The fibrillation at first is of the coarse variety, but with time it becomes finer and ultimately flat as the muscle gradually degenerates and its co-ordination and contractibility become more impaired. Some degree of heart-block is not uncommon.

III. In Aortic Aneurysm a *diastolic* murmur is sometimes heard if the aortic ring shares in the dilatation of the aorta.

IV. An Austin Flint murmur is a presystolic apical murmur occasionally heard with aortic regurgitation. It is diagnosed from that due to mitral stenosis by its not being followed by an accentuated first sound, by the position of the cardiac impulse, and by the absence of the other signs of mitral stenosis.

V. Regurgitation through the pulmonary artery is rare; it may be produced by congenital malformation of the heart, or by severe pulmonary hypertension.

VI. Tricuspid Stenosis is very rare, but it is occasionally seen in young women, and is recognised by (i.) a presystolic murmur, heard loudest over the fifth right costal cartilage, close to the sternum. (ii.) Œdema occurs early otherwise the symptoms and signs are those of tricuspid regurgitation (§ 59, VI). Dyspnœa is less than the degree of venous and hepatic distension would seem to warrant. Orthopnœa is absent. Acquired tricuspid stenosis or pulmonary stenosis may exist singly or together in cases of malignant argentaffin (carcinoid) tumours of the lower ileum. The chief symptoms are attacks of flushing after meals, shortness of breath and sometimes even asthma, with diarrhœa (§ 571).

Fallacies in the Diagnosis of Diastolic Murmurs.—1. A diastolic murmur due to *aortic regurgitation* may be heard at the *apex*. It must not be mistaken for that of mitral stenosis. In addition to the fact that the aortic murmur is heard louder at the base than at the apex, it has a rushing character, whereas a mitral diastolic murmur is low-pitched and rumbling, and the character of the pulse and the blood pressure is different.

2. *Mitral stenosis* is sometimes hard to detect in the stage of auricular fibrillation, when the characteristic murmur may be *altogether absent*. It may, then, be strongly suspected when there is—(i.) a loud, clear, sharp first sound at the apex, with marked

accentuation of the pulmonary second sound; or (ii.) hypertrophy of the right ventricle, basal congestion and hæmoptysis, especially if the second sound is split.

C. **Double Murmurs** may be produced by a combination of any of the above systolic and diastolic murmurs.

(a) Double murmurs most audible at the **base** (other than hæmic):

I. COMBINED AORTIC STENOSIS AND REGURGITATION is the most common condition, and causes a loud double to and fro murmur, heard best in the second right interspace.

II. ANEURYSM OF THE AORTA may be attended by a double murmur having the same characters as in disease of the aortic valves. This is heard loudest in the second right interspace, but it may also be heard at the back, to the left of the fourth dorsal vertebra.

III. A double murmur occasionally occurs in the DILATED AORTA of the -aged, but with less marked features.

IV. A double murmur, loudest in the pulmonary area, usually indicates CONGENITAL HEART DISEASE, especially with patent ductus arteriosus.

(b) A double murmur most audible at the **apex** may be heard when both MITRAL STENOSIS and REGURGITATION are present. It consists of a typical presystolic murmur running up to the first sound, immediately followed by a systolic mitral murmur which is conducted outwards to the axilla. In other cases, the systolic murmur is followed by a mid-diastolic mitral stenotic murmur.

FALLACIES IN THE DIAGNOSIS OF DOUBLE MURMURS.—1. When a double murmur can be heard both *at the base and apex*, do not take for granted that mitral regurgitation exist as well as aortic disease. Remember that a systolic mitral and a systolic aortic may be alike in character, and that aortic murmurs can often be heard at the apex, as well as the base. To arrive at a conclusion is often difficult, but one must rely on the position in which the murmur is loudest, and on the other features which distinguish mitral and aortic lesions.

2. When a *double aortic* murmur is present, the lesion may be regurgitation, or stenosis, or both together. A diagnosis is made by examining the pulse (§ 87), the time of the thrill, if one is present, and the position of the apex beat. In regurgitation the apex is displaced farther downwards and outwards than in any other form of valve disease. In aortic stenosis the left ventricular wall is hypertrophied, with but little enlargement of the cavity; but as emphysema is so often associated with it, the apex may be hard to find.

3. Murmurs of *pericardial friction* may easily be mistaken for a double aortic murmur; but whereas endocardial murmurs begin synchronously with the first or second sounds, the rub of pericardial friction often lags slightly behind them.

4. *Hæmic, cardio-pulmonary* and exocardial murmurs are occasionally double.

§ 61. SYMPTOMS RESULTING FROM CARDIAC VALVULAR DISEASE.—The first effect of valvular disease is *hypertrophy* of the heart, as already mentioned, and so long as there is adequate compensatory hypertrophy there may be no concomitant symptoms at all.

But, sooner or later, in most cases hypertrophy gives way to *dilatation*, and then a series of characteristic symptoms ensue. Those special to each form of valvular lesion have been referred to in the preceding section.

Certain *general symptoms are common to all forms of chronic valvular disease* when this has produced myocardial failure.

1. *Breathlessness* on walking uphill, or even on very slight exertion, is a constant feature. No serious enfeeblement of the heart wall or disturbance of its function can exist without this symptom; and it cannot be too much insisted on that breathlessness is not only a symptom, but, in general terms, is the most accurate measure of the extent of the cardiac failure.

2. *Œdema* occurs early in mitral, late in aortic, disease.

3. *Palpitation* is of less diagnostic import, for it generally occurs without organic heart change.

4. *Pain* is by no means always present in cardiac dilatation, but few cases run their entire course without some præcordial discomfort. Anginal pain is a fairly common feature of aortic disease; it is due to interference with the coronary blood flow.

5. *Insomnia*, in advanced cases, is frequently troublesome, and in aortic regurgitation may be the first symptom of failure. Sometimes the patient, when dropping off to sleep, suddenly starts with the terror of suffocation and gasps for breath. *Headache* and *delirium* are also met in cardiac failure. The former is often due to variations in the blood pressure. Delirium in heart disease is usually due to cerebral anoxæmia, resulting from slowing of the circulation rate (see § 35).

6. *Embolism* may occur, as described under Subacute Endocarditis (§ 50a), but without evidence of general infection. It is most frequent in mitral stenosis with auricular fibrillation, and can occur in aortic disease. Emboli commonly lodge in one of the middle cerebral arteries.

The chief ETIOLOGY OF CARDIAC VALVULAR DISEASE in *youth* is rheumatic endocarditis, which has a special tendency to attack the mitral valve. In *advancing years*, the commonest cause is an atheromatous degeneration (§ 58). Rarer causes are: infective endocarditis (§ 50) and syphilis. The latter attacks only the aortic valve.

1. *Acute Endocarditis* of rheumatic origin is by far the most frequent cause, and a large majority of " heart cases " date their symptoms from an attack of that disease in youth or early adult life.

2. *Chronic Endocarditis may come on insidiously*. Syphilis causes aortic regurgitation between the ages of 40 and 60, often in association with arteriosclerosis. Chronic rheumatic endocarditis more often supervenes upon acute endocarditis—attacks of which may have been overlooked. Rheumatic heart infection may begin during rheumatic fever, chorea, rheumatic tonsillitis or scarlet fever, and may be of insidious onset.

3. *Degenerative* changes (*e.g.*, atheroma) are the lesions chiefly met with after middle life. They affect especially the aortic orifice, either by injuring the valves or by causing dilatation of the aorta, which, extending to the situation of the valves, prevents them from meeting during diastole.

4. Any prolonged *high blood pressure*—*e.g.*, that which accompanies arteriosclerosis —may lead to valvular strain, usually aortic. Persistent obstruction in the lungs

(*e.g.*, chronic bronchitis), or in the general systemic circulation, may have the same effect as persistent high tension on the right or left side of the heart respectively.

5. *Congenital* conditions are referred to in § 59.

Prognosis. In a case of chronic heart disease the fundamental factor is the heart muscle. Is the heart muscle handicapped ? If so, is the handicap removable ? If not, is a handicap likely to arise in the future ? These questions must all be answered in any one case. In actual practice the prognosis is good in proportion to *the amount of exercise a patient can take without producing breathlessness*. The factors which influence the function of the heart muscle are toxins, metabolic factors, oxygen supply and certain mechanical considerations, which include occupation or exertion, valvular defects and cardiac irregularities.

Toxins. Diphtheria, influenza, pneumonia, typhoid fever and certain septic foci produce a myocarditis which completely recovers if the patient survives the disease. Acute rheumatism not only produces permanent myocardial changes; it is apt to recur repeatedly during a patient's life, thus injuring the heart muscle ever more severely. If, however, the rheumatic process ceases, and if mitral stenosis has not been produced, a complete functional recovery is possible. Alcoholic excess and uræmia also damage the myocardium. If toxæmia of any kind is present, the myocardium will fail as a result of increased work, and the severity of the failure will be in proportion to the amount of toxæmia and the amount of work. A healthy, non-toxæmic heart muscle will never fail, whatever the severity of the exertion undertaken. The factors which cause an athlete to be " rowed out " are not myocardial, but vasomotor and nervous.

Metabolic factors producing myocardial failure are hyper- and hypo-thyroidism and beri-beri. Complete cure is here possible.

Oxygen supply to the myocardium is deficient in anæmia and in coronary disease. In the former case the prognosis depends upon the removability of the cause. The prognosis in coronary disease depends upon the following factors: (i.) with advancing years the collateral coronary anastomoses become freer; (ii.) coronary disease is often very localised, but it may or may not be part of a generalised arteriosclerosis; and (iii.) any individual coronary lesion tends to be progressive. Thus a coronary thrombosis in a man of 50, who has no hypertension, may heal and leave him with no dyspnœa; then a complete recovery is possible and the prognosis is good. On the other hand, a man with cardiac pain on exertion, due to coronary sclerosis and associated with hypertension, will be likely to lose ground progressively. Pulsus alternans, gallop rhythm and Cheyne-Stokes' breathing are bad signs.

Mechanical factors. The *valvular* lesions which seriously hamper cardiac efficiency are mitral stenosis and aortic incompetence. In mitral stenosis an increasing check is placed upon the amount of blood allowed to enter the left ventricle, and since this chamber can only expel what it receives the cardiac output is progressively reduced. Aortic incompetence is a mechanical handicap, for the left ventricle has extra work to do per beat, the diastolic coronary flow to the myocardium is less efficient, and the propulsive effect on the circulation of the aortic recoil is lost; also the factors which cause injury to the aortic cusps are apt to obstruct the mouths of the coronary vessels. The prognosis in aortic stenosis is better. Cardiac irregularities chiefly cut down the circulation rate by the associated tachycardia, which reduces the diastolic time and thus interferes with ventricular filling.

The prognosis in *valvular lesions* depends upon the myocardial condition, and the size of the valvular defect. A case of arrested aortic valvulitis, from rheumatism or syphilis, may live a healthy life for many years. As a brief generalisation the least dangerous valvular defect is mitral regurgitation; next in order come aortic stenosis and mitral stenosis. But in every case the etiological factor must be taken into account. The extent of the lesion can be best gauged from the size of the heart chamber affected by it. The enlargement of the left ventricle is proportional to the extent of the lesion in aortic stenosis or regurgitation and in mitral regurgitation. Hypertrophy of the right ventricle from valvulitis is only found clinically in advanced cases of mitral stenosis. Hypertrophy is a compensatory function; dilatation is a bad omen.

As regards individual examples: in *aortic regurgitation*, a good prognosis may be given in young rheumatic individuals with a good exercise tolerance, a not unduly large heart, a slow resting pulse rate and a normal diastolic blood pressure with a comparatively small pulse pressure. A relatively bad prognosis should be given in aortic regurgitation when the case is of syphilitic origin, where the heart is considerably enlarged, the apex beat weak (not heaving in character), where the pulse is rapid, where the systolic pressure is high but tending to fall, and the diastolic pressure low; when the patient is sleepless, gets vertigo on changing his position or after exercise, when the heart is irregular, whether the irregularity be due to extra systoles, to alternation (failing contractility), or to auricular fibrillation. Associated conditions, such as pregnancy, of course, add to the gravity of the prognosis.

In *mitral stenosis*, the prognosis is excellent when the lesion is operable (§ 62, p. 109); it is relatively good in inoperable cases when the patient is capable of leading a sheltered life, when the pulse is regular and of good volume, when there is no marked dyspnœa or cyanosis, no raised pulse rate, and a relatively good exercise tolerance. The prognosis is bad when there is marked cyanosis and dyspnœa on mild exertion, or orthopnœa; when the blood pressure is very low, the pulse is rapid and irregular, the liver is palpable, and when there are crepitations at the bases of the lungs and œdema of the feet.

The occupation, sex and temperament of the individual are of importance. If the patient is peacefully occupied with work which he can carry out in his own way, in his own time, the prognosis may be relatively good, but if he has to work against time, especially at an occupation that he is not used to, the prognosis becomes relatively bad. The placid individual who takes things as they come and does not worry, usually lives longer than the worrying person who meets trouble half-way. Generally speaking, the prognosis is better in women than in men, but here again it is largely a question of the lives they lead and the amount of rest they are able to take.

The prognosis of *Heart Disease as affected by Pregnancy* demands special notice. In pregnancy the maternal heart is loaded (1) owing to the increased nutritive demands of the fœtus, (2) by the increased maternal blood volume after the third month, and (3) by the mechanical embarrassment caused by the growing uterus. The former of these operate from early in pregnancy; the latter becomes of increasing importance as pregnancy proceeds. In conditions such as inoperable mitral stenosis with pulmonary hypertension, special care must be taken. In the case of aortic regurgitation, where the left heart is under a strain, the early months of pregnancy are attended with no particular risk, but towards the end of pregnancy (the 8th and 9th months) the risk of failure is gradually increased. Furthermore, after delivery it is essential to keep the patient still and to bandage the splanchnic area, as sudden vaso-motor collapse is liable to occur. With proper precautions heart cases stand pregnancy well. Decision as to the safety of pregnancy is a matter of experienced judgment and varies with individual cases. Briefly, it may be said that if there are no symptoms or signs of failure, pregnancy can be considered. If such symptoms have previously existed, pregnancy is possible but is a definite risk. Mitral valvotomy is sometimes performed in early pregnancy. If signs of failure are present, pregnancy must not occur, or must be terminated.

§ 62. The **Treatment** OF CHRONIC HEART DISEASE (including Myocardial Degeneration and Valvular Disease) may be considered under four heads: (a) When compensation is fully established; (b) when compensation begins to fail; (c) when compensation has broken down. (d) Surgical treatment has, in recent years, proved of great help.

(a) When there is efficient compensation, no symptoms are present and no active treatment is needed, but much may be done to avoid the supervention of cardiac failure and to prolong the patient's life. Patients with chronic heart disease should be instructed to lead quiet, regular and orderly lives. With regard to exercise, it may be said, in general terms, that the patient himself is the best judge, provided always that he does not exert himself sufficiently to cause undue dyspnœa or præcordial pain. Some sports are preferable to others; thus cricket, tennis and golf may often be enjoyed, whilst football, racing and rowing must generally be forbidden. Climbing, especially to high altitudes, must be disallowed. Alcohol, tobacco and tea are all myocardial poisons if taken to excess, and should be used only in strict moderation. The skin should be kept active by the daily bath, and the bowels regular by purgatives when necessary. Whenever possible, a means of livelihood should be chosen in which the heart is subjected to but little strain. A sedentary occupation, with moderate exercise in the intervals, is more suitable than one which entails earning a living literally by the sweat of the brow. Lifting or carrying heavy weights, climbing ladders, wielding heavy hammers, and physical labour in constrained positions, are liable to overtax the powers for compensation of the cardiac muscle. Meals should be regular and heavy meals should be avoided.   The diet should be easily assimilable, and contain only a moderate amount of fluid and little salt.   A small quantity of stimulant with meals may be called for, but should not be used unnecessarily, because of the reaction afterwards, and of the tendency to excess which exists in cardiac cases.

(b) When compensation is beginning to fail, the condition of the heart should be noted frequently; rest, drugs, and exercises being prescribed in accordance with the variations in the circulation and the capability of response to treatment by the cardiac muscle.

Drugs.—In cardiac failure, especially in auricular fibrillation, when the pulse becomes feeble, rapid, and irregular, *digitalis is par excellence* the remedy.   It is especially indicated in mitral stenosis or regurgitation. It is unnecessary when there is full compensatory hypertrophy and the pulse is fairly strong, regular and slow, or if vomiting is present.   By its action on the vagal nerve endings in the Bundle of His, in auricular fibrillation it reduces the number of auricular impulses reaching the ventricle.   Its action is not quite so efficacious if fever is present.   There are two methods of administering it—massive or intensive dosage, and maintenance dosage.   When a patient is acutely ill with heart failure and auricular fibrillation, digoxin 1 mg. in normal saline 10 ml. should be injected intravenously.   It can be repeated in 6 hours.   In a patient less ill digoxin can be given by mouth in doses of 1 mg., 4-hourly, for three doses.   After these emergency measures, a maintenance dose of digitalis folia is given, gr. 1 four times or three times daily according to circumstances.   The two things to watch are the heart rate and for signs of digitalis overdose.   The apex rate, not the pulse rate, is the only safe guide to the correct dose of digitalis in auricular fibrillation, owing to the apex-pulse deficiency which occurs.   No nurse should be allowed to record the pulse figures in these cases who cannot count the heart rate by stethoscope; pulse figures alone are valueless.   The result to be obtained is a reduction of the heart rate to 70–80 per minute.   The signs of overdose to watch for, in order of severity, are: reduced urinary output, coupled beats, nausea, vomiting, headache and visual disturbance.

When digitalis is required and there is no urgency, the most useful preparations of digitalis are digitalis præparata B.P. (digitalis folia), 1 gr. being equal to 10 minims of the tincture, or digitoxinum (B.P.C.) which is similar to Nativelle's digitaline.   When a rapid action is desired, the most useful drug is digoxin B.P. (0·25 mg.), one tablet being equal to 1½ gr. of digitalis præparata.   Digoxin has removed one of the chief deficiencies in digitalis medication, namely, the slowness of its action.   It may be given in doses up to 1 mg. intravenously.   Strophanthin has an action similar to that of digitalis, and can also be used intravenously.   It must never be so given to a patient who recently has been taking digitalis, as sudden death has been known to occur.   Digitalis can be continued indefinitely, as tolerance is not acquired.   In all conditions with a failing myocardium, it has a definite effect by improving contractility.

In very acute cases of heart failure recourse is often had to rapidly acting stimulants, such as brandy, nikethamide B.P. 4 ml. intravenously, or leptazol B.P. (cardiazol) subcutaneously, but it is questionable whether any direct cardiac effect is produced by them: these preparations act on the vaso-constrictor and respiratory centres and not on the heart. Strychnine is useless as a cardiac stimulant. In *aortic valvular disease* and in the early stages of *mitral stenosis*, digitalis is not so valuable; but in the later stages of these diseases, when compensation begins to fail and especially when auricular fibrillation is present, digitalis gives relief. Aminophylline B.P. (Cardophylin) intravenously once a day is a useful drug for failure due to arteriosclerosis.

The various symptoms may be met by appropriate remedies. For *pulmonary congestion*, venesection is a most efficacious form of treatment; injections of mersalyl are especially helpful. Phenobarbitone is valuable for anxiety and restlessness, but in cases with cerebral arteriosclerosis it is apt to cause mental changes and even delirium. For paroxysms of *dyspnœa*, morphia, aminophylline (0·24 G. in 10 ml. of sterile water, intravenously, daily for 7 days), or oxygen inhalations by mask or nasal catheter are useful. *Cough* is relieved by drinks of hot milk and by drugs such as codein or small doses of opium. For *palpitation*, alcohol is a valuable sedative. The quantity should always be moderate. Other causes of palpitation should be treated by the appropriate remedies (§ 34). For *sleeplessness*, in more acute cases, opium or a hypodermic injection of morphia is most useful, and should be given without hesitation. In children or in cases where the insomnia is not obstinate, other drugs may be employed, such as potassium bromide, phenobarbitone and paraldehyde. Chloral is harmless. The *hæmoptysis* of heart disease is best left alone. Digitalis must be stopped for 24 hours if it causes vomiting, and then it can be resumed in smaller doses. For the treatment of *pain* and syncopal attacks, *vide* §§ 33 and 35.

Massage and Systematised Exercises.—At one time complete rest was regarded as imperative for all forms of cardiac disease. But the advance of physiological knowledge has shown what an important part the skeletal muscles play in the circulation of the blood. When the patient *is confined to bed* regular leg exercises should be done morning and night, each leg being firmly flexed and strongly extended twelve times. The purpose is to stimulate circulation in the leg veins at regular intervals in order to prevent silent clots from forming, these being a source of the severe complication of pulmonary embolism. When *the patient is ambulatory* once more, compensation having been established, slowly increasing and graduated exercise is of the utmost benefit and should be continued indefinitely unless undue fatigue or shortness of breath supervene. In this way the cardiac recovery will be best stimulated. In cases of early failure who are still ambulatory, much good can be done by reducing excessive weight (see § 18). Breathing exercises, by helping the venous return, are valuable in chronic heart disease.

(c) When compensation has broken down and marked cardiac failure is present, absolute rest is necessary. The patient is usually unable to lie down, but has to be propped up with pillows, and in severe cases sleep can be obtained only when the legs are hanging down. A special "heart" bed is valuable in such cases, as the degree of dorsal support and dependence of the legs can be adjusted to each case. In severe failure of the right heart, as indicated by distended jugular veins, cyanosis, the liver dullness extending well below the costal margin and the cardiac dullness extending far to the right, *venesection* is called for, and brings prompt relief. The rapid removal of from 10 to 20 oz. of blood is usually sufficient; this may be repeated. Diuretics are valuable in the treatment of cardiac œdema. Inject. mersalyl is one of the most useful remedies and usually renders tapping unnecessary; the injection can be repeated each 2–7 days. See § 29 for the use of diuretics. The diet should contain no added salt. Œdema may be treated by draining the legs with Southey's tubes (§ 29) or by multiple superficial incisions, asepsis being maintained by penicillin cream and sterile dressings. Aspiration of a pleural effusion or paracentesis abdominis may be necessary. Pleural effusions are common in congestive heart failure: treatment by removal of the fluid will increase the expanding area of the lung, decrease the anoxæmia and benefit the myocardium. They should be looked for, and removed by aspiration even though comparatively small. Diaphoretics are of no use in cardiac œdema. Digitalis is of especial value, even in heart conditions with sinus rhythm; it augments the force of contraction and therefore the emptying of the cardiac chambers.

The prolonged use of propyl thiouracil B.P. has proved successful in reducing the basal metabolic rate of cardiac patients, and thus lightening the burden of the heart. It has been used for repeated attacks of congestive failure in myocardial degeneration. It is also useful in carefully chosen cases of anginal pain of organic origin; for this sympathectomy has also been performed (§ 51).

(d) The *Surgical Treatment* of certain types of heart disease can give excellent results. Mitral valvotomy of cases of mitral stenosis in expert hands gives a mortality of under 5 per cent. The valve is reached through the left auricular appendix and the commissures separated either by digital pressure, or by a special dilator. This operation is indicated where there are clear signs both of mitral stenosis and of pulmonary hypertension, and when the patient's disability is considerable or rapidly increasing, but is contra-indicated when there is considerable cardiac enlargement or mitral regurgitation. The operation may have to be repeated more than once in the course of years. The other cases particularly amenable to surgery are of *congenital* origin. A patent ductus arteriosus is approached most frequently from the back: it is ligatured, transfixed and tied and in some cases divided. The operation is practically free from risk in skilled hands, and after such treatment the enlarged heart and an increased pulse pressure return to normal. Should an infected ductus prove not to be amenable to antibiotics, this treatment can prove curative. The narrowed valve of pure pulmonary stenosis can be approached through the right ventricle and a dilator or valvulotome used to dilate the stenosed orifice. The results are satisfactory but the pulmonary murmur and some degree of right ventricular hypertrophy generally persist. Various blind operations have been tried for an atrial septal defect, but these measures are likely to be discarded as the position of the defect is not easy to localise and the defect may be multiple: hypothermia and anæsthesia of the cooled patient and " the cardiac pump " now enable open operations to be performed in this and in other conditions.

§ 63. Group E. We now turn to the consideration of those cardiac disorders the recognition of which depends upon **Alterations in the Rate or Rhythm of the Pulse.** In all cases *it is essential to compare the radial pulse with the heart sounds,* and to observe the pulsation in the veins of the neck.

The Electrocardiograph (§ 44) may be required to make an exact study of a case presenting pulse alterations; but it is often possible to make a correct diagnosis without their aid.

I. With an occasional PAUSE in the radial pulse . . .
- Premature Beat (Extrasystole) (§ 64).
- Incomplete Heart Block (§ 71).
- Sino-auricular Block (§ 64).

II. With RHYTHMIC alteration of rate DEPENDENT ON RESPIRATION . . . .
- Sinus Arrhythmia (§ 65).

III. With INCREASED rate . .
- Tachycardia, Physiological (§ 84).
- Paroxysmal Auricular Tachycardia (§ 66).
- Auricular Flutter (§ 67).
- Paroxysmal Ventricular Tachycardia (§ 68).
- Auricular Fibrillation (§ 69).

IV. With DISORDERLY RHYTHM .
- Auricular Fibrillation (§ 69) or Multiple Premature Beats (§ 64).

V. With DECREASED rate . .
- Bradycardia (§ 85).
- Complete Heart Block (§ 71).

VI. COUPLING of the Pulse Beats .
- Premature Beats (§ 64).
- Pulsus Alternans (§ 73).
- Extreme Dicrotism (§ 72).

The various causes of altered rate and rhythm of the pulse, other than cardiac disease, are considered in § 84 *et seq.* Here we consider only the cardiac conditions to which attention may first be called, and in which the diagnosis may be largely made, by alterations in the pulse rate and rhythm.

A PAUSE IN THE PULSE, which is OTHERWISE REGULAR, is due to three conditions: PREMATURE BEATS, HEART BLOCK and SINO-AURICULAR BLOCK. The first of these is very common, the second somewhat rare, and the third very rare. The pause in the pulse caused by premature beats is due to the fact that the ventricle is prematurely stimulated early in diastole, and the output from it is therefore generally insufficient to produce a pulse wave. Following the premature beat there is a compensatory pause. During the pause in the pulse, as felt at the wrist, the stethoscope, if placed over the heart, can detect the sound of the premature beat. This differentiates premature beats from heart block and sino-auricular block.

I. *There is an occasional pause in the radial pulse, during which the heart gives a short premature beat which can be heard over the præcordium.* The condition is PREMATURE BEAT.

§ 64. **Premature beats** (Syn. Ectopic beats, Extrasystoles) are of frequent occurrence in healthy persons, but are more common in later life. They are due to local irritability of the myocardium, causing early contraction in some part of the heart; and are distinguished from auricular fibrillation by their disappearance when the heart rate is increased by any cause, *e.g.*, exercise, excitement or sniffing amyl nitrite.

The normal beat of the heart always starts at the most irritable point, normally the sino-auricular node. Should any other point of the heart become more irritable it initiates the contraction; such a beat is said to be ectopic in origin, and inasmuch as the contraction occurs earlier in the cardiac cycle than the normal beat, it is called *premature*. Ectopic

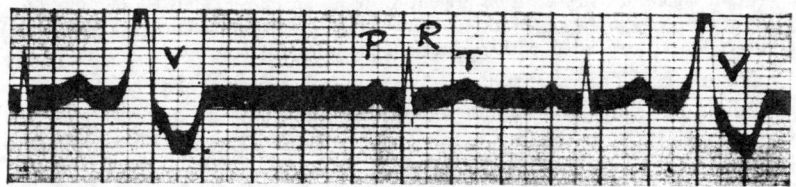

FIG. 38.—Premature ventricular beats (V). Note the prematurity and the large amplitude of the complexes.

beats may arise either in the auricular, nodal or junctional tissue (*i.e.*, the tissue between auricles and ventricles) or in the right or left ventricles. Ectopic auricular beats give rise to a ventricular contraction of normal type. Should the ectopic beat start in the nodal tissue, it travels upwards towards the auricles and downwards towards the ventricles, so that the auricles and ventricles contract more or less simultaneously.

Symptoms. The patient may or may not be conscious of the altered heart beat. The symptoms are palpitation, a catch in the breath, a thump, a sinking sensation, or even a sudden momentary stab of præcordial pain. They are often a source of needless anxiety to the patient.

Broadly speaking, the *causes* of local irritability which give rise to premature beats or extrasystoles are of (1) extrinsic or extra-cardiac, or of (2) intrinsic or cardiac origin. Extrinsic, *e.g.*, a distended stomach causing premature beats starting in either the right ventricle or auricle: such beats disappear on relief of the distension. In the eighth month of pregnancy the heart is often irregular, due to the distended abdomen.

Some common intrinsic causes of local irritability are: (1) Toxæmia; (2) physical effort; (3) inflammation; (4) degeneration.

(1) The connection between premature beats and *toxæmia* is seen with such conditions as malaria, typhoid, influenza, excessive tobacco, etc. Thyrotoxicosis, an abnormal susceptibility to coffee or tea, and digitalis poisoning are also common causes. Septic foci may be causal. Generally speaking, all parts of the heart are involved, so that the irregularity is considerable, sometimes the auricles, sometimes the right and at other times the left ventricle showing premature beats. The abuse of tobacco as producing cardiac irregularities is well known and has been a recognised method of evading military service.

(2) Rarely premature beats appear or increase only after physical effort, and are then suggestive of myocardial damage. Any irregularity of the heart which develops with or after exercise, whether due to premature beats, auricular fibrillation, auricular flutter or any other cause, must always be looked upon as due to some definite myocardial disability. In auricular fibrillation, the rhythm is more irregular *during* exercise.

(3) *Inflammation.*—In acute myocarditis premature beats are common. In chronic forms of myocardial disease they frequently occur independently of any endocardial or pericardial involvement. If auricular, they often precede fibrillation; if ventricular, they are often associated with acute local or diffuse myocardial disease. The association between premature beats and inflammation is often well seen in the course of an attack of rheumatic fever. The patient, perhaps, has well-marked signs of endocarditis or pericarditis, but as far as one can tell the myocardium has escaped damage. The heart then becomes irregular, and owing to the development of premature beats, one knows that the inflammation has involved the myocardium.

(4) In *myocardial degeneration* premature beats most commonly occur after fifty years of age; they are frequent antecedents of such conditions as auricular fibrillation or heart block, associated with generalised myocardial change.

Prognosis.—The essential point to remember first is that the majority of individuals who have ventricular premature beats do not suffer at the time or subsequently from heart failure or gross disease. The prognosis in all cases with premature beats must be decided independently of the presence of this sign.

Treatment.—Symptoms produced by premature beats normally require simple reassurance. They are often abolished by reducing smoking, and avoiding heavy meals and strong coffee. If they persist in spite of these measures, it may be necessary to give a mixture containing quinidine sulphate gr. 2 or 3, atropine sulphate gr. $\frac{1}{150}$, acid. sulph. dil. ℳ 10 in aq. chlorof. ad. $\frac{1}{2}$ fl. oz., t.d.s., p.c. For ventricular premature beats tab. procainamide is often helpful.

The first stage of **heart block** (§ 71), in which the only change is lengthening of the " P–R " interval, is not diagnosable clinically (Fig. 16). The second stage is that of an occasionally dropped beat, the " P–R " interval lengthening from normal progressively, until eventually an auricular stimulus fails to reach the ventricle. A ventricular beat then drops out. In this case the pause is completely silent (Fig. 17). The common causes of this condition are myocardial ischæmia, acute rheumatism, pneumonia, diphtheria, and occasionally other febrile states.

Sino-auricular block is a rare condition of no especial clinical significance, in which there is a complete obliteration of the whole of a cardiac cycle, both auricular and ventricular beats being equally affected. It is sometimes accompanied by other evidences of excessive vagal tone.

II. *The patient is* YOUNG, *and presents a* REGULARLY RECURRING *alteration of the pulse rate, usually dependent upon* RESPIRATION. *The condition is* SINUS ARRHYTHMIA.

§ 65. Sinus Arrhythmia is a condition in which the mechanism of the heart beat remains in all respects normal.

Signs.—The pulse rate increases with inspiration, but there is no difference between the strength of any two successive beats. The regular waxing and waning of the heart rate is accentuated when the patient breathes deeply. Auscultation reveals no alteration in the heart sounds. This irregularity is without symptoms.

Causes.—The condition is common in the young and during convalescence from diseases in which the heart rate has been rapid. It is of vagal origin in individuals in whom there is exaggeration of the normal inspiratory increase and expiratory slowing of pulse rate.

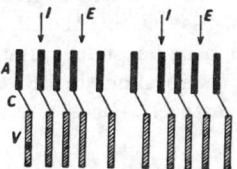

FIG. 39.—Sinus arrhythmia. The heart mechanism, auricular contraction (A), conduction (C) and ventricular contraction (V), is normal. The heart rate during inspiration (I) is increased, and during expiration (E) is slowed.

Prognosis.—The condition is of little importance; it ceases when the pulse rate quickens from any cause, *e.g.*, after exercise. When found after fevers, it is a good sign, inasmuch as it suggests the absence of extensive damage to the heart wall. No treatment is indicated.

§ 66. III. *The Cardiac conditions in which an Increased Rate forms the most striking feature are:* PAROXYSMAL AURICULAR TACHYCARDIA, AURICULAR FLUTTER, PAROXYSMAL VENTRICULAR TACHYCARDIA, AURICULAR FIBRILLATION.

In the majority of cases of regular TACHYCARDIA the increase is physiological in character. In two conditions, paroxysmal tachycardia and auricular flutter, the heart beat starts from a new focus.

In PHYSIOLOGICAL TACHYCARDIA the pulse rate is (i.) affected by posture, falling 10 to 30 beats when the patient passes from a standing to a recumbent position; (ii.) the pulse rate increases with exercise, and is affected by emotion, meals, fever, and sleep; (iii.) the onset and termination are gradual; (iv.) electrocardiograms are normal; (v.) jugular tracings show no exaggeration of the force of the auricle. The causes of this form of tachycardia are dealt with in § 84.

The pulse rate is REGULAR, 130 *to* 200 *a minute; the rate is unaffected by exercise or posture. The condition is usually* PAROXYSMAL AURICULAR TACHYCARDIA: *otherwise it is* AURICULAR FLUTTER OR PAROXYSMAL VENTRICULAR TACHYCARDIA.

Paroxysmal Auricular Tachycardia is a term reserved for cases of rapid action of the heart presenting the following characters: (1) the onset of the tachycardia is abrupt; (2) the duration varies from seconds to days;

(3) the relief is sudden, and the pulse returns to its normal rate in the course of a few beats, which are often irregular in force and rhythm. During the paroxysm violent jugular pulsation may be visible. The majority of attacks occur in healthy individuals.

The *symptoms* complained of by the patient depend upon the duration of the paroxysm. Many of the short paroxysms, lasting a few hours, are accompanied only by a fluttering or throbbing sensation in the chest or at the root of the neck, and a feeling of lassitude. Some attacks cause anginal pain. When the attack is prolonged over several days, grave cardiac embarrassment with dilatation, cyanosis, œdema of lungs, and engorgement and enlargement of the liver occur, especially if the heart is already diseased. Occasionally there is great distress and discomfort. The general disturbance of the patient, the rapidity of the pulse, and the severity of the abdominal pain dependent upon the engorgement of the liver may be so extreme as to simulate an acute abdominal condition calling for surgical interference. Cases are on record of exploratory

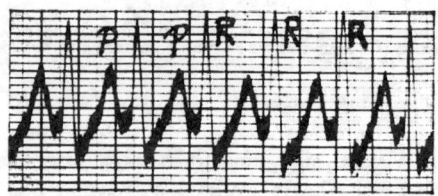

FIG. 40.—Paroxysmal auricular tachycardia. The " P " waves are abnormal in shape showing an ectopic origin, and at a rapid rate. The " QRS " waves are normal.

laparotomy having been performed owing to such an error of diagnosis. The rapid disappearance of abdominal symptoms on cessation of the tachycardia is a striking feature. The immediate *prognosis* depends chiefly upon the presence or absence of dilatation of the heart. The most severe symptoms disappear almost immediately if the heart muscle is healthy.

Etiology.—The condition is due to sudden rhythmic activity of an ectopic focus in the auricle, which for a time overcomes and replaces the normal activity of the sino-auricular node. It is most common in young adults, but may occur in early childhood or old age. The attacks may be excited by exertion, emotion, flatulence, or change of posture. Usually no underlying disease of the heart can be found, but in some cases there is myocardial disease, the consequence of rheumatism, scarlet fever, syphilis or coronary disease (see § 69, Etiology). Often no valvular lesion is present; if valvular murmurs are present they become unrecognisable during the paroxysm.

The *diagnosis* from tachycardia of purely *nervous* origin depends upon: (i.) the abrupt onset and relief; (ii.) the presence of violent jugular pulsation; (iii.) the occasional presence of a few premature beats in the intervals between the paroxysms. Many attacks of so-called " Paroxysmal Tachycardia " are really paroxysms of Auricular Fibrillation or Auricular Flutter (see below) which can only be recognised by the electrocardiogram.

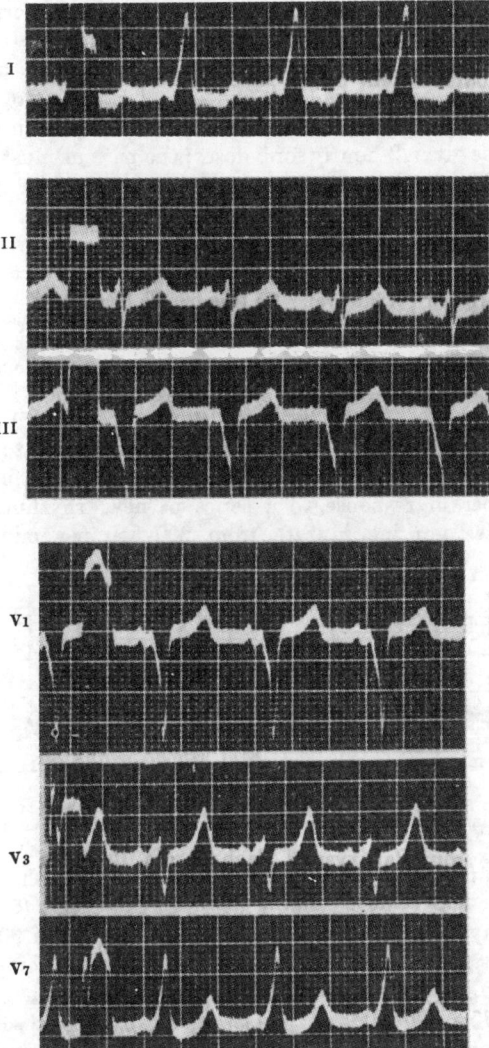

Fig. 41.—E.C.G. Tracings from a case of the WOLFF-PARKINSON-WHITE SYNDROME. The short PR interval of 0·10 sec. is followed by the ventricular pattern of a Left Bundle Branch Block.

Treatment.—The brief paroxysms which produce no subjective symptoms call for no treatment. For the prolonged attacks the patients often discover for themselves some simple procedure which increases vagal tone and cuts them short, viz., holding the breath, compressing an eyeball, taking a cold drink, or the assumption of some special posture. If these fail pressure over the carotid sinus or compression of the abdomen with a tight binder may be successful. Acetylcholine in the form of carbachol B.P. (Doryl) intravenously will often cut short an attack; 0·25 mg. diluted in 10 ml. of N. saline is given very slowly into a vein until the attack stops.

Should embarrassment of the right heart become extreme, digitalis in full doses (see § 62) can be tried. Alternatively quinidine sulphate gr. 3 to 5 can be given 2-hourly for 5 doses; the patient must be recumbent. Prophylactically, quinidine sulphate in doses of gr. 2 or 3 t.d.s., p.c., is a safe and useful remedy.

The *Wolff-Parkinson-White Syndrome* causes paroxysmal auricular tachycardia in approximately 50 per cent. of cases. *Diagnosis* is only obtained by electrocardiographic records which show the pattern of a bundle branch block together with a considerably shortened PR interval. No true bundle block is present as the interval between the beginning of the P-wave and the end of the QRS is normal (Fig. 41). The decreased PR interval is believed to be due to an aberrant conduction pathway between the auricles and ventricles which bypasses the AV node. The *Prognosis* in most cases is excellent. *Treatment* is as for paroxysmal auricular tachycardia.

§ 67. Auricular Flutter.[1]—This name has been given to a condition in which " the normal beats of the auricle are submerged by contractions of this chamber in response to a series of new, rhythmic, and pathological impulses varying in rate from 200–350 per minute " (Lewis).

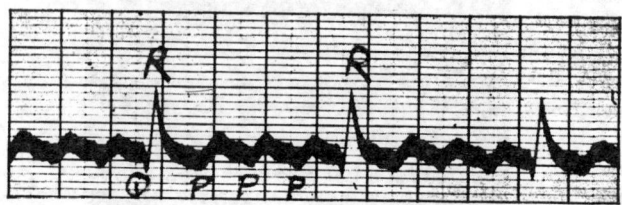

FIG. 42.—Auricular flutter. The auricular waves are undulatory at the rate of 300, and the ventricle responds only to every 4th auricular beat. One of the " P " waves is periodically obscured by the " QRS " waves.

Flutter differs from Paroxysmal Tachycardia in that the auricular rate is much higher and there is some degree of heart block (§ 69—Etiology); the auricle may, for instance, be beating at the rate of 300 per minute, while the ventricle responds with only 150 beats per minute. In other cases a higher grade of heart block (4–1) may be present, and the pulse rate be about 75 and regular. The rate of the auricle is absolutely regular; that of the ventricle may be regular or irregular, depending upon the constancy of the degree of heart block present (Fig. 42).

Symptoms and Signs.—The symptoms of auricular flutter are generally those of heart failure; palpitation is sometimes complained of and the

---

[1] Flutter has been placed under this heading because it is usually associated with a regular ventricular pulse. When varying grades of heart block are present this regularity in rate disappears, but in contrast to the pulse of auricular fibrillation regularity in force and volume persists.

pulse rate is found to be unexpectedly feeble and rapid. For the certain recognition of the disorder electrocardiographic records are necessary, but its existence may be suspected when (i.) the pulse rate is 130–160, regular (except for occasional momentary intermissions), and the rate is maintained for long periods; syncopal attacks sometimes occur; (ii.) the ventricular rate shows no quickening with exercise or slowing on lying down. This constancy of the rate on alteration of posture and with exercise is an important diagnostic feature. However it will often alter abruptly with pressure over the carotid sinus (in contradistinction to ventricular tachycardia). (iii.) A visible jugular pulse of greater rate than the apex should lead one to suspect auricular flutter.

Etiology.—The condition is usually associated with chronic myocardial degeneration, but occasionally accompanies mitral stenosis. The patients are often past middle life, and are subjects of arteriosclerosis. The irregularity is occasionally produced by quinidine when given in auricular fibrillation.

Prognosis.—The duration of the condition varies. It may occur in recurrent but brief attacks (paroxysmal auricular flutter) or may be a chronic condition which persists for years. This long duration is a further diagnostic point of great importance. There is a danger of the ventricle suddenly assuming a rate equal to that of the auricle—a condition which can lead to syncopal attacks which may be fatal.

Treatment.—Digitalis præparata (digitalis folia) in 2-gr. doses four times a day will often effect a cure; it acts by producing auricular fibrillation (see below). If the drug is then withdrawn, fibrillation may suddenly cease and the heart resume its normal rhythm. Even if digitalis fails to produce fibrillation, it may be relied upon to reduce the ventricular rate. If large doses of the drug are given, the period of fibrillation may be cut short. Quinidine sulphate can be used as an alternative method of treatment, as described in § 69.

§ 68. Paroxysmal Ventricular Tachycardia.—Ventricular premature beats are common (§ 64). When from a similar focus in the ventricular muscle there arise,

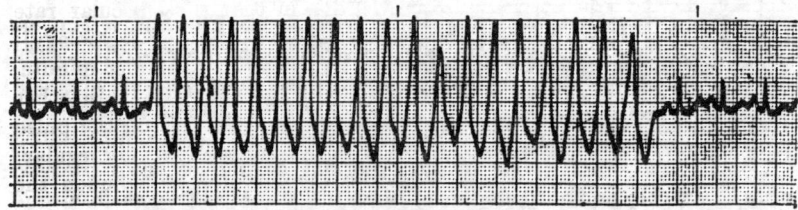

FIG. 43.—A short attack of Paroxysmal Ventricular Tachycardia.

not one, but a rapid and regular succession of such impulses the condition is paroxysmal ventricular tachycardia (Fig. 43).

Symptoms.—The heart rate is high (150–200 per minute), the rhythm as observed clinically is regular. The patient is frequently distressed, anginal pain may be felt in the middle of the chest, perhaps radiating to the arms; and the blood pressure is often lowered.   If the attack lasts more than 24 hours congestive failure may appear.

Etiology.—The condition is generally associated with clinical or electrocardiographic evidence of disease of the heart muscle, usually caused by coronary arteriosclerosis.

The *Prognosis* is more serious than in the other three types of paroxysmal tachycardia.

Treatment.—Quinidine sulphate is given 2 hourly in 3-gr. doses to a maximum of eight doses per day.   This should not be given for more than three successive days. Should quinidine therapy fail, procainamide hydrochlor. may be given orally in doses of G. 0·50 every 2 hours for eight doses.   In cases of emergency procainamide hydrochlor. may be given slowly intravenously (100–200 mg. per minute to a total of 2·0 G.).   The speed of administration can be even slower than this.   The blood pressure should be taken every minute during this therapy and the patient watched carefully for hypotension and twitching of the muscles: if these appear the injection must be stopped.

IV.   *The heart rate is* COMPLETELY IRREGULAR *in rhythm and in volume; in failure it may beat at a rate as high as* 180 *per minute; the condition is probably* AURICULAR FIBRILLATION.

§ 69. **Auricular Fibrillation** is recognisable by (i.) Complete irregularity of the pulse; (ii.) the difference between the apex and the pulse rates; (iii.) increase in the irregularity by exercise; (iv.) absence of the " P " wave on the electrocardiogram (Figs. 14, 44). (v.) The blood pressure always varies from beat to beat.   Furthermore, auricular fibrillation is almost invariably associated with (vi.) cardiac enlargement. (vii.) Auricular fibrillation is sometimes paroxysmal in character, the attacks lasting from a few minutes to hours, days, or even weeks: permanent fibrillation usually supervenes later.

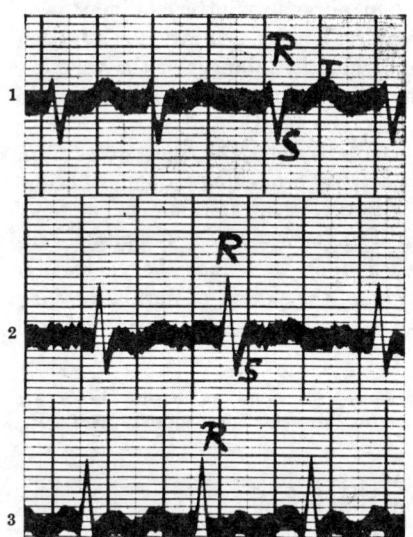

FIG. 44.—Right-sided preponderance. " S " is deepest in lead 1, and " R " is tallest in lead 3. (Auricular fibrillation is present.)

Etiology.—The auricle is composed of a number of intimately connected muscle fibres, so much so that some people regard them as forming a syncytium; and a normal systole of the auricle is initiated at the sino-auricular node, and the stimulus travels from one muscle fibre to another, and gives a systematic and co-ordinate contraction of the auricle from above downwards, *i.e.*, from the sino-auricular to the auriculo-ventricular node.   The older view is that in auricular fibrillation and in auricular flutter the underlying process is a " circus movement " in which the sino-auricular node ceases to function and is replaced by a stimulus which makes a circuit of the muscle surrounding one of the large venous orifices 400–500 times a minute. The auricular muscle derives its stimulation from this circus movement in an entirely irregular fashion, for much of the auricular muscle is refractory to such a rate of stimulation. The rate of circus movement in auricular fibrillation at 400–500 times per minute is faster than in auricular flutter (200–350 per minute) because the path of the circus movement in fibrillation is shorter than in flutter. A more recent view is that the auricular impulses are derived from one or more foci and not from a circus movement (Prinzmetal). In either case co-ordinate auricular contraction no longer occurs, but individual bundles of fibres, or even individual fibres, contract inco-ordinately, so that the whole auricular wall appears to be trembling or quivering in a state of diastole. The ventricle therefore receives impulses at very irregular intervals, and so the force and the rhythm of the ventricle varies from beat to beat. The stronger of these stimuli, at irregular intervals, traverse the Bundle of His and excite a ventricular contraction. According to the number of auricular stimuli which are transmitted to the ventricles, the rate of these will be fast or slow; the apex rate may vary between 180 and 40 per minute. Auricular fibrillation usually occurs: (1) secondary to valvular disease, especially mitral stenosis; (2) in myocardial degeneration, *e.g.*, cardio-vascular sclerosis; (3) in toxic conditions, *e.g.*, Graves disease; (4) in the course of acute inflammatory conditions, *e.g.*, acute carditis; (5) very rarely as a result of syphilis.

The *prognosis* depends chiefly upon (1) whether the underlying cause is removable or not. In myocardial degeneration the cause is not removable but progressive; the prognosis is consequently bad. In Graves' disease, provided the muscle is only in the toxic and not in the degenerative stage, removal of part of the thyroid will remove the hyperthyroidism and the auricular fibrillation will cease. In mitral stenosis the immediately exciting cause of the fibrillation is a rise of pressure in the auricles. (2) The condition of the ventricular muscle. If the auricular fibrillation is due to a more or less local condition of the auricle, the outlook is comparatively good. But if the cause of the fibrillation has seriously affected the ventricular muscle, the prognosis is bad. (3) The extent to which the ventricle is overstimulated by the erratically acting auricle. Obviously the greater the ventricular rate and the larger the number of ineffective beats, the greater the over-work of the ventricle and the worse the outlook. (4) Where the cause cannot be removed, how far it is possible to control the fibrillation. For example, with many cases of mitral stenosis, it may not be possible to stop the fibrillation, but it may be possible to control it by treatment so that the ventricular rate is slowed and the number of ineffective beats few. In such cases the prognosis is good, the fibrillation making little difference to the conditions of life.

Treatment.—It is thus obvious that the treatment of auricular fibrillation first lies in attempting to remove the underlying cause. In some cases this is comparatively easy, in others it may be impossible. In hyperthyroidism it can be stopped by removing part of the over-active thyroid. In mitral stenosis, on the other hand, the removal of the cause may be impossible. If it is impossible to stop the actual fibrillation, it is usually possible to control its effect on the ventricle. This is done by giving the patient that dose of digitalis which will keep the heart rate, at rest, between 70 and 80. If the heart rate is already as slow as this, digitalis is not needed. If there are signs of failure the patient must be treated in bed according to the scheme described above (see § 62). Digitalis must be continued, if needed, so long as the fibrillation remains, *i.e.*, usually for the rest of the patient's life.

Quinidine, an isomer of quinine, is sometimes useful in stopping auricular fibrillation. Contra-indications for its use are established mitral stenosis, signs of congestive failure, and marked cardiac enlargement. Where fibrillation is known to have persisted for many months, quinidine is generally not used. Thyrotoxic and early arteriosclerotic cases are the most suitable. Before quinidine treatment digitalis can be stopped; during quinidine treatment patients must be nursed flat, strictly confined to bed, and must not be allowed to sit up, for the drug is a myocardial poison. Dosage is as follows: gr. 2 twice daily, p.c., for one day, to exclude the possibility of hypersensitivity to the drug, and on successive days eight 2-hourly doses of gr. 2, 3 and 4, the final total daily dose being gr. 32. This final dose can be maintained for 2 or 3 more days, and is then stopped. If the auricular fibrillation ceases during treatment the course can be stopped, and a maintenance dose of gr. 2 or 3 t.d.s., p.c., continued for 2-3 months. In cases where auricular fibrillation is paroxysmal, a dose of 3-5 gr. t.d.s. will usually prevent attacks.

Quinidine sulphate acts as a myocardial depressant, and slows the rate of conduction as well as increasing the refractory period of the heart muscle. When the latter effect predominates, auricular fibrillation ceases.

V. *Conditions of the heart which are associated with a* SLOW PULSE.

§ 70. **Slow pulse**—between 40 or 50 or below—occurs in four more or less common conditions. (1) Personal idiosyncrasy; (2) The heart of the well-trained athlete; (3) With digitalis therapy; (4) Conditions of complete or partial heart block.

(1) In the bradycardia of the athlete, the subject usually looks and seems physically very fit: on exercise he shows no symptoms of distress; and his pulse rate, instead of being actually increased, suddenly doubles.

(2) Bradycardia may occur in conditions of lowered metabolism, such as inanition, exposure to cold, and myxœdema. It is also seen in some toxic states, as in jaundice.

(3) Digitalis may cause it in three ways—by producing heart block, by producing premature beats which fail to reach the arterial pulse, and by central vagal stimulation. In vagotonic conditions (*e.g.*, in increased intracranial pressure) and in shock bradycardia is often seen.

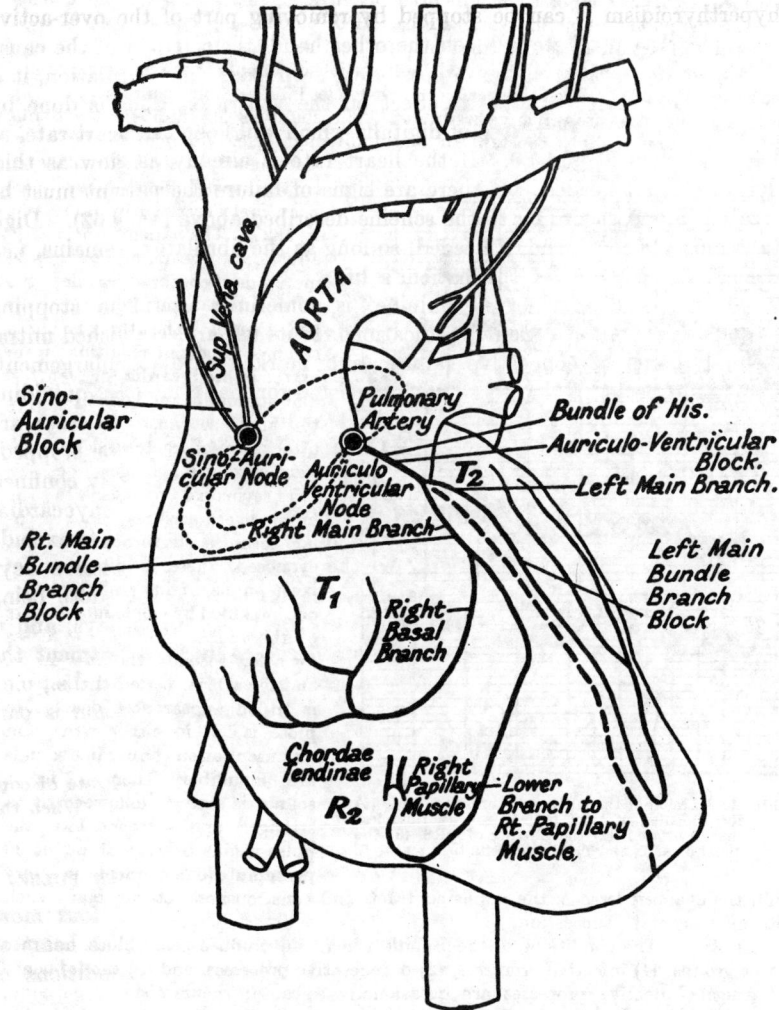

Fig. 45.—Diagram illustrating the positions of the lesions in the different varieties of Heart Block.

(4) In complete or partial *heart block* (when affecting the main Bundle of His) the rate is unaffected by exercise and signs of cardio-vascular degeneration are frequently present.

§ 71. Heart Block.—Conductivity is specialised in the Bundle system described in the introduction to this chapter. Any part of this conducting tract may be damaged, a whole series of conditions arising therefrom (Fig. 45). The varieties are:—

1. AURICULO-VENTRICULAR (Main-stem) block. When the Bundle of His is

damaged, either partial or complete auriculo-ventricular block occurs. The damage may be temporary or permanent, and partial or complete.

Partial Heart Block is described in § 44 (and see Figs. 16, 17).

Complete Heart Block implies total interruption of impulse between auricles and ventricles (Fig. 18). When this occurs the ventricles initiate their own rhythm. This is regular, and at a rate which varies from 24–36 (usually 28–30) in different patients, but remains remarkably constant in any individual case. *Symptoms.*—It is not infrequently associated with syncopal attacks—**Stokes-Adams' Disease**, first described by R. Adams in 1827. The patients are usually advanced in years, and have even more marked bradycardia, the pulse rate ranging from 20 to 30 per minute. The attack is due to cerebral anæmia resulting from extreme bradycardia or ventricular standstill, and lasts from four to thirty seconds. The shorter attacks are characterised by transient dizziness, longer ones by brief syncopal periods. In the more severe seizures the breathing becomes stertorous, the face cyanosed, there is dilatation of both pupils, rigidity of the body, accompanied by clonic movements of the limbs. The pulse ceases for a few seconds, the jaw drops, and for a brief period the patient is to all appearances dead. No pulse is felt in either wrist and on auscultation the cardiac sounds are inaudible. Then a feeble sound is heard followed by a stronger, and a second later the pulse begins beating at about 30 per minute (one can feel the artery fill), the cyanosis lessens, the pupils contract, and consciousness returns. Many such fits may occur in succession.

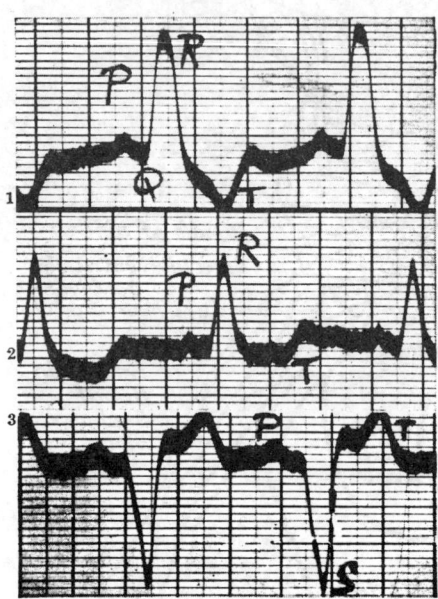

FIG. 46.—Lesion of the left bundle branch. Note (1) the widening of QRS to 0·12 sec. (normal less than 0·10 sec.), (2) the slurring of QRS, (3) the direction of T_1 and T_3, *i.e.*, opposite to R and to S.

Etiology.—The conditions of the Bundle which can produce heart block fall into three groups: (1) infective processes, (2) degenerative processes, and (3) the influence of drugs. Infective processes are occasionally a cause: rheumatism, diphtheria, pneumonia, influenza and scarlet fever. Degenerative processes include fibrosis, the result of old rheumatic fibrotic processes, interference with nutrition through disease of the coronary vessels, and tertiary syphilitic lesions of the heart muscle itself. Digitalis has a pronounced action in lowering conductivity of the Bundle, an effect which is most marked when the Bundle is already diseased, and which is usefully employed in the treatment of auricular fibrillation.

The *Prognosis* in complete heart block depends upon the presence of dyspnœa and other signs and symptoms of failure. Life is often prolonged for years, for the slow heart rate saves the heart muscle.

Treatment.—The attacks may be prevented by the subcutaneous injection of adrenalin ($\frac{1}{2}$–1 ml.) which in all probability acts directly on the Bundle of His via the sympathetic. Sublingual isoprenaline sulph. is also efficacious. Ephedrine sulph. in doses of gr. $\frac{1}{2}$ or gr. 1 three or four times a day by mouth or prednisolone are also used. If tertiary syphilis is present it must be treated.

2. SINO-AURICULAR (Supra-auricular) block. Here the stimulus appears to be blocked in the sino-auricular node, when the whole heart is silent and misses a beat (§ 64).

3. BUNDLE BRANCH BLOCK is a condition in which either the right or the left division of the bundle is interrupted by disease. Since the auricular impulse can travel freely through the main stem and the opposite intact branch of the Bundle,

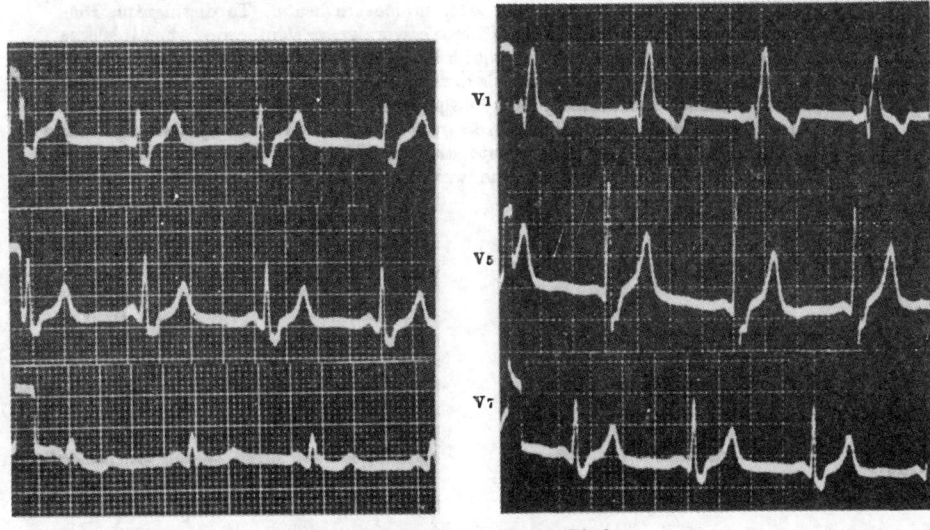

FIG. 47.—Right Bundle Branch Block.

the ventricular rate is undisturbed and is not slowed. *Symptoms* do not arise from this condition. *Diagnosis* is only possible by the Electrocardiogram (Figs. 46, 47). *Etiology.*—Bundle block not infrequently occurs in coronary atheroma, with aortic regurgitation, in coronary thrombosis, in chronic lung affections and in certain cases immediately prior to death. *Treatment* is of the cause. No special treatment for this type of block is required.

§ 72. *The Heart-beats occur in couples, with a pause after every alternate beat.*

This condition may be apparent or real, and may be due to:

(1) Regularly recurring PREMATURE BEATS; a common cause of which is DIGITALIS overdose. (Fig. 48.)

(2) PULSUS ALTERNANS. (Fig. 48.)

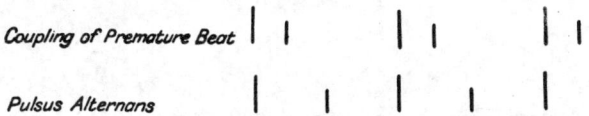

FIG. 48.—In Premature Beat the interval between the beats is unequal; in Pulsus Alternans the interval is equal.

(3) Extreme DICROTISM produces an appearance of coupling, but is distinguished from that due to premature contractions by the fact that

the apparent second beat occurs synchronously with the closure of the aortic valves, and is unaccompanied by a systolic heart sound. It occurs where the diastolic pressure is low but the aortic valve competent (§ 89).

§ 73. **Pulsus Alternans** is a condition in which every second ventricular beat is feebler than its predecessor and the rhythm remains regular. This sign is evidence of exhaustion of contractility and is usually of grave prognostic significance: it may be constant, or only appear occasionally after premature beats. To distinguish from a coupled pulse see Fig. 48. The condition is of very grave significance when it occurs with a slowly acting heart. With a quick pulse rate it need not be regarded with such apprehension, but its appearance is always a warning sign of cardiac exhaustion. Pulsus alternans is most readily shown in a pulse tracing, but can be easily diagnosed by the sphygmomanometer. If the pressure is raised above the systolic figure and allowed slowly to fall, only the alternate stronger beats will at first be heard by the stethoscope. At a lower pressure the weaker beats, evenly spaced between the stronger ones, then appear.

CHAPTER IV

INTRATHORACIC TUMOURS INCLUDING ANEURYSM OF THE THORACIC AORTA

Anatomy.—The mediastinum is the irregular space in the chest which lies between the two pleural sacs. For descriptive purposes it is divided into four parts—viz., the *middle mediastinum*, which is occupied by the heart and pericardial sac; the *anterior*, which is the space in front; the *posterior*, the space behind; and the *superior*, the space above the pericardial sac. The most important structures contained in these spaces are: The thymus or its remains; the arch of the aorta with its branches (innominate, left subclavian, and left carotid); the superior and inferior venæ cavæ, with the innominate and azygos veins; the pulmonary vessels, the trachea and bronchi; the vagus, recurrent laryngeal, phrenic, and splanchnic nerves; the cardiac and pulmonary plexuses; the roots of the lungs; the œsophagus, thoracic duct, lymphatic glands and vessels, and loose cellular tissue (Fig. 11). The lymphatic glands are important on account of the occurrence of enlargement in certain diseases to form a mediastinal tumour.

In recent years there has been a great change as to the frequency and the type of tumours within the chest. New growths of the bronchus now form by far the largest group of causes whereas aneurysm of the thoracic aorta is becoming a rarity. Early diagnosis of the type of tumour present has become much more accurate as the result of ancillary methods of investigation, particularly with X-rays.

PART A. SYMPTOMATOLOGY

The CARDINAL SYMPTOMS of mediastinal tumours are **Pain, Cough, Breathlessness** and a **Husky Voice.** Other symptoms include **Enlarged Veins** on the Chest Wall or in the neck, **Cyanosis, Dysphagia, Pyrexia** and **Anæmia.**

§ 77. **Pain** is a common early symptom. It may be located in the front or back of the chest and may radiate to one or both arms or to the abdomen. The types of pain are :—

(1) A persistent dull ache, worse on lying down, is often one of the first symptoms. It occurs with carcinoma of the bronchus, enlarged glands due to primary or secondary malignant disease as well as with other slowly growing tumours.

(2) A neuralgic pain occurs when there is pressure on the intercostal nerves: or it may be of a dull boring character when due to erosion of bone, as with an aneurysm of the ascending or descending thoracic aorta.

(3) A sharp stabbing pleuritic pain, made worse by coughing and deep breathing, may be an early symptom especially when the cause is pulmonary in origin. (See also § 103.)

125

(4) Pain and discomfort on swallowing occur when the tumour is œsophageal in origin, or when a new growth of the cardiac end of the stomach involves the lower œsophagus. In this latter case the pain, instead of being in the midline of the chest, may be located in the front or back of the left lower chest.

(5) Sudden severe pain in the chest accompanied by collapse is a symptom of a dissecting aneurysm of the aorta (§ 81).

The **Cough** is usually dry, but may be moist and accompanied by sputum when there is irritation of the bronchus. Mediastinal growths often cause the cough to commence when lying down at night, and to be accompanied by a sense of suffocation. A brassy or " gander " cough results from pressure on the trachea—when compression is marked tracheal stridor accompanies this characteristic cough. Hæmoptysis may occur.

The symptoms of mediastinal tumour which are due to **pressure** on the various structures around are as follows:

Breathlessness appears sooner or later in almost all cases. Stridulous breathing, which resembles tubular breathing heard without the aid of a stethoscope, indicates pressure upon the trachea and larger bronchi. The breathlessness is often paroxysmal, resembling asthma when there is pressure upon the heart or cardiac plexuses.

A **husky voice** is usually the result of involvement of the left recurrent laryngeal nerve. It is accompanied by abductor paralysis of the vocal cord.

Engorged veins in the neck with a compensatory enlargement of veins on the front of the chest and abdomen indicate obstruction of the superior vena cava. The face, neck and one or both arms may be œdematous and **cyanosed,** the extent of these signs depending on the anatomical position of the lesion in relation to the left or right innominate vein or the superior vena cava. The commonest cause of these signs is carcinoma of an upper lobe bronchus. Owing to its short course the inferior vena cava is scarcely ever involved by intrathoracic tumours.

Dysphagia from narrowing of the œsophagus is chiefly present with primary disease of the organ itself, or of the cardiac end of the stomach. Owing to its mobility, it is rarely a symptom of aortic aneurysm or of other tumours in the posterior mediastinum. A combination of coughing and vomiting up food immediately it is swallowed is the symptom of a fistula between the œsophagus and the trachea or main bronchus.

Pyrexia and **Anæmia** are fairly common with most mediastinal tumours. A low-grade temperature may be caused by the tumour itself: it is higher when there is secondary infection behind an obstructed bronchus. A persistent or a periodic temperature is almost invariable in mediastinal Hodgkin's disease.

PART B. PHYSICAL EXAMINATION

After taking a careful history, not only of the symptoms described above but also of the general health of the patient, a detailed physical examination of the chest should follow. The method of performing this is described under Diseases of the Lungs and Pleuræ (Chapter VI). However, in Mediastinal Tumour the signs can be classified as (*a*) the Signs of Displacement of Organs; (*b*) the Physical Signs of a Tumour and (*c*) Certain Signs special to the different kinds of Tumour.

§ 78. (*a*) The **Displacement of Organs** should be carefully looked for. The *trachea* should be palpated as it runs behind the manubrium sterni. It will be shifted to the affected side when there is collapse of an upper lobe bronchus, but will travel to the opposite side when it is being displaced by a large tumour. The *apex beat of the heart* may be displaced to the left or to the right of its normal position, usually in association with involvement of the lungs and pleurae. When a tumour compresses a main bronchus and produces *collapse of a part or the whole of one lung*, the apex beat moves to the affected side in association with signs of pulmonary collapse—reduced movement, an impaired percussion note, with reduced or absent breath sounds. The trachea and the heart are moved to the opposite side not only by a large tumour but also by the occurrence of a secondary pleural effusion.

(*b*) The **Physical Signs of a Tumour** may appear on the front or the back of the chest. They consist of (1) Dullness to percussion, corresponding to the position of the tumour. Normally percussion over the upper part of the sternum gives a more resonant note than over the lower part, but when a tumour lies behind the upper sternum this area becomes less resonant than lower down. (2) Auscultatory signs differ with the position and nature of the tumour. When it is solid the breath sounds will be tubular over it and there may be increased conduction of the heart sounds. Additional signs are: (3) Unequal pupils may appear owing to involvement of the first dorsal sympathetic nerve fibres or the sympathetic ganglia adjacent to the neck of the first rib. Usually the pupil on the affected side is contracted from paralysis of the sympathetic with an accompanying enophthalmos, ptosis of the upper eyelid and a malar flush (Horner's Syndrome). (4) Laryngoscopic examination will reveal recurrent laryngeal nerve paralysis. On the left side the nerve is usually involved as it hooks round the aortic arch, by carcinoma and occasionally by tuberculosis or an aortic aneurysm. (5) In every case a search should be made for enlarged superficial glands in the neck or axillæ and for liver enlargement due to deposits.

(*c*) The Signs Special to the different kinds of Tumour are described in §§ 81 *et seq.*, 138.

SPECIAL INVESTIGATIONS include Radiological Examination, Examination of the Blood, Sputum or Pleural fluid and Instrumental Methods. *Radiological Examination* must invariably be undertaken when a mediastinal tumour is suspected. The chest must be screened in the postero-anterior (and sometimes also in the antero-posterior position) as well as in the right and left oblique positions. A permanent record should always include a film taken in the postero-anterior and lateral positions. By this means the position and outline of the tumour, the presence or absence of expansile or of transmitted pulsation, the displacement of other organs, the presence of a pleural effusion and diaphragmatic paralysis are detected. In some cases it is valuable to examine the œsophagus and the fundus of the stomach with a barium sulphate emulsion, to perform bronchography or to take tomographic views in the postero-anterior or lateral positions.

Blood investigations may include a complete blood count, the erythrocyte sedimentation rate and serological tests for syphilis.

The *Sputum* and a *Pleural Effusion* may reveal the nature of any primary disease, or of a secondary infection, and may show characteristic malignant cells (§§ 119, 138, 1213).

Instrumental Methods include examination by bronchoscopy or œsophagoscopy. These should not be routine but undertaken with due regard to the risks involved and the information likely to be afforded. Although of great value in cases suspected to be due to carcinoma of the bronchus or of the œsophagus they may be highly dangerous in a case of aortic aneurysm.

PART C: DISEASES OF THE MEDIASTINUM: THEIR DIAGNOSIS, PROGNOSIS AND TREATMENT

Classification. There are eight clinical groups of tumours:—

Common.	*Rare* (in Great Britain).
I. Malignant Tumours.	V. Innocent Mediastinal Tumours.
II. Enlarged Mediastinal Glands.	VI. Suppurative Mediastinitis.
III. Retro-sternal Enlargement of the Thyroid Gland.	VII. Gummatous Mediastinitis.
IV. Aortic Aneurysm.	VIII. Enlarged Thymus.

The patient has pain or discomfort in the chest, A PERSISTENT COUGH, *often associated with* SHORTNESS OF BREATH *and there is* ABNORMAL DULLNESS *to percussion—the disease is likely to be due to a* MEDIASTINAL TUMOUR.

§ 79. I. **Malignant Tumours** form by far the largest group. PRIMARY growths are usually due to *carcinoma* of the bronchus which has recently become much more frequent (§ 138). Symptoms arise not only from the initial disease but by massive invasion of the mediastinal glands and its spread to the pleura. Carcinoma of the œsophagus causes symptoms in the gullet and rarely produces signs of mediastinal involvement. *Sarcoma,* in the form of lymphosarcoma and less commonly endothelial sarcoma, produces pressure on the mediastinal structures and may give the signs of a large mass especially in the superior mediastinum. In carcinoma and sarcoma the lymph glands above the clavicle usually enlarge at an early stage. SECONDARY growths in the lungs and in the mediastinal glands arise from carcinoma of the breast and from abdominal sources.

II. **Enlarged Mediastinal Glands** cause paroxysms of coughing, " croupy " or like whooping-cough especially at night, and if large enough may produce stridulous breathing from pressure on the trachea or larger bronchi. There are usually few physical signs but there may be impairment of percussion posteriorly in the upper half of the interscapular space and occasionally there is dullness over the upper half of the sternum. The *causes* of enlarged bronchial glands are:

(a) As described above, *malignant disease* of the glands is the most common cause.

(b) *Tuberculosis* is more common in children, or in adults of the non-immune races. With a primary infection the glands are the chief seat of the disease. Rarely the glands caseate and may form an abscess which opens into a bronchus. (Compare VI below.) Constitutional symptoms include cough, pyrexia, anorexia and night sweats.

(c) *Hodgkin's disease* (Lymphadenoma) may start in the mediastinal glands, and is then difficult to diagnose from lymphosarcoma. (See also § 584.)

(d) *Bronchitis* and the *pneumonia* which complicates measles, influenza and whooping-cough, are often attended by enlargement of the bronchial glands, which may occasionally be recognised in children.

(e) *Whooping-cough*, without bronchitis or other disease of the lungs, may give rise to swelling of the bronchial glands, although the condition may be hard to make out. Some observers consider that it is the pressure of these glands which causes the paroxysms of whooping-cough at night.

(f) *Sarcoidosis* produces few mediastinal symptoms and is usually recognised by X-ray examination. The mediastinal glands are never very large but persist for months or years. There may be a low-grade pyrexia, the erythrocyte sedimentation rate is usually high and there may be other signs of the disease (§§ 141, 710).

III. When an ENLARGED THYROID grows behind the sternum it often produces pressure on the trachea with a sense of suffocation and shortness of breath. This occurs especially with a colloid goitre and sometimes with an adenomatous goitre.

If there is **abnormal dullness** *near the base of the heart, which is accompanied by* PULSATION, *and on auscultation, there is a* REINFORCED OR RINGING SECOND HEART SOUND—*perhaps a systolic or diastolic murmur—the disease is probably* ANEURYSM OF THE AORTA.

IV. § 80. **Intrathoracic Aneurysm.**—In regard to the anatomy of this disease, the student should study Fig. 11 (p. 52). Since the introduction of penicillin for the treatment of syphilis, this condition has become comparatively rare.

All three parts—the ascending, transverse or descending portions of the thoracic aorta—may be affected. The dilatation may be of fusiform shape, or less frequently saccular. The fusiform aneurysm gives few physical signs: the saccular aneurysm produces many more symptoms and signs of a tumour for it compresses or displaces some organs and erodes hard structures such as bones and cartilages. According to its position, aneurysm of the aorta may be very easy or difficult to detect. When it involves the ascending aorta, near the front of the chest, it is so revealed by definite *physical signs*: but when the transverse or descending portions are involved and the tumour extends backwards, there may be no physical signs and even *pressure symptoms* may be obscure.

Symptoms common to aortic aneurysm in all positions will be considered first, as these will probably first attract our notice. We shall then turn to certain others special to the ascending, transverse and descending parts of the aorta respectively.

Symptoms COMMON TO ALL POSITIONS:

1. Dyspnœa is often one of the earliest complaints. When the aneurysm presses on the trachea, as in aneurysm of the aortic arch, it is persistent and stridulous in character. When dyspnœa is due to narrowed orifices of the coronary arteries it is often paroxysmal. Orthopnœa of a marked degree may be present.

2. A gander cough with a characteristic brassy quality is often present. Paralysis of the left vocal cord due to pressure on the left recurrent laryngeal nerve is common, causing hoarseness or even aphonia.

3. Pain in the chest or back is frequently worse at night or on exertion. Short of definite anginal attacks, patients are liable to feelings of suffocation, constriction or " spasm " in the chest. Such attacks are often brought on by movements of the neck. When the coronary orifices are involved pain may be in the form of angina of effort; when there is pressure on nerves it may be neuralgic, and when due to erosion of the bone it is of a dull boring character.

4. Palpation of the chest may reveal two signs. A diastolic shock is felt over the aortic base synchronously with the second sound: or systolic pulsation may be seen or felt locally over the front of the chest—especially if the patient is sat forwards.

5. A ringing aortic second sound is much more frequent with aneurysms of the first part of the aorta.

6. Unequal pulses may be detected: it occurs when the aneurysm is so placed as to cause a difference in arterial pressure in the great vessels arising from the aorta. The sign is not, however, diagnostic for atheroma of the great vessels may cause it.

7. Unequal pupils may be due to unequal blood pressures in the iris, from inequality of the carotid blood pressures. It is more commonly due to irritation of the sympathetic nerve causing dilatation of the pupil on the same side, or later on to paralysis of the sympathetic as part of Horner's syndrome.

8. The heart may be displaced when the aneurysm is large, usually to the left.

9. Hæmoptysis may occur: it is slight when due to congestion of the lungs and profuse with a leak from the aneurysm itself.

10. Left ventricular failure and later right ventricular failure may occur.

(a) Symptoms peculiar to aneurysm of the **ascending** or **first part of the arch**. In marked cases the *Physical Signs* are unmistakable. (i.) Inspection often reveals visible pulsation over the right upper intercostal spaces. (ii.) Palpation may give the feeling of a systolic thrill, or of a diastolic shock unless the aortic ring is stretched by the aneurysm. An expansile suprasternal pulsation and a tracheal tug may be palpable. (iii.) By percussion, dullness is detected to the right of the upper part of the sternum, continuous with the praecordial dullness. (iv.) On auscultation, a systolic murmur may or may not be heard. Since the aortic ring is frequently involved, all the signs and symptoms of aortic incompetence may also be present (see § 60). (v.) Pressure on the right bronchus leads to signs of partial or complete collapse of the right lung; and pressure on the superior vena cava causes œdema of the neck and arms together with the development of a collateral circulation on the front of the chest. The right recurrent laryngeal nerve is rarely involved and then there is right laryngeal paralysis.

(b) Symptoms of aneurysm of the **aortic arch** are often very similar to those of other intrathoracic tumours. (i.) Symptoms (2), (5), (6) and (7) above are usually marked. (ii.) The dyspnœa may be paroxysmal or continuous, with inspiratory stridor, owing to pressure on the, trachea. (iii.) Pressure on the left bronchus may lead to diminished breath sounds in the left lung, partial collapse or bronchiectasis. (iv.) Tracheal tugging is a characteristic sign of aneurysm in this situation. Standing beside the patient, whose head is held level and straight, the examiner defines the cricoid with finger and thumb, and lifts it upwards without backward pressure, away from the thorax. If the aorta is in close contact with the bronchial tree, either by pressure of an aneurysm or by adhering to it by growth, a systolic downward tracheal tug will be felt. (v.) There may be a thrill on palpating the suprasternal notch and dullness on percussion over the manubrium.

(c) Aneurysm affecting the **descending aorta** may be very difficult to diagnose. (i.) Pain in the back and dysphagia are the most constant symptoms. The pain may pass to the side, following the course of an intercostal nerve. It is due to erosion of the vertebræ, which can be demonstrated radiologically. (ii.) Other pressure symptoms are dysphagia, from pressure upon the œsophagus; wasting, from pressure upon the thoracic duct, and signs in the left lung, from pressure upon its bronchi. (iii.) The most diagnostic sign when present is the " Lateral Thoracic Jerk " (Bourne).[1] The whole thorax is jerked to the left during systole.

[1] The *Lancet*, 1932, II, 68.

This can best be seen by inspection from the foot of the bed. The jerk is caused by the fact that the ventricles, the aneurysm, and the vertebral column are in direct propinquity, and a thrust is thus transmitted laterally to the left chest wall from the left side of the vertebral bodies when the first two structures become hardened during systole. (iv.) If the swelling enlarges, physical signs on auscultation and percussion may become apparent in the left (occasionally the right) scapular region; and in advanced cases there may even be a pulsating swelling without the knowledge of the patient. Osler found that in some cases there is absence of pulsation in the femoral arteries.

Etiology.—(1) Aortic aneurysm is far more frequent in men than in women, especially between the ages of thirty-five and fifty. (2) It is more frequent among soldiers, blacksmiths and others who do laborious work, probably due to the fact that they are subjected to sudden and severe muscular exertion and heart-strain. (3) Syphilis is the sole cause of aneurysm of the ascending aorta and accounts for the majority of cases of thoracic aortic aneurysm, and for many of those of the abdominal aorta.   Atheroma is the cause in the remaining cases: it generally produces a fusiform aneurysm, and is responsible for a small number of cases of aneurysm of the descending thoracic aorta and of a higher percentage of aneurysms of the abdominal aorta (§ 263). (4) Some cases of aneurysm date from an injury as an exciting or secondary cause.

Diagnosis.—The diagnosis of an aneurysm is sometimes difficult in the early stages. *Mediastinal growths* may have the same pressure symptoms as aneurysm. Pressure upon the veins is more common with growth than with aneurysm, and there are no physical signs referable to the heart, no murmur on auscultation over the dull region, the area of dullness is usually not so limited or defined, there is no expansile pulsation over the tumour, and there are signs of collateral venous circulation. The course of mediastinal tumours rarely lasts longer than eighteen months. X-ray examination reveals an expansile pulsating tumour in connection with, or seen to be arising from, the thoracic aorta. Under no circumstances should paracentesis be attempted. A Wassermann or Kahn test also helps to distinguish aortic syphilis and tumour. The diagnosis from *cardiac valvular disease* is made by the pressure symptoms. Moreover, aneurysm does not cause cardiac enlargement unless there is secondary aortic incompetence. Some of the local signs of a fusiform aneurysm may be produced by a *dilated and rigid aorta*, but here the pressure symptoms are wanting. The *throbbing aorta* of hypertension and of aortic regurgitation, as felt in the suprasternal notch, is apt to be mistaken for aortic aneurysm: the throbbing aorta in Graves' disease and severe cases of anæmia may also give rise to difficulty.

Prognosis.—Treatment can do much to prolong life, and the patient may live a good many years if his occupation does not necessitate overexertion. Death may occur from rupture, congestive failure or complications. Rupture usually leads to a sudden copious hæmorrhage, which terminates life; but sometimes there is a slight leakage, which may recur each few days. With aneurysm of the *ascending* aorta rupture usually takes place into the pericardium, pulmonary artery, or superior vena cava; with aneurysm of the *transverse* arch, into the trachea (a frequent situation) or bronchi; and, when the *descending* aorta is involved, the blood usually finds its way into the pleura or œsophagus. The process may be so gradual that there is no sudden onset of symptoms, such as dyspnœa, cyanosis, or bleeding, and death may not occur for some time. The severity of any case is measured by the amount of dyspnœa present and the rapidity of the evolution of symptoms. Other consequences or complications are usually due to the effects of pressure—such as collapse of the lung or a low form of pneumonia, hydrothorax and œdema of the head and neck.

Treatment will depend on the stage at which the diagnosis is made. In early cases, a full course of antisyphilitic treatment may be very helpful in arresting the course of this disease. The patient must be kept in bed for 2 months. To avoid the dangers of the Jarisch–Herxheimer reaction it is necessary to give an initial course of potassium iodide (in increasing doses up to 45–60 gr. t.i.d.) and weekly injections of metallic bismuth (0·2 G.) for 4 weeks. Then a full course of procaine penicillin (600,000 units daily) should be given for 4 weeks. After an interval of one month the course of penicillin should be repeated. Strenuous physical and mental work must be avoided subsequently. In late cases penicillin has little effect and treatment should be directed to the complications and especially heart failure. For the pain, morphia injections are used; if of anginal character, nitroglycerin. Even if the dyspnœa is very urgent, tracheotomy is not called for. If there be an external swelling, some elastic support is needed. Phenobarbitone is valuable for palpitation. For venous distension or severe dyspnœa, venesection may be performed. Surgical measures have been adopted from time to time in the treatment of superficial aneurysms, but they are not free from danger and have proved of little value.

§ 81. A **Dissecting Aneurysm** occurs most frequently in the thoracic aorta, usually in its ascending portion some little distance from the aortic valve. An abnormal channel forms between the intima and the media and may extend upwards or downwards—in the latter case the blood may find its way back into the normal aortic lumen producing a " false aorta." The condition occurs in elderly persons, much more commonly in men than women.

Symptoms.—The two presenting symptoms are pain and/or shock. In 50 per cent. of cases there is no pain. (i.) The sudden agonising pain is occasionally so abrupt that the patient thinks he has been kicked in the back. The pain is usually felt in the mid-dorsal region and may extend forwards around the lower chest and downwards towards the legs. (ii.) Shock is usually severe and the blood pressure may be unrecordable. The patient is very collapsed, grey and cyanosed, sweating and often develops a slight temperature and leucocytosis. When the pulses return there may be ischæmia in one arm. Extension of the false channel causes a variety of symptoms: when into the pericardium it causes sudden death, when it involves the mouth of the innominate or carotid arteries it produces hemiparesis or hemiplegia, and when it involves the subclavian or common iliac arteries it causes pain, numbness and coldness of the corresponding limb. Spread into the pleura produces a blood-stained effusion and into the renal arteries results in hæmaturia or anuria. The physical signs are variable and often not diagnostic, but diminution or loss of pulsation in one or both of the brachial or femoral arteries is highly suggestive: secondary aortic regurgitation may develop.

Diagnosis is from coronary thrombosis or an acute abdominal condition, such as a perforated peptic ulcer. An antero-posterior chest film may show diagnostic widening of the aortic shadow.

Etiology.—The condition arises from degenerative changes in the subintimal structures of the aorta. The immediate cause is a transverse tear in the inner coat, caused by local necrosis or by the biochemical changes associated with atherosclerosis.

The *Prognosis* is bad and death commonly occurs within a few hours from extension into the pericardium, pleura or mediastinum. A few cases recover when secondary involvement of the main branches of the aorta does not supervene.

Treatment is by the use of morphia and supporting measures combined with good nursing.

V. INNOCENT MEDIASTINAL TUMOURS are rare. They include (1) cysts of congenital origin—dermoid, teratomatous and pleuro-pericardial cysts. The last is not uncommon but rarely causes symptoms, being discovered on routine X-ray examination. (2) Hydatid cysts. (3) Lipoma, fibroma, neurofibroma and enchondroma, the latter growing from the sternum.

VI. SUPPURATIVE MEDIASTINITIS in an acute or chronic form and perhaps producing an abscess of the mediastinum is a rare condition which may affect the anterior or posterior mediastinum, or both. (i.) The most prominent symptom is pain in the front or back of the chest. (ii.) Pyrexia is present, usually intermittent, with the rigors, sweats and weakness which attend all serious inflammations. (iii.) Dullness, with œdema and redness, may be present over the upper part of the sternum if the disease be in the anterior mediastinum. Pulsation communicated from the aorta may be present, and lead to a diagnosis of aneurysm, but the pulsation is not expansile, and fluctuation may be felt. (iv.) The presence of leucocytosis is an important diagnostic feature. The causes of acute mediastinitis are trauma from a perforating wound, an impacted dental plate in the œsophagus and occasionally from the passage of an œsophagoscope or a bougie: other cases are due to carcinoma of the œsophagus or bronchus. The chronic form is usually due to tuberculous disease, rarely to actinomycosis. It may rupture in various directions.

VII. Diffuse GUMMATOUS MEDIASTINITIS, especially affecting the mediastinum, may give all the symptoms and signs of a tumour. The Wassermann reaction and the response to antisyphilitic remedies are diagnostic.

VIII. ENLARGED THYMUS.—A certain degree of enlargement is normal to childhood, and may cause dullness over the manubrium. It begins to decrease after the second year of life, and should have disappeared by adult life. An enlarged thymus is also frequently found in myasthenia gravis, Graves' disease, and rarely in Addison's disease, myxœdema and rickets. Simple inflammation, œdema and tubercle may affect the gland. Tumours may occur—thymoma, cysts, sarcoma, rarely epithelioma.

The *diagnosis* of an intrathoracic tumour is made by a careful consideration of all the facts, and is greatly helped by X-ray screening and taking films in different positions. X-ray tomography can materially aid. When a tumour is accompanied by a blood-stained pleural effusion, malignancy is usually present.

Prognosis.—In cases of intrathoracic tumours which are large enough to produce symptoms the prognosis is unfavourable. Moreover, all of these conditions entail much suffering to the patient. Malignant tumours are fatal in six to twelve months, depending upon the site and progress of the growth. Innocent tumours may last for a long time or may be removable surgically. Syphilitic, tuberculous and simple inflammatory glandular enlargements may recover under treatment, but even in these no confident prognosis of recovery can be given in any case. Suppurative mediastinitis may open externally or into the pleura, and run a course of a few days or weeks only; other cases are chronic, and last for years, or lead to pulmonary gangrene and other serious complications when the pus burrows into adjoining organs. An enlarged thymus may lead to sudden death from pressure upon the trachea.

Treatment in intrathoracic tumour is almost wholly palliative. For treatment of carcinoma of the bronchus see § 138, and for aneurysm, see § 80. Abscesses, hydatids, dermoids or growths connected with the sternum should be dealt with by the surgeon. X-ray and radium applications should be used in glandular and malignant tumours when necessary. Penicillin and other forms of chemotherapy are indicated for infective conditions.

CHAPTER V

THE PULSE AND ARTERIES

§ 82. The Meaning of " The Pulse."—The pulse is the wave of increased pressure which passes along the arteries with each contraction of the heart. It is important to distinguish between the transmission of pressure within the arteries and the movement of the blood itself.

The clinical features to be studied in palpation of the pulse are its (1) frequency, (2) rhythm, (3) force, (4) volume, (5) tension and character, and (6) the state of the arterial wall. These features depend on the frequency and rhythm of contraction of the left ventricle, on the strength of the contractions and on the output at each beat. They also depend on the elasticity of the arteries and the peripheral resistance encountered by the flow of blood, especially in the arterioles and capillaries. On account of the peripheral resistance the pulse generally ceases at the arterioles, but when the arterioles are relaxed the pulse is often transmitted through the capillaries and may even appear in the veins. *Capillary pulsation* is thus to be seen in a healthy person who has taken exercise on a hot day, and it is a clinical feature of aortic regurgitation (§ 60). In the great veins near the heart a pulse is normally present. Visible *venous pulsation* is to be seen in the veins at the base of the neck in congestive heart failure, and is due to tricuspid regurgitation (§ 59). Venous pulsation is sometimes seen in the veins on the backs of the hands in Graves' disease.

§ 83. Clinical Investigation.—Examination of the pulse provides evidence of great value both as to the state of the circulatory system and the general condition of the subject. Whatever examination is to be made, palpation of the pulse is the first observation to make. If the subject is nervous or emotionally disturbed, or has lately hurried, the observation is repeated later when the pulse has settled. For accurate record the pulse is always taken under similar conditions as to posture, time of day, relation to meals, etc. The radial pulse is generally chosen, since it is easily accessible and lies against bone (the radius). If it is aberrant, the opposite radial artery is palpated. Whenever disease of the cardiovascular system is suspected, both radial pulses should be felt simultaneously and carefully compared. The pulse can also be felt in other arteries near the surface, such as the temporal, facial, dorsalis pedis and posterior tibial arteries, and in the abdominal aorta. To feel the radial pulse three fingers are placed over the course of the artery, the index finger nearest the heart. Allowance is made for the thickness of the subcutaneous tissues.

The special features of the pulse may be brought out more clearly by holding the forearm up when palpating the pulse. The main points

136

to note have been mentioned in § 41.   After noting the frequency, rhythm and character of the pulse (the term character refers to the nature of the pulse wave, its rise, summit and fall), the tension is estimated by the amount of pressure exercised by the forefinger in order to obliterate the pulse wave and prevent it reaching the middle finger.   In case there is a return pulse wave through the palmar arches it may be necessary at the same time to obliterate the pulse with the third finger.   Finally, after obliterating the pulse by pressure with all three fingers, the wall of the artery is felt by rolling the empty vessel under them.

The SPHYGMOGRAPH is an instrument employed to obtain a record on smoked paper of the characters of the pulse.   With Dudgeon's instrument strapped to the wrist, a system of levers magnifies the pulse wave and records a tracing.

The SPHYGMOGRAM or sphygmographic tracing is useful as a graphic record of the pulse, but its readings can never be quite accurate.   Fig. 49a is a normal pulse tracing.   Fig. 49b shows the principal named parts of which it consists.   The first or *percussion wave* is caused by the arrival of the pulse in the artery under the sphygmograph.   Its form is determined by the output per beat of the ventricle, the rate

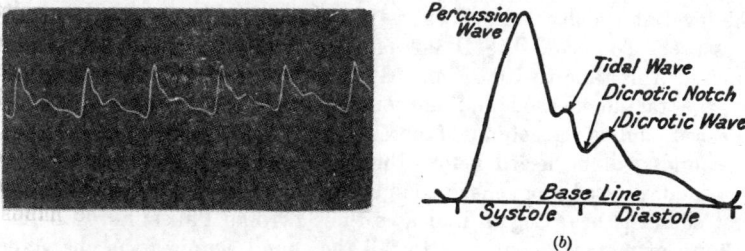

FIG. 49.

(a)—NORMAL PULSE TRACING, taken with Dudgeon's Sphygmograph. (b)—NORMAL PULSE TRACING magnified, with the names of the principal parts.   The dicrotic (or aortic) notch indicates the closure of the aortic valves, and therefore the termination of the ventricular systole and the commencement of the ventricular diastole.   The diastolic line is that part of the tracing from the dicrotic notch to the next percussion wave.

at which the blood is ejected from the ventricle into the aorta, the peripheral resistance and the extensibility of the arterial walls.   The percussion wave is abrupt and the pulse is sudden when the diastolic pressure is low and the ventricle has little resistance to overcome in discharging its contents.   The *tidal wave* represents, according to Crighton Bramwell, the summation of the outgoing percussion wave, and waves reflected back from the periphery of the arterial field.   It is prominent in aortic stenosis and hypertension, for in both conditions ventricular pressure is well maintained throughout systole: the summation of the percussion and the reflected waves may cause the tidal wave to be higher than the percussion wave producing an anacrotic pulse.   In aortic regurgitation, on the other hand, the ventricle ejects most of its contents during the early part of systole, because of the lower diastolic pressure. During the latter part of systole the ventricular output is much reduced, the falling pressure tends to neutralise the wave reflected from the periphery.   Hence the tidal wave is inconspicuous.   The *dicrotic wave* indicates the rebound of blood against the closed aortic valve.   It is most marked with a forcibly beating heart, a low peripheral resistance and an elastic arterial wall.

Many instruments have been devised for the **measurement of the blood pressure.**   For practical purposes only the aneroid and the mercurial manometers need be considered. The former is portable, but should be checked against a mercurial manometer from time to time. The sphygmomanometer type of mercurial manometer, reading up to 260 or 300 mm., is the more reliable. The column of mercury should be open to direct atmospheric pressure and unspillable. The armlet is at least 5 inches (12 cm.) wide, and tapers after the first 18 inches. The cuff is better made of fabric than leather, because fabric is more easily adjusted. The armlet is wrapped round the patient's upper arm well above the bend of the elbow. The second turn fixes the upper limit of the armlet, the third turn fixes its lower limit so that, when the rubber bag contained in the armlet is inflated, an even pressure over the whole width of the armlet will be exerted. The sphygmomanometer is placed at about the level of the heart and the patient's arm extended on the bed or couch. To record the Systolic blood pressure, the pressure in the mercury column is quickly raised above the level at which pulsation is felt by the fingers placed over the radial artery. By turning the screw-cap attached to the pump, the column of mercury is immediately allowed to fall gently and the level at which the first beat is felt in the radial artery is the systolic pressure. To record the Diastolic blood pressure the armlet is again inflated, this time to 10–15 mm. Hg. above the systolic level determined by the tactile method and no sound is heard. The pressure is again released, and as the column of mercury falls, four different tones, or phases of sound, will be heard before there is complete silence. (1) The first phase consists of short sharp sounds, and the mercury level at which the first sound is heard again indicates the Systolic Pressure. (2) As the column of mercury continues to fall the sound acquires the character of a murmur. This phase is often of short duration and is usually followed by the *silent phase*. (3) Then comes the third phase with loud and clear sounds; this is the longest and most distinct phase. (4) The clear sounds suddenly become dull and distant; the level of the mercury column at which this occurs is the Diastolic Pressure.

The Systolic Pressure indicates the maximum work of the heart. The Diastolic Pressure may be regarded as representing the resistance to be overcome by the heart when the aortic valves are opened: it is the more constant, more significant and less liable to alter with nervous influence.

In practice the blood pressure is often recorded in even numbers. There is a considerable variation in the figures for normal subjects and fluctuations readily occur (see *Fallacies*). Readings are usually taken sitting or lying down and after the patient's confidence has been gained. The figures for normal adults are usually within the range 100–140 mm. systolic and 60–90 mm. diastolic. In young infants the figures are around 66 mm. systolic and 40 mm. diastolic. The blood pressure in adolescence and early adult life is often somewhat raised. It returns to normal with maturity. The average reading in 150 young soldiers aged 23 to 27, in the fourteenth week of training, was 135 mm. Hg systolic and 80 mm.

Hg diastolic. The systolic pressure tends to increase with advancing years. The saying that the systolic pressure should not exceed 100 plus the age is not very accurate. Old people often have nearly normal systolic pressures and many live to good age with a relatively high systolic pressure. In general terms, a systolic pressure above 170 mm. Hg or a diastolic above 90 mm. Hg is pathological. Pressures below these levels may, however, be too high for the particular individual and of clinical importance.

The following figures give the average found in several thousand actual readings. The range of the normal limit is not more than 15 mm. above or below. Age 21–30: 124 (*systolic*), 82 (*diastolic*); 31–40: 126 and 84; 41–50: 130 and 86; 51–60: 134 and 90.

Fallacies. (1) Although it is possible to take the systolic blood by auscultation, incorrect readings may be obtained when a long silent gap is present. A silent gap may, for example, occur between 160 and 140 mm. Hg when the systolic pressure is 200 mm. Hg. If the auditory method alone is used and the cuff is inflated to a pressure of 150 mm. Hg the systolic blood pressure may be recorded as 140 mm. Hg instead of 200 mm. Hg. This error can never occur if the tactile method of recording is always used.

(2) In a nervous subject, the systolic pressure as taken by auscultation frequently gives higher figures than the tactile reading. Even with the latter method the initial systolic reading may be considerably higher than the true value: if a nervous factor is suspected the patient should be allowed to relax on a couch for five minutes and a fresh reading taken. More accurate figures are obtained in such patients if readings are taken in the patient's own home than in a busy clinic. Recent excitement or exertion and fatigue may also give figures higher than normal.

(3) In grossly obese patients with huge upper arms, a larger armlet than the usual 5-inch variety is needed. The narrower armlet in common use will cause fictitiously high readings to be recorded. This error accounts in part for the high blood pressure readings noted in obese patients, the benign course taken and the apparent fall of blood pressure with weight reduction. Weight loss in the grossly obese with benign hypertension also causes a true fall in the blood pressure.

The PULSE PRESSURE is the difference between the systolic and the diastolic pressure, *e.g.*, with 120 mm. Hg systolic and 80 mm. Hg diastolic, the pulse pressure = 40 mm. A high pulse pressure may be caused by a lowered peripheral resistance, by aortic incompetence (§ 60) and by loss of elasticity in the arterial system. A lowered peripheral resistance due to vaso-dilatation occurs physiologically in warm weather and during exercise; it occurs pathologically in febrile states, thyrotoxicosis, in arterio-venous shunts as with arterio-venous aneurysms, with highly vascular growths, Paget's disease of bone and in many other conditions. With a decreased peripheral resistance not only does the diastolic pressure fall but the systolic pressure rises consequent on the increased return to the heart.

§ 84. Rapid Pulse (Tachycardia).—The rapidity or frequency of the heart beat varies considerably within the range of normal health due to variations in the rate of impulse production in the normal-pace-maker (the sino-auricular node). This is called sinus tachycardia. The normal pulse rate is about 70 per minute. A few people have pulse rates under 60 or over 80, but such must not be accepted as within normal limits without careful consideration. Rarely a pulse rate of 50 or just under, or of 90 or just over, is compatible with perfect *health*. The pulse tends to be faster in the female than in the male. It varies at different ages. In the fœtus and new-born infant its average rate is 140 per minute; under 1 year, 120; under 3 years, 100; from 7 to 14, 90; from 14 to 21, 80; from 21 to 65, 70; in old age, 80 per minute. The pulse is *normally* more rapid during the menstrual period and menopause, in the evenings and after meals. After a severe illness and in asthenic states the pulse more easily becomes rapid. When the tachycardia is due to *simple causes*, not the result of myocardial changes, the number of the beats falls ten to twenty per minute when the patient alters his position from standing to lying. Exercise, emotion, meals, fever and sleep modify the rate, and the electrocardiogram is normal. These features differentiate simple tachycardia from Paroxysmal Auricular Tachycardia, in which the pulse-rate is unaffected by posture, exercise, etc. (§ 66).

The **pathological** causes of sinus tachycardia are numerous. (1) *Pyrexia* is the most common. (2) Early *tuberculosis* should always be borne in mind. Any other *bacterial* infection is a common cause, *e.g.*, streptococcal and pneumococcal infections, whether generalised or focal. Pulse frequency is increased in the acute specific fevers, especially in scarlet fever. (3) Of *endogenous toxæmias*: (i.) Graves' disease is the most common; close observation for larval forms of this disease should be made in any obscure case of tachycardia; (ii.) uræmia; (iii.) malignant disease, especially when undergoing degenerative changes; (iv.) all blood diseases with moderate and severe anæmia. (4) *Exogenous toxæmia* includes a large variety of drugs and poisons, such as tobacco, alcohol, tea, coffee, thyroid extract, belladonna and atropine. (5) *Nervous states*, including ordinary emotional disturbance, often of trivial kind; neurasthenia, anxiety neurosis and neuro-circulatory asthenia are common causes in which the border-line between physiological and pathological disturbance is hard to define. (6) Most forms of *heart disease*, toxic, inflammatory or degenerative, and whether acute or chronic. Increased pulse frequency is an important sign of heart failure. Forms of tachycardia in which the stimulus for contraction arises from an abnormal focus are described in § 66.

§ 85. **Slow Pulse** (Bradycardia). A slow pulse should be verified by counting the frequency of heart beats on listening to the apex. A frequency of 60 per minute or under requires careful consideration, as it may be the first indication of serious organic disease such as heart block or cerebral tumour. Bradycardia may be a personal idiosyncrasy and is compatible with perfect *health*. It is sometimes familial. A slow heart rate is an advantage because it allows of an increased cardiac output without increase of heart rate. In a group of 28 Marathon runners examined by Bramwell and Ellis the average heart rate was 58, and

4 of these had heart rates under 50, while only 9 had heart rates over 60. In healthy subjects bradycardia is due to a slow rate of impulse production in the sino-auricular node. It is known as *sinus bradycardia.*

Pathologically, sinus bradycardia may be (1) the result of *reflex* nervous *effects,* via the vagus nerve; *e.g.,* with an overactive carotid sinus. (2) Bradycardia is one of the cardinal features of myxœdema, and other states of *lowered metabolism,* such as exposure to cold, starvation, anorexia nervosa, cachexia and melancholia except in the terminal stages of these conditions. It is associated with a low basal metabolic rate. (3) *Toxic conditions:* (a) endogenous, such as jaundice, diabetes and uræmia, and (b) exogenous, such as may be due to digitalis, strophanthus and opium. At first tobacco may slow the heart. (4) Bradycardia is not uncommon in *convalescence* from acute infection, *e.g.,* influenza, and in exhaustion states. A pulse rate low in proportion to the fever is found with infections by the typhoid and salmonella groups, *E. coli,* and sometimes staphylococcal infections and influenza. (5) *Increased intracranial pressure* of whatever etiology. A slow and irregular pulse may occur in meningitis. Bradycardia in heart disease is generally due to heart block (§ 71). *Temporary slowing* of the pulse rate occurs with pressure on the vagus in the neck, and characteristically in an ordinary fainting attack (vaso-vagal slowing).

§ 86. The **Irregular Pulse,** apart from *Sinus arrhythmia,* indicates an abnormal action of the heart. Pulse irregularities are dealt with in § 41, and the heart conditions responsible for them in § 63. A few additional points may be noted here. Sinus arrhythmia (§ 65), which is probably due to rhythmic alterations in vagal tone, is most common in young persons and is physiological. Bramwell has observed the association of pronounced sinus arrhythmia with a liability to simple fainting attacks, and he attributes both to an over-active vagal mechanism. *Premature beats* (§ 64), unless very frequent, can be recognised by a regular pulse interrupted by an occasional irregularity recurring rarely, or say once in every 5 to 10 beats. The diagnosis is made by auscultation of the heart, and confirmed by electrocardiogram, especially if intrinsic disease of the heart is suspected. *Auricular fibrillation* (§ 69) is recognised by the irregularity in which no two beats or intervals are alike: exercise considerably exaggerates this irregularity and also the rate of the heart, whereas premature beats usually disappear with increased frequency of the heart beat.

In auricular fibrillation the apex and pulse rates must be counted at the same time. The pulse rate is generally less than the apex beat—and the difference between the two rates (the " pulse deficit ") is represented thus, $A/p. = 124/92$. With recovery the pulse deficit becomes less, and it disappears when every ventricular beat reaches the radial artery.

§ 87. The **Quality of the Pulse** may also change in various valvular diseases of the heart. A collapsing or Corrigan pulse occurs with aortic incompetence (§ 60), whereas a slow rising anacrotic or plateau pulse, *pulsus tardus*, occurs in aortic stenosis when there is little or no regurgitation through the stiffened valves. It is due to the ventricle being forced to empty its contents more slowly, and so throughout the ejection phase of systole the rate of discharge of blood into the aorta is much more uniform. Mitral stenosis causes a small pulse, *pulsus parvus*, but if mitral incompetence is marked, the pulse is full and may tend to take on the collapsing quality of aortic incompetence.

Pulsus alternans denotes alternate weaker and stronger ventricular contractions. It is occasionally diagnosed by recognising an alternate weaker and stronger pulse, but it is readily diagnosed when taking the systolic pressure by the auditory method (and see § 73).

In *pulsus paradoxus* there is considerable, or almost complete, disappearance of the pulse with deep inspiration. In the normal person during deep inspiration and deep expiration there is a waxing and waning of the venous return to the heart leading to a slightly stronger ventricular output during inspiration with a slightly increased pulse volume and pulse pressure. When a large pericardial effusion or constrictive pericarditis impedes the filling of the auricles, the output of the left ventricle is reduced during deep inspiration and increased with expiration resulting in waning and waxing of the pulse volume and pulse pressure.

The *dicrotic pulse* is due to a marked dicrotic wave. It is said to simulate coupled beats, but once felt it is quite distinctive. It is common in asthenic states with a full soft pulse, as in typhoid fever.

Pulseless disease (Takayashu's disease) occurs more commonly in Japan than elsewhere, as the result of progressive obliterative endarteritis of the vessels to the head, neck and arms, producing absent brachial and radial pulses. *Symptoms.—* The disease chiefly affects young women. There may be (i.) syncopal attacks, fits, strokes and psychological changes due to cerebral ischæmia; (ii.) degeneration of the retina or the iris with opacities in the lens or cornea; (iii.) ischæmic atrophy of the skin of the face and of the gums; (iv.) fatigue of the arms after slight use; (v.) cardiac hypertrophy; (vi.) usually low pyrexia, tachycardia and a high sedimentation rate. *Treatment* is purely symptomatic.

§ 88. The term **Blood Pressure** refers to the tension in the *systemic arterial system*, and usually to the pressure in the brachial artery. It depends on two main factors—(1) the peripheral resistance, which is of cardinal importance; (2) the output of the left ventricle. Any gross variation in blood pressure is due to alteration of one or both of these factors.

The *pulmonary blood pressure* has, with the advent of cardiac surgery, become of importance. It can be measured by cardiac catheterisation (p. 59) and in the healthy adult averages 16 mm. (systolic) and 7 mm. (diastolic). In disease it may be considerably above the upper limits of normal (30 mm. systolic, 15 mm. diastolic). An increased pulmonary pressure is indicated by an accentuated pulmonary second sound, signs of hypertrophy of the right ventricle (§ 54) and by the presence of right axis deviation in the electrocardiogram (Fig. 32). The pressure is raised in left ventricular failure, mitral stenosis, many forms of congenital heart disease and in arteriolar sclerosis of the pulmonary vessels. It rises suddenly when a large pulmonary embolus becomes impacted—acute cor pulmonale.

The *venous blood pressure* undergoes a general increase in right sided or congestive heart failure.   There is a local engorgement of veins behind a local obstructive lesion.

High Blood Pressure (Syn. Hypertension, Hyperpiesis,[1]) is due to many different causes.   It is a physical sign and not a disease *sui generis*.   For the methods of measuring the blood pressure, see § 83.   In a healthy adult the resting blood pressure is fairly constant, but the limits of normal variation are wide, namely—systolic, 100–146 mm., and diastolic, 64–84 mm.   In older people the systolic pressure may be as high as 160 mm., but persistent pressures above 170 mm. systolic and 90 mm. diastolic indicate the presence of arterial disease and are certainly pathological (§ 83).

TEMPORARY HYPERTENSION (Symptomatic hypertension) occurs during exercise and with emotional disturbances.   It is also seen during acute attacks of gout, with a disturbance of the cerebral circulation (*e.g.*, increased intracranial pressure, cerebral thrombosis) and in *paroxysmal* attacks.

In *Paroxysmal hypertension* due to a tumour of the suprarenal medulla (pheochromocytoma) the blood pressure may reach very high levels.   It is due to the liberation of large quantities of nor-adrenaline and adrenaline from the pheochromocytoma: and often causes attacks of sweating, trembling, palpitation and sometimes acute left ventricular failure.   For *Diagnosis* see § 97.

PERSISTENT HYPERTENSION can be classified as follows:—

(1) *Essential (or primary) hypertension*.   In clinical practice 95 per cent. of hypertensive patients over the age of 35 years fall into this group.   The condition is due to a generalised increase in peripheral resistance throughout the body, the cause of which is largely unknown.   It is described in § 96.

(2) *Secondary hypertension* is due to a number of causes.

(i.) *With Renal Disease*.   In any case of persistent hypertension, the urine must be examined for albumen, red cells and for casts (§ 396).   Even when the urine is normal and renal function adequate, intravenous pyelography and renal biopsy may show changes in the kidneys.   The blood pressure is raised in the acute phase of diffuse glomerular nephritis, chronic diffuse nephritis, toxæmia of pregnancy, polycystic disease of the kidneys and often in chronic pyelonephritis.

Hydronephrosis, renal calculus, renal tuberculosis, hypernephroma, fibrosis of the kidneys, and impaired blood supply from occlusion of the renal artery (*e.g.*, by severe arteriosclerosis or aneurysm) also can cause renal hypertension.   When unilateral, removal of the diseased kidney may allow return of the blood pressure to normal, provided the other kidney is healthy.   Interference with emptying of the bladder (*e.g.*, by an enlarged prostate) may produce persistent hypertension.

---

[1] *Hyperpiesis* is a state of hypertension, whatever the cause, and may be temporary (as with emotion) or persistent.   *Hyperpiesia* is a clinical condition associated with arterial disease (diffuse hyperplastic sclerosis § 95).

The blood pressure is usually not raised in acute focal nephritis, nephrotic nephritis, nephrosis or amyloid disease of the kidneys.

(ii.) *Endocrine causes.*

Thyroid deficiency and especially myxœdema are often accompanied by hypertension. Thyrotoxicosis produces an elevated systolic pressure but the diastolic pressure is normal or lowered; the high pulse pressure is the result of peripheral vaso-dilatation and the increased cardiac output.

Cushing's Syndrome may cause persistent (even malignant) hypertension. It is usually due to a benign tumour of the suprarenal cortex but can be due to a malignant tumour or to a basophil adenoma of the pituitary gland. Permanent or paroxysmal hypertension can be caused by a tumour of the suprarenal medulla (pheochromocytoma) *vide supra.*

Primary aldosteronism is a rare condition due to a suprarenal cortical adenoma with hyper-secretion of aldosterone. There is a combination of fairly mild hypertension with attacks of muscular weakness or paralysis in association with marked reduction of the serum potassium (§ 547a). It is remedied by removal of the adenoma.

(iii.) *Coarctation of the Aorta* is often first suspected when hypertension is found in a young person: the femoral pulses should be felt as a routine in such cases (§ 59).

(iv.) *Polycythæmia* (§ 31) and *polyarteritis* (§ 98) are rare.

When a definite cause for hypertension exists, such as a chromaffin tumour of the adrenal medulla, the raised blood pressure is referred to as symptomatic hypertension, for removal may lead to a relatively normal blood pressure. In all cases where no definite factor is found, other than heredity, the condition is called essential hypertension (hyperpiesia).

§ 89. Low Blood Pressure (Syn. Hypotension) in an adult is indicated by a systolic blood pressure persistently below 90–100 mm. To the examining finger the pulse is soft and is easily obliterated; when the patient is erect, the rate is rapid, and falls 30 or 40 beats when he lies down. *Symptoms* are often absent. When present, headache, giddiness and sometimes syncope may be complained of, especially when rising from a recumbent posture: depression, lassitude and undue fatigue are usual. In cases of " postural hypotension," the systolic blood pressure is 20–30 mm. less when the patient is standing than when lying down.

Etiology.—In *health* a persistent state of low blood pressure is sometimes a hereditary condition. It may be aggravated by meals, a warm bath or moist heat. In *disease*, the chief causes are (a) Cardiac disease, especially left ventricular failure, such as occurs in coronary thrombosis and toxic myocarditis with diphtheria; (b) General conditions: (i.) suprarenal atrophy or tuberculosis (Addison's disease); (ii.) pulmonary tuberculosis; (iii.) cachexia and malnutrition; (iv.) shock, collapse, hæmorrhage or dehydration; (v.) exhaustion due to mental or physical overstrain; or following asthenic types of fever, especially typhoid and influenza; (vi.) occasionally with certain types of advanced renal disease and with senile arteriosclerosis.

The *treatment* depends upon the cause. The diet should be nourishing and easily digestible. Free purgation, very hot baths and prolonged standing should be avoided. Adequate mental and physical rest should be given and later graduated exercises, abdominal exercises and if necessary an abdominal belt to support the splanchnic area. Vaso-constrictors (including ephedrine hydrochloride) may be used, provided the myocardium is not seriously damaged. Alcohol must be used with caution. See also Addison's disease (§ 576). Collapse is dealt with in § 35 and § 239.

§ 90. **The Pulse in Relation to Prognosis and Treatment of Disease.** Examination of the pulse affords valuable information both as to the general condition of the patient and the state of the cardio-vascular system. Indeed there is so much to be learnt from palpation of the pulse by the experienced finger that it should always be the first step in the general examination of a patient. The pulse frequency in *febrile diseases* should be charted four-hourly, so that it may be read in conjunction with the temperature and respiration rate. In an adult the pulse frequency increases 8 to 10 beats per minute for each degree rise of temperature. A pulse frequency increased out of proportion to the rise of temperature may be an indication of a *toxic myocarditis*, and a pulse rate over 130 per minute in *pneumonia* is evidence of severe toxæmia. In a *child*, the increase of pulse frequency with each degree rise of temperature is greater, namely 12 to 15 beats per minute.

Slowing of the *pulse frequency* in relation to *fever* may be an indication of heart block. A sudden drop of temperature, pulse and respiration rates together takes place at the crisis in pneumonia; but a fall of temperature without a fall in pulse rate, or perhaps even a slight increase of pulse rate, is evidence of a complication. In *abdominal conditions* the pulse rate may decide a diagnosis between inflammation (rapid pulse) and colic (slow pulse). A fall in temperature with an increase of pulse frequency occurs with intestinal hæmorrhage, in perforation of the bowel, and with profuse diarrhœa complicating typhoid fever. The pulse rate may be of outstanding importance in the diagnosis and treatment of appendicitis; in a doubtful case, when the patient looks ill, has indefinite abdominal discomfort but no localised pain, and a soft abdomen, an increasing pulse rate observed half-hourly may be the deciding factor for immediate operation: this is considered in detail in § 239. Again, in a patient recovering from a severe *hæmatemesis* the temperature tends to oscillate about normal with an occasional rise to 99° or 99·4°; the pulse rate may be 100–110, gradually falling to 80. With recovery the temperature gradually becomes subnormal at a steady level, and the pulse drops to 70–80. A rise in pulse rate will accompany further hæmorrhage, and thus provide an indication for more cautious treatment, or if the hæmoglobin is already low, it may determine treatment by blood transfusion. The pulse rate in *afebrile toxic states* is to some extent a measure of the degree of toxæmia, as in alcoholic poisoning, especially delirium tremens. In *Graves' disease* the pulse rate (especially during sleep) and the height of the pulse pressure with the patient at rest in bed provide a fair index of the basal metabolic rate and the toxæmia. (See Tachycardia, § 84, for other toxæmias to which these observations also apply.) Pulse frequency to the extent that it is a measure of the *degree of toxæmia* thus provides important information as to prognosis and treatment. A rapidly rising pulse rate is a common terminal event in both febrile and afebrile diseases. A transient increased frequency is some measure of *emotional* reaction. The pulse rate in response to *exercise* and the time taken for its return to normal tells us something of cardiac efficiency. Variations in pulse volume are also of great importance. A full bounding pulse is characteristic of an acute febrile illness and asthenic state. In contrast is the small thready pulse which is felt in all states of shock, both medical and surgical. The pulse in relation to heart disease is discussed in §§ 41, 45.

ARTERIAL DISEASE

PART A

§ 91. SYMPTOMATOLOGY. The symptoms of arterial disease *per se* depend in the first place on changes in the function and structure of the blood vessels, and in the second place on the effects of these changes on the activity of the organs which the affected blood vessels supply. The symptoms vary according to whether the vascular affection is general or local, and necessarily according to the part which is chiefly affected. The CARDINAL LOCAL symptoms of active arterial disease are **pain** and **decreased function** of the ischæmic area. With sudden complete occlusion of an artery there is an abrupt onset of continuous pain and loss of use of the affected part. Thus in sudden coronary occlusion there is severe chest pain, with a decreased cardiac output and even sudden death. Relative ischæmia may occur as an artery narrows gradually or obstruction is incomplete, the pain being due to failure of the blood supply to meet extra demands of muscular activity. Thus in angina pectoris, whether due to atherosclerosis or to spasm of the coronary vessels, and in intermittent claudication in the legs (well-named angina cruris) there is the same history of pain brought on by exercise and relieved by rest. The amount of pain produced by ischæmia varies with the site affected: in cerebral vascular occlusion there may be little or no pain even though a large area of nervous tissue is involved: on occasions arteriosclerotic disease may be the cause of dyspeptic symptoms. The GENERAL symptoms depend upon the variety and location of the arterial disease. See Part C.

PART B

§ 92. The PHYSICAL EXAMINATION of the arteries has been described in the preceding pages which deal with the pulse. The condition of the arteries can be gauged by inspection of the retinal vessels, by palpation of the superficial arteries, by blood pressure observation and by X-ray examination which will show the size of the aorta, and calcification whether present in the aorta or in vessels of smaller calibre such as the limb arteries. Finally, an examination of all the systems is necessary, for evidence of changes due to vascular disease: the urine in particular is important in showing evidence of changes in the capillaries of the glomeruli.

Physical Signs. (i.) Hæmorrhage is the cardinal sign of arterial disease. The common sites are from the nose (epistaxis), uterus (menorrhagia), in the eyes (retinal hæmorrhages or hæmorrhage into the vitreous: conjunctival hæmorrhage has not this significance), and kidneys (microscopic and some-times macroscopic hæmaturia). Hæmorrhages from the lungs (hæmoptysis), from the stomach (hæmatemesis) and bowels (melæna), are occasionally seen. Such hæmorrhages may be the forerunners of more serious events. Thus epistaxis may precede a cerebral accident, such as hæmorrhage or throm-bosis, and is sometimes the first sign of incipient psychosis due to cerebral arteriosclerosis. (ii.) Visible or palpable thickening or tortuosity of visible (retinal) vessels or palpable vessels, such as the temporal, radial, brachial, and sometimes the carotid and other arteries, indicates arteriosclerosis. This thickening of a palpable artery may be due to hypertrophy of the media in response to hypertension. In such a case on post-mortem examination the thickened artery may be found healthy except for the hypertrophy of its walls, which may involve the intima as well as the media. In other cases the thickening and tortuosity of the vessel felt by palpation may be due to hyperplastic and degenerative changes. (iii.) The loss of elasticity in the arterial system in medial sclerosis is recognised by an increase of pulse pressure. (iv.) A rise in the diastolic pressure, as occurs in persistent hypertension due to arteriolar sclerosis, also causes a loss of elasticity and increase in pulse pressure. (v.) Accentuation of the aortic second sound is heard in hypertension, sclerosis of the ascending aorta and syphilitic aneurysm of the ascending aorta without aortic incompetence. Similarly pulmonary hypertension will cause accentuation of the pulmonary second sound. (vi.) Calcification in the vessels can be demonstrated by radiography. (vii.) Obstruction of an artery may be partial or complete. Narrowing of the larger arteries such as the carotid or femoral vessels by atherosclerosis causes the pulse to be reduced distally and may give rise to a local systolic murmur which can be heard with a stethoscope. Complete obstruction abolishes the arterial pulse and, unless a sufficient collateral circulation is present, causes tissue necrosis or gangrene (§§ 586, 587, 902). The cause may be (*a*) thrombosis due to atherosclerosis or to syphilitic endarteritis (especially of the cerebral vessels) and (*b*) embolism.

The arteries are commonly held to be more prone to disease than are the veins, but it is not as yet known in what proportion of cases major vascular accidents, such as hæmorrhage or thrombosis, are located in the arteries, capillaries or veins. In those areas that are more available for observation, such as the vessels of the nasal septum and retina, capillary and venous accidents are certainly of importance.

Arteriography demonstrates partial or complete obstruction of a main artery and of its chief branches, and the collateral circulation present. It is performed by injecting a radio-opaque and relatively innocuous substance such as diodone, B.P., into the main artery and taking a rapid series of X-rays (Fig. 170).

PART C

The DISEASES OF THE ARTERIES which admit of clinical recognition are as follows:

I. Arteriosclerosis, a term used to describe a group of degenerative diseases. The following pathological types are recognised: (*a*) Atherosclerosis, (*b*) Medial sclerosis, including the Mönckeberg type, (*c*) Arteriolar sclerosis (§ 95) and Hypertension (§ 96).

II. Thrombo-angiitis obliterans (§ 586).

III. Polyarteritis nodosa.

IV. Chronic and acute endarteritis.

V. Aneurysmal dilatation.

VI. Complications such as embolism and thrombosis.

VII. Functional diseases of the arteries.

§ 93. I. *a.* **Atherosclerosis** (Syn. Atheroma, Intimal Sclerosis) starts as a patchy thickening of the intima of the larger arteries. It is often found in early adult life, but becomes more marked after middle age and then becomes more or less widespread.

There is first a localised hyperplasia in the deeper layers of the tunica intima, best seen in the abdominal aorta and its larger branches. At post-mortem this appears as a circular or oval patch of pale grey tissue. It may undergo fatty degeneration (when it appears yellowish in colour) and subsequent calcification. Alternatively it undergoes necrosis and caseation: when the necrotic process involves the superficial layers of the intima and the endothelial lining of the vessel wall an atheromatous ulcer is formed.

The process is closely related to a disorder of lipoid metabolism. It can occur at a very early age in diabetes, and is usually more advanced in obese persons, with myxœdema and in nephrosis.

§ 94. I. *b.* **Mönckeberg's Medial Sclerosis** is a diffuse form of arterial disease which occurs after 50 years of age. It is characterised by fibrosis, fatty degeneration and later calcification of the muscle coats of the larger arteries of the limbs and their branches, and it does not involve the aorta. It is the result of ageing and it causes lengthening, tortuosity and hardening of the arteries but it does not diminish their calibre. It occurs in a more advanced form in the legs, and it is especially here that calcification often in the form of encircling plaques or rings can be demonstrated on X-ray films.

The Clinical Results of Atheroma and Medial Sclerosis. These two conditions are commonly associated, but the degree of atheroma and of medial sclerosis in any particular subject may vary considerably. Thus it is common in old people to see gross signs of medial sclerosis with thickened tortuous brachial, radial and temporal arteries and a raised systolic pressure, causing no ill effects over many years.

The *Symptoms of Arteriosclerosis* are more commonly the results of atheroma than of medial sclerosis. During life there is no known method of demonstrating atheroma *per se* but it produces a wide and varied group of clinical syndromes: (i.) Narrowing of the lumen or actual thrombosis of the arteries, when affecting the coronary vessels, may cause angina pectoris or coronary thrombosis, in the cerebral vessels the symptoms of cerebral arteriosclerosis, transient or permanent paresis, cerebral softening, senile psychosis and other cerebral changes. In the legs anoxia may develop during activity causing muscle cramps (intermittent claudication): particularly in diabetic persons gangrene of the toes and feet may occur. (ii.) Especially in the presence of hypertension, the weakened vessel walls may give way and cause cerebral hæmorrhage: and in the aorta an atheromatous plaque in the presence of an idiopathic cystic medial necrosis may be the starting point of a dissecting aneurysm. (iii.) Besides the more dramatic effects produced by thrombosis and rupture, narrowing of the lumen in atheromatous vessels may lead to impaired vitality and degeneration in the organs they supply; hence various forms of dyspepsia (including anorexia, flatulence and colic) due to arteriosclerosis of the splanchnic vessels, and the various forms of senile psychosis in cerebral arteriosclerosis. (iv.) Many of the signs of old age, such as loss of weight, diminished vitality (asthenia), ready fatigue and a poor peripheral circulation are due to generalised arterial disease (§ 574). (v.) Diseased arteries are liable to functional disturbances and hence the symptoms of giddiness and of senile syncope (§ 833) which may occur.

The *physical signs* due to vascular disease *per se* have already been referred to: (i.) the thickening of the palpable arteries, (ii.) the irregularity of calibre of the retinal vessels with deviation of the veins and obstruction to the blood flow in them at the arterio-venous crossings (§ 96, *Signs*). (iii.) Increased pulse pressure, generally associated with a rise in systolic pressure, and (iv.) an alteration in the second aortic sound.

Diagnosis.—The signs and symptoms of vascular disease already described in detail provide the diagnosis of arteriosclerosis, but whether the patient who has arteriosclerosis is or is not suffering from it, will depend on the signs and symptoms of activity of the disease. This is to be judged in the first place by the presence or absence of hæmorrhages and pain, and in the second place on an evaluation of symptoms referable to organs other than blood vessels, and the opinion as to what extent such symptoms are determined by a disorder in structure or function of the vessels which supply them.

Etiology of Arteriosclerosis (Atheroma and Medial Sclerosis).— (i.) *Heredity*. As Osler said, certain families seem to " inherit bad tubing." A history of arterial degeneration causing " strokes," angina, high blood pressure or " sudden death " is common; and sometimes " anticipation " occurs, so that subsequent generations show the essential changes at earlier ages. (ii.) *Age*. Medial sclerosis is a disease of old age. Atheroma can occur much earlier and has even been seen in childhood. Age is chiefly of importance in providing a longer opportunity for the causes of atheroma, whatever they may be, to have their effect. (iii.) *Constitution*. Dietetic, metabolic, endocrine, infective or toxic and other factors not yet understood, may all play a part. In general terms there is an association between arteriosclerosis and obesity, gout, myxœdema and osteo-arthritis. (iv.) Diabetes mellitus, especially when poorly controlled, hastens arteriosclerosis. The Mönckeberg type of arteriosclerosis is chiefly found in patients suffering from diabetes mellitus. (v.) Marked atheroma can occur in certain rare metabolic disorders associated with considerable hypercholesterolæmia and the process can be partially reversed by a reduced dietary intake of cholesterol. (vi.) Hypertension of sufficient degree and duration will cause a " work hypertrophy " of the arteries, followed later by medial sclerosis. There is evidence that mechanical strain may be a factor in the production of atheroma: thus atheroma tends to be marked in hypertension and is found in the pulmonary arteries when the pressure is raised by mitral stenosis.

Prognosis.—The question of prognosis depends firstly on the activity or quiescence of the arterial disease; and secondly on the degree of cardiac and renal involvement If there are signs of heart failure the prognosis is necessarily guarded, and with the development of retinitis and severe kidney involvement it becomes grave. The thickening of the artery, and indeed many of the structural changes which characterise arteriosclerosis, are largely the result of recovery and repair. The structural pathology of arteriosclerosis is to some extent comparable with that of fibroid phthisis, in which type of tuberculosis the lesion may be active, but the process of repair keeps pace with it or dominates it. If it is realised that the process of repair may keep pace with the smouldering vascular lesion, and perhaps overtake it, it will be readily understood how often patients have arteriosclerosis without at any time suffering from it.

Treatment.—Arterial disease cannot be arrested and no specific remedies are known. When a condition which aggravates the disease is found (*e.g.*, obesity, diabetes mellitus, oversmoking) this must be corrected. Otherwise the results of the disease processes must be treated. Nevertheless much can be done to improve the health and prolong the life of the patients. It is unwise to tell the patient that he is suffering from " hardened arteries " although the relatives may need to be told. Medial sclerosis and a moderate degree of hypertension (with a systolic pressure to 170 mm.) are compatible with a long life and need no special treatment. *Activity* should not be restricted unless essential, for this often proves irksome.

Although it is obviously wise that the patient should avoid sudden or prolonged strenuous exertion, especially if these produce symptoms such as giddiness, breathlessness, or undue fatigue, it is better for a person to continue at work provided it is within the limits of his strength. A longer night in bed or an hour on a couch between lunch and dinner will usually give the extra rest needed. Regular *exercise* in the open air, such as walking or golf, is very helpful. Residence in a warmer climate during the winter months is certainly beneficial, and also provides a change of environment. The *diet* should be plain, varied and easily digestible, with an optimum of vitamins B and C. Some patients seem to benefit by reducing animal protein in their diet; fish, chicken or meat taken once a day may be prescribed. The empirical restriction of meat and of salt has recently received support from the adverse effect of giving meat and sodium chloride to dogs with experimentally produced hypertension. In some where there are symptoms or signs of active disease, especially if it is likely to be of recent origin, intensive treatment may be tried with two to four weeks' rest in bed on a low calorie diet, together with sedatives. Removal of *excess weight* is often of great benefit. Large meals and over-eating are always to be avoided and alcohol taken in strict moderation. *Constipation* must be corrected by vegetable laxatives or magnesia and paraffin, but habitual loose stools are weakening. The *activity of the skin* is aided by suitable clothing, a daily warm bath and in some cases a weekly Turkish bath. An *infection* is often badly tolerated; thus patients feel much better when septic teeth or an infected urine have been treated; and it has often been noted that a coronary or cerebral thrombosis may supervene a week or so after an attack of influenza or of bronchitis in an arteriosclerotic subject. *Drugs* are chiefly of value in symptomatic treatment. Small doses of aspirin, phenobarbitone, chloral or whisky at bedtime secure peaceful sleep. Digitalis may be needed for myocardial damage. Phenobarbitone, meprobamate or a small dose of chloro-promazine relieves restlessness and nervous tension. Lastly treatment will have to be directed to the control in the various organs of the body of structural changes which are due to arteriosclerosis. *Gangrene* in the extremities (§ 587) and progressive occlusion in carotid stenosis (§ 903) may be delayed by suitable measures and sometimes by the regular use of anti-coagulant drugs. *Associated conditions* which hasten the progress of arteriosclerosis, especially gout, diabetes mellitus, myxœdema and obesity, must be controlled by suitable treatment. Various *surgical methods* of reconstructing or recanalising diseased arteries are now being used.

§ 95. I. c. **Diffuse Arteriolar Sclerosis** (Syn. Diffuse Hyperplastic Sclerosis, Arterio-capillary Fibrosis) is the structural equivalent of persistent hypertension.

Functional Pathology.—Increased peripheral resistance is the cause of persistent hypertension. It is determined by narrowing of the very small arteries and arterioles, and is accompanied by an increased force of the heart beat. This means increased work for the heart and leads to left ventricular hypertrophy. The blood flow to the periphery is thus maintained in spite of the contraction of the vascular bed. Neither increased output of the heart, nor an increased flow of blood, nor increased viscosity, contribute materially to persistent hypertension. Goldblatt, by constricting the renal arteries of dogs, was the first to show that renal ischæmia produced hypertension. According to Page, the reduction of arterial pulsation in the kidney is of cardinal importance. The ischæmic kidney secretes a substance known as renin which acts on a protein-like substance (renin activator) in the blood plasma to form a heat-stable pressor substance called angiotonin (Page and Helmer). The action of angiotonin is directly on the arterioles and not on the heart. As to the mechanism by which angiotonin and like substances cause arteriolar hypertonus, it has been shown that nervous mechanisms have no part; although the pressor substance is quite distinct from adrenalin, integrity of the adrenal cortex is necessary to allow of the production of hypertension. The production of renal hypertension is not related in any way to interference with the excretory function of the kidney and hypertension can be produced by constricting one renal artery only. Arteriolosclerotic changes due to the hypertension may then be found in the opposite kidney, while these changes do not occur in the kidney whose blood supply is reduced by the clamp. If the clamped kidney is now removed the blood pressure may return to normal, or the ischæmic changes induced in the opposite kidney may perpetuate the hypertension. The problem is made more complicated because after removal of both kidneys hypertension may persist. An extrarenal factor must, therefore, be present even in cases of renal hypertension (Wilson).

In an animal in which persistent hypertension, comparable with benign hypertension in the human subject, has been produced by an alteration of the intrarenal circulation in one kidney, removal of the other kidney may determine the development of a condition comparable with malignant hypertension in man. The same transition from benign to malignant hypertension may be determined on occasion by the large addition of sodium chloride or meat to the animal's basic diet. This observation gives some support to the adoption of a vegetarian diet and restricted sodium chloride intake in certain cases of human hypertension. Although the over-production of renin may be a factor in the hypertension of renal disease it is very unlikely to be associated with the etiology of primary essential hypertension in man.

Structural Pathology.—In contrast to atheroma, which is *localised*, the lesion in arteriolar sclerosis (hyperpiesia) is *diffuse*. In contrast to arteriosclerosis, in which the lesion affects the media as well as the intima, in arteriolar sclerosis the intimal thickening (or hyperplasia) is the distinctive pathological feature. The coincident thickening of the media is explained in terms of physiological response to the persistent hypertension always found in this form of arterial disease. Further, in arteriosclerosis the main incidence of the lesion is in the conducting arteries, whereas in arteriolar sclerosis it is in the arterioles. The lesion is characterised by the following pathological features. In the terminal arterioles there is intimal thickening due to endothelial or subendothelial proliferation of cells, followed by an increase of hyaline substance and fibrous connective tissue. The process may go on to complete closure of the lumen, and in the terminal stage there is fatty degeneration of the thickened intima, so that in cross section the lumen of an arteriole appears blocked by a plug of fat. In the parent vessel from which the terminal arteriole springs, there is the same intimal thickening accompanied by an increase in thickness and number of strands which form the internal elastic lamina, at the same time an increase of fibrous tissue. There is little or no fatty change in the arteries of this size. In serial sections the marked fatty degeneration of the terminal arterioles may be seen to stop short at their off-shoot from the parent vessel (Jores). The initial hyperplasia is accompanied by hypertrophy of the media, and this may be a prominent feature and widely distributed. In any organ the distribution of the lesion is partial, some vessels being more affected than others, and in the arterioles the lesion may be complete in some, whereas others escape. The organ distribution is characteristic. The lesion is always found in the kidneys or spleen, and generally in both. It is commonly found in the brain, pancreas, and suprarenals, and rarely in the liver or digestive tract; it does not occur as a complete lesion in the heart or skeletal muscle.

§ 96. Essential Hypertension.—Persistent hypertension without kidney disease was first recognised in this country by Sir Clifford Allbutt, who called it hyperpiesia. Allbutt maintained that hyperpiesia pursues its course and ends in a cerebral catastrophe or cardiac defeat, or life is terminated by intercurrent disease, but that at no stage of the disease does uræmia develop. The clinical syndrome described by Allbutt as hyperpiesia is now known as Essential Hypertension.

Essential hypertension is diagnosed in a case of persistent hypertension in which kidney disease (renal hypertension) and other known causes of secondary hypertension have been excluded (§ 88). It is subdivided into benign and malignant types according to the severity of the condition. It is now known that benign hypertension may (in 10 per cent. of cases) become malignant.

Benign Hypertension. *Symptoms.*—There may be none, especially in the early stage of the disease. Whereas some patients have a variety of symptoms before they seek advice, others develop symptoms only when they have been informed that they have " high blood pressure," as the expression of an anxiety state. The symptoms commonly met are (i.) loss of energy, ready fatigue, insomnia and nervous exhaustion. (ii.) Headache is often occipital but may be vertical or frontal and is sometimes paroxysmal. (iii.) Dizziness and vertigo, often with sudden change of position, palpitation, or a sense of faintness are common. Other symptoms arise as a result of the complications of hypertension. (iv.) Hæmorrhage, from the nose (epistaxis), into the retina or the occurrence of a cerebral hæmorrhage are frequent. (v.) Incipient left ventricular failure causes shortness of breath on exertion. (vi.) Nocturnal dyspnœa (cardiac asthma) is due to paroxysmal attacks of acute left ventricular failure. In turn this may lead to right-sided (congestive) heart failure. (vii.) Angina pectoris is fairly common in cases of hypertension: auricular fibrillation is rare and only occurs if there is myocardial ischæmia.

Signs.—(i.) In established cases the blood pressure is persistently 180 mm. systolic and 100 mm. diastolic, or over; it may be much higher, reaching 260 mm. systolic and 120 mm. diastolic or more. (ii.) There is left ventricular hypertrophy, recognised by the cardiac impulse which is forceful and sustained, an increase in the area of cardiac dullness, and a lengthening and lowered tone of the first sound at the apex. Or it is recognised by an increase in the size of the heart in a radiogram and by left axis deviation in the electrocardiogram. (iii.) The second aortic sound is accentuated. (iv.) The radial pulse is hard and resists compression. The artery is generally felt to be thickened, and it may be tortuous. (v.) The changes in the retina are of the greatest importance and have been divided into four grades (Keith and Wagener). Grade I changes consist of narrowing, tortuosity and irregularity of the retinal arteries. In Grade II, the changes are more marked and there is nipping of the veins where the arteries cross in front of them. Grade III changes include the presence of exudates and hæmorrhages. Grade IV is characterised by papillœdema which shows the hypertension has entered the malignant phase. (vi.) The urine is normal, apart from the presence in some cases of a trace of albumin, and a small number of granular and hyaline casts. Renal function is normal. As was pointed out by Sir Clifford Allbutt, there is no anæmia or other effect of a chronic toxæmia. In fact, in benign essential hypertension the patient is often over-weight and plethoric. The complexion is a good colour in contrast to the pale and muddy complexion of chronic renal disease accompanied by persistent hypertension.

The *differential diagnosis* of hyperpiesia is from the various forms of urinary disease on the one hand and symptomatic hypertension on the other. *Urinary disease* is excluded by the absence of a history of kidney disease or its symptoms, a normal or practically normal urine, normal renal function and pyelography. *Symptomatic hypertension,* such as may be due to heart failure or endocrine disturbance, is diagnosed by recognising the etiological factors, and the diagnosis is confirmed by response to treatment and the progress of the patient.

Etiology.—Apart from the fact that heredity is an important factor, in many cases the etiology is ill-defined. (i.) *General causes* include modern city life, worry, anxiety and prolonged mental strain, especially when combined with sleeplessness and lack of regular exercise. (ii.) *Obesity* due to over-eating or drinking. Following weight reduction the hypertension is much less and may disappear. (iii.) At the climacteric or after removal of both ovaries hypertension is seen; the associated rapid gain in weight is an important causal factor and the blood pressure frequently drops when weight reduction is accomplished. (iv.) *Diabetes mellitus* and hypertension often occur together. (v.) *Gout* and *osteo-arthritis* are often associated with hypertension. (vi.) *Chronic alcoholism* and *chronic lead poisoning* are exogenous causes.

Prognosis.—It is uncommon for established high blood pressure to return to normal in the absence of treatment. Nevertheless this may happen on occasion as after coronary thrombosis or treatment for obesity. In the majority of cases the disease in its general course is slowly progressive, with periods of activity alternating with periods of quiescence. Many cases pursue a benign course and in these progress of the disease is very slow. The blood pressure may become established at a moderately high level, such as 210 mm. systolic and 100–110 mm. diastolic, with a period of good health for four to ten years; during this time the patient lives in good health with little limitation of his or her activities, and perhaps dies of intercurrent disease or natural causes. After such a quiescent phase and for no accountable reason the disease then suddenly takes on a progressive form. In others, particularly when the diastolic pressure is 130 mm. or over (and the systolic pressure 260 mm. or more), the disease tends to progress more rapidly. Severe ventricular strain, shown by gallop rhythm and pulsus alternans with attacks of left ventricular failure ("cardiac asthma"), is always ominous. The disease ends fatally from heart failure or coronary disease in about 60 per cent. of cases; from apoplexy in 19 per cent.; from renal failure in 8 per cent. and from intercurrent disease in 12 per cent. (Bell and Clawson).

Treatment in the first place is as outlined in § 94 for arterial disease. Moderation in the hours of work, additional rest and sleep, the avoidance of mental and physical overwork and stress, the correction of obesity and of constipation and a regular life with small meals, aided by a sedative (such as a barbiturate) when necessary, will do much to lower the height of the blood pressure.

When conservative treatment on the above lines fails, and in severe cases, other medicinal or surgical treatment may be advised. It must be emphasised that the majority of patients with benign hypertension need no more than an adjustment of their daily regime, reassurance and periodic medical assessment. Modern *hypotensive drugs* are, however, indicated in certain patients, (i.) those with a diastolic pressure of 130 mm. or over; (ii.) those with evidence of left ventricular embarrassment; (iii.) when the disease is entering the malignant phase; (iv.) occasionally in patients with persistent symptoms due to arterial disease with hypertension who cannot obtain relief by other methods.

Hypotensive drugs fall into three main groups. (i.) Ganglionic blocking drugs are the most effective. They paralyse the sympathetic and the parasympathetic ganglia alike. Those in common use are pentolinium tartrate (Ansolysen) and the more powerful mecamylamine hydrochlor. (Inversine) and pempidine tartrate (Perolysen, Tenormal). They remain by far the best treatment for controlling the blood pressure in malignant hypertension but have unpleasant side effects due to their action on the parasympathetic ganglia, causing dryness of the mouth, blurred vision, constipation and occasionally paralytic ileus, effects which can be lessened by neostigmine methylsulphate (Prostigmin). (ii.) Methyldopa (Aldomet) has many fewer side effects. It fails in malignant hypertension, but is especially valuable in moderate hypertension. It acts even when the patient is supine and interferes with the formation of noradrenaline in the tissues and at the nerve-endings. (iii.) Drugs which prevent the release of noradrenaline at the sympathetic nerve endings, but which do not affect the parasympathetic system, are a little less effective than methyldopa. Two are in common use, guanethidine sulphate (Ismelin) and less often bretylium tosylate (Darenthin). Whichever drug is chosen the initial dose is small and is gradually increased, for the range of dose necessary to reduce the blood pressure varies from patient to patient. The chlorothiazide group of diuretics (§ 29) and the rauwolfia alkaloids potentiate the hypotensive drugs, but because the first of these causes potassium loss by the kidneys, supplementary potassium chloride must be given especially when digitalis is being used. The hypotensive drugs lower the blood pressure when the patient is reclining, but produce a much greater fall when standing; the dose required should therefore be estimated when in the upright position and the postural hypotensive effect utilised at night by sleeping with extra pillows. Tolerance to the drugs is often acquired and necessitates corresponding adjustment of dosage.

Dorsi-lumbar sympathectomy should be reserved for those patients in whom medicinal treatment is either ineffective or too irksome, the latter being usually due to the side effects of the ganglion blocking drugs. Adrenalectomy has been reported to give good results in cases of severe hypertension. Lastly, treatment by severe sodium restriction is the basis of the Kempner rice diet.

§ 97. **Malignant Hypertension** may suddenly declare itself after an insidious onset, as judged by symptoms, over a period of a few weeks or months. It also occurs in severe cases of eclampsia.

Structural pathology.—The changes observed are those already described in diffuse arteriolar sclerosis (§ 95). In malignant hypertension these changes are over-shadowed and partly obliterated by fibrinoid degeneration of arterioles and acute arteriolar necrosis, and in the more rapid and severe cases hyperplasia may be negligible or absent.

Symptoms.—The disease is recognised by the presence of papillœdema with or without retinal exudates or hæmorrhages, or by a hæmorrhage elsewhere, such as hæmaturia, hæmoptysis, hæmatemesis and so on. It is suspected when the diastolic pressure is 130 mm. Hg or over. In addition to macroscopic or microscopic hæmaturia renal involvement is registered by albuminuria, cylindruria and urea retention (§ 401). Left ventricular stress or failure may be marked. At the same time, the patient's general condition deteriorates. There is malaise, loss of strength, energy and body-weight, often loss of appetite and anæmia.

Diagnostic importance must be attached to papillœdema with which retinal hæmorrhages, exudates and arterial narrowing are seen. This indicates a condition of hypertensive encephalopathy (p. 157, § 851).

Diagnosis is from chronic nephritis and hypertension. Although malignant hypertension has in the past been regarded as of relatively short duration, many cases of chronic nephritis are now known to terminate with the clinical features of malignant hypertension.

Prognosis.—When malignant hypertension is clearly established with retinopathy, renal involvement and anæmia the disease generally ends fatally in six months to two years, unless treatment is rapidly successful in lowering the blood pressure.

Treatment is on the same lines as that described for benign hypertension, but must be pushed. In elderly patients with a poor myocardium, vigorous treatment with hypotensive drugs must be used, the initial doses being injected. In younger patients additional measures are by dorsi-lumbar sympathectomy and adrenalectomy. A raised blood urea is no contra-indication to these forms of treatment but a rapidly rising blood urea denotes a hopeless prognosis and the hypotensive therapy in these cases often precipitates uræmia and death.

HYPERTENSIVE CEREBRAL ATTACKS (Syn. Hypertensive Encephalopathy) are a cerebral form of this. *Symptoms* are sudden headache, drowsiness, coma or convulsions, vomiting and albuminuria. The retinal arterioles are constricted, retinal hæmorrhages, exudates and papillœdema suddenly appear. The systolic pressure may rise rapidly in a few hours by as much as 100 mg. Hg. The C.S.F. pressure is raised and there is cerebral œdema. *Diagnosis* is from a cerebral vascular complication of benign hypertension and from carotid or basilar artery stenosis (§ 851).

Treatment is by the vigorous use of the ganglion blocking drugs: when vomiting is present inject hexamethonium bromide 25 mg. or pentolinium tartrate 10 mg. intramusc. and repeat in 8–12 hours. A raised C.S.F. pressure is an indication for the removal of 10–20 ml. of C.S.F. Restlessness is controlled by the injection of heroin hydrochloride gr. ⅛–¼.

A **Phæochromocytoma** is a rare but important cause of malignant hypertension. The tumour is usually in the suprarenal medulla but may exist in chromaffin tissue along the abdominal aorta or accompanying the abdominal sympathetic ganglia. It secretes excess of noradrenaline and to a lesser extent adrenaline.

Symptoms.—Severe hypertension may be paroxysmal or continuous. In *paroxysmal* cases the blood pressure suddenly rises to 300 mm. or higher accompanied by intense headache, substernal pain, forceful beating of the heart, profuse sweating with cold hands, and sometimes left ventricular failure. After an attack lasting half an hour or more the patient takes several days to recover. In *continuous* cases the hypertension is of the severe or malignant type.

Diagnosis.—This may be confirmed by several different tests. (1) The urine contains an excess of catechol amines during the hypertensive phases in over 70 per cent. of cases: and (2) since noradrenaline and adrenaline are converted to vanilmandelic acid, estimation of the 24-hour output of this is a useful index (normal 1·0–6·0 mg./per day). (3) Phentolamine methanesulphonate (Rogitine) antagonises the pressor effect of adrenaline and noradrenaline and so produces a fall in the systolic blood pressure of more than 35 mm. within two minutes of an intravenous injection of 5 mg. (4) Histamine acid phosphate (0·02 mg. intravenously) produces a lowered blood pressure in normal persons, but in this condition causes a sudden and even dangerous rise to over 300 mm. within 1–3 minutes. (5) Perirenal insufflation of oxygen to demonstrate the tumour can be helpful but may precipitate a hypertensive crisis (§ 394).

Treatment.—When the diagnosis has been confirmed the hypertension can be controlled by phentolamine methanesulphonate 30 mg. in 1 litre of 10 per cent. dextrose intravenously. Surgical removal of the tumour is curative; the right suprarenal is the common site of this. When at operation the tumour cannot be visualised gentle pressure of the suspected site produces a sudden rise in blood pressure which is diagnostic.

§ 98. III. Polyarteritis Nodosa (Syn. Periarteritis Nodosa) is a collagen disease of the smaller arteries and arterioles which is usually generalised and produces widespread effects.

Symptoms.—The onset may be acute or subacute. In the generalised variety, the patient feels progressively weak and ill, loses weight and later shows mental apathy. There is an irregular temperature with tachycardia. (i.) Headache and vague pains in the limbs suggest a diagnosis of rheumatism or rheumatoid arthritis; (ii.) chest symptoms comprise shortness of breath, cough, sputum and sometimes hæmoptysis, and these are often associated with rales or consolidation of the lungs; (iii.) abdominal pain may occur, and thromboses in the abdominal organs at times give rise to gastrointestinal hæmorrhages or even perforation; (iv.) pericarditis or myocardial infarction may be found; (v.) polyneuritis is fairly common; (vi.) skin rashes include macular rashes, various types of erythema and purpura. The urine almost invariably contains albumen, casts and red cells, and uræmia with or without hypertension is common. A blood count shows a more or less severe degree of anæmia, with a polymorph leucocytosis and an eosinophilia, particularly in cases with pulmonary changes. The erythrocyte sedimentation rate is usually very high; blood cultures are invariably sterile. In a proportion of cases, one or more palpable skin nodules, the size of a millet seed or a pea, materially aid diagnosis. The *diagnosis* may be confirmed by biopsy of a skin nodule, or of voluntary muscle in which the characteristic vascular changes can be found.

Etiology.—The disease is believed to be a widespread reaction to a bacterial antigen hypersensitivity often originating in the respiratory tract: in some cases the reaction may be to a chemical antigen. The essential lesion is a whitish-grey nodule consisting of aggregations of polymorphonuclear cells, together with eosinophils and monocytes. The earliest change is in the adventitia. There is necrosis of the media and proliferation of the intima. Thromboses with infarction and even aneurysms are complications of this lesion.

The *Prognosis* used to be considered invariably fatal sooner or later, but after a period of many months, recovery can ensue spontaneously. Remissions and relapses are common. Death is usually due to renal or left ventricular failure or to a cerebral vascular lesion. *Treatment* is with cortisone, prednisolone or ACTH. Cortisone in full doses (100–300 mg. daily by mouth) may arrest the disease: it needs to be given for a long period of time and in larger doses during relapses.

Temporal Arteritis is a special type of periarteritis nodosa in which the disease is particularly prominent in one or both temporal arteries. It usually occurs in the elderly. *Symptoms.*—There is a persistent temporal headache, usually on both sides of the head. This is associated with a tender swelling and redness over one or both arteries; pulsation often ceases due to thrombosis and the pain then disappears. Similar changes occur in other arteries in the head with a more generalised headache. Loss of vision may be cortical and due to posterior cerebral arteritis, or may be ocular with papillœdema, retinal hæmorrhages and exudates often in association with partial or complete occlusion of the central artery of the retina. Optic atrophy may follow. The constitutional symptoms and signs of periarteritis nodosa are usually present.

The *Etiology* is unknown. As compared with periarteritis nodosa it is much less common to obtain evidence of a preceding bacterial infection.

Prognosis.—On the whole this is favourable, and many recover with no residual disabilities. The *Treatment* is the same as for periarteritis nodosa. Local resection produces a dramatic relief from pain.

§ 99. IV. Chronic and Acute Endarteritis, due to syphilis and other causes, is recognised by its pathological effects (cerebral softening, aneurysm and gangrene). Acute endarteritis has pathological rather than clinical significance. It is common in arteries at the base of chronic ulcers, such as the perforating ulcers of tabes, syringomyelia and diabetes, in new growths, both malignant and benign, in the terminal branches of the coronary arteries in patients dying of rheumatic carditis, in tuberculous, actinomycotic and lymphadenomatous lesions. Syphilis affects the arteries in two ways: (1) a proliferation of the intima of small vessels reduces their lumen and interferes with the nutrition of the parts supplied by these vessels (syphilitic endarteritis). This condition also predisposes to thrombosis in the affected vessel, and explains many cases of cerebral thrombosis. (2) A weakening of the muscular coats of the large vessels is seen typically in syphilitic mesaortitis and is brought about probably by obliterative changes in the vasa vasorum. With this is commonly associated a proliferation of the intima, especially of the first part of the aorta: it may lead to extensive scarring, and often causes anginal pain when the mouths of the coronary vessels are affected.

V. Aneurysmal Dilatation of the Arteries belongs to surgery, excepting aneurysm of the thoracic aorta (see § 80), the abdominal aorta (§ 263), and the cerebral arteries (§§ 853, 1047).

VI. Complications of vascular disease are: (*a*) **Hæmorrhage** from an artery weakened by disease; (*b*) **Thrombosis,** the coagulation of blood in the living vessels, results either from local vascular disease or an altered blood state; (*c*) **Embolism,** *i.e.,* the blocking of an artery by an embolus, which may result from heart disease, especially infective endocarditis (§ 50) and mitral stenosis with auricular fibrillation; or may be secondary to thrombosis; (*d*) **Stenosis,** as in the carotid artery, may give hemiplegic symptoms. *Diagnosis* is confirmed by carotid angiography and the condition may be remedied surgically (§ 903). Embolism and Thrombosis are dealt with elsewhere. See, for example, §§ 580, 587, 589, Phlebitis and Localised Œdema.

§ 100. VII. Functional Diseases of the Arteries and Arterioles produce a variety of syndromes, the causes of which are largely unknown. Yet patients are very conscious of the unpleasant nature of the symptoms they produce. Under this heading can be placed Raynaud's disease, migraine, alternate flushing and pallor (" flush-storms "), dead hands, cold hands and feet, chilblains, various other erythematous conditions, paroxysms of copious urination, acroparæsthesia, erythromelalgia, feelings of tingling, itching, throbbing, and actual swelling of the limbs. These are all described elsewhere. (See § 585 *et seq.*)

CHAPTER VI

THE LUNGS AND PLEURÆ

ILLNESSES arising in the respiratory tract account for over 25 per cent. of the cases seen in medical practice in Great Britain today. Upper respiratory tract disease is more common in children and lower respiratory illnesses in adults. These various ailments may arise from a primary respiratory infection, or be a complication of an acute general disease as in the acute specific fevers and other infective disorders. Overcrowding in badly ventilated atmospheres greatly increases the risk of infection from person to person.

PART A. SYMPTOMATOLOGY

The **Cardinal Symptoms** of diseases of the lungs are **cough, breathlessness, sputum,** and sometimes **pain in the chest** and **hæmoptysis.** The general symptoms are pyrexia, sweating, emaciation and debility. The right side of the heart suffers sooner or later in all serious or prolonged pulmonary diseases owing to interference with the pulmonary circulation.

§ 101. Concerning **Cough,** if it is attended by expectoration (as in 1 to 4 below), it points to definite changes either in the lungs, bronchi, or upper respiratory passages. If without expectoration (as in 5 to 9 below), it may point to simple congestion of the throat or larynx, to the presence of pleurisy, to the early stage of some pulmonary disorder, or to some source of reflex irritation. The *Causes of Cough* are as follows:

1. The commonest form is the recurring WHEEZY cough, attended by expectoration, so typical of bronchitis.

2. PAROXYSMAL cough, usually without much expectoration, occurs during attacks of *asthma,* and with *carcinoma of the bronchus* and other *mediastinal tumours.* Paroxysms of cough followed by vomiting are met especially in *whooping cough* and in advanced *phthisis.* A paroxysmal cough accompanied by purulent sputum is often due to *bronchiectasis* and more rarely to rupture into a bronchus of an empyema, or of a lung or liver abscess. (See also 8 on p. 161.)

3. The HAWKING cough of throat affections is very characteristic, and is met with in catarrhal *pharyngitis, chronic laryngitis* and *tracheitis,* especially in cigarette smokers. It also occurs in *nervous* subjects. A similar type of cough may be found in cases of chronic nasal catarrh associated with *infection of the accessory nasal sinuses,* especially the maxillary antrum: a constant hawking cough, with occasional severe paroxysms, is often present, and is relieved only by drainage of the antrum.

4. The IRRITABLE and mainly dry cough, most marked in the early morning and on going to bed, is especially associated with *early phthisis.*

160

5. A NIGHT cough may be due to chronic congestion of the pharynx, which is rarely associated with a *long uvula.*

6. The long BARKING or nervous cough of *hysteria* is very characteristic. It is unattended by expectoration.

7. The SHORT SUPPRESSED cough associated with *pleurisy* is so characteristic as to be almost diagnostic; it is unattended by expectoration unless pneumonia is present.

8. The GANDER, OR BRASSY cough associated with *aneurysm* and other *mediastinal tumours* is typical, and when once heard is readily recognised.

9. The REFLEX cough, due to irritation in the area of the vagus nerve, may be caused by (i.) *gastro-intestinal* disorders, such as dyspepsia, or worms in children; (ii.) *pericarditis*; (iii.) *ear* troubles, such as impacted wax; (iv.) *abdominal.* disease with irritation of the diaphragm—*e.g.,* by subphrenic or liver abscess.

The *Diagnosis* of these varieties of cough is important in practice, since they arise from, and may be seen in, affections other than those of the lungs. When a short dry cough is set up by going into the cold, it may be due to pharyngeal congestion or irritation. In simple throat affections the cough comes on in paroxysms, especially after talking. In chronic irritation of the larynx or trachea the cough is often worst in the early morning, when a paroxysm is induced by the effort to bring up a little glairy mucus; the face is congested, there is difficult inspiration and even vomiting.

The *Treatment* of cough depends upon the cause, but in general terms, irritable coughs should be treated by a linctus such as linct. simplex, linct. scillæ opiatus, linct. codeinæ or a linctus containing heroin gr. $\frac{1}{32} - \frac{1}{24}$; by various medicated lozenges (trochisci) such as the B.P. liquorice, morphia and ipecacuanha, or krameria and cocaine lozenge; or by bromides. Smoking cigarettes and mouth breathing should be avoided. Coughs associated with tenacious sputum, which is difficult to expectorate, should be treated not by sedatives, but by alkaline mixtures, with or without the addition of small doses, *e.g.,* gr. 3 of potassium iodide, to loosen the sputum.

§ 102. **Breathlessness,** or dyspnœa, is another symptom of lung affections. The causes of breathlessness are dealt with in more detail in the symptomatology of cardiac disorders (§ 26). The types of breathlessness special to respiratory disorders are:

1. Breathlessness attended by SNIFFING and NASAL BUBBLING is caused by *nasal* or *naso-pharyngeal catarrh.* The obstruction in the nose or mouth in these conditions may cause considerable stertor at nighttime.

2. Dyspnœa attended by considerable WHEEZING or rhonchi in the chest is characteristic of *bronchitis,* accompanied usually by emphysema.

3. STRIDULOUS respiration, in which the stridor attends both inspiration and expiration, is caused by obstruction in, or *pressure* upon, the trachea or larynx. It is accompanied in severe cases by drawing in of

C.M.—G

the epigastrium and lower costal cartilages during inspiration (§§ 171, 176 and 177).

4. PAINFUL dyspnœa occurs when the pain of *dry pleurisy* is sufficiently severe to prevent any more than a very shallow breath at each inspiration.

5. CONTINUOUS dyspnœa may be a prominent symptom of gross disease in the chest, such as with *emphysema* or a large *pleural effusion*: in this the embarrassment of respiration is mainly due to the reduction in respiratory capacity. The dyspnœa associated with extensive *fibrosis of the lung* from any cause, or with *collapse* following *obstruction of the bronchus*, *e.g.*, by malignant disease, may be considerable: dyspnœa is often one of the chief symptoms in the last mentioned, and is often disproportionate to the physical signs of disease present.

6. A rapid respiration with altered PULSE-RESPIRATION RATIO is very suggestive of *pneumonia*. Especially in children there is seen in this disease a characteristic working of the alæ nasi.

7. PAROXYSMAL dyspnœa is present in asthmatic attacks, but is often an indication of *cardiac disorder* (§ 27).

8. The SUDDEN and URGENT dyspnœa of *spontaneous pneumothorax* is a dramatic clinical phenomenon (§ 126).

§ 103. **Pain in the Chest** is usually present with affections of the pleura but otherwise it is not a constant symptom in pulmonary disorders. The various causes of pain in the chest are enumerated in § 33. The following are the chief types of pain met in diseases of the lungs:

(i.) The SHARP, cutting, stitch-like pain of *pleurisy* occurs on one or other side of the chest before the effusion separates the inflamed surfaces. It is greatly aggravated by drawing a long breath: respiration therefore becomes very shallow. This is undoubtedly the commonest of the pulmonary causes of pain in the chest, and this symptom in *pneumonia* indicates involvement of the pleura. It must be remembered, however, that in some *subdiaphragmatic diseases*—*e.g.*, of the liver, spleen or colon —pain is also felt on deep inspiration. One of the most intense forms of pain in the chest is due to *diaphragmatic pleurisy*. When it originates in the central part of the diaphragm it is referred via the phrenic nerve to the tip of one or both shoulders, but when it involves the lateral portion of the diaphragm it is referred along the costal margin and via the intercostal nerves to the abdominal wall. It then may also cause abdominal rigidity and hiccough and give rise to difficulty in diagnosis, since it may suggest the presence of acute abdominal disease. (ii.) A SORENESS behind the upper part of the sternum attends the onset of *acute tracheitis* and *bronchitis*. (iii.) SUDDEN severe pain, followed by considerable pulmonary distress and general collapse, occurs with the onset of *pneumothorax*. (iv.) SUDDEN pain, often attended by hæmoptysis, marks the occurrence of *embolism* of the lung or rupture of an aneurysm into the lung. (v.) *Cancer* of the lung may or may not be accompanied by pain, according to its proximity to the pleura or other sensitive structures. (vi.) *Mediastinal tumours*, including aortic aneurysm (§ 80), give rise sooner or later to pain in the chest. (vii.) Slight pain in the upper intercostal spaces is a frequent symptom in early phthisis: a similar pain is also found in some cases of lung abscess, the site varying according to the position of the abscess.

The presence of **sputum** is an important sign; its naked-eye appearance may lead to the diagnosis of certain lung diseases. It must be examined by the physician, and it is therefore described in § 111. Let it be remembered that children usually swallow sputum; as also do some adults. Secretions from the pharynx must not be mistaken for sputum from the bronchi or lungs. The amount of coughing required to void the sputum may aid diagnosis—*e.g.*, in the early stages of bronchitis a considerable amount of coughing results in only a little tenacious sputum, whereas in the later stages a moderate degree of coughing brings up much frothy muco-purulent sputum.

§ 104. **Hæmoptysis** means the spitting of blood ($\alpha\iota\mu o$, blood; $\pi\tau\acute{v}\omega$, I spit), but the term is confined to the expectoration of blood from the lower respiratory tract—the larynx, trachea, bronchi or the lungs. The blood may be present in several different forms: (*a*) streaks of blood largely separate from the sputum; (*b*) intimately mixed with the sputum forming a blood-stained frothy secretion; or (*c*) it may be more copious giving rise to small clots or a more profuse hæmorrhage. A clear distinction of these different varieties is important in diagnosis and in treatment. After any fairly profuse hæmorrhage it is usual for the patient to have pyrexia for a few days, due to the breakdown products of the blood in the respiratory passages.

The *fallacies* with regard to this symptom are very important. When a patient comes with a history of having " brought up blood," it may at first be difficult to determine whether the blood has come from the lungs, from the stomach (hæmatemesis), or from the upper respiratory passages (nose, throat, etc.)—" false hæmoptysis." In the so-called spurious hæmoptysis, small quantities of thin reddish fluid containing red corpuscles are coughed up; its source is usually from spongy gums or the mucous membrane of the cheeks or pharynx. Although in many such cases the bleeding is genuine, the possibility of deliberate malingering must be borne in mind.

The differentiation of the various forms of blood-spitting is given more fully under Hæmatemesis (§ 272), but the following points are mentioned here as being characteristic of the issue of blood from the lungs: (i.) It is not infrequently preceded and accompanied by a tickling cough (if the blood be large in quantity it may excite retching on touching the pharynx); (ii.) the patient usually continues to cough up blood for some time afterwards; (iii.) the blood has a bright red colour, is alkaline and frothy (if very profuse, it may be without froth, and clots may be present); (iv.) physical signs of disease of the lungs are often, though not always, present—they may be absent in the hæmoptysis of early phthisis; (v.) the antecedent history of the patient may point to pulmonary tuberculosis, to cardiac disease or to a bronchial neoplasm, these being undoubtedly the most common causes of hæmoptysis. The above details are given for guidance; in actual practice the distinction between hæmoptysis and hæmatemesis seldom presents real difficulty if care is taken to obtain an accurate history; the descriptions of hæmoptysis given by patients themselves are remarkably constant:—"I felt something suddenly come up in my throat and it was blood."—These or similar words constitute a common statement volunteered by patients. The persistence of stained sputum for a day or two after the initial attack affords further strong presumptive evidence of true hæmoptysis. The amount of blood expectorated at once may be slight, and the bleeding may be protracted or recurrent; or there may be copious bleeding at one time, and the attack can be fatal within a few minutes. The main causes of hæmoptysis are:

I. PHTHISIS. This is by far the commonest cause, at any rate in young adults, and it is a reasonable clinical rule that definite blood spitting in a young adult, however small in quantity, should be assumed to be due to pulmonary tuberculosis until it has been proved to originate from some other cause. The hæmoptysis of phthisis may occur either in the early or in the advanced stage of the disease; in either case it may be small or very large in amount. When the disease is advanced, and bleeding occurs from rupture of an eroded vessel, the issue may be rapidly fatal, though death seldom occurs with such suddenness as in rupture of an aortic aneurysm (q.v.). Tuberculosis of the lungs may be recognised by: (i.) the previous history of the patient; and (ii.) evidence of congestion, consolidation or excavation of the lung. Nevertheless, the most careful physical examination may fail to reveal any obvious signs; sputum tests and especially X-ray examination are essential before the presence of tuberculosis can be ruled out.

II. MITRAL STENOSIS. Here the pulmonary blood pressure is raised and the lungs are congested owing to obstruction at the mitral valve. The patient's cardiac condition is usually known before the hæmoptysis, but in some cases hæmoptysis may be the first symptom which occasions a visit to the doctor. An erroneous diagnosis of phthisis has often been made in these circumstances, even in the absence of tubercle bacilli from the sputum, and when characteristic cardiac signs are present.

III. In BRONCHIECTASIS there may be recurrent hæmoptysis from granulation tissue lining the cavities. As in phthisis, this may occur at any stage of the disease, but is a prominent and occasionally severe symptom in the so-called "dry bronchiectasis." In this, between the attacks of hæmorrhage, the patient may be free from symptoms and physical signs, and only X-ray examination (after the introduction of iodised oil into the bronchi) reveals the cause (see § 145).

IV. In PRIMARY MALIGNANT DISEASE of the bronchus there may be hæmoptysis, seldom severe, except in the advanced stages; even then much hæmorrhage is uncommon. Repeated small hæmorrhages in a patient of middle-age, or especially one of more advanced years, should raise the suspicion of malignant disease in some portion of the respiratory tract. *Adenoma* of the bronchus may be the cause of recurrent hæmoptysis.

V. Various PULMONARY DISEASES other than phthisis may be attended by expectoration of blood of varying amount. In *acute tracheo-bronchitis* the sputum may contain streaks of blood from time to time; in *spirochætal bronchitis* the hæmorrhage is likely to be much more definite and pronounced. In *pneumonia* blood in the sputum is a frequent characteristic, the amount varying with the type and bacteriology of the disease. The rusty sputum which is such a diagnostic feature of the pure pneumococcal lobar pneumonia differs from the expectoration of some of the acute broncho-pneumonic conditions following influenza, especially those associated with a hæmolytic streptococcus; in these the whole lung becomes sodden, and almost pure blood may be coughed up in large quantities throughout the acute stage. In *chronic bronchitis* with emphysema the sputum may at times be blood-streaked. *Gangrene, abscess, sporotrichosis* and other *fungal* infections, and *hydatid* disease may cause bleeding. *Pulmonary distomatosis* is the cause of so-called endemic hæmoptysis in Japan.

§ 105. VI. **Pulmonary Infarction** is very common and is present in 10 per cent. of routine autopsies. It is usually due to an embolus lodging in one of the branches of the pulmonary artery, but can occur with primary thrombosis of the pulmonary vessels. The size of the embolus varies greatly: on the one hand it may form a large coiled embolus which completely blocks the main pulmonary artery near its bifurcation, causing sudden unexpected death—"*pulmonary apoplexy.*" On the other hand it may cause a small area of peripheral infarction, usually at the base of the lung. Embolism may recur in the course of a few hours or days: single large emboli or repeated small emboli cause acute pulmonary hypertension.

When *large emboli* are dislodged from distant parts, the patient may die suddenly at the moment of impaction of the clot in a main branch of the pulmonary artery. In such cases there may be no premonitory symptoms, even the existence of a clot being unsuspected. *Emboli of intermediate size* cause sudden dyspnœa, pleural pain and collapse with a rapid thin pulse, sweating, a fall of systemic blood pressure and *acute cor pulmonale* with a rise in jugular venous pressure. The patient becomes cyanosed, at the moment of infarction there is often a sudden reflexly-induced desire to defæcate and later the patient often coughs up sputum which is uniformly blood-stained. There are usually signs of consolidation at one or other lung base (more usually on the right side), often followed by a blood-stained pleural effusion. X-ray examination is most informative when performed 24 hours later and usually reveals a cone-shaped or a spherical area of consolidation, a raised dome to the diaphragm or a small pleural effusion. *Small emboli* may be difficult to locate in the lungs and may only be suspected when sudden dyspnœa arises. They are not necessarily accompanied by hæmoptysis.

Etiology.—Pulmonary infarction is encountered much more often in the elderly and in those with chronic diseases such as cancer or other debilitating causes. It is common in patients with severe chronic heart failure of all kinds (§ 55). The embolus may arise *centrally* in the heart especially in those with mitral stenosis or auricular fibrillation, or it may originate *peripherally* as the result of thrombo-phlebitis in the pelvic veins (often following an abdominal or pelvic operation, or childbirth) or from the deep calf veins. There may be premonitory signs of such changes in the veins, with a slight rise of temperature, tachycardia and local swelling or tenderness in the calf.

Treatment consists of bed rest for four or more weeks, and if emboli recur anticoagulants such as phenindione B.P. (Dindevan) are essential —see § 52. Morphia or other sedatives and oxygen may be required. An antibiotic such as penicillin for a few days will help to prevent the occurrence of infection and even of an abscess in the devitalised area of the lung. *Surgical* intervention by tying the femoral vein or even the inferior vena cava is occasionally necessary: pulmonary embolectomy in severe cases is only possible when skilled surgical treatment is at hand immediately the need arises. *Prophylaxis* consists in giving breathing and leg exercises to all patients (especially the elderly) as soon as they have recovered from an operation or an acute illness: they should then be got out of bed and made more mobile as soon as possible.

VII. Rupture of an ANEURYSM into the trachea or bronchus is usually followed by immediate death, the preceding hæmoptysis being of the most dramatic and appalling character, though in some cases there may be a considerable leakage for several days before the final issue (§ 80). Apart from such instances of fatal hæmoptysis, a slight degree of blood-spitting is common; hence the occurrence of occasional mild hæmoptysis, if associated with a history of substernal pain, should raise suspicion as to the presence of an aneurysm.

VIII. ULCERATION and NÆVI in some part of the upper respiratory tract (throat, larynx, trachea, etc.). In rare circumstances bleeding from this source may be considerable, but as a general rule hæmoptysis due to local ulceration or nævi of the upper respiratory passages is small in amount, but apt to be recurrent. The diagnosis depends upon thorough and complete investigation of the respiratory tract, including bronchoscopic examination. It is often dangerous to conclude that hæmoptysis is due to local causes in the throat; the diagnosis of varicose veins of the pharynx is seldom justified or substantiated, and patients who have been told that their blood-spitting originates from enlarged veins at the back of the throat are usually found on subsequent investigation to be suffering from phthisis, a bronchial carcinoma or some other serious organic disease.

IX. TRAUMA can cause hæmoptysis as the result of a foreign body, or a fractured rib penetrating the chest wall. Apart from these, simple contusion of the lung may occur and if the bruised area becomes infected traumatic pneumonia may develop. The possibility of an injury causing hæmoptysis from already existing disease, such as a previously unrecognised tuberculous cavity, should be remembered.

X. Purpura, polycythæmia vera, Ayerza's disease, hæmophilia, scurvy, leukæmia and some other BLOOD CONDITIONS may be attended by bleeding from the lungs. These causes are rare, but when present are usually recognised, though at first they may not be obvious. Hæmoptysis has been recorded in severe cases of the acute specific fevers.

XI. CARDIO-VASCULAR and RENAL DISEASE. Hæmoptysis occurs in subjects of *arterial* and *renal* disease. Hæmorrhages from bronchial arteries have been described in cases of chronic interstitial nephritis. It is certain that hæmoptysis may occur in some patients with a *high systemic blood pressure*, in whom no serious disease of the lungs exists. Though this cannot be described as common, it is perhaps less rare than is supposed.

XII. VICARIOUS MENSTRUATION as a cause of hæmoptysis has been described as occurring shortly before the menstrual period is due, normal menstruation being absent or greatly diminished. It must be insisted that vicarious menstruation is a very rare cause of hæmoptysis; this diagnosis should not be an excuse for failure to carry out the most complete investigation in cases of hæmoptysis of uncertain origin.

Diagnosis. Although the cause of hæmoptysis may in many instances be obvious on ordinary clinical examination, in other cases it can only be determined after prolonged, even elaborate, investigation. First a careful history of the case should be taken. This must be followed by bacteriological and cytological examination of the sputum and a routine chest X-ray in postero-anterior and lateral planes: the latter may demonstrate a lesion lying behind the heart or other mediastinal structures. If these simpler measures do not reveal the presence of disease in the heart or lungs, it is necessary to introduce a radio-opaque iodised liquid (such as lipiodol) into the bronchi (§ 110) or to examine with the laryngoscope and the bronchoscope. If a definite diagnosis is still not possible the patient should be kept under regular observation with X-ray control for another twelve months.

The *Prognosis* depends upon the cause. Hæmoptysis must be regarded as a serious symptom, at any rate in the first place, and a patient should never be informed that it is of little or no account until complete investigation has elicited not only the cause of the symptom, but the relative severity of the underlying disease. The hæmoptysis of phthisis is of importance chiefly from a diagnostic standpoint; its prognostic significance is less obvious, and even in cases of active tuberculosis of the lungs the occurrence of hæmorrhage should not *per se* be taken as necessarily indicating a grave outlook. It is often the first symptom in an early case. It must be regarded as an indication for complete and exhaustive examination by modern methods, the ultimate prognosis depending on the evidence thus acquired. Following hæmoptysis from a primary source in one area, it is common to find physical signs and X-ray evidence of aspiration of blood into another area of lung—usually at a lung base. Such an occurrence must not prevent a search for the original cause of the bleeding.

Treatment.—The patient is usually very frightened by the appearance of blood from the chest and reassurance, combined with the use of sedative drugs, is then necessary. The patient should be put to bed in a recumbent position, with one or two pillows for comfort, but absolute rest should not be enforced as it is desirable to move sufficiently to permit the coughing up of blood from the bronchi. When the side of the chest from which the blood is coming can be identified, it is better to lie on this side to help immobilise the affected area and lessen the chance of aspiration into healthy areas of the lungs. (*a*) For *profuse hæmorrhage* the most effective remedy is a hypodermic injection of morphia (gr. $\frac{1}{6}$–$\frac{1}{4}$), repeated in 4–6 hours if necessary: this quietens the patient and lessens his alarm. If the bleeding continues, 10 ml. of 1·0 per cent. freshly prepared solution of Congo-red (intravenously) has often proved of value—to avoid reactions it must have been passed through a fine filter. Sometimes the intravenous injection of calcium gluconate (20 ml. of a 10 per cent. solution) appears to stop the hæmorrhage. Intramuscular injections of emetine (gr. $\frac{1}{2}$ each 6 hours) are sometimes useful. Where the hæmorrhage is due to extensive tuberculosis of the lung and if it be definitely known that it is coming from one side, collapse of the affected lung by artificial pneumothorax may be the only effective remedy. In these circumstances one must introduce a much larger amount of air (perhaps up to 1,500 ml. altogether, or even more) than is ordinarily given in the course of pneumothorax therapy; such a procedure has obvious disadvantages, which can only be disregarded in view of the extreme urgency of the situation. To prevent secondary infection of the blood remaining in the bronchial tree it is advisable to give a routine course of antibiotic for about 5 days. (*b*) When hæmoptysis occurs in *small quantity*, bed rest alone may be sufficient. The hæmorrhage of congestion due to cardiac disease should not be checked, unless excessive, as it relieves the pulmonary congestion. Once the cause of hæmoptysis has been defined, *surgical measures* are sometimes necessary.

PART B. PHYSICAL EXAMINATION

Examination of a patient suffering from disease referable to the organs of respiration includes: (*a*) an accurate history; (*b*) recording the temperature, pulse rate and the weight; (*c*) careful physical examination of the chest; (*d*) examination of the upper respiratory passages; (*e*) X-ray examination of the chest; (*f*) pathological examination of sputum, blood, pleural fluids, etc.; (*g*) bronchoscopic examination. Especially when a primary bronchial neoplasm is suspected these methods of investigation may be followed by further X-ray examination after partial collapse of a lung with a pneumothorax, or by exploratory thoracotomy. It is not suggested that X-ray examination and/or instrumental examination of the respiratory tract are necessary in every case (*e.g.*, of uncomplicated recurrent bronchitis); but modern techniques have come to play an increasing part in the diagnosis and treatment of chest disease. The history usually gives a fair guide to the extent of examination required; time spent in obtaining a comprehensive account of the symptomatology is not wasted and often avoids unnecessary duplication of special tests. Physical signs, although valuable as part of the total evidence, can only give information as to relatively gross structural changes.

The temperature and the pulse rate are often raised in acute chest diseases, and in some chronic conditions such as pulmonary tuberculosis. A record of the weight will show whether there has been a gain or loss in recent months and may be useful for comparison with subsequent weighings.

The PHYSICAL EXAMINATION OF THE LUNGS is carried out by means of Inspection, Palpation, Percussion and Auscultation.

§ 106. Inspection.—The inspection of the chest must be carried out in a good light, and the patient must be instructed to stand or sit erect, or, if in bed, to lie flat and evenly and to breathe deeply. After noting the movements from the front, examine the back, then look from behind over the clavicles in order to make out the slighter distortions or inequalities of the chest. By inspection we note (1) the rate and character of the breathing; (2) the position of the apex beat of the heart (§ 39); (3) the shape and size of the chest. The chief landmarks of the chest are mentioned in § 38. Posteriorly the chest is divided into the suprascapular, scapular, and infrascapular regions. The scapular region is divided by the scapular spine, into the infra- and supra-spinous regions. The names sufficiently indicate the positions of the various regions.

(1) *Rate and Character of the Breathing.*—The rate varies normally from 15 to 20 per minute, or one-fourth the rate of the pulse; any change in this proportion, or pulse-respiration ratio, should be observed. Notice whether the breathing is rapid, slow, deep, shallow or irregular. The respiration should be counted without the patient's knowledge—while counting the breathing, it is a good plan to feel the radial artery as if you were examining the pulse. Both sides of the chest should move equally. *Any diminution of movement of any part of the chest points to disuse of the underlying lung from disease,* whether new (pleurisy and pneumonia) or old (fibrosis or collapse). Instead of the normal concavity of the intercostal spaces there is flattening or convexity when pleural fluid is present. Drawing in of the interspaces on both sides during inspiration is indicative of some interference with the free entry of air into the lungs (inspiratory dyspnœa) due to obstruction of the larynx or trachea. The grunting expiration of broncho-pneumonia in children should be especially noted. It is convenient also at this stage to observe whether the alæ nasi are moving. *Cheyne-Stokes'* breathing is a special type of rhythmical irregularity of breathing (see § 28). When movement of the chest causes pain as in pleurisy, or when the muscles of the chest wall are paralysed, there is abdominal breathing. When the diaphragm is

out of action, as in certain abdominal conditions, there is exaggerated heaving of the thorax and noisy respiration.

(2) The *position of the apex* beat of the heart gives an important clue to many diseases of the lungs. Thus effusion and pneumothorax cause it to be displaced to the opposite side; fibrosis or collapse draw it over to the same side; emphysema masks it.

(3) *The Shape and Size of the Chest.*—A cross-section of the *healthy* adult chest gives almost the form of an ellipse, the longer diameter being from side to side. In the child it is more circular in shape. The chest should appear symmetrical, although in reality the right side is slightly larger than the left. There should be no marked hollowing anywhere; the clavicle should form only a moderate prominence. The circumference of the chest varies with the height of the individual, but it should average about 34 to 35 inches for a man 5 feet 6 inches in height. With deep inspiration it should expand 1½ to 2 inches or more.

The shape of the chest varies considerably in different persons. The long narrow *asthenic* chest in those of slight build is associated with a narrow vertical-shaped heart. At the other extreme is the *broad* chest with a relatively horizontal heart in the person of " stocky " and usually muscular build. The association of the former with a tendency to phthisis is no longer accepted for the occurrence of pulmonary tuberculosis is independent of the shape of the chest. The *barrel-shaped* chest is still common: it is traditionally associated with emphysema but it may occur in normal persons. In this condition the chest is wide from side to side and from front to back, the lower ribs are raised and become more horizontal and the epigastric angle is unusually wide. The *rachitic* chest with its vertical parasternal grooves and horizontal Harrison's sulcus is now much less commonly seen. The *pigeon-breast* is the name given to a deformity in which the lower end of the sternum bulges forward to form a central prominence, the front end of the ribs bending forward to meet the sternum. It is usually the result of juvenile rickets or of recurrent respiratory disease in childhood. The opposite condition is represented by the congenital deformity of a *funnel-shaped* chest in which there is a deep hollow at the lower end of the sternum and in the upper epigastrium. When severe this causes the heart to be flattened between the sternum in front and the vertebral column behind, or to be displaced into the left chest. The apparent cardiac enlargement is often associated with a systolic murmur, and must be distinguished from that of true cardiac disease.

More important than the general shape and cross-section of the chest are any irregular or *asymmetrical abnormalities*, among which we should look for *hollowing, prominence* or *contraction*.

(a) *Localised Hollowing* or " flattening " of the infraclavicular region may indicate chronic tuberculosis or any other disease in which fibrosis and lung contraction occur.

(b) *Undue Prominence on one side* of the ribs anteriorly may be due to: (i.) Scoliosis—*i.e.*, lateral curvature of the spine, the convexity of the chest being in the opposite direction. (ii.) Large intrathoracic tumours, including aneurysm, effusion, abscess or air (pneumothorax) in the chest. (iii.) If the precordial area be prominent, it may be the result of cardiac disease in early youth, before the ribs were fully developed. (iv.) An enlarged liver or spleen, abdominal tumour or abscess may also cause a bulging of the lower ribs on the right and left sides respectively. Other causes are: (v.) Subcutaneous emphysema or a localised deposit of fat or other tumour. (vi.) Localised muscular over-development, as in athletes.

(c) *Contraction* of an *entire side* of the chest may be due to (i.) fibrosis of the lung from whatever cause; (ii.) pulmonary collapse; (iii.) a thickened pleura, such as follows a previous empyema; (iv.) the operation of thoracoplasty.

During inspection of the lungs it is convenient to note at the same time if there is any abnormal pulsation in the aortic region (see aneurysm), whether the veins in the neck are engorged and pulsating, the size of the thyroid gland, the presence of cyanosis of the face and hands, or clubbing of the fingers.

Clubbing of the fingers is seen in diseases of the lung in association with pulmonary fibrosis, bronchiectasis, lung abscess, empyema and sometimes with carcinoma of the lung or mediastinum.

§ 107. Palpation is the next step in the routine examination of the lungs. The position of the apex beat should be confirmed and any displacement of the trachea noted. The amount of movement of the two sides of the chest with respiration is estimated better by palpation than by inspection. This is important in the diagnosis of consolidation at one apex, and in the detection of fluid, tumour, or other cause of deficient activity of one lung or part of a lung. By palpation *Vocal Fremitus* (V.F.), or the vibration of the voice, can be felt. In the normal person the voice sounds produced in the larynx are transmitted through the air columns in the trachea and bronchi to the surface of the chest wall. The V.F. is marked in the adult man but may be scarcely appreciable in women or children with high-pitched voices. The normal V.F. is slightly greater at the right than at the left apex. Towards the bases it is less intense but almost equal. This test is of the greatest value in differentiating solid and fluid. Thus the V.F. is *increased* where there is consolidation of the lung, as in pneumonia or phthisis, whereas it is *diminished* or absent when the lung is separated from the chest wall by fluid or air, or when the air passages are occluded, as in obstruction of a bronchus.[1] Not only is the V.F. a valuable differential sign, but its degree of diminu-

---

[1] The absence of vocal resonance on auscultation over a pleural effusion is due to the fact that the lung, being displaced by the fluid, is usually above the level at which the chest-piece of the stethoscope is applied. It is true that water conducts sound better than air when the source of the sound and the auditory reception apparatus are both below the water level, but when sound waves reach an air–water or a water–air surface, few are transmitted.

tion is a useful measure of the *amount* of fluid present in cases of pleural effusion.   In bronchitis the rhonchi can be felt, *rhonchial fremitus*; and in pleurisy and pericarditis *friction* may be distinctly felt by the hand. A broken rib, a pointing empyema, subcutaneous emphysema and external tumours are made out by palpation.

§ 108. **Percussion** is, after palpation, the next step in the examination of the chest.   Begin at the apex and percuss *alternate sides* at exactly

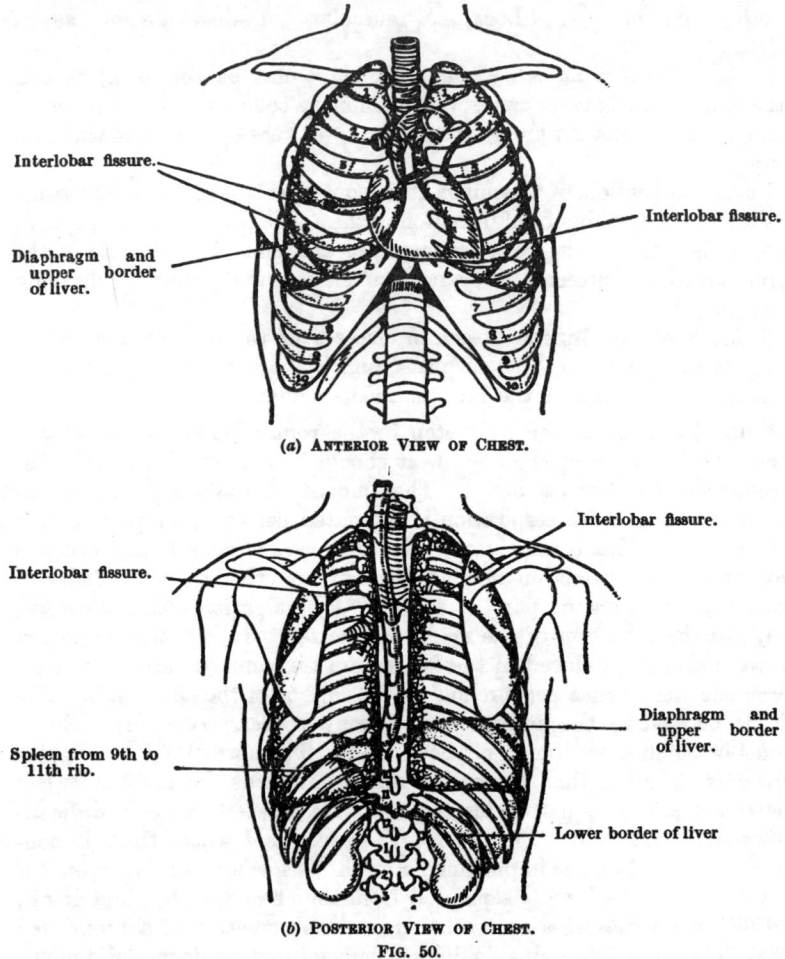

(a) ANTERIOR VIEW OF CHEST.

(b) POSTERIOR VIEW OF CHEST.

FIG. 50.

corresponding points in order *to compare the healthy and unhealthy sides*, and thus work gradually downwards.   Place the index or middle finger *firmly* and *flat* against the chest, in a horizontal position.   Then strike upon it with the tip of the middle finger of the right hand.   The blow should come from the wrist, not the elbow, and should be short and sharp. Except for the percussion of deep structures (*e.g.*, the dome of the liver) heavy percussion should not be employed.

When examining the *back* of the chest (Fig. 50), the patient should be instructed to cross his arms and bend a little forward so that the scapulæ are drawn out of the way. The normal resonance of the lung extends posteriorly to the upper border of the eleventh rib on the right side, and to the lower border of the eleventh rib on the left side. On deep inspiration the resonance extends over an inch lower, and during deep expiration over an inch higher. Owing to the thickness of the scapular muscles the note over the scapulæ may be markedly impaired in muscular people. For examination of the *sides* of the chest the patient should be told to put his hands on the top of his head.

The normal pulmonary note can only be learned by practice and experience, and the student should *frequently practise first on normal chests*, so as to accustom himself to the normal resonance.

The normal percussion note is resonant. It is *dull* or flat when the lung tissue is solid, as in pneumonia; or when the chest contains fluid, as in pleural effusion, or with a thickened pleura or a tumour. When a note is said to be dull, it means that the pitch is raised and the volume of the note diminished. Between a dull note and one that is resonant there are all stages of *impaired resonance*. The percussion note is *hyper-resonant*, sometimes tympanitic, whenever the lung tissue is unduly open —*i.e.*, too full of air, as in emphysema, or when there is air in the pleura (pneumothorax). When one part of the lung is floating above a pleural effusion (which compresses the lower part of the lung), the percussion note is unduly resonant. This so-called *Skodaic resonance* may be tympanitic (drum-like) in character, somewhat resembling the note normally obtained over the stomach.

Increased Resistance is another quality which can be observed in the process of percussion as above described. It is greatest over fluid, but is present also in consolidation. This sign is used especially by those whose auditory appreciation is imperfect. Subtle differences cannot be appreciated by this means.

§ 109. Auscultation.—In auscultation there are four things to observe: (*a*) The intensity and the quality of the vesicular murmur (V.M.); (*b*) the relative length of inspiration and expiration; (*c*) the presence of adventitious sounds within or outside the lungs; and (*d*) the voice sounds or vocal resonance (V.R.).

(*a*) The normal CHARACTER OF THE BREATH SOUNDS—*i.e.*, the *vesicular murmur* (V.M.)—should be listened to in healthy chests as often as possible. Away from the apex and larger bronchi it has a soft whiffing character and there is no appreciable pause between the inspiratory and the expiratory phases. The breath sounds audible over the right apex are more pronounced than on the left side because of the presence of the eparterial bronchus on this side (cf. p. 177, fallacies no. 9). The difference varies with the age and the build of the patient. The V.M. is normally very

loud in children, and when a loud V.M. is met with in adults, it is called
"*puerile* breathing." The V.M. is diminished when the lung is under-
ventilated by a diseased process. A decreased V.M. over a particular
area therefore represents a deficient local air entry and over fluid it is
usually absent: the commonest cause of a general decrease of V.M. in
both lungs is pulmonary emphysema. *Bronchial breathing* differs from
vesicular breathing in three main respects: (i.) it is much harsher and
more prolonged; (ii.) inspiration and expiration are of approximately equal
length and character, or the expiratory phase may be obviously prolonged;
(iii.) there is an appreciable interval between the inspiratory and the

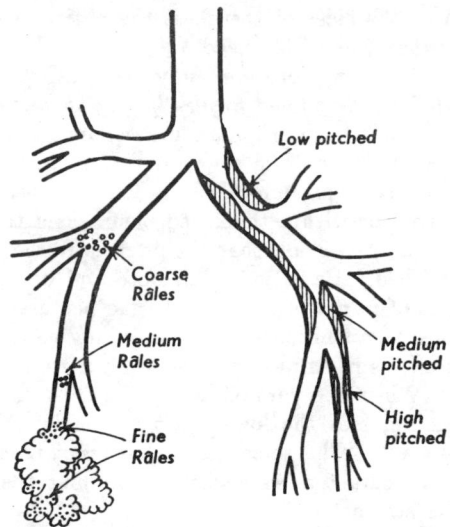

Fig. 51.—Diagram to show the production of rhonchi on right, by narrowing of the tubes, and of
râles on left by moisture in the bronchial tubes. Fine râles, also known as crepitations, occur
in the smallest bronchioles and possibly in the vesicles, especially near the lung bases.

expiratory phases. Bronchial breathing can be heard *normally* by listening over the upper segment of the sternum, or near the fourth dorsal
vertebra at the back. In other areas the breath sounds are bronchial
when the lung is solid, as in tuberculosis, pneumonia, or collapse from any
cause; the sound produced in the glottis is conveyed down the bronchi and
smaller tubes direct to the ear, owing to the increased conductivity of the
solid tissue. In pleural effusion bronchial breathing is sometimes heard,
especially near the angle of the scapula; the effusion causes a collapse
of the lung so that the bronchial quality present in the nearest bronchus
is well conducted to the surface (Fig. 55).

The terms "bronchial" and "tubular" breathing are sometimes
taught as synonymous; it is more accurate to describe three kinds of
bronchial breathing: (i.) high-pitched or tubular breathing; (ii.) medium-

pitched or true bronchial breathing; and (iii.) low-pitched or cavernous breathing. This is the variety normally heard over the trachea and in other areas it is heard when the sound produced in a dilated bronchus or cavity is conveyed to the surface.

Amphoric breathing is a sound like air entering a bell-jar, and is sometimes heard over a pneumothorax or a very large cavity.

(*b*) Heard through the stethoscope, the inspiratory sound is normally three times as long as the expiratory sound, which follows it without a pause. The *process* of expiration is much longer than inspiration, but through the stethoscope most of the former is unheard because the velocity of the air-current is low. *Expiration is prolonged* in any disease which involves a loss of elasticity of the lung tissue, such as emphysema, or an increase in conductivity, as in consolidation.

(*c*) The presence or absence of ADVENTITIOUS SOUNDS has next to be noted. These may be either dry or moist.

DRY SOUNDS.—*Pleural friction* is produced by the two inflamed and roughened surfaces of the pleura rubbing together. The sound has been likened to the creaking of leather. It is generally heard both in inspiration and in expiration, is often intensified by pressure with the stethoscope and by deep breathing, and is not abolished by coughing.

MOIST SOUNDS are of two varieties:

(1) *Rhonchi* are continuous sounds produced when the lumen of the bronchial tubes is narrowed (i.) by swelling of the mucosa, (ii.) by adherent sticky mucus (as in bronchitis), or (iii.) by spasm of the bronchial muscle as in asthma. They occur during inspiration (inspiratory rhonchi), during expiration (expiratory rhonchi) or in both phases of respiration— expiratory rhonchi being especially characteristic of asthma. When low-pitched they are described as *sonorous* (produced in the larger tubes), when high-pitched as *sibilant* or *whistling* (when the small tubes are concerned) with an intermediate variety of medium-pitched rhonchi.

(2) *Râles* are discontinuous moist sounds due to the presence of mucus or other fluid in the bronchial tubes. Unlike rhonchi they are chiefly audible during inspiration. Râles are of three main varieties, according to the size of the tubes involved and the amount of fluid present, viz. coarse, medium and fine râles. *Coarse râles* are produced in the medium-sized bronchi when there is much sticky mucus or muco-pus present, as in an area of resolving pneumonia or in bronchiectatic cavities. These latter have sometimes been termed *leathery* râles. *Medium* râles are due to mucus in the smaller bronchial tubes. *Fine râles* (*crepitations*) occur when there is excess of moisture in the terminal bronchioles and perhaps in the alveoli; during inspiration the alveoli open up for otherwise their walls are kept in apposition by a thin layer of moist secretion. They have been likened to the sound produced by the rustling of tissue-paper near the ear. When râles are few and difficult to detect, they may become clearer when the patient draws a deep inspiration immediately after a slight cough (post-tussic râles). Râles sometimes resemble friction

sounds, but are distinguished by being audible only during inspiration and by being altered by coughing.

(*d*) The VOICE SOUNDS, or vocal resonance (V.R.). (i.) When the patient speaks, the vocal resonance is INCREASED (*bronchophony*) if the conductivity of the lung substance is rendered greater by consolidation, such as that produced by tuberculosis or pneumonia. If this be so great that even whispered words are distinctly conducted, it is known as *whispering pectoriloquy*. (ii.) The vocal resonance is DIMINISHED when a layer of fluid or air intervenes between the lung and the chest wall (*e.g.*, in pleural effusion and pneumothorax), or when there is a thickened pleura. Nevertheless, in a pleural effusion, at the upper level of the fluid, the higher tones of the voice sounds are sometimes conducted, and have been likened to the bleating of a goat (hence called *Ægophony*). Transference of the voice sounds depends upon patency of the bronchi; in any condition therefore in which there is gross obstruction of the bronchus or its main divisions, *e.g.*, by a growth, the vocal resonance is diminished or lost.

The COIN or BELL sound is a sign of some value. To elicit this, a large coin is laid flat on the chest and is tapped by another coin; the mouthpiece of the stethoscope is placed some distance away, but not on the same rib or over the stomach. A bell sound is pathognomonic of pneumothorax.

Clinically, diseases of the lungs may be conveniently divided into those with **dullness on percussion,** those in which the percussion note is **normal,** and those in which it is **hyper-resonant.** Those with **dullness** may be subdivided into two groups—those in which the dullness is due to CONSOLIDATION, and those in which it is due to FLUID. The clinical features by which solidification of the lung is distinguished from fluid in the chest are so important that they are given in tabular form.

TABLE V.—DIFFERENTIATION OF SOLID LUNG FROM FLUID
IN THE CHEST

	Consolidation of Lung.	Pleural Effusion.
INSPECTION ..	Movement impaired. May be flattening over the part (if infraclavicular region).	Movement impaired. May be bulging (of intercostal spaces).
PALPATION ..	V.F. INCREASED.	V.F. DIMINISHED or absent.
PERCUSSION ..	Resonance impaired.	Absolutely dull over fluid.
AUSCULTATION	BREATHING BRONCHIAL. V.R. INCREASED.	V.M. ABSENT OR WEAK. V.R. DIMINISHED.
HEART	In normal position (pneumonia), or pulled towards affected side (fibrosis or collapse).	Displaced to the opposite side.

Fallacies in Diagnosis of Diseases of the Chest.—This list includes the most important fallacies, but it is impossible to make it exhaustive.

1. Care should be taken to hold the chest piece firmly and flat on the skin.

2. When the chest wall is very thin the sounds heard on auscultation are proportionately loud. The percussion note is also more resonant, and it is consequently easy to fall into the error of supposing that emphysema is present. In children

the breath sounds are always more distinct than in adults, and are more readily conducted, so that adventitious sounds having their origin on one side may even be heard quite plainly on the other.

3. A chest wall with excess of muscular development, subcutaneous fat or œdema will give rise to error if it is not borne in mind that the sounds on percussion and auscultation are alike deadened and indistinct. The sounds heard over the scapular region are always less distinct than those heard elsewhere. When a patient does not breathe deeply, owing to enfeeblement or pain on movement of the chest, or when the chest wall is very fat, the breath sounds may be almost inaudible.

4. The presence of much hair on the chest, as it is rubbed by the stethoscope, gives rise to sounds like fine crepitations.

5. The sounds in the subcutaneous and fascial tissues around the scapula often lead to mistaken diagnosis of pleurisy at the apex (scapular creak).

6. It is well to remember that dullness on percussion does not necessarily mean that there is fluid or consolidation present. It may also be caused by a thickened pleura and by a tumour. The latter may be outside the chest, but pushing up into the thorax—*e.g.*, hepatic or splenic enlargement, subdiaphragmatic abscess.

7. Tumours of the chest wall will sometimes lead to the impression that there is some difference in the size of the two sides of the thorax, and this difference may be referred to a pathological condition of the chest contents. The swelling caused by subcutaneous emphysema or blood clot, both of which may follow an accident, gives rise to a faint crepitation which may be easily mistaken for the signs of injury to the lung beneath.

8. When one lung has been long out of action, as in fibroid phthisis, the other undergoes compensatory enlargement and encroaches on the affected side of the chest. The hypertrophied lung gives rise to sounds identical with those of emphysema.

9. The breath sounds are better heard and the percussion note is higher at the right than at the left apex, owing to the presence of the eparterial bronchus on the right side. The area over which the bronchial quality can be detected is also larger.

10. Atrophy of the muscular tissues about one shoulder leads to an apparent flattening on that side very like that seen in phthisis.

11. Dextro-cardia is very rare, but it is necessary to be on one's guard lest it be rashly supposed that the heart is displaced by effusion or by some tumour.

12. Finally, it is well to remember that the presence of lung signs usually found in association with acute disease must always be interpreted with due regard to the constitutional condition and co-existing signs of disease in other organs.

13. Distension of the abdominal organs as in ærophagy, eventration of the diaphragm, and occasionally a large diaphragmatic hernia (§ 234) may produce a tympanitic note on percussion of the lower part of the left side of the chest and simulate hyper-resonance of the lungs. This also occurs when the lungs have been drawn up by adhesions or fibroid contraction or when one half of the diaphragm is paralysed.

§ 110. Radiology of the Chest.—

X-ray examination often reveals the presence of disease in the chest when other methods of examination give a negative result. Its value is best exemplified in early pulmonary tuberculosis, indubitable evidence of which may be furnished by a radiogram when the most careful and competent clinician has been unable to detect any abnormal physical signs. Good radiological work is essential for the diagnosis of many cases of bronchiectasis and of new growths of the bronchi and lungs. Not only in diagnosis is X-ray important; in treatment, and especially in that following thoracic surgery, it is a *sine qua non*. For ideal work in a difficult case the investigation should be carried out by the physician, surgeon and radiologist co-operating in a team. For practical purposes the physician must often interpret his own radiograms.

METHODS OF X-RAY EXAMINATION OF THE CHEST are as follows:—

1. Examination with the *fluorescent screen* is an important preliminary. This enables the lungs and heart to be viewed in postero-anterior, oblique and lateral directions, to see any abnormality in the mediastinum or in the movements of the diaphragm and to observe various other features which cannot be demonstrated by radiography alone.

2. The ordinary *X-ray film* exposed in a postero-anterior direction at a distance of 6 feet may suffice to demonstrate many details of disease such as early tuberculous infiltration of the lungs. Certain opacities lying behind the heart or other mediastinal structures are hidden from view in a film taken in this one plane, and it is therefore often necessary to expose a second film in a lateral plane (Figs. 53a and 53b).

3. *Bronchography* is performed by the introduction of iodine as a radio-opaque contrast medium into the bronchi. Provided the patient is not iodine-sensitive, iodised oil B.P. (lipiodol, containing 40 per cent. of iodine in poppy seed oil) or propyliodone B.P. as an oily or aqueous injection, is introduced into the trachea and bronchi. This is usually performed by passing a small catheter through one side of the nose and the larynx after application of a suitable local anæsthetic, or occasionally by insertion of a needle through the crico-thyroid membrane. By positioning the patient the radio-opaque solution can be made to enter the different areas of the lungs. X-ray films exposed in different planes (bronchograms) give details of the pathological changes in the bronchi. This method is particularly helpful in demonstrating the existence of cylindrical or saccular dilatation of the bronchial tubes (bronchiectasis), the exact size and position of cavities, sinuses, etc. in the lungs and bronchi, as well as bronchial obstruction due to new growths. Iodised oil can also be used to demonstrate the ramifications of a sinus through the chest wall, as after an operation for empyema.

4. A *Barium Meal* examination may be useful for the investigation of new growths pressing on the œsophagus, or in cases of œsophago-bronchial fistula.

Mass Miniature Radiography has materially advanced the preventive treatment of chest disease. With a 35-mm. ciné film in a specially designed apparatus, the radiologist can examine a large number of individuals in rapid succession: these miniature films are subsequently projected on a screen, and in the enlarged image it is possible to detect definite or suspicious abnormalities. Any individual revealing abnormalities in the miniature film is subsequently X-rayed on a standard apparatus with a 15″ × 12″ film, and submitted to such clinical, bacteriological and other investigations as are necessary to establish a diagnosis:—this should not be made from the miniature film alone. In very large numbers of ostensibly healthy individuals thus examined in numerous surveys, a small but definite proportion have shown lesions of the lungs, heart or mediastinum (and see § 131).

Tomography. In a special form of X-ray apparatus the tube, instead of being fixed, moves across an arc during the exposure; a corresponding synchronous movement of the cassette containing the film takes place in the opposite direction. As a result certain of the rays pass always through one point on the film, the remainder passing through different points and giving an image which is blurred or even invisible while the fixed point image is distinct. For this reason, and as the focal point of the tube can be altered so as to centre the fixed rays at different depths of the chest, it is possible, by taking a series of radiographs (tomograms), accurately to delineate various details which are not seen in the ordinary flat radiograph, *e.g.*, to demonstrate growths or to obtain more exact localisation of cavities in the lung. The tomograph has a limited sphere of application, but within that sphere its value is inestimable.

§ 111. **Examination of the Sputum** is essential in all diseases of the chest. Patients should be instructed to expectorate into a sputum mug or other suitable container so that the physician can examine the material

PLATE I

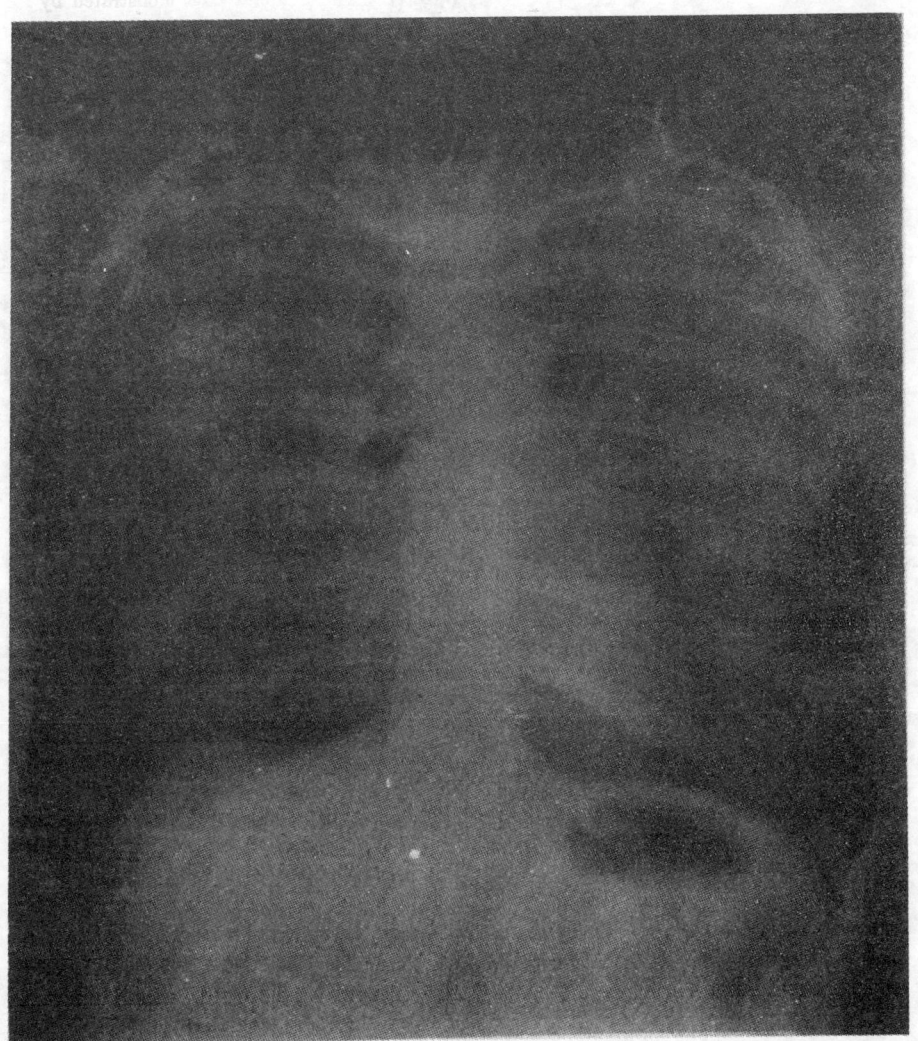

FIG. 52.—X-RAY FILM OF THE CHEST of a healthy woman, taken in a postero-anterior direction. (The breast shadows produce the slight shadowing just above the domes of the diaphragm.)

PLATE II

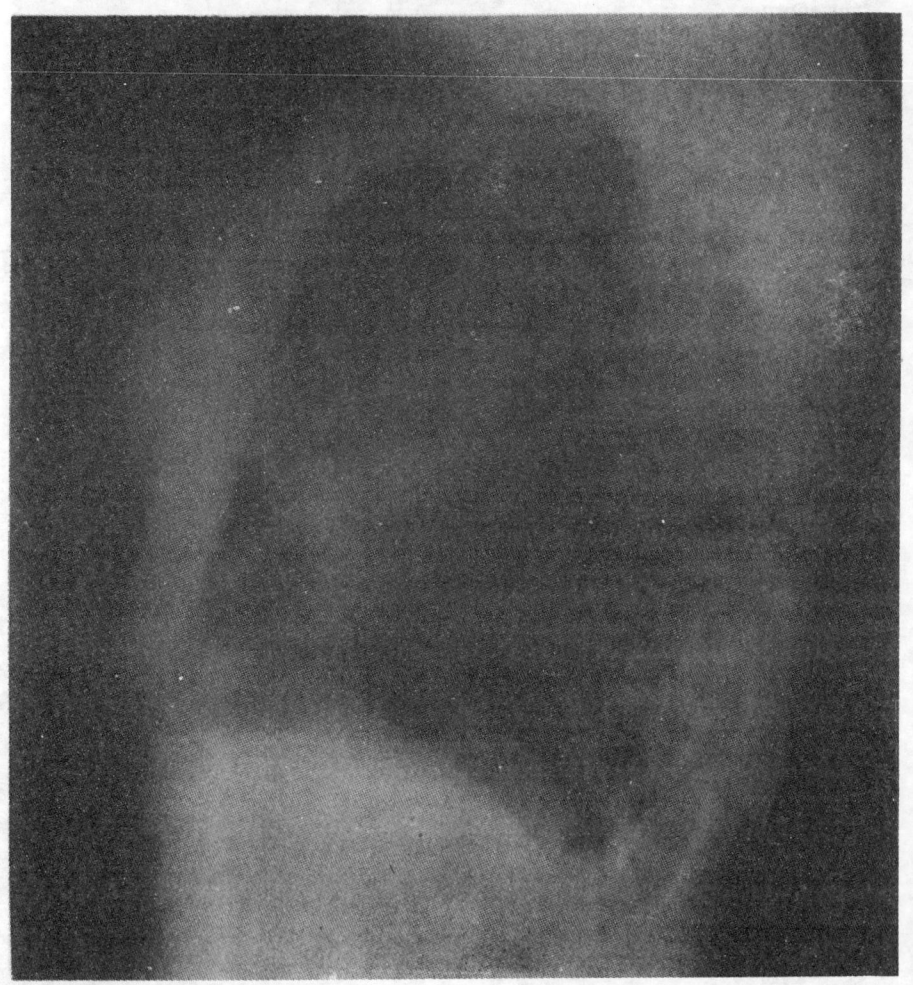

FIG. 53.—X-RAY FILM OF THE CHEST of a healthy woman, taken in a lateral direction.

coughed up. Sputum, as distinct from saliva and post-nasal secretions, is in part or in whole frothy. Sputum should be examined for its quantity in the twenty-four hours and for its NAKED EYE APPEARANCE. In town-dwellers and in those with dusty occupations, the sputum is dark or even black from the presence of carbonaceous or other particles. Note whether the sputum is thin and watery, thick and tenacious, whether it is coloured by the presence of pus or of blood and also note any unusual odour. Sputum may be classified as watery, mucoid, muco-purulent or purulent. *Watery sputum*, often stained with blood, is sometimes expectorated in large quantities in acute œdema of the lungs. *Mucoid* sputum is white, clear and frothy and indicates a mild catarrhal process in the bronchi. *Muco-purulent* sputum is thicker, greenish or yellowish and contains pus indicating that the infection is more severe. *Purulent* sputum often occurs in large amounts in cases of lung abscess, tuberculous or bronchi-ectatic cavities, or when a subphrenic abscess or an empyema bursts into the lung. Extremely *fœtid* purulent sputum is obtained when gas-forming organisms are present in gangrene of the lung or in advanced cases of bronchiectasis. The sputum is coughed up in thick tenacious muco-purulent masses, which float on the surface like coins (" *nummular sputum* ") in acute bronchitis and when the lung is breaking down in phthisis. *Rusty-sputum* is characteristic of lobar pneumonia: the sputum is extremely viscid and large portions of it are uniformly stained with dark red blood. More or less *pure blood*, either in a fresh state or slightly altered to a brownish-red colour, is easily identifiable (hæmoptysis). *Casts* of the bronchial tubes, which can be seen by the naked eye, are expec-torated in asthma, acute plastic bronchitis and occasionally in bronchial pneumonia, and shreds of membrane may be seen in diphtheria. Hydatid cysts, resembling empty gooseberry-skins, are expectorated in that rare condition hydatid disease of the lungs, or when hydatid of the liver ruptures into them. " Anchovy sauce " coloured sputum is characteristic of abscess of the liver which has burst into the lung (§ 336).

MICROSCOPIC AND BACTERIOLOGICAL EXAMINATION OF THE SPUTUM is most informative and should be performed as a routine in all but the most straightforward case. The *type of cell* present indicates whether the specimen comes from the mouth (squamous epithelial cells) or from the chest (pus cells and sometimes eosinophilic cells). *Elastic tissue*, especially in gangrene or abscess of the lung, can be identified by special staining methods. Various *bacteria* may be found—pneumococci, strepto-cocci (non-hæmolytic or hæmolytic), staphylococci, tubercle or hæmophilus bacilli (including *H. influenzæ* and *H. pertussis*), spirochætes and on rare occasions many other bacilli. The *fungæ* of candida albicans, actino-mycosis, blastomycosis and aspergillosis are being increasingly identified. It is not sufficient to isolate these infecting organisms: it is important also to test in the laboratory their sensitivity to the different antibiotics, to the sulphonamides, and in the case of the tubercle bacillus to strepto-mycin, P.A.S. and isoniazid. Various *parasites* such as streptothrix, echinococcus, distoma pulmonale and yeasts are sometimes found. *Mites* have been recorded in some cases of asthma.

In cases of primary bronchial carcinoma, special staining methods in the hands of an experienced cytologist may reveal carcinoma cells, either singly or in groups, in the sputum and in pleural effusions (and see §§ 138, 1213). For this examination fresh samples of sputum should be examined as soon as possible by staining smears with methylene blue, Leishman's stain or with Dudgeon's or Papanicolaou's technique.

A **Pleural Biopsy** may be performed when a pleural effusion is present, using a " Harefield " needle as described by Abrams (§ 1201). The specimen may reveal a characteristic histological appearance of tuberculosis or of malignant disease.

§ 112. Bronchoscopy is playing a most important part in the diagnosis and treatment of chest diseases: at times the bronchoscope is indispensable, but it should only be used by the expert. Apart from those cases in which the presence of a foreign body is known or suspected, it may give vital information in an obscure case of hæmoptysis. In bronchial neoplasms the diagnosis can often be confirmed and a biopsy undertaken. When no intra-bronchial mass is visible, broncho-stenosis due to extrinsic pressure from a neoplasm may be recognised; and a widened angle of bifurcation of the trachea at the carina, due to a large lymph node infiltrated by secondary growth, may decide between exploratory thoracotomy and palliative X-radiation. As a means of treatment, it may be possible via the bronchoscope to extract inspissated mucus plugging a bronchus in a patient with pulmonary collapse; and even to remove an innocent intrabronchial neoplasm (*e.g.*, adenoma).

PULMONARY VENTILATION FUNCTION TESTS are valuable in recording statistically the amount of air which can be inhaled and exhaled by a particular patient in comparison with the normal person. The values are diminished, sometimes greatly, by disease such as pulmonary fibrosis, emphysema, those conditions which impede free diaphragmatic movements and by cardiac disorders. The two principal methods used are:—

(i.) *The Vital Capacity* which measures the maximum volume of air which can be expired after taking a very deep breath. The air is blown through a spirometer and the best of three values recorded. The figure obtained can be compared with the normal values as recorded in tables: they decrease with age, vary with stature and are higher in men than in women. In the normal person a fairly close approximation is obtained by multiplying the height in cm. by 25 (for men) and by 20 (for women), so that a man of 160 cm. should have an average vital capacity of 160×25 ml., i.e., 4,000 ml.

(ii.) *The Maximum Breathing Capacity* is a better index of the function of the pulmonary ventilation for it measures the volume and also the speed of ventilation. It is usually recorded with a spirometer bell on a moving drum over a period of a few seconds, and is expressed in terms of litres/minute. The average for men is 125–150 litres and for women 100 litres/minute.

PART C. DISEASES OF THE LUNGS AND PLEURÆ: THEIR
DIAGNOSIS, PROGNOSIS, AND TREATMENT

§ 113. Classification.—For practical purposes, diseases of the lungs and pleuræ may be divided into ACUTE and CHRONIC, and each of these may be subdivided into those without dullness, those with dullness, and those with hyper-resonance.

Acute.	Chronic.

WITHOUT DULLNESS.

I. Acute Bronchitis. § 115.
II. Dry Pleurisy. § 116.
III. Acute Miliary Tuberculosis (Pulmonary form). § 117.
IV. Whooping-cough. § 494.
V. Acute Pulmonary Œdema. § 118.

I. Chronic Bronchitis (and Plastic Bronchitis). §§ 129, 130.

WITH DULLNESS.

I. Pleurisy with effusion. § 119.
(and Empyema). § 120.
II. Lobar Pneumonia. § 121.
III. Broncho-pneumonia. § 122.
IV. Acute Pneumonic Phthisis. § 124.
V. Acute massive collapse. § 125.
VI. Pulmonary Infarction. § 105.

Common.

I. Chronic Tuberculosis[1] (and Fibroid Phthisis). §§ 131, 132.
II. Hydrothorax. § 133.
III. Pulmonary Congestion (Hypostasis). § 134.
IV. Fibrosis and Bronchiectasis. §§ 135, 145.
V. Thickened Pleura. § 137.
VI. Malignant disease of the Bronchus. §§ 79 and 138.
VII. Secondary malignant disease of the Lung. § 138.
VIII. Collapse of the Lung. § 139.

Rare.

IX. Hydatid cyst. § 140.
X. Sarcoidosis. § 141.
XI. Syphilitic disease. § 142.

WITH HYPER-RESONANCE.

I. Pneumothorax.[2] § 126.

I. Emphysema. § 143.

One acute disease tends to be **Paroxysmal.**

I. Asthma. § 127.

Diseases suggested by the character of the sputum.

I. Bronchiectasis. § 145.
II. Abscess and Gangrene of the Lung. § 146.
III–IV. Actinomycosis and other diseases due to fungi and parasites. §§ 147, 148.

---

[1] There is no dullness in the early stages of the disease.
[2] Spontaneous pneumothorax is sometimes an acute incident in a chronic disease—tuberculosis.

§ 114. The **Routine Procedure** here resembles in principle that used in diseases of the heart. First, *What is the patient's leading symptom ?* If suffering from lung disease, his cardinal symptom will be one of those mentioned in section A: cough and breathlessness are the most common.

Secondly, follow this up with a few questions to ascertain the *history of his illness,* and especially whether *the disease be acute or chronic.* Other important points are whether the patient has been exposed to a " chill," and whether there is any " lung disease " in the family. Do not use the word " consumption "; it may frighten your patient unnecessarily.

Thirdly, the *general physical state of the patient* should be noted. Is he breathless, does he appear wasted and is the voice affected (§ 164). In most acute conditions and in some chronic conditions the temperature is raised and there may be a rise in the pulse rate. These should be recorded, together with the patient's weight. Observe also the alæ nasi and the colour of the face and lips—are they congested (polycythæmia) or cyanosed. It is convenient at this stage to look for clubbing of the fingers (§ 106).

Fourthly, proceed to the PHYSICAL EXAMINATION OF THE LUNGS. The chest should always be stripped, and it is more convenient to examine the patient in a standing or sitting posture, if he be not too ill. The routine method is as follows:

1. Ascertain whether there is any increased rate or other modification in the breathing, or any alteration in the shape of the chest (by *inspection,* and, if necessary, by measurement). Note whether any part of the chest shows decreased movement.

2. Find the position of the apex beat.

3. Test the vocal fremitus by *palpation.*

4. Ascertain if there be any dullness or hyper-resonance (by *percussion*).

5. Listen to the breath and voice sounds, and then to any adventitious sounds which may be present.

6. The sputum should be inspected, and, if necessary, examined by the pathologist in further detail.

7. X-ray examination must be insisted on when necessary; in the diagnosis of many chest diseases the physician is more and more dependent on radiological evidence.

If the illness developed gradually and is of some standing, and unattended by obvious constitutional disturbance, then turn to **Chronic Pulmonary Disorders** (§ 128).

If the illness came on recently and suddenly, accompanied by fever, quickened respiration, coated tongue, and with marked malaise, then the case is one of the **Acute Pulmonary Diseases,** below.

There is one disease of the lungs, ASTHMA, which comes on in sudden acute attacks from time to time; it is **chronic,** with **acute exacerbations.**

ACUTE DISEASES

We now proceed to percuss the chest.

The acute diseases without alteration in the percussion note, *i.e.*, **without dullness,** are: ACUTE BRONCHITIS; DRY PLEURISY; ACUTE MILIARY TUBERCULOSIS; WHOOPING-COUGH; and ACUTE PULMONARY ŒDEMA. ASTHMA is of a paroxysmal nature.

I. *The patient complains of a* cough, *with frothy or purulent expectoration, and his temperature is elevated; there is* no alteration *in the percussion note but on auscultating the chest, loud* RHONCHI *and* RÂLES *are heard. The disease is* ACUTE BRONCHITIS.

§ 115. **Acute Bronchitis,** or inflammation of the bronchial tubes, is certainly the most common acute disease of the lungs in this climate. It is much more common in childhood and after middle age, and attacks are much more likely to occur in the winter and spring months of the year.

Symptoms.—The disease commonly commences with symptoms of an upper respiratory infection and a slight sore throat. In the course of a day or so it affects the trachea and larger bronchi, with a feeling of soreness behind the sternum, tightness in the chest, a frequent and mainly dry cough and a rise in temperature. The voice may become husky. The sputum is at first thick and scanty and later becomes more copious,

TABLE VI.—DIAGNOSIS OF COMMON ACUTE DISEASES OF THE LUNGS AND PLEURÆ

	Percussion Note.	Auscultation.
Acute Bronchitis	Normal	V.M. and V.R. normal; Loud râles and rhonchi.
Dry Pleurisy	Normal	V.R. normal. R.M. normal, or may be diminished in intensity owing to restriction of inspiratory movements due to pain; Pleural friction.
Acute Pulmonary Tuberculosis	Normal, or scattered areas of impaired note	V.M. diminished; crepitations later.
Pleurisy with effusion ..	Dull	V.M., V.R. and V.F. diminished; Pleural friction at early and late stage.
Lobar Pneumonia	Dull	V.R. and V.F. increased: Bronchial breathing.
Broncho-pneumonia ..	Scattered areas of impaired note	Fine crepitations and scattered areas of bronchial breathing.

muco-purulent and is more easily coughed up. The severity of the infection varies: in milder cases and when only the large bronchi are affected, the patient may not feel ill, the temperature is scarcely raised and he may continue at work. More commonly a few days in bed are necessary until the temperature settles; the disease lasts 7–10 days and a slight morning cough persists for another week or so. In cases of great severity, such as may occur in epidemics or with aerial pollution with smoke (" smog "), there is a severe purulent bronchitis affecting the larger and the smaller tubes, a high swinging temperature (to 104°–105°), severe dyspnœa, cyanosis and prostration. The sputum may be streaked with blood. Especially at the extremes of life death may occur, or recovery will take 4–8 weeks.

Physical Signs.—The percussion note is unaltered unless, as so frequently happens, emphysema is also present, in which case the chest is unduly resonant. On auscultation, when only the larger bronchi are involved, there may be little more than a few râles over the lower lobes of the lungs. In cases of greater severity, the vesicular murmur is obscured over the whole chest by loud rhonchi and coarse râles (see Fig. 51): high-pitched rhonchi are a sign that the smaller tubes are affected. On palpation rhonchial fremitus can frequently be felt. A variable degree of bronchospasm may be found in more severely dyspnœic cases. As the condition resolves the râles take on more of a bubbling character: the lung bases are the last to clear. X-ray examination often shows some increase in the peribronchial shadows.

Etiology.—(i.) Acute bronchitis may follow exposure to cold producing " a chill." (ii.) In the majority of cases there is an infection of the upper respiratory passages causing the symptoms of coryza. The primary infection, with a superimposed secondary infection, spreads to the trachea and bronchi. (iii.) The severity of the secondary infection depends on the resistance of the patient and on the type of organism present. Those commonly found are *Strep. viridans*, *M. catarrhalis*, *H. influenzæ*, *pneumococci* and sometimes *Staph. aureus* and *Strep. hæmolyticus*. (iv.) Bronchitis accompanies many of the specific fevers and is invariably present in measles and whooping-cough; it is commonly met in infections with viruses such as those of influenza, and in typhoid-fever. (v.) It is now clearly recognised to be the result of exposure to chemical agents. During World War I an acute and often fatal type followed exposure to chlorine, phosgene and to mustard gas. In city-dwellers living in smoke-laden atmospheres sulphur dioxide acts as a severe bronchial irritant: the " smog " which descended on London for three days in December 1952 probably caused 3,000–4,000 deaths. Certain occupations which expose people to irritating vapours and small particles of dust also predispose. (vi.) It is common among those who are exposed to all weathers (*e.g.*, mariners). (vii.) Patients with congenital heart disease and mitral stenosis with pulmonary congestion readily develop acute bronchitis. (viii.) A rare form of bronchitis, due to a fluke, is met with in the East (§ 148 and p. 428, Table XIX).

The *Diagnosis* is usually not difficult: a history of previous attacks and the presence of rhonchi are characteristic. *Pulmonary tuberculosis* may follow an acute respiratory infection: it should be suspected when the signs are more marked at one or both lung apices, when the symptoms and signs are unduly persistent and sputum examination should confirm the diagnosis. *Whooping-cough* and *measles* present acute catarrhal symptoms with pyrexia and sometimes occur in adults. The " *capillary*

bronchitis " of children is really a form of *broncho-pneumonia* (*q.v.*); the
constitutional symptoms and the dyspnœa are much more marked, dullness
to percussion may or may not be present, and the differentiation from
simple acute bronchitis is not always easy.

The *Prognosis* is much more favourable in recent years since the discovery of the sulpha drugs and the antibiotics.   Mild attacks should clear
up in 7–10 days and more severe attacks in 3–4 weeks.   The condition
is much more dangerous in infancy and in old age partly because the
powers of resistance are not so good and partly the result of the greater
difficulties of expectoration.   Enfeebled infants and old people may not
have the strength to cough up thick purulent sputum: smaller or larger
areas of atelectasis may develop if this produces a persistent block in a
bronchus.   Recurrent attacks are likely to be followed by chronic bronchitis and by emphysema.

Treatment.—The patient should remain in bed until the temperature
falls, in a warm room at 65° F without draughts but with adequate ventilation.   In the presence of dyspnœa the patient should be supported
in the upright position.   A very dry atmosphere tends to promote much
unnecessary cough and inhalations of steam containing benzoin or menthol
(vapor benzoin B.P.C. or vapor menthol with benzoin N.F.) a teaspoonful
to one pint of hot water 2–3 times daily are helpful, especially in the
presence of an upper respiratory infection.   When the neck and the
upper part of the chest are sore due to tracheitis, the application of
camphorated liniment B.P. or of a kaolin poultice is comforting.   The
diet should be as plentiful as the patient wishes: copious *hot* drinks help
to promote secretion from the respiratory passages.   Mist. sodii chloridi
co. (B.P.C.) given in a tumblerful of *hot* water and sipped slowly twice
daily is often helpful.   A linctus such as linctus scillæ co. (B.P.C.), linct.
codeinæ (B.P.C.) or even linct. diamorphinæ (gr. $\frac{1}{24}$ in ♏ 60) are to be
preferred in the earlier stages when secretion is scanty: later an expectorant
mixture such as mist. potassii iodidi et ammon. (B.P.C.) or mist. ammon.
et ipecacuanhæ (B.P.C.) helps to promote secretion.   When bronchial spasm
is marked anti-spasmodic drugs are also indicated (§ 127).   Sleep, which
is particularly important in elderly subjects, may be secured by a dose
of linctus at bedtime, perhaps combined with a barbiturate.   Morphine
is better avoided and should never be given to elderly bronchitic subjects.
The routine administration of antibiotics is to be deprecated: however,
they are necessary when there is considerable toxæmia, much thick sputum
in elderly subjects, and in those with previous chronic lung disease such
as fibrotic changes.   Occasionally the use of oxygen is valuable (§ 121).
Adequate convalescence must be insisted upon.   *Prophylaxis* is especially
important in those who are subject to recurrent attacks.   Those who
have retired from work should seek a suitable climate (§ 129).   The use
of a reliable bacterial vaccine during the winter months can be most
helpful, but it is most important to give a booster dose each 4 weeks
until the liability to recurrence has passed.   Particularly in elderly

subjects the author has found prophylactic sulphonamide therapy of considerable value: for this purpose give tab. sulphadimidine (B.P.) G. 1 each morning or twice daily.

II. *The patient complains of sharp* PAIN *in the chest on inspiration; he has a short dry cough, and his temperature is moderately elevated; on auscultation,* FRICTION *sounds are heard. The disease is* DRY PLEURISY.

§ 116. **Dry Pleurisy** is inflammation of the pleura without effusion. In this disease there is a fibrinous exudation on the visceral and parietal layers of the pleura, and a tendency to the formation of adhesions and to the effusion of fluid.

Symptoms.—The most obvious symptom is pain in the chest, usually affecting only one side. The pain, which is caused by the rubbing together of the inflamed pleural surfaces, often occurs quite suddenly: it is variously described as a sharp stabbing pain, or as a stitch-like or knife-like pain, and characteristically " catches " during inspiration. It is also aggravated by coughing, yawning and by other movements of the chest wall. A short dry cough, reflexly produced by the pleural irritation, is usually present. Constitutional symptoms are seldom great and the patient may not even take to his bed. The temperature is usually raised, but rarely exceeds 100° or 101° F. Dyspnœa is unusual, but the patient may be afraid to breathe on account of the severity of the pain. For the distribution of pain in diaphragmatic pleurisy see § 103.

Physical Signs.—(i.) The cardinal sign is the auscultation of a pleural friction rub (§ 109), which may on occasions be palpable. When pain is severe, and particularly at the onset, the rub may be heard with difficulty: at the site of pain, only superficial dry crepitant sounds are detected: with diaphragmatic pleurisy no rub is audible. The loud creaking sound is often better heard after two or three days when deeper breaths are possible because the inflamed surfaces are protected by a thin layer of fibrin. A rub is differentiated from a rhonchus by being intensified by pressure with the stethoscope and by being unaltered by coughing. (ii.) On inspection movement of the affected side of the chest is decreased. The percussion note and vocal resonance are unaffected but the air entry is limited by the pain of inspiration. Usually the inflammation undergoes resolution: when an effusion takes place the pain and pleural friction disappear.

Etiology.—(i.) Inflammation is usually the result of extension from disease of the underlying lung, such as with pneumonia, tuberculosis, infarction or carcinoma. (ii.) Especially on the right side it may be due to disease of the liver or of the subphrenic space. (iii.) Undoubtedly a large number of cases of pleurisy are tuberculous in origin, especially if recurrent; this fact should always be remembered. Acute pleurisy, with or without effusion, occurring in a young adult, should be regarded as tuberculous in origin, unless it can be definitely proved to be due to some other infective agent. (iv.) It may occur as a complication of an infective disease such as influenza, scarlet fever, measles, rheumatic fever or septicæmia. (v.) It may be the result of a fractured rib. (vi.) Dry pleurisy is sometimes found in the advanced stages of chronic nephritis.

The *Diagnosis* from *fibrositis* (pleurodynia) may be difficult. Local injection of the muscles with 2 per cent. procaine solution will decide the point. The rhonchi heard in *bronchitis* must be distinguished from a pleural rub (*vide supra*). In epidemics of *Bornholm disease* (§ 509) there is a raised temperature (102–104° F), severe pain in one or both sides of the chest wall and a pleural rub may be present. *Herpes Zoster* is associated with marked cutaneous hyperæsthesia and later on the herpetic ˜esicles appear. A *scapular* creak (§ 109) between the fasciæ of the muscles of the upper scapular area may be mistaken for a pleural rub. The *left-submammary pain* met in anxiety states is more persistent and unrelated to breathing. In every case of dry pleurisy a radiogram must be taken to see if there is evidence of tuberculosis or other intra-pulmonary disease, and the X-ray should be repeated at intervals of 2–3 months for a period of one year.

Prognosis.—It is not in itself a serious condition and readily yields to treatment; but sometimes effusion occurs (Pleural Effusion, § 119). When this effusion becomes purulent (§ 120) the prognosis is graver. A frequent result of no great importance is thickening and adhesions of the pleura.

Treatment.—The patient should remain in bed until the temperature has settled. Relief from pain is afforded by strapping the affected side of the chest so as to limit the costal movements of respiration: two pieces of non-elastic strapping should be applied at the end of expiration, the strapping passing across the middle line in front and behind for 2 inches. Otherwise a kaolin poultice may be used. Aspirin gr. 10, tab. codein. co., or aspirin with Dover's powder gr. 10 may be helpful. With very severe pain as when accompanying pneumonia, morphia may be needed. Other measures which have been used are a local injection of procaine hydrochlor. (2 per cent.) into the pleura, or separation of the two pleural surfaces with 20–30 ml. of air via an artificial pneumothorax apparatus. The treatment of pulmonary tuberculosis is discussed later (§ 131).

III. *The patient exhibits the signs of subacute bronchitis. He becomes progressively and ultimately gravely ill, has a* HIGH TEMPERATURE *and may* PASS INTO THE TYPHOID STATE. *The disease is* ACUTE MILIARY TUBERCULOSIS.

§ 117. Acute Miliary Tuberculosis (Syn. Acute Phthisis, Galloping Consumption) is almost invariably the result of the hæmatogenous dissemination of tubercle bacilli throughout the body. It is more common in children or young adults, but may be met in adults with established tuberculosis in the lungs or in other organs. The clinical picture may be chiefly pulmonary, although in childhood this may be overshadowed by the symptoms of tuberculous meningitis.

Symptoms.—The disease is insidious in onset with progressive weakness, drowsiness and emaciation. Some weeks before physical signs appear the thermometer may show the typical intermittent pyrexia so characteristic of tuberculosis, with a normal morning temperature and an evening rise to 101–103° F (see Fig. 153, a chart showing the typical course of the temperature). As the disease progresses the remissions are likely to be less, the fever being more of the continuous type. In some cases the inverse type is present, when the temperature is higher in the morning than in the evening. Tachycardia is present at an early stage often in excess of that due to the pyrexia. In the pulmonary form of acute generalised tuberculosis dyspnœa and sometimes cyanosis develop out of all proportion to the physical signs—the cyanosis being a very characteristic feature. Some cough and sputum are present with night sweats. Progressive weakness and emaciation are the rule, and in the third or fourth week the patient may develop the symptoms of the typhoid state or of meningitis.

The *Physical Signs* referable to the lungs are indefinite, or resemble at first those of bronchitis. Initially there is no alteration in the percussion note, but later careful percussion may reveal scattered areas of impaired resonance, especially in the lower lobes, due to small areas of broncho-pneumonia. Auscultation at first gives little help but in a week or so it reveals fine râles: later still it may show areas of weak breath sounds or of tubular breathing and the râles become coarser.

The *Diagnosis* in the early stages is extremely difficult. To differentiate from other forms of bronchitis and broncho-pneumonia, we have to rely upon the disproportionate emaciation and cyanosis, the character of the temperature, and the patchy distribution of the physical signs in tuberculosis. In other cases the disease is almost indistinguishable from typhoid fever except for the marked predominance of the pulmonary signs and the absence of the roseola; the Widal test is negative. Diagnosis is confirmed by finding tubercle bacilli in the sputum, the stomach washings, the fæces (in small children), or in the cerebro-spinal fluid when meningitis is present: their absence does not exclude acute tuberculosis. Choroidal tubercles (§ 1137) may be found with the ophthalmoscope. X-ray examination of the lungs may reveal the characteristic " *snowstorm* " appearance of miliary tuberculosis (Fig. 54).

Etiology.—The disease may occur at any age, but is commonest in infants, in young adults, and in those with a tuberculous family history. Acute general tuberculosis may originate from a primary focus, such as a tuberculous joint which had been considered cured. The disease may follow measles or whooping-cough in children.

Prognosis.—Without treatment the disease is invariably fatal. With modern methods of chemotherapy the infection can be overcome in 50 per cent. of late cases and in at least 70-80 per cent. of cases coming under treatment at an early stage.

Treatment is with good nursing care combined with inject. streptomycin, *p*-aminosalicylic acid (P.A.S.) and isoniazid (§ 131). The latter drug, which diffuses freely into the cerebro-spinal fluid, has proved a useful addition to the first two.

IV. *The patient, a child, has* PAROXYSMS *of coughing which terminate in a* WHOOP, *and frequently in* VOMITING; *there is some fever, but the only signs in the lungs are those of a little bronchial catarrh. The disease is* WHOOPING-COUGH.

Whooping-cough (Pertussis) is an acute infectious disease and is described in § 494.

V. *The patient is suddenly seized with acute dyspnœa, becomes cyanosed and copious frothy sputum may flow from the mouth and nose. The disease is* ACUTE PULMONARY ŒDEMA.

§ 118. Acute Pulmonary Œdema. *Symptoms.*—The characteristic features are the sudden onset of acute dyspnœa, a cough and rattling in the chest, the attacks often occurring in the middle of the night. The sputum is frothy, and in the more severe attacks may be copious and even blood-stained (rose-coloured). The attacks cause the patient to sit up in bed or to go to an open window in an effort to breathe. Severe attacks are often terrifying, the face becomes very pale, the body drips with sweat and cyanosis is marked. The temperature is subnormal, the breathing rapid and shallow, the pulse fast and feeble; and the jugular veins become engorged. An attack may last minutes or hours and recurrence is common.

and in the same type is present, when the temperature is higher in the morning than at night.

PLATE III

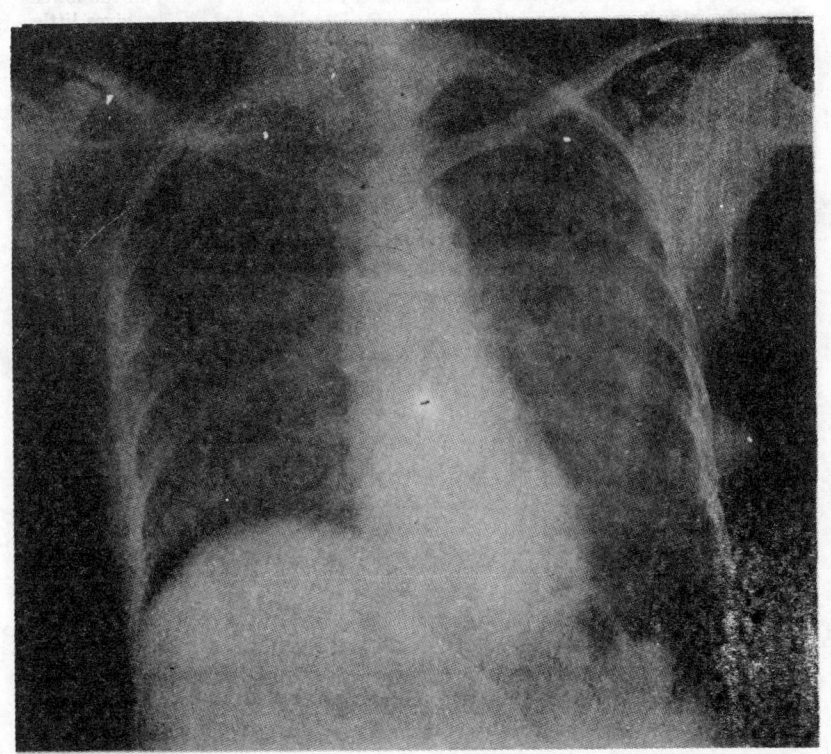

FIG. 54.—CHEST X-RAY showing MILIARY TUBERCULOSIS in a woman of 50 years of age.

The *Physical Signs* in the chest consist of numerous bubbling râles and crepitations with dullness at the base due to pulmonary collapse.

Etiology.—The primary cause is usually acute left ventricular failure (" cardiac asthma "), due to hypertension, acute coronary thrombosis, mitral stenosis, or to disease of the aortic valves. Less frequent causes are the inhalation of irritant gases, a fulminating strep. hæmolyticus infection during an attack of influenza, failure of the medullary centre in association with a cerebral tumour, thrombosis or hæmorrhage, excessive increase in the blood volume with infusions of saline or with blood transfusion, giant urticaria, a large pulmonary infarction or shortly after a lung operation, *e.g.*, thoracoplasty.

Treatment.—The patient should be propped into an upright position in a chair or in a cardiac bed with the legs in a dependent position. Constant nursing care is essential. Relief is often obtained following the intravenous injection of aminophylline G. 0·25 and the administration of oxygen. Full doses of atropine may be helpful. In severe cases it may be necessary to inject morphine gr. ⅙-¼ and to apply suction through an intratracheal catheter (after local anæsthesia of the throat and larynx). Venesection of fl. oz. 15–20 may be helpful in cases of hypertension and aortic disease. When attacks recur frequently they may be prevented by a salt-free diet, regular injections of mersalyl or by a tablet of morphia under the tongue at bedtime.

We now turn to the **Acute Diseases with Dullness on Percussion.**— I. PLEURISY WITH EFFUSION (Serous or Purulent); II. LOBAR PNEUMONIA; III. BRONCHO-PNEUMONIA; IV. ACUTE PNEUMONIC PHTHISIS; and V. ACUTE POST-OPERATIVE MASSIVE COLLAPSE.

I. *The patient has a* DRY COUGH, *with moderate fever and other constitutional symptoms. The lower part of the chest is* DULL *on one side, and over this area the* VOCAL FREMITUS *and* RESONANCE *are* DIMINISHED *or* ABSENT. *The heart is displaced towards the healthy side. The disease is* PLEURISY *with* EFFUSION.

§ 119. Acute Pleurisy with Effusion.—When describing acute Dry Pleurisy (§ 116) it was pointed out that the disease may undergo resolution or result in adhesions. It may also go on to effusion.

Symptoms.—There is usually a history of a more or less acute onset with pain (§ 116), but as the disease progresses, and the surfaces of the pleura are separated by fluid, pain becomes less and less marked. Occasionally the onset is insidious, and a considerable amount of fluid accumulates in the pleural cavity without any history of initial pain. In young adults in whom tuberculosis is a common cause, there is often a history of previous malaise, and the onset of the effusion is ushered in by a sudden rise of temperature to 103°–104° F and even by a mild rigor: the temperature continues in a remittent manner so characteristic of tuberculosis over a period of weeks or even months. In these cases night sweats are frequent. A dry cough, without sputum, is common in the early stages. Some breathlessness may be present, and the patient may find it difficult to lie on the sound side, because the action of the healthy lung is thereby impeded, but even with a large amount of fluid this may not be a prominent feature.

Physical Signs (see Fig. 55).—(i.) Inspection shows diminished movement and sometimes fullness or bulging of the chest wall and intercostal spaces. (ii.) On palpation, the vocal fremitus is found to be diminished or absent over the fluid. (iii.) Percussion reveals absolute dullness over the areas of the fluid. The level of dullness rises to the axilla, a sign which is best demonstrated posteriorly: this is in contrast to consolidation or collapse of a part of the lung where the dullness posteriorly falls to the axilla. Above the level of the fluid, if the lung be otherwise healthy, there is a hyper-resonant note (Skodaic resonance). (iv.) On auscultation over the fluid, the breath sounds are absent; the vocal resonance is greatly impaired or lost. High-pitched bronchial breathing and bronchophony are commonly heard just above the level of the fluid, over the compressed

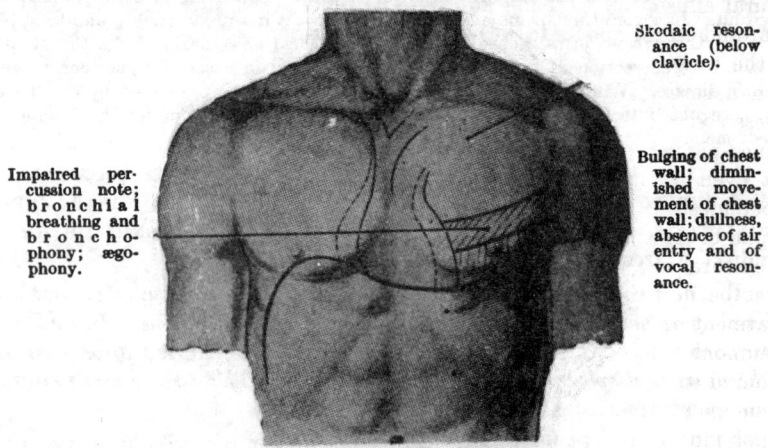

Skodaic reson-
ance (below
clavicle).

Impaired per-
cussion note;
bronchial
breathing and
broncho-
phony; ægo-
phony.

Bulging of chest
wall; dimin-
ished move-
ment of chest
wall; dullness,
absence of air
entry and of
vocal reson-
ance.

FIG. 55.—Physical signs of Pleurisy with effusion

lung (especially in children). At the upper margin of the fluid posteriorly —perhaps just about the angle of the scapula—only certain overtones of the voice are transmitted, and they produce, therefore, a sound like the bleating of a goat (ægophony). (v.) When the effusion is large it causes displacement of the heart and even of the trachea, sometimes to a considerable extent. The position of the apex beat is therefore of cardinal importance in determining the presence of fluid in the chest and its amount. A large effusion also causes congestive râles at the base of the opposite lung, with considerable dyspnœa. Grocco's triangle is an area of paravertebral dullness in the right chest posteriorly, caused by a large left-sided effusion displacing the heart to the opposite side.

As the fluid absorbs the temperature gradually drops, the upper level of the dullness falls and the apex beat of the heart moves back towards its normal position. When the fluid has absorbed the pleural surfaces again come into contact and a painless pleural rub can be heard once more.

The *diagnosis* of pleurisy in its earlier stages is referred to under Dry Pleurisy. The differentiation of the physical signs of fluid in the chest, as compared with those of consolidation of the lung, is so important that it is given in Table V (§ 109). Radiology of a chest with a pleural effusion shows a uniformly opaque area gradually fading into the normal lung markings: when the amount of fluid is considerable the heart is seen to be displaced towards the opposite side. When only a small amount of fluid is present it first obliterates the costo-phrenic angle. Exploratory puncture is essential to determine both the presence and the character of fluid in the pleural cavity.

Etiology.—(i.) Tuberculosis is by far the commonest cause of a sudden pleural effusion in a young adult. The fluid in such cases is commonly clear and straw-coloured: the cells are predominantly lymphocytes, though in the early stages some polymorphs may be present. Young patients with a serous lymphocytic effusion should be regarded as tuberculous unless some other cause can be proved; culture on special media and/or guinea-pig inoculation of the deposit often reveals tubercle bacilli (§ 1203), but even a negative result with the guinea-pig test does not exclude tuberculosis. (ii.) Since pneumonia is now treated routinely with the sulpha-drugs or with the antibiotics, a pleural effusion (frequently sterile on culture) is often found when the temperature has settled. This variety must be differentiated from that due to tuberculosis for the prolonged treatment required for the latter variety is not necessary. The post-pneumonic variety is differentiated by the acute onset often with rusty-coloured sputum, the rapid subsidence of the temperature within 2–3 days when an antibiotic has been administered and the persistent presence of polymorphonuclear cells in the effusion. Furthermore, unless bacteria are found on culture, the effusion does not recur after aspiration. (iii.) The occurrence of a pleural effusion in a middle-aged or elderly patient should raise the suspicion of malignant disease, especially when it is blood-stained. In such cases enlarged glands may be found in the neck or axilla. The fluid usually recurs after aspiration and carcinoma cells may be found by special staining methods or by pleural biopsy (§ 111). In a few instances of acute tuberculous effusions the fluid is blood-stained; in the majority of cases a sanguineous pleural effusion is pathognomonic of new growth. (iv.) Other causes are following a fairly large pulmonary infarction: or with an inflammatory condition under the diaphragm such as with a subphrenic abscess or an amœbic abscess of the liver (see also § 133, Hydrothorax).

Prognosis.—This depends on the cause. Many tuberculous effusions will absorb if left alone but the adjacent pleural surfaces usually become permanently adherent. When all the fluid has been removed in the first stages of a tuberculous effusion, miliary tuberculosis has sometimes followed. If on the other hand the effusion is allowed to persist unchanged for many weeks a very thick pleura often persists indefinitely (§ 137). Any young adult should be examined and X-rayed regularly for two years after the occurrence of a tuberculous effusion, in case tuberculosis develops later.

Obliterative Pleurisy.—Occasionally, after gradual absorption of a pleural effusion, the formation of multiple adhesions results in a partial or complete obliteration of the pleural cavity. This is a common sequel of effusion occurring during a course of artificial pneumothorax therapy, and arrests this treatment. In such cases, provided no uncollapsed cavities remain in the lung, an obliterative pleurisy may sometimes be an entirely beneficial end-result. The physical signs of this condition are those of thickened pleura. (See § 137.)

An *Interlobar Pleural Effusion* is due to the causes mentioned above but particularly to the post-pneumonic group. There are usually no physical signs of such a collection of fluid, the diagnosis being made only by radiography.

Treatment.—This depends entirely on the cause. (i.) For tuberculous cases, the patient must be kept strictly in bed until the temperature has finally settled. Patients usually prefer to sit up, supported by pillows. Following a diagnostic puncture of the chest, general nursing measures and treatment with streptomycin, together with P.A.S. or with isoniazid (§ 131), must be instituted and continued for a period of 6–12 months. Many still consider that aspiration, other than the removal of 20 ml. for diagnosis, is unnecessary: it may even prove dangerous unless the patient is under the influence of tuberculous antibiotic therapy. However, when the fluid has persisted unchanged for 4 weeks or more, it is wise to remove at least 10–20 fl. oz. after which the remainder will probably be absorbed in a reasonably short time. Other authorities institute vigorous chemotherapy and aspirate at the end of a week of this, removing all the fluid possible over the course of 2–3 days: if the fluid recurs in spite of this, streptomycin is injected into the pleural cavity each time aspiration is repeated. Replacement of the fluid by air is rarely performed nowadays. (ii.) A post-pneumonic effusion should be removed as soon as the diagnosis is made, unless the fluid is showing signs of rapid spontaneous absorption. If the fluid is not sterile, 100,000–500,000 units of penicillin should be inserted into the pleural cavity before the aspirating needle is withdrawn and intramusc. penicillin given. (iii.) Malignant pleural effusions should be aspirated when they are large enough to cause symptoms; radio-active gold inserted into the pleura has been used in an attempt to limit the recurrence of such effusions. As a general rule it is inadvisable to delay paracentesis and aspiration under the following conditions: (i.) a large effusion (*e.g.*, with dullness extending upward as far as the third rib); (ii.) cardiac embarrassment, as evidenced by cyanosis, palpitation and a rapid pulse; (iii.) respiratory embarrassment, shown by urgent dyspnœa and paroxysmal attacks of coughing; (iv.) effusion in the other pleura, or œdema of the other lung; (v.) if the fluid is not sterile.

Paracentesis thoracis.—When possible the patient should be sat up, well supported with pillows; the hand on the affected side is placed on the opposite shoulder.

The usual site of puncture is the 8th space in the post-scapular line—or at a site where localised dullness is maximal. An intradermal injection of 2 per cent. procaine is made at the intended site of puncture with a hypodermic syringe and needle. The needle is withdrawn, then thrust through this now anæsthetic skin area, and on slowly through the tissues of the intercostal space until the pleura is reached; the piston of the syringe is pushed down as the needle advances. Thus the track of the needle is anæsthetised with a fine stream of procaine. Then an exploring needle, attached to 20 ml. glass record syringe, is pushed vertically through the anæsthetised area, gentle suction being maintained all the time. If there is fluid in the pleural cavity, it will enter the barrel as soon as the needle reaches it. Perforation of the lung is indicated if air or frothy bright red blood is sucked into the syringe; in such a case the needle is withdrawn, the blood driven out and the process repeated, with the needle inserted in another direction.

Aspiration of a pleural effusion is usually performed by the method just outlined. When a large quantity of fluid has to be withdrawn it is necessary to use a syringe fitted with a two-way tap or otherwise a syringe with a double action. The side tube is connected by sterile tubing with a receptacle. Alternatively *siphonage* can be used for removal of the fluid, but is seldom so efficacious. A trocar and cannula are introduced through the chest wall, and after withdrawing the trocar a long rubber tube filled with sterile saline is connected with the cannula: the other end of the tube empties into a dish at a lower level. In either case aspiration can be continued until the patient is conscious of slight discomfort. If cough or pain occur, it is wiser to cease; it is unwise to remove more than 20 fl. oz. at a time. At the conclusion, after withdrawing the needle or cannula, cover the puncture wound with gauze soaked in collodion.

I*a*. *The physical signs are those of pleurisy with* EFFUSION, *but it does not clear up in due course, and the patient continues to have an* INTERMITTENT HIGH TEMPERATURE *with* SWEATINGS *and* SHIVERINGS. *The disease is probably* EMPYEMA.

§ 120. **Empyema** is a collection of purulent or sero-purulent fluid within the pleural cavity. It often follows a serous effusion, but it may be purulent from the beginning. The pneumococcus is the organism most commonly found.

The *Symptoms* and *Physical Signs* are similar to those of serous effusion (*q.v., supra*), with certain others in addition—viz.: (1) It may be found that the fluid *does not clear up* as a serous effusion should do, and thus the presence of pus may be suspected. (2) Whenever pus forms, in the pleura or elsewhere, it is normally characterised by the occurrence of an intermittent pyrexia and occasional rigors. When, however, the patient is under the influence of full doses of one of the antibiotics, there may be little or no temperature and the presence of pus and even virulent organisms may be overlooked. (3) Œdema of the integument, the pointing of an abscess in an intercostal space, or even in the groin (*empyema necessitatis*), or copious expectoration of pus, may occur if an empyema is overlooked. The modern knowledge of the radiograph and the wider use of the exploring needle have made these accidents less frequent. (4) Clubbing of the fingers, especially in children, is a valuable sign which may come on very rapidly in empyema. (5) The history commonly reveals one of the following *causes* of empyema:

(i.) Lobar pneumonia is by far the commonest cause, especially in children; (ii.) abscess of the lung (often with a fungating carcinoma of a bronchus), of the spine or from a perforated œsophagus; suppurative conditions of the pericardium, mediastinum, or respiratory tract; (iii.) tuberculosis in any form in the thorax; (iv.) an abscess under the diaphragm, especially a subphrenic abscess, perinephric abscess or a hepatic abscess; (v.) pyæmia or from the acute specific fevers; (vi.) any wound from without, permitting the introduction of organisms, or careless paracentesis.

(6) In doubtful cases a leucocyte count should always be made, since in the absence of acute lobar pneumonia more than 20,000 leucocytes per cu.mm. would strongly favour the diagnosis of empyema.   (7) Diagnostic puncture is essential when pus is suspected, though there are two fallacies in this method: first, in rare cases the fluid may be too thick to come through the needle; or, again, the pus may be encysted between the lobes of the lung.   In any case, a pathological examination of the material at the point of the needle will assist the diagnosis.   Although the commonest organism found is the pneumococcus, a streptococcus is not unusual. Other organisms occasionally met are the staphylococcus, *B. coli*, *H. influenzæ* and the streptothrix actinomycosis.

An *interlobar empyema* has become rare since the use of modern drugs for the treatment of pneumonia.   It is often not suspected until the patient, who is recovering from pneumonia, suddenly coughs up pus due to rupture of the abscess.   X-rays are most helpful in localising the lesion.

Prognosis.—Empyema is always serious, and may run a somewhat prolonged course of some months.   Cases of pure pneumococcal empyema are much more favourable than those due to streptococci or staphylococci, either alone or with the tubercle bacillus.   Operation, adequate drainage, and strict aseptic precautions, both at the operation and at the subsequent dressings, are the points in treatment which most favourably influence prognosis.   If left to itself, the results vary: sometimes there is compression and destruction of the lung; sometimes, as above mentioned, the pus opens into the lung, the pericardium, through the chest wall or burrows in other directions; or the condition may lead to pyæmia.

Treatment.—A pneumococcal empyema is usually treated at first with daily aspiration and the insertion of penicillin (500,000 units in 10 ml. of normal saline) combined with parenteral penicillin injections.   If, however, the pus is thick when it is first discovered or if aspiration is not rapidly successful, the abscess must be drained by sub-periosteal rib resection.   A streptococcal empyema is treated on similar lines: with this condition drainage must never be performed until the fluid is frankly purulent, because operation in the sero-purulent stage is attended by a very high mortality.   In tuberculous cases open operation is avoided whenever possible and anti-tuberculous drugs must be administered for at least 12 months.

The after-treatment of empyema is designed to promote expansion of the lung and is most important.   When operation has been performed the establishment of air-tight drainage is very helpful, the tube leading from the wound being connected with an under-water drain. Whichever method is used, during convalescence breathing exercises are of the utmost value: they must be supervised by an expert, who will ensure the maximum degree of movement of the affected side, movements of the contralateral side being restricted by the masseuse.

II. *The patient is* SUDDENLY TAKEN ILL *with a* SHIVERING ATTACK OR RIGOR: *the* TEMPERATURE RISES RAPIDLY *to* 102°–104° *with a* DRY COUGH *and often* PLEURITIC PAIN. *The sputum becomes rusty; there are* SIGNS OF CONSOLIDATION *at the base of one lung. The disease is* ACUTE LOBAR PNEUMONIA.

§ 121. Pneumonia—*i.e.*, inflammation of the pulmonary tissue proper, or parenchymatous inflammation—occurs in two forms. The *first* and more acute is, from its area of distribution, termed " Lobar Pneumonia."

The second, termed " Broncho-pneumonia," is a much less clearly defined entity. It is not in anatomically defined areas as is lobar pneumonia, but is scattered through one or more lobes of the lungs in a patchy or lobular manner. Broncho-pneumonia is due to a number of different pathological processes, with a corresponding variation in the symptoms and signs; see § 122.

Especially in children this traditional distinction cannot always be maintained, for some cases exhibit certain features of both varieties. Since the advent of chemotherapy it is becoming of increasing importance to differentiate the pneumonias, particularly those of the broncho-pneumonic and atypical varieties, according to the nature of the infecting organisms as a guide to rational treatment by specific drugs.

Acute Lobar Pneumonia occurs at any age, but is most commonly seen in those between 15 and 40 years of age and particularly in the autumn and winter.

Symptoms.—It commences suddenly with well-marked constitutional symptoms, such as shivering and often a rigor, headache, backache and, in children, convulsions or vomiting. The temperature during the rigor rises to 103–105° F. The aspect of a patient with lobar pneumonia is very characteristic (§ 7). The face is flushed, anxious and a little cyanosed and herpes appears around the mouth. There is pain in the affected side of the chest due to pleural involvement, a short cough, rapid shallow breathing and a little clear viscid sputum which becomes rust-coloured on the second or third day. The pulse-respiration ratio is 3 to 1 or 2½ to 1, instead of the normal 4 to 1: the alæ nasi often dilate with each inspiration. The urine is scanty and concentrated. The patient becomes more and more distressed and sleepless and in a short time delirium may develop.

In patients untreated by penicillin or the sulphonamides the fever persists at 104°–105° for an average of 7–8 days (and on rare occasions for 11–12 days). The patient continues to be extremely ill, with a hot dry skin, a painful cough, considerable sleeplessness and exhaustion, and takes little nourishment. About the *seventh* or *eighth* day the fever, as also the pulse and respiration rate, in favourable cases, terminates by crisis, falling to normal in the course of a few hours. This is accompanied by marked general improvement; the pulse-respiration ratio returns to normal, and a critical sweating or diarrhœa may occur. Pseudo-crises occasionally occur, but these are distinguished from true crises by the fact that the pulse and respiration do not return to normal. In some cases the temperature falls by lysis. The whole illness lasts about two or three weeks.

In patients treated by penicillin, by other suitable antibiotics or by the sulphonamides the illness is very much shorter. The temperature begins to fall within 12 hours after commencing treatment (a little later with

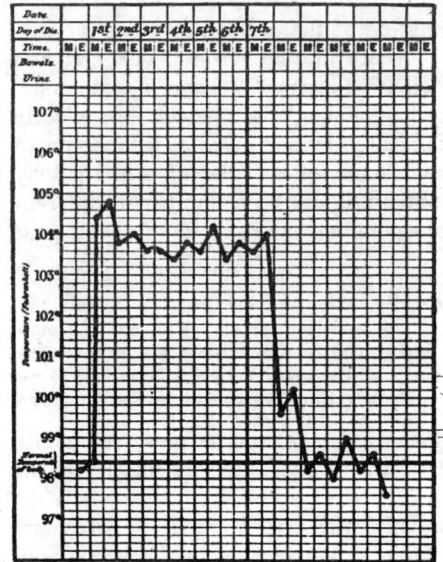

FIG. 53.—ACUTE LOBAR PNEUMONIA, showing typical crisis on the seventh day. George H., aged thirty-five, was taken ill very suddenly with shivering and acute pain in the side. (No chemotherapy was given.)

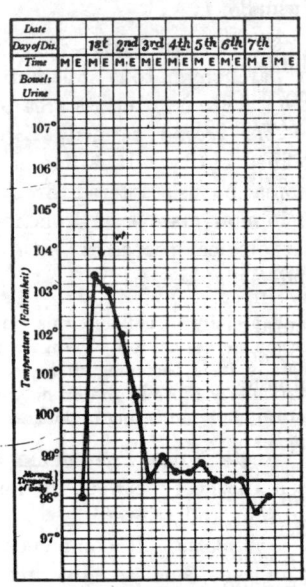

FIG. 57.—ACUTE LOBAR PNEUMONIA in a woman of 40; tetracycline 0·5 g. 6-hourly was started where indicated by arrow.

sulphonamides) and becomes normal within 36 hours, with a corresponding improvement in the general condition of the patient.

The *Physical Signs* are limited to one lung or to one lobe, commonly the right lower lobe. It is only in rare cases that both lungs are involved ("double pneumonia"). *At the onset* there is reduced movement of the affected side of the chest. For the first day or so there is no dullness to percussion but as a rule there is slight impairment of the percussion note. On auscultation the breath sounds are weak and fine rustling crepitations are heard. As the inflammatory exudate increases the lung becomes solid on the second or third day. A pleural rub is often heard, and over the solid area we get all the *signs of consolidation* (§ 109) with bronchial breathing. When penicillin is started early in the illness these signs of consolidation are not so fully developed. On occasions rhonchi may be heard in other areas. In either case soon after the fever has settled coarse moist râles (redux crepitations) are heard, and the normal percussion resonance and breath sounds gradually return.

Central Pneumonia.—The symptoms are the same as have just been described, but even in untreated patients, the physical signs of consolidation do not appear until very late (7–10 days) or not at all. This is due to the fact that the actual lesion in the lung is deep-seated and only spreads to the surface much later, if at all: for this reason pleuritic pain is usually absent. X-ray examination, however, reveals the condition.

Apical Pneumonia occurs most frequently in children. There is consolidation of the upper lobe of one lung: cerebral symptoms and particularly those of meningismus are prominent.

Diagnosis.—The classical features of lobar pneumonia are the sudden onset, the labial herpes, a persistent temperature of 103–104° F with little diurnal variation, the rusty sputum and the subsequent solidification of one or more lobes of the lung. Acute pleurisy with *effusion* is recognised by the data given in the table of diagnosis between consolidation of the lungs and fluid in the pleura (§ 109): but let it be remembered that, especially in cases treated with antibiotics, some fluid often collects in the pleural cavity when the underlying lung is solid with pneumonia. *Bronchopneumonia* (see Table VII, page 203). A *bronchial carcinoma* causes pulmonary consolidation and collapse, often with a raised temperature and hæmoptysis. The onset is, however, more gradual, the temperature does not settle to normal and the lung signs persist even in the presence of full doses of penicillin. *Pulmonary infarction* (§ 105) causes sudden pleuritic pain, followed by a low-grade temperature and often blood-stained sputum with signs of consolidation at a lung base; there is usually evidence of a cause for the formation of a clot which has given rise to embolism. The sudden onset of acute pneumonia resembles that of *scarlet fever*, *erysipelas*, and *small-pox*, but the absence of rusty sputum and altered pulse-respiration ratio distinguishes them. There is a pneumonic form of *acute pulmonary tuberculosis* which has to be borne in mind (§ 124); also various *aberrant forms of pneumonia* (§ 123); and acute exacerbations in *bronchiectasis*. Especially in children, apical pneumonia may cause meningismus with headache and neck stiffness which can be confused with *meningitis*; and basal pneumonia may at its onset simulate *abdominal inflammation*, pain being referred to the abdomen and lung signs being absent (§§ 238, 248). In such cases a diminished respiratory murmur at one lung base and an increased respiratory rate are signs of great value.

Etiology.—The disease is a specific infectious illness, the causal organism being a Gram-positive diplococcus, the pneumococcus of Fraenkel. Infection occurs by inhalation through the larger bronchi and the organism then spreads from the hilar area to the affected lobe or lobes via the peribronchial lymphatics. Although healthy men are often attacked, debilitating conditions such as a chill, exposure, diabetes and chronic alcoholism can all act as predisposing causes. A blow on the chest may determine an attack (*traumatic pneumonia*). Although some 32 types of pneumococci have been isolated, most cases are due to types I, II and III. Type III is more virulent than types I and II and does not excite such a high leucocytosis. In severe cases there is often a bacteræmia in the earlier stages and the organism can be isolated by blood culture.

Prognosis.—The case mortality of all ages combined used to vary between 20 and 40 per cent., but the advent of the sulphonamides and subsequently of penicillin treatment has reduced this to well under 5 per cent. Instead of lasting on an average 7–8 days, treatment with these drugs causes the temperature to drop to within one degree of normal in 36–48 hours, with corresponding improvement in the patient's clinical condition (Fig. 57). The prognosis is worse when the natural resistance of the patient is low; pneumonia is especially serious in chronic alcoholics and in diabetics (in both of these a positive blood culture is often obtained), in children under one year and in elderly persons particularly when they are suffering from emphysema, chronic bronchitis and other debilitating conditions. The prognosis is greatly improved by early and adequate treatment with one of the specific remedies: children from 3 to 10 years of age nearly always recover and in those between the ages of 5 and 45 years the death rate is about 1 per cent. Unfavourable features include extensive involvement of the lung (the outlook being worse when both lungs are involved), marked cyanosis, considerable delirium, an unduly low temperature, marked tachycardia especially when the pulse rate exceeds the systolic blood pressure in mms., and signs of peripheral circulatory failure. A mild toxic hepatitis with jaundice, albuminuria, paralytic ileus and (in the elderly) paroxysmal auricular fibrillation may occur. *Complications* of serious import include pneumococcal septicæmia, meningitis, pericarditis or endocarditis, and the occurrence of secondary infection with organisms such as the streptococcus, staphylococcus, or *H. influenzæ*, all of which should come under control with adequate and early chemotherapy. The lung condition should have cleared completely and even radiographically in 4–6 weeks, but may take longer in small children and elderly subjects. When there is delayed resolution some other condition such as carcinoma of the bronchus or empyema must be suspected.

Treatment.—The first essential is to send a specimen of sputum for bacteriological examination: the early mucoid sputum usually gives a pure growth of pneumococci and in elderly or debilitated subjects will reveal any secondary invading organisms. It is no longer necessary to type the pneumococcus, as in the days when serum therapy was used. *Chemotherapy.*—The pneumococcus is very sensitive to the sulphonamides, to penicillin and to many other antibiotics such as chlortetracycline B.P. (Aureomycin), chloramphenicol B.P. (Chloromycetin), tetracycline (Achromycin) and oxytetracycline B.P. (Terramycin). On the grounds of therapeutic efficiency there is little to choose between these, but penicillin or sulphadimidine produce much less drug toxicity and alimentary disturbance, and are a great deal cheaper than the tetracyclines. Penicillin cannot be given if the patient is penicillin-sensitive. The usual procedure when using penicillin is to give benzylpenicillin B.P. (soluble penicillin) 500,000 units 8 or 12-hourly, or procaine benzylpenicillin B.P. (procaine penicillin G) 600,000 units daily with soluble penicillin 250,000 units with the first dose. To prevent complications these doses must be continued until the temperature has been normal for three days: smaller doses once a day are desirable for a further three days. When sulphonamide therapy is chosen, either sulphadimidine B.P. (sulphamethazine) or trisulphonamide (Sulphatriad) is equally effective: an initial dose of G. 4 is followed by G. 1 four-hourly until the temperature has settled, after which G. 1 is given eight-hourly for another 4–5 days. Of the tetracyclines, tetracycline itself has the fewest side-effects. When the patient is very ill it is often wise to give penicillin, with sulphadimidine or tetracycline in addition: and when the temperature has not largely settled after 48 hours of such treatment and the bacteriological result shows a secondary infection with an organism (such as staphylococcus or *H. influenzæ*) which is insensitive to these drugs, another suitable antibiotic must be chosen (Table XXXI). (For doses for children see Table XXXII.)

General Treatment.—The administration of penicillin and/or a sulphonamide cannot be regarded as a substitute for the general measures which must be observed in all cases of pneumonia. The patient's strength must be maintained by rest in bed, good nursing, relief from pain and adequate sleep. Fresh air at a temperature of 62–65° F is much to be preferred to a vitiated atmosphere. Patients usually prefer to be nursed sitting up with three or four pillows but their own wishes should be considered over this. They should be kept warm with blankets and hot-water bottles, as necessary. The bowels need to be cleared by an initial dose of a mild aperient. The diet should be light with fruit drinks, milk, broths and jellies totalling 3–4 pints in 24 hours. Sugar can be added to the drinks when it is acceptable. Once the temperature has fallen, a light solid diet is often possible. *Relief from pain* with its accompanying anxiety is best obtained by an initial dose of inject. papaveretum B.P.C. (Omnopon) gr. ⅓ for an adult: this produces less depression of the respiratory centre and less tendency to vomiting than does inject. morphine gr. ¼. The injection may need to be repeated. Other measures used are the local application of a kaolin poultice, strapping or even a local anæsthetic to the pleura (§ 116). If *cough* is troublesome in the early stages a linctus such as of codeine or diamorphine will prove helpful. *Sleep* is of cardinal importance—no patient with pneumonia should be allowed to lie awake at night, tossing in bed from side to side. Apart from the administration of papaveretum or morphine, a quick tepid sponge to the skin when the temperature is over 103° is a great comfort. Hypnotics may be used: inject. sod. phenobarbitone gr. 3, tab. sod. amylobarbitone gr. 3–4½, chloral hydrate and potass. bromide gr. 25 of each and well diluted, or paraldehyde ℳ 120 covered by a little alcohol and with orange juice are most helpful. When there is extreme restlessness and even *delirium*, as in alcoholic patients or in those with extreme toxæmia, apart from increased doses of the chemotherapeutic agents, give chloral hydrate and potassium bromide in doses of 30–45 gr. of each, and to alcoholics also give 6–10 fl. oz. of whisky a day. An injection of paraldehyde (4–6 ml. intramuscularly) is of particular help in very noisy or alcoholic patients. Delirium is usually an indication of cerebral anoxia and when this symptom or when *cyanosis* is present it is essential to give oxygen by inhalation. The object is to obtain a concentration of 40–60 per cent., either in an oxygen tent, or with a mask such as the B.L.B. mask or a polymask with an oxygen flow rate of 5–7 litres a minute. It is preferable to bubble the oxygen through warm water to moisten it before inhalation. When cyanosis is slight morphia may be used, but it may prove lethal if given when cyanosis is marked, particularly in elderly patients who also have bronchitis. *Engorgement of the right side of the heart* is indicated not only by cyanosis but by distension of the neck veins and some tenderness and enlargement of the liver. Oxygen is of help; rapid venesection of 10–15 fl. oz. of blood is of special value in elderly or plethoric individuals. *Peripheral circulatory collapse* is a serious but happily a rare sign, and is due to intense toxæmia. For this give large doses of antibiotics, oxygen, plenty of fluid with sugar by mouth and injections of mephenteramine (Mephine) or metaraminol (Aramine) added to a slow intravenous drip or intramusc., or inject. nikethamide 5 ml. *Auricular fibrillation* must be vigorously treated with intravenous digoxin followed by a suitable digitalis preparation by mouth: usually the rhythm returns to normal as the temperature falls. The routine use of digitalis in elderly subjects with pneumonia (other than those with auricular fibrillation), although preferred by some, is not justified by the results. *Acute dilatation of the stomach* with vomiting and abdominal distension may require aspiration of the stomach and intravenous fluids together with the injection of posterior pituitary extract, and meteorism with intestinal paresis will indicate the additional necessity of turpentine fl. oz. ½ in an enema: later on a flatus tube may be needed. Unresolved pneumonia is treated by breathing exercises and by local short-wave diathermy. Prophylaxis comprises care of the mouth, teeth and naso-pharynx, and the use of pneumococcal and influenzal vaccines.

III. *The illness has come on* LESS SUDDENLY *than in lobar pneumonia; there is* COUGH, *with frothy expectoration; the physical signs of* CONSOLIDATION *are* MORE PATCHY *and accompanied by* SIGNS OF BRONCHITIS. *The disease is probably* BRONCHO-PNEUMONIA.

§ 122. **Acute Broncho-pneumonia** is also an acute parenchymatous inflammation of the lungs, but it runs a very different course to that of acute lobar pneumonia. The inflammatory process does not involve the whole of one or more lobes but occurs in patches with intervening normal or emphysematous areas. These may be scattered unequally through both lungs or may chiefly involve one portion of a lung (inhalation pneumonia): there is usually accompanying bronchitis, hence the name.   The disease varies in its symptoms and signs according to the pathological process and the type of organism present.   Thus although influenzal pneumonia may occur at any age, broncho-pneumonia secondary to bronchitis is much more likely to occur in small children (especially with measles or whooping-cough) and in elderly patients as a complication of chronic bronchitis.

Symptoms.—These usually come on much more gradually than in lobar pneumonia, but vary with the type of invading organism.   There may be a history of an initial upper respiratory infection or " cold " followed by bronchitis with slight fever, general malaise, a cough and some shortness of breath.   After an interval and when the infection has reached the smaller tubes, the patient becomes more distressed with a higher temperature (about 100° F in the mornings and 101–103° in the evenings), accompanied by a shallow cough, dyspnœa and muco-purulent sputum: pleural pain is rare.   He looks much more ill: the pulse is rapid, the face is pale instead of flushed, there is distressed breathing and often cyanosis.   Children take no interest in their surroundings, their whole attention appearing to be devoted to the effort and the rapidity of breathing.   Extensive broncho-pneumonia in old people is equally serious: they show evidence of heart failure with marked anoxia and cyanosis, and when these become extreme restlessness, drowsiness and finally delirium ensue.   Without the help of chemotherapy the temperature will remain raised for 2 or 3 weeks, but with suitable chemotherapy the temperature subsides over a period of one or two weeks.

Physical Signs.—The lungs show evidence of bronchitis, with râles and rhonchi which are especially marked at the lung bases.   Signs of consolidation are not so marked as in lobar pneumonia: there are reduced breath sounds and occasional areas of tubular breathing, but dullness to percussion and the signs of consolidation which are so clearly elicited in patients with lobar pneumonia, are not made out unless the areas of broncho-pneumonic consolidation become more or less confluent.   The chief auscultatory signs in children consist of *intensely loud*, " consonating " râles, and rhonchi.   The " capillary-bronchitis " of infants is really an indication of broncho-pneumonia.

Etiology.—Broncho-pneumonia is much more common in the winter and spring months.   *In Infants and Small Children*, the cases fall into two groups.   In *Primary* broncho-pneumonia the infecting agent is usually the pneumococcus which, as in pneumococcal lobar pneumonia, causes a sudden rise of temperature to 104°–105° F often with a convulsion and vomiting.   The child looks very ill: the alæ nasi are working and the ribs often sucked in during inspiration.   Signs of consolidation are more easy to elicit than in the other varieties of broncho-pneumonia.   *Secondary* broncho-pneumonia arises as a complication of measles, whooping-cough and of debilitating conditions such as marasmus or steatorrhœa.   *In*

Adults broncho-pneumonia is especially seen complicating chronic debilitating conditions, such as chronic renal disease, chronic cardiac disease, or bed-lying, as from fracture of the femur in old people; elderly patients often die of pneumonia as a terminal event in senile decay. *Aspiration or deglutition (septic) pneumonia* occurs when solid food particles or liquids are aspirated with the larynx, trachea and larger bronchi. There are a large number of different causes such as (i.) with cancer of the throat, larynx or of the œsophagus causing a fistula into the air passages, or due to a spill-over of food in achalasia of the œsophagus or from a pharyngeal pouch: congenital malformation is an occasional cause in infants; (ii.) in neurological states with coma due to any cause, following an epileptic fit, in bulbar palsy or post-diphtheritic paralysis; (iii.) following the aspiration of blood during a dental extraction, hæmoptysis and when infected material from a quinzy, a lung abscess or bronchiectasis enters normal lung tissue; (iv.) with post-operative vomiting, after tracheotomy and particularly after operations on the nose, mouth or tongue. When these are undertaken under general anæsthesia, especial care must be taken to keep the head lowered and attention paid to the drainage of blood and the removal of all solid particles of tissue.

Rarer types of Broncho-pneumonia occur with a variety of other specific bacterial lung infections. They are less common than those already described and are identified by culture of the sputum. They are:—

H. Influenzæ and B. Friedländer are becoming increasingly recognised as primary or secondary infections in the lungs: they are identified only by sputum cultures. Friedländer's bacillus may produce a mild attack following aspiration of the organism from the nose, but on occasions it can cause a severe type of pneumonia leading to abscess formation, or to subsequent fibrosis.

Staphylococcal pneumonia is often the result of a staphylococcal pyæmia from a distant site such as a carbuncle, a perinephric abscess, a renal carbuncle, osteomyelitis or mastoiditis. It can occur as a secondary infection in the course of bronchopneumonia due to other causes. *Symptoms.*—The infection may be acute, with headaches and rigors: it often assumes a sub-acute form, and it produces localised areas of consolidation in the lungs. There is a great tendency to the development of abscesses. The X-ray appearances are often suggestive and bacteriological examination of the sputum is diagnostic.

Streptococcal pneumonia.—Attention was dramatically focused on this by the very severe cases of pneumonia seen towards the end of World War I. Associated with the widespread epidemic of influenza the lungs were invaded by a virulent β-hæmolytic streptococcal infection. The outcome was often rapidly fatal. Happily this has not occurred with any great frequency since. Infections with streptococcus viridans and other non-hæmolytic streptococci are now more common than the hæmolytic streptococcal variety. *Symptoms.*—In many cases of acute streptococcal pneumonia the onset is similar in its suddenness to that of the pure pneumococcal (lobar) type, but the subsequent picture often differs considerably from that above described under lobar pneumonia. Early features in these streptococcal cases are the greater toxæmia, the high temperature, the mental apathy, pallor and often cyanosis, sometimes apparent before the occurrence of appreciable physical signs in the chest. There is a particular tendency to cause a streptococcal empyema.

Typhoid, anthrax and plague may cause pneumonia during the course of each of these infections.

Tuberculous pneumonia is discussed in § 124.

Diagnosis of Broncho-Pneumonia.—The principal diagnostic features are the catarrhal symptoms, the dyspnœa and frequent cyanosis, and the toxæmic appearance of the patient. Patients with bronchitis are usually much less ill than are those with broncho-pneumonia. The diagnosis from *lobar pneumonia* is given in Table VII. The pulmonary signs of *measles, whooping-cough, bronchitis* and *psittacosis* resemble broncho-pneumonia in its early stages, and it may not be easy to diagnose these several diseases until the rash of the one or the whoop of the other appears. When the diagnosis is in doubt an X-ray film often helps. In any case the important point is to differentiate the acute pneumonias according to the

TABLE VII.—DIFFERENTIATION BETWEEN A TYPICAL CASE
(untreated by chemotherapy) OF

	LOBAR PNEUMONIA	*and*	LOBULAR OR BRONCHO-PNEUMONIA.
Onset	Sudden, with rigors.		Gradual, and preceded by bronchitis.
Course of Temperature	Continuous.		Remittent.
Defervescence ..	Crisis usually by seventh day.		By lysis in two to four weeks.
Percussion ..	Dullness in one lung, usually the base.		Scattered patches of dullness in both lungs.
Auscultation ..	(i.) Fine crepitations. (ii.) Consolidation signs in a day or two.		Fine crepitations and signs of consolidation over dull areas, though obscured by rhonchi and bronchitic râles.
Sputum	Rusty.		Frothy and muco-purulent.
Respiration ..	Pulse-respiration ratio 3 : 1 or 2½ : 1.		Less marked difference of pulse-respiration ratio.

nature of the infecting organisms as a guide to accurate chemotherapy. In children who have repeated attacks, the possibility of fibrocystic disease of the pancreas (" mucosis ") and of agammaglobulinæmia should be considered. Tuberculous broncho-pneumonia is described in § 124 and the aberrant pneumonia in § 123.

Prognosis.—Prior to the advent of drugs of the sulphonamide group the case mortality in children under five varied from 30 to 50 per cent.; the younger the child the more fatal was the disease, and under the age of 6 months 90 per cent. of cases were lethal. The sooner the disease is recognised and treated by the appropriate antibiotic the more likely is the patient to recover: a considerable improvement should be shown within 48 hours of commencing therapy. Other factors are the virulence of the infection and the age of the patient. Broncho-pneumonia is often superimposed on some other disease, and a factor of importance is the nature of the antecedent condition. A well-recognised sequel is pulmonary fibrosis, which is especially common in broncho-pneumonia occurring in whooping-cough and measles. The aspiration and deglutition pneumonias are often fatal.

Treatment.—The general principles are the same as those described in acute lobar pneumonia (§ 121). Children need to be placed in an oxygen tent at an early stage. Adults may need Dover's powder or linctus heroin if their nights are rendered sleepless. For the reduction of excessive fever tepid sponging may be invaluable. Pneumococcal, streptococcal and staphylococcal pneumonias usually respond to penicillin, but when the organisms are penicillin-resistant (especially with staphylococci) intramusc. methicillin (Celbenin), one of the tetracyclines or erythromycin must be prescribed. *H. influenzæ* does not respond to penicillin but is very susceptible to inject. streptomycin and to the tetracyclines (especially to chloramphenicol); *B. Friedlander* infections are usually responsive to a combination of these same drugs. In severely ill patients, oxygen administration through a tracheostomy often with assisted positive and negative ventilation of the lungs, may be life saving.

§ 123. Atypical Acute Pneumonias (including *Primary Atypical Pneumonia*). We have seen that in acute lobar pneumonia, pleurisy and in most cases of broncho-pneumonia due to pyogenic bacteria the course of the disease and the physical signs in the lungs are characteristic. But it is important to remember that these same conditions may occur secondary to, or as part of, some general disorder. In these circumstances some of the symptoms or physical signs may be wanting or irregular, and it may not be possible to arrive at a diagnosis, except by passing in review the whole history of the case, and by making a thorough and systematic examination of all the other organs. The bacteriology of the infection can usually be identified by examination of the sputum or by lung puncture. There are, however, a large number of cases which do not conform to this regular pattern, it may not be possible to recognise the causal organism, there is no leucocytosis and there is usually no response to administration of penicillin or the sulphonamides. They usually do respond to the tetracyclines. Most of these cases fall into one of the following groups:

1. *Virus infections.* (a) The virus of *psittacosis* was the first to be described in association with atypical pneumonia: cases arose in those handling exotic birds (especially budgerigars) and gave rise to a serious pandemic in 1929–30. It is now known that similar virus infections can be transferred to man from pigeons, chickens, canaries, finches, mice and cats, and that infection can also be transferred from man to man without animal contact. These infections have been given the group name Ornithosis. *Symptoms.*—Although in mild cases only an upper respiratory tract infection ensues, a severe case often at first resembles typhoid fever until bilateral broncho-pneumonia occurs a few days later. *Diagnosis* is with a complement-fixation test using a group specific antigen. The virus may be detected in the sputum (as in psittacosis, § 507): the cold agglutination test is usually negative. X-ray of the chest shows a bilateral basal " ground-glass " type of consolidation. *Treatment* with the tetracyclines and especially with chloramphenicol B.P. is usually successful.

(b) *Primary Virus Pneumonia* (Syn. Primary Atypical Pneumonia) is the name given to another group which is now more common than orni-

thosis.   It occurs in epidemics, especially in the winter and spring months.
Symptoms.—The onset is with a dry paroxysmal cough, headache, muscle
pains and a temperature of 101–103° F with a relatively slow pulse and
respiration rate.   There may be a pleuritic chest pain and some blood-
streaked sputum.   The chest signs are few: there may be a localised area
of consolidation or the only physical sign may be the presence of localised
post-tussic râles towards the lung bases.   The temperature usually settles
in 7–12 days but in more severe cases persists for 3 weeks.   The X-ray
findings vary: there may be a localised opacity or a diffuse haze spreading
out from the hilum, but in other cases widely disseminated lesions occur
which may resemble miliary tuberculosis.   The *Diagnosis* is suggested
by the much greater constitutional symptoms and the relatively few lung
signs: it may be aided by a rising titre of the cold-agglutinins in the plasma
during the second–fourth weeks, but in some epidemics this is only found
in 10 per cent. of cases.   *Treatment* is again with the tetracycline drugs
to combat the secondary infection.

(c) The viruses of *Influenza* may give rise to pneumonia but the lung
changes are more commonly due to a secondary bacterial invasion.

2. *Pneumonia due to Localised Aspiration.*   When material heavily
infected with pyogenic organisms is inhaled it causes pulmonary suppuration (§ 146).   However, during the course of a nasal or bronchial
cold many patients appear to aspirate infected mucus into the bronchial
tree: these plugs of mucus produce an area of collapse in one of the basal
lung segments, which Scadding has named " aspiration pneumonia."
Even if the original cold was viral in origin, there is no reason to believe
the pneumonia is of virus origin, and the serological tests obtained in cases
of virus pneumonia are negative.   *Symptoms* arise a few days after a
" cold " and especially when this occurs during severe physical exertion.
There is often little fever, patients are often ambulant and the *diagnosis*
is made by X-ray examination.   When more severe symptoms arise there
is increasing malaise, a temperature of 100–101° F and some pleuritic
pain.   *Treatment* is by antibiotics, and physiotherapy with vigorous
percussion of the chest combined with breathing exercises.

3. *Bronchial Obstruction* may first show itself by the occurrence of
an area of pneumonic consolidation in a lobe or segment of a lobe of the
lung.   Such an obstruction may be due to a bronchial carcinoma or
adenoma, a foreign body, enlarged hilar glands or a bronchial stricture.
Symptoms.—The collapsed lung behind the obstruction becomes airless,
solid and often develops a suppurative pneumonia.   The infection responds
only in part to penicillin and the fact that the temperature does not settle
to normal (it often recurs when penicillin is withdrawn) and the lung
remains solid, calls for further investigation by radiology and bronchoscopy.

4. **Rickettsial Pneumonia** occurs with Q fever.   It is rare but is met in sporadic
outbreaks in many countries, including Great Britain.   *Symptoms.*—The onset is
insidious with headache, malaise, anorexia, nausea and vomiting with a variable rash.
After the third day chest symptoms arise.   X-ray shows one or more soft shadows

in the lungs which clear spontaneously and do not usually require treatment with the tetracyclines. Agglutinins and complement-fixing antibodies are present in the serum after the eighth day (and see § 483).

5. **Rare Causes** of atypical pneumonia are (i.) *Systemic Lupus Erythematosus*. This may produce broncho-pneumonic lesions, usually towards the lung bases, with a high temperature and sometimes dry or wet pleurisy. Sooner or later there are other manifestations of the cause: L.E. cells are often found in the peripheral blood, the bone marrow or in the effusion. (ii.) The pulmonary form of *polyarteritis nodosa* is usually of a more chronic nature, but pneumonic lesions occur. (iii.) *Wegener's granulomatosis* bears resemblances to polyarteritis nodosa. It occurs in middle-age with symptoms of an upper respiratory infection followed by ulceration: persistent pyrexia accompanies signs in the lungs of consolidation and sometimes cavitation, unaffected by antibiotics. A hæmorrhagic vesicular rash is common. Death occurs from broncho-pneumonia or uræmia after an average period of five months. (iv.) *Pulmonary aspergillosis* should be thought of (§ 147).

The term *pneumonitis*, introduced originally in the United States of America, was intended to cover a wide range of conditions characterised by the presence of an area or areas of localised consolidation in the lung. Such conditions, although inflammatory in origin, are not examples of pneumonia in the ordinary sense of the term, and do not give any typical clinical picture with a definite clinical course. The term is a useful one to denote the nature of the underlying pathological process, but it should not be supposed that pneumonitis indicates a clearly defined clinical entity.

§ 124. IV. **Acute Pneumonic Phthisis** (Syn. Acute Caseous Pneumonia) is more common in children than in adults. The disease is caused by rupture of a caseating tuberculous focus into a bronchus. This more commonly produces a general dissemination of the organism through the entire bronchial tree, and sets up tuberculous broncho-pneumonia. Occasionally only one lobe is involved to produce a tuberculous lobar pneumonia. Some cases follow a hæmoptysis or dissemination while under a general anæsthetic. The *Symptoms* and physical signs are those of pneumonia and may start suddenly with a rapid rise in temperature and pain in the chest. The temperature, however, does not respond to penicillin or to the tetracyclines: it begins to swing much more at the end of the first week and the course of the disease becomes prolonged for many weeks. This is followed by physical signs of breaking down in the lung, purulent expectoration, night sweats, hæmoptysis and the finding of tubercle bacilli in the sputum. Although the outlook has been greatly improved by modern therapy, the disease is still serious.

§ 125. V. **Acute Massive Collapse** of the lung is usually post-operative, but can occur after trauma to the chest, with inhalation of a foreign body, and occasionally from other causes. The most important factor producing this is obstruction of a bronchus by viscid secretion—most cases of so-called post-operative pneumonia are due to massive collapse. The *Symptoms* come on acutely with sudden pain in the chest, severe dyspnœa, cyanosis, shock and the patient looks very ill. The *Physical Signs* resemble those of pneumonia, but owing to the obstructed bronchi, bronchial breathing is rare and the voice sounds are reduced. The displacement of the heart and often the trachea to the affected side should make the diagnosis clear: if need be this can be confirmed radiographically. *Treatment* consists in loosening post-operative bandages for short periods, encouraging deep breathing with 7 per cent. carbon dioxide in 93 per cent. oxygen several times a day, and the administration of an expectorant mixture containing potassium iodide. Percussion by a physiotherapist over the affected lobe may help to dislodge the mucus and prophylactic penicillin injections serve to prevent the formation of pus behind the obstruction. Sometimes removal of the obstructing plug of sputum, mucus, etc., through a broncho-scope is necessary.

We now turn to the **acute disease with hyper-resonance on percussion**—viz., Pneumothorax. Bear in mind that an acute disease may supervene upon a chronic condition accompanied by hyper-resonance—*e.g.*, when acute bronchitis supervenes on emphysema (see Table VIII, § 142).

The patient SUDDENLY *develops* SEVERE PAIN *on one side of the chest, with marked* RESPIRATORY DISTRESS *and there may be* COLLAPSE *and* CYANOSIS. *One side of the chest scarcely moves with respiration, there is* HYPER-RESONANCE *and* ABSENCE OF BREATH SOUNDS *in the corresponding lung, and the* HEART AND TRACHEA *are* DISPLACED *to the opposite side. The disease is* SPONTANEOUS PNEUMOTHORAX.

§ 126. **Pneumothorax** is a term used to denote the presence of air in the pleural cavity, the air having gained admission by perforation of the pleura, either from within or from without. An effusion may form (hydro-pneumothorax) which, after a time, may become infected (pyopneumo-thorax). Occasionally the fluid consists of almost pure blood (hæmo-pneumothorax). A recurrence on one or more occasions is not unusual.

The *Symptoms* vary greatly in severity, depending on the amount of air that enters the pleura and on the condition of the opposite lung: when this is extensively diseased the symptoms are much more urgent. On the other hand if the amount of air in the pleura is small and the opposite lung healthy, symptoms are minimal and the condition may only be recognised by X-ray examination. Three groups of cases are met:

(*a*) Severe symptoms occur when the pneumothorax is large. The patient complains of very sudden severe pain on one side of the chest, accompanied by great shortness of breath, and his breathing is rapid and shallow. He becomes very anxious and collapsed, with sweating, and cyanosis may develop. The pulse becomes rapid, weak and even thready with considerable fall in the blood pressure. In the worst cases death may occur in a few minutes.

(*b*) There is a sudden pleuritic pain in the chest with some shortness of breath on exertion. There may be a slight dry cough; but there is no collapse, shock or cyanosis.

(*c*) There may be pain on one side of the chest or this may be absent. There are no other symptoms and there are no physical signs of abnor-mality, but a routine X-ray of the chest reveals a small amount of air separating the two layers of pleura, perhaps localised to one area by disease in the lung.

The sudden onset of symptoms is often apparently the result of strenuous physical effort, e.g., throwing a cricket ball. The degree of severity should not be judged so much by the amount of pain as by the degree of disability and distress: these depend on the amount of air which gets into the pleural cavity and the resulting degree of displacement of the heart and mediastinum. Once symptoms have commenced, they get worse for a day or so unless treatment is instituted. There is often a slight rise in temperature over the next 3–4 days.

The Physical Signs in a typical case consist of: (i.) A fullness or bulging of the chest on the affected side, with little movement even with a deep breath; (ii.) palpation confirms the lack of movement and reveals diminished tactile vocal fremitus; (iii.) percussion usually gives a hyper-resonant note which is often described as " boxy " or tympanitic, but if the air in the pleura is under tension this may be reduced or absent; (iv.) on auscultation the respiratory murmur is reduced or absent; amphoric breathing may be heard over the lower half of the chest behind; the vocal resonance is usually diminished, but pectoriloquy and bronchophony are sometimes present. A localised area of amphoric breathing can sometimes be detected posteriorly: this is believed to correspond with the aperture in the lung which has produced the pneumothorax; (v.) the heart and trachea are displaced to the opposite side. The apex beat may be difficult to locate: with a left-sided pneumothorax it may be well to the right of the sternal border and with a right-sided pneumothorax it may be found in the left axilla. When the pneumothorax is on the right side the hyper-resonance due to the air in the pleural cavity extends well down over the liver dullness. The " coin " or " bell " sound is the sound with a ringing quality, produced when the chest is tapped with two coins in one area and the stethoscope is placed on the chest at a distance from this. Especially when there is a small hydrothorax, a high-pitched tinkling sound is imparted to râles heard during breathing.

Diagnosis.—In many cases the diagnosis is clear, especially in the presence of sudden pain on one side of the chest, accompanied by dyspnœa in a young man. The physical signs are usually conclusive—especially the absence of air entry into one lung with displacement of the heart and mediastinum to the opposite side. X-ray examination in one or more planes demonstrates the two pleural surfaces, separated by a clear space in which no lung markings are visible. When the amount of air is considerable the lung is seen to be collapsed against the hilum. A fibroid lung causes the mediastinum to be displaced to the diseased side and the opposite lung is hyper-resonant due to emphysema: but with this hyper-resonance there is an increased movement of the one side of the chest and the underlying breath sounds are exaggerated. Senile emphysema causes poor movement on both sides of the chest, and although the apex beat of the heart may be difficult to locate, the trachea is central and

PLATE IV

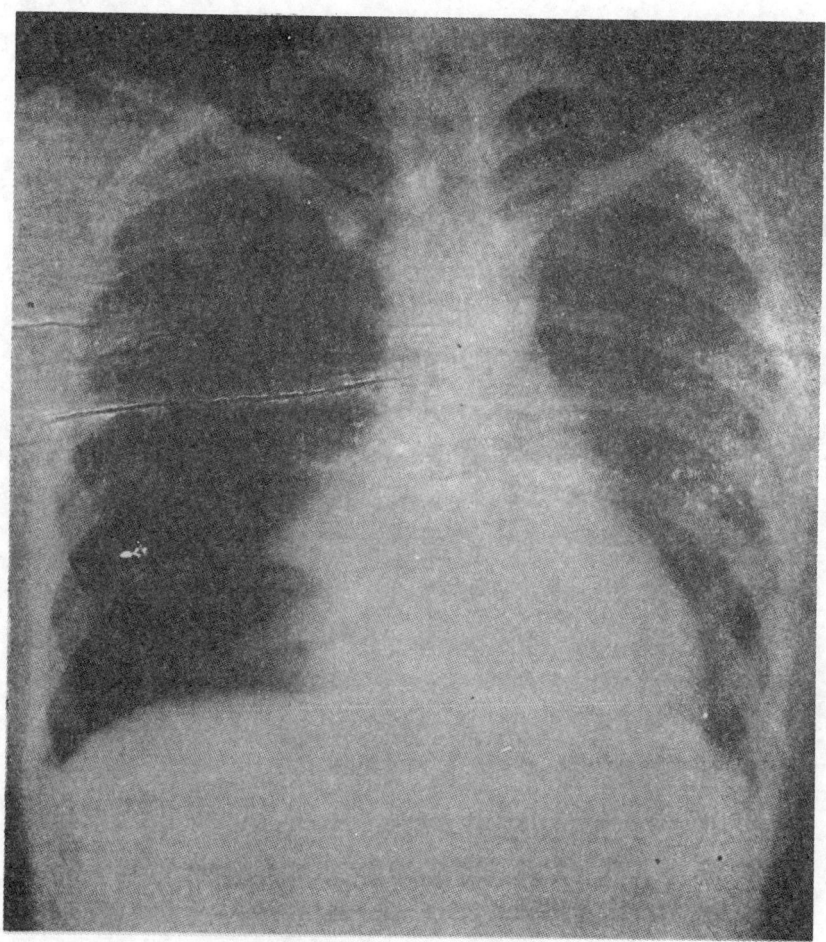

FIG. 58.—CHEST X-RAY demonstrating a large PNEUMOTHORAX on the right side. There are no lung markings in the right chest and the collapsed lung lies adjacent to the right border of the heart.

a hyper-resonant percussion note is present on both sides. A *large cavity* or a *large cyst in the lung* may cause difficulty but there is no sudden onset of pain or dyspnœa. A large *diaphragmatic hernia* or *eventration of the diaphragm* produces a tympanic note in the left lower axilla and at the left lung base, but borborygmi may be clearly heard and radiology of the chest with possibly a barium meal should decide the diagnosis. A sudden *coronary occlusion* usually occurs at a later age. It causes sudden severe pain in the chest, dyspnœa, collapse and even early death, but there are no unilateral lung signs in this condition. *Pulmonary embolism* should not cause difficulty if this possibility is borne in mind.

Etiology.—(i.) The commonest cause of spontaneous pneumothorax in young healthy individuals is the rupture of an emphysematous bulla in the subpleural area of the lung. Such emphysematous bullæ may or may not be associated with scarring from an old tuberculous focus. (ii.) A less common cause is pulmonary tuberculosis, when a caseous focus or a small cavity just under the pleura ruptures. It is important to distinguish these two varieties for active tuberculosis, perhaps first discovered when a spontaneous pneumothorax occurs, needs prolonged active treatment. The tuberculous variety differs from the non-tuberculous in that tuberculosis is much more likely when there is a hydropneumothorax: once the early temperature has settled the blood sedimentation is still raised and X-ray examination is likely to reveal tuberculosis especially when the lung has re-expanded. (iii.) A fractured rib, a stab or bullet wound and sometimes needling the chest (especially with a wide bore needle) may lead to perforation of the lung. (iv.) Less common causes are gangrene of the lung, or an abscess connected with the spine or liver bursting into the pleural cavity.

The *Prognosis* is uncertain soon after the pneumothorax has occurred and may be grave when the amount of air in the pleural cavity is sufficient to cause severe dyspnœa, cyanosis and collapse. The degree of dyspnœa is greatly increased if the opposite lung is already diseased. The *immediate* risk is greatly increased when the opening through the pleura is valvular: this rare condition allows more air to enter but none to escape so that air accumulates rapidly and under pressure ("tension pneumothorax"). With the rapid increase in the symptoms there is soon death from respiratory or heart failure—unless the condition is immediately recognised and relieved by inserting a needle into the chest. More commonly the opening allows air to pass to and fro for a while and then it closes spontaneously: the air in the pleural cavity absorbs over the next 3–4 weeks and recovery is complete. When infection of the pleural cavity occurs with pyogenic organisms or with tubercle bacilli a pyopneumothorax occurs and on the rare occasions when blood is present there is a hæmopneumothorax: both these carry a much worse prognosis. The *cause* of the condition is also important for pneumothorax resulting from late phthisis or gangrene of the lung is often fatal; but that which occasionally complicates whooping-cough, pneumonia, early phthisis, and injury, usually results in recovery.

Treatment.—In most cases all that is required is that the patient should be kept in bed until the air has largely absorbed: an upright or semi-recumbent position is usually the more comfortable. When there is no cyanosis but anxiety is marked, an injection of morphia (gr. ¼) is helpful. Provided the condition proves to be non-tuberculous no further treatment is required. However, if at the commencement shock is severe, the usual remedies are indicated, and oxygen may help if there is marked cyanosis. When there is evidence of a tension pneumothorax or when the amount of air in the pleural cavity is great, it is urgently necessary to insert a wide-bored needle: as soon as possible afterwards this should be connected by sterile rubber tubing with an under-water drain at the bedside. More accurate control is obtained with an artificial pneumo-thorax apparatus, but it is unwise to empty the pleura completely for the aperture in a fully expanded lung heals more slowly. With a severe tension pneumothorax it may be necessary to connect the pleural cavity with an electrical suction pump for 48 hours, after which pleural adhesions often form and close the aperture. Rarely thoracotomy may be required to seal the opening. The treatment of pus in the pleura is described under empyema (§ 120). In recurrent cases of pneumothorax various mildly irritant solutions such as camphor (0·5 per cent. in arachis oil) or weak silver nitrate solutions may be inserted to produce permanent adherence of the pleural surfaces but these are not always successful.

A **Hydropneumothorax** resembles closely spontaneous pneumothorax and is especially common in the presence of a tuberculous focus in the lung. A small quantity of fluid first fills the costo-phrenic angle and later fills the lower part of the chest, the fluid moving with the position of the patient. As seen radiologically the upper level of the fluid is always horizontal, unlike the upper level in a pleural effusion.

The *Symptoms* are those of a pneumothorax but the patient may be conscious of the fluid flapping about in the chest on movement. The most characteristic sign is the *succession splash*—a fact which was well known to Hippocrates. It may be heard by placing one's ear against the chest whilst moving the patient's body from side to side.

Treatment is of the primary cause, especially with tuberculosis. If the fluid is present in more than a very small quantity it should be aspirated and in any case it needs a full bacteriological examination.

A **Hæmopneumothorax** is rare. The symptoms and signs are those of a hydropneumothorax but the patient will be noticed to become unduly pale and shocked due to the hæmorrhage. The *diagnosis* is confirmed by aspirating almost pure blood from the lower part of the chest; the blood remains fluid for several days. The cause may be an external perforating wound of the chest wall or a fractured rib. Some cases are due to tuberculosis, to new growths or to an aneurysm of the aorta.

Treatment must be to the cause: blood must be removed by aspiration and prophylactic penicillin is advisable.

Cysts of the Lung have been recognised more commonly since the

routine use of X-rays. *Large balloon-like cysts* are congenital in origin
and produce the symptoms and signs of a chronic pneumothorax. If
urgent symptoms ensue they must be punctured with a needle and
subsequently be removed surgically. Small cysts may be multiple. They
can be congenital, or acquired as the result of bronchiectasis with a valvular
opening due to a partially occluded bronchus. Any cyst in the lung
may contain fluid which can become purulent.

*One disease of the lungs does not belong to the acute or to the chronic
category, but is* **paroxysmal**: IT OCCURS AS SUDDEN ATTACKS OF DIFFICULT
BREATHING WITH CONSIDERABLE WHEEZING, *but usually* WITHOUT RISE
OF TEMPERATURE—ASTHMA.

§ 127. **Asthma** is characterised by paroxysmal attacks of dyspnœa,
with a short inspiratory effort and prolonged expiration. The cause is
a narrowing of the trachea, bronchi and bronchioles which is especially
marked during expiration. It may occur at any age and in severe cases
there is much distress and cyanosis. In patients afflicted with this disease there is often a family history of allergy, *e.g.*, attacks of asthma, hay
fever, migraine or giant urticaria.

Symptoms.—The leading characteristic of this disease is its paroxysmal
nature. A person who is subject to asthma may be perfectly well one
minute, and half an hour later may be in the throes of a violent attack.
The onset is often in the early hours of the morning, the patient waking
with a feeling of tightness in the chest; he begins to cough, to gasp for
breath and to wheeze and if the attack is severe he may get out of bed
and stand by an open window, while clinging to surrounding objects in
order to bring into play the accessory muscles of respiration. As a
paroxysm develops and breathing becomes more difficult, the patient
becomes increasingly alarmed. An attack may last minutes, hours or
days and when prolonged is termed *status asthmaticus*. As the attack
subsides breathing becomes gradually easier, the patient often coughs up
plugs of mucoid sputum and then rapidly recovers.

There are many interesting features in this disease such as a personal
history of skin eruptions (urticaria, prurigo and eczema), these often
alternating with paroxysms of asthma. As an attack subsides large
quantities of urine may be passed.

Physical Signs.—During an attack the patient sits upright in bed
struggling for breath. On inspection the chest is seen to be maintained
in a position of inspiration, undergoing but little expansion with the
short inspirations: to aid breathing the accessory muscles of respiration
(such as the sterno-mastoids, scalenes and pectorals) are in continual
action and as each short breath is taken there is marked sucking in of the
supra-clavicular hollows. The lips, the cheeks and the nail beds and
later the skin as a whole become increasingly cyanosed and the jugular
veins distended. The percussion note is hyper-resonant, especially so
when after many attacks emphysema also supervenes. On auscultation
the inspiratory effort is shortened and may be hardly audible; expiration

is markedly prolonged. Loud sibilant rhonchi and coarse râles replace the normal vesicular murmurs—these rhonchi may be so loud as to be heard across the room. The cough and sputum become more prominent as an attack subsides: unless there is coincident bronchitis the sputum is clear and mucoid and contains the " perles " of Laennec—small plugs of inspissated mucus wrapped round by more liquid mucus: in some patients the sputum contains large numbers of eosinophil cells. In between attacks the chest is often normal: after repeated attacks in childhood a characteristic chest deformity develops and in adults emphysema is found. In uncomplicated asthma, the chest X-ray shows no especial features.

Etiology.—The primary condition is an overaction of the vagal nerve mechanism, producing constriction of the bronchial muscle which is distributed around the whole of the bronchial tree.

In the normal person the lumen of the trachea and bronchi enlarges during inspiration, and becomes smaller during expiration. During an attack of asthma these

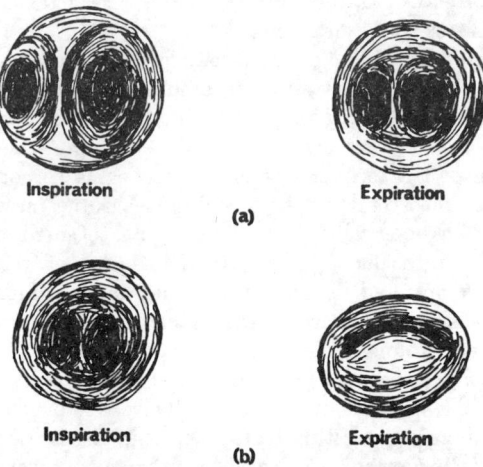

FIG. 59.—Diagram of the appearances through a bronchoscope of the trachea and two main bronchi; (*a*) in a normal person; (*b*) during an acute attack of asthma showing the great narrowing of the trachea. (After W. A. Lell.)

changes are greatly exaggerated: during expiration not only does the bronchial muscle contract vigorously but (as seen through a bronchoscope) the lumen of the trachea and larger bronchi is greatly narrowed by collapse of the less rigid posterior wall, mainly due to the force used in expiration. Furthermore the mucous membrane of the trachea and main bronchi becomes markedly swollen due to congestion, œdema and even multiple small hæmorrhages, so that the mucosa is thrown into folds: at the same time the internal surface is covered by liquid and later by thick tenacious mucus. These changes are maximal at the orifices of the broncho-pulmonary segments. In status asthmaticus the combined effect of the bronchial spasm, the thickening of the mucous membrane and the internal coating of mucus is to reduce the lumen of the trachea and bronchi to ¼–⅓ normal; the lumen is smaller still during expiration and many of the bronchi are temporarily blocked altogether by the inspissated secretion. Repeated attacks of asthma produce more permanent hypertrophy of the bronchial muscle and of the mucous membrane.

The causes contributing to attacks of asthma can be divided into two groups:

A. *Predisposing Causes*, the chief of which are: (i.) an inherited tendency with a family and often a personal history of allergy. Careful enquiry may reveal asthma, hay-fever, urticaria, Besnier's prurigo, infantile eczema or migraine. (ii.) A most important cause is the psychological factor. Most asthmatics have sensitive, intelligent and dynamic personalities and attacks may follow anxiety, frustration, overwork, fatigue and sleeplessness. (iii.) Any cause of lowered health tends to bring on attacks. (iv.) Endocrine causes may play a part in some women, in whom attacks occur particularly before menstruation, and become more frequent about the time of the menopause.

B. Among the *Exciting Causes* of attacks we can recognise (i.) hypersensitivity to a variety of allergens. The best example is hay asthma: a person who has hay fever develops also hay asthma at the height of the hay fever season. In general, patients are sensitive to (*a*) inhaled allergens —pollens, animal hair and dandruff (such as from horses, dogs or cats), feathers, house dust, various moulds and orris-root (face powder); (*b*) ingested allergens such as wheat, milk, chocolate or potatoes; (*c*) some micro-organisms. Certain gram-negative bacilli have been especially incriminated. The spores of fungal infections (especially *Aspergillus fumigatus*) can cause allergy and so give rise to asthma in those handling hay and straw in which this organism multiplies. Certain mites can be causal. (*d*) Drugs and chemicals are occasional causes. Aspirin is the commonest drug: iodine and gum-acacia (used by printers) may induce attacks. Food idiosyncrasy usually results in allergic manifestations (and even asthma) before the age of 4 whereas inhaled allergens usually cause asthma after this age. (ii.) Infections of the bronchial tree such as give rise to bronchitis, tuberculosis or pulmonary suppuration (*e.g.*, bronchiectasis) are important. At all ages and especially in the elderly, a bronchitic infection is particularly liable to bring on asthma. (iii.) Reflex causes play a part. Many patients have a nocturnal attack after a large supper or in association with constipation. (iv.) Conditions of the nasal passages, such as polypi, hypertrophic rhinitis and nasal sinusitis, are often found. These may be part of the allergic diathesis but the elimination of infection in the sinuses is of great help. (v.) Certain little understood climatic conditions play a part. Thus one patient may have attacks in dry weather and another in damp weather: one patient may be troubled by asthma when living in London and another develop attacks when leaving London and seeking a high altitude. A warm, dry, equable climate well above sea level suits the majority. Although there are many exceptions, broadly speaking asthmatic patients can often be divided into those with pure allergic asthma, young persons who in attacks have no rise of temperature and who cough up mucoid sputum; and those with chronic bronchial asthma, a condition seen after middle age when attacks occur with a respiratory infection, in association with pyrexia and a purulent sputum. There is no single cause for the occurrence of asthma: attacks occur when three, four or more of the above groups of predisposing and exciting causes summate. From the point of view of treatment some causes cannot be eliminated (*e.g.*, the family tendency, and the constitutional and the psychological make-up of the patient), but others can be got rid of (*e.g.*, fatigue, hypersensitivity to drugs or to orris) and when a sufficient number of contributing causes has been eliminated attacks cease, at least for a while.

Diagnosis usually presents no difficulty especially when the patient is seen in the throes of an attack. In allergic asthma the blood often shows a marked eosinophilia. *Chronic bronchitis* causes wheezing and shortness of breath and there may be an element of superadded bronchial spasm especially in the winter months. The disease tends to be less paroxysmal and more chronic. Nocturnal *cardiac dyspnœa* has been called cardiac asthma; it is the result of left ventricular failure (§ 55) and is not asthmatic in origin. *Renal dyspnœa* has in the past been termed renal asthma. Other evidence of advanced chronic nephritis is readily found. *Pulmonary tuberculosis* is occasionally present with asthma and it may be that the patient is allergic to tuberculin. It is wise to X-ray the chest of all patients with asthma to exclude this and to exclude a *bronchial carcinoma* or other *mediastinal tumour*. *Hysterical hyper-ventilation* of the lungs can be confused with asthma, but does not cause wheezing or the production of a cough: often the early symptoms of tetany result from washing out too much CO_2 (§ 1030) with tingling in the finger tips: tetany never occurs in true asthma.

The various substances to which the patient may be susceptible can be tested for by applying prepared solutions containing extracts of the different allergens to the skin and scratching or pricking the surface but without drawing blood. Alternatively 0·01–0·02 ml. may be injected intradermally. Twenty minutes later the results are compared with that of an injection of a control solution of the solvent, a positive response being indicated by marked erythema or erythema with a central wheal. While giving a useful indication of allergy to various inhalants, foods, etc., the results must not be taken too literally but must be taken in conjunction with the overall clinical picture.

Prognosis.—It is rare for sudden death due to right heart failure to occur in an attack. Children frequently grow out of the disease about puberty. Adults never lose the tendency to attacks but may be free for years: frequent recurrences are followed by emphysema, bronchitis and embarrassment of the right heart.

Treatment.—The remedies used are such as relax the bronchial muscle, either directly or by stimulating the sympathetic nerves.

(a) *During the Attack.* The antispasmodics which abort or control a *mild attack* are legion: what suits one patient may not suit another, but in any case the earlier the remedy is given the more effective it will be. For this reason a patient often has to be taught to give his own injections. Suitable preparations are tab. ephedrine hydrochlor. gr. ½, tab. isoprenaline sulph. mg. 10–20 dissolved slowly under the tongue, inject. adrenaline B.P. ℳ 3–8 (subcut.): an inhalation of adrenaline and atropine co. B.P.C. or of isoprenaline sulph. co. B.P.C. through a suitable inhaler (of the Deedon or Rybar variety).   If these remedies fail adrenaline and posterior pituitary extract may be combined for injection as in Kadamysin (0·5–1·0 ml.) or Pitrenalin.   Morphine in elderly patients with bronchitic asthma often proves fatal: in younger patients it is rarely used nowadays partly because of the risk of drug addiction.   Intravenous pethidine hydrochlor. 50–100 mg. is a useful stand-by but is also a drug of addiction.   Asthma cigarettes containing stramonium, potassium nitrate and belladonna should be discouraged, as their frequent use tends to produce chronic bronchitis.   For a *severe attack* or for *status asthmaticus* the first and safest remedy is intravenous aminophylline B.P. (Cardophylin) 0·25–0·50 G. in 10 ml. of distilled water given over a period of 3–5 minutes: a rectal suppository of aminophylline (0·5 G.) is also often helpful.   If intravenous aminophylline is not available, give intravenous pethidine hydrochlor. 100 mg.   Hurst's method consists of filling a 2·0 ml. syringe with adrenaline solution B.P., and giving ℳ 1 each half-minute until the attack has ceased or until the whole dose has been given: it is important to withdraw the piston of the syringe immediately after insertion as adrenaline injected into a vein is dangerous.   Once the attack has ceased the slowly absorbed inject. adrenaline muconate (0·5–1·0 ml.) will prevent a recurrence.   In obstinate cases valuable remedies are hydrocortisone acetate (alcohol-free) 100–200 mg. in 20 ml. N. saline given slowly into a vein, corticotrophin B.P. (ACTH) 12·5–25 mg. intramuscularly each 6 hours, or cortisone acetate by mouth or intramuscularly 25·0–37·5 mg. each 6 hours for 24 hours followed by 25 mg. q.d.s. for a week and with decreasing doses subsequently.   Tab. prednisolone 5 mg. q.d.s. for a week can replace the cortisone.   During severe attacks reassurance, with a period in hospital or in a nursing home, is often immediately salutary; in any case constant nursing care is usually required and oxygen inhalations are helpful. Particularly in the elderly, persistent severe asthma is associated with a severe bronchitic infection: simultaneously with the bronchial dilator drugs it is then necessary to give wide spectrum antibiotics such as inject. penicillin with streptomycin, or the tetracyclines.   Sometimes aspiration through a bronchoscope is necessary.   To loosen secretion and promote bronchial drainage it has long been the custom to administer expectorant mixtures containing potassium iodide with stramonium or lobelia but these are only helpful once bronchial dilatation has been achieved and the attack is subsiding.

(b) *Between the Attacks* and to try and prevent recurrence, it is necessary to assess the importance of the various factors discussed under etiology and to mitigate or eliminate as many of the predisposing and exciting causes as possible. The patient's general health and anxiety, worry, overwork and other psychological factors must receive particular attention. Reflex causes need treatment and the patient should avoid large bulky meals at any time and especially after 4.0 p.m. The nose should be examined for chronic sinusitis and for polypi but operations should only be performed when they are indicated on the grounds of general health. Patients with nocturnal asthma should not suddenly go from a hot room to a cold bedroom—the bedroom should be warmed beforehand and adequate ventilation ensured at night. In these cases a simple hypnotic at bedtime such as aspirin, tab. codeine co., chloral and bromide, linctus diphenhydramine hydrochlor. (Benylin) or the combination of a barbiturate with antispasmodics as in tab. Franol, caps. Amesec or caps. Monotheamine and Amytal are of help; as is a rectal suppository of aminophylline. The effect of locality on the disease can only be ascertained by experience; though, with many exceptions, the smoke and fog of towns are detrimental. When the results of skin testing are known it is wise to avoid contact with known allergens to which the patient is susceptible: thus sensitivity to feathers should be combated by elimination of feathers in pillows, eiderdowns and beds, replacing the feather pillow by kapok (unless the patient is also kapok sensitive) or by a rubber pillow; those sensitive to orris root should avoid this, and those sensitive to wheat should try avoiding wheaten flour. Specific desensitisation has usually been disappointing. Non-specific desensitisation may be tried by injecting Armour's No. 2 peptone intramusc. (7½ per cent. solution), or intravenously (5 per cent. solution), starting with 0·3 ml. and increasing to 2·5 ml., each third or fourth day. Weekly intramuscular injections of 10 ml. of the patient's own blood have often resulted in considerable benefit, without the occurrence of untoward reactions. When the asthma is mainly associated with acute bronchitis, the treatment is that of the primary disease. Potassium iodide is especially useful in liquefying the sputum, and if small doses (3 grains) are not sufficient, much larger doses may be employed. The antispasmodic drugs are again very useful. Some benefit from the use of an autogenous vaccine or regular daily doses of tab. sulphadimidine G. 1. Controlled breathing exercises to encourage relaxation and expiration, under the supervision of a physiotherapist, can be very helpful. In children, regular doses of glucose, and avoidance of undue excitement or mental strain, are advisable.

Pulmonary Eosinophilia is the name given to a group of cases characterised by X-ray evidence of scattered pulmonary infiltration with marked eosinophilia. The symptoms include cough, dyspnœa, sometimes asthma and a variable degree of constitutional disturbance: many cases have a personal or family history of allergy. *Löffler's syndrome* is a benign transitory form of this condition: *tropical eosinophilia* (of unknown origin) is a more severe variety and some cases are due to *polyarteritis nodosa*. Tropical eosinophilia readily responds to intravenous neoarsphenamine B.P.

CHRONIC DISEASES OF THE LUNGS AND PLEURÆ

128. Classification.—Chronic disorders of the lungs and pleuræ may follow an acute attack of the conditions described in the previous sections, as when chronic bronchitis and emphysema succeed attacks of acute bronchitis. But many of the chronic diseases of the lungs, such as pulmonary tuberculosis, start insidiously, and attention may not be directed to the lungs for a considerable time.

The chronic diseases, like the acute, may be classified, *for clinical purposes*, according to the results of percussion. It is convenient in actual practice, although unscientific from the point of view of classification, to make a subsidiary group in which the sputum is highly offensive or has some other characteristic feature.

(A) **Chronic Disease** in which the **Percussion Note is unaltered:**

(B) **Chronic Diseases** attended by **Impaired** or **Dull Percussion Note:**

(*a*) *The commoner* diseases presenting dullness, *usually in regular and defined areas either at the base or apex*, are—

(*b*) The diseases presenting dullness, *usually not* in regular and *defined areas at base and apex*, are—

(C) **Chronic Diseases** attended by **Hyper-resonance:**

(D) **Diseases** suggested by the **Character of the Sputum:**

[1] Pneumothorax usually comes on acutely, but it may be part of a chronic illness.

GROUP A.—The patient's symptoms point to **chronic disease of the lungs,** and on examining the chest there is **no alteration in the percussion note.**

I. *The patient has a chronic cough; there is no elevation of temperature, and on auscultation* RHONCHI *and* RÂLES *are heard over the chest. The disease is* CHRONIC BRONCHITIS.

§ 129. Chronic Bronchitis signifies a chronic inflammation of the bronchial tubes. It commonly commences after the age of 40 and is nearly five times more common in men than women. Many cases start after an acute respiratory infection, especially after pneumonia or influenza, but in an equal number the onset is insidious.

Symptoms.—The common symptoms are a chronic cough and the expectoration of mucoid sputum: sooner or later, especially with the advent of emphysema, breathlessness on exertion appears. In the warmer summer months the patient is comparatively well and may lose all symptoms, but in damp, cold and foggy weather the symptoms return, and with a fresh catarrhal infection an acute attack of bronchitis supervenes. In the course of a few years the cough and sputum become more persistent and may last the whole year round: the patient becomes more and more breathless, and in the presence of superadded emphysema, marked pulmonary hypertension results; particularly following an acute attack of bronchitis or of broncho-pneumonia right-sided heart failure supervenes and is the common cause of death.

Physical Signs.—In the later stages these patients present a characteristic appearance: they are often stout in build, with a florid and slightly cyanosed complexion; they have a short, thick neck with pulsating jugular veins. The breathing is short, the respiration wheezy and the chest barrel-shaped with emphysema. In the absence of complications there are no febrile or constitutional symptoms—chronic bronchitic patients often have a subnormal temperature. Physical examination of the chest shows poor movement on both sides. Palpation confirms this and may reveal rhonchial fremitus. On percussion the note is either normal or hyper-resonant in proportion to the degree of emphysema present. Auscultation reveals some prolongation of expiration: at times the chest may be dry but on other occasions there are sonorous and sibilant rhonchi, and râles when the smaller tubes are involved. Some patients also show a considerable degree of bronchospasm (§ 127).

The *Diagnosis* is usually not difficult. The history of onset following an acute respiratory illness, or with a gradual onset and with winter exacerbations, is most helpful. Except in the course of acute attacks patients with chronic bronchitis tend to gain weight largely because of their enforced inactivity. The X-ray appearances show exaggerated peribronchial markings and evidence of emphysema, but there are no areas of consolidation. In *chronic phthisis* there may be local signs especially at one or both apices, some weight loss, the X-ray film shows evidence of infiltration in the soft tissues of the lungs and the sputum may reveal the presence of tubercle bacilli. It is important to remember that bronchitis and emphysema may mask the physical signs of chronic tuberculosis. *Bronchial neoplasms* often cause loss of weight and blood-stained sputum, and the X-ray findings are often confirmatory. *Heart failure*, especially in association with mitral stenosis, causes attacks of acute congestion of the bases of the lungs especially during the winter months: the main physical finding in the lungs is the presence of numerous basal râles and generalised rhonchi are less in evidence. *Bronchiectasis* may be associated with chronic bronchitis: the signs of consolidation and fibrosis, usually at one or both lung bases, the clubbed fingers and the purulent and even fœtid bronchitis aid diagnosis.

Etiology.—Although in the healthy person the nose and naso-pharynx show the constant presence of catarrhal organisms such as *N. catarrhalis, Streptococcus viridans* and certain *viruses*, the respiratory tract below the larynx is remarkably free of pathogenic organisms. This is the result of constant disinfection by the ciliary action of the mucous membrane. When there is irritation of the lower respiratory tract by chemical agents or by infection, there is usually a flow of mucus which not only encourages the further growth of organisms but impedes ciliary action. Sooner or later permanent changes in the mucous membrane make a return to normality impossible.

Chronic bronchitis may be primary or secondary in origin. Primary cases may follow recurrent infections especially with pneumococci, influenza virus A and to a less extent staphylococci and streptococcus hæmolyticus. However, in recent years more and more emphasis has been placed on the influence of air pollution by noxious gases, dust and smoke: this explains why it is five times more common in industrial than in non-industrial cities. It is also more common in heavy cigarette smokers and in mouth-breathers. Secondary bronchitis occurs after measles and whooping-cough, as a complication of obesity, gout, chronic nephritis, with chronic nasal sinusitis and in those whose lungs have been scarred by fibrosis following healed pulmonary tuberculosis, pneumoconiosis or sarcoidosis.

There are five recognised *Varieties* of this disease: (i.) *Bronchitis* with *winter cough*, attended by slight or abundant expectoration, mucous or muco-purulent, sometimes fibrinous, sometimes containing streaks of blood. (ii.) *Dry Bronchitis* (*catarrhe-sec* of Laennec) is attended by a frequent cough and soreness of the chest, but little or no secretion; it is of a very obstinate character, and occurs mostly in elderly people of a gouty diathesis. (iii.) *Purulent* and/or *fœtid bronchitis* and bronchiolitis (*catarrhe-suffoquant* of Laennec) is characterised by expectoration of large quantities of purulent and offensive sputum; and is associated with bronchial dilatation (*cf.* bronchiectasis). (iv.) *Bronchorrhœa* signifies expectoration of very large amounts of sputum, often of a thin clear nature or else thick and ropy. It is a symptom rather than a disease entity, and is often associated with bronchiectasis (*q.v.*). (v.) *Plastic Bronchitis* (see § 130).

Prognosis.—Children with chronic bronchitis often recover completely around puberty. Adults seldom entirely recover, though they may live for a great many years especially if the heart is fairly healthy, and care is taken to avoid exposure and contact with those with respiratory infections. Even so, many of these sufferers lead a very restricted and even a semi-invalid existence, with a chronic cough, sleepless nights and increasing respiratory insufficiency due to emphysema, bronchitic asthma and pulmonary congestion: in trades and industries it accounts for 15 per cent. of premature retirement from work. The death rate from chronic bronchitis in Great Britain rises steeply after the age of 60 in both sexes, and has been little affected by the greatly increased use of antibiotics in recent years. On the other hand it is nearly five times higher in the poorer classes (Class V) as compared with the better social classes (Class I) —overcrowding and an unsuitable environment being the main causes of this. In any individual case the following factors render the prognosis much more serious: (i.) when acute attacks of muco-purulent bronchitis and bronchiolitis occur, due usually to *H. influenzæ*; (ii.) co-existing obesity, chronic nephritis and cardio-vascular degeneration make the outlook somewhat less favourable; (iii.) the prognosis is grave when there is evidence of right-sided cardiac failure, such as great breathlessness, cyanosis, engorgement of the liver and veins of the neck, and ascites.

Treatment.—In acute exacerbations the treatment is that of acute bronchitis (§ 115). In between these acute episodes the patient must avoid chill and exposure, as far as possible must avoid smoky and dusty occupations, must keep away from crowded places (*e.g.*, cinemas) especially during epidemics of respiratory illness, and must strictly limit smoking (especially of cigarettes) or become a non-smoker. Any impediment to nasal breathing should be removed and nasal sinusitis corrected. Those who have retired from work should endeavour to seek a warm and equable climate such as in the South-west of England or in the Channel Islands, avoiding fogs and damp atmospheres. Other important points in treatment are: (i.) to endeavour to repress an excessive cough since this increases the work of the right heart and aggravates emphysema. For this purpose a sedative linctus such as linctus codeinæ or even linctus diamorphinæ is required and throat pastilles such as troch. glycyrrhizæ (B.P.C.) may help. (ii.) When the cough is irritant but dry, give remedies to promote secretion such as mist. sodii chloridi co. (B.P.C.) in hot water or one containing potassium iodide such as mist. pot. iod. ammon. (B.P.C.). (iii.) When there is much spasm of the tubes lobelia, iodide, ephedrine, and other remedies for asthma are to be tried. (iv.) Measures to prevent dilatation and failure of the right ventricle are called for sooner or later where dyspnœa and other cardiac symptoms are present. (v.) Obesity must be corrected and (vi.) in suitable cases tab. sulphadimidine G. 1 each morning or twice daily during the winter months and vaccines have been found useful.

§ 130. **Plastic Bronchitis** is inflammation of the bronchi, with the formation of fibro-plastic casts, which are expectorated by a severe bou⁺ of coughing.

Symptoms.—The symptoms consist of (i.) violent attacks of coughing, with pain in the chest, severe expiratory dyspnœa and cyanosis, followed by (ii.) the expectoration of a fibrinous cast of a bronchus with immediate relief of symptoms. (iii.) The patient generally suffers from chronic bronchitis, and a little hæmoptysis may follow the expulsion of a cast. (iv.) Sometimes there are no constitutional symptoms, but slight pyrexia may be present. Such symptoms supervening in a case of chronic bronchitis lead us to suspect the condition.

Physical Signs may be absent. If present, they are those of an obstructed bronchus —an absent or diminished respiratory murmur, accompanied by impaired percussion note. Whistling rhonchi or " flapping " sounds may be heard.

Etiology.—The disease is twice as common in men as in women. It may occur at any age in subjects of chronic bronchitis.

Prognosis.—The condition is more serious than simple bronchitis. Two varieties have been described: (1) An acute form, lasting for some weeks; and (2) a chronic form, recurring at intervals for years, in the course of chronic bronchitis. Each attack may last for some weeks, and the casts may be coughed up daily. The condition occasionally leads to a fatal issue.

The *Treatment* differs but little from that of bronchitis. The removal of the membrane may be promoted by the administration of potassium iodide in order to liquefy the sputum: the inhalation of a weak solution of sodium bicarbonate atomised by means of a spray, in order to dissolve the mucin in the cast, has been advised by some. Removal via a bronchoscope is sometimes required.

GROUP B.—We now turn to those chronic diseases of the lungs which are accompanied by **dullness on percussion.** (*a*) The *common* diseases in which the dullness occurs, usually in regular and fairly DEFINED AREAS at base or apex, are: I. CHRONIC PULMONARY TUBERCULOSIS; II. HYDRO-THORAX; III. PULMONARY CONGESTION OR ŒDEMA.

I. *The patient complains of a* PERSISTENT COUGH *with* CONSTITUTIONAL SYMPTOMS, *especially loss of energy and loss of weight. Examination of the chest may show* SIGNS OF CONSOLIDATION, *most marked at the* APEX *of the lung; there is* INTERMITTENT PYREXIA, *and the sputum may contain tubercle bacilli. The disease is* CHRONIC PULMONARY TUBERCULOSIS (*Phthisis*).

§ 131. **Chronic Pulmonary Tuberculosis** (Phthisis). The word phthisis is not satisfactory because it only indicates one of the symptoms—viz., the wasting ($\varphi\theta\iota\nu\omega$, I waste). Pulmonary tuberculosis has been recognised as a clinical entity since the days of Hippocrates (460–370 B.C.) and the tubercle bacillus was discovered by Robert Koch in 1882. Members of civilised races, among whom the disease has long been endemic, have gradually acquired an increased resistance to the tubercle bacillus because (i.) of improved conditions of housing, of work and of nutrition; (ii.) almost everyone comes into contact with the disease and so receives a minute dose of bacilli which, in the majority, is not sufficient to cause disease and therefore gives an acquired immunity; and (iii.) because the most susceptible families have not survived. The figures for the annual death-rate per million persons in England and Wales over the last 100 years are most impressive:

			All forms of Tuberculosis.	Pulmonary Tuberculosis.
1851–60..	..	..	3,623	2,665
1901–10..	..	..	1,648	1,157
1945–49..	..	..	523	448
1961 ..	..	..	72	65

The continued fall in the last ten years has been accentuated by two other factors: (i.) the earlier diagnosis of pulmonary tuberculosis by mass miniature radiography, often before the development of symptoms or signs; and (ii.) the much more effective treatment with new drugs.

Pathological Processes.—A brief account will help to explain the clinical phenomena concerned. Pulmonary tuberculosis is caused mainly by the human form of Koch's bacillus and is spread by direct contact: in England and Wales in 1955 it was estimated that there were about 45,000 infectors with a positive sputum, each expectorating at least 25,000 tubercle bacilli per ml. of sputum. At birth the infant, even of a tuberculous mother, is not infected, and there is abundant evidence that such children are no more liable to the disease than other children, provided they are kept clear of external sources of infection. The first infection of the lung by tubercle bacilli occurs as a result of inhaling droplets of infected sputum or particles of infected dust: the bacilli are unable to penetrate the bronchial mucous membrane, and as they are very small they reach the peripheral part of the lung tissue. The bacilli are picked up by phagocytic cells and carried a very short distance to the nearest of many minute patches of lymphoid tissue scattered through the interstitial tissue. Here they lodge and form the *primary focus* of infection (Ghon's focus): this is always situated just under the pleural surface of the lung, usually in the middle or lower zone. As the lung has little or no resistance, the bacilli are carried through the lymphatics to the corresponding regional lymph gland: these glands enlarge to a size much greater than that of the primary focus. The Ghon's focus and the hilar glands usually heal by fibrosis and subsequent calcification; but if the dose of bacilli is large or the resistance very low (as in young children) the Ghon's focus or the lymph glands may break down and initiate either a local spread of bacilli (usually in the same lobe of the lung) or a general spread through the blood-stream, giving rise to peripheral foci in, for example, a bone or a kidney, or even generalised (miliary) tuberculosis.

In the vast majority of cases there is no clinical evidence of the primary infection, but there develops a state of allergy, after which a further dose of bacilli will call forth a type of local reaction not seen with the first inoculation (Koch's phenomenon). This local reaction forms the basis of the Mantoux test (§ 525). When a *second infection* occurs this local allergy confines the bacilli to the site of re-infection, tends to destroy them and prevent their entrance into the body. Allergy does not imply that there is an increased resistance in the body as a whole, but if small repeated minimal infections do occur, then an increased immunity does develop. Second infections (post-primary infections) occur mainly as a result of re-infection from without, although on occasions they may be due to reactivation and spread from the primary focus. The secondary lesions in the lungs occur most commonly in the subapical regions: this time the bacilli are arrested at the point of re-infection producing a local lesion known as an Assmann focus. This focus may (i.) be very small—" a minimal lesion "—which often gives no clinical indication of its presence although it can be seen on an X-ray (Fig. 60). These minimal lesions may disappear, may be replaced by fibrous tissue which calcifies, but in some cases they develop into an active focus of disease. (ii.) Soon after re-infection the local Assmann focus may cease the develop-

PLATE V

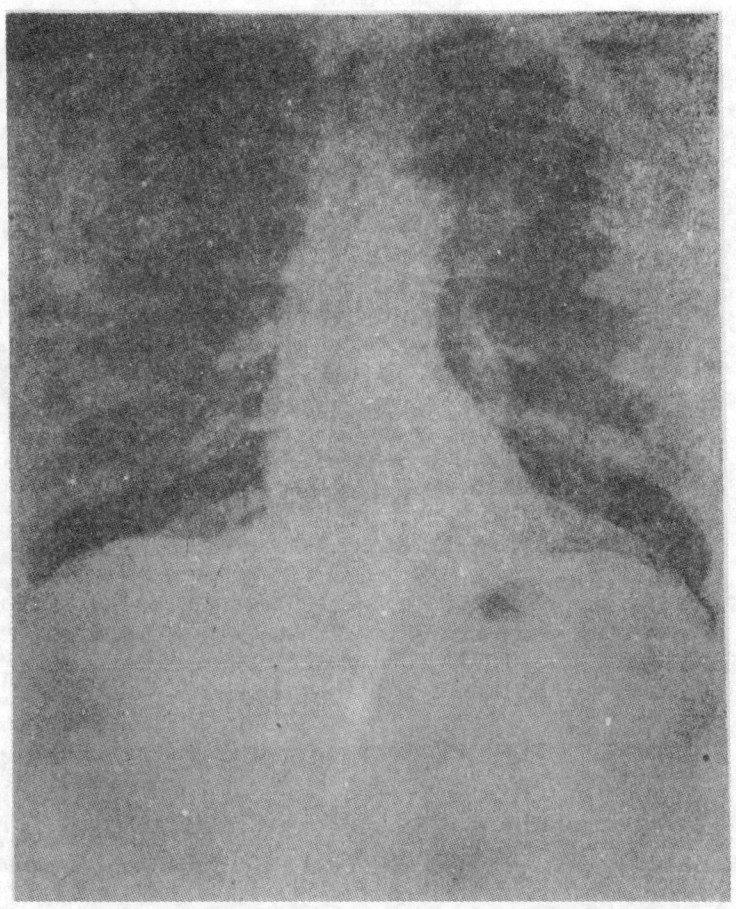

FIG. 60.—X-RAY FILM OF CHEST, showing a MINIMAL LESION of TUBERCULOSIS (Assmann's focus) in the Right Upper Lobe. The subapical position, in the second intercostal space, is typical.

PLATE VI

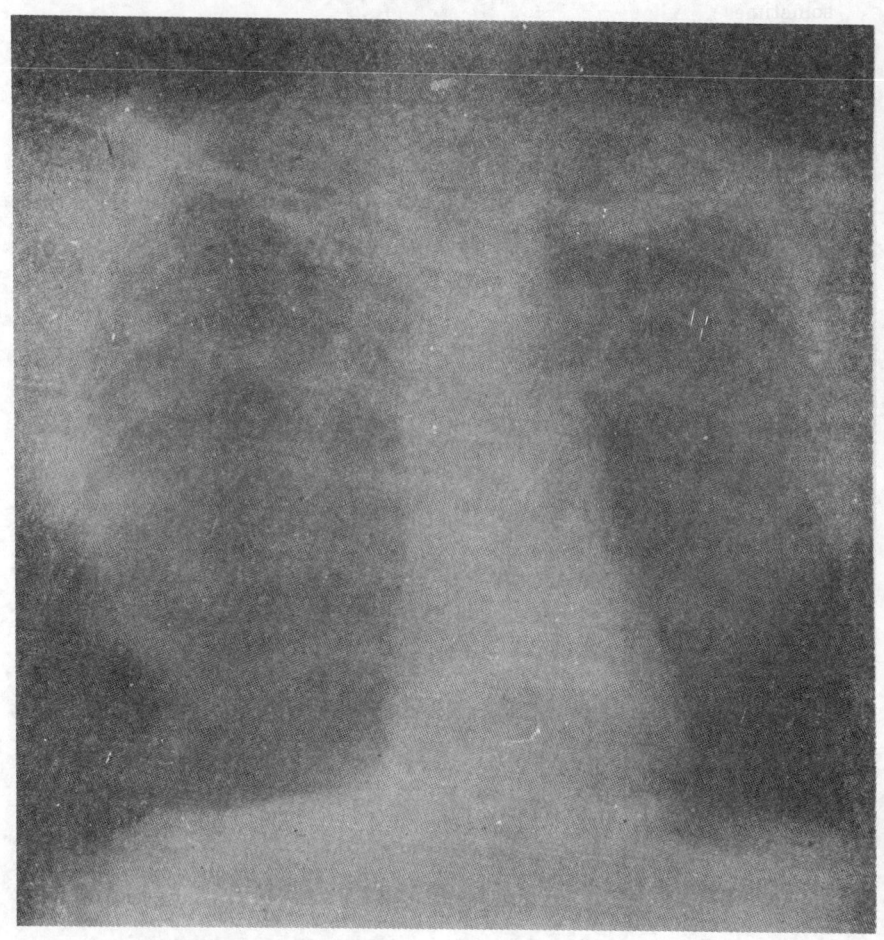

FIG. 61.—CHEST X-RAY of a man aged 49, showing chronic FIBROCASEOUS TUBERCULOSIS in the Upper Zones of both lungs. The sputum contained large numbers of tubercle bacilli.

ment of clinical pulmonary tuberculosis or, if rupture into a vein occurs, of miliary tuberculosis. Greatly affecting these tissue reactions in the lungs is the general resistance of the patient—the virulence of the human type of bacilli varies little. Any condition of malnutrition or excessive fatigue may predispose to bacillary invasion (see Etiology).

Symptoms.—The disease is mainly a chronic one, and its onset is sometimes insidious. It is more amenable to treatment in the early stage, and since the introduction of modern methods of treatment early recognition of the disease has become of paramount importance.

(a) *Early Stages.*—It must be remembered that in a considerable number of early cases of active pulmonary tuberculosis there may be no symptoms, the disease only being recognised by radiography.

Clinically the symptoms can be divided into Pulmonary and Constitutional Symptoms. *Pulmonary Symptoms* are (i.) a persistent dry cough, perhaps appearing to follow " a cold." A cough is not invariably complained of in the early stages, but careful questioning will often elicit the fact of its presence, especially in the early morning. (ii.) Sputum is often absent at first. Most children and many adults swallow their sputum, but can be made to collect an early morning specimen for testing when requested to do so. Such specimens are usually mucoid and are small in quantity. (iii.) Hæmoptysis is often present and may be the first symptom to draw the patient's attention to the lungs (§ 104). The amount of blood is very variable, sometimes being copious (even 2 or 3 pints), sometimes in the form of small clots and sometimes it consists of a blood-streaking of the sputum. (iv.) Pain in the chest is usually due to localised dry pleurisy. A lymphocytic pleural effusion may be the first sign of disease (§ 119), and many patients with this develop obvious pulmonary tuberculosis within a few months. (v.) Shortness of breath on exertion in the early stages does not mean extensive pulmonary disease but is an indication of toxæmia. It is much more marked in the presence of a pleural effusion or a pneumothorax. (vi.) Acute pneumonic tuberculosis with a sputum loaded with acid-fast bacilli is sometimes the first sign (§ 124). *Constitutional Symptoms* affect a number of different systems of the body. (i.) There is often a complaint of undue tiredness at the end of the day's work, perhaps with a frontal headache. (ii.) Night sweats, especially in a young person, are very suggestive of active disease. A slight perspiration at night may occur in many on occasions, but repeated profuse night-sweating, perhaps sufficient to need a change of night-clothes, is strongly suspicious of pulmonary tuberculosis. (iii.) Slight persistent loss of weight is of considerable importance, particularly in a person whose weight is normally steady or is increasing during a period of growth. (iv.) Dyspepsia may increase this tendency to weight loss. There is often some loss of appetite and a feeling of fullness after a small meal. (v.) Palpitation may be complained of. (vi.) In young women amenorrhœa can be an early symptom, but many women become pregnant even in the presence of active tuberculosis.

The *Physical Signs* of early disease are often difficult to detect. While not in any way decrying the great value of X-rays, there is no question but that the greater the care taken, the more likely are suspicious or definite signs to be found in the chest. It is unfortunate that, even among chest physicians, it is becoming more and more the custom to try to elicit physical signs in a perfunctory manner and to rely solely on X-ray appearances. The patient's chest should be completely stripped and he should be taken to a room where there is good lighting and quiet prevails. Inspection may reveal a little flattening below one clavicle, or an exaggerated hollow above the clavicle: and when the back of the chest is examined the muscle of the trapezius above the spine of the scapula may be thinned by wasting. Palpation often reveals decreased expansion of the upper part of the chest on one or both sides. Percussion above or below the clavicle, but particularly *on* the clavicle, may reveal a flatter and rather less resonant note than usual, or than on the opposite side. Auscultation may show a weakened respiratory murmur at one apex: but it is most important to listen for persistent râles or crepitations after each of a series of short coughs, for these moist sounds not previously audible may then become evident. These auscultatory signs can often be heard best at the apex, behind, by placing the patient's hand on his opposite shoulder and listening to that part of the lung, which will thus be *uncovered by the scapula*.

Four *Special Investigations* should be performed when there is any suspicion, from the history or from the physical signs, that pulmonary tuberculosis may be present. The *temperature* is an indication of great importance, for an active tuberculous process is usually associated with pyrexia, however slight. A single evening reading may be of some help, but if there is a persistent evening rise of temperature on a succession of nights, at 6.0 p.m., 8.0 p.m. or 10 p.m. when taking the reading with the minute thermometer in place for five minutes, this is most important. A regular 4-hourly chart shows that with early disease in the lung, there is usually an *intermittent* temperature, normal or subnormal in the morning and raised in the late afternoon or in the evening; in rare instances this is reversed. With the rise of temperature there is usually tachycardia: it is unusual to find the pulse rate below 70 in the evening, after a day's work, in a young patient with active disease. The *sputum* should be repeatedly examined for tubercle bacilli the presence of which is diagnostic: the early morning specimen is the most likely to contain the bacilli. In repeatedly negative cases bacilli may be found by examining the early morning gastric washings, or sometimes the stools, and special cultural methods (§ 1203) or guinea-pig inoculations are often necessary. However, the absence of bacilli, even after several examinations, does not necessarily indicate the absence of pulmonary tuberculosis. *X-ray examination* by an expert is ABSOLUTELY ESSENTIAL in all cases of hæmoptysis or of cough lasting more than three weeks. Not only should a straight postero-anterior film be taken, but it is often helpful to take a special apical view, with the clavicles well raised in the lordotic stance, to examine the upper lobes of the lungs when no longer covered by the clavicles.   The *erythrocyte sedimentation rate* is usually, but not invariably, raised in those with active tuberculosis of the lungs and the increase or decrease in the values each few weeks is a useful guide to the activity of the disease in the same patient.

Epituberculosis is the name applied to collapse of a lobe or a segment of the lung due to early tuberculosis.   It is a disease of children usually discovered by X-ray examination.   Originally believed to be the result of external pressure by an enlarged hilar gland it is now recognised that other cases are due to an exudative lesion or to tuberculous bronchopneumonia affecting a lobe or segment of lung.

(b) *Later Stages.*—The *Pulmonary Symptoms* are similar to those in the early stages but are more advanced.   (i.) The cough is much louder and more persistent by day and later on at night.   (ii.) The sputum becomes more copious and nummular in appearance.   This is characteristic of active disease with caseation and sometimes cavitation.   The sputum floats on the surface of the water in the sputum-mug and appears to consist of a number of discrete " coins "—disc-like aggregations of mucopurulent material.   In advanced cases with secondary infection or with bronchiectasis the sputum becomes frankly purulent and sometimes offensive-smelling.   (iii.) One or a succession of brisk hæmoptyses are the result of hæmorrhage from a vessel whose wall has been weakened, often by aneurysmal formation in a cavity.   Such hæmoptyses can prove fatal.   (iv.) Shortness of breath even at rest becomes increasingly severe as the pulmonary tissue becomes destroyed by disease.   The *Constitutional Symptoms* of particular importance are the amount of the *loss of weight* and of the *appetite* of the patient—those with advanced disease find it very difficult to eat a sufficiency of food and even to manage solid food in any quantity.

The *Physical Signs* of more advanced disease are of a wide variety: in the main they are those of consolidation, fibrosis and often cavitation. They are most marked in the upper lobe of the lung but may be present in the apex of the lower lobe, on one or both sides.   Inspection shows a much greater wasting of the muscles and often sinking in of the chest wall, with a greatly diminished expansion of the lung on deep breathing. Palpation confirms this lack of movement and usually shows an increased tactile local fremitus.   Percussion gives a much less resonant note than normal or even a dull note over the upper lobes in front and/or behind, and often also at the apex of the inner wall of the axilla.   Auscultation reveals that the respiratory movement is replaced by a large number of coarse râles which often possess an explosive or crackling quality: and again the vocal resonance is markedly increased.   When fibrosis is much more marked on the one side, not only are the physical signs much more obvious on this side, but the trachea and the heart move across to the affected side.   If, on the other hand, the disease is due to recent bronchopneumonia or to pneumoric consolidation superimposed on a chronic lesion, the signs of solid lung may be local or widespread without such extensive signs of fibrosis. Fibrosis and the often-associated clubbing of the fingers always indicate a long-standing lesion. Emphasis must be given to the fact that many of these signs are hidden when there is any considerable degree of emphysema.

The presence or absence of a CAVITY is in the majority of cases impossible to diagnose with certainty by physical examination alone. The percussion note is usually dull, but varies with circumstances. Thus the note may be resonant when the cavity is very large, or lies very superficially. When the cavity is large and superficial, and the communicating bronchus remains patent, a characteristic note, almost tympanitic, is obtained on percussion whilst the patient keeps his mouth open. This is known as the " cracked-pot " sound (*bruit de pot felé*). The breathing is bronchial, cavernous or amphoric; post-tussic suction is occasionally heard after a cough. Râles are usually also heard.

A *tuberculous tracheo-bronchitis* occurs in about one-third of all cases of pulmonary tuberculosis. There are no characteristic symptoms and the disease is discovered by bronchoscopy. It is often the result of perforation of the bronchial wall by ulceration: it may result in a bronchial spread of the disease, in obstruction of the smaller bronchi and in subsequent bronchiectasis.

The same *Special Investigations* must be undertaken, as are described with early tuberculous disease of the lung. The *temperature* may not be raised in a patient with chronic disease and with a high resistance: but when there is spread to a healthy lung area, often with local pneumonic consolidation, the temperature is elevated. The *sputum* is much more likely to reveal tubercle bacilli, often in very large numbers. *X-ray examination* is again essential and the findings need to be read in conjunction with the history and the physical examination. A great variety of changes are revealed especially in the upper lobes or in the apices of the lower lobes. There may be scattered shadows, some of sufficiently long standing to be calcified: or areas of consolidation and fibrosis intermingled with emphysema or with cavitation. Some areas of soft shadowing are due to recent broncho-pneumonic spread, *e.g.*, from an upper lobe to the lower lobe on the same or on the opposite side. Areas of local disease and confirmation of cavitation are often best revealed by tomography. Hæmoptysis followed by the inhalation of blood gives a finely speckled appearance corresponding to the lobule or lobules which the blood has entered: if the blood contains tubercle bacilli these areas may persist, setting up new areas of tuberculosis. Miliary tuberculosis is revealed as " a snow-storm " effect, its extent depending on the degree of miliary dissemination: it is either part of a generalised tuberculous septicæmia or the result of local spread in the lungs when tubercle bacilli have entered the main pulmonary artery or one or its branches. Many of these varied X-ray appearances may be hidden by the uniform opacity created by a tuberculous effusion or empyema which usually collects in the lower part of the pleural sac.

The *Diagnosis* of Pulmonary Tuberculosis is especially difficult in the early stages. Other causes of cough (§ 101), of hæmoptysis (§ 104) and of debility (Chapter XVI) need to be differentiated. When the condition begins with dyspepsia, it is very liable to be overlooked unless the physician is aware of this mode of commencement. Repeated X-ray exposures for diagnostic purposes may be necessary and have little effect in producing a radiation hazard. A *bronchial carcinoma* usually starts at a later age, but in other respects it may mimic pulmonary tuberculosis involving one lobe or one segment of a lobe; it may appear to follow pneumonia, often produces a cough, a rise of temperature and hæmoptysis and it may be the cause of cavitation and of a pleural effusion. *Sarcoidosis* (§ 141) produces a coarse mottling in the lung fields with considerable enlargement of the hilar glands and a very high erythrocyte sedimentation rate, a condition which was previously often diagnosed as chronic miliary tuberculosis. *Polyarteritis nodosa* (§ 98) is a rare collagen disease, usually seen in conjunction with polyarthritis in young or middle-aged adults. The lung symptoms and signs may appear several months before the other varied systemic signs show themselves. A cough, sputum (sometimes blood-stained) and breathlessness are associated with pyrexia, infiltration and even cavitation of the lungs and a very high E.S.R. There may be a granuloma in the nose or middle ear: over 50 per cent. of cases show an eosinophilia. Tubercle bacilli are never found in the sputum, there is no response to anti-tuberculous drugs but the corticosteroids (*e.g.*, tab. prednisolone 40 mg. daily) usually produce a rapid clearing of the symptoms and signs. Various fungal infections which can simulate pulmonary tuberculosis are *moniliasis* (usually due to candida albicans), *aspergillosis* and *blastomycosis* (see § 147).

Classification.—Reference has been made to (*a*) the earlier stages and (*b*) the later stages of this disease, and a brief account of the symptomatology and physical signs has been given under each heading. The primary classification which has now been accepted by the Ministry of Health is *Class A*, persons from whom tubercle bacilli have never been identified, and *Class B*, those in whom tubercle bacilli have been found at some time—in the sputum, fæces, urine, other excreta or in effusions. A further subdivision of adult cases into three main groups conforms closely to the actual clinical facts: (1) *ambulant afebrile*, (2) *resting afebrile—ambulant febrile*, (3) *resting febrile*, conforms more closely to the actual clinical facts. The extent of the lung lesion is of importance, although extensive disease may exist with but little constitutional disturbance. X-ray examination at intervals can and does reveal the development of fresh lesions in patients who are practically without symptoms, and who not only are afebrile but may even be increasing in weight. The age of the patient, the length of time during which manifest clinical disease has developed, the amount of sputum and its content of tubercle bacilli, the character of the adventitious shadows in the radiogram, etc., are also points to be taken into account in the assessment of any individual case.

Etiology.—The primary cause of the disease is infection by the human type of the tubercle bacillus: in recent years 3-6 per cent. of cases have been found to be due to the bovine type of organism. The period of infectivity is about 6 weeks, as shown by the time taken after infection for a negative tuberculin reactor to develop a positive reaction: this is also the time after infection when erythema nodosum (§ 706) shows itself.

Invasion by the tubercle bacillus produces different effects on different individuals: the younger the person the more serious is the disease, so that infants and small children are particularly susceptible. The usual age at which the disease appears clinically is between sixteen and thirty: young women are more often affected at this younger age period, but in recent years there has also been an increasing incidence in Great Britain among elderly men. Of major importance is the dose of tubercle bacilli inhaled at any one time for a large dose more easily overwhelms the resistance of the human body.

Recently there has been increasing evidence that the genetic factor of racial and familial resistance/susceptibility plays a much greater part than was at one time thought likely—a view which has been greatly strengthened by the findings of the Prophit Committee of the Royal College of Physicians of London. There is some correlation between the degree of reaction to tuberculin and the liability to develop pulmonary tuberculosis. Whereas a negative Mantoux reaction among young children, in nurses and in medical students, indicates that they have a lowered resistance to infection, those with a very high cutaneous susceptibility (and a strong positive Mantoux reaction) are also more likely to develop clinical tuberculosis than are those who give a weak positive reaction.

Conditions which favour active disease are any state of malnutrition such as arises from insufficient food, diabetes mellitus and chronic alcoholism. It is a curious circumstance that pregnant women offer a high resistance; a phthisical subject becoming pregnant will frequently improve until after her confinement, when an exacerbation of the disease will often occur. Some cases are first recognised when basal pneumonia occurs after general anæsthesia. Excessive exposure to artificial or natural sunlight has sometimes precipitated an attack: so does the administration of adrenocorticotrophic hormone and the various corticosteroids. Unhealthy surroundings play an important part in the spread of tuberculosis; indoor occupations in over-crowded and ill-ventilated rooms are especially dangerous. Those who work in a silica-laden atmosphere are also more prone to pulmonary tuberculosis (see Silicosis, § 136).

Prognosis.—1. Many of the factors influencing this have already been discussed. To summarise they are: the age of the patient, the disease being more virulent in children, young adults and rather more so in elderly men; the type of disease present—cases with miliary and with broncho-pneumonic tuberculosis are particularly severe whereas those with chronic fibroid disease of the lungs may live for many years; the presence of tubercle bacilli in the sputum means the disease is more serious than in those with consistently negative results, and those whose sputum becomes negative under treatment have a much more favourable outcome than those whose sputum remains consistently positive; cavitation in the lungs always means the disease is more difficult to heal; constitutional disorders which greatly aggravate the disease are malnutrition, chronic alcoholism, diabetes mellitus and recent pregnancy; and last but not least there is the ability and determination of the individual patient to undertake adequate treatment.

2. The *prognosis in individual cases* has been greatly improved in recent years by four advances in treatment: (a) early diagnosis; (b) chemotherapy; (c) rest and open-air treatment; (d) surgical measures of collapsetherapy or of excision of diseased areas in the lungs. The type of disease, its rate of progress and its distribution are all important: a correct prognosis cannot always be made until the patient's reaction to treatment has been observed.

3. *Untoward Symptoms.*—(i.) The severity of the toxæmia and the activity of the tuberculous process can be judged by the degree of fever and by the extent of its daily variations. The pulse rate is also important, and, quite apart from the temperature chart, is valuable as a measure of toxæmia. Increase of weight and a falling erythrocyte sedimentation rate during treatment are good signs. (ii.) The extent of the disease must be judged by the physical signs elicited and by the X-ray appearances. Serial X-rays each month or two often show whether the disease is spreading or is being arrested by the treatment given. (iii.) Hæmoptysis does not appear to bear any constant relation to prognosis, though profuse hæmorrhage weakens the patient considerably, and may be fatal; it is occasionally followed by extension of the disease.

4. *Complications* add to the gravity of the disease. The commonest are: (1) Pleurisy is very frequent and its adhesions may be beneficial in preventing spontaneous pneumothorax. On the other hand a tuberculous abscess in the pleura (empyema) is a serious event; (2) tuberculosis may occur in other areas—the peritoneum, meninges, the kidney, and the intestine giving rise to ulceration of the terminal ileum and cæcum with an exhausting diarrhœa. Tuberculous pericarditis is rare; (3) a tuberculous ischio-rectal abscess may arise from swallowed tubercle bacilli; (4) involvement of the larynx undoubtedly influences the prognosis adversely; (5) bronchiectasis results from destruction and fibrosis of tuberculous areas in the bronchi—a pyogenic infection of the cavities produces profound toxæmia; (6) thrombo-phlebitis is a less common complication; (7) erythema nodosum (§ 706).

The *Treatment* of pulmonary tuberculosis has undergone revolutionary changes in the last ten years, mainly as a result of effective antibiotic therapy. No longer is it necessary to concentrate solely on raising the patient's resistance to tubercle bacilli for now it is possible to attack and to destroy the bacilli themselves. Even the need for routine sanatorium treatment is questioned by some authorities. It is not yet possible to foretell what regime of treatment will ultimately prove to be most beneficial, but at the present time the most important principles can be classified under the headings (a) Institutional and general measures; (b) Chemotherapy; (c) Surgical measures; (d) Symptomatic treatment and (e) Rehabilitation of the patient.

(a) *Institutional Treatment.*—The five main indications for a sanatorium regime or for other institutional care are when: (i.) the pulmonary disease is open (with a positive sputum test); (ii.) there is cavitation of the lung; (iii.) the patient is febrile; (iv.) there are symptoms or signs which need assessment; (v.) the home conditions are such that the patient cannot be cared for at home. During residence in a chest hospital it is also possible to teach the patient the *general measures* necessary for his welfare. These include (i.) a period of bed-rest so long as he is pyrexial —but complete rest is no longer obligatory and various occupations and diversions while in bed are now allowed; (ii.) the insistence on adequate ventilation. Although there is now much less stress on the importance of " open-air " treatment in chalets, etc., fresh air does help to stimulate the appetite, it helps to create a sense of well-being, it lessens the chance of the introduction of other respiratory infections such as influenza and it is most effective in overcoming the discomforts of severe night sweats; (iii.) the diet should be of high calorie value when there has been loss of weight, with a varied and pleasing combination of foods which should include milk, butter, eggs, cheese, fruit, meat and fish; (iv.) instructions can be given as to the collection and disposal of sputum, handkerchiefs, etc., and how to avoid infecting others; (v.) when coughing is in any way aggravated by smoking this must be strictly curtailed or stopped. It is wise to insist on the patient giving up smoking altogether when there is pulmonary cavitation or tuberculous laryngitis. After a preliminary period in a chest hospital it is often possible to continue treatment at home provided the patient is afebrile, the sputum is negative and all lung cavities have closed. The patient must, however, continue to have the regular care of the chest physician and the family doctor and have the help of a health visitor (see Fig. 62).

(*b*) *Chemotherapy* has become of major importance in the treatment of all forms of tuberculosis. The three drugs in common use are inject. streptomycin sulphate, the sodium salt of *p*-amino-salicylic acid (P.A.S.) and isoniazid B.P.C. (isonicotinic acid hydrazide). If only one of these three drugs is administered at a time strains of tubercle bacilli may develop which are resistant to the drug, but if two or more drugs a e given simultaneously this only occurs in 1 in 1,000 patients. Therefore, in a newly-diagnosed patient, at least two specimens of sputum should be collected, the tubercle bacillus in each specimen cultured and its sensitivity tested to each of the three drugs: culture of the sputum at monthly intervals during treatment will detect the subsequent emergence of a drug-resistant strain. Streptomycin sulphate is administered in a single daily dose of 1·0 G. (in children 30 mg. per kilo a day): the main drawback is that, particularly after the age of 40, daily injections often give rise to toxic damage to the vestibular nerve with symptoms of giddiness and unsteadiness in walking. For this reason the dose in middle-aged and elderly patients is now usually not above 1·0 G. three times a week. P.A.S. is bacteriostatic and not bactericidal, at least *in vitro*: its main advantage is its power to prevent the development of drug-resistant strains. The dose is 3–5 G. q.i.d., in rice-paper cachets—unfortunately the larger dose often causes nausea, vomiting and even diarrhœa. Both streptomycin and P.A.S. can give rise to drug-fever and skin rashes, and P.A.S. can cause toxic hepatitis, exfoliative dermatitis and occasionally a goitre to develop. Isoniazid is well tolerated in doses of 100 mg. b.d. (in children 3·0–5·0 mg./kilo a day) and only occasionally gives rise to toxic polyneuritis or psychiatric changes. The evidence at present indicates that the combination of streptomycin with isoniazid 100 mg. b.d. is slightly preferable to streptomycin with P.A.S. 5 G. q.i.d., especially in improving the general condition of the patient: the Therapeutic Trials Committee of the Medical Research Council has recently reported that streptomycin with isoniazid 100 mg. b.d. is equalled in therapeutic efficiency by P.A.S. 5 G. q.i.d. with isoniazid 100 mg. b.d.

The usual regime therefore recommended is, for young adults, inject. streptomycin 1 G. a day (and to patients over 40 years old, 1 G. three times a week), in each case giving also P.A.S. 4 G. t.i.d. with isoniazid 100 mg. b.d. for the first 8 weeks. Once the results of sensitivity tests of the bacilli in at least two specimens of sputum are known, then the drug to which the tubercle bacilli are not sensitive is omitted and the other two drugs continued: but when P.A.S. is used in combination with one other drug the dose should be raised to 5 G. q.i.d. When, as is usually found, the bacilli are sensitive to all three drugs, the P.A.S. is stopped so long as the patient is in hospital, but when he is fit to return home a combination of isoniazid and P.A.S. is often more convenient. The duration of treatment with these drugs has not yet been decided but all are agreed that continuous treatment must be given for at least 12 months— otherwise a relapse within 2 years of stopping treatment is likely to occur. Some authorities believe that to prevent relapse the chosen drugs should be continued indefinitely. This is certainly advisable when a lesion (such as a cavity) persists and when surgery is not possible either because it is refused by the patient or because the respiratory reserve of the patient makes it inadvisable.

The main indications for chemotherapy are: (i.) in patients with a positive sputum or with cavitation. It must be continued for at least 12 months after sputum tests have become consistently negative or after the last cavity has closed. Such treatment results in the abolition of at least 60 per cent. of cavities. (ii.) Whenever pulmonary tuberculosis is the cause of fever, toxaemia and pulmonary infiltration even in the absence of a positive sputum test. (iii.) Most chest physicians believe drug treatment is necessary when there is X-ray evidence of a " minimal lesion " even in the absence of fever, toxaemia or a raised erythrocyte sedimentation reaction: most of these patients can continue at work but bed rest is necessary when there is a raised temperature. (iv.) In children with evidence of primary tuberculosis—and the younger the child the greater the need for this treatment. In fact Heaf now advises a three-month course of isoniazid with P.A.S. for all children under 10 years who have a positive tuberculin reaction and who have not had B.C.G. vaccine, even in the absence of a positive X-ray finding. The only type of disease which does not respond well to chemotherapy is that associated with considerable fibrosis; some cases with a chronic tuberculous abscess of the lung are also resistant.   The place of cortisone therapy in pulmonary tuberculosis is not yet decided, but good results have been recorded in severely ill patients and in those who have developed drug reactions with streptomycin or P.A.S.

(c) *Surgical Measures* are used much more freely than in former years, but only after the patient has had 6–9 months' trial of medical treatment.   When chest surgery is contemplated consultation with a thoracic surgeon is imperative.   The two chief procedures are lung resection and thoracoplasty, the former tending to replace the latter.   *Lung resection* consists of the removal of one or more pulmonary segments, of lobectomy or of pneumonectomy, the aim of the surgeon being to remove the minimal amount consistent with excision of the diseased area.   Cases that do well are those with a positive sputum or a cavity not responding to drug therapy and those with dense fibrotic lesions, bronchial stenosis or bronchiectasis.   *Thoracoplasty* is usually reserved for local fibrotic lesions in the upper lobe, or for patients with an apical cavity and a positive sputum test which persist after adequate drug treatment.   Prior to any chest operation the patient must have had at least 6 months of chemotherapy, which in itself often lessens the amount of diseased lung which requires removal: and after operation such treatment must be continued for another 6–12 months to prevent relapse.   The operative risk of these procedures is now very low; in a recent series the mortality being for segmental resection 1·3 per cent., for thoracoplasty 2 per cent. and for lobectomy 4 per cent.

Until recently *artificial pneumothorax* or an artificial *pneumo-peritoneum* combined with phrenic nerve paralysis performed a most useful service by inducing collapse and rest of a diseased lung area.   There was always an element of risk with A.P. therapy such as air embolism or the rupture of a cavity to form a tuberculous empyema.   These procedures have largely been abandoned in the last 5 years in favour of chemotherapy and subsequent lung resection where necessary.   In chronic bronchitis with an apical cavity, the operation of *apical plombage*, involving extra-fascial stripping and the insertion into the extrapleural space of plastic balls, has been reported to give good results.

(d) *Symptomatic Treatment* is much less often required now that the causal organism can be combated.   (1) When cough is troublesome it can be relieved by a throat lozenge, a sedative linctus such as linct. codeinæ B.P.C. or linct. diamorphinæ (containing heroin grs. $\frac{1}{24}-\frac{1}{32}$ in each dose), perhaps in combination with a barbiturate at bedtime.   (2) Night sweats are seldom troublesome if there is free exposure to fresh air.   A pill containing dry extract of belladonna gr. $\frac{1}{4}$ may be of service.   (3) Diarrhœa is exhausting and must be combated with a low residue diet and a mixture containing tincture of morphine and kaolin.   (4) Vomiting is sometimes a very troublesome symptom, and there are three kinds of vomiting which admit of three different methods of treatment.   (*a*) If preceded by nausea, it points to disorder of the stomach, and should be treated by bismuth, etc., on the usual lines.   (*b*) If the vomiting be preceded and caused by coughing, it is a good plan to give hot drinks just before a meal, in order to encourage expectoration and get the paroxysms of coughing over before the meal is begun.   (*c*) If neither of these ·is successful, vomiting may sometimes be relieved by opium; sometimes it is controlled by the will. (5) The treatment of hæmoptysis is given in § 104 and of tuberculous laryngitis in § 172.

(*e*) *Rehabilitation* of the patient involves co-operation between the patient, his employer, the family doctor, the chest physician and often the rehabilitation officer of the Ministry of Labour.   The majority of patients who have recovered from the active stage of disease are able to return to work, while still on drug treatment and under regular observation at a chest clinic.   They are no longer a danger to their fellow-men when they have become sputum-negative as a result of the measures outlined above.   Unless the job is particularly arduous or otherwise unsuitable, it is always desirable that patients should return to their previous employment—learning a new job is not easy and often involves a lowered income.

Preventive Measures are of major importance in avoiding the spread of the disease and in the protection of susceptible individuals. The need for these is shown by the weekly notification in England and Wales of over 500 new cases of respiratory tuberculosis and about 70 new cases of other forms of tuberculosis even at the present time.   Preventive measures come under three main categories: (1) the special chest clinics and the public health organisation, (2) the education of the layman, (3) the stamping out of bovine tuberculosis.

(1) Tuberculosis is a notifiable infectious disease and as such all medical practitioners are under an obligation to inform the local medical officer of health of any new case that they see.   All suspected or reported cases are seen by a chest physician and hospital in-patient treatment is arranged for all sputum-positive cases.   Contacts in the family circle and sometimes at work are also seen to detect the occurrence of recent infection.   Closely linked with these special chest clinics is the mass miniature X-ray service set up under the Ministry of Health for the regular chest X-ray examination of the population: any suspicious X-ray shadow is followed up by taking a life-size film and where necessary subsequent reference of the person to a chest physician.   By these means an endeavour is being made to eliminate infectious cases from the general community, to detect early cases before the sputum becomes positive, and to follow up and rehabilitate arrested cases to prevent a relapse.   Furthermore, the local health authorities and the chest physicians perform a most useful service by tuberculin-testing those who are in close contact with the disease (family contacts, doctors, nurses and others working in hospitals) so that those who are tuberculin-negative reactors can be given the benefit of

immunisation by the inoculation of Bacillus Calmette-Guérin vaccine (B.C.G.). This consists of living bacilli derived from a pathogenic strain of bovine tubercle bacilli attenuated by repeated sub-culture over a period of more than 10 years: in a series of children of school-leaving age followed for 4 years the vaccine has been found to reduce the incidence of tuberculosis from 1·7 to 0·37 per thousand children, but the total duration of the immunity following vaccination is not yet known.

Other public health measures which have greatly contributed to control of the disease are the clearance of slum-areas, the prevention of overcrowded housing conditions, the insistence on adequate ventilation in shops, factories and places of entertainment, and giving special priority for rehousing tuberculous families.

(2) Education of the general public is concerned to make known the ways in which disease is spread—by coughing, sneezing, and in the case of tuberculous parents by kissing their children. The proper disposal of sputum from infected patients is of great importance, the patient being instructed to spit only into some portable receptacle containing a disinfectant such as lysol, or into paper sputum cups or handkerchiefs which can be burned. The public is also becoming increasingly aware of the advantage of regular examination by mass miniature X-ray of the chest. For those undergoing treatment for pulmonary tuberculosis special monetary allowances are available through the Ministry of National Insurance.

(3) Bovine tuberculosis has in the past been the cause of the majority of cases of disease in the lymphatic glands, bones, joints and in the abdomen: and about 2·3 per cent. of cases of pulmonary tuberculosis were bovine in origin. Great efforts have been made to avoid the human consumption of milk and meat from tuberculous cattle: this has been done by tuberculin testing the animals, eliminating all those that have given a positive reaction and so building up tubercle-free herds. Milk from all sources is treated by pasteurisation to kill tubercle and all other pathogenic bacteria. These methods have already produced a gratifying reduction of disease, particularly in the younger and more susceptible members of the community (see Table on p. 222).

Chronic miliary tuberculosis was described some years ago as a condition with X-ray shadows in the lungs comparable to the acute variety. It is now doubtful whether such a condition really exists, for most if not all the cases were due to sarcoidosis, which has only comparatively recently been recognised as a separate clinical entity.

§ 132. Fibroid Tuberculosis is a very chronic form of pulmonary disease. It is a tuberculo-fibroid process occurring for the most part in elderly subjects, running a protracted course, and terminating in contraction of the lung. It should be differentiated from other forms of chronic fibrosis of the lung (§ 136).

Symptoms.—The disease is essentially of insidious onset and long duration. For many years the patient complains of a chronic cough which is especially troublesome in the morning. The other symptoms are progressive shortness of breath, clubbed fingers, slowly increasing weakness and emaciation, with little or no fever.

The *Physical Signs* begin and are almost always most marked at the apex. *Both lungs* are usually affected (which contrasts with interstitial pneumonia), but the signs of disease become more advanced on one side. There is impairment of the chest movement and contraction of one side of the chest with signs of consolidation of one or more segments or lobes of the underlying lung. The heart, trachea and other viscera are displaced to the more affected side. Hæmoptysis sometimes occurs, and the tubercle bacillus may be discovered on careful and repeated examination of the sputum or by guinea-pig inoculation.

The *Diagnosis* from other forms of pulmonary tuberculosis is made by the age of the patient and the extremely protracted course of this disease. The physical signs and symptoms of non-tuberculous *pulmonary fibrosis* and *sarcoidosis* resemble it closely and the diagnosis can only be inferred by (i.) the history, (ii.) the absence of tubercle bacilli after frequent sputum examinations, (iii.) the more usual localisation in one lung.

Etiology.—Fibroid phthisis is more frequently met with at and after middle life. It may follow chronic bronchitis, broncho-pneumonia, or repeated attacks of pleurisy. In true Fibroid Tuberculosis the tubercle bacillus is primarily deposited in a healthy lung in the same manner as in chronic pulmonary tuberculosis, and then causes an indolent fibroid reaction often succeeded by calcification.

Prognosis.—Its course is very protracted. Sometimes acute tuberculosis supervenes. The chief complications are bronchiectasis, compensatory emphysema of the lungs, lardaceous disease of other organs and cardiac failure. In general terms the prognosis and *Treatment* are similar to those of chronic pulmonary tuberculosis.

II. *The patient complains of breathlessness; on examining the chest, dullness is found at one or both* **bases,** *and* SIGNS OF FLUID *are detected there. The disease is* HYDROTHORAX.

§ 133. **Hydrothorax** is a chronic collection of serous fluid in the pleural cavity, differing from the effusion of pleurisy in being non-inflammatory.

Symptoms.—The onset is usually gradual, and as hydrothorax is always a secondary condition, the symptoms may be masked by the presence of generalised œdema in other areas. On this account it is remarkable how often hydrothorax is overlooked. Dyspnœa is usually present and its degree depends in large measure on the amount of fluid present. In the absence of inflammation, pain, a pleural rub and pyrexia are usually absent. In rare cases the fluid collects with great rapidity. The sudden onset of signs of fluid in the chest, accompanied by shock or collapse, in a case which has previously presented the symptoms of aneurysm, points to the occurrence of hæmorrhage into the pleural cavity (hæmothorax).

The *Physical Signs* are those of fluid in the lower parts of one or both pleural cavities (*vide* §§ 109 and 119).

Diagnosis.—The disease has to be diagnosed from other disorders giving rise to dullness on percussion (§ 113). When there is any doubt as to the cause, it is very helpful to remove a little fluid for pathological examination. The cell count is of less value than is the protein content of the fluid: in a passive exudate the protein is about 1 per cent. whereas in an inflammatory effusion it is nearer 5 per cent.: malignant disease gives intermediate values and often produces a uniformly blood-stained effusion. Repeated cytological examination reveals carcinoma cells in about 60 per cent. of cases (§ 1213).

Etiology.—(i.) The commonest cause is a combination of right- and left-sided heart failure so that the hydrothorax is part of a cardiac œdema. Often the right pleura is solely or chiefly affected, perhaps due to pressure by the distended right auricle on the pulmonary veins. Sometimes only left ventricular failure is present. (ii.) Malignant disease in the chest is the next in frequency. This may be due to a primary bronchial carcinoma, to a mediastinal tumour or to secondary malignant disease arising from a primary focus situated almost anywhere in the body. *Meigs' Syndrome* is a very rare condition of hydrothorax and hydroperitoneum arising from an ovarian fibroma and is cured when this is removed. (iii.) Hydrothorax may form part of the *general* dropsy of subacute nephritis, in which circumstance both pleuræ are usually involved. Here the hydrothorax is of no very great importance *per se*, but the onset of dyspnœa in nephritis should always direct our attention to the pleuræ. (iv.) An aneurysm pressing on the intrathoracic veins is a rare cause.

Prognosis.—The disease is essentially chronic, the duration depending very much upon the cause. In general terms the prognosis of the condition is unfavourable. The patient should be carefully watched for the occurrence of intermitting pyrexia indicative of empyema.

Treatment.—Paracentesis (§ 119) should be performed when the amount of fluid is such as to cause symptoms: in congestive heart failure it is wise to undertake this early. Tapping may be repeated indefinitely. Diuretics or circulatory stimulants are useful. Otherwise treatment must be directed to the primary condition (see also § 119).

III. *The patient complains of breathlessness; on examining the chest, an* IMPAIRED PERCUSSION NOTE *is found at one or both* bases, *and on auscultation* CREPITATIONS *are heard. The disease is* PULMONARY CONGESTION, HYPOSTASIS OR ŒDEMA.

§ 134. **Hypostasis of the Lung** (Pulmonary Congestion or Œdema) is a serous exudation into and around the air vesicles. It is synonymous with the term "hypostatic congestion," or, as it is sometimes called, "hypostatic pneumonia." It is present at the end of many serious disorders and is frequently accompanied by fluid in the pleural cavities (§ 133).

Symptoms.—(i.) It is never a primary condition, the causes being similar to those of hydrothorax (§ 133). The onset is always insidious, and it is only by careful watching that it can be detected. (ii.) A considerable amount of dyspnœa is present, which may amount to orthopnœa. (iii.) There is a frothy mucous expectoration, not infrequently tinged with blood.

The *Physical Signs* are somewhat indefinite but they are found, as is implied by the term " hypostatic," chiefly at the bases of both lungs. The percussion note is impaired, the expansion and the air entry at the lung bases are diminished and there are abundant fine crepitations which take on a much coarser quality as the condition advances.   Any rise of temperature that may be present is due to the primary or causal condition or to the development of broncho-pneumonia in the hypostatic areas.

Diagnosis.—The condition is diagnosed from true *pneumonia* by the gradual onset, the absence of any marked pyrexia or signs of consolidation and the recognition of the cause of the condition.

Etiology.—(i.) The disease is most frequent in elderly people, especially when bed-ridden.   (ii.) It is common for a day or so after any abdominal operation due to poor movement of the diaphragm.   (iii.) Cardiac disease, especially mitral stenosis and left ventricular failure, lead to pulmonary hypertension and so cause pulmonary œdema, sometimes acutely (§ 118). (iv.) When present at only one lung base it may be due to inflammation under the diaphragm, such as with a subphrenic, hepatic or perinephric abscess.   (v.) In subacute nephritis œdema of the lungs occurs as part of a generalised dropsy.   (vi.) Tumours pressing on the veins within the mediastinum may result in pulmonary œdema.

Prognosis.—The presence at the lung bases of poor ventilation with a few crepitations in whose who are confined to bed for short periods is of little significance.   In others and especially in elderly bed-ridden patients with little vitality it may be a very serious sign as it indicates failing general health and heart failure.

Treatment.—The indications are to relieve the cause whenever possible and to stimulate the use of the lung bases.   In elderly people who are liable to develop pulmonary œdema very easily, and in post-operative cases, it is well to keep the patient sitting up in bed in the Trendelenberg position, to roll them from side to side and to encourage deep breathing exercises.   Then as soon as possible, éven in the case of fracture and other surgical illnesses, the patient should be sat out of bed and encouraged to take short walks.   Stimulating expectorant mixtures containing ammonium carbonate help to free the lung bases of sticky mucoid secretions.   The mercurial and other diuretics are of value in many cases and when auricular fibrillation is present digitalis is useful (§ 62).   Should acute pulmonary œdema supervene, see § 118.

GROUP B.—We now turn to the chronic diseases attended by **dullness on percussion,** which does NOT always occur in regular and DEFINED AREAS AT BASE OR APEX.   The *common* diseases in this group are: IV. PULMONARY FIBROSIS; V. THICKENED PLEURA; VI and VII. NEOPLASMS.

§ 135. IV. **Pulmonary Fibrosis** may be localised or diffuse, and may involve one or more pulmonary segments or lobes, or even the greater part of one or both lungs depending on the cause. (A) The localised variety is due to a local cause, generally infective in origin. (B) The diffuse type is the result of the inhalation of irritant dusts (as in the pneumoconioses) or may be due to rare systemic diseases.

(A) *The patient complains that for a number of years there has been* INCREASING SHORTNESS OF BREATH, *associated with a* COUGH *and* SPUTUM WHICH IS OFTEN PURULENT. *There are local signs of* CONSOLIDATION *and* CONTRACTION *in the lung and* CLUBBING OF THE FINGERS *is usually present. The disease is* FIBROID LUNG.

§ 136. **Fibroid Lung** (Syn. Chronic Interstitial Pneumonia) is the name given to localised fibrosis in one or more areas, often associated with bronchiectasis (§ 145). A common cause is *chronic pulmonary tuberculosis* in middle-aged and elderly patients who have a very high resistance to the tubercle bacillus, in which case the disease tends to be more marked in the upper lobes of the lungs (see Fibroid Tuberculosis, § 132). There is also a *non-tuberculous* variety which usually commences at an earlier age and which is more often met in the middle or the lower lobes of the lungs.

Symptoms.—The prominent symptom is shortness of breath, at first only on exertion but later occurring even when at rest, the result of a progressive diminution of respiratory function. Many of these patients are forced to give up work at a relatively early age. There is usually a cough, particularly with change of position and therefore marked on waking, and the sputum resulting from this is often purulent and is always more copious when derived from bronchiectatic cavities (§ 145). Particularly in the winter months there are recurrent respiratory infections which lead to increasing cyanosis. Sooner or later the signs of right-sided heart failure are likely to develop.

Physical Signs.—The patient is usually of spare build with a rather sunken face on which dilated vessels make their appearance. The *chest signs* are: (i.) some wasting of the corresponding pectoral muscles, a flattening or hollowing of the chest wall and little or no expansion with a deep breath; (ii.) palpation confirms the lack of movement and usually shows an increased tactile vocal fremitus; (iii.) there is a very impaired or a dull percussion note over the fibrotic area; and (iv.) over this same area there is little evidence of the normal vesicular murmur. This is replaced by bronchial breathing, or when cavitation of any size is present there may be cavernous or amphoric breathing. In the presence of bronchitic or bronchiectatic changes, persistent rhonchi and râles are audible. With unilateral fibroid changes the opposite lung shows the signs of compensatory emphysema. A characteristic feature of unilateral pulmonary fibrosis is the marked displacement of the heart and of the trachea to the affected side, so that the cardiac impulse may, with disease of the lower lobe of the left lung, be found far out in the left axilla; and with disease of the right lung it may be close to or behind the sternum. *Other signs* invariably found are (i.) accompanying the contracted chest wall there is scoliosis of the dorsal spine, the concavity of the spinous processes being towards the diseased lung, and (ii.) a marked clubbing of the fingers. X-ray examination confirms these physical findings and shows a dense shadowing corresponding to the fibrous tissue in the lung: cavitation is occasionally visible in the area of diseased lung and the diaphragm is drawn well up into the chest on the one side.

Diagnosis is in most cases straightforward. The important differentiation is to identify the *tuberculous* cases as these may be heavily infective to others. A tuberculous cause should be suspected when the disease involves one or both upper lobes of the lungs; when the sputum is mucoid rather than purulent, and confirmation is obtained by finding tubercle bacilli. A *pneumothorax* on the side of the healthy lung is sometimes wrongly diagnosed because of the hyper-resonance on that side and the fact that the apex of the heart is moved to the opposite side, but obviously the diseased lung is on the side which shows little or no movement of the chest wall and no vesicular murmur.

Etiology.—(i.) In young people the commonest cause is following acute *broncho-pneumonia*, especially that associated with measles or whooping-cough: the inflammatory process becomes chronic and fails to resolve. (ii.) A chronic pleural effusion, a slowly clearing empyema and repeated attacks of *pleurisy* may be attended by a subpleural fibrosis (thickened pleura (§ 137), and dense bands of fibrous tissue may extend into the lung. (iii.) Persistent *collapse* of a part or whole of a lung may result from an unsuspected foreign-body or from pressure due to enlarged glands, etc. (iv.) *Syphilitic disease* of the lung is rare, except as a congenital manifestation in infancy, in which circumstances the change consists of a fibroid induration of the lung. Gummata also occur.

Treatment is solely concerned with the complications arising for no treatment of the fibrosis *per se* is possible. When bronchiectasis is a troublesome feature, surgical procedures are sometimes indicated.

(B) *The patient complains of* BREATHLESSNESS *which has gradually progressed over a number of years: there is a* SLIGHT COUGH *but* LITTLE SPUTUM. *The* LUNGS *show signs of* EMPHYSEMA. *Except in the advanced stages there are no local signs of fibrosis but* X-RAY EXAMINATION *shows a considerable degree of* DIFFUSE FIBROSIS *and sometimes* NODULES. *The disease is* DIFFUSE FIBROSIS OF THE LUNGS *which may be* OCCUPATIONAL *in origin.*

This group of diseases has received considerable attention during the last few decades. The striking clinical feature is the shortness of breath: the diagnosis is almost impossible without the aid of chest X-rays. The changes are the result of (*a*) the inhalation of dust by industrial workers (*Pneumoconiosis*). By far the most hazardous is Silicosis, although a proportion of those engaged as Coal-miners, as Asbestos-workers (Asbestosis) and in handling Beryllium are also subject to lung damage. (*b*) Rarer non-industrial causes include Sarcoidosis, diffuse Systemic Sclerosis, some cases of Hæmosiderosis and after intensive X-ray treatment of the lungs.

(*a*) **Pneumoconiosis** arises after exposure of the lungs to various dusts for a long period of years. Apart from the fibrotic lung changes and the shortness of breath these cause, there is a tendency to bronchitis, emphysema and polycythæmia; and chronic fibroid pulmonary tuberculosis develops especially with silicosis. In the later stages right-sided heart failure or a terminal broncho-pneumonia develops.

Silicosis is the result of inhalation of silicon dioxide during the process of mining hard ores, or in industries which involve sandblasting, chipping granite, grinding, buffing or moulding metals with sandstone or glass-making. The silica inhaled into the alveoli of the lungs is carried by phagocytes into the interstices and aggregates of these form the basis of the silicotic nodules and massive fibrosis: these are clearly seen by X-ray, especially in the upper parts of the lungs (Fig. 63). Usually the patient has been exposed to the dust for an average of 30 years.

Pneumoconiosis of Coal-miners (Anthracosilicosis) is partly due to silicosis but the dust from hard coal and anthracite is also injurious. X-rays show an initial fine mottling, most marked in the upper and middle lobes, succeeded in later years by chronic fibrosis.

Asbestosis arises after an average of seven years' exposure to the dust. Asbestos is mainly a silicate of magnesium and of iron and is used in many trades and to make protective fabrics. The pulmonary changes are first seen in the lower lobes and radiologically appear as a very fine shadowing resembling ground-glass. Microscopically asbestos bodies are found in the sputum. There is a tendency to pulmonary tuberculosis, to carcinoma of the bronchus and to malignant mesothelioma of the pleura.

Treatment consists in the early recognition of the pulmonary changes and of complications such as pulmonary tuberculosis by regular X-ray examination. This ensures a change of employment before the lungs are extensively diseased. All these occupational diseases are compulsorily notifiable. Preventive measures depend on the industry concerned; they consist of adequate ventilation, sprays of water on to the dust and the wearing of dust-masks.

Chronic Beryllium Poisoning is in a separate category from the above: it occurs in those engaged in mining beryllium ore, preparing it for incorporation into steel or various alloys and in coating fluorescent lamps. It can cause chronic changes in the lungs including diffuse fibrosis and emphysema, as well as acute tracheo-bronchitis and lesions of the skin and conjunctivæ.

(*b*) NON-INDUSTRIAL DISEASES which may be accompanied by diffuse fibrotic changes in the lungs are rare. Intensive deep X-ray therapy to the lungs and sarcoidosis (§ 141) may be causal, but diffuse systemic sclerosis (§ 751) and hæmosiderosis are very rare.

The **Hamman-Rich Syndrome** is of unknown origin. *Symptoms.*—At between 40–50 years of age there is intermittent or severe dyspnœa, cough, cyanosis, poly-

PLATE VII

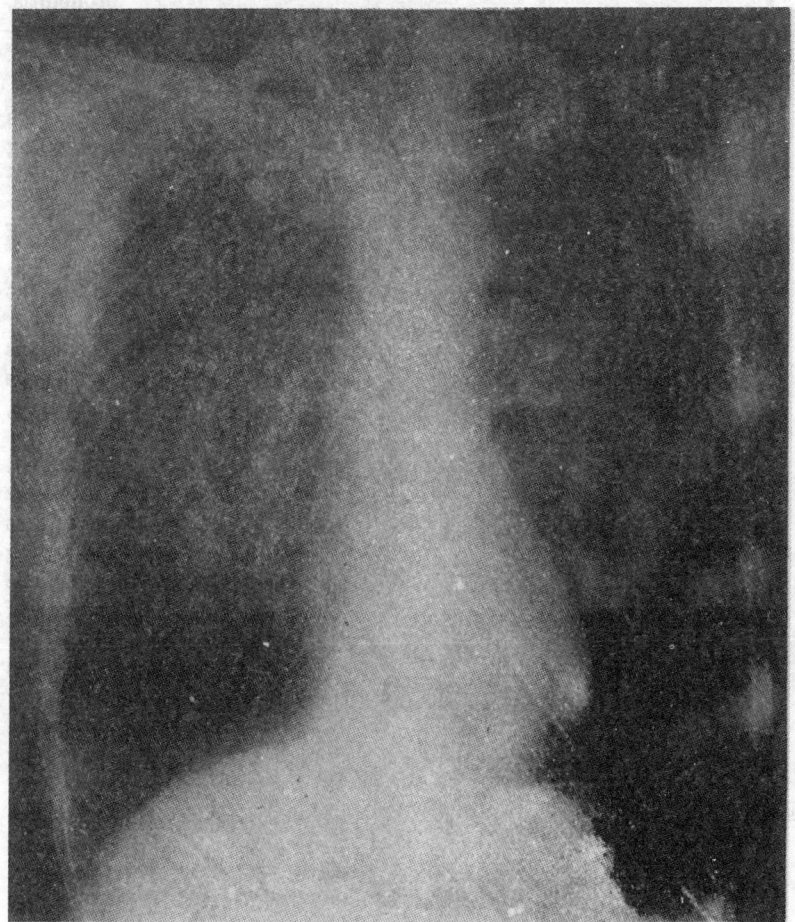

Fig. 62.—X-RAY FILM OF CHEST showing WELL-CALCIFIED SHADOWS in the Upper Lobes of both lungs. The patient had been treated in a Sanatorium 20 years previously for PULMONARY TUBERCULOSIS, which is now healed and symptomless.

PLATE VIII

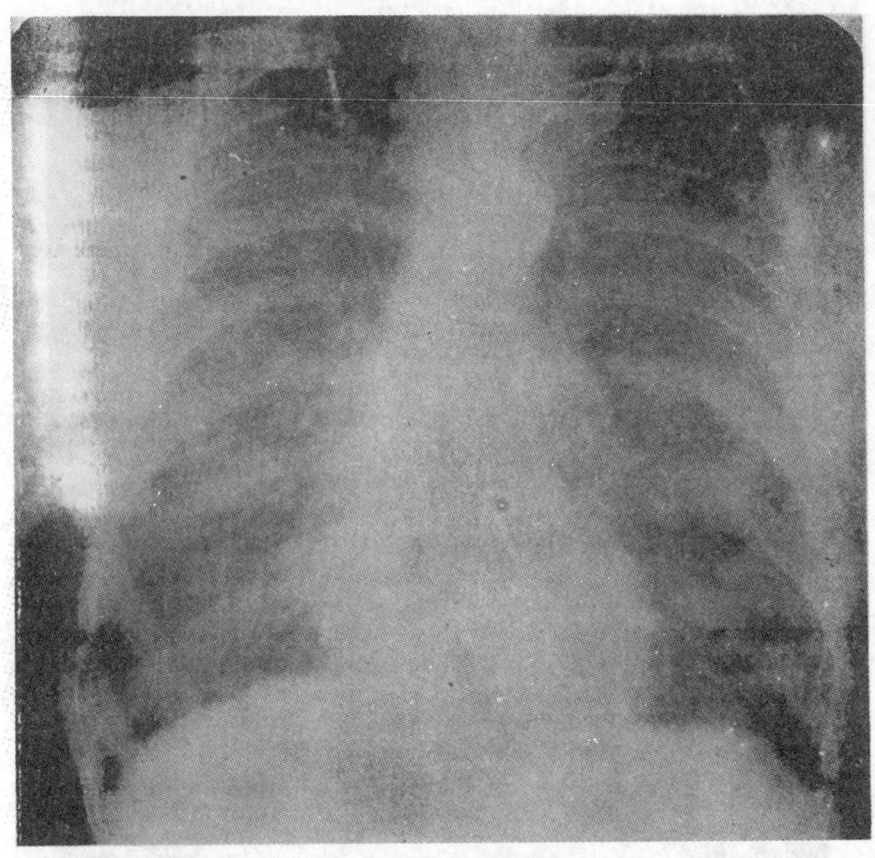

FIG. 63.—CHEST X-RAY showing well-defined nodules of SILICOSIS throughout the lung fields. There is also considerable diffuse pulmonary fibrosis.

cythæmia, clubbed fingers and later cor pulmonale. The X-ray changes confirm. There is a defect in the oxygen exchange in the alveoli in this progressive disease. *Treatment* is symptomatic.

§ **137.** V. **Thickened Pleura** is a condition which sometimes succeeds recurrent dry pleurisy. It is much more common following a chronic empyema, a persistent pleural effusion or a hæmothorax. It is important to recognise it, lest it should be mistaken for some more serious condition, though it is difficult to diagnose. *Physical Signs.*—When the pleura is very thick there is (i.) diminished movement over the affected area of the chest; (ii.) dullness on percussion; (iii.) localised enfeeblement of the respiratory murmur; and (iv.) diminished vocal fremitus and resonance.

The *diagnosis* is arrived at (i.) by the history of the case—*e.g.*, there has been an attack of pleurisy or pneumonia in the past—and (ii.) by the characteristic sensation of going through very thick dense tissue when a needle is inserted. The condition is often discovered only by chance, when the patient seeks advice for other ailments. X-ray examination shows a uniformly dense shadow and if the condition is basal there is restricted movement of the diaphragm: calcified plaques are often seen in the pleura. *Treatment* is not required and usually the condition is of little consequence.

§ **138.** VI. **Malignant Disease of the Bronchus,** frequently known as cancer of the lung, has become very much more common during the last 40 years; in England and Wales the yearly deaths have risen from 250 in 1911–1919 to 12,241 in 1950 and 23,774 in 1962, and the rate continues to rise by about 8 per cent. per annum. It is five times more common in men than in women, and is now the commonest cause of cancer in men and accounts for 1 in 18 of all deaths among males. The disease is almost entirely due to carcinoma of the bronchus, sarcoma being rare: beginning in the bronchial mucous membrane, it spreads to the parenchyma of the lung and forms a large intrathoracic tumour.

Symptoms vary greatly from one patient to another, depending on the site of the tumour and the effect it has on surrounding structures. In the majority of cases it commences near the hilum of the lung; especially when the growth starts more peripherally it may be silent for several months. *Common symptoms* are (i.) a persistent cough, which may not attract attention as a large number of patients are heavy cigarette smokers; (ii.) Pain of pleuritic type or behind the sternum. The first of these may be due to pleural involvement by the growth, but a number are due to infection behind the growth. The retrosternal pain is of a more indefinite but persistent character; (iii.) Unexplained hæmoptysis in a middle-aged or elderly man is common; (iv.) Shortness of breath appears early and is out of proportion to the signs found on examination; (v.) When a bronchus is occluded by growth infection arises distal to the block and the symptoms and signs at first suggest pneumonic consolidation. Later an abscess may form in the lung; (vi.) A recurrent pleural effusion in a patient of middle age, with no history of tuberculosis, is a suspicious sign, especially if on exploration the fluid is found to be uniformly blood-stained; (vii.) The first sign may be due to metastases, with enlargement of glands in the lower neck or the inner wall of the axilla, or the symptoms of a cerebral tumour; (viii.) The recent occurrence of localised wheezing may indicate partial bronchial obstruction. *Invasion of other structures in the chest* may occur early or late and produce (ix.) Left recurrent laryngeal nerve paralysis with a particular type of husky voice (§ 176); (x.) Compression of the superior vena cava causes œdema and cyanosis of the face and neck, with distended jugular veins, and (xi.) When the tumour involves the apex of the lung it causes pain in the corresponding side of the neck and arm. *Rare symptoms* include dysphagia from pressure on the œsophagus; neurological changes due to motor or sensory poly-neuritis or subacute cerebral or cerebellar degeneration; cardiac enlarge-ment with arrhythmia due to invasion of the heart and pericardium. Loss of energy occurs early, loss of weight may be relatively late.

Physical Signs.—In the early stages there may be no signs, just as there may be no symptoms of disease. When there is occlusion of one of the larger bronchi there are signs of a collapsed lobe of the lung with reduced movement of the chest, dullness to percussion, absent air-entry and often reduced vocal resonance in association with deviation of the heart and/or trachea to the affected side. When a pleural effusion is present there are the corresponding signs of fluid and the heart and trachea are displaced to the opposite side of the chest: a combination of collapse of part of the lung with fluid overlying this is not unusual. Pulmonary osteo-arthropathy is occasionally observed.

Pancoast's tumour is not due to a special variety of carcinoma, but is the name given to a carcinoma of the apical or sub-apical segment of the upper lobe. It causes pain in the arm due to invasion of the first thoracic nerve root, pain in the lower neck due to erosion of the vertebral end of the first three ribs and Horner's syndrome due to cervical sympathetic nerve involvement.

Diagnosis may be difficult in the earlier stages. The symptoms which should suggest this diagnosis are an increased cough, pain, recent wheezing and shortness of breath, especially when these are aggravated by change of position. Hæmoptysis often brings the patient for medical attention. A routine mass-miniature chest X-ray may help to make an earlier diag-nosis possible, by revealing an abnormal shadow before symptoms arise: in this case the patient needs either to be under regular supervision with monthly skiagrams, or if the suspicion is a strong one full investigation is immediately required. The diagnosis from unresolved pneumonia re-quires particular care, but any case of pneumonia which is slow in clearing in spite of giving an antibiotic, especially in a man over 45 years of age, should be regarded with suspicion. A diagnosis of senile tuberculosis in a patient with unilateral symptoms and signs should be open to doubt unless tubercle bacilli are found.

Special Investigations.—A growth in the larger tubes is usually visible

PLATE IX

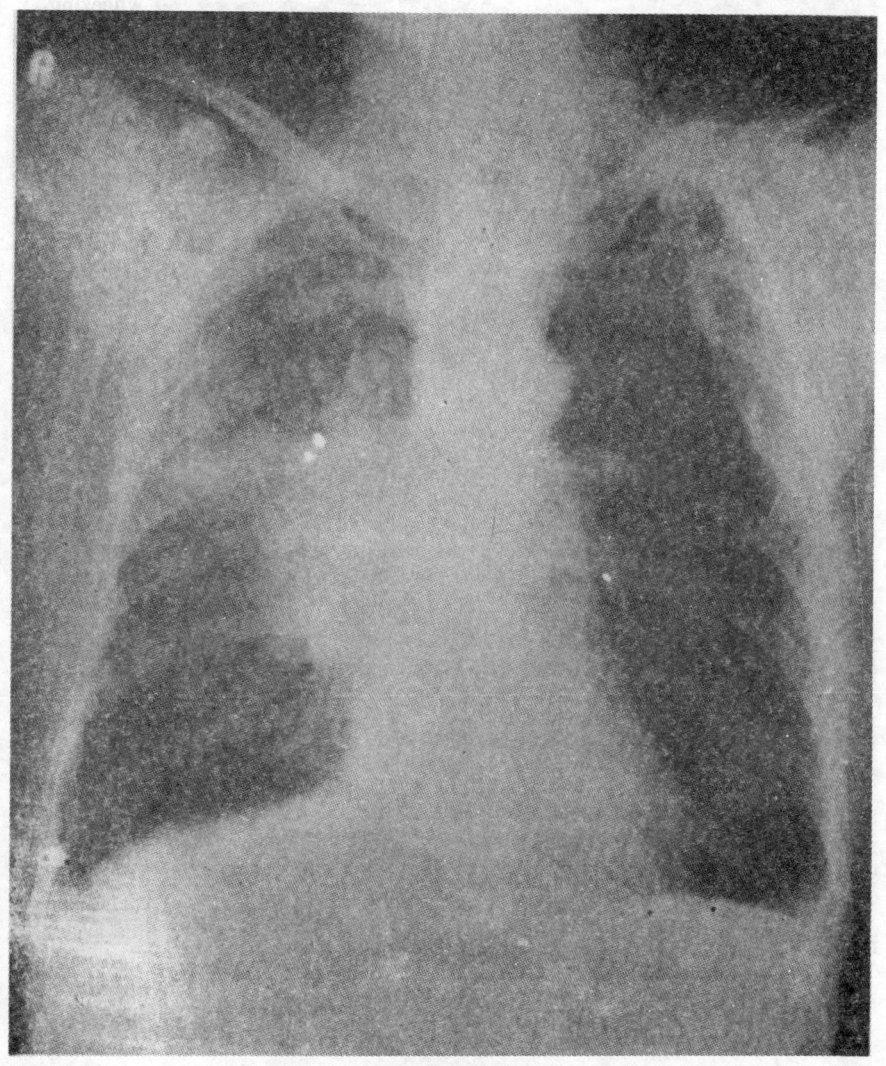

FIG. 64.—X-RAY FILM OF CARCINOMA OF BRONCHUS, spreading from the hilum outwards into the Right Lung.

PLATE X

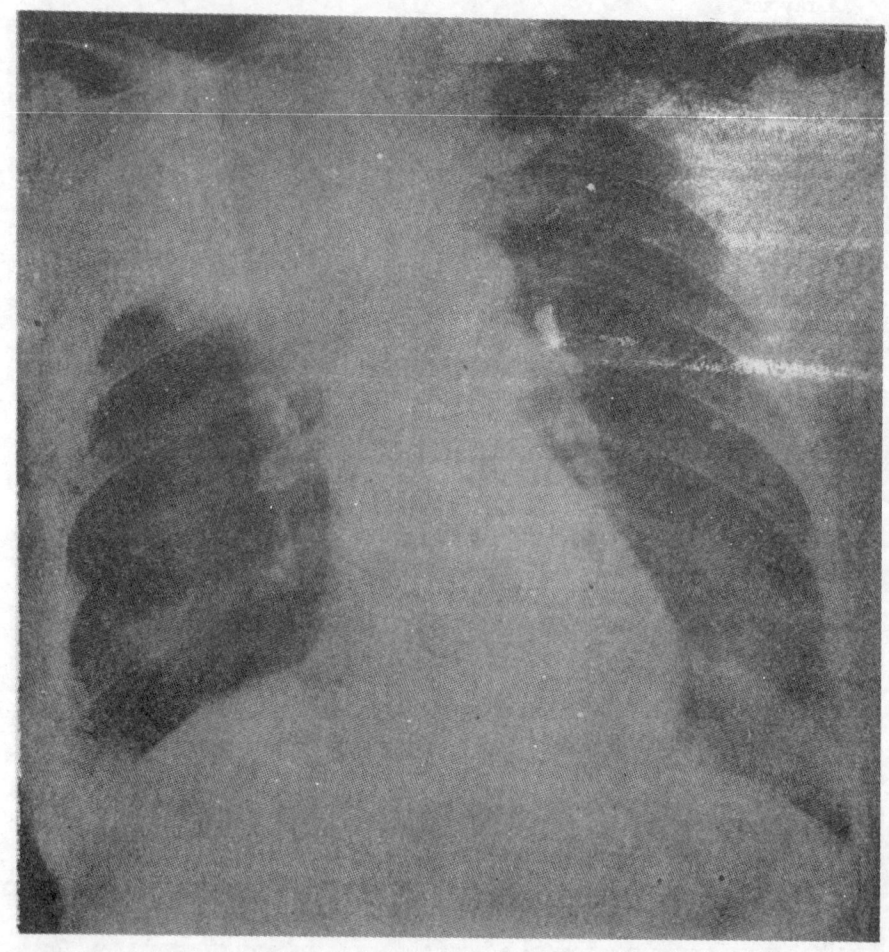

FIG. 65.—X-RAY FILM of the chest of a patient with a CARCINOMA OF THE BRONCHUS, producing complete collapse of the Right Upper Lobe.

with a bronchoscope. Examination with this instrument is therefore essential: it may also demonstrate a deformity at the carina due to pressure of an enlarged gland, and it often permits removal of a small portion of suspicious material for biopsy. In the larger as well as the smaller bronchi X-ray screening aided by films taken in different positions helps to localise an abnormal shadow: narrowing or occlusion of the bronchi even in the more peripheral parts of the lung fields may be revealed by tomography or X-ray after the injection of iodised oil into the trachea (bronchography). In a recent series of cases the original X-ray appearances were those of pulmonary collapse in 64 per cent., a hilar shadow in 17 per cent., a cavity resembling a chronic lung abscess in 10 per cent. and a solitary mass in the lung field in 4 per cent. (Figs. 64, 65). Malignant cells can be found in the sputum or in a pleural effusion in about 60 per cent. of cases if a series of specimens are examined by an expert cytologist, using special staining methods (§ 1213); when there is a pleural effusion pleural biopsy may help (§ 1201). When a doubt still exists, exploratory thoracotomy is justifiable if the condition of the patient allows this.

Etiology.—Bronchial carcinoma is rare before 45, the commonest age in men being between 65 and 75 years of age. The increased incidence is almost certainly the result of chronic irritation of the bronchial mucosa and the disease not infrequently complicates long-standing chronic bronchitis and possibly chronic pulmonary tuberculosis. The factors believed, in the present state of our knowledge, to be causal or contributory are (i.) cigarette smoking. Statistics from seven different countries agree that heavy cigarette smokers are much more liable than non-smokers, the incidence being roughly proportional to the smoking habits of those affected. Some observers have found the death-rate 40 times higher in heavy smokers than in non-smokers. The risk is halved if heavy cigarette smokers give up smoking when 40 years of age. Cigar and pipe smokers are much less heavily afflicted, but filter-tipped cigarettes do not materially lessen the incidence. The carcinogenetic agent responsible is not yet known: it is not nicotine but five possible substances have been isolated, capable of causing cancer in animals. The 3 : 4-benzpyrene present is a well-known carcinogenetic agent. (ii.) The fact that non-smokers can still develop cancer of the bronchus shows that other factors also play a part. Atmospheric pollution is almost certainly one of these, for deaths from the disease are three times higher in thickly populated cities than in rural areas: perhaps diesel-exhaust fumes play a part. (iii.) A relatively small number of cases are due to industrial hazards. Men working with nickel, hæmatite, chromate, with gas-retorts and those handling asbestos are rather more susceptible.

Prognosis.—At least 75–80 per cent. of cases when first seen are beyond radical treatment, which means that every endeavour must be made to facilitate an earlier diagnosis. Of the patients operated upon about 20 per cent. survive more than 5 years, so that the chance of a patient when first seen by the physician being alive in 5 years' time is about

5 per cent. There are three main histological types: (i.) the highly malignant and largely anaplastic oat-celled tumour; (ii.) the squamous-celled
carcinoma which spreads less widely but tends to necrose centrally to
form an abscess, and (iii.) the adeno-carcinoma. Only the first two of
these types seem to be etiologically related to cigarette-smoking.

Treatment.—Surgical treatment gives the only hope of eradication of
the disease: it is usually reserved for patients under 65 years of age who
are in a good physical condition and without evidence of spread beyond
the lung. The operation of resecting large areas of the contents of the chest
has now been largely abandoned. On the other hand radical lobectomy
or pneumonectomy, including a block dissection of the mediastinal glands,
is more often successful. The majority of patients when first seen are
not suitable for these measures, in which case a palliative lobectomy for
a breaking-down growth may make the patient more comfortable. Deep
X-ray therapy may give temporary relief from an exhausting cough or
recurrent hæmoptysis but produces a severe constitutional reaction. Antibiotics may aid when there is secondary infection in a growth. In the
advanced stages methadone, pethidine or morphine are often required
and the Brompton Hospital " cocktail " (morphine $\frac{1}{6}$–$\frac{1}{4}$ gr., cocaine hydrochlor. $\frac{1}{8}$ gr. with gin 1 fl. oz.) may give symptomatic relief.

VII. **Secondary Malignant Disease of the Lung** occurs as numerous,
scattered, more or less circumscribed nodules, and is always secondary to
cancer of the breast or abdominal organs. Sarcoma of any part of the
body may give rise to secondary deposits in the lungs.

Symptoms.—The most common symptoms are increasing dyspnœa,
cough, and cyanosis. Much respiratory distress occurs when a large area
of lung tissue has become involved. Miliary carcinomatosis, which is
usually secondary to carcinoma of other organs, especially the stomach,
causes great dyspnœa and cyanosis (Assmann). Whereas hæmoptysis is
common with primary malignant disease, it is very unusual with secondary
deposits. The *physical signs* are often very indefinite. When a large
surface of the pleura is involved, the first sign may be an effusion into
the pleura; on exploration the fluid may be found to be hæmorrhagic.
X-ray examination may show one or more " cannon-ball " tumours
(Fig. 66): when there is only a single opacity it may be due to a primary
carcinoma of the bronchus and should be treated as such.

We now turn to the less common and the rare chronic diseases
attended by **dullness on percussion,** not always in regular or DEFINED
AREAS AT BASE OR APEX. These are: VIII. COLLAPSE OF THE LUNG;
IX. HYDATID CYST; X. SARCOIDOSIS; XI. SYPHILIS OF THE LUNG; XII.
Some of the DISEASES DUE TO FUNGI AND PARASITES.

§ 139. VIII. **Collapse of the Lung,** or **Atelectasis,** is a condition in which
the lung tissue is in an unexpanded state. The term " atelectasis " is
usually applied to lung tissue which has never properly expanded, a

PLATE XI

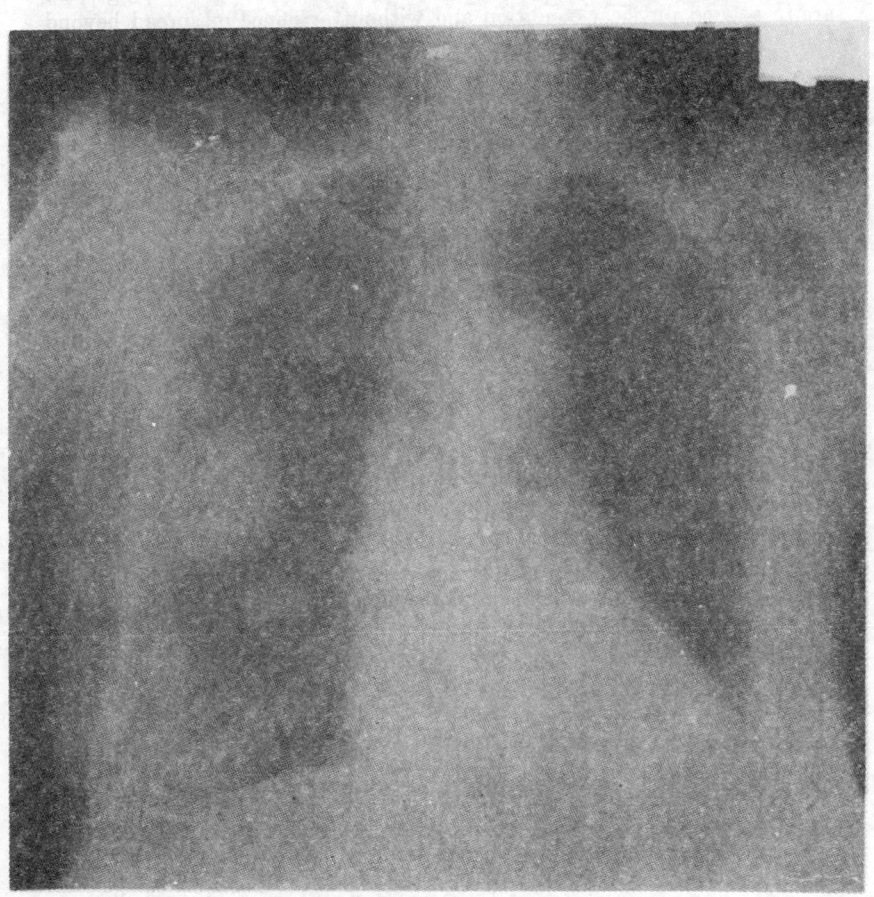

FIG. 66.—X-RAY FILM of chest showing circular shadows in the Right Lung, due to SECONDARY DEPOSITS from a CARCINOMA OF CERVIX UTERI.

PLATE XII

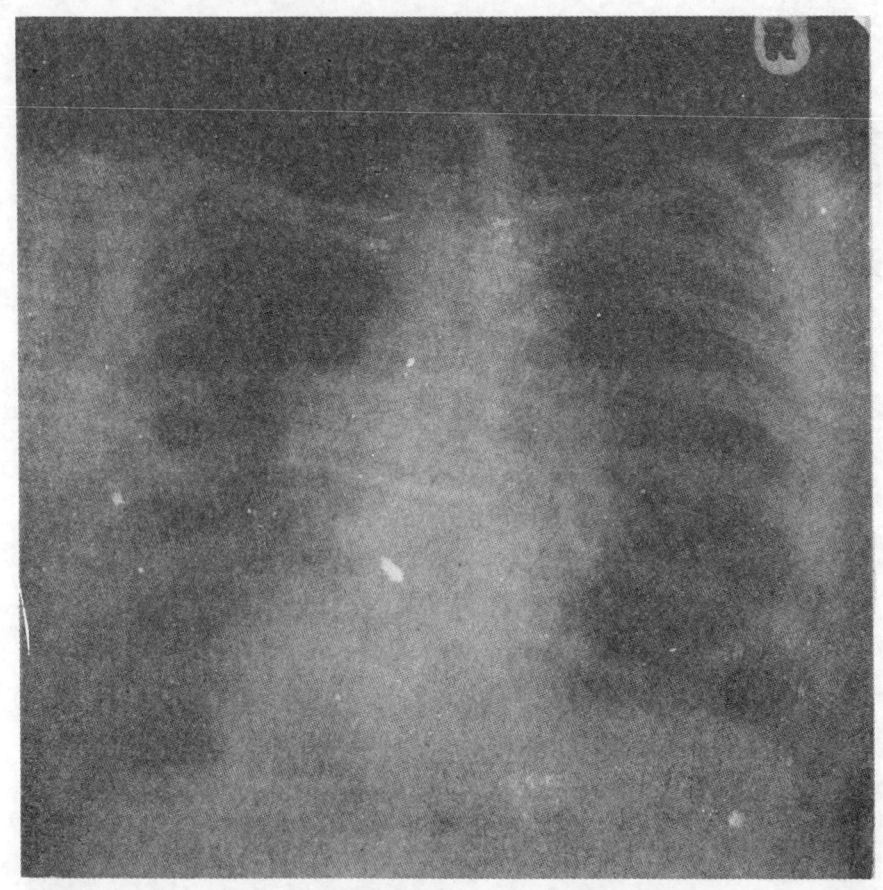

FIG. 67.—CHEST X-RAY of a woman aged 47 suffering from SARCOIDOSIS OF THE LUNGS. There is mottling of the lung fields with considerable enlargement of the hilar lymph glands.

congenital condition, due to imperfect development. The term " collapse of the lung " is applied to lung tissue which has previously expanded, but in which the air vesicles have subsequently collapsed.

Atelectasis is a *congenital* condition. The *symptoms* occurring in the new-born child consist of cyanosis, with shallow, rapid respiration. The lower part of the chest is drawn in by each respiration. On auscultation, the respiratory murmur is found to be very faint.

Collapse of the lung complicates the primary disease which has led to its occurrence. Acute massive collapse such as occurs after abdominal operations is described in § 125. A more chronic condition should be suspected when the breathing is more embarrassed than can be accounted for by the concurrent disease in the chest. The physical signs vary considerably with the degree of collapse. Thus:

(a) In *complete* collapse of a part of the lung, as, for instance, in collapse due to compression or complete obstruction of a main bronchus, there is reduced movement of the chest wall, impairment of the percussion note, with a diminution or absence of the breath sounds and of the vocal resonance and fremitus.

(b) Where the collapse is only *partial* in degree—*e.g.*, where the bronchi remain patent, as occurs sometimes when the lung is compressed by pleural or pericardial effusion—there are signs resembling those of consolidation (§ 109), except that the percussion note is not so dull and the breath sounds, though bronchial in character, are somewhat feeble.

(c) Where the collapse is *slight* and limited, the chief sign is an enfeebled respiratory murmur. During deep inspiration fine rustling crepitations are heard, due to the expansion of the collapsed vesicles.

If the collapse is extensive the heart and mediastinum are drawn over to the side of the lesion.

The *Diagnosis* is made usually by the existence of a causal condition. It will be observed that the signs of partial collapse resemble the signs of consolidation and those due to slight collapse resemble early pneumonia, but in neither of these is the position of the heart and trachea altered. Radiography may give valuable confirmation of the condition and may help to reveal the cause; the airless portion of the lung appears as a more or less homogeneous opacity. Localised collapse may be recognised by X-ray examination. Routine X-ray examinations show that localised pulmonary collapse, without symptoms, is much more frequent than was originally supposed. It is particularly common in children, despite the absence of obvious clinical manifestations of disease.

Etiology.—Common causes are: (a) those due to *obstruction* such as (i.) a foreign body or a thick plug of secretion in the lumen (see § 123, (2)); (ii.) carcinoma, adenoma or stricture within a bronchus; (iii.) pressure from outside the bronchus as by a growth, aneurysm or an enlarged gland. (b) An *active* collapse occurs when the usual negative intrathoracic pressure disappears with a pneumothorax. (c) *Compression* of the lung may be produced by pleural or pericardial effusion, an enlarged heart or tumours of the mediastinum. The condition may be the result of gross spinal curvature. (d) *Paralysis* of the intercostal muscles or diaphragm as in acute poliomyelitis. (e) *Injury* to the chest wall with or without involvement of the thoracic contents, especially by high velocity projectiles, is a fertile cause of collapse of lung either on the same or the opposite side.

In *adults* collapse is most often met with as the result of pleural effusion or tumours in the chest; in *children*, as the result of bronchitis or slight catarrhal affections of the respiratory tract.

Prognosis.—The course of the disease depends very much upon the cause. Recovery as a rule soon takes place after compression by effusion, obstruction or stricture of the bronchi, and throat affections.

Treatment must be directed to removal of the cause, and especially to the use of measures which will remove obstructing secretions from the bronchi: antibiotics may help this. In persistent cases bronchoscopy may be needed to identify the cause and to clear the air-way. Respiratory exercises should be given (and see § 125).

§ 140. IX. Hydatid of the lung and pleura is much more common in the Argentine and Australia than in this country. Generally cysts are single and tend to involve the base of the lung, especially on the right side. Clinically they remain latent in 75 per cent. of cases till the supervention of some complication such as hæmoptysis, rupture or suppuration. A history of the expectoration of " grape skins " is pathognomonic; cough is frequent. The physical signs resemble those of a pleural effusion, but the area of dullness is localised and has a rounded outline. Apical hydatid simulates tuberculosis, but the pulse is slower and fever less marked.

The *Diagnosis* of deep cysts is often impossible until X-ray reveals the characteristic spherical shadow surrounded by translucent lung tissue. Eosinophilia is generally absent, but the Casoni intradermal test is almost invariably positive, the complement fixation and precipitin tests less frequently so. The sputum may contain hydatid elements such as hooklets, scolices or laminated membrane.

The *Prognosis* largely depends on the presence or absence of complications. Many cases undergo spontaneous cure by rupture into a bronchus; others may be drowned in the process or develop laryngeal obstruction. Rupture into the pulmonary artery or heart is fatal. Secondary infection may lead to pulmonary abscess or empyema. Cysts of the liver frequently coexist (§ 347).

Treatment is by thoracotomy, incision and evacuation of the cyst content with or without drainage. Aspiration is dangerous owing to the danger of flooding the bronchial tree.

§ 141. X. Sarcoidosis (Besnier-Boeck-Schauman Disease).—Much attention has been directed in recent years to the pulmonary manifestations of this generalised disease which may involve almost any part of the body. The organs most commonly affected are the skin (§ 710), the lungs, the lymph glands, the liver, and the iris and choroid of the eyes: less commonly affected areas are the mucous membranes of the nose and throat, the parotid and lachrymal glands (see Mikulicz's syndrome, § 9), the bones, spleen, kidneys, gastro-intestinal tract, the myocardium and the central nervous system (§ 889).

In the chest the most constant feature is enlargement of the hilar glands. In addition, there is a general reticulosis which may progress to an interstitial fibrosis of the lungs with a tendency to nodulation. Occasionally, diffuse and confluent parenchymatous infiltrations are seen throughout the lung-fields.

Symptoms.—The disease is of insidious onset and occurs particularly in those between 20 and 40 years of age: patients may be symptomless, the condition being discovered by routine X-ray examination. The most frequent chest symptom is dyspnœa: there may be slight constitutional disturbance, *e.g.*, pyrexia, lassitude and anorexia, with occasional cough. If the condition progresses to an extensive fibrosis, dyspnœa is likely to become more severe. The radiological picture is of bilateral enlargement of the hilar glands: less commonly there is a fine miliary infiltration of the lungs with peribronchial thickening. Later a fine diffuse fibrosis makes its appearance. Skin manifestations occur in 50 per cent. of cases.

Etiology.—Sarcoidosis is almost certainly of infective origin and presents granulomatous lesions in the affected organs: histologically there are collections of pale staining epithelioid cells among which giant-cells occur. The main distinction between these lesions and tubercles is the absence of caseation and of tubercle bacilli. The three chief hypotheses as to the pathogenesis of these lesions are that they are (*a*) due to tuberculosis of an atypical and anergic form, since the Mantoux reaction is negative; (*b*) a non-specific tissue response called forth by a variety of pathogenic organisms such as the tubercle and lepra bacilli; (*c*) a manifestation of a generalised systemic disease, allied to the collagen diseases such as polyarteritis nodosa and lupus erythematosus.

The *Diagnosis* is from miliary tuberculosis, silicosis, chronic beryllium poisoning and from miliary carcinomatosis. In an X-ray the enlargement of the hilar glands is the most constant and reliable feature: this is often found by mass miniature X-ray without any symptoms being present. The blood shows a very high erythrocyte sedimentation rate with an altered albumen/globulin ratio in the serum: there is often a mild anæmia, with no leucocytosis but occasionally monocytes or eosinophils are in excess. The diagnosis is established by (i.) the chest X-ray; (ii.) biopsy of a skin lesion or a lymph gland; (iii.) X-ray of the small bones of the hands which may show rarefaction and later punched-out areas in the medulla without a periosteal reaction; (iv.) the high E.S.R. is helpful; (v.) the Kveim test is positive in over 80 per cent. of cases. An extract from a cutaneous nodule of a proven case when injected intradermally produces a local skin nodule and sometimes ulceration, after an interval of 1, 2 or more weeks: it is wise to confirm the diagnosis by biopsy of the induced lesion.

The *Prognosis* is usually favourable, the disease pursuing a chronic course and tending to recovery. Progressive pulmonary fibrosis leads to cor pulmonale, and left ventricular failure occurs when the disease affects the myocardium. In about 10 per cent. of cases pulmonary tuberculosis develops and the Mantoux reaction becomes positive.

Treatment.—Often no treatment is needed. Drugs have little influence on the disease. Treatment with prednisolone 5 mg. q.i.d. is advisable when there is involvement of the eyes, the myocardium, or when the X-ray shows miliary pulmonary changes: to prevent pulmonary tuberculosis arising, simultaneous administration of P.A.S. and isoniazid is recommended.

§ 142. XI. Syphilis of the Lung.—In *infants* this disease may take one of two forms: (*a*) The pneumonic condition of lung, found in infants, usually still-born, is regarded as an interstitial pneumonia of syphilitic origin. (*b*) Gummata are occasionally met with in the lungs of infants who are the subjects of hereditary syphilis; still more rarely they are met with in adults. Dyspnœa is usually the only symptom. The signs are those of consolidation and collapse. In *adults* it is extremely rare: it may cause broncho-pneumonia, bronchiectasis, and may lead to extensive infiltration and breaking down, or to fibrosis. For mediastinal gummata see § 81. VII.

XII. DISEASES DUE TO FUNGI AND PARASITES are recognised on examination of the sputum, and are referred to in §§ 147 and 148.

GROUP C.—CHRONIC DISEASES attended by **Hyper-resonance** on percussion: I. In the majority of cases it is present equally on the two sides and is due to EMPHYSEMA. Other conditions which give rise to it are: II. PNEUMOTHORAX (§ 126); III. SKODAIC RESONANCE above the level of an effusion (§ 108 and Fig. 55). The diagnosis is given in the form of a table (Table VIII).

TABLE VIII.—CAUSES OF HYPER-RESONANCE

Cause.	Hyper-resonance.	Auscultation.	Other Diagnostic Features.
I. Emphysema.	Bilateral and universal.	R.M. distinct but weak and expiration prolonged; signs of bronchitis, if present.	Barrel-shaped chest, cardiac dullness obscured.
II. Pneumothorax. An acute condition.	Hyper-resonance always unilateral, though it may extend beyond middle line.	Absence of R.M. and V.F. over affected area; sometimes amphoric breathing and bell sound.	Heart and trachea moved to opposite side.
III. Skodaic Resonance. —i.e., the high-pitched note above a large *pleural effusion*, when the lung is otherwise healthy.	Unilateral; level may shift with position of patient.	Loud R.M.; V.F. felt above the fluid level.	History of pleurisy; signs of fluid in lower part of chest; heart and trachea moved to opposite side.

I. *The patient is probably an* ELDERLY MAN *who has complained of increasing* BREATHLESSNESS *for some years. He is subject to recurrent bronchitis or asthma. There is* **hyper-resonance** *of* **both** *lungs and the chest is barrel-shaped. The disease is* HYPERTROPHIC EMPHYSEMA.

§ 143. Hypertrophic Emphysema is a common disease of the lungs, occurring in later middle life and in the elderly, and much more often in men than in women. It is a chronic progressive condition in which the air vesicles become hyper-distended and the walls separating the vesicles inelastic, thinned and even ruptured. This reduces the capillary bed in the alveoli with corresponding diminution in the ærating surface; and as the lungs are deficient in their elastic recoil, the chest remains in a permanent position of over-distension.

Symptoms.—(1) The onset is imperceptible but gradually shortness of breath becomes evident, at first on exertion and later even at rest, causing dyspnœa and orthopnœa. (2) There is usually a history of chronic cough due to bronchitis, or of asthma; after a series of attacks of either of these the breathlessness becomes more marked. (3) With the passage of time the symptoms of bronchitis become more persistent, not only in the cold foggy winter months but even in the summer. (4) A sense of lassitude and ready fatigue is noticeable. (5) The breathlessness becomes much worse when the right side of the heart begins to fail: emphysema with chronic bronchitis is the commonest cause of right heart failure at and after middle age.

Physical Signs.—The *general appearance* of the patient is often characteristic. The face is congested and the appearances polycythæmic.

He has a short thick " bull neck " with raised clavicles, and in the later stages the jugular veins are distended. On *inspecting the chest* the breathing is a little quicker and shallower than normal. The chest is barrel-shaped: the ribs are raised and the dorsal spine kyphotic so the antero-posterior diameter of the chest is increased. In many cases there is a reduced expansion of the chest on deep breathing from $2\frac{1}{2}$–3 inches or more to 1–$1\frac{1}{2}$ inches or less. Palpation confirms the lack of expansion and as the borders of the heart are covered by expanded lung tissue it is usually impossible to feel the apex of the heart—even localisation of the apex by auscultation may be difficult. Percussion gives a high pitched note over the whole of both lungs: since the over-distended lung covers the heart and the upper border of the liver the hyper-resonance extends over these areas. On auscultation the vesicular murmur is weak, expiration is distinctly prolonged and bronchitic râles and bronchospasm are often present. In the normal person diaphragmatic movements contribute about 40 per cent. to the filling and emptying of the lungs but in emphysema there is only a small excursion of the diaphragm and little movement of the abdominal wall. By *X-ray examination* there is seen to be an abnormal translucency of the lungs combined with a characteristic shape of the chest, widely spaced ribs, greatly diminished movements of the diaphragm and sometimes emphysematous bullæ are found: but care should be taken not to make a diagnosis of emphysema on the strength of an over-exposed chest film. Pulmonary ventilation tests show a reduction of the vital capacity and of the maximum breathing capacity (§ 112) roughly in proportion to the severity of the disease.

Diagnosis.—The cardinal symptom is shortness of breath and emphysema should never be diagnosed in the absence of this. *Pneumothorax* also produces hyper-resonance to percussion, but the condition is unilateral, and of acute onset. *Chronic myocardial degeneration* causes shortness of breath and later the signs of right heart failure in an elderly subject. This condition may co-exist with emphysema but when the heart is diseased it is also considerably enlarged as shown by radiological examination.

Etiology.—The *cause* is not known with certainty, but some factors are known to be important. (1) There is a loss of elasticity in the lungs, partly on account of age, so that the elastic recoil of the lungs which normally causes them to empty becomes increasingly deficient. This may help to explain the tendency of emphysema to have a family incidence. There is evidence that such degenerative changes may in part be due to sclerosis of the nutritive bronchial arteries. (2) Any obstruction to expiration materially contributes. The act of coughing is performed against a partially closed larynx and causes the intra-alveolar pressure to rise suddenly to 20–30 cm. of water. Therefore chronic bronchitis, with its cough and narrowed bronchial lumen (§ 129), and the bronchospasm of asthma (§ 127) are important causative factors. (3) In emphysema the distribution of inspired air is not uniform: there is an area in the lungs (the " poorly ventilated space ") which takes little part in the normal gaseous interchanges. The *compensatory mechanisms* which take place in emphysema are (1) polycythæmia; (2) an increased output of the left and of the right heart. The greater pressure in the jugular veins, the right auricle, right ventricle and pulmonary artery is part of this compensatory process; (3) the respiratory centre acquires an increased tolerance to carbon dioxide.

Prognosis.—Patients with emphysema may live to a good age and provided it is only moderate in degree it does not necessarily shorten life, though it predisposes to, and adds to, the seriousness of other pulmonary disorders. The gravity of any particular case is dependent on the amount of bronchitis or of asthma, and particularly whether there is evidence of right heart failure.

Treatment.—The indications are: (i.) to relieve any cause of coughing. Excessive smoking must cease and steps be taken to relieve the cough of bronchitis (§ 129); (ii.) bronchospasm is almost invariably present and may be severe in cases of recurrent asthma. Small regular doses of ephedrine often relieve this and other suitable measures are described in § 127; (iii.) to aid the emptying of the alveoli, expiratory breathing exercises are of service and when the abdominal wall is slack and diaphragmatic movements particularly weak, wearing an elastic abdominal support (" emphysema belt ") is of help; (iv.) obesity should be corrected for this reduces the oxygen requirements of the body and may increase the efficiency of the respiratory mechanism; (v.) the right side of the heart is enlarged by hypertrophy (cor pulmonale) but when symptoms and signs of right heart failure occur these must receive attention (§ 62). Oxygen inhalation tends to relieve cyanosis but in advanced cases prolonged administration may be dangerous. In emphysema the respiratory centre is relatively insensitive to carbon dioxide and oxygen-lack plays an important part in stimulating it: if oxygen is given for a long period, the stimulant effect of oxygen deficiency is absent and carbon dioxide accumulates giving rise to CO_2 intoxication, with drowsiness, delirium, coma and death. Therefore it is wise to give oxygen only for 15 minutes at a time each hour; (vi.) sleep is most important but morphia can be very dangerous.

§ 144. Other Types of Emphysema are:

Atrophic Emphysema occurs in old people as a result of degenerative changes. There is some shortness of breath on exertion; but there is no barrel-shaped chest and although the breath sounds are weak the lungs are not enlarged and do not overlap the præ ordial area and the liver dullness.

Compensatory Emphysema is present as dilated air vesicles in the same lung around areas of obstruction or scarring, and in the opposite lung in conditions such as pneumothorax, a collapsed or a fibroid lung. There is hyper-resonance over the area affected which is in marked contrast to the dullness to percussion over an area of solid lung.

Mediastinal Emphysema occurs when air escapes from a ruptured air vesicle into the interstitial tissues. It is usually first detected when it spreads to the subcutaneous areas of the lower neck or around the site of a recent pleural puncture and gives a characteristic crackling feeling when a finger is pressed over the part. The air is prevented from involving the face by the platysma muscle. The causes are (i.) traumatic, such as arise from a fractured rib or a penetrating wound of the chest wall; (ii.) spontaneous in association with a violent cough as in whooping-cough or occasionally with pneumonia. The air is spontaneously absorbed in 2–3 days once the cause has been remedied.

GROUP D.—There are three chronic pulmonary conditions in which the percussion note varies considerably in different cases, but the **character of the sputum** suggests their presence—viz.: I. BRONCHIECTASIS AND FŒTID BRONCHITIS; II. GANGRENE AND ABSCESS OF THE LUNG (*vide* § 111). In Abscess the sputum is not invariably offensive. III. ACTINOMYCOSIS and other diseases due to fungi and parasites affecting the lung can usually be diagnosed only by examination of the sputum.

The patient gives a history of recurrent attacks of pulmonary consolidation and now complains of a cough with PURULENT SPUTUM *which may be* OFFENSIVE. *There may be* HÆMOPTYSIS. *The lungs show evidence of localised fibrosis especially in the lower lobes and leathery râles are present. The disease is* **bronchiectasis.**

§ 145. I. Bronchiectasis is a cylindrical or saccular dilatation of the bronchial tubes: when the smaller tubes are involved it is sometimes known as bronchiolectasis. It is always secondary to some other pathological process and is not strictly speaking a disease *sui generis*. The situation of the dilatation depends on the cause but it is more common in the lower than in the upper lobes. It occurs at any age and may be met in small children or in middle-aged or elderly adults. It can exist for some time without sputum but sooner or later infection occurs.

Symptoms.—The most characteristic is a persistent but paroxysmal cough with sputum. In typical cases there are bouts of coughing at intervals varying from a few hours to a day or so accompanied by the expectoration of sputum. The cough and sputum are often started by some change of position and are therefore frequent when the patient wakes in the morning. The amount of sputum is at first small but in advanced cases the total amount expectorated during 24 hours may be considerable (up to 20 fl. oz. or more). The sputum is purulent due to secondary infection, and sooner or later may become extremely fœtid and offensive owing to stagnation and to the presence of saprophytic and/or anærobic organisms. In later cases, and occasionally even at an early stage, there is a characteristic sweet sickly odour to the breath and to the sputum, of which the patient may be acutely conscious. This fœtor depends on the presence of putrefactive bacteria in the sputum. On standing, the sputum divides into three more or less distinct layers, the upper one frothy and muco-purulent, the middle more fluid and the lower one chiefly pus, in which may be found numerous organisms including spirochætes, crystals of fatty acids and foul-smelling yellowish Dittrich's plugs which consist of leucocytes, fat and epithelial cells. Hæmoptysis, occasionally an early symptom, may occur at any stage, and in advanced cases may be considerable, often causing a diagnosis of phthisis. Shortness of breath is not usually marked, but acute respiratory infections are common especially in the winter months and then broncho-pneumonia is likely to arise. *Constitutional symptoms* depend on the severity of the disease: in advanced cases the chronic infection present causes recurrent fever, general lassitude, loss of appetite and some loss of weight.

The *Physical Signs* of bronchiectasis as such may be absent: thus when it exists in association with the inflammatory process and the scarring of pulmonary tuberculosis, the signs are those of the fibrotic or fibrocaseous changes of this disease. When, however, as often happens bronchiectasis occurs in a fibrotic area in the lower lobe of one or both lungs, there are signs of consolidation and fibrosis (§ 136) in association with sticky or "leathery" râles which persist after coughing. When there are comparatively large cavities present, after emptying by posturing the patient, the corresponding signs (§ 109) may be found. Clubbing of the fingers is almost always present, and varies in extent according to the degree of infection and toxæmia.

Diagnosis.—Chronic cough, aggravated by movement or change of posture, and accompanied by the typical offensive sputum, is usually sufficient to distinguish the presence of bronchiectasis, especially when accompanied by the physical signs of fibrosis and cavitation. In earlier cases, where there is little structural damage to the lung tissue, and little infection, the diagnosis may only be established by radiology; even a plain X-ray film may fail to show appearances which are pathognomonic but when the bronchi are filled with iodised oil the appearances are unmistakable (*vide* Fig. 68). The bronchi are crowded together and instead of tapering as they spread to the periphery they show cylindrical or saccular dilatation. It is sometimes difficult to distinguish bronchiectasis from abscess of the lung, especially as the two conditions are frequently associated and are often part of one pathological process (see § 146).

Dry (hæmorrhagic) bronchiectasis (Syn.: Silent Bronchiectasis). In this form of the disease, which is now recognised as a clinical entity, infection has not occurred, and consequently the clinical picture above described does not appear. The condition is characterised by hæmoptysis of varying severity occurring at intervals; between these attacks the patient exhibits neither symptoms nor abnormal physical signs. This variety of bronchiectasis, which is one of the possible causes of sudden hæmoptysis, is only demonstrable by bronchography.

Polycystic disease of the lung resembles bronchiectasis or, rather, bronchiolectasis. It may be congenital in origin: however, many cases in adults are due to acquired causes. In this latter group, often known as "honeycomb lung," the disease may be localised or widespread: it is probably due to obliteration of some bronchioles and compensatory dilatation of neighbouring bronchioles, which form multiple cysts. There are many causes, including eosinophilic granuloma, sarcoidosis and berylliosis. *Symptoms* may be absent, or there may be cough, sputum, shortness of breath and

PLATE XIII

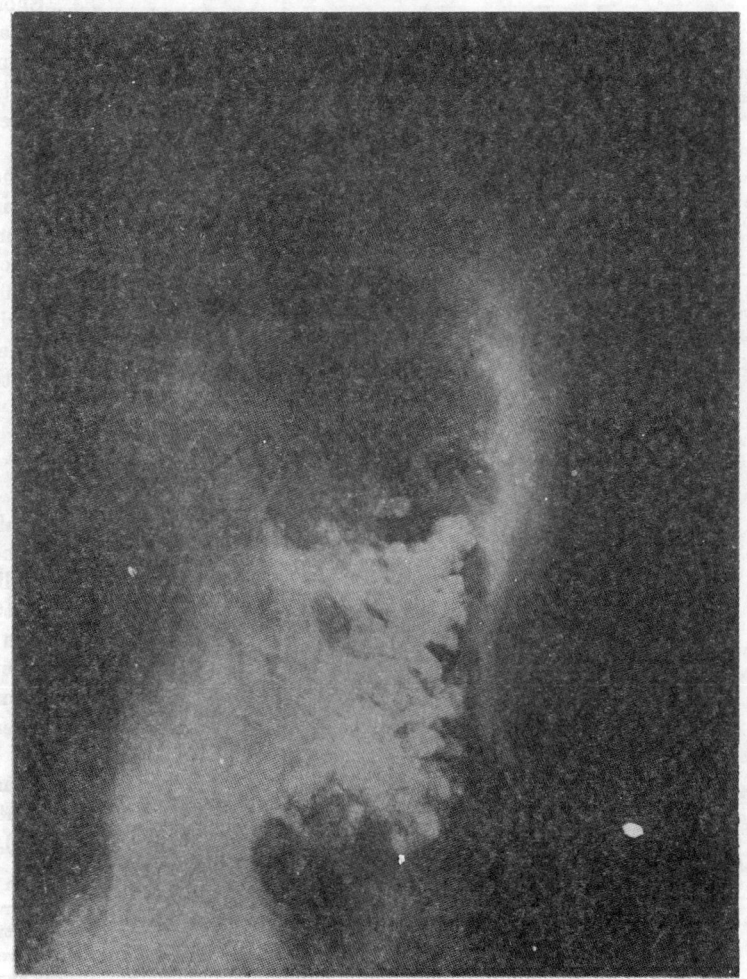

FIG. 68.-CHEST X-RAY showing left basal BRONCHIECTASIS. The dilated bronchi have been
outlined by iodised oil (Bronchography).

PLATE XIV

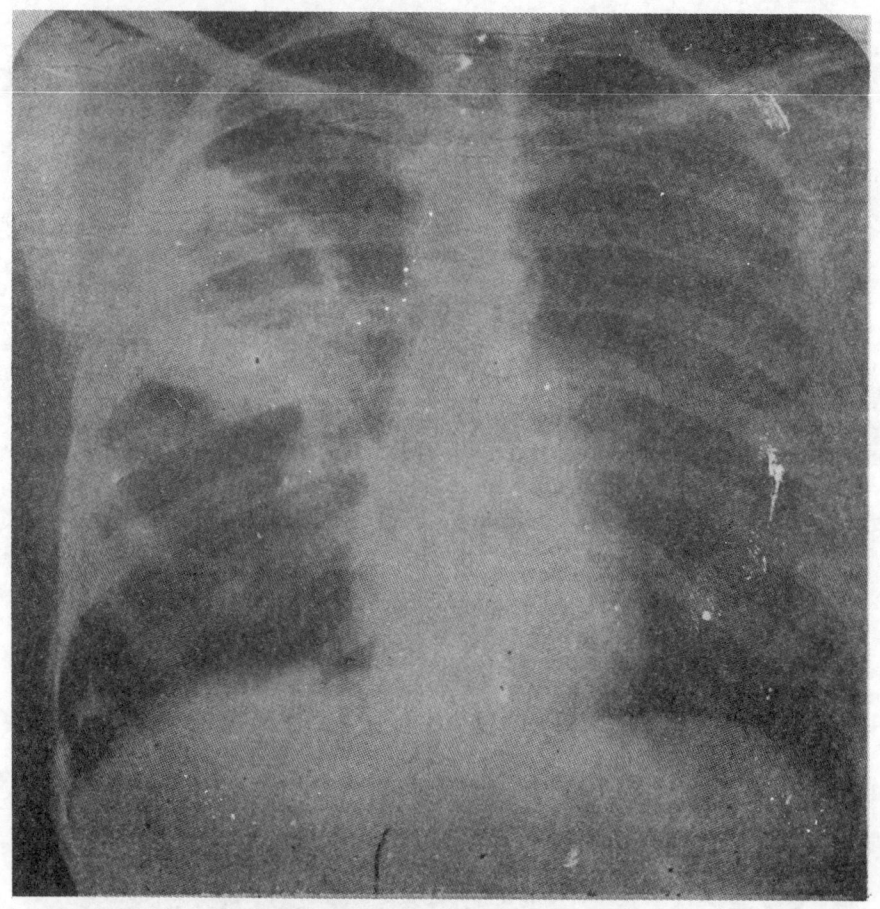

FIG. 60.—CHEST X-RAY showing an ABSCESS CAVITY in the Right Lung. The ringed opacity, within which is shown a horizontal fluid level with air above, is diagnostic.

recurrent hæmoptyses. The X-ray appearances are characteristic and give rise to the so-called " soap-bubble " lung.

Solitary cysts of the lung are frequently recognised on X-ray examination and are congenital. In small children a tension cyst may suddenly enlarge and cause severe dyspnœa. Although *Symptoms* are usually absent hæmorrhage and infection of the cysts may arise.

Etiology.—Bronchiectasis is almost invariably accompanied by pulmonary fibrosis. There are at least three major causes which contribute to the pathogenesis of this condition. (1) The most important is a blocked bronchus leading to pulmonary collapse: by bronchography it has in many cases been possible to demonstrate dilated bronchi within such a collapsed lobe. (2) There is some weakening of the bronchial wall due to infective processes. (3) Once the disease has commenced there may be the additional factor of increased intra-bronchial pressure due to excessive coughing or to asthmatic spasm. (4) A more doubtful factor is the traction of fibrous tissue. The conditions which particularly give rise to bronchiectasis are periodic infections of the lower respiratory tract with plugs of mucus or muco-pus producing atelectasis, especially with measles, whooping-cough or unresolved pneumonia and with bronchial obstruction due to a foreign body, neoplasm, chronic tuberculosis, aneurysm, or syphilitic stricture. It is also seen in association with a thickened pleura and following empyema.

The *Prognosis* depends on the stage reached. Some early cases clear up completely and a bronchogram will confirm this. Once the disease has become advanced with much foul sputum and recurrent fresh infections the condition is permanent and tends to progress as adjacent healthy tissue becomes involved. The *Complications* which may occur are attacks of broncho-pneumonia, abscess or gangrene. of the lung, a cerebral abscess or pyæmia: a fatal hæmorrhage from the lung is rare. Pulmonary osteoarthropathy is sometimes seen.

Treatment.—Conservative Treatment. The first aim is to promote bronchial drainage of the areas of lung involved: when the site and extent of the cavities are known, postural drainage over the side of the bed or in a Nelson bed should be undertaken daily: the position of the patient must be arranged so that the infected area is uppermost and this position is maintained for 20–30 minutes twice a day. Stimulating expectorants such as Mist. ammoniæ et senegæ help to liquefy the sputum. To produce a deodorant and antiseptic effect liberal inhalations of creosote may be used: this is best performed with a creosote vapour bath. Patients (whose eyes are protected by closely fitting goggles) are placed in a more or less air-tight room in which crude creosote is volatilised by placing it in a shallow iron dish which is supported on a stout ring and heated by a Bunsen burner. Terebene or creosote (refined) may be given by mouth in capsules (3 to 5 minims of the oil) three times a day. Especially when an acute pyrexial bout supervenes antibiotics should be given by injection, after bacteriological culture and sensitivity tests have been performed:

penicillin inhalations are not so often used now as formerly. In established cases *Surgical Treatment* is the only method of eradicating the disease. When the condition of the patient allows, lobectomy or pneumonectomy are the operations of choice, but they are not performed until the patient has had a few weeks of treatment to build up the general health first.

§ 146. II. Abscess and Gangrene of the Lung have become much more rare in recent years, partly because early chemotherapy has become the routine treatment of infective conditions in general and also because of the great improvement in methods of anæsthesia. For practical purposes it is convenient to consider abscess and gangrene of the lung under one heading. The distribution of lung abscess may be single or multiple. Single abscesses are more often found in the right lung than in the left, and in the lower more often than in the upper lobe.

Symptoms.—The onset is often indefinite, though (i.) cough may be an early and prominent symptom. (ii.) The patient is obviously ill and is running a high and remitting or intermitting temperature characteristic of loculated pus. (iii.) Following the sudden coughing up of a considerable quantity of thick sputum, which may be offensive or blood-stained, there is an immediate drop in temperature due to the abscess discharging into a bronchus. (iv.) Pain is variable and only occurs when the pleura is involved. (v.) Clubbing of the fingers develops rapidly in many cases.

The *Physical Signs* are those of consolidation, but when the abscess is situated deep in the lung they are indefinite or absent. When the abscess is superficial and has recently drained by rupturing into a bronchus, there may be the signs of cavitation. There is usually little or no displacement of the heart and mediastinum.

The *Diagnosis* is greatly helped by X-ray examination. In the earlier stages, before there is extensive breaking down of the lung, the skiagram may show only a dense homogeneous opacity. If a definite cavity has formed, it may be possible to see a fluid level, which remains horizontal in spite of changes in the position of the patient. This phenomenon is practically diagnostic of abscess (Fig. 69). Generally there is a high polymorph leucocytosis. It is not always easy to differentiate this condition from *bronchiectasis*, and indeed bronchiectasis may spread into the surrounding lung tissue and form a lung abscess: usually there is a previous history of the symptoms of bronchiectasis, even extending over a number of years, and bronchiectatic dilatation can be identified by bronchography (Fig. 68). Radio-opaque substances do not usually enter the cavity of a lung abscess. An *interlobar empyema* is almost impossible to differentiate from an abscess in the lung, although it may be suspected when the abscess is in the plane of an interlobar fissure. A *tuberculous abscess* is usually placed in the upper part of the affected lobe of the lung, and tubercle bacilli should be readily detected.

Etiology.—It is difficult to draw a sharp line of demarcation between lung abscess and gangrene; both result from invasion of the lung tissue by pathogenic organisms, and the consequent damage varies in character and extent according to (a) the nature of the invading organisms; (b) the virulence-resistance ratio of the individual; (c) the blood supply of the particular part affected. In the case of rapid and extensive necrosis of the lung parenchyma, for which the term gangrene should really be reserved, the effects of an unusually virulent toxin are probably aided by the vascular occlusion which accompanies the process.

The main causes of intrapulmonary suppuration (abscess and gangrene) are: (i.) aspiration of infected material into the lower respiratory tract (see Aspiration Pneumonia, § 123); (ii.) embolism containing micro-organisms, as in pyæmia following lateral sinus thrombosis or from pelvic suppuration. Right-sided infective endocarditis is a rare cause; with emboli the abscesses are often multiple; (iii.) following the occurrence of a pulmonary infarct; (iv.) complicating pneumonia which has not responded to antibiotic measures; (v.) an underlying bronchial carcinoma is a cause in about 20 per cent. of cases; (vi.) as a spread from bronchiectasis, carcinoma of the œsophagus or suppurative mediastinitis; (vii.) a liver abscess (especially the " tropical abscess ") or a suppurating hydatid may rupture into the lung; (viii.) following a perforating wound of the chest wall. Any of the well-known pathogenic organisms may be present: streptococci, staphylococci, pneumococci, spirochætes and various saprophytic organisms. Anærobic organisms should always be sought for, especially in cases of acute and rapid gangrenous necrosis of the lung.

The *Prognosis* has been greatly improved by the use of massive doses of penicillin and of the other antibiotics. Complications have also become rare but rupture into the pleura causes a pyopneumothorax and metastatic cerebral abscesses may occur.

Treatment.—The main indications are to identify the organisms responsible, by ærobic and anærobic cultures of sputum and of the blood, and to prescribe full doses of the appropriate antibiotic. Penicillin can be started in doses of 2 million units b.d. pending the results of the pathological examinations. Many abscesses rupture spontaneously into a bronchus: when the site of suppuration is known, prolonged posturing in the most suitable position and on a special bed for many hours in the day must be adopted. To facilitate this drainage aspiration through the broncho-scope may be necessary and bronchoscope examination is particularly necessary when there is a suspicion that a solitary abscess is due to a bronchial carcinoma. *Surgical measures* are much less commonly needed since most abscesses respond to chemotherapy: but they are still needed when antibiotics are ineffective, or when there is a new growth or a persistent slough of dead tissue present.

§ 147. III. Actinomycosis may affect the pleura or the lung, imitating the signs of empyema, pneumonia (§ 121), phthisis, or bronchiectasis. In the absence of cutaneous or other lesions it is rarely diagnosed except by an examination of the sputum, when the little yellow pellets containing the ray fungus are visible. The streptothrix may be cultured anærobically. The disease usually responds to penicillin in combination with a sulphonamide and potassium iodide.

Moniliasis, due to infection with the thrush fungus *Candida albicans,* has long been known to affect the mouth (§ 210), the vagina (p. 618) and the intestine. Invasion of the lungs has become much more frequent since treatment with penicillin and the tetracyclines has become routine for cases of pneumonia and purulent bronchitis. The fungus is insensitive to these drugs and establishes itself as a persistent secondary invading organism. In the lungs and bronchi it is usually a harmless saprophyte: rarely it may cause a cough, sputum, pyrexia, sweating and sometimes hæmoptysis. With these symptoms there may be unilateral or bilateral infiltration, leading occasionally to cavitation and fibrosis, which closely simulates pulmonary tuberculosis.

Aspergillosis is due to the fungus *Aspergillus fumigatus* or sometimes to *A. nidulans* and is more common than was originally believed. It occurs as a primary infection among pigeon fanciers, who chew the seeds containing the fungus and transfer them from their own mouths to the birds; it produces a cough and greenish or reddish sputum, hæmoptysis, prolonged fever and asthmatic attacks with signs of bronchitis, broncho-pneumonia or of chronic fibrosis. It is distinguished from pulmonary tuberculosis by direct examination and by culture of the sputum. Secondary invasion of bronchiectatic cavities or as a terminal complication of cachetic states may occur. *Treatment.*—The organisms are penicillin-resistant and should be treated with large doses of potassium iodide.

Blastomycosis or **Torulosis** is due to a yeast-like organism, *Torula histolytica* (*Cryptococcus neoformans*), which can be seen in smears or cultured from the sputum. The portal of entry is unknown. The *Symptoms* produced are usually due to invasion of the lungs, of the brain and meninges, causing a subacute or chronic meningitis, or of the bones. Involvement of the lungs causes a cough with mucoid sputum and dense areas of consolidation resembling those of tuberculosis or neoplasm. *Treatment* with the usual antibiotics and P.A.S. is useless, but Amphotericin B is proving more effective.

Histoplasmosis is due to the fungus *Histoplasma capsulatum,* an infection which is much more common in the U.S.A. than in Great Britain. In man the chief portal of entry is via the respiratory system. Two main varieties exist—the primary pulmonary form and the type in which the fungus is widely disseminated. *Symptoms.* —In the *pulmonary* variety there is a dry cough, pyrexia, headache, backache, joint pains but with few chest signs; in the most severe cases there is X-ray evidence of bilateral pneumonitis which heals slowly over many months with fibrosis, calcification and enlarged hilar glands. The disease closely resembles pulmonary tuberculosis. The *disseminated* variety is especially common and lethal in young children. Patients show persistent irregular fever with miliary or patchy pneumonitis, and there may be enlargement of the liver, spleen, lymph glands and signs of suprarenal failure. *Diagnosis* is by the complement fixation test (positive in the 3rd–4th week), the histoplasmin skin reaction (1 in 1,000 dilution positive after 2–3 days): and the organism may be cultured from the sputum, blood or bone marrow. The *prognosis* is excellent in the primary pulmonary variety; but when dissemination occurs 75 per cent. of cases may prove fatal. *Treatment* is with the antibiotic Amphotericin B (intramusc.) combined with tab. trisulphonamide. Steroids tend to produce dissemination and are dangerous.

COCCIDIOIDOMYCOSIS, also common in the U.S.A. and due to the inhalation of spores of the fungus, gives a low-grade fever and an influenzal-like illness, often with Erythema nodosum and E. multiforme; sometimes cavitation of the lung or a pleural effusion are found. The *diagnosis* is aided by the specific skin reaction to the fungus antigen. *Treatment* is as for histoplasmosis, but natural resolution of the pulmonary lesions is usual, independent of active measures.

SPOROTRICHOSIS is very rare. The fungus commonly enters the skin through an abrasion, and causes abscesses in many different organs, including the lungs. Treatment is with potassium iodide and griseofulvin.

Various OTHER FUNGI have been identified in association with broncho-pulmonary inflammations, *e.g.*, *geotrichum*. The presence of MITES has also been identified with asthmatic and other respiratory symptoms.

PSITTACOSIS, Q FEVER, ANTHRAX, PLAGUE, GLANDERS and DISTOMA may affect the lungs, and can be recognised only by the sputum and concurrent signs. Psittacosis (§§ 123, 507) often resembles pneumonia. ASCARIS infections may be hard to diagnose in the early stages.

§ 148. IV. **Paragonimiasis,** caused by *Paragonimus westermani*, the common lung fluke of Japan and China, gives rise to pulmonary symptoms, including cough and hæmoptysis. The physical signs may suggest bronchiectasis, broncho-pneumonia or pleurisy, the diagnosis being made by finding operculated eggs in the rusty-brown sputum or in the fæces. Diarrhœa and Jacksonian epilepsy due to involvement of the intestine and brain may occur. No specific drug treatment is known.

CHAPTER VII

THE UPPER RESPIRATORY PASSAGES AND THE THYROID GLAND

THE mucous membrane of the nose and throat performs a most important function in that it warms the inspired air and filters out small particles of dust and injurious bacteria. In health it is the normal habitat of a variety of organisms such as *Streptococcus viridans*, *Micrococcus catarrhalis*, diphtheroids and certain viruses. In disease the mucous membranes often become the site of an air-borne infection which causes local and constitutional diseases. Apart from such infective processes, other pathological reactions such as œdema, hæmorrhage, ulceration or new growth occur as part of a general or of a local condition. Because it is easily inspected, the throat may give much valuable information to aid diagnosis; examination of the nose and throat constitutes an essential part in the investigation of a wide variety of different conditions.

This chapter deals with the symptoms referable to the **pharynx** (§ 151), the **larynx** (§ 164), the **nasal cavities** (§ 178) and the **thyroid gland** (§ 184).

THE THROAT

§ 151. **Symptomatology.**—" The throat " may be said to consist of the fauces, tonsils, palate, pharynx and larynx, and we are here concerned with the investigation of these structures. The symptoms indicating disease of these parts are principally two—namely, SORE THROAT and HOARSENESS. The examination of the mouth and tongue is described under Disorders of Digestive Tract (Chapter VIII).

(*a*) SORE THROAT is indicative mainly of disease of the *pharynx*, tonsils and adjacent structures. If the patient complains of " sore throat," turn to § 153.

(*b*) HOARSENESS AND OTHER ALTERATIONS OF THE VOICE are indicative of some affection of the *larynx* (§ 164). If NASAL INTONATION OR NASAL DISCHARGE be present, turn to § 178.

There are also several minor symptoms which arise in conjunction with these, such as a dryness accompanied by a tickling sensation, or an excessive secretion which leads to " hawking " and " coughing." Thus it happens that we may be consulted for what the patient believes to be pulmonary disease, when in reality the lungs are perfectly healthy. Dyspnœa and dysphagia may also be produced by local conditions of the throat and larynx. " Globus," a paroxysmal sensation as of a ball in, or constriction of, the throat is a symptom of hysteria.

§ 152. **Clinical Investigation.**—The anatomy and relations of the throat are indicated in Fig. 70; the various parts may be investigated by (*a*) direct, and (*b*) indirect (*i.e.*, laryngoscopic) examination.

(*a*) For the DIRECT EXAMINATION of the fauces and neighbouring structures all that is necessary is a good light and a spatula or spoon to depress the tongue. If direct light is not available—as, for instance, when the patient is in bed—a head mirror can be used (*vide infra*). The patient should be instructed *not to strain*, and to "*breathe quietly in and out.*" The posterior wall may be seen by directing the patient to say "Ha—ah,"

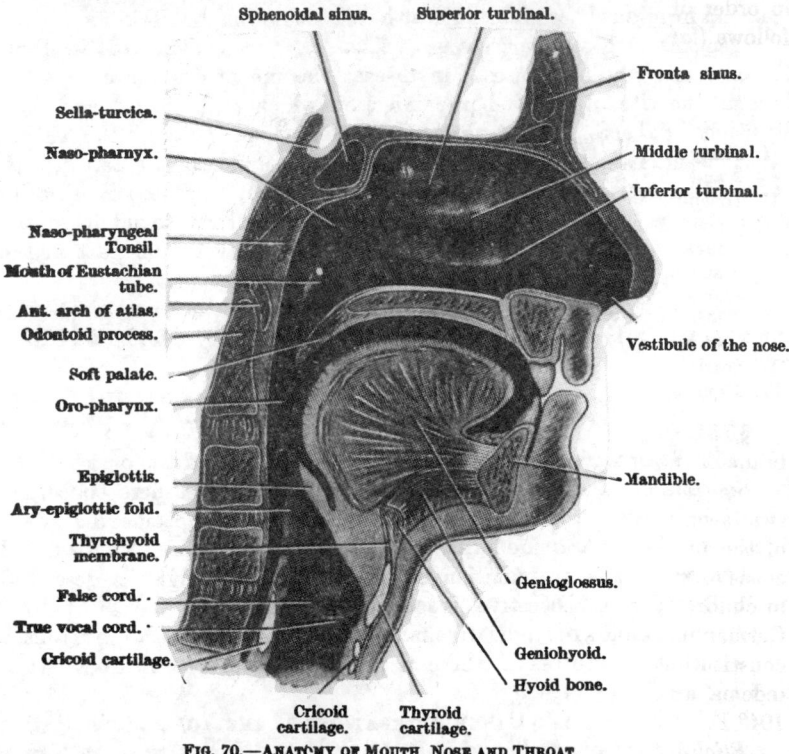

Sphenoidal sinus.   Superior turbinal.

Fronta sinus.

Sella-turcica.

Naso-pharynx.

Middle turbinal.

Inferior turbinal.

Naso-pharyngeal Tonsil.

Mouth of Eustachian tube.

Ant. arch of atlas.

Odontoid process.

Vestibule of the nose.

Soft palate.

Oro-pharynx.

Epiglottis.

Ary-epiglottic fold.

Mandible.

Thyrohyoid membrane.

False cord.

Genioglossus.

True vocal cord.

Cricoid cartilage.

Geniohyoid.

Hyoid bone.

Cricoid cartilage.   Thyroid cartilage.

FIG. 70.—ANATOMY OF MOUTH, NOSE AND THROAT.

by which procedure the soft palate is raised. Note should be made of the colour of the mucous membrane, the presence of exudation or ulceration, of granulations in the pharynx, of mucous patches (syphilis), bulging of the pharyngeal walls; also of paralysis or weakness of the tongue, palate or pharynx. The size and length of the uvula should be observed; an *elongated uvula* may rarely be the cause of a chronic cough coming on, or getting worse at night or when he lies down, and of symptoms such as the sensation of a foreign body and constant hemming and hawking. The symptoms frequently ascribed to a long or "relaxed" uvula are often due to pharyngeal or post-nasal catarrh which, indeed, may be the cause of the elongation. Treatment should be directed to any catarrh or sepsis in the upper air-passages, with the use of local astringent paints and lozenges. When conservative treatment has failed, part of the uvula may be amputated, but this is rarely done nowadays.

(b) The INDIRECT OR LARYNGOSCOPIC EXAMINATION of the throat is described in § 164.

§ 153. Classification, Diagnosi:, Prognosis and Treatment.—Sore Throat is a symptom common to nearly all diseases of the throat. Mentioned in order of frequency, the diseases which give rise to sore throat are as follows (*laryngeal affections being excluded for the present*; see § 164):

TABLE IX

Commoner Causes.	Rarer Causes.
I. Pharyngitis, including several acute and chronic varieties.	V. Retro-pharyngeal abscess.
II. Tonsillitis (acute parenchymatous, acute follicular, quinsy, glandular fever, and more rarely Vincent's angina, agranulocytic angina, and acute leukæmia). Chronic tonsillitis (including keratosis of the tonsils).	VI. Acute Septic Pharyngitis and Laryngitis.
	VII. Carcinoma and other new growths.
	VIII. Tuberculosis.
	IX. Syphilis.
III. Scarlet fever.	X. Other acute specific fevers.
IV. Diphtheria.	

§ 154. I. Acute Pharyngitis is an inflammation of the mucous membrane of the pharynx and soft palate, and to a certain extent of the tonsils.

Symptoms.—In *mild* cases it may cause only slight discomfort in swallowing, a dry throat, a tickling and hawking cough, and on examination of the throat only a moderate congestion can be seen. The commonest cause of this mild form is a febrile catarrh due to the common cold (coryza): in children it may occur as an early symptom of scarlet fever, measles or German measles. In *more severe* cases there is also complaint of dysphagia, constitutional symptoms are more pronounced, and locally there may be œdema and marked congestion. The temperature varies from 100° to 104° F.

Etiology.—The majority of cases are due to a *virus* infection, often in an epidemic form. Three different types are now recognised, each running a course of 4–5 days. (i.) There is acute pharyngitis and fever only. (ii.) There is acute pharyngitis, conjunctivitis and cervical adenitis with no spread below the pharynx. (iii.) The acute pharyngitis is accompanied by involvement of the lower respiratory passages, with laryngitis, tracheitis, bronchitis and sometimes pneumonia. Conjunctivitis and cervical adenitis are not a feature of this group. Another variety is that due to the *influenzal viruses*: this also occurs in epidemic form but differs from those just described by the presence of marked constitutional symptoms, sweating and aches and pains in the limbs. Less often an acute streptococcal infection can be causal.

Treatment consists in remaining indoors for a day or so, giving aspirin to relieve the soreness, and avoiding smoking. In the more severe forms treatment should be that of acute tonsillitis.

Chronic Pharyngitis exists in several forms:

(a) The *Catarrhal* variety presents the same symptoms as the acute variety, in a milder degree, and extending over a longer period of time. It is often known as Relaxed or Relapsing Sore Throat, on account of the chronic congestion of the parts and the consequent predisposition to the repeated occurrence of subacute attacks. It forms one variety of clergyman's or school-teacher's sore throat.

(b) The *Granular* form is a further stage of the catarrhal variety, with the addition of visible granulations on the pharyngeal walls due to the grouping of masses of lymphoid cells round the openings of the ducts of the mucous glands.

(c) *Follicular* pharyngitis occurs when the ducts become obstructed and dilated so that yellow cheesy matter collects and periodically is discharged. These rather dense plugs may be mistaken for the secretion of an acute infection: they may cause no symptoms but, especially in cold damp weather or when the general health is below par, a chronic soreness with hawking and a persistent cough may arise.

(d) *Atrophic* pharyngitis (pharyngitis sicca) occurs when the mucous glands have atrophied. The throat then becomes dry and rather shiny.

(e) *Keratosis pharyngis* occurs only in adults. It is a harmless condition in which yellowish-white spikes protrude from the surface of the lymphoid tissue of the pharynx. It is most noticeable on the tonsils (see § 155).

Etiology.—Local causes. (1) The commonest causes are excessive smoking, chronic alcoholism or infection arising from carious teeth or pyorrhœa. (2) Post-nasal discharge due to sinusitis or chronic rhinitis infects the pharynx and causes congestion by the constant effort to get rid of it. (3) Persistent mouth-breathing aggravates the condition: this may be due to habit or to nasal obstruction. (4) Overuse of the throat and wrong methods of voice production cause clergyman's and school-teacher's throat. (5) The bristle of a tooth-brush or a fish bone impacted in the pharynx may be an unsuspected cause. *General causes* contributing to the condition are (6) Overcrowding in insufficiently ventilated rooms, exposure to cold and damp, and the presence of dust or irritating vapours at work. (7) General ill-health predisposes especially to granular pharyngitis, so that in some persons the throat constitutes a veritable barometer of the state of their health. Cases arise due to poor feeding, tuberculosis and anæmia (see the Plummer-Vinson syndrome, § 226). On the other hand a surfeit of food or alcohol such as give rise to obesity or gout is also causal. (8) The pharyngitis of influenza is slow to disappear and is accompanied by a very irritating cough.

*Prognosis.—*This depends on the cause and whether it can be removed. All the chronic forms have a great *tendency to relapse.*

Treatment must be primarily directed to the cause: local treatment is a secondary consideration. Any sepsis in the nose, teeth or tonsils needs to be adequately treated. All causes of local irritation such as persistent mouth-breathing, working in a dusty atmosphere, smoking and alcohol must be avoided. The general health should be improved, anæmia corrected and obesity overcome. Excessive secretion may be removed by a gargle of a warm solution of bicarbonate of soda. For a "relaxed throat" Mandl's paint, or a spray containing menthol 1 in 50 of paroleine, are good applications. Later astringent paints should be used such as one containing argentoprotein B.P. (protargol) 10 per cent. The most efficient treatment for the granular forms of pharyngitis, where gargles are of little use, is painting with protargol: the galvano-cautery may be applied to the individual granulations. For an irritating cough a linctus of codein, methadone or diamorphine may be necessary. In any case overtreatment of the local condition must be avoided, lest the patient's attention be unduly focused on his throat and a functional overlay perpetuated.

(*f*) **Adenoids** may be regarded as a form of chronic pharyngitis limited to the nasopharynx: they are often associated with chronic enlargement of the tonsils. The hypertrophied mass of lymphoid tissue which constitute adenoids may fill a large part of the naso-pharynx. They occur particularly in young children and tend spontaneously to disappear after puberty: the disease often runs in families.

Symptoms.—(1) During the day the child cannot breathe through the nose: it therefore persistently breathes with its mouth open even when it has not a common cold. The voice develops a dull or nasal twang. (2) At night there is disturbed sleep, snoring and restlessness so the child is unrefreshed on waking. (3) The expression becomes vacant and in the course of time the alæ nasi fall in, the palate may be high from a diminished pressure in the nose and a pigeon-breast may follow. (4) The condition is a common cause of recurrent head colds, with enlargement of the upper cervical glands: such catarrhal infections may contribute to recurrent laryngitis, tracheitis and bronchitis. (5) Middle ear catarrh and subsequent deafness may ensue: these further contribute to lack of mental concentration and backwardness at school. (6) Rarely a condition of congenital hypertrophy of adenoids is met: this causes feeding difficulties in children for they cannot feed at the breast or from a bottle and need spoon-feeding. Chronic malnutrition may ensue. (7) In a child who co-operates the adenoids may be seen with a post-nasal mirror: otherwise they can be felt as a soft cushion in the naso-pharynx under general anæsthesia.

The *Diagnosis* is from the less common condition of chronic allergic rhinitis: in this there is often early morning sneezing and the nasal obstruction may get worse in the afternoon, the child being susceptible to the dust of a school class-room. The nasal mucous membrane in allergy is glistening and pale, there is much less tendency to recurrent infections and to otitis media and the patient may not benefit by the removal of any adenoids present. An infection of the nasal antra may cause adenoids to develop and must be looked for and dealt with: X-ray examination aids the diagnosis of concurrent sinusitis.

Treatment of adenoids when small in amount is by attending to the general health, giving open-air exercise and by the establishment of nose-breathing. The correction of sinusitis may cause adenoids to decrease in size. When large in amount they must be thoroughly removed under general anæsthesia.

§ 155. II. **Tonsillitis** is met with clinically in acute and chronic forms. The acute variety may be the forerunner of a number of severe constitutional diseases such as scarlet fever, measles, rheumatic fever, acute nephritis, septicæmia or acute mastoiditis.

(a) **Acute Parenchymatous Tonsillitis.**—The whole substance of each tonsil is inflamed and appears red and swollen.

(b) **Acute Follicular Tonsillitis.**—The inflammation is often more severe and the crypts become filled with fibrin, leucocytes, bacteria, etc. The tonsils are not so swollen as in (a), but their surface is studded with yellow dots which may be wiped off without bleeding.

The *Symptoms* are the same in both varieties. There is a complaint of a sore throat and pain on swallowing may be severe. The tongue is heavily furred and the cervical glands on both sides are enlarged and tender. Constitutional symptoms are usually marked: at the onset the temperature rises to 100°–104° F and there may be a mild rigor. Headache, pains in the limbs and general malaise occur. In *children* there may be no complaint of soreness in the throat even with a severe local infection: with a rapid rise of temperature a convulsion may take place. Also there may be abdominal pain when the lymphoid tissue in and around the appendix is simultaneously affected.

The *Diagnosis* of both forms of tonsillitis from scarlet fever and diphtheria is sometimes a matter of difficulty, but one of great importance. It is given in the form of a table (X, p. 267). The onset of measles is associated with a sore throat and sometimes a follicular tonsillitis (§ 481).

Etiology.—In health a number of different organisms are found in the tonsils including the *Streptococcus viridans*, non-hæmolytic streptococci, *N. catarrhalis*, pneumococci, hæmophilus organisms and sometimes staphylococci and *B. coli*. (1) In tonsillitis the commonest pathogenic organism is the *Streptococcus hæmolyticus* (Lancefield Group A), although the *Staphylococcus aureus*, *Streptococcus viridans* and other organisms may be the exciting cause. Such infections, especially with *Strep. hæmolyticus*, may occur as a local epidemic due to droplet infection—especially where a number of young persons are in closed communities as at school, or when sleeping in ill-ventilated rooms as in overcrowded dormitories or hospitals and in the sleeping quarters of ships. (2) The tonsils are also acutely inflamed as a part of a general pharyngitis in the common "cold," with influenza and in other virus diseases. (3) Fish-bones and bristles of a tooth-brush sometimes give rise to one-sided tonsillitis.

Prognosis.—Acute tonsillitis, without complications, is a frequent, sometimes troublesome, but rarely fatal, disease. Sometimes the patient continues at work; usually he is totally incapacitated. The infection is always much more severe when the general resistance is lowered by other diseases such as hyperthyroidism, chronic nephritis or anæmia.

Treatment.—The patient must be put to bed and given as liberal a diet as the febrile condition and the discomfort on swallowing will allow. When there is any doubt as to the nature of the infecting organism a swab of the throat must be taken for bacteriological examination on a direct smear and by culture before any drugs are administered. In *mild cases,* aspirin suspended in water by pulv. tragacanthæ co. is very comforting. In *more severe* cases, tab. phenoxymethylpenicillin (penicillin V) 120–240 mgm. 4-hourly or inject. benzylpenicillin B.P. (soluble penicillin) 500,000 units b.d. are required. An alternative treatment is with tab. sulphadimidine (B.P.) 2 G. initially followed by 1 G. six-hourly: this may be combined with penicillin or used alone when the patient is penicillin-sensitive. Other antibiotics are sometimes used.

(c) **Quinsy or Peritonsillar Abscess.**—In this condition, which occurs usually after tonsillitis but occasionally primarily, an abscess forms just outside the capsule of the tonsil, as a rule only on one side. Severe pain is felt in the throat and swallowing may be almost impossible. The pain radiates to the ear and down the neck. The temperature may be high (103° F); the patient looks toxic and speech is thick and muffled. Trismus often makes examination difficult. The anterior pillar of the fauces and the soft palate on the affected side are very red and œdematous and bulge forwards, while the tonsil is pushed inwards. Much sticky mucus is present. The cervical glands on the corresponding side of the neck are enlarged and tender.

Treatment.—Penicillin injections should be given. If the abscess is pointing or does not respond to the penicillin within 24–36 hours it should be opened by inserting a fine-pointed pair of sinus forceps into the abscess, and slightly opening the blades. Enter at the point of maximum swelling and softening. A guarded scalpel, with plaster wound round the blade to within half an inch of the point, may be used instead of the forceps. No anæsthetic should be used, other than cocaine locally, lest the cough reflex be abolished and pus inhaled.

(d) **Glandular Fever** is particularly common in young adults. It causes (i.) a sore throat, with general reddening of the fauces and tonsils, enlargement of lymphatic glands and often some enlargement of the spleen. On the palate multiple tiny petechiæ occur. (ii.) In the anginose variety, after 1–2 weeks of malaise and fever, the throat becomes sore and a membrane indistinguishable from that of diphtheria forms on one or both tonsils. There is much peritonsillar œdema and cervical adenitis (§ 498).

Diphtheria bacilli cannot be cultured from the membrane, and a rash with the typical blood changes helps to confirm the diagnosis.

(e) An uncommon form of acute tonsillitis is known as **Vincent's Angina.** It is often mistaken for diphtheria; it can occur during convalescence from diphtheria, and *vice versa.* As a rule only one tonsil is affected, occasionally both. It is characterised by one or more patches of exudation, often presenting a necrotic appearance, on the tonsil or adjacent anterior pillar, and sometimes encroaching on the palate. Later a deep ragged excavation may form. The pellicle is not easily detachable, and leaves a shallow ulcerated surface, the healing of which may be somewhat tedious. It is attended by some pyrexia and constitutional disturbance, usually slight. There is characteristic fœtor of the breath. A smear from the affected surface contains Vincent's organisms—a large fusiform bacillus which stains with the aniline dyes, but will not grow on ordinary culture media, and a delicate mobile spirochæte. Both these organisms may be found in ordinary ulcerative stomatitis, in carious teeth, and in some cases of severe scarlet fever. The *Treatment* of choice is with penicillin injections combined with sucking troch. penicillin B.P.: salvarsan powder may be applied locally.

(f) **Agranulocytic Angina** (Agranulocytosis, malignant neutropenia) is an uncommon but serious disorder. It occurs as a rule about middle age: women are much more susceptible than men. In *acute cases* there is first soreness of the throat, and malaise with pyrexia. The disease rapidly progresses and there is necrotic ulceration of the tonsils, fauces, buccal mucous membrane, and sometimes the vagina and any part of the intestinal tract, but especially the rectum. In the absence of polymorph cells in the blood, any invading micro-organism produces widespread local invasion of tissues as well as septicæmia. Prostration is marked and the patient commonly dies in a few days. A *chronic type* may also occur with recurrent mild attacks of sore throat, malaise and fever, often occurring at the menstrual periods. The blood picture is characteristic. The total white count is very low (it may be only a few hundred) and the polymorphonuclear granulocytes (neutrophils, eosinophils and basophils) are much reduced in number (absolutely and relatively), and may be absent. This is due to their non-formation by the bone marrow. Sternal bone marrow biopsy shows either that no cells of the granular series are formed at all, or that myeloblasts and myelocytes are present in large numbers but are unable to mature to form polymorphs (see p. 793).

Etiology.—Although spontaneous cases occur, the condition is more common after the use of certain drugs, especially amidopyrine and thiouracil, and sometimes after arsphenamines, troxidone, phenylbutazone, dinitrophenol, the nitrogen mustard and the sulphonamide groups and compounds of heavy metals.

Treatment.—(1) First eliminate possible causes, *e.g.*, drugs; (2) Penicillin injections are essential to prevent bacterial invasion; (3) To overcome the agranulocytosis stimulate the formation of granulocytes by full doses of corticotrophin B.P. (ACTH) or by cortisone. Nuclein derivatives may be tried, *e.g.*, pentnucleotide, injected daily intramuscularly in doses of 20–40 ml. in divided doses until the white count rises. In certain cases intravenous pyridoxine 100–200 mg. daily is helpful; (4) Repeated transfusions of fresh blood may be required; (5) Treat local lesions with mouth washes (*e.g.*, hydrogen peroxide) and sprays.

(g) **Acute leukæmia** may cause a membranous form of acute tonsillitis as one of its earlier manifestations (§ 554).

Chronic Tonsillitis is a condition about which there has been much controversy. In the past the tonsils have often been removed, especially from children, without sufficient evidence of disease to justify this.

Symptoms.—There is often a history of recurrent attacks of sore throat with pyrexia at frequent intervals, *e.g.*, three attacks a year: with each of these the glands at the angles of the jaws become temporarily enlarged.

Sometimes it develops insidiously. The size of the tonsils is no criterion of disease; infected tonsils may be enlarged, or small and fibrotic. Those remaining after incomplete removal are especially dangerous. The crypts of diseased tonsils may contain epithelial débris and pus, the pillars of the fauces remain chronically injected and there is enlargement of the upper cervical glands.

(a) In *adults* with a crypt infection of the insidious type the patient may be unaware of any throat trouble; he may have a chronic toxæmia, leading to arthritis, neuritis, nephritis and diminished vitality. (b) In *children*, the condition is indicated by local and general symptoms. *Local:* running nose, muco-purulent rhinitis, post-nasal discharge, fœtid breath, enlarged cervical glands, unilateral or bilateral otorrhœa, associated with a history of frequent colds, sore throats and other infections, particularly exan-themata.

Diagnosis.—Particularly in children chronic enlargement of the tonsils is associated with enlarged adenoids (§ 154). This hypertrophic type occurs especially in the presence of dental sepsis, or persistent mouth-breathing, and also in the " catarrhal diathesis." In this latter condition the children are over-weight, subject to recurrent catarrh, and have a bright malar flush which gives the appearance of good health. In adults the diagnosis of chronic tonsillar infection is made by the history of repeated sore throats and especially of a quinsy, by the local physical signs in the tonsils and the upper cervical glands and by the constitutional symptoms present. In cases of doubt bacteriological examination of the secretion from the crypts of the tonsil may reveal a pathogenic organism.

Etiology.—Tonsils are much more commonly inflamed in children who live in overcrowded and ill-ventilated rooms with lack of sunlight. They are also secondarily inflamed when there is infection in the mouth from broken dental stumps or pyorrhœa: once this dental sepsis has been removed they usually recover. Tuberculous glands in the upper part of the neck are often due to a tuberculous focus in the tonsils.

Course and Prognosis.—Enlarged tonsils in children often resolve during adolescence. Chronic tonsillitis renders the patient liable to repeated attacks of acute tonsillitis and coryza and is a common source of recurrent pharyngitis, leading to otitis media and deafness. The mental and physical development of the child is more likely to be hindered by the presence of adenoids, which interfere with the respiration. In adults chronic tonsillar sepsis may be the cause of general ill-health and local conditions such as infective polyarthritis or irido-cyclitis.

Treatment in mild cases consists in sending the young patient 'for a period of convalescence in healthy surroundings: iron and cod-liver oil may aid. In more troublesome cases and after reviewing carefully the local condition of the tonsils in relation to the general health of the individual, removal is often indicated in adults as well as in children. This must be performed thoroughly, preferably by dissection. On the other hand routine tonsillectomy for conditions such as otitis media, rheumatic fever or chorea, in children who have no evidence of local tonsillar infection, is to be deplored—in fact chorea recurs much more frequently after tonsillectomy than in children in whom the operation has not been performed. The *principal indications for tonsillectomy in children* are: (1) a history of recurrent tonsillitis; (2) in the absence of dental sepsis the presence of engorgement or of a granular appearance of the anterior pillars of the fauces and the uvula; (3) chronic enlargement of the glands at the angles of the jaws in between attacks of acute tonsillitis; (4) tuberculous cervical adenitis; (5) failure of the child to thrive, often with a poor appetite, with local evidence of tonsillar sepsis; (6) obstructed swallowing due to the size of the tonsils; (7) some cases of recurrent middle ear infection.

Keratosis of the Tonsils is liable to be confused with chronic follicular tonsillitis. It occurs only in adults, and is a harmless condition in which there are creamy coloured spikes of epithelial débris projecting from the surface of the tonsils. These contain only the normal throat organisms and often a mycelium. *Symptoms* are absent although the patient may be alarmed by the appearance of the tonsils. No *treatment* is required.

§ 156. III. In **Scarlet Fever** (§ 477) the tonsil is generally the chief site of inflammation in the throat. Both scarlet fever and acute tonsillitis start more or less suddenly, with constitutional symptoms, and thus the diagnosis is often difficult. There are four distinguishing features of scarlet fever—viz.: (i.) The diffuse *scarlet* colour of the soft palate and pharynx, with complete immunity of the larynx; (ii.) sudden onset of the illness with high fever and often vomiting; (iii.) on the second day the rash; and (iv.) about the third day the " strawberry " tongue (see Table X and § 477).

§ 157. IV. The sore throat of **Diphtheria** (§ 497) may be recognised at once if there be an ashen-grey patch of exudation *upon the soft palate.* When this is absent, and the membrane is on one or both tonsils, there may be difficulty in diagnosing between diphtheria and follicular tonsillitis or Vincent's angina. In diphtheria the large size and the colour of the patches (grey with surrounding red areolæ), the raised, sharply defined margin, the difficulty of removing them, and the raw bleeding surface left, enable us to come to a conclusion. The membrane may become blackish with a very offensive odour, and hæmorrhages may occur. There may be considerable swelling of the tissues of the fauces and of the neck (" bull-neck "). The onset is more insidious, the pyrexia less marked, but the prostration is greater in diphtheria. A muco-purulent or hæmorrhagic discharge from the nose is characteristic of diphtheria. Albuminuria is frequent with acute tonsillitis as well as with diphtheria. When other diagnostic features are absent, the presence of *one* large patch on a tonsil, instead of several small patches, is in favour of diphtheria. A swab will reveal the presence of the bacillus. Vincent's angina usually affects only one tonsil (§ 155). Diphtheria is now rare in the British Isles owing to immunisation in childhood.

TABLE X

Tonsillitis.	Scarlet Fever.	Diphtheria.
	(a) LOCAL SIGNS.	
Swelling and redness chiefly confined to one or both tonsils. In the follicular form, tonsils covered with sticky mucus, with numerous small, separate yellow spots of secretion on one or both, which are easily removable. Nothing on soft palate.	Diffuse *bright* redness of throat and palate generally. The tonsils swollen, and may be covered with mucus and *sometimes* with multiple yellow points. Nothing on soft palate in ordinary cases.	Ashy-grey patch or patches on tonsils, uvula and *soft palate* (latter situation is pathognomonic). Patches *larger* than in follicular tonsillitis; they consist of membrane surrounded by red areolæ; difficult to remove, leaving raw surface. Characteristic smell. *C. diphtheriæ* (K.L.B.) bacillus in membrane. Sometimes a muco-purulent, acrid *nasal discharge*. Comparative absence of pain.
	(b) GENERAL SYMPTOMS.	
(i.) Onset moderately sudden, with moderate fever. (ii.) Temperature may be very high, but local symptoms are usually more troublesome than general symptoms.	(i.) Onset with fever and usually vomiting. (ii.) Temperature may be high. Local symptoms a subordinate feature. (iii.) Rash on first or second day. (iv.) Strawberry and cream tongue about third day.	(i.) Onset insidious. Early and marked enlargement of cervical glands. (ii.) Temperature usually low during whole course. (iii.) Paralytic sequelæ sometimes.

The less frequent causes of Sore Throat are—RETRO-PHARYNGEAL ABSCESS, ACUTE SEPTIC PHARYNGITIS AND LARYNGITIS, NEOPLASTIC, TUBERCULOUS and SYPHILITIC ULCERATIONS and ACUTE SPECIFIC FEVERS.

§ 158. V. A **Retro-pharyngeal Abscess** is situated in the areolar tissue between the pharynx and the spine. It may develop insidiously, or the onset may be comparatively sudden. It is known by (1) the rigidity of the neck, with difficulty of swallowing, alteration of the voice, laryngeal obstruction and inspiratory stridor; (2) evidence of swelling in the posterior pharyngeal wall on inspection and palpation, by which means it is diagnosed from other causes of dyspnœa in children.

Etiology.—Acute cases are met mostly in young enfeebled and undernourished children. They are due to the formation of an abscess in the retro-pharyngeal lymphatic glands following an acute infection in the nose or throat.

Treatment.—The acute abscess should be opened at once, through the mouth, no anæsthetic being given. The child is held with the head down, and the pus removed by a suction apparatus.

Chronic retro-pharyngeal abscess is much less common and is almost always due to tuberculous disease of the bodies of the cervical vertebræ. The abscess tends to point in the posterior triangle, where it should be opened.

§ 159. VI. Acute Septic Pharyngitis and Laryngitis (Syn. Phlegmonous Sore Throat)—and ANGINA LUDOVICI (when the inflammation is chiefly external, in the neck).—This very severe disease may start *inside* the throat, with symptoms of sudden pain, accompanied by considerable swelling, leading to severe dyspnœa, stridor, aphonia and complete dysphagia in a few hours. There is much œdema around the fauces, followed by a brawny infiltration of the skin of the neck, spreading from under the jaw to the tongue and larynx. In some cases there is hæmorrhagic necrosis of the tonsils and surrounding parts, suggesting agranulocytic angina or diphtheria gravis. Sometimes the infiltration starts *externally*, and rapidly invades the internal structures. There is considerable constitutional disturbance, and a temperature of 102° to 105° F. Fluctuation in the centre of the œdematous area indicates pus formation. There is often an accompanying septicæmia which causes pleurisy, pneumonia, pericarditis and meningitis. Especially in debilitated and alcoholic subjects, the disease rapidly progresses, and death takes place in 12 to 48 hours from heart failure, coma or asphyxia from œdema of the larynx. Suppurative forms are often fatal. There is a more chronic form in which induration is in excess of pus formation; this may continue indefinitely until the pus is found and drained.

Etiology.—The condition, happily, is rare; it is usually streptococcal in origin. (1) It sometimes arises in association with scarlet fever, erysipelas and small-pox (in former times being a common cause of death in this disease), or other acute specific fevers. (2) Dental suppuration or an alveolar abscess often forms the source from which rapid infiltration starts. (3) It may arise in people apparently in good health, and has then been attributed to the entrance of infection by the tonsils, or through the socket of an extracted tooth. (4) It occurs in some cases of acute leukæmia and in agranulocytosis.

Treatment.—The indications are to control the inflammation, and to keep up the strength of the heart. Large doses of penicillin injections and one of the sulphonamides must be given. The general lines indicated in the treatment of acute tonsillitis should be followed. Use hot or cold applications to the neck. Remove carious teeth or stumps. Free and early incisions should be made if there is pus formation, and tracheostomy is necessary if the dyspnœa is increasing.

ACUTE ŒDEMA of the throat may be part of the above disease when the œdema is secondary to septic infection; or it may be part of a general œdema or due to giant urticaria. It is dangerous, as it may spread to the larynx and cause death by suffocation (§ 167).

§ 160. VII. CARCINOMA commonly affects the pharynx, more often in men than in women. No part of the pharynx is immune, but most frequently the pyriform sinus, the ary-epiglottic fold or the epiglottis and base of the tongue and tonsil are involved. The main complaint is of soreness, and later, of difficulty in swallowing. Pain may be felt in the throat and may be referred to the ear. Hoarseness, fits of coughing and a blood-stained sputum may be complained of. Metastases in lymphatic glands occur comparatively early and may be the first sign of disease. Frequently patients come for treatment when the condition is already advanced. SARCOMA is rare. The diagnostic features are more or less the same as those mentioned for the tongue (§ 217). Deep X-ray therapy, radium and surgical removal (sometimes by diathermy) are all employed with increasingly satisfactory results.

§ 161. VIII. TUBERCULOUS ULCERS of the pharynx occur as secondary lesions. (1) They resemble syphilitic ulcers, but there is pallor of the mucous membrane, and a characteristic " worm-eaten " appearance of the pharyngeal wall: pain is usually severe. (2) *Their course is not nearly so rapidly progressive.* (3) It may be possible to obtain the tubercle bacillus from the scrapings; and (4) there are usually other manifestations of tubercle, especially in the lungs. *Lupus* is uncommon. For treatment, see Tuberculosis of the Larynx (§ 172).

§ 162. IX. Syphilitic Sore Throat and **Syphilitic Ulcers** are very characteristic. This and the other *secondary* manifestations of syphilis develop about 3–6 weeks after the appearance of the chancre, but they may appear much later. Symptoms may be slight but there is usually some pain and dryness in the throat and sometimes marked soreness on swallowing. The symptoms last for some weeks. (1) Syphilitic *erythema* is the most constant change. Dusky red patches, isolated or symmetrical, appear on the soft palate, tonsil or pharynx. The whole throat may be involved. (2) *Mucous patches* (snail-tracks) appear later as grey-white, translucent or milky areas of variable size, surrounded by a narrow red areola. They are seen on the uvula, the pillars of the fauces, the tonsil and the soft palate and tend to be symmetrical. (3) All the lymphoid tissue in the throat enlarges. *Primary chancre* of the tonsil does occur, though rarely. Symptoms are slight, and it is characterised by great enlargement of the tonsil and the glands on the corresponding side of the neck. Spirochætes may be recovered from the small ulcer or erosion usually present.

Tertiary syphilitic ulcers usually cause little pain; their favourite position is the soft and hard palate, the tongue, the fauces and tonsil, and the posterior pharyngeal wall. They are usually preceded by gummatous swellings. (1) The ulcers are deep, with a ragged floor, sharply cut edges, and covered with thick yellow-grey secretion. (2) They are progressive, and in course of time will destroy the hard palate or any other parts they invade. (3) They leave characteristic stellate cicatrices, which are indisputable evidence of the disease.

§ 163. X. ACUTE SPECIFIC FEVERS other than those mentioned above, such as typhoid, give rise to inflammation and ulceration of the throat. In variola, for example, the pustules often form upon the palate, fauces and buccal mucous membrane, leaving superficial circular ulcers. An examination of the throat is often useful as an aid to the diagnosis between measles, scarlet fever and small-pox. The first named always affects the *larynx*, rarely the pharynx; scarlet fever always affects the *pharynx*, and very rarely the larynx; whereas small-pox affects them *both about equally*. Patches of *Lichen planus* may be found on the palate even before the disease occurs on the skin, and the eruption of varicella may be found in that situation. Other patches may be due to *thrush, herpes* or *pemphigus*.

THE LARYNX

§ 164. **Symptoms and Clinical Investigation.**—It will be remembered that the two cardinal SYMPTOMS of diseases of the throat (used in its widest sense) were (*a*) Sore Throat, and (*b*) Alterations of the Voice. Both of these may be present in disorders of the larynx, but it is the latter especially which indicates derangements of the organ of voice. Diseases of the larynx are also sometimes indicated by Cough, Hawking, Dysphagia, Dyspnœa and actual Pain. But in some cases all of these may be absent; there may, indeed, be pronounced disease of the larynx (*e.g.*, paralysis or papilloma) without any *subjective* symptoms.

The CLINICAL INVESTIGATION of the larynx (laryngoscopy) is a procedure of considerable technical nicety, and requires practice. The necessary appliances are a good steady light, a *reflecting mirror* mounted on a band (an electric light attached to a head-band may be used instead), and a small circular *throat-mirror* mounted on a handle at an angle of 135°. The light should be placed on a level with, and a little behind, the patient's left ear. The operator takes his seat directly opposite; and it is advisable that his seat should be a little higher than that of the patient. Having directed the patient to open his mouth and " breathe quietly in and out," the first step is to adjust the *reflecting* mirror in order thoroughly to illuminate the back of the pharynx. The focal length of the head-mirror is generally 8 to 14 inches, and this should represent the distance of the mirror from the patient's pharynx. Having warmed the throat-mirror over a small flame to prevent condensation from the breath, ask the patient to protrude the tongue: then hold the tongue gently, with the left hand, in a piece of gauze. Take care not to hurt the under surface of the tongue against the teeth of the lower jaw. Then test the warmth of the throat-mirror against your cheek or the back of your hand, and, having pushed the patient's head a little backwards by pressing your right thumb against the upper teeth, introduce the mirror with the right hand, *taking care to avoid touching the top of the tongue.* Push the mirror obliquely upwards against the soft palate just over its junction with the uvula (Fig. 70,

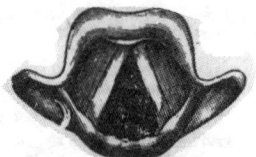

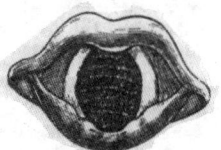

FIG. 71.—Quiet Inspira-
tion.   FIG. 72.—Forced Inspiration.

§ 152). A good view of the vocal cords should be obtained by slightly lowering or raising the handle. In children and persons with very sensitive throats it is sometimes advisable to render the pharynx less sensitive before laryngoscopy by a spray of a 5 per cent. solution of cocaine hydrochloride, or by a dose of phenobarbitone during the preceding 24 hours.

In normal conditions the *epiglottis*, which is in reality anterior, appears at the *upper part of the mirror.* The *vocal cords*, which are of a pearly white colour, are close together at their anterior or epiglottic ends; and at their posterior ends are widely divergent during quiet respiration. Posteriorly they appear to terminate in two prominent knobs seen at the lower edge of the mirror, which mark the position of the *arytenoid cartilages* (Figs. 71 and 72). The *ary-epiglottic folds* stretch on each side from the arytenoids to the sides of the epiglottis. To the outer side of the cords appear the ventricular bands or false cords of mucous membrane. With a little practice, and under favourable circumstances, the bifurcation of the trachea may be seen.

DIRECT LARYNGOSCOPY, with or without anæsthesia (general or local), allows of careful examination of the larynx and has almost entirely replaced indirect laryngoscopy for the performance of intralaryngeal operations. Direct laryngoscopy is also used to expose the larynx preliminary to the introduction of the bronchoscope. By means of the *bronchoscope* (§ 112) the interior of the bronchi may be directly examined. When a foreign body has entered the air-passages, the patient should immediately be X-rayed, then examined by one who is expert in bronchoscopy.

In LARYNGOSCOPY there are FOUR POINTS to be investigated:

(a) The *colour* of the vocal cords and the parts around. Redness of the vocal cords is evidence of LARYNGITIS, sometimes of ulceration or new growth.

(b) The presence of *ulceration*. Ulceration is often due to MALIGNANT disease.

(c) The presence of any *swelling*. This may be caused by inflammatory reaction, *e.g.*, tuberculosis, or to New Growths (innocent or malignant).

(d) Whether the vocal cords move normally or not.

§ 165. Classification. It has been mentioned that there may be no *subjective symptoms* with disease of the larynx, and therefore it is well to adopt as a basis of classification the *physical signs* discovered by laryngoscopy. However, when symptoms are present there is always some ALTERATION OF THE VOICE (except with bilateral abductor paralysis, in which there may be dyspnœa and stridor without much alteration of the voice). The principal diseases giving rise to such **alterations of the voice** or **dysphonia** may be grouped as follows:

TABLE XI

I. LARYNGITIS—

  (a) *Acute Laryngitis*, including also—

    Œdema of the larynx.
    Foreign Bodies in the Larynx or Trachea.

  (b) *Chronic Laryngitis*, including also—

    Perichondritis.
    Congenital Laryngeal Stridor.
    Early Tuberculosis.

II. ULCERATION of the Larynx—

  (a) Tuberculous Ulceration,
  (b) Syphilitic Ulceration,
  (c) Malignant Ulceration.

III. NEW GROWTHS—

  (a) Benign,
  (b) Malignant.

IV. PARALYSIS of the Vocal Cords—

  (a) Organic,
  (b) Functional.

V. SPASM of the Vocal Cords—

  Laryngismus Stridulus (§ 177).

VI. Diseases of the PHARYNX (§ 153); VII. Diseases of the NOSE (§ 178); VIII. Some severe PULMONARY affections; and IX. Certain NEUROSES also cause alterations in the voice.

I. *The patient complains of huskiness or loss of voice, a comparatively dry cough, soreness on swallowing, and there are local signs of congestion of the vocal cords. The disease is* LARYNGITIS, *of which there are two varieties,* ACUTE *and* CHRONIC.

§ 166. Acute Laryngitis comes on fairly rapidly and usually runs its course in a week. As a rule it is not a serious affection, but in children it may be alarming—a slight laryngitis coming on suddenly is **a frequent**

cause of what mothers describe as " croup." The child wakes up suddenly
in the night with loud inspiratory stridor, due to spasm, followed by an
attack of coughing. This symptom is technically known as *laryngitis
stridulosa*, and is not to be confused with laryngismus stridulus (see § 177).
Simple laryngitis is differentiated from membranous croup (laryngeal
diphtheria) by the good general condition of the child, the sudden onset of the former condition and by the general redness of the larynx.

Etiology.—The chief cause of acute laryngitis is exposure to cold—
especially when combined with overuse and wrong production of the voice
(*e.g.*, actors, music-hall artists, etc.). It is frequently a part of the
" common cold." Diphtheria or measles may start in the larynx. Persons
who suffer from chronic laryngitis (*q.v.*) or nasal obstruction are predisposed
to attacks. A foreign body in the larynx or trachea is a cause of irritation
which may produce symptoms resembling simple laryngitis.

Prognosis.—The affection is troublesome and apt to recur. When
occurring during the course of the specific fevers, the prognosis is less
favourable, because œdema of the larynx may supervene.

Treatment.—All use of the voice must be forbidden. The patient must
be kept in a warm, moist atmosphere, and should use warm inhalations
(Vapores N.F.) such as tr. benzoin co. ℳ 60 to the pint of hot water.
Warm compresses or fomentations should be applied externally, and warm
mucilaginous and alkaline drinks freely taken. The most efficacious
medicine is one containing small doses of potassium iodide. See also
formulæ in § 115. For laryngitis stridulosa, apply hot sponges to the
throat, and give tinct. ipecac. in teaspoonful doses, with warm water,
every ten minutes until emesis ensues. If much swelling is present,
spraying with cocaine and adrenaline is valuable. In more severe cases
one of the sulphonamides or an antibiotic should be given.

§ 167. **Œdema of the larynx,** or œdematous laryngitis, is a clinical phenomenon,
not a definite disease. It is often called œdema glottidis, but the mucous membrane
of the glottis is too adherent to allow much swelling; it occurs above and below the
cords affecting the epiglottis and submucous tissue of the larynx. The onset is usually
sudden, and attended by considerable dyspnœa, dysphagia, and inspiratory stridor.
The diagnosis is usually simple, on account of the swelling which can be seen and felt
on palpation at the back of the tongue. If this be absent, some difficulty may be
experienced, but the sudden onset of laryngeal dyspnœa should bring the disease to
our minds. It may arise either as a primary or as a secondary affection. As a
primary disease it may come on as part of an acute septic inflammation of the throat,
or it may be part of angioneurotic œdema (§ 652) (see Acute Œdema of the Tongue
(§ 216)). It may occur as a *secondary* condition in association with (1) one of the
various causes of acute or chronic laryngitis; (2) a general anasarca; (3) injury of the
glottis by boiling or caustic liquids, etc. Its rapid onset is the chief source of danger,
but if the patient does not shortly succumb to asphyxia, recovery generally takes place
in a few days.

The *Treatment* consists in the use of ice internally and externally. In severe cases
a 20 per cent. cocaine spray or a local application of adrenaline with ephedrine should
be tried; and if this be unsuccessful, tracheostomy must be performed without delay.
In infective conditions give penicillin and one of the sulphonamides, and in allergic
cases administer inject. promethazine hydrochlor. (Phenergan) 50 mg. or inject.
chlorpheniramine (Piriton) 10 mg.

§ 168. **The Inhalation of a Foreign Body** will give rise to varying symptoms depending on its size and nature. A *large* foreign body will be arrested *in the larynx* and death from asphyxia will rapidly ensue unless it is removed or immediate tracheotomy is carried out. A *small* foreign body is likely to pass into the trachea or one of the lower bronchi (usually the right).

Symptoms.—If a small foreign body is arrested in the larynx it will produce hoarseness or loss of voice and possibly some degree of dyspnœa. With a foreign body in the bronchus the symptoms differ markedly, depending on the nature of the material. There is usually some cough on inhalation, followed by a quiescent period. Later, cough will reappear and with it expectoration and possibly dyspnœa. *Non-vegetable foreign bodies* (pins, beads, etc.) on inhalation into the bronchus cause a cough of short duration and then may produce no symptoms for a considerable time—sometimes years: sooner or later, however, the cough returns. The bronchial obstruction produces collapse below the foreign body, and the collapsed lung becomes infected, giving rise to expectoration and, later, hæmoptysis: a lung abscess or bronchiectasis will eventually result. Unexplained attacks of cough and fever with unilateral chest disease should make one suspect the presence of a foreign body. X-ray examination and investigation by the introduction of iodised oil B.P. (lipiodol) and, if necessary, bronchoscopy should be carried out. *Vegetable foreign bodies* (peanuts, orange- and apple-pips, etc.) in the trachea or a bronchus soon give rise to acute tracheo-bronchitis: an asthmatic type of wheeze may be heard at the patient's open mouth. Obstructive emphysema of the lung tissue below the foreign body may be produced, followed later by atelectasis with expectoration, dyspnœa, and pyrexia. X-ray examination will show no foreign body, but may show the emphysema or atelectasis. In cases where there is a reasonable suspicion of a foreign body, bronchoscopy should be carried out. In untreated cases lung abscess and eventually death will result.

Treatment.—The foreign body should be removed by direct laryngoscopy or bronchoscopy.

§ 169. **Chronic Laryngitis** is troublesome on account of the perpetual hoarseness and discomfort in the throat with a liability to acute laryngitis. Laryngoscopy reveals a general redness of the larynx with a pink colour of the vocal cords.

Etiology.—Its causes are (1) repeated acute attacks; (2) excessive speaking, singing, teaching, overuse with faulty production of the voice (actors, clergymen, teachers, etc.); (3) masons and others exposed to dusty air; (4) nasal obstruction and mouth-breathing; (5) tubercle, syphilis and new growths, evidences of which should always be sought for in cases of intractable laryngitis. These usually go on to ulceration (p. 274). (6) Spread of inflammation from adjacent parts. Many cases of chronic laryngitis are associated with a granular condition of the pharynx. Nasal sinusitis is a common cause, often overlooked. (7) Any cause of general ill-health predisposes.

Treatment.—The indications are to avoid the cause and to relieve the local congestion. The removal of the cause is most important, and often most difficult to accomplish, for the living of many of these patients depends upon the daily excessive use of the voice. Much may be done to prevent and relieve the condition by proper voice-production and breathing exercises. This affection is common among teachers, and they ought to be specially trained to obviate this defect. Nasal sinus infection is very common and necessitates appropriate treatment. The avoidance of tobacco and alcohol will aid, and residence in a dry climate will often accomplish a speedy cure. Locally, painting with strong astringent remedies, such as zinc chloride (1 in 16) or silver nitrate (1 in 24 or 1 in 16), are useful. These strong applications should not be made more than twice a week; weaker solutions can be applied more frequently. The patient himself may use sprays of alum (1 per cent.), zinc sulphate ($\frac{1}{2}$ per cent.), menthol (1 per cent. in paroleine), or argyrol (10 per cent.), two or three times daily, or inhalations of turpentine, creosote, iodine, menthol, etc., for fifteen minutes three times a day.

§ 170. **Perichondritis** is uncommon and is an inflammation of the perichondrium of the laryngeal cartilages. If considerable, it may lead to necrosis of the cartilages and abscess of the larynx. The differential features, besides loss of voice or hoarseness, are dull aching pain and acute tenderness. These may be accompanied by swelling in the neck. As regards its *Etiology*, apart from traumatism, it is rarely due to a primary cause. It more often occurs secondary to syphilitic or tuberculous laryngitis or to malignant disease, especially after treatment by radium or deep X-ray. It may also follow typhoid and other specific fevers.

Prognosis and Treatment.—It is a serious disease, for even in the mild forms the voice is rarely restored. Stenosis of the larynx may result. If there be much swelling the dyspnœa is very marked, and the patient may die from pneumonia or, in the suppurating forms, from pyæmia. Abscess and fistula may follow. Tracheotomy may be required: large doses of penicillin should be injected as early as possible.

§ 171. **Congenital Laryngeal Stridor** is a rare form of laryngeal stridor commencing at or soon after birth and generally passing off by the age of two years. It is due to a congenital malformation of the vestibule of the larynx, the epiglottis being folded on itself and the ary-epiglottic folds thus being approximated. Stridor is marked on inspiration, slight or absent on expiration. It is worse when the child is startled or excited, and may be absent during sleep. Cyanosis is rare and although there may be retraction of the thorax and abdomen the child is usually in good health. The cry and voice are normal. When bronchitis occurs it is unusually severe. As a rule no *treatment* is required; small doses of chloral or potassium bromide help to quieten a restive child and to lessen attacks.

II. **Ulceration** *of the larynx is met in* TUBERCULOSIS *and* SYPHILIS *and, in persons past middle life,* MALIGNANT DISEASE. *The simple erosions present in* CATARRHAL LARYNGITIS *hardly amount to ulceration. Ulceration is also found in the later stages of* LUPUS *and* LEPROSY, *usually when cutaneous lesions are present.*

§ 172. (*a*) **Tuberculous Laryngitis** should always be suspected when a patient complains of constant hoarseness. This form of laryngitis is recognised by (1) the general pallor of the pharyngeal and especially the palatal mucous membrane; (2) a thickening or swelling most marked over the arytenoids, aryteno-epiglottic folds or the epiglottis; (3) redness and thickening of the vocal cords; (4) the occurrence of irregular, slowly growing ulcers, usually bilateral; and (5) the history or presence of pulmonary uberculosis.

The *Prognosis* has greatly improved in recent years; previously recovery was practically unknown.

Treatment is primarily directed to the accompanying tuberculosis of the lungs (§ 131). Absolute rest from speech, a warm, dry climate, and sanatorium treatment, are essential. Creosote in doses of 1 to 5 ℳ is recommended. In certain cases the application of the galvano-cautery is useful. For the pain, which may be severe enough to cause dysphagia, orthocaine B.P. (Orthoform), or benzocaine B.P. (Anæsthesin), gr. 3–5, may be inhaled into the larynx from a Leduc's tube; or the larynx may be sprayed with 10 per cent. cocaine. Alcohol has been injected into the superior laryngeal nerve with excellent results.

§ 173. (b) **Chronic Syphilitic Laryngitis.**—The laryngitis accompanying secondary syphilis may resemble simple catarrh, with the addition of whitish patches (§ 158). But that which occurs in the later stages nearly always takes the form of ulceration. The intensity of hyperæmia, the irritability, and the profuseness of the purulent discharge are features of syphilitic ulceration. It is distinguished from tuberculous ulceration by (1) the bright red colour of the mucous membrane; (2) the presence of a deep, *rapidly growing ulcer*, with bright yellow surface, regular edges, often undermined, sometimes unilateral; (3) a history of syphilis and a positive blood Wassermann test.

Prognosis and Treatment.—This form of laryngitis is twice as rapid as, and far more destructive than that due to tuberculosis, and is liable to involve the cartilages (*vide* Perichondritis). Even when arrested considerable stenosis may result. *Treatment* is with large doses of injected penicillin.

(c) **Malignant Disease** and (usually in other countries) **Leprosy** give rise to ulceration of the larynx (see below).

III. **New Growths.**—*The diagnosis between* **malignant** *and* **benign** *growths does not usually present any difficulty.* SYPHILIS *and* TUBERCLE *may very closely simulate new growths, especially malignant ones. The history of the case and a general examination are helpful.*

§ 174. (a) **Carcinoma** of the larynx occurs chiefly in men. The growth may be (1) *Extrinsic*, growing on the epiglottis, arytenoids, ary-epiglottic folds, pyriform sinuses and the pharyngeal surface of the cricoid, or (2) *Intrinsic*, arising from the vocal cords, the ventricle and false cords, the interarytenoid region and the subglottic area. The *extrinsic* variety rapidly passes on to ulceration, with soreness or pain and perhaps hæmorrhage; secondary enlargement of the glands follows. Death ensues unless early treatment is instituted. Laryngectomy, pharyngo-laryngectomy or radiation therapy are available. *Intrinsic* cancer, on the other hand, is of slow growth, and low malignancy. It usually starts in the vocal cord, and causes a persistent huskiness. Every case of persistent hoarseness occurring in men over middle age should be sent to a laryngologist for examination. The diagnosis is often difficult, but a one-sided sessile lesion in a patient, especially if he is a man over forty, should raise suspicion, and the case should be watched carefully. When in doubt as to the exact diagnosis a small portion should be removed for microscopic examination by direct laryngoscopy. If the disease is malignant, ulceration will probably appear and the growth will spread along the cord. The movement of the affected cord will sooner or later be impaired. The operation of laryngo-fissure affords 80 per cent. of cures in these cases if seen early. X-ray and radium therapy, and especially exposure to a cobalt beam, afford excellent results in many cases.

§ 175. (*b*) **Benign New Growths** are usually papillomata, fibromata or hæmangiomata. These are almost always unilateral and are pedunculated rather than sessile. They occur as a rule in children or young adults, whilst malignant disease is unusual before the age of forty. If the growth is on the vocal cord or prevents the cords meeting properly, hoarseness will result; otherwise there may be no symptoms. Papillomata may be multiple and may cause stridor, especially in children. A form of chronic laryngitis is what is known as **singer's nodes.** These affect the inner margins of the vocal cords at the junction of their anterior and middle thirds. They are distinguished from other nodules by their involvement of both sides symmetrically. In **Pachydermia Laryngis** there are more or less symmetrical small swellings situated at the *posterior* ends of the cords; there is often a nipple on one cord which fits into a crater on the other. **Leprosy** may affect the larynx. Benign growths often cause but little inconvenience. They are easily removable by direct laryngoscopy.

IV. **Paralysis of the Vocal Cords** *can only be detected by inspecting carefully both the* POSITION *and the* MOBILITY *of the cords during* (i.) *rest,* (ii.) *phonation and* (iii.) *deep inspiration.*

§ 176. **Paralysis of the Vocal Cords.**—The larynx is supplied by two nerves, the superior laryngeal and the recurrent laryngeal branches of the vagus. The former supplies the crico-thyroid or tensor muscle and the mucous membrane of the larynx, while the recurrent laryngeal supplies all the other muscles. In progressive lesions of the recurrent nerve the abductors are paralysed first, and later on the adductors.

The Signs of Laryngeal Paralysis.—It is very rarely that a single muscle is paralysed; the paralysis nearly always affects a physiological group of muscles—*i.e.*, the glottis-openers (abductor paralysis) or glottis-closers (adductor paralysis) on one or both sides. Paralysis is often accompanied by more or less catarrh, which modifies the appearance somewhat, but the evidences of laryngeal paralysis depend upon the position and mobility of the cords during phonation and respiration. The symptoms are given in Table XII.

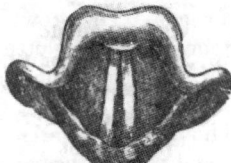 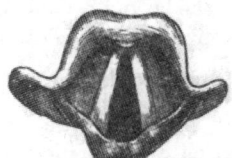 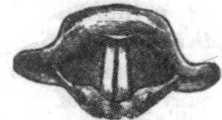

FIG. 73.—MODERATE AD-DUCTION.—The appearance seen during REST.

FIG. 74.—CADAVERIC POSITION of cords.

FIG. 75.—Typical position during PHONATION of high notes.

Normally, during rest the cords are midway between open and closed (Fig. 73); during phonation they are approximated so that practically no space is left between them (Fig. 75); during deep inspiration they are widely opened (Fig. 72).

When the cords are normal during phonation, but do not move out on inspiration, there is bilateral paralysis of the glottis-openers—*bilateral abductor paralysis* (Fig. 76). If both cords move during phonation, but one of them fails to move out fully during inspiration, there is *unilateral abductor paralysis* (Fig. 77).

When the cords neither move to the middle line with attempted phonation, nor move as far outwards as normal during deep inspiration, but remain midway between the two more or less in the so-called cadaveric position (Fig. 74), there is *total bilateral paralysis of* adductors and abductors (Fig. 78).

If during phonation and inspiration one cord remains immobile, there is *total unilateral paralysis.*

If there is aphonia, and on laryngoscopic examination the cords do not meet properly during attempted phonation, although they move outwards with inspiration, there is *bilateral adductor paralysis* (Figs. 79 and 80).

The *Etiology* of laryngeal paralyses differs considerably in the various forms. They may arise from **organic or functional** conditions, but each is so characteristic that it can be readily identified. *Abductor paralysis*, whether unilateral or bilateral, is always organic in origin. If the left vocal cord cannot be abducted, it is almost certainly due to pressure on the left recurrent laryngeal, and this is frequently due to a mediastinal neoplasm. *Adductor paralysis* is always bilateral and functional in origin.

TABLE XII.—LARYNGEAL PARALYSES

(From Gowers, slightly modified.)

Lesion.	Symptoms.	Signs.
Bilateral abductor (opener) paralysis.	Voice little changed; cough normal; inspiration difficult and long, and attended with loud stridor.	Both cords near together; not separated during inspiration, but even drawn nearer together.
Unilateral abductor (opener) paralysis.	Symptoms inconclusive; little affection of voice or cough. Brassy cough sometimes.	One cord near the middle not moving during inspiration, the other normal.
Bilateral complete paralysis.	Weak voice; no cough; stridor only on deep inspiration.	Both cords moderately abducted and motionless (*i.e.*, the cadaveric position).
Unilateral complete paralysis.	Voice low-pitched and hoarse; no cough; stridor absent.	One cord moderately abducted and motionless, the other moving freely, and even beyond the middle line in phonation.
Bilateral adductor (closer) paralysis.	No voice; normal cough; no stridor or dyspnœa.	Cords normal in position, and moving normally during respiration, but not brought together on an attempt at phonation.

(*a*) BILATERAL ABDUCTOR PARALYSIS (Fig. 76) may be due to—

(i.) The earlier stages of *pressure* upon both recurrent laryngeal nerves, as by mediastinal tumour, œsophageal carcinoma or malignant neoplasm of the thyroid gland.

(ii.) *Central Causes*, as in lesions affecting the medulla or base of the brain, bulbar paralysis, disseminated sclerosis, syringobulbia, thrombosis, tumours, tabes dorsalis, chronic forms of meningitis (especially syphilitic pachymeningitis), etc.

(iii.) *Peripheral* causes (rare), such as neuritis from toxins (diphtheria, alcoholism, influenza), certain drugs (*e.g.*, lead, arsenic). Myasthenia gravis may produce the same lesion. It sometimes follows damage to the recurrent laryngeal nerve during thyroid gland operations.

(*b*) UNILATERAL ABDUCTOR PARALYSIS (Fig. 77) is due to the same causes acting on one side only. Thus, if on the *left side*, it is commonly due to aortic aneurysm, mediastinal tumour, or cancer of the bronchus or œsophagus: if on the *right side*, the commonest cause is cancer of the œsophagus, and (rarely) a thickened pleura. Pressure upon the vagus in the neck, as by an enlarged thyroid, or cervical glands, may affect one or both sides. Damage to one recurrent laryngeal nerve may occur during thyroid operations. (Very occasionally ankylosis of the crico-arytenoid joint is a cause: this may result from rheumatism, tuberculosis, trauma and other causes.)

(*c*) TOTAL (AB- and ADDUCTOR) BILATERAL PARALYSIS (Fig. 78) is always of organic origin. It may arise from any of the causes mentioned under Bilateral Abductor Paralysis, but is most frequently of *central* origin. It occurs later in the disease than abductor paralysis, the abductor fibres in the nerve being the first to be affected.

(*d*) TOTAL (AB- and ADDUCTOR) UNILATERAL PARALYSIS is due to the same causes as mentioned under unilateral abductor paralysis—*i.e.*, usually involvement of the recurrent laryngeal nerve. This condition, however, occurs at a later stage in the case, unilateral abductor paralysis being a feature of the earlier stage. Total paralysis is sometimes called " recurrent paralysis," because it is due to paralysis of the recurrent laryngeal nerve.

(e) BILATERAL ADDUCTOR PARALYSIS (Figs. 79 and 80) is always *functional* (viz., unconnected with *gross lesions*): (1) hysterical; (2) simple catarrh, or overuse of the voice; (3) general weakness, as in anæmia. But the first of these is by far the most common.

Diagnosis.—Careful investigation of the neck, chest and the œsophagus should be made in all cases and the cranial nerves should be examined.

Prognosis.—Laryngeal paralysis is generally only a minor element in the case. When occurring alone,

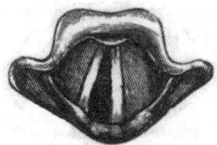

FIG. 76.—BILATERAL ABDUCTOR PARALYSIS.—The patient is able to oppose the cords during phonation, but *the cords do not move outwards during deep inspiration* (as in Figs. 71 and 72).

The same appearance as the above is sometimes produced by acute laryngeal catarrh, but the cords would be pink instead of white.

however, the prognosis in adductor paralysis is good, because it is always of functional origin. In all forms the prognosis depends upon whether the cause is re movable or not. Sometimes paralysis arising fr [.] syphilis is remediable if treated early.

Treatment.—Hysterical paralysis shoul[.] be treated on lines laid down in § 1173. Strong ' ism or static electricity to the larynx is sometimes indicated, the patient being instructed to call out loudly. In organic paralyses the prognosis depends upon the cause. Syphilitic remedies should receive a fair trial. In organic cases, if dyspnœa be severe, tracheostomy must be performed. Operations to improve the airway are sometimes performed (Woodman's operation and then the tracheostomy tube may be discarded).

ILLUSTRATIONS OF LARYNGEAL PARALYSIS.—It should be remembered, in studying these illustrations, that to test the motor power of the vocal cords it is necessary

PATIENT'S RIGHT

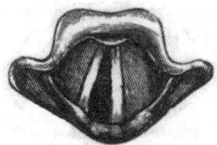

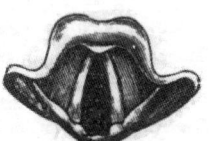

FIG. 77.—LEFT ABDUCTOR, or glottisopener, paralysis.—DURING INSPIRATION the *left cord* remains fixed, instead of moving outwards as does the right cord. This occurs in early paralysis of the recurrent laryngeal nerve of ORGANIC ORIGIN—*e.g.*, aneurysm.

FIG. 78.—TOTAL BILATERAL paralysis.—DURING INSPIRATION AND DURING PHONATION *oth cords* are immobile, and remain in what is practically the cadaveric position. Always of ORGANIC origin, and frequently central.

PATIENT'S LEFT

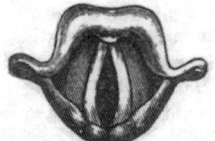

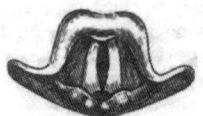

FIG. 79.

FIG. 80.

FIGS. 79 and 80.—PARTIAL BILATERAL ADDUCTOR, or glottis-closer, paralysis.—It is the condition commonly met with in hysterical or FUNCTIONAL aphonia. DURING PHONATION the cords close anteriorly and posteriorly, but leave an elliptical space between them. Two muscles help to close the glottis—the crico-thyroid in front, and the arytenoideus behind. If the CRICO-THYROID is mainly affected, the condition depicted in Fig. 79 is seen, and it is met with in functional aphonia and exhaustion. The ARYTENOIDEUS closes the posterior angle, and when this is paralysed the posterior angle remains open (Fig. 80). Both of these forms are met with in acute and chronic laryngitis, and are generally independent of any actual nerve lesion, excepting perhaps peripheral neuritis and some rare cases due to a local lesion affecting the recurrent laryngeal nerve of both sides.

to make the patient INSPIRE deeply to OPEN the cords, then to PHONATE, so as to CLOSE the cords, for a given position of the cords conveys no information unless it is first known which of these acts the patient is performing.

In laryngeal paralysis it is very important to decide whether a functional or organic cause is in operation, and the following hints should be remembered:

1. Glottis-closer (adductor) paralysis is functional; glottis-Opener (abductor) paralysis Organic.
2. Bilateral paralysis is often functional; One-sided paralysis is Organic.
3. Left Abductor (glottis-opener) paralysis suggests Aneurysm or new growth.

V. SPASM OF THE LARYNGEAL MUSCLES, *and consequent* INSPIRATORY DYSPNŒA, *is not a very common occurrence, except in the form of Laryngismus Stridulus, a disease almost confined to childhood. It may arise when a foreign body passes into the larynx, and may occasionally occur in adults who are the subjects of acute laryngitis. Inspiratory dyspnœa may also arise in Bilateral Abductor Paralysis.*

§ 177. Laryngismus Stridulus or Nervous Croup (Syn. Laryngeal tetany, spasmus glottidis, spasmodic croup, child-crowing) is a form of paroxysmal inspiratory dyspnœa. It occurs in young children and is considered to be due either to a spasm of nervous origin or to the indrawing by a more than usually deep breath, of unusually soft and yielding laryngeal tissues, so that the glottis is obstructed. The whole attack lasts from a few seconds to a minute or two. The child may become cyanosed or the spasm may spread to other muscles and give rise to general convulsions. Rarely it terminates fatally. The attack usually comes on at night and starts with a few crowing inspirations followed by a period of apnœa. Attacks tend to recur, and their severity may increase at each recurrence. On the other hand, if the attacks are slight, they may gradually disappear as the child grows older. In the intervals the child is free from cough or hoarseness, and the larynx appears healthy.

Etiology.—It is a manifestation of infantile tetany (§ 1030), and may be associated with infantile convulsions. It is practically confined to children of from four months to two years old, and is twice as common in boys. It is more frequent in the spring-time, and it is often hereditary. In older subjects laryngeal spasm and inspiratory dyspnœa occur sometimes in tabes dorsalis, when it forms the laryngeal crisis of that disease. Its rarer causes are epilepsy, hysteria, tetany, parathyroid deficiency, chorea, reflex irritation of the vagus or its recurrent laryngeal branch from mediastinal growths, a growth or foreign body in the larynx.

The *Diagnosis* is not difficult, though it is well to bear in mind the possibility of a foreign body in the throat, larynx or trachea. There are, however, three pathological conditions to which the term "croup" is loosely applied and which are also characterised by a PAROXYSMAL INSPIRATORY DYSPNŒA.

1. *Laryngismus stridulus* is the non-inflammatory nervous affection described above. It is recognised by the absence of cough, hoarseness and other symptoms referable to the larynx in the intervals between the attacks. There is often a history of similar attacks.

2. *Catarrhal Laryngitis* (laryngitis stridulosa, false croup) is often associated with attacks of dyspnœa, coming on usually at night in children under ten who are suffering from cough and hoarseness during the day. It may last for an hour or so. It is due to the collection of thick secretion, to the relatively small size of the child's larynx, and to the readiness with which swelling occurs (§ 166). In addition, the nervous system of a child is more unstable.

3. *Membranous Croup*, or laryngeal diphtheria.—This is true diphtheria, and is attended by the constitutional and other symptoms of that disease. A non-diphtheritic membranous croup may occur. A severe injury (*e.g.*, drinking out of a boiling kettle) may certainly result in a membranous or " diphtheritic " inflammation of the mucous membrane.

Treatment of Laryngismus Stridulus.—(*a*) *For the Attacks.*—Mild cases require no treatment except rest and warmth. In severe cases cold water may be dashed in the face, or the patient plunged into a hot bath, or alternately hot and cold, or cold water douches applied. Inhalation of 2–3 drops of chloroform relieves it promptly. Artificial respiration may revive, even after apparent death. In the rare cases in which the spasm is prolonged and continuous, tracheostomy may be necessary. (*b*) *For the Intervals.*—The patient should be kept quiet, and any stimuli conducive to an attack should be avoided. Reflex causes of irritation should be sought for in the gums (*e.g.*, teething), the alimentary canal (*e.g.*, worms or gastric disorder), the lungs and elsewhere (*vide* causes). The general treatment of rickets should be adopted, and it is worth bearing in mind that children taken into the country very often cease to have these attacks. Calcium salts, vitamin D_2, bromides and chloral in small doses allay the irritability of the nervous system, on which the condition mainly depends.

VI. and VII. **Diseases of the Pharynx** (*ante*) **and of the Nose** (*post*) *are generally attended by a certain amount of hoarseness and alteration of the voice.* Nasal disorders give to the voice a characteristic nasal twang.

THE NASAL CAVITIES

§ 178. **Symptoms and Physical Examination.**—Diseases of the nose will be considered under three cardinal SYMPTOMS: *Inodorous discharge* from the nose (Rhinorrhœa); *foul discharge* from the nose (Ozæna); *mouth-breathing* and snoring (Obstruction of one or both Nostrils). *Bleeding* from the nose also occurs in some nasal disorders, but it is *not* a cardinal symptom. It is perhaps more generally associated with some constitutional or general derangement. *Sneezing, tickling* in the nose and *sniffing* may also be present; the quality of the *voice* may be altered, particularly in nasal obstruction; and the sense of *smell* is always disturbed to some extent. In some instances, headache, vertigo and other nervous derangements are met in association with disorders of the nose, especially when the free transit of air through the nasal passages is interfered with, and the air pressure within the tympanum disturbed. Various *constitutional* *symptoms* may result from septic conditions of the nose or the adjacent sinuses, and not infrequently a patient suffers from general toxæmia for a long time before our attention is directed to the true source of his troubles. The sense of smell and its disturbances are dealt with in Chapter XX.

Clinical Investigation.—Rhinoscopy or examination of the nose may be effected through the anterior nares (anterior rhinoscopy), and the posterior nares (posterior rhinoscopy); and by digital examination posteriorly.

ANTERIOR RHINOSCOPY.—First examine the anterior nares for any obvious disorder, such as fissures, ulcers, scars from ulcers, any narrowing of the nares, or a deviation of the septum; secondly, introduce a speculum, using either a direct light or one reflected from a mirror on the forehead, as in laryngoscopy. In this way an examination of the inferior turbinate bone can be made, to see if it be hypertrophied. The inferior or middle meatus should be examined for polypi or alteration in the mucous membrane. If, as frequently happens, the anterior part of the inferior turbinate is hypertrophied, and hides the view, this may be reduced by swabbing out with a cotton-wool pledget soaked in a 10 per cent. solution of cocaine.

POSTERIOR RHINOSCOPY is effected by depressing the tongue with a spatula and introducing a warmed postnasal mirror (like a very small laryngeal mirror) which should be placed facing upwards, below and behind the posterior edge of the soft palate. It is important to avoid touching either the dorsum of the tongue or the posterior wall of the pharynx. The patient should be instructed to breathe gently all the while through the nose. This depresses the soft palate and widens the field of observation. By moving the mirror slightly in different directions we are able to examine the posterior nares and turbinate bones, the inner end of the Eustachian tube for any swelling, and Luschka's tonsil (*cf.* Fig. 70). The pharyngeal or Luschka's tonsil is a mass of lymphoid tissue on the pharyngeal roof and posterior wall above and between the Eustachian tubes; when in a condition of hyperplasia it forms the cushion-like growth of post-nasal adenoids (§ 154).

Information may also be derived by passing the finger behind the soft palate; for this it is generally necessary to spray the pharynx with a cocaine solution (5–10 per cent.). In young children, POSTERIOR RHINOSCOPY is often difficult. A DIGITAL EXAMINATION may be effected by introducing the forefinger behind the soft palate and guiding it along the wall up to the roof of the pharynx. If skilfully done, this causes little more than an unpleasant surprise. Digital examination nowadays is rarely performed except under general anæsthesia.

TRANSILLUMINATION of the antra is a useful aid to diagnosis.—A bright light is placed in the mouth and with the room dark a crescent of light appears over the lower eyelids. With an infected antrum, the normal crescent will be absent on that side. Similarly the light may be placed on the floor of the frontal sinus. X-RAY EXAMINATION OF THE SINUSES is extremely helpful; disease in any sinus causes an opacity.

Our *first* inquiries concerning any given case of suspected disease of the nose should be relative to the LEADING SYMPTOM, especially whether there be any nasal discharge, and whether it is inodorous or foul smelling. We cannot depend upon the patient's statement on this point, because often the disease which causes a foul discharge may blunt the sense of smell. *Secondly*, we must investigate the HISTORY, and whether any of the other symptoms above mentioned were present. *Thirdly*, we proceed to the PHYSICAL EXAMINATION. Test whether the patient can breathe freely through each nostril separately; then examine the anterior and the posterior nares.

Classification.—Diseases of the nose, like those of the throat, are best classified by the PHYSICAL SIGNS met on examination—viz., **nasal discharge, nasal obstruction, epistaxis**—and their **causes.**

(*a*) ACUTE and SUBACUTE INODOROUS DISCHARGES (Acute Rhinorrhœa) —the causes of which are—

    I. Acute Rhinitis; II. Acute Sinusitis; III. Allergic Rhinitis; IV. Hay Fever; *Subacute causes:* V. Diphtheria, and other fevers; VI. Syphilis (snuffles); VII. Glanders; VIII. Myiasis.

(*b*) CHRONIC INODOROUS DISCHARGES (Chronic Rhinorrhœa)—the causes of which are—

    I. Chronic Simple Rhinitis; II. Chronic Hypertrophic Rhinitis; III. Postnasal Catarrh; IV. Chronic Sinusitis and Polypi; V. Cerebro-spinal Rhinorrhœa.

(*c*) CHRONIC OFFENSIVE DISCHARGES (Ozæna), which have for causes—

    I. Chronic Sinusitis; II. Atrophic Rhinitis; III. New growths and foreign body; IV. Ulcerations and Bone Disease—Syphilis, Tuberculosis and Lupus.

(*d*) NASAL OBSTRUCTION (Snoring and mouth-breathing)—the causes of which are—

    I. Adenoids; II. Allergic Rhinitis (§ 179); III. Hay Fever (§ 179); IV. Polypi; V. Deviated Septum; VI. Hypertrophy of Turbinate; VII. Foreign body and Neoplasms; VIII. Hæmatoma and Abscess of the septum.

(*e*) EPISTAXIS, the causes of which may be Local or General.

§ 179. Acute (or recurrent) **Inodorous Discharge from the Nose (Rhinorrhœa).**—*The patient complains of an* ACUTE ODOURLESS DISCHARGE FROM THE NOSE, *which should be confirmed as the disease may have blunted the sense of smell. The commonest causes at any age are* ACUTE CORYZA *and* SINUSITIS. *Apart from this,* CONGENITAL SYPHILIS *should be suspected in infancy;* DIPHTHERIA *in childhood.*

I. **Acute Rhinitis** may be set up by *irritation* of any kind, as by the vapour or dust of some trade, or by any injury. For instance, a profuse discharge from one nostril in a child should make us suspect his having inserted a pea, marble or other *foreign body*, although the history may be wanting. But its commonest cause is a " cold."

Acute Coryza (Syn. " Cold in the Head ") is not serious but is extremely common in temperate climates and occurs in widespread epidemics. Recent statistics of the Registrar-General show it to be the commonest cause of absence from work among males in Great Britain. Some persons are much more susceptible than others.

Symptoms.—The patient first complains of a slight sore throat and stuffiness in the nose, sometimes associated with a tendency to sneezing and conjunctivitis: herpes labialis may be present. A steadily increasing mucoid catarrhal secretion develops in the nose and within 24–48 hours this becomes muco-purulent and finally purulent. The mucous membrane of the nose and throat is generally reddened and later covered by secretion which can be seen in the post-nasal space. The sense of smell and of taste is frequently lost and nasal breathing may become impossible—especially in children. Constitutional symptoms vary in different persons: early on there may be a dull frontal headache; the temperature rises to 99°–100° F and there is a variable degree of general malaise: with higher temperatures pains in the limbs and in the back may occur. After 4 to 7 days the temperature subsides, secretion in the nose lessens and the mucosa becomes covered by a relatively dry secretion of pus. The severity of the complaint varies greatly from person to person: in some it remains localised to the nose and throat, but especially in children and elderly persons it may give rise to infection of the lower respiratory tract and even to pneumonia. The immunity following an attack is relatively short. (See also Acute Pharyngitis, § 154.)

Diagnosis is from other types of respiratory catarrh. *Influenza* causes much more constitutional upset with a temperature of 100°–103° F, severe headaches and aching in the limbs. *Measles* should be suspected in children, especially when an epidemic is prevalent. *Allergic rhinitis* causes recurrent swelling of the nasal mucosa but the mucous membrane is often pale, there is no dried secretion present and it does not cause fever.

Etiology.—The primary cause is a virus of which seven varieties have been identified; it spreads by droplet infection as a result of sneezing, coughing and speaking. Only human beings and anthropoid apes are susceptible. The symptoms caused by the virus are relatively mild: the majority are probably due to the subsequent secondary infection as a result of an increase of virulence of the normal inhabitants of the nose and throat—*Strep. viridans, N. catarrhalis,* or due to super-added infection with other streptococci, staphylococci and hæmophilus organisms. It is predisposed to by cold and damp weather, by adenoids and septic tonsils, sinus trouble and other causes of chronic rhinitis.

Prognosis and Complications.—The whole illness usually lasts between 4 and 10 days: by itself it is of little consequence to the person affected, but in susceptible persons the complications may be numerous. They induce maxillary or frontal sinusitis, Eustachian catarrh, otitis media, tracheitis, bronchitis and broncho-pneumonia. Even when there are no symptoms, X-ray examination may show evidence of primary atypical pneumonia (§ 123).

Treatment of an attack ideally is to insist on the patient spending two or three days in bed as soon as it occurs—but few will do this. As the disease is highly infectious to others, those affected must be taught to use a handkerchief—otherwise they project the infecting organism many feet into the surrounding air. Aspirin or Dover's powder is helpful as are inhalations containing tinct. benzoin. co. Some find relief to the swollen mucous membrane by the use of antihistamine drugs. Antibiotics should only be used when complications arise. It is better not to use vasoconstrictor drugs in nasal sprays or drops.

Prophylactic treatment.—Anti-catarrhal vaccines cannot protect the individual from the primary virus infection but may be of great help in preventing the troubles caused by secondary infecting catarrhal organisms. Other measures consist in avoiding closed spaces, *e.g.*, cinemas during epidemics, correcting diseased conditions of the nasal sinuses, tonsils and adenoids and teaching every child to breathe correctly through the nose.

II. **Acute Sinusitis** commonly occurs as a result of an attack of Acute Rhinitis, or during the course of influenza. (For other causes, see § 181, I.) The symptoms are nasal discharge and obstruction. In the case of the *maxillary* sinus pain may be felt in the cheek; with *frontal* sinusitis, severe frontal headache is felt. With *ethmoiditis* there is pain behind the eyes; occasionally orbital cellulitis with proptosis arises and severe complications may ensue. With *sphenoidal* sinusitis the characteristic headache is occipital or vertical; see § 181, I, and p. 1083.

Treatment should aim at favouring drainage from the affected sinus. The application of cocaine and adrenalin, argyrol 10 per cent. or protargol 10 per cent., or the use of ephedrine hydrochloride (1 per cent. in normal saline) in a spray is often extremely useful. Inhalations with menthol or tinct. benzoin co. are helpful. In severe cases the sulphonamides and penicillin should be given. Short-wave diathermy is of value. In the case of the maxillary sinus, puncture and lavage may be necessary, and if the condition fails to clear up, an operation to establish drainage may be called for.

III. **Allergic Rhinitis** (Syn. Allergic or Paroxysmal Rhinorrhœa) is becoming more commonly recognised. It may occur at any time of the year and although usually starting between 15 and 30 years of age it occurs in younger children: it tends to die away after middle age.

Symptoms.—(i.) The patient complains of irritation of the nose with paroxysmal attacks of sneezing, especially on getting up in the morning or when going into a hot or smokey atmosphere. (ii.) The nose becomes partially or completely blocked. (iii.) In some cases a profuse watery discharge (paroxysmal rhinorrhœa) occurs, sufficient to soak several handkerchiefs in the space of an hour or so. (iv.) On examination of the nose, especially during attacks, the mucous membrane is very sensitive to the touch and is swollen, pale pink and glistening: the clear watery secretion contains a high proportion of eosinophils. In the course of time polypi may form especially in the middle meatus of the nose.

Diagnosis is helped by the paroxysmal nature of the symptoms. X-ray examination of the nasal sinuses often shows a swollen mucous membrane. In the *common cold* there is an initial sore throat and the symptoms persist for 3–5 days without intermission. *Hay fever* is a special variety of allergic rhinitis with a definite seasonal incidence.

Etiology.—As in the other forms of allergy the important causal factors are the inherited tendency, emotional factors and immediate precipitating causes (§ 127). In allergic rhinitis these latter include animal emanations and feathers, vegetable particles such as orris-root (in face powder), certain flowers, moulds and fungi (as in dry-rot), house-dust, and on occasions articles of diet and drugs (especially aspirin). Secondary infections and sinusitis aggravate the condition.

Treatment is difficult and a cure is rarely possible: at the best alleviation of symptoms is all that can be hoped for. The usual measures used are (1) the administration of antihistamine drugs: at bedtime a capsule of diphenhydramine hydroch. B.P.C. (Benadryl) 50 mg. or tab. promethazine hydrochlor. B.P. (phenergan) 25 mg. alleviates the early morning symptoms and helps to ensure sleep. During the day, drugs with a less marked hypnotic effect are used—such as tab. phenindamine tartrate B.P.C. (Thephorin) 25 mg. or tab. chlorpheniramine maleate (Piriton) 4 mg.; (2) ephedrine nasal drops (B.P.C.) and antazoline compound drops (Antistin-privine) when applied in the head-down position and phenylephrine hydrochlor. (Neophryn) as a nasal spray are of help; (3) zinc ionisation is sometimes used and large nasal polypi may need operative removal. Surgical treatment should be as conservative as possible. *Prophylaxis* is by finding and removing the sensitising agent when possible and by keeping the general health at a high level.

IV. **Hay Fever** is a particular type of allergic rhinitis, which also affects the conjunctivæ and often the throat due to hypersensitivity to grass pollen. It comes on fairly regularly in April, May, June or August of each year, depending on the particular pollens to which the patient is ˙ sensitive (in this country usually to timothy grass).

Symptoms may start between the age of 4 and 20 years, tend to recur each year, but usually die away by middle life. (i.) There is intense irritation of the eyes, nose and back of the throat; (ii.) considerable paroxysmal sneezing occurs, often with (iii.) periodic profuse watery discharge from the nose and eyes; (iv.) headache, mental depression and exhaustion may be present; (v.) hay asthma, with bronchial spasm, may occur in the worst cases. Symptoms are always aggravated on hot windy days, and markedly relieved in cool and wet weather. *Examination* reveals marked nasal obstruction, with a general swelling of the mucous membrane of the nose, which is pale and often " water-logged." The eyes prick and the conjunctivæ are reddened and may water.

Etiology.—The condition is due to an allergic state, often with an inherited disposition to other allergic manifestations. An attack is always precipitated by contact with the particular allergens. In Great Britain, when due to tree pollens, symptoms usually commence in the spring, when due to grass pollens they often start in the first two weeks of June (some grasses pollinate in July and August) and when due to shrub pollens (*e.g.*, privet), autumn flowers and moulds they start in September or October. The particular causal agents can be recognised by performing skin tests, using the prick method (§ 127).

Treatment.—The first indication is to avoid the cause: in severe cases residence by the sea or at an altitude may be necessary. A course of desensitising injections of a vaccine composed of the pollens to which the patient is most sensitive is best given before the hay-fever season commences: it should be repeated each year and in many cases gradually produces permanent desensitisation. The various remedies described in the treatment of allergic rhinitis are helpful. Recently hydrocortisone nasal drops (2 mg. in 1 ml. normal saline) and also prednisolone phosphate (1 mg. in 1 ml.) have been found to be very effective. For the conjunctivitis prescribe dark glasses and advise the use of Estevin drops, or eyedrops containing liq. adrenalin. (B.P.) 1 in 8,000 with or without zinc sulphate ¼ per cent.

Subacute causes. V. DIPHTHERIA.—There is an anterior nasal discharge, often blood-stained, with excoriation of the nostrils and upper lip. Nasal obstruction is present but constitutional symptoms are slight; the condition is often present for some weeks before advice is sought; meanwhile the patient is a carrier and infectious to others. A greyish-white membrane is seen on the septum and inferior turbinals; diphtheria bacilli are found in the membrane and can be cultured.

VI. "**The Snuffles.**"—In infants a few weeks old, congenital syphilis is usually attended by profuse nasal catarrh, known familiarly as the "Snuffles." Syphilitic snuffles is obvious in the presence of a purulent rhinitis and other associated symptoms. Respiration is noisy and the discharge is usually blood-stained. (See § 181. IV.*b*.)

VII. GLANDERS.—The copious discharge of viscid semi-purulent matter from the nostrils is one of the earliest symptoms of Farcy, or Chronic Glanders (§ 491).

VIII. **Myiasis** is chiefly met in tropical countries. It is due to the presence of maggots. The eggs from which they hatch are laid by a fly on the nasal mucous membrane, usually while the patient is asleep. Inhalation or local application of pure chloroform is the usual remedy, but insufflations of calomel are also successful.

§ 180. In **Chronic Nasal Discharges** *it is still more difficult to draw the line between odorous and inodorous discharges, since many of the conditions, though odourless at the outset, become offensive later on, and it is generally necessary to pass in review all the conditions mentioned in this section and* § 181. The following are the chief causes of INODOROUS DISCHARGE:

I. **Chronic Rhinitis** is a chronic inflammatory condition of the mucous membrane of the nose, attended by increased secretion, and usually by thickening. It occurs in three forms: (*a*) SIMPLE: (*b*) HYPERTROPHIC (*infra*); (*c*) ATROPHIC (§ 181). The first two give rise to an *inodorous*, but the ATROPHIC to an *odorous* discharge.

CHRONIC SIMPLE RHINITIS is a chronic, congested, and sometimes later on, hypertrophied state of the mucous lining of the nose, with a continuous mucous or muco-purulent discharge. There is generally some nasal obstruction, giving rise to altered voice and snoring.

Etiology.—(i.) It is *predisposed to* by pulmonary disease, alcoholism and the tuberculous diathesis. There is often an allergic basis. It may be *determined* by (ii.) oversmoking; (iii.) recurrent attacks of neglected coryza; (iv.) injury caused by an unsuspected foreign body, in which case the condition is generally confined to one side; or (v.) constant irritation of dust and noxious vapours—*e.g.*, in masons, fustian-cutters. (vi.) It is often associated with adenoids, enlarged tonsils, a deflected septum, and other causes of obstruction in the nose. (vii.) Unsuspected antral or sinus trouble. (viii.) Prolonged use of vaso-constrictor drugs as drops or in a spray (rhinitis medicamentosa).

Prognosis.—The disease is chronic, and requires prolonged treatment. The chief fear is that middle-ear catarrh may result from the extension of the inflammation up the Eustachian tube. Even apart from this, it is very important to treat these cases in children, because the condition interferes with the respiratory functions of the body.

Treatment.—In the early stages alkaline washes—sod. chloride, gr. 10, sod. bicarb., gr. 10, and borax, gr. 5 to fl. oz. 1—should be sniffed up or given by the nasal douche. This is followed later on by a spray of menthol and eucalyptol (gr. x. to fl. oz. 1 of paroleine), or argyrol (10 per cent.). Constitutional treatment is necessary, by means of tonics, cod-liver oil and other sources of vitamin A. Alcohol should be avoided, and a high and dry climate should be sought. In some cases, treatment by short-wave diathermy or the cautery is helpful.

II. **Chronic Hypertrophic Rhinitis** is a special form distinguished from the preceding by the fact that there is considerable hyperplasia of the nasal mucous membrane, especially over the inferior turbinate bone at its anterior and posterior ends. It presents the same symptoms as the preceding, but in a greater degree. Even in slight cases it is apt to be accompanied by headache and mental depression. It is frequently associated with adenoids. The *Prognosis* is on the whole less favourable. The *Treatment* is much the same, but more active measures are indicated—sometimes cauterisation and sometimes surgery.

III. **Post-nasal Catarrh** is usually due to some definite cause in the nose, or to pharyngitis. Occasionally a localised catarrhal inflammation of the naso-pharynx is responsible. *Treatment* should be directed to the primary cause if this can be found; otherwise follow on the lines advised for Chronic Rhinitis.

IV. **Chronic Sinusitis** and **Nasal Polypi** often produce an inodorous muco-purulent discharge. The conditions are dealt with later, § 181, I, and § 182, II.

V. **Cerebro-spinal Rhinorrhœa** is a continual dripping of a watery, clear fluid (cerebro-spinal fluid) from the nose, due to the formation after injury or disease of a communication between the nasal cavity and the sub-arachnoid space. The fluid passes through the cribriform plate of the ethmoid. Its nature is at once recognised by the fact that it reduces Fehling's solution. The flow sometimes ceases spontaneously. By the insertion of a fascial graft the deficiency may be closed. The danger of meningeal infection is considerable and so long as the rhinorrhœa persists penicillin or some other antibiotic must be administered.

§ 181. **Ozæna** or a **Chronic Offensive Discharge** *from the nose may occur in the later stages of* MANY OF THE CONDITIONS *mentioned in the preceding section. But the chief causes of foul discharge from the nose are as follows: the commonest and foulest occurring in* ATROPHIC RHINITIS *in the young;* SYPHILITIC DISEASE *in middle life; and* CANCER *in the aged.*

Foreign bodies (*which have already been referred to*) *may cause one-sided ozæna, and are described under Nasal Obstrvction* (§ 182), *which is their leading symptom. It is here necessary to give some detailed account of*—Chronic Sinusitis; Atrophic Rhinitis; and Ulcerations and Bone disease.

I. **Chronic Sinusitis** may occur in any or all of the accessory nasal sinuses. It is usually due to an extension of infection from the nasal cavities. Chronic maxillary sinusitis is the commonest form; sinus infections may be overlooked for months or years.

Symptoms. (i.) The most constant and cardinal symptom is discharge from one nostril, which is occasionally foul smelling. (ii.) Sometimes discharge is not noticed and nasal obstruction is the main complaint. (iii.) Pain may be localised over the area of the involved sinus, or may be referred to the various parts of the skull, particularly when acute attacks of sinusitis supervene (§ 179). (iv.) Various constitutional symptoms, due to septic absorption, may be the sole manifestation of sinus disease. Headache, lassitude, occasional elevations of temperature and nervous and vaso-motor symptoms are amongst the commonest. They generally have a periodic or paroxysmal character. Facial neuralgia may result from sinus disease. (v.) If overlooked or neglected, sinusitis may excite middle-ear catarrh (with tinnitus, deafness, etc.), recurrent nasal catarrh and nasal polypi: cases of chronic sinusitis are often associated with asthma, recurrent bronchitis, bronchiectasis and sometimes with giant urticaria.

Physical Signs.—(i.) Pus is present in the nose, draining from the affected sinus. It is seen in the middle meatus under the middle turbinate when it comes from the maxillary antrum, or from the frontal or anterior ethmoidal sinuses: and flows over the middle turbinate and down to the pharynx when it is derived from the posterior ethmoidal cells and sphenoidal sinuses. (ii.) Transillumination (by putting a bright light in the mouth) shows an absence of the characteristic crescent of light through the lower eyelid, when one antrum is diseased. (iii.) X-ray examination shows an opacity in the affected sinuses, and sometimes a fluid level is seen in a diseased antrum (Figs. 81, 82). (iv.) Diagnostic puncture and lavage will further confirm the presence of pus.

Etiology.—Acute Rhinitis or " cold in the head " is probably the most frequent cause. Influenza is responsible for many cases. It may arise

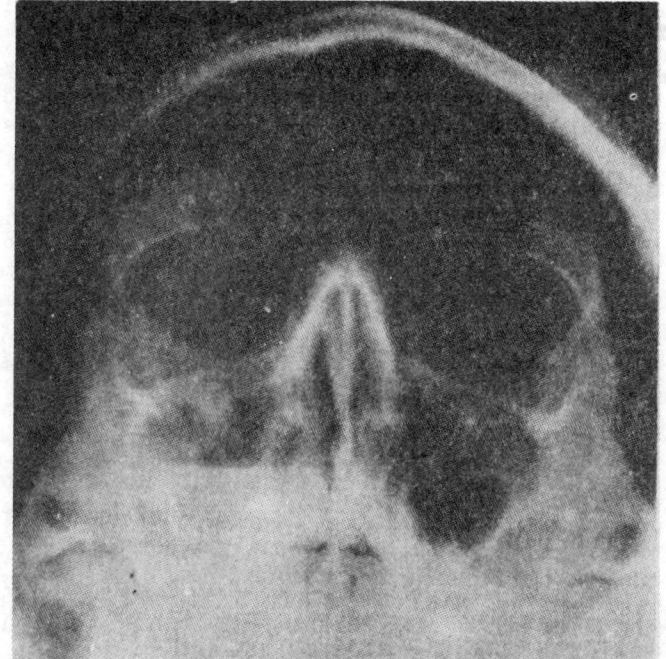

FIG. 81.

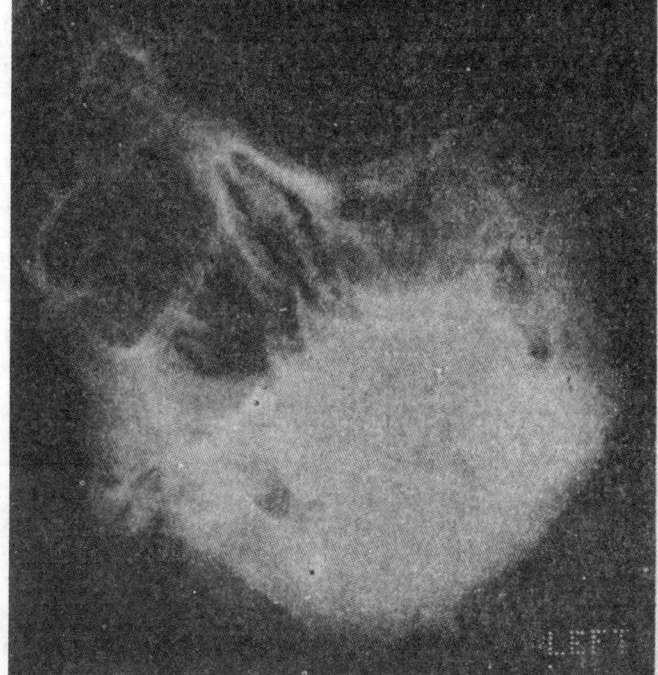

FIG. 82.

FIGS. 81 and 82.—Fig. 81 shows a uniform opacity in the lower half of the Right Antrum. Fig. 82 demonstrates that this is fluid as the upper margin remains horizontal on tilting the head.

C.M.—L

in the course of any of the acute specific fevers, and after injury or operation on the nose. Infection of the maxillary sinus frequently follows dental disease or the extraction of the second premolar and the first two molar teeth in the upper jaw.

Prognosis.—Chronic sinusitis is intractable, but very rarely fatal.

Treatment.—Relief is given by inhalations of 25 per cent. menthol in spirit, 10 drops to a pint of boiling water, by ephedrine in a spray or drops or by alkaline douches. Short-wave diathermy is often valuable. Operation may be needed to establish drainage, before a cure is possible.

II. **Atrophic Rhinitis**, also known as ozæna, is characterised by (i.) a thick, foul discharge, which is sometimes profuse, sometimes scanty; (ii.) the nasal cavities are often large, and the bridge of the nose broad and sometimes depressed. The mucous membrane is thin, pale, and covered with crusts, hard, adherent and decomposing. Sometimes it is unilateral—*e.g.*, in cases of deviated septum. A certain amount of chronic pharyngitis is usually present. (iii.) The breath has a foul odour, which is not detected by the patient, as the sense of smell is blunted. It is *Diagnosed* from the other causes of ozæna by the absence of ulceration, the presence of atrophied mucous membranes and wide cavities.

Etiology.—(i.) It is commoner in the young and in women. It usually starts before sixteen years of age. (ii.) Unilateral atrophic rhinitis is mostly due to some local cause, such as deviated septum or sinus disease, the narrower side being healthy. (iii.) The exciting causes of bilateral atrophic rhinitis are obscure. It is much less common than it was some years ago, and its disappearance seems to have occurred with the general improvement in the nation's health. (iv.) In some cases it follows too extensive operative interference.

Prognosis.—Prolonged treatment is necessary, and even this is not very hopeful if the disease be advanced. The disorder is generally most marked at about twenty years of age; it becomes less troublesome at middle age, and, as it gradually disappears with advancing years, we may presume that it tends slowly to spontaneous cure.

Treatment.—Alkaline and antiseptic douches and sprays are indicated, as in § 180. To stimulate the mucous membrane, nasal tampons of cotton-wool, soaked in 25 per cent. glucose in pure glycerine, are used. These are useful in unilateral rhinitis, as they ensure respiration through the narrower cavity. The instillation of œstrin into the nose is said to help. Constitutional treatment is also advisable. Vaccines assist certain cases. Various operations such as cartilage grafting have been devised to narrow the nose, and while they do not cure, considerable improvement may result.

III. **Neoplasms and Polypi** (§ 182, II), and **Impacted Foreign Body** (§ 179, I, and § 182, V), are referred to elsewhere.

IV. **Ulcerations and Bone Disease** attacking the nose are mostly of traumatic or syphilitic origin. Neoplasms in the later stages ulcerate, but in the earlier stages give rise to discharge and Nasal Obstruction. Leprosy is also a cause.

(*a*) **Simple perforation** of the nasal septum causes a small perforation in the front of the cartilage: it is probably due to the habit of nose-picking.

(*b*) **Syphilitic Rhinitis.**—In the early stages of syphilitic infection we may get an acute catarrh with superficial ulceration, which is the condition found in children with congenital syphilis, known as " snuffles." In the later stages gummata form in various situations, which *rapidly involve the bone* and other parts; the discharge then becomes very foul. Perforation of the septum often occurs. The ulcers have the same characters as those affecting the throat (*q.v.*). There is a positive Wassermann reaction.

(*c*) **Tuberculosis** of the nose is extremely rare except in the form of Lupus, which is now infrequent. It is more common in women than in men, and occurs most often between the age of 15 and 30 years. The anterior part of the septum and the adjacent part of the inferior turbinal present characteristic apple-jelly-like nodules. Perforation of the cartilage of the septum, sometimes crusting and fœtor may result. The progress of the disease is very slow—much slower than with syphilis.

Diagnosis.—Atrophic rhinitis is distinguished from these ulcerations by the pallor and thinning of the mucous membrane, the absence of visible ulcers, and the absence of a history of syphilis or tuberculosis respectively.

The *Prognosis* of nasal ulceration is fairly good if the patient comes under treatment early, otherwise it leads to considerable destruction of tissue. Lupus Vulgaris may slowly lead to the destruction of the *alæ* of the nose, but syphilis results in the most extensive destruction of the *bones* both of the septum and the palate; the bridge of the nose falls in, and the anterior nares may be represented by a single gaping orifice. It is this extensive and rapid destruction which is so pathognomonic of nasal syphilis.

Treatment.—Alkaline sprays are useful palliatives, but surgical measures may be called for if the bone is involved. All dead bone must eventually be removed. Penicillin injections or neoarsphenamine with large doses of potassium iodide lead to rapid healing of syphilitic ulcerations. For Lupus, in the early stage, general and local light treatment is useful. The galvano-cautery or diathermy may be needed in more advanced cases. Isoniazid is the drug of choice: it may be combined with inject. streptomycin or P.A.S.: or calciferol may be given (§ 709).

§ 182. Nasal Obstruction, Snoring and Mouth-breathing.—*Nasal obstruction may be partial or complete, and it may exist on one or both sides. It is met with in a greater or less degree in nearly all of the various nasal conditions previously discussed, and it is a marked feature in* ALLERGIC RHINITIS (§ 179, III), HAY FEVER (§ 179, IV) *and* CHRONIC HYPERTROPHIC RHINITIS (§ 180, II). *Its commonest cause in children is* ADENOIDS (§ 154). *It is also a cardinal symptom in* NASAL POLYPI, DEVIATION OR SPUR OF THE SEPTUM, COLLAPSE OF THE ALÆ NASI, FOREIGN BODIES, NEOPLASMS, HÆMATOMA *and* ABSCESS *of the* SEPTUM.

Effects.—Apart from the inconvenience of snoring, nasal obstruction renders the individual prone to pharyngitis, stomatitis, bronchitis and other results of entry of cold air into the lungs without its being properly warmed and filtered by its passage through the nose. . Other consequences are a nasal quality of the voice, distortion of the chest (when arising early in life), and impeded respiratory functions of the body generally. The ultimate results are quite out of proportion to the degree of local disease.

I. **Adenoids** are very common and are the most frequent cause of mouth-breathing and snoring in children. They are described in § 154.

II. **Polypi,** or pedunculated tumours, are commonly found in the nose. Polypi are of three kinds: (*a*) MUCOUS; (*b*) NASO-PHARYNGEAL; and (*c*) MALIGNANT.

(*a*) Mucous Polypi are frequent. They may occur early in life; but are more common after puberty and in men than women. They are not neoplasms but œdematous mucosa associated with disease of the ethmoidal sinuses. They may be unilateral, but more frequently bilateral. The extent of polypi formation may vary from a few small beads along the under surface of the middle turbinate to enormous masses completely filling both nostrils. There is often an allergic diathesis: if carefully looked for they may be found in many cases of asthma, hay fever and spasmodic rhinorrhœa. In most cases their detection is not difficult; they appear as long, pedunculated, pale grey, glistening bodies.

Antro-choanal polypus is due to chronic infection in the maxillary sinus. The polypus grows out of the antrum and passes back to the naso-pharynx, where it may be seen with the post-nasal mirror. It usually resembles a mucous polypus, but it may be rather pink in colour.

(b) Naso-pharyngeal polypus, or fibroma of the naso-pharynx, a rare but serious disease, grows from the periosteum of the naso-pharynx. It may expand the bones of the face and produce the deformity known as " frog-face." The main symptoms are: nasal obstruction, discharge, headache and epistaxis. They are considered benign tumours because they do not disseminate or involve glands, although they tend to recur locally.

(c) Malignant growths or polypi are not common in the nose and naso-pharynx, but carcinoma and sarcoma do occur. They grow rapidly and cause " frog-face," glands in the neck, pain, deafness and a hæmorrhagic and offensive discharge.

Simple polypi may occur as a result of septic infection in cases of malignant disease of the ethmoid and antrum. These neoplasms may assume a polypoid appearance but are generally fleshy and bleed readily.

Prognosis and Treatment.—Simple polypi usually recur when removed with a snare. With the judicious use of cocaine this operation is easy and painless. Radical surgical treatment of the ethmoidal labyrinth is the only curative measure. Antro-choanal polypus may be removed by the snare but no satisfactory result is gained unless the antrum is at the same time opened and drained. The fibroma and malignant growths require operations of some magnitude and the skilled use of X-rays, radium or exposure to a cobalt beam.

III. **Deflected Septum and Nasal Spur.**—The nasal septum is rarely quite in the median line, but the displacement is often considerable. Sometimes it results from injury. Various consequences may ensue, such as hypertrophied turbinate on one side, atrophic rhinitis on the other. When an angle is formed in the septum nasi, it is spoken of as a " spur," and this is most readily dealt with by the surgeon.

IV. **Hypertrophied Turbinate** is met with usually either as part of, or a consequence of, chronic hypertrophic rhinitis or nasal allergy. It may occur on one or both sides, and in either case in narrow nostrils produces partial obstruction, snoring and mouth-breathing. *Treatment* should first be directed to the causative disease in the nose. Applications of the galvano-cautery are often useful and very rarely partial removal may be required.

V. **Foreign Bodies** within the nose, and **Malignant Neoplasms,** especially of the ethmoid and antrum, may also produce *unilateral* nasal obstruction and discharge. Epiphora is common even before a local swelling appears.

VI. **Hæmatoma of the septum** is almost always due to trauma. The septum swells so as to occlude both nostrils. If not drained, the contents suppurate and *abscess* results.

§ 183. **Epistaxis** (bleeding from the nose) may be a symptom of nasal disease, but if in any appreciable quantity it is usually evidence of some general disorder. Frequently both general and local causes are in operation. The *nasal cavities should be carefully examined.* The blood-vessels give way in this situation (sometimes as a kind of safety valve) merely because they are thin-walled, numerous, near the surface, and liable to traumata great and small. So much is this the case that the diminished atmospheric pressure on high mountains may produce nose bleeding.

(*a*) LOCAL CAUSES, in which the hæmorrhage consists usually of little more than streaks, may arise from any marked congestion of the mucous membranes, such as that which accompanies adenoids, polypi, acute rhinitis, multiple telangiectases, a foreign body or myiasis; or as a consequence of a blow, applied either directly to the nose or to the base of the skull. Any destructive disorder—such as new growths, especially malignant, syphilitic, tuberculous or other ulcerations (which if small are *very apt to be overlooked*)—may be attended by recurrent bleeding. When small in quantity the blood often passes backwards into the throat and is swallowed, or it may be coughed up and be mistaken for hæmatemesis or hæmoptysis.

(*b*) With CONSTITUTIONAL CAUSES the bleeding is usually, although not always, of larger quantity, and it may, indeed, be so profuse as to endanger life. In this group the blood comes from a spot near the anterior part of the septum. Among the *predisposing causes*, there is in certain individuals an idiopathic family tendency to bleed from the mucous surfaces (not amounting to hæmophilia) with or without a wound. Epistaxis is more frequent in children, especially in boys. It is also met in the aged, but only when vascular disease and some other conditions about to be mentioned exist. The constitutional causes may be grouped under (*a*) *Alterations in the Cardio-vascular System*, (*b*) *Blood Diseases* and (*c*) *Specific Fevers*.

(*a*) Epistaxis occurring for the first time in an apparently healthy person over forty years of age should always give rise to the suspicion of chronic nephritis or hypertension. A considerable number of patients, after repeated admissions to hospital for epistaxis, finally come in to die of cerebral hæmorrhage. Epistaxis frequently occurs with cardiac valvular disease, emphysema, chronic bronchitis, thoracic tumours, and cirrhosis of the liver: also with extremes of temperature, after violent exercise, with the menstrual period, mountaineering and in aeroplanes.

(*b*) *Blood Diseases·* Purpura, hæmophilia, scurvy, leukæmia, anæmia (simple and pernicious), deficiency of blood platelets (thrombocytopenia).

(*c*) *The Specific Fevers* especially responsible are typhoid, acute rheumatism, and the hæmorrhagic forms of the exanthemata. It is in children a frequent prodromal manifestation of whooping-cough and other fevers.

Prognosis.—Slight epistaxis in children is of no consequence, but when occurring for the first time in persons at or past middle life it should receive serious attention. Inquiry should always be made as to whether it has occurred previously because, as above mentioned, certain persons have this tendency, and in these the symptom is not important.

Treatment.—Epistaxis which accompanies nephritis and the congestion of cardiac and pulmonary disease should not be checked unless the amount be profuse. In such cases the epistaxis is usually preceded by headache, and is accompanied by high blood pressure. In all cases of epistaxis, examine the blood pressure. So long as this remains high or moderate no harm can accrue from the epistaxis.

(*a*) The treatment of *the attack* resolves itself into checking the hæmorrhage. The patient should be kept perfectly quiet, sitting up in bed, the head being cool, the feet warm. With the head tilted slightly to one side, palatal movements should be restricted by instructing the patient to breathe through the mouth, with a dental prop or cork between the teeth (Trotter). Morphia should be given if the hæmorrhage is severe. Pressure should be kept up over the anterior part of the septum with the thumb and forefinger externally. The cautery, at a dull-red heat, may be applied to the bleeding spot. Other useful measures consist of using an adrenalin spray, or in severe cases packing the nose for not more than 24 hours with ribbon gauze soaked in adrenalin or adrenalin and cocaine (5 per cent.). Rarely is it necessary to tie, by operation, the anterior ethmoidal artery or even the external carotid artery. Serious anæmia may be suspected when there is extreme pallor of the skin and mucosa; this can be confirmed by a blood examination. In such a case it may be necessary to resort to blood transfusion (§ 547).

(*b*) *Between the attacks a thorough investigation* of the nasal and post-nasal cavities must be made. A deflection of the septum near the front of the nose on which dust or face-powder collects may be responsible and require correction. Minute lesions are easily overlooked. Vaseline, lanoline or ung. aquosum (B.P.) introduced into the nostril often helps to prevent attacks: this is most useful where children are prone to epistaxis.

THE THYROID GLAND

This gland is anatomically connected with the upper respiratory passages, but is physiologically quite separate. Its activity is largely controlled by the thyroid-stimulating hormone (TSH) of the anterior pituitary gland. Deficiency of TSH leads to underaction of the thyroid gland, whereas excess may produce hyperthyroidism. Iodine is an essential component of the active principle of the thyroid gland, thyroxine. In the cells of the thyroid iodine unites with tyrosine to form diiodo-tyrosine: this conjugates to form tetraiodotyrosine and then *l*-thyroxine, which is stored in a close combination with protein in the colloid vesicles as thyroglobulin. When required, the *l*-thyroxine is set free again and some is converted to triiodothyronine, both of which have been identified in the bloodstream and are active in the tissues. Excessive production of the thyroid hormones is normally self-limiting because of their inhibiting effect on the TSH of the pituitary. When the thyroid secretion is increased it stimulates the sympathetic nervous system, in part by acting on the suprarenal medulla. Together, these stimulate the liver to liberate glycogen, which circulates as glucose. The thyroid is in close relationship with the other ductless glands, especially the suprarenal, pancreas, and ovary. In health it enlarges at puberty, during menstruation, sexual excitement, pregnancy, lactation, and in the presence of most acute specific fevers, notably rheumatic fever. An unusual degree of enlargement at puberty is not pathological unless constitutional symptoms are present.

Symptomatology.—There are two opposite clinical conditions which may arise from disorder of the thyroid gland. In one there is a *diminished* thyroid action, a condition of *Hypothyroidism*, the symptoms of which (lethargy, lowered vitality, and impaired growth and development) are similar in kind but less in degree to those of Myxœdema and Cretinism. The other condition is one of *increased* (or perverted) thyroid action or *Hyperthyroidism* (thyrotoxicosis): this, with the exception of the proptosis, can be produced by the administration of thyroid extract or thyroxine in large doses to normal people. It is important to remember that the size of the gland does not necessarily aid diagnosis, for enlargement of the gland is consistent with diminution of its function; while what appears to be a small gland may be functionally very active.

§ 184. Physical Examination. Special Tests and Classification.—There are but two physical signs referable to the thyroid gland—the size, *i.e.*, enlargement or diminution of volume, and altered consistency. When the change in volume is only slight it is difficult, if not impossible, to estimate it with accuracy, because it is partially covered by muscles, and is intimately connected with the trachea and other deeper structures. The patient should be instructed to let his head fall forwards and *to swallow* whilst we endeavour to palpate the gland. The thyroid rises during deglutition as does no other tumour in the neck. Pathological enlargement is referred to as a goitre. Note whether the enlargement is regular and diffuse, or irregular and localised. Some idea may be obtained of the progress of a case by measuring the neck from time to time, always exactly at the same level.

When the thyroid fails to develop normally, part of the thyroid tissue may be left at the base of the tongue. There it forms a painless, soft swelling in the mid-line, which may not attract notice until it enlarges at puberty or later. If the swelling be removed, myxœdema or hypothyroidism will follow in the event of there being no other thyroid tissue.

Special Tests of Thyroid Function. Three tests are in common use:

1. *The Basal Metabolic Rate* is a measure of the body metabolism under standard resting conditions: it is now performed by estimating the oxygen requirement per minute per sq. metre of body surface, using a closed-circuit portable Benedict apparatus (§ 1214). The normal range on the Aub-Du Bois standards is plus 15 per cent. to minus 10 per cent. *Fallacies:* apart from thyroid disease, high values may be obtained in leukæmia, polycythæmia, Cushing's syndrome, acromegaly, diabetes mellitus, heart failure, Paget's disease, in late pregnancy and during lactation. Mild sedation lowers the value in anxiety states but not in hyperthyroidism.

2. *The Radio-active Iodine Uptake* of the thyroid measures the activity of the gland by the proportior of iodine which it absorbs. In the normal person, between 23 and 64 per cent. of a given dose is absorbed by the gland: in hyperthyroidism the gland takes up much greater amounts and correspondingly less is excreted in the urine. The reverse occurs in myxœdema. For the test I^{131} is given by mouth and the amount absorbed by the gland up to 4 hours later is measured by a Geiger counter. The protein-bound I^{131} level is a measure of the iodine in the serum proteins and in hyperthyroidism exceeds 0·4 per cent. of the dose per litre of plasma.

3. *Protein-bound Iodine.*—This estimation is technically difficult but gives an accurate index of the level of the circulating hormones. Levels above 7·5 μg. per cent indicate hyperthyroidism and below 3 μg. hypothyroidism.

Fallacies.—All these three tests give misleading results if medicines containing iodine or iodides, or iodine containing X-ray contrast media, have been given even weeks beforehand.

Classification.—*Enlargement* of the thyroid is due to seven common and several rare causes. *Diminution* of the gland occurs in two well-marked types.

(A) **An Enlargement of the thyroid** is—at some stage of the malady—the essential or pathognomonic feature in—

COMMONER CAUSES.

REGULAR ENLARGEMENTS:

without toxic symptoms ..	Parenchymatous Goitre. § 185.
with toxic symptoms	.. Graves' Disease, or Exophthalmic Goitre. § 186.
with myxœdema	Lymphadenoid Goitre. § 187 (rarer than the above).

IRREGULAR *or* NODULAR ENLARGEMENTS:

without toxic symptoms ..	Simple Adenoma. § 188.
	Colloid Goitre. § 189.
	New Growths. § 190.
with toxic symptoms ..	Toxic Adenoma. § 191.

RARE CAUSES are: Anæmias; Specific fevers; Leukæmia; Hæmorrhage; Granulomata and parasitic diseases; Reidel's disease; Menopausal goitre; Cretinism; Acromegaly (some forms).

(B) **Atrophy of the thyroid**—or at any rate a diminution of its function (and usually of its size)—is the essential feature in two diseases.

I. Cretinism ..	..	..	..	..	§ 192
II. Myxœdema ..	..	..	..	..	§ 575

It therefore follows that:

1. Increased or disordered thyroid secretion gives rise to profound disturbance of the general health, and neuro-vascular irritability (Graves' disease).

2. An innocent enlargement of the thyroid, unaccompanied by increased or disordered thyroid secretion, has no effect on the metabolism (as in many cases of simple goitre).

3. Simple absence or diminution of the thyroid secretion (*a*) when it is congenital or comes on in early life, causes deficient development both mentally and physically (*i.e.*, cretinism); and (*b*) when it supervenes in adult life, causes lethargy and deficient vitality (myxœdema).

(A) *There is a* UNIFORM ENLARGEMENT OF THE THYROID GLAND, WITHOUT TOXIC SYMPTOMS: *the patient is between the* AGES OF 5 AND 20. *The disease is* PARENCHYMATOUS GOITRE.

§ 185. Parenchymatous Goitre.

—This condition arises especially in endemic areas in England, as well as abroad (especially in Switzerland and certain parts of India). It also occurs sporadically. It starts in childhood or may appear at or near puberty and last to adult life. It affects women more than men.

Symptoms.—(i.) The patient is noticed to have a uniform smooth and rather soft enlargement of the thyroid gland, of small or moderate degree. One lobe or the isthmus of the gland may be enlarged more than the remainder. (ii.) The general health is good, but the patient is often somewhat anæmic. (iii.) Otherwise the symptoms are those of hypothyroidism rather than of hyperthyroidism. (iv.) If the enlargement lasts to adult life, it becomes a colloid or adenomatous goitre.

It may be *Diagnosed* from other tumours in the neck by the fact that it invariably rises with the larynx during deglutition. The enlargement generally increases steadily, but it is rare that there is any danger from tracheal obstruction and asphyxia.

The *Etiology* of the condition is not fully understood. The disease is primarily due to a deficient uptake of iodine by the cells of the thyroid gland with a resulting insufficient production of thyroxine: the thyroid-stimulating hormone of the pituitary therefore overacts to produce an increased size of the thyroid. The known causes are (i.) shortage of iodine in the food or drinking water. This accounts for the condition being endemic in certain districts in England and especially in parts of Switzerland, the U.S.A. and in the Himalayas. The work of McClendon and Hathaway showed that most forms of goitre were caused by deficiency of iodine. In ordinary diet iodine is obtained from milk, butter, fruits and leafy vegetables; vegetables lose two-thirds of their iodine content in cooking and when fish is canned its iodine content is lost. (ii.) There is an inability of the intestine to absorb the available iodine: one cause of this is when the drinking water is very hard and contains an excess of calcium. (iii.) In other cases although the amount of iodine absorbed is adequate, the thyroid may not be able to utilise it; certain foods, and drugs such as the perchlorates, thiouracil derivatives, the sulphonamides and para-amino-salicylic acid, are known to act in this way.

Treatment.—In early cases it is often sufficient to give iodine in the form of potassium iodide gr. 1 or liq. iodi aquosus B.P. (Lugol's solution) ℳ 3 daily. When the condition is more advanced thyroid gr. 1–2 a day should be added to suppress the TSH of the pituitary. Surgical treatment is necessary if pressure symptoms occur. *Prophylaxis* (as advised by a Medical Research Council Report), and especially where endemic goitre is prevalent, is secured by adding 1 part of potassium iodide to 100,000 parts of all common table salt.

There is ENLARGEMENT *of* BOTH LOBES *of the* THYROID *with* PROPTOSIS, TACHYCARDIA *and* NERVOUS SYMPTOMS; *the patient is usually a* YOUNG WOMAN. *The disease is* EXOPHTHALMIC GOITRE.

§ 186. Graves' Disease (Syns.: Primary Thyrotoxicosis, Exophthalmic Goitre, Basedow's disease). Usually the onset is insidious, but it may start acutely, or acute symptoms may arise in a mild case, after sudden shock or acute focal infections (*thyrotoxic crisis*). The disease is due to over-secretion of thyroxine producing a raised metabolic rate.

Symptoms.—1. *Cardio-vascular* disturbances are among the earliest and most important symptoms. They are never absent, and may precede other symptoms by some months: (i.) Præcordial palpitation. (ii.) Tachycardia is present during rest and sleep; a raised pulse rate during sleep aids diagnosis, as psychological causes are thus excluded. The heart rate may be 100 or more at rest, and may rise to 150 or over on slight exertion or emotion. (iii.) The pulse is forcible and the systolic blood pressure raised, with a corresponding rise in the pulse pressure. (iv.) Shortness of breath on exertion is usual: paroxysmal dyspnœa and a distressing sense of suffocation are sometimes present. (v.) At first the heart is hypertrophied, with a widespread forcible cardiac impulse; later myocardial degeneration with corresponding electrocardiographic changes, premature beats, and in severe cases auricular fibrillation ensue.

(2) *Nervous* disturbances are always present. They are very variable: thus (i.) there is almost invariably restlessness, nervousness, irritability and insomnia. Especially in those with a psychopathic tendency there may be hysterical attacks, excitement alternating with depression and even acute mania. (ii.) Neuralgic headache, vertigo and hypersensitivity to sudden noises. (iii.) The muscles are hypertonic and the tendon reflexes exaggerated but ill-sustained. (iv.) There is always a fine vibratile tremor of the outstretched fingers and often of the protruded tongue. (v.) There are many types of vaso-motor disturbances. Intolerance of heat is usual and there may be sudden perspiration. The hands are hot and sweating even at rest. (vi.) Skin changes include pigmentation and sometimes leucoderma. Loss of hair is often complained of.

(3) *Thyroid Enlargement* is present at some stage of the disease, though it is rarely the first symptom noticed by the patient. Although the whole thyroid is enlarged, one lobe may be larger than the other. It is always more marked in women of 15–30. In older subjects the degree of enlargement may be slight. The degree of enlargement varies considerably in different cases, and is by no means proportionate to the other symptoms, because the symptoms depend more upon the histological changes than the degree of enlargement: some of the enlargement is due to the increased vascularity which produces a hum on auscultation over the gland. Mechanical effects of thyroid enlargement may be present (see §§ 79, III, 188), and occasionally alteration in the voice occurs.

(4) *Exophthalmos* (proptosis or protrusion of the eyeballs) is present in a varying degree, though sometimes not until late in the disease (Fig. 3,

§ 11). It is best detected by seating the patient in a chair, standing behind, and looking down the forehead. As a rule no changes can be detected in the fundi. Later on, ulceration of the cornea occasionally takes place, either from neurotrophic causes or from deficient protection (§ 1111). Even when true exophthalmos is absent, the retraction of the upper lids contributes to a characteristic strained or startled expression.

Four signs of Graves' disease referable to the eyes bear the names of different physicians. *Von Graefe's* sign is a condition in which the upper eyelid lags behind the eyeball when looking downwards, exposing the white sclerotic. *Mœbius's* sign is a deficient convergence of the two eyes when looking at a near point. *Stellwag's* sign is a deficiency of blinking as an involuntary act. *Abadie's* sign is an involuntary twitching or spasm of the levator palpebræ superioris. All except the first are present only in advanced cases, and are not therefore of great diagnostic value.

(5) The *general health* is always disturbed. In spite of a large appetite some loss of weight is always present due to the raised metabolic rate: sometimes 2–3 stone may be lost in as many months especially when the basal metabolic rate is raised to 75 per cent. or more. Diarrhœa is often present and aggravates the weight loss. Lack of energy and undue fatigue are usually present. The menses are decreased or absent and abortion is fairly common. There is no anæmia, but a decrease in the total white cell count with a relative lymphocytosis is usual. The blood cholesterol is decreased. Glycosuria may occur because of a lowered sugar tolerance or a lowered renal threshold: true diabetes mellitus may develop and then weight loss is much more rapid.

In certain patients the cardiac symptoms predominate. In these cases (*formes frustes*, masked hyperthyroidism), the patient is usually older and complains of palpitation. There is a rapid, forcible apex beat, high pulse pressure and often auricular fibrillation: the thyroid may be little altered in size but is of firm consistence, exophthalmos is usually absent; some tremor of the outstretched fingers and vascular symptoms are present.

Diagnosis.—The chief diagnostic points are the emotional excitability, the characteristic facies and often exophthalmos, the rapid forceful heart action, the tremor of the outstretched fingers, the intolerance of heat and undue sweating, and the loss of weight. In a young person *pulmonary tuberculosis* will also produce tachycardia, palpitation, loss of weight and ready fatigue: a chest X-ray is often necessary to differentiate these. An *anxiety state* and especially that form known as neuro-circulatory asthenia (§ 34) also gives rise to irritability, præcordial palpitation, tachycardia, shortness of breath and ready fatigue. However, in this condition the thyroid gland is not enlarged, the pulse rate settles to normal during sleep, undue perspiration is confined to the hands and to the axillæ and the basal metabolic rate is not raised.

Confirmation of the diagnosis of hyperthyroidism is obtained by (i.) the basal metabolic rate being above normal (§ 1214); (ii.) the protein-bound iodine of the serum is above the normal maximum of 7·5 μg. per 100 ml.; (iii.) the administration of a suitable oral tracer dose of radio-active iodine I¹³¹ (usually about 40 microcuries). In hyperthyroidism a Geiger counter shows an excessive uptake of the I¹³¹ by the thyroid, a diminished urinary excretion and the radio-active protein-bound iodine is above 0·4 per cent. of the dose administered per litre of plasma. All these tests are invalidated by recent doses of iodine.

Etiology.—Although the immediate cause is oversecretion of thyroxine, in some this is due to overstimulation of the thyroid by the thyroid-stimulating hormone of the anterior pituitary. Exophthalmos is believed to be due to oversecretion of a pituitary hormone (§ 1114). Although nearly 90 per cent. of cases are women, especially of the child-bearing age, cases occur in children and in the elderly. Locality has no known influence. Heredity sometimes plays a part. Other members of the family often show nervous instability or even disordered thyroid action. Fright, anxiety, love affairs, and mental overwork are potent factors in determining the disease. Toxæmia (oral sepsis, etc.) undoubtedly aggravates the condition.

Prognosis.—Without treatment the disease usually lasts for years, waxing and waning in severity each few months: ultimately it shortens life; if the duration be prolonged the disease will certainly produce cardio-vascular degeneration. The prognosis is worse when the heart is appreciably enlarged, when auricular fibrillation ensues and with marked mental changes. Improvement is judged by the general excitability lessening, by a lowered resting pulse rate and a gain in weight. Even after recovery relapse may occur. Upper lid-lag or true exophthalmos often persists: following treatment by operative removal of the thyroid or by other methods progressive exophthalmos and ophthalmoplegia (malignant exophthalmos) may arise (§ 1114). Myxœdema may develop in later years.

Treatment.—In early cases more rest and sleep are essential: a short period of rest in bed with freedom from fuss and worry, preferably in the country, is most helpful. Treatment in a general hospital ward is therefore undesirable, especially as these patients are very susceptible to infections such as an epidemic sore throat. The diet should be of high calorie value to counteract the loss of weight. Sleep is most important, and sedative doses of phenobarbitone, chloral and potassium bromide should be used when necessary. All sources of toxæmia must be sought for and eliminated as soon as the patient's condition permits. Liquor iodi aquosus (Lugol's solution) 5–10 minims in milk, twice daily, appears to hasten the cure, but should be given in short courses of 3–4 weeks rather than for longer periods.

In more severe cases three lines of treatment are available. (1) *Medical treatment* on the lines just indicated is reinforced by specific drug therapy. (*a*) Thiouracil has been abandoned due to the risk of sudden agranulocytosis: this complication is much less common with methyl-thiouracil and is almost unknown with propyl-thiouracil—and other side-effects such as drug-fever and skin rashes are less frequent. This latter is given as tab. propyl thiouracil 30–60 mg. t.d.s., gradually reducing the dose after

3–4 weeks to 10–50 mg. daily—a dose which must be continued for at least 12 months, and even then relapse may occur when it is stopped. During propyl-thiouracil treatment the thyroid gland may enlarge further and exophthalmos become a little worse—these subside when treatment is stopped. The thiouracil compounds prevent iodine joining with tyrosine to form diiodotyrosine—therefore iodine and iodides must not be given simultaneously. (b) Tab. carbimazole B.P. (Neomercazole) is almost free of undesirable side-effects. It probably acts by blocking the ability of the thyroid to concentrate iodine. The initial dose is 10–15 mg. t.d.s., gradually reduced to 2·5–5·0 mg. daily as the hyperthyroidism comes under control. (c) Potassium perchlorate is slower in action: it is also largely free of side-effects but can cause gastric irritation. It also prevents iodine being concentrated in the gland: initial doses are 0·2 G. q.i.d., reduced after 4 weeks to 0·2 G. b.d.: iodine preparations must again be avoided. (2) *Surgical treatment* follows control of the acute symptoms by a course of medical treatment with propyl-thiouracil or carbimazole: in either case a 5–7 day course of liq. iodi aquosus B.P. (Lugol's iodine) is given immediately before operation. Three-quarters to seven-eighths of the gland is removed and in expert hands it is attended by a very low mortality. Surgery is indicated when the gland is greatly enlarged and is producing pressure symptoms and when myocarditis is developing. (3) *Radio-active iodine* in a single therapeutic dose of 3–10 millicuries orally is a simple procedure and is becoming increasingly popular. The iodine is concentrated in the thyroid and the *beta* rays produce a local involution of the gland. The effect does not show itself for 3–4 weeks: a second dose may be given after 3–4 months if found necessary for it is not usual to administer too large a dose initially for fear of producing myxœdema. This treatment is especially useful if a patient relapses after previous thyroidectomy. In young women there is said to be a possible danger of damaging the ovaries or of producing a thyroid carcinoma 20 or more years after: some therefore only give I^{131} to women over 45 years of age, but so far there is little evidence of these late effects.

Whichever treatment is used, the chief complication which develops within 2–4 months is progressive exophthalmos with ophthalmoplegia and papillœdema (see § 1114).

There is RECENT ENLARGEMENT *of the whole or of part* OF THE THYROID *in a* WOMAN OF 40–65 YEARS; *the swelling is* VERY FIRM; *sooner or later the patient presents signs of* MYXŒDEMA—*the disease is* LYMPHADENOID GOITRE.

§ 187. **Lymphadenoid Goitre** (Hashimoto's disease) is being diagnosed more often as a result of specific tests.

Symptoms.—The goitre is frequently of recent origin, usually in a woman at or after middle age, and it is usually symmetrical although it may involve only one lobe. The gland is very firm but it is not fixed to surrounding structures as is a carcinoma. When first seen the patient is either euthyroid or already presents the symptoms of myxœdema. Later, pressure symptoms such as dysphagia or a sense of constriction in the neck may arise.

Diagnosis and Etiology.—The condition is due to a local destructive effect in the thyroid due to an auto-immune (antigen-antibody) response to the patient's own thyroglobulin. As the swollen gland becomes more fibrotic myxœdema develops. When only part of the gland is involved diagnosis from carcinoma is effected by finding a greater uptake of tracer doses of radio-active iodine (I^{131}) over the swelling than in the rest of the gland (in carcinoma the converse is usual); and the radio-active protein-bound I^{131} is high at 48 hours even with clinical myxœdema. Needle-biopsy is a valuable diagnostic aid. Other tests are: (i.) the erythrocyte sedimentation rate and the blood cholesterol are high; (ii.) the serum flocculation values are raised (with a normally functioning liver); (iii.) a specific precipitin test between the patient's serum and thyroglobulin is positive and (iv.) there is a positive complement fixation test between the heat-inactivated serum of the patient and a saline extract of normal thyroid. Positive serological tests are sometimes obtained in other diseases of the thyroid.

Treatment is by the oral administration of thyroid. Not only does the clinical condition of the patient improve but within a few weeks the thyroid swelling disappears and the blood and serological findings revert to normal.

Irregular *or* Nodular Enlargements

The patient is a middle-aged *or* elderly *person (usually a woman), with a* nodular swelling *in the* thyroid gland; *otherwise she is in good health. The condition is* Simple Adenoma.

§ 188. Simple Adenoma.—This common condition comes on later in life than those mentioned above.

Symptoms.—(i.) There are one or more smooth firm nodules in the substance of the thyroid gland which very slowly enlarge over a period of years. (ii.) There are no toxic symptoms, but anxiety may be caused by the size of the swelling. (iii.) If the swellings are large enough there is pressure upon or displacement of the trachea, and occasionally of other structures in the neck. When the swelling is retro-sternal there may be shortness of breath, an irritating cough especially when lying down, and other symptoms of a mediastinal tumour (§ 77). (iv.) Some of the swellings may be soft and even cystic due to colloid degeneration or hæmorrhage.

Etiology.—This innocent type of new growth is the result of focal hyperplasia in a gland previously damaged by chronic parenchymatous changes or by focal inflammation. A single adenoma occurring in younger adults may arise from an embryonic cell rest: this " fœtal adenoma " is particularly liable to malignancy.

Treatment.—No treatment is necessary or desirable provided pressure symptoms are absent; otherwise surgical intervention is needed.

The thyroid gland *is* enlarged throughout *and may be* enormous;

there are IRREGULAR LARGE CYSTIC SWELLINGS.   *The condition is probably*
COLLOID GOITRE.

§ 189. **Colloid Goitre.**—Colloid change may arise in a simple parenchy-matous goitre in areas where the disease is endemic, or it may be sporadic. *Symptoms.*—(i.) The gland slowly enlarges and may form a tumour involving all parts of the gland and weighing many pounds.   (ii.) It occurs generally in adolescent girls, but persists into adult life.   (iii.) The surface is firm, but not hard, and localised cystic swellings can often be clearly distinguished.   (iv.) The enlargement frequently surrounds the trachea, causing atrophy of the tracheal rings.   Pressure on the trachea produces feelings of suffocation, and on the œsophagus difficulty in swallowing. (v.) The patient usually shows the early symptoms and signs of hypothyroidism.

Treatment.—If necessary for cosmetic reasons, or if pressure symptoms are troublesome, one or both lobes of the gland will have to be surgically removed.   Thyroid will probably have to be prescribed later.

There is a SMALL *or* MEDIUM-SIZED MASS *of almost* STONY HARDNESS *in one part of the thyroid gland; with* ENLARGED CERVICAL GLANDS *and/or signs of* MALIGNANT DEPOSITS ELSEWHERE.   *The condition is* MALIGNANT DISEASE.

§ 190. **Malignant Disease** of the thyroid gland is known by (i.) a very hard mass in the gland; (ii.) this has recently increased in size and become fixed to surrounding structures; (iii.) the lymphatic glands in the posterior triangles of the neck are involved early. (iv.) Invasion of adjacent parts produces recurrent laryngeal paralysis, tracheal stridor, and/or dysphagia. (v.) When the primary growth is small, and found only after careful examination, the patient may show signs of deposits elsewhere in the body, particularly in the bones, with spontaneous fractures; (vi.) anæmia of the leuco-erythroblastic type occurs when the bone marrow is involved. *Diagnosis* may be aided by obtaining a specimen for microscopy by needle-biopsy.

Treatment is surgical when the condition is diagnosed before metastatic deposits develop.   Administration of radio-active iodine helps in those rare cases which can be shown to concentrate tracer doses of I^{131} in the gland.   In some, deep X-ray therapy is beneficial.

There is ENLARGEMENT OF THE THYROID, *diffuse or localised, which has* LASTED FOR YEARS *before the appearance of symptoms of hyperthyroidism; the patient is usually a woman of* MIDDLE AGE—*the disease is* TOXIC ADENOMA.

§ 191. **Toxic Adenoma** (Syns. Secondary Graves' disease, secondary thyrotoxi-cosis) is a condition in which the enlargement of the thyroid may be diffuse or localised, sometimes of considerable size, continuing for years before the appearance of symptoms suggestive of hyperthyroidism.

Symptoms.—(i.) The patient is usually a woman of middle age. (ii.) **Cardiac** symptoms usually predominate.   Palpitation, tachycardia and shortness of breath on exertion are early symptoms.   Sometimes the patient first seeks advice on account of the symptoms of myocardial degeneration, or when auricular fibrillation and heart failure are already present. (iii.) There are few nervous signs such as tremor, etc. (iv.) Exophthalmos is slight or absent. (v.) The condition is not improved by the administration of iodine, whereas in primary Graves' disease iodine brings about dramatic early improvement.

Treatment consists in the adoption of every measure which can improve the health, such as adequate rest and removal of sources of sepsis and toxæmia.   Iodine is better avoided except pre-operatively: drugs of the thiouracil series diminish symptoms, but are not as beneficial as in primary thyrotoxicosis. X-ray treatment is not advisable but radio-iodine therapy is often helpful; surgery is indicated in most cases, especially when carditis is present.

Rarer Causes of Thyroid Enlargement

ENLARGEMENT OF THE THYROID is also met with (i.) in anæmias, and (ii.) in subacute thyroiditis, which may occur with the acute specific fevers. It may go on to abscess formation, as in typhoid fever. (iii.) Rarely, it enlarges during the course of leukæmia. (iv.) Acute hæmorrhage may occur in the gland. (v.) Syphilis, tubercle, lymphadenoma, actinomycosis and parasitic diseases. (vi.) **Riedel's disease** is a chronic inflammation which leads to the slow formation of a hard mass of fibrous tissue which is fixed to surrounding structures, and becomes dangerous to life from pressure upon the trachea. It is often aggravated by prolonged iodine administration; surgical treatment may be required when dyspnœa and dysphagia are marked. (vii.) **Menopausal** goitre is a soft, uniform enlargement of the thyroid, which sometimes occurs in women near the menopause; it is accompanied by a mild degree of hypothyroidism and it may pass on to myxœdema if the general health of the patient is not treated. (viii.) In some types of cretinism defective thyroid activity is associated. (ix.) In acromegaly the thyroid is sometimes enlarged.

(B) *Diseases in which the thyroid may be* DIMINISHED *in size.—viz.*, I. CRETINISM, II. MYXŒDEMA. *The latter is described elsewhere, since the leading symptom is General Debility.*

§ 192. I. **Cretinism** is a condition of dwarfism and deformity attended by mental imbecility, due to an absence or perversion of the thyroid secretion, and is endemic in certain districts. In advanced and typical cases the face is characteristically broad and flat, the tongue protrudes from the mouth, the eyes are wide apart, and the head is brachycephalic (*i.e.*, broad transversely). The skin and hair are dry and coarse, and the mental condition is extremely backward. In severe cases the body may be so dwarfed that a person of twenty is the size of a child of five. X-ray reveals delayed epiphyseal formation. The limbs are shortened, the neck stunted; pads of fat are present above the clavicles; the hands are short and square (spade-like), the abdomen prominent and an umbilical hernia is often present. Constipation is an early and persistent symptom. Puberty is delayed indefinitely. The thyroid may be enlarged, small, or absent. In *juvenile myxœdema* development occurs normally till a certain age, then suddenly ceases, with signs resembling adult myxœdema. This usually follows an infection, such as measles.

Etiology.—Cretinism is endemic in certain districts, *e.g.*, the valleys of Switzerland, Northern Italy and India. Some of these cases have a large thyroid, but in such patients the cretinism preceded the development of the goitre. Sporadic cases, with an atrophic thyroid, are found in healthy families. In other cases the cretin is the child of goitrous parents; in some of these families of goitrous cretins there is an absence of essential thyroid enzymes which leads to an insufficient production of thyroxine.

Prognosis.—The patient may grow up capable of doing light manual work, or may remain an idiot. Under treatment begun early, the child may recover completely, but in other cases, although the body is greatly improved, the mind does not improve in proportion.

Treatment.—Thyroid B.P., beginning with ½-gr. doses, causes a rapid and remarkable change. The skin becomes soft, the general conformation normal, and if the treatment has not been too long delayed, the mind assumes its natural vigour. The patient must *continue* to take thyroid all his life, or else he will relapse. A case showing the remarkable efficacy of this treatment is figured in § 19, FIGS. 9A, B and C.

II. Typical MYXŒDEMA is described in detail elsewhere (§ 575). It should be remembered that there are minor degrees of thyroid insufficiency which, though falling short of typical cretinism or fully developed myx-œdema, are nevertheless sufficient to account for many of the minor troubles for which patients seek advice. In adults, especially in women about the menopause, increase of weight (especially deposits on the back of the neck and the shoulders), falling hair, intolerance of cold, constipation, muscular fatigue, a slow pulse, a dry skin with a tendency to chronic eruptions, are all suspicious features. In younger women premature greyness is also suggestive. Rarefaction amounting to complete absence of the outer two-thirds of the eyebrow is a fairly constant sign. The treatment is started with thyroid B.P. in very small doses—$\frac{1}{8}$ to $\frac{1}{4}$ gr. daily—and the dose increased until the symptoms go and the basal metabolism becomes normal (Figs. 1 and 2).

CHAPTER VIII

THE MOUTH, TONGUE AND ŒSOPHAGUS

THE MOUTH

(Lips, Breath, Saliva, Teeth, and Gums.)

INSTRUCTIVE information is afforded by a thorough examination of the mouth. Anæmia, lead and bismuth poisoning, scurvy and leukæmia may be recognised from an inspection of the mouth. Many of the indications of syphilis, hereditary or acquired, are here revealed. Make a thorough examination of the LIPS, the BREATH, the SALIVA, the TEETH and GUMS and pay particular attention to the TONGUE. The symptoms referable to these structures are considered below.

§ 200. The Lips.—The points to observe are any alteration in colour, dryness, swelling and whether they are inflamed (cheilitis), cracked, fissured or ulcerated. The *colour changes* most often seen are the pallor of anæmia, and the cyanosis of right-sided heart failure and of other conditions (§ 30). *Dry* lips are the result of climatic conditions, a febrile state and a gastro-intestinal disorder. A dry *cracked* lip is seen in nervous people who lick and bite their lips or are exposed to cold winds: it is also seen in those who dribble saliva and may result from hypersensitivity to denture material. *Swelling* of the lips may be due to injury, to neighbouring inflammation such as herpes, to urticaria or angio-neurotic œdema, to lymphatic obstruction after cellulitis and sometimes to an unknown cause. It is also seen in acromegaly. *Inflammation* is the result of a simple infection (usually streptococcal). In *exfoliative cheilitis* there is persistent vesiculation and crusting of the lips, usually due to hyper-sensitivity to the pigment (often eosin) in lipsticks. *Angular stomatitis* (perlèche) occurs with a streptococcal or fungal infection at the corners of the mouth: there is initially redness followed by fissuring and crusting —this is most common with iron-deficiency anæmia and vitamin B deficiency. *Stellate fissures* around the lips are an almost infallible sign of syphilis, especially when surrounded by a dull red infiltration: this infiltra-tion distinguishes a syphilitic fissure from perlèche. *Ulceration* may be due to a primary syphilitic chancre and in the elderly man to epithelioma. The *scars* left by syphilitic fissures, usually congenital, are white and stellate. (And see § 11.) *Treatment* depends on the cause. A simple lip salve (such as lanoline) protects the lips: chloramphenicol cream (1·0 per cent.) is effective when there is a local infection and a vitamin B complex, and iron therapy are often indicated.

§ 201. The Breath should normally be quite free from any kind of odour. Offensiveness of the breath (halitosis) may arise from several sources: (1) A want of cleanliness *in the mouth*, particles of decomposing food, pyorrhœa, stomatitis, septic teeth and dental caries. (2) Septic *tonsils*, and other *throat* infections. (3) Some disorders of the *liver* and of the *alimentary canal* especially when offensive volatile products of fat digestion are absorbed from the small intestine; and with the disordered digestion in *fevers*. (4) Some *diseases of the nose, antrum* and *sinuses*; it always accompanies ozæna. (5) A large cavity in the *lungs*, especially if *bronchiectatic*, fœtid bronchitis and gangrene of the lungs produce a putrid odour (§§ 145, 146). The sickly odour of bronchiectasis may be intermittent, lasting a few days and gradually disappearing. (6) Certain general conditions are attended by a more or less characteristic odour of the breath. Thus, in *ketosis* it is sweet; in acute *alcoholism* it is alcoholic or ethereal. In *uræmia* it is often urinous. (7) Certain *drugs* cause a characteristic odour in the breath—*e.g.*, turpentine (a resinous odour), chloral (odour of chloroform), bismuth (odour of garlic), paraldehyde and opium (odour of the drugs). Alcohol, ether, chloroform and other volatile substances are partly excreted by the breath. (8) When a patient states that he is persistently aware of his offensive breath this is usually the result of an *obsessional neurosis* (§ 1175); those suffering from halitosis are rarely conscious of the smell of their own breath. A **Bad Taste** in the mouth accompanies most of the conditions which give rise to foul breath.

Treatment is by attempting to rectify the cause. With digestive disorders, reducing the intake of fat to 40–60 G. a day and the free administration of tab. chlorophyll may be effective.

§ 202. The Saliva may be *increased* (ptyalism) (i.) in inflammation of the mouth as in stomatitis, and during dentition; (ii.) in chronic gastritis there may be such a profuse flow of saliva during the night that it gives rise in the morning to vomiting of clear alkaline fluid (waterbrash or pyrosis). Salivation may occur after a heavy meal, especially with exercise when the stomach is loaded, or after certain foods, such as excess of sugar or sour fruit. (iii.) During pregnancy, in mania, hydrophobia and some other nervous diseases; (iv.) after the administration of mercury, physostigmine, iodides, bitters and sometimes alkalies and acids. The saliva may *appear to be increased*, owing to defective swallowing, in bulbar paralysis, myasthenia gravis, encephalitis lethargica and other paralytic conditions; and with sore throat or other causes of difficult swallowing. " Dry mouth " (xerostomia) occurs with deficiency of saliva. The saliva is *decreased* in dehydration, especially (i.) in certain fevers, (ii.) in diabetes, (iii.) severe diarrhœa, (iv.) chronic nephritis, (v.) after atropine, morphine or stramonium, and (vi.) with emotions of fear or nervousness. (vii.) Sometimes it is associated with calculus of the salivary glands and with old age. (And see § 210.)

Thirst (polydipsia) accompanies all febrile conditions. It is met with also in diabetes mellitus and diabetes insipidus, after various causes of loss of fluid, *e.g.*, diarrhœa, excessive perspiration, hæmorrhage and vomiting, chronic interstitial nephritis, after a diet excessively salted, and with dyspepsia and gastritis.

§ 203. **The Palate** may be " cleft " from childhood, otherwise a hole in this situation may be the result of a badly performed tonsillectomy or is evidence of past syphilis. The *soft* palate shares in the diseases of the fauces (§ 153). It is a favourite position for the membrane of diphtheria, which distinguishes it from follicular tonsillitis. The *hard* palate is sometimes involved in the diseases of the floor of the nose. A swelling here is commonly due to the presence of pus originating from the lateral incisor, second premolar or first molar tooth, to a gumma or, rarely, to the pointing of an antral abscess.

§ 204. **The Teeth** are subject to a certain amount of variation, even in health. The *average* dates of the eruption of the temporary and permanent teeth are as follows:

TABLE XIII

Temporary or " Milk " Teeth.	*Permanent Teeth.*
6th to 8th month, central incisors.	6th year, first molars.
8th to 10th month, lateral incisors.	7th ,, central incisors.
12th to 14th month, first molars.	8th ,, lateral incisors.
18th to 20th month, canines.	10th ,, first premolar.
2 to 2½ years, second molars.	11th ,, second premolar.
	11th to 12th year, canines.
	12th to 13th ,, second molars.
	17th to 25th ,, third molars.

One quarter of the mouth may be represented diagrammatically thus:

Teeth	I.	I.	C.	M.	M.		Teeth ..	I.	I.	C.	PM.	PM.	M.	M.	M.
Month of eruption }	6	9	18	12	24		Year of eruption }	7	8	11	10	11	6	12	24

The normal order of eruption of teeth may be represented thus: MILK teeth, 6, 9, 18, 12, 24 MONTHS; and PERMANENT teeth, 7, 8, 11, 10, 11; 6, 12, 24 YEARS. These details are worth remembering, because defective or deficient teeth are a frequent cause of faulty digestion. Every Mongol has an irregular order of dentition.

Septic teeth, dental caries and pyorrhœa alveolaris are common causes of dyspepsia and serious ill-health. The causes of dental caries are still debated. It is *predisposed* to by some underlying systemic factor and by deficiency of calcification of the tooth substance; to overcome the latter various preparations containing calcium and vitamin D can now be prescribed. The fluoridation of drinking water probably helps to resist dental caries. The *exciting* cause is apparently the presence of acid-producing organisms which multiply in the food débris around the teeth. Soft, pulpy, sweet and farinaceous foods encourage the growth of these organisms. Hence the importance of adequate cleansing of the teeth after such food: otherwise every meal should finish with firm raw fruit, such as an apple or some other hard food which requires thorough mastication. X-ray examination helps to reveal dental caries.

The permanent teeth are altered in appearance by constitutional upsets occurring at the time of calcification. They present transverse ridges or lines of pits in the enamel as a result of exanthematous fevers or rickets. Those affected are the incisors, canines or first molars. " Hutchinson's teeth " are due to congenital syphilis—the upper incisors are narrowest at the free edge, which shows a semilunar notch; the molars are dome-shaped, and all the teeth are spaced and liable to caries owing to calcium deficiency (Fig. 4). The face often presents a typical syphilitic facies. The onset of acromegaly and of Paget's disease may sometimes be detected by the alteration of the " bite " of the teeth owing to an unequal increase in the size of the jaws.

§ 205. **Toothache** (odontalgia) is produced by acute or chronic inflammation of the tooth pulp or of the periodontal membrane. Irritation of the tooth pulp is due to (1) presence of a carious cavity, (2) exposure of dentine or cementum with or without caries, (3) filling too near the pulp, (4) a blow on a sound tooth. The pain is neuralgic in character, and intensified by extremes of temperature. It ceases on the death of the pulp and is followed by inflammation of the periodontal membrane (periodontitis) due to the passage of infection through the apex. The tooth then becomes tender on pressure. Later the gum shows signs of extension of the inflammatory process and the formation of pus. The lymphatic glands draining the area are enlarged and tender and diffuse swelling of the neighbouring soft tissues ensues. Situations in which an alveolar abscess may point are (1) usually in the mucous membrane overlying the affected tooth; (2) the palate, especially arising from lateral incisor, premolar and molar teeth; (3) antral cavity, from any tooth whose roots are in proximity to the antral floor; (4) on the face along the lower border of the mandible from lower premolar and molar teeth.

NEURALGIC PAIN, either local or referred from one jaw to the other, but never across the mid-line, may also be due to impacted teeth, chronic apical abscesses, odontomes, fragments of root remaining after incomplete extraction and to empyema and growths of the antrum. A not uncommon cause of neuralgia is pressure by a lower denture on the mental nerve exposed by extensive loss of bone subsequent to the extraction of heavily infected teeth.

The *treatment* belongs to the dental surgeon. Temporary relief of pain due to a carious tooth is obtained by applying a pledglet of cotton wool soaked in clove oil. If the tooth is tender on tapping, indicating periodontitis, hot mouthwashes such as carbolic (1–200) are advantageous, with or without the application of counter-irritants such as equal parts of the tinctures of aconite and iodine to the over-lying gum.

For Trigeminal Neuralgia and Dental Causalgia, see § 817.

SWELLINGS OF THE JAWS. *Fluid swellings* are regular and smooth, enlarging the outer wall of the jaw as they increase in size. The most common are cysts, such as a dental cyst on a dead tooth or a dentigerous cyst on an unerupted tooth. Innocent *solid swellings* include fibroma, chondroma, osteoma and solid odontomes, but sarcoma and carcinoma occur.

SWELLINGS OF THE SOFT TISSUES. Acute inflammatory swellings of the tissues overlying the jaws, and often spreading downwards in the neck, are nearly always caused by an alveolar abscess. *Treatment* is by removal of the offending tooth, but if this does not produce adequate drainage incision is needed to release the pus. *Actinomycosis* may simulate the results of an acute alveolar abscess. The swelling associated with the cellulitis of this infection is typically hard and board-like and is accompanied by little pyrexia. Later, areas soften and discharge pus containing the typical sulphur granules. The organisms are usually sensitive to penicillin which needs to be given in large doses over many weeks.

TRISMUS of local origin may be due to a fracture of the body or the ramus of the mandible, or to the extension of the inflammation from an alveolar abscess or a septic wisdom tooth to the surrounding muscles.

The **Gums.** Examination of the gums gives important clues, apart from the pallor of anæmia, in the diagnosis of disease. The effect of administering metallic substances manifests itself in the appearance of the gums; bismuth and lead produce a blue line which is seen below the free margin of the gums, due to deposit in the gum tissue itself. Various forms of stomatitis accompanying constitutional conditions, such as leukæmia, scurvy, purpura, agranulocytosis, syphilis, are described in § 211. Pigmented patches are seen with Addison's disease.

TUMOURS of the gums and mucous membranes are quite common and include: (1) polypus due to local irritation; (2) epulis, usually pedunculated, growing from the junction of the periosteum with the periodontal membrane; (3) papilloma—all of which are treated by excision; and (4) epithelioma and sarcoma; (5) gumma.

Oral Sepsis includes affections of the teeth, gums and alveolar bone.

§ 206. Dental infections present two different forms: (1) *Closed infection* —i.e., where there is no drainage and where toxins are absorbed directly by the blood-stream from apical abscesses, granulomata and cysts on dead teeth. This type of infection may be serious because it is unsuspected and revealed only by radiographic examination, there being usually no local clinical signs. It may be responsible for joint, muscle, eye, heart and numerous other lesions. Dead teeth which are apparently normal on X-ray examination are commonly infected and must be regarded with suspicion. When all the teeth have been extracted " residual infection " may persist in the alveolar bone. This can be eliminated in mild cases by the application of diathermy or infra-red rays often combined with a suitable antibiotic: in severe cases curetting the infected areas is necessary. (2) *Open infection*—i.e., where drainage permits the swallowing of the products of the inflammation, as in cases of broken roots and carious teeth, infection of the gums, alveolus and mucous membranes of the mouth.

§ 207. Inflammation of the Gums—Gingivitis.

Symptoms.—The gum margins are slightly swollen, reddened, and bleed easily; they appear to have a smooth, glossy surface. Clinical and X-ray examinations do not reveal involvement of the periodontal membrane or alveolus.

Etiology.—The commonest cause is lack of oral hygiene, food stagnating round the teeth and gums. Putrefaction occurs, followed by infection. Deposits of tartar act as a predisposing factor. Prolonged administration of mercury, bismuth, arsenic, gold and epanutin are also common causes. It may also be associated with general diseases such as diabetes and nephritis and commonly occurs at the third to fourth month of pregnancy.

Treatment consists in the maintenance of strict oral hygiene. It is essential to clean the teeth regularly and to use floss silk between the teeth to remove débris. Deposits of tartar must be removed from around the teeth by the dental surgeon. The regular use of a warm mouth wash of hydrogen peroxide (2 vols.) promotes cleanliness. Under normal conditions the disease can be completely eliminated.

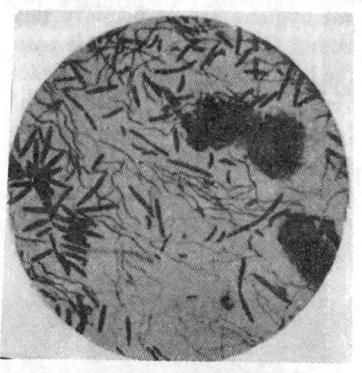

FIG. 83.—PHOTO-MICROGRAPH OF SMEAR OF GUM AFFECTED BY VINCENT'S INFECTION, SHOWING FUSIFORM BACILLI AND SPIRILLÆ.

§ 208. Ulcerative Gingivitis (Vincent's Infection) is due to infection of

the gum margins by fusiform bacilli and spirillæ in symbiosis.

Symptoms.—The gums are inflamed and sore, with yellowish marginal ulcers. The breath is offensive and the tongue coated. The onset and spread of the disease are rapid, the tonsils are often involved. Constitutional symptoms may be severe, with pyrexia and enlargement of the submaxillary and cervical glands. The disease is highly contagious and there are often epidemics in institutions. A smear taken from around the gums, when stained and examined microscopically, confirms the diagnosis.

Treatment consists in isolating the patient in severe cases. As the organisms producing the disease are penicillin-sensitive, the lesions disappear within 2-3 days if tablets containing 1,000 units of penicillin (B.P.) are allowed to dissolve slowly in the mouth every two hours. Meanwhile, no antiseptic mouthwashes must be used, but the mouth may be irrigated with warm saline. When the ulcers have healed any local factors predisposing to gingivitis must be treated, otherwise the disease is likely to recur.

§ 209. Inflammation of the Gums and Alveolus—Pyorrhœa Alveolaris.—

If untreated, the infection of gingivitis spreads to the periodontal membrane and the supporting alveolus. The bone becomes infected and subsequently resorbed.

Symptoms.—The gum margins are usually engorged and swollen; there are pockets of varying depth around the teeth from which pus can often be expressed. The breath may be offensive and the swallowing of pus may be an exciting factor in the formation of gastric or duodenal disorders. X-ray examination shows evidence of destruction of the periodontal membrane and alveolus.

Treatment.—When the loss of alveolar bone is not extensive, skilled dental treatment can accomplish much. Removal of all tartar and strict oral hygiene are of primary importance. The gum forming the pockets around the affected teeth is resected. With advanced disease and extensive loss of alveolar bone, extraction of the teeth is necessary, especially if it is suspected that the condition may be producing lesions in other parts of the body. It is unwise to remove many teeth at one operation; it is often necessary to extract only one at a time. The injection of 100,000 units of penicillin half an hour before the extraction and again an hour later is often of advantage, especially when the patient has a rheumatic heart lesion.

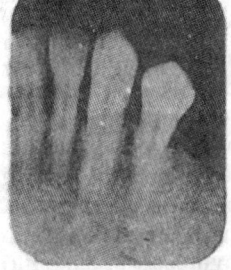

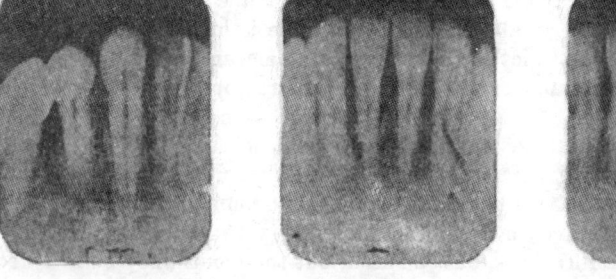

FIG. 84.

FIG. 85.

FIGS. 84 and 85. RADIOGRAPHS to illustrate (Fig. 84) chronic apical abscesses, with destruction of the periodontal membrane and lamina dura around the apices of the teeth, and infection of surrounding bone: (Fig. 85) destruction of periodontal membrane and alveolus around the necks of the teeth typical of pyorrhœa alveolaris.

§ 219. **Inflammation of the Mucous Membrane of the Mouth—Stomatitis.**—In this condition there is a more or less widespread inflammation of the cheeks, the tongue, the floor of the mouth or the palate. There is a variable degree of discomfort and pain associated with redness, swelling and tenderness. In severe cases the lips may be swollen, there is an offensive odour to the breath, excessive salivation and the upper cervical lymph glands are enlarged and tender. There are several varieties:

(a) *Catarrhal Stomatitis* causes few symptoms and is not serious. There is a patchy redness and a little swelling of the mucous membrane, often due to dirty or loose dentures and sometimes associated with catarrh of the nose and throat. A similar condition is seen following the prolonged administration of penicillin and especially of the tetracycline drugs. *Treatment* consists in remedying the cause: a mouthwash of weak hydrogen peroxide or containing glyc. thymol co. (B.P.C.) may help.

(b) *Ulcerative (Vincent's) Stomatitis* is due to spread from ulcerative gingivitis (§ 208). The more widespread inflammation in the mouth causes more severe symptoms. Bacteriological diagnosis and the treatment are those of the gingivitis; in severe cases intramuscular injections of penicillin may also be required.

(c) *Herpetic Stomatitis* is probably due to a virus. It is a painful condition with crops of vesicles which subsequently burst: sometimes the vesicles are hæmorrhagic. The diagnosis is from *pemphigus*: in the early stages of this much more serious disease the flaccid bullæ are not surrounded by a red margin and there are usually lesions elsewhere (§ 681). *Treatment* of the lesions is by painting either with gentian violet (1·0 per cent.) or preferably with aureomycin hydrochlor. (1·0 per cent.) in equal parts of glycerin and water.

(d) *Aphthous Stomatitis* is common, especially in young women. There are crops of small vesicles with a red base and a sharply defined circular margin. When the vesicles rupture they leave very painful ulcers with a greyish-yellow surface. These may make mastication difficult: the pain is aggravated by any acid food or drink. The lesions occur on the inside of the lips, the cheeks, gums, on the under surface of the tongue and sometimes on the palate: the crops are much more frequent before the menses. The condition is believed to be due to a virus. Apart from the local lesion in the mouth the patient may complain of no other symptoms; although there are usually no digestive complaints, aphthous ulceration is very common with tropical sprue and idiopathic steatorrhœa. *Treatment* of the lesions is by cauterisation with a silver nitrate stick, or preferably by slowly dissolving in the mouth in the area of ulceration tab. sodium hydrocortisone hemisuccinate (2·5 mg. in a lactose base): these tablets should be taken 3–4 times a day for 36–48 hours until the ulcers heal. *Preventive treatment* is by improving the general health with more fresh air, exercise and sleep, correcting anæmia however slight and sometimes inj. cyanocobalamin (1,000 μg. twice a week for 3–4 weeks) helps.

(e) *Parasitic Stomatitis* or *Thrush* occurs at any age. It usually starts on the cheek or the side of the tongue, but may invade the lips and the whole of the inside of the mouth and pharynx. The mucous membrane shows a number of white membranous patches which coalesce to form large areas. The typical lesion resembles " milk curds " and when removed with a piece of gauze there is a large red area beneath. Unless the condition is advanced the patient usually complains of no symptoms: the ulceration and the salivation seen in other forms of stomatitis are absent. The *diagnosis* is usually made by the appearances in the mouth. In children excoriations may be seen around the anus, and the mother thinks the " thrush has gone through the child." Occasionally it attacks the skin of adults, spreading rapidly over groins, abdomen and axillæ; it is usually mistaken for eczema intertrigo, but readily yields to a weak solution of iodine. Rarely, the nails are affected. (For moniliasis of the respiratory tract see § 147.)

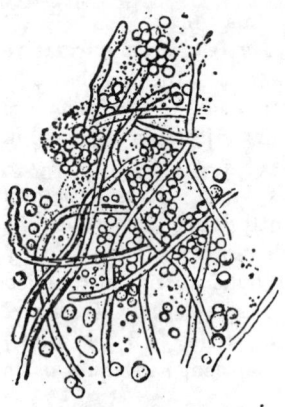

FIG. 86.—CANDIDA ALBICANS OR THRUSH FUNGUS.

Etiology.—The lesions are due to the fungus *Candida* (*Monilia*) *Albicans* (Fig. 86) found by microscopy. In babies the condition is especially seen with the use of dirty feeding-teats and feeding-bottles in badly cared for and often undernourished children. In middle age it is met in those who are taking little food and especially following hæmatemesis. In the aged it is seen in patients with senility, carcinoma and other wasting diseases. The common factors causing thrush are dehydration, deficient mastication and swallowing, lack of cleanliness in the mouth and not infrequently the prolonged use of antibiotics. Acute suppurative parotitis is a troublesome complication.

Treatment.—Penicillin is not effective. Glycerinum boracis applied with surgical gauze or on a soft toothbrush rubs off the white patches and exerts a mild antiseptic effect: in more severe cases painting with gentian violet (1·0 per cent.) once each day is useful. A better remedy is the local application of a suspension of nystatin (100,000 units per ml.) or a solution of amphotericin B (15 mg. in 100 ml. of sterile water) antibiotics to which the fungus is sensitive. *Prevention* is by washing the mouth after every meal and by giving adults apples or pineapple chunks to chew so as to encourage the flow of saliva.

(*f*) *Gangrenous Stomatitis* (Cancrum Oris) is now rare. It may be seen in neglected young children suffering from measles and other acute specific fevers. There is acute inflammation, usually starting on the cheek or lip, followed by ulceration with a surrounding brawny induration: this is followed by sloughing, with a gross loss of tissue and perforation of the cheek. The patient is very ill with a high fever and often develops broncho-pneumonia and gangrene in other parts of the body (noma pudendi).

Treatment is by the free administration of penicillin or the appropriate antibiotic to which the infecting organisms are most sensitive, combined with free excision of the ulcerated area; and later a plastic repair to replace the lost tissue.

§ **211.** Certain GENERAL CONDITIONS and DISEASES OF THE SKIN may manifest themselves in the mouth. These are:

(i.) The *rashes* of small-pox, chicken-pox, measles and herpes. In measles, the spots, first described by Koplik, appear on the inner sides of the cheeks, opposite the bicuspid or molar teeth, before the skin eruption occurs. They appear as a greyish-white stippling on a slightly raised purplish base, and afford considerable aid in the early diagnosis of the disease. With Wood's glass under ultra-violet light they are readily seen.

(ii.) *Drugs* must always be thought of as a possible cause of stomatitis and gingivitis. Those commonly responsible are sodium phenytoin (epanutin), gold and bismuth injections, phenobarbitone, phosphorus and the prolonged use of mercury. Mercurial stomatitis, now uncommon, produces fœtor of the breath, with swollen bleeding gums, and later ulceration spreading to the cheeks, tongue and floor of the mouth. Phosphorus produces ulcerative stomatitis, with necrosis of the jaw. Prolonged use of the antibiotics produces a red, raw and very sore mouth often accompanied by considerable thirst and diarrhœa.

(iii.) *Lichen planus* and *leucoplakia* are two common types of hyperkeratosis which occur in the mouth. Lichen planus may affect the mucous membrane of the mouth and tongue long before it appears on the skin: it is usually symptomless but shows as a typical " white lace " appearance with poorly defined margins. Leukoplakia (§ 215, II) produces a denser raised white area on the tongue, cheeks and hard palate; these may become fissured and later malignant.

(iv.) *Lupus erythematosus* usually manifests itself as red areas denuded of surface epithelium: the skin lesions commonly precede those in the mouth.

(v.) *Erythema multiforme* is also usually first seen on the skin. In the mouth it produces a moist ulcerative lesion. In Erythema multiforme major (the *Stevens-Johnson syndrome*) the skin lesion is associated with extensive ulceration in the mouth and vagina and when the cornea is involved it usually results in blindness: pyrexia and constitutional symptoms are marked.

(vi.) *Pemphigus vulgaris* appears as flaccid bullæ without a surrounding red margin: when the bullæ rupture the lesions tend to coalesce. Bullæ are also present on the skin and in other areas.

(vii.) *Behcet's syndrome* produces ulcerative lesions of the mouth, conjunctiva and of the genitalia with nodules in the skin.

(viii.) *Purpuric* lesions occur as in other areas.

(ix.) *Acute leukæmia* (often of the acute monocytic type) produces swollen purple-coloured gums with small nodules which readily ulcerate. Not infrequently such cases are treated without any suspicion of their true nature. The degree of swelling is usually much greater than in lesions due to infection.

(x.) *Agranulocytosis* (§ 155*f*) causes in the mouth yellow sloughs of varying size with well-defined margins, often in areas from which an extraction has recently been performed.

(xi.) *Scurvy* is associated with soft spongy hæmorrhagic gums and gingival inflammation.

(xii.) *Foot-and-Mouth Disease* (Syn.: epidemic stomatitis; aphthous fever) is an acute infectious disease attacking pigs, sheep, cattle and other domestic animals. Epidemics have been reported in which the disease was transmitted to man, with symptoms of fever, gastro-intestinal derangement and vesicles on the lips, mouth and pharynx, and sometimes near the nails of fingers and toes.

(xiii.) With *Espundia*, in S. America, oro-pharyngeal ulceration follows the primary skin lesion, which is due to a type of Leishmann-Donovan body, transmitted by a bug. Tartar emetic is specific for this condition.

§ 212. **Oral Syphilis** may affect the mouth: (*a*) the primary lesion may, on rare occasions, show itself on the lip, gums and tongue; (*b*) the mucous patches, secondary lesions, occur on the inner side of the cheeks and the edge of the tongue; ulceration may follow, producing typical " snail-track " ulcers (§ 162). (*c*) The gummata of the tertiary stage, with typical deep, excavated ulcers, are sometimes seen (§ 738). For leukoplakia see § 215, II.

THE TONGUE

Apart from the local diseases which may affect the tongue, its appearance aids in the diagnosis and prognosis of certain general diseases. Examination should be made of its surface as regards (*a*) furring, moisture and dryness; (*b*) its colour, and other alterations of the surface; (*c*) the presence of white patches; (*d*) altered size, warts, growths and fissures; (*e*) ulcers; (*f*) note also the method of protrusion. A mother sometimes speaks of her child being " *tongue-tied* " when the frenum is too short: in some cases this is really so, or the structure may be attached to the tongue too far forward, but it exists much less frequently than parents suppose.

§ 213. (*a*) **Furring and Moisture of the Tongue.**—In health the tongue is clean and moist, although a slight deposit over its posterior third is not unusual. *Furring* occurs when the greater part of the tongue is covered by a white or greyish layer; when a thick brown and dry crust forms over the surface, the tongue is said to be *coated*. Furring or coating therefore occurs with (i.) local irritation or *sepsis in the mouth*—excessive tobacco smoking, tonsillitis or pharyngitis, dental caries, gingivitis or pyorrhœa. An unpleasant taste in the mouth, or unpleasant breath (halitosis, § 201), may accompany such conditions. (ii.) In most *febrile states* some degree of furring is the rule. Its degree is often in proportion to the toxæmia present and it is therefore a guide to prognosis; with defervescence of fever the tongue cleans. Special importance attaches to the tongue in typhoid fever. In the first week the dorsum is covered with a thin dirty-white fur, but soon the tip and the edges begin to clear so that by the third week the fur has disappeared, and the tongue becomes glazed and dry, or red and smooth. In scarlet fever the fur with the initial tonsillitis rapidly strips, especially from tip and edges, so that by the fourth day there is a bright red raw tongue, with prominent fungiform papillæ (strawberry tongue, § 477). In measles the tongue is dry and heavily coated at first, but later it peels, leaving a papillated tongue very similar to that of scarlet fever. In typhus the tongue is at first flabby and coated with a thick brown layer; later it becomes extremely dry, often tremulous, and in severe cases dark and shrivelled. (iii.) The condition of the tongue gives much help in the diagnosis of *abdominal conditions*. In acute gastritis and enteritis, the tongue is heavily coated, and is associated with heartburn and an unpleasant taste in the mouth, whereas in chronic gastritis, cirrhosis of the liver, atonic and gouty dyspepsia, the tongue shows a thin white coating, is large, pale and flabby, with a broad tip and indented edges. A red tongue, with sharp red tip and edges, in which the hyperæmic papillæ contrast strongly with the slight white coating in the centre, is found in diabetes and hyperchlorhydria. In acute appendicitis, the tongue is almost invariably furred at an early stage, and later is coated and dry, especially when peritonitis follows. (iv.) *Toxic absorption* usually produces furring. The commonest cause is constipation, which may be " occult." Any bacterial focus, *e.g.*, intestinal obstruction, pyelitis, sinusitis or chemical poisoning—*e.g.*, chronic alcoholism, chronic arsenical poisoning—act similarly. (v.) *Deficient secretion of saliva* causes a tongue which is dry and often furred. A dry tongue, in the absence of fever, indicates a lack of appetite (except in diabetes mellitus) or a depletion of water, as in diabetes insipidus, after profuse perspiration, diarrhœa (especially cholera) or vomiting. In asthenic states the tongue becomes very dry and coated, *e.g.*, coma, abdominal cancer, advanced phthisis. (vi.) In these extreme conditions a *denuded red tongue* generally follows as the crust falls off—the tongue is red, shining, smooth, dry and often cracked. It is found in the advanced stages of any chronic ailment, and indicates a grave prognosis; it is also seen in patients treated with long courses of penicillin, the tetracyclines and other antibiotics. Aphthous stomatitis or thrush may supervene. (vii.) A rare condition, *black* or " hairy " tongue, is due to elongation of the papillæ at the back of the tongue; they resemble dark hairs. The hyperplasia of the papillæ permits growth of organisms, usually a streptothrix variety. Dequalinium chloride (0·5 per cent.) in propylene glycol, applied with a toothbrush t.d.s. for 4 weeks, has cured some cases.

§ 214. (b) **Other Characters of the Surface of the Tongue.**—The *colour* of the tongue is an important indication of the state of the blood. It is *pale* in all anæmic conditions except when the tongue is also inflamed. With the modern use of cosmetics in women, the colour of the tongue is a much more reliable indication of anæmia than is the colour of the lips, cheeks or even conjunctivæ. The tongue is stained *black* when a patient takes iron mixtures. *Blueness* occurs in cyanotic states, and during nitrous oxide anæsthesia. *Excessive redness* occurs (i.) with polycythæmia, (ii.) scarlet fever, typhoid, advanced cachectic conditions, and hyperchlorhydria (see § 213); (iii.) with acute or chronic inflammatory changes (glossitis). In the early stages the papillæ hypertrophy, but later atrophy, and the tongue becomes *smooth* or *bald*. This may occur in local patches; later, the whole tongue is involved and still later *fissuring* occurs, from the contraction of subepithelial scar tissue. There may be local *ulceration*, *tenderness* or *soreness* with streptococcal invasion along the margins, especially with oral sepsis or in association with achylia gastrica, pernicious anæmia, subacute combined degeneration, sprue, pellagra and other allied conditions. Diffuse soreness of the tongue and cheek with no visible lesion may be met in cancerphobia. The " Geographic " tongue and leukoplakia are described in § 215 and the " Plicated " tongue in § 216.

The *treatment* of these conditions is to remedy the cause. In persistent furring local conditions are often overlooked and an abdominal cause sought for. It is an old saying that a red tongue requires alkalies and a white tongue acids. A dry tongue indicates either dehydration, or no appetite and deficient gastric secretions, therefore the patient should be fed on fluids, soups, jellies and other foods requiring little digestive power. In painful conditions of the tongue, condiments, acid, rough and irritating foods must be forbidden: some cases of chronic glossitis respond to an intensive course of inject. cyanocobalamin (1,000 μ g. two or three times a week for 8–9 doses). Local painting with silver nitrate 4 per cent. is sometimes used.

§ 215. (c) **White Patches** are not infrequently met with on the tongue, and may

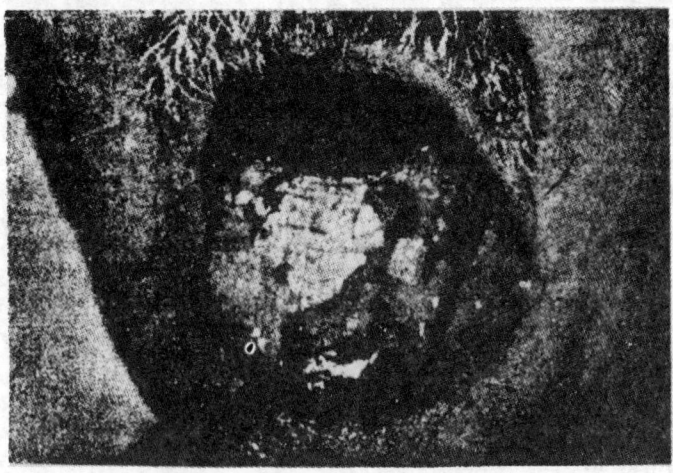

FIG. 87.—LEUCOPLAKIA OF THE TONGUE.

result from: I. Thrush; II. Leucoplakia; III. Geographical tongue; IV. **Aphthous Stomatitis** (§ 210); V. Syphilitic Patches (§ 162).

I. In THRUSH (parasitic stomatitis) there are white membranous patches, like milk curd, sometimes with an areola round them (see § 210e).

II. LEUCOPLAKIA LINGUÆ is a term applied to flat, whitish patches on the tongue. At first the areas are red and sensitive, with hypertrophy of the papillæ; later these atrophy and become slate coloured or white due to a heaping up of the epithelium. The disease may appear in small patches or may involve a considerable area. The patches may also invade the cheeks, gums and palate, and give rise to discomfort and tenderness (§ 211, iii). This condition is variously attributed to excessive smoking, jagged teeth, drinking strong spirit, and syphilis. Syphilis is the usual cause in cases which show a glazed and atrophic tongue. In 30 per cent. of these cases malignant disease supervenes. The *Treatment* is, as a rule, very unsatisfactory, unless the disease be met in the early stages. A mouthwash, consisting of bicarbonate of soda (1 in 24), sometimes relieves the symptoms. The tongue should be periodically examined for evidence of malignant changes. Antisyphilitic remedies should be tried, but are not often successful. Alcohol, smoking and other irritants must be avoided.

III. In GEOGRAPHICAL or "Mapped" tongue the normal desquamation of the tongue takes place irregularly, with the formation of more or less circular patches surrounded by margins of slightly proliferating whitish-grey epithelium. Although the cause is unknown it indicates impaired health. It may persist for long periods or disappear spontaneously.

§ 216. (d) **Alterations in the Size of the Tongue.** An Enlarged Tongue may be due to ACUTE SWELLING, HYPERTROPHY, MACROGLOSSIA and TUMOURS.

ACUTE SWELLING OF THE TONGUE may be due to (I) *Acute Glossitis* or (II) *Acute Œdema*. In both the tongue rapidly enlarges, and may even protrude beyond the teeth. Much pain is present, and difficulty in swallowing and speaking.

(I) ACUTE GLOSSITIS may be due to local causes—*e.g.*, the sting of an insect, streptococcal infection from the teeth or throat, biting or wound of the tongue, acute ulcers or to constitutional conditions—*e.g.*, mercurial salivation and acute specific diseases, such as erysipelas and pneumonia. It may be, like Angina Ludovici (§ 159), of an erysipeloid nature. The onset is rapid, though not so rapid as in acute œdema; the swelling may extend to the neck, and involve the glands. *Treatment.*—In severe cases give ice to suck and cold compresses to the neck. Penicillin injections and tracheostomy may be necessary.

(II) ACUTE ŒDEMA OF THE TONGUE is serious, because of its liability to involve the glottis. It may be associated with urticaria and angio-neurotic œdema. The œdema comes on suddenly; in the course of a few hours the tongue may protrude from the mouth. The swelling rapidly extends to the throat, nose, and down the œsophagus and trachea. There is inability to speak, to swallow, sometimes even to breathe. It is *diagnosed* from simple acute glossitis by (i.) its rapid advent; (ii.) the rapid extension to the throat and other parts; (iii.) the presence sometimes of urticaria, or a history of sensitiveness to some article of food (§ 652).

Prognosis and Treatment.—The disease comes on rapidly, and runs a very rapid course, subsiding in the course of 24 hours. It is apt to cause suffocation. Prompt measures are necessary. Adrenalin B.P. should be repeatedly painted on the tongue and injected (0·25 to 1·0 ml.). Inject. promethazine (Phenergan) 50 mg., inject. chlorpheniramine (Piriton) 10 mg. or caps. diphenhydramin (Benadryl) may be very helpful. The practitioner must be ready to perform tracheostomy if necessary.

HYPERTROPHY AND MACROGLOSSIA. Simple hypertrophy occurs in cretinism, myxœdema, acromegaly, mongolism and with acquired syphilitic lesions. MACROGLOSSIA is a congenital condition of an enormously enlarged tongue due to an overgrowth of the lymphatic, muscular, arterio-venous or neurofibromatous tissues. If persistent application of mild caustics or the galvano-cautery fails to relieve the condition, operation must be resorted to.

TUMOURS of the tongue are rare; for diagnosis and treatment of these a surgical work must be consulted. Overgrowth of the *lymphoid tissue* at the base of the tongue (the "lingual tonsil") is found in local septic conditions and acute blood diseases. Rarely, *thyroid tissue* remains at the base of the tongue as a developmental defect.

A **Small Tongue** which is tremulous occurs in hyperthyroidism. ATROPHY of the tongue (microglossia) usually arises from nerve lesions (§ 1088).

Warts are simple or syphilitic. *Simple* warts are distinguishable by the fact that they are soft; they are raised, and often pedunculated, and there is but little secretion. The glands are not shotty to the touch. *Syphilitic* warts are hard, with infiltration; they are never pedunculated, secretion is present, and the glands in the neck and elsewhere are shotty.

Fissures may be congenital, simple or syphilitic. The *congenital* variety (Plicated Tongue) shows deep sulci irregularly crossing the surface. It has no significance, but when food débris lodges in a very deep fold local hygiene may be necessary. The *simple* fissure can generally be accounted for by some such cause as the irritation of a ragged tooth, and are never infiltrated. On pinching *syphilitic* fissures between the fingers, infiltration is felt. CICATRICES.—Simple ulceration rarely leaves a scar, but if so, it is never hard. Hard, stellate scars invariably indicate syphilis.

§ 217. (*e*) **Ulcers of the Tongue** may be Simple, Malignant, Syphilitic or Tuberculous.

I. SIMPLE ULCERS of the tongue are known by their superficial character, by the presence of some local cause, such as a jagged tooth or other local irritation. They also occur in chronic glossitis and ulcerative stomatitis (§ 210). The *frenum* is apt to be ulcerated in whooping-cough, due to friction against the lower teeth; this is a useful aid in diagnosis.

II. A MALIGNANT ULCER is known by (i.) its site, usually on the side of the tongue; (ii.) its hard, raised, everted edges, and uneven warty base, with foul discharge and tendency to hæmorrhage; (iii.) the induration around, and the early involvement of the glands; and (iv.) the early impairment of the movements of the tongue with great pain. These characters in an advanced case render the diagnosis from syphilis relatively easy. In an early stage the diagnosis may be very difficult. In that stage a cancerous ulcer has flat sloping edges and scanty secretion, *its progress is very slow*, and it does not yield to iodides. Before an ulcer has existed for any length of time, a Wassermann test should be made and a piece excised for microscopic examination.

III. SYPHILITIC ULCERS are of two kinds: (*a*) superficial, (*b*) deep.

(*a*) *Superficial Syphilitic Ulcers* of the tongue are met usually at the side, or in the form of fissures on the dorsum (*cp.* § 162) or superficial circular " punched-out " ulcers.

(*b*) *Deep Syphilitic Ulcers* are preceded by the formation of a roundish nodule (a gumma) which ulcerates. They are recognised by (i.) their site, which is usually on the centre of the dorsum; (ii.) their raised, ragged and sometimes undermined edges; (iii.) the yellow slough which covers the base; and (iv.) the fact that they leave deep stellate scars. Syphilitic ulcers are usually multiple; difficulty in diagnosis arises in the case of a single ulcer as to whether it be syphilitic or cancerous. Syphilitic ulceration is differentiated by (1) the relative absence of surrounding induration, and consequently less interference with the movements of the tongue; (2) the dorsal site; (3) less glandular enlargement, and the glands have a shotty feel; (4) the age of the patient, malignant ulcers rarely occurring before forty; (5) little or no pain; and (6) a history of syphilis, a positive Wassermann reaction and the lesion *heals with iodide of potassium*.

IV. TUBERCULOUS ULCERS are not common. They are superficial, with a yellowish discharge usually near the tip, and they only occur in advanced stages of tuberculosis of the lung or throat. The tubercle bacillus may be found in the scrapings and a biopsy is usually confirmatory.

Prognosis.—Simple ulcers are easily dealt with, but other ulcers of the tongue are dangerous chiefly from their liability to hæmorrhage and because of the important structures around. The diagnosis of malignant from syphilitic lesions is as important as it is difficult, for however advanced the latter may be, they yield to appropriate remedies, but the former are necessarily fatal unless removed early. The deep ulcers often seen in advanced syphilitic glossitis are dangerous, as the deeper parts may be affected by malignant change.

The Treatment consists in removing local sources of irritation. In syphilitic cases, potassium iodide in large doses, and the normal anti-syphilitic remedies, must be given. Malignant disease must be treated surgically or by radium.

(*f*) **The Method of Protrusion of the Tongue.**—The tongue usually protrudes evenly between the teeth, and is equally developed in its two halves. In health there may be constant slight deviation to one or other side, of no organic significance. *Tremor* of the protruded tongue occurs in paralysis agitans, general paralysis of the insane, chronic alcoholism, hyperthyroidism, and lead and mercury poisoning. Coarse *jerky movements* are one of the early signs of rheumatic chorea. *Deviation* of the tongue to the paralysed side, forming a sickle-shaped tongue, occurs in hemiplegia or unilateral hypoglossal paralysis. *Failure to protrude* is evidence of an organic lesion involving the nerve supply or the muscles of both sides of the tongue. *Fasciculation (fibrillary twitching) and wasting* should also be looked for (and see § 842).

THE ŒSOPHAGUS

Anatomy.—The œsophagus starts at the cricoid cartilage, opposite the sixth cervical vertebra, and ends opposite a point between the ninth and tenth dorsal vertebræ, a distance of 10 inches.

§ 218. Symptomatology.—The **Cardinal Symptoms** arising in the œsophagus are **discomfort** or **pain** in the mid-line of the chest, **dysphagia**—*i.e.*, difficulty in swallowing, **heartburn, acid regurgitation** or **water-brash.** **Bleeding** sometimes occurs from the lower end of the œsophagus. Of these dysphagia is by far the most important.

Pain or discomfort is felt behind the sternum when there is an obstructive lesion. The pain is usually felt just above the level of the block. Thus an obstruction at the lower end of the œsophagus usually causes pain behind the xiphisternum, whereas a mid-œsophageal obstruction produces pain in the middle of the sternum and often between the scapulæ.

Dysphagia.—In analysing this symptom there are certain features which aid diagnosis:

First, does the difficulty apply to both liquids and solids ? This gives us an idea of the *degree* of the obstruction. *Secondly*, does the food return ? and if so, after what interval ? This is sometimes a guide to the *seat* of the obstruction. Obstruction of the *œsophagus* has to be distinguished

C.M.—M

from obstruction at the pyloric end of the *stomach* (i.) by the easy way
in which food regurgitates as compared with the vomiting which accompanies pyloric obstruction; and (ii.) by the absence of acidity or bile or
evidence of digestion in the material returned. *Thirdly*, is there any
pain ? Its situation aids diagnosis of the position of the lesion. Is it
present only after the ingestion of food ? Constant pain may occur in
malignant disease. *Fourthly*, what is the duration of the dysphagia ?
Has it been persistent, and become progressively worse ? The last named
is the leading feature of organic, as distinguished from functional, dysphagia
which is frequently intermittent, and by no means progressive. *Fifthly*,
is there any regurgitation through the nose ? This feature implies paralytic
dysphagia, with paralysis of the soft palate. *Sixthly*, is there loss of
weight, or any symptom referable to other organs ? Emaciation coming
on early in a patient beyond middle life is characteristic of carcinoma.

Heartburn is a burning sensation passing up the mid-line of the chest
from the epigastrium for a variable distance—sometimes even to the
pharynx. It is due to regurgitation of the contents of the stomach into
the lower end of the œsophagus: such regurgitation is usually symptomless.
Heartburn is much more likely to arise when there is also inflammation
of the lower œsophagus (œsophagitis). When the inflammation becomes
more severe there may also be pain due to temporary spasm of the cardia.
Heartburn particularly occurs (i.) in association with hyperchlorhydria,
with which there may be a duodenal ulcer: but it can occur even with
achlorhydria of the gastric contents. It is frequent in diseases of the
gall-bladder; (ii.) also in association with raised intra-abdominal pressure.
It becomes very common in the later months of pregnancy and may
occur with obesity—especially after a large meal; (iii.) with a sliding
hiatus hernia of the stomach. In this condition it is often a leading
symptom. Regurgitation of the gastric contents is especially liable to
occur when the patient bends down, or lies flat in bed at night.

Acid regurgitation or " acid risings," when the acid contents of the
lower œsophagus suddenly fill the mouth, often co-exists with heartburn.
As it is usually due to primary disease in the upper abdomen, it is described
in § 273.

Water-brash (Pyrosis) occurs when the mouth suddenly fills with a
tasteless fluid, which is chiefly the result of an excessive salivary secretion.
The clear slightly alkaline fluid may be due to sudden reflex overactivity
of the salivary glands resulting from a dyspeptic condition in the stomach
or duodenum, or it may be fluid which has collected in the œsophagus
during the night when the cardiac sphincter is largely closed. (Some of
this fluid may be the result of ciliary action in the bronchi and trachea for
even in healthy people 100 ml. of bronchial secretion are transferred to the
œsophagus each 24 hours.) Sometimes the œsophageal fluid is expelled
without any kind of straining, but more often there is some early morning
retching: this is particularly noticeable with alcoholism.

Bleeding may be in small quantities, mixed with secretion, when there is subacute œsophagitis or a neoplasm. Much more copious bleeding occurs from a ruptured œsophageal varix (§ 260), or when the lower end of the œsophagus contains cell rests of gastric mucous membrane which cause a true gastric ulcer above the cardia.

§ 219. Physical Examination.—Patients may complain that they have *difficulty in swallowing*, yet the condition may not be true dysphagia. Thus, for example, tenderness and painful lesions of the mouth, throat and larynx may make it impossible to take solid or liquid food. The hysterical symptom *globus* may be mistaken for dysphagia; the patient complains of a sense of constriction in the throat or high in the epigastrium, or of a " ball rising up in the throat " (§ 1173). A careful *inspection* of the throat should be made with and without a tongue depressor and a laryngeal mirror. The dysphagia may arise from tonsillitis or other pharyngeal or laryngeal conditions. Paralysis of the palate which succeeds diphtheria, or the paralysis of the face, tongue and palate in bulbar palsy, may thus be detected. Any swelling should be carefully examined, such as retro-pharyngeal abscess, tumour or foreign body in this situation. A toothbrush bristle in the pharynx can cause serious difficulty in swallowing. In children dysphagia is often due to pain on swallowing; in adults tuberculous laryngitis is now a rare cause.

SPECIAL EXAMINATIONS.—In cases of dysphagia a skilled *X-ray examination* is necessary. First, the chest should be examined with the fluorescent screen and with X-ray films. These enable us to identify extra-œsophageal causes of dysphagia such as aneurysm, mediastinal tumour, etc. Then an opaque meal is given: a thick emulsion allows more detail to be made out, especially if the patient is lying down or in the Trendelenberg position. On the screen the progress of the meal is watched and any obstruction noted; its characteristics will usually make the diagnosis clear.

The *œsophagoscope* is most useful in skilled hands. With it the exact site of any obstruction may be viewed, and when doubt exists as to its nature, a piece of tissue may be removed for microscopical examination. Early œsophagoscopic examination for any œsophageal symptom, however slight, probably offers the best chance in the future for improvement in the results of treatment. The œsophagoscope is also used for (i.) the removal of foreign bodies, (ii.) the treatment of malignant stricture by the introduction of Souttar's tubes, radon seeds or radium, (iii.) the treatment by dilatation of non-malignant strictures. The use of the bougie is dangerous: bouginage should only be performed under direct vision through an œsophagoscope.

DISEASES OF THE ŒSOPHAGUS

§ 220. Classification.—The œsophagus is not amenable to physical examination and even the cervical portion is deep-seated. Therefore the first indication of disease is the nature of the symptoms complained of. For *clinical purposes* the diseases can be classified in two groups.

(A.) Those with **Dysphagia** .. .. § 221
(B.) Those with recurrent or persistent **Heartburn** .. § 232

GROUP A. **Causes of Dysphagia.**—The COMMONER CAUSES are—

I. Cancer of the œsophagus .. .. § 221
II. Achalasia of the cardiac orifice .. .. .. § 222
III. A tumour pressing upon the œsophagus from the outside .. .. § 223
IV. Cardio-vascular disorders .. .. § 224
V. Foreign bodies, acute œsophagitis, and simple stricture .. .. § 225
VI. Plummer-Vinson syndrome .. .. .. § 226

LESS FREQUENT CAUSES are—

VII. Functional dysphagia .. .. § 227
VIII. Paralysis of the pharynx .. .. § 228
IX. Pharyngeal crises .. .. § 229
X. Diverticulum or pouch of the pharynx .. .. .. § 230
XI. Congenitally short œsophagus .. .. § 231
XII. Congenital atresia of the œsophagus .. .. § 232

When a patient complains of DIFFICULTY IN SWALLOWING, *or that the food returns to his mouth, the practitioner should first think of* CANCER, *secondly of* ACHALASIA.

§ 221. **Malignant Disease** of the œsophagus is in the large majority of cases due to a squamous epithelioma—sometimes to an adeno-carcinoma in the wall—which goes on to ulceration, and forms a stricture from 1 to 4 inches long; or it may be due to extension upwards of malignant disease at the cardiac end of the stomach. Rarely the growth is sarcomatous. It is important to emphasise that any œsophageal symptom, even the slightest, should be carefully investigated. Dysphagia is a late symptom of cancer of the œsophagus. A lumen of 5 mm. is sufficient to swallow chewed food. The favourite sites of malignant stricture are in the three areas where the lumen is narrowest and therefore where thermal, mechanical and chemical irritation from food or drink would have a maximal effect; these three areas are opposite the cricoid cartilage, 6 inches from the teeth (this is especially common in women—post-cricoid carcinoma); opposite the bifurcation of the trachea, 10 inches; and at the lower end of the œsophagus, 16 inches from the teeth. The last of these is the commonest site, most cases being in men.

Symptoms.—(i.) The patient is past middle life. (ii.) The dysphagia becomes steadily and progressively worse; in rare cases it may be intermittent. At first a difficulty exists only with solids which the patient tries to wash down with a little fluid; later fluids will not pass and are returned in an undigested state immediately after swallowing. The vomit contains a good deal of mucus, often has an unpleasant smell and may contair. streaks of blood. In some cases sudden complete obstruction to swallowing occurs when a large piece of food blocks the narrowed lumen. There may have been no previous symptoms. The duration of the whole illness rarely exceeds 12–18 months. (iii.) Loss of weight and other evidence of cachexia occur quite early in the illness, owing to deficient nourishment. Dehydration and thirst become troublesome. (iv.) There is usually no evidence of metastasis, but there may be enlarged glands, especially above the left clavicle. (v.) Pain is relatively late but persistent. (vi.) Sometimes there is a dry cough independent of but aggravated by food. It may be slight or very severe. (vii.) When the cervical œsophagus is involved, a bout of coughing immediately follows the taking of food and weakness or loss of voice may occur from recurrent laryngeal paralysis. (viii.) A fistula into the trachea or left bronchus or a peri-œsophageal abscess may form. (ix.) X-ray examination with a thickened barium swallow shows a very narrowed area in the œsophagus due to encroachment by the growth on the lumen. (x.) Œsophagoscopy and biopsy clinch the diagnosis.

'Fig. 88.—X-ray of the middle of the Œsophagus during a barium swallow; there is deformity and obstruction due to a Carcinoma.

Prognosis. — Without treatment patients rarely live more than 12 to 18 months. With modern radiotherapeutic and surgical techniques the period of survival has been lengthened but not more than 5 per cent. survive more than 5 years. The outlook is best with growths of the lower end of the œsophagus: resection of this area together with the cardiac end of the stomach in expert hands gives a 5-year survival of 15–20 per cent. of patients operated upon. Most patients die of the complications of inanition and the length of survival depends to a large extent on nutrition.

Treatment.—The treatment of choice of growths of the upper third of the œsophagus is by deep X-ray therapy or the use of the Cobalt bomb. Radical cure by surgical removal is being increasingly used for malignant disease of the lower third.   When the disease is in the middle third radio-therapy of the average case gives rather better results than surgery: resection of the diseased area with a supra-aortic œsophago-gastric an-astomosis is now often performed but the operative mortality is high. Inoperable cases are those where there is invasion of the lung or trachea, or evidence of metastases: then the insertion of a Souttar's tube through an œsophagoscope may give much relief, the tube being replaced by another after some months.   Octyl nitrite inhalations during a meal may make swallowing easier for a while.   Food should be finely divided or minced: milky foods and chocolate are taken easily.   In advanced cases with metastases and marked loss of weight with dehydration, gastrostomy may help temporarily: morphia should be used freely for pain in the terminal stages.

Fibroma and *Myoma*, and other benign growths in the œsophagus, sessile or pedunculated, are very rare.   They may cause no trouble, or only vague and trifling symptoms.   Their discovery is usually accidental.

§ 222. II. **Achalasia** (sometimes called Cardiospasm) is a condition in which there is a narrowed segment at the lower end of the œsophagus, and in which simple stricture and new growth can be excluded.   The site of the obstruction is between the point where the œsophagus passes through the diaphragm and its entry into the stomach; in this area the mucous membrane is sometimes inflamed.

Symptoms.—(i.) Achalasia can occur at any age but is usually met in men between the ages of 30 to 50.   (ii.) The food is felt to stick at the lower end of the œsophagus and pain may be felt behind the xiphisternum. (iii.) At a variable time after a meal, the food may pass on into the stomach or it may be vomited in an undigested condition.   (iv.) At first there is rather rapid loss of weight, but after a time this ceases and the weight remains stationary.

Diagnosis.—On X-ray examination, the barium meal does not pass into the stomach but accumulates above this in a tremendously distended and rather coiled œsophagus.   The amount of dilatation is much greater than is found from any other cause of dysphagia.   A height of about 8 inches of barium collects above the sphincter, and if still more barium (or food) is taken, the weight of the food is often sufficient for the obstruc-tion to be overcome until the level is reduced to the original height. Achalasia is differentiated from stricture or new growth by passing a heavy tube filled with mercury: this forces the sphincter open, and if the tube be moved up and down, it is not gripped by spasm of muscle fibres.

The *Etiology* of the condition is not yet settled; there is a failure of the muscle fibres at the lower end of the œsophagus to relax (hence the name achalasia), with degeneration of the cells of Auerbach's plexus of the

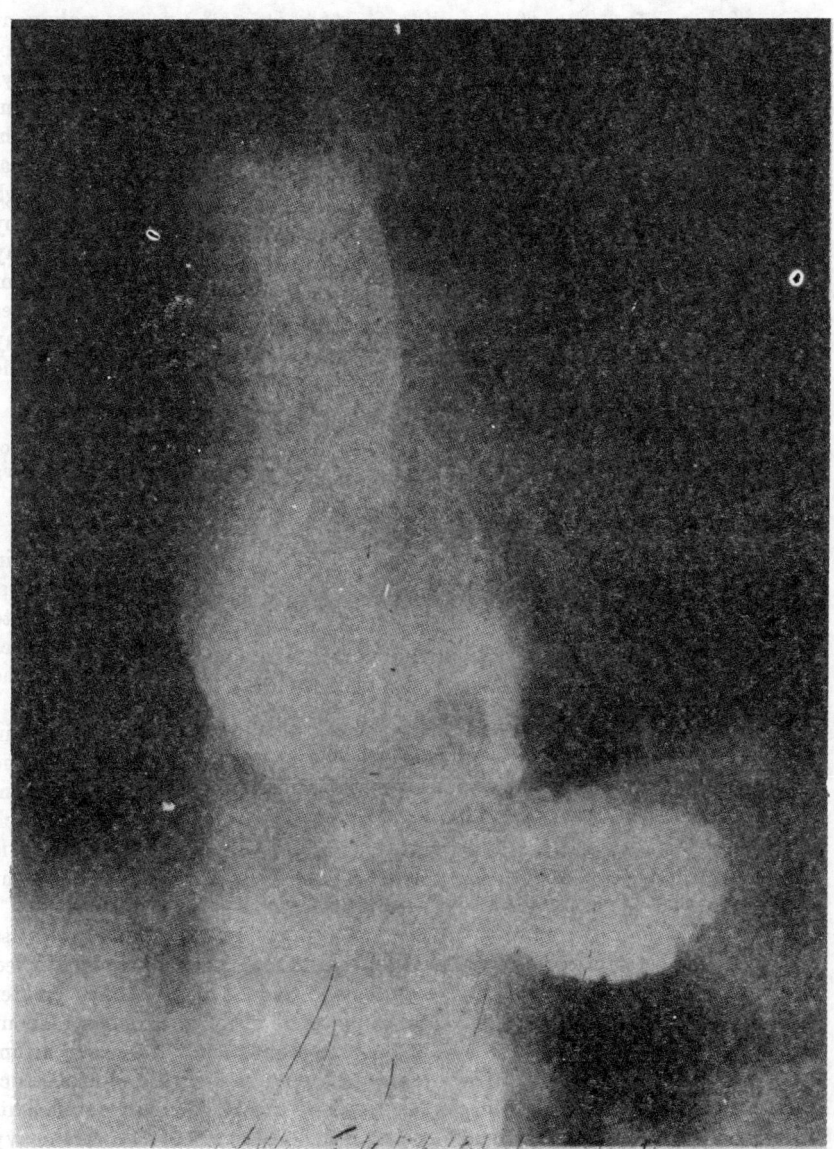

FIG. 89.—X-RAY OF THE ŒSOPHAGUS IN ACHALASIA. The enormously dilated middle and lower portions of the Œsophagus is characteristic.

œsophagus. The onset is sometimes sudden and psychosomatic causes may play a part when the condition follows a nervous shock.

Prognosis.—Once under treatment, most patients live for years but in a lowered state of health. Aspiration of the œsophageal contents into the larynx may cause pneumonia and sometimes bronchiectasis.

Treatment is by a high calorie diet of relatively soft foods. A heavy rubber tube filled with mercury should be passed just before meals. At first this must be done before every meal, but as the symptoms are relieved, it is required less and less often, until, in most cases, once a week or once a fortnight suffices. This method of treatment has been largely replaced by hydrostatic dilatation with a rubber bag placed at the level of the sphincter: this stretches the muscle fibres and even ruptures some of them. In obstinate cases Heller's operation of dividing the muscle fibres is much to be preferred to excision of the area as this often leads to œsophagitis.

§ 223. III. **Pressure** upon the gullet from outside is a fairly common cause of dysphagia. Any intrathoracic tumour may, by its pressure, narrow the lumen of the gullet. Other tumours are cancer of a neighbouring organ, enlargement of the bronchial glands, lympho-sarcoma or other mediastinal tumour, goitre, pericardial effusion and diverticulum of the pharynx filled with food (§ 230). The features common to all such tumours are the slowly progressive character of the dysphagia, the symptoms of pressure on other viscera, and the physical signs of the tumour in question. The differential features vary according to the nature and position of the tumour. The *Treatment* is that of the primary disease.

§ 224. IV. CARDIO-VASCULAR DISORDERS, which occasionally cause dysphagia, are a saccular aneurysm of the descending aorta, a large left auricle due to mitral stenosis and a large pericardial effusion. The *signs* of these conditions usually determine the cause.

In *aortic aneurysm* the amount of dysphagia is rarely very great at any time, although it is slowly progressive (§ 80). Rest in bed generally improves the dysphagia. The physical signs of aneurysm are commonly absent on account of its deep-seated position.

§ 225. V. **Foreign bodies. Acute Œsophagitis and Simple Stricture.**— The commonest foreign bodies to be swallowed and to lodge in the œsophagus are a meat or fish bone, a large piece of meat or a denture: a needle or a pin may stick in a fold of mucous membrane. These set up acute localised œsophagitis which comes on very suddenly and causes difficulty and pain on swallowing in one localised area. The patient may have forgotten the incident which led to the lodgement of the foreign body. Acute œsophagitis also occurs after the passage of the œsophagoscope or gastroscope, and may follow purposeful or accidental swallowing of a *corrosive substance* or of *boiling water*—in this case the mouth is also involved. The maximum damage occurs at the three narrowest portions of the œsophagus—opposite the cricoid cartilage, at the level of the tracheal bifurcation and at the lower end; the acute œdema and ulceration produced cause severe painful dysphagia and mucus, pus and blood may be vomited. *Simple (non-malignant) strictures* of the œsophagus which follow the removal of the foreign body occur at several levels (especially at the lower end) after swallowing corrosive or boiling liquids; they also occur in the lower 1–2 cm. after chronic œsophageal reflux and ulceration (§ 233) or very rarely are syphilitic. Dilatation takes place above a stricture: weight loss may be considerable and the patient may die of inanition or of aspiration pneumonia.

The *Diagnosis* rests on the history and on careful examination of the œsophagus with a barium swallow and with the œsophagoscope. With multiple strictures the instrument may only show the uppermost area of narrowing as the lower areas cannot be visualised.

Prognosis depends very much on the cause and the severity of the local injury. Foreign bodies need prompt attention, otherwise they may perforate and produce mediastinitis. A mediastinal abscess may also follow the use of the gastroscope or swallowing corrosive fluids. The formation of a stricture is always a serious complication.

Treatment of acute œsophagitis is by removing any foreign body through an œsophagoscope, treating pain with morphia hypodermically or by sucking cocaine lozenges, and combating shock. Thirst may be allayed with spoonfuls of iced water in which small doses of opium, cocaine and milk may be administered, and later a more varied fluid diet can be given. If the patient cannot swallow, intravenous fluids are necessary and in any case chemotherapy should be used to control infection. When a stricture is liable to form, this must be prevented at as early a stage as possible: thus after swallowing a corrosive substance, on the tenth to the fourteenth day a start should be made by passing a bougie under direct vision, or with a weighted mercury tube.

§ 226. VI. The **Plummer-Vinson Syndrome** is almost confined to women of middle age.

Symptoms.—The dysphagia is usually associated with an iron-deficiency anæmia (§ 549), which usually precedes the dysphagia by many months or years: there is a smooth bald tongue, throat and pharynx, koilonychia and often perlèche and an achlorhydria. Very occasionally there is pernicious anæmia instead. The condition predisposes to post-cricoid carcinoma in a high proportion of cases.

Etiology.—The atrophic state of the mucous membrane is associated with a decreased sensitivity: therefore the reflex arc which causes relaxation of the pharyngo-œsophageal sphincter at the commencement of swallowing does not function properly.

Treatment.—The anæmia should be treated by massive doses of iron and vitamin B complex or riboflavin, or by inj. cyanocobalamin if pernicious anæmia is present. The passage of the œsophagoscope usually relieves the dysphagia.

We now turn to the **rarer causes of Dysphagia.**

§ 227. VII. Functional Dysphagia is rare. When it occurs it may be associated with hysteria and other functional neuroses. Its differential features are fairly characteristic: (i.) The dysphagia is never progressive. It may come on somewhat suddenly, dating perhaps from an emotional shock or trouble, and it is very often intermittent, the patient being well enough in the intervals. Sometimes solids can be taken, while fluids are regurgitated, or *vice versa.* (ii.) It may be accompanied by considerable loss of weight; in other cases the patient sometimes appears to be in perfect health, a feature in which it differs from all other causes of dysphagia. There is usually little or no pain, and never any bleeding. (iii.) The dysphagia may last intermittently for years. (iv.) The passage of the œsophagoscope, or mercury bougie, or flexible stomach tube, generally results in curing the condition, at least for a time. (v.) The patient is usually of the female sex, and often presents other evidences of hysteria; but it occurs also in males. There is often great fear of malignant disease. (vi.) X-ray examination reveals no organic disease.

Diagnosis.—Care must be taken to exclude organic disease, and especially the Plummer-Vinson syndrome.

Treatment.—The passage of the œsophagoscope serves to exclude organic disease and to reassure the patient. The psychopathic personality of the individual needs treatment and valerian or tab. meprobamate are useful.

§ 228. VIII. Pharyngeal Paralysis.—Paralysis of the *pharyngeal constrictors* is not uncommon as an accompaniment and complication of diphtheria. Difficulty of swallowing under these circumstances may be one of the first evidences of diphtheritic paralysis. It also occurs in polioencephalitis, syphilitic pachymeningitis, syringobulbia, bulbar paralysis, polyneuritis and myasthenia gravis. Thrombosis, hæmorrhage and new growth at the base of the brain are other causes. It differs from the other causes of dysphagia in being attended by regurgitation of fluids through the nose, owing to the paralysis of the soft palate. There is often associated paralysis of the tongue.

Treatment.—Feeding must be through a nasal tube: a rubber tube (size 6) or a latex tube is passed through the nose: milk and milky foods, milk and eggs, chocolate, etc., may have sugar or malt added to increase the calorie value. In less severe cases, semi-solid foods are swallowed more easily than solids or liquids.

§ 229. IX. The Pharyngeal Crises of Tabes Dorsalis are violent gulping movements of the pharynx associated with eating or drinking. There is dysphagia with a feeling of a lump in the throat, with or without pain.

§ 230. X. Diverticulum, or a Pouch of the Pharynx.—(i.) A *pressure* diverticulum forms by herniation of the mucous membrane through the muscular wall. These pouches usually arise in the lowest part of the pharynx, probably from inco-ordination of the muscles of the pharynx and the cricopharyngeus guarding the entrance to the œsophagus. (ii.) A *traction* diverticulum of the œsophagus is due to adhesions between the œsophagus and neighbouring glands, pulling out the œsophageal wall as they contract. This variety does not usually cause symptoms.

The *symptoms* are: (i.) Regurgitation of food after an interval varying from a few minutes to a few hours after ingestion. It is apt to be mistaken for persistent vomiting, but the ease with which the food is returned, and the absence of acid in it, should make us suspect this condition. (ii.) The regurgitation gradually increases in amount, and the breath is sometimes foul from the decomposition of food in the gradually enlarging pouch. (iii.) Sometimes the pouch forms a definite tumour in the neck. (iv.) X-ray reveals the pouch. *Treatment* may necessitate surgical removal.

§ 231. XI. A Short Œsophagus with partial intrathoracic stomach (hiatus hernia, § 234) is an uncommon cause of dysphagia. The patient has symptoms of œsophagitis, with regurgitation and discomfort after a meal, which is relieved in one special position. In some cases the symptoms are those of dyspepsia only. The condition can be diagnosed by X-ray examination of the œsophagus and of the stomach in the Trendelenberg position.

§ 232. XII. Congenital Atresia of the œsophagus causes a recurrent cough and vomiting immediately the child is fed. Progressive loss of weight and dehydration rapidly ensue, and aspiration of the vomit into the chest causes collapse of part of a lung and pneumonia. A barium swallow should not be tried for this same reason: a small rubber tube is held up 3–3½ in. from the gums and 0·5 ml. of iodised oil shows the position of the upper pouch. *Treatment* is by effecting an anastomosis within the first 1–2 days of birth, immediately the diagnosis is made.

GROUP B.   **Causes of Chronic Heartburn.**

1. Chronic Œsophagitis .. .. § 233
2. Hiatus Hernia of the Stomach .. .. .. § 234

The patient complains of recurrent attacks of a BURNING PAIN (*heartburn*) BENEATH THE LOWER PART OF THE STERNUM *and* FOOD APPEARS TO STICK THERE *immediately after swallowing: there may be a complaint of* DISTENSION *in the left hypochondrium,* air-swallowing, VOMITING OF BLOOD *and loss of weight. The disease may be* CHRONIC ŒSOPHAGITIS *with or without simple peptic ulceration.*

§ 233. Chronic Œsophagitis has become more commonly recognised in recent years as a cause of symptoms which have previously been labelled as functional. The condition is commonest in men of middle age.

Symptoms.—(i.) At first there is a burning pain behind the lower end of the sternum shortly after swallowing a solid bolus, or after drinking very hot tea or alcoholic spirits. The pain may at first be intermittent but later becomes more continuous so that the patient is afraid to eat solid food: he therefore goes on to a liquid diet with antacid powders which he finds give relief. (ii.) There is often considerable swallowing of saliva and air which cause distension and even pain in the left upper abdomen. (iii.) In others, there is marked spasm of the lower end of the œsophagus with regurgitation of alkaline fluid into the mouth during the daytime. (iv.) The initial condition of simple inflammation may result in the formation of one or more *peptic ulcers* a little above the cardia, and there may be a minor or more severe degree of bleeding causing hæmatemesis, melæna and anæmia. Loss of weight may occur due to insufficient food intake but it is not usually so marked as in carcinoma.

Diagnosis.—The symptoms closely resemble those of a *peptic ulcer in the stomach or duodenum*, but with œsophagitis the pain is higher up (beneath the lower sternum) and often to the left of the lower dorsal vertebræ—instead of in the lumbar area. *X-ray examination* in the erect position may fail to reveal the condition. To visualise the lower œsophagus accurately the bolus must be fairly solid and preferably swallowed while the patient lies horizontally. A series of film exposures may then reveal thickened irregular folds of mucous membrane in the lower third of the œsophagus, and sometimes an ulcer niche can be seen—often protected by spasm a little higher up. To distinguish a carcinoma, *œsophagoscopy* by an expert, with removal of a small portion of the mucous membrane for biopsy, is often essential. The affected area of mucous membrane is seen to be generally reddened, thickened and even superficially eroded.

Etiology.—Œsophageal regurgitation (reflux) usually has no effect and leaves the mucous membrane intact. Symptoms occur when gastric juice regurgitates freely into the lower end of the œsophagus and is not neutralised; then simple inflammation, ulceration, even fibrosis and stricture follow. Two factors are of especial importance: (i.) the concentration of acid and the simultaneous action particularly of pepsin. Therefore symptoms often arise when there is a high gastric or a duodenal ulcer, or gall-bladder disease; the damage occurs chiefly at night when the patient is recumbent and when no saliva is being swallowed. Some cases are due to the lower end of the œsophagus being lined with gastric mucous membrane. (ii.) The second cause is an incompetent cardiac sphincter. This is due to *mechanical* causes, particularly a hiatus hernia of the sliding type, or to *increased intra-abdominal* or *intra-gastric pressure* (as with obesity, pregnancy, tight corsets, persistent vomiting, pyloric or intestinal obstruction). If the condition becomes severe or very obstinate it may give rise to a fibrous stricture of the lower 2 cm. of the œsophagus and a shortened œsophagus may result: sometimes perforation occurs.

Treatment is by giving frequent small quantities of a liquid diet combined with sucking antacid tablets slowly in the mouth—a tablet containing magnesium trisilicate and milk powder is especially useful. The patient should always rest and sleep sitting up with three or four pillows. This treatment must be persisted in until the patient is sympom-free and also until X-ray re-examination shows healing to be complete. Œsophagoscopy and dilatation may be helpful. In cases not responding to this treatment operative measures may be needed.

§ 234. **Hiatus Hernia of the Stomach** (Syn. Intrathoracic Stomach) gives rise to symptoms very like those of chronic œsophagitis, with which it frequently co-exists. On the other hand it is much more common in women than in men, especially in association with obesity. Many patients with radiographic evidence of hiatus hernia are completely symptomless —especially when œsophagitis is absent.

Symptoms.—(i.) There are usually the symptoms of œsophagitis with recurrent heartburn by day when stooping, and by night when lying flat in bed, especially after a large supper. Also there is a complaint of distension in the upper abdomen when half-way through a meal; ærophagy may be marked. (ii.) Pain in the lower sternal or in the præcordial area, sometimes radiating to the neck or arms, often produces a fear of angina pectoris. Other patients have attacks of paroxysmal tachycardia. (iii.) Recurrent hæmatemesis and/or melæna may occur. More insidious bleeding, with positive tests in the stool, sometimes causes symptoms of anæmia of obscure origin. (iv.) Some loss of weight is usual. (v.) Physical signs are usually absent.

Diagnosis depends largely on the characteristic symptoms in a person over 40, and should be confirmed with a barium meal, the patient being examined in the prone or supine position with a small firm pillow or balloon exerting pressure on the upper abdomen. Although the condition is often present by itself, in a considerable proportion of cases there is at the same time a gastric or duodenal ulcer or gall-stones are present. *Carcinoma* of the lower œsophagus or of the fundus of the stomach also causes pain behind the xiphisternum and anæmia, but the symptoms are of more recent onset and dysphagia and loss of weight are more marked. *Cardiac disease* and especially cardiac infarction are more likely to produce shortness of breath and gives electrocardiograph signs. *Eventration* of the diaphragm can be recognised by X-ray.

Etiology.—A hiatus hernia can produce symptoms at any age. In the normal person the œsophageal opening in the diaphragm is closed by a sling of muscle fibres encircling the cardia, producing a sphincteric action, aided by the oblique entry of the œsophagus into the stomach and by interdigitation of the gastric folds just below the cardia. Two types of hiatus hernia are recognised: (i.) the sliding hernia is the more common and is produced when a portion of the stomach (with the cardia) is drawn

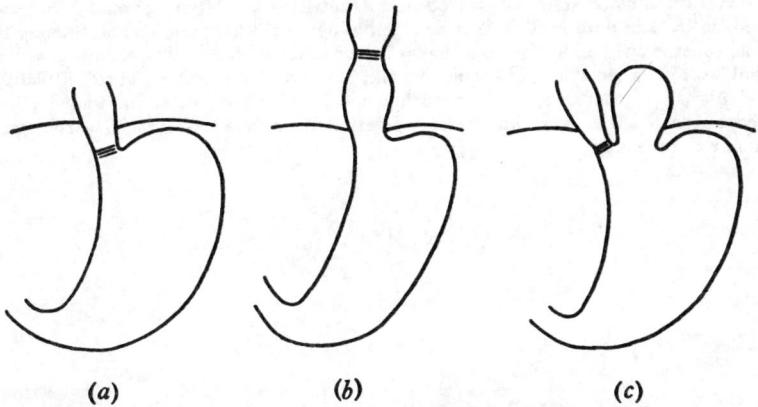

(a)   (b)   (c)

Fig. 90.—Hiatus Hernia. Diagram of (a) Normal stomach with the cardia below the diaphragm; the œsophagus enters the stomach obliquely. (b) Sliding hiatus hernia; a shortened œsophagus with the cardia and a portion of the stomach above the diaphragm. (c) Para-œsophageal hiatus hernia. The cardia is intact and below the diaphragm, but a portion of the fundus of the stomach has entered the chest. In each case the cardia is shaded.

up into the chest. This may be due to a congenitally short œsophagus or secondary to scarring from chronic œsophagitis. The œsophagus runs almost vertically into the stomach, the cardia is often incompetent, and then symptoms of œsophagitis arise (*q.v.*) with heartburn, epigastric pain, flatulence, vomiting, hæmatemesis and sometimes dysphagia. (ii.) The para-œsophageal or rolling hernia is less common, a portion of the fundus of the stomach passing through the diaphragmatic opening while the cardia remains closed and in its normal position below the diaphragm. Here obesity, previous pregnancies, trauma, a chronic cough and kypho-scoliosis play a part. As the sphincter is intact the symptoms of œsophagitis do not occur—and the main complaints are of substernal discomfort, belching, intermittent dysphagia and recurrent hæmorrhage producing an iron-deficiency anæmia.

Treatment.—The chief medical measures are (i.) the relief of symptoms produced by the resulting chronic œsophagitis (§ 233); (ii.) meals should be small in volume but of increased frequency—dry meals are best; (iii.) the last meal of the day should be particularly small in size and taken 4–5 hours before bedtime; (iv.) obesity and a chronic cough should be avoided; and (v.) tight abdominal belts and corsets must be removed. Surgical treatment may be necessary and measures used by different authorities include partial gastrectomy and vagotomy (to reduce gastric secretion), pyloroplasty, drawing the intrathoracic stomach into the abdomen and suturing it to the abdominal wall, as well as occasionally resecting the lower œsophagus and effecting an anastomosis. Repair of the hiatal opening often leads to recovery or great improvement but recurrence may occur.

Infants may be born with a *congenital hiatus hernia*. This condition, which is being much more commonly diagnosed, causes early effortless vomiting of material which is often blood-stained. It leads to malnutrition and often anæmia. *Diagnosis* is made by a barium meal. *Treatment* is by giving thickened feeds and nursing the child constantly in an upright position as in a special cot-chair. The condition usually rectifies itself when the child begins to walk, but severe cases may lead to œsophagitis and fibrosis of the lower end, producing one form of congenital shortening of the œsophagus (§ 231). For this reason operation on severe cases at an early age is preferred by many.

CHAPTER IX

THE ABDOMEN

THE abdomen contains a large number of very important organs and structures, but just as their physiology and pathology are in some instances obscure, so are the means at our disposal for their thorough clinical investigation also imperfect. It is in this region that we have to deal with symptoms which on the one hand may be of trivial order, or on the other of extreme gravity; symptoms and conditions the issue of which will largely depend on the promptitude, knowledge, and skill of the medical practitioner and upon his adequate comprehension of their true meaning.[1]

PART A. SYMPTOMATOLOGY

§ 238. **Local Symptoms.**—The symptoms referable to disease situated within the abdomen are necessarily of the widest and most varied kind, but there are only three which are sufficiently constant to be regarded as cardinal symptoms, all of which are referable to the abdomen itself— viz., ABDOMINAL PAIN, GENERALISED ENLARGEMENT and LOCALISED TUMOUR.

VOMITING is a fairly constant accompaniment of all acute abdominal conditions, whether the stomach is involved in the lesion or not. Its causes are discussed in § 271.

The presence of DIARRHŒA and CONSTIPATION depends very largely on whether the intestinal canal is affected, and these are fully dealt with in Chapter XI. The other symptoms also depend largely upon which of the abdominal organs is affected, with one important exception—viz., "INDIGESTION." In all chronic abdominal disorders, no matter which organ is affected, we are often consulted for "INDIGESTION"; in fact, nausea and all the other symptoms of pronounced dyspepsia may be due to disease quite unconnected with the stomach, and located, for instance, within the appendix, gall-bladder, colon, kidneys, prostate, liver, lungs, pancreas, uterus or other organs.

ABDOMINAL PAIN, if acute and sudden, is a medical emergency of the most important kind; if chronic, it presents many difficult questions for diagnosis. It therefore merits the most careful study and analysis (§ 242). The diseases *outside the abdomen* which may cause it are:

1. *Coronary thrombosis, pericarditis* and *paroxysmal tachycardia* have been mistaken for a condition requiring laparotomy.

---

[1] Although in one particular patient there is usually only one pathological process at work, it must not be overlooked that a patient with tabes dorsalis may also be suffering from a perforated peptic ulcer, or that a patient with pneumonia does occasionally develop acute appendicitis at the same time.

2. *Diaphragmatic pleurisy*, a basal pneumonia or blast injuries involving the chest may give rise to acute abdominal pain of sudden onset (often referred to the corresponding iliac region), and to abdominal rigidity and other symptoms of acute peritonitis, which can only be differentiated by the pulse-respiration ratio and the concurrent symptoms.

3. *Root pains* from the spinal nerves may be referred to the abdomen. In this way spinal caries (especially in children), a spinal tumour, or the crises of locomotor ataxy may be mistaken for various abdominal diseases.

4. An *abscess* in the abdominal wall, a bruise, or a ruptured muscle may be similarly mistaken, but these should present no difficulty. *Fibrositis* of the abdominal wall has led to mistaken diagnoses of appendicitis and ovaritis, or of the diaphragm to confusion with an upper abdominal lesion.

5. *Diabetic coma* is occasionally heralded by pain simulating appendicitis.

ABDOMINAL ENLARGEMENT and ABDOMINAL TUMOUR are considered in Part C.

The **General** or **Remote Symptoms** met with in abdominal disorders are of an extremely varied nature, and our endeavour should be to associate correctly these symptoms with the abdominal organ which is affected.

§ 239. **Shock** (or **Collapse**) is a frequent general symptom in acute abdominal disease; it is a condition of extreme prostration. Shock and collapse are clinically identical. There is paresis of all the muscles, voluntary and involuntary (muscles of the limbs, of respiration, of the heart and arteries), and a rapid fall in blood pressure. The *Symptoms* may be arranged under the following headings: (1) The skin (especially of the extremities) is pale, cold, clammy or sweating; the surface temperature is 2° F or more under normal; the pupils are dilated, and react slowly to light. (2) The circulation and respiration are feeble, the pulse being rapid, of low volume and often scarcely perceptible. (3) The temperature is subnormal. (4) Restlessness, air hunger and marked pallor are present in shock accompanied by profuse hæmorrhage. (5) There is apathy, but the intellect is clear. The urine and other secretions are diminished or suppressed. The patient may die, or may pass into a reaction stage, with slight pyrexia and sometimes vomiting.

Diagnosis.—In *coma* the mind is completely obscured, and the respiration laboured and stertorous. Save for the vital functions, all is in abeyance. (See § 850 *et seq.*) In *syncope* consciousness is generally lost, but the condition is transient.

The *Causes* of shock may be divided into those of sudden and those of gradual onset. The depth of shock varies with the causative lesion.

Surgical shock is frequently divided into primary and secondary stages: the former comes on rapidly and is believed to be due to afferent nervous impulses acting on the brain, producing paresis of the vaso-motor centre and dilatation especially in the splanchnic vessels. Secondary shock is much more insidious and more dangerous: it is the result of loss of blood plasma through the capillary walls, often in association with pooling stagnant blood in a dilated capillary bed: later it is followed by absorption of toxic products from the site of injury.

(a) OF SUDDEN ONSET (often due to primary shock). These may be subdivided into: (1) Those due to *external injury*. (i.) Traumatic shock such as gunshot wounds and accidents. The amount of shock varies, especially with the extent of hæmorrhage, and to a less extent with the amount of injury. (ii.) Fractures of long bones produce an amount of shock out of proportion to the apparent injury. (iii.) Severe burns, especially on the trunk. (iv.) Head injuries with concussion. (v.) From electrical currents. (vi.) Certain narcotic poisons (hydrocyanic acid, carbon monoxide, § 577). (2) Those due to *internal causes*. (i.) Profuse internal hæmorrhage as with hæmatemesis, ruptured ectopic gestation. (ii.) Perforation of an abdominal viscus with extravasation of its contents into the peritoneum. (iii.) Rupture or torsion of an abdominal organ. (iv.) Very severe acute pain, as with renal or biliary colic. (v.) Sudden intestinal obstruction. (vi.) Pulmonary or other embolism. (vii.) A large spontaneous pneumothorax. (viii.) Coronary thrombosis. (ix.) Cerebral hæmorrhage. (x.) With acute pancreatitis (§ 357) or acute suprarenal hæmorrhage (§ 245).

(b) OF GRADUAL ONSET: (i.) Peritonitis and other abdominal inflammations. (ii.) Delayed hæmorrhage from trauma on the 7th–10th day, *e.g.*, from a ruptured liver, spleen or kidney, and following sudden movement or even an enema. (iii.) Profuse diarrhœa and vomiting. (iv.) Sudden and severe emotion (terror, grief, etc.). (v.) Privation and exposure to extremes of heat and cold. (vi.) Sea and air sickness. (vii.) Blast and crush injuries associated with renal failure. Other *toxic causes* include (viii.) Post-anæsthetic and post-operative shock. (ix.) An overdose of hypnotic and anæsthetic drugs. (x.) Poisoning by irritants (oxalic acid, arsenic, phosphorus). (xi.) Food poisoning. (xii.) Anaphylaxis (§§ 524, 652). (xiii.) The asthenic types of fever such as may attend typhoid and yellow fever. (xiv.) The termination of many diseases described in the chapter on debility.

Diagnosis.—When a patient is found in a state of collapse or shock, the physician has to diagnose the *cause* of the condition. After applying restoratives he should inquire: first, whether there is a history of injury, hæmorrhage or emotional disturbance, etc.; secondly, if the patient was in good health up to the time of onset of the condition, so as to exclude group (b); thirdly, what food the patient has recently taken, remembering the possibility of poison. Finally, he should examine all the viscera, especially the heart and abdominal organs, beginning at the part which is or has been the seat of pain.

Etiology.—The main factors producing shock vary from case to case, and with the cause. The most important are: (i.) hæmorrhage; (ii.) circulatory failure; (iii.) severe pain; (iv.) dehydration; (v.) prolonged exposure; (vi.) the mental reactions of the patient, including loss of consciousness; (vii.) the absorption of toxic products.

The reduction of blood volume is a most important factor: with hæmorrhage this is due to the loss of whole blood, but in extensive burns, crush injuries, diabetic coma, severe diarrhœa and vomiting and other conditions of dehydration it is the blood plasma which is decreased.

The immediate *Treatment* consists in dealing with the cause: *e.g.*, blood loss must be stopped, an injured or fractured limb immobilised. When pain is severe this should be combined with an injection of morphine, and by the application of warmth with hot-water bottles and warm blankets, or by an electric cradle. The head should be lowered, the feet raised and even the legs bandaged from below upwards following severe hæmorrhage. In mild cases, and if there is no abdominal injury, brandy may be given by mouth. Stimulants such as injections of nikethamide (Coramine) 1–2 ml., leptazol (Cardiazol) ½–1 ml., and adrenalin may be repeated. When blood loss has been marked, transfusion of whole blood (½–2 litres or more) is essential. In severe cases with extensive burns, crush injuries and in the presence of dehydration, isotonic blood serum or plasma (½–2 litres) should be given intravenously, or failing these dextran (6·0 per cent.); these may be supplemented by isotonic gum-saline or dextrose (5·0 per cent.) intravenously, or normal saline or isotonic glucose per rectum. Only after recovery from primary shock, and when the fall of blood pressure has been corrected, should the patient be operated on.

SHOCK (COLLAPSE) AND PULSE-TEMPERATURE RATIO.—In connection with the general symptoms of abdominal diseases, two facts need special mention—(1) Profound primary shock is common at the onset of acute abdominal conditions. A subnormal temperature is one of the symptoms of shock, and for this reason it is often present in the early stage of abdominal trouble, and it rarely ranges very high even in the gravest abdominal conditions. In acute peritonitis, for instance, an extensive inflammatory process affects the peritoneum, which acting alone might produce a temperature of 105° F or more, but by reason of the secondary shock it is rarely more than 102° or 103° F. (2) *In the pulse*, however, *we find our best guide to the severity of trouble within the abdomen.* In all acute diseases, other than abdominal, we find a rough general proportion between the height of the temperature and the rate of the pulse. Thus, a temperature of 100° F will correspond roughly with a pulse of 100, 101° with 110, 102° with 120, 103° with 130, and so on—an increase of about 10 for every 1° F. But in acute abdominal conditions this is not so. The pulse-temperature ratio is disturbed, for although the pulse rate increases with the severity of the abdominal condition, the temperature never increases proportionately. Indeed, in many of the worst cases, the temperature is one or more degrees below normal. The pulse, however, is usually a good guide, and one may say (1) that if the pulse remains under 100 nothing very serious has happened within the abdomen; and (2) that the rate of the pulse and the pulse-temperature ratio are great aids to the diagnosis, and in some sense measures, of acute abdominal disorder, especially when peritonitis is suspected. In assessing a patient's condition due regard must be paid also to the effects of anxiety on the pulse rate.

PART B. PHYSICAL EXAMINATION

§ **240.** In the examination of the abdomen we must proceed systematically, as in the examination of the thorax, by INSPECTION, PALPATION, PERCUSSION, MEASUREMᴱNᴛ and occasionally AUSCULTATION; though of all these measures palpation by the educated hand is at the present time the most valuable means we have. X-RAYS assist in many cases.

1. CAREFUL inspection OF THE ABDOMEN should on no account be omitted; much can be learned from this. Sometimes it is desirable to view the abdomen from the foot of the bed, or by bending over the patient's feet, so as to view the abdomen from below. The mere fact of *enlargement* may thus be verified, and whether the enlargement be generalised and uniform, or whether it be localised or asymmetrical. Notice whether the umbilicus is centrally situated, and also whether the surface presents dilated veins, such as occur in abdominal cancer, or when the portal vein or inferior vena cava is obstructed. Dilatation of the abdominal veins is met with chiefly in three conditions: (1) In liver cirrhosis, these veins being part of the collateral circulation which gradually becomes established (§ 260); (2) the veins, without being much dilated or prominent, are unduly apparent in cases of advanced abdominal carcinoma. (3) Extreme dilatation and varicosity of the superficial veins occur only when the inferior vena cava is obstructed. This is generally due to a tumour in or around the posterior border of the liver where the vena cava passes through it. The veins of the legs and testes generally share to a less extent in the dilatation. Notice also whether there is any fistula, thickening or infiltration round the umbilicus such as occasionally occur in cancer and tuberculous peritonitis. An abdominal enlargement due to the presence of air or gas is rounded anteriorly, but when due to fluid it is usually flattened in front and the flanks bulge; when there is obstruction of the large intestine the flanks bulge; whereas in obstruction of the small intestine low down the swelling occupies the centre of the abdomen. Incidentally you may notice the presence or absence of the white lines (lineæ albicantes) left by a previous pregnancy, and of scars left by a previous operation. The presence of a hernia or of tumours of the wall (increased by coughing) may be recognised. The amount of *movement* of the abdominal wall with inspiration should be noticed, for diminished or absent movement constitutes an important sign of general peritonitis. With local peritonitis, the abdominal wall over that area may not move, whilst elsewhere abdominal respiratory movement is normal. Pulsation seen in the epigastrium is often normal, but may be due to the right ventricle or an engorged liver secondary to heart failure. Sometimes aortic pulsation is unduly visible, especially in thin neurotic dyspeptic women, or it may be transmitted by a pyloric tumour lying over the aorta. Occasionally the pulsation is due to an abdominal aneurysm. *Visible peristalsis* should be looked for and

should be provoked by gently flicking the abdomen or, in the case of a child, giving a feed; if present, its position and direction should be noted. The REGIONAL ANATOMY OF THE ABDOMEN is important as a guide to the seat of disease (Fig. 91).

2. **Palpation.**—With practice, experience and a knowledge of anatomy a great deal can be learned by careful palpation. To relax the abdominal muscles the patient should lie on his back with his neck and shoulders supported and his arms lying comfortably by his sides. He should have the legs extended loosely or have the knees drawn up, and should be instructed to breathe quietly through his mouth. The hand should be warm, otherwise the patient may flinch. Palpation may be (a) superficial and (b) deep. Superficial palpation should be carried out first; test for hyperæsthesia by picking up a fold of the skin and subcutaneous tissue from each of the four quadrants in turn. If hyperæsthesia is present the patient may complain of soreness, or show pain by his expression. Hyperæsthesia of the underlying segments of the abdominal wall is revealed by repeatedly stroking the overlying skin; where it is present the reflex is brisker and is maintained for a longer time than on the normal side. For deep palpation the hand should always be laid *flat* on the abdominal wall; do not use the tips, but only the pads of the fingers, for the tips stimulate the recti muscles to contract. Then by gently dipping the fingers, by flexing the metacarpo-phalangeal joints, we ascertain (1) the presence of deep tenderness or (2) of a tumour; (3) the boundaries of some of the solid organs. Bimanual palpation should be employed in feeling the kidneys, spleen and pelvic organs. Relaxation is obtained in others by an anæsthetic such as gas and oxygen or sodium thiopentone B.P. (Pentothal) in adults, and ethyl chloride in children. Much obesity is another obstacle to palpation. Palpation reveals the presence of localised resistance and tenderness which denote underlying inflammation, but it must be remembered that in severe toxæmia this reflex rigidity may be very slight: morphia and the corticosteroids also lessen or abolish these signs. Tumours and flatulence are detected by palpation; the movement of fluid within the abdomen conveys a thrill (§ 259). The palpation and percussion boundaries of the different organs are described in later chapters.

Gastric Succussion or *Splashing* is made out by placing one hand on each side of the stomach, and suddenly pressing inwards the finger-tips of each hand alternately: listening over the stomach at the same time with a stethoscope materially aids this sign. Otherwise it can be detected by vigorously rolling the patient from side to side. Splashing can be *normally* elicited during the process of digestion—*i.e.*, during the first hour or two after a meal, especially if much fluid has been taken. But if succussion can be elicited after that time, it suggests that there is delayed emptying of the stomach.

3. **Percussion** of the abdomen is carried out with the same precautions as in the case of heart and lungs. The liver and spleen give a dull note on percussion. A full bladder or an ovarian cyst is dull with a horseshoe-

shaped area of resonance above it. By this means we ascertain the
presence of solid and fluid, which are dull, or of gas, which is resonant.
When the fluid is free the dullness alters with the position of the patient
and gives a percussion wave or thrill.

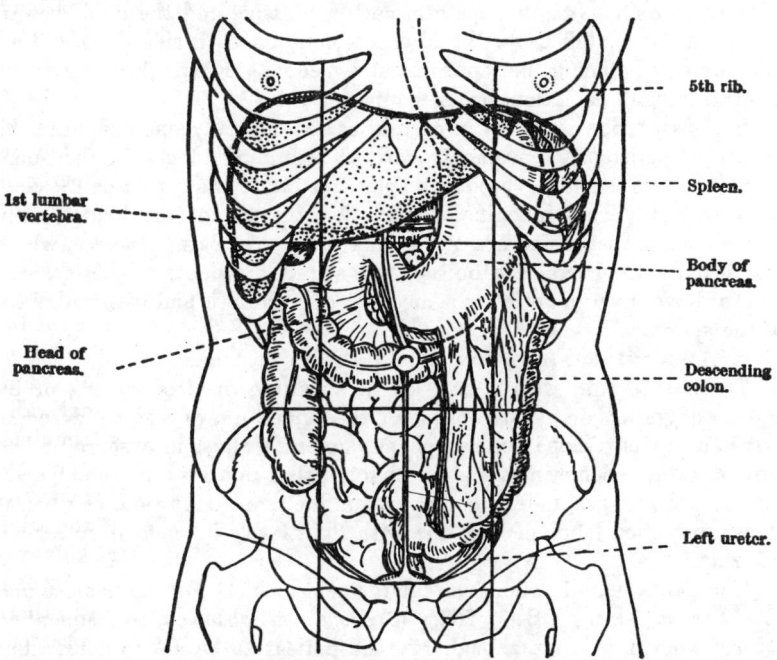

FIG. 91.—REGIONS OF THE ABDOMEN.

For purposes of convenience the abdomen is divided into nine regions. These are bounded by
(a) two imaginary lateral vertical lines running upwards from the mid-point between the symphysis
pubis and the anterior superior iliac spine below, to the ribs above; and (b) two imaginary horizontal
lines. The upper lies mid-way between the symphysis pubis and the suprasternal notch (transpyloric plane running through the first lumbar vertebra and usually coinciding with the tips of the
ninth costal cartilages): the lower crosses at the level of the iliac crests.
Their names and the organs they contain are as follows:

Right Hypochondriac.	*Epigastric Region.*	*Left Hypochondriac.*
The right lobe of the liver and the gall-bladder, upper part of the right kidney, and the right suprarenal.	The left lobe and lobulus Spigelii of the liver, and part of the fundus and body of the stomach.	Part of the fundus and body of the stomach, the spleen and tail of the pancreas, the splenic flexure of the colon, upper half of the left kidney and the left suprarenal.
	Umbilical Region.	
	The middle and pyloric end of the stomach, the first, second and proximal portion of the third part of the duodenum, the head and body of the pancreas, the middle of the transverse colon, part of the great omentum and mesentery, and some convolutions of the jejunum and ileum.	
Right Lumbar.		*Left Lumbar.*
The ascending and proximal part of the transverse colon, lower part of the right kidney, and some convolutions of the small intestine.		Descending colon, part of the omentum, lower part of the left kidney, and some convolutions of the small intestines.
	Hypogastric Region.	
	Convolutions of the small intestines and the bladder in children and in adults when distended, the appendix, the pelvic colon, and the uterus during pregnancy.	
Right Iliac.		*Left Iliac.*
The cæcum, ovary and ureter.		Sigmoid flexure of the colon, ureter and ovary.

4. By **measurement** we ascertain the amount of increase or decrease in size. As a general rule, horizontal measurement should be taken at the level of the umbilicus, and it should be recorded for future reference. In order to ascertain whether the enlargement is symmetrical, we measure from the umbilicus to the ensiform cartilage above and the pubis below, and from the umbilicus to the anterior spine on each side. These four measurements should be approximately equal. From these data we ascertain slight deviations from symmetry.

5. **Auscultation** is useful in certain cases: normally one can hear the results of peristaltic movements with the gurgling of gas in the small intestine or as it passes through a sphincter (as at the cardia or the ileo-cæcal valve). With intestinal obstruction the sounds are louder, they occur in short rushes and are of a higher pitch. In paralytic ileus, which may occur with general peritonitis, these sounds disappear. Friction may be heard over liver or spleen in some cases of peritonitis and with embolism of the spleen.

6. A RECTAL EXAMINATION should always be made.

7. EXAMINATION with X-rays (with a barium meal or enema, or by cholecystography or pyelography): or the skilled use of a sigmoidoscope, cystoscope, gastroscope and œsophagoscope may assist in obscure and in chronic cases. Sometimes a plain abdominal X-ray film may be of help, *e.g.*, by showing gas under the diaphragm due to a perforation, or when it shows distended loops of intestine with fluid levels in them in intestinal obstruction.

The FALLACIES of abdominal enlargement are: (1) *Fat in the omentum.* (2) *Phantom tumour.* See § 262. (3) *Pendulous abdomen*, so frequent in elderly women, is often thought by the patient to be a " tumour," but is due to weakness of the muscles. (4) In *rachitic children* the weakness of the abdominal muscles combined with gaseous distension produce the appearance of an enlarged abdomen. (5) Extreme lordosis (and see § 262).

PART C. ABDOMINAL DISORDERS: THEIR DIAGNOSIS, PROGNOSIS AND TREATMENT

§ 241. **Routine Procedure and Classification.**—Having *first* ascertained that the patient's leading symptom is one of those referred to above (§ 238), we *secondly* inquire into the history, and especially whether the condition came on acutely and suddenly, or is chronic and long-standing. The procedure to be adopted in acute cases, and in chronic cases, is given under their respective headings. *Thirdly*, proceed to the physical examination of the abdomen, the routine method in ordinary cases consisting of (1) Inspection; (2) Palpation; (3) Percussion; and (4) Measurement. In any doubtful case the rectum, vagina, hernial orifices, urine and fæces must be examined. The fallacies mentioned in § 240 must be borne in mind.

If **severe abdominal pain,** which came on **suddenly** and acutely, be the leading symptom, first turn to § 242.

If **abdominal pain** of some duration and running a **chronic** course be the leading symptom, turn to § 250.

If there be a **generalised abdominal enlargement,** turn to § 257.

If there be **localised tumour,** turn to § 262.

§ 242. Acute Abdominal Pain, coming on **suddenly,** or supervening on chronic abdominal pain, includes amongst its causes some of the most serious conditions with which a physician or surgeon can have to deal.

The *causes* of abdominal pain may be conveniently classified thus:

A. ABDOMINAL PAIN coming on **suddenly, with shock.**

  I. Perforation of some organ or cyst (perforative peritonitis) §§ 243, 244
  II. Internal hæmorrhage .. .. § 245
  III. Acute intestinal obstruction (strangulated hernia, intussusception, internal strangulation, volvulus and paralytic ileus) §§ 244, 326
  IV. Torsion of ovarian cyst; V. embolism of the mesenteric artery;
      VI. acute pancreatitis; VII. Acute dilatation of the stomach § 246
  VIII. Severe acute gastro-enteritis .. .. § 280

B. ABDOMINAL PAIN coming on **suddenly, without shock.**

  IX. Colic (intestinal, renal, biliary, appendicular), and pyloric spasm § 247
  X. Appendicitis (some cases) .. .. § 248
  XI. Pancreatic calculus; floating kidney; splenic embolism; and some other obscure organic affections .. .. .. § 249
  XII. Root or referred pain .. .. § 249

In the first seven the acute abdominal pain is usually ATTENDED BY SHOCK, but not in the last four. This, however, is only relative, and in any doubtful case the whole should be passed in review.

In order to ascertain which of these causes is in operation, and in view of the gravity of some of these cases, it will be desirable to consider the METHOD OF PROCEDURE in some detail.

1. Regarding the *cardinal* or *leading* symptoms, inquire carefully, as in all cases of " pain," concerning its position, character, intensity and duration. The position of the pain is not always a guide to the organ affected, for it rapidly tends to become generalised; but the direction in which it is referred is of great help in the diagnosis of the four kinds of colic. Moreover, local disease may be accompanied by generalised pain (which may later settle down locally), and widespread disease may give rise to a localised pain. Inquire whether it is associated with other symptoms (*e.g.,* vomiting). Whenever the three symptoms, ABDOMINAL PAIN, VOMITING and SHOCK, come on together suddenly, the condition is very probably due to PERFORATION (which will later be accompanied by PERITONITIS), INTERNAL HÆMORRHAGE or INTESTINAL OBSTRUCTION.

2. As to the *History of the Illness,* it is useful to note whether there have been previous attacks of pain; and whether there has been any illness or operation in times gone by which indicates ulceration or other derangement of the abdominal organs. The occupation may shed some light on the cause—*e.g.,* sudden muscular strain, working with lead. The description of the mode of onset may assist—*e.g.,* " something was felt to give

way," and it should especially be noted whether the pain was acute at its onset or whether it worked up to a climax later.

3. In the *Examination of the Patient*—(i.) the *age* is an important aid in the diagnosis of the cause of the pain. In childhood there is very probably some intestinal affection, such as enteritis or colic, intussusception, strangulated hernia, or a congenital abnormality; in adolescents and young adults, appendicitis may have to be considered. In adults we think of hernia, ulcer of the stomach and tabetic crises; after middle life and in old age we think of cancer, volvulus or diverticulitis. (ii.) The *sex* may aid us, for in young females we may suspect an ulcer of the stomach even without previous symptoms; and in older women, biliary colic, salpingitis, torsion of an ovarian cyst, the rupture of an ectopic (extra-uterine) pregnancy, frequently overlooked, or gall-stones. (iii.) The presence of *rigidity*, as shown by resistance to palpation, or of *tenderness*, is of considerable aid; they point to the existence of underlying inflammation. (iv.) *All the organs* of the abdomen must be as carefully and as thoroughly examined as circumstances will permit. Never forget to examine per rectum and vagina, because local tenderness, a pelvic abscess, hæmatoma or tumour may throw considerable light upon the case. (v.) The patient's *general symptoms* must also be carefully investigated. If the temperature *and the pulse* be normal, we can exclude serious conditions such as an abscess, perforation or acute peritonitis. The temperature alone is not a sufficient guide in this respect (see § 239), but in general terms no serious acute abdominal condition exists without the *pulse rate* exceeding 90 or 100. If the patient is very emaciated, in adults we must bear in mind malignant disease, and in children the presence of tubercle. Examine the tongue for dryness and furring: the urine for sugar, crystals or pus: and do not forget to examine the chest (see § 238).

If the pain, which is severe and has come on suddenly, is **attended by marked shock,** first turn to § 243. If it is **unattended by shock,** turn first to § 247. It must be remembered, however, that any severe pain will cause a certain amount of prostration.

GROUP A. I. *The patient complains of very severe* **abdominal pain,** *which has come on* **suddenly,** *followed by* SHOCK *and repeated* VOMITING *of small amounts. Later,* ABDOMINAL DISTENSION *develops. The case is one of* PERFORATION *with* PERITONITIS.

§ 243. **Perforation of the Alimentary Canal, or Rupture of an Abscess, Cyst or a Solid Organ** (which shortly develops into Perforative Peritonitis). (1) *Ulcers* of the stomach or duodenum are especially liable to perforate. Other ulcers which may perforate are: ulcer of the lower part of the ileum (due to tuberculosis or typhoid fever), ulcer of the cæcum, ulcer of the large intestine, especially the sigmoid (usually cancerous, dysenteric or with ulcerative colitis). (2) *Abscesses* of the appendix (§ 248), sigmoid diverticulitis, liver, gall-bladder, kidney or other organs, or of mesenteric glands. (3) *Cysts which may rupture* are pancreatic, ovarian and parovarian cysts, and sometimes simple or hydatid cysts of the liver, kidney or other organs.

A ruptured bladder produces similar symptoms. (4) *Rupture of a solid organ* is usually followed by internal hæmorrhage (§ 245) and causes similar symptoms.

The *immediate symptoms* of the perforation in the order of occurrence are (1) very severe sudden abdominal pain, which is the cardinal symptom, accompanied by (2) primary shock, with an ashen pallid face showing a cold clammy sweat; the temperature is subnormal and the pulse of low volume: then (3) vomiting occurs. As the patient recovers from the initial shock the inexperienced physician may be deceived until the *symptoms* of *general perforative peritonitis* set in; (4) the pain remains severe and becomes generalised; (5) toxæmia produces a condition of secondary shock with rising temperature and pulse rate; (6) vomiting of small quantities becomes incessant. Later the material becomes alkaline to litmus and even fæcal; (7) the eyes become sunken and the tongue furred and dry; (8) there is board-like rigidity of the abdomen and, a little later, (9) constipation and moderate abdominal distension from paralytic ileus; (10) the blood shows a marked and progressive leucocytosis.

The commonest causes are acute perforative appendicitis and perforation of a peptic ulcer. This latter may be taken as a type. We should inquire for a history of dyspepsia and other symptoms (§ 281), but in not a few cases rupture has occurred without previous symptoms of any kind whatever. On examination the thighs are flexed, there is tenderness, a board-like rigidity of the muscles, most marked in the epigastrium, and a tympanitic note over the whole abdomen. The disappearance of the liver dullness in the mid-axillary line denotes free gas, and is usually due to ruptured peptic ulcer. After a few hours there is a deceptive *latent period* during which all symptoms of discomfort are diminished. A *stage of reaction* occurs several hours later, when symptoms of secondary shock are found, with acute peritonitis (§ 244), generalised or localised. There is increased abdominal distension, vomiting and tenderness, with decreased rigidity and a rising pulse rate. In a perforated duodenal ulcer the pain may spread to the right iliac fossa, simulating appendicitis. Three degrees of severity occur with perforation: (*a*) When there are adhesions the peritonitis may be localised or partial; (*b*) when there are no adhesions, but a small leakage, it may be only moderately sudden in its onset; (*c*) when the leakage is large it is extremely sudden and severe in its onset. In typhoid fever the symptoms and signs of perforation in the third week may be few (see § 496).

Diagnosis of perforative peritonitis is from diaphragmatic pleurisy and basal pneumonia, in which the pulse-respiration ratio is disturbed; also from coronary thrombosis (§ 52) and from tabetic crises (§ 1022). The presence by X-ray of a small quantity of gas under the diaphragm indicates a perforative lesion.

Treatment and Prognosis.—Laparotomy should be performed at once. If the deceptive latent period leads one to believe the patient is recovering, in a few hours general peritonitis will have set in, but operation is still indicated, with or without drainage. In cases where patients have been operated upon within the first 12 hours the prognosis is good; if after 24 hours, it is serious. The after-treatment depends on the cause. In the case of rupture consequent on injury internal hæmorrhage may take place with a rapidly fatal result, but even in such cases early laparotomy and blood transfusion should be performed.

§ 244. Acute Peritonitis is rarely a primary disease, but its onset is usually sudden, especially after a perforation.

Symptoms.—(1) The aspect is very characteristic; the countenance has an anxious pinched look, the cheeks pale, and the skin cold and clammy. The posture of the patient is also characteristic, as he lies on his back with his legs drawn up to fix the abdominal muscles. (2) The pain is severe and constant, but liable to exacerbations on account of the intestinal peristalsis and the passage of wind along the bowel.[1] It is increased by any movement, even by the respiratory movements; consequently the respiration is thoracic; (3) vomiting is persistent. (4) There is acute tenderness on pressure, so much so that the weight of the bed-clothes can hardly be borne. (5) The abdomen is rigid and immobile. (6) Pyrexia is sometimes ushered in with rigors, and is attended by a small, thin, rapid pulse of 100 to 140 per minute. The temperature is elevated only 2° or 3° F above normal, and maintained there continuously, unless pyæmia be present, in which case there are rapid variations of wide range. In some cases—*e.g.*, perforation—it may be subnormal at first (*vide supra*). (7) Leucocytosis is found. There is marked prostration, as in all abdominal inflammations, and a great tendency to secondary surgical shock. Even from the beginning there is constipation: hiccough is often present, and if persistent is a bad sign, as in all abdominal disorders. There is diminution and even suppression of urine. Death occurs from toxæmia in uncomplicated cases but the mind remains clear until the end.

In acute localised peritonitis the symptoms are those of acute general peritonitis, but are less severe, and result in the formation of a localised abscess.

The *Causes* of acute peritonitis may be grouped under seven headings: (i.) *Acute appendicitis* is the most common (§ 248). There may be extension of inflammation from other organs in the abdomen—especially diverticulitis and otherwise gonorrhœal salpingitis, typhoid, dysenteric and actinomycotic conditions of the intestine, or tuberculosis of other organs.

(ii.) *Perforation of* or *slow leakage from some part of the alimentary canal,* which had previously become thin by ulceration—simple ulcer of the stomach or duodenum (malignant ulcer rarely perforates because of the infiltration around), typhoid or tuberculous ulcer of the ileum, etc. (see Perforative Peritonitis). Slow leakage from a gastric ulcer may cause a subphrenic abscess or abscess in the lesser sac.

(iii.) *Rupture* of an organ or of an abdominal cyst, such as an ovarian

---

[1] Acute peritonitis, which complicates typhoid fever, is of a latent character, and unaccompanied by pain. This and puerperal peritonitis are the only exceptions.

cyst, or of an abscess of the appendix, of the Fallopian tube, or rupture of the gall-bladder, etc. (§ 243).

(iv.) *Injury or Operation.*—In cases occurring in women without obvious cause, the possibility of criminal procedure for abortion should always be remembered. As regards surgical operations on the abdomen, modern experience has shown that it is not the actual injury but faulty technique, permitting the introduction of septic organisms, which produces peritonitis.

(v.) Various *Blood Infections*—*e.g.*, pneumococcal (usually in females), streptococcal, staphylococcal, and gonococcal. *Idiopathic Peritonitis* was the name formerly employed when no cause could be discovered. Peritonitis may also complicate scarlatina, dysentery, and the other acute specific fevers. *Puerperal Peritonitis* arises when septic organisms enter through the infected uterine surface. *Bacillus coli communis* may produce peritonitis either as part of a general septicæmia, or primarily.

(vi.) Any condition such as *volvulus* or *intussusception*, in which there is injury of the intestinal wall, may be a cause of peritonitis, local or general.

(vii.) Local peritonitis from *Crohn's disease.*

Diagnosis of acute general peritonitis is from four diseases: (1) *Acute intestinal obstruction*, in which the constipation is absolute and no flatus is passed, even after repeated enemata; there is usually no pyrexia, and the constitutional disturbance is usually less. (2) In *colic*, although the pain is also very severe, there is an absence of rigidity, and pressure may give relief. Pyrexia and shock are absent, and the pulse is normal. (3) In *catarrhal enteritis* there is pain, and there may be vomiting and tenderness on pressure, but in this disease there is profuse diarrhœa. (4) In certain cases of *hysteria*, acute peritonitus may be very accurately simulated, though the temperature and pulse are normal, there is very little shock and no leucocytosis, and evidence of a hysterical state is present.

The *Prognosis* of general peritonitis is always very serious. As regards etiology, perforative peritonitis, formerly considered the gravest, is probably now the most hopeful if promptly dealt with. Surgery has done much for the rescue of such cases, and undoubtedly the most favourable of them is that due to appendicitis. Patients with this disease, if diagnosed early and properly managed, should hardly ever be lost. The prognosis in any particular case depends therefore on (i.) the time elapsing before operation, (ii.) the cause and the severity of the shock due to toxæmia, and (iii.) adequate drainage.

Treatment.—The treatment of acute peritonitis depends upon whether it is general or local. If *general*, the only rational treatment is by operation, with drainage, immediately a diagnosis has been made. A fatal issue is almost invariable in cases not operated upon, because the condition is rarely primary, and a definite local lesion is usually present. Antibiotics are of help both therapeutically and for prophylaxis: they should be started before the results of bacteriological tests are known. When there is vomiting or gastric lavage is being used, injections will be essential. Penicillin with streptomycin should be given twice daily in full doses (intramusc.):

alternatively chlortetracycline B.P. (Aureomycin) 0·5 G. by mouth or intravenously (5·0 per cent. in N. saline) should be given 6-hourly, the doses being reduced as recovery occurs. Otherwise tetracycline B.P. may be used. In *local* peritonitis medical treatment is indicated in the early stages, but even then only with the co-operation of a surgical colleague. Medical treatment comprises keeping the patient in bed in the Fowler position and relieving symptoms. The diet should be fluid, consisting of fruit drinks with glucose, soups, jelly, milk, to which stimulants (*e.g.*, brandy) may be added according to the condition of the pulse. Rectal or intravenous feeding with 5 per cent. solution of dextrose may be necessary and antibiotics given (*vide supra*). Severe cases with much vomiting are treated by continuous aspiration through a Ryle's tube in the stomach, or a Miller-Abbott tube in the duodenum, fluids being administered solely per rectum and intravenously. Local applications may give relief, especially heat in the form of fomentations. Once a diagnosis has been arrived at, morphia is a most valuable drug, for it relieves the pain, and reduces the peristalsis of the bowel, and so gives local rest. If there is any doubt as to the advisability of a surgical operation, either at once or later, morphia must be withheld, for by masking the symptoms it may lead to a continuation of medical treatment when operation is called for. It is therefore of use chiefly in local peritonitis, or in general peritonitis where an operation is not permissible. Purgatives may be dangerous, but the lower bowel should be cleared by means of enemata. The hiccough may be relieved by giving ice to suck, by liq. iodi mitis ℳiii in a little water, by injections of morphia.or chlorpromazine, or chloral per rectum (§ 273).

II. *The patient complains of* **sudden abdominal pain** *and vomiting, and shows* **severe shock,** *pallor, restlessness, air-hunger and subnormal temperature, with a rapid running pulse of low volume—the condition is* INTERNAL HÆMORRHAGE.

§ 245. In **Internal Hæmorrhage** *shock* is the striking feature, and the patient may become very anæmic in a few hours. Pain is not marked, and vomiting, although present at the onset, is not diagnostic. Local tenderness may serve as a guide to the cause of the hæmorrhage. The most important causes are: (1) a ruptured ectopic pregnancy. There may be a history of a missed or abnormal last menstrual period, and on examination a boggy mass is felt in the pouch of Douglas (§ 446). (2) Injuries to the abdominal organs, and especially traumatic rupture of the spleen, liver or kidneys: hæmorrhage may follow immediately after the injury, or may be delayed to the 7th–10th day. (3) A leaking abdominal aneurysm is a rare cause.

(4) **Acute Hæmorrhagic Pancreatitis** is a special variety of acute pancreatitis (§§ 246, 357), in which auto-digestion may lead to extensive internal hæmorrhage.

(5) **Acute hæmorrhage into the suprarenal capsules** produces symptoms similar to those of acute hæmorrhage into the pancreas. There is sudden epigastric and lumbar pain, with vomiting, shock, marked dyspnœa and cyanosis. Death may occur in a few days. Or there may be delirium convulsions or coma, or extreme muscular

weakness for some days before death. It is rarely diagnosed during life. When it occurs as part of a meningococcal septicæmia with purpura, it is known as the Waterhouse-Friderichsen Syndrome. In newly-born infants it occurs as part of a hæmorrhagic diathesis.

Treatment.—Blood transfusion is usually a primary consideration. As soon as possible operation must be undertaken in order to stop the hæmorrhage. With suprarenal hæmorrhage, give injections of vitamin K and of cortisone. In any case of internal hæmorrhage it is important to remember that the primary hæmorrhage may cease from clotting or encapsulation, but recur subsequently from disintegration of blood clot from sepsis.

III. *The patient complains of* **acute abdominal pain with shock,** *attended by* URGENT AND COPIOUS VOMITING (*at first food, then bile, and later, material which is alkaline to litmus, and finally fæcal*). *There is* ABDOMINAL DISTENSION *and* INABILITY TO PASS FLATUS *even after repeated enemata—the condition is* ACUTE INTESTINAL OBSTRUCTION.

Acute Intestinal Obstruction—*i.e.*, obstruction coming on suddenly, is always a matter of serious importance, and every practitioner should be thoroughly acquainted with its several causes. The diagnosis and the various causes are fully dealt with under Intestinal Disorders in § 326.

§ 246. *The patient complains of* **acute abdominal pain,** *with more or less* **shock;** *the temperature is probably normal or subnormal, but the symptoms do not quite conform to any of the preceding*—some of the **rarer causes** are probably in operation, such as the following:

IV. **Torsion of an Ovarian Cyst** is known when the signs of such a cyst are associated with the onset of sudden pain and tenderness of the cyst.

V. In **Embolism of the Mesenteric Artery,** a cause of embolism, such as auricular fibrillation or endocarditis, is present. It is rarely diagnosed during life. The absence of symptoms pointing to the other causes, and the presence of melæna, may lead one to suspect embolism. Embolism of the spleen may also cause severe symptoms.

VI. **Acute Hæmorrhagic Pancreatitis** is more common in middle age. It causes sudden severe pain in the epigastrium extending to the back, with vomiting, relatively little rigidity, but circulatory collapse and cyanosis are marked (§ 357).

VII. **Acute Dilatation of the Stomach** sometimes occurs a few days after an abdominal operation. Acute pain, vomiting, and collapse occur; the outline of the distended stomach can be seen in the left hypochondrium. *Treatment* is by continuous gastric suction through a Ryle's tube combined with intravenous feeding (and see § 271).

GROUP B. IX. *The patient, while apparently in good health, complains of* **acute abdominal pain,** *which has come on* **suddenly, without** *definite* **shock;** *the pulse does* NOT EXCEED 100; *there may be* VOMITING *and constipation.* The case is probably one form of COLIC, though APPENDICITIS, ROOT OR REFERRED PAIN, and some OTHER AFFECTIONS may start in this way.

§ 247. Colic is a somewhat vague term applied to spasmodic paroxysmal pain situated in the abdomen. There are **intestinal, biliary, renal** and **appendicular colic.** All have the following features: (1) The pain is extremely severe (in the first three, less so in appendicular colic), and sudden in its onset; (2) the patient is " doubled up " with pain, restless, or rolling about in a " cold sweat "; (3) often there is reflex vomiting from the severity of the pain; (4) the face is pale and " anxious," and in severe cases the pulse is rapid and feeble, though it rarely exceeds 100; (5) *the temperature is neither above nor below normal*; (6) there are no physical signs of disease in the abdomen, and the pain may even be relieved by pressure.

(*a*) **Intestinal Colic** is due to distension and spasm of the bowel. The colic of the small intestine is characteristically twisting, paroxysmal, and is referred to the epigastrium or umbilicus; colic of the colon is referred to the hypogastrium. In intestinal colic a hardening of the bowel may be appreciated by the palpating hand. It is relieved by pressure, which distinguishes it from peritonitis. The abdomen may be distended with flatus. Sometimes it is followed or accompanied by diarrhœa and vomiting, as in gastro-enteritis, or by constipation, as in lead colic. Colic may be the first sign of lead-poisoning, accompanied by a slow, hard pulse, with other signs of plumbism, such as a blue line on the gums; a history of working with lead may be obtainable (§ 568). Colic is a frequent early symptom of *diverticulitis* (§ 328). The *heat cramp* (§ 510) of miners and workers in stokeholds may resemble abdominal colic. Cramp may also be experienced in high or low atmospheric pressures.

(*b*) In **Biliary Colic,** due to the passage of a gall-stone into the cystic or common bile duct, the pain starts in the right hypochondrium: it often radiates round the 9th segment to the angle of either scápula, or reflexly it occurs along the root of the neck or at the tip of the shoulders. A dull pain continues during the intervals between the spasms and may be felt in the right iliac fossa. After a few hours or a day or two jaundice and bile in the urine may follow. A history of previous attacks assists the diagnosis.

(*c*) **Renal Colic** is due to the movement of a calculus, crystals, muco-pus or blood-clot in the pelvis of the kidney or along the ureter. The pain starts in the loin or in the upper lateral abdomen, and radiates *downwards* to the groin and testicle of the same side, which is often retracted. It may last for a day or two. Sometimes pain is referred to the opposite kidney. During the attack there is rigidity in the loin and often some tenderness over the kidney; micturition is frequent; sometimes there is hæmaturia or strangury. For some time after the colic an exaggerated cremasteric reflex persists. There is probably a history of previous attacks, or of gravel, blood or pus in the urine.

(*d*) **Appendicular Colic** is due to an obstruction in the appendix, by a concretion, kink or stenosis from a previous attack; distal to the obstruction acute inflammation may develop. The pain occurs in the right iliac fossa, is never very severe, and is accompanied by some rigidity and localised tenderness over MacBurney's point; in children it may be referred to the epigastric or umbilical regions.

Pyloric Spasm, especially with a duodenal ulcer, can give attacks of

TABLE XIV.—DIAGNOSIS OF COLIC

	Character and Distribution of Pain.	Associated Symptoms.	Age and Sex of Patient.
Intestinal.	Twisting, around umbilicus, paroxysmal; relieved by pressure.	Constipation (or diarrhœa). No jaundice.	Any age or sex. Sometimes evidence of plumbism.
Biliary.	In right hypochondrium, shooting upwards to right or left shoulder, constant, but also in paroxysms.	Jaundice may supervene. Other hepatic symptoms may be present.	Stout married women over forty.
Renal.	In loin shooting down to groin and testicle or labium of same side.	Crystals or other urinary change, pus or hæmaturia. No jaundice. Sometimes frequent micturition or strangury.	Usually male. Children and adults.
Appendicular colic.	In right iliac fossa.	May be vomiting; local tenderness and rigidity.	Any age; both sexes.

acute paroxysmal pain in the upper abdomen, and more rarely **Spasm of the Cystic Duct** can cause acute pain arising from the gall bladder.

The *Diagnosis* of the forms of colic is given above. An X-ray examination should be made when more than one attack occurs.

Prognosis.—The course of an attack of colic is short and severe.

Treatment.—For all forms of colic give local applications of hot fomentations, a kaolin poultice; injections of morphia (gr. ⅙ to ¼), and atropin (gr. $\frac{1}{60}$), of pethidine (50–100 mg.) or of ephedrine (gr. ½–1) may be necessary to alleviate the extreme pain. Large draughts of warm water should be taken. Especially with intestinal colic an enema should be given, followed by suitable purgatives. For lead-poisoning, see § 568. Hepatic colic is dealt with under gall-stone (§ 353) and renal colic in § 413.

X. *The* **Abdominal Pain** *is constant, but liable to exacerbations, especially after exercise; there is* NAUSEA *or* VOMITING, *with some elevation of the temperature; there is* RIGIDITY *and* TENDERNESS *in the right iliac region; the pulse is rapid. The disease is probably* ACUTE APPENDICITIS.

§ **248.** **Acute Appendicitis** may consist simply of (*a*) a catarrhal inflammation of the vermiform appendix, which is relatively benign: or (*b*) a virulent form with ulceration, gangrene and local or diffuse peritonitis.

Symptoms.—In a typical *acute attack of appendicitis* there are six symptoms which, occurring in this sequence, point to appendicitis—pain, vomiting, tenderness, local rigidity, a quickened pulse and leucocytosis. (1) The chief symptom is *pain*, coming on acutely, first referred to the umbilicus or epigastrium, and later becoming localised to the right iliac fossa. (2) *Vomiting* may be urgent at the onset of an attack; when it continues for many days the prognosis is unfavourable. (3) On examination, the most marked features are tenderness, rigidity, and later a local swelling. The *tenderness* may be manifest as cutaneous tenderness on picking up the skin in the right iliac fossa between fingers and thumb. There is also deep tenderness on palpation, particularly well marked at

" MacBurney's point," *i.e.*, at the junction of the outer and middle thirds of a line joining the right anterior superior iliac spine and the umbilicus. A third point of tenderness is often found on rectal examination in the right anterior wall of the rectum, particularly with the pelvic position of the appendix. The *rigidity* causes the abdomen as a whole to show a poor respiratory excursion: on palpation there is guarding of the muscles, particularly of the lower right segment of the rectus abdominis. (4) There may be a local *swelling* or an indefinite tumour with dullness to percussion. These are due to local peritonitis or to abscess formation; they may also be found on rectal examination. (5) The *pulse* is quick and thready and its rate forms the best single indication of the acuteness of an attack. The temperature is rarely above 99°–100°, and this disturbance of the pulse-temperature ratio is an important diagnostic aid (§ 90). The disease is rarely ushered in by a rigor. The fever often falls and the pain goes with the onset of gangrene or with spreading peritonitis, but the pulse, except in rare cases, remains rapid. (6) The tongue is almost always coated. Constipation is usually present, so that the case may be mistaken for intestinal obstruction; but sometimes the attack is ushered in with diarrhœa. The urine is scanty; with pelvic appendicitis the bladder is irritable, and often there is diarrhœa. (7) On listening with a stethoscope no gurgling sounds are heard, owing to spasm of the ileo-cæcal sphincter associated with inflammation around. (8) Leucocytosis of 15,000 to 20,000 per c.mm. occurs. (9) Paralytic ileus is usually a late event.

Types of Acute Appendicitis.—(i.) *Catarrhal* inflammation is mild and localised to the appendix. It may subside completely, but usually some degree of inflammation remains which causes local discomfort and vague dyspeptic symptoms. (ii.) Recurrent attacks of this nature cause fibrous thickening in the wall and retention of secretion forming a *mucocœle* of the appendix. Then (iii.) a subsequent attack of inflammation produces an abscess in the tip of the appendix. (iv.) *Ulceration and gangrene* of the appendix are due to a more virulent infection, arising behind the obstruction of a stercolith, in a mucocœle, or by obstruction of the lumen by external adhesions. Gangrene is usually due to septic thrombosis of the blood supply to the appendix. (v.) An *abscess* which forms in the lumen may perforate. If the reaction of the peritoneum is vigorous and the organisms not too virulent, a local peritonitis results: the abscess can resolve and the inflammation give a mass of local adhesions. (vi.) In other cases the abscess enlarges and may finally rupture into the bowel or bladder, may descend into the pelvis or point externally above Poupart's ligament (when it is often mistaken for a psoas abscess). (vii.) Sometimes the inflammation extends to the cæcum (typhlitis) or to the surrounding tissues (perityphlitis). (viii.) When the organisms are very virulent, a fulminating general peritonitis is likely to arise.

Aberrant types.—With a retrocæcal appendicitis pain may be referred to the loin, or down the right thigh, in each case leading to flexion of the hip from psoas spasm. If the appendix happens to be a long one with the tip lying in the left side of the pelvis, there may be pain, tenderness and rigidity entirely confined to the left iliac fossa.

Course and Prognosis.—With an acute attack there are three possible events—recovery, local abscess formation, or general peritonitis. (1) In a favourable case the temperature falls about the third day, the swelling disappears, pain and other symptoms subside, and the patient may be well in ten days. In other cases slight fever persists for a few weeks, and there is left an indurated swelling due to the omentum. The patient may go about for months or years with chronic appendicitis, and suffer only vague pains, general malaise and dyspeptic symptoms. At any time, however, the acute symptoms may recur. (2) When the general symptoms show no improvement by the second day, and the local swelling progressively increases, it is probable that an abscess is forming. (3) Perforation, with generalised peritonitis, may occur at any time. The general symptoms in such cases are much more severe, vomiting persists, and the abdomen is distended and motionless by the second or third day. There is no disease in which it is more dangerous to hazard a prognosis. An apparently convalescent case may develop general peritonitis and die within 24 hours; on the other hand, a case presenting every sign of a large and extending abscess may clear up entirely and prove free from any subsequent attack. Apart from the great improvement in the prognosis when immediate operation is performed, the only indications of value when forming an opinion are the condition of the patient as regards shock, collapse, and age. The younger the subject, the more grave the prognosis. In pregnancy, appendicitis is serious. *Complications.*—Apart from local and general peritonitis the complications most to be feared are the formation of a subphrenic, perinephric or pelvic abscess: or implication of the liver by spread along the vessels and lymphatics leading to portal pyæmia. Any previous appendicular inflammation which has not been treated surgically may act as a focal point of infection, causing arthritis, iritis, etc.

Etiology.—Two main types of appendicitis are often recognisable. In the first there is obstruction to the lumen of the appendix and the stasis leads to inflammation. In the second there is a blood-stream infection of the appendix, often from a catarrhal condition of the naso-pharynx or tonsils.

Treatment.—Operative measures must be undertaken as a routine and a surgeon should see the patient as soon as possible. The largest proportion of recoveries is recorded in patients operated on within twelve hours of the onset of symptoms which permit a correct diagnosis to be made. In any given case it is often very difficult to tell whether the disease is already subsiding or whether it is advancing; even when gangrene is developing the signs may subside and the pulse rate return to normal. A leucocyte count which rises to 20,000 is always a sign of danger. Especially in children the rapid progress of the disease to a stage at which general peritonitis is present often proves fatal. Sometimes the patient is not seen until an abscess has already developed; even so drainage of the abscess with simultaneous removal of the appendix should be the operation of choice.   In the presence of a severe infection full doses of antibiotics are essential (intramusc. streptomycin 12-hourly and/or intravenous chlortetracycline B.P.—Aureomycin—10 ml. of a 5·0 per cent. solution in N. saline 6-hourly).   If delay in undertaking operation is necessary or if operation is refused, the patient should be put to bed in the Fowler position and nothing but fluids given by mouth: pur̄ gatives are especially dangerous but injections of antibiotics are helpful. Morphine or pethidine should never be given until the diagnosis has been firmly established as analgesics hide the presence of the disease and of its complications; once the diagnosis has been settled a small dose may be employed to relieve pain pending operation being performed.

§ **249.**   Among the **rarer causes of acute abdominal pain** without shock are :

XI. Of various OBSCURE ORGANIC AFFECTIONS of the abdomen, evidenced at first only by pain, two may be mentioned: PANCREATIC CALCULUS and OBTURATOR HERNIA, in both of which the only symptom for some time is pain coming on SUDDENLY without shock.   In the former the pain may be extremely severe, and of a paroxysmal character, situated just below the umbilicus; later on it can be associated with fat in the fæces, emaciation and glycosuria.

Attacks of KETOSIS in children are associated with pyrexia, headache, abdominal pain and vomiting (§ 271). URÆMIA and PYELITIS can give similar symptoms.

DISLOCATED or FLOATING KIDNEY may be attended by a constant (chronic) pain, or give rise to severe attacks (Dietl's crises, § 254), hardly distinguishable from intestinal or renal colic.

DIVERTICULITIS may cause attacks of acute abdominal pain in the left iliac fossa (§ 328).

INTESTINAL WORMS (§ 323) can cause abdominal pain, pyrexia and constitutional symptoms which must not be confused with acute appendicitis, especially in children.

TORSION OF AN UNDESCENDED TESTIS should be suspected when a testicle is found to be absent from the scrotum.

OSTEOMYELITIS OF THE ILIUM or OF THE SACRAL VERTEBRÆ shows persistent pain, pyrexia and leucocytosis.

In SPLENIC EMBOLISM the pain is generally sudden in onset, but is not usually very severe or lasting, and is referred to the splenic region.   Its most common cause is acute or subacute endocarditis, evidences of which are present.

HENOCH'S PURPURA, angio-neurotic œdema and periarteritis nodosa, may have acute recurring attacks of colic simulating intussusception (and see § 595).

ENLARGED GLANDS may cause symptoms resembling appendicitis.   They may be tuberculous, or associated with typhoid or glandular fever, or with streptococcal throats.

In a number of other organic affections the pain comes on gradually, and is of a chronic character.   Acute pain occurring in attacks of varying duration is met with in cases of MUCOUS COLITIS, OVARITIS and PANCREATITIS: also with ANEURYSM OF THE ABDOMINAL AORTA, with a FLOATING RIB and in CROHN'S DISEASE (§ 312c). DIABETIC COMA is sometimes heralded by pain, usually in the epigastrium, which may be very severe (§ 238): exaggerated abdominal breathing is a useful diagnostic aid.

The causes of abdominal pain which originate from organs outside the abdomen are discussed in § 238.

XII. In ROOT PAIN or in REFERRED PAIN abdominal pain may come on suddenly and acutely, and may be for a long time the only symptom.

1. *Nervous dyspepsia* is one of the most typical forms of referred pain. The pain is severe, periodic, but usually relieved rather than aggravated by food or by pressure. The skin may, however, be very sensitive to the flick of a handkerchief.

2. The gastric and vesical crises in association with *tabes dorsalis*.

3. At the onset of *acute poliomyelitis*, pain may be referred to the abdominal wall.

4. *Spasm* or *colic* of any hollow viscus may occur without organic derangement or discoverable nervous cause, especially in nervous subjects. The commonest type is colospasm (§ 313).

5. The neuralgia which accompanies or follows *herpes zoster.*

6. *Coronary thrombosis* causes pain to be referred more to the abdomen than to the chest, but is recognised by the circulatory disturbances (§ 52).

7. *Basal pneumonia, diaphragmatic pleurisy* and *blast injuries to the lung* can cause abdominal pain with rigidity.

8. *Migraine* is certainly met with, alternating with abdominal pain.

9. *Acute glaucoma* is an occasional cause (§ 1110).

§ **250. Chronic Abdominal Pain** comes and goes at first, then BECOMES CONTINUOUS with PERIODIC EXACERBATIONS. Here we do not deal with pain which points definitely to lesions of the stomach, liver, spleen or intestines: these are considered in their respective chapters. Abdominal pain is the leading or only symptom in the following conditions:

I. Chronic appendicitis	§ 250a
II. Chronic intestinal obstruction (malignant stricture, simple stricture, pressure by a tumour)	§ 327
III. Chronic peritonitis	§ 251
IV. Visceroptosis	§ 252
V. Spastic colon, chronic or mucous colitis	§ 313
VI. Diverticula of the Jejunum or Ileum	§ 253
VII. Movable Kidney	§ 254
VIII. Pain following previous abdominal operations	§ 255
IX. Obscure visceral and spinal disease	§ 256
X. Pancreatic disease	§ 357 *et seq.*

The history must be thoroughly investigated, and every organ carefully examined. Three features may afford us important clues:

1. The POSITION, character, degree and constancy of the *pain*, and the presence of *tenderness* must be observed. (i.) If the pain and tenderness be *generalised*, one may suspect Tubercle or Cancer of the Peritoneum. (ii.) If they be situated chiefly in the *lower abdomen*, one may suspect Appendicitis or disease of the Intestine, Bladder, Ovary, Fallopian tubes or Uterus. (iii.) If the pain be chiefly in the *upper abdomen*, Gastric, Duodenal, Liver, Gall-bladder or Pancreatic disease. Thorough and REPEATED EXAMINATIONS of the *abdomen, rectum* and *vagina* are nearly always necessary. The *urine* also should be repeatedly examined for blood, pus and crystals, and the *fæces* (§ 303) for gall-stones. Occult blood (§ 303) and chemical changes of the fæces may be very helpful. If there be general abdominal enlargement, turn to § 257; if a localised tumour, turn to § 262. X-ray or special instrumental examinations (§ 240) may yield important information.

2. The AGE of the patient, and the history and duration of the illness, should be inquired into. In *children* perhaps the commonest of the obscure causes of chronic abdominal pain are constipation, dietetic errors, intestinal worms, tuberculosis of the peritoneum and Meckel's diverticulum; in the *aged* cancer of some organ.

3. The STATE OF THE BOWELS, both previous to and at the time of examination. In I., II., and III. above there is constipation, while in some of the other causes there is diarrhœa or irregularity of the bowels.

I. § 250a. **Chronic Appendicitis** occurs in two typical forms: Chronic, and Recurrent or Subacute Appendicitis. (*a*) In CHRONIC APPENDICITIS (1) the chief symptom is pain starting from the right iliac fossa, or radiating from the umbilicus or epigastrium to this region. It occurs particularly after food, but the typical time-relationship of gastric or duodenal ulcer is absent, and strict dieting affords only partial relief. The pain is characteristically aggravated by over-exertion. (2) Hæmatemesis may occur from an acute gastric or duodenal ulcer, secondary to the appendicular sepsis. (3) Nausea may occur, apart from vomiting, and sometimes there is alternating diarrhœa and constipation, and (4) a history of general malaise. (5) X-ray will reveal tenderness, fixation or deformities and defects of filling, with prolonged retention of barium in the lumen. One form of chronic appendicitis is due to malignant disease, tuberculosis or actinomycosis of the cæcum or appendix. Another is due to stricture of the lumen with formation of mucocœle of the appendix.

(*b*) RECURRENT APPENDICITIS has recurring subacute attacks. Here the course of the disease is essentially chronic, and is often associated with colitis. The patient may have months of apparent health, but in most cases a fresh attack of inflammation occurs sooner or later. It is wise to operate if circumstances permit.

II. *In addition to* **chronic abdominal pain,** *there is a history of* CON-STIPATION, *steadily increasing to* COMPLETE STOPPAGE *of the bowels and* DISTENSION. VOMITING *gradually becomes more severe.* The case is probably one of CHRONIC INTESTINAL OBSTRUCTION *with supervention of acute symptoms.*

In CHRONIC INTESTINAL OBSTRUCTION (§ 327) the abdominal pain is more or less generalised and intermittent. The constipation may at first have alternated with diarrhœa, but after a time it is so complete that not even flatus can be passed. Vomiting, at first of food, and later of alkaline or even fæculent matter, a rapid pulse, and other constitutional symptoms ensue if the condition is not relieved. The commonest causes are Malignant Stricture, Simple Stricture, Peritoneal bands, Diverticulitis, Pressure of a Tumour, Volvulus and Impacted Contents.

III. *The* **abdominal pain** *is* **chronic** *and* GENERALISED; *it is attended by* CONSTITUTIONAL SYMPTOMS, *and some* ABDOMINAL ENLARGEMENT *or other local signs.* The disease is probably CHRONIC PERITONITIS.

§ 251. **Chronic Peritonitis** runs a slow and chronic course, and is usually attended by a certain amount of generalised pain. There is a simple or idiopathic chronic peritonitis, but three more frequent forms are: (*a*) That due to **tuberculosis,** and (*b*) that due to **cancer**—two conditions which, by the way, are most frequently met with at the opposite extremes of life, and present a marked contrast both in their clinical and anatomical features; (*c*) Rupture of a papilliferous ovarian cyst (§§ 243, 261).

CHRONIC TUBERCULOUS PERITONITIS is known by (1) the patient is young; (2) pain and tenderness; (3) localised hard masses or a general doughy feeling; (4) often fluid, and (5) always emaciation and fever. Hence the disease is discussed under the heading of emaciation (§ 573). CHRONIC CANCEROUS PERITONITIS (Malignant Peritonitis) is always attended by much pain, constant and also in paroxysms. There is a great tendency to the rapid formation in the abdominal cavity of fluid which is nearly always tinged with blood. It arises especially in late middle or advanced life. In typical cases its recognition is easy on account of the age, acute pain, and ascites (under which heading it is described, § 260). SARCOMA of the peritoneum is rare.

CHRONIC PERITONITIS of the simple or idiopathic type is very difficult to diagnose in the majority of cases, because of the extreme variability and vagueness of the symptoms. (1) Pain and tenderness, sometimes localised, are present, worse at times and with exertion; (2) dyspepsia, often constipation, sometimes vomiting; (3) malaise with pyrexia from time to time; (4) ascites is sometimes present; in others it is absent, and the abdomen is quite flat; (5) palpation may detect localised thickenings and areas of resistance which convey a doughy sensation on palpation. Perihepatitis (sugar-loaf liver) may be present (§ 335).

Etiology.—(1) After an attack of acute peritonitis; (2) inflammation of any organ may cause localised peritonitis; (3) after paracentesis without strict asepsis; (4) post-operative cases may be due to talc from the surgeon's gloves or to a foreign-body left behind at operation; (5) idiopathic, due to unknown causes. It may occur with chronic nephritis, with cirrhosis of the liver, and with other general conditions, in which two or more of the serous membranes (pleura, pericardium) become simultaneously affected (polyserositis).

The *Diagnosis* has often to be made by a process of exclusion, especially when there is no history of acute peritonitis or of inflammation of any organ. Sometimes it is indistinguishable from tuberculous and cancerous peritonitis. Abdominal pain simulating colic may be due to peritoneal adhesions. When ascites reappears after repeated tappings peritonitis is usually present.

The *Prognosis* as to life is good in mild cases, though chronic invalidism is apt to ensue. Subacute attacks are liable to occur, and there may be great exhaustion and emaciation from involvement of some part of the alimentary canal, or from the formation of local abscess. Adhesions may lead to intestinal obstruction. When associated with advanced hepatic or renal disease, the prognosis is grave.

Treatment.—Rest and supporting belts may give relief. When ascites is present prescribe a low salt diet and give diuretics. Paracentesis and surgical treatment may be required (§ 260).

IV. § 252. Visceroptosis (Synonyms: Glénard's disease, enteroptosis)

is a condition with ptosis or downward displacement of one or all of the abdominal organs. It may be compatible with perfect health and yet its presence may be shown by X-ray examination. In other cases, especially in thin nervous women, it is accompanied by poor muscle tone of the anterior abdominal wall with a bulging of the lower abdomen on standing. It is considerably aggravated by loss of the intra-abdominal supporting fatty tissue and by any further loss of weight. The *symptoms* which are usually present on rising from the lying position, or after standing for some time, comprise: (1) pain, a dragging sensation or "sinking feelings" in the abdomen; (2) lumbar backache; (3) vaso-motor disturbances with palpitation and dizziness; (4) dyspepsia, sometimes nausea and vomiting with delayed gastric emptying, simulating a gastric ulcer; (5) constipation which may alternate with diarrhœa; (6) headache, fatigue and general lethargy; (7) nervousness and insomnia; (8) anæmia is common; (9) sometimes Dietl's crises are present (§ 421), and in other cases there is duodenal ileus of the superior mesenteric type (§ 271). Palpation of the abdomen reveals a gurgling cæcum lying low in the right iliac fossa and a tender mobile right kidney.

The *Diagnosis* may be from a gastric ulcer or anorexia nervosa in a young woman, or from malignant disease in older persons. The dumping syndrome following a partial gastrectomy gives similar symptoms (§ 289). The diagnosis should not be made unless X-ray examination has failed to reveal any other cause for the symptoms, but has shown the greater curvature of the stomach to lie low in the pelvis, a mobile and elongated duodenum, a dilated and prolapsed cæcum, the transverse colon low in pelvis, and an elongated pelvic colon. When X-ray examination is not available, the condition is usually detected by percussion and palpation of the abdomen, and inspection in the upright position.

Treatment.—In severe cases an initial period of a few days' rest in bed in the supine position relieves the symptoms; in any case the patient should be instructed to get a long night's rest in bed, aided when necessary by a simple hypnotic, as well as to rest on a couch each afternoon. The diet should be of a high calorific value with extra vitamins, and often dry meals with fluids taken between meals aid. The correction of anæmia by iron preparations and the injection of a few weekly doses of cyanocobalamin B.P. materially lessen the symptoms. Constipation should be relieved by an emulsion containing liquid paraffin or paraffin-agar. Abdominal exercises performed regularly each day, if necessary under the guidance of a trained physiotherapist, will serve to correct the poor condition of the abdominal muscles. A well-fitting and correctly applied support, such as an elastic corset or a Curtis spring belt, aids mechanically by holding in better position the dropped viscera, and relieves the pain and dragging sensations. The symptoms usually disappear when a satisfactory gain in weight and correction of the anæmia have been achieved. Operations to fix the viscera in position are rarely successful and should be avoided.

V. Spastic Colon (Syn. Chronic or Mucous Colitis) is a condition seen much more commonly in women, with recurrent or chronic abdominal pain and irregularity of the bowels. There is a persistent state of anxiety which may lead to chronic invalidism (see § 313).

VI. § 253. **Diverticula of the Jejunum or Ileum** are common as single or multiple lesions in late middle life. *Symptoms* are often absent. Those which occur are recurrent attacks of abdominal pain, a feeling of distension, and sometimes steatorrhœa or a megaloblastic anæmia. *Diagnosis* is by X-ray examination of the small intestine. *Treatment* is by repeated intermittent doses of a tetracycline to control infection in the bowel; operative removal is rarely necessary.

VII. § 254. **Movable Kidney** (Dropped or Floating Kidney, according to the degree of mobility).—This condition is by no means uncommon in women and does not usually give rise to symptoms unless the degree of mobility is considerable. It is often accompanied by visceroptosis (§ 252).

The *Physical Signs* are usually discovered by palpation of the abdomen, with the patient lying down. The method of palpating the kidneys is given in § 394. The kidney comes down more during inspiration with the patient in the erect or sitting posture than when lying down. After a little practice the patient will be able to lean forward and relax the muscles, which is an important aid to the observer. The left kidney rarely falls below the umbilicus, but the right one may be displaced into the iliac fossa, and even into the pelvis.

Symptoms.—In a few cases two kinds of pain may be experienced: (a) A constant dull, dragging pain in the back, or perhaps only an uneasiness in the loin, radiating down to the groin and inner side of the thigh, relieved by rest; (b) Attacks like renal colic may be followed by the passage of urine in large quantities, occasionally with albumin and blood, due to vascular engorgement of the kidney—" Dietl's crises " (§ 421). Sometimes hydronephrosis results. Neurasthenia, with mental depression, often accompanies this condition.

Etiology.—A much larger percentage of women than of men have a movable kidney: it often follows pregnancy. A fall or strain will also displace the organ. It occurs more often in tall, narrow-chested than in short people. Rapid loss of fat, or lowering of the intra-abdominal pressure, such as occurs after delivery, are frequent causes.

Treatment.—Patients should not be told of this condition unless symptoms arise. The main methods of treatment are those used in visceroptosis (§ 252); especially important are reassurance, fattening the patient, abdominal exercises and sleeping in a horizontal position. An abdominal belt with a specially fitted renal pad is advocated by some. When neurasthenic symptoms are present valerian and pheno-barbitone may help.

VIII. § 255. **Pain Following Previous Abdominal Operations.**—After previous operations intra-abdominal adhesions may form or nerves supplying the abdominal wall itself may be involved in the scar tissue and give rise to persistent pain. The latter variety may be differentiated by using a local anæsthetic to block the intercostal nerves before they reach the abdominal wall. If this relieves the pain, a more permanent effect may be obtained by the subsequent blocking of nerve impulses with 2–3 ml. of 90 per cent. alcohol: local radium to the scar tissue gives relief.

IX. § 256. **Obscure Visceral or Spinal Disease.**—(a) In cases of chronic pain, GENERALISED OVER THE ABDOMEN, and in the absence of constipation, diarrhœa or any of the causes mentioned under § 249 onwards, one might suspect cancer of the intestines, of the pancreas or of the kidney, or malignant peritonitis, Addison's disease of the suprarenals, in which epigastric pain is a constant symptom, " rheumatism " of the abdominal muscles, visceroptosis or movable kidney. In many cases the pain is an expression of a psychoneurotic anxiety state. Children may suffer from recurrent attacks of abdominal pain due to worms: but often no cause can be found. Such cases should be treated by avoiding purgatives and giving digestible foods and enemata.

(b) In diseases of the spine the pain is frequently referred to the FRONT OF THE ABDOMEN, and among the more obscure causes may be mentioned abdominal aneurysm pressing on the spine, and cancer myelomatosis or caries of the vertebræ. The first of these occurs mostly in male adults, and caries occurs in children. In the latter the child frequently refers to the pain as " stomach-ache," worse after sneezing or running about. The girdle pain due to a spinal cord tumour, chronic and acute myelitis, acute poliomyelitis and the prodromal stages of the exanthemata should also be borne in mind.

(c) If the patient complains of PAIN SITUATED CHIEFLY IN THE LOWER ABDOMEN, one may suspect diseases of the intestine or rectum, appendicitis (§§ 248, 250a), cancer or other diseases of the bladder or uterus, psoas abscess, lymphatic gland enlargement, and pelvic peritonitis (in which the pain shoots down the legs), extra-uterine pregnancy, pyosalpinx, dysmenorrhœa and all its causes, pelvic displacements, cancer or tubercle of the prostate or testes, sacro-iliac arthritis and obturator hernia. The fatigue pains of debilitated women may be referred to one or other iliac region.

(*d*) PAIN SITUATED CHIEFLY IN THE UPPER ABDOMEN may be due to various diseases of the stomach, duodenum, liver or gall-bladder, and spleen. In lesions of organs in this region pain is often referred to the scapula or to the root of the neck. Among the painful affections of the *stomach* may be mentioned gastric (or duodenal) ulcer, gastritis (acute or chronic), cancer of the stomach, which in its most usual form, scirrhous of the pylorus, is commonly difficult to diagnose in its early stages. Among the painful diseases of the *liver and gall-bladder*, perhaps passive congestion, cancer, gall-stones, chronic cholecystitis and perihepatitis are the commonest; hydatid is difficult to diagnose though it is rarely painful. Abscess of the liver should be suspected in those who have resided in tropical countries. Painful diseases of the *spleen* are not common, the chief being infarction, but the capsule is sometimes the seat of perisplenitis: enlargement of the organ aids diagnosis (§ 362).

GENERALISED ABDOMINAL ENLARGEMENT

Difficulty in the diagnosis of the cause of abdominal enlargement can often arise in cases of obesity, constipation, pregnancy, venous congestion, atony or ptosis of the abdominal organs. And see Fallacies, § 240, for the less common sources of error.

§ 257. Classification.—Generalised abdominal enlargement occurs under five conditions:

I. Gaseous distension of the stomach and intestine; occasionally
    gas in the peritoneum .. .. § 258
II. Fluid free in the peritoneum (ascites) .. .. § 260
III. A cystic collection of fluid in the abdomen .. .. .. § 261
IV. Solid abdominal tumours .. .. §§ 262, 263
V. The later stages of pregnancy .. .. § 451

The **Routine Procedure,** as previously described (§ 240), should be by Inspection, Palpation, Percussion, Measurement and Auscultation.

If a **hard tumour** can be felt in any part, turn first to § 262.

If the abdomen is quite **soft to palpation** and **resonant** all over, turn first to § 258.

If the abdomen is **dull to percussion** in the flanks and presents a fluid thrill, turn first to § 260.

If the abdomen is **resonant in the flanks** and **dull in front,** turn first to § 261.

I. *The abdomen is* **uniformly enlarged;** *it is* SOFT *and yielding to palpation; percussion, systematically conducted over the whole area, gives a* RESONANT *note.* The swelling is probably due to GASEOUS DISTENSION.

§ 258. Gaseous (Flatulent) Distension (Syn. Tympanites) occurs when the stomach and/or intestines are over-filled with gas. It should be remembered that flatulent distension may accompany and render obscure a *small quantity of fluid in the peritoneum.*

The *Causes* of gaseous enlargement are:

(i.) Atonic and other forms of DYSPEPSIA and AEROPHAGY (air swallowing) are the most frequent causes of flatulent distension. It is usually intermittent, and generally greatest after meals (§ 281).

(ii.) In ATONY OF THE COLON the bowels are constipated, and the patient is liable to "colicky" pains; constitutional symptoms are usually few (§ 324).

(iii.) In INTESTINAL OBSTRUCTION there is considerable abdominal distension, accompanied by pain, vomiting and other general constitutional disturbance (§§ 326 and 327).

(iv.) PARALYTIC ILEUS causes general distension of the abdomen (§ 326).

(v.) ACUTE DILATATION and ACUTE VOLVULUS OF THE STOMACH causes distension in the left hypochondrium and persistent copious vomiting (§§ 246, 271).

(vi.) In TUBERCULOUS PERITONITIS there is a tendency to the formation of intestinal adhesions and *flatulent distension.* Moreover, the distended abdomen has a doughy feel and here and there a patch of dullness on percussion, which is quite characteristic (§ 573).

(vii.) "PHANTOM TUMOUR" may assume the shape of a generalised more or less resonant enlargement, but it more often resembles a localised tumour (§ 262). It disappears during anæsthesia.

Gas in the Peritoneal Cavity gives much the same signs as tympanites, but there is extreme distension, and hyper-resonance all over to such a degree that the normal dullness of the liver and spleen is obscured. It is met after perforation or rupture of some part of the alimentary canal. The patient is shocked, and presents all the symptoms associated with perforation (§ 243). A few hours after the occurrence of the perforation a delusive lull occurs in the shock and other symptoms, only to be succeeded by a fatal exacerbation. Perforation of a peptic ulcer is the commonest cause. An early diagnosis can be made by finding gas under the diaphragm on an X-ray film.

II. *There is* **uniform abdominal enlargement,** *which is soft and yielding to palpation and* DULL TO PERCUSSION *in parts; a* FLUID THRILL *is present.* There is FLUID WITHIN THE ABDOMEN.

§ 259. When there is **Fluid in the Peritoneal Cavity,** either free or encysted, the abdomen is soft to palpation, dull to percussion in parts (either in the flanks or in front), and measurements show it to be enlarged.

When the fluid is in any quantity, two special signs can be elicited. (1) *Fluid thrill.*—A thrill can be transmitted from one hand to the other, through the surface of the fluid. Place the left hand over one side of the dull portion, and tap sharply with the fingers of the right hand over the opposite side; an impulse or thrill will be felt by the left hand when fluid is present. To prevent the wave or impulse from travelling across the abdominal wall, instead of through the fluid, an assistant should place the edge of his hand vertically on the umbilicus. (2) In some cases of free fluid in the peritoneum, on suddenly dipping the fingers over a solid organ (*e.g.,* the liver), a characteristic sensation, due to displacement of fluid, can be felt. Neither of these signs can be elicited with a gaseous enlargement or a solid tumour. In *obese persons* considerable difficulty arises in the detection of fluid.

The fluid may be either (a) FREE in the peritoneal cavity, when it is termed ascites; or (b) enclosed in a CYST, such as an ovarian cyst.

(a) If FREE in the peritoneal cavity, it will obey the law of all fluids, and *shift with the position of the patient.* Thus in ascites (§ 260) when the patient lies on his back both flanks are dull to percussion, and the epigastric region is resonant; then, if the patient turns on one side the uppermost flank which before was dull is now resonant, while the epigastric region, if there is much fluid, is dull (shifting dullness). Much may be learned from the character of the fluid withdrawn by a cannula. Ascitic fluid is usually straw-coloured, with much albumen. Hæmorrhagic fluid usually means cancer (§ 1203).

(b) If the fluid is ENCYSTED—*e.g.*, ovarian cyst, we can still elicit the fluctuation and the percussion tests just referred to, but the level of the dullness will not alter with the position of the patient (§ 261). In many cases fluctuation can be felt on bimanual examination. In every case a catheter should be passed to avoid mistaking a distended bladder.

There is a **generalised uniform enlargement** *of the abdomen, which gives all the* SIGNS OF FLUID, *and the fluid* ALTERS ITS LEVEL *with the position of the patient.* The condition is ASCITES.

§ 260. Ascites is a term applied to an effusion of fluid within the peritoneum. The physical signs of fluid have been described above. It is very difficult to detect a small quantity of fluid in the peritoneum (less than 1½–2 litres), but its existence is rendered probable (i.) by the dullness on percussion of the umbilical region with the patient on his hands and knees; (ii.) by finding that when the patient turns from one side to the other, the flank which was dull is now resonant. On rectal examination fluid may be detected at an early stage when it has gravitated to the pelvis, and it may be detected here when it is insufficient to give other signs.

Ascites may have to be *Diagnosed* from any of the cystic conditions mentioned below (§ 261), but certainly the most frequent and important source of difficulty is *ovarian cyst* (Table XV, p. 366). Occasionally peritoneal adhesions may confine the fluid to one part of the abdomen, and then the fluid does not shift with the position of the patient. A greatly distended urinary bladder may simulate ascites, but the passage of a catheter readily excludes this fallacy.

The other *Symptoms* which accompany ascites belong to two categories: (1) Those due to pressure within the abdomen—*e.g.*, œdema of the feet and legs, from pressure on the inferior vena cava and its branches; later on dilatation of the surface veins of the anterior abdominal wall may occur from the same cause; albuminuria from pressure on the renal veins, and dyspnœa from undue elevation of the diaphragm (and often an accompanying pleural effusion). (2) There are evidences of the condition which has caused the ascites. The temperature is generally normal, except in chronic peritonitis.

The *Causes of Ascites* are six in number. In reference to the diagnosis of these causes, if there be any œdema of the ankles, it is important to ascertain whether this œdema or the ascites came first. For instance, when PORTAL OBSTRUCTION is in operation, the œdema of the feet will have started subsequent to the ascites; in HEART or LUNG disease it will have preceded the ascites; whereas in RENAL DISEASE they will have started about the same time. ASCITES with well-marked JAUNDICE in an old person is extremely likely to mean CANCER OF THE LIVER or peritoneum. ASCITES with a SALLOW skin in a MIDDLE-AGED person is most probably due to ALCOHOLIC CIRRHOSIS of the liver. For Ascites due to TUBERCULOUS PERITONITIS see § 573.

I. **Portal Obstruction** (with concurrent Portal Hypertension) is recognised in two ways: (*a*) By a history or presence of the *symptoms* of portal obstruction (of which ascites is only one); and (*b*) the presence or a history of one of the *causes* of portal obstruction.

(*a*) The SYMPTOMS of portal obstruction, in the order in which they usually appear, are as follows: (1) A liability to attacks of flatulence and of gastric and intestinal catarrh, as evidenced by abdominal pain, flatulent dyspepsia, alternating diarrhœa and constipation. (2) Vomiting of mucus streaked with blood, especially before breakfast. (3) Hæmorrhage, sometimes in very large quantity, from enlarged anastomatic veins in the lower end of the œsophagus or in the fundus of the stomach (œsophageal varices). (4) Bleeding from hæmorrhoids is also common. (5) Congestion, and therefore enlargement of the spleen follows. (6) ASCITES is one of the later results. (7) Œdema of the legs also appears subsequent to the ascites, largely due to pressure on the large veins in the abdominal cavity by the ascitic fluid. (8) Albumen in the urine may arise in the same way, or from concurrent disease of the kidney; in the former case the albuminuria may disappear after paracentesis. (9) Enlargement of the veins of the abdominal wall from the establishment of a collateral circulation may occur.

(*b*) The CAUSES of portal obstruction may be grouped into (α) diseases within the liver, or (β) diseases outside it.

(α) *Diseases within the Liver.*—Cancer is the chief cause; it produces portal obstruction usually by the pressure of the enlarged glands in the fissure, or by masses protruding from the liver. *Chronic Interstitial Hepatitis (Atrophic cirrhosis)* is usually due to previous infective hepatitis or to alcoholism, there being a history of the cause. Simple ascites without marked jaundice or other obvious symptoms is suggestive of cirrhosis. A large *gumma* at the portal fissure may obstruct the portal vein. *Perihepatitis* sometimes produces ascites by thickening of the capsule (sugar-loaf liver). Ascites only very rarely accompanies *hepatic congestion*, and never fatty liver, hydatid or abscess.

(β) The causes of portal obstruction *outside the liver* are: (1) *Cancer* of the stomach or pancreas, and various other tumours pressing on the vein. (2) Enlargement of the *glands* in the fissure of the liver (cancer, tubercle, syphilis or lymphadenoma). (3) *Thrombosis* of the portal vein is rare: when it occurs the signs of portal obstruction develop rapidly. *Etiology.*—Ascites due to portal obstruction is due to (i.) the portal hypertension; (ii.) the lowered plasma albumen content resulting from liver disease; (iii.) in cirrhosis the excessive level of aldosterone in the blood causes sodium retention.

II. In **Heart Disease,** either primary (*e.g.*, mitral disease and cardiac dilatation) or secondary to lung disease, the ascites is generally part of the œdema affecting the cellular tissues and other serous cavities of the body. Here œdema of the feet *will have preceded the ascites*, the heart will be considerably enlarged and there will be a history of shortness of breath and perhaps cough. Examination of the heart will reveal the nature of the disease.

III. In **Kidney Disease** ascites may be part of a General Œdema affecting the face, limbs, peritoneum, pleuræ and pericardium. The fact that the dropsy started in all of these situations about the same time suggests this cause. Albuminuria is frequently enough a consequence of the pressure of the ascitic fluid, but the presence of epithelial casts almost certainly indicates that the renal disease was primary. It usually takes the form of acute or subacute parenchymatous nephritis, rarely amyloid or granular kidney.

IV. **Chronic Peritonitis** is another cause of fluid in the peritoneum. An idiopathic form of chronic peritonitis is sometimes described, but it is practically never met with apart from a deposit of tubercle (in the YOUNG), § 573, or of cancer (in the AGED), § 251.

V. **Chylous Ascites,** with fat globules suspended in the fluid, is rare: it occurs when the thoracic duct is obstructed by malignant disease or after trauma. In tropical countries it is more often due to *Filaria bancrofti*. PSEUDO-CHYLOUS ASCITES is more common: the fluid is milky, due to a lipoid-globulin complex. It is seen in malignant, tuberculous and nephrotic cases and in hepatic cirrhosis.

The *Prognosis and Treatment of Ascites* are very largely those of the causal condition. The *Prognosis of Ascites due to portal obstruction* depends very much on the nature of the intra- or extra-hepatic lesion which has produced it, as given above and in Chapter XII The degree of the obstruction is measured by the amount of ascites and other symptoms present, and by the amount and frequency of the hæmorrhage that has taken place from the gastro-intestinal tract. Life may be prolonged for many years even when a considerable amount of ascites has accrued, provided it has come on slowly, and time has thus been afforded for the gradual establishment of a collateral circulation through the surface veins of the abdomen and other collateral channels. It is in this sense that repeated tappings are good, for in this way time is gained for the establishment of collateral circulation. In cases of alcoholic cirrhosis the patient must become a strict teetotaller, otherwise he cannot live longer than six to twelve months, for ascites indicates an advanced condition of cirrhosis; cases treated early may recover.

The *Treatment of Ascites*, like its prognosis, must depend upon its cause (*q.v.*). The treatment of *ascites due to portal obstruction*, and to some extent that of other forms, is as follows: (1) Diuretics may be successful in causing fluid absorption and excretion. Chlorothiazide (Saluric), hydrochlorothiazide (Hydrosaluric) and chlorthalidone (Hygroton) are often effective. (2) When the plasma albumen is low a high protein diet is essential; a salt-free diet helps to prevent re-accumulation of fluid. (3) Paracentesis is generally necessary sooner or later. Some physicians say it should be put off until it is called for by the urgency of dyspnœa. In cancer this is certainly a good rule, but in cirrhosis of the liver it is best to perform paracentesis at once in all cases where there is much fluid, unrelieved by medicinal measures. Often diuretics which were useless before, are efficacious after drainage, because the renal blood flow is greatly improved. Sometimes recovery takes place after repeated paracentesis, because time is thus afforded for the establishment of the collateral circulation. It is best to use a *small* trocar with the tube conducted to a pail, so that the peritoneum may gradually empty itself. To relieve portal hypertension, porto-caval anastomosis is less commonly performed nowadays; in the Talma-Morison operation the omentum is transplanted between the layers of the abdominal wall to facilitate anastomosis between the vessels of the portal and the systemic circulations.

III. *There is a* **generalised abdominal enlargement** *which gives all the* SIGNS OF FLUID (§ 259); *but the fluid does* NOT ALTER ITS LEVEL *with the position of the patient.* There is ENCYSTED FLUID IN THE ABDOMEN.

By far the commonest of such cystic tumours is an OVARIAN CYST. Other and less common cystic abdominal tumours are PREGNANCY WITH HYDRAMNIOS, CYSTIC FIBROMA of the uterus, HYDRO- and PYO-NEPHROSIS, PANCREATIC or MESENTERIC CYST, a large HYDATID, a MUCOCŒLE of the GALL-BLADDER and an ENCYSTED ASCITES.

§ 261. I. **An Ovarian Cyst** is centrally situated, and grows from below upwards. It is attached to the pelvic organs, it can be moved laterally but not upwards. The enlargement is fairly uniform, and gives all the signs of fluid (§ 259). But the level does not alter with the position of the patient; and whereas the umbilical region is dull on percussion (" horse-shoe shaped dullness "), the flanks are resonant. On palpation it is tense and elastic, and in malignant ovarian cysts nodules can be felt in the walls. Ballottement between the two hands on combined abdominal and pelvic examination is often a most useful sign.

The features associated with a cyst are (1) a history of it having grown upwards from the pelvis, and (2) these tumours (unlike encysted ascites) may be of very rapid growth, and reach quite a large size in three or four months. (3) There have usually been menstrual irregularities, though by no means always. (4) The cyst may be clearly felt by bimanual examination of the pelvis. There may have been no general symptoms of any

TABLE XV

DIFFERENTIAL DIAGNOSIS OF ASCITES AND AN OVARIAN CYST

	Ascites.	*Ovarian Cyst.*
Inspection.	Flanks bulge, front flat.[1]	Flanks flat, front bulges.
Percussion.	Flanks dull, front resonant. On turning, upper flank becomes resonant.	Flanks resonant, front dull. No alteration of dullness on turning.
Measurement.	Umbilicus to xiphoid greater than umbilicus to pubes. Circumference at umbilicus greater than slightly below. Navel to iliac spine same both sides.	Umbilicus to xiphoid less than umbilicus to pubes. Circumference at umbilicus less than slightly below. Navel to iliac spine greater one side than the other.

kind, but generally some pain and local discomfort have been complained of. Often when the cyst contains pus there is little or no fever. When there is a history of attacks of pain, it generally indicates adhesions, an

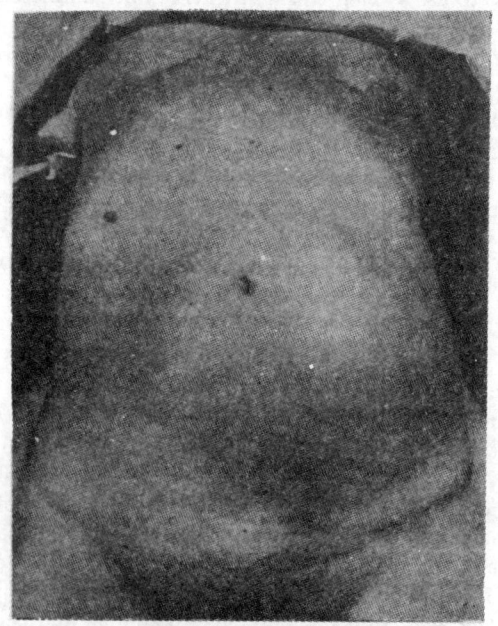

FIG. 92.—OVARIAN CYST.

important matter to the operator. An examination of the uterus usually reveals nothing. A malignant papilliferous cyst is indicated by (1) the presence of nodules in the walls; (2) the age of the patient, a history of emaciation, and severe pain; (3) later ascites and œdema of the legs.

[1] Bulging in front may occur in cases with a large and acute effusion.

Diagnosis.—In the *earlier stages* the diagnosis of an ovarian tumour is sometimes difficult. It is an elastic, movable and globular swelling; the uterus is not enlarged and can be defined as quite separate from the tumour. In this stage it may have to be diagnosed from *hydro-* or *pyosalpinx*. Pelvic *peritonitis* and *cellulitis* and *pelvic hæmatocele* form a swelling which is very firmly fixed in the pelvic cavity and accompanied by constitutional symptoms. In *extra-uterine fœtation* there will be morning sickness, a patulous os uteri, and other symptoms of pregnancy, with an empty uterus, and a positive Zondek-Aschheim Test.

In the *later stages* ovarian cysts have to be diagnosed from all the conditions mentioned below.

II. PREGNANCY WITH HYDRAMNIOS and a thin uterine wall is sometimes very difficult to diagnose from an ovarian cyst, for both develop very rapidly. Experienced clinicians have been known to fail in the differentiation. The symptoms of pregnancy (see § 451), the exactly central position of the tumour, and the softened cervix, may aid. The test for pregnancy and, later, an X-ray examination, settle the diagnosis. *Hydatid mole* presents similar difficulties, but it is fortunately rare.

III. A LARGE CYSTIC FIBROID of the uterus, especially of the subperitoneal (pedunculated) variety, may produce the signs of a fluid tumour. It is recognised by (1) its connection with the uterus, which is enlarged; (2) its slow growth, which may extend over many years; and (3) menorrhagia in some cases.

IV. A HYDRO- or PYO-NEPHROSIS, a dilated GALL-BLADDER, a large PANCREATIC, OMENTAL or MESENTERIC CYST, a large PERITYPHLITIC ABSCESS or a LARGE HYDATID CYST of the spleen or liver, may on rare occasions produce the appearance of a general fluid enlargement of the abdomen, and may require to be diagnosed from ovarian cyst; but they are nearly always *asymmetrical*. They grow from, and their percussion dullness is continuous with, the organs whence they rise; they are referred to among Abdominal Tumours (§ 263).

V. ENCYSTED ASCITES is not common. It may result from previous peritonitis, of which there will probably be a history. More frequently, perhaps, it results from tuberculosis or cancer of the peritoneum (§ 251). In all of these there is a want of symmetry in the enlargement and in the fluid, an absence of the associated symptoms of ovarian tumour, and a history or other evidences of the cause in operation.

VI. PNEUMOCOCCAL PERITONITIS in children may form an encysted swelling, but this is accompanied by a swinging temperature.

The *Prognosis* of ovarian tumour is always serious, though in the non-malignant form it may be quiescent for some years. If not treated, a cyst may (1) rupture and produce peritonitis; (2) it may become infected; (3) the pedicle may become twisted; (4) hæmorrhage may take place into its cavity; (5) occasionally it bursts into the bowel with sinus formation.

The *Treatment* is entirely surgical. The earlier the cyst is removed the better. It is well to do this before the occurrence of attacks of pain indicate inflammatory adhesions.

ABDOMINAL TUMOURS

§ **262. Method of Procedure.**—We now turn to the second group of abdominal enlargements—namely, those in which the enlargement has originated in, or is localised to, one part—*i.e.*, Abdominal Tumours. It is only by repeated and careful examination that mistakes can be avoided in the diagnosis of abdominal tumours. The same methods are adopted here as in general enlargement (§§ 242, 257). (1) *Inspection* in the recumbent, and sometimes in the erect, posture *should never be omitted*; (2) *Palpation* to determine its size, position, borders, mobility and texture. This requires a flat hand previously warmed and with the patient's abdominal muscles thoroughly relaxed by a suitable posture; (3) *Percussion,* to define the resonance or dullness of the tumour; (4) Careful *Measurement* made and recorded, both for the comparison of one part with another, and to note the progress made by the growth; (5) *Auscultation,* which is especially useful in the diagnosis of late pregnancy; and (6) *Examination under an anæsthetic* is sometimes required.

 Fallacies of Abdominal Tumours.—(1) *Obesity* may offer a serious obstacle to the examination of abdominal enlargements or tumours. In these cases the umbilicus is usually depressed. The only way to arrive at a correct decision is to place the hand flat upon the abdomen and then dip the fingers suddenly and forcibly inwards.

 (2) The presence of *fluid* within the abdomen, together with a solid tumour, may prevent our discovering or examining the latter thoroughly. It is best to re-examine after paracentesis has been performed.

 (3) *Pregnancy* and a *distended bladder* are frequent sources of error.

 (4) *Gas in the intestine* causes enlargement in the lower abdomen, with marked resonance to percussion.

 (5) *Fæcal accumulations* may simulate malignant and other tumours, though they can generally be indented by the fingers. They are always situated in some part of the large bowel. Give a course of purgatives and/or repeated enemas.

 (6) A "*phantom tumour*" is a swelling (usually tympanitic, sometimes dull), produced by irregular muscular contraction of one or both recti muscles, and it is remarkable how precisely it may simulate a solid tumour. It is apt to appear and disappear suddenly, hence the name. The condition is met for the most part in young hysterical women, and is usually beyond the control of the patient. It is a frequent cause of error in diagnosis. The patient should be placed in a position of perfect ease for the relaxation of all the muscles of the body, with the knees drawn up and the neck slightly bent. Sometimes an anæsthetic is required in order to establish the diagnosis.

 (7) The *liver* occasionally presents an extra lobe (§ 263. I.). Displaced or movable organs may be mistaken for tumours.

 Having excluded these fallacies, and being satisfied as to the existence of an abdominal tumour, there are five points to which our attention should be directed:

 1. The first and most important question is the *locality of the tumour,* in which region is it situated, or where did it start ?

 2. To ascertain with *which organ it is connected,* consider what organs are located in the region occupied by the tumour, and then see if it

be structurally continuous by palpation and percussion with one of these.

3. If it *moves with the breathing* of the patient we know that it must be connected with the diaphragm, or some organ depressed by it during respiration, such as the spleen, liver, gall-bladder, stomach, intestines, kidney or omentum. If fixed, it is a tumour of the pancreas, aorta, lymphatic glands, or some other organ unaffected by respiration, or bound down by adhesions.

4. Inquire for a *history of any disease* or functional disturbance of the abdominal organs—*e.g.*, in the case of the kidney, whether the urine contains, or has contained, blood or pus; or perhaps there has been jaundice, pointing to hepatic disease. Inquire also whether the tumour is constantly present or appears intermittently.

5. The diagnosis of the *nature of the tumour* depends very largely upon its history and the age and sex of the patient. Tense cystic tumours are extremely difficult to differentiate from solid growths, but we can try to obtain the percussion and fluctuation tests (§ 259). There is also another question which very frequently presents itself for consideration—viz., is the tumour benign or malignant ? The general symptoms of malignant disease (cancer) are discussed in § 571; but the age of the patient, and the rapid course and lethal tendencies of the disease, are the chief means of differentiating it.

IV. § 263. *If there is a visible or palpable* tumour *in the abdomen, ascertain which* REGION *the tumour chiefly* OCCUPIES *or* ORIGINATED *in, and refer to that region in the following summary. Having identified* ITS ORIGIN *in this way, reference must be made to the diseases of the organ affected to ascertain the* NATURE *of the tumour.*

I. RIGHT HYPOCHONDRIUM.—The commonest tumours in this position are those of the *liver*, especially cancer and enlargement of the organ. The features which HEPATIC TUMOURS present in common, in addition to their position, are: (1) They are not covered in front by resonant bowel, and their dullness is continuous with that of the liver; (2) they move with respiration; and (3) there are ascites, jaundice or other evidences of liver derangement. It must not be forgotten that hepatic tumours may be simulated when there is perihepatitis (§ 335) (and see Diagnosis of Hepatic Enlargements, p 493 *et seq.*); Riedel's lobe (see below) is another fallacy. A distended GALL-BLADDER (*e.g.*, by cholecystitis) is recognisable as a tense pear-shaped swelling below the ninth costal cartilage. There is only occasionally a history of biliary colic but often a history of " chills " (biliary fever, § 354). It is distinguished from the kidney by the fact that the colon passes over the kidney. Tumours in this region may also be connected with the *duodenum* or *right kidney* (see II. and IV.).

Riedel's Lobe of the Liver.—In certain cases, sometimes associated with gall-stones retained within the gall-bladder, a tongue-shaped process projects downwards from the right lobe of the liver. It may reach as far as the iliac crest, or even to the iliac fossa. Frequently the condition has been incorrectly diagnosed before operation. It has most often been mistaken for a floating kidney, and has also been taken for distended gall-bladder, hydatid cyst, renal or omental tumour. It is sometimes tender, its shape more or less that of a pear. Under anæsthesia its connection with the liver may possibly be made out. By X-ray its shadow may obscure the pyelogram of a normal right renal pelvis, leading to the mistaken diagnosis of renal tumour.

Suprarenal Tumours become manifest in the right or left hypochondrium, and are difficult to distinguish from tumours of the liver, gall-bladder, kidney and spleen. THE LOCAL SYMPTOMS consist of: (i.) Pain radiating across the abdomen and to the back; (ii.) pain referred to the shoulder tip; (iii.) emaciation, with nervous depression, and digestive disturbance; (iv.) a tumour felt beneath the costal margin, at first movable with respiration, but soon becoming fixed; it can be felt posteriorly in the costo-vertebral angle; (v.) absence of urinary and gall-bladder symptoms. Early diagnosis is aided by excretion urography, the tumour depressing the corresponding kidney and giving filling defects in the renal pelvis. The injection of air into the loin, followed by a skiagram, has also revealed tumours of the adrenal—a procedure to be undertaken only by experts. GENERAL SYMPTOMS depend on the type of tumour and whether it arises in the medulla or in the cortex.

(A) The important **Medullary Tumours** are (a) the pheochromocytoma which is associated with hypertensive properties (§ 97), and (b) the neuroblastomata. The latter arises chiefly in children; a striking feature is their extensive metastases. In the *Hutchinson syndrome* they arise in the left adrenal and form metastases in bones, especially the ribs, skull, lungs and liver; exophthalmos and ecchymosis of the left eye may be the first sign. In the *Pepper syndrome* the tumour arises in the right adrenal, usually in the first year of life; metastases occur mainly in the liver and become enormous.

(B) **Cortical Tumours** may be due to adrenal hyperplasia, an adenoma and sometimes a carcinoma. The clinical effects depend on (i.) the degree of hyperplasia or malignancy and (ii.) whether the tumour secretes an excess of the androgenic hormone to produce virilism, of the glucocorticoid (17-hydroxycorticosteroid) hormones (especially hydrocortisone) to give rise to Cushing's syndrome or of aldosterone (Conn's syndrome). Mixed cases occur.

Virilism (the adreno-genital syndrome) occurs in the female. The *Symptoms* are more marked when they arise before puberty. There is a general mascularisation with (i.) hirsuties—an excessive growth of hair on the chin, the upper lip, the sides of the face as well as the forearms, thighs, legs and trunk; (ii.) the muscular development is that of the male, with broad shoulders and narrow hips; (iii.) masculine voice changes are present; (iv.) there are decreased female sex characters, e.g., amenorrhœa, either primary or secondary, deficient mammary glands and sometimes an enlarged clitoris. In many of these cases adiposity also occurs. The urine contains excessive quantities of 17-ketosteroids, and the adrenal tumour is characterised by a positive Ponceau-Fuchsin staining reaction (Vines). A malignant tumour in the male is rare but may produce feminisation.

Cushing's Syndrome is also more common in the female and can occur at any age —usually between 15–45. The *Symptoms* are: (i.) adiposity of the trunk, sparing the limbs; (ii.) a plethoric complexion; (iii.) kyphosis and rounded shoulders; (iv.) osteoporosis especially of the spine, with backache; (v.) general weakness, depression and sometimes a frank psychosis; (vi.) hypertension; (vii.) a reduced sugar tolerance and even diabetes mellitus. Increased amounts of hydrocortisone (above 18 µg. per 100 ml.) can be demonstrated in the blood, and in the urine of these patients. Some also show androgenic effects with hirsuties, etc. The cause is usually hypertrophy of the adrenal cortex, sometimes an adrenal adenoma, occasionally a carcinoma; rarely a chromophobe adenoma of the pituitary is causal.

Conn's Syndrome mainly occurs in adults, due to one or more small tumours; these cause excessive loss of potassium via the kidneys. Recurrent attacks of muscular weakness or paralysis are associated with other symptoms and signs of hypo-kalæmia (p. 813), tetany, moderate or severe hypertension, excessive thirst and headache. The urine contains large amounts of aldosterone; pyelonephritis is a frequent complication.

Treatment of tumours of the cortex is by removing one or part of both suprarenals. In florid cases total adrenalectomy is sometimes performed, followed by replacement therapy with a gluco-corticoid such as cortisone.

II. In the EPIGASTRIC REGION tumours may be connected with the liver (*vide supra*); but the first tumour which would occur to one's mind would be CANCER OF THE STOMACH—*i.e.*, a hard, irregular swelling attended by vomiting, "coffee-ground" in character. The commonest form of malignant disease of the stomach, however, is scirrhous of the pylorus, in which visible peristalsis, copious vomiting at long intervals, and other gastric symptoms appear before any swelling can be detected (§ 293).

Pancreatic cysts may cause a fluctuating swelling in the epigastrium, but their detection is extremely difficult. There may be a history of pain, and symptoms of pancreatic disease (see § 360). Cysts of the *small omental sac* present a similar swelling. *Pulsation in the epigastrium* may be due to hypertrophied right ventricle but is usually normal; rarely it is caused by abdominal aneurysm.

III. In the LEFT HYPOCHONDRIUM tumours of the SPLEEN originate and sometimes attain an enormous size (§ 362). They move with respiration, and they make their way forward in *front* of the colon towards the umbilicus. A splenic tumour can generally be moved forwards by getting the hand behind it, a fact which distinguishes it from tumour of the left kidney, and it presents the characteristic splenic notch. It resembles tumour of the left lobe of the liver, but the latter cannot be displaced downwards by the hand. Other tumours in this position may be connected with the *stomach, pancreas, liver, kidney* and *sigmoid flexure*.

IV. The LUMBAR REGION may be the starting place for RENAL TUMOURS, which are characterised by four features: (i.) Their comparative fixity during respiration. (ii.) Dullness in one flank, and, unless both kidneys are involved, resonance in the other. (iii.) They are *always resonant in front*, because as they make their way forwards and downwards they push the colon in front of them; and (iv.) there is no resonant part between the dullness of a renal tumour and the spine, as there would be in the case of a splenic tumour. In many the rounded and reniform shape of the kidney is retained. They are distinguished from hepatic tumours by the dullness in the flank not being continuous with that of the liver, and by the presence or history of blood, pus or other urinary changes. The commoner forms of renal tumours are hydro- and pyo-nephrosis, congenital cystic kidney, renal sarcoma (commonest tumour in children), and peri-nephric abscess. A perinephric abscess tends to point backwards. *Pyo-* or *Hydro-nephrosis* are cystic tumours, containing urine *with* or *without* pus respectively (§ 432). Hydro-nephrosis may be almost painless, not tender, and unattended by subjective or constitutional symptoms; pyo-nephrosis is always tender, and attended by hectic fever (unless the abscess is chronic). Hydatid of the kidney may only be evidenced by swelling; sometimes it gives a thrill on percussion. Other tumours in the lumbar regions may be connected with the *ascending* and *descending colon*.

Movable or *Floating Kidney* is one of the most frequent of abdominal tumours, especially on the right side. It descends with inspiration, slips back into position during expiration, and may be found as low as the iliac fossa. Its mobility and rounded or reniform shape are characteristic, but not always easily detected. There is a characteristic pain of a dull aching, or dragging character in the back, increased by exertion.

V. The LEFT ILIAC REGION may be the seat of a tumour caused by CANCER of the SIGMOID FLEXURE, and this is the most frequent position in the bowel for cancerous growth. Cancer and other *tumours of the large intestines* are distinguished generally by their free mobility (unless fixed by adhesions). They are, when cancerous (far the commonest neoplasm of the intestines), attended by irregularity of the bowels, generally alternating constipation and diarrhœa. The commonest starting-point for primary cancer of the bowel is the sigmoid flexure; but before a cancerous swelling can be detected in the left iliac region the patient will have been troubled with recurrent diarrhœa and pain, sometimes bleeding. The local symptoms are followed in course of time by œdema of the leg or sciatica. A primary growth in the lower sigmoid colon is often difficult to palpate in the abdomen or per rectum. In *cancer* of the peritoneum the intestines may become matted together, and although fluctuation may be detected, there may be little fluid in the peritoneal cavity. Sarcoma and carcinoid (argentaffin) tumours (§ 328) of the *small intestines* are rare and usually only diagnosed by laparotomy. The prognosis of cancer is given in Chapter XVI. While diverticulosis may occur in any part of the alimentary canal, *diverticulitis* may show a swelling due to adhesive peri-diverticulitis or abscess formation which is difficult to distinguish from cancer. (See § 328.)

VI. The RIGHT ILIAC REGION is the position in which APPENDICITIS is usually manifested; it is fully described under "Abdominal Pain" (§ 248). *Intussusception* of the bowel, which occurs mostly in childhood, generally arises in this region, but the tumour is most commonly felt under the liver (§§ 326, 328). *Pelvic peritonitis* may form a firm swelling in either iliac region. Its other features are (i.) vaginal examination reveals a tender swelling in the corresponding fornix, pushing the uterus to the opposite side; (ii.) there is a history of acute pain and fever at the onset, frequently following childbirth or abortion (§§ 453, 454). *Cancer, tuberculosis* and *gumma of the cœcum*, contrary to what we might expect, often constitute a *movable* tumour in the iliac region, and are apt to be mistaken for a mass of fæces. Cancer or *actinomycosis* of the cæcum may be attended by suppuration, so giving rise to abscess with pyrexia. The history of such cases may run a long course, and resemble appendicitis. Enlarged *glands* and *Crohn's disease* may be mistaken for appendicitis. Iliac *abscess* in Pott's disease may point in this region. A movable right kidney may simulate a tumour.

VII. The UMBILICAL REGION is the starting place of tumours connected with the pancreas, duodenum, mesenteric glands and aorta, all of which are *immobile during respiration*; though a tumour in this position is far more often connected with the stomach, liver, or transverse colon, which *move with respiration.* Enlargement of the *mesenteric glands* may be sometimes detected in spare subjects by grasping the two sides of the abdomen either between the two hands or the finger and thumb of one hand. When large enough to form a tumour, they are fixed and matted together.

Aneurysm of the Abdominal Aorta is a pulsatile and expansile swelling, immobile during respiration. In thin subjects a thrill may be felt, and a murmur heard. In auscultating the abdominal aorta we must be careful not to produce a murmur by pressure of the stethoscope. It is attended always by a severe fixed neuralgic pain in the spine. It is important to differentiate an aneurysm from a swelling in front of the vessel to which the pulsation has been communicated. An endeavour should be made to grasp the swelling on each side, so as to confirm the expansile nature of the tumour.

Pulsating Abdominal Aorta (throbbing in the abdomen).—Dyspeptic subjects and thin nervous females are often troubled with marked pulsation of the abdominal aorta, which is sometimes obvious both to the patient and the doctor. There is in this affection great local discomfort, and even pain, with marked pulsation, obvious to both inspection and palpation. The diagnosis from aneurysm rests partly on the fact that the pulsation is not limited to any part of the aorta, and partly that such rapid and violent action of the heart is not common in aneurysm.

VIII. The HYPOGASTRIC REGION is the situation whence BLADDER, UTERINE, OVARIAN and TUBAL TUMOURS grow. *Ovarian tumours* (which are nearly always cystic) are usually characterised in the *early stages* by their free mobility, unless they are malignant, and their rapid growth (§ 261). *Tumours of the bladder* are usually rendered sufficiently obvious by changes in the urine and by passing a catheter. *Tumours of the uterus* are similarly revealed by uterine symptoms, excepting perhaps some subperitoneal fibroids. These may reach a large size without any symptoms at all; their origin and relations are detected by bimanual examination. *Pregnancy* causes a symmetrical enlargement starting from the hypogastric region about the third month of gestation. Among the rarer tumours are pelvic hydatid and pelvic hæmatocele.

The NATURE, PROGNOSIS and TREATMENT of these various abdominal tumours are discussed under the organs with which they are connected.

§ 264. **Flattening or Recession of the Abdomen** is not a sign of any great importance. " Ventre plat, enfant il y a " is a French expression signifying that the abdominal wall slightly recedes during the first two or three months of pregnancy. It is met with in abstinence from food, and in wasting disorders, such as with dehydration, cancer and tuberculosis. It may be present also in intestinal, hepatic and renal colic, and as a consequence of excessive purging or vomiting. A hollow or " boat-shaped " abdomen is often characteristic of meningitis in infants. It may also occur when acute general peritonitis is present, especially in children.

CHAPTER X

THE STOMACH AND DUODENUM

Surface Anatomy of the Stomach. (Fig. 91 and § 240.) The cardiac orifice lies behind the seventh left costal cartilage 2¼ inches from the mid-line. The fundus occupies the left dome of the diaphragm and lies behind the apex of the heart. As this part of the stomach always contains gas, it is resonant (Traube's space). The body of the stomach is more or less vertical, and turns sharply into the pyloric antrum. The pylorus lies opposite the first lumbar vertebra in the transpyloric plane just to the right of the mid-line. The greater curvature is extremely variable and depends on the state of filling; it may reach below the umbilicus in normal conditions.

It is to be noted that the alimentary tract, apart from the mouth, pharynx and rectum, is not subject to direct examination by ordinary methods. Much progress has followed the use of test meals (§ 277) and examination by X-ray; and in expert hands the œsophagus and stomach, and the sigmoid may be brought into direct vision by œsophagoscopy, gastroscopy and sigmoidoscopy. In ordinary practice we are largely dependent upon subjective symptoms in the investigation of disorders of the stomach. However, the patient's sensations before and after meals are not necessarily related to his stomach, for gastric symptoms are frequently not of gastric origin, but associated with disease of the heart, kidney, lungs, gall-bladder, duodenum, appendix or glands of internal secretion. On the other hand, diseases of the stomach produce widespread effects in the general economy. The nutrition, of course, fails; but, apart from this, those suffering from gastric disorders often complain of lack of energy and depression. In chronic disorders of the stomach the functions of the nervous system may be so profoundly disturbed by neurasthenic and other symptoms that the physician may overlook the primary cause of the mischief—namely, malassimilation of food. The stomach and digestion are influenced by two sets of nerves—the sympathetic and vagus; their relationship and equilibrium may be disturbed by (1) reflex conditions, (2) asthenia of the nervous system, (3) endocrine secretions and (4) emotions.

PART A. SYMPTOMATOLOGY

The symptoms which reveal disorders of the stomach may be **local** (viz., epigastric pain or discomfort, nausea or vomiting, hæmatemesis, dryness or bad taste in the mouth, thirst, flatulence, hiccough, altered appetite, heartburn, water-brash); or **general** and **remote** (viz., cardiac symptoms, various nervous derangements, skin symptoms and emaciation).

Among the **Local Symptoms** of gastric disorder, PAIN OR DISCOMFORT AFTER FOOD, and NAUSEA OR VOMITING, are the most constant and important—*i.e.*, the cardinal symptoms. HÆMATEMESIS is less frequent, but more serious. Other local symptoms are also of value in diagnosis.

§ 270. **Gastric Pain,** or discomfort, in diseases of the stomach, is a most important *local* feature. Although it is not in every case sufficiently constant in its characters to enable us to establish the diagnosis, nevertheless it merits close study. In some cases it is altogether absent (even when simple ulcer or malignant disease exists), but when present, the features which should be noted are its *position*, its *character*, its *degree*, its *constancy*, and above all, its *relation to the taking of food.*

Its *Position* is usually over the epigastrium, but pain is very frequently complained of between the shoulders, and severe pain in the back may also occur. A localised pain with tenderness occurs with ulcer. In *character* it varies considerably. Sometimes it is like a dull weight or a feeling of distension, such as occurs in nervous dyspepsia and chronic gastritis; or it may be of a burning character, as in hyperchlorhydria; or it may resemble abdominal cramp, as in spasm of the pylorus (§ 247), or in some cases of nervous dyspepsia. Sharp or lancinating pain which persists usually attends ulcer or cancer of the stomach.

Its *Relation to Food* is by far the most important feature of the pain in gastric diseases: (*a*) *It comes on at once* and lasts a variable time in nervous (atonic) dyspepsia, in acute and chronic gastritis and in malignant disease. With a simple ulcer pain may come on soon or as long as two hours after the meal, varying with the site of the ulcer; the pain is at once relieved by vomiting—a characteristic feature; and solids usually give more pain than liquids. In gastric ulcer the sequence generally is food, ease, pain, ease till food is taken again. (*b*) When pain *comes on an hour or more after food*, it is due to excessive acidity, either from hypersecretion or fermentation (organic acids). In hypersecretion, pain is relieved by taking food and alkalies. Pain coming on late after food is common in duodenal ulcer (hunger pain), and the sequence tends to be food, ease, pain lasting until the next meal. A similar pain may be caused by a diseased appendix or gall-stones. (*c*) Pain *coming on without time relation to food* is characteristic of nervous dyspepsia, and is met with in carcinoma of the stomach. If deep pressure *over the seat of pain* relieves it, the condition is probably functional, not organic.

Fallacies.—Pain of the acute type may be mistaken for *biliary colic*, but in that condition the pain is greater on the right side, and is sometimes followed by jaundice. In *hepatic* disorders, pain is more often limited to the right hypochondrium. The spine should always be examined for *caries*, especially when stomach pain is complained of by children. The pain in such cases is referred to the terminations of the intercostal nerves; this also occurs in *herpes zoster*. The gastric crises of *tabes dorsalis* may be mistaken for simple gastritis. Pain in the *chest* (§ 33) must not be mistaken for abdominal pain. *Hiatus hernia* (§ 234) and other causes of *dysphagia* must be thought of. *True angina pectoris* and *coronary thrombosis* can be mistaken for that type of dyspepsia in which the stomach is distended with gas and hampers the heart's action. In acute *pancreatitis* there is extreme pain of sudden onset in the epigastrium with severe shock, and the case may terminate fatally in a few days (§§ 246, 357). Other pancreatic diseases are also attended by pain in the situation of the stomach.

§ 271. Nausea or Vomiting is, after pain, the most frequent and most definite symptom of stomach disorders. Its causes may be grouped under four headings: (*a*) Local, (*b*) Cerebral, (*c*) Reflex and (*d*) Toxic. Water-brash (§ 218) is sometimes spoken of by the laity as " vomiting," but is not true vomiting. Regurgitation from a dilated œsophagus (§ 218) or œsophageal pouch is another fallacy; the food returns easily and is not acid in reaction. Prolonged coughing may induce vomiting; patients may complain of vomiting, and the physician may be led in consequence to treat the stomach instead of the lungs.

(*a*) LOCAL CAUSES of vomiting include: (1) *Errors of diet*, such as shell-fish, infected food, excess of alcoholic, fatty and other irritating foods; the vomiting of the peccant material occurs soon after ingestion. (2) *Irritant and corrosive poisons* and *emetics* also speedily give rise to vomiting. The diagnosis of this cause is aided by (i.) an examination of the vomit, which should *always be preserved*; it may smell of phosphorus (which is luminous in the dark), or of carbolic, or other acids. (ii.) An examination of the mouth for any corrosive action. (iii.) The occurrence later of the toxic effects peculiar to the several poisons; and (iv.) a history of poisoning obtained from the patient or his friends. (3) Overdoses of some drugs, such as digitalis, are often overlooked. (4) *Fermentation* of the contents of the stomach, such as that met with in dilatation due to pyloric obstruction, when the vomiting may occur only once each day or so—often in the late evening or middle of the night; the vomited matter is copious, frothy, and contains sarcinæ and yeasts. (5) *Diseases* such as acute gastritis, carcinoma and simple ulcer, especially when they cause obstruction, are usually accompanied by vomiting. In chronic gastritis of alcoholic origin mucus from the œsophagus and stomach (§ 282) is vomited chiefly in the early morning.

(6) **Acute Dilatation of the Stomach** comes on more or less suddenly in children or in adults who are ill and toxæmic, especially after acute abdominal operations or with pneumonia.

Symptoms.—(i.) Vomiting is frequent but only partially empties the stomach. (ii.) There is progressive distension of the upper abdomen and particularly of the stomach which becomes more and more atonic. (iii.) Air-swallowing often adds considerably to the distension, and if this is sufficiently severe, a mechanical condition of acute duodenal ileus (see below) is an added complication. (iv.) Shock and collapse supervene.

Diagnosis.—X-ray examination helps by showing a stomach excessively filled with gas displacing the left dome of the diaphragm upwards.

Treatment is by repeated aspiration of the stomach (*e.g.*, each half-hour) through a Ryle's tube: nothing must be given by mouth, intravenous feeding with dextrose-saline being used instead. In a few days the stomach usually recovers its tone and fluids can be given by mouth, aspiration being used before the next feed to determine how much is still being retained in the stomach.

(7) **Acute Volvulus of the Stomach** occurs when the stomach rotates around its longitudinal (cardio-pyloric) or its transverse axis—in this latter case the pyloric end of the stomach usually comes to lie in front of the lower end of the œsophagus. *Kinking* of the stomach produces similar symptoms when the fundus is overfilled with gas and falls backwards. There may be a history of previous minor attacks.

Symptoms.—(i.) Pain in the epigastrium of increasing severity is the first symptom. The pain may radiate to the left lower chest. (ii.) There is a severe full feeling with much retching, vomiting and tympanites. (iii.) The left upper abdomen becomes progressively ballooned. (iv.) Collapse and shock ensue.

Diagnosis.—A plain X-ray examination shows a very distended stomach filled with gas and liquid displacing the left diaphragm upwards. Confirmation is obtained by the great difficulty in passing a stomach tube.

Etiology.—Excessive air-swallowing and sometimes the too liberal use of sodium bicarbonate are the main precipitating factors, and patients with minor attacks must guard against these.

Treatment.—It may be impossible to pass a Ryle's tube and adopt treatment as for acute dilatation of the stomach: in this case and if the symptoms are severe, an emergency laparotomy must be performed and the stomach punctured to empty it.

(8) **Acute duodenal ileus,** an obstructive condition of the third part of the duodenum due to compression by the superior mesenteric vessels, occurs with dilatation of the stomach, profuse vomiting, epigastric distension and later severe prostration. It must be treated on the same lines as acute dilatation of the stomach, with continuous gastric suction by a tube left in the stomach, and with the foot of the bed raised. (See also §§ 294, 326.)

(9) **Congenital Hypertrophic Stenosis of the Pylorus** causes persistent vomiting and marasmus in young infants, more commonly in boys than girls. *Symptoms* commonly begin about the end of the second week of life—(i.) projectile vomiting, which cannot be stopped; (ii.) progressive loss of weight; (iii.) constipation; and later (iv.) visible peristalsis of the stomach is seen just after a feed. (v.) A small hard nodule (the hypertrophied pylorus) may be palpated under the upper part of the right rectus. Careful feeding, gastric lavage, and atropine methonitrate (Eumydrin), beginning with 0·5 ml. and increasing by 0·5 ml. to 2·5–3·0 ml. of 1/10,000 solution half an hour before meals q.i.d., often effect a cure. Toxic symptoms, such as abdominal distension, bouts of fever, dilatation of the pupils, indicate a reduced dose. Rammstedt's operation of dividing longitudinally the hypertrophied muscle of the sphincter gives good results, but it must not be left as a last resource.

(b) VOMITING DUE TO A CEREBRAL CONDITION. 1. In *Migraine* (*Bilious Headache*) the patient often awakens with a headache, and vomits only mucus and bile (merely an indication that the vomiting is urgent, or that the stomach is empty). A history of previous attacks is usual (and see § 812).

2. *Organic Cerebral Disease* is another important cause of vomiting —e.g., tumour, early meningitis, abscess. This is recognised by: (i.) The vomiting occurs without relation to food; (ii.) it is urgent and projectile; (iii.) there may not be nausea; (iv.) the vomiting may be excited by simple change of posture; (v.) the presence of other cerebral symptoms, such as vertigo and perhaps papillœdema (§ 1127). Vomiting may also attend the gastric " crises " of *tabes dorsalis*; it occurs at intervals, and is usually severe. It is recognised by the absence of the ankle and

knee jerks and the presence of other symptoms of the disease (§ 1022). Vomiting associated with *glaucoma* (§ 1110) is easily overlooked.

3. *Mountain sickness* is due to anoxia. This used to contribute to *aviator's sickness*, but the modern developments of air-pressurised travel have shown that in the latter other factors are more important. Acceleration both vertically and laterally affects the semicircular canals; swaying and visual stimuli from rapidly passing objects may contribute as in *train, sea and car sickness*. These latter may affect young children and in car sickness the closed atmosphere, car smell as well as psychological factors from apprehension, boredom and the drumming of engines all play a part. Even so, famous admirals are known who have never been free from sea-sickness.

4. *Ménière's syndrome* also causes vomiting due to a labyrinthine disturbance (§ 831).

5. *Hysterical Vomiting* occurs when the patient (usually a woman) faces an insoluble mental problem or has had a frightening mental upset. Vomiting usually occurs directly after a meal, or even at the sight of food, no matter what its quantity or quality may be; or perhaps digestible articles like milk will cause vomiting, while indigestible foods like pickles may be retained. Pain is usually absent. Anorexia nervosa (§ 569) is a severe variety of this.

(c) REFLEX VOMITING from *visceral irritation* may be met in a great many abdominal disorders, such as peritonitis, pancreatitis, intestinal, biliary or renal colic; in all stages of intestinal obstruction, in strangulated hernia, and with intestinal new growths. In the last named the attention of the physician is often drawn from the true source of trouble. It occurs also with pregnancy, uterine and ovarian disorders. Pharyngeal irritation, especially in alcoholics and smokers, leads to prolonged hawking often followed by vomiting.

(d) TOXIC CAUSES are uræmia and jaundice and the onset of some of the acute specific fevers. The vomiting of Addison's disease, hyperthyroidism and pernicious anæmia comes under this heading. Certain cases of vomiting in pregnancy are due to toxæmia. After anæsthetics vomiting may be urgent; sometimes this is due to blood in the stomach, and will cease when it is expelled or washed out.

Diagnosis.—A careful history of the factors which induce vomiting and a complete physical examination are essential. Early morning vomiting of small amounts occurs especially in the early months of pregnancy, with a raised intracranial pressure, with uræmia and with alcoholic gastritis. When the vomiting is more copious and occurs late in the day, or during the early hours of the night and follows epigastric pain, there is probably a gastric or duodenal ulcer or pyloric obstruction. Fæcal vomiting indicates intestinal obstruction.

The *Treatment* of vomiting must be directed to its cause, but there are certain measures which can be applied to relieve the symptom. The patient should be kept at rest in the horizontal position, and without

food, or only given milk in small quantities at a time, and iced water.
Milk diluted with barley-water, whey, or citrated milk are given where
ordinary milk is not retained. Washing out the stomach with normal
saline may give relief. Among the remedies which may be used are
kaolin, bismuth carbonate, hydrocyanic acid or liq. iodi mitis (in a teaspoonful of water). In more severe cases chlorpromazine B.P. (Largactil)
50 mg. or antihistamine drugs such as promethazine hydrochlor. (Phenergan) 25–50 mg. or chlorpheniramine (Piriton) 10 mg. by mouth or
intramuscular injection are very effective. With *travel sickness*, in the
course of time sufferers usually become less troubled. Passengers are
helped by lying supine in a quiet place with the eyes open; a barbiturate
such as quinalbaritone B.P. (Seconal), an antihistamine such as tab.
meclozine (Ancolan) 25–50 mg. or tab. cyclizine (Marzine) 25–50 mg.
once to three times daily, or a tablet or injection of the drugs just mentioned, or hyoscine hydrobromide gr. $\frac{1}{100}$ are all most helpful. Bromides
and valerian aid nervous vomiting.

Cyclical or Recurrent Vomiting, " acidosis," is a common condition
in children. The attacks may occur at regular intervals of a few weeks.
Predisposing causes: (i.) there is often a family history of the same condition or of allergy or migraine; (ii.) thin, highly-strung, lordotic children
are much more susceptible. Precipitating causes: (i.) constipation, over-
eating of fatty foods, eggs, chocolates; (ii.) over-fatigue, excitement, overstrain at school, riding in cars and trains; (iii.) the onset of any infection,
commonly in the throat or at the onset of one of the specific fevers; when
arising in the appendix the differential diagnosis may be difficult and a
surgeon should be consulted. The condition is associated with defective
function of the liver. An attack comes on suddenly, with headache,
pallor, repeated vomiting and retching, followed by abdominal pain, some
pyrexia, drowsiness, and if the vomiting persists, dehydration and a rapid
thready pulse; the breath smells sweet from the presence of acetone, and
acetone and diacetic acid are found in the urine (Ketosis, § 384). Cases
have been mistaken for meningitis and for acute abdominal conditions.

Treatment.—The child should be kept at rest in a darkened room, and
the bowels freed with magnesia or an enema. Frequent small sips of
glucose in water or in a fruit drink (1–2 oz. to 1 pint) must be given by
mouth, with small doses of alkaline carbonates and citrates. In severe
cases rectal or intravenous glucose may have to be used. Any associated
infection must be treated. To prevent attacks, the above-mentioned
predisposing conditions must be dealt with.

§ 272. **Hæmatemesis** (Vomiting of Blood).—Bleeding from the stomach,
unless in slight quantity, is usually accompanied by nausea and vomiting.
In the first place, it is important to decide whether the blood really comes
from the stomach and œsophagus.

Sources of Fallacy.—(1) Blood from the *lungs* may be mistaken for
blood from the stomach (see Hæmoptysis, § 104). (2) *Epistaxis*, the blood

running down the gullet and being vomited, is a common fallacy in
children, in whom the blood is apt to be swallowed. This may follow
operations on the tonsils or teeth. Epistaxis is recognised by making the
patient blow his nose: there are no abdominal symptoms. (3) Blood
from the *fauces* or *gums*, especially when the gums are spongy, or when
pyorrhœa alveolaris exists, may give rise to a sanguineous vomiting or
expectoration, the cause of which is very apt to be overlooked even by
competent observers; but the blood is mixed with saliva, and is rarely
large in amount. (4) Blood from a fracture of the base of the skull and
from œsophageal disease may also be swallowed and vomited. On the
other hand, *hæmorrhage from the stomach* is (i.) preceded by a feeling
of faintness and nausea, and (ii.) followed by melæna (tarry stools).
(iii.) Blood from the stomach is mixed with food; when the quantity is
large (*e.g.*, in ulcer) it is usually red and may be clotted: when in small
amounts it is partially digested beforehand and mostly brown (" coffee-
grounds "). (iv.) There is no history or local sign of pulmonary disease,
and there may be a previous history of disease of the stomach, duodenum
or liver.

The *Causes of Hæmatemesis* may be roughly divided into (*a*) those
which produce a slight or protracted hæmorrhage, and (*b*) those which
give rise to a large quantity at one time.

(*a*) **Slight or Protracted Hæmorrhage** occurs chiefly in Chronic Gastritis
and Cancer. A temporary irritation or congestion of the stomach produced
by irritating articles in the food or by urgent vomiting (*e.g.*, with migraine),
may be attended by *streaks* of blood in the vomit. A smaller hæmorrhage
may occur in cases described in group (*b*) below.

I. Chronic Gastritis is known by (i.) vomiting in the morning—
often viscid mucus streaked with blood—or at other times. (ii.) It
may be accompanied by, and due to, disease of the liver (cirrhosis), or
advanced cardiac disease, and is found especially in alcoholic subjects
(see § 282).

II. Cancer of the Stomach or Œsophagus is recognised by: (i.) The
patient is usually beyond middle age; (ii.) pain is complained of—severe,
constant, and generally worse after food; (iii.) the blood vomited is *rarely
copious*, but typically " *coffee-ground* " in character, and may recur for
weeks; (iv.) the hæmatemesis is followed by melæna unless the blood is
scanty, and occult blood is usually present in the fæces; (v.) there is
progressive cachexia; (vi.) an abdominal tumour or evidence of cancer
elsewhere *may* be found (see also § 293).

(*b*) A **Large Hæmorrhage** at one time may occur in Ulcer of the
Stomach or Duodenum, Hiatus Hernia of the Stomach, after taking certain
Drugs and Chemical Irritants, Portal Cirrhosis of the Liver, Splenic Anæmia,
Gastrostaxis, Purpura or Chronic Nephritis.

III. Peptic Ulcer, of the Stomach or Duodenum, or of the
Jejunum after Gastro-enterostomy.—(i.) The bleeding is copious, the
vomit is often bright red, after being brown at first, and melæna follows;

(ii.) there is usually a history of indigestion, sometimes of operation; but hæmatemesis may occur in the previously healthy.

IV. A HIATUS HERNIA OF THE STOMACH, A PEPTIC ULCER IN THE LOWER ŒSOPHAGUS and CHRONIC ŒSOPHAGITIS (§ 233) are all causes of small or large hæmatemesis.

V. DRUGS AND CHEMICAL IRRITANTS. The commonest is acetylsalicylic acid (aspirin); when swallowed in lumps or tablets which lodge between folds of mucous membrane an acute erosion occurs: calcium aspirin does not do this. Some individuals are especially susceptible to aspirin, perhaps because it prolongs the bleeding time. Phenylbutazone B.P. (Butazolidin), cortisone and its derivatives and ACTH all cause bleeding from small pre-existing peptic ulcers. Strong alkalies, mineral acids or mechanical injuries from articles which have been swallowed are less common causes.

VI. ATROPHIC CIRRHOSIS OF THE LIVER causes portal obstruction so that a collateral circulation (with lower œsophageal varices) develops (§ 342). A tumour pressing on the portal vein and thrombosis of the portal or splenic veins are rare but acute causes of the same condition. The hæmatemesis may be slight, but it is more often very copious—the most copious met with, as it is of venous origin, from ulceration of the œsophageal varices.

VII. SPLENIC ENLARGEMENT in the early stage of splenic anæmia, even before the liver is involved (§ 559).

VIII. PATHOLOGICAL CONDITIONS OF THE BLOOD AND BLOOD VESSELS such as with nephritis, yellow fever, malignant forms of the specific fevers, purpura, leukæmia, hæmophilia and hereditary telangiectasia.

IX. GASTROSTAXIS.—Under this title are included cases of hæmatemesis, occurring usually in young anæmic women, due to small acute gastric ulcers or erosions, especially in the posterior part of the fundus of the stomach adjacent to the lesser curvature. Hypertrophic gastric rugæ may be seen with the gastroscope.

X. ANEURYSM OF THE AORTA, or of one of its branches, leaking into the œsophagus or third part of the duodenum. This is known by (i.) possibly a previous history of aneurysmal symptoms (§ 80); (ii.) the blood is copious; (iii.) sudden death usually occurs; but in certain other cases there is a small recurrent leakage from the aneurysm for a few days or weeks preceding death.

Diagnosis of the cause may be difficult. (1) Always enquire for a history suggestive of peptic ulcer in the lower œsophagus, stomach or duodenum; and remember to ask the nature of any drugs or medicines recently consumed. Local pain and tenderness in the epigastrium due to a peptic ulcer often disappear when hæmatemesis occurs; (2) examine the liver, especially for cirrhosis, and feel for an enlarged spleen; (3) ascertain the approximate quantity of vomited blood, and then review the case, remembering the possibility of simulation in neurosis. (4) When a lesion of the lower œsophagus is suspected, œsophagoscopy may be necessary. (5) It is unwise to perform a barium meal X-ray sooner than 12–14 days after even a moderate hæmatemesis for the examination and deep palpation may cause bleeding to recommence and if surgical procedures are suddenly required the barium sulphate adds to the difficulties at a subsequent operation.

Prognosis.—Hæmatemesis is usually a serious symptom, but its gravity depends upon the cause and the severity of the blood loss. The commonest cause is from a chronic ulcer of the stomach with a mortality of about 10 per cent.: acute ulcers usually stop bleeding more quickly, but they can cause dangerous hæmorrhage. The severity of the blood loss can be judged by the degree of shock and pallor, and is always worse when there is a rapid thready pulse, a low blood pressure, repeated vomiting of blood and melæna with recurrent diarrhœic stools. A quarter- or half-hourly pulse rate which is steadily rising indicates that the loss of blood is continuing. The prognosis is always worse in elderly debilitated patients (usually men), and when there is concurrent renal or myocardial failure. A blood urea value of above 150 mg. per cent. is always a bad sign, even when there is no pre-existing renal disease.

Treatment.—The indications are: (i.) to stop the hæmorrhage. The patient must be kept absolutely at rest in the horizontal position. An ice bag should be placed over the epigastrium. Morphia hypodermically is the best hæmostatic and relieves anxiety: it must be repeated to allay restlessness. (ii.) When shock is at all severe, blood transfusion by the drip method (30–40 drops a minute) is necessary. A fall in the hæmoglobin value is not a good measure of the need for blood transfusion since in acute hæmorrhage, although the blood volume falls, hæmo-dilution is relatively slow: blood volume estimations are much more valuable but time-consuming. Unless the blood volume is known it is inadvisable to give more than 2 pints of blood at a time for fear of restarting the hæmorrhage, unless bleeding continues and shock remains severe. If blood is not immediately available intravenous dextran (6 per cent.) should be used. When bleeding and shock are not severe, blood transfusion is often resorted to unnecessarily especially in young subjects: rectal glucose-saline and early mouth feeding are sufficient. (iii.) If there is repeated vomiting it is not practicable to give much by mouth at first: some allow sips of iced water or ice wrapped in muslin to be sucked. Then iced citrated milk should be given for 12 hours, followed by 3 pints of citrated milk each 24 hours to prevent starvation and dehydration and to keep gastric acidity low. Within 3 days at the outside it is desirable to start a Gastric 1 diet (§ 296. III) together with antacid medicines (§ 288). Meulengracht has advised much more liberal feeding (§ 296. III). (iv.) Aperients or enemas must never be given until after the lapse of several days. Liquid paraffin by mouth or rectal washouts are permissible. (v.) General treatment must include scrupulous care in the toilet of the mouth to prevent parotitis, and the subsequent administration of iron. (vi.) If hæmorrhage recurs after 36–48 hours of treatment, surgery is necessary as often there is an open artery in the base of the ulcer. (vii.) For hæmatemesis due to bleeding from œsophageal varices, give intravenously 20 units of post. pituitary extract in 10 ml. of 5 per cent. dextrose over a period of 20 minutes; this lowers the portal pressure and can be repeated 4-hourly. Œsophageal tamponage is on trial: a balloon is inserted just beyond the cardiac sphincter and by keeping it inflated the increased pressure in the portal circulation is prevented from distending the varices (and see § 342).

§ 273. The **other Local Symptoms** of gastric disorder are :

1. BAD TASTE IN THE MOUTH, most noticeable in the morning, and DRYNESS OF THE LIPS are often complained of in gastric disorders. Sleeping with the mouth open must be excluded.

2. HALITOSIS (foul breath) is often due to causes outside the digestive tract (§ 201). A *tainted breath* may also be due to dental caries, pyorrhœa and septic tonsils.

3. THIRST occurs in dyspeptic conditions with acute dilatation of the stomach, inflammatory stomach lesions, and with persistent vomiting.

4. FLATULENCE is a distension of the stomach or intestines by gas, which may be brought up by the mouth or passed by rectum.

Symptoms due to flatulence may be *local* with discomfort, distension and hiccough, or *remote* with palpitation and cardiac irregularity.

Etiology.—Gastric flatulence (ærophagy) is a common symptom in ptyalism, chronic gastritis, gall-bladder dyspepsia, œsophageal hiatus hernia and in some nervous individuals without gastric derangement in whom there is repeated swallowing of air and subsequent noisy " belching " of gas. It may be the result of pure hysteria especially in women. Intestinal flatulence may be the result of swallowed air, of excessive fermentation of starches and sugars, of constipation or diarrhœa, and of redundant relaxed large bowel from excessive use of aperients; paralytic ileus, cœliac disease and sprue give a flatulent distension of the abdomen often without any complaint from the patient.

Treatment necessitates removing the cause. Carminatives such as brandy, spir. ammon. aromat., ginger, peppermint and phenol may aid: magnesia helps the flow of bile as well as emptying the small and large intestines, and so Gregory's powder is particularly helpful. Charcoal, atropine and similar preparations (Trasentin) aid intestinal flatulence.

5. " HEARTBURN " and ACID ERUCTATIONS often occur together. Heartburn is a burning sensation passing up from the epigastrium to the pharynx due to partial regurgitation of the gastric contents into the lower end of the œsophagus (§§ 218, 233); sometimes mouthfuls of acid fluid are brought up at the same time.

Causes.—Superacidity, or " acid risings," may be of two kinds. (a) *Organic acids* are met with in diseases where there is *deficient* gastric secretion—some forms of atonic dyspepsia, chronic gastritis, cancer, and dilatation of the stomach. HCl is a germicide, and when from any cause it is absent, bacteria flourish; fermentation ensues within a *few hours* after food, and is accompanied by pain in the epigastrium. The three principal acids are butyric, lactic and acetic.

(b) Hyperchlorhydria, or *excessive secretion of HCl*, is met with in one form of acute dyspepsia, and is usually present with duodenal ulcer. Here, the pain or " gnawing " occurs *before* meals, and is temporarily relieved by food (see also § 283).

(c) In pregnancy it may be a persistent symptom, and is often relieved by acid nitro-hydrochlor. dil. 15 ℳ, spir. chlorof. 10 ℳ in water after food.

6. HICCOUGH.—Normally the opening of the glottis synchronises with the contraction of the diaphragm, and consequently there is no hindrance to the free entry of air. Hiccough is caused by a spasm of the diaphragm (usually on one side only) which occurs at irregular intervals and sometimes at the moment of closure of the glottic aperture. The characteristic cough is then heard. The important causes of persistent hiccough are: (1) *Gastro-intestinal.* There is reflex stimulation of the phrenic nerve by (i) gastric dilatation after too large a meal or excess of swallowed air; (ii) gastric irritation due to excess of hot peppery foods, alcohol and tobacco; (iii) intestinal dilatation and flatulence with simple constipation, intestinal obstruction and paralytic ileus. They are common after operations on the prostate, bladder and colon. (2) In *acute peritonitis* whether local or general especially when gastro-intestinal paralysis becomes marked. (3) With *subphrenic irritation* due to an abscess or hiatus hernia. (4) Diseases of the *thoracic viscera* especially diaphragmatic pleurisy and with mediastinal tumours. (5) *Neurological causes* include cerebral tumour and meningitis. *Encephalitis Lethargica* may show itself first with persistent hiccough. Persistent hiccough may also arise from central or peripheral irritation of the phrenic nerve by spinal tumours. EPIDEMIC HICCOUGH, probably an infection of the central nervous system, clears up spontaneously, without sequelæ. (6) *Toxic* conditions such as uræmia (a common cause) or liver failure, and sometimes with influenza, malaria and gout. (7) *Psychoneurotic* causes sometimes appear to be contributory. Whatever the cause, patients are usually very alarmed and need reassurance.

Prognosis.—Hiccough is not as a rule a serious symptom. In abdominal disease it is of grave import. In the terminal stages of uræmia, meningitis or cerebral tumour, persistent hiccough may herald exitus. Epidemic hiccough may resist all treatment; it exhausts the patient, and may be the immediate cause of death.

Treatment.—The simplest forms of treatment are those directed to producing definite physiological contractions of the diaphragm. These are such well-known methods as sipping water and holding the breath, or inhaling CO_2. Anything which gives rise to a feeling of suffocation may cause a forcible contraction of the diaphragm, and so stop the spasm; for this reason tickling the nares and taking snuff have been tried, often with success. The hiccough due to dyspepsia is readily cured with bicarbonate of soda, by peppermint (as in crême de menthe), and that of

colonic distension by colonic lavage. If these measures fail, or if the
hiccough recurs frequently, a thorough investigation is called for. When
no causal condition can be found and the hiccough continues to be severe
inject. morphine or inj. chlorpromazine (Largactil) may be needed. Otherwise give sedative drugs by the mouth, or, if necessary, by the rectum;
barbiturates, or $\frac{1}{10}$ gr. apomorphine (subcutaneously) are successful.
Peripheral stimuli, such as blisters to the epigastrium, pinching the lobe
of the ear, forcible pulling forward of the tongue, and digital pressure
on the vagus in the neck, may be tried; and the abdomen may be bound
tightly with a bandage or with adhesive strapping. A general anæsthetic
may have to be administered and if all else fails division of the phrenic
nerve may be necessary.

7. " WATER-BRASH " (Pyrosis) is the name given to a clear alkaline
fluid expelled from the mouth in gushes (§ 218). It is met in many
dyspeptic conditions, and fairly often with *peptic ulcer.*

8. ANOREXIA (Loss of Appetite) is not always an indication of stomach
disease, as it is present in many general constitutional disturbances, such
as infectious fevers, tuberculosis and malignant disease. Its chief clinical
importance lies in its presence in the early stage of *gastric cancer.* In
cancer and *chronic gastritis* there is sometimes no appetite before a meal
or a premature feeling of fullness after a few mouthfuls. In *ulcer* there
is sometimes a fear of taking food. HYSTERICAL ANOREXIA (Anorexia
Nervosa) is known by: (i.) general failure of appetite or refusal to eat;
(ii.) pronounced loss of weight; (iii.) constipation; (iv.) slow pulse;
(v.) growth of downy hair on limbs and face; (vi.) cold blue extremities:
(vii.) it occurs mostly in young females, in whom there is amenorrhœa,
depression and restlessness; (viii.) careful investigation reveals no organic
condition (see §§ 569, 1173).

INCREASED APPETITE is often met, as Shakespeare pointed out, in
gastric disorders. It is found in some cases of chronic gastritis and dilated
stomach, in acromegaly, pregnancy and during convalescence. A FALSE
APPETITE which is satisfied with the first few mouthfuls of food is sometimes met in subacute and chronic gastritis, owing to irritation of the
mucous membrane. A RAVENOUS APPETITE, bulimia, is seen in diabetes,
in gastric neuroses, after acute gastritis, in wasting disorders such as sprue,
in phthisis, intestinal worms and Graves' disease. PERVERTED APPETITE,
excessive fondness for acids and sweets, or desire to eat objects such as
chalk, pencils or hair, may occur in hysteria and pregnancy.

§ 274. General or Remote Symptoms are usual.

1. GENERAL MALAISE and a sense of ill-health and incapacity for work
are among the earliest and most constant accompaniments of all derangements of the digestion, whether functional or organic. The dark rim
beneath the eyes, and the sallow " earthy " complexion, so frequently
associated with town-dwellers, are quite as often due to dyspepsia, just
as this latter is often due to defective teeth or to the insufficient use of
them. EMACIATION is not common in gastric disorder, though in chronic

cases there is some loss of flesh. It appears early in cancer of the stomach, and is severe in anorexia nervosa.

2. The CARDIAC SYMPTOMS met with in dyspepsia are palpitation, pain in the region of the heart (angina innocens); dyspnœa, syncope and vertigo; intermission of the cardiac rhythm. Cough may occur, due to pharyngeal catarrh or reflex irritation. Collectively, these symptoms may give rise to the impression that the case is one of cardiac valvular disease, although the heart may be structurally healthy (Roemheld's syndrome).

3. FUNCTIONAL DISTURBANCE OF NERVOUS SYSTEM.—*Headache and depression of spirits* are frequently met in all forms of dyspepsia. A sense of general ill-health and irritability of temper out of all proportion to the local mischief attend most gastric disorders, and, where stomach symptoms are not prominent, may lead the physician away from the true cause. Many of the symptoms of *neurasthenia* may result from gastric disorder.

4. DIARRHŒA may accompany stomach disease when the gastric contents are of an irritating nature, and when achlorhydria is present (gastrogenous diarrhœa). CONSTIPATION is usually found with simple ulcer, cancer, and chronic gastritis. But a more usual condition is an IRREGULARITY of the bowels, accompanied by borborygmi (rumbling in the bowels).

5. The URINE often exhibits signs which reveal disturbances of metabolism. The commonest of these is an excess of URATES; in other cases PHOSPHATES and OXALATES are found. In these circumstances dyspepsia is a predisposing cause of renal and vesical calculus.

6. SKIN SYMPTOMS.—General *pruritus* may accompany some forms of gastric derangement. *Flushing* of the face after meals is met in gastric disorders, especially in women. Acne rosacea is common with dyspepsia. *Urticaria* occurs in certain individuals after eating indigestible articles, and with several forms of gastric disorder (§ 652).

7. THE DUMPING SYNDROME which follows partial gastrectomy, is described in § 289.

PART B. PHYSICAL EXAMINATION

Disorders of the stomach are investigated by Inspection, Palpation, Percussion, Auscultation, X-ray examination after an opaque meal, the Gastroscope, Examination of material vomited or withdrawn from the stomach by a tube, by Test Meals and by Fæcal Analysis.

§ 275. **Inspection.**—(1) The *Teeth* in all cases must be closely examined. Common causes of indigestion are bolting the food, defective or absent teeth, septic tonsils and other forms of oral sepsis. See §§ 204 and 209.

(2) The *Tongue* and its diseases have been described (§ 213). At one time the tongue was thought to indicate the state of the stomach, but it is a more certain indication of the patient's general condition. But even in this, allowance has to be made for certain variations—namely: (i.) a coated tongue is normal to some, even in health, and a clean tongue

in others may be associated with disease; (ii.) certain diets—*e.g.*, milk—produce a coated tongue; and (iii.) certain habits—*e.g.*, smoking and alcoholism—also coat the tongue. The mouth may show signs of poisoning by corrosive acids.

(3) Inspection of the epigastric region may reveal a tumour, or the peristaltic movements of a dilated stomach. Aortic pulsation may be transmitted by a pyloric tumour, although no bulging is visible.

(4) In skilled hands the flexible gastroscope may be employed to examine the interior surface of the stomach. Alterations in the mucous membrane, mucus secretion, hæmorrhages, ulceration or neoplasm may be seen and specimens for biopsy taken.

Palpation and Percussion are described in Chapter IX on the Abdomen (§ 240).

§ 276. The **Motor Functions** of the Stomach and Intestinal Tract are most accurately investigated by X-ray examination after an opaque meal.

There is considerable individual variation. Delay in the alimentary canal may be tested by giving a teaspoonful of charcoal the night before a test breakfast. Charcoal so given should appear in the fæces in 36 to 48 hours. If it does not appear on the second morning, the presence of charcoal in the evacuation after an enema shows delay in the lower colon; if it is not present, the delay is higher up. This test is not very accurate.

X-RAY EXAMINATION is carried out with the fluorescent screen after giving the patient a suitable suspension of barium sulphate to drink. Radiograms taken can be studied afterwards. The *barium meal* is seen passing down the œsophagus and any obstruction or diverticulum is noted. The outline, position, tone and the rate and character of the peristaltic movements of the stomach are observed, the time at which it is empty, and the passage through the pylorus and duodenum. Irregularity of outline may be seen with a growth of the stomach, or when the barium lodges in the crater of an ulcer: with an ulcer local tenderness may be found. During the filling or emptying of the stomach, the folds of mucous membrane are defined, and give valuable information. The normal shape of the duodenal cap is characteristic, and is altered by ulcer, adhesions or pressure from without, as by a distended gall-bladder. The position and mobility of the lower ileum and cæcum are observed, and the appendix may be seen filled. The passage of the barium through the colon is watched at intervals. Normally the stomach empties in 2 to 4 hours; the terminal ileum and cæcum begin to fill about the same time. The terminal ileum should be clear of material 4 hours after the stomach is empty, and the colon should be clear in 72 hours. Abnormal appearances of the stomach, duodenum and colon are seen in Figs. 93 to 98. With a *barium enema*, the colon is observed filled and after evacuation, and if necessary with air inflation.

§ 277. Examination of Stomach Contents.[1]—First, as to the CHEMISTRY OF DIGESTION, and the practical information to be derived from clinical examination of the stomach contents. *Four processes* normally take place in the stomach: (1) The conversion of starch into sugar, begun in the mouth, is carried a stage further; (2) proteins are changed into peptones; (3) fat globules are set free from their envelopes; (4) milk is curdled. Delay in digestion may be caused by (1) deficient peristalsis of the stomach walls, (2) deficient quality or quantity of the gastric juice, (3) the consumption of indigestible articles, or (4) the dilution of the gastric juice by drinking too much fluid at meal-time.

The gastric juice contains HCl, water, pepsin, rennin, mineral salts, a *little* mucus,

---

[1] It is not possible here to give more than a brief outline of this important subject.

and Castle's intrinsic factor (§ 548).   Pepsin and rennin exist in the secretory cells only as zymogens, which, on secretion into the stomach, become active ferments or enzymes. In the healthy state, as the result of digestion, about 30 ml. of fluid should be obtained from the stomach one hour or so after a test-meal (*vide infra*), straw-coloured, without much odour, without organic acid, and with about 0·2 per cent. of free HCl.

As regards *hydrochloric acid*, much depends on the time of examination. *Hyperchlorhydria* has come to be somewhat loosely used for " excessive acidity," and thus to be confused with the acidity of fermentation (due to organic acids).   On the other hand, after a meal, a negative result on testing for HCl would indicate the absence of peptic activity, as this acid is required for the normal digestive action of pepsin.   Excess of HCl is distinctive of pyloric or duodenal ulcer.   HCl is diminished in catarrhal conditions of the mucous membrane, in many anæmias, in the majority of cases of malignant disease, during pregnancy, and in states of nervous exhaustion.

Three organic acids are met in the presence of fermentation in the stomach, *lactic acid*, *butyric acid* and *acetic acid*.   *Lactic acid* is easily recognised on testing with Uffelman's reagent (*vide infra*), and is the only one of diagnostic importance.   It is normally absent in the gastric juice after digestion has proceeded for one hour, but traces may be found, due to the ingestion of lactic acid in certain foods, or to fermentation in the mouth.   Fermentation occurs when HCl is deficient or when there is delayed emptying of the stomach: lactic acid is most frequently found in cases of gastric carcinoma with achlorhydria.

The secretion of *pepsin* is not interfered with, unless there be destruction of the glands of the stomach.   An acid secretion without peptic activity does not occur.

Examination of Gastric Contents after a Test-meal is a useful method of investigating the secretion and emptying of the stomach.   The gastric contents should be tested in all doubtful cases of digestive disturbance.

The **fractional test-meal** yields information as to the gastric secretion, the emptying of the stomach and the neutralisation of excessive acid by the reflux of alkaline duodenal contents.   A soft rubber tube (Ryle), with an oval perforated bulb at the end, is swallowed, any resting contents are withdrawn with a small glass syringe, and then a pint of test gruel is drunk with the tube in position.   (The gruel is made with two tablespoonfuls of breakfast oatmeal mixed with one quart of water, and boiled down to one pint and strained.)   The tube is kept in position whilst the patient reads quietly.   During the next 2–3 hours, at intervals of a quarter of an hour, about 10 ml. are drawn up and placed in a numbered test tube.   If four or five tubes have shown no acid with congo-red indicator, histamine may be injected subcutaneously (0·25 mg. histamine or 1 mg. histamine acid phosphate), in order to excite secretion.   The contents of the test tubes are separately examined and a curve plotted.   Record the appearance, smell, consistency and presence of excess of mucus, bile, or blood in each specimen.   MICROSCOPICALLY, we can detect fat globules, starch cells, vegetable and muscle fibres, residues of delayed emptying, cells of the mucous membrane, torulæ cerevisiæ or sarcinæ, and pus cells.   Epithelial cells may be in excess in carcinoma. The Oppler-Boas bacillus may sometimes be seen on examination under the high-power lens.   CHEMICALLY, the stomach contents are normally acid, although 4 per cent. of otherwise normal people have no acid in the gastric juice.   The normal free acid is *free hydrochloric acid*, much of which is loosely combined with proteins.   In the absence of free HCl, the acid present is due to organic acids, such as lactic and butyric acids produced by fermentation in the stomach (*e.g.*, in gastric carcinoma), and this is combined with protein.   The sum of the free acid and the combined acid gives the *total acidity*.

To estimate the *free hydrochloric acid*, titrate 5 ml. of the filtered gastric contents with N/10 solution of caustic soda, using a 1 per cent. solution of dimethylamido-azobenzol as the indicator, and add the alkali till the pink colour is discharged.   Then add phenolphthalein as an indicator, and add more NaOH till the red colour of the phenolphthalein is developed.   The amount of alkali added in the first instance is a measure of the amount of free HCl present, and the total amount of alkali added is a measure of the free + combined acid, *i.e.*, the total acidity. The results are usually expressed in terms of ml. N/10 NaOH per 100 ml. gastric juice, and in the fractional method of gastric analysis, may be plotted in the form of a graph.

Lactic acid may be detected by adding Uffelmann's reagent (made by mixing a little 5 per cent. solution of carbolic acid with a few drops of liquor ferri perchloridi). The blue colour is discharged by lactic acid and a yellow colour is produced.

The *emptying time* of the stomach is indicated by noting when no more juice can be aspirated. Normally the stomach is empty in 2–4 hours, and if a large residue is aspirated at 3 hours, delayed emptying is present.

Regular *aspiration of the stomach contents for a period of 24 hours* reveals excessive acidity during the night in patients with a duodenal ulcer: normally the gastric acidity is much lower during sleep.

Tubeless gastric analysis is carried out by giving caffeine sodium benzoate 0·5 G. as a gastric stimulant on an empty stomach. One hour later the bladder is emptied and the patient takes a cation-exchange resin in combination with quinine 2·0 G. (Diagnex): in the presence of HCl the quinine is freed, absorbed and the amount found in the urine after 2 hours is estimated. This test serves to detect cases of achlorhydria, but gives no quantitative estimate of the HCl secreted.

PART C. DISEASES OF THE STOMACH, THEIR DIFFERENTIATION, PROGNOSIS AND TREATMENT

§ 278. Routine Investigation. FIRST: We must identify the patient's LEADING SYMPTOMS as being referable to gastric disorder (see Part A).

SECONDLY: Inquire as to the HISTORY, and especially whether the symptoms came on *acutely* and recently, or whether, as is more usual, the illness came on insidiously, and has run a *chronic* course. Much depends on the skill and method with which the history is elicited. Inquire particularly as to pain or discomfort and its relation to meals, and as to the other symptoms mentioned in Part A.

THIRDLY: Proceed to the PHYSICAL EXAMINATION, and ascertain whether there be any localised tenderness and pain, and whether any tumour or other abnormality be present.

FINALLY: where an organic lesion of the œsophagus, stomach or duodenum is suspected from the symptoms and signs thus obtained, it is essential to have performed the appropriate investigations with a barium meal X-ray, gastroscope, fractional test-meal, etc. In many cases the blood should be examined for anæmia and the stools analysed (§ 303).

If the patient's symptoms have come on gradually, and lasted a considerable time, turn to **Chronic Disorders** of the Stomach (§ 281).

If, on the other hand, the symptoms have begun somewhat suddenly and recently, the case is probably one of the two **Acute Disorders** of the Stomach: I. ACUTE DYSPEPSIA; or, II. ACUTE GASTRITIS.

I. *The patient—whose temperature is normal—complains of* NAUSEA, GASTRIC DISCOMFORT, *headache and depression, which have come on suddenly; there is a little epigastric tenderness.* The disease is probably ACUTE DYSPEPSIA.

§ 279. Acute Dyspepsia (" Bilious Attack," " Congestion of the Liver ") consists of a sudden disturbance of the digestion in a previously healthy person, such as occurs in association with surfeit, high living or other errors in diet, overwork and worry.

The *Symptoms*, which come on suddenly, are: (1) Pain, or a feeling of oppression or distension in the epigastrium, occasionally accompanied by slight tenderness on pressure. (2) Nausea and vomiting often follow. (3) Headache, depression, anorexia, coated tongue, constipation, scanty urine loaded with urates. (4) The illness is sometimes preceded and accompanied by drowsiness, and there is often a history of previous attacks.

Diagnosis.—Acute gastritis is a similar condition in which the constitutional symptoms are more apparent, the duration of the illness considerably longer, and the *tenderness much more marked*. Irritant poisoning comes on more suddenly with urgent vomiting (§ 271). *Migraine* also produces recurrent attacks, characterised by headache (often unilateral), fortification spectra, nausea and vomiting. Similar symptoms may usher in certain infectious diseases.

Etiology.—(1) Too large a meal, especially after previous fatigue. (2) Errors in diet, such as excess of alcohol (which retards digestion), fats, ice, and many other articles which vary with the idiosyncrasy of the individual. (3) Fits of temper, disappointment or worry.

Prognosis and Treatment.—Acute dyspepsia usually passes off in two or three days. (1) If pain be present, assist vomiting by mild emetics, such as copious draughts of salt and water, tickling the fauces, etc. Violent emetics aggravate the condition. (2) Calomel gr. 3 or blue pill, and milk diet for a day or two, generally relieve. (3) Mixtures containing bismuth carbonate and sodium bicarbonate may then be prescribed.

II. *The patient complains of considerable* PAIN *or discomfort, and* TENDERNESS IN THE EPIGASTRIUM, *with nausea or vomiting, all of which have come on rather suddenly*. The disease is probably ACUTE GASTRITIS.

§ 280. Acute or Subacute Gastritis is relatively a much more serious disorder than the foregoing. It consists of a sudden derangement of digestion due to inflammation of the mucosa of the stomach.

Symptoms.—(1) Pain, intense and burning, or a feeling of distension in the epigastrium, coming on directly after food, and accompanied by tenderness on pressure. (2) Vomiting, not always immediately after a meal, of undigested food and mucus, sometimes with streaks of blood. (3) Malaise, anorexia, slight pyrexia, headache, depression and other constitutional symptoms may be present, attended sometimes by great prostration, thirst, furred or coated tongue. (4) Diarrhœa may ensue after a day or two.

The *Diagnosis* may have to be made from acute dyspepsia (§ 279), and from other causes of vomiting (§ 271).

Etiology.—(1) In the majority of cases simple acute gastritis is caused by errors in diet; alcohol or an excessive quantity of normal food also causes it. (2) Local epidemics may be caused by food infected with *staphylococcus aureus* or salmonella organisms. (3) Irritant poisons (*e.g.*, arsenic, phosphorus, lysol, etc.). In long-continued vomiting, without apparent cause, poisoning should be suspected, and the vomited matters examined. (4) In some cases, gout and other constitutional conditions predispose to or determine an attack. Heart, lung and liver diseases are predisposing causes.

Prognosis.—Recovery generally takes place in about three to six days, the affection rarely lasting longer than eight or ten days. It may go on to chronic gastritis. Death rarely takes place, excepting from irritant poisoning or in cases of membranous gastritis.

Treatment.—The indications are: (1) To remove any irritant that may be present in the stomach. This can be done by promoting vomiting, especially if the epigastric pain continues. The stomach may be washed out with saline or a weak solution of bicarbonate of soda. It may be desirable to give a purgative, such as calomel gr. 3 (if there is vomiting, gr. ½ hourly), followed by a seidlitz powder next morning. Hot fomentations or a mustard leaf to the epigastrium may relieve the pain. (2) The stomach needs rest by 12 or 24 hours' abstinence from food, followed by fruit juice and glucose, and then milk in small quantities. Later on, bismuth combined with opium is the best treatment. The milk diet should be supplemented only very gradually.

CHRONIC DISORDERS OF THE STOMACH

§ 281. *The patient, whose temperature is normal, complains of " Chronic Indigestion"*—i.e., *pain or discomfort in some way connected with his food, which has probably come on gradually, and may have lasted a long time.*

Note the relationship of the discomfort or pain to food and examine for tenderness. Guidance may be obtained from the summary on p. 392 (Table XVI).

Many disorders **unconnected with the stomach** may give rise to symptoms of chronic indigestion; among these the following may be mentioned: Pulmonary tuberculosis (of which dyspepsia is often the earliest symptom), Appendicitis, Colitis, Anæmia, Abdominal Tumour, Cardiac, Hepatic, Renal or Uterine Disease, various Nervous Disorders, and Pancreatic Disease (rare).

In patients in whom no organic disease can be found, an **Anxiety State** is an increasingly common cause of acute and of chronic dyspepsia. But it must not be forgotten that many digestive disorders (including gastritis and ulceration) are the direct result of psychoneurotic stresses; or that patients with organic gastro-duodenal lesions may develop a functional overlay when they become anxious as to the cause of their symptoms. The need for thorough investigation in all such cases is obvious (and see §§ 1171, 1172).

TABLE XVI

The patient complains of SUBSTERNAL PAIN on SWALLOWING FOOD	Dysphagia ..	§§ 218, 220
The discomfort FOLLOWS MEALS, and *is* RELIEVED by *vomiting and belching*	Chronic gastritis ..	§ 282
There is DISCOMFORT and PAIN, RELIEVED by *alkalies and by food*	Acid gastritis	§ 283
There is PAIN, AGGRAVATED BY FOOD, and there is TENDERNESS *on the left*	Gastric ulcer .. or gastro-jejunal ulcer	§§ 286, 287 § 290
The pain is RELIEVED BY FOOD and there is TENDERNESS *on the right*	Duodenal ulcer ..	§ 288
The pain, 3-4 hours after food, is associated with NAUSEA, VOMITING and DISTENSION *on the right*	Chronic duodenal ileus	§ 291
There is CONSTANT DISTENSION in the epigastrium and *attacks of pain on the right side*	Duodenal diverticulum	§ 292
There is pain, which is constant and AGGRAVATED BY FOOD; there is FLATULENCE and NAUSEA, UNRELIEVED *by* BELCHING	Cholecystitis	§ 354
There is DISCOMFORT following meals, variable in position, with FLATUS which passes downwards	Colitis	§ 312
There is PAIN which FOLLOWS EFFORT	Angina pectoris ..	§ 51
There is severe and INTERMITTENT PAIN, *not connected* with FOOD or EFFORT	Gall-stones and tabetic crises ..	§§ 353, 1022
Pain is more or less CONSTANT, with DISTENSION, FLATULENCE and EMACIATION:		
Cancer of the stomach	.. ..	§ 293
Chronic dilatation of the stomach	.. .. ..	§ 294
There is HEARTBURN on lying or stooping, PAIN under the left lower ribs and sometimes HÆMATEMESIS	Hiatus hernia	§ 234

I. *The patient complains of* CHRONIC INDIGESTION, *and the epigastric pain or discomfort comes on* SOON AFTER A MEAL. The disease is probably CHRONIC GASTRITIS.

§ 282. **Chronic Gastritis** is a common form of chronic dyspepsia. It was formerly called atonic or nervous dyspepsia. The *symptoms* are: (1) Pain or distress, usually in the epigastrium, coming on immediately or very shortly after food—especially fried and greasy food. The pain may be in the back or shoot up to the shoulders; or there may be no definite pain, only a feeling of weight or distension. It may be accompanied by tenderness and is often relieved by eructations of wind. (2) The appetite is usually diminished; it may be good, but ceases quickly after beginning the meal. Often breakfast is well taken, lunch not so well, and later meals worse. (3) There is a bad taste in the mouth. The tongue is flabby, dry and indented by the teeth. (4) There is a tendency to eructation and heartburn; nausea, even vomiting may occur, but not frequently. (5) There are languor, headache, depression, disturbed sleep, fatigue, and discomfort and drowsiness after meals. There may be palpitation, dyspnœa and other cardiac symptoms: sometimes acne rosacea and urticaria.

There are three stages: First, a simple *congestion*, in which the hydrochloric acid is diminished. The second stage is one of *mucous catarrh*, in which there is a large secretion of mucus, and hydrochloric acid is almost completely absent. In the third stage there is *atrophy* of the mucous membrane; hydrochloric acid, pepsin and mucus are much reduced or are now absent. Iron deficiency (hypochromic) and nutritional anæmia, and Addisonian or other macrocytic anæmias may be associated with this stage; malignant disease may follow in after years.

Diagnosis.—The subjective symptoms are not characteristic, and chronic gastritis may be secondary to disease elsewhere in the body. Some

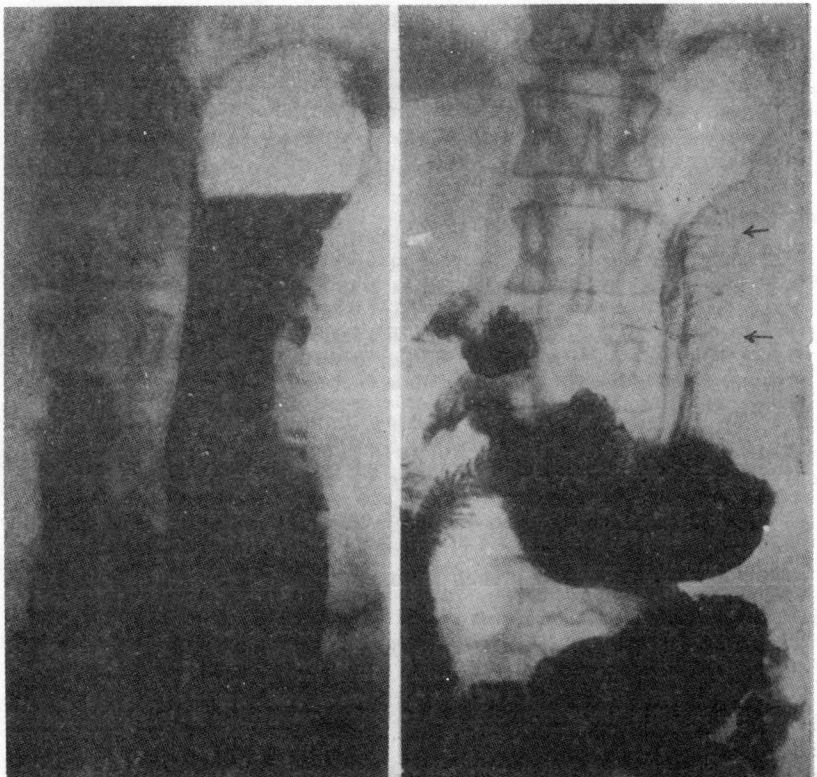

FIG. 93. *Right.*—Hypertrophic gastritis of greater curvature, showing the feathered appearance indicated by arrows. *Left.*—The same with the stomach filled.

forms of chronic gastritis do not give rise to digestive symptoms, the patient complaining only of weakness and exhaustion. Test meal, gastroscopic and X-ray examinations are necessary for the diagnosis of the state of the stomach. The strial picture of the stomach shows thickening or thinning of the mucosal folds. Intragastric biopsy has shown that the extent of gastritis is parallel with the amount of hydrochloric acid secreted in response to an injection of histamine. There is excess of mucus and usually diminution of hydrochloric acid. Alcoholic and acid gastritis are special varieties (see II and III below). The important stomach conditions to be differentiated are *gastric ulcer* in the young and middle-aged, and *cancer of the stomach* after the age of 40 and especially in later years (see Table XVII, p. 399). *Achylia gastrica* is the late stage of chronic gastritis and may be accompanied by acne rosacea, visceroptosis and ileal stasis; it also occurs in Addisonian anæmia. Gastritis is often accompanied by gall-bladder disease, appendicitis, chronic colitis and other abdominal conditions.

Etiology.—(1) Errors of diet, excess of fats and condiments; (2) defective teeth and inadequate mastication; (3) the abuse of alcohol and sometimes of tobacco; (4) accompanying either local disease of the stomach (ulcer, hiatus hernia, cancer, pyloric obstruction) or cholecystitis, gall-stones and chronic pancreatitis; (5) acute or chronic febrile illnesses, sepsis, anæmia, infections of the mouth and tonsils; (6) dyspepsia is often the earliest symptom met in pulmonary tuberculosis; (7) circulatory diseases, early hypertension and chronic nephritis.

Syphilis of the Stomach is now rare in Great Britain, but is met abroad. It is a tertiary manifestation of the disease, especially in middle-aged men. The *Symptoms* resemble closely those of chronic gastritis, with epigastric pain shortly after taking food often followed by vomiting and loss of weight. Radiography shows rigidity and deformity of the gastric outline, which is easily confused with carcinoma. However, the Wassermann reaction is strongly positive and the symptoms and X-ray findings rapidly respond to anti-syphilitic measures.

II. *In addition to other symptoms of* CHRONIC INDIGESTION, *the patient has much nausea, and* VOMITS MUCUS IN THE MORNING, *occasionally streaked with blood. The disease is probably* ALCOHOLIC GASTRITIS.

Alcoholic Gastritis is produced by persistent dietetic errors, especially alcoholic excesses, and is aggravated by the changes in the œsophagus and venous congestion arising from cirrhosis of the liver.

III. *The patient complains of* BOUTS OF INDIGESTION, *in which the discomfort does* NOT *come on* SOON AFTER A MEAL, *is followed by* VOMITING OF ACID FLUID, *and is* RELIEVED BY FOOD *and by alkalies. The discomfort consists of* SINKING FEELINGS *in the epigastrium, or* HUNGER PAINS. *The disease is probably* ACID GASTRITIS.

§ 283. Acid Gastritis (Acid Dyspepsia, Hyperchlorhydria) is due to causes which bring about directly or reflexly excessive secretion of gastric juice, or retention with pyloric spasm. Among these are nervous strain and worry—especially business stress from travelling and interviews; alcohol, tobacco and condiments; colitis, appendicitis, cholelithiasis, gastric or duodenal ulcer, and duodenal diverticulum. In *achylia gastrica* there may be acid eructations, but these are due to organic acids formed by fermentation.

The *Prognosis of Gastritis* depends on the cause and the duration of the symptoms. It is never fatal, but often renders life wretched for the sufferer. If met early, treatment should be thorough; if untreated, dilata-

tion of the stomach, general malnutrition and neurasthenia may develop.
Simple alcoholic gastritis soon recovers. The outlook is more grave when
due to general toxic states or when there is irremovable venous obstruction.
Treatment of Gastritis.—(1) Remove the cause. Correct faulty habits
of chewing and bolting the food, remove infected teeth and provide
efficient dentures, treat any catarrh of the nose or infection of the tonsils.
(2) Give advice as to arrangement of work, holidays and relief of stress.
(3) Reduce or prohibit alcohol and tobacco. (4) Local treatment: Gastric
lavage with water or sod. bicarb. (gr. 60 to Ōi); hydrogen peroxide (℞ 30
to Ōi) may be used. (5) Substitution therapy with hydrochloric acid,
℞ xv with bitters before meals in suitable cases; in achylia give ℞ 60 of
dilute hydrochloric acid in a tumbler of diluted orange juice to be sipped
with meals. (6) Diet does not depend on the character of the gastric
secretion (§ 296. I and II). Small dry meals of simple but varied foods,
avoiding condiments as a rule, are best. Give vitamin B as wheat germ
or Marmite, or by a suitable injection. (7) Symptomatic treatment: For
the pain, bismuth or magnesium carbonate, dilute hydrocyanic acid; for
fermentation and acidity, sodium phenolsulphonate (B.P.C.) and alkalies
two or three hours after a meal. Mucous vomiting is relieved by draughts
of hot water, with alkalies, before breakfast. For flatulence, sodium
bicarbonate gr. 20 in a cupful of hot water, with tincture of ginger ℞ 20,
give great relief. Some find helpful pepsin, lactopeptine, takadiastase or
other artificial digestives. (8) General measures. Attention to the
general health is necessary. A holiday from work, with regulated exercise and diet, and the treatment of sleeplessness, may be required at the
beginning. Abdominal exercises to improve muscle tone are important
curative measures. Rest before and after meals is excellent in nervous
cases. In acid gastritis, olive oil ℞ 60 before meals or atropine gr. ₁/₁₅₀
inhibits secretion.

IV. *The patient complains of* NAUSEA, FULLNESS *and* ERUCTATIONS,
*having no definite relation to the taking of food, and careful investigation
reveals* NO STRUCTURAL DISORDER OF THE STOMACH. *The case is probably
one of* NERVOUS DYSPEPSIA.

§ 284. Nervous Dyspepsia was formerly a frequent diagnosis, but
modern investigations have shown that these symptoms are usually due
to gastritis or to disease elsewhere in the abdomen. The constant discomfort and distress of gastric disorders bring about a neurasthenic and
depressed state. On the other hand, flatulence is common in anxiety
neurosis. Anxiety and worry cause spasm, and therefore delay. By
means of the fractional test-meal and X-ray examination it has been
discovered that with strong emotional states digestion may stand still
for the first hour or more; then if the cause be suddenly removed, digestion proceeds rapidly from that moment. But it is not wise to diagnose
gastric neurosis until all clinical and special investigations have been
carried out to exclude organic disease. Air swallowing and rumination are

not gastric diseases, but bad habits, and are to be treated by explanation and psychotherapy.

V. *The patient complains of* INDIGESTION. *The* PAIN COMES ON DAILY, WITH CONSTANT RELATION TO FOOD. *It is* RELIEVED *by* LIQUID FOOD *and by* ALKALIES. *There is* TENDERNESS ON PRESSURE. *The disease is probably an* ULCER.

§ 285. Simple or Peptic Ulcer is extremely common. It is reliably estimated to be present in 5·8 per cent. of men and in 1·9 per cent. of women in Great Britain at any one time. It may be acute or chronic, and may be situated in the stomach, or the duodenum as far as the ampulla of Vater. It may also occur where there is aberrant gastric mucous membrane as in the lower end of the œsophagus and in Meckel's diverticulum. The ulcers probably arise by peptic digestion of areas of mucous membrane which have been injured by local trauma, by toxins swallowed from the mouth or pharynx, or absorbed from septic foci elsewhere in the body. Such abrasions are perpetuated by large doses of corticosteroid drugs and by ACTH, with the production of an ulcer. Such ulcers are also caused by solid lumps of aspirin as well as by phenylbutazone B.P. They tend to heal readily unless there is gastric stasis and superacidity, when they become chronic, erode the wall of the viscus and may invade adjacent organs.

V*a*. *The patient complains of severe* PAIN, PRODUCED BY FOOD *and* RELIEVED BY VOMITING, *the vomit sometimes containing a quantity of blood.* The disease is ACUTE ULCER OF THE STOMACH.

§ 286. Acute Peptic Ulcer is less common than formerly. It occurs in the second and third decades of life. The ulcers are usually small and may be multiple. In many cases there may be no symptoms and spontaneous healing occurs. There are three very characteristic features, to which the symptoms of chronic dyspepsia may be added:

(1) *Pain* of a distending or boring character in the epigastrium, (2) *aggravated by food*, and accompanied by tenderness. A small, very tender area is sometimes present, and is characteristic. (3) The pain is *relieved by vomiting*; the vomited matter may contain an excess of hydrochloric acid. (4) Hæmatemesis, which may be profuse, often occurs without pain or other symptoms. (5) The appetite is usually normal or decreased and the patient avoids food because of the pain it produces. There is generally constipation and anæmia, and often a history of inadequate food and lack of fresh air. In many cases there may be no symptoms until profuse hæmorrhage or perforation suddenly occurs.

The *Diagnosis* is not difficult if pain, an area of tenderness, and hæmatemesis be present. Confirmation is made with X-ray and gastroscopy. Chronic appendicitis may simulate the disease. See Table XVII.

Treatment of Acute Ulcer.—In all but the mildest cases the patient must rest in bed. In cases of perforation immediate laparotomy is the best treatment. Where there is recent hæmorrhage or intractable vomiting, iced citrated milk is started as soon as possible, followed by 3 pints of milk in 24 hours. (See treatment of hæmatemesis, § 272.) Suitable diets are given in § 296. III. All foci of infection—teeth, tonsils, appendix, gall-bladder—must be removed later. Chronic inflammation of the appendix must be remembered.

V*b*. *The patient is a* MIDDLE-AGED *or* ELDERLY MAN *or a* YOUNG *or* MIDDLE-AGED WOMAN *who is enfeebled by illness or anxiety, and who complains of* INDIGESTION *at* REGULAR INTERVALS AFTER FOOD, *which is* RELIEVED BY *taking* LIGHT FOOD, BY VOMITING *and* BY ANTACIDS. *The disease is probably* CHRONIC GASTRIC ULCER.

§ 287. A **Chronic Gastric Ulcer** usually occurs as a single lesion on or adjacent to the lesser curvature, on the posterior wall or in the pyloric antrum: sometimes a chronic ulcer is present simultaneously in the duodenum. It occurs with equal frequency in men and women but is seen two or three times more often in those of the lower social classes who are poorly fed.

Symptoms.—The patient is often thin and miserable and may complain of recurrent attacks, each few weeks or months, of (1) " Chronic indigestion." (2) Attacks of pain in the epigastrium, left upper abdomen or back, come on half an hour to two hours after a meal and pass off before the next meal: the higher the ulcer in the stomach the sooner does the pain come on after food. (3) The pain is often described as an aching or gnawing pain, and is located to a definite area of the upper abdomen. (4) The appetite is poor or may be restrained, the patient being afraid to take solid food and feeling better when resting and on light food. (5) Nausea and vomiting may occur, and the latter is sometimes induced by the patient to obtain relief. (6) Antacid mixtures and powders almost invariably relieve the pain. (7) Hæmatemesis is not common but when it occurs it is severe. Constipation is usual.

Physical signs.—Particularly during a bout of pain, deep pressure in the mid-line of the epigastrium usually indicates a definite local area of tenderness. In some cases, there is guarding of the left upper rectus abdominis, and deep tenderness may be elicited over the actual site of the ulcer.

The *diagnosis* is not difficult when the characteristic pain with epigastric tenderness is present, but pain after food, relieved by emptying the stomach, with occasional vomiting of blood, may occur in other diseases. The pain may be continuous if there are local complications such as adhesions to surrounding organs or chronic perforation. Every case of " chronic dyspepsia " should be investigated. The test-meal and efficient X-ray examination are the chief means of coming to a diagnosis. The stomach contents usually show increased free hydrochloric acid and total acidity, except where an atrophic gastritis is present. In the X-ray examination the crater of the ulcer projecting into the wall of the stomach may be filled by the barium emulsion and there is often spasm of the circular muscle which produces an incisura opposite the ulcer; at the

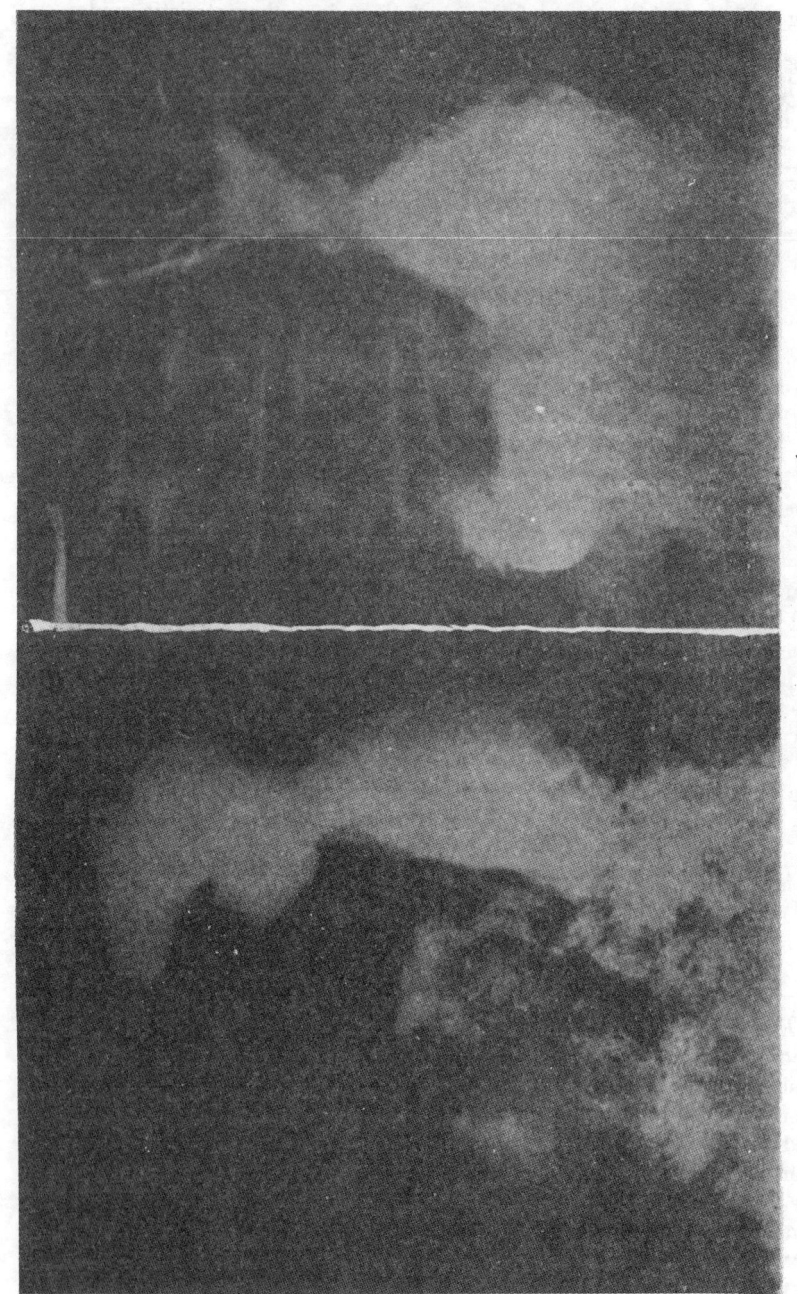

FIG. 94.—GASTRIC ULCER on lesser curvature of the stomach.
Left, before treatment; *Right*, after treatment.

filling and emptying stages of the meal there is a characteristic spider-form of the striæ of mucous membrane converging towards the ulcer. In the hands of experts the ulcer may be shown with the gastroscope (Table XVII).

TABLE XVII

	CHRONIC GASTRIC ULCER.	MALIGNANT DISEASE.	CHRONIC GASTRITIS.
Pain ..	1½–2 hours after food.	Constant discomfort.	Shortly after food.
Aggravated by	Large meals and condiments.	Meat.	Fried foods.
Appetite ..	Usually good.	Anorexia often severe.	Poor.
Duration of symptoms.	For months or years.	Recent, and not responding to treatment.	Often long-standing.
Vomiting ..	Not frequent; relieves pain.	Often large quantity every few days.	Morning vomiting of mucus, especially with alcohol.
Hæmatemesis	Occasional but profuse; therefore bright red.	A continuous oozing; therefore "coffee-ground" in character.	Rare; and only streaks, unless in the venous congestion due to heart disease.
Tumour ..	None.	Present, though may not be palpable; secondary deposits may be recognisable in liver, peritoneum, glands, etc., later.	None.
Age	Thirty to fifty.	Usually men over forty.	Any age.
Course ..	Recovery if well treated; with relaxation of regime, relapses occur.	Fatal in one or two years if not removed.	Liable to pass on to a chronic dyspepsia.

Etiology.—The primary condition is probably one of gastritis; superimposed on this are other factors such as fatigue, overwork, worry, oral sepsis, or irregular meals, which cause the inflamed gastric mucosa to ulcerate. Two groups of patients may be found: (1) Young or middle-aged women debilitated by overwork in poor surroundings, poor food or after infectious diseases. They are usually anæmic, thin and easily tired. The ulcer may be part of a general gastritis. (2) Middle-aged and elderly men who have pyorrhœa or have lost their teeth. In these cases, also, overwork or excess of tobacco smoking may contribute. In some instances the ulcer symptoms may be masked by tiredness and a sense of exhaustion. The *prognosis* is usually favourable if treatment is carried out early, and the general condition of the patient medically and socially attended to. If untreated, perforation into the peritoneal cavity or hæmorrhage may occur; in healing, cicatrisation may lead to distortion or stricture of the stomach (hour-glass) or of the pylorus (stenosis). Death occasionally results from hæmorrhage and in a small proportion of cáses of chronic ulcer of the stomach cancer may develop in the site of the ulcer. *Treatment* is described in § 288.

Vc. *The patient is a healthy-looking* ACTIVE MAN, *who* FOR YEARS HAS HAD ATTACKS OF ACIDITY *after overwork, worry or indigestible food: he* DEVELOPS PAIN 3–4 HOURS AFTER FOOD *or in the night:* RELIEVED *by* TAKING FOOD OR ANTACIDS. *The disease is* CHRONIC DUODENAL ULCER.

§ 288. Chronic Duodenal Ulcer is eight times as frequent in males as in females. The *symptoms* often begin at the age of 20–35, and tend to come in attacks after dietetic errors, overwork, worry or exposure. The first attack may only last a few days or a week or so with a long period of freedom until the next presents itself. In the course of time the duration of each attack becomes longer and the periods of freedom shorter. (1) Epigastric pain, sometimes intense, and usually of nagging or gnawing type, comes on when the stomach is empty 3–4 hours after food—the so-called " hunger-pain," which frequently wakes the patient at about 2 a.m. and is almost immediately relieved by food. The pain tends to come at a regular time each day or during the night. (2) Vomiting is sometimes complained of, especially in a particularly severe bout of pain: it is due to pylorospasm, and after the stomach is emptied, relief is immediately obtained. (3) The pain may radiate to the back, and become more constant when the ulcer burrows into the head of the pancreas. (4) Sudden intestinal hæmorrhage may occur, evidenced by melæna, and sometimes preceded or accompanied by hæmatemesis. (5) Perforation may occur, after mild early symptoms.

Physical signs always increase during one of the recurrences of symptoms. There may be rigidity, or resistance to palpation, in the right upper quadrant of the abdomen. Deep tenderness is usually present in the mid-line just above the umbilicus, and/or locally over the site of the ulcer in the first part of the duodenum. *X-ray examination* reveals either pyloric spasm and delay, or the stomach contents rush through with rapid emptying of the stomach; a series of radiograms, rapidly taken, may reveal characteristic irregularity of the duodenal cap (Fig. 95). Hyperchlorhydria is usual.

Diagnosis.—In typical cases, the characteristic pain makes the diagnosis easy. Chronic gastric ulcer, stone in the gall-bladder or kidney, and chronic appendicitis are to be differentiated. The diagnosis is confirmed best with the X-rays. A fractional test-meal showing superacidity and the discovery of occult blood in the fæces may help in obscure cases. Similar symptoms, but with left-sided pain, may accompany ulceration occurring after gastro-enterostomy (see § 290).

Etiology.—Duodenal ulcers occur especially in energetic ambitious young men who tend to overwork and to eat irregular and often hurried meals. Attacks often follow periods of acute anxiety or other emotional stresses: some occupations are contributory, as in bus drivers, waiters, medical practitioners and high-powered business executives. There is often a strong family tendency.

Prognosis.—Medical treatment is usually successful, but it must be adequate. Insufficient treatment is the cause of non-success, as the

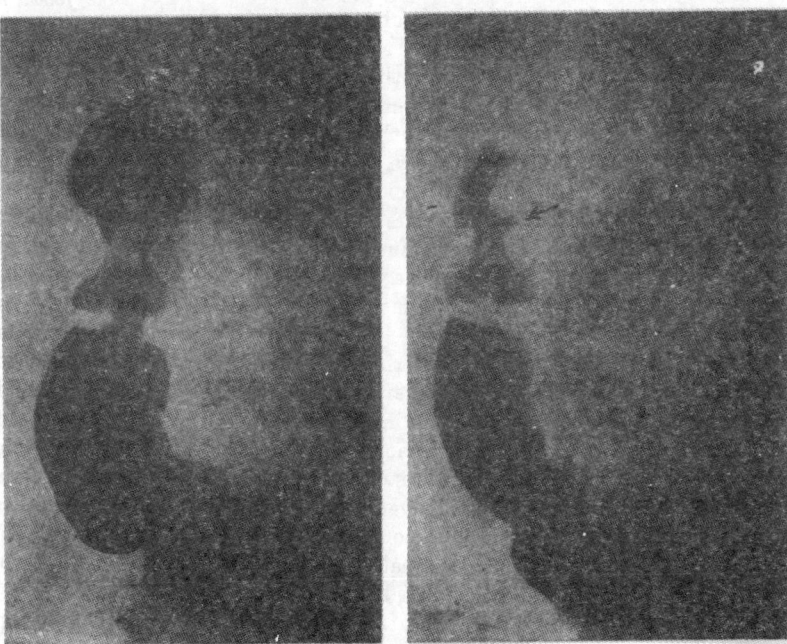

Fig. 95.—A Deformed Duodenal Cap with an Opaque Spot in the Centre.
The right-hand illustration shows the same duodenal cap (in the second left oblique view). The ulcer (see arrow) can be seen as a spur on the posterior surface, with opposing spasm.

ulcer readily heals superficially, but tends to relapse easily unless time is given to allow healing to take place throughout. Perforation, hæmorrhage and persistence or recurrence of symptoms after thorough medical treatment are indications for surgical interference.

Medical Treatment of Chronic Gastric and Duodenal Ulcers. The indications are to (1) give the patient mental and physical rest, (2) administer a sufficiency of nourishing food which will call for little digestive effort, (3) reduce the superacidity of the gastric juice and (4) eliminate all sources of sepsis. (1) It should be stipulated that the patient be in bed 4–6 weeks, followed by slowly getting up and not returning to work for at least 3 months. (2) The food given will be such as will neutralise the stomach acid, will excite little secretion and of a bulk which will not distend the organ. Diet in the initial stages consists chiefly of milk of which 3–4 pints are consumed in the 24 hours: it may be diluted, citrated or mixed with egg as unboiled custard: feeds should be given at least every 2 hours during the day, with 1–2 feeds during the night, and many prefer that the milk be sipped continuously all the waking hours, or be administered by a continuous nasal drip directly into the stomach. In 1–2 weeks, depending on the cessation of symptoms, cereals, bread and butter, biscuits, rusks and butter, steamed white fish, tender or minced meat or chicken, well-boiled rice and milk puddings are gradually added; and at the end of 3–4 weeks a light invalid diet is reached (and see § 296. III). All mechanical and chemical irritants in the diet should be avoided: to prevent deficiency of vitamin C, small amounts of orange juice, grape-juice or ascorbic acid are necessary. From the first, olive or arachis oil 1–2 teaspoonfuls are given several times a day: this may be flavoured with peppermint water. (3) The superacidity of the gastric juices and thirst are remedied by antacids which neutralise the gastric secretion: teaspoonful doses of a powder containing bismuth carbonate 1 part, sodium bicarbonate 2 parts, magnesium carbonate 1 part, calcium carbonate 1 part, can be given half an hour after a meal: the proportions of bismuth carbonate and magnesium carbonate are varied so that constipation is avoided. It must be remembered that if too much sod. bicarb. is used for too long a period, alkalæmia and even uræmia may occur. Magnesium trisilicate and colloidal aluminium hydroxide are also powerful antacids. Olive oil, cream and tincture of belladonna ℳ 3–5 twice or thrice daily restrict the acid secretion. Alcohol and smoking are forbidden until the ulcer has healed, and even then only allowed in moderation after meals. (4) All foci of infection, *e.g.*, septic teeth, infected tonsils, or chronic appendicitis, must be treated. Adequate mastication must be insisted on and artificial teeth fitted where necessary. The progress of healing may be determined by repeating the barium meal each 4–5 weeks, or by observation with the gastroscope.

Certain *complications* are liable to occur: any return of symptoms is an indication to resume a fluid diet. For pain or vomiting due to pylorospasm inj. atropine gr. $\frac{1}{150}$ and tinct. belladonnæ should be given: opiates are not advisable. Constipation is avoided by varying the composition of the antacid powder, by mist. magnes. hydrox., by liquid paraffin or a plain paraffin emulsion. Anxiety and restlessness are treated by small doses of amylobarbitone or phenobarbitone, and sleeplessness by the first of these. For the treatment of hæmorrhage see § 272. Perforation should be treated by omitting all food and medicine by mouth, and usually by immediate operation (§ 243); occasionally perforation with adhesion to the posterior abdominal wall subsides without operation.

Treatment should continue for 3 months on the strict lines laid down above, followed by a careful diet with regular 2-hourly, small, easily digested meals for 6 months or more (see post-ulcer diet, § 296. III).

Part of this time should be spent on holiday before returning to work. The results of medical treatment, when fully carried out as outlined above, are usually satisfactory, four out of five patients becoming symptom-free and able to resume work. However, there is a tendency to relapse as the result of recurrence of the stress conditions which contributed to the onset of the ulcer, or of an intercurrent infection such as influenza, so that not more than one-third of the patients followed up remain well. Unless the conditions at home and at work can be made so easy that a careful regimen can be maintained, consideration must be given as to whether surgery will give a better outlook.

The indications for operation are (i.) to treat obstinate cases recurring after full medical treatment; (ii.) to permit the patient to live and to work comfortably by removing the ulcer-bearing area of the stomach and duodenum and to lower gastric acidity, by partial gastrectomy; (iii.) perforation; (iv.) repeated hæmatemesis; (v.) pyloric stenosis or hour-glass stomach are often treated by gastro-jejunostomy. The *operation* of choice for both gastric and duodenal ulcers is partial gastrectomy: this has an operative mortality of about 2 per cent. and removes the pyloric end and a variable amount of the body of the stomach. (Excision of the prepyloric region removes the source of the hormone " gastrin " which plays an important part in the secretion of gastric juice.) Other operations which are less frequently performed are pyloroplasty with vagotomy, or (for duodenal ulcer) gastro-duodenostomy with vagotomy. These give a rapid and permanent relief of ulcer symptoms in most cases, and abolish superacidity. Gastro-jejunostomy is performed when operative difficulties arise such as with extensive duodenal adhesions. Partial gastrectomy is often followed by " the dumping syndrome "; and in after years by an iron-deficiency anæmia, or sometimes a megalocytic anæmia when the B_{12} reserves of the body are exhausted.

§ 289. **The Dumping Syndrome** only occurs in patients who have recently had partial gastrectomy performed. It occurs at all ages and is met much more commonly in recent years because of the increasing use of this operation as treatment for a chronic peptic ulcer.

Symptoms occur in a large number of patients when they first get out of bed after this operation: in the great majority the symptoms disappear in the course of weeks, but a small number of patients have the symptoms for months or even years. Especially on standing up after a meal there is an urgent sense of great weakness, nausea, sweating and ready fatigue; these may be accompanied by palpitation, vomiting of bile and sometimes by diarrhœa and occasionally by the symptoms of hypoglycæmia. Loss of weight and, especially in women, an iron-deficiency anæmia with a vitamin deficiency may occur. The symptoms rapidly ameliorate on lying down immediately after a meal: an anxiety neurosis often develops.

Diagnosis.—The sudden onset of symptoms shortly after partial gastrectomy is characteristic. It is important to exclude other diseases which may have been overlooked—such as of the gall-bladder, or a hiatus hernia.

Etiology.—The cause is rapid emptying of a small stomach into the proximal loops of small intestine immediately after taking food. The symptoms are most common with a wide stoma and are much less severe, and often do not occur at all if a valvular opening between the stomach and small intestine is made, as with a Bilroth I or Lake anastomosis. Particularly with a diet of high carbohydrate content (which is rapidly digested to create a high osmotic pressure in the jejunal contents), there is a rapid flow of fluid from the blood plasma into the small intestine—which may well be the immediate cause of the trouble.

Prognosis.—Symptoms recede with the course of time, but in about 3 per cent. of patients they persist for years.

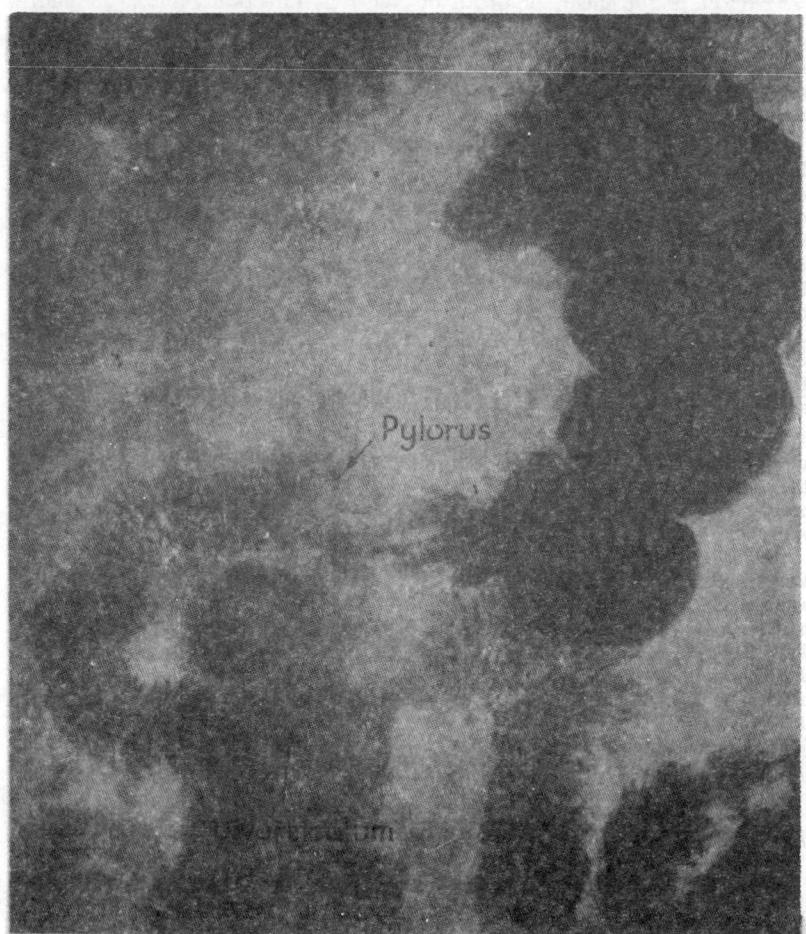

Fig. 96.—DUODENAL DIVERTICULUM; large mushroom-shaped diverticulum in the third part of duodenum.

Treatment.—Medical treatment is by giving a high-calorie diet with extra protein and fat but with a low carbohydrate content. Solid food should be dry and fluid should be taken between meals; great relief is afforded by lying down after all large meals. The patient is encouraged to gain weight. Iron-deficiency anæmia and vitamin deficiencies should be corrected. Tanner advises olive oil or trying xylocaine viscous 10 ml. before meals. In very obstinate cases the gastro-jejunal anastomosis may need to be undone and converted into a gastro-duodenal anastomosis.

§ 290. V*d*. A **Gastro-jejunal** or **Jejunal ulcer** may occur close to the site of the anastomosis of a gastro-enterostomy and sometimes after a partial gastrectomy: in almost every case superacidity of the gastric juices is still present. These ulcers are much more common in men than in women. The *symptoms* resemble those of duodenal ulcer but the hunger-pain occurs shortly after meals, is on the *left side* and may be referred to the flank and local tenderness is to the left of the umbilicus. X-ray or gastroscopy confirms the presence of an ulcer. Perforation may occur into the peritoneal cavity, but more usually the ulcer spreads into the gastro-colic omentum and if neglected a gastro-colic fistula may result. Hæmorrhage gives rise to hæmatemesis and melæna. Rest and diet as for peptic ulcer will usually relieve. Further surgery is often required with partial gastrectomy and abdominal vagotomy, and sometimes even almost total gastrectomy.

§ 291. V*e*. **Chronic Duodenal Ileus** occurs especially in visceroptotic patients who have lost weight or who lack abdominal muscle tone; it may follow a wasting illness, or a complicated childbirth. *Symptoms* are in many ways similar to those of a duodenal ulcer (which may co-exist). Pain 3 to 4 hours after food, distension, nausea and repeated vomiting occur. Anorexia, malaise, depression, migrainous headaches and other nervous symptoms may be present. *Diagnosis* is usually only possible by a barium meal, when the duodenum, lying to the right of the mid-line, is seen to be distended, to show to and fro peristalsis, and much delay in emptying. *Treatment.*— A period of rest in bed (with the foot of the bed raised, or lying on the face) is necessary. Abdominal exercises, massage and faradism to the abdominal muscles; small, frequent, nourishing meals, a supporting abdominal belt, and later, a change of environment help (and see § 252).

§ 292. VI. Duodenal Diverticula occur: (i.) in the first part of the duodenum in men as pouches formed by the contraction of adhesions from a previous ulcer; (ii.) in the second part (commonly in women) as a dilatation of the terminations of the pancreatic ducts; (iii.) in the third part as a result of a hernial protrusion through the wall (Fig. 96)—this type is often symptomless.

Symptoms.—(i.) The patient is usually past middle age; (ii.) the symptoms resemble those of chronic duodenal ulcer, but without periods of well-being; (iii.) attacks of severe bursting pain in the right hypochondrium may occur as the result of inflammation of the pouch; (iv.) hæmorrhage with sometimes severe melæna may occur. The *diagnosis* is made by X-ray examination. *Treatment* consists in giving a bland diet containing no hard or indigestible pieces; liquid paraffin or olive oil ((♏ 60) two or three times a day before meals, to which bismuth carbonate (gr. 15) may be added if there is pain. In severe cases surgery may be indicated. Good results have followed, but the operation is serious because the pouches are usually embedded in the head of the pancreas.

P AIN *is more or less* CONSTANT *with* DISTENSION *and* FLATULENCE; *the disease is probably* CANCER *or* DILATATION *of the* STOMACH.

VII. *The patient, who is in middle or advanced life, presents more* CACHEXIA *than could be accounted for by dyspepsia, and vomits from time to time "* COFFEE-GROUND *" material.* There is probable MALIGNANT DISEASE OF THE STOMACH. Gastric symptoms beginning in a patient of middle age or over should always be regarded as suspicious of cancer.

§ 293. Cancer of the Stomach (Synonym: Carcinoma ventriculi).— The clinical history rarely extends beyond one or two years. The *Early Symptoms* depend largely on the situation of the disease. (i.) Loss of appetite, especially for meat and bulky foods, is usual. (ii.) A sense of epigastric discomfort, flatulence and fullness occur during the meal, or immediately afterwards, and may be associated with belching foul-smelling gas. (iii.) Pain is not a prominent symptom in the early stages. It is situated in the epigastrium or back, radiates in different directions, and is usually accompanied by tenderness but no rigidity. It is increased rather than diminished by taking food, and is sometimes continuous and independent of meals. (iv.) Vomiting may occur early or late, and usually indicates obstruction in some part of the stomach. Generally it takes place some time after the ingestion of food, the interval depending on

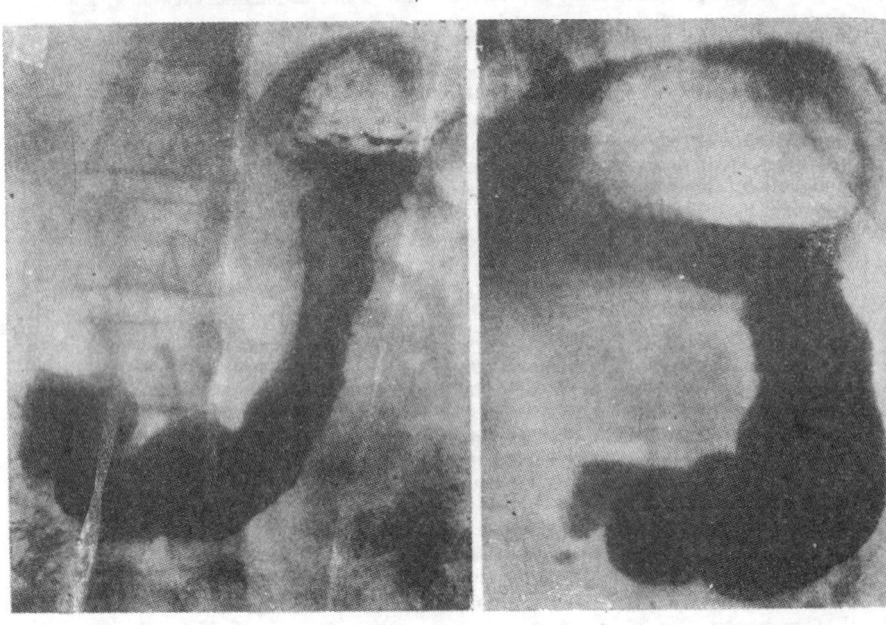

FIG. 97.—CANCER OF THE BODY OF THE STOMACH, with partial and with complete filling with barium sulphate emulsion. Note that the filled stomach does not expand.

the position of the lesion: thus, if at the cardiac end, the interval is short: if at the pylorus it may be hours after taking food. Sometimes the vomiting occurs every two or three days. An examination of the vomited matter often shows diminution or absence of hydrochloric acid and the presence of lactic acid: altered blood is often seen in the form of " coffee-grounds." (v.) Some degree of anæmia is present in practically all cases by the time advice is sought. Sometimes this is severe, and may be of megalocytic type as in pernicious anæmia. The E.S.R. is raised. (vi.) Loss of general strength and energy, and an insidious loss of weight, are present at an early stage in most cases. Less frequent early symptoms include: (vii.) Brisk hæmatemesis or melæna occurs in less than 5 per cent. of cases. (viii.) Sudden perforation is unusual. (ix.) Persistent diarrhœa associated with " a leather-bottle stomach " is sometimes met.

(x.) Acanthosis nigricans, unexplained phlebitis, polyneuritis and even Korsakoff's syndrome may be the first expression of the disease. *Late Symptoms:* (xi.) Cachexia becomes marked, anæmia prominent, and the sallowness of the skin may suggest pernicious anæmia or even jaundice. (xii.) The appetite fails, with profound anorexia and wasting. (xiii.) Vomiting occurs as a fairly constant sign: even the body of the stomach may be sufficiently obstructed to make the reception and passage of food difficult. (xiv.) A tumour is present sooner or later in two-thirds of the

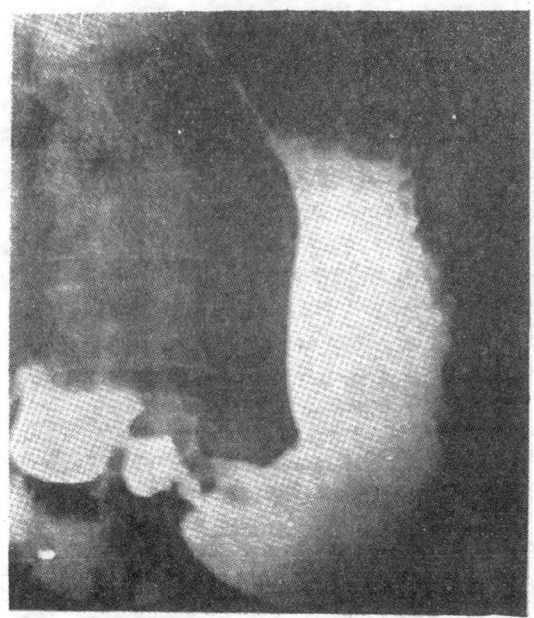

FIG. 98.—CANCER OF THE PREPYLORIC PORTION OF THE STOMACH.

cases. Transmitted aortic pulsation, and slight fullness or rigidity of the upper end of the right rectus, may be present without a palpable tumour. When the cancer is deposited in the pylorus, it may cause adhesions which prevent the tumour from coming forward. The great majority of gastric tumours come forward to the left of the middle line. It is usually stated that whereas hepatic tumours move, gastric tumours usually do not move with respiration: but this feature has many exceptions. One of greater importance is the alternate appearance and disappearance of the tumour. At first it is extremely mobile, but later it becomes fixed by adhesions: this is also the reason why perforation is rare. (xv.) Metastases occur in the pelvi-rectal pouch, in the ovary as a Krukenberg tumour, in the liver, or in the glands above the clavicles. (xvi.) Occasionally a gastro-colic fistula forms, producing intractable diarrhœa. In many cases, however, there are no symptoms referable to the stomach, and the diagnosis is only made at autopsy.

Diagnosis.—The disease should always be suspected when gastric symptoms first occur after the age of 40 years: and especially when there is only partial relief of the symptoms and the ulcer fails to heal on a strict ulcer regime. Radiology is essential if an early diagnosis is to be made. There is a characteristic irregular outline of the stomach wall, with rigidity, and defective or absent peristalsis. With cancer of the body, there is a tube-like stomach with food rushing through; in pyloric cancer there is obstruction and dilatation. Simple ulcers of the stomach are usually adjacent to the middle of the lesser curvature: many chronic ulcers in the prepyloric area and most ulcers in the fundus and adjacent to the greater curvature are malignant. A fractional test-meal may give a normal acid curve: often free HCl is absent, the total acidity is normal or low, and blood is present: organic acids (such as lactic acid) and sarcinæ are present when there is gastric dilatation. The fæces show occult blood persisting even when the patient is on a strict ulcer regime. Gastroscopy greatly aids diagnosis. If emaciation be rapid, and gastric symptoms resist treatment, cancer should be strongly suspected. *Dyspepsia* and *chronic gastritis* have pain directly related to food: for these, and *Simple ulcer* of the stomach, see Table XVII, p. 399. For Simple pyloric stricture, see Dilatation. *Tumour of the pylorus* or stomach has to be diagnosed from tumour in the neighbouring regions (§ 263). Thus a growth on the back of the stomach may resemble a kidney tumour. *Addison's disease* and other cachectic conditions must be excluded (Chapter XVI). *Pernicious anæmia* is sometimes strongly suggested by the colour of the patient, but in this disease there is not a corresponding amount of emaciation, and the blood-picture is different.

Etiology.—(1) Cancer of the stomach is more common in men. (2) It is rarely met with under 40, although cases occur under 30. (3) Simple ulcer and chronic gastritis appear to predispose. (4) There is an inherited tendency in 20 per cent. of cases.

The *Prognosis* is very grave. The duration is rarely longer than six to eighteen months after the first definite symptoms appear. Death is the invariable result unless surgical measures are adopted early. The symptoms upon which one relies most in the diagnosis in these cases, anorexia and emaciation, appear to be those which also best measure the longevity of the patient. Death generally takes place by inanition, but almost as often it occurs suddenly by the involvement of important structures, and it would be unwise to assume that because the patient does not waste he will not die soon. Partial gastrectomy is successful if undertaken early, but of those diagnosed by X-ray and judged fit for surgery, only about half are capable of removal. A clinical diagnosis without X-rays and test-meal is rarely made early enough; the chance for successful treatment lies in the early investigation of cases of dyspepsia.

Treatment.—Early surgical treatment affords most hope of success.

Apart from this the indications are to support the strength and relieve
the symptoms. The former may be accomplished by easily digestible or
predigested food (§ 296. XX), and by the use of pepsin and hydrochloric
acid. For the latter consult § 294, Dilatation. For the flatulence and
pain, give opium or morphia hypodermically.

VIII. *The patient presents symptoms of* CHRONIC INDIGESTION, *and
on physical examination there is* SPLASHING, *or the* AREA OF THE GASTRIC
RESONANCE *is increased, or there are* FOOD RESIDUES *before breakfast.* The
disease is probably GASTRIC DILATATION or ATONY.

§ 294. Gastric Dilatation may be due to two main causes, (a) Motor
Insufficiency or Hypotonia; (b) Pyloric Obstruction.

(a) GASTRIC HYPOTONIA occurs independently of pyloric obstruction.
There is delay in emptying the stomach, often associated with gastroptosis.
The condition is most common in women of poor physique, between the
ages of 30 and 50.

Symptoms.—(1) The patient is of the asthenic type with general loss
of muscle tone, and often backache. There is vague dyspepsia, or discomfort in the upper or mid-abdomen, which is usually worse after meals.
(2) Flatulence and aerophagy often accompany this dyspepsia. (3) True
pain is absent. (4) Prolonged lassitude follows a moderate-sized meal.
(5) A disinclination for food is often associated with some loss of weight
and constipation. (6) Depression and anxiety are often superadded.

Physical signs.—(1) The tone of the abdominal wall is poor. (2) Gastric
splashing or succussion can be demonstrated several hours after a meal
(§ 240). (3) Food residues can be detected six or more hours after a
previous meal, and in extreme cases a fractional test-meal will show food
residues in the fasting stomach juice next morning. (4) A barium meal
examination affords a ready method of detecting the degree of gastric
atony, and will measure the amount of gastric delay. (5) A fractional
test-meal usually shows a low acid content in the gastric juice, and delayed
emptying.

Diagnosis.—It is important to exclude organic disease in the body as
a whole and in the stomach by a thorough physical examination and
by a barium meal X-ray of the stomach. This will set a firm foundation
for treatment, and will be especially reassuring to the patient.

Etiology.—(1) Acute infectious diseases such as typhoid, influenza and
pneumonia contribute by virtue of their toxins. (2) Chronic states of
malnutrition such as are associated with anæmia, tuberculosis and neurasthenia predispose. (3) An ill-balanced diet, with irregular meals and
especially lack of vitamin B, leads to defective muscle tone. (4) Depression
and chronic anxiety states are potent predisposing factors. (5) There is
a definite correlation between the motor activity of the stomach and
the athletic capacity of the individual—lack of regular walking exercise is
undoubtedly detrimental.

Prognosis.—The disease is always troublesome and liable to relapse.

If diagnosed and treated early and thoroughly, and if contributing factors such as anæmia can be remedied, a cure is possible.

Treatment.—The indications are: (1) To relieve anxieties and improve the living conditions. (2) To keep the stomach as empty as possible. This may be done by diets No. I or III, § 296. (3) Give concentrated or predigested foods with very little fluid. Little carbohydrate, not at the same meal as animal food, is preferable. Give vitamin B in the form of wheat germ, a teaspoonful twice or thrice daily, or by weekly subcutaneous injection. (4) Promote digestion: *vide* § 283. (5) Adequate rest and sleep are essential: lying on the right side for ½–1 hour after the bigger meals/promotes emptying of the stomach. (6) A lower abdominal support may aid. (7) Regular exercise, and local abdominal exercises, massage and faradism help to improve the hypotonia.

(b) In PYLORIC OBSTRUCTION there is difficulty in emptying the stomach due to organic obstruction in the prepyloric canal or at the pyloric sphincter. Radiology has demonstrated two distinct types: in the first, due to temporary or minor pyloric obstruction, the vigorous peristalsis of the stomach keeps the stomach small and nearly empty. In the second type, with more obstruction, peristalsis is largely absent and the stomach remains as a dilated sac containing many pints of fluid and food residues.

Symptoms.—*Early Cases.* (1) Epigastric pain is present, due to exaggerated gastric peristalsis. It is often of colicky type (*vide* pyloric spasm, § 247). (2) Vomiting of relatively small amounts produces a vomitus containing partially digested food, with an acid reaction, but no bile. (3) Loss of weight and constipation mainly depend on the amount of vomiting. (4) There are symptoms of the cause of the obstruction, *e.g.*, duodenal ulcer, pyloric carcinoma. Physical examination may reveal (5) fullness in the left upper abdomen, (6) visible peristalsis (passing from left to right) in the epigastric region, which is more obvious after a meal and may be started by palpating or sharply flicking the abdominal wall. (7) A pyloric tumour may be felt. *Later Cases.* (1) There is vomiting, particularly towards the end of the day, or at intervals of two or three days, of acid, sour-smelling, frothy material, on which a scum forms on standing. The quantity vomited may amount to several pints. (2) Decomposition and fermentation in the stomach give autotoxic symptoms and the symptoms of chronic gastritis: (3) loss of weight and constipation are marked: (4) dehydration may ensue. (5) In severe cases, tetany and alkalosis are sequelæ. Physical examination reveals, in addition to the wasting, (6) a dry tongue and poor volume pulse: (7) the distended atonic stomach may form a prominence in the left upper abdomen: (8) through a stomach tube, a large residue may be withdrawn.

Diagnosis.—To diagnose the cause and extent of the obstruction, X-ray examination is essential. If there is much gastric retention, the stomach may have to be emptied by a stomach tube, to prevent the barium emulsion being unduly diluted, and so obscuring the examination.

Etiology.—The causes are (1) spasm of the pyloric sphincter secondary to a duodenal ulcer, and rarely as a reflex phenomenon due to other causes, *e.g.*, chronic appendicitis: (2) pyloric stenosis may occur from cicatrisation of a simple ulcer of the duodenal or prepyloric areas. (3) Obstruction due to a scirrhous cancer (§ 293). (4) Pressure from without, *e.g.*, enlarged glands in the portal fissure, or due to a band of adhesions, is rare. (5) For congenital hypertrophic pyloric stenosis, see § 271.

Treatment.—(1) The main indication is to treat the various causes of the condition. (2) Gastric lavage may be necessary as an adjunct to other treatment, or before operation: it may be carried out once or twice daily, and particularly in the evening. Normal saline or water is best: add bicarbonate of soda (gr. 60–Ōi) or hydrogen peroxide (℔ 30–Ōi) to dissolve any mucus present. (3) To prevent fermentation, the symptoms of which are very troublesome, carbolic acid (1 to 3 minims), thymol (5 gr.), or sodium sulphocarbolate (20 gr.), are given preferably in a tumbler of water between meals. After lavage, calomel ($\frac{1}{6}$ gr. t.i.d.) may be given with advantage. (4) Prevent dehydration by the administration of fluids rectally, subcutaneously or intravenously. (5) Inj. atropinæ gr. $\frac{1}{100}$, or tinct. belladonnæ, ℔ 10, 4–5 times a day, is most helpful in overcoming pyloric spasm. (6) Surgical treatment is essential in all cases of pyloric stenosis, of pyloric neoplasm producing obstruction, and in cases of pyloro-spasm not responding to medical measures.

§ 295. **Gastroptosis** is a condition in which the stomach has dropped from its position. The symptoms and signs are apt to be confused with Gastric Dilatation, with which it may be associated. The condition is often part of a general visceroptosis (§ 252), and is most clearly demonstrated by a barium meal. Intestinal stasis is usually also present, and hence an aggravated state of neurasthenia is frequently associated with the condition. *Treatment* is on the lines of visceroptosis (*q.v.*).

Dietaries and Invalid Foods

§ 296. Less food is required in old age than in youth, and with a sedentary life than with an active or outdoor one. For a person in health three meals a day are usually sufficient; but when a man is unable, from illness, to take more than a very small quantity at a time, he may require to take it more often. Dietetic errors are a fruitful source of dyspepsia and gastritis. Too frequent meals, habitual over-feeding, bolting the food, and irregularity of the meals will in time derange any stomach. A diet lacking or deficient in vitamins (especially vitamin B) leads to atony of the muscles of the digestive canal. Vitamin B is supplied by wheat germ, yeast (marmite) and wholemeal bread. Deficiency of food, and long restriction to the same kind of food, induce dyspepsia by affording no stimulus to excite the secretions; and a frequent cause of failure to relieve dyspepsia is disregard of this latter fact. In anæmic cases, starchy foods, especially potatoes and new bread, do not afford sufficient stimulus for the gastric functions; proteins such as tender and underdone meat are more readily digested. It is often a good rule to begin treatment by cutting down the amount rather than by entirely prohibiting the use of certain articles of diet. The frequent use of condiments, spices, strong tea, and of alcohol especially, leads to chronic gastritis; while dyspepsia is induced by imperfect mastication, bolting of meals, an idiosyncrasy to fats, too much fluid with meals, hard mental or physical work immediately after eating, too cold or too hot food, or food which is badly prepared. Excess of tobacco-smoking and constipation are certainly causes of dyspepsia. Greasy and fried foods are bad in dyspepsia, because the gastric juice cannot penetrate the coating of fat. Pastry and other rich carbohydrate foods are a source of dyspepsia, especially when eaten at the same meal as protein.

Without appropriate dietetic rules our best efforts may fail, especially in the treatment of gastro-intestinal disorders, and other diseases which depend on the proper elaboration and assimilation of food. A few specimen dietaries are therefore given.

I. The following menu is a guide for drawing up a diet for mild cases of dyspepsia or chronic gastritis: *Breakfast.*—Boiled or steamed sole, whiting or flounder; or a slice of crisp grilled bacon or a soft-boiled egg; a slice of dry toast or of bread (not new) and butter; marmalade jelly or honey. *Beverage.*—One cup of cocoa or of milk and water, sipped after eating. *Luncheon.*—Chicken or tender meat, with bread, creamed potato and a little tender, well-boiled vegetable, such as spinach, vegetable marrow or young French beans. For sweets and dessert, a plain biscuit or milk pudding. *Beverage.*—Half a tumbler of water sipped *after* eating. *Afternoon Tea.*—A cup of marmite, bouillon, or of weak tea with milk, and a slice of wholemeal bread and butter, sponge cake. *Supper* (two courses only).—Vegetable soup, fish of the kinds allowed for breakfast, without potatoes. Or a slice of tender bird or meat, such as saddle or loin of mutton, or the thick part of an underdone chop with crumbled stale bread; custard, junket or jelly, or a little well-stewed fruit. *Beverage.*—Half a tumbler of water, with from one to two tablespoonfuls of spirit if desired.

Condiments and stimulants are good in some forms of dyspepsia, but must be avoided in chronic gastritis, as tending to irritate the mucous membrane. The patient should abstain from salted and cured meats, sweets, pastry, raw vegetables, cheese (except cream cheese), fried foods, strong tea and coffee.

II. In **Superacidity** fried foods, game, vinegar, jam, condiments and alcohol should be avoided. The food should consist of soft, well-cooked, finely cut up or minced fish, meat or poultry, eggs and cream cheese; fats, olive oil if it can be taken, plain butter not made into sauces, ice cream; mashed potato, rice, macaroni; weak tea—not coffee—or plain water, preferably after meals. Weak meat or vegetable soups may be allowed. Milk is often difficult. If there is delay in the stomach, meals should be taken dry. Sometimes it is necessary to give food more frequently than three times a day. The patient should not sit at an ordinary table with others eating appetising food. *Early Morning.*—Weak tea and milk, without sugar, or tumbler of hot water. *Breakfast.*—Eggs (boiled, poached or scrambled), cold ham or bacon, crisp toast, plenty of unsalted butter; and a cup of weak tea after the food is taken. *Lunch.*—Fish or well-cooked meat which may be minced, little mashed potato, rice or macaroni; suet or baked castle or stiff milk pudding, toast, butter and cream, tumbler of water after food. *Tea.*—Cup of weak tea with milk and no sugar, little bread and butter or rusk and butter. *Supper* as lunch, with addition of fruit juice or jelly or purée. Half to one ounce of olive oil half an hour before lunch and supper, if it can be taken.

III. **Peptic ulcer.** SIPPY DIET (modified). *First week,* or until the patient has been free of symptoms for at least 3 days: 3 oz. milk, citrated milk, milk and cream, or with a raw egg stirred in, each 2 hours while awake and an extra feed may be given at night. *Second week.*—Breakfast: 1 egg, 1 oz. toast, ⅓ oz. butter, 4 oz. milk. Mid-morning: glass of milk and rusk. Noon dinner: 2 oz. minced or pounded beef or chicken, 1 oz. toast, ¼ oz. butter. 2 p.m.: 1 egg in 3 oz. milk. 4 p.m. tea: 1 oz. thin bread and butter, without crusts, 3 oz. milk. 7 p.m. supper: 1 oz. well-boiled rice or macaroni, ¼ oz. butter, 1 oz. toast, 3 oz. milk. 9 p.m.: 6 oz. of Benger's, Allenbury's, etc. A tablespoonful of olive oil at 11.30 a.m. and 6.30 p.m. *Third to fifth weeks.*—Breakfast: egg (poached, boiled or scrambled), or steamed or boiled fish, toast, butter, milk. Mid-morning: milk and biscuit. Noon: chicken or mince, mashed potato, dry toast, butter, boiled milk pudding. 2 p.m.: milk or egg and milk. Tea: toast or bread and butter, sponge cake, milk. 7 p.m.: steamed fish, toast and butter, macaroni or vermicelli; milk pudding, junket or custard. Bedtime: milk, Benger's, etc. Then a *post-ulcer diet.*—Breakfast: porridge, fish, cold fat ham, egg, toast, butter, cream, flavoured milk or weak tea. Dinner: chicken, tender mutton, lamb or beef, potato, sieved green or mashed root vegetables, milk or light steamed pudding, cream, cream cheese and biscuit. Tea: bread and butter, sponge cake, milk and water or weak tea. Supper: fish, chicken or sweetbread, potato, sieved green vegetables, macaroni, milk pudding or milk shape, toast, butter, cream. In these diets with fresh milk, there is plenty of vitamin C; to avoid deficiency a little diluted orange juice or tab. ascorbic acid (B.P.) may be given each day. On the whole, fruit is better avoided for several weeks, and should be as a purée, or as fruit juice alone, or in jelly.

MEULENGRACHT DIET. Two-hourly feeds with four light meals a day. *Early morning*—milk or milky tea. *Breakfast*—strained oatmeal porridge and milk, eggs, rusks, biscuits or bread (toasted), butter. *Mid-morning*—milk with rusk or biscuit, or milk soup with vegetable stick. *Mid-day*—minced chicken, rabbit, beef, mutton, pounded fish, or soufflé, brains, tripe or sweetbread; mashed potato, sieved spinach or greens or mashed carrot, parsnip or turnip; junket or milk pudding. *Tea*—milky tea, bread or biscuits, butter, jelly or honey. *Supper*—as at mid-day. *Bedtime*—milk with biscuit, Ovaltine, Benger's or other invalid food. Milk in the night if awake.

IV. **Diet for Cholecystitis** and protective diet in convalescence from infective hepatitis. Adequate protein and carbohydrate are needed; fats should be restricted, only butter and milk fats being allowed. Foods to be *avoided* are: Fried foods, twice-cooked meats, made-up dishes, fried fats; pork, sausages, hard meat or gristle, liver, pastry, ice-cream, cream, cream cheeses; baked beans, nuts, sultanas; wholemeal bread, Ryvita or Vita-weat. *The patient can eat:* Toasted breakfast cereals, toast, white or brown bread, plain cake; butter (sparingly); white fish (sole, plaice, whiting or turbot); tender veal, lamb, beef, mutton, ham, tongue (not fatty); chicken, poultry of any kind if well cooked; soups without hard vegetable matter; asparagus, heads of cauliflower or broccoli, young brussels sprouts; French beans, young peas; very ripe pears, juice of grapes, tomatoes, baked apple, oranges or grapefruit juice, bananas (avoid skins and pips); small portions of mashed potato, rice, ground rice, sago, tapioca puddings; porridge in small quantities; honey, marmalade, golden syrup; weak tea or coffee. It is better to drink between meals rather than with meals. Casilan or another casein hydrolysate, methionine or other amino-acid preparation may be added.

V. **Constipation.**—The first thing in the morning drink a tumbler of plain water, hot or cold, or eat an apple, pear, bunch of grapes, banana, orange, etc. *Breakfast.*—Coffee, not too strong, with a little milk; stone-ground flour or wholemeal bread with plenty of butter, honey or treacle; or well-cooked oatmeal, Kellogg's All-Bran or wheat germ, with cream or treacle. *Lunch.*—Sardines or olives in oil; fish, chicken or roast meat; vegetables, greens and salad; cream cheese, wholemeal bread and butter; fresh or stewed fruit with cream. *Tea.*—Coffee and milk, wholemeal bread, butter. *Dinner.*—Vegetable soup, fish or egg dish, vegetables and salads; suet pudding; fruit, wholemeal bread and butter. Lactose may be used instead of ordinary sugar. Cultures of *B. acidophilus* in milk can be taken once or twice a day. Fluids may be taken freely with meals, and half to one ounce of liquid paraffin or emulsion night and morning for a limited time. Some do better with bassorin or agar-agar preparations, psyllium or other vegetable seeds.

VI. Diet for Obesity (§ 18).

—A *simple Reducing Diet* is as follows:—

The following articles must not be taken: butter, cream, ice-cream, fat of meat, duck, pork, sausages; fried foods or twice-cooked foods of any kind; salmon or herrings; cheese, pies, cakes, bread, sugar or tinned fruit; beer.

The patient can eat: lean meat, lean of ham, and tongue; eggs; boiled or steamed fish (except above); moderate quantity of potatoes; fresh fruit, including grapefruit; fresh green foods *ad lib.*; salads, cooked green foods, vegetable soups; Ryvita and Vita-weat biscuits; sugarless jam or marmalade; $\frac{1}{2}$ pint of milk allowed daily; saccharin allowed for sweetening.

Strict Reducing Diet (Calorie value 1,000). Foods to be *avoided* are: sweets, chocolates, sugar, potatoes, cakes, pastry, puddings, jam, marmalade, honey, syrup, fruits preserved in syrup, fried foods, sausages, thickened soups and sauces, beer, salad oil or dressing. Salt should be taken sparingly. *The patient can eat: Breakfast.* —Milk 2$\frac{1}{2}$ oz. for tea or coffee, no sugar, bread 1 oz., butter or margarine $\frac{1}{4}$ oz., 1 egg boiled or poached, fruit or tomatoes 4 oz. Alternatives: replace 1 egg by one of the following in the quantity stated:—grilled lean bacon 1 oz.; kidney 2 oz.; baked kipper 3 oz.; baked haddock 3 oz. plus margarine $\frac{1}{4}$ oz.; herring baked in vinegar 2 oz.; Bemax 1 oz. with milk from day's ration. *Lunch.*—Lean mutton, veal, ham 2 oz.; or chicken, rabbit, liver, corned beef 2 oz.; or tinned salmon, pilchards or sardines (no oil) 2 oz.; carrots, onions, swedes, turnips or leeks 5 oz.; any fresh fruit or melon 5 oz. *Tea.*—Bread 1 oz.; butter $\frac{1}{4}$ oz.; milk 2$\frac{1}{2}$ oz. for tea (no sugar). *Dinner.*—White fish or tripe or sweetbread 4 oz.; or lean meat or liver (as for lunch) 1$\frac{1}{2}$ oz.; or cheese 1 oz.; any fresh fruit or melon 4 oz.; bread 1 oz. and butter $\frac{1}{4}$ oz. At *bedtime.*—Milk 5 oz. Saccharin may be used in tea or for cooking.

VII. Diet in Nephritis.

(A) **Acute.**—A preliminary period of almost complete renal rest must be given, especially when anorexia or nausea is present. *Diet: Stage I.* 1$\frac{1}{2}$ pints of fluid a day; water, barley water, Imperial drink, orangeade or lemonade with glucose added in the proportion of 4–6 oz. per pint, grape-juice or tomato-juice, and toffee if acceptable. This is continued until the hæmaturia has diminished, the blood pressure has fallen and the "critical diuresis" set in—usually a matter of three to four days; after this time the diet may be increased to *Stage II.* 2–2$\frac{1}{4}$ pints of fluid a day—milk $\frac{1}{2}$ pint, weak tea, barley water, glucose-orangeade or lemonade, Imperial drink, 1 orange, 1 small tomato, grapes, stewed fruit, 2 oz. of wholemeal bread with unsalted butter, 2 oz. of potatoes, porridge, milk puddings, honey, marmalade, jam and $\frac{1}{2}$ oz. of cream. (Fruit and vegetables to count as an equivalent weight of water.) After ten to fourteen days it is usually possible to increase further to *Stage III.* 3 pints of fluid a day—milk 1 pint, weak tea, barley water, orangeade or lemonade, grapefruit, oranges, grapes, tomatoes, *ad lib.*, stewed fruit, milk puddings, cereal foods such as grapenuts, porridge, bread, cakes, fresh butter, cream, honey, jam, marmalade, steamed fish, potatoes, greens and salads. *Foods to be entirely forbidden:* Soups, Bovril, beef-tea, liver, brains, sweetbread, alcohol, acid foods such as vinegar, and spices. *Foods to be avoided until œdema has disappeared:* Salt (in cooked food and at table). *To be avoided until blood pressure lowered:* Meat, bacon, ham, poultry and salt.

(B) **Subacute Nephritis** *with Œdema.*—The total fluid intake, including fruit and vegetables, should not exceed the daily output of urine, but cannot be reduced below 35 oz. a day. Adexolin, 2 capsules, should be taken daily. Salt-free bread or same toasted 6 oz.; white fish, preferably fresh-water trout 6 oz.; mutton, veal, lamb, lean ham or chicken 10 oz.; skimmed milk flavoured with weak tea or coffee (1 pint a day); sugar, honey, jam, marmalade *ad lib.*, rice or other cereal 1 oz., made into milk pudding; flaked cereals *ad lib.*, grapes, tomatoes, apples, oranges, stewed fruit 10 oz.; salt-free butter $\frac{1}{2}$ oz. a day. *Approximate Values*—Protein content, 150 G.; fat, 45 G.; carbohydrate, 300 G.; NaCl, 2·5–3·0 G.; calories, 2,100.

Karell Diet.—*Days* 1–7.—Milk, 7 oz., at 8 a.m., 12 noon, 4 p.m. and 8 p.m. Total salt is 1·3 G. *Day* 8.—Add at 10 a.m. a softly-cooked egg and one slice of toast. Total salt is 1·78 G. *Day* 9.—Add 2 oz. vegetables such as asparagus, celery, cauliflower or carrot, and two teaspoonfuls of cornflour to the milk taken at noon, to form milk soup. Add one slice of toast at 4.30 p.m. Total salt is 1·89 G. *Days* 10–12.— Add one egg, 1 oz. rice (weighed raw) and 2 oz. vegetables. Total salt is 2·41 G.

(C) **Chronic Nephritis** *with Blood Urea over* 100 *milligrammes per cent.*—Total fluid intake, 3–5 pints per day: Weak tea, barley water, lemonade, orangeade, grapefruit juice. Also glucose in the proportions of 4–6 oz. to the pint, with grape juice and tomato juice; cream, ½–1 oz. daily. After three or four days of such a regime, usually the blood urea has fallen to lower limits and then a higher protein diet should be given and a greater fluid intake should be possible.

Chronic Nephritis *with Blood Urea over* 80 *milligrammes per cent.*—Total fluid intake, 3–5 pints of fluid daily, consisting of weak tea or coffee, milk (½ pint), lemonade, orangeade; bread or biscuits (5 oz.), butter (2 oz.), porridge or cereal foods such as flaked wheat or flaked rice (2 oz.), milk puddings, cream (1 oz.), cake; jam, honey or marmalade (½ oz.), sugar (2 oz.), green vegetables and salads *ad lib.*; potatoes (5 oz.), fish, meat or chicken (2 oz.), or one egg. Approximate content: Protein, 37 G.; fat, 69 G.; carbohydrate, 212 G.; calories, 1,600. Unrestricted Foods: Green vegetables, salads, fruits, sugar, honey, jam, arrowroot, butter.

Chronic Nephritis *with Blood Urea between* 40 *and* 80 *milligrammes per cent.*— Total fluid intake, 3–3½ pints a day (*i.e.*, average normal amount). Bread or cake or biscuits (10 oz.); milk (½ pint); white fish (4 oz.) or one egg; meat or chicken (3 oz.). Unrestricted Foods: Green vegetables, potatoes, salads, fruit, sugar, honey, jam, marmalade, oatmeal, cereal foods such as flaked wheat or flaked rice or other cereal preparations, milk puddings, butter, cream. Approximate protein value = 72 G.; approximate caloric value, 2,200. *Foods to be avoided:* Condiments, spices, meat extracts, brains, liver, sweetbreads.

VIII. **Diabetic Diets.**—It is no longer considered necessary to weigh the amounts of protein and fat at each meal, but it is still very important that the diabetic patient should consume a fixed quantity of carbohydrate each day, the amount for an adult varying between 100–200 G. (with averages between 150–180 G.) daily. Suitable systems (based on the Lawrence line ration scheme) are as follows:—

(A) For **overweight diabetics**, the weight must be reduced by a diet low in calories (usually 1,000) and not more than 100 G. of carbohydrate each day. This is continued until the desired reduction in weight has been obtained. Such a diet is set out above (p. 414). After the desired weight reduction has been produced, a diet as for mild diabetics should be followed so as to prevent a relapse.

(B) For **mild diabetics** without obesity a diet of 120–160 G. of carbohydrate daily is usually satisfactory, the protein and fat being rather small " average " helpings which need not be weighed. Lawrence's Simple Diabetic Diet is:—

FOODS FORBIDDEN, unless specially allowed, are sugar, jams, sweets, flour, cakes, pastry, puddings, tinned and dried fruits, figs, dates, grapes, pineapple, beer, stout, cider, port, sweet minerals (lemonade, ginger-beer, ginger-ale, tonic water), sausages, " diabetic preparations "—bread, biscuits, sweets.

FOODS TO BE TAKEN ONLY IN THE EXACT AMOUNTS ALLOWED (below) are: bread or toast and biscuits, porridge, rice and tapioca, potatoes, peas and beans, fresh fruit, milk. Do not use sugar, flour or breadcrumbs in cooking.

FOODS ALLOWED are *Liquids*: tea, coffee, water, soda, fresh lemonade, clear soups, beef-tea, Bovril, etc. Consult a doctor about alcohol if wanted. *Seasoning:* saccharin for sweetening, salt, pepper, vinegar, mustard, oil, unsweetened pickles. *Protein and Fats*: small or average helpings of animal foods (fresh or tinned), such as beef, veal, mutton, pork, bacon, ham, liver, kidney, tripe, etc., poultry, game, fish, shell-fish, cheese. *Fats*, such as meat fats, butter, margarine, cream, olive oil. *Carbohydrates:* unlimited amounts of these VEGETABLES—asparagus, artichokes (green), brussels sprouts, cabbage, cauliflower, celery, chicory, cress, cucumber, egg-plant, endive, French beans, greens, horse-radish, Kohlrabi, lettuce, marrow, mushrooms, olives, onions, pawpaw, pumpkin, radishes, scarlet runners, seakale, spinach, tomato, turnips. Also unlimited amounts of these FRUITS—red currants, cranberries, lemons, stewing gooseberries and rhubarb. *In addition*, one helping (5 G. carbohydrate) twice a day of *one* of the following:—Three tablespoonfuls of carrots, Jerusalem artichokes, leeks, swedes; these stewed fruits, apples, apricots, blackberries, black currants, cherries, damsons, greengages, pears, plums; or ½ grapefruit; or 12 cherries, or small slice of melon, or 12 almonds, or 6 walnuts or 6 brazil nuts.

The following EXACT PORTIONS (each about 10 G. carbohydrate) must be accurately weighed or measured:

Portions.

Breakfast	..	..	..	..	..	..
Lunch ..	..	..	..—	..	..	..
Tea ..	..	..	..	..	..	..
Supper ..	..	..	..	..	..	..

Total 11–15 a day.

Each of the following is One Portion (10 G. carbohydrate).

Bread (⅔ oz.), size of measure supplied.[1]
Potato (size of hen's egg).
Peas or beans, cooked, 2 dessertspoons.
Oatmeal, rice or tapioca, 1 dessertspoon, measured uncooked.
Milk, teacup (7 oz.).
2 plain or semi-sweet biscuits.

1½ sections Vita-weat, Ryvita.
3 tablespoons any breakfast cereal.
¼ lb. apple or pear.
2 oranges (small), peaches or plums.
Small banana: 6 small prunes.
Ovaltine, Horlick's, Benger's, 2 teaspoons.
Jam, honey, marmalade, 1 teaspoon.

(C) For **severe diabetics** who require either two doses of an insulin preparation or a single injection of one or two varieties of insulin each day, the carbohydrate intake is 120–180 G. a day and some authorities prefer to give a more rigid intake of protein and fat (10 red lines on the Lawrence Scheme, equivalent to 75 G. of protein and 90 G. of fat). Most physicians, however, advise *small helpings* of protein and fat with strict attention to the consumption of carbohydrate. The scheme for mild diabetics (B above) is suitable, but six meals a day are necessary, so that the following EXACT PORTIONS (each of 10 G. carbohydrate) must be accurately weighed or measured:—

Portions.

Breakfast	..	..	..	..	..	..
11 a.m.	..	..	..	..	..	..
Lunch ..	..	..	..	..	..	..
Tea	..	..	..	..	..	..
Supper ..	..	..	..	..	..	..
Bedtime	..	..	..	..	..	..

Total 12–18 a day distributed in accordance with the type of insulin injected (§ 423 and Table XXIV).

IX. **Milk Diet.**—The basis of the diet is 8–10 oz. milk every 3 hours from 7 a.m. to 10 p.m., with additional feeds if the patient is awake in the night. The milk may be hot or cold, citrated, junket, or mixed with 2 oz. barley water or lime water, one tablespoonful of cream, or flavoured with vegetable soup stock, tea, coffee, cocoa, Ovaltine, ground rice, sago, or one of the invalid foods, if there is no special contraindication. The addition of 1 oz. bread, three rusks or plain biscuits, and ⅓ oz. of butter for some meals is allowed.

X. **Predigested Foods** are indicated in dilatation of the stomach, cancer, and advanced cases of chronic gastritis. Benger's *Liquor Pancreaticus* is the usual ferment employed, because the pancreas contains both a proteolytic and a diastatic ferment. *Taka-diastase* is a valuable aid in the digestion of farinaceous foods The patient takes it with his food at the commencement of the meal.

---

[1] Obtainable from Messrs. H. K. Lewis & Co. Ltd., 136 Gower Street, London, W.C.1.

1. *Peptonised Milk.*—One pint new milk.   One tube Fairchild's Zymine peptonising powder.   Five oz. cold water.   Method: Mix peptonising powder with cold water, add to milk heated to 105° F; keep at this temperature for the time ordered (5 to 30 minutes).   Bring rapidly to the boil to stop peptonising process.

2. *Peptonised Beef-Tea.*—Half a pound of finely minced lean beef is mixed with a pint of water and 20 gr. of sod. bicarb.   This is simmered for an hour.   When it has cooled down to a lukewarm temperature, the peptonising powder is added.   The mixture is then set aside for three hours, and occasionally stirred.   At the end of this time the liquid portions are decanted and boiled for a few seconds.

3. *Other foods* can be similarly prepared.

4. *Nutrient Enemata.*—Glucose alone is of practical use.

XI. **Beef-Tea.**—Cut up a pound of lean beef into pieces the size of dice; put it into a covered jar with 2 pints of cold water and a pinch of salt.   Let it warm gradually, and simmer for a couple of hours, care being taken that *it does not boil.*

XII. **Improved Beef-Tea.**—Three-quarters of a pound of steak, scraped or passed through a mincing machine, and pounded; ¾ pint of cold water; one piece of sugar, one pinch of salt, one teaspoonful of tapioca; simmered for three hours.

XIII. **Artificial Protein Foods.**—Beef-tea and other meat preparations do not contain the nutritive constituents of meat, except in small quantities, but may be useful as stimulants of gastric secretion.   *Peptonised albumin* (or peptonised meat) is more nourishing, but the taste of peptone is very bitter and nasty.   The *albumoses* are intermediate between albumin and peptone.   They are freely soluble, tasteless and readily digested and absorbed.   *Plasmon* is another artificial protein food.   It is prepared from milk, and contains casein in a soluble form.   It is a nutriment of some value.   *Casein hydrolysate* can be given by mouth or intravenously.

XIV. **Diet for Oxaluria** (after Poulton).   Figures in brackets indicate oxalic acid content in mg. per cent.   Foods with high oxalic acid content must be *avoided.* Tea (1,380); cocoa powder (640); chocolate (90); sorrel (2,000); spinach (830); rhubarb (410); dry figs (100); beetroot and potatoes (40); parsnips (39); spring onions (55); red and black currants (70); bilberries and raspberries (42).   Foods to be *taken sparingly* are: broad beans (39); French beans (20); lettuce (30); green peas (36); oranges (28); gooseberries (27).   A smaller amount of oxalic acid is found in endive, tomatoes, strawberries, plums, carrots and beetroot.   It is advisable also to avoid foods with high purine content.

XV. **Diet for Gout.**—A low purine diet is essential: it is also advisable to exclude foods with a high oxalate content.   Articles to be *avoided* are: chocolate, cocoa, strong coffee and tea, port, sherry, gin, burgundy, beer and stout, barley, oatmeal, shell-fish, most meat—especially kidneys, liver, sausages, sweetbread, fish roe, caviare, rich sauces and pastry.   Also broad beans, brussels sprouts, butter beans, haricot beans, lentils, peas, radishes, spinach, sorrel, raspberries and rhubarb.   Foods *taken sparingly* include: simply cooked meat or fish, bacon rashers, mutton, poultry, ham, boiled ox tongue, oysters.   Also cider, whisky and brandy.   Fats can be taken in small amount: butter, cheese, cream, dripping, suet.   Foods *allowed* include: milk, bread, eggs, milk puddings, fruit and vegetables (other than above), nuts, cereals, sugar, jam, honey, marmalade.

XVI. **Diet for Tropical Sprue** (Hamilton Fairley).—*High Protein, Low Fat, Low Carbohydrate Diet.*—A gluten-free flour is also useful.

Breakfast (8 *to* 9 *a.m.*).—Lightly boiled or poached eggs; underdone lean chop or steak; filleted, boiled or steamed fish—whiting, sole, plaice, haddock; thin toast, and butter in moderation; weak tea; stewed fruit: apples, rhubarb; honey or jam in small quantity; also butter.   11 *a.m.*—½ pint of milk, if desired, and if it agrees.

Lunch.—Chicken or vegetable soup; underdone grilled steak; roast or boiled chicken; liver cooked in various ways; cold beef or mutton, but fat not to be eaten.   Vegetables: spinach, marrow, cauliflower, French beans, celery, young peas, boiled onions; salad of lettuce and tomato; boiled potatoes in small quantity. Custard, junket, milk jellies, and jelly with fruit, such as bananas, etc. Baked apples. Small quantity of cream allowed. Fresh fruits such as oranges, Canary bananas, pears, peaches, grapes, raspberries, strawberries, melons, grapefruit. Rusks or toast allowed. *Tea,* 4 *p.m.*—Weak China tea, Madeira cake or sponge cake, dry toast and butter, Marie or water biscuits. *Dinner,* 7 *p.m.*—Chicken, rabbit, brains, sweetbread, tripe, cold lean meat; lettuce and tomato salad or other vegetables mentioned, but no potatoes; custard, junket, baked apple, stewed fruit or fruit in jelly, and a small quantity of fresh cream; rusks or toast and butter allowed.

Articles to be avoided.—Avoid overdone and twice-cooked meat and articles fried or cooked in fat. Condiments, like pepper, mustard, chillies, sauces, chutneys, curries and spiced food. Game, duck and fat fish, such as salmon, trout, mackerel and herrings. Fresh bread, grease, fat, salad oil dressings and sauces of all kinds, suet puddings, cakes with icing, raisins and pastry. Sweets and chocolates. Alcoholic drinks and mineral waters.

Note.—Smoking in moderation is allowed once convalescence has been established.

XVII. **Diet for Idiopathic Steatorrhœa and Cœliac Disease** (Gluten-free). The glutens of wheat and rye have an inhibitory effect on the absorption of other food-substances, of iron and the vitamins. The protein deficiency is made up by adding animal protein. A useful diet is:—*Breakfast.*—Oatmeal porridge, cornflakes, puffed rice with milk, egg, bacon, haddock, kedgeree, gluten-free bread or biscuit, butter, marmalade or preserves; tea or coffee with milk and sugar. *Lunch.*—Soup from bone or vegetable stock, fresh meat, liver, kidney, fish or ham, fresh vegetables, fresh or tinned fruit, sago or rice pudding, custard from custard powder, jelly, ice-cream, blancmange and fruit. *High-tea.*—Omelette, bacon and egg, herring or meat, toasted gluten-free bread,[1] cheese, butter, savoury, greens or preserves, cakes or biscuits made from gluten-free flour. *Bedtime.*—Milk with tea or cocoa, fruit juice. Supplements of ascorbic acid 30 mg. daily, vitamin B by mouth daily or by injection twice a week, folic acid, vitamin D and ferrous sulphate are needed.

XVIII. **Diet in fevers** should consist mainly of nourishing fluids, water, barley-water, orangeade or lemonade with glucose (1–2 oz. per pint), lemon and barley-water, weak tea and other fruit juices allowed *ad lib.*, with milk ($\frac{1}{2}$–2 pints daily), egg and milk, Oxo, Bovril, meat or chicken broth, calves-foot jelly. Especially if there is high fever or much sweating, the total fluid intake should be 3–5 pints daily. Milk may be diluted with half to two-thirds of water, soda-water or barley-water. If curds are passed, the milk may be peptonised, or sodium citrate may be added in the proportion of gr. 2 to the ounce of milk. Lime water may be used instead if diarrhœa be present. If milk is not well tolerated, whey or cream may be given, or the yolks of eggs or egg-flip. Where intestinal infection is present, meat extracts and jellies are better avoided. Some invalid foods are given below. Iced water is agreeable, but generally increases the thirst.

XIX. **Milk, Egg and Brandy.**—Scald some new milk, but do not let it boil. Put it into a jug, and the jug into a dish of boiling water. When the surface looks filmy, it is sufficiently done, and should be put away in a cool place in the same vessel. When quite cold, beat up a fresh egg with a fork in a tumbler, with a lump of sugar; beat quite to a froth, add a dessertspoonful of brandy and fill the tumbler with scalded milk.

XX. **Whey.**—Into a vessel of warm milk put sufficient quantity of rennet to cause curdling, and strain off the liquid, which is then ready for use.

XXI. **Imperial Drink.**—Acid potassium tartrate 60 grains, oil of lemon 3 drops, flavoured with sugar or saccharine 1 grain, and dissolved in a pint of boiling water.

---

[1] Gluten-free flour is made by Energen Foods Co. Ltd., Willesden, London, N.W.10.

CHAPTER XI

THE INTESTINAL CANAL

Anatomy and Physiology.—The intestinal canal is 25 to 30 feet in length. Excluding the duodenum, which measures only 10 inches, the upper four-fifths forms the small intestine and the lower one-fifth the large intestine. The small intestine consists of a proximal portion, the jejunum, and a distal portion, the ileum: the digestive processes commenced in the mouth, stomach and duodenum continue throughout the small intestine, the churning or segmental movements ensuring an intimate mixture of the food with the digestive juices and the subsequent absorption of the products so produced. The main process of digestion and absorption occurs in the jejunum so that, for example, glucose and most of the fat is absorbed in the first 3–4 feet; this activity of the jejunum is made possible by the mucous membrane being thrown into large circular folds and also by the presence of enormous numbers of minute villi on the surface. The activity of this area is shown by the replacement of its epithelium each 36–48 hours by new epithelial cells produced in the bottom of the crypts of Lieberküln, the cells ascending the villi and being lost at the tips. Following these major processes of absorption short peristaltic waves transfer the liquid remainder gradually to the ileum. Corresponding to the lesser importance of the ileum in the process of absorption, the crescentic folds gradually disappear and the villi are much smaller in size. Even so important substances (such as Vitamin B 12) are absorbed almost entirely in the ileum.

Under the influence of peristaltic waves which take place at varying intervals, the contents of the small intestine slowly fill the cæcum and ascending colon; in those with an ileostomy it is found that approximately 2 litres of material of a thin porridgy consistency pass through the ileo-cæcal valve each 24 hours. In the ascending colon a considerable absorption of water and of sodium chloride takes place; this causes the contents of the transverse and descending colon to be much more solid. Further peristalsis transfers the contents of the proximal colon into the middle and lower portions of the large intestine where the greater part of the remaining soluble constituents are absorbed. The residue forms the fæcal contents of the sigmoid colon: these are evacuated once or twice daily by a mass reflex (the gastro-colic reflex) through the rectum during defæcation.

The importance of the small intestine to the human economy is shown by the fact that whereas persons can live a healthy life after the complete surgical removal of the stomach or of the large intestine, life is considerably shortened if more than a relatively small portion of the jejunum or ileum is removed. Although the small intestine is so inaccessible to examination, great advances are being made by investigation of the X-ray appearances, by sampling the contents via a tube lying at different levels and by removing small areas of the surface for microscopic examination. Examination of the stools, by the naked eye and by chemical and bacteriological methods, is necessary in any suspected disease of the intestine and in many cases of simple malnutrition.

A striking feature about diseases of the intestines is the disproportionate amount of prostration which accompanies them. When a patient is attacked by a slight but sudden diarrhœa or abdominal pain, the feeling of exhaustion, which in some cases may amount almost to collapse, is out of all proportion to the local disorder. This disproportionate degree of prostration or collapse is especially seen in early life, when " diarrhœa " is found to be one of the chief causes of death in children under two years of age. Again, among the acute specific fevers fatal collapse and prostration often occur in those in which the chief lesion is in the intestinal canal —in cholera, dysentery, and typhoid fever. This may be due in part to the large vascular bed in the abdominal cavity, and to the extensive surface through which toxins can be absorbed.

PART A. SYMPTOMATOLOGY

§ 301. The cardinal symptoms of intestinal disorder are ABDOMINAL PAIN, DIARRHŒA, CONSTIPATION and INTESTINAL DISCOMFORT.

ABDOMINAL PAIN is frequently present, especially in the more acute conditions, and may be due to many causes arising within the abdomen (see § 241). DIARRHŒA and CONSTIPATION are dealt with in Part C.

INTESTINAL DISCOMFORT may be due to colic, peritoneal pain or strangulation, or distension with wind, accompanied by borborygmi. It is a marked feature in COLOSPASM, which occurs in two conditions: (i.) reflex as from adhesions after appendicitis or operation, with gall-stones, and in the early stages of diverticulosis; (ii.) with worry, tense brain work and anxiety, associated with depression (visceral neurosis) (§ 313).

The GENERAL or REMOTE symptoms, such as loss of appetite from toxæmia and discomfort, are sometimes (especially in acute cases) of a very severe character, in view of the profound PROSTRATION which is associated with some intestinal disorders. PYREXIA is not usually a marked feature (see § 239). In the more chronic forms of intestinal disease EMACIATION is apt to ensue from malnutrition. The SALLOW SKIN of intestinal toxæmia is well known. Various PSYCHONEUROSES are sometimes, as in gastric diseases, associated with disorders of the intestinal canal.

PART B. PHYSICAL EXAMINATION

§ 302. The physical investigation of the intestinal canal must be accomplished by an EXAMINATION OF THE ABDOMEN AND OF THE FÆCES. In all cases of abdominal disease a RECTAL EXAMINATION should be made. X-RAY and SIGMOIDOSCOPIC EXAMINATIONS are called for in some cases.

Examination of the Abdomen.—PALPATION and PERCUSSION will enable us to make out any general swelling or local tumour. The tenderness which often accompanies intestinal disorders may also be elicited. A loaded cæcum, descending colon, or the *scybala* present within the colon, may be felt; these should not be mistaken for the nodules of cancer or other tumour. Their mobility is a very deceptive feature, and the occasional association of diarrhœa may delude us. Their disappearance after active purgation or a course of enemas, is the only certain method of diagnosis. The reader is referred to § 240 for further details as to examination of the abdomen.

§ 303. An **Examination of the Stools** is always important, and sometimes absolutely necessary for the diagnosis of intestinal disorders. A great deal of information can also be thus obtained with regard to diseases of the other abdominal viscera. The fæces should be examined *first* as to their physical properties—size, consistence, colour, shape, odour and reaction; *secondly*, for undigested food and other substances, such as mucus, gall-stones, or parasites; *thirdly*, for the presence of blood or pus; *fourthly*, by microscopy. *Lastly*, culture of the stools is often of great value. One can rarely rely on a patient's statement, even as to the colour and appearance of the stools; they should be inspected by the physician. Early disease of the pancreas and intestinal canal can be detected by thorough investigation. For the detailed techniques of the pathological examinations the student should consult standard text-books.

It is preferable to see the fæces in bulk, the patient having used a night-stool. He should pass urine before going to stool. A large wide-mouthed glass jar, closed at the top by a stopper, is a convenient receptacle for their preservation. Nothing should be added to the motion until the doctor has examined it.

Physical Properties of the Stools.—(1) The *Consistency* is normally solid or semi-solid and the form roughly cylindrical. On an ordinary diet about 3–6 oz. are passed daily, but when fat is inadequately absorbed, as in sprue, the bulk is much increased. (*a*) When passed in hard, dry, roundish balls they are known as *scybala*, this condition being due to defective intake of fluid or its excessive absorption by a " greedy " colon. Scybala are generally coated with mucus and sometimes the irritation they cause sets up a spurious diarrhœa which may alternate with constipation. (*b*) *Pencil-like* stools may result from spasm of the anal sphincter, possibly associated with fissure, while *ribbon-like* stools may be produced by colospasm or stricture of the rectum resulting from cancer or lymphogranuloma inguinale. (*c*) *Uniformly fluid* stools are common in lesions of the small intestine like typhoid, sprue and tuberculous or simple enteritis: in lesions of the large bowel the evacuations are generally more fæcal, solid and slimy; but fluid motions from the small intestine may be passed rapidly through a dysenteric or ulcerated colon.

(2) The *Colour* of the fæces varies normally from light to dark brown, due to stercobilin, chlorophyll and other pigments; the depth of colour affords a fair index of the amount of bile passing into the intestinal canal. As diarrhœa progresses they become lighter in colour. *Pale-coloured stools* may be due to (*a*) obstruction to the entrance of bile into the intestine as in jaundice; (*b*) dilution of the stool as in cholera; (*c*) excess of unabsorbed fat; (*d*) a milk diet. Characteristic naked eye appearances are: (i.) *Clay-coloured* stools, found in obstructive jaundice, and pale, bulky, acid stools occur with steatorrhœa, due either to defective pancreatic secretion or defective fat absorption, as in tropical sprue, non-tropical sprue and cœliac disease; (ii.) *tarry stools*, dark coloured or black, due to blood entering the alimentary canal *high up*, as in duodenal ulcer. Black

stools are also seen in patients taking iron, bismuth and charcoal; (iii.) "*red-currant jelly*" or "*strawberry ice*" stools are seen in intussusception. (iv.) *Streaks of blood* may be present with local lesions such as hæmorrhoids or a rectal polyp, and fresh blood in conditions such as ulcerative colitis, cancer of the bowel or acute dysentery, when it is generally associated with mucus. *Mucopurulent* stools are also met in the latter disease. Other characteristic stools are: (v.) the *green* stools of dyspeptic diarrhœa and enteritis of infancy and after calomel; (vi.) the odourless, colourless "rice-water" stools of cholera, alkaline in reaction and containing flocculi of mucus and epithelium; (vii.) the frothy, acid, yellow stools resulting from excessive carbohydrate fermentation (the gaseous stool characteristic of sprue has a similar origin); (viii.) the soft, brown, offensive, alkaline stool of protein putrefaction; (ix.) the bilious "pea-soup" stools of typhoid.

(3) The *Odour* of the stools is due to skatol and indol, and is largely governed by the amount of meat ingested. A characteristic foul smell accompanies severe ulceration. An ammoniacal odour originates from contamination with urine.

(4) The *Reaction* of the fæces is normally amphoteric; with excess of protein it is alkaline, and of starchy foods and fats (steatorrhœa) distinctly acid. The stool should be tested soon after being passed by moistening litmus paper with distilled water and rubbing a small portion of the stool on the paper; the colour reaction is seen on the other side.

VARIOUS SUBSTANCES may be found:—

1. UNDIGESTED PARTICLES OF FOOD, if in excess, are indicative of imperfect digestion (gastric or intestinal), and, unless the food has been excessive, denote especially intestinal or pancreatic disease (see also p. 424 and § 356). In children this feature usually indicates overfeeding. Small, hard concretions, consisting of phosphates and other matter, are sometimes found. By noting those articles of diet (meat, vegetable, fruit or carbohydrate) which pass for the most part undigested, the physician learns which the patient should reduce.

2. MUCUS in the fæces is often overlooked unless specially sought. To discover it satisfactorily *water must be added* to the fæces, when any mucus present will be seen floating about like small pieces of jelly. The presence of mucus in small amount is of no consequence; it is usual in constipation. When in quantity, and intimately *mixed with the fæces*, it indicates catarrh of the *small* intestine. When in *isolated masses* it signifies the presence of catarrh of the large bowel. In membranous, or mucous, colitis, *long cylinders* of mucus are passed, sometimes without much fæces.

3. BLOOD in the stools may appear either in streaks or in quantity, when from the rectum or large bowel. If it comes from the stomach or small intestines, it will have undergone partial digestion and gives to the stools a tarry appearance (melæna). In either case it reddens the water in which the stool is placed, and gives the characteristic spectrum. The *causes* are dealt with below (§ 321). *Occult* blood must be tested for in cases of suspected oozing from an ulcerated surface.

OCCULT BLOOD TEST in fæces. The patient should be given a purge three days before the intended investigation, and take a hæmoglobin-free diet—milk and milk puddings, bread and butter, eggs, cheese, potatoes, fruit, tea, coffee or cocoa. Meat, meat extracts, liver or liver extracts, soups, poultry, game, fish and green vegetables, must not be given. A charcoal biscuit given at the beginning of the diet will indicate when a fæcal specimen may be collected. During this period a soft toothbrush should be used, lest bleeding from the gums occur. A series of tests over consecutive weeks is of importance where the result is positive. If each is positive the diagnosis is in favour of malignant ulceration; if the positive result is intermittent it is in favour of simple ulceration.

To a piece of fæces of the size of a walnut, add 5 ml. each of glacial acetic acid and water, preferably in a large " boiling-tube." Break up the fæces thoroughly with a glass rod, add an equal quantity of ether, and stir well. The ether extracts all the blood pigments, and if it does not rise spontaneously to the surface add water till it does. Decant the ethereal extract and divide it into two parts. To the first apply the guaiacum or benzidine test (§ 382). To the other add a quarter of its volume of conc. HCl, and shake. The acid hæmatin dissolves in the ether layer at the top, while the acid hæmatoporphyrin dissolves in the watery layer underneath. These pigments may be examined for by the spectroscope. If the bleeding is from the lower colon, the blood is not appreciably altered, and a positive guaiacum reaction and the presence of acid hæmatin is shown. If the blood is from a high level (*e.g.*, stomach or duodenum), only acid hæmatoporphyrin will be present; but when the bleeding is considerable, some undigested acid hæmatin will be present in addition.

4. PUS always indicates *ulceration* of the rectum or colon, which may be due to ulcerative colitis or proctitis, dysentery, cancer or tuberculosis (§ 310). Pus is difficult to detect when diarrhœa is present. When in large quantity, pus indicates an abscess bursting into the bowel, such as a pelvic or ischio-rectal abscess.

5. GALL-STONES may be found by mixing the stools with water, and passing the mixture through muslin or a fine sieve. Gall-stones sink in water when recently passed, though they float when dried. They are often friable, and any suspicious particles should be examined under the microscope for cholesterin.

6. WORMS, see Tables XVIII and XIX, § 304 and § 323.

7. Various FLY LARVÆ are common; generally they are deposited after defæcation, but sometimes man swallows the eggs and larvæ develop later in the gut, giving rise to intestinal myiasis; gastro-intestinal and toxic symptoms may result. A dose of castor oil is generally effective; if not, thymol, santonin or turpentine may be subsequently administered.

SPECIAL INVESTIGATIONS of the Intestine are often essential for accurate diagnosis. The most important are:

A. Microscopic Examination of the Stool for parasites and for abnormal organisms as well as for excess of undigested food residues.

B. X-ray Examination.

C. Instrumental Examination by Proctoscopy, Sigmoidoscopy, Biopsy, etc.

A. **Microscopic Examination** of the fæces (Fig. 99) is often necessary to diagnose pathogenic protozoa and helminthic ova. As a routine a loopful of mucus or fæces should be rubbed up on slides, with (1) warm physiological saline (0·9 per cent.);

(2) Lugol's iodine solution, and cover slips applied. Smears stained by Gram's method may also be made. NORMALLY, under the microscope, a few undigested starch granules, fat cells and partially digested muscle fibres may be observed, also crystals of fatty acids, oxalate of lime and other calcium salts. Hæmatoidin, phosphates, cholesterol and Charcot-Leyden crystals are rare. Various bacteria, cocci and yeasts are found, as well as occasional epithelial cells.

1. *Abnormal* constituents to look for first are: ova, segments of tapeworms, flukes and nematodes (§ 304).

2. Amongst the *undigested food products* note any excess of muscle fibres, starch granules and fat. STARCH GRANULES stain blue with iodine, and if their presence is pathological the stools are usually acid and show signs of fermentation (gas bubbles) and the presence of yeasts. With starch indigestion excessive gas is formed in fermentation tubes in the incubator. Where digestion of PROTEIN is defective there

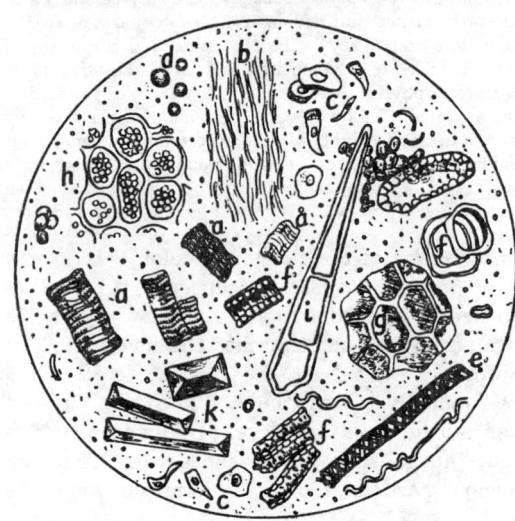

FIG. 99.—MICROSCOPIC ELEMENTS OF NORMAL FÆCES: a, a' muscle fibres; b, connective tissue; c, epithelial cells; d, white blood corpuscles; e, spiral vessels of plants; f—h, vegetable cells; i, plant hairs; k, triple phosphate crystals. Scattered among these elements are micro-organisms and débris.

is an excess of undigested muscle fibres showing cross striations and frayed ends: the stools are generally brown, offensive and alkaline. Neutral FAT droplets are soluble in ether and stain with Sudan III; fatty acids show up as sheaves of colourless, acicular crystals, while soaps form greasy amorphous masses which dissolve on heating. On a normal diet with a fat intake varying between 50 G. and 120 G. a day the fæcal fat should not exceed 6 G. in 24 hours. To ensure reliable results for fat analysis the patient must be on a normally balanced diet for at least three days previously, and without liquid paraffin. Excess of fat amounting to 30–80 per cent. of the dried fæces indicates: (1) defective bile secretion; (2) disease of the pancreas (§ 356) with defective external secretion; (3) intestinal disease interfering with absorption. In (1), as in obstructive jaundice, there is lack of bile salts with resulting defective absorption; the fat, however, is mainly split. In (2), as in chronic pancreatitis, fat may fail to be adequately split owing to the diminution of lipase in the pancreatic juice. In (3) splitting is adequate, the excess of fat resulting from malabsorption; this may occur in tropical sprue (§ 318), idiopathic steatorrhœa, cœliac disease of infants, gastro-colic and gastro-jejuno-colic fistula, and in lymphadenoma, lymphosarcoma and tuberculosis involving the mesenteric lymph glands (and see § 316).

3. Various *bacteria* are found in a fresh stool: those normally present are *B. coli* and streptococcus fæcalis. In disease many varieties of abnormal organisms are

found by direct or by cultural examination. Thus in food poisoning there may be abnormal types or *B. coli*, salmonella organisms or *Staphylococcus aureus*; other pathogenic bacteria are those of the Salmonella-typhoid group, *V. choleræ* and *M. tuberculosis*. In bacillary dysentery it is important to obtain cultures at as early a stage as possible (§ 1201). The bacterial flora of the stool is altered by diet and purgation, and especially by the administration of the sulpha-drugs and the antibiotics; these may cause the appearance of excessive numbers of fungi, especially *Candida albicans*.

4. *Intestinal sand* consists of fine granules of calcium salts and silica formed around an organic nucleus, or of granules from pears or other fruit. 5. *Charcot-Leyden*

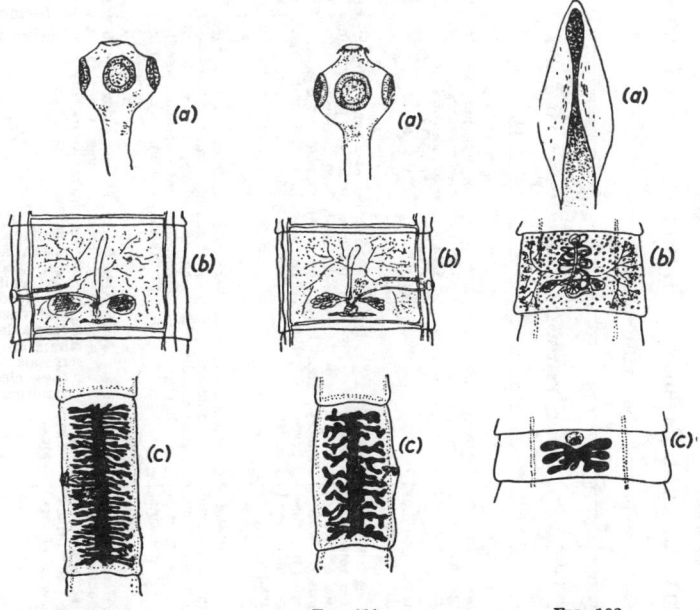

FIG. 100.   FIG. 101.   FIG. 102.

FIG. 100.—*Tænia saginata.* (a) Head × 10; (b) maturing segment showing reproductive system × 3; (c) segment, showing central stem uterus with 15 *to* 30 *lateral dichotomous* branches, × 3.
FIG. 101.—*Tænia solium.* (a) Head × 10; (b) maturing segment showing reproductive system × 3; (c) segment, showing central uterus with 7 *to* 10 *lateral ramifying* branches, × 3.
FIG. 102.—*Diphyllobothrium latum.* (a) Head × 10; (b) maturing segment showing reproductive system × 3; (c) segment, showing *rosette-shaped* uterus, × 3.

crystals are common in amœbiasis, but also occur in ankylostomiasis and mucous colitis.

§ **304. Certain Intestinal Parasites** and their ova, described in Tables XVIII, and XIX, may be found in the fæces (Figs. 100 to 108). In addition, the operculated eggs of certain intestinal and liver flukes are met in tropical countries. Segments of tapeworms often appear in the stools: held between two glass slides and examined with a hand lens they are identified by the number of lateral branches each side of the central uterine stem. *T. saginata* has fifteen or more, but *T. solium* never exceeds twelve. The cysticercus stage of the latter parasite may involve the muscles and brain: epilepsy may result (§ 867). The segments of *Diphyllobothrium latum*, the tapeworm of Central Europe, possess a rosette-shaped uterus. Eggs of the common roundworm (*Ascaris lumbricoides*), of the whipworm (*Trichuris trichiura*), and of the

TABLE XVIII.—THE PRINCIPAL PATHOGENIC HELMINTHS OF THE INTESTINE

For treatment, refer to § 323.

SPECIFIC NAME.	CHIEF CHARACTERISTICS OF WORMS AND HABITAT.	CLINICAL FEATURES.	OVA OR EMBRYO; CHIEF CHARACTERISTICS, AND WHERE FOUND.	ANIMAL HOSTS, ETC.
CESTODES. **Tænia saginata.** (Tapeworm in man.) Fig. 100.	14 to 24 ft. long. Head, 4 suckers, no hooklets. Segments, over 1,000, show central stem uterus with 15 to 30 lateral *dichotomous* branches. Fastens itself to mucosa of small intestine in man.	Segments passed per rectum.	Recognised by segments containing ova discharged in fæces. Ova similar to those of *T. solium.* Cystic stage in beef (35μ × 25μ).	Cattle the intermediate hosts. Found in Great Britain. Widespread geographical distribution. Man infested by eating underdone beef.
Tænia solium. (Tapeworm in man.) Fig. 101. (Cysticercosis also in man.)	About 7 to 10 ft. long. Head, 4 suckers, and double row of 26 hooklets. Segments, about 850, show central stem uterus with 7 to 10 lateral *ramifying* branches. Fastens to mucous membrane of small intestine in man.	Ditto—from adult worm. Epilepsy from embryo (Cysticercosis).	Recognised by segments containing ova discharged per rectum. A six-hooked embryo inside ovum which, eaten by pig, bores its way into the flesh. Ova spherical; 35μ in diameter.	Pig the intermediate host. Adult worm takes 3 months to develop in man, who becomes infested by eating ", measly pork." Man may also act as intermediate host, ingestion of eggs leading to Cysticercosis.
Diphyllobothrium latum or **Bobothriocephalus latus.** Fig. 102.	16 to 25 ft. long. Head clubshaped, with long lateral grooves. No hooklets or suckers. About 3,000 segments; uterus, rosette-shaped. Found in intestinal canal of man.	Occasionally anæmia of pernicious type. Intestinal disorder in children.	Segments containing ova discharged per rectum. Sometimes ova discharged alone; brown shelled with a lid at one end, broadly oval (70μ × 45μ).	Ova hatch on reaching water. Swallowed by a *Cyclops* which is eaten by a fish (intermediary host). Chiefly found in Switzerland and other parts of Europe, also in U.S.A.
Echinococcus granulosus or **Tænia echinococcus.** (Hydatid cyst in man; tapeworm of dog.) Fig. 112.	¼ in. to ¾ in. long. Head pointed, with 4 suckers; double row of hooklets. Has 4 segments, the 4th longer than all others. Found in intestinal canal of dogs, wolves or jackals.	Hydatid cysts form in liver, or other organs in man, sheep, cattle and pigs.	Ova found in fæces of dog or wolf. Embryo becomes encysted in various organs, especially liver and lungs.	Man, sheep and cattle are intermediary hosts. Man becomes infected from contaminated food or water, or from contact with dogs to whose coats and mouths ova may be adherent. Found chiefly in Australia, New Zealand, Argentine and Iceland; occasional cases occur in Great Britain and elsewhere.

NEMATODES. **Enterobius vermicularis.** **Oxyuris vermicularis.** (Threadworm.) Fig. 105.	F. = 8–13 mm.; M. = 2–5 mm. in length. Found in large intestine, chiefly the rectum.	Reflex irritation. Worms tend to migrate at night, and cause itching of anus and genitals.	Worms emerge from anus at night to lay eggs in sticky masses on peri-anal skin. Fingers contaminated by scratching cause reinfection. Ova ($50\mu \times 20\mu$) thin-shelled, planoconvex and contain coiled embryo.	Often trouble children. Found in all countries.
Strongyloides stercoralis.	Only female worms found in intestine—1 in. long. Males develop outside body from rhabditiform larvæ.	Early—dermatitis and lung symptoms. Later—sometimes diarrhœa and urticaria.	Thin-shelled, oval eggs ($60\mu \times 30\mu$) which hatch out free rhabditiform larvæ passed in fæces.	Sexual cycle outside human body. The rhabditiform larvæ differ from ancylostome larvæ in being free and having a short præœsophageal mouth.
Ancylostoma duodenale. (Old world hookworm.) Fig. 108.	M. = 8–10 mm.; F. = 12–18 mm.; buccal cavity large and contains two pairs of ventral teeth; attached to mucosa of jejunum.	Hypochromic anæmia; eosinophilia: œdema: serous effusions: epigastric discomfort.	Ova = $60\mu \times 40\mu$, thin, transparent shell showing 2–8 stages of segmentation. Ova found in fæces, rhabditiform larvæ rarely.	Man is infected by filariform larvæ in the soil penetrating human skin. Widespread geographical distribution.
Necator americanus.	M. = 7–9 mm.; F. = 9–12 mm. The buccal cavity is small with a less effective biting apparatus.	Ditto.	Ova = $70\mu \times 36\mu$ slightly narrower and longer than *A. duodenale.* Found in fæces.	Ditto.
Ascaris lumbricoides. (Roundworm.) Fig. 106.	M. = 6 in.; F. = 12 in. Inhabits the small intestine of man.	Early—urticaria and ascaris larval pneumonia. Later—produce symptoms by toxic, reflex and mechanical means.	Ova are yellow elliptical with thick outer shell showing excrescences ($60\mu \times 45\mu$).	World-wide distribution; very common in children, also adults. May wander widely in human host.
Trichuris trichiura or **Trichocephalus dispar.** (Whipworm.) Fig. 107.	Length = 1¼ in. found in cæcum; anterior portion thread-like.	Generally none. May be dysenteric symptoms in children.	Ova brown, barrel-shaped with terminal knobs ($50\mu \times 23\mu$).	Cosmopolitan distribution. Man is infected by swallowing embryonated eggs.

TABLE XIX.—SOMATIC HELMINTHIC INFESTATIONS OF MAN

SPECIFIC NAME.	CHIEF CHARACTERISTICS OF WORM AND HABITAT.	CLINICAL FEATURES.	OVA OR EMBRYO; CHIEF CHARACTERISTICS, AND WHERE FOUND.	LIFE CYCLE AND GEOGRAPHICAL DISTRIBUTION.
TREMATODES. Schistosoma haematobium. (Vesical Schistosomiasis.) Fig. 194. Syn., Vesical bilharziasis.	M. = 10-15 mm.; F. = 20 mm. Female lives mainly in gynaecophoric canal of male in portal veins and pelvic venous plexuses.	Terminal hematuria, frequency, perineal, penile and loin pain. Eosinophilia.	Terminal spined ova (120-160μ × 40-60μ) containing a ciliated miracidium passed in urine.	Africa, Syria, Arabia and Mesopotamia. Intermediary host mainly *Bulinus* species of snail; man infected by cercariæ penetrating skin while bathing.
Schistosoma mansoni. (Intestinal Schistosomiasis.) Syn., Intestinal bilharziasis.	M. = 12-20 mm.; F. = 12-16 mm. Worms inhabit portal and mesenteric veins.	Schistosomal dysentery, papillomatosis of colon common. Sometimes cirrhosis and splenomegaly. Eosinophilia, anemia.	Lateral spined ova (140-165μ × 60-70μ) containing a ciliated miracidium passed in faeces.	Africa, South America. Intermediary host mainly *Planorbis* species of snail. Infection ditto.
Schistosoma japonicum. (Japanese Schistosomiasis.)	M. = 12-20 mm.; F. = 18-26 mm. Worms inhabit portal and mesenteric veins.	Ditto.; also cerebral symptoms.	Ova (70 × 100μ-50 × 65μ). Have a lateral knob; passed in faeces.	China and Japan. Intermediary host mainly Katayama and *Oncomelania* species of snail. Infection ditto.
Clonorchis sinensis.[1] (Liver fluke.)	Adult is a spatulate fluke (10-20 mm. × 2-5 mm.). Found in the bile ducts of man.	Anorexia, epigastric pain, diarrhœa, enlarged liver and ascites.	Oval, brownish ova (30μ × 15μ) with an operculum, found in faeces.	Common in Japan and China. Life cycle is through a snail and fish which has to be eaten by man.
Paragonimus westermani. (Distoma ringeri) (Lung fluke.)	Adult flukes (7·5 mm.-12·0 mm. × 4-6 mm.). Live in bronchi, where they produce cystic swellings and dilatation.	Cough, hemoptysis; physical signs like bronchiectasis and broncho-pneumonia. Causes "endemic hemoptysis" of Japan.	Broad, oval operculated ova (100μ × 60μ). Appear in brown, rusty sputum; sometimes in faeces also.	Life cycle through a snail, and crabs or crayfish.

[1] Fasciola hepatica, the common liver fluke of sheep and other mammals, rarely affects man.
T. solium and E. granulosus also produce somatic infestations in man (vide Table XVIII, p. 428).

NEMATODES.				
Wuchereria bancrofti.	Worms resemble fine cat-gut. M. = 30-40 mm. F. = 75-100 mm. Inhabit lymphatics and discharge embryos, appearing in the blood stream at night.	Transient painful red swellings in arms, legs, scrotum, etc., with eosinophilia and occasionally mild fever; later lymphangitis, elephantiasis, chyluria, etc.	Embryos appear in blood at night; possess a loose sheath (280-320μ × 7·5-10μ). In Pacific filaria is non-periodic.	Mosquito (Anopheline, culicine or aëdine) is the intermediary host. In Pacific the vector is Aedes variegatus; bites in day time.
Wuchereria malayi. (Syn., Filaria malayi.)	Adult worm resembles W. bancrofti. Embryos are nocturnal.	Similar but less severe.	Sheathed embryos (200-250μ × 5-6μ) in blood.	Mosquito (various species of Mansonioides) is the intermediary host.
Loa loa or Filaria loa	Worms inhabit subcutaneous and retro-peritoneal tissues. M. = 30-34 mm. F. = 50-70 mm.	Painless Calabar swellings; worms cross conjunctiva producing conjunctivitis. Marked eosinophilia.	Sheathed embryos (250-300μ × 6-8μ) appear in blood from 9 a.m. to 9 p.m., i.e., diurnal periodicity.	Transmitted by mangrove fly (Chrysops species) feeding in day time. Occurs in West Africa.
Onchocerca volvulus. (Onchocerciasis.)	Adult male and female worms occur encapsulated in fibrous tissue nodules in subcutaneous tissue.	Subcutaneous nodules. Dermal lesions. Ocular lesions: blindness. Eosinophilia.	Sheathless embryos occur in local lesions and in skin; not found in peripheral blood.	Transmitted by black fly—(Simulium)—in Tropical Africa and Central America.
Dracunculus medinensis. (Guinea-worm.)	Adult female measures 40-80 cm. Inhabits the subcutaneous tissues producing a local ulcer through which embryos are discharged.	Urticaria; anaphylactoid features; local vesicle and ulcer; local abscess, cellulitis, etc.	Larvae are reflexly ejaculated by female worm; they are filariform, actively motile, measuring 500-750μ × 15-25μ.	Larvae escape into water and undergo development in a water-fleas, Cyclops; man becomes infected by drinking water containing it. Occurs in India, Africa, Arabia, etc.
Trichinella spiralis. (Syn., Trichina spiralis.)	Adults inhabit the intestine and liberate embryos which migrate to muscles. M. = 1·4-1·6 mm. F. = 3-4 mm.	Gastric and intestinal symptoms followed by fever, eosinophilia and myositis of affected muscles.	Embryos (100μ × 6μ) may be found in laked blood, or identified in piece of muscle removed at biopsy.	Rats act as reservoir hosts. Infection acquired by eating underdone pork in which larvae are encysted.

threadworm (*Enterobius vermicularis, Oxyuris vermicularis*) may be found in stools throughout the world. The latter's eggs are best demonstrable, however, by the use of a peri-anal swab. The ova of *Ancylostoma duodenale* and *Necator americanus*, and the larvæ of *Strongyloides stercoralis*, are frequent in stools in the tropics. For symptoms and treatment, see § 323. The eggs of *Schistosoma mansoni*, with a lateral spine, and of *S. japonicum*, with a lateral knob, occur in the mucous coating of the stool, and the terminal-spined eggs of *S. hæmatobium* are found in the urine. Biopsies of the rectal mucous membrane are often found to contain the ova in each of these infections.

Entamœba histolytica, the cause of amœbic dysentery and tropical liver abscess,

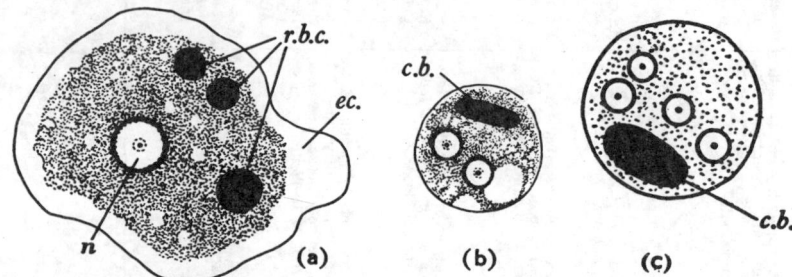

FIG. 103.—*E. histolytica* with hyaline ectoplasm (ec) and ingested red blood cells; the nucleus (n) has a central karyosome in the middle of which is a central granule of chromatin. (b) The same organism in stage of encystment with two nuclei and chromatoid body (c.b.). (c) Matuer cyst with four nuclei and chromatoid body.

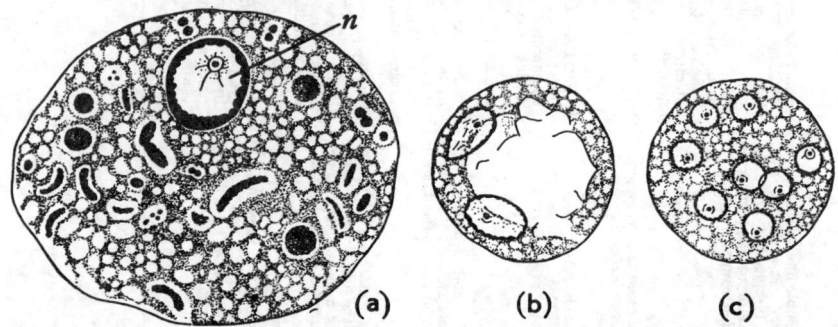

IG. 104.—*E. coli* is, usually larger than E. histolytica but has no clearly defined ectoplasm. It contains various bacteria, yeasts, starch grains in the endoplasm, but no red blood cells. The nucleus has an eccentric karyosome. (b) The same organism with two nuclei as it becomes encysted and with large glycogen vacuole. (c) Mature cyst with 8 nuclei.

must be distinguished from other amœbæ, e.g., *E. coli, Iodamœba bütschlii, Endolimax nana* and *Dientamœba fragilis*. Mucus from a warm, freshly-passed stool is mixed with saline and examined microscopically; diagnosis of *E. histolytica* depends on the presence of an actively motile amœba containing ingested red blood corpuscles. Their *cysts* occur in the solid fæces and are best demonstrated by mounting in a weak solution of iodine; spherical and less than 14μ in diameter, they characteristically have a diffuse glycogen mass, chromidial bodies, and one to four nuclei with central karyosomes.

Various flagellates, including *Giardia intestinalis* (Lamblia), are not uncommon, but unless in large numbers their pathogenicity is doubtful. A ciliate, *Balantidium coli*, gives rise to ulceration of the large bowel which may end fatally.

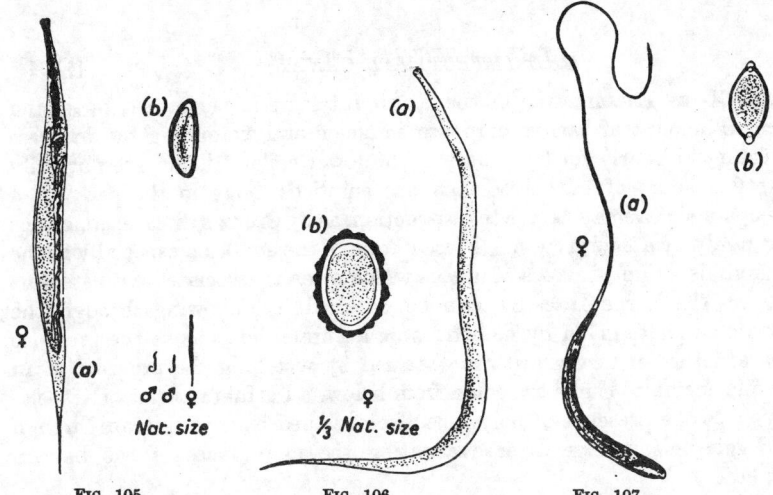

FIG. 105.   FIG. 106.   FIG. 107.

FIG. 105.—*Oxyuris vermicularis.*
    (*a*) Female × 8, also two male worms and female natural size; (*b*) egg × 30.
FIG. 106.—*Ascaris lumbricoides* (Round Worm).
          (*a*) Female, one-third natural size; (*b*) egg × 200.
FIG. 107.—*Trichuris trichiura* (Tricocephalus dispar, " Whip-worm ").
          (*a*) Female × 30; (*b*) egg × 170.

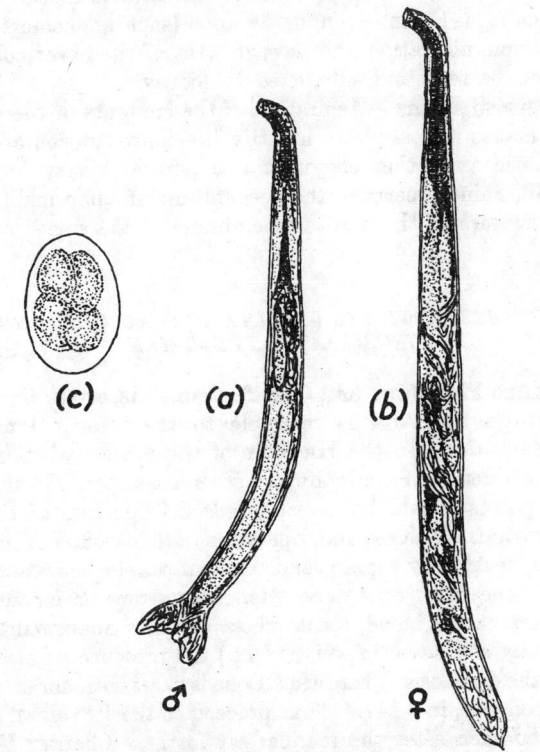

FIG. 108.—*Ancylostomum duodenale.*
(*a*) Male × 5; (*b*) female × 5; (*c*) egg × 170.

B. **X-ray Examination** of the Small Intestine is performed by giving a small amount of barium sulphate emulsion and examining the progress of the meal hourly for 5-6 hours. The lower coils of ileum are normally empty 4 hours after the stomach has emptied: delay in the passage of the opaque meal may be due to obstruction, as by Crohn's disease, adhesions and rarely by a new growth. Flocculation of the emulsion especially in the jejunum is a sign of excess of mucus which often is associated with steatorrhœa. The Large Intestine can be outlined by following through the barium sulphate given by mouth: more accurate detail as to the presence of a stricture or new growth is obtained by watching the progress of an opaque enema as it fills the colon from below. Useful information, especially as to the presence of polypi, is also obtained by injecting air through a Higginson's syringe after evacuating the main mass of the barium sulphate.

C. **Proctoscopy** enables us to examine the appearance of the mucous membrane of the anus and the lower rectum while **sigmoidoscopy** also allows the examination of the interior of the upper rectum and of the lower few inches of the sigmoid colon. A preliminary wash-out may be necessary if there is much stool present, but anæsthesia is rarely required. By such means local lesions around the anus (such as hæmorrhoids or a fissure) and simple ulceration and new growths of the lower colon and of the rectum can be seen and submitted to biopsy.

D. **Other Investigations.**—Aspiration of the contents of the duodenum and jejunum makes it possible to identify the concentration and activity of the pancreatic and other enzymes, and peroral biopsy by a special instrument (M. Shiner) permits the recognition of abnormalities in the histological structure of the mucous membrane of the small intestine.

PART C.   DISEASES OF THE INTESTINAL CANAL, THEIR DIAGNOSIS,
PROGNOSIS AND TREATMENT

§ 305. Routine Procedure, and Classification.—Ascertain first that the patient's Leading Symptom is referable to the intestinal canal; and secondly, by inquiries into the History of the illness, whether it came on *acutely* and suddenly, or gradually in a *chronic* manner. In the History, the following points should be investigated: (i.) duration of the present symptoms, previous diseases and operations; (ii.) residence in tropical climates; (iii.) fever; (iv.) pain and uncomfortable sensations in the intestine; (v.) tenesmus; (vi.) defæcation; frequency or incontinence of fæces; (vii.) presence of blood, steatorrhœa or other abnormalities; (viii.) the appetite; any alteration in weight; (ix.) the presence of gastric symptoms may aid the diagnosis. Intestinal Colic is dealt with under abdominal pain without collapse, in § 247. Next proceed to the Physical Examination of the abdomen after the manner set forth in Chapter IX (§ 240). If, in the course of these inquiries, definite disease is suspected in any particular organ, reference should afterwards be made to the appropriate chapter.

A. **Diarrhœa** is the leading symptom:
If *acute*, or attended by choleraic or dysen-
teric symptoms .. .. turn to §§ 307–311
If *chronic* .. ..·. .. „ „ §§ 312–318
B. There is **Tenesmus** without diarrhœa .. .. „ „ § 319
or there is Rectal Spasm .. .. „ „ § 320
C. **Blood** or some other **alteration in the stools** is
the leading feature .. .. .. „ „ §§ 321–322
D. **Constipation** is the leading symptom .. „ „ § 324
E. **Intestinal Flatulence** is the principal feature „ „ § 325
F. **Stoppage in the Bowels** is complete .. .. „ „ § 326
G. **Pain in the Left Iliac Fossa** which may be
associated with **Fever** and **Constipation** „ „ § 328

§ **306. Diarrhœa** is the frequent occurrence of loose or liquid motions; it is the *watery consistence* of the stools which is the chief characteristic. The *size* of each stool may vary greatly from a few mls. to over a litre of liquid each time the bowel is emptied. A frequent call to stool may arise from some local irritation (see Tenesmus), without any alteration in the consistency or form of the stool. This source of fallacy should be guarded against by careful inquiry.

Examination of the fæces (§ 303) may show the situation of the disease. Thus, for instance, when the stools are coloured with bile, and contain undigested food, and *small pieces of mucus intimately mixed* with the fæces, catarrh of the small intestine may be suspected. When mucus or " slime " occurs in *larger masses*, in " strings " or " casts," it points to disease of the large intestine.

§ **307.** In **Acute Diarrhœa** there is usually a good deal of pain and tenesmus (straining at stool); the tongue is usually furred, there is thirst,

TABLE XX.—CAUSES OF ACUTE DIARRHŒA

COMMON.	RARE.
I. Intestinal Infections especially with Dysentery bacilli.	VI. Typhoid and other toxic conditions.
II. Unsuitable food.	VII. " Chill."
III. Water.	VIII. Acute ulcerative colitis.
IV. Intestinal parasites.	IX. Some causes of chronic diarrhœa.
V. Infantile diarrhœa.	X. Cholera.

and may be vomiting. Profuse vomiting and prostration indicate some violent irritant, or serious organic lesion of the bowel or peritoneum. In profuse diarrhœa the temperature is usually subnormal, and the urine diminished. Severe diarrhœa sooner or later leads to dehydration with shortage of water, sodium chloride and sometimes of potassium. Scybala retained in the intestines may give rise to attacks of diarrhœa alternating with constipation. The possibility of a " controlling appendix " is also to be considered.

§ 308. I. An Acute Infection of the alimentary tract is a common cause of *diarrhœa, abdominal colic* **with pyrexia.** (*a*) The most frequent form is due to the bacillary dysenteries: these are infections with Shigella organisms (*S. flexneri, S. shigæ, S. sonnei, S. boydii* and *S. schmitzii*). (*b*) Cases of gastro-enteritis are caused by infection with *Salmonella* organisms, less commonly by (*c*) *Staphylococcus aureus* and sometimes (*d*) by other organisms. (*e*) A virus origin may account for a large number of cases in which no satisfactory bacterial cause can be identified. In every case culture of the stools, the vomit and sometimes of the blood is essential: agglutination tests may be helpful later.

(*a*) *The patient, who may be living abroad, complains of more or less* SUDDEN DIARRHŒA *with* MUCUS *and sometimes* BLOOD IN THE STOOLS; CONSTITUTIONAL SYMPTOMS *with pyrexia, headache and abdominal pain are present and dehydration may follow.* *The disease is likely to be* ACUTE BACILLARY DYSENTERY.

§ 309. Acute Bacillary Dysentery, although more common in tropical and subtropical climates, has become one of the biggest epidemiological problems in Great Britain during the past few years; in 1960, there were 43,000 cases notified in England and Wales.

Symptoms.—After an incubation period of 1 to 7 days there is a sudden onset with fairly high fever, nausea, vomiting and headache, followed by colicky abdominal pain, tenesmus and the frequent passage of small stools, 5 to 50 times daily. As toxæmia increases the cheeks become flushed, the pulse rapid, the tongue coated. Dehydration produces restlessness, mental confusion, thirst, dry brown tongue, pinched features, sunken eyes, collapsed veins, and in infants a depressed fontanelle. The stools soon lose their fæcal character and consist of odourless, gelatinous mucus mixed with bright red blood, later becoming muco-purulent; with recovery bile-stained fæcal matter reappears. Localised abdominal pain and tenderness are infrequent in the absence of peritoneal involvement; and though some rigidity of the abdominal muscles may at first be present, the contracted sigmoid can later be palpated. Arthritis and iritis may occur. Fulminating and severe Shiga cases die of toxæmia or dehydration with subnormal temperature, but with appropriate treatment the average case becomes apyrexial within 7 days; renal failure sometimes occurs associated with glomerulo-nephritis from dehydration and toxæmia. For *treatment* see § 315.

SONNE DYSENTERY forms 95–98 per cent. of cases of Shigella dysentery in England and Wales. It occurs at all ages but is much more common in children and often causes local epidemics, especially in closed or semi-closed communities. Spread is by food or by personal contact. The *diagnosis* is by culture of a specimen of the stool or of a rectal swab. Most cases recover with appropriate *treatment* (see § 315).

(*b*) *Gastroenteritis due to Salmonella infections. Symptoms.*—After an incubation period of 12–36 hours, this is of rather sudden onset with diarrhœa and abdominal colic, especially in hot weather. The stools are loose, soon become watery and often offensive. Headache, malaise and a temperature up to 100° F for 2–5 days are sometimes associated with nausea and vomiting. In more severe cases there may be chills and even rigors, with a blood-stream invasion causing localised abscesses, cholangitis and rarely meningitis and endocarditis.

Etiology.—The commonest organism is *Salm. typhi-murium* (*B. ærtryche*) and less commonly *Salm. enteriditis* (Gærtner). Local epidemics may occur and the infection is common in cows, pigs, rodents and poultry. Human beings are infected by a large number of foods, especially processed meats, milk, custard, ice-cream and imported duck eggs. Recovery is the rule. Although the symptoms subside in 1–2 weeks the organism may persist in the intestine for up to 9 weeks.

Treatment is by bed-rest and glucose with half-normal saline until the acute symptoms subside. Tetracycline B.P. or chloramphenicol B.P. (0·5 G. 4- or 6-hourly) are most effective. The patient must be isolated, and the stools disinfected until stool tests show the infection to have been overcome.

(*c*) *Severe diarrhœa and vomiting with prostration within* 2–4 *hours* of ingestion are caused by *a toxin*, produced in food by *Staphylococcus aureus*. A temperature of 100–101° F, dehydration, collapse, a low blood pressure and an appearance of impending death are followed by an almost equally sudden recovery. The cause is usually a *Staph. aureus* infection on the finger of the cook who prepares the food (perhaps from a whitlow or from a discharging ear). The foods contaminated are usually cooked meats, or pies containing meat and starches. The toxin is not destroyed by cooking. A similar condition is sometimes produced by *Salmonella toxins* in food after the organisms have been killed by heat. *Treatment* is symptomatic.

(*d*) *Outbreaks of gastro-enteritis due to other organisms* are usually milder with little or no nausea or vomiting but with some diarrhœa. Bacteriological examination of the material vomited or of the stools shows organisms such as the clostridia—*Cl. perfringens* (*Cl. welchii*), specific types of *E. coli* and *E. paracoli, Strep. fæcalis, B. proteus, A. ærogenes* and *B. cerus*. The first or diarrhœic stage of *trichinosis* should be considered in pork-eating countries (§ 606); in cases of acute diarrhœa in which trichinosis is suspected, the worm should be sought in the fæces. *Botulism* produces neurological symptoms (§ 1068).

(*e*) In many cases of gastro-enteritis no causal organisms can be discovered. These occur in outbreaks especially in children and young adults and comprise 40 per cent. of all outbreaks investigated. *Symptoms.*—

Headache, giddiness, nausea, vomiting, diarrhœa and abdominal pain are associated with a transient pyrexia (100° F). These cases are often labelled as " gastric influenza," as they are frequently associated with upper respiratory infections. A virus origin appears probable in many of these epidemics. Recovery is the rule.

§ 310. II. *In all cases of acute diarrhœa and intestinal colic* coming on suddenly in a healthy person, **when there is no pyrexia,** the food taken should be inquired into. The physician should patiently consider every article taken at every meal during the preceding 24 hours. Indigestible food such as unripe or decomposing fruit, too much raw vegetable, food poisoning by fungi, plants, vegetables, certain fish and shell-fish and personal idiosyncrasies and allergies may be causal. It should be borne in mind that one of the irritant poisons may have been introduced into the food accidentally or designedly. The diarrhœa which precedes the intestinal obstruction caused by *intussusception* in children frequently follows a heavy meal of indigestible articles; and diarrhœa is itself a cause of intussusception.

III. The quality of the **water** is often responsible for diarrhœa, acute or chronic. This is frequently the case in malarial districts in the summer and autumn, especially when the temperature is high. Soft water containing much peat from the mountains may be a cause.

IV. Of the **intestinal parasites**, worms often cause diarrhœa, especially in children, who may have had uneasy abdominal sensations, night terrors, picking of the nose, itching of the anus, vulvo-vaginitis; but sometimes they are discovered in the stools when there have been no symptoms (§ 323).

LAMBLIA INTESTINALIS (Giardia) is a frequent inhabitant of the small intestine: small numbers of organisms are not pathogenic, but very large numbers can cause recurrent attacks of acute diarrhœa, with mucus and some blood in the stools. *Treatment:* mepacrine hydrochloride B.P. 0·1 G. t.d.s. by mouth for five days is a certain cure.

V. **Infantile Diarrhœa** occurs in at least three well-recognised clinical forms: (i.) Acute Catarrhal or Dyspeptic Diarrhœa; (ii.) Inflammatory Diarrhœa or Entero-colitis; and (iii.) Epidemic Diarrhœa or " summer diarrhœa " (including Infantile Cholera)—mentioned in progressive order of severity.

(i.) In ACUTE CATARRHAL (dyspeptic) DIARRHŒA the stools are offensive, at first yellow, then greenish, slimy and mixed with curds of undigested food. Vomiting may or may not be present. It is usually transient if adequately treated.

(ii.) In INFANTILE INFLAMMATORY DIARRHŒA (Entero-colitis) the stools are green, slimy and often contain mucus and streaks of blood; there is some fever at the beginning, and abdominal distension. The stools vary with the predominant infection; they are acid and frothy in the fermentative type, alkaline and green in the putrefactive variety. The inflammation attacks chiefly the colon; consequently there is tenderness on pressure over the region of the colon. Dehydration and prostration are great when much vomiting occurs. Adults also are sometimes affected. It lasts only one to three weeks if treated correctly.

(iii.) EPIDEMIC DIARRHŒA is met with chiefly in childhood and infancy. It is no longer a disease of the summer months of the year, and is attended by catarrh of the mucous membrane of the bowel. The *symptoms* of a severe attack may start insidiously or suddenly. They are: watery stools which are foul smelling, green in colour and containing mucus—becoming paler as they become choleriac in type; vomiting; acute abdominal pain with prostration and collapse especially when there is rapid dehydration; the temperature is elevated at first but may become subnormal later although hyperpyrexia may occur terminally; when toxæmia is severe there is stupor leading to coma and even convulsions. Death may occur in a few hours or within a day or so; recovery is often protracted.

Etiology of Infantile Diarrhœa.—These diseases affect chiefly hand-fed and over-fed children, in warm weather, being probably in part due to dirty feeding-bottles, teats, sour milk, etc. Most of the cases occur in children under six months old. Dietetic errors account for some cases, but the cause of *Epidemic Diarrhœa* is usually an infection. Outbreaks occur sporadically at any time of the year, especially among infants in hospital wards and in maternity homes. Some cases are due to dysentery bacillary infection of *Shiga*, *Flexner* or *Sonne* types, or to Morgan's bacillus; in others to the food-poisoning bacteria (*B. enteritidis of Gærtner* and *B. ærtrycke*) and to specific types of *E. coli* or to *Staph. aureus*. In many epidemics no causal organism can be identified and a virus infection is probable.

In the *Treatment of Infantile Diarrhœa* (1) first free the gastro-intestinal tract of all irritant materials; small doses of calomel (gr. $\frac{1}{10}$), grey powder (gr. $\frac{1}{4}$), castor oil or gr. 2–5 sodium sulphate in water every 2 or 3 hours, until the stools become healthy; (2) give half-normal saline for the first 12–24 hours; and later, (3) 2-hourly feeds of breast-milk, whey, half-cream dried milk or condensed milk—in each case diluted with half-normal saline. In the fermentative type, use only a small amount of sugar, or a non-fermentable sugar such as dextri-maltose or lactose; subsequent additions to the diet must be made very cautiously. When vomiting is troublesome, gastric lavage with saline solution (not bicarbonate) should be used; then give whey (§ 296. XX). When diarrhœa is persistent, give phthalyl-sulphathiazole, sulphasuccidine or one of the tetracyclines and combine with astringents. In mild chronic cases, give protein milk, such as sprulac, or milk protein such as soluble casein or casec. In more severe cases colonic lavage with warm normal saline removes irritant material. Albumen or barley water can be tried, and brandy, arrowroot and an astringent mixture are useful (bismuth carbonate 2 gr., calcium carbonate 3 gr., tincture catechu 5 min., glycerin 10 min., water to 60 min.). If used cautiously, nepenthe ($\mathtext{M}$ iii t.d.s. at 6 months) is valuable. Dehydration is a serious complication and must be combated with water by mouth or saline by rectal, subcutaneous, intraperitoneal or continuous-drip intravenous methods.   For collapse give a transfusion of human blood plasma; nikethamide B.P. (Coramine) and a warm mustard bath are the best stimulants.

VI. **Typhoid** and other **Toxic Conditions.**—Diarrhœa is usual in typhoid fever, and may occur in measles and the other eruptive fevers (especially at their onset), some cases of Graves' disease, chronic renal disease, uræmia and pyæmia.   Sometimes it appears at the termination of acute illness, as in pneumonia.   (And see chronic causes, § 312.)

VII. A chill to the surface of the body in some individuals will determine an attack of acute diarrhœa.

VIII. **Acute Ulcerative Colitis** is usually of sudden onset, with diarrhœa, and abdominal pain occurring in paroxysms.   The stools are dark, offensive, and contain mucus and blood.   There is tenderness over the colon, and its ascending portion is usually distended.   The tongue is furred at first, and the breath very offensive.   Pyrexia is present, to 101°–102°. The commonest complications are exhaustion, anæmia, profuse hæmorrhage; less common are perforation and peritonitis.   Sigmoidoscopy shows a uniformly inflamed mucosa with exudate, necrosis' of membrane, and often ulceration.   It is a more acute form of chronic ulcerative colitis (§ 314), the chronic form being much more common.   Its etiology is unknown and it must be differentiated from bacillary and sometimes amœbic dysentery.

IX. In cases of acute diarrhœa in which the cause is obscure, reference should be made to the other **Causes** of **Chronic Diarrhœa,** any of which may from time to time give rise to an acute attack.   It should not be forgotten that acute diarrhœa often follows the prolonged administration of antibiotic drugs and especially the tetracyclines.   **Dysentery** (§ 308) and **Cholera** (§ 311) are the commonest causes of diarrhœa in tropical climates, and are occasionally met in this country.

Prognosis of Acute Diarrhœa.—The causes of acute diarrhœa are for the most part removable; and though exhausted by the attack, the patient generally makes a good recovery.   Acute Epidemic Diarrhœa in children, however, is a more fatal affection, and it leads to a high death-rate in infancy.   The prognosis in any given case depends upon (i.) the cause; (ii.) the severity of the symptoms and the evidences of dehydration; (iii.) the state of the hygienic surroundings; and (iv.) the response to treatment.   Infantile cholera is usually fatal.   Dyspeptic diarrhœa may be cured in a few weeks, but if untreated, is apt to go on to catarrhal or mucous colitis.   Without treatment all forms of epidemic diarrhœa, even in adults, are serious.   Should symptoms of prostration or collapse ensue, the outlook is bad; but it is only at the two extremes of life that this disease is so grave.   Ulcerative colitis is serious; death may occur from complications, exhaustion, anæmia or relapses.

General Treatment of Acute Diarrhœa.—The indications are (a) to remove any irritating matters left in the intestinal canal; (b) to provide absolute rest in bed and warmth to the abdomen; and (c) to check excessive diarrhœa. (a) Thus, simple acute diarrhœa following the eating of bad food is readily arrested by giving castor oil, ½ fl. oz., with tr. opii, ℥ x, followed by a simple bismuth salicylate mixture. No food is allowed for a day, but as much water as desired is drunk: half-normal saline by mouth is essential when dehydration is severe. Then arrowroot made with water is given, and a gradual return to ordinary diet, beginning with milk and milk puddings. For some time all irritating skins, seeds, vegetable cellulose and raw fruits may not be taken. After the acute stage is over, if the condition threatens to become chronic, other drugs are used. Opium checks diarrhœa; it can be given in the form of Tr. chloroformi et morphinæ, B.P./'85, ℥ 5–10. Catechu, kino, chalk and tannin are excellent astringents. Bismuth carbonate or kaolin (up to 3–4 G. daily) soothe the congested mucous membrane. For offensive stools give salol, calomel or charcoal. A short course of intestinal antiseptics is often useful—sulphasuccidine, phthalylsulphathiazole—or antibiotics such as the tetracyclines. For putrefactive diarrhœa, protein foods should be avoided; B. acidophilus helps to implant a healthier intestinal flora. In fermentative diarrhœa carbohydrates must be restricted; sugar, bread and flour are usually digested; but rice, tapioca, bananas, root vegetables, especially potatoes, should be avoided for a time, and a diastase preparation taken. In more obstinate cases of diarrhœa colonic irrigations may be required; saline or permanganate douches, introduced slowly and without pressure, give excellent results in some cases. Where there is much loss of fluid, dextrose-saline or plasma infusions may have to be given to prevent collapse. The treatment of acute ulcerative colitis is similar to that of the chronic form and is therefore dealt with in § 314. IV.

The patient complains of ACUTE DIARRHŒA, *coming on very suddenly, and attended with severe* COLLAPSE, *abdominal* CRAMPS, *and " rice-water " stools. The disease is probably* CHOLERA.

§ 311. X. Cholera (Synonym: Asiatic Cholera) is a disease caused by *Vibrio choleræ*; it begins with urgent vomiting, purging and colourless evacuations, cramps and a tendency to collapse, and which, if not fatal in the first stage, is attended by secondary fever. The period of incubation is usually three to six days, but it may vary between one and ten. There are three well-marked stages:
(a) *Stage of evacuation,* which lasts from 2 to 12 hours, or longer. The patient is *suddenly* seized with violent vomiting, profuse diarrhœa and later cramp. The stools, after the first few, are colourless and opaque, resembling rice-water, and containing flakes of columnar epithelium and casts of villi, and the *comma-shaped bacillus*. There are severe cramps in the fingers, toes and abdominal muscles, great exhaustion, small and weak pulse, and coldness of the body. (b) The *algid stage*, cold stage, or stage of collapse, lasts a few hours to a few days according to the severity of the case. The patient looks like a corpse; the surface temperature falls, and the skin becomes a deadly livid hue; the pulse cannot be felt at the wrist. The temperature is most remarkable, for in the rectum it may be as high as 105° F, while in the axilla it is only 90° F. During this stage the purging ceases, but the vomiting and cramps persist. The mind remains clear. There is suppression of urine and bile. (c) *Stage of reaction*.—The pulse returns, the temperature rises, the bile reappears, the urine is scanty and deficient in urea. The temperature goes up, and may be attended by

typhoid symptoms. The bowels are confined. There may be erythematous, urticarial and other eruptions upon the skin. This stage is followed by great weakness. Fluid and salt loss is important in this disease. Diarrhœa and vomiting both produce salt depletion, decreased blood volume with increased viscosity of blood and de-hydration of the tissues. Polycythæmia and leucocytosis also result from concentration. The blood chemistry shows reduced blood chloride, diminished plasma alkalinity, phosphate retention and increased blood urea, with decreased urinary output. Finally the weakened heart fails to pump the viscous blood through the kidneys and anuria with acidosis results.

The *Diagnosis* is easy in severe cases on account of the extreme suddenness and severity of the symptoms. The copious colourless evacuations are characteristic of cholera. Conditions which resemble it are acute poisoning by arsenic, croton oil, and other irritants, ptomaine poisoning, and certain cases of malignant malaria. The identification of the bacillus renders the diagnosis certain.

Etiology.—The disease occurs in great epidemics, but has not visited this country, except sporadically, since 1895–6–7. In India it is endemic. As regards age, none are exempt. All epidemics in this country have occurred in the autumn and the end of the summer. The exciting cause is the specific organism, which must be introduced into the alimentary canal. As with typhoid, the disease is usually communicated by drinking water contaminated by evacuations from the bowels and stomach, and requires the same preventive measures (§ 525 *et seq.*). It may be conveyed in other ways, as by flies, through *want of cleanliness*. One attack does not confer immunity.

Prognosis.—The earlier cases of an epidemic are the most fatal. The mortality rate varies from 30–70 per cent. in different epidemics. Aged and debilitated people, young children and alcoholics do badly. New methods of treatment have reduced the mortality by half. In the reaction stage uræmic coma, hyperpyrexia, or the typhoid state may cause death. *Untoward Symptoms* are blood in the evacuations, long stage of collapse, restlessness, extreme cyanosis and absence of the pulse at wrist. Favourable signs are a perceptible pulse in the algid stage, the early occurrence of reaction, cessation of cramp, secretion of urine and the occurrence of sleep. *Complications* include pneumonia, occurring in the reaction stage, bronchitis, pleurisy, parotitis, bed-sores, inflammation of the pharynx, genitals or bladder, corneal ulcers and gangrene of the fingers, toes, scrotum or penis.

There are two rare *varieties*: (1) Choleraic diarrhœa, or " cholerine "—resembling autumnal diarrhœa occurring during an epidemic of cholera. (2) Dry cholera or cholera sicca, where there has been no vomiting or diarrhœa, the patient dying of collapse before these have had time to develop. At autopsy the intestines contain much fluid.

Treatment.—Rest in bed and warmth are essential. To save life intravenous saline, hypertonic at first, is given at once and usually it is necessary to cut down to the vein. The hypertonic solution contains sodium chloride 9·0 G. in one pint of pyrogen-free distilled water. The first pint is given in 5 to 10 minutes, the second in 20 minutes and each subsequent pint in 4 hours. Isotonic saline is given interspersed with the hypertonic saline for the first 24 hours; the ratio of hypertonic to isotonic saline being about 2 : 1. On the next day usually isotonic saline alone will suffice. Great care must be taken not to overload the patient with fluid. The aim is to restore the systolic blood pressure to about 100 mm. Hg and the specific gravity of the blood to normal. If the urinary chloride rises, hypotonic saline may be substituted for isotonic. Complete bed-rest and warmth are essential. Light kaolin in massive doses is given when it can be retained. Sulphaguinidine or chloramphenicol are advocated but are little use while severe vomiting is present. In convalescence rest is still essential to avoid the recurrence of vascular collapse. Only sips of water and saline are given at first, but the diet is very gradually built up as the patient improves. Morphia is not now used. A *prophylactic vaccine* gives partial immunity for several months. The attack rate in the uninoculated is 2·4 times greater than in the inoculated.

§ 312. Chronic Diarrhœa.—The term chronic diarrhœa signifies the occurrence of frequent *loose* evacuations, say three or more in the 24 hours, extending over a period of weeks, months or even years (as in Sprue). It is usually, though not necessarily, attended by tenesmus. The stools should be examined (§ 303) and the anus and rectum carefully inspected. Tenesmus points to disease of the rectum.

TABLE XXI.—CAUSES OF CHRONIC DIARRHŒA

GROUP A. COMMON.	GROUP B. LESS COMMON.
I. Acute causes becoming chronic.	IX. Steatorrhœa (§ 316):—
II. Ulceration, other than ulcerative colitis.	(a) Idiopathic and cœliac disease, § 317.
III. Colon spasm (mucous colitis), § 313.	(b) Tropical sprue, § 318.
IV. Chronic ulcerative colitis, § 314.	(c) Pancreatic disease, §§ 359, 360.
V. Nervous diarrhœa.	(d) With jaundice.
VI. Local conditions about anus.	(e) After operation and with fistula.
VII. Portal obstruction or congestion.	(f) Amyloid disease.
VIII. Dysenteric diarrhœa, § 315.	(g) Other causes.
	X. Senile diarrhœa.
	XI. Mineral poisons (e.g., arsenic).
	XII. Gastrogenous diarrhœa.
	XIII. Constitutional causes.

GROUP A.—We must first consider the *more common* diseases which cause **Chronic Diarrhœa.**

I. Chronic Diarrhœa may be due to some of the same causes as **Acute Diarrhœa** (Table XX). In children think of worms or bad feeding; and in adults, errors in diet, carbohydrate dyspepsia, ulceration and chronic irritant poisoning.

II. **Ulceration of some part of the Intestinal Canal** is a not infrequent cause of diarrhœa. In England the ulcerating lesions which may affect the intestine are: (1) Ulcer of the lower part of the ileum may be due to tuberculosis, typhoid fever or Crohn's disease. (2) Ulcer of the cæcum may arise from the pressure of inspissated fæces or some foreign body —e.g., a toothbrush bristle—which has been swallowed. (3) Ulcer of the appendix may similarly arise from foreign bodies or as part of appendicitis (§ 248). (4) Simple ulcerative colitis (§ 314. IV). (5) Cancer of the bowel may produce an ulcer, the most frequent situation being the sigmoid. (6) Ulcer of the rectum is generally of malignant origin; it is attended by the passage of blood and pus and stricture may result. Mainly in tropical areas, lymphogranuloma inguinale can cause chronic ulceration and stricture formation. (7) Ulcers of the large intestine and rectum occur in dysentery. These may contract on healing and produce stricture. (8) Ulceration may follow prolonged constipation with atony of the colon. (9) A submucous streptococcal infection may cause chronic diarrhœa with precipitate stools, as may chronic nephritis, severe anæmia, and other wasting diseases.

The commonest causes of ulceration in this country are ULCERATIVE COLITIS, CANCER, REGIONAL ILEITIS, TUBERCULOSIS, sometimes LYMPHO-GRANULOMA INGUINALE, and in tropical climates DYSENTERY (§ 315).

a. ULCERATIVE COLITIS (§ 310. VIII and § 314. IV) causes one of the most intractable forms of chronic diarrhœa.

b. INTESTINAL CANCER presents the following features: (i.) The patient is usually over fifty; (ii.) diarrhœa and anæmia due to hæmorrhage are common if the disease is in the cæcum or ascending colon: obstructive symptoms and diarrhœa alternating with constipation if in the descending or sigmoid colon; (iii.) paroxysmal abdominal pain is frequent; (iv.) tenesmus indicates a lesion in the rectum; (v.) a tumour may be palpable through the abdominal wall, or by rectal examination. It is most difficult of access when in the lower sigmoid colon; and may then (vi.) be within reach of the sigmoidoscope. (vii.) Cancerous cachexia often accompanies. (viii.) Pyrexia and leucocytosis may be due to ulceration. (ix.) The stools vary; they may contain blood in considerable quantity, but invariably occult blood. (x.) X-ray with a barium enema may show a characteristic filling defect (Fig. 109). And see § 327. Cancer of the small intestine is rare.

c. Regional Ileitis (Crohn's Disease) is fairly common. It mainly affects the terminal ileum and may also involve the cæcum and ascending colon, especially in young adults. *Symptoms* resemble those of appendicitis or ulcerative colitis. There is recurring colicky pain around the umbilicus or in the R.I.F., often worse after meals. The attacks are associated with diarrhœa and sometimes with vomiting, borborygmi and a low-grade rise of temperature. Examination shows tenderness internal to the cæcum and a sausage-shaped tumour may be felt in the abdomen or per rectum. In some a number of areas are involved, even in the jejunum with "skip areas" between; such cases may lead to steatorrhœa with the mal-absorption syndrome (§§ 316, 318).

Diagnosis is with a small barium meal which shows a narrowed area of small intestine, with distended loops proximal to this: later the lumen may be narrowed to a mere linear shadow. A barium enema helps to reveal spread of the disease to the proximal colon and the barium sulphate which runs back through the ileo-cæcal sphincter may show the condition of the terminal ileum. Ulceration of the mucous membrane leads to positive occult blood tests; the Mantoux test is usually negative. The differential diagnosis is from ileo-cæcal tuberculosis, subacute appendicitis, new growth and actinomycosis.

The *Etiology* is unknown. There is a non-specific inflammatory reaction in the affected area, with giant cells and fibrosis, but tubercle bacilli have not been demonstrated. There may be considerable peritoneal reaction leading to matting of the affected coils and the neighbouring lymph glands are enlarged.

Prognosis.—Many early cases gradually recover with medical treatment. Fistula may form between the affected loops and other coils of the small intestine, the large intestine, the bladder or on to the surface.

Treatment may be surgical with excision of the affected segment, but 45 per cent. show recurrence after 2 years and 78 per cent. after 10 years. In early cases, and particularly when there is extensive involvement of the jejunum as shown by steatorrhœa, a low residue diet, the corticosteroids, streptomycin combined with isoniazid or P.A.S. should be used instead.

d. TUBERCULOSIS of the lungs may be attended by diarrhœa, even without ulceration of the bowel. Multiple ulcers due to tuberculosis may be found in the lower ileum, and less commonly in the rectum, where the symptoms mimic ulcerative colitis (see Ulcerative proctitis, § 321. VIII). It is much less common now that pulmonary tuberculosis is so much more readily controlled. Tuberculous ulceration of the bowel is recognised by (i.) evidences of tuberculosis in the lungs or other parts of the body; (ii.) the presence of night sweats and intermittent pyrexia; (iii.) the stools are watery, and there is rarely any pain; (iv.) tubercle bacilli may be demonstrated in the stools by appropriate staining methods. Relief follows treatment with inj. streptomycin with sodium aminosalicylate B.P. (P.A.S.) or isoniazid B.P.

e. In LYMPHOGRANULOMA INGUINALE (Syn. Lymphogranuloma Venereum) there may be ulceration with stricture of the rectum, especially in women. Most cases acquire the infection abroad (§ 582), but the disease is occasionally seen in the white population of Great Britain and of the U.S.A. The rectum is converted into a narrow ulcerated tube, especially 1–3 in. above the anus. Syphilis may co-exist but the rectal lesion is now believed to be due solely to L. inguinale. The *symptoms* are (i.) the passage of blood, pus and mucus, (ii.) increasing constipation, (iii.) fistulæ may form and polypoid swelling occur around the anus. The *diagnosis* is by the complement fixation reaction (above 1 in 20) and by Frei's test. *Treatment* is by a prolonged course of the sulphonamides or the tetracyclines. Surgical measures and excision may be required later.

§ 313. III. Colon Spasm (Syn., Chronic or Mucous Colitis) is more common in young and middle-aged women. It can cause many years of ill-health, and needs much patience in treatment.

Symptoms.—(i.) There is persistent abdominal pain and discomfort of a nagging or burning character, especially in the left iliac fossa: the pain is liable to colicky exacerbations, which may be most marked *after* a bowel evacuation. (ii.) There are attacks of obstinate constipation during which the stools may be hard, scybalous and ribbon-like, alternating with attacks of diarrhœa, brought on by slight dietetic errors, by nervous causes, or by the misuse of aperients. (iii.) During the attacks of diarrhœa, mucus may be passed in masses, shreds or casts several inches long: the stools often contain intestinal sand but not blood. (iv.) There may be intestinal flatulence and abdominal distension due to excessive carbohydrate fermentation. (v.) *B. coli* may infect the urinary tract. (vi.) Nervous prostration, insomnia, ready fatigue and loss of weight are almost always present and may be the presenting symptoms. (vii.) Examination may reveal a distended cæcum while the colon is felt as a tender contracted tube in spasm. The patient often accurately delineates the colon along its whole course. Eczema of the umbilicus may co-exist. The sigmoidoscope aids diagnosis in obscure cases.

Diagnosis.—The disease is distinguished from ulcerative colitis by the presence of blood in this latter condition, and from carcinoma coli by the length of history and the type of stool. A barium enema and sigmoidoscopy may be necessary to exclude organic disease and to reassure the patient. A barium meal shows a normal outline to the large intestine but the descending and sigmoid colon may be markedly narrowed.

Etiology.—It is primarily a nervous disorder and attacks are caused by overwork, worry and are often worse in cold weather. The prolonged use of purgatives greatly aggravates the condition and promotes the formation of large masses of mucus.

Treatment must be directed to the underlying nervous make-up of the individual. Diverticulosis and diverticulitis often result, in later years. Reassurance after a thorough examination is essential: fatigue and overwork should be avoided, and often an unhappy home environment requires correction. The diet needs to be liberal except that coarse roughage is better avoided: it is a mistake to use a diet with too little residue and some fruit and vegetables as purée are valuable for their cellulose content. Agar and liquid paraffin emulsions and isogel granules aid normal peristalsis, but drastic purgatives must be avoided. At all times, the patient must be discouraged from examining the stools. Vitamin B preparations may be of help. Taka-diastase is useful when und'gested starch appears in excessive quantities in the stool. Adequate warm clothing covering the abdomen is essential, and when visceroptosis is also present, a suitable abdominal belt aids. Excessive smoking must be avoided and some are benefited by giving up smoking altogether. The most useful drugs are belladonna or atropine methonitrate (Eumydrin) combined with phenobarbitone or the bromides. Although an initial colon lavage may help by removing excess of mucus, the repeated use of lavage or enemata is harmful.

§ 314. IV. Chronic Ulcerative Colitis is usually insidious in onset, but may follow the acute variety (§ 310, VIII). It occurs most commonly in young adults, but may occur later. There is a great tendency to remissions and relapses.

Symptoms.—At first these comprise (i.) diarrhœa with the passage of watery stools containing fairly bright red blood and mucus intimately mixed with the fæces; (ii.) lower abdominal flatulence, discomfort and often colic before the bowels act; (iii.) rectal discomfort and tenesmus indicate involvement of the lowermost portion of the bowel. In more severe cases, or as the disease worsens, (iv.) the number of stools may increase to 20–30 a day, blood and muco-pus being passed by day and by night. This leads to (v.) considerable exhaustion, often dehydration, marked weight loss and anæmia—even to 30 per cent. of hæmoglobin; (vi.) there is a remitting temperature as high as 103°–104° F; (vii.) hypochlorhydria is common.

The *Diagnosis* depends on: (i.) Sigmoidoscopy. At first the middle and upper rectum are hyperæmic and bleed easily when touched by the instrument: at this stage the mucous membrane is œdematous and glistens. A well-established, case shows a uniformly inflamed, granular mucosa bleeding readily on pressure with miliary or larger-sized ulcers; the lumen of the rectum and large bowel is narrowed, its walls rigid and thickened so that ballooning with air becomes painful and difficult. (ii.) X-ray reveals a shortened, tubular bowel with complete loss of haustration; if deep ulcers exist the outline of the colon is feathery and moth-eaten in appearance. The disease must be differentiated from simple ulcerative proctitis, carcinoma of the colon or rectum, and chronic amœbic dysentery.

Etiology.—In the absence of any single bacterial or other causal agent, the condition is commonly regarded as being psychogenic in origin. It occurs especially in hypersensitive individuals and the onset and relapses frequently follow emotional trauma. The condition often begins as a granular proctitis which tends to ascend to the pelvic and descending colon and in extreme cases the cæcum. The lesions are at first confined to the mucous and submucous coats; when gross ulceration occurs there is an inflammatory necrosis of the blood vessels, causing the disease to extend more deeply into the muscle coats with resulting spasm and an X-ray appearance of stricture: true fibrosis with stricture formation is rare. In a proportion of cases the ileo-cæcal sphincter is incompetent and the lower ileum is also involved.

Prognosis.—Intermissions are common, apparent recovery being followed by relapses extending over many years. Complications include hæmorrhage, acute or chronic perforation, polyposis, ischio-rectal abscess, arthritis, pyoderma and in chronic cases carcinoma of high malignancy. Fatty infiltration of the liver is common and hepatic cirrhosis may ensue.

Treatment is necessarily prolonged and requires great patience. An understanding and confident attitude on the part of the physician is of great value. (i.) The patient should be kept strictly in bed until the condition has healed. As progress is made, the abdominal discomfort, fever and diarrhœa disappear, the stools become more formed and visible blood, pus and mucus are absent from the stools: healing is not complete until confirmed by sigmoidoscopic examination. (ii.) The diet must be ample and varied: a high calorie, high protein, low vegetable residue diet should be given and supplements of vitamins B and C added. (iii.) A mixture containing tinct. opii ℳ 10, tinct. belladonna ℳ 7½ with bismuth carbonate is often helpful in controlling the diarrhœa. (iv.) A short course of tetracycline is often of help in the acute phases, but the tendency of the antibiotics to cause diarrhœa when given for long periods must be remembered. Long courses of sulphasuccidine or phthalyl-sulphathiazole (1-2 G. q.i.d. for many weeks or months), until the diarrhœa ceases, are often of great value; many prefer salazopyrin in similar doses. Septic foci must be suitably dealt with, but there is little evidence that either sera or vaccines are of any help. (v.) For the anæmia one or more blood transfusions are often of remarkable value; oral preparations of iron rarely help. (vi.) A Medical Research Council therapeutic trial has shown that especially in the first attack and in acute relapses large doses of cortisone (initially 300 mg. a day) are of great help: inject. corticotrophin (initially 90 units a day) is even more effective: simultaneous administration of an antibiotic or of a sulphonamide is necessary.   Such patients also require potass. citrate 1 G. q.d.s. to prevent potassium depletion.   The risk of a silent perforation of the intestine must be borne in mind.   (vii.) Courses of colonic lavage on alternate days, for 10–14 days, are sometimes given— first, sodium bicarbonate solution (60 gr. to 1 pint) or normal saline is used to remove as much fæces and mucus as possible: this is followed by chiniofon B.P. (Yatren 1 per cent.), tannic acid (1/500), Protargol or Albargin (1/1,000) or potassium permanganate (1/5,000) for their astringent and antiseptic effects.   Others now use the local rectal instillation of hydrocortisone hemisuccinate sodium 100 mg. dissolved in 120 ml. of normal saline by a slow rectal drip, daily for 2 weeks.

Surgical measures are being used more commonly in certain cases.   The indications are: for cases which have failed to respond to adequate medical treatment, in those subject to severe relapses or severe anæmia, for acute or chronic perforation, when ileitis is marked or when polyposis is present with the risk of malignant change.   Complete colectomy with ileo-sigmoid or ileo-rectal anastomosis is preferable when the rectum is healthy— otherwise a temporary or permanent ileostomy is necessary.

Chronic Segmental Colitis resembling chronic ulcerative colitis has been recently described.   The disease does not start in the rectum but is present on one or more areas of the ascending, transverse, descending or sigmoid colon.   The common symptom is diarrhœa, with blood-stained stools in half the cases: there is cramp-like abdominal pain and intermittent fever, sometimes with complications in the joints and in the skin: later malignant changes are much less frequent.

V. Nervous Diarrhœa may continue for years; it has the following characteristics: (i.) The motions are often quite healthy.   There is usually no pain or tenesmus.   The diarrhœa is recurring or intermittent, occurring in the early morning, or when the patient is " nervous."   Sometimes it follows each meal (lienteric diarrhœa).   (ii.) Diet has little or no influence; the attacks are determined by mental emotion or bodily fatigue.   The administration of nux vomica, belladonna and bromides is more efficacious than astringents.

The crises of LOCOMOTOR ATAXY sometimes take the form of acute diarrhœa, with or without pain.   In HYSTERIA acute attacks of diarrhœa, with noisy borborygmi, may occur, determined in the same way as other hysterical attacks.

VI. Fissure of the Anus, slight ulcers or abrasions, or even an inflamed pile, may cause a chronic diarrhœa.   Actually there is underlying retention of stool (constipation), and the diarrhœa is " false diarrhœa."

VII. Obstruction in the Portal Circulation produces diarrhœa, due to the congestion of the intestinal wall.   It is recognised by: (i.) A previous history of heart disease, or of intemperance and alcoholic dyspepsia; (ii.) other signs of liver or cardiac disease; (iii.) other evidences of portal obstruction, such as ascites, piles and a large spleen (§ 260); (iv.) there is little or no pain, and the stools are liquid and dark, occasionally bloody.   The Treatment requires caution, because the diarrhœa and hæmorrhage of themselves relieve the condition by diminishing the venous engorgement.   (i.) If the diarrhœa has not lasted long, a dose of calomel will relieve the portal congestion, and so cure the diarrhœa.   (ii.) Bismuth and opium, with caution, are the most useful for checking the diarrhœa.

In the tropics **Diarrhœa** is a common complaint; it may merely indicate some simple intestinal derangement due to bad food or indiscretion of diet. On the other hand, many serious intestinal diseases such as cholera, typhoid and sprue may begin with diarrhœa; the appearance of mucus, pus and blood in the stools, however, indicates that the trouble, which may be due to a number of different causes, probably arises in the large bowel.

The patient, who is living or has lived abroad, complains of severe DIARRHŒA, WITH BLOOD, MUCUS *and perhaps* PUS *in the stools.* The disease is probably CHRONIC DYSENTERY.

§ 315. VIII. Subacute and Chronic Dysentery is a colonic inflammation, often leading to necrosis and ulceration of the mucosa, due to certain specific bacilli, protozoa or helminths, and characterised by the frequent passage of stools containing mucus, blood and pus.   Three main types occur: (1) SUBACUTE and CHRONIC BACILLARY DYSENTERY, due to a number of different micro-organisms; (2) PROTOZOAL DYSENTERY, due to (a) *Entamœba histolytica*, (b) *Balantidium coli*, (c) malignant tertian malaria and (d) kala-azar; (3) HELMINTHIC DYSENTERY, associated with (a) blood flukes: *Schistosoma mansoni*, *S. japonicum*, (b) the intestinal nematode *Œsophagostomum apiostomum*, (c) *Trichuris trichiura* in children (§ 315c).

(1) Chronic Bacillary Dysentery may follow an acute attack (§ 309) or be subacute from the onset.   Generally there is frequent defæcation, rectal discomfort or tenesmus, muco-pus and blood in the fæces.   During exacerbations abdominal colic and fever may recur.   Emaciation, asthenia, secondary anæmia and often œdema of the limbs follow.   The thickened, spastic descending colon is palpable.

Diagnosis.—Sigmoidoscopy reveals superficial ulcers in the rectum and lower colon: in more severe cases granulation tissue is also present.   Dysentery bacilli may be isolated from the fæces, and in a large proportion of cases by taking a direct swab from an ulcer during sigmoidoscopy.   When they are absent the condition may be ulcerative colitis (§§ 310, 314).   *Carcinoma* is excluded by sigmoidoscopy and by a barium enema.

Etiology.—The specific organisms are *Shigella shigæ*, various types of *S. flexneri* and of *S. boydii*, *S. schmitzii* and *S. sonnei*.   Shiga dysentery is mainly a tropical malady; the others may occur in Europe, especially in military barracks, prisons, asylums and in certain outbreaks of summer diarrhœa in children.   The disease is spread by water and food contaminated by carriers, or by infected flies.

Treatment of Acute and Chronic Bacillary Dysentery.   The *sulphonamide compounds* are of the greatest value.   Give by mouth sulphaguanidine, 6–8 G. initially, followed by 3–4 G. 4-hourly until the stools are less than five per day; then 8-hourly until the stools are normal, the total course not to exceed 10 days.   This drug is effective and safe in patients initially dehydrated.   Succinyl sulphathiazole 20 G. daily, or phthalyl-sulphathiazole 20 G. daily, in divided doses at 3-hourly intervals, have been advocated, as also have the absorbable sulphonamides, *e.g.*, sulphadiazine 1 G. 4-hourly.   In severe cases with much toxæmia, where *S. shigæ* infection is proved or suspected, concentrated Shiga anti-toxin (100,000 units or more) should be given intravenously as early as possible and repeated in 12 hours if indicated.   *Dehydration* is treated by fluids liberally by mouth and if necessary by intravenous infusions of saline or 5 per cent. dextrose-saline.   In severe cases with circulatory failure serum, plasma or blood *transfusions* may be of value.   The *diet* should be fluid for the first day or two, then gradually increased to a high calorie, high vitamin diet, but maintaining a low residue throughout.   Symptomatic relief of griping or tenderness will be obtained with warmth to the abdomen, or tinct. opii. Sometimes the organism is sulphonamide resistant. In such cases only are antibiotics justified, *e.g.*, Aureomycin 0·5 G. 6-hourly for 7 days. Streptomycin orally 1–2 G. daily for 4 days is very successful in the treatment of *S. sonnei* infections, which are usually sulphonamide resistant.

(2) PROTOZOAL DYSENTERY. (*a*) **Amœbic Dysentery** is characterised by afebrile diarrhœa with several voluminous fœtid stools daily, containing brownish mucus and dark red blood; tenesmus occurs if the rectum be involved. In 10 per cent. of patients the condition is more acute, fever is present and the bowels may act a dozen times in the 24 hours. Palpation reveals a thickened, tender colon; sigmoidoscopy may show typical painless, yellow, amœbic ulcers surrounded by a zone of hyperæmia, and healthy intervening mucosa. *Entamœba histolytica* can be found by examining the fresh material obtained by swabbing or lightly curetting the base of the ulcer. The disease is acquired by swallowing the cysts in contaminated water and food, especially vegetables, infected from convalescent or contact carriers.

Diagnosis.—The actively motile amœba containing red blood corpuscles is found in the mucoid exudate in acute cases, and the cysts in the solid fæces of chronic cases (Fig. 103). Ulceration is almost always confined to the large intestine, and often involves the muscular coats. Complications include intestinal hæmorrhage, perforation with peritonitis, retro-colic abscess and post-dysenteric adhesions, and *amœboma* (a chronic amœbic granuloma) often closely simulating neoplasm. Amœbic liver disease is at first associated with fever, enlarged, tender liver and slight leucocytosis, and later with rigors, sweating, shoulder pain, and involvement of the base of the right lung (§ 336). Amœbiasis of the lung is occasionally found; involvement of the brain, spleen and abdominal wall is rare.

Treatment.—Patients require a low-residue diet and must be kept in bed during treatment with emetine as it is a myocardial poison. For *intestinal* infection, each night emetine bismuth iodide (E.B.I.) gr. 3 in gelatin-coated capsules is given on an empty stomach, preceded one hour beforehand by phenobarbitone gr. 1 and butobarbitone gr. 1½. The E.B.I. is given for 10–12 nights, and the patient must stay in bed until the third day after the treatment has ended. E.B.I. alone is as efficacious as any combination of drugs. The tetracycline group of antibiotics are less effective but are alternatives to E.B.I.; the latter should not be given to patients with heart disease or those severely malnourished. In very severe acute amœbic dysentery symptoms are quickly controlled by emetine hydrochloride gr. 1 intramuscularly daily for 3 days, followed by E.B.I. for only 7–9 days. Patients *without dysenteric symptoms*, but whose fæces contain *E. histolytica cysts* and no exudate, can be given ambulatory treatment such as Diodoquin 2 G. daily for 3 weeks, carbarsone (B.P.), stovarsol (B.P.) 0·25 G. b.d. or Entamide 0·5 G. t.i.d., all by mouth. A radical cure rate of about 80 per cent. may be expected with any of these.

For amœbic *liver disease* give emetine hydrochloride gr. 1 intramuscularly daily for up to 10 days, and if pus is present it requires aspiration. Open operation is only performed if secondary infection necessitates it, or in the rare case in which the left lobe of the liver contains an abscess. Chloroquine is greatly concentrated in the liver and lungs and can be used in place of, or after, emetine in the treatment of amœbiasis of these organs. The dose of chloroquine phosphate is 0·25 G. t.d.s. for 21 days. Two important points should be remembered: the antibiotics will not cure amœbic liver disease and emetine overdosage is dangerous.

(*b*) **Balantidial Dysentery** occurs in people who handle pigs. There are frequent muco-sanguineous stools and anæmia; many cases remain latent. Ulcers form in the colon and may perforate. Clinically, this condition is indistinguishable from amœbic ulceration, the diagnosis being made by microscopical examination of the stools or of material curetted from the ulcers during sigmoidoscopy. *Balantidium coli*, in vegetative forms or cysts, may occur in the excreta.

Treatment is with tab. oxytetracycline dihydrate B.P. (Tetracycline) 2 G. daily for 7 days.

(c) **Malarial Dysentery.**—Malignant tertian malaria (*Plasmodium falciparum*) may manifest itself by severe diarrhœa, with occasionally blood and mucus, producing a syndrome indistinguishable clinically from bacillary dysentery; the condition originates from obstruction in the capillaries by clumps of agglutinated corpuscles infected with parasites. Sigmoidoscopy in the milder cases shows a diffuse or patchy hyperæmia; in severe cases scattered hæmorrhagic areas are seen in the hyperæmic bowel wall, and these may go on to actual necrosis. The *diagnosis* is made by finding the parasites in blood smears and by the associated clinical features, such as splenomegaly, anæmia and fever.

(d) **Kala-azar Dysentery.**—In kala-azar, diarrhœa is a not uncommon complication; *Leishmania* may be found in the intestinal villi or polypoid tissue formed in the gut wall. Occasionally a dysenteric-like syndrome with the passage of blood and mucus supervenes, which may prove to be due either to kala-azar itself or to a superadded bacillary dysentery infection.

(3) HELMINTHIC DYSENTERY.—(a) **Schistosomal dysentery,** especially at first, is characterised by diarrhœa or loose motions containing mucus and blood; later there are often solid stools coated with mucus containing the lateral spined ova of *S. mansoni* or the lateral knobbed ova of *S. japonicum*. Occasionally the terminal spined ova of *S. hæmatobium* may be found (Fig. 134), though this species rarely gives rise to dysenteric features. Tenesmus, loss of weight and secondary anæmia may follow: many cases remain latent. Subacute or chronic schistosomal appendicitis, colonic and rectal papillomata, fistulæ, and a periportal cirrhosis of the liver may develop; the latter may be associated with an enlarged spleen (Egyptian splenomegaly). Involvement of the Central Nervous System may occur in *S. japonicum* infections (§ 896). Proctoscopy or sigmoidoscopy reveals minute nodules and ova are often best found on examination of small snips of rectal mucous membrane. Eosinophilia is not constant. The schistosomal complement-fixation reaction is often useful when ova are difficult to find but is unreliable in long-standing infections.

Treatment.—Trivalent antimonial compounds are specific. Sodium antimony tartrate intravenously on alternate days for one month is frequently used; give an initial dose of gr. $\frac{1}{4}$ and increase in successive doses by gr. $\frac{1}{4}$, to a maximum of gr. $2\frac{1}{2}$. Recently a short intensive course of a total dosage of gr. i per 12 lb. body weight (12 mg./kg.) divided into 6 doses has been advocated, 3 doses being given at 3-hourly intervals on two successive days: each dose is dissolved in 10 ml. of 5 per cent. dextrose solution and injected not faster than 2 ml. per minute. Cough, vomiting or rheumatic-like pains may follow administration of this drug. Other drugs which are easier to give but which are less effective are: Stibophen (6·3 per cent. solution) in doses of 1·5 ml., 3·5 ml. and then 5 ml. intramusc. on alternate days to a total of 60 ml.: Anthiomaline (6 per cent. solution) 4 ml. intramusc. on alternate days to a total of 60 ml.; Miracil in doses of 1–2 G. b.d. by mouth for three days and repeated a month later.

(b) *Dysentery due to Œsophagostomiasis.*—The nematode parasite, *Œsophagostomum apiostomum,* commonly affects men in Northern Nigeria. Its embryos embed themselves in the walls of the colon and become enclosed in fibrous tissue nodules; as they approach maturity they escape into the lumen, often leaving behind an ulcerated area, and finally attach themselves to the mucosal lining of the gut. Diarrhœa with blood and mucus may result, and peritonitis is an occasional complication. The eggs, which resemble ancylostome ova, are passed in the stool. Tetrachlorethylene or carbon tetrachloride cures the disease. (See Ancylostomiasis, § 563.)

(c) *Dysentery due to* **Trichuris trichiura.** Very heavy infections (over 100,000 ova per G. of fæces on the Stoll count) are sometimes found in children of poor families, associated with chronic dysentery and often rectal prolapse. The condition responds to dithiazanine iodide (Telmid) 100 mg. per 10 lb. body weight per day, in three divided doses for seven days.

GROUP B. We now turn to the *less common* diseases which cause **Chronic Diarrhœa.** They are IX. the various causes of STEATORRHŒA; X. SENILE DIARRHŒA; XI. MINERAL POISONS; XII. GASTROGENOUS DIARRHŒA; and XIII. Various CONSTITUTIONAL CAUSES.

The patient complains of passing PALE BULKY STOOLS *which look " greasy."* *There may be attacks of* CHRONIC DIARRHŒA *and there is loss of weight. The condition is* STEATORRHŒA.

§ 316. IX. Steatorrhœa is the principal finding in the *Malabsorption Syndrome* which may result not only from the deficient absorption of fats but also of carbohydrates, proteins, calcium, iron, the hæmatinic factor, folic acid and vitamins.

The *Symptoms* vary considerably from case to case, depending partly on the cause. (1) Attention may first be drawn to the character of the stools. They may be pale, bulky and fatty in appearance and often float in water. (2) There may be 2–5 stools a day. (3) The stools may be gassy, there may be borborygmi and gaseous distension of the abdomen causing much abdominal enlargement. (4) Loss of weight and of energy are frequent. However, abdominal symptoms may be largely absent, with no diarrhœa, and yet examination of the stool shows the presence of steatorrhœa. In such cases the early symptoms may be those caused by the associated deficiencies of absorption in the small intestine. (5) Anæmia may be the result of a deficient absorption of iron (from the duodenum), of folic acid (from the upper jejunum) or of cyanocobalamin (from the ileum). (6) Vitamin A deficiency gives rise to xerophthalmia and skin changes, vitamin B deficiency to a sore tongue, polyneuritis, œdema and the pellagra syndrome (§ 633), vitamin C lack to scurvy, failure of absorption of vitamin D and of calcium to osteoporosis and rickets (§ 608), vitamin K deficiency to an abnormal bleeding tendency and to a low plasma prothrombin content.

The *Diagnosis* of steatorrhœa depends on an examination of the stool. Two tests are available. (1) Fat taken in the food is almost entirely digested and absorbed: when a diet containing between 60 and 150 G. of fat a day results in the passage of more than 6 G. of fæcal fat a day over a three-day period, steatorrhœa is present. (N.B. Liquid paraffin must be avoided over this period.) (2) *The labelled-fat absorption test* is becoming popular. To prevent an action of the radio-iodine on the patient's thyroid gland, potassium iodide (100 mg.) is given daily for a week starting the evening before the test. At breakfast on the day of the test a capsule of olive oil labelled with I^{131} (30 microcuries) is given, immediately followed by a meal containing 15 grammes of fat, and by a normal lunch and tea. After taking the labelled fat, for 6 hours at hourly intervals, 10 ml. of blood is taken into bottles containing heparin; and the whole of the stool is collected in polythene bags for the next 72 hours. In the normal individual the plasma radio-iodine level rises, usually within a 6-hour period, to contain more than 4 per cent. per litre of the given dose: while in malabsorption there is generally less than 2 per cent. throughout. Normal individials excrete less than 2 per cent. of the labelled fat in the stool, whereas in malabsorption the excretion is more than this and may reach 90 per cent.

Many cases show a very poor absorption of sugar so that a glucose tolerance curve after glucose 50 G. gives a low or even a flat curve: sometimes deficient absorption of protein causes a low plasma albumen content. Achlorhydria or a histamine refractory achylia gastrica may be present.

The *Etiology* can be classified as follows:—

(1) A primary defect of absorption exists in the small intestine and especially in the jejunum. This may be due to

　　Widespread atrophic changes in the villi—idiopathic steatorrhœa (§ 317).
　　Tropical sprue (§ 318) and in infants cœliac disease (§ 317).
　　Disease of the coats of the small intestine as with amyloid disease (§ 318. IXf).

Obstruction of the lacteals by Tuberculosis, Lymphosarcoma or Reticulo-sarcoma.

Local chronic obstruction of the small intestine with inflammatory changes above the obstruction as with Crohn's disease, tuberculosis, simple stricture or annular carcinoma.

Surgical conditions such as following widespread resections or short-circuiting of the small intestine, or fistula formation such as with a gastro-jejuno-colic fistula.

(2) A deficiency of biliary secretion particularly in obstructive jaundice (§ 330).

(3) A deficiency of pancreatic secretion such as occurs with pancreatic calculi, or carcinoma or (in infants) fibrocystic disease (mucosis). These conditions may be diagnosed by radiological evidence of pancreatic calculi or by finding a deficiency of pancreatic enzymes in samples obtained via a duodenal tube.

(4) After the operation of partial or total gastrectomy there is an inadequate mixing of the food with the pancreatic and biliary secretions.

(5) Rarely there is an abnormal bacterial flora in the small intestine resulting from a stagnant loop or pouch produced by previous operation or by diverticula of the small bowel.

The *Prognosis* varies with the cause and the rate of progress of the disease. Many cases live for years, but sooner or later a semi-invalid existence may be reached.

Treatment is primarily that of the cause where possible. In general (i.) the diet should possess a low fat, high protein content with the carbohydrates largely derived from sucrose or glucose. Gluten-free diets are especially successful with cœliac disease and idiopathic steatorrhœa; (ii.) vitamin A in doses of 50,000 I.U. a day is indicated for night-blindness and xerophthalmia, vitamin B complex for patients with glossitis, pellagra or peripheral neuritis and folic acid and/or inj. cyanocobalamin for macrocytic anæmia, vitamin D in doses of 25,000–50,000 I.U. daily is required for osteomalacia and tetany, and vitamin K in oral doses of 4–8 mg. a day will usually check a hæmorrhagic tendency. Calcium lactate 4 G. t.d.s. before meals helps to correct a calcium deficiency. (iii.) Pancreatic enzymes help to replace a lack of the corresponding ferments.

§ 317. IXa. Idiopathic Steatorrhœa (Syn. Non-tropical Sprue) is becoming much more commonly recognised as being associated with failure of the small intestinal canal to absorb a variety of essential food substances.

Symptoms.—(i.) There may be intermittent bouts of loose or watery stools for a few days, perhaps with constipation in between. The diarrhœa may be precipitated by an unduly fatty meal, or by physical or nervous stresses. (ii.) The abdomen is not often distended with gas as it is with cœliac disease. (iii.) There is loss of weight and of energy. (iv.) In some the main symptoms may be those of macrocytic anæmia, cramps and tetany, osteoporosis, an undue tendency to bleeding, the results of vitamin deficiencies mentioned in § 316. (v.) Clubbing of the fingers is often present.

Diagnosis is made by peroral small intestinal biopsy (§ 304) and finding partial or more or less complete atrophy of the villi (and see p. 419). The excess of fat in the stool is mainly as split fat.

The *Etiology* is unknown but a familial tendency is common. A considerable proportion have had cœliac disease in childhood.

Treatment.—The elimination of the gluten in wheat and rye flour gives a considerable improvement in the symptoms of a large number of patients with lessening of the anæmia. (For details of the diet see § 296. XVII.) In many cases it is necessary to restrict the intake of fats to 50–60 G. a day and to give folic acid 5 mg. t.d.s.

Cœliac disease is a rare form of recurrent diarrhœa with steatorrhœa, usually commencing insidiously between the age of 6 and 24 months.

Symptoms.—(i.) There is a failure to gain weight with loss of appetite; (ii.) diarrhœa commences: the stools are large, pale and very offensive, and may become frothy; (iii.) the abdomen becomes distended with gas; (iv.) loss of weight continues, the large abdomen contrasting markedly with the flat wasted buttocks; (v.) complications include a failure to grow (infantilism), often rickets, anæmia which is usually due to iron-deficiency (occasionally it is megalocytic), scurvy and infantile tetany.

Diagnosis.—The steatorrhœa is due to a large excess of split fat, amounting to 40–60 per cent. of the dried weight of stool. In fibrocystic disease of the pancreas (mucosis) the failure to thrive dates from birth and the pancreatic enzymes are absent in samples of the duodenal juices.

Etiology.—Recent work has shown that the gluten content of certain cereals (especially wheat and also rye) interferes with the absorption of split fat from the upper part of the small intestine with the formation of a large amount of short-chain fatty acids. The absorption of vitamins A, C, D is also affected and calcium is lost in the stool in combination with the fatty acids. The malabsorption appears to be due to a glutamine containing peptide derived from these two cereals. Cœliac children show an excess of glutamine in their blood.

Prognosis.—If untreated the disease runs a chronic course with periodic exacerbations, marked stunting of growth and sometimes death from intercurrent infection: even in untreated cases recovery tends to occur in later life. The outlook has been greatly improved by modern therapeutic methods.

Treatment is by the administration of a gluten-free diet (§ 296. XVII): once treatment is under way it is no longer necessary to decrease the fat of the diet. Supplements of vitamins A, C, D and of iron may be necessary for a while. After 12–18 months gluten-containing articles of diet may be added cautiously, and if no ill-effects are produced ordinary wheaten-flour products may be further added until finally a normal diet is consumed.

§ 318. IX*b.* **Tropical Sprue** is a disease of unknown etiology which is now curable. It particularly affects adult people of European descent in India, Ceylon and the parts of Asia further East. It is still confused with " idiopathic steatorrhœa " which has a sporadic world-wide distribution, is usually less easily cured and therefore more chronic. Sprue is associated with derangement of the gastro-intestinal tract, characterised by deficient absorption of fat, glucose, certain vitamins and calcium; the secretion of the intrinsic hæmatopoietic factor is often also defective.

Symptoms.—(i.) Apyrexial morning diarrhœa with bulky, acid, pale, frothy, fatty stools. (ii.) Inflammatory lesions of the mouth; the tongue is tender, shows patches of inflammation, and later becomes pale and atrophic with disappearance of the papillæ. Aphthous ulcers may involve the lingual or buccal mucosa. (iii.) Anæmia, which may be severe; this is almost always megalocytic in type with an increase in the average diameter of the corpuscles. The marrow shows megaloblastic and normoblastic hyperplasia. (iv.) Asthenia with low blood pressure. (v.) Emaciation and wasting; the skin becomes dry and wrinkled and sometimes brown pigmentation occurs over the forehead and malar eminences. (vi.) Intestinal flatulence; occasionally vomiting and dyspepsia. (vii.) In advanced cases neuritis, œdema of the feet, cramp and tetany may occur occasionally. (viii.) Physical examination shows a distended abdomen with thin abdominal parietes.

Diagnosis.—Tropical sprue has to be diagnosed from idiopathic steatorrhœa, chronic pancreatitis, carcinoma of the pancreas, gastro-colic fistula, tuberculosis and lymphadenoma involving the mesenteric lymph glands and from all other types of megalocytic anæmia. Biochemical and radiological investigations often assist. Sprue shows a high fæcal fat which is adequately split, and low gastric acidity; with the aid of histamine, however, 78 per cent. secrete acid. Blood analysis often shows lowered calcium, slight increase in plasma bilirubin and delayed or low glucose tolerance curve, due to malabsorption of glucose. A barium meal X-ray (using a special non-flocculating barium sulphate) shows irregular clumping of the barium sulphate in the small intestine—the so-called " deficiency pattern."

Prognosis.—With adequate treatment the symptoms readily come under control; the disease is now curable, provided treatment is persevered with for a period of months. A proportion of patients relapse while in the tropics but it is now permissible to allow patients to remain in the tropics so long as they continue under medical observation. However, the elderly are wise to leave tropical districts permanently.

Treatment.—It is necessary to give a high protein, low fat, low carbohydrate diet to all patients. The majority of cases obtain a remission while on a sprue diet (§ 296. XVI) so long as it is combined with one of the tetracycline group of antibiotics. Severely ill patients need bed rest and should be given a more strict diet in which red meat is the main source of protein, or alternatively a defatted, dried milk known as " sprulac " may be substituted. Crude liver extract, equivalent to 1½ lb. of whole liver daily, should be given orally or intramuscularly; in severe cases, where large doses of liver are so beneficial, oral and intramuscular liver extract therapy may be combined. In many cases good initial results are obtained with folic acid 20 mg. daily for a week, followed by a daily maintenance dose of 5 mg., but liver may be required to complete the response. A suitable diet with liver extract has made it possible to restore the majority of sprue cases to normal health in two months. Relapses may follow indiscretions in diet or an infection such as influenza. Nicotinic acid, 50 mg. t.i.d., is indicated when oral symptoms are severe, riboflavin 3 mg. daily for angular stomatitis, acid hydrochlor. dil. ℍ 30–60 t.i.d. with meals for achlorhydria and calcium lactate gr. 30 t.i.d. for calcium deficiency.

IX*c*. **Pancreatic Disease** is associated with chronic diarrhœa, with pale stools containing a large excess of unsplit fat (§§ 359, 360).

IX*d*. **Obstructive Jaundice** also causes the stools to be bulky, pale and a little loose (§ 330).

IX*e*. **Partial or total Gastrectomy, Gastro-enterostomy, Resection of the Small Intestine, Partial Colectomy** and especially a **Gastro-colic or Entero-colic Fistula** produce diarrhœa and anæmia with malabsorption of the food substances and steatorrhœa. Especially with a fistula there is progressive emaciation for which operative treatment is usually required.

IX*f*. **Amyloid Disease** of the intestines gives rise to a most intractable form of chronic diarrhœa and steatorrhœa. Indeed, this is the common mode of death in amyloid disease of the viscera. The characteristics here are: (i.) A history of long-standing purulent discharge, of rheumatoid disease or of syphilis; (ii.) great pallor of the skin, accompanied by evidences of lardaceous disease in the spleen, liver and kidney; (iii.) the stools are generally liquid and extremely offensive, sometimes attended by hæmorrhage. The *Treatment* is very unsatisfactory. Opium does no harm, even when there is amyloid disease of the kidney, as there is no tendency to uræmia.

IX*g*. Other *causes* of steatorrhœa include Crohn's disease, multiple diverticula, carcinoma or a carcinoid tumour of the small intestine. *Whipple's disease* (intestinal lipodystrophy) is a rare form of the malabsorption syndrome occurring chiefly in men of 40–65 years. There are attacks of intermittent diarrhœa with fatty stools, anæmia, œdema, ascites, intermittent fever and often rheumatoid polyarthritis. The primary condition appears to be in the submucous coats of the small intestine where large mononuclear cells are filled with a foamy cytoplasm of a muco-protein nature. Death is usual within five years; the corticosteroids may help treatment.

X. **Senile Diarrhœa** occurs in persons over sixty or seventy, and is very chronic in its course, but the patient suffers little. Careful examination for organic disease should be made before concluding that the condition is simple senile diarrhœa. Most remedies fail to relieve it; it may exist for years without emaciation or danger to life.

XI. **Mineral Poisons,** and especially arsenic and antimony, in small and continued doses, may cause persistent diarrhœa.

XII. **Gastrogenous diarrhœa** may occur in cases of achylia gastrica, even when it is not associated with pernicious anæmia. It ceases when 30 to 60 drops of dilute hydrochloric acid are taken in a tumblerful of water with meals.

XIII. *Constitutional causes* are hyperthyroidism, Addison's disease, excessive tobacco smoking in susceptible persons, chronic renal disease, diabetes mellitus, anaphylaxis, and exhausting or wasting diseases of any kind.

§ 319. Tenesmus literally means straining at stool (τείνω, to strain or stretch); but in its widest sense it may be taken to mean any local rectal sensation of " bearing down " which results either in constant desire to go to stool, or straining when at stool. The latter may lead to prolapse of the rectum, especially in children. Diarrhœa is always attended by more or less tenesmus, but tenesmus is not always attended by diarrhœa. (1) Ascertain if the tenesmus is accompanied by diarrhœa—*i.e.*, are the motions frequent and liquid? If so, refer to the section on Diarrhœa, § 306. (2) Examine the motions; note their consistence and any abnormal constituents such as mucus and blood. (3) Search for any local anal or rectal condition such as fissures, piles, polypi or ulcers. All the pelvic organs should also be thoroughly investigated, especially in women, in whom the symptom is commoner than in men.

Causes.—Tenesmus (not necessarily accompanied by diarrhœa) may arise from four groups of causes:

1. Various conditions of the ANUS—pruritus, eczema or fissure—may be overlooked for a long time. Piles also, if internal, may be difficult to detect, even by the examining finger, but streaks of bright blood will appear in the motions from time to time.

2. Various RECTAL CONDITIONS, especially carcinoma, simple ulceration (proctitis, § 321) or (rarely) stricture. The former are attended by pus or blood, or both. The latter (usually due to lymphogranuloma venereum (§ 312. IIe)) is attended by tape-like stools. In the aged, always suspect cancer of the rectum and examine for impacted fæces. Prolonged use of purgatives or constant use of enemas may result in straining at stool and prolapse of the rectum. An impacted fish-bone is a rare cause.

3. PRESSURE on, or irritation of, THE RECTUM FROM WITHOUT, such as may be caused by chronic congestion, retroversion or other disease of the uterus. Ischio-rectal abscess, pelvic hæmatocœle and various ovarian and Fallopian tube lesions in women, and congestion or new growth of the prostate in men, are common causes. Any bladder disease, such as stone—a frequent cause of tenesmus in children, and apt to result in prolapse of the rectum—or new growths or chronic cystitis may cause this distressing condition. Menstruation and the later stages of pregnancy may be attended by a certain amount of tenesmus.

4. In HYSTERICAL AND NERVOUS SUBJECTS any fright or other emotion may at once determine tenesmus, which the patient calls " diarrhœa." In tabes dorsalis the " rectal crises " may take the form of tenesmus.

Treatment.—The indications are (1) the removal of the cause, the treatment of piles and other causal conditions being described elsewhere; (2) the relief of local congestion or irritation of the rectum. In any case, morphia, bismuth, belladonna, or cocaine or allied drugs in the form either of suppositories or ointments inserted by an applicator, will relieve the distress from which the patient suffers.

§ 320. In Proctalgia Fugax the patient has recurrent severe cramp-like pain in the rectum and perineum, which usually wakens him up at night; it may last three to ten minutes or even longer. Rectal examination is negative. The pain is regarded as due to rectal or anal spasm or arising in the levator ani; some medical sufferers regard it as an allergic symptom or attribute it to venous engorgement. In women it occurs near the menstrual period.

Treatment.—The pain is usually relieved by a small meal which excites a gastro-colic reflex: otherwise insert the finger or suppos. bism. subgall. (B.P.C.) or inject the rectum with air or warm enemata. Sometimes attacks cease when the patient gives up smoking.

§ 321. **Blood in the Stools** is met with, as we have seen, in dysentery and some cases of simple diarrhœa; it may occur in other conditions. The presence of blood in the stools may be recognised by the reddening of the water in which the stool is placed, or by the spectroscope (§ 303). Clinically, blood in the stools may present two widely different characters: (a) When the blood is of *bright crimson colour* and is on the surface of the stool, it indicates either that the bleeding comes from the rectum or the lower part of the large bowel; or, if it comes from the upper part of the intestinal canal, that it is too large in amount to be acted upon by the intestinal secretion. (b) *Melæna (tar-coloured stools)* is met when hæmor-rhage in moderate quantity has taken place in the stomach or the upper part of the alimentary tract, in which case the digestive fluids of the stomach and intestine acting on the blood give it a tarry appearance. The causes of these two conditions are to some extent interchangeable, for what will produce a large hæmorrhage at one time may at another produce only a little. Bleeding, even if small in quantity, should never be neglected; often slight intermittent bleeding is the first sign of a malignant growth somewhere in the gastro-intestinal tract.

(a) **Bright Red Blood** may be due to lesions of the lower part of the alimentary canal. Of these several causes are referable to the anus or rectum, and are discovered on local examination or by proctoscopy.

I. Hæmorrhoids, or Piles, are undoubtedly the commonest cause of blood in the stools. The blood is generally met in streaks only, but the quantity may at other times be very large (§ 322).

II. Prolapse of the Rectal Mucous Membrane, either acute or chronic, with contraction of the anal sphincter, may cause the appearance of bright blood, usually after a motion.

III. Fissure of the Anus may also produce streaks of blood. It is not infrequent, and is recognised by excruciating pain during and after defæcation. The irritation it causes may give rise to a variety of false diarrhœa. The fissure can always be seen by *careful* examination. There may be a history of trauma.

IV. In Carcinoma of the Rectum or Colon the blood is usually mixed with the stool, and may be intermittent. A sudden and very severe hæmorrhage from the rectum may be the first sign of carcinoma. An innocent polyp may cause hæmorrhage; in adults they are often multiple and should be looked on as a precancerous condition and removed. Diverti-culosis of the sigmoid colon is a common condition, but it rarely causes bleeding; remember that it may co-exist with a new growth. Careful digital and sigmoidoscopic examinations should be made.

V. A discharge of blood-stained mucus, coming on somewhat suddenly in an infant, is highly suggestive of INTESTINAL INTUSSUSCEPTION, which is one of the causes of acute obstruction (§ 326).

VI. RECTAL POLYPI are met chiefly in children.

VII. TYPHOID and TUBERCULOUS ULCERATION sometimes produce profuse discharges of bright red blood, coming from the lower end of the small intestine. Other evidences of these affections are present.

VIII. **Proctitis** may be simple, traumatic or infective (gonorrhœal, syphilitic, tuberculous or pyogenic). *Simple proctitis* occurs in association with chronic constipation or the repeated use of soapy enemata. *Ulcerative proctitis* is usually present in the upper part of the rectum, and may spread to the sigmoid and progress to ulcerative colitis. It can only be diagnosed with certainty by proctoscopic examination. Lympho-granuloma inguinale is a cause of ulcerative proctitis and rectal stricture (90 per cent. of cases are women): and see § 312. IIe.

The leading *symptoms* are tenesmus and painful defæcation, sometimes discharge of blood and mucus *after* the passage of normally formed stools. *Treatment* is by avoiding hard vegetable residues in the diet, keeping the stools soft and the use of mild astringent retention enemata: a course of hydrocortisone acetate enemata (0·2 per cent.) or hydrocortisome hemisuccinate suppositories is often of great help.

IX. ULCERATIVE COLITIS (§ 310. VIII, § 314. IV) occasionally causes severe hæmorrhage, more usually repeated small hæmorrhages.

X. SCHISTOSOMA MANSONI and HÆMATOBIUM infestations cause a spurious dysentery with polypoid masses in the rectum. They are described in § 315 (3). *Schistosoma japonicum*, a third species, causes Katayama disease or Schistosomiasis of the Far East.

XI. Various GENERAL BLOOD CONDITIONS may give rise to hæmorrhage coming from the rectum or elsewhere in the alimentary canal in varying amount. This occurs in purpura, primary thrombocytopenia, multiple telangiectasia, scurvy, agranulocytosis, hæmorrhagic forms of the specific fevers, acute yellow atrophy of the liver and leukæmia.

(*b*) **Melæna** (*tarry stools*) is met when bleeding takes place in moderate quantity from the stomach, or high up in the alimentary tract. 60 ml. of blood can cause a tarry stool. Its causes are:

1. When coming FROM THE STOMACH, it may be associated with profuse *hæmatemesis* (§ 272); the commonest causes of hæmatemesis are peptic ulcer and hepatic cirrhosis. Melæna occurs often without hæmatemesis in duodenal ulcer and in hiatus hernia of the stomach.

2. PORTAL OBSTRUCTION (§ 260) is a frequent cause of melæna, especially that form due to peri-portal cirrhosis of the liver. It may also occur with advanced cardiac disease. In either case the hæmorrhage·is a natural safety-valve, and relieves the engorged state of the portal circulation.

3. CANCEROUS, TUBERCULOUS and other ULCERATIONS of the small intestine (see §§ 310 and 312), Crohn's disease, lardaceous disease of the bowel, mesenteric thrombosis or embolism, may produce melæna.

4. The GENERAL BLOOD CONDITIONS above named, when the hæmorrhage is small in amount, are attended by tarry instead of bright red stools. *Melæna neonatorum* is a rare condition in which there is a passage of blood in new-born children (see § 567. V).

5. ANCYLOSTOMIASIS is a possible cause of melæna in Egypt and other foreign countries (§ 563) but generally it is only revealed by tests for occult blood.

The *Treatment* of melæna should be directed to the cause, but the general principles are those laid down for hæmatemesis (§ 272). Worms are dealt with in § 323. For melæna neonatorum, see § 567. V.

§ 322. **Hæmorrhoids,** or Piles, are varicose rectal veins. This varicosity forms a swelling of variable size, which may be altogether within the anus (internal piles), or partly internal and partly external. Internal piles may in some cases be seen, when the patient strains down, as small purple swellings protruding through the sphincter.

Symptoms.—(1) Streaks of *bright red* blood occur in the stools, usually dripping after the bowel has acted; sometimes as much as ¼ pint of blood may be passed at a time. (2) There may be pain on defæcation, the pain continuing for some time after the passage of a stool. When a pile becomes inflamed, or strangulated by the sphincter, severe pain and discomfort are experienced, and the patient may have to remain in bed. Pain may be referred to other parts of the body—*e.g.*, to the testicles or bladder. (3) Constipation nearly always accompanies piles, due partly to mechanical obstruction, and partly to the pain caused by defæcation. (4) Pruritus is often troublesome. (5) In severe cases constitutional symptoms develop due to severe anæmia.

Etiology.—(1) Habitual constipation is undoubtedly the most common cause of hæmorrhoids, particularly in women, who in early life are so apt to contract this habit. (2) Portal obstruction is itself a cause of piles, and in all cases we should seek for the other symptoms of this lesion (§ 260). (3) Alcohol causes portal congestion, and thus becomes a cause of piles. (4) Sedentary occupations and deficient exercise. (5) Various local conditions, such as sitting on a cold seat or soft cushions which constrict the inferior hæmorrhoidal veins, uterine displacements, pregnancy, carcinoma of the rectum, pelvic and other tumours.

Prognosis.—Hæmorrhoids are not serious, but may be extremely troublesome, by the constant loss of blood, by their liability to repeated attacks of inflammation and thrombosis, and by the pain they cause.

Treatment.—Much may be done by three simple means: (1) The avoidance of alcohol (especially malt liquors) and sugar; (2) keeping the piles scrupulously clean, and (3) the bowels regularly and loosely open. Prolapsed piles must be replaced at once. Rich food, wines and other causes of hepatic congestion must be forbidden. Confection of senna (B.P.C.) with an occasional cholagogue at night is good; paraffin is apt to cause the piles to descend. Local applications should be simple. The old-fashioned gall and opium ointment is now replaced by hamamelis, with bismuth, morphia or cocaine for the pain, if necessary, or calamine powder on a pad of lint: Suppos. bismuth subgallate co. B.P.C. is very useful. Liquid hazeline is excellent, and is best applied on a strip of lint inserted within the anus, and left there; or a suppository may be employed, containing gr. 1 to 3 of hamamelis, and morphia gr. ⅛, if requisite. Inflamed piles are very painful, and are best treated by warm hip-baths, frequent bathing, warm fomentations with opium, belladonna or cocaine. Surgical removal is sometimes called for, but a cure may be obtained by a peri-venous injection of the subcutaneous tissues around the pile. Use 5 ml. of a solution containing phenol 20 gr., menthol 1 gr., almond oil to 1 fluid oz. Thrombosis is caused, and healing by scar. A strangulated pile may be incised radially under local anæsthesia, and the clot evacuated: this effects a cure.

A PERI-ANAL HÆMATOMA may be mistaken for a pile. It causes a local swelling and pruritis, and is best treated by simple incision and evacuation of the clot. Gas-gangrene infection is very rare, but is invariably fatal.

§ 323. Intestinal Worms often cause no symptoms. They are common in children, in inmates of mental hospitals and in adults who come from the tropics. The mor-phology, symptoms and habitat of various parasitic helminths are described in Tables XVIII and XIX, p. 426 et seq. Threadworms (Fig. 105) and roundworms (Fig. 106) are the most common in Britain.

Symptoms are often absent. They may result from reflex disturbances, mechanical action, helminthic toxins or anaphylaxis. They include (1) abdominal pain, some-times paroxysmal in character, (2) capricious or ravenous appetite associated with (3) loss of weight, (4) irregularity of the bowels or diarrhœa, (5) such reflex disturb-ances as grinding of the teeth at night, enuresis, strabismus and even convulsions. (6) Erythema, urticaria and eosinophilia result from helminthic toxins or anaphylaxis. Skin hypersensitiveness to helminthic protein is manifest by rapid wheal formation following intradermal injection of saline extracts of the different parasites. The roundworm, Ascaris lumbricoides, may produce helminthic pneumonia during the first week of infection owing to embryos traversing the lungs. Later, after the worms reach the small intestine, the above-mentioned symptoms may appear and occasion-ally severe manifestations such as: perforation of the bowel with generalised peritonitis or localised abscess with a fistula from which the worm is discharged, intestinal obstruction from masses of worms impacted near the ileo-cæcal valve, obstructive jaundice due to worms obstructing the common bile duct, or cholecystitis, liver abscess or œdema of the glottis associated with worms in these regions. Thread-worms (Enterobius vermicularis or Oxyuris vermicularis) inhabit the colon and migrate through the anus at night, producing pruritis and eczema ani, bladder irritability, sometimes vulvitis and vaginal discharge, and even catarrhal appendicitis. Toxocara worms are helminths recently demonstrated in the fæces of 20 per cent. of London dogs and cats (Woodruff). After ingestion by man the eggs develop into larvæ which migrate in the tissues; they do not mature but stimulate small granulomata when they die. Lesions in the retina may cause blindness, in the lungs a wheezy bronchitis with mottling, and they can cause meningo-encephalitis; an allergic response causes unexplained eosinophilia. An alcoholic extract produces a diagnostic skin reaction in those infected. Whip-worms (Trichuris trichiura or Trichocephalus dispar) inhabit the colon, appendix and terminal ileum: the eggs have characteristic knobs. Strongyloides stercoralis is a common tropical parasite, the females living in the jejunum and duodenum, occasionally invading the bile ducts and stomach: the eggs hatch out rhabditiform larvæ which are found in the fæces. Dermatitis and lung symptoms may appear a few days after exposure; later, in severe cases, there is epigastric discomfort and diarrhœa. Urticaria, œdema and occult blood may be present. Ancylostomes are dealt with in § 563. Heterophyes heterophyes is a minute intestinal fluke infesting man in Egypt; by means of a sucker it clings to the mucosa and causes indigestion and diarrhœa. Diagnosis depends on finding the eggs in the stools, or the parasites themselves after straining the fæces through muslin.

Five different TAPEWORMS may inhabit the intestine of man—*Tænia saginata*, the beef tapeworm; *Tænia solium*, the pork tapeworm, which has now been eliminated in Great Britain; and *Diphyllobothrium latum* (*Dibothriocephalus latus*), the broad-fish tapeworm which undergoes development first in the water flea, *Cyclops*, and later in fish, man becoming infected by eating underdone fish. There are also two unimportant dwarf tapeworms—*Hymenolepis nana* and *H. diminuta*.

Symptoms may be absent or there may be (1) gastro-intestinal symptoms; (2) reflex disturbances, especially in children, and occasionally (3) megaloblastic anæmia with *D. latum*. The cysticercus stage of *T. solium* is occasionally found in man, especially in India, producing encapsuled nodules in the muscles, subcutaneous tissues and organs, including the brain; in the latter case epilepsy may result several years after infection, symptoms being associated with the death of the cysts (§ 867).

Diagnosis of the cysticercus stage of *T. solium* is made by biopsy of a cyst, or X-ray examination may show calcified cysts in muscle tissue. The prognosis is bad if the brain be involved (§ 867). The cyst stage of *Echinococcus granulosus*, the small tapeworm of the dog, may affect man, especially involving the liver (see § 347) and lungs (see § 140), causing hydatid disease.

Treatment.—*Roundworm:* in the tropics ancylostome infection often co-exists and both worms are treated together. A saline purge is given overnight; next morning oil of chenopodium (1 ml.) and tetrachlorethylene (4 ml.) are given together followed in 2 hours by another saline purge. Hexylresorcinol (1 G. for an adult) is effective and safe, but the capsules must not be bitten or they will burn the mouth. The piperazine compounds are non-toxic and effective both for roundworms and for *threadworms*. They are now the drugs of choice for children with these infections. The dose of piperazine adipate or citrate is 600 mg. t.d.s. for seven days for an adult (300 mg. t.d.s. for children under six years). This should be repeated after one week's interval when treating threadworms. Oxytetracycline (terramycin) is also very effective. To prevent reinfection, patients should wear drawers and gloves at night to prevent scratching; the nails should be cut short; a mercurial ointment may be applied to the anus. The hands should be scrubbed and the buttocks cleaned with antiseptic soap on rising and whenever there is any chance of their being soiled by contact with contaminated clothing, skin or excreta. The other children in the family should be examined and all positive cases treated simultaneously. There is now a satisfactory treatment for *Trichuris* and *Strongyloides*. Slight infections are best left untreated but dithiazanine iodide (Telmid) 200 mg. t.d.s. for seven days often eradicates the former, and the same dosage for 21 days the latter. For *Heterophyes* tetrachlorethylene, beta-naphthol or thymol is effective. The treatment of *Tapeworm* infestations has three stages: (1) no solid food is given for 48 hours and no fluids either for the last 12 hours. This empties the small intestine. (2) On the third morning at 7 a.m. give extractum filicis liquidum 30 minims in gelatine capsules or emulsion; this is repeated three or four times during the next hour; the total adult dose is ℳ 90–120. (3) At 10 a.m. sodium or magnesium sulphate (½ oz.) is given and all the motions sieved against a black background to identify the head; if this is not removed recurrence is inevitable. Castor oil must never be given with filix mas, as the active principle, filicic acid, is soluble in it and dangerous toxic effects result. When vomiting is likely the anthelminthic may be administered through a duodenal tube. Mepacrine 1·0 G. can be given in place of filix mas. Dichlorphen is very effective for *Tænia saginata*. It is lethal to the tapeworm in doses of 500 mg./16 lb. body weight (maximum dose 6·0 G.) and does not require preliminary preparation. It is not advised for *T. solium* since destruction and digestion of the worm may lead to auto-infestation with the ova released. Surgical treatment will be necessary in *hydatid* disease, and rarely for intestinal perforation or obstruction due to ascaris infection, but in the last case medical conservative treatment, consisting of duodenal suction and a piperazine salt, 3 G. by a duodenal tube, will usually render it unnecessary.

§ 324. Constipation is insufficient action of the bowels, delay in the passage of the contents of the intestine, causing hard, dry fæces (scybala). Organic disease within or outside the intestinal canal must be carefully excluded before diagnosing a case as one of simple constipation. *Causes.*— (1) The usual cause is insufficient or incomplete movement of the mass of contents collected in the proximal colon. (2) In about a fourth of cases the delay is in the sigmoid colon and rectum (dyschezia). (3) A third form occurs when spasm of the colon prevents the mass movement from forwarding the contents through the region of the spasm (spastic constipation). (4) In elderly patients and those with feeble musculature there may be delay or absence of initiation of the mass movement. (5) A rarer type is due to lack of residue from too complete absorption of water and ingested food. A simple test for delay consists in giving a tablespoonful of powdered charcoal at night; it should normally have completely disappeared from the stools within 72 hours.

The *Symptoms* which accompany or result from constipation are sufficiently familiar—at first headache, languor and depression, followed by a furred, coated tongue, dyspepsia, sallow or pigmented skin, anæmia, sleeplessness and eruptions, usually of an urticarial or erythematous nature. The temperature may rise a degree or so in certain conditions from temporary constipation, and even up to 102° F. The retention of hard fæcal masses may give rise to an alternating diarrhœa, which leads to error in diagnosis (false diarrhœa). Habitual constipation may give rise to hæmorrhoids, and even to a distended ulcerated colon or atony of the colon. In women, in whom the condition is more common than in men, chronic constipation aggravates any pelvic disease. In both sexes varicose veins, œdema of the legs, sciatica, especially on the left side, and numbness of the legs may occur; these are more usually associated with diverticulitis (§ 328). In some cases ptosis of part of the intestine may ensue, leading to further delay of the bowel contents.

For purposes of treatment we may consider the *Causes* of simple or uncomplicated cases of constipation under three headings:

(a) **Errors of Diet.**

    (i.) Too bland food—*e.g.*, no vegetables, too little food with coarse residue.
    (ii.) Too dry food—*e.g.*, deficient fluid ingesta.
    (iii.) Too rough and irritating food, in certain cases of colon spasm.
    (iv.) Too little or poor food, deficiency of vitamins.

(b) **Causes of Defective Peristalsis,** other than errors of diet.

    (i.) Sedentary habits.
    (ii.) Depressing emotions, anxiety, worry, etc., cause spasm, as in "spastic colon." Catarrh of the colon may co-exist.
    (iii.) Old age and other conditions, such as anæmia with poor general tone.
    (iv.) Prolonged disregard of the calls of nature, with dilatation of rectum and pelvic colon consequent on blunted sensation.
    (v.) Weak abdominal muscles.
    (vi.) Atony of the colon, with or without colitis.
    (vii.) Some febrile states.

(viii) Endocrine disorder, especially deficient activity of thyroid and pituitary.

(ix) Disease of brain or cord, such as tabes and cerebral tumour.

(x) Drugs, such as opium, iron, lead.

(c) **Deficiency of Bile, or Intestinal Secretions.**

(i.) Functional inactivity of the liver.

(ii.) Profuse vomiting.

(iii.) Excessive loss of fluid by skin or kidneys.

(iv.) Astringents and certain drugs. Hard waters also act in this way.

Diagnosis.—As chronic constipation may lead to the troublesome consequences mentioned above, we must first *find the cause*. With the patient lying down and the muscles well relaxed, examine the abdomen to see if the colon be distended or loaded; place one hand at the back, and press it forwards between the iliac crest and the last rib to meet the other hand, which is placed flat on the anterior abdominal wall. Always make a rectal examination. An X-ray examination and sigmoidoscopy assist in deciding the presence or absence of mechanical obstruction, and the position of chief delay in the passage of the intestinal contents. Having excluded local causes by a thorough examination, we should consider the various causes above mentioned.

The *Treatment* of constipation comes under the following headings. (1) *Dietetic.*—Increase the amount of fluid taken—*e.g.*, by sipping a tumbler of cold water slowly whilst dressing in the morning and undressing at night. Avoid large quantities of milk, eggs, cheese or hard water. To provide bulk and stimulus, where there is no spasm, but chiefly dyschezia, foods to be eaten include oatmeal, wholemeal or brown bread, green and raw vegetables, onions, figs, prunes and ripe fruits (see § 296. V). A teaspoonful or tablespoonful of salad-oil at mealtimes aids this diet. Where there is colonic spasm, give smooth food with little residue. (2) *Lubricants* may be used for short periods; paraffin, plain or in emulsion, bassorin, psyllium seeds, Isogel and agar-agar preparations, provide bulk without irritating material, an important point in cases of spasm. (3) Inculcate *regular habits*. As stated above, in about one-fourth of the cases of simple constipation the delay is in the sigmoid and the upper rectum; hence it is important, even when there is no inclination to go to stool, that an attempt should be made at a regular hour daily, for 10 minutes by the watch, trying at regular intervals but being careful not to strain so hard as to cause pain in the abdomen or in the head. The squatting position aids, and lessens strain. If there is no result, a glycerine suppository should be inserted, and after waiting 10–15 minutes another effort made. That failing, a soap and water enema is given on the second day. (4) *Active exercise* is advisable except when uterine or ovarian disease or colonic spasm is present; many systematic exercises are now taught which strengthen the abdominal and pelvic muscles. (5) Abdominal *massage* is useful; gently " rolling " the abdominal wall, or rolling a 7-pound shot-ball over the abdomen in the direction of the hands of the clock. (6) With signs of *endocrine deficiency*, as of the thyroid, replacement therapy greatly aids constipation. Bile extracts are efficacious in other cases.

(7) *Drugs.*—To avoid prolonged use of drugs give methodical trial of the measures above mentioned. For occasional constipation, senna with the evening meal and a seidlitz-powder in the morning are the most harmless. Phenolphthalein is an excellent preparation for temporary use but is not advisable for continued use. Cascara, aloes and senna may be used frequently. A useful vegetable pill is pil. colocynth co., pil. rhei co., āā gr. I., hyoscyami, gr. ½; one or two at bedtime. Another good formula is tr. nuc. vom., tr. belladonna, āā ℳ 5; tr. hyoscyam. ℳ 10, ext. casc. sag. liq. ad ℳ 60. Nux vomica in small doses promotes peristalsis; belladonna is especially useful to relax spasm of the colon and in simple dyschezia. Salines given daily for some weeks will often re-establish the functions of a sluggish intestine. These may be given in the form of the mineral waters, such as Carlsbad, or their equivalents, which contain 20-60 gr. of sulphate of soda, sometimes with alkalies. They are best given on an empty stomach. An excellent aperient for children is cascara and malt mixed together in the proportion of 10 to 20 ℳ of the ext. casc. sagrad. liq. to the teaspoonful of malt. (8) *Enemata* are used in conditions of atony of the descending and pelvic colon, and dilated rectum—1 or 2 pints of plain water may be given, at gradually increasing intervals. Half an ounce of glycerine is an effective enema, but it should not be used longer than a few weeks, for it tends to irritate the rectum. In cases of very prolonged constipation, ⅛ to ¼ pint of olive oil may be given every night. If this be injected very slowly, it is retained, and after a course of one or two weeks the bowel often resumes its functions. (9) *Lumbar sympathectomy*, including the removal of the presacral plexus, may succeed in very obstinate cases, where these measures fail, and where evacuations occur at long intervals or only with enemata.

Colon irrigation with normal saline is often necessary where hard masses can be felt in the cæcum. One or two pints at a time, at body temperature, are introduced slowly under a pressure of not more than two feet, and are immediately evacuated. This is repeated until the washing is returned clear. It is best preceded by injection of 3 fl. oz. of warm olive oil to be retained for a few hours. Carried out daily for a week, then in alternate days, and later once a week, this is very effective in clearing the colon of accumulated fæces. Gradually the bowel resumes its normal functioning. The only type of case in which this is not very satisfactory is that in which there is considerable ptosis and as a result the whole of the saline is not evacuated at once. The repeated calls to stool are annoying, and frequently this type of patient complains of depression and increase of toxic symptoms.

Hirschsprung's Disease (megacolon) is a condition of atony and dilatation of the colon of congenital origin: it is ten times more frequent in boys than girls.

Symptoms.—There is obstinate constipation from the first weeks of life, and subsequently gross abdominal distension, tympanites with visible dilatation of coils of the bowel, auto-intoxication and emaciation. If early childhood is survived, complications such as peritonitis and intestinal obstruction may ensue. The disease is often fatal in the absence of treatment.

The *Diagnosis* can be made only by the history and obvious signs of a distended colon. A barium enema shows enormously dilated and redundant bowel. A similar condition may be acquired by prolonged bad habits.

Etiology.—The cause is a failure of development cells of the parasympathetic nervous system (Auerbach's plexus) in a short segment of the bowel with resultant excessive tone and lack of peristalsis in this area. The colon proximal to the block becomes extremely dilated and hypertrophied. The region involved is either that of the lower sigmoid colon or the rectum.

Treatment.—Conservative treatment is by the use of large enemata combined with neostigmine 5–10 mg. t.i.d. The operation of lumbar sympathectomy has now been superseded by recto-sigmoidectomy with resection of the aganglionic area of the bowel (Swenson's operation): in most cases an anastomosis is carried out between the colon and the anal canal 1–2 cm. short of the muco-cutaneous junction leaving the anal sphincter intact. Subsequent to operation enemata are often required for a while to educate the mechanism of defæcation.

§ 325. **Intestinal Flatulence** may be due to fermentation of carbo-hydrates, especially in the colon, but more often to interference with the absorption of air which has been swallowed with food or drink. Anything which causes congestion of the intestinal veins will delay the absorption of the intestinal gases, and give rise to distension and flatulence, such as heart failure and pulmonary disease, portal congestion and local venous block, as in volvulus and intestinal obstruction.

Symptoms.—There is a sense of fullness with discomfort which may be painful, relief being obtained by loosening the clothing, eructation or passing flatus. Breathing may become embarrassed and palpitation, hiccups or irregularity of the heart occur.

Treatment consists in reducing the vegetables and cellulose of the diet, and giving charcoal biscuits and carminatives. When constipation is present, Gregory's powder is most useful. Pituitary extract or neostigmine may be used, by injection: to relieve spasm give trasentin, tablets of phenobarbitone, or atropine.

The patient complains of SUDDEN STOPPAGE OF THE BOWELS *with inability to pass even flatus,* ABDOMINAL PAIN *and* VOMITING *which gradually becomes stercoraceous; there is increasing abdominal distension, and a tendency to* SHOCK. The case is one of ACUTE INTESTINAL OBSTRUCTION.

§ 326. **Acute Intestinal Obstruction** is one of the most serious medical or surgical emergencies.

The *Symptoms* common to all forms of acute obstruction are— (1) complete constipation, not even flatus being passed. Absolute constipation can be assumed only when flatus cannot be passed even after repeated enemata. (2) Pain may be acute at first, and referred to the umbilicus, though later it may be superseded by colicky pains, owing to the peristalsis of the bowel trying to overcome the obstruction. There is not usually much tenderness. (3) Vomiting is a prominent symptom from the onset. It is copious and projectile, first of food, then bile, and later material which is alkaline to litmus and finally fæcal. It comes on earlier, is more urgent, and becomes more rapidly stercoraceous in proportion as the obstruction has taken place high up in the intestines. (4) Abdominal distension is generally present; it is more in the flanks with obstruction to the colon, and more central with obstruction to the small intestine. (5) Peristalsis may be visible. (6) Constitutional symptoms gradually supervene, with prostration and a thready, *rapid pulse.* These also are more urgent when the small intestine is involved. The urine is diminished in proportion as the obstruction is near the stomach, for then the vomiting is more urgent. (7) Tetany can occur in high obstruction of the small intestine.

Diagnosis.—When summoned to a case presenting these three symptoms—stoppage of the bowels, vomiting and acute abdominal pain—the first step is to identify the case as one of acute intestinal obstruction. In *colic* (renal, hepatic or intestinal) all of these three symptoms may be present, but the patient's general condition is not so serious. Moreover, the position of the pain in renal and hepatic colic is characteristic (see § 247). In *acute peritonitis* there is great tenderness over the abdomen, thoracic respiration and some fever (see also § 244). But when there is *perforation* into the *peritoneum* shock is present, at first without fever, and perforation is diagnosed with difficulty only by (i.) the pain is constant and there is local tenderness; (ii.) the passage of wind by the bowel; (iii.) the collapse being much greater even than that in acute obstruction; and (iv.) a possible history of the condition which has resulted in perforation or rupture (consult also § 243). It is sometimes impossible to diagnose between these two conditions, and an exploratory operation should be undertaken without delay.

Causes of Intestinal Obstruction.—It is of some importance to ascertain the cause, for the prognosis and treatment differ somewhat in each case. (*a*) In *acute* intestinal obstruction, in which the symptoms come on *suddenly* in a person previously healthy, there are four *common* causes: (1) External hernia; (II) internal strangulation; (III) paralytic ileus; (IV) intussusception. (*b*) Sometimes, however, acute will supervene on chronic obstruction, and the *common causes of chronic obstruction* (§ 327) are four in number: (I) Malignant stricture of the bowel; (II) diverticulitis; (III) simple stricture; and (IV) pressure of a tumour.

Features special to the several causes of acute intestinal obstruction.

I. EXTERNAL HERNIA must always be looked for: it is known by the presence of a tumour in the femoral, inguinal or umbilical region. No impulse on coughing is present. Obturator hernia is very rare, and is usually only discovered at operation. A femoral hernia, especially of the Richter type in a fat woman, can be easily overlooked.

II. INTERNAL HERNIA OR STRANGULATION—*e.g.*, by bands of adhesion—is known by (i.) the urgency of the symptoms; (ii.) the patient is an adult, with (iii.) a history of old peritonitis or previous operation. VOLVULUS (or twisting of the bowel) may be indistinguishable from the preceding—indeed, it practically results in strangulation—but (i.) it occurs in men over forty, usually with a history of chronic constipation; (ii.) abdominal distension may be great; (iii.) sometimes a tumour is felt over the sigmoid flexure, the usual site of volvulus.

Internal strangulation may also arise from (1) adhesion of the end of the appendix vermiformis through which a knuckle of the bowel gets nipped. (2) Adhesions of the bowel. (3) Congenital deficiencies in the mesentery or bowel, or the foramen of Winslow.   (4) A persistent Meckel's diverticulum.

III. **Paralytic ileus** is a severe complication which usually follows a surgical operation. It may complicate pneumonia or follow the use of ganglion blocking drugs (§ 96). It may be defined as a condition of "intestinal inertia," in which the intestine is incapable of muscular action, and becomes distended with gas. Its pathology is not settled; it may be caused by injury to the wall of the gut, by interference with its blood supply or the nervous visceral connections.

Symptoms.—A *mild form* is met after most major abdominal operations and is manifested by constipation, gas and windy spasms; there may be some contraction of the sphincters. This occurs after the first 24 hours, with moderate distension, usually relieved at the end of the 3rd day by an enema. *Severe* paralytic ileus sets in about the 2nd or 3rd day, with pain, vomiting, distension and absolute constipation. The pain is a dull ache, not colicky, and there is complete cessation of peristalsis so that bowel sounds are not audible even on auscultation with the stethoscope. Vomiting is persistent and copious. It may last 3 to 4 days and then clear up, but if unrelieved death takes place about the 3rd, 4th or 5th day. Much fluid loss and also a potassium deficiency are contributory causes.

It must be *diagnosed* from mechanical adhesive obstruction. The latter occurs later, from the 3rd to the 7th day. It has the same insidious onset; vomiting becomes progressive, and the material is alkaline to litmus, but there is usually colicky pain and peristalsis may be detected.

Treatment.—At the end of 24 hours ox-bile or turpentine enemata should be given and a flatus tube left in. Nothing should be given by mouth; the stomach should be kept empty by repeated aspiration through a Ryle's tube, and the fluid intake kept up by a continuous dextrose-saline infusion intravenously. Heat to the abdomen and morphia (gr. $\frac{1}{12}$–$\frac{1}{8}$ 4-hourly for five or more doses) are beneficial. If these are unsuccessful, carbachol B.P. subcutaneously (0·25–0·50 mg.) or neostigmine 15 mg. repeated two or three times, and followed by a glycerine enema often helps. Should these methods fail, a spinal anæsthetic should be given, and if no result follows, operation is necessary. Only in desperate cases should ileostomy be performed.

IV. ACUTE INTUSSUSCEPTION is the commonest cause in childhood. Following a local swelling of the lymphoid tissue of the bowel (with a low-grade temperature) peristalsis causes this to invaginate into the bowel below. In more than half the cases the lower part of the ileum becomes invaginated into the cæcum, in a third some other part of the ileum and in about one-eighth some part of the colon, is implicated. Unless dealt with surgically death usually occurs from perforation or collapse; rarely the invaginated portion sloughs and separates about the eighth or tenth day, the two edges are welded together and spontaneous recovery occurs. Intussusception is known by (i.) severe pain and vomiting; (ii.) a rectal discharge of *blood and mucus* with a red jelly appearance; (iii.) a sausage-shaped tumour may be felt, altering in position, on palpating the abdomen, and in extreme cases the invaginated portion of bowel is felt *per rectum*; and (iv.) the patient is usually a previously healthy boy under two years of age.

The **rarer causes** of acute obstruction are three in number:

V. IMPACTION IN THE BOWEL of a large GALL-STONE which has escaped from the gall-bladder by ulceration into the bowel. The obstruction is high up in the small intestine, and consequently (1) the pain and constitutional symptoms are of extreme severity, and of very sudden onset. (2) The patient is usually a woman at or beyond middle age. (3) There may be a history of biliary colic, and in all cases there is a history of localised peritonitis some weeks or months before the attack. (4) The symptoms may intermit, from the stone shifting its position.

VI. Obstruction of the bowel may sometimes be due to an EXTRAVASATION OF BLOOD into the coats of the intestine: this occurs in purpura, hæmophilia and other blood disorders. Such cases are recognised by evidences of hæmorrhage in other positions—melæna, epistaxis, purpura or a history of urticaria or angioneurotic œdema (§ 652). An embolus in the mesenteric artery is a rare cause.

VII. Among the still rarer causes of obstruction may be mentioned masses of roundworms (Trousseau), impaction of too much cellulose, orange-peel, etc., hair-balls, concretions of ammonio-phosphate of magnesium (a frequent cause in horses, though rare in man), and other foreign bodies in the intestine.

Clinical Investigation and Diagnosis of the Cause of Obstruction.— If the case occurs in a child, and there is a history of sudden onset, it is almost certainly intussusception; in an old person suspect growth, impacted fæces, diverticulitis or volvulus; in a young adult suspect strangulation or hernia. If the vomiting comes on early and is urgent, it points to a tight constriction *high up* in the intestinal tract. So also after the onset of obstruction high up there may be a movement of the bowels. If the distension is chiefly in the centre of the abdomen, the obstruction is probably above the ileo-cæcal valve; if it is chiefly in the flanks, the obstruction is below the valve; if more in the right than in the left flank, the obstruction is probably in the splenic flexure.

When called to such a case, first examine for swelling in the positions of external herniæ. If the abdomen be distended, and presents visible waves of peristalsis, inquire as to the causes of chronic obstruction (*infra*), as the case is probably an acute supervening upon a chronic obstruction. Always *examine per rectum*, for in acute intussusception the invaginated part of the bowel may be felt *per rectum*, and there may be a discharge of blood and mucus; or a growth or other cause of chronic obstruction may thus be discovered. Next inquire into the past history—*e.g.*, for operation or peritonitis (as this is a cause of internal strangulation), or for appendicitis or hepatic colic. Then examine the abdomen by palpation and percussion for tumour or tenderness. If the abdomen is distended only on one side, the site of the obstruction may be localised.

Prognosis.—The prognosis of obstruction of the bowels is always serious. Death occurs in the natural course either from (1) gangrene and rupture of the bowel, or (2) exhaustion and collapse. At the present day the prognosis almost entirely depends upon the *stage at which the case comes under notice*, the age of the patient and the treatment adopted. All acute cases require early surgical interference, and a surgeon should be summoned at once. As regards the *Causes*, obstruction from a gall-stone is perhaps the most serious, then femoral hernia, internal strangulation and intussusception. Among the gradual causes, carcinoma of the bowel gives the gravest prognosis, and paralytic ileus the most favourable. Cases of obstruction high up are less favourable than those in the large bowel.

Treatment.—Acute intestinal obstruction is one of those serious conditions that demand the resources of both a physician and a surgeon, who should jointly undertake the management of a case. The indications are (1) to ascertain the cause; (2) to endeavour to remove the obstruction; and (3) in the meantime to support the strength and relieve the pain by controlling the peristalsis upon which it depends. Enemata of soapy water to which olive oil, glycerine or oxbile is added may be given in all cases; purgatives by mouth should be avoided. Warmth is applied to the abdomen in the form of hot fomentations, turpentine, belladonna or opium stupes. The question of the administration of opium is debated (see Appendicitis), but, generally speaking, for the relief of the pain morphia may be given as soon as the diagnosis is certain. The diet should consist of fluids, such as iced milk, beef-tea and stimulants, given in small quantities, and frequently. Intravenous dextrose-saline is needed to correct dehydration.

Except in cases due to faecal impaction, operation is required in most cases and should not be delayed. At laparotomy the cause can be readily identified by the distension of the bowel proximal to the obstruction and the collapse distally. The simpler the operation the better: adhesions and bands can be divided, an intussusception reduced and a gall-stone or other foreign body removed. When a growth is found in the large intestine a caecostomy or colostomy proximal to the obstruction may allow a subsequent operation for removal. Generally speaking a segment of *small* intestine should be removed at the time of laparotomy and an immediate anastomosis performed: but with obstruction of the *large* intestine this is inadvisable as the suture line has such a great tendency to give way and to cause leakage.

The patient complains of CONSTIPATION *progressively increasing*, ABDOMINAL PAIN, *and from time to time* VOMITING; *there is general ill-health.* The case is one of CHRONIC INTESTINAL OBSTRUCTION.

§ 327. In **Chronic Intestinal Obstruction** (1) the abdominal pain is generalised, intermittent and of increasing severity. (2) There is constipation, or a history of alternate constipation and diarrhœa culminating in complete stoppage; and (3) abdominal distension in most cases, and peristalsis in some, may be visible. The chief causes are four in number:

I. MALIGNANT STRICTURE by new growth in the wall of the bowel— *e.g.*, cancer. Its most common situations are the colon, especially the sigmoid flexure, and the rectum. This cause of obstruction may be recognised by (1) the presence of a tumour or stricture which may be felt on examination *per rectum*, and the distension of the abdomen being mostly in the flanks. When the tumour is situated higher up than the sigmoid flexure, it may generally be felt through the abdominal wall;

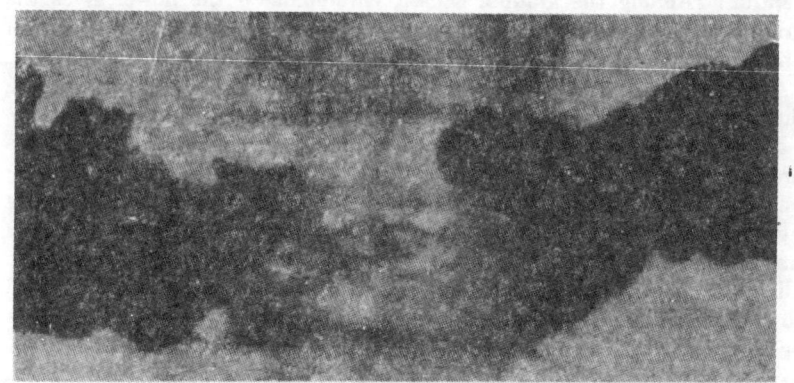

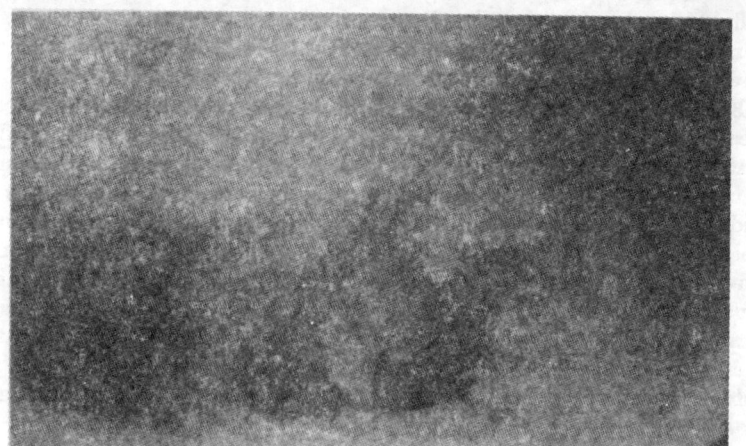

FIG. 109.—BARIUM ENEMA.—A. Carcinoma of transverse colon; could possibly be confused with a filling defect caused by pressure from spine. B. Oblique view after air inflation, showing the absence of relaxation of the indurated part.

and when situated in the sigmoid flexure, it may be inspected by a sigmoidoscope. (2) When the sigmoid flexure or rectum is affected, the illness may be preceded by sciatica on the left side. (3) The age of the patient, the passage of blood, and perhaps cancerous cachexia or deposits in the liver aid in the diagnosis. (4) X-ray with a barium enema combined with air insufflation will show a filling defect (Fig. 109). A barium meal may precipitate an acute obstruction.

A man of middle age or over who has suffered from FLATULENCE, ABDOMINAL DISCOMFORT *and* IRREGULARITY OF THE BOWELS—*usually constipation—for some time, has an attack of* PAIN IN THE LEFT ILIAC FOSSA *with some fever; the disease may be* DIVERTICULITIS.

§ **328. II. Diverticulitis** of the colon is a fairly common complication of diverticulosis. Patients are usually above middle age and often obese. For some years there may have been irregularity of the bowels, with a

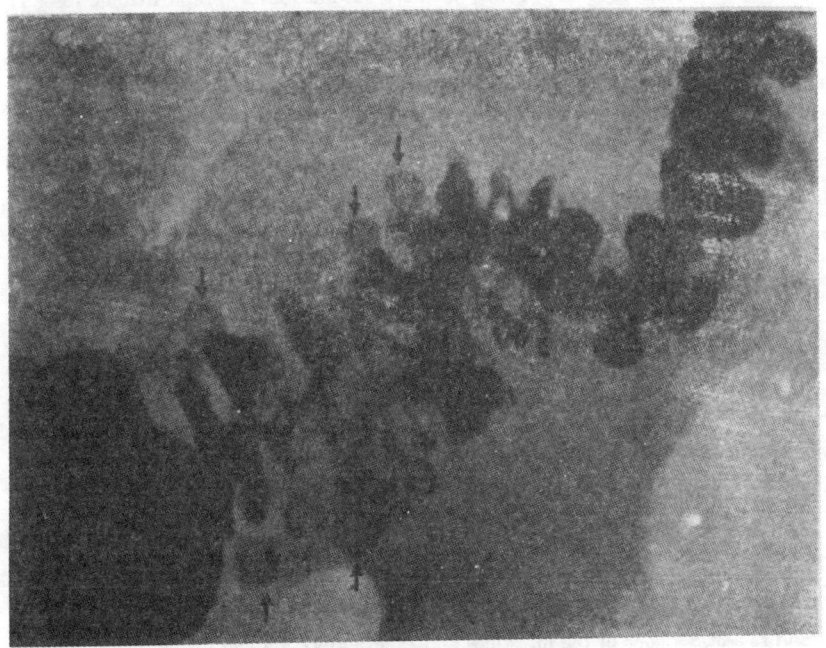

FIG. 110.—DIVERTICULITIS OF SIGMOID COLON.

tendency to constipation, abdominal discomfort and attacks of diarrhœa which are ascribed to indigestible foods. Sometimes there is a little mucus but rarely blood in the stool. There is (i.) some degree of fever, occasional rigors and often leucocytosis; (ii.) tenderness and rigidity in the left iliac fossa; (iii.) sometimes a local mass is felt, due to simple inflammation or abscess formation; (iv.) irritation of the bladder with frequency of micturition and sometimes cystitis.

For *Diagnosis* of these cases, see also § 326. Diverticulitis has to be diagnosed from *cancer* of the colon and *appendicitis*. It must not be forgotten that diverticulosis and a carcinoma of the colon may be present at the same time. X-ray after a barium enema shows a contracted and irregular lumen of the bowel in the sigmoid region and diverticula scattered throughout the rest of the colon. Complications are: local peritonitis from peri-diverticulitis, perforation with acute or chronic peritonitis, obstruction or the formation of a fistula into the bladder or the vagina.

Treatment: (a) during the acute attack, consists of bed, fluid and semi-solid diet, poultices or other forms of heat to the abdomen, liquid paraffin by mouth and by injection into the bowel. Succinylsulphathiazole B.P. or the tetracycline group of antibiotics help to overcome infective complications. (b) Between the attacks, the diet should be fuller, but must contain nothing hard or indigestible; liquid paraffin should be taken by mouth two or three times a day. Belladonna preparations lessen intestinal spasm. A course of intestinal douches with normal saline, given at low pressure, may be necessary, to clear away the accumulation of fæces and soothe the bowel. The rectal injection of 3 fl. oz. of warm olive oil two or three times a week, the patient lying on the left side and retaining it as long as possible, is of considerable value. Operation is sometimes necessary.

III. SIMPLE—*i.e.*, NON-MALIGNANT STRICTURE of the intestine may arise in consequence of amœbic dysentery, Crohn's disease, diverticulosis of the colon or chronic ulcerative colitis (§ 314). Lymphogranuloma venereum is a rare cause.

IV. PRESSURE ON THE BOWEL by a tumour; post-operative, tuberculous or other adhesions, or an enlargement of some viscus such as the uterus. This cause is recognised by the physical signs of tumour or enlargement respectively.

Rarer Causes of chronic intestinal obstruction are:

V. CHRONIC PERITONITIS (§ 251) causes a matting together of the intestines, and intestinal obstruction may result. Cancerous peritonitis is attended by considerable pain and the effusion of much fluid; but in tuberculous peritonitis (§ 573) there are mostly adhesions, less pain, and less fluid. Localised peritonitis occurs as a result of diverticulitis, usually in the left lower abdomen. Another cause is the result of high super-voltage radiotherapy (above 5,000 rœntgen units in 7–8 weeks): this can give rise to chronic peritonitis with adhesions producing intestinal obstruction, ulcerative and sclerotic lesions of the intestines and even perforation and fistula formation.

VI. CARCINOID (Argentaffin) tumours of the small intestine and appendix produce chronic obstruction and are of low-grade malignancy. They are derived from the Kulchitsky cells which secrete 5-hydro-oxytryptamine into the blood-stream. Even when the liver is invaded by deposits the patient may live for several years. *Diagnosis* is usually made only at operation and by subsequent histological examination (and see § 571).

VII. CHRONIC INTUSSUSCEPTION is thus known: (1) It occurs usually in children; (2) tenesmus is present; (3) a tumour may be felt similar to that met in acute intussusception; and (4) there is usually no great distension (see also Acute Intussusception, above).

VIII. HIRSCHSPRUNG'S DISEASE (§ 324).

Prognosis.—In all forms the symptoms of acute obstruction are apt at any time to supervene, from impaction of fæces above the narrowed lumen of the gut, but apart from this the prospect differs considerably in the various causes. A cancerous stricture is the most, diverticulitis the least, serious. The course of a tumour varies with its nature. Chronic intussusception *may* spontaneously resolve, the invaginated part sloughing off and being passed by the rectum, but the outlook is always grave.

Treatment.—In most cases surgery is ultimately necessary, but at first the treatment consists in watching the patient until a diagnosis can be formed with as much accuracy as possible, giving digestible food, preferably such as leaves but little residue, and relieving pain by opium and hot external applications. For simple *stricture of the rectum* gradual dilatation by bougies may be tried. In *chronic intussusception* operation is advisable. In *cancerous stricture* where radical removal is impossible life may be prolonged by colostomy; the longer the operation is delayed, the worse is the prognosis. It should never be delayed until vomiting has begun.

CHAPTER XII

THE LIVER

THE liver is the largest gland in the body and the fact that it can contain a fourth of the blood in the body shows the important role it plays in the metabolism of the body. All the blood passing from the stomach and intestines circulates through the liver, after which it joins the general circulation considerably altered in its composition. The pancreas and the liver work in close co-operation, the pancreatic internal secretion passing direct to the liver. The liver aids in preparing proteins, carbohydrates and fats for the tissues. Other important functions of the liver are: the manufacture and the storage of glycogen; a detoxicating action by arresting poisons and bacteria absorbed from the intestinal tract, and converting certain noxious chemical substances—indol and skatol—into innocuous compounds; the elaboration of the products of protein metabolism into urea and uric acid; the excretion of bile salts and pigments, cholesterol, various toxins, drugs and antibiotics; the regulation of the body content of water, salt and hormones as well as of the blood volume; the storage of the anti-anæmic factor against pernicious anæmia, and the production of prothrombin and fibrinogen, both necessary for blood clotting. The Küpffer cells form part of the reticulo-endothelial system. The liver has considerable reserve and much power of regeneration; approximately one-tenth of the normal parenchyma is adequate to maintain its various functions.

PART A. SYMPTOMATOLOGY

The symptoms due to disorders of the liver are not so clearly defined as those of cardiac or pulmonary diseases. The cardinal symptoms of *structural* disease of the liver are PAIN IN THE HEPATIC REGION, JAUNDICE, and a group of symptoms due to PORTAL OBSTRUCTION, which includes Ascites. When the liver cells become gradually destroyed, as in hepatitis, serious disturbance of the general health ensues, and in the later stages of that and of some other hepatic disorders LETHARGY passing into COMA supervenes. Functional derangement of the liver is attended by DEPRESSION and vague DIGESTIVE DISTURBANCES.

§ 329. **Pain and Tenderness over the Liver** occur in PERIHEPATITIS and in any other condition which involves or stretches the capsule, as in heart failure. The pain may radiate upwards towards the right scapula. The onset of pain in the course of a liver complaint may therefore be of considerable importance; for example, in hydatid of the liver the natural course of which is painless, it would point to a danger of inflammation and possible rupture of the cyst. When the upper surface of the liver is involved, the pain is very often *referred to the right shoulder*; it is, indeed, a symptom of phrenic (diaphragmatic) irritation. The most severe form of pain, however, is that which occurs with the passage of GALL-STONES (*biliary colic*). Pain may be completely absent in hepatic disorder. In many cases of disease or enlargement of the liver there is, however,

472

a feeling of weight or fullness in the right hypochondrium, accompanied by an inability to lie on the left side.

Hepatic pain may be *simulated* by Pleurodynia ("rheumatism of the intercostal muscles"), Intercostal Neuralgia, Herpes Zoster, Pleurisy, Dyspepsia and various gastric conditions, and by Intestinal or Renal Colic.

§ 330. Jaundice is the term applied to the yellow pigmentation of the skin and other tissues due to the rise in plasma bilirubin. In the earlier stages it is very difficult to recognise jaundice by artificial light. It appears first in the blood then in the urine, in which increased urobilin, bile pigments and salts may be detected (§ 383), next in the conjunctivæ, then in the skin uniformly.

FALLACIES.—The yellow coloration of the conjunctivæ differentiates jaundice from all similar pigmentations of the skin. (1) Excess of *subconjunctival fat* may simulate jaundice, but this is readily distinguished by its unequal distribution. (2) The *sallowness* of the skin in anæmia is distinguished by the absence of bile in the urine and of yellowness of the conjunctivæ. (3) The *cachexia* of carcinoma, malaria, tuberculosis and certain other forms of visceral disease, is differentiated in the same way. (4) The *bronzing* of the skin in Addison's disease is hardly likely to be mistaken for jaundice. (5) Long-continued *mepacrine* administration colours the skin (but not the sclerotics) yellow. (6) *Santonin* and *rhubarb*, administered internally, colour the urine, but do not give the reactions for bile pigment in that fluid. (7) Carotenæmia (§ 772) may be mistaken.

Jaundice is classified as follows: (a) Obstructive; (b) Toxic or infective; and (c) Hæmolytic. Pure instances of these varieties are rare; even with obstructive jaundice, damage to liver cells follows.

(a) Clinically, **Obstructive Jaundice** is distinguished by the colour of the stools, which are pale, slate- or clay-coloured, due to the absence of bile pigment in the intestinal canal. There is increased intestinal putrefaction and steatorrhœa, due to the increase of soaps and fatty acids in the stools. The urine is high-coloured and contains bile pigment. The serum bilirubin steadily rises and gives a direct van den Bergh reaction (§ 333); the serum alkaline phosphatase is increased; the flocculation tests and serum proteins are unaltered unless there is also liver cell damage; the bile salts and cholesterol in the blood are also increased and the coagulation time is prolonged. Pruritus is often severe. Leucocytosis is present in advanced obstructive jaundice, but not in mild cases unaccompanied by inflammation or suppuration.

Obstructive jaundice may be produced in four ways:

I. FOREIGN BODIES within the bile-duct, such as (1) gall-stones and inspissated bile; (2) hydatids, roundworms, Fasciola and other parasites.

II. INFLAMMATION of the bile-ducts (cholangitis).

III. STRICTURE, or obliteration of the duct owing to (1) congenital absence; (2) ulceration or a primary carcinoma of the bile-duct, which may produce obstruction by the swelling around, or lead to stricture; (3) cicatrisation after operation; (4) chronic pancreatitis; and (5) perihepatitis.

IV. TUMOURS pressing on the duct, such as (1) cancer and other tumours of the liver; (2) enlargement of the glands in the transverse fissure of the liver (porta hepatis); (3) tumours of the stomach, pancreas, kidney, great omentum.

(*b*) In **Toxic** or **Infective Jaundice** some bile usually reaches the intestine, so that the stools are not always clay-coloured, and severe damage to the liver may occur without marked jaundice. The blood in toxic jaundice gives an indirect or a biphasic van den Bergh reaction and special tests may be performed which show evidence of liver-cell damage (§ 333). The urine contains excess urobilin; the serum albumin is lower and the serum globulin (especially the gamma-globulin) increased; the concentration of serum transaminase is markedly raised and is often the first sign of disease, but the serum alkaline phosphatase is only a little higher than normal. Pruritus is not severe. This form of jaundice causes swelling of the liver cells, and later retention of bile pigment and salts in the blood. The damage may be mild and recovery complete; or severe, as in acute yellow atrophy of the liver, with only partial recovery, leaving some degree of cirrhosis. The *causes* of toxic jaundice are: (1) viral, bacterial or protozoal poisons such as occur in infective hepatitis, pneumonia, septicæmia, typhoid, typhus, syphilis, spirochætosis ictero-hæmorrhagica; relapsing fever, malaria, yellow and other tropical fevers; (2) chemical poisons such as trinitrotoluene, tetrachlorethane (poisons affecting munition workers), carbon tetrachloride, phosphorus, arsenobenzol derivatives, nitrobenzene, gold salts, cinchophen B.P. (atophan), dinitrophenol, ether and chloroform; (3) toxæmias as in pregnancy; (4) chronic heart disease with congestion of the liver.

(*c*) In **Hæmolytic Jaundice** (i.) the fæces are of normal colour; usually there is no bilirubin or bile salts in the urine, but much urobilin or urobilinogen (§ 383). The spleen is usually enlarged and there may be perisplenitis. (ii.) There is a delayed direct and an indirect van den Bergh reaction. (iii.) This form of jaundice is caused by increased blood destruction and is of extrahepatic origin. Its *causes* are: (A) an increased fragility of the red blood corpuscles, usually of hereditary origin, as in acholuric jaundice, sickle-celled anæmia and Cooley's anæmia; (B) the development of an abnormal hæmolytic tendency, of acquired origin (§§ 547, 553, 565); (C) increased destructive agents; (1) animal poisons, such as snake-venom; (2) streptococcal infections; (3) pernicious anæmia; (4) specific hæmolysis as in transfusion with blood from incompatible donors. The icteric index is much increased (§ 333). Physiologically, this form occurs in the jaundice of the newly-born.

Of all these causes of jaundice, *gall-stones* and *infective hepatitis are the most common*.

To *diagnose* the type of jaundice (see Table XXII): 1. EXAMINE THE FÆCES, which are slate- or clay-coloured in complete obstruction, and of normal colour in hæmolytic jaundice. The presence of fat or parasites may assist in diagnosing the cause. But it must be remembered, as possible *fallacies*, that the fæces may become stained if mixed with urine;

and that the bile-duct may be only partially obstructed, and enough bile may thus escape to colour the fæces.

2. EXAMINE THE URINE for bile pigments and salts (§ 383).

3. Inquire as to the HISTORY OF THE ATTACK. Jaundice coming on suddenly, especially in a middle-aged woman previously in good health, almost invariably indicates obstruction by gall-stones. The intensity of the jaundice varies from week to week as the stones pass. Jaundice coming on slowly, and ultimately becoming intense, is generally due to a tumour pressing on the common bile-duct, and is most often seen in association with cancer. Severe jaundice persisting some weeks is almost certainly obstructive. Occupation in a munition factory, or previous intravenous treatment with arsenobenzol derivatives, renders easy a diagnosis of the cause. A history of previous temporary attacks points in adult life to gall-stones; in youth, to infective hepatitis.

4. EXAMINE THE HEPATIC REGION CAREFULLY. If the liver is enlarged, cancer is the most probable cause; interstitial hepatitis is less common. If the gall-bladder is enlarged, cancer is more probable than stone. If ascites be present, the diagnosis rests between cancer and cirrhosis.

5. Inquire as to PAIN AND CONSTITUTIONAL SYMPTOMS. Pain of a spasmodic and severe character accompanies jaundice due to gall-stones and cancer. It is more constant and dull in character in congestion of the liver and catarrh of the bile-ducts. The temperature is not often

TABLE XXII.—DIFFERENTIATION OF TYPES OF JAUNDICE

	Obstructive.	Toxic or Infective.	Hæmolytic.
Onset	Stormy.	Quiet.	Chronic.
Colour of skin ..	Yellow, orange or greenish.	Yellow, orange or greenish.	Light yellow—" lemon yellow."
Distribution of pigment	Seen in conjunctivæ before skin.	Seen in skin before conjunctivæ.	Conjunctivæ rarely affected.
Irritation of skin ..	Usually severe.	May be present.	Not present.
Colour of stools ..	Pale.	Normal or pale.	Normal.
Urine	Bile pigments present.	Often no bile pigments: urobilin present.	No bile pigments: urobilin present.
Liver	Large or very large.	Large, normal or small.	A little large or normal.
Gall bladder	May be palpable.	Not palpable.	Not palpable.
Spleen	Rarely palpable.	Rarely palpable.	Often palpable.
Anæmia	May or may not be present.	Usually not severe.	Severe.
Sedimentation rate	Usually normal.	Normal or increased.	Much increased.
Serum alkaline phosphatase	Increased.	Little increased.	Little increased.
Turbidity tests ..	Negative.	Positive.	Variable.
Albumen, globulin and ratio	Normal.	Low albumen: raised gamma-globulin.	Normal.
Prothrombin level	Normal until late in disease.	Decreased.	Normal; fragility of red cells may be increased.
Van den Bergh reaction (serum bilirubin)	Steadily rising serum bilirubin and direct reaction	Moderate serum bilirubin and indirect reaction.	High serum bilirubin. and no direct reaction.

elevated, but it may be so in infective hepatitis, jaundice due to poisons in the blood, pyæmic hepatitis, tuberculous affections, and local pus formation, such as liver abscess. Cerebral symptoms are rarely present, except when a fatal termination is at hand, unless the jaundice occurs in the course of pneumonia, fevers, or in acute yellow atrophy of the liver.

6. EXAMINE THE BLOOD with the van den Bergh test; estimate the plasma protein, the serum transaminase and alkaline phosphatase and carry out the flocculation tests (§ 333). Coombs test may be helpful.

The *Prognosis* and *Treatment* of jaundice depend on its causal diseases (*q.v.*). When bile pigment disappears from the urine and returns in the stools the attack is subsiding, though it may be some weeks before the skin clears. Plenty of milk, preferably skimmed of excess cream and diluted or citrated, is the staple diet (§ 296. IV); extra amino-acids such as in casein digest or as methionine are advocated but are often nauseous. Fluids must be taken freely, and glucose (and perhaps insulin) given when the liver cells are damaged. The flatulent dyspepsia and many of the concurrent symptoms may be relieved by the administration of extract of ox-gall (gr. 5 to 15) with meals, together with alkalies and carminatives after meals such as mistura rhei co. (B.P.C.). A suitable purgative may be necessary. Injections of mersalyl, 1–2 ml., with tab. chlorothiazide 0·5 G. are used for the associated ascites. Paracentesis may be necessary. The itching of jaundice is often a most troublesome symptom, but it can generally be relieved by calcium salts, by methyl testosterone 0·25 mg. sublingually each day, by ergotamine tartrate 1 mg. t.i.d., or by sodium thiosulphate in doses of 10 gr. in saline intravenously; local treatment with alkaline lotions or bran baths, or bathing in potassium permanganate 40–60 gr. to 30 gallons of water, is beneficial. Phenobarbitone helps. Vitamin K and blood transfusion are given for bleeding. Great care is needed to secure efficient sterilisation of needles and syringes after use with jaundiced patients (§ 1200).

By the time jaundice appears in a MUNITION WORKER the condition is serious. Symptoms of acute toxæmia may develop, with delirium, coma and death. Prophylaxis consists in strict cleanliness of hands and food, abundance of milk and glucose, and intermission of work in the trinitrotoluene department.

§ 330a. Icterus Neonatorum is usually PHYSIOLOGICAL. This variety is a mild transitory form of jaundice which affects a very large number (estimated by various observers at from 50 to 75 per cent.) of new-born infants. It appears usually on the second or third day of life, is not generally very intense, and rarely lasts longer than one or two weeks. The fæces are normal in colour, and apart from the jaundice the infant presents no other symptoms. The condition is almost invariably present in premature infants. The circulating bilirubin is in the unconjugated form and gives an indirect van den Bergh reaction only, and there are no bile pigments in the urine. There is an increased breakdown of red cells as they rapidly fall from 6·5 millions per c.mm. at birth to 4·5 million at the end of the first week; and the enzyme which converts unconjugated bilirubin into conjugated bilirubin (bilirubin glucuronide) does not function fully for the first week after birth. Coombs test on the infant's red cells is negative. No *treatment* is required.

SEVERE JAUNDICE in the new-born has a much graver prognosis. (1) *Icterus Gravis Neonatorum* is a severe form which affects several members of a family, and if untreated is fatal in 50–75 per cent. of cases: usually the first and second members of a family are exempt. It is recognised by (i.) being present at birth or within the first 24 hours after birth; (ii.) the accompanying severe anæmia which may be masked by the deepening jaundice: the blood shows excessive numbers of nucleated red cells which persist for 3–4 weeks (erythroblastæmia); (iii.) the child's serum gives an indirect positive van den Bergh test only and there is no bilirubin in the urine; (iv.) the infant becomes increasingly drowsy; (v.) there is enlargement of the liver and spleen; (vi.) purpura may develop. *Diagnosis.*—At birth the infant's red cells, obtained from the umbilical cord, show a positive Coombs test. *Etiology.*—Approximately 90 per cent. of cases are due to the mother's red cells being Rh-negative but the infant has Rh-positive red cells inherited from the father; the mother having had one or two previous Rh-positive infants, or having had a prev.ous transfusion with Rh-positive blood, has formed antibodies (hæmolysins) which destroy the infant's red cells (see §§ 547, 567. IV–V). A warning that this is likely to occur shortly after birth is given when, during the later weeks of pregnancy, there is an increase in the maternal Rh-antibody in the blood of an Rh-negative mother. About 10 per cent. of cases are due to ABO incompatibilities, especially if the mother is group O and the child group A or B; other rare blood groups sometimes play a part.

Prognosis.—In cases where the serum bilirubin has been above 20 mg. per cent. during the stage of jaundice, damage to the brain may later cause spasticity, athetosis or mental defects (Kernicterus).

Treatment.—Mild cases recover with simple treatment: they are helped by giving oral magnesium sulphate or hydrarg. cum creta which aid removal of inspissated bile. However, as soon as the child's hæmoglobin is below 100 per cent. (Haldane) or the serum bilirubin above 5·0 mg. per cent., an exchange-transfusion must be given, preferably during the first 2 days of life while the umbilical vein is still patent. This is perfor ned by removing small quantities of blood from the umbilical vein, replacing it with Rh-negative blood, until 80 per cent. of the infant's blood has been replaced —this usually necessitates giving 80–100 ml. of blood/lb. body weight (p. 810). Since this method has been used more than 90 per cent. of infants recover completely.

(2) *Infective jaundice* may be due to neonatal infection, especially of the umbilicus, causing multiple small abscesses in the liver. Some cases are due to an unknown cause—possibly virus in origin.

(3) *Congenital absence of the bile-ducts* is distinguished by obstructive jaundice starting in the second or third weeks of life, with very pale stools, a biphasic van den Bergh reaction and a high plasma alkaline phosphatase. It leads to a large liver and biliary cirrhosis. Hæmorrhages from various sites are common, and unless operative measures are successful, death is inevitable about the fourth to the sixth month.

(4) *Galactosæmia* and *Congenital Syphilis* are rare causes.

(5) *Vitamin K* overdoses can be causal.

§ 331. Acholuric Jaundice (Synonym: Hereditary Spherocytosis). *Symptoms* may be absent; it is a notable point in connection with the disease that the patients are often able to go about their work as if they were not the subjects of any abnormality. Symptoms when present can occur at any age, at birth, in young children or in adults. There is jaundice, weakness, a variable degree of anæmia, and splenomegaly which may be extreme. These are liable to exacerbations in which the jaundice grows deeper, the anæmia and weakness become more profound, and the general malaise may be associated with fever and perhaps vomiting. Attacks seem to be especially determined by an acute infection or by cold. Gall-stones composed of bile pigment may form and cause obstructive jaundice; intractable ulceration of the legs is less common. The blood changes are characteristic: the red cells, usually 3-4 millions, are small in diameter but more globular (spherocytes) and are abnormally fragile—a point which clinches the diagnosis (§ 543). A constant high reticulocyte count (10–50 per cent.) is also characteristic. The blood also contains an excess of bilirubin, whereas the urine contains only urobilin. The van den Bergh test (§ 333) shows a strong indirect reaction. The colour of the fæces is normal.

Etiology.—The disease is congenital and occurs in families, the abnormality in the red cells being transmitted as a Mendelian dominant by affected members of either sex.

The *Prognosis* is good as regards life, though cure is not to be expected. Death may occur during the hæmolytic crises or from biliary tract complications.

Treatment.—It is important to avoid cold and infections. Unless symptoms arise, no treatment is needed. When a patient develops severe anæmia, often in the form of hæmolytic crises, blood transfusions are necessary. Subsequent splenectomy greatly reduces the hæmolytic tendency even though the increased fragility and spherocytosis persist after the operation. Gall-stones usually also require surgical treatment.

PART B. PHYSICAL EXAMINATION

The liver lies chiefly in the right hypochondrium; the left lobe extends across the epigastrium above the stomach (Figs. 91, 111).

The gall-bladder is dealt with on p. 500. See Figs. 114 and 115.

The routine methods of examination of the liver consist of INSPECTION, PALPATION and PERCUSSION. Examination of the urine and fæces and hepatic EFFICIENCY TESTS are necessary in many cases. X-ray examination may assist in the diagnosis of obscure cases—*e.g.*, hydatid and abscess.

§ 332. Inspection may show an altered symmetry of the abdomen. In a thin subject the lower edge of the enlarged liver may be seen moving with respiration. The presence or the absence of *jaundice* should always be noted; if slight, it may be seen only in the conjunctivæ and urine and on observing by daylight. Poor expansion of the lower chest occurs with inflammatory disease of the liver. Note also if there are multiple small *telangiectases* on the skin generally, or dilated venules and capillaries on the face or enlargement of the veins of the abdominal wall, such as occur with cirrhosis and portal obstruction. Look to see whether the outer margins of the palms of the hands are red and congested ("liver palms").

Palpation.—All the directions given in § 240 for the palpation of the abdomen must be followed when palpating the liver. The knees should be drawn up and the shoulders supported. Standing on the right side of the patient, place the palmar surface of the hands, previously warmed, on the right side of the abdomen, immediately above the iliac crest, pressing firmly yet gently inwards. The pads of the fingers should be inclined slightly upwards and inwards towards the median line, and should be pressed firmly down, working little by little upwards towards the costal margin. In this way the pads of the fingers, always held perfectly flat, will come in contact with the margin of the organ if it be enlarged. But if it is not enlarged, the liver can only be felt below the xiphisternum, for laterally it lies altogether beneath the costal margin in the adult. In young children the liver is proportionately larger, and the lower edge is normally palpated below the costal margin. If the liver is enlarged, try to feel its surface and consistency by gently dipping the fingers down. Notice if its surface is smooth (as in fatty liver), irregular, or simply rough ("hobnail"), and if it is tender. Umbilicated nodules may be felt in cancer of the liver. When there is fluid in the peritoneal cavity (ascites), the method of suddenly " dipping " the fingers is also useful; anything but gentle use of the finger tips only excites contraction of the abdominal muscles, and so frustrates our object.   Expansile pulsation of the whole liver is felt in cardiac disease with tricuspid regurgitation.   The rectum should be examined in all cases of suspected liver disease.   For examination of the *gall-bladder* see § 351.

Percussion should be light so as to elicit the absolute dullness of the organ.   In percussing the upper margin, begin where there is a good lung note above, and percuss down from rib to rib in the nipple, mid-axillary and scapular lines.   Then repeat the process from space to space.   In defining the lower edge, still lighter percussion should be used,

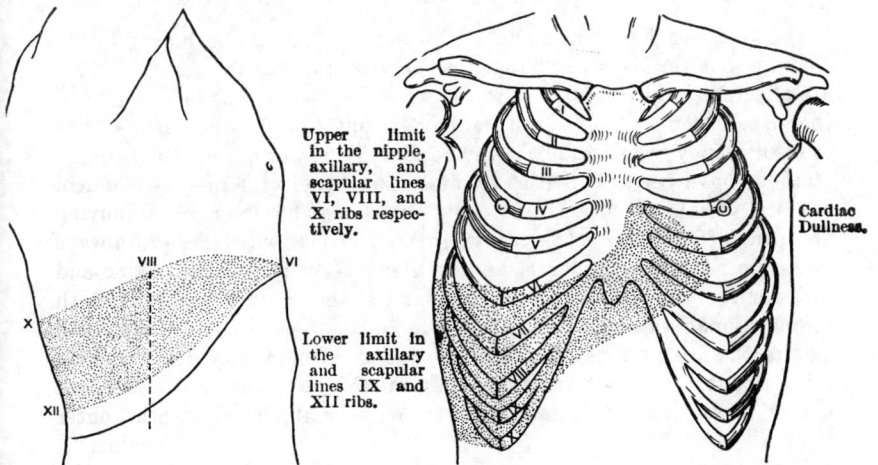

FIG. 111.—AREA OF LIVER AND CARDIAC DULLNESS.—The dullness corresponds to the shaded area.

and the examination should proceed from the tympanitic note of the intestine upwards towards the hepatic region.   But the more certain method of detecting the lower edge is by palpation.

The normal boundaries of the liver are given in Figs. 91, 111.   The *absolute* dullness measures on an average about 2 *inches in the mid-sternal line and* 5-6 *inches in the right nipple line*.

X-RAY EXAMINATION helps to confirm the position and shape of the upper margin of the liver.

FALLACIES.—The physician should never feel satisfied with mapping out the liver once only, because the organ may be temporarily affected by many varying conditions, and the *percussion* boundaries by no means always give a true index.   Thus the lower edge may be masked by the dullness of the stomach after a full meal, by an accumulation of fæces in the colon, by a thickened omentum, by great rigidity of the muscles or by œdema of the abdominal walls.

Apparent *diminution* of the liver may arise from (i.) distension of the stomach or intestines with gas; or (ii.) emphysema of the lungs or pneumothorax which obscures the *upper* border very much.   Great diminution or absolute loss of the liver dullness, owing to gas in the peritoneal cavity, is a diagnostic feature of perforation of the stomach or intestine.

Apparent *enlargement*, when attention is paid solely to the lower edge of the organ, may be due to a *displacement* of the liver downwards by (i.) pleural effusion, empyema or pneumothorax; (ii.) intrathoracic tumours; or (iii.) enlargement of the heart or hydro-pericardium. These and other fallacies may arise from paying attention solely to the *lower edge* of the organ; and, finally, the liver may in rare cases be dropped or "*floating*." "Riedel's lobe" is mentioned under Abdominal Tumours (§ 263). Tumour or enlargement of the *gall-bladder* may be percussed as a dullness extending down from the liver towards the umbilicus.

Fluid in the Peritoneum (Ascites) is a frequent accompaniment of some hepatic disorders, and its presence or its absence must always be carefully noted. The methods of investigating Ascites have already been given (§ 259 and § 260), in which PORTAL OBSTRUCTION is dealt with in full.

§ 333. Liver Function Tests. It was noted at the beginning of this chapter that the liver has numerous functions: in disease not all of these are affected simultaneously or to the same degree. It has been estimated that 80–90 per cent. of the liver may be put out of action before signs of insufficiency occur, and it has a considerable power of repairing damage. Methods have been devised to estimate the capacity of the liver to carry out its various functions. Broadly speaking the liver tests may be grouped into (*a*) those that show an interference with the clearance of bile from the liver, the larger and smaller bile-ducts and the gall-bladder (obstructive jaundice) and (*b*) those that test the damage to the liver cells (parenchymatous liver disease). There is, however, some overlapping, *e.g.*, in the later stages of obstructive jaundice there is evidence of liver-cell damage. It is never wise to rely on the results of any single test: one or more of the liver function tests may be abnormal with a healthy liver.

(1) The *van den Bergh test* is helpful with both these groups. It detects small amounts of bile pigment (bilirubin) in the blood even before any clinical sign of jaundice is evident. Bilirubin, formed by the reticulo-endothelial cells of the liver, is fat-soluble (not water-soluble) and is free or non-conjugated. This fat-soluble bilirubin is converted into two conjugated water-soluble pigments (sometimes called pigments I and II). The first is bilirubin mono-glucuronide, the conversion taking place in the liver and in other sites; the second is bilirubin di-glucuronide which is formed only in the liver.

For the VAN DEN BERGH (DIAZO) REACTION two solutions are required. (1) Concentrated HCl 15 ml., sulphanilic acid 1 G., distilled water 1,000 ml. (2) Sod. nitrite 0·5 G., distilled water to 100 ml. Mix 25 ml. of (1) with 0·75 ml. of (2) shortly before use. For the *direct reaction*, 1 ml. of blood serum is mixed with 0·5 ml. reagent. A violet colour begins at once and attains its maximum in 10–30 seconds. This reaction occurs with bile and with serum bilirubin as in obstructive jaundice. The colour change may be delayed for 1–15 minutes or even longer. It may be reddish at first, slowly or rapidly changing to blue (*biphasic*).

The *indirect reaction* is tested by adding to the mixture of 1 ml. of serum and 0·5 ml. of diazo reagent, 2·5 ml. of 96 per cent. alcohol and 1 ml. saturated ammonium sulphate and centrifuging. A reddish-violet hue results, rapidly attaining its maximum. This indirect reaction occurs with hæmolytic jaundice or with liver damage (hæmo-hepatogenous jaundice) and is valuable in assessing the progress of the illness.

For the *quantitative estimation* of bilirubin, the colour reaction is compared in a colorimeter with a standard solution of cobalt sulphate in water or of methyl red in acetic acid: in normal persons the value is not above 0·5 mg. (1 unit). It is of value in detecting latent jaundice, and in assessing the progress of a case of manifest jaundice. In the interpretation of the results, it is now recognised that neither the direct van den Bergh reaction nor its modifications enables the distinction to be made between hepatogenous jaundice and that due to obstruction. Even in hæmolytic jaundice the test may be unreliable owing to the presence of intercurrent damage to the liver cells.

(2) The *icteric index* is not so valuable. It is obtained by matching the yellow colour of the serum, mainly due to bilirubin, with the colour of a potassium bichromate solution. The normal is between 4 and 6. Clinical jaundice gives values above 16, latent jaundice between 6 and 16.

(3) Tests for Interference with Bile Elimination (Obstructive Jaundice) are: (i.) The *Serum Alkaline Phosphatase* is excreted in the bile. The normal value of 3–13 units (King and Armstrong) may be increased by obstruction of the bile-ducts to 30 units or more. The value is raised to a less extent in hepatitis but not in hæmolytic jaundice.

(ii.) The *van den Bergh Reaction* is discussed above: and demonstration by X-ray of the gall-bladder and larger bile-ducts by cholecystography and cholangiography in § 351.

(4) Tests of Liver-cell Damage (Parenchymatous Disease) depend on which functions of the cells are under investigation. Those in common use include:—

(i.) *Plasma Proteins.* In health the plasma albumen is about 4 G. per cent. (range 3·4–6·7 G. %) and the plasma globulin 2 G. per cent. (range 1·2–2·9 G. %). In hepatitis the albumen is reduced and the globulin increased so that the albumen globulin ratio of about 2 : 1 (range 4 : 1 to 1·2 : 1) becomes about 1·0 : 1·0 or even reversed.

(ii.) The *Transaminase Enzymes* are liberated from liver cells when they are damaged and the amount present in the serum is a rough quantitative measure of the extent of disease. Although both enzymes are increased, the serum glutamic pyruvic transaminase (SGPT) is probably a better measure of cell damage (normal limits 8–32 units/ml. at 20° C.) than is the serum glutamic oxaloacetic transaminase (SGOT).

(iii.) *Flocculation (Turbidity) tests.* The alteration of globulins, especially beta (β) and gamma (γ) globulin, alters the stability of the plasma so that these tests become positive. The chief are (*a*) the thymol turbidity test (normal 0–4 units); (*b*) the cephalin-cholesterol flocculation and less commonly (*c*) the Takata-Ara test with alkaline mercuric chloride. These tests may be abnormal due to other causes, when the liver is functioning satisfactorily.

(iv.) *Electrophoresis* shows there is an alteration of the pattern of plasma protein distribution in the electrical field, so that in the early stages the β and γ globulin bands become more marked, and in advanced disease the γ band is especially prominent.

(v.) The *Erythrocyte Sedimentation Rate* is increased (§ 1210).

(vi.) The *Prothrombin time* may be considerably lengthened when the liver is unable to produce prothrombin (§ 543).

(vii.) *Bromsulphthalein and rose-bengal* are excreted by the liver cells. The former, if injected in amounts of 5 mg. per kg. of body weight, is wholly excreted within half an hour in normal people, but excretion is delayed in cases of liver damage. Rose-bengal, 10 ml. of 1 per cent. intravenously, disappears from the serum in 10 minutes after injection. These tests are of no value in obstructive jaundice.

(viii.) The *Lævulose and Galactose Tolerance tests* and the *Hippuric acid (Quick) test* are no longer used.

(5) The Urine should be examined for bile pigment and for urobilin. Bile pigment (bilirubin) gives a yellow froth. *Fouchet's test* detects small amounts of bilirubin (§ 383). Urobilin (§ 383) is absent in complete obstruction of the

bile-ducts, but is present when the obstruction is incomplete as well as with hepato-cellular damage. In liver disorders the urine often contains excess of urates. The *ammonia-urea ratio* is an important test. One of the main functions of the liver is to convert ammonium salts into urea. If the liver function is inadequate, the formation of urea is decreased, and the resulting excess of ammonium salts and diminution of urea in the blood is reflected in the urine. The normal ratio of ammonium salts to urea is determined in a 24 hours' specimen of urine, and is 4 per cent. In liver insufficiency, this may rise to 30–40 per cent. This estimation is rapidly performed and is a useful index by which to gauge from day to day the effect of treatment.

(6) LIVER BIOPSY at laparotomy or by needle aspiration is of great help in giving information as to the histological changes present (§ 1201).

(7) X-RAY EXAMINATION OF THE PORTAL VEIN (portal venography) is useful in cases of portal obstruction and portal hypertension. In this procedure 30 ml. of 70 per cent. diodone is introduced into the spleen under local anæsthesia and films are exposed immediately afterwards.

Routine Procedure.—FIRST: Ascertain *what is the patient's Leading Symptom*. The symptoms of disorder of the liver we discussed in Part A. —*e.g.*, gastric disturbance, pain (or a feeling of weight or discomfort in the hepatic region) and jaundice. If there be severe and paroxysmal pain, turn first to biliary colic (§ 353).

SECONDLY: Learn the *History* of the patient's illness, eliciting the facts in chronological order, and in this way ascertain also whether the disease be *acute* or *chronic*.

THIRDLY: THE EXAMINATION OF THE LIVER must next be made. The routine method is given in §§ 329–332.

Ascertain: 1. Whether the liver is *enlarged*, locally or generally, or *diminished* (by abdominal palpation and percussion in the nipple line), and whether there is any *pain, tenderness* or other abnormality; 2. Whether there is any *fluid* in the peritoneum; 3. If there is any *jaundice*. 4. Examine *the urine* for bile pigments, urates, etc. 5. In certain cases the *liver function tests* and *X-ray examination* must be carried out.

Classification.—For clinical purposes, diseases of the liver may be conveniently divided into ACUTE and CHRONIC Disorders.

If the illness is one of long standing, and has come on insidiously, the reader should turn to **Chronic Diseases of the Liver** (§ 340).

ACUTE DISEASES OF THE LIVER

If the illness has come on more or less suddenly, and is attended by considerable malaise and other constitutional symptoms, it is one of the **acute diseases of the liver,** probably: I. ACUTE OR SUBACUTE HEPATITIS: I*a*. INFECTIVE HEPATITIS; I*b*. ACUTE OR SUBACUTE YELLOW ATROPHY; I*c*. WEIL'S DISEASE. The less common acute diseases are: II. PERIHEPATITIS; III. ABSCESS; IV. ACTINOMYCOSIS; V. DISTOMIASIS.

I. *The patient, after a short spell of* LASSITUDE, ANOREXIA *and* VOMITING, *becomes* JAUNDICED *and usually* PYREXIAL. *The disease is* ACUTE or SUBACUTE HEPATITIS, *and is due to interference with the function of the liver cells, due to viral, bacterial, chemical or protozoal causes.* It may be mild (CATARRHAL JAUNDICE), *or severe* (ACUTE YELLOW ATROPHY), *or due to* WEIL'S DISEASE.

§ 334. Iα. **Acute Infective Hepatitis,** previously known as *Catarrhal Jaundice,* occurs in sporadic or epidemic fashion, particularly in the autumn. It is milder in children than in adults, and one attack usually confers immunity. In recent years it has become increasingly common.

Symptoms usually begin with a *pre-icteric stage*: (1) Anorexia is constant, and all solid food is refused for 2–3 days. (2) Nausea usually accompanies but vomiting is unusual. (3) Frontal headache, malaise and disinclination for any work are usually present. (4) A feeling of uneasiness or weight in the epigastrium is sometimes accompanied by actual pain. (5) Constipation is much more common than diarrhœa. (6) There is fever for 3–4 days, sometimes only to 99°, more usually to 101° and occasionally higher, during which time the pulse is relatively slow. As the temperature falls the *icteric phase* is reached. (7) Jaundice occurs between 1 and 8 days from the start of the illness. It is accompanied by pale stools, bile-stained urine and often by pruritus. The depth of the jaundice is very variable, and so is its duration, which may be as short as a week, or may persist for even 2 months. (8) At the onset of jaundice the temperature usually settles to normal and the appetite simultaneously returns. (9) At an early stage the liver is often enlarged and firm, 1–2 finger breadths below the right costal margin, and the spleen is usually palpable. (10) Occasionally the skin rashes of macular, urticarial or purpuric type occur even in the pre-icteric stage. (11) The urine is concentrated and contains bile pigment and urobilin. The van den Bergh test gives at first a biphasic and later an indirect positive result. (12) Leucocytosis never occurs and a polymorph leucopenia is usual.

During the course of an epidemic, cases may reveal only the symptoms of the pre-icteric stage, and jaundice may never develop: even the serum bilirubin is not necessarily raised in such cases.

Etiology.—The disease is due to inflammation and a variable degree of necrosis of the liver cells. Three related varieties are recognised. (1) *Primary infective hepatitis,* in which an agent (probably a virus) is transmitted from an infected person by droplet infection from the nose, and from the fæces and urine. The incubation period is usually 17–35 days, and more than one member of a family may be involved. (2) *Homologous serum jaundice* occurs when human serum containing an icterogenic agent is used for blood transfusion, or to convey immunity against measles, mumps or yellow fever. Convalescent serum from cases of measles and mumps, and pooled human serum used in the preparation of yellow fever vaccine as well as tattooing, have produced liver damage, without or with jaundice, in a large number of subjects, after an incubation period of 2–8 months (average 3 months). This type of hepatitis has been transmitted from the serum and from the nose of persons in the pre-icteric and early icteric stages, to volunteers who were inoculated subcutaneously or intranasally. (3) *Post-arsphenamine jaundice* rarely occurs in the first two weeks after the initial dose, and this is probably chemical in origin. Much more often an icterogenic agent is transmitted by a syringe contaminated by blood from a previous patient (*Syringe jaundice*), and produces hepatitis 12–19 weeks later: this agent is not readily destroyed when syringes are " sterilised " by boiling (§ 1200), and can be transmitted to a third person by the subcutaneous inoculation of infected serum.   Jaundice subsequent to the injection of gold salts, neoarsphenamine, and other chemicals is usually also due to " syringe jaundice."

Whereas an attack of infective hepatitis provides almost complete immunity against a second attack, post-vaccinal yellow fever jaundice does not confer immunity against a subsequent attack of infective hepatitis, suggesting that infective hepatitis and homologous serum jaundice are due to related but separate agents.

Diagnosis.—In *infective hepatitis*, pain is never severe and is often absent, bile is absent from the stools only for a short time although they remain pale for a longer period, the spleen is often palpable and the gall-bladder is never enlarged: leucopenia is the rule.   The serum proteins are altered, the albumen/globulin ratio becoming lowered through increase of the globulin.   The unstable gamma-globulins give positive flocculation tests (§ 333).   In *gall-stones* the onset is usually with severe biliary colic, jaundice is often deep and the stools persistently clay-coloured: the spleen is not palpable.   *Cancer* occurs in middle-aged or elderly persons; jaundice is often insidious in onset and lasts for many months.   Jaundice following abdominal inflammation may be due to *abscess of the liver*.   *Post-arsphenamine jaundice*, and those varieties following *blood transfusions* and *human serum inoculations*, may occur at any age and give a history of the cause, whereas primary infective hepatitis is essentially a disease of the young. *Pneumococcal* and *Streptococcal infections* and *glandular fever* occasionally give rise to jaundice.

Prognosis.—Most cases clear up completely within 6–8 weeks, but there is a danger of relapse especially after alcohol and excessive exercise. Cirrhosis of the liver ensues in 0·5–1·0 per cent. of cases.

Treatment.—The patient should be kept warm in bed for at least 2 weeks.   Until the appetite returns, the diet should consist mainly of a large amount of fluid (such as fruit drinks) with plenty of glucose or sucrose and animal protein: it is important to avoid irritating substances, fats and all alcohol.   Insulin, 5 units, may be injected twice a day.   A rectal drip of glucose-saline may be given.   Methionine and casein digests do not benefit cases of infective hepatitis, but may modify attacks of post-arsphenamine jaundice.   A brisk mercurial purge, followed by a saline twice a week, relieves the congestion of the intestines and the liver.   In *fulminant* cases with much vomiting it is wise to give intravenously 3–4 litres of 10 per cent. dextrose combined with 200 mg. hydrocortisone each 24 hours.   To prevent relapse, patients should not be allowed to return to work until the indirect van den Bergh in the blood is under 1 unit: they should avoid all alcohol for 4–6 months.

Prophylaxis is by giving an injection of gamma-globulin—this gives immunity for 6 months.

§ **334a.** I*b*. **Acute or Subacute Yellow Atrophy** (Syn. Severe Acute Hepatitis, Icterus Gravis) is a rare disease characterised by extensive necrosis of the liver cells, jaundice and cerebral symptoms and usually ending fatally.   Some cases are due to a severe form of infective hepatitis and others are the result of chemical poisons. A very severe form is associated with toxæmia of pregnancy.

Symptoms.—(i.) The premonitory symptoms may be slight, resembling infective hepatitis, and are associated with temporary enlargement of the liver. There is increasing tenderness over the liver. (ii.) In a few days or weeks severe symptoms set in, with deepening jaundice, headache, confusion and delirium (or sometimes a state of excitement); the patient finally passes into coma (cholæmia). (iii.) Hæmorrhages occur from the stomach, bowel and kidney, and there may be petechiæ under the skin. (iv.) Fever is usually absent during the course of the illness, but at the end it may be high. (v.) With the onset of the severe symptoms the liver dullness begins to diminish rapidly. The spleen is usually enlarged. (vi.) The urine contains bile, albumen, blood and sometimes acetone. (vii.) Liver function tests show evidence of severe cellular damage. (viii.) In the most severe cases, as in the toxæmias of pregnancy, early collapse, with tachycardia, prostration and death, may take place before jaundice is apparent.

Diagnosis.—Acute Yellow Atrophy is not likely to be mistaken for any other liver disease after the acute symptoms set in. In phosphorus poisoning the liver is enlarged, and signs of irritant poisoning precede the onset of the jaundice.

Etiology.—Predisposing Causes.—(i.) Acute Yellow Atrophy is most common under middle age, though rare in children; and (ii.) in women, especially during pregnancy often accompanying eclampsia. (iii.) Dissipation and excesses predispose. *Exciting Causes.*—(1) It may complicate fevers, such as typhoid fever, streptococcal infections and influenza. It is found in (2) those inhaling trinitrotoluene and carbon tetrachloride; (3) delayed chloroform poisoning and poisoning with phosphorus, iproniazid or cinchophen (atophan); and (4) in some cases of secondary syphilis. (5) It may follow the passage of a gall-stone. (6) In a large number of cases no cause can be found, but a virus infection is suspected.

Prognosis.—The disease is often fatal. After the severe symptoms set in the patient may die in a comatose condition within a week. Pregnant women usually abort. Recovery may take place, followed by cirrhosis of the liver (interstitial hepatitis).

The *Treatment* is very disappointing. The disease is treated as under infective hepatitis (§ 334) by intravenous feeding with 3-4 litres a day of 10 per cent. dextrose and with protein hydrolysates (such as Aminosol vitrum). Hydrocortisone (200 mg. i.v. each day) helps to protect the liver cells. In some cases, especially those due to carbon tetrachloride, calcium gluconate i.v. may aid.

LEPTOSPIROSIS is the term applied to those diseases caused by spirochætal organisms of the genus Leptospira.

§ 334b. Ic. Weil's Disease (Synonym: Spirochætosis Ictero-hæmorrhagica) is caused by *L. ictero-hæmorrhagica.*

Symptoms.—There is a sudden onset of fever with toxæmic symptoms, and in more severe cases, with jaundice and renal involvement. The incubation period varies from 6 to 12 days. The onset is with rigor, headache and frequently vomiting, followed by backache, joint pains, tenderness of the muscles and severe prostration. Sore throat is common. The blood pressure is low, the tongue furred, the face flushed and the conjunctivæ injected. The temperature generally oscillates between 102° and 104° F. and then begins to fall by lysis: it is generally 7 to 14 days before the temperature is normal. Jaundice appears from the 4th to the 6th day in about 50 per cent. of cases and may be intense.

The stools are light or even clay coloured. The urine is scanty, contains bile pigment and bile salts, protein and sometimes red blood corpuscles. The van den Bergh reaction often gives a direct biphasic reaction and bilirubinæmia is increased. The blood urea is raised to 60-300 mg. per 100 ml. A leucocytosis is the rule, varying from 12,000 to 30,000 per c.mm., with neutrophil polymorphonuclears increased to 80 per cent. Skin petechiæ, epistaxis, melæna and hæmorrhage from other mucous membranes are not infrequent, and herpes is common.

The outstanding feature of the physical examination is the extreme tenderness of the muscles, especially those of the legs, neck and abdomen. Abdominal rigidity may suggest an acute abdomen. The liver is generally enlarged and tender and splenomegaly may be present. Later, nocturnal delirium, a typhoid state, muscular twitchings and convulsions may develop and the patient die with anuria and uræmia. In other instances cholæmia, associated with increasing jaundice, hiccough, Cheyne-Stokes' respiration and coma, terminates the picture. Meningeal symptoms predominate in some cases; the cerebro-spinal fluid then contains polymorph leucocytes, lymphocytes, increased quantities of globulin and sometimes also leptospiræ. In about 50 per cent. of cases jaundice does not appear and kidney involvement is slight; the fever may only last 2 to 4 days, and unless the occupation of the patient suggests the need of laboratory investigations the condition will be missed.

Diagnosis.—Features of importance include an occupational relationship to rats or immersion in infected water, profound prostration, extreme tenderness of the muscles, jaundice appearing about the 5th day, hæmorrhages, proteinuria and leucocytosis. At the onset, *meningitis*, later, *infective hepatitis*, may be suspected: the latter does not cause leucocytosis. In the tropics *yellow fever* and *relapsing fever* complicated by jaundice may prove confusing. During the first week leptospiræ can be demonstrated by blood cultures or by the intraperitoneal inoculation of blood into guinea-pigs. Triple centrifugation of citrated blood may show leptospiræ in the deposit, with dark ground illumination. The agglutination test becomes positive in the second week and from the third week onwards leptospiræ can be isolated from the urine.

Etiology.—The causative organism, *Leptospira ictero-hæmorrhagica*, is carried by the rat which passes it in the urine, so infecting water. Human beings are infected during bathing or immersion accidents, by mouth or through abrasions of the skin; hence canal workers, bargemen, rat catchers, miners, sewer workers, fish curers and farmers run most risk.

Treatment.—The patient should be kept in bed on a diet with plenty of glucose, but with a reduced protein content. When vomiting is troublesome, intravenous feeding is necessary. Specific treatment is with leptospiral antiserum (B.P.C.) 60–100 ml. (intravenously or intramusc.) each day, starting as early as possible. Inject. penicillin 5 mega-units is combined with chlortetracycline (B.P.) or oxytetracycline, B.P. (4–6 G.), daily, these doses being reduced as improvement occurs. *Preventive treatment* consists of rat destruction, avoidance of bathing in infected water and the protection of skin abrasions in workers whose occupation brings them in contact with rat-infected slime.

Other Forms of Leptospirosis are: **Canicola fever,** due to *L. canicola*, is a disease of dogs and sometimes, in a mild form, of men; *L. hebdomadis*, carried by the vole, causes a mild disease in man in the Far East; and **Swamp fever** is caused by *L. grippo-typhosa* in eastern Europe. The symptoms, diagnosis and treatment of these varieties are as for Weil's disease.

The less common **Acute Disorders** of the Liver remain to be considered, viz., PERIHEPATITIS and ABSCESS OF THE LIVER.

II. *The patient complains of* PAIN AND TENDERNESS *in the hepatic region, aggravated by movement. There is* NO JAUNDICE, *and other hepatic symptoms are absent but* ASCITES *develops.* The disease is probably PERIHEPATITIS.

§ 335. **Perihepatitis** is inflammation of the capsule of the liver, which becomes opaque and thickened (sugar-loaf liver), and by its contraction may lead to considerable distortion of the shape of the liver.

Symptoms.—(i.) Acute attacks usually set in suddenly, with pain in the hepatic region, radiating to the shoulder, and there is tenderness, increased on movement, pressure or cough. (ii.) Fever is absent as a rule, and the patient may appear to be in his usual health. (iii.) Friction may be felt or heard. (iv.) Unless some other disease is present, there is no jaundice. Recurrent attacks lead to thickening of the capsule, recurring ascites, necessitating repeated tapping, and occasionally jaundice. The puckered liver, with its thickened, rounded, distorted edge, can sometimes be made out.

Diagnosis.—The characteristic pain and the absence of jaundice differentiate it from many other liver diseases. Cases of gall-stones or gumma of the liver may at times be mistaken for perihepatitis. Other signs of syphilis aid diagnosis.

Etiology.—The cause may be (i.) an associated general peritonitis such as is due to tuberculosis; (ii.) a local peritonitis or other inflammation due to a perforated peptic ulcer, subphrenic abscess or cholecystitis, or (iii.) part of an inflammation of the liver itself and due to syphilis, cirrhosis, a tumour or abscess.

Prognosis.—Simple cases tend to recover. In those which have lasted for a long time a certain amount of cirrhosis of the liver ensues. Portal obstruction may ultimately result from puckering at the fissure, and considerable distortion of the liver and ascites may follow.

Treatment.—The diet must be spare, and the patient must be kept warm. Salines are given, with blue pill and rhubarb. Externally, hot fomentations and kaolin poultices give relief, and if the pain is severe, leeches are recommended. The cause when known must be treated.

III. *There is* ENLARGEMENT *of the liver, accompanied by* PAIN *and tenderness, and the boundaries of the area of dullness are* IRREGULAR; *there are* SHIVERINGS, SWEATING *and* INTERMITTENT PYREXIA. The disease is ABSCESS OF THE LIVER.

§ 336. Abscess of the Liver.—Solitary or multiple collections of pus may occur in the liver, due to septic infection, to suppuration of the bile channels (cholangitis), or portal vein (portal pyæmia), or more rarely to suppuration of pre-existing lesions, such as hydatids or gummata. "Tropical" abscess occurs after amœbic infection of the colon, a common cause in the tropics; it is usually solitary, whilst pyæmic abscesses are generally multiple.

Symptoms.—(i.) The onset is usually *acute*, except in the tropical form, with pain and tenderness of the liver, accompanied perhaps by a dry cough, shallow respiration and digestive disturbance. The pain is affected by respiration, and may be worst when the patient lies on the left side. (ii.) The liver is enlarged, and the enlargement may extend downwards, or more often upwards, even to the nipple. There may be fluctuation. (iii.) Jaundice is rarely present. (iv.) Constitutional symptoms are severe. There is usually high fever, continuous at first, then with increasing oscillations. Rigors and sweats are common. Later, the patient falls into a state of delirium, with emaciation, vomiting and diarrhœa.

Besides the acute type just described, there is a variety with an *insidious* onset. As amœbic hepatitis gradually develops into frank abscess formation, there is general failure of health, and periods of continuous, remitting or intermitting fever, sometimes followed by intervals of apyrexia. Cough and dull aching over the liver and in the right shoulder may be present from the beginning. *Amœbic abscess of the liver* affects the right half of the liver in 85 per cent. of cases and is usually associated with physical signs at the base of the right lung; there may be a history of dysentery, while cysts of *Entamœba histolytica* may or may not be found in the fæces. Compensatory hypertrophy of the left half of the liver commonly occurs with destructive lesions implicating the right side.

Diagnosis.—(i.) The pain and pyrexia distinguish abscess from *hydatid* (when not in a suppurating condition). (ii.) A distended and *inflamed gall-bladder* may be palpable. Suppurative pylephlebitis, septic cholangitis, hepatic carcinoma and a breaking down gumma may simulate abscess. (iii.) Abscess is often mistaken for severe *malaria*. But malaria is amenable to mepacrine and quinine, the elevations of temperature are periodic, and each paroxysm has three stages. (iv.) Hepatic abscess may be diagnosed from other swellings of the liver by exploratory aspiration, revealing the chocolate "anchovy sauce" thick, tenacious pus. (v.) Physical signs suggestive of collapse or consolidation at the base of the right lung so frequently accompany liver abscess that their presence is an important aid to diagnosis. (vi.) X-ray shows upward enlargement of the liver (when the right lobe is involved), limited movement of the diaphragm, and sometimes local bulging due to a pointing abscess.

The insidious cases of liver abscess are always difficult to diagnose. No history of dysentery may be obtained and several examinations of the stools may be negative; furthermore liver function tests are usually normal. In amœbic hepatitis there is often more fever than the total white count would suggest. With amœbic abscess the counts mostly range from 12,000 to 16,000 per c.mm., the polymorphonuclears 65 to 75 per cent. Where secondary streptococcal or staphylococcal infection supervenes, the leucocytes rise to 20,000–30,000 per c.mm. and the polymorphonuclear cells to 80–90 per cent. of the total; these counts also hold for pyæmic abscesses. Always suspect hepatic amœbiasis in a patient with obscure pyrexia coming from a tropical country.

Etiology.—Hepatic abscess, single or multiple, is facilitated by thrombosis of radicles of the portal vein causing focal necrosis. It may arise from—(i.) cholangitis following obstruction of the common bile-duct; (ii.) amœbic hepatitis which may give rise to one large abscess, consisting of necrotic liver tissue which is sterile except for the presence of the amœbæ; such an abscess may become secondarily infected with streptococci, etc.; (iii.) portal pyæmia, especially in cases of old-standing suppuration of the appendix and of the pelvic organs; (iv.) suppuration in a pre-existing focus of disease—*e.g.*, hydatid, gumma, tuberculous abscess, actinomycosis or malignant growth; (v.) septicæmia is a rare cause.

Prognosis.—(1) The case mortality is high, except in tropical liver abscess. Death usually takes place in three weeks in cases with multiple abscesses. The pyrexia increases, and the patient dies in the typhoid state. The abscess may burst into the peritoneum, pericardium, or alimentary canal, with a fatal issue, or it may open externally and gradually heal by free discharge. Frequently the abscess, especially a " tropical " abscess, bursts into the right lung or the pleura. The patient develops a severe cough, with signs of consolidation of the right pulmonary base, and the abscess contents are brought up as a red-coloured sputum. Recovery may result in hepatic fibrosis, or the continued discharge may lead to death from exhaustion or lardaceous disease.

Treatment.—For multiple pyogenic abscesses, penicillin in large doses with streptomycin, or tetracycline should be tried. Where amœbic hepatitis or abscess is suspected treat it as such (§ 315 (2)). Absolute rest in bed is necessary. If the condition does not clear up, exploratory puncture of the liver should be made under local anæsthesia; if pus is discovered it should be aspirated as often as necessary and large doses of penicillin and/or one of the tetracycline drugs administered. Incision and drainage are rarely performed nowadays. If the stools still contain cysts, the treatment outlined for amœbiasis should be instituted (§ 315 (2)).

§ 337. IV. Actinomycosis of the Liver is a condition which may be mistaken for abscess of the liver. It is due to absorption of the ray fungus from the intestines, and starts as one or more foci in the liver substance, which slowly enlarge and may undergo suppuration.

The *Symptoms* consist of vague uneasiness referable to the liver, with gradually increasing enlargement—at first uniform, later unequal, the organ becoming prominent in one place. Exploration with a needle may yield no results; but if the tumour is laid open, the characteristic greenish fluid with yellow specks containing the ray fungus clinches the diagnosis. Actinomycosis often responds favourably to large doses of penicillin, with a sulphonamide and potassium iodide (gr. 40–60 daily).

§ 338. V. Distomiasis of the Liver is commonly found in the Far East, due to *Clonorchis sinensis*, while more rarely *Fasciola hepatica*—the sheep fluke—may affect man. In these diseases the bile-ducts are invaded with flukes, leading to thickening and dilatation of the ducts and cirrhosis of the liver. Mild infections may be symptomless, but the more severe cases present anorexia, epigastric pain, hepatomegaly, diarrhœa, wasting, œdema, ascites and jaundice. Secondary bacterial infection may produce fatal cholangitis or liver abscess. The *Diagnosis* is made by finding the operculated eggs in the fæces, associated with eosinophilia in the blood.

Treatment.—Carbon tetrachloride 3 ml. in a gelatine capsule is sometimes effective; and favourable reports have been recorded as to the value of emetine injections (1 gr. daily for 10 days). A course of antimony sodium tartrate or organic compounds of antimony may be given intravenously.

§ **339. Subphrenic Abscess.**—The *Symptoms* resemble those of tropical liver abscess. When occurring above the right lobe, the liver dullness is continued up in the axilla, perhaps as far as the level of the nipple, and is convex or dome-shaped upwards. The base of the right lung shows signs of congestion, and there are evidences of pleurisy at one or both bases.

Etiology.—The most common causes are appendicitis and ruptured peptic ulcer. Other causes are extension of hepatic abscess, empyema perforating the diaphragm, extension of pelvic abscess, and local tuberculous or (rarely) cancerous processes.

Diagnosis.—In a case of suspected abscess exploratory puncture may be performed, sometimes under general anæsthesia. The needle should not penetrate beyond 3½ inches, so as to avoid puncturing the portal vein. In a right-sided *empyema* of the chest the upper border of the dullness, when continuous with that of the liver, is concave, being higher towards the spine. In *hepatic abscess* the liver is tender and enlarged below the costal margin, but it is often impossible to distinguish subphrenic from hepatic abscess. A variety containing air so greatly resembles pneumothorax that it is called *pyopneumothorax subphrenicus.*

The *Prognosis* is good if surgical treatment is carried out thoroughly and in time.

CHRONIC DISEASES OF THE LIVER

§ **340. Routine Procedure.**—It will be remembered (§ 332) in the physical examination of a patient suspected to be suffering from hepatic disease that the *first* and most important question to investigate is whether there is *any alteration in size,* especially enlargement *of the liver* (by palpation and with the help of percussion). (2) For reasons which will be apparent below, the next question is whether there is any *pain or tenderness* in the organ. And then (3) is there any *jaundice*? (4) Is there any *ascites*? (5) In every case of suspected liver disease the spleen (§ 361), the stools, and the urine should be carefully examined.

The numerous *fallacies* in the alteration of the size of the liver dullness must be carefully studied (§ 332).

Classification.—Chronic diseases of the liver are divided into those in which the **size of the liver is unchanged** and those in which it is altered, either **diminished or enlarged;** the latter again being divided according to the presence or absence of pain over the liver.

A. The organ is **Normal in size** in:—
Functional derangement of the liver   ..   ..   ..   § 341

B. The organ is **Diminished in size** in:—
Portal cirrhosis or Chronic hepatitis   ..   ..   ..   § 342

C. The organ is **Increased in size:**—

(*a*) WITHOUT PAIN OR TENDERNESS:
I. Hypertrophic cirrhosis (bacterial and toxic); I*a*. Biliary

cirrhosis; I*b*. Right-sided heart failure; I*c*. Chronic
syphilitic disease; I*d*. Cirrhosis of biliary obstruction;

A. The liver is normal in size. *The patient complains of* LETHARGY,
vague digestive disturbances, sleepiness after meals, furred indented tongue,
CONSTIPATION, *headaches, and there is frequently a deposit of* URATES IN
THE URINE *on cooling.* There is probably FUNCTIONAL DERANGEMENT
OF THE LIVER.

§ 341. Functional Derangement of the Liver.[1]—The liver is the largest
organ in the body and has many functions, which may become deranged
together or separately. Usually one or two functions are more severely
affected. See liver tests (§ 333).

The common complaint, "My liver is sluggish," is often equivalent
to saying that the bowels do not act properly, but in some cases other
parts of the digestive system may be at fault. The causes of this complaint may be temporary or continuous. Help may be obtained by
consulting the following classification.

I. TEMPORARY:
Acute dyspepsia, "bilious attack" (§ 279).
Migraine (§ 812).
Onset of colds, febricula.
Excess of food, alcohol or mental stress (§§ 282–284).

Errors of diet, especially rich, sweet, greasy foods, with highly-flavoured
sauces and alcoholic beverages, *i.e.,* indigestible and excessive food rather
than plain food. Alcohol *combined with sugar* (*e.g.,* port and other fruity
wines) is especially injurious; or taken in the form of undiluted spirit,
e.g., cocktails, particularly on an empty stomach, is more harmful than
dilute alcohol at meal-times.

II. CONTINUOUS:

Constipation (§ 324).	Colitis (§§ 310, 312).
Cholecystitis (§ 354).	Acidosis (§ 271).
Chronic appendicitis (§ 250*n*).	Psychoneurosis (§ 1171).
Gastritis (§ 282).	

[1] The introductory remarks at the head of this chapter may be referred to in this
connection.

B. *The liver is* **diminished in size**; *if the surface can be felt it is* HARD AND UNEVEN (*hobnail*); ASCITES *is probably present, but no very distinct jaundice; the patient is subject to* HÆMORRHOIDS, *and* HÆMORRHAGES *from the stomach and bowel.* The disease is PORTAL CIRRHOSIS (CHRONIC INTERSTITIAL HEPATITIS).

§ 342. Portal Cirrhosis of the Liver (Lænnec's Cirrhosis or Interstitial Fibrosis of the Liver) is a form of chronic hepatitis. In the earlier stages there may be some enlargement due to fatty degeneration or cloudy swelling of the liver cells; this becomes considerable if the patient is seen during an acute bout of alcoholism. Later there is an increase of the interstitial fibrous tissue, leading to portal obstruction and portal hypertension, hæmorrhoids and œsophageal or umbilical varices, and eventually ascites. It may follow infective hepatitis or occur insidiously in spirit drinkers, and affects men between 35 and 60 years old. Whereas it used to be thought to be the result of chronic alcoholism it is now recognised to be more commonly due to other causes.

Symptoms.—(1) The onset is slow and may extend over years. There is a feeling of uneasiness and weight in the hepatic region, accompanied by hepatic enlargement. Gastric and other symptoms of alcoholic gastritis such as a capricious appetite, morning sickness and headaches after meals may be complained of. The tongue becomes furred, the breath fœtid. Some degree of asthenia and loss of weight follow. (2) Later the liver becomes small and hard and the surface is often nodular or " hobnail." At this stage the patient's facies shows dilated venules and capillaries in the cheeks. Spider nævi may be seen in the neck, arms and trunk above the level of the nipples. The palms of the hands show a diffuse erythema (" liver palms "). (3) Clubbing of the fingers is sometimes seen. (4) The sclerotics develop a slatey-blue sheen and jaundice appears in about one in three cases. (5) Symptoms of portal obstruction occur (§ 260) and hæmatemesis with melæna from œsophageal varices may be the first obvious symptom. The spleen enlarges, sometimes to a considerable size. Hæmorrhoids also appear. Ascites (which is present in 80 per cent. of the cases) may be very considerable in amount: when the ascites recurs after paracentesis, chronic peritonitis has probably supervened. (6) There is an increased tendency to hæmorrhage as a result of prothrombin deficiency. (7) Impotence, sterility, disappearance of the secondary sexual hair and a low 17-ketosteroid excretion in the urine are found. In alcoholic men gynæcomastia (due to failure of the liver to destroy œstrogens) and Dupuytren's contracture are seen. (8) In the concluding stages when the cells of the liver have been largely destroyed various neurological symptoms develop. The patient periodically becomes either confused and drowsy, or euphoric and excited; the outstretched hands and fingers show a flapping tremor and a cogwheel rigidity may be found. The disorientated and confused mental state becomes more prominent, stupor, coma and a muttering delirium (cholæmia) develop, the tendon reflexes are lost and the plantars become extensor.

Diagnosis.—The clinical picture of a middle-aged man, with a history of chronic dyspepsia, a congested facies, liver palms, hæmatemesis, recurrent ascites and a small hard liver and an enlarged spleen, readily identifies this disease. In the early stages estimation of the degree of liver damage can be aided by liver function tests (§ 333). *Cancer* of the liver is only difficult to diagnose from cirrhosis in the early stages; but usually it runs a more rapid course, and is accompanied by more pain, and more intense jaundice. The spleen is not usually enlarged in cancer. In *passive congestion* of the liver with ascites there are evidences of a cause, such as heart or lung disease. In the absence of ascites early cirrhosis may be mistaken for the other causes of liver enlargement. The enlargement of the spleen in atrophic cirrhosis may lead to the primary condition being overlooked. The liver is reduced in size in *starvation*. *Chronic peritonitis* with effusion may not be recognised as such until the organs can be palpated after paracentesis.

Etiology.—Peri-portal cirrhosis of the liver used to be regarded as the result of alcoholic poisoning. Although alcohol plays a part in a number of cases, and spirits taken on an empty stomach are particularly injurious, the condition may develop in those who are strict teetotallers. A previous attack of infective hepatitis is a more important cause and then cirrhosis usually develops within 3 years. Other factors are a lack of animal protein, an excess of fat in the diet and vitamin B deficiency. Syphilis, malaria, chronic dysentery, bilharzia and many bacterial infections may predispose. In poisoning by T.N.T., carbon tetrachloride and tetrachlorethane, the process is subacute or even acute. Banti's syndrome is an occasional cause (§ 559). The occurrence of hæmatemesis is the result of the formation of a collateral anastomosis with large dilated varices in the œsophagus and in the fundus of the stomach. The cerebral symptoms are regarded as being due to the formation of nitrogenous substances (especially ammonia) in the intestines by bacterial action, these by-passing the liver via the collateral circulation, instead of being detoxicated in this organ. The cerebral changes are aggravated by the anæmia of a gastro-intestinal hæmorrhage and are accompanied by electro-encephalographic abnormalities. For cirrhosis with hepato-lenticular degeneration see § 917. In 40 per cent. of cases no antecedent cause for cirrhosis can be found.

Prognosis.—The disease has a slower and more insidious onset than hypertrophic cirrhosis (below), and is in most cases a more serious condition. If the patient is seen before signs of portal hypertension supervene much can be done; if later, the prognosis is grave. The outlook is more favourable in patients who are young and where the general health is good. With treatment the condition may remain stationary for years. *Untoward Symptoms.*—Although restoration to comparative health has occurred after the development of ascites, with the onset and recurrence of rapid ascites the end is in view, the patient rarely living more than a few months. Pleurisy, renal disease, or tuberculous or pneumococcal peritonitis are occasional complications. Primary carcinoma of the liver occurs with advanced cirrhosis, particularly in men.

Treatment in the early stages is practically the same as that employed for chronic congestion of the liver, and chronic gastritis (§§ 348 and 283). (i.) The habits of the patient must be corrected and the diet adjusted to give a high-protein and a low-fat content (§ 296. IV); methionine and choline chloride (2 G. āā daily) have been advocated. Glucose and insulin aid. Alcohol must be avoided at all times and regular exercise taken. (ii.) For hæmorrhage, post-pituitary extract i.v. (§ 272), blood transfusions and vitamin K injections are required. If bleeding continues balloon tamponage to compress the varices may be of temporary benefit (§ 272). Recurrent hæmorrhage necessitates surgical resection of the varicose site in the lower œsophagus and cardiac end of the stomach, with subsequent end-to-end anastomosis. (iii.) Relief of portal hypertension is obtained by portocaval anastomosis. This operation is only undertaken when liver damage is slight and when there is little ascites—it is now less commonly performed than formerly. (iv.) Ascites may be lessened by a low salt diet and with diuretics such as chlorthalidone (Hygroton), spironolactone (Aldactone) or inject. mersalyl, but repeated paracentesis is often required. (v.) The neurological symptoms are treated by rectifying the anæmia with transfusions, reducing the protein intake to lower levels, giving dextrose-saline intravenously when dehydration is present and reducing the bacterial changes in the intestine with oxytetracycline B.P. 0·25 G. q.d.s. or with neomycin.

C. We now turn to those chronic liver diseases in which **the size of the liver is increased.** These may be divided into two groups—those WITHOUT PAIN AND TENDERNESS are described immediately below. If the enlargement is attended WITH PAIN AND TENDERNESS, turn to § 348.

There are five diseases with **enlargement** of the liver **without pain and tenderness:** I. HYPERTROPHIC CIRRHOSIS; II. FATTY LIVER; III. VON GIERKE'S DISEASE; IV. AMYLOID LIVER; and V. HYDATID and other rare diseases. In INFECTIVE HEPATITIS (§ 334), CHRONIC CHOLELITHIASIS, and some other disorders, the liver is somewhat enlarged, but this is not their main feature.

Other rare causes of PAINLESS ENLARGEMENT of the liver are chronic blood diseases, notably LEUKÆMIA and SPLENIC ANÆMIA, ACHOLURIC JAUNDICE (§ 331), KALA-AZAR and MALARIA (§ 343, I*f*). TUMOURS (§ 350) may be unaccompanied by pain in the early stages.

I. *The* **liver is enlarged** *and* **painless;** *its surface is hard,* JAUNDICE IS PRESENT, *but little or no ascites, and there is a long history of failing health.* The disease is probably HYPERTROPHIC CIRRHOSIS.

§ 343. **Hypertrophic Cirrhosis of the Liver** is a term employed in a generic or clinical sense to indicate a progressive enlargement of the liver due to an increase in the connective tissue of the organ with a tendency to jaundice. The condition occurs in at least six different forms.

I*a*. BILIARY CIRRHOSIS (Chronic Infective Cholangitis) is a condition occurring principally in young adults.

Symptoms.—(1) There is a history of two or more attacks of acute hepatitis in preceding months. (2) The liver is uniformly, and often considerably, enlarged, hard and sometimes rough. (3) The spleen is considerably enlarged. (4) Recurring attacks of jaundice occur, with pyrexia even to 103° F, during which the urine contains bile and the stools are pale or clay-coloured. During these subacute exacerbations, the liver and spleen enlarge further, and the liver may become tender, with a feeling of a dull weight in the hepatic region. (5) In spite of the intense jaundice there are few or no signs of portal obstruction, and ascites is rarely, if ever, present. (6) Hæmorrhages, purpura and telangiectases may occur.

Diagnosis.—From *portal cirrhosis* it is known by the absence of signs of portal obstruction (§ 260). *Fatty* and *amyloid* livers are not accompanied by jaundice. *Cancer* has a more rapid and painful course.

Etiology.—The condition appears to be due to a subacute or chronic inflammation around the bile-ducts, leading to partial obstruction. It is probably infective in origin; a similar condition may arise following chronic biliary obstruction, *e.g.*, with gall-stones in the common bile-duct.

Prognosis.—Sometimes patients die within twelve months, with an acute onset of hepatic failure (cholæmia), but most live for a number of years, with signs of progressive liver damage. In children the general health may appear unaffected for a long period.

Treatment is as for Hepatitis (§ 334). Mercurial inunction of the abdominal wall, or calomel, gr. $\frac{1}{16}$ to $\frac{1}{4}$ t.i.d. for three days, with intervals of three days, continued for some months has good results. Glucose and insulin aid restoration of liver function. A prolonged course of penicillin should be tried. Drainage of the gall-bladder has cured some cases.

I*b*. CIRRHOSIS OF BILIARY OBSTRUCTION.—Hypertrophic cirrhosis has been produced experimentally in one half of the liver by ligature of one hepatic duct, and it is met with clinically in association with gall-stones, tumours or glands pressing on the bile-ducts. There is a history of repeated attacks of biliary colic, enlargement of the liver, with jaundice of some years' duration. The spleen is only slightly enlarged. The acholic stools aid the diagnosis of this form of hypertrophic cirrhosis.

I*c*. RIGHT-SIDED HEART FAILURE results, as we have seen, in very considerable congestion of the liver. Long-continued passive engorgement of the liver gives rise to changes known as the " nutmeg liver," accompanied by enlargement of the organ; and this may be attended by a considerable degree of fibrosis. The diagnosis depends on the presence of cardiac valvular disease and other features (see Passive Congestion, § 348).

I*d*. CHRONIC SYPHILITIC DISEASE of the liver generally takes the form of a diffuse hypertrophic fibrosis; or it may be met with in the form of *gummata*. Hepatic fibrosis may result from both hereditary and acquired syphilis, though the gummatous form is commoner in the latter: both are becoming rare. In the inherited variety two forms of fibrosis occur. In one there is fine diffuse fibrosis between the individual cells (pericellular cirrhosis), and this variety is usually accompanied by an enlarged spleen. The liver is smooth and firm. In the other, coarse fibrosis with perihepatitis occurs, as in the acquired disease.

The *Symptoms* are variable. The liver is moderately enlarged; there is not much tendency to jaundice or to portal obstruction excepting in the final stages. There may be actual pain, especially when the capsule of the liver is involved; but as a rule there are only indefinite sensations of illness, accompanied in the gummatous cases by a low form of intermittent pyrexia. In the gummatous form nodular projections may possibly be made out on the surface of the organ. The presence of such projections, accompanied by intermitting fever and a history of syphilis in a young or middle-aged adult, makes the diagnosis practically certain. In the absence of a syphilitic history the occurrence of pain and local tenderness at intervals points to syphilitic rather than to alcoholic cirrhosis, because *perihepatitis and the involvement of the capsule* are prominent features of syphilitic cirrhosis. In the diagnosis from cancer we have mainly to rely on the Wassermann reaction, the response to therapy and the (usual) absence of jaundice and ascites in syphilitic disease.

The *Prognosis*, as a rule, is good, if the nature of the disease be discovered and it be treated adequately with antisyphilitic remedies.

I*e*. HÆMOCHROMATOSIS (Syn. Bronzed Diabetes) is a rare condition almost confined to men. The *symptoms* are (i.) a slow progressive enlargement of the liver but without jaundice; the spleen is also enlarged; (ii.) the skin becomes thinned and takes on a bronzed or slatey colour: the pigmentation differs from that of Addison's disease in that it usually avoids the oral mucous membrane and appears on parts exposed to light rather than to pressure and friction. The pigment contains iron (§ 577). (iii.) In most cases there is diabetes with glycosuria which is often severe; (iv.) the blood pressure may be low. *Etiology.*—The disease is due to a disorder of iron metabolism which leads to excess deposition of hæmosiderin especially in the liver, pancreas, the skin and the suprarenals. It is usually the result of excessive absorption of dietary iron but may follow large numbers of blood transfusions. The serum iron content is much higher than normal and this and a skin biopsy aid diagnosis. The *treatment* is that of the liver disease and the stabilisation of the diabetes. Repeated venesections to remove iron are often helpful. With adequate treatment patients often live for many years.

I*f*. TROPICAL CIRRHOSIS.—Many parasitic infections involve the liver, but only a few produce actual cirrhosis. Malaria may induce hepatitis and biliary pigment stones, but it is doubtful if a true malarial cirrhosis ever occurs; kala-azar parasites, however, may produce it. Biliary cirrhosis is found in clonorchiasis and bilharzial peri-portal cirrhosis with *S. mansoni* and *S. japonicum*. Though hepatomegaly with occasional jaundice occurs, ascites is rare. And see Abscess of liver (§ 336).

II. The **enlargement of the liver** *is* PAINLESS *and uniform; the surface is smooth and soft; there is* NO JAUNDICE OR ASCITES, *and the* SPLEEN IS NOT ENLARGED; *there is a history of alcoholism, phthisis, or other toxæmia.* The disease is probably FATTY LIVER.

§ 344. **Fatty Liver** is a condition in which fat is deposited in the hepatic cells, commencing in the periphery of the lobules. It is nearly always associated with some other disease.

Symptoms.—(1) The liver is enlarged uniformly and is quite smooth. (2) Pain, jaundice and portal obstruction are absent. (3) The accompanying symptoms are due to the cause of the fatty liver, and may consist, therefore, of asthenia, anæmia, etc. (4) The history of a *Cause* is important—viz., (i.) Chronic wasting disease, such as phthisis. (ii.) Fatty liver appears in association with fatty heart (*q.v.*) and general obesity. (iii.) It often accompanies chronic alcoholism; and a mixed degeneration with fat and fibrosis is not uncommon.

The *Diagnosis* from the painful enlargements of the liver is not difficult. In amyloid liver there are also signs of amyloid disease of the spleen or kidney.

The *Prognosis* and *Treatment* depend upon the cause.

§ 345. III. **Von Gierke's Disease** is a rare congenital, and sometimes familial, cause of enlarged liver, usually seen in the young, due to excessive glycogen accumulation in the liver, kidneys, heart and other organs. Adrenalin does not produce the usual rise in blood sugar.

IV. *The* **enlargement of the liver** *is* UNIFORM *and* PAINLESS; *the surface is smooth and hard; there is* NO JAUNDICE, NO ASCITES; *the* SPLEEN IS ENLARGED; *there is a history of prolonged purulent discharge, rheumatoid arthritis, phthisis, or constitutional syphilis.* The disease is AMYLOID DEGENERATION.

§ 346. Amyloid Liver (Syn. Lardaceous Disease of the Liver, Secondary Amyloidosis) is a condition in which the liver tissue is replaced by amyloid material, which starts in the capillaries and smaller arteries of the organ, leading sometimes to an immense enlargement.

Symptoms.—(1) The liver is enlarged uniformly and smoothly, and feels firm; (2) pain, jaundice and portal obstruction are absent; (3) the constitutional symptoms are due to the causal condition, and to amyloid disease of other organs—especially the spleen, the kidneys, the intestine, the adrenal glands and the skin.

Diagnosis.—The presence or history of a cause may render the diagnosis of amyloid disease comparatively easy. A positive diagnosis should not be made unless over 90 per cent. of congo red (injected intravenously) is removed from the serum within an hour. Confirmation is often obtained by biopsy of a piece of gum, using the staining reactions classical of amyloid, but even in established cases this test may be negative. *Primary amyloidosis* does not usually produce clinical involvement of the liver, but affects selectively the muscles (including the cardiac muscle), or the lungs, or sometimes the kidneys, or the skin with a brown pigmentation. There is rarely a recognisable etiology for this primary type, although multiple myeloma may co-exist.

Etiology.—(i.) Long suppuration and purulent discharge, as from chronic osteomyelitis; (ii.) rheumatoid arthritis; (iii.) syphilis; and (iv.) tuberculosis disease of the lungs or elsewhere. Amyloid liver has become much rarer since chronic suppuration has been obviated by improved surgical methods and by antibiotics.

The *Prognosis* depends upon the amount of amyloid disease elsewhere. Diarrhœa, indicating amyloid changes in the intestines, abundant pale urine with albuminuria indicating amyloid disease of the kidneys, are untoward signs. If the cause is remediable, as by surgical treatment, the liver may decrease in size. Otherwise progressive amyloidosis is usually fatal within two years.

Treatment.—The indications are (i.) to remove the cause, and (ii.) to keep up the strength. The former is attained by anti-syphilitic treatment in the case of syphilis, and by surgical treatment in the case of long-standing discharges. The corticosteroids combined with an antibiotic may be helpful.

V. *The* **enlargement of the liver** *is* PAINLESS, *but* NOT UNIFORM, *and the upper margin of the liver dullness is perhaps* ARCHED; *there is no jaundice or ascites and the spleen is not enlarged; a thrill may be felt on percussion.* The disease is HYDATID CYST.

§ 347. Hydatid of the Liver depends on the presence in the liver of the parasite, *Echinococcus granulosus*, rare in this country, though common in Australia, New Zealand, the Argentine, Greece, and Iceland, where dogs live in close association with man.

Symptoms.—(i.) There is a slowly increasing enlargement of the liver, which is smooth, globular and elastic, sometimes fluctuating. The right chest may be bulged outwards, with dullness in the axilla. When the fingers of the left hand are laid on the tumour and tapped with those of the right hand, the " hydatid fremitus," or " thrill," is felt in some cases. (ii.) Pain is absent unless the tumour is very near the surface, when pain may be present, because *the liver capsule* is involved. (iii.) No constitutional symptoms appear unless the tumour presses upon the surrounding structures, or becomes inflamed and

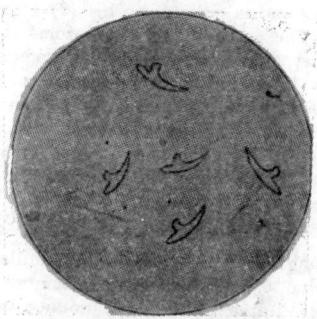

FIG. 112.—Hooklets, from a HYDATID CYST in man, magnified about 150 times. These form the crown of hooklets around the anterior end of the scolex, and are absolutely distinctive of hydatid fluid.

suppurates. (iv.) Rupture into the peritoneal cavity may be followed by anaphylactic shock and urticaria, and later by the growth of secondary cysts. Jaundice may occasionally be caused by cysts obstructing the bile-ducts.

Etiology.—The parasite enters the intestine of man with food or water contaminated by fæces containing the ova of the *Echinococcus granulosis* (*Tænia echinococcus*), a tapeworm which infests the dog. The embryo is carried to the liver, where it encysts and grows, the liver tissues forming a fibrous capsule (the adventitia). The cyst so developed has a lining membrane composed of an endogenous germinal-layer and an exogenous hyaline layer, and contains a clear fluid. The endogenous layer buds the tiny brood-capsules in which scolices or embryonic heads develop, each with a crown of hooklets. Daughter and grand-daughter cysts may also be formed.

Diagnosis.—*Abscess* of the liver produces pain and fever, and on aspiration yields purulent material like anchovy sauce. *Pleural effusion* on the right side, leading to dullness in the axilla, may resemble hydatid. In such cases a *bulging* outwards of the lower ribs over the liver points to the presence of hydatid. A *renal cyst* has resonance in front, due to the colon. A history of residence in Australia, the Argentine, etc., should lead one to suspect hydatid in cases of slowly increasing enlargement of the liver, *with few other symptoms*. The symptoms of suppurating hydatid cyst of the liver are very like those of inflammation of the gall-bladder. X-rays are of value in diagnosis. Hydatid cyst fluid is pathognomonic, although exploratory puncture entails serious risk, as it may set scolices free, which subsequently form secondary cysts (see Fig. 112 and Table XVIII). X-ray of the lungs may reveal unsuspected hydatid cysts in the chest. The blood sometimes shows eosinophilia, and the serum gives the complement fixation reaction with a suitable antigen in 70 per cent. of cases. Infested patients react to an intradermal injection of hydatid fluid (Casoni); it is a group reaction for infection with tapeworm, for in cysticercosis similar positive reactions are occasionally recorded.

Prognosis.—The patient may live for several years with no other symptoms than a slow increase in the size of the liver. The prognosis must be guarded even when the cyst is safely removed for other cysts may develop later. A cyst may remain quiescent for twelve years or more without losing its potentiality for mischief. The cyst may suppurate, giving rise to the symptoms of liver abscess, or pyæmia may be set up. When a cyst leaks into the surrounding tissues, anaphylactic symptoms may occur—collapse, vomiting and urticaria associated with eosinophilia. Sometimes death occurs by the sudden rupture of the cyst into the pleura or peritoneum.

Treatment.—Hydatid cysts most often involve the inferior aspect of the right half of the liver and are generally accessible through an anterior abdominal incision. A transpleural route may be necessary for cysts impinging on the diaphragm. After opening the abdomen, packing off and locating the cyst, aspirate the fluid and inject 6 to 10 ml. of pure commercial formalin. Subsequently the adventitia is incised and daughter cysts removed. The cyst cavity is filled with saline and the adventitia sutured together, where possible. Drainage is better avoided.

There are three diseases in which **enlargement of the liver** is attended **with pain and tenderness ;** I. Chronic Passive Congestion, II. Cancer of the Liver, and III. Abscess of the Liver. In chronic cholelithiasis and several acute disorders the liver may be slightly enlarged and tender.

I. *The* **enlargement** *is moderate, smooth and uniform,* painful *and* tender; *some jaundice and ascites may be present, the* spleen is slightly enlarged, *and there are signs of congestion of the abdominal viscera.* The disease is probably Chronic Congestion of the Liver.

§ 348. Chronic Passive Congestion of the liver is a condition in which the enlargement is due to right-sided heart failure.

Symptoms.—(i.) The liver is tender, and a sensation of weight and fullness is complained of in the hepatic region. Expansile pulsation synchronous with the heart may be conveyed to the palpating hand when the tricuspid valve is incompetent, but as the organ becomes firmer this is lost. (ii.) Signs of general venous obstruction appear with ascites, œdema of the legs, albuminuria, gastro-intestinal symptoms and slight enlargement of the spleen. Some degree of jaundice may occur.

Etiology.—Passive congestion is the result of any backward pressure due to obstruction or failure of the circulation. In most cases this is caused by heart or lung disease, and especially mitral stenosis.

The *Diagnosis* is often aided by the recognition of the heart disease on which it depends. In some cases of *ascites* with anasarca of the legs, we may find both *hepatic enlargement* and *albuminuria*, and a difficulty may arise as to which was the primary cause of the condition—heart, liver or renal disease. The difficulty is increased if extensive bronchitis prevents accurate auscultation of the heart. In such cases, *the liver* may be excluded as the primary cause, if the œdema in the legs clearly preceded the ascites. The presence of hepatic enlargement is then a sign of great value as helping to exclude *renal disease*, because enlargement of the liver is not a usual sequence of kidney disease, although it is a fairly constant result of *cardiac* valvular disease. The enlarged liver quickly decreases in size when congestive heart failure is relieved.

Prognosis.—The prognosis depends on the cause of the congestion; the state of the heart is generally the measure upon which the patient's chance of a longer or shorter life depends. In mitral stenosis an enlarged liver with ascites is less grave than in mitral regurgitation, because it normally occurs at an earlier stage in stenosis. It is most serious in aortic disease, as it indicates concurrent mitral and tricuspid insufficiency.

The *Treatment* is that of the cause, and our attention must be directed to the heart and lungs. Purgatives and light foods are necessary in order to relieve the strain on the portal system. Venesection may be indicated.

II. The **enlargement of the liver** is IRREGULAR; *the* PAIN *and tenderness may be great;* JAUNDICE *and* ASCITES *are present; the spleen is not enlarged; the patient is middle-aged or advanced in years, feeble and emaciated.* The disease is CANCER OF THE LIVER.

§ **349. Cancer** of the liver is usually secondary to disease elsewhere. It is rare before thirty-five.

Symptoms.—(i.) Pain is an almost constant feature of cancer of the liver; it is continuous, with exacerbations, and is independent of food or posture. A certain amount of tenderness develops. (ii.) The enlargement of the liver is irregular and may become enormous in size, and often umbilicated nodules may be made out. These are of a hard consistence, and increase rapidly. There is also less commonly diffuse cancer, in which there are no nodules, and in which the liver is only slightly and uniformly enlarged. (iii.) Jaundice is usually present, *sooner or later*, and becomes intense and progressive; deep jaundice persisting over five to seven weeks in an old person should indeed always lead one to suspect cancer. Ascites generally occurs either from involvement of the glands in the fissure, or of the peritoneum. The spleen is not enlarged. (iv.) The general health of the patient is bad, and emaciation and cachexia may be present before any local signs are discovered. Cancer may be present in another part of the body. Fever may occur at intervals, and a polymorph leucocytosis (sometimes considerable) is usual. Rectal examination may reveal malignant glands in the pelvis.

Diagnosis.—Jaundice is rarely entirely absent in cases of cancer of the liver: this and the cachexia alone may justify a diagnosis. The diagnosis from *cirrhosis* may be difficult when nodular enlargement cannot be made out, and when considerable ascites is present. In cirrhosis there is little or no pain and tenderness, the history of the illness is of longer duration, the spleen may be enlarged, and the jaundice is not so intense. The *inflammatory thickening* under the liver after a long history of gallstones may resemble cancer, and can be distinguished only when time shows little or no increase in the enlargement. In doubtful cases, the abdomen should be thoroughly examined after removal of the ascitic fluid. *Syphilitic* liver has not so much pain and tenderness, is of slower growth, and rarely produces ascites.

Etiology.—Cancer of the liver is usually secondary to a carcinoma or sarcoma elsewhere in the body. It is liable to spread to the liver (a) via the portal bloodstream or the abdominal lymphatics, from primary disease in the stomach, colon, pancreas or other abdominal organs. (b) It may invade the liver via the systemic blood vessels from a primary site in the breasts, lungs, testicles, etc. (c) There may be a direct extension from disease of the stomach or gall-bladder. (d) Primary cancer of the liver may follow cirrhosis.

Prognosis.—Cancer of the liver is usually fatal within six to twelve months, death taking place from exhaustion. Untoward symptoms are rapid enlargement, ascites or respiratory difficulties due to extension of the disease to the lungs and pleura. The degree of malignancy varies in different cases—some live for a surprisingly long period even when the liver is very large as with malignant carcinoid tumours (§ 571).

Treatment can be palliative only. Treatment of ascites makes the patient more comfortable. Chlorpromazine or morphia is administered for the pain, and attention must be given to the relief of the symptoms of gastric distress, and to aid nutrition. With rest and care there may be periods during which the disease makes no progress, and which hold out to the patient false hopes of his ultimate recovery. Partial hepatectomy has sometimes been successfully performed.

III. **Abscess of the Liver** also produces considerable hepatic enlargement, which is PAINFUL and TENDER. It has already been described among the Acute Diseases, § 336; but sometimes it runs a very chronic course.

§ 350. **Tumours of the Liver** other than CANCER (§ 349), HYDATID (§ 347) and GUMMA (§ 343. Id), are more rare. Their presence is manifested by *enlargement of the* *organ*, which may be regular or irregular, accompanied in some cases by constitutional symptoms. When, as in some cases of ACTINOMYCOSIS and FASCIOLA HEPATICA (*Distoma hepaticum*) (§§ 337, 338), they assume an inflammatory form, pyrexia is present. SARCOMA OF THE LIVER is occasionally met with—*e.g.* Lymphosarcoma—but it is most often secondary to deposits elsewhere, and the liver condition is only a subordinate part of the case. The patient may be younger than in the other forms of malignant disease. An ADENOMA of the liver is usually asymptomatic, but it may cause a single large swelling in the substance of the liver. A HÆMANGIOMA may be single or multiple. It is usually of small size and located in the left lobe of the liver: it produces no symptoms and is detected when nodularity of the surface of the liver is discovered. Calcification in the substance of the tumour may help diagnosis. Chondrosarcoma, Melanosarcoma, Tuberculosis, Lymphadenoma and Fibroma occur very rarely. Riedel's lobe is often mistaken for a tumour (§ 263).

THE GALL-BLADDER

PART A. SYMPTOMATOLOGY

§ 351. The cardinal symptoms commonly associated with gall-bladder disease are **pain** or **discomfort in the upper abdomen** and back, **flatulence, nausea** or **vomiting.** Occasionally **constitutional symptoms** are also present. Pain or discomfort is usually epigastric, often worse on the right side, and may be related to meals. It varies from a dull ache to acute paroxysms of colicky pain, as when a calculus becomes impacted in the neck of the gall-bladder or in the cystic duct. The pain is often referred to the lower right ribs, the angle of the right scapula or between the scapulæ. Flatulence in the abdomen may be severe; it produces a sense of fullness, so that the patient loosens the clothing. Nausea is rarely present before a meal, but after a few mouthfuls of food the patient may feel so distended and nauseated that he cannot eat more. Vomiting may be occasional, or in attacks, associated with the other symptoms. With colic it is usually severe. A characteristic feature of gall-bladder disease is the aggravation of the symptoms by food containing eggs, cream and animal fats, so that the patients avoid these foods. Pyrexia and other constitutional manifestations accompany catarrhal or suppurative processes in the gall-bladder. **Jaundice** is present when there is obstruction of the hepatic or common bile ducts.

PART B. PHYSICAL EXAMINATION

When examining the gall-bladder one must ensure that the abdominal wall is entirely relaxed. With the patient in the supine position and the knees drawn up, palpate gently with the fingers laid flat on the abdominal wall, the patient breathing quietly all the time. Occasionally more satisfactory results are obtained by making the patient sit and lean forward with the knees flexed, completely relaxed, whilst one palpates with the tips of the fingers under the right costal margin. The gall-bladder may be best felt when a deep breath is taken; when enlarged it is felt as a tender globular swelling coming forward at the tip of the ninth right costal cartilage. It usually remains just under the surface of the anterior abdominal wall, moves freely downwards with respiration, but cannot be moved laterally; when very large it is dull to percussion and may extend even to the right iliac fossa. With cancer of this organ, the surface becomes hard and nodular (and see § 263. I). Even when the gall-bladder is not large enough to be felt, with inflammation the upper right rectus muscle shows rigidity. If the lower hepatic margin in the right hypochondrium be divided into outer, inner and middle segments, when the patient takes a deep breath he flinches and his face expresses pain on deep palpation of th middle segment but not with palpation of the other segments. In d:s :ases of the gall-bladder it is essential to examine the back, as refer..d :reas of tenderness may be met (a) over the 11th and 12th right ribs, (b' over the 5th–8th dorsal spines or (c) over the paravertebral muscles be .n the scapulæ, especially over the right side. A friction rub is occa: o· liy audible over the gall-bladder.

Special Investigations of the Gall-bladder and Bile-ducts may be undertaken by:—(a) X-RAY EXAMINATION. (i.) A *plain X-ray* film usually reveals gall-stones if they contain calcium. (ii.) *Cholecystography* (Graham-Cole test) is performed by giving iodine compounds which are excreted by the liver and concentrated in the gall-bladder. Iodophthalein B.P. or the less toxic iopanoic acid B.P. (Telepaque) may be used. When it is taken by mouth, radiograms 12 hours later reveal the degree of filling; if a fatty meal is then given, a further plate reveals the degree of emptying.

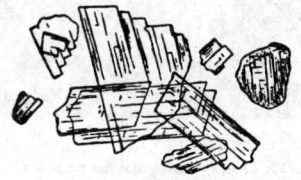

FIG. 113. — Cholesterol Crystals. Microscopic appearance presented by fragments of gall-stones in the fæces or from the duodenum.

If the gall-bladder does not fill, a fat-free diet is given, and the dose repeated 24 hours later. (iii.) *Cholecystangiography* outlines the hepatic and common bile-ducts and is particularly useful when the condition of the ducts has to be investigated after cholecystectomy; the gall-bladder shadow is rather less dense than with the method used for cholecystography. Iodipamide methylglucamine (Biligrafin intravenous) is used as a 30 per cent. solution and a series of X-ray films taken between 30 and 150 minutes later. Normal filling and emptying are occasionally compatible with a diseased gall-bladder, but as a rule improper filling and emptying, especially after the intravenous method, indicate a pathological condition. Non-opaque stones may be visualised only when they are surrounded by opaque substance (Fig. 114b).

(b) DUODENAL INTUBATION. By introducing a long rubber tube into the duodenum, especially after a period of starvation, a sample of resting duodenal contents may be obtained; if then 20 ml. of warm olive oil or of sterile peptone (10 per cent.) are introduced through the tube, a profuse flow of bile from the gall-bladder may be obtained within a few minutes and a sample aspirated; this is examined for micro-organisms (especially *B. coli* and those of the typhoid group), cholesterol crystals (which may be deformed when gall-stones are present) (Fig. 113), for lipoid globules (from a " strawberry gall-bladder "), and for pus cells. If achlorhydria is present, the results must be viewed with caution.

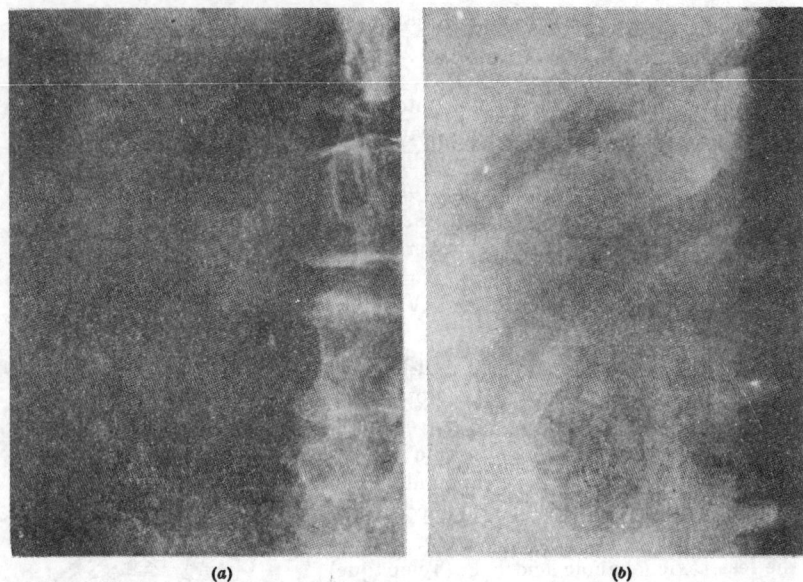

(a)   (b)

FIG. 114 (a) shows opaque gall-stones. FIG. 114 (b) is a cholecystogram showing facetted gall-stones displacing the Iodophthalein.

PART C. DISEASES OF THE GALL-BLADDER

Gall-bladder Disease may be: **Acute**—I. ACUTE CHOLECYSTITIS, II. GALL-STONE COLIC; or **Chronic**—III. CHRONIC CHOLECYSTITIS, IV. CANCER OF THE GALL-BLADDER.

I. *The patient complains of* PAIN *in the* GALL-BLADDER REGION; *the pain is* PAROXYSMAL, *or* DULL AND CONTINUOUS, *and* RADIATES TO THE RIGHT SHOULDER. *There is* TENDERNESS *over the* GALL-BLADDER, *vomiting and some fever. The disease is* ACUTE CHOLECYSTITIS.

§ 352. **Acute Cholecystitis** may be catarrhal, suppurative (empyema of the gall-bladder) or gangrenous according to the severity of the infection.

Symptoms.—(1) Local pain in the right hypochondrium and epigastrium.   (2) Pain is spasmodic or dull and continuous, and radiates through to the back and right shoulder-tip.   (3) Tenderness in the right upper abdomen; this becomes localised below the tip of the ninth costal cartilage. (4) Rigidity of this area; if the muscles are relaxed, the enlarged gall-bladder may be felt. (5) Symptoms may be mild, like dyspepsia, or severe with vomiting, jaundice, rigors and much general disturbance.

Etiology.—Predisposing: (1) stagnation of bile; (2) calculi of solitary cholesterol type; (3) foreign bodies, worms and ova in the gall-bladder; and (4) previous attacks. The *exciting cause* is infection, which may come from the tonsils or teeth; or follow pneumonia, influenza or typhoid fever, gastric, duodenal or appendicular disease.

*Diagnosis.—*Absence of jaundice is not a point against cholecystitis. In *gall-stone colic* the pain is more severe, while local signs of tenderness, paralytic distension of intestines and palpable gall-bladder favour cholecystitis. Leucocytosis is rare with gall-stones, unless accompanied by cholecystitis. In perforated *duodenal ulcer* there may be a history of characteristic indigestion. In *acute pyelonephritis,* pus and *B. coli* are found in the urine. *Appendicitis* may cause difficulty; appendicitis and cholecystitis may co-exist. Right *diaphragmatic pleurisy* or *basal pneumonia, herpes zoster* and *intercostal neuralgia* must be excluded.

*Prognosis.—*The attack may subside or pass into chronic cholecystitis. If it proceeds to suppuration or gangrene, the gall-bladder may rupture and produce local or general peritonitis so that life is endangered.

*Treatment.—*The patient should be in bed on milk or light diet. The local application of a kaolin poultice may be used, or morphia may be required for the pain. Vomiting may be relieved by bismuth carbonate, hydrocyanic acid or an effervescing mixture. In mild cases salicylate of soda and hexamine with alkalies are useful as antiseptics. A drachm of magnesium sulphate taken in a dessertspoonful of water, fasting, in the morning, and followed after an hour by a pint of hot water or weak tea, and also olive oil ℳ 120 between meals, act as a stimulus to gall-bladder evacuation. In more severe cases, injections of penicillin or of streptomycin, or administration of one of the tetracyclines, give good results. If fever and rigors persist, operation on the third or fourth day is indicated. In cholecystitis, even without gall-stones, drainage is not sufficient to cure and the gall-bladder should be removed.

II. *The patient, usually an elderly female, is suddenly seized with* PAROXYSMS OF SEVERE PAIN *in the hepatic region, and in the course of twelve to twenty-four hours she may become* JAUNDICED, *the stools becoming clay-coloured.* The attack is one of BILIARY COLIC.

§ 353. **Gall-stones** and **Biliary Colic.**—Gall-stones are concretions which form in some part of the biliary passages, most commonly in the gall-bladder. CHOLELITHIASIS is the condition in which gall-stones are developed. When gall-stones move along any of the ducts, they give rise to Biliary Colic.

GALL-STONES may be *metabolic,* consisting of deposits of cholesterol or bile pigment, or *infective,* of mixed composition. They vary in size from a sand-grain to a golf-ball. When solitary, they are round or oval in contour. The facets or flattenings of their surface are caused by the pressure of one against the other; this indicates that there has been more than one stone in the gall-bladder or bile-ducts. The colour varies from yellow to dark brown; their chief physical characteristics are the smooth " soapy " surface, the ready way in which they crumble between the thumb and finger (though sometimes they are very hard), and their lightness as compared with renal calculi. They generally consist chiefly of cholesterol mixed with calcium and bile pigment, but are sometimes pure cholesterol, pure bilirubin, or pure calcium carbonate. Cholesterol is contained and held in solution by bile salts in normal bile. When from various causes the liver is unable to produce the bile salts in sufficient quantity, there is a high cholesterol content in the blood and bile, with eventual deposition of cholesterol and formation of gall-stones. Normal individuals can eat food containing cholesterol, because more bile salts are produced by the liver and hold the cholesterol in solution. With other individuals this capacity is defective. The foods which increase the cholesterol content of the blood are: egg yolk, butter, cream, liver, kidney, pancreas, brain and meat fats.

Biliary Colic.—Symptoms may be absent when the stone is at rest, but when it begins to move (i.) the pain is agonising; it starts in the epigastrium and shoots into the right hypochondriac region towards the spine and up to the right shoulder-tip, but rarely passes downwards. The paroxysm is usually so severe that the patient is in a state of partial collapse, with vomiting, hiccough, subnormal temperature, and a quick, weak pulse. Sometimes there is a rigor, and the temperature rises a few degrees. Between the paroxysms of acute pain there is a constant dull aching and tenderness over the hepatic region. The attack lasts from a few hours to a few days. (ii.) The liver may be enlarged and if a stone becomes impacted in the hepatic duct the enlargement may be considerable. (iii.) Jaundice usually appears 12 to 24 hours after the paroxysm, and lasts from a few days to a few weeks. It is most intense when the stone is impacted in the common duct, and may give rise to severe pruritus.

The *Symptoms* which arise vary somewhat with the *position of the gall-stone* (Fig. 115). Thus: (i.) If a stone is impacted in the *common duct* there are biliary colic, obstructive jaundice and sometimes a distended gall-bladder, and if the impaction continues the liver becomes enlarged. (ii.) If a gall-stone is impacted in the neck of the gall-bladder (*i.e.*, in the *cystic duct*), *biliary colic without jaundice* is present. In time the gall-bladder may be distended with mucus, and form a definite abdominal tumour (mucocœle), but more often the chronic irritation of many calculi leads to chronic fibrosis of the gall-bladder which prevents its becoming enlarged. Considerable distension of the gall-bladder is not usually associated with the presence of many gall-stones, but more often with cancer of the pancreas or chronic pancreatitis.

(iii.) A stone impacted in the *hepatic duct* is rare. It causes biliary colic and jaundice, but the gall-bladder is not distended. (iv.) Stones occasionally form in the *radicles of the hepatic ducts,* and give rise to indefinite symptoms, sometimes without pain, and usually without jaundice. (v.) Sometimes small particles of cholesterol (biliary sand) in the *gall-bladder* give rise to recurring paroxysms of pain, unaccompanied by other symptoms, eluding diagnosis. (vi.) The stones may become encysted, but more often, without surgical intervention, abscess and fistula result.

Diagnosis of Biliary Colic.—It is distinguished from the two other forms of colic in Table XIV, § 247. The severity of the pain and its paroxysmal character usually distinguish it from other acute diseases of the liver. *Pseudo-biliary colic* is sometimes met in nervous women. The diagnosis from *cancer* of the liver may be very difficult. Both occur at the same age, and both cause jaundice; further, cancer of the gall-bladder may follow after years of trouble from gall-stones. In cancer, jaundice steadily becomes more intense. It must be remembered that in some cases gall-stones are passed without colic, but with jaundice; consequently, *recurring attacks* of jaundice in an elderly woman should lead one to suspect gall-stones. A radiogram may show gall-stones, but a negative plate

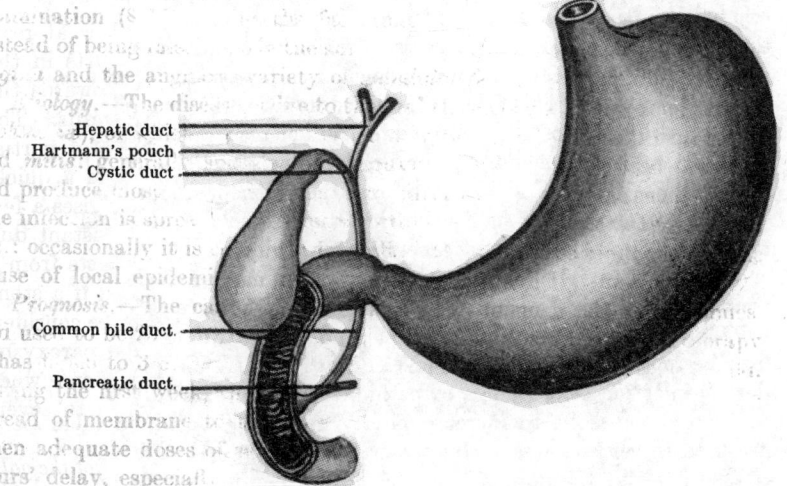

Hepatic duct
Hartmann's pouch
Cystic duct

Common bile duct.

Pancreatic duct.

Fig. 115.—The Stomach and Duodenum opened to show the ducts in connection with the Liver and Pancreas.

is not conclusive. Negative shadows may be defined in the opaque gall-bladder with the Graham-Cole test (Cholecystography, p. 501). In all suspected cases the stools should be carefully examined for stones. *The presence of ascites* points to cancer, which rarely exists long without peritoneal effusion.

Gall-stones at rest in the Gall-bladder occur often in elderly women: they give rise to *Symptoms* the cause of which may be difficult to diagnose. They are the symptoms of cholecystitis (§§ 352, 354) which precedes or accompanies gall-stone formation. They consist of (1) flatulence, especially after fats, (2) pain referred to the right upper abdomen and shoulder-tip, (3) subcostal ache, especially when chilled.

Etiology of Gall-stones.—(i.) They usually occur after the age of 50 but are sometimes seen at a much younger age; (ii.) are much commoner in women, especially in multiparæ, and (iii.) in stout persons of sedentary habit whose diet is rich in fat and sugar. (iv.) There is often a history of gout, asthma or migraine. (v.) They may follow cholecystitis due to typhoid, coli or streptococcal infection, or any cause of stagnation of bile in the gall-bladder. (vi.) The colic is often determined by a sudden strain, by motoring or by an overloaded stomach especially with rich fatty food.

Course and Prognosis.—The prognosis as to recovery from an attack of biliary colic is excellent, but recurrence may be expected. A stone usually forms in the gall-bladder and becomes impacted for a time in the neck of the cystic duct, giving rise to biliary colic without jaundice. It may then pass down the common duct, and cause jaundice. This rarely lasts more than a few weeks, but cases have been reported where it lasted two years. Impaction with infection is followed by: (i.) *Ulceration* of the ducts, with pyrexia, or abscesses of the liver and bile-ducts (cholangitis), and consequent subacute pyæmia; (ii.) *perforation* into adjacent tissues, leading, for example, to fatal peritonitis; (iii.) inflammation and *abscess* (empyema) of the gall-bladder, which may open externally, perforate into the peritoneum, or rupture into the intestines; (iv.) formation of *fistula* between the gall-bladder and the colon or duodenum, through which stones can pass of such a size that they may cause intestinal obstruction. (v.) *Cancer* may supervene in later years.

Treatment.—*During the attack* treatment aims at relieving spasm and controlling pain. If mild, a tablet of trinitrin may give relief. If severe, belladonna is the drug of choice: a dose of 15 minims of the tincture may be repeated after 2 hours, or a full dose of atropine given. A hypodermic injection of morphine or pethidine may be necessary for the pain, but morphine tends to increase biliary spasm. Chloroform inhalations are used in severe cases. Hot water with gr. 60 of bicarbonate of soda to he pint aids the flow of bile, and hot turpentine stupes relieve pain. So letimes an attack of pain is warded off by a hot bath (100° F).

Between the attacks the diet must be supervised. Foods containing cholesterol must be omitted, therefore forbid most animal fats, especially if cooked. A little butter is allowed, but no cream or yolk of egg, no kidney, liver, brain, sweetbread or the fat of meat, pork, goose and duck. (For specimen diet see § 296. IV.) To flush out the biliary passages, the liver can be made to secrete more bile by administering bile acids, potassium and magnesium salts, salicylates and oil of peppermint: particularly powerful is dehydrocholic acid (decholin): Carlsbad Sprudel salt is popular, as it is rich in potassium salts. When it is desirable to cause the gall-bladder to contract and empty itself (gall-bladder drainage), give magnesium sulphate in doses of gr. 30 to 60 in concentrated solution before breakfast, and olive oil between meals. Where there is hyperchlorhydria, a tablespoonful of olive oil with a small dose of tincture of belladonna is useful, given before meals. Penicillin and/or streptomycin injections, or the tetracyclines, help to sterilise an infected biliary tract. Felamine is a useful preparation, in 5-gr. tablets twice or thrice daily. Surgery is indicated where there is suppuration, when the gall-bladder remains distended, the common duct is blocked, or biliary colic frequently recurs. The old practice of giving large amounts of olive oil does not remove gall-stones; the resulting masses passed in the fæces are aggregations of fatty acid crystals, not the gall-stones.

CHRONIC DISEASES OF THE GALL-BLADDER

III. *The patient, a young or middle-aged adult, complains of* FULLNESS, *weight or oppression* IN THE EPIGASTRIUM *about half an hour after meals,* WORSE AFTER GREASY *or* ACID FOOD. *Relief is obtained by belching, and cessation almost at once by vomiting. There is* CHILLINESS *or* SHIVERING *in the evenings, and a shoulder ache or stabbing* PAIN *in the* RIGHT SIDE *with a deep breath.* The disease is probably CHRONIC CHOLECYSTITIS.

§ 354. **Chronic Cholecystitis** is one of the commonest of all abdominal diseases, and is often undiagnosed in the early stages when medical treatment is available. It may follow acute cholecystitis, it may precede or accompany gall-stones, or it may be chronic from the onset, brought on by sedentary habits which predispose to stagnation of bile and infection. The infection, usually blood-borne, is first seated in the wall of the gall-bladder. Cholesterol metabolism is interfered with, hypercholesterolæmia follows, and the mucosa of the gall-bladder becomes engorged with cholesterol (" strawberry gall-bladder "). Cholesterol stones form in the lumen followed by infection of the contents of the gall-bladder; at this stage are formed the mixed gall-stones of cholesterol, bile pigments and calcium.

Symptoms.—(1) Continual flatulent dyspepsia, fullness or oppression in the epigastrium, coming on soon after food; (2) worse after fruit, eggs, cooked fats, pork, pastry, pickles or heavy meals; (3) relieved by belching and ceasing almost at once after vomiting; (4) distension or tightness relieved by bending forwards, flexing the right thigh on the abdomen or loosening the clothing; (5) acidity or heartburn, sometimes a gush of saliva into the mouth; (6) chilliness or " gooseflesh," especially in the evenings. Attacks of " biliary fever," *i.e.*, shivering, nausea, vomiting, diarrhœa and faintness, with slight rise of temperature, may occur at intervals for months or years, especially after exertion. (7) Aching in the right shoulder or stabbing pain with tenderness at the angle of the right scapula. Tenderness may occur in the areas supplied by the seventh to ninth thoracic segments, the areas which supply the sympathetic nerves to the gall-bladder and bile-ducts. (8) There may be congestion and œdema at the right base. (9) There is sometimes reflex gastric hyperchlorhydria, but the stomach juices are usually sub-acid. (10) Remote symptoms from the gall-bladder as a source of infection are chronic infective arthritis, fibrositis, phlebitis, anæmia or myocardial degeneration with palpitation, extrasystoles and breathlessness on exertion.

Etiology.—Chronic cholecystitis may occur at any age, but is frequent in the young. It follows (1) biliary stasis from sedentary habits, insufficient exercise or constipation; (2) infection, which takes place usually (*a*) by the blood-stream, but may spread (*b*) by direct extension from pre-existing hepatitis by way of the lymphatics, or (*c*) by ascent up the bile-ducts from the duodenum, and (3) disturbance in cholesterol metabolism.

Diagnosis.—Persistence of symptoms of flatulence (" wind ") is characteristic of chronic cholecystitis. In cases with reflex superacidity of stomach contents, symptoms may resemble those of *duodenal ulcer.* The pain, coming long after meals or in the early morning, is relieved by food and alkalies; but with gall-bladder disease the pain is less regular and is made worse by fats. *Spastic gall-bladder* has much the same symptoms, but is relieved by belladonna (Newman). In *intercostal neuralgia*, the tenderness is in the abdominal parietes, not deep: and with a painful *slipping costal cartilage*, there is local tenderness of the costal margin. With X-ray, there may be (*a*) opacity in the gall-bladder region; (*b*) irregularity and fixation of the hepatic flexure; (*c*) with cholecystography, non-filling or irregular filling points to a diseased gall-bladder; negative shadows of stones may be seen. A barium meal will demonstrate any lesion in the adjacent pylorus or duodenum. Duodenal intubation may show pus cells or bacteria (§ 351). The symptoms may resemble those of *psychoneurosis* and a careful inquiry into the environment and former history of the patient will help in diagnosis.

Course and Prognosis.—Gall-bladder disease must be thought of as a focus of infection in " toxæmic " states. If neglected, cholecystitis may lead to gall-stones, empyema or cancer of the gall-bladder.

Treatment.—Indications are (1) to prevent the stagnation of bile by exercise, plenty of fluids, magnesium sulphate, gr. 60 in water fl. oz. 2, first thing in the morning; (2) reduce bile cholesterol by a dietary of vegetables and carbohydrates, avoiding cream, egg-yolk, sweetbreads, brain, liver, kidneys and large meals; (3) treat infective foci by removal of diseased teeth or tonsils and attention to the bowel, appendix, pelvic organs and nasal sinuses. Sodium salicylate or hexamine combined with sodium bicarbonate and potassium citrate act as mild disinfectants of the biliary tract. Since the infection is intramural, drainage alone at operation will not effect a cure, and the gall-bladder should be removed. In older people palliative treatment should be recommended and a course of penicillin and/or streptomycin injections tried; in younger patients, operation.

IV. *The patient, a stout woman of sedentary habits, between fifty and sixty, who has suffered for years with " windy spasm " or mild colic, has a* CONSTANT OPPRESSION OR DISCOMFORT *in the* RIGHT HYPOCHONDRIUM, *loses weight and appetite, is* JAUNDICED *and has a palpable* TUMOUR IN THE GALL BLADDER REGION. The disease is probably CANCER OF THE GALL-BLADDER.

§ 355. **Cancer of the Gall-bladder** is uncommon. It is closely associated with cholelithiasis. Calculi are found in 70–90 per cent. of cases, and primary carcinoma of the gall-bladder occurs in 4–14 per cent. of all cases of cholelithiasis. It is much more common in women than in men (4 : 1).

Symptoms.—(1) The symptoms preceding the onset of carcinoma of the gall-bladder are those of the pre-existing cholelithiasis and cholecystitis. Biliary colic may occur, but usually there is only discomfort and heaviness in the right upper abdomen. (2) A tumour may be felt, at first round and smooth, but later nodular and hard. It moves with respiration. (3) Jaundice follows from pressure on the ducts by secondary glands or from catarrh. (4) Ascites occurs from pressure on the portal vein or secondary growths in the peritoneum.

Diagnosis.—The presence of a hard, nodular, progressively increasing tumour in the gall-bladder region of an elderly woman is suggestive. Gall-stones may cause inflammatory thickening round the gall-bladder, but enlargement of the gall-bladder is in favour of growth. Jaundice may come on suddenly with diarrhœa and vomiting, simulating infective hepatitis, but is progressive. Carcinoma of the stomach or hepatic flexure of the colon may cause confusion.

Treatment.—Extirpation by total removal offers the only hope of recovery. Medical treatment must be merely palliative.

THE PANCREAS

This lies as a retro-peritoneal organ across the back of the abdomen on a level with the first and second lumbar vertebræ—the major part of it lies in the epigastrium. The main duct traverses the gland from left to right and immediately after leaving the pancreas joins the common bile-duct to enter the second part of the duodenum at the Ampulla of Vater. The accessory duct, of comparatively small size, drains the head of the pancreas and, after communicating with the main duct, enters the duodenum a little higher.

The main functions of the pancreas are (i.) to produce an external secretion, the pancreatic juice; (ii.) also to secrete insulin directly into the blood-stream. The pancreatic juice, by virtue of the water and sodium bicarbonate contained in it, neutralises the hydrochloric acid as it enters the duodenum from the stomach. The juice also contains enzymes which help in the digestion of fats (lipase), proteins (trypsin) and carbohydrates (pancreatic amylase or diastase, and maltase). These enzymes are in an inactive form in the pancreatic cells but become activated, especially when in contact with succus entericus or with bile. Insulin in small amounts is secreted the whole time (basal secretion), but in much larger amounts after a meal as soon as glucose is absorbed from the small intestine. It is derived from the beta-cells of the islets of Langerhans, which are much more numerous in the tail of the pancreas and in the adjacent portion of the body of the gland. The function of the secretion from the alpha-cells of the islets (glucagon) is not fully understood; it appears to antagonise the effects of insulin in the body.

After total pancreatectomy, such as may be performed for carcinoma, the external secretion may be replaced by extracts of the pancreatic juice in an enteric coating; the patient will also need the injection of 40–50 units of insulin a day.

PART A. SYMPTOMATOLOGY

Fortunately, diseases of the pancreas are relatively uncommon for they are difficult to recognise. Even gross disease usually fails to give symptoms directly referable to the organ itself. Most of the symptoms are the indirect result of the absence of the pancreatic juice or of the production of insulin.

The *Symptoms* produced by pancreatic disorders depend on the nature of the disease, but among the commonest are: (1) Pain in the upper abdomen, situated in the epigastrium or in the right or left hypochondrium, often associated with upper lumbar pain; (2) progressive loss of weight commences early in association with general debility and depression; (3) obstructive jaundice is present in a proportion of cases; (4) diarrhœa is associated with the passage of bulky, pale and fatty stools; (5) other digestive disturbances, not regularly related to meals, include nausea, anorexia and vomiting.

PART B. PHYSICAL EXAMINATION

Owing to its deeply-seated position in the upper abdomen it is impossible to palpate the pancreas. Even a large carcinoma is only occasionally palpable. A tumour may be felt in the upper abdomen following acute or subacute pancreatitis, and in the former a proportion of cases subsequently show a greenish-blue discoloration in the left loin and sometimes around the umbilicus, due to hæmorrhagic extravasation. Disorder of the pancreatic function is usually revealed with certain pancreatic function tests.

§ 356. Tests of Pancreatic Function.—There is no one satisfactory test because the pancreas is concerned with the secretion of the pancreatic juice on the one hand and the secretion of insulin on the other: the disturbance of pancreatic function partly depends on the portion of the organ involved—whether it be the head, the body or the tail of the pancreas. Those in common use are:

(1) *Examination of the Fæces.*—When pancreatic juice is deficient, the proper digestion of fats and of muscle protein is affected. The amount of undigested starch granules is altered by the amount consumed, the activity of the ptyalin of the saliva and of the amylase of the succus entericus, and the rate of passage of the food to such an extent as to make this entirely unreliable. The two tests in use are:—

(a) The FAT should be looked for with the naked eye. *But before doing any examination or tests on the stool, liquid paraffin and all similar oils must be excluded from the diet for at least three days.* When in considerable excess the stool is pale, greasy and fatty-looking, loose but not watery and floats on the surface of water in the pan. Steatorrhœa may be due to many causes, the chief of which comprise the absence of the fat-splitting lipase of the pancreatic juice, or the failure of absorption after the ferment has acted (see Steatorrhœa, § 316). Therefore when a pale greasy-looking stool is passed, it should be examined (i.) microscopically. With deficient pancreatic lipase there is a large excess of oil globules (which stain with appropriate dyes) but there is no excess of fatty acid crystals or soap plaques. (ii.) Quantitative analysis of the stool. On a normal diet containing between 60-150 G. of fat a day over a 3-day period (with no liquid paraffin), the total amount of fat does not exceed 6 G. a day. In pancreatic steatorrhœa, further detailed analysis shows the unsplit fat is above 25 per cent. of the dried fæces (it may rise to 60–80 per cent.) and the proportion of unsplit fat exceeds 25 per cent. of the total fat present.

(b) UNDIGESTED MUSCLE FIBRES. When a normal person is on a diet containing animal protein, a certain number of partially digested muscle fibres are seen. These are more numerous in the presence of diarrhœa (Fig. 116a, b, c, d, e). When, however, nuclei are present, the transverse striations are well seen and even the ends of the muscle fibres are fragmented and irregular, creatorrhœa pointing to a definite deficiency of pancreatic trypsin. The absence of these features is not diagnostic for other protein-splitting ferments may cause the muscle fibres to be partially digested.

(2) *Urinary Diastase (Amylase).*—The starch-splitting ferment of the pancreas becomes activated if concentrated bile releases the ferment from its precursor amylopsin: this occurs especially when bile flows up the pancreatic duct in acute and subacute pancreatitis. Normally, an average of 20 units per ml. is excreted daily in the urine; but in these diseases it is above 100 units per ml. and it may even rise to 1,000–2,000 units. When in doubt as to the renal efficiency, a simultaneous estimation of the blood urea is advisable as there is much less diastase in the urine when renal activity is impaired.

The test measures the amount of starch digested in a given time by a definite quantity of urine. A 24-hours' sample of urine is required, and is made just acid to litmus, also (i.) 0·1 per cent. of soluble starch; (ii.) 0·9 per cent. solution of NaCl; and (iii.) a weak solution of iodine. Ten test-tubes are numbered 1 to 10. With a 1 ml. pipette, place in tube No. 1, 0·9 ml. urine; and then in tubes 2–5, 0·6 ml., 0·4 ml., 0·2 ml. and 0·1 ml. respectively. For further dilutions of the urine dilute some of the original urine ten times with the saline solution, and into

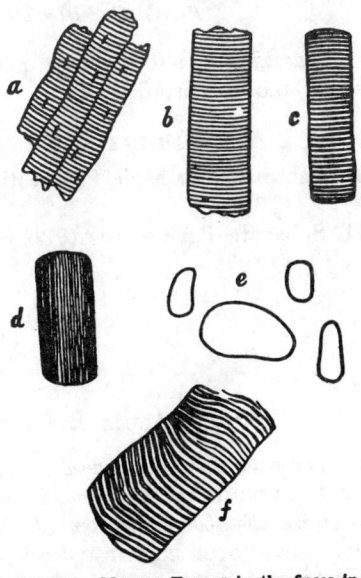

FIG. 116.—MUSCLE FIBRES in the fæces in various stages of digestion (a–e); (f) is a vegetable fibre.

tubes 6–10 place 0·9 ml., 0·6 ml., 0·4 ml., 0·2 ml. and 0·1 ml. of the diluted urine. Fill each tube with saline solution to 1 ml. The tubes now contain 0·9, 0·6, 0·4, 0·2, 0·1, 0·09, 0·06, 0·04, 0·02 and 0·01 ml. of the original urine. Add to each tube 2 ml. of the starch solution, shake, and incubate or stand in a water bath at 37° for half an hour. Then remove the tubes to cold water and immediately add 2–3 drops of the iodine solution to each tube, and shake. Notice when the change occurs from the blue to the slight pink tinge. The first tube showing this contains just enough diastase to digest the starch. Divide 2 (the number of ml. of starch) by the number of ml. of urine in that tube. Suppose it was tube No. 7. Then

$$\frac{2}{0·06} = 33 \text{ units of diastase.}$$

(3) The *Serum Diastase (Amylase)* is sometimes estimated, particularly when there is also renal inadequacy. The normal value of 80–180 units (Somogyi method) is raised in acute pancreatitis even to 300–1,000 units per 100 ml.

(4) The *Duodenal Contents* can be aspirated via a duodenal tube and a rough guide as to the amount of pancreatic enzymes obtained. Owing to the difficulty of the method any exact measurement is impossible but complete absence in congenital cystic disease of the pancreas is valuable confirmation of the diagnosis.

(5) *Sugar tolerance* curves after 50 G. glucose (Fig. 135) may show reduced tolerance and high blood sugars, when pancreatic function is deficient, but as most of the islets are in the tail and diseases usually involve the head and body of the pancreas, glyco-suria and diabetes mellitus are uncommon. With islet-cell tumours and excessive insulin production, hypoglycæmia and a greatly increased sugar tolerance result (§ 425).

(6) *Loëwi's test:* three drops of 1 in 1,000 adrenalin dropped on the conjunctiva, and repeated five minutes later. If the pupil dilates in half to one hour, one can conclude that there is irritability of the sympathetic, which is frequent with pancreatic disease, but there are other causes.

PART C. DISEASES OF THE PANCREAS

Classification.—For clinical purposes these may be divided into ACUTE and CHRONIC Disorders.

ACUTE DISEASES.	CHRONIC DISEASES.
I. Acute Hæmorrhagic Pancreatitis (§ 357)	III. Carcinoma (§ 359)
II. Subacute Pancreatitis (§ 358)	IV. Chronic Pancreatitis (§ 360)
	V. Pancreatic cysts (§ 360)
	VI. Pancreatic calculi (§ 360)
	VII. Islet cell tumours (§ 360)
	VIII. Hæmochromatosis (§ 343. I*e*)
	IX. Fibrocystic disease of Infants and young Children (§ 360)

ACUTE DISEASES OF THE PANCREAS

The patient is middle-aged or elderly and is suddenly seized with VIOLENT UPPER ABDOMINAL PAIN, *sometimes passing to the lumbar region. Vomiting is severe, the abdomen distended, the bowels constipated and* SEVERE SHOCK *with* VASO-MOTOR COLLAPSE *develops. The condition is likely to be* ACUTE HÆMORRHAGIC PANCREATITIS.

§ 357. I. **Acute Hæmorrhagic Pancreatitis** (Syn., Acute Pancreatic Necrosis) is a rare condition which is twice as common in middle-aged or elderly women as in men. There may be a previous history of gall-stones or of similar but less severe attacks. The onset often follows a large meal with alcohol.

Symptoms.—(1) The pain is very sudden in onset, persistent and severe, in the mid-line or to the left or right of the upper abdomen; (2) pain in the lumbar area of the back is often present but much less in intensity; (3) severe and repeated vomiting (never fæcal) is present, but the bowels are constipated and soon bowel sounds cannot be heard by auscultation, and there is some tympanitic abdominal distension; (4) marked upper abdominal tenderness with a less degree of rigidity are present; (5) vaso-motor collapse with a thin thready pulse, low blood pressure, profuse sweating and some cyanosis develop; (6) the temperature is usually sub-normal but may be slightly raised; (7) the later development of a brownish-green discoloration around the umbilicus or in the lumbar area, when present, is almost diagnostic. The skin as a whole becomes mildly icteric if the inflammatory reaction around the common bile-duct is severe enough.

The *Diagnosis* is confirmed by a very high content of diastase in the urine and in the serum (§ 356); glycosuria and a raised blood sugar value may also be found. A *coronary occlusion* with epigastric pain and circulatory collapse is not accompanied by a raised diastase value but does give a high serum transaminase result (§ 52). *Perforation of a peptic ulcer* is accompanied by a greater degree of rigidity and by X-ray evidence of gas under the diaphragm. *Uræmia* can give rise to upper abdominal pain, vomiting and paralytic ileus but the pain is much less severe and the blood urea is high.

Etiology.—The cause is obstruction at the sphincter of Oddi where the common bile-duct and the main pancreatic duct enter the second part of the duodenum. Bile is forced under pressure up the pancreatic duct and activates the precursors of the pancreatic enzymes, setting free the active enzymes which produce autolysis and a hæmorrhagic necrosis. The inflammatory reaction occurs in the retro-peritoneal tissues of the upper abdomen; fat necrosis in the omentum follows. The commonest cause of the obstruction is an impacted gall-stone, sometimes a pancreatic calculus, but when no obvious cause is found, spasm of the sphincter is said to be causal. If the bile is infected, *Acute Suppurative Pancreatitis* quickly ensues but *Gangrenous Pancreatitis* is rare.

Prognosis.—The mortality rate is 10–15 per cent. Severe cases may die rapidly but in less severe cases recovery is the rule.

Treatment.—The main indications are (1) to treat the collapse and shock by warmth, blood or plasma transfusion and intravenous dextrose-saline combined with noradrenalin, nikethamide and other restorative measures; (2) give nothing by mouth to avoid stimulating the biliary and pancreatic juices, and continuous gastric suction is advisable; (3) pain must be relieved with full doses of morphia combined with atropine and, to lessen the effect of morphia in producing spasm of the sphincter of Oddi, some give glyceryl trinitrate to suck or octyl nitrite to inhale; (4) penicillin and streptomycin or otherwise chlortetracycline (Aureomycin) are injected to lessen the danger of suppuration; (5) when general peritonitis ensues operation and drainage of the pancreatic area may be considered but this entails considerable risk in such a severely shocked patient.

§ 358. II. **Subacute Pancreatitis** (Syn., Subacute Necrosis of the Pancreas) is similar to the acute variety but less severe in type: the inflammatory reaction in the pancreas causes œdema but little or no hæmorrhage. It tends to be recurrent, to produce pain in the upper abdomen but with little or no shock, although temporary jaundice is more commonly found during the acute phases. After a series of attacks, chronic fibrosis and dysfunction of the pancreas occurs, and diabetes mellitus is not uncommon. The *treatment* is on the lines of the acute attack.

C.M.—S

With Mumps a special variety may arise. At the end of the first week the temperature rises again, with headache, nausea, vomiting, epigastric pain and tenderness, backache and often profuse sweating. It runs a favourable course and the symptoms subside in 4 to 5 days.

CHRONIC DISEASES OF THE PANCREAS

The patient is probably a man at or after middle age who complains of persistent PAIN IN THE UPPER ABDOMEN AND BACK, *marked* LOSS OF WEIGHT *and perhaps* OBSTRUCTIVE JAUNDICE *with a palpable gall-bladder.* The disease is likely to be CARCINOMA OF THE PANCREAS.

§ 359. III. Carcinoma of the Pancreas is not uncommon and can be very difficult to recognise as it manifests itself in so many different ways. The mode of onset depends in part on whether the head of the pancreas is first involved (three-quarters of the cases) or whether it starts in the body or tail. The cardinal *Symptoms* are: (1) a dull pain, which has not been previously present, develops in the upper abdomen and extends to the back even as high as the scapula. The pain gradually gets worse, especially at night, and is somewhat relieved by sitting forward (to relieve the pressure on the nerve plexuses behind the peritoneum); (2) loss of weight occurs at an early stage and becomes progressively more severe, and anæmia develops. When the disease affects the head of the pancreas (3) an obstructive type of jaundice, intense and persistent, is seen in 70 per cent. of cases, for the common bile-duct usually passes through the pancreas: the gall-bladder is then enlarged and palpable; (4) melæna and sometimes hæmatemesis occur when the growth ulcerates into the duodenum; (5) steatorrhœa with pale stools and diarrhœa may develop. (6) Ascites is due to secondary deposits or to pressure on the portal vein. Other symptoms which are occasionally met are (7) glycosuria and a raised blood sugar; (8) a form of thrombosis migrans occurs in the veins in different parts of the body due to the excess of circulating pancreatic ferments; (9) a fixed tumour may be felt below the liver; (10) although secondary deposits are not common at an early stage, sometimes they metastasise widely in the peritoneum as well as in the chest and skin (11) severe anxiety and restlessness develop in some cases.

Diagnosis can be extremely difficult and when a hidden carcinoma is suspected a primary growth of the pancreas (particularly in the body or tail) should be considered. Epigastric pain, rapid early wasting and perhaps obstructive jaundice are strongly suggestive. Pancreatic function tests (§ 356) may show deficiency, but even in advanced cases the diastase index and the state of fat digestion in the stools may be normal. The absence of stercobilin in the stool favours complete bile-duct obstruction by a growth rather than by a calculus. A barium meal may show displacement or narrowing of the first and particularly the second part of the duodenum by a growth in the head of the pancreas. *Chronic pancreatitis* with a hard fibrotic mass in the head of the pancreas in combination with obstructive jaundice can cause difficulty even at laparotomy: it is so important to differentiate these that a small piece taken for biopsy is justifiable. *Infective hepatitis, cirrhosis of the liver, carcinoma of the pyloric end of the stomach and of the common bile-duct* may cause confusion. Even when there are extensive liver deposits from a pancreatic growth the erythrocyte sedimentation rate is often normal or near normal in contrast to the effects of most other metastatic liver growths.

Etiology.—The commonest form is a scirrhous carcinoma. When in the head of the pancreas it produces few secondary growths at an early stage, whereas a growth of the tail metastasises early.

Prognosis.—In cancer of the pancreas death usually occurs soon after the onset of jaundice, or within six weeks after ascites sets in. The complications are: (i.) Symptoms due to pressure on the neighbouring organs—intestine, pylorus or portal vein; (ii.) sudden hæmorrhage into the alimentary tract or the peritoneal cavity; (iii.) pulmonary embolism.

Treatment.—In favourable cases, radical removal of the growth has been undertaken, by partial or complete resection of the pancreas. The latter involves simultaneous removal of the pyloric end of the stomach, the duodenum and of the spleen combined with anastomosis of the common bile-duct, the pancreatic duct and the stomach to the jejunum—but this formidable operation has a mortality rate of at least 25 per cent. In those with severe obstructive jaundice with its attendant pruritus, palliative anastomosis of the enlarged gall-bladder to the stomach or the jejunum is much simpler. The administration of pancreatic extracts may aid digestion. Deep X-ray therapy is not helpful.

§ 360. IV. Chronic Pancreatitis is a fibrosis of the organ which may follow repeated attacks of subacute pancreatitis, or it may be latent and the onset insidious.

Symptoms. are: (1) Usually there are recurrent attacks of pain and tenderness above and to the right of the umbilicus. The pain may be referred to the lumbar regions and to the left scapula—each attack lasting a few days; (2) mild attacks of obstructive jaundice may accompany the pain. In other cases obstruction of the common bile-duct is progressively severe and painless—it is then accompanied by an enlarged gall-bladder and the enlarged liver may become cirrhotic; (3) discomfort and distension in the upper and middle abdomen are associated with steatorrhœa and emaciation of lesser or greater severity; (4) diabetes is rare.

The *Diagnosis* is difficult in the early stages, especially from carcinoma of the head of the pancreas and other causes of obstructive jaundice. A *duodenal ulcer* on the posterior wall can cause local pancreatitis, but the pain is usually relieved by antacids and X-ray examination will confirm the ulcer.

Treatment is by the removal of the cause, especially if this be a gall-stone at the ampulla of the Vater (see § 353). Anastomosis of the gall-bladder to the jejunum relieves obstructive jaundice and lessens the steatorrhœa. Pancreatic ferments may help.

V. PANCREATIC CYSTS are of three types: (a) the very rare true cyst which contains pancreatic ferments—due to obstruction or obliteration of the duct by pancreatic calculi or cicatrical contraction; (b) the false cysts containing no ferments. These follow acute pancreatitis or more commonly occur after injury: in fact most false cysts are not in the pancreas but are traumatic effusions into the lesser sac. The swelling appears above the stomach or sometimes between the stomach and the colon and *does not move with respiration*. When very large it appears to fill the whole abdomen and may be difficult to differentiate from an ovarian cyst. Fatty diarrhœa is rare. (c) Multiple cysts also occur with polycystic disease of the kidneys (§ 432). *Treatment.*—Surgical removal is necessary when the size of the cyst warrants this.

VI. Pancreatic Calculi are rare. They consist of small concretions of calcium carbonate and calcium phosphate, lying in the main ducts. They are caused by chronic inflammation of the ducts and cause sudden attacks of pain in the epigastric and lumbar areas when they shift their position. Otherwise they are painless. They are visible on X-ray examination. *Treatment.*—Removal is only indicated in the presence of severe symptoms.

VII. ISLET-CELL TUMOURS produce hypoglycæmia (§ 425).

VIII. HÆMOCHROMATOSIS is a disorder of iron metabolism which affects principally the liver, the spleen, the skin and the pancreas (§ 343. Ie). Diabetes mellitus often accompanies the pancreatic disorder (§ 423).

IX. Fibrocystic Disease of Infants and Young Children (Syn., Mucoviscidosis) has become recognised much more frequently in recent years. It is a recessively inherited congenital anomaly of mucous secretion—the mucus being much more viscid and tenacious than usual.

Symptoms therefore affect principally the pancreas, the gastro-intestinal tract and the lungs. (1) Retention of mucus in the small pancreatic ducts causes flattening and atrophy of the cells. Sometimes the retained trypsin is activated locally, giving an inflammatory reaction and later pancreatic fibrosis. The islet tissues are not affected. (2) Similar changes in the intestine interfere with absorption, and in the sublingual glands may cause enlargement. The result is extreme emaciation in spite of a voracious appetite, with the distended abdomen and the large bulky offensive stools of steatorrhœa. (3) The retained bronchial mucus causes bronchiectasis and fibrosis of the lungs with atelectasis, emphysema and clubbed fingers. Attacks of broncho-pneumonia are sooner or later fatal.

The *Diagnosis* in the presence of steatorrhœa and recurrent bronchial infections is confirmed by the absence of pancreatic ferments removed via a duodenal tube. The sweat shows an excessive loss of sodium chloride.

Prognosis. A large number die in the first weeks of life. Some survive and lead a semi-invalid existence for a number of years. Cirrhosis of the liver may co-exist.

Treatment cannot remove the primary cause. The diet should be as for steatorrhœa (§ 296. XVII). Antibiotics need to be used prophylactically and for the control of respiratory infections.

THE SPLEEN

The spleen remains an organ of mystery. This applies both to its physiology and pathology. Its *functions* are not fully understood; it does not produce external secretions, nor act like other endocrine glands such as the thyroid, adrenals and pituitary. The spleen, like the lymph glands, forms part of the reticulo-endothelial system which is widely distributed throughout the body. After removal and in certain diseases of the spleen other parts of the reticulo-endothelial system may take over some of its functions. In fœtal life the spleen is one of the major sites of production of red and white cells: in certain conditions it resumes this function, and in most cases where such myeloid transformation or metaplasia takes place, it becomes enlarged. In the adult the spleen and lymph glands form lymphocytes and monocytes

and may be concerned with the product on of certain antibodies and other immunological entities. The spleen also plays a part in the removal from the circulation of
senile red cells and of certain pigments and in conditions such as malaria it concentrates the parasites. During digestive activity it enlarges, just like the other
abdominal organs; after hæmorrhage it contracts, adding its reserve of red cells to
the circulation. How it does this is not certain; unlike animals such as the cat its
capsule has very few muscle fibres.

The spleen may show various congenital abnormalities. Accessory spleens, or
splenunculi, are very common, particularly in the region of the tail of the pancreas.
These are especially important when splenectomy is considered necessary, as they may
in due course enlarge and assume the character and functions of the spleen. They
should therefore be removed at splenectomy. Occasionally the spleen is replaced by
a cluster of splenunculi. Sometimes it is completely absent and this may be found
only at autopsy.

PART A. SYMPTOMATOLOGY

§ 361. **Local Pain and Discomfort** may be caused by enlargement of
the spleen. Acute pain may be due to infarction of part of its substance,
or to perisplenitis when inflammation has occurred. Pyrexia and vomiting
often accompany these conditions. The liver and spleen frequently
become enlarged together, sometimes as a result of a common cause.
In great **enlargement** of the spleen the patient is inconvenienced merely
by the size of the organ and may not suffer any other symptoms; on the
other hand pressure symptoms may develop. Its size is not necessarily
a measure of the severity of the disease nor of its duration. The other
symptom most often associated with disease of the spleen is **anæmia**,
with its *pallor* of the skin, *weakness* and *changes in the blood cells*. These
are discussed elsewhere (§ 535 et seq.).

PART B. PHYSICAL EXAMINATION

The normal spleen lies in the left hypochondrium between the upper
border of the ninth and the lower border of the eleventh ribs, roughly
between the mid-axillary and scapular lines. It extends obliquely forwards and downwards almost to the costal margin. It is completely
covered by the ribs and its upper third is overlapped by the lung.

Enlargement of the spleen cannot in most cases be detected clinically
unless it is at least three times the normal size: in healthy adults it weighs
100–200 G. (3–7 oz.). With progressive increase in size the anterior edge
and particularly the lower pole of the spleen tend to advance towards
the umbilicus. A *notch* in its anterior border distinguishes a large spleen
from other swellings; it is rarely absent even in the very large spleen of
myeloid leukæmia.

Inspection of the abdomen can only lead to a suspicion of splenic
enlargement when it is gross.

Palpation of the spleen should be carried out as follows:—The patient
should lie on his back and the examiner should tand on his right side.

The left hand is placed over the lower ribs in the posterior axillary line: during inspiration this should help to tilt the spleen forwards and upwards. The right hand is placed flat on the abdomen with the finger tips just below the costal margin: then gently dip the fingers into the abdomen to feel the edge of the spleen and its notch. A deep breath considerably aids this. The size of the spleen is best recorded diagrammatically in relation to the costal margin and to the umbilicus.

The CHARACTER of the enlarged spleen may vary. In acute conditions such as septicæmia or typhoid fever the spleen is soft, but when the disease is more chronic as in chronic passive congestion or in pernicious anæmia the spleen is firm. Fibrosis occurs in diseases such as Hodgkin's disease or Banti's disease and this causes a hard consistency.

Percussion of the spleen is often difficult and rarely accurate. It is best to percuss along the eleventh rib and in expiration, as less lung substance is then likely to interfere (Fig. 50, § 108).

Auscultation of the splenic area may yield a peritoneal rub when a recent infarct of the spleen has occurred.

Fallacies.—The spleen may be displaced downwards in conditions such as pleural effusion, emphysema and rickets and this may simulate enlargement. The dullness of the spleen may appear to be increased when there is consolidation of the lung or a pleural effusion. A diminished area of dullness in the splenic area is caused by emphysema of the lungs and by the accumulation of gas in the stomach or intestines.

§ 362. SPLENIC ENLARGEMENT is characterised by: (1) the splenic notch which is felt on the anterior border; (2) the fact that the mass moves with respiration unless it is bound down by adhesions, and (3) it is dull to percussion. (The colon lies deep to it, but in front of a mass arising in the kidney.) Furthermore (4) it is felt just beneath the abdominal wall; (5) it is impossible to palpate above it because the spleen descends from beneath the costal margin; (6) an enlarged spleen rarely crosses the midline above the umbilicus; (7) an area of dullness due to splenic enlargement resembles in outline that of the spleen; (8) its smooth, firm surface distinguishes splenic enlargement from masses arising in the peritoneum, stomach, intestines, etc. Irregular enlargement of the spleen is very rare and should only be diagnosed after disease of other organs has been excluded.

Splenic enlargement or tumour may have to be distinguished from:— (1) *A left renal tumour* or an unusually mobile kidney. The resonant intestines lie in front of such a mass and there is no resonance in the flank. Also an enlarged left kidney is pushed forward on to the examining fingers when the left hand is placed medially in the left flank, whereas a splenic tumour only comes forward when pressure is applied in the lateral part of the left flank. (2) *Enlargement of the left lobe of the liver.* Dullness is continuous with that of the liver, while splenic dullness rarely reaches the mid-line. (3) *Carcinoma of the stomach.* In this case dullness is less defined and less absolute and the splenic notch is absent. (4) An *ovarian or uterine tumour* will have grown from below upwards. The palpating hand cannot be pushed between the mass and the pelvis, as it can with a splenic enlargement. It can be felt on pelvic examination. (5) An *accumulation of fæces* has an irregular outline, a doughy consistency and is likely to be removed by a course of purgatives or enemata. (6) A *retro-peritoneal mass* (or the "*lateral cell mass*") does not possess a notch and does not move on respiration. (7) *Aneurysm of the abdominal aorta,* if large enough to be mistaken for the spleen, causes pain in the back and shows expansile pulsation. (8) *Carcinoma of the splenic flexure of the colon* is variable in size and causes intestinal symptoms. (9) *Perinephric, subphrenic* or other diseases occasionally give rise to diagnostic difficulties as may *adrenal* or *pancreatic tumours,* or localised granulomatous masses from such causes as *tuberculosis* or *bilharziasis.*

PART C. DISEASES OF THE SPLEEN

§ 363. Excepting only absence and atrophy, diseases of the spleen give rise to **enlargement** and its recognition is therefore important. It is detected by palpation and percussion. When the spleen is greatly enlarged it causes dyspnœa and gastro-intestinal disturbances merely as pressure symptoms. Vomiting, pyrexia and occasionally diarrhœa develop and acute pain may be caused by perisplenitis (§ 520). Pressure upwards can cause collapse of the base of the left lung.

Enlargement of the Spleen occurs in association with:—

I. Acute infections.
II. Chronic infections.
III. Portal obstruction or congestion.
IV. Disorders of the blood.

V. Parasitic and tropical diseases.
VI. Relative enlargement occurs in infancy and childhood.
VII. Irregularity of the surface of the spleen.

Method of Procedure.—The patient rarely seeks advice for symptoms directly pointing to the spleen. It is often found to be enlarged when the patient is examined for other reasons. The finding of a large spleen gives valuable clues in the diagnosis of many diseases.

A careful HISTORY is always important. Residence abroad may point to malaria; fever and shivering suggest some infection.

The patient's AGE should be recorded. Certain conditions such as rickets are commoner in childhood.

The TEMPERATURE and particularly a temperature chart helps in the diagnosis of infection and in some blood dyscrasias.

EXAMINATION OF OTHER ORGANS and particularly of the LIVER may make diagnosis easier. A normal spleen in the presence of a large liver and jaundice suggests gall-stones or malignant disease. If both liver and spleen are large congestion, obstruction or early cirrhosis of the liver may be present. A very large spleen in the presence of a moderately enlarged liver strongly favours one of the disorders of the hæmopoietic system, which may be more accurately diagnosed by an *examination of the blood* (§ 537) or other investigations, such as lymph gland biopsy.

I. **Acute Infections.**—Slight enlargement of the spleen is a common finding in almost all cases of acute infection. In the acute specific fevers this offers little clinical or prognostic guidance. The enlarged spleen is soft, particularly in *typhoid, typhus* and *abortus* fevers, and there are no local symptoms. An ABSCESS in the spleen sometimes develops, especially in typhoid, and local tenderness and pain occur. These symptoms may also arise during the course of some systemic disorder and be due to necrosis and suppuration commencing in an area of INFARCTION caused by embolism or in a splenic cyst or tumour. The infarction causes (i.) acute sudden pain and (ii.) local tenderness due to perisplenitis and peritoneal irritation. It is usually due to cardiac disease such as auricular fibrillation, acute endocarditis or to pyæmia. In gross enlargement of the spleen, such as occurs in leukæmia, attacks of ACUTE CAPSULITIS occur; they are mostly caused by local areas of necrosis. These acute attacks may be recognised by an audible friction rub over the splenic area, due to localised peritonitis.

The *diagnosis* of acute infection with splenic enlargement may be very difficult and often needs patient investigation. Until a definite diagnosis is made, rest in bed, attention to the bowels and hot applications to the splenic area will reduce tenderness and pain. If, however, the attacks do not subside and the local condition becomes aggravated, laparotomy and sometimes splenectomy may become necessary. In most cases attacks resolve in a few days and leave adhesions which may cause trouble later on.

II. **Chronic Infections.**—(1) CONGESTIVE CARDIAC FAILURE, auricular fibrillation and SUBACUTE INFECTIVE ENDOCARDITIS (§ 50a) cause chronic enlargement of the spleen, partly due to chronic passive congestion and partly to the accompanying septicæmia. Cardiac disease may also give rise to embolism and the resulting splenic infarcts cause acute symptoms. It is often difficult to distinguish *splenic anæmia* (§ 559) from these conditions, but the difference is important since certain patients with splenic anæmia benefit from splenectomy, while the operation should not be performed in endocarditis. ABSCESS of the spleen may sometimes develop as a late consequence of infarction.

(2) SYPHILIS in the secondary stage often causes the spleen to become palpable. In the tertiary stage both spleen and liver enlarge and ascites and anæmia may develop.

(3) TUBERCULOSIS may affect the spleen in various forms: (i.) as miliary tuberculosis, (ii.) as a " cold " tuberculous abscess, (iii.) as tuberculomata and (iv.) in tuberculous peritonitis where splenic capsulitis may occur. In almost all cases the existence of the infection will be apparent elsewhere: thus the chronic miliary form may be revealed by radiographic examination of the lungs. Tuberculosis rarely occurs as a primary disease of the spleen; if it does, chemotherapy and/or splenectomy offers a reasonable chance of cure. In some cases of tuberculosis of the spleen instead of the

more usual anæmia, a different blood picture may occur: it may be similar to polycythæmia or occasionally even to myeloid leukæmia and not infrequently a leuco-erythroblastic reaction occurs.

(4) In BOECK'S SARCOIDOSIS the enlargement of the spleen which occurs resembles that of tuberculosis.

(5) In CHRONIC SEPTIC SPLENOMEGALY which in tropical countries follows dysentery and other intestinal disorders, the presence of leucocytosis distinguishes it from splenic anæmia.

(6) AMYLOID DISEASE sometimes affects the spleen which may become large. It is usually associated with chronic suppuration or rheumatoid arthritis (§§ 346, 409); there may be amyloid disease of the liver and diarrhœa due to intestinal involvement.

III. **Portal Obstruction or Congestion** of whatever cause and whatever degree leads to congestion in the splanchnic area which includes the spleen. Therefore the spleen is enlarged in:—

(1) CHRONIC CARDIAC or CHRONIC PULMONARY DISEASE which gives rise to back pressure in the venous systems and to chronic passive congestion.

In (2) THROMBOSIS OF THE INFERIOR VENA CAVA the obstruction is absolute, at least for some time, before some canalisation takes place. The spleen enlarges considerably and it may become difficult to distinguish it from splenic anæmia (§ 559).

(3) CIRRHOSIS OF THE LIVER (§ 342) is often associated with splenic enlargement.

(4) TERTIARY SYPHILIS causes fibrosis, but both liver and spleen may be slightly enlarged.

(5) TORSION of the splenic pedicle, a rare occurrence, may cause sudden splenomegaly and the increased weight of the spleen may in turn displace the organ downwards.

§ **364.** IV. **Disorders of the Blood** are predominantly diseases of the myeloid and lymphatic tissues. A fuller description is contained in later paragraphs. The acute attacks of perisplenitis or capsulitis mentioned earlier may occur in any of these disorders.

(1) PERNICIOUS ANÆMIA in about half the patients and (2) IRON-DEFICIENCY ANÆMIA in a smaller proportion of patients cause some enlargement of the spleen, usually of moderate degree.

(3) MYELOID LEUKÆMIA (§ 556) causes the spleen to be enormous, but in (4) LYMPHATIC LEUKÆMIA it may also reach the pelvis.

(5) HODGKIN'S DISEASE (§ 584) is a disease in which groups of lymph glands are usually also found.

(6) SPLENIC ANÆMIA (§ 559) is an entity not clearly defined. The spleen is usually very large.

(7) ACHOLURIC JAUNDICE (§ 331), a congenital form of hæmolytic anæmia characterised by frequent increase in size of the spleen, has a family incidence and almost diagnostic blood changes.

(8) SICKLE-CELL ANÆMIA (§ 564) and certain cases of THROMBO-CYTOPENIC PURPURA (§ 767) are also associated with splenic enlargement.

(9) POLYCYTHÆMIA RUBRA VERA (§ 31) shows cyanosis, weakness and increases in the numbers of red and white cells.

(10) GAUCHER'S DISEASE (cerebroside lipoidosis), NIEMAN-PICK'S DIS-EASE (phosphatide lipoidosis) and HAND-SCHÜLLER-CHRISTIAN'S DISEASE (cholesterol lipoidosis) are associated with a spleen which may be of considerable size (§ 544).

(11) MYELOID METAPLASIA with or without OSTEOSCLEROSIS or MYELO-FIBROSIS and certain types of RETICULOSIS also cause splenic enlargement (§ 559).

V. Tropical Diseases.—MALARIA and KALA-AZAR are the most common. In acute malaria the enlargement is not very great, but after many attacks it may be enormous. A history of attacks of malaria occurring in a person who has been abroad leads one to suspect the cause of the splenic enlargement; but the diagnosis is made certain by finding the parasite in the blood. Anæmia is common, and periodic fever occurring on alternate days or every third day is suggestive of malaria. In kala-azar the spleen is usually large, and is rendered the more prominent by the emaciation of the subject. The diagnosis rests on the discovery of the parasite by blood culture on rabbit blood agar medium incubated at room tempera-ture, or in the material obtained by liver, sternal or spleen puncture, while the formal-gel reaction in the serum is characteristic. Only occa-sionally is it possible to demonstrate Leishman-Donovan bodies by microscopic examination of blood smears. TRYPANOSOMIASIS and RELAPSING FEVER may also cause splenic enlargement, while spleno-megaly is not uncommonly associated with INTESTINAL BILHARZIA in Japan (S. japonica) and Egypt (S. mansoni).

VI. In Infancy and Childhood it must be remembered that the spleen enlarges more readily than in adults and on slighter provocation. RICKETS (§ 608) may cause slight enlargement of the spleen, to which the associated catarrh of mucous membranes may contribute. CONGENITAL SYPHILIS and the infantile types of TUBERCULOSIS can be diagnosed by evidence of the disease elsewhere. In syphilis the liver is usually enlarged also. In the infantile form of KALA-AZAR, previously common in the Eastern Mediterranean area, and COOLEY'S ANÆMIA (thalassæmia) the spleen reaches a very large size (§ 567. VII). In CONGENITAL ABNORMALITIES OF THE HEART associated with cyanosis the spleen is large. ERYTHRÆMIC MYELOSIS and MYELOID LEUKÆMIA occasionally occur in children.

VII. Irregularity of the Surface of the enlarged spleen is in most cases due to cysts or tumours, the exact nature of which is not usually revealed until laparotomy is carried out. LYMPHOSARCOMA, RETICULUM CELL SARCOMA and HÆMANGIOMA are the commoner of a rare group of tumours. Secondary carcinomatosis is even rarer. HODGKIN'S DISEASE may cause nodular splenic enlargement.

HYDATID DISEASE of the spleen may be cystic. It is accompanied by marked eosinophilia in somebody who has been abroad, by positive serum and intradermal tests and by finding of cysts in other parts of the body. CONGENITAL CYSTS and CONGENITAL POLYCYSTIC DISEASE are rare.

The *Prognosis* and *Treatment* of splenic enlargement depend on the nature of the cause. With localised pain the patient will need rest in bed and strapping of the splenic area reduces irritation and the danger of rupture; sedatives may be required. The treatment of malarial splenic enlargement (" Ague Cake ") must include anti-malarial drugs. In syphilitic splenomegaly penicillin and arsenicals have been helpful. In a certain number of cases splenectomy (§ 366) improves the patient's general health without necessarily curing the disease.

§ 365. **Wandering Spleen** (Splenoptosis) may simulate splenic enlargement, but it can also be mistaken for a floating kidney. The presence of the splenic notch, the position in front of the colon and its mobility will help diagnosis.

Atrophy of the Spleen is rare. Congenital atrophy or complete agenesis are occasional incidental necropsy findings. Atrophy may be due to CIRRHOSIS of the Spleen particularly in the later stages of the disease, or due to SYPHILIS, which causes diffuse fibrosis or gives rise to a gumma-like lesion which may resemble cartilage.

§ 366. SPLENECTOMY should not be undertaken lightly and only if it is reasonably certain that the bone marrow is sufficiently active. It would, for instance, be disastrous if in a case of myelofibrosis the spleen, which may then be the chief area of the production of blood cells, be removed and the patient die of aplastic anæmia. In order to guard against such complications, it is wise to examine the bone marrow by puncture (§ 1201) before splenectomy is carried out.

Splenectomy is indicated under the following conditions:—(i.) Rupture, torsion or extensive infarction, provided this latter is not part of the general embolic phenomena of bacterial endocarditis. Rupture is rare in typhoid or in glandular fevers. (ii.) Most cases of acholuric jaundice (hereditary spherocytosis), splenic anæmia and thrombocytopenic purpura benefit to some extent from splenectomy. In the latter case, if the patient is a woman, splenectomy should be performed during the middle of the menstrual cycle, since the danger of hæmorrhage is much increased during or near the menstrual period. In some similar disorders, (iii.) often referred to as *hypersplenism*, complicated by a hæmolytic anæmia or a hæmolytic crisis, often with granulopenia and/or thrombocytopenia, splenectomy may also be of benefit. (iv.) Abscesses, tumours and single cysts of the spleen. (v.) Persistent attacks of perisplenitis not responding to other forms of treatment. (vi.) If the size and weight of the spleen is such that the patient is embarrassed cosmetically or if the size interferes with other bodily functions. (vii.) Certain cases of portal hypertension benefit by splenectomy by reducing the flow of blood through the portal veins. This may apply to Banti's disease and to certain types of cirrhosis of the liver. (viii.) Cases of pernicious anæmia, Hodgkin's disease, polycythæmia vera and leukæmia do not benefit from splenectomy, but the operation does not reduce the prognosis.

Splenectomy is performed when it is clear that the enlarged spleen or its underlying condition impairs the health and working ability of the patient. The operation should be performed before any adhesions are caused by attacks of perisplenitis, as they may make the operation more difficult and more dangerous. Adequate pre-operative preparation may have to include blood transfusion, particularly when anæmia has been present for long. Sometimes much useful information may be gained by making smear preparations of the freshly cut spleen and the spleen should always be examined microscopically. At splenectomy it is also useful to remove for biopsy a small piece of liver which may yield very important information without inconvenience to the surgeon or patient. Post-operatively a common complication is collapse of the left lower lobe of the lung; this may be avoided by breathing exercises. In most cases of anæmia treated by splenectomy the number of reticulocytes rises temporarily after the operation: also many late normoblasts and red cells containing Howell–Jolly bodies appear in the blood. The number of white cells and of platelets also rises temporarily and when platelet showers occur the dangers of thrombosis must be borne in mind.

CHAPTER XIII

THE KIDNEYS AND URINARY TRACT

§ **367.** *Applied Physiology and Anatomy.* A proper understanding of the pathological processes in the kidneys is facilitated by recalling certain physiological facts. The unit of the kidney is the nephron, comprising the glomerulus, the proximal and distal convoluted tubules and the collecting tubule. In the normal person, each 24 hours the *glomeruli* filter off approx. 150–200 litres of a fluid similar to the blood plasma (but with less protein, § 396), under the pressure in the glomerular capillaries. The *proximal convoluted tubules* absorb all the dextrose and protein, approx. 85 per cent. of the water and electrolytes, most of the amino-acids and nearly 50 per cent. of the urea received from the glomeruli. The *distal convoluted tubules* therefore receive 25–30 litres of fluid. These tubules are more selective: they regulate the final volume of urine secreted (usually 1·5 litres a day but in health varying between 0·75 and 25 litres according to the body requirements): they determine the further amounts of sodium, calcium, chloride and other essential solutes to be absorbed: they secrete potassium and they regulate the acidity of the urine. A concentrated residue is left to be carried away by the *collecting tubules*, this containing the final waste products.

The kidneys therefore keep the osmotic pressure of the extra-cellular fluids of the body constant and so prevent sudden changes in the water content of the body cells. When the volume of extra-cellular fluid falls, the kidneys retain water and sodium by increasing still further the absorbing power of the distal convoluted tubules. These are under the influence of (*a*) the anti-diuretic hormone of the pituitary and (*b*) the adrenal corticosteroids (especially aldosterone): the ADH increases the absorption of water and aldosterone increases the absorption of sodium. (With an excess of extra-cellular fluid these mechanisms are reversed.) The primary centres regulating the secretion of ADH and the corticosteroids are probably located in the hypothalamus. Disorders of these regulating mechanisms may well be responsible for the different types of œdema. To accomplish these physiological processes, only a small proportion of the one million nephrons present in each kidney are in action at a time for short periods.

In diseased conditions there may be a generalised inflammation or degeneration of the nephrons (nephritis or nephrosis), or a patchy destruction of groups of them owing to narrowing or obliteration of their blood supply (arteriosclerosis).[1] Such is the enormous reserve power of the kidneys that a large part may be destroyed and yet the remainder can carry out the necessary work; but the reserve power is diminished. With further destruction each remaining nephron is called into continuous activity. To maintain the action of the glomeruli, the blood pressure rises. The blood is still cleared of waste products (*e.g.*, urea) to a normal extent, but, as the power of the absorbing mechanism of the tubules is diminished, a larger volume of the dilute urine passes down them. With still further damage to the nephrons, less fluid is filtered by the glomeruli,

[1] Richard Bright in 1836 described the acute and chronic forms of inflammation of the kidneys, associated with albuminuria and hyperpiesia. Unfortunately the term chronic Bright's disease is still sometimes loosely and incorrectly applied to high arterial pressure and its associated symptoms, and so is better avoided.

auu so the blood now contains an excess of waste products (uræmia) and the volume of urine falls.

When the glomeruli are inflamed, albumen and even blood leak into the urine, as in acute nephritis. Some forms of renal disease are associated with general œdema and with intense albuminuria; modern research suggests that the primary defects are not in the kidneys, but in the composition of the blood and in the semipermeability of the capillaries throughout the body (in which the renal capillaries share). The loss of such a large quantity of albumen from the blood may so lower the osmotic pressure of the blood plasma that fluid is attracted from the blood into the tissues with the production of œdema: sodium chloride retention contributes to this. The cardinal features of renal disease are therefore best seen by examination of the urine, aided later by examination of the blood and the tissues. In practice it is not always possible to separate kidney diseases proper from disorders of other parts of the urinary tract, because changes in the urine are common to them all. It will be necessary, therefore, to refer to disorders of the bladder, prostate and urethra for diagnostic purposes, though their treatment is often mainly surgical.

PART A. SYMPTOMATOLOGY

One of the chief functions of the kidneys is the elimination of nitrogenous waste. When this is interfered with by structural or functional disease, a toxic condition results, which is known as uræmia. Other functions are the removal of water, acid products and excess of sugar from the blood, and to maintain the optimum concentration of electrolytes in the tissues.

As a consequence of the deep-seated position of these organs, the local symptoms referable to the kidney are, except in cases of Tumour or Displacement, of subordinate importance. The most constant and CARDINAL SYMPTOM of kidney disorders is some **Alteration in the Urine,** which, as an indication of renal disease, corresponds to the physical signs in other organs, and is dealt with in PART B of this chapter. The cardinal symptoms next in order of importance are **Pallor of the Surface** and **Œdema. Pain** and **symptoms connected with the passing of urine** may also be present. **General Symptoms,** due to toxæmia resulting from the retention of nitrogenous waste and to a disturbance of the water and electrolyte balance generally accompany these diseases.

Pallor of the Surface and Malaise are very constant features of all organic kidney diseases. To the experienced eye the pallor differs from that of anæmia in a manner somewhat difficult to describe. The skin has a " waxy " hue, a simile which is still further exemplified when dropsy is present. It affects the whole body, but is always most evident in the face. In chronic interstitial nephritis the pallor has a greyish hue. The diagnosis from other causes of pallor will be found in Chapter XVI, § 535.

§ 368. Renal Œdema (or Dropsy) is of *general* distribution, in which respect it differs from cardiac œdema, which starts in the *legs* or most dependent parts, and from hepatic dropsy, which starts in the *abdomen* (§ 29). It is, however, most evident in the loose cellular tissue—*e.g.*, around the eyelids, where it is most marked on first waking in the morning. Towards evening the ankles become œdematous, or, as the patient may express it, " a ridge is present around the top of the boot." In severe cases the eyes may be almost closed by the swollen lids (Fig. 133), and at the same time there may be signs of fluid in the serous cavities—the peritoneum, pleura and pericardium. Œdema of the solid organs also occurs in severe cases, and death may be produced by pulmonary œdema. Œdema glottidis is another serious though less frequent complication.

Œdema is not an equally constant feature in all diseases of the kidney. In *acute nephritis* it is often present, and it is seen in *subacute parenchymatous nephritis* and in *nephrosis*. But in *chronic nephritis* and *lardaceous kidney* it is comparatively rare; in the former it may occur late in the course of the disease, when it is generally due either to cardiac failure, to recrudescence of the subacute nephritis, or to secondary inflammation of the serous membranes. In uncomplicated *pyelitis* and *neoplasms* fluid retention is not present.

§ 369. Pain in the Kidney.—Many serious diseases of the renal substance are unaccompanied by any pain or local symptoms. A sense of dull aching in the loins may be present at the onset of acute nephritis and is frequent with pyelitis, pyelonephritis, pyonephrosis and oxaluria. Pain may be very severe when a renal calculus is present (Renal Colic, §§ 247, 413). Various tumours of the kidney are accompanied by pain, and perinephric abscesses are associated with lumbar pain and tenderness. A pain of gradually increasing intensity in the renal area on one side, which finally becomes very severe, but is relieved suddenly with the passage of a large quantity of urine, suggests Dietl's crisis (§ 421). A dull, dragging pain in the lumbar region, relieved by rest in the recumbent posture, occurs with movable kidney; it is usually on the affected side, and is liable to acute exacerbations resembling renal colic. The lumbar pain of renal disease must not be mistaken for the backache due to congestion of the female generative organs, nor for lumbago, in which the pain is usually of sudden onset, is not confined to one side, and may be accompanied by other signs of rheumatism. Less frequent causes of lumbar pain are dealt with in § 461.

Symptoms *connected with the passing of urine* are: increased frequency of micturition (§§ 430 and 460), incontinence of urine (§ 429), inability to pass urine (retention § 427, suppression § 428), the passage of large quantities of urine (§ 421) or the passage of blood (§ 411).

§ 370. Uræmia is a term used to describe the symptoms arising from renal failure. It was originally intended to indicate the retention of nitrogenous products in the blood and tissues, but, as indicated in § 367, it is now more widely recognised that in health the kidneys also regulate the amount of extra-cellular fluid, its acid-base equilibrium and its content of inorganic substances. Therefore renal failure produces widespread effects in most of the organs of the body. Uræmia is more common as a result of progressive renal failure of *Chronic* type, but sometimes it arises *Acutely.*

§ 371. **Chronic Renal Failure** can be divided into (1) an early stage and (2) a late stage (established uræmia).

(1) *Early Stage* ("Incipient uræmia"). The effects are partly renal but are mainly due to hypertension and its associated vascular changes. The renal symptoms are the result of decreased absorption in the renal tubules causing the 24-hour volume of urine to be increased. At this stage a common symptom is (i.) Polyuria and especially nocturia. To compensate for the renal damage the blood pressure rises so as to produce an increased filtration pressure in the glomeruli. Changes in the vessel walls follow; thickening of the arteries due to hypertrophy of the muscular coat is followed by degenerative changes in the vessel walls. In consequence further symptoms arise: (ii.) Breathlessness. At first present only on exertion, it is associated with hypertrophy of the left ventricle and an accentuated aortic second sound. Later, signs of left ventricular failure may occur (§ 55), the resulting pulmonary œdema aggravating the breathlessness. (iii.) Headache accompanies most forms of renal disease, especially that which terminates in uræmia: chronic interstitial nephritis is a frequent cause of headache in advanced life. (iv.) Mental disturbances such as lack of power of concentration, forgetfulness and irritability may be present as early symptoms. (v.) Vertigo, tinnitus and various neuralgias may also be complained of. (vi.) Insomnia in the aged is another common symptom of chronic renal disease. The patient readily drops off to sleep, but as readily awakes, and may do so a dozen times every night. (vii.) Hæmorrhages sometimes occur in chronic renal disease, a consequence of the high pressure, combined in most cases with a diseased state of the blood-vessels. Epistaxis may be the first symptom which leads to the discovery of chronic renal disease. Bleeding from the stomach or intestines, and purpura, sometimes occur. *Cerebral hæmorrhage is the most frequent cause of death* in chronic interstitial nephritis. (viii.) Ocular changes may be so characteristic that a diagnosis may be made by their presence. Albuminuric retinitis is diagnosed by typical alterations in the fundi, with loss of visual acuity—œdema and swelling of the retina, papillitis, flame-shaped hæmorrhages, and white areas of degeneration. Changes in the arteries may also be seen (§§ 1132, 1134, Plate XXI). (ix.) Even though the patient remains at work, there is loss of mental and physical vigour, and wasting of muscular and subcutaneous tissues.

(2) *Late Stage* ("Established uræmia"). This gives rise to a considerable variety of biochemical changes together with toxæmia.

There is a retention of nitrogenous bodies (urea, uric acid, creatinine); of acids (especially sodium acid phosphate), causing respiratory symptoms;

of phosphate (with a rise in blood phosphate and often a lowering of calcium), producing neuromuscular irritability and even tetany. Excessive loss of potassium (potassium-losing nephritis) causes muscular weakness and even paralysis. Added to these are the cerebral changes consequent on hyperpiesis—cerebral œdema, vascular spasm or occlusion (see hypertensive cerebral attacks, § 97) producing convulsions, amaurosis, headaches, drowsiness, etc. Terminal malignant hypertension occurs in over 50 per cent. of cases of chronic nephritis. The term uræmia therefore is used to indicate a symptom complex which may show many different features, depending on the chemical state of the blood and the condition of the cerebral vessels.

Symptoms.—(i.) Persistent headache. (ii.) Restlessness, twitching, muscular cramps and tremors are frequent: the latter may be complained of by the patient or noticed by the doctor. True tetany is sometimes seen. (iii.) Drowsiness during the day, with sleeplessness or "cat-sleeps" (dropping off for a few minutes at a time) at night. Disorientation, stupor and later uræmic coma often supervene, with or without muttering delirium. Sometimes convulsions occur before death. (iv.) Uræmic dyspnœa is in part due to the cardio-vascular changes mentioned earlier, partly to left ventricular failure, and also due to retention of acid products together with an altered sensitivity of the respiratory centre. The various types are: (a) *Paroxysmal*; the attacks coming on chiefly at night, and resembling asthma ("uræmic asthma"). The patient sits up in bed gasping for breath, but there is no cyanosis, and the mind is clear. The breathing is often noisy, with a characteristic hissing quality (Addison). (b) *Continuous*, or continuous alternating with paroxysmal. (c) *Cheyne-Stokes' Respiration* (§ 28) may last for weeks. The pulse slows in the apnœic periods, and there is alternate contraction and dilatation of the pupil, the contraction occurring during the period of apnœa. (v.) Gastro-intestinal disturbances such as thirst, anorexia, nausea, vomiting, hiccough and often epigastric pain may be present, and diarrhœa, sometimes with ulcerative colitis, may occur towards the end. (vi.) Dehydration is partly due to the renal disease and partly to general nutritional failure. Wasting follows and in the terminal stages is very marked. (vii.) There is often a uriniferous odour in the breath and a metallic taste in the mouth. (viii.) Præcordial pain due to dry pericarditis is not unusual. (ix.) A severe grade of anæmia (even to 20 per cent. hæmoglobin) is common. This is mainly due to a toxic effect on the bone marrow, but is aggravated by hæmorrhages from the nose (epistaxis), gums, bronchial mucosa and gastro-intestinal and urinary tracts. (x.) The ocular changes (§ 1132 and Plate XXI) become more advanced. (xi.) A low form of bronchitis or pneumonia is a common complication of nephritis. (xii.) Renal disease may be complicated by various skin affections other than dropsy and the cellulitis which is liable to affect œdematous limbs. Amongst these may be mentioned eczema, urticaria, and various forms of erythema and purpura. Generalised irritation of the skin is frequent, and crystals of urea (" urea frost ") may be deposited on the face.   (xiii.) Finally the volume of urine falls (oliguria) and anuria may follow.

Bone changes occur in very chronic varieties of uræmia.   (i.) Especially in children during the more active periods of growth there may be retardation of ossification and of bone growth with the epiphyseal and metaphyseal changes of renal rickets (§ 608). (ii.) Subperiosteal cortical erosions in the phalanges, along the cortex of the long bones near the joints and occasionally cyst formation.   These are associated with hypertrophied parathyroid glands (secondary hyperparathyroidism).   (iii.) Occasionally sclerosis of the vertebral bodies, the skull and the long bones is seen.   (iv.) There may be metastatic calcification in the smaller arteries, in the muscles and subcutaneous tissues as well as in the kidneys (nephrocalcinosis).

§ 372. **Acute Renal Failure** is the result of acute infective or toxic damage to the kidneys (§ 397); in many cases there is gross diminution in the blood supply to the glomeruli (renal ischæmia) which may result in acute tubular necrosis—a condition which can also arise from a direct chemical poisoning of the renal tubules (§ 428).

The retention of water and of electrolytes (especially sodium chloride) leads to water-intoxication of the brain and other tissues: this is aggravated by the tendency to force fluids on the patient and if a diuresis results, sodium chloride depletion ensues as the tubules are unable to absorb this substance.   Although the blood urea rises, in fatal cases the disturbances of water and electrolyte balances are much more important than the accumulation of nitrogenous bodies.   Failure of hydrogen ion excretion leads to acidæmia.

Symptoms.—(1) The 24-hour volume of urine falls, with oliguria, so that only 1–2 fl. oz. are secreted: complete anuria is rare.   (2) Generalised œdema is usual and pulmonary œdema especially common.   (3) Mental symptoms follow, with stupor, muscular twitchings and even epileptic convulsions.   (4) Anorexia, nausea and vomiting are often present.

An acute fulminating form of uræmia occasionally occurs.   It may supervene at any stage of the foregoing or may come on abruptly in an apparently healthy person (small white kidney, § 405. 2 (*d*)).   Its leading symptoms are (i.) low muttering delirium, (ii.) stupor, passing into coma, with or without convulsions, (iii.) a hissing type of respiration.

Extra-renal Uræmia occurs, especially in elderly subjects, when the kidneys are relatively healthy.   It is seen when the renal blood flow is greatly diminished by hæmorrhage, shock, circulatory failure or dehydration.   Following melæna it is often marked as a result of the excessive breakdown of protein and the absorption of nitrogenous material from the intestine (gastric uræmia).   Severe alkalosis, *e.g.*, due to the administration of large doses of sodium bicarbonate in the treatment of peptic ulcers, and repeated vomiting are other causes.

Etiology of Acute and Chronic Renal Failure and Uræmia.   These may occur in almost any disease of the kidney.   In acute and subacute nephritis and in chronic pyelonephritis uræmia is the usual form of death; in chronic glomerulo-tubular nephritis cerebral hæmorrhage is a more common cause.   In tuberculous, calculous and polycystic disease, in hydronephrosis and consecutive nephritis, in active or passive congestion, and in lardaceous disease (rarely), mentioned in order of frequency, it is also apt to supervene. Acute uræmia may occur in patients with previous chronic renal disease (1) when vomiting and diarrhœa cause salt depletion which cannot be compensated because the renal tubules can no longer retain sodium efficiently; and (2) in an acute exacerbation of chronic pyelonephritis. Moreover, complete suppression of urine may produce death associated with symptoms of what is called *latent uræmia* (§ 428), in those relatively rare cases of removal of a solitary kidney, or obstruction of both ureters.

Diagnosis.—The presence of any albumen with casts in the urine indicates renal damage. The earlier stages of renal failure are best diagnosed by performing one or more of the renal efficiency tests (§ 389): in the later stages examination of the blood, especially for its urea content, will decide the diagnosis, a value over 120–150 mg. per cent. usually being diagnostic. The differential diagnosis of uræmic coma is dealt with in §§ 850, 855.

Prognosis.—This depends on the extent of renal damage and how far it can be removed. In chronic nephritis where the kidneys are permanently and irremediably damaged, the prognosis is grave: whereas if uræmia is secondary to obstruction (*e.g.*, enlarged prostate) or some other cause which can be removed, the prognosis is correspondingly improved. Untoward symptoms are a greatly reduced 24-hour quantity of urine, severe anæmia, emaciation, drowsiness, uræmic dyspnœa, toxic myocardial changes, vomiting or diarrhœa, and a blood urea which is rising in spite of treatment. A safe rule is that, once retinal changes are present, the patient will not survive more than 18 months.

Treatment depends on the cause and on the symptoms and signs present. It is of considerable help in rectifying abnormalities in the electrolytes to have the sodium, potassium, chloride and alkali-reserve of the serum estimated each few days; in any case periodic blood urea analyses are required, and in the presence of œdema an occasional evaluation of the serum albumen and globulin is helpful.

When *chronic uræmia* is developing the treatment is that of chronic nephritis (§ 408). In the later stages (1) the diet should be of as high a calorie value as possible (at least 2,000 cals. a day) to lessen breakdown of tissue protein. The protein of the diet should be lowered in proportion as the blood urea rises (for suitable diets see § 296. VII, C) and when the blood urea is above 80 mg. per cent. the protein intake should be 40 G. a day. (2) The fluid intake needs to be about 5 pints (3 litres) a day unless there is œdema or salt depletion; if the urinary volume is small, it is often wise to reduce the fluid intake to correspond to the urinary volume of the previous 24 hours, adding 600 ml. to allow for the loss of water in the breath, the stools and via the skin, with an extra allowance to compensate for vomiting. Glucose should be added freely to the liquid given, whenever possible. (3) Sodium depletion is rectified by giving sodium chloride orally or intravenously, or isotonic sodium lactate: potassium is often in excess in the plasma, but in cases of potassium-losing nephritis potassium chloride 3–6 G. a day are required.   (4) Convulsions may be due to sodium depletion, and when calcium shortage is present, 20 ml. of 10 per cent. calcium gluconate intravenously is helpful.   In older subjects with severe hypertension venesection ($\frac{1}{2}$–1 pint) can be used unless anæmia is present, but intramuscular or intravenous hypotensive drugs (§ 96) are now more commonly given.   To control fits, morphia in small doses and intramuscular injections of paraldehyde (3–5 ml.) are often required.   (5) Vomiting is lessened by inject. chlorpromazine B.P. (6) For uræmic dyspnœa with a low alkali reserve, these same sedatives combined with sodium bicarbonate (3–6 G. a day until the urine is faintly alkaline) or isotonic sodium lactate (1·9 per cent.) intravenously are necessary.   (7) Benzyl-penicillin in full doses, or occasionally tetracycline 0·25 G. 12-hourly, is necessary to control infections which are very likely to arise in the lungs, the urinary tract and elsewhere.   (8) It is unwise to restrict the fluid intake or to lower the blood pressure excessively in chronic uræmia, as these defeat the attempt at compensation by the kidneys.   In those cases where the heart shows evidence of failure, supporting measures must be undertaken (and see § 62).   (9) Whether retinopathy is present or not, when the systolic blood pressure reaches 200 mm. or more, it is wise to try and lower the pressure by hypotensive drugs (§ 96). This tends to lessen progressive renal damage and may considerably prolong the expectation of life.

In *acute uræmia* following crush injuries or other causes of acute toxic tubular damage, the volume of urine secreted is very small.   Then Bull's regime should be followed and a 24-hour fluid intake and output chart carefully kept.   No protein can be given.   (1) During each 24 hours of the *oliguric period* (and for two days after the urine reaches 1 litre a day) give a basic intake of 500 ml. of 50 per cent. glucose by a continuous intragastric drip via a polythene tube.   To this add all vomitus after filtering through lint.   (2) In addition to this, it is necessary to measure each 24 hours the volume of vomitus not already returned via the intragastric tube, the volume of urine passed and of liquid lost by diarrhœa.   These three added together are replaced by an equal amount of a solution containing sod. bicarbonate 1 G., sod. chloride 3 G., glucose 100 G. with water to 1 litre, also given via the intragastric drip each 24 hours. (These have replaced the earlier intragastric glucose solution with arachis oil.)   (3) In the presence of much diarrhœa and/or vomiting, Bull advises a continuous intravenous drip via a polythene cannula and gives each 24 hours 500 ml. of 50 per cent. dextrose, together with an equivalent amount of the following to replace the measured fluid loss in the urine, vomit and diarrhœic stools—sod. lactate (1·9 per cent.) 150 ml., isotonic saline 350 ml., dextrose (5 per cent.) to 1,000 ml.   (4) During the *early diuretic* phase, two days after the urinary volume exceeds 1 litre in 24 hours, the intragastric or intravenous tube is withdrawn and in its place fruit juice, tea, coffee and water of a volume equivalent to the urinary volume plus 500 ml. are given; toast, jam, boiled sweets and juicy fruits are given liberally (the fluid of the fruit forming part of the total fluid intake); and to these are added each day potass. chloride 1 G. sod. bicarbonate 1 G., and sodium chloride 3 G. for each litre of urine passed.   This regime needs to be continued until the blood urea has fallen below 100 mg. per cent.   (5) Penicillin 1 mega unit is followed by 0·25 mega units daily, and (6) a single dose of an anabolic steroid such as nandrolone (Durabolin) or norethandrolone (Nilevar) helps to prevent breakdown of tissue protein.

PART B. PHYSICAL EXAMINATION

§ 373. The **Examination of the Urine** corresponds, in renal diseases, to the physical examination of other organs.

We examine it by (a) observing its *physical characters* (§ 374)—viz., its appearance (*i.e.*, its colour, and whether it is clear or cloudy)—its odour, reaction, specific gravity; the presence and characters of any deposit; and its diurnal quantity. (b) Then by *chemical analysis* (§ 379) we ascertain the presence or absence of albumen, the presence or absence of sugar and other substances, according to circumstances. (c) A *microscopic examination* (§ 391) has to be made of any deposit which may be present. (d) The *kidney efficiency* tests consist in part of examination of the urine, and in part of examination of the blood. The blood examinations, usually conducted by skilled laboratory workers (§ 389), are of special value in the detection of kidney disease where albuminuria is slight or sometimes absent. *It is important in all cases—not only in cases of suspected renal disease—to observe and to record the condition of the urine when the patient is first seen, even when the symptoms do not suggest renal disease.*

(a) Physical Characters of the Urine

§ 374. **Appearance.**—The colour of the urine depends upon the proportion of pigments present. The chief pigments are urochrome and urobilin, the antecedents of which are the blood and bile pigments; but there are many others.

The urine varies from a pale yellow to a deep amber, according to the DEGREE OF DILUTION of the pigments: and, as the latter are fairly constant in quantity, a *dark urine* is commonly associated with a smaller diurnal quantity and a higher specific gravity than a pale urine. The urine is concentrated in excessive perspiration, acute nephritis, pyrexial states, and with diminished fluid intake, as in diarrhœa or vomiting. On the other hand, in certain diseases with *polyuria* the urine is *pale*, as in chronic nephritis, and in diabetes. With a large intake, in diabetes insipidus, and other conditions, the urine may be as colourless as water.

The colour of the urine may be altered by ABNORMAL PRODUCTS. Thus:—*a dark orange colour to brown* is due to the presence of bile pigments or urobilinogen (§ 383); a *red* colour, which may be a dark red or porter colour or only a mere " smokiness," to the presence of blood (§ 382); a *blackish brown* colour to melanin and certain oxyacids, which cause the urine to darken on exposure (§ 386); a *bright green* urine may be associated with chloroma; an intense *grass-green* fluorescence follows the ingestion of fluorescein-coloured sweets (fluoresceinuria). *Milky* urine is found with chyluria and multiple myeloma. Various DRUGS affect the colour of the urine. A *dark olive-green* or *black colour* may be due to the absorption of phenol or after administration of creosote, salicylates, salol, tar, resorcin or naphthol. The colour is explained by the presence of hydroquinone, which turns crimson on the addition of ferric chloride. A *port-wine colour* is due to porphyrins (§ 415). A *reddish-brown colour* may be due to rhubarb, senna or chrysophanic acid taken internally—these turn red on the addition of alkali. A *bright yellow colour* follows the administration of mepacrine and santonin; and an *orange colour* of phenindione. A *colourless* urine is said to result from tannin taken by the mouth, and a *reddish* hue from hæmatoxylin. A *coloured* urine, from the presence of eosin, methylene blue or other dye, may result from coloured sweets or cakes or certain proprietary pills.

Urinary Deposits and Cloudiness will be described in § 390.

§ 375. **Reaction.**—The urine should be tested soon after being passed. In normal urine an *acid reaction* is usual from the presence of acid phosphate of sodium. On standing, decomposition takes place, the urea being transformed into ammonium carbonate $(NH_2)_2CO + 2H_2O = (NH_4)_2CO_3$, and hence the reaction becomes alkaline.

The same change takes place within the bladder in many cases of chronic cystitis. *Alkalinity* occurs in normal urine on waking and after meals—the " alkaline tide "—due to the disodium phosphate (Na_2HPO_4) replacing the acid salt, or when alkalies are administered. A *neutral* reaction may occur under the same conditions. The reaction of the urine is often expressed in terms of pH values, with extremes in health from pH 4·7 (acid urine) to pH 8·0 (alkaline urine), the neutral point being at pH 7·2.

§ 376. **Specific Gravity.**—This is most conveniently measured in the specimen passed on waking, as it has been collecting over a period of 8–10 hours. The instrument, a urinometer, must not touch the sides of the vessel, and the graduated stem should be read along the surface of the fluid, not at the place where it is raised along the stem by capillarity. When enough urine is not obtainable, and a glass bead urinometer is not accessible, mix the urine with one, two or three times its own bulk of water and multiply the last two figures of the specific gravity by two, three or four, respectively. For example, a mixture of one ounce of urine with *three* ounces of distilled water gives a specific gravity of 1005; the specific gravity of the urine is 1020 (0·005 × 4 = 0·020).

The average specific gravity of the urine in health varies between 1015 and 1025. It depends chiefly upon the percentages of urea and salts (especially chlorides) present. Extractives and pigments play only a small part: and—since the salts are fairly constant—the specific gravity, *in the absence of sugar*, gives a fair measure of the urea present in a given sample. In the absence of sugar and of albumen, a specific gravity above 1018 usually indicates a satisfactory renal function, especially when the 24-hour volume is less than 700 ml. The specific gravity is low in granular, lardaceous and polycystic kidney disease; high in acute and subacute nephritis, passive congestion and with glycosuria.

§ 377. The normal **odour** of freshly-passed urine is described as "aromatic"; it is very different from the ammoniacal odour of decomposing urine. It may smell of volatile sulphides due to the presence of some bacteria, notably *E. coli communis*, and also when cystinuria is present, especially after the urine has stood for a while.

§ 378. **The Diurnal Quantity** varies considerably within the range of health. Normally, 40 to 50 oz. (1½ litres) are passed per diem, but the quantity depends upon the amount of fluid drunk and of protein consumed, the action of the skin, the presence of fever or diarrhœa and the activity of the renal circulation. Polyuria indicates a supernormal and oliguria a subnormal volume in the 24 hours. In order to measure the 24-hour output and for some other purposes, collect all the urine passed, for example, from 8 A.M. Monday to 8 A.M. Tuesday. The patient should pass water *at* 8 A.M. *on Monday morning*, and this should be thrown away. All that is passed after that hour, together with what is passed *at* 8 A.M. *on Tuesday*, should be collected in one clean vessel. During the whole time it is necessary to pass water *before* going to stool, and to add this to the total collected. At 8 A.M. on Tuesday, after passing urine and adding it to that previously passed, the whole should be stirred and measured. A specimen from this should be put into a clean bottle (say 10 fl. oz.), suitably labelled (also giving the total quantity passed in 24 hours) and sent for examination immediately. A few drops of chloroform or toluene will preserve it.

(b) *Chemical Examination of the Urine. Abnormal Constituents.*

In disease the most important abnormal substances for which the urine has to be tested chemically are albumen, sugar, blood, bile, acetoacetic acid, acetone and pus.

§ 379. **Albumen** is the most frequent of the pathological constituents of the urine. The variety of " albumen " usually present is serum albumen and serum globulin and for this reason some prefer the term proteinuria;

but because of its smaller molecular size more albumen than globulin is lost from the plasma in renal disease. The chief tests for albumen are: (1) boiling; (2) cold nitric acid; (3) Esbach's Test.

1. *Boiling.*—After testing with litmus, adjust the reaction (by the addition of alkali or 2 per cent. acetic acid) until slightly acid; then boil. A generalised white precipitate forms on boiling if albumen is present, and is not dissolved by further addition of acetic acid. It is always best to boil the upper part of a column of urine to compare it with the lower.

The *Fallacies* of this test are: (i.) Phosphates may be precipitated by heat alone if the urine be faintly acid, neutral, or alkaline, but the acetic acid dissolves these whereas it increases the albuminous precipitate. (ii.) Excess of acid redissolves the albumen; undue natural acidity may have the same effect; all of which prove how essential it is to adjust the reaction correctly in the first place. (iii.) In acid urines a cloud sometimes appears, not on boiling only, as albumen would do, but when the acid is added, due to mucus. (iv.) If the urine is not quite clear, it may be necessary to filter it. If turbid from bacteria it can be centrifuged; otherwise add a trace of NaOH, and the deposit of phosphates which occurs will carry the bacteria down with it. Filter and acidify again before testing.

2. *Cold Salicylsulphonic Acid Test.*—To 5 ml. of urine (filtered if necessary) add 7 or 8 drops of salicylsulphonic acid (25 per cent.). Depending on the amount of albumen present, a white haze or a dense white cloud will appear. This is a very quick and reliable test.

The *Fallacies* of the test are: (i.) Bence-Jones' protein also gives a precipitate, whereas in the boiling test it has redissolved. (ii.) Uroselectan in the urine gives a false-positive reaction in the form of a white crystalline precipitate.

3. *Esbach's Test.*—Add Esbach's solution[1] to the urine by a pipette. A precipitate indicates the presence of albumen. Alkaloids and albumoses may also be precipitated, but disappear on heating.

4. The *Paper Test* is carried out with a paper strip (Albustix) containing tetra-bromphenol blue with a citrate buffer. A positive reaction occurs when the strip changes from yellow to green or blue, depending on the concentration. It detects albumen, globulin, hæmoglobin and Bence-Jones' protein.

The *quantitative estimation* of albumen may be determined by one of two methods:—

(i.) *Esbach's albuminometer* is a tube graduated for measuring the grammes per litre of albumen. Urine taken from 24 hours' collection is poured into the tube up to the mark U, and the reagent is added up to the mark R. After mixing, the tube is set aside for 24 hours, and the precipitate falls to the bottom. The level to which this reaches is then noted, and the number on the glass indicates the grammes per litre of albumen present. *Fallacies.*—(1) This method is not reliable, if the specific gravity of the urine is over 1015. The urine should be diluted to 1015 or below, and a calculation made afterwards by multiplying the result by the number of times of dilution. (2) If the patient is taking alkaline salts, the urine must be first acidified before adding the reagent.

(ii.) *Salicylsulphonic acid* (3 per cent.) 3 ml. is added to urine 1 ml. in a special tube and, after shaking, the turbidity reached 5 minutes later is compared with that in a rack of similar tubes containing standard amounts of albumen. If in large amounts the urine may need to be diluted beforehand ten or a hundred times. The results are expressed in mg. per cent.

Electrophoresis is used to identify the relative amounts of plasma albumen and of plasma globulins (α_1, α_2, β and γ globulins) in the urine, as in the blood plasma (§ 543).

§ 380. **Mucin** is precipitated, as above mentioned, by adding dilute acetic acid which precipitates it in the cold; the precipitate is not redissolved by excess of

---

[1] Picric acid, 1 part; citric acid, 2 parts; water, 100 parts.

acetic acid. Mucin is dissolved in alkaline urine. Excess of mucus indicates irritation of the bladder or genito-urinary tract, or a vaginal or uterine discharge.

§ 381. Sugar is present in normal urine to the extent of 0·1 per cent., but the reagents used to detect an abnormal amount do not give a reaction with this normal trace of sugar. Glycosuria (sugar in the urine) is most commonly due to the presence of glucose (dextrose), as in Diabetes Mellitus (§ 423), but may be due to lactose in certain cases.

QUALITATIVE TESTS FOR GLYCOSURIA (glucose, lactose or pentose).

(1) *Benedict's Test.*—The reagent consists of copper sulphate 17·3 G. sod. cit. 173 G. sod. carb. (anhyd.) 100 G. aq. dest. ad. 1,000 ml. Add 8 drops of urine to 2 ml. of the reagent and boil for 2 minutes. If a reducing sugar is present a red or greenish-yellow precipitate forms. When the test is done in this manner, a reduction is only given by a reducing sugar.

(2) *Fehling's Test.*—Fehling's solution is an alkaline solution of potassiotartrate of copper, so prepared that 10 ml. is reduced by 0·05 gramme of glucose. As it will alter on keeping, it should be boiled before use, to make certain that no precipitate forms before adding the urine (it is better to keep the copper solution and the alkali solution in separate bottles, mixing them just before use). Add an equal quantity of urine which is boiled in a separate tube, bring the whole to the boil and allow to stand—the boiling must not be prolonged. If glucose or some other readily oxidisable substance is added, the blue cupric hydrate on gentle heating is reduced, and falls as a *red* or *yellow* precipitate of cuprous hydrate (Cu_2O, H_2O), which on longer boiling becomes red cuprous oxide (Cu_2O).

Fallacies.—(i.) The urine to be tested must be freed from albumen, and (ii.) it must not be ammoniacal. (iii.) Other reducing agents may occasionally give the reaction. After the administration of chloroform, chloral and some other drugs, a reaction is obtained resembling that due to sugar, due to glucuronic acid. Lactose, uric acid and urates, ammonium salts, hippuric acid, creatinine, oxyacids and the products of certain drugs, such as carbolic or benzoic acids, may be sources of fallacy. It is well to control the result by the Fermentation Test.

(3) The *Clinitest Method* avoids the need of external heat; it is performed by measuring 5 drops of urine and 10 drops of water in a test-tube and adding 1 tab. Clinitest copper sulphate, citric acid, sodium hydroxide and sodium carbonate. After boiling there is a change from a blue solution to an orange or dark greenish-brown colour which indicates sugar.

Lactose is only present in the urine during the later months of pregnancy, and during lactation. To distinguish between glucose and lactose, two tests may be used : (1) *Fermentation Test.*—Glucose is the only substance occurring in urine which is fermented by yeast. Lactose is not fermented. See that the urine is acid. Pour it into a test-tube, and insert a piece of yeast; invert the tube over a saucer of water (or mercury) and place in a warm place (*e.g.*, on the mantelpiece). Have a control tube beside it with normal urine and a piece of yeast. If glucose is present, bubbles of CO_2 form and collect at the top of the tube. (2) *Phenyl-Hydrazine Test.*—To a third of a test-tube of urine add enough phenyl-hydrazine hydrochloride to cover a sixpence, sodium acetate to cover a shilling, and a few drops of glacial acetic acid ; boil in a water-bath for half an hour. Cool by placing the tube in cold water. In the case of glucose a mass of yellow crystals forms, which under the microscope appear as fine yellow needles arranged as in a " wheatsheaf." In the case of lactose, yellow balls with fluffy edges are seen.

Pentosuria, due to a rare error of metabolism, causes a reduction of the alkaline copper solutions, but does not give the fermentation test, and the crystals found with phenyl-hydrazine hydrochloride are different from those produced by glucose and lactose. It may be tested for by Bial's reagent.

Galactosuria occurs particularly in the rare condition of congenital galactosæmia (§ 424). Galactose does not reduce Benedict's solution very strongly and is non-fermentible with yeast. It is best identified in the urine by paper chromatography.

Paper Chromatography is a useful laboratory method of identifying the nature of the various reducing substances which may be met in urine (§ 386).

QUANTITATIVE ESTIMATION OF GLUCOSE.—An approximate estimate of the amount of glucose present in urine may be formed if it is remembered that the specific gravity of a 1 per cent. solution is 1003. Thus, if from the depths of pigments present, it is judged that the specific gravity should be 1010, whereas the urinometer shows it actually to be 1031, the amount of sugar present is approximately $\dfrac{1031 - 1010}{3} = 7$ per cent. *Benedict's Method.*—The urine should be a sample taken from the total collection in 24 hours. Fill a burette with urine, diluted if necessary. Also measure 25 ml. of Benedict's *quantitative* solution into a conical flask, add 4 G. of anhydrous sodium carbonate and bring to the boil. The urine is run into the boiling solution until the blue colour is discharged and only a white precipitate remains. The solution must be kept boiling between each addition from the burette. 25 ml. of Benedict's solution are reduced by 0·05 G. glucose. Read off the amount of urine required for complete reduction and calculate. Suppose 60 ml. of urine, which has been diluted 20 times, are required to decolorise the 25 ml. of Benedict's solution, then 60/20 = 3 ml. contain 0·05 G. glucose. From this the percentage of glucose present can be calculated.

If lactose is the reducing sugar present, when calculating the results remember that 10 parts of lactose have the same reducing power as 7 parts of glucose.

§ 382. Blood in the urine imparts a characteristic smoky colour and may be present largely (*a*) in the form of red blood corpuscles (hæmaturia), some usually being broken up by the acidity of the urine, or (*b*) only in the form of free hæmoglobin (hæmoglobinuria). A darker colour of different shades may also be imparted to the urine by Methæmoglobinuria, Hæmato-porphyrinuria, Alcaptonuria and Carbolic Acid. To identify these use the spectroscope.

Microscopic Examination of the centrifuged deposit of a fresh specimen of urine will identify red cells in small numbers. Much larger quantities are necessary to give the chemical tests for blood.

Chemical Test for Blood.—Add a few drops of *freshly* prepared tr. guaiaci to the urine (which has been previously boiled and cooled) and shake; then add excess of ozonic alcohol or ozonic ether. A blue line appears at the junction of the fluids. The same reaction may be obtained by using filter- or blotting-paper. Allow a drop of each of the reagents to fall on the paper beside a drop of the urine, noticing the colour at the junction of the three drops. *Fallacies.*—Saliva gives the same reaction, and so do iodides, in patients taking these salts. Pus gives a green-blue colour with guaiacum alone. Tincture of guaiacum must be freshly prepared, and it is best to dissolve a little of the resin in rectified spirit just before use.

The *Occultest* detects hæmoglobin by producing a blue colour with oxidised o-tolidine. On the test paper provided place 1 drop of urine and then 1 tablet in the centre of the moist area: 2 drops of water on the tablet cause a blue colour to develop around it within 2 minutes when blood is present.

Hæmoglobinuria is always present with hæmaturia, because the corpuscles break up. Its presence *alone* is rare, and can only be proved by examining the centrifugalised deposit of absolutely fresh urine under the microscope and finding *no red cells*, although hæmoglobin is present. Some of the hæmoglobin is converted into methæmoglobin. (See also § 414.)

Methæmoglobinuria.—The characteristic smoky colour of the urine in hæmaturia of renal origin depends largely on methæmoglobin, a substance formed from hæmoglobin by the action of acid urine. (See § 411.) It is recognised by the spectroscope.

Porphyrins in large amounts in the urine impart a " port-wine " colour to the urine (§ 415). The different varieties which may be met need examination by an expert.

§ 383. **Bile** is present in the urine in cases of obstructive jaundice, and can be detected even before the skin becomes yellow. Both bile pigments and bile salts are present early in jaundice, but later only the pigments are present in many cases, probably because the liver ceases to manufacture the salts. A greenish-orange colour of the urine betrays the presence of bile if in more than slight amount.

Bile pigments may be tested for by: (1) *Gemlin's Test.*—Run fuming nitric acid down the side of a test-tube containing urine. As the bile-pigment oxidises, rings of colour form red, violet and green at the top; the green indicates bile. (2) *Marechal's Test.*—Add a few drops of very diluted solution of iodine to the surface of the urine in a test-tube: a green reaction is obtained. (3) *Fouchet's Test* is more delicate than these first two. Mix 10 ml. of urine (acidified if necessary) to 5 ml. of 10 per cent. barium chloride and filter. Spread the filter paper on to another fresh sheet and add to the precipitate 1 drop of Fouchet's reagent (trichloracetic acid 25 G., 10 per cent. ferric chloride 10 ml., and distilled water 100 ml.). A positive reaction is shown by the development of a greenish-blue colour.

Bile Salts are tested for by *Hay's Test.* Sprinkle flowers of sulphur on the surface of the urine in a wide-mouthed vessel (not a test-tube). If bile salts are present, the sulphur sinks, instead of floating as on normal urine, because the surface tension of a fluid containing bile salts is lowered. For the same reason urine containing bile salts gives a yellow or greenish froth when shaken in a test-tube.

Urobilinogen is present in small amounts in normal urine, but in cases of hepatic deficiency or of hæmolytic anæmia is in excess of normal, giving the urine a brighter yellow or yellowish-brown tinge. It rapidly disappears in urine on standing, being converted to urobilin.

To test, fresh urine must be used. Use Ehrlich's aldehyde reagent (*p*-dimethyl aminobenzaldehyde 10 G., conc. hydrochloric acid 100 ml., distilled water to 300 ml.). To 10 ml. urine add 1 ml. reagent, and if urobilinogen is in excess of normal a cherry-red colour develops within three minutes: this is hastened by gently warming.

Urobilin is absent in normal urine, but is slowly formed from urobilinogen on standing: when large quantities of urobilinogen are passed in pathological conditions, some urobilin probably accompanies it.

To test.—The colourless chromogen is converted into urobilin by 2 drops of liq. iodi mit. (B.P.); after acidifying with HCl, the spectroscope will detect an absorption band between the green and blue.

§ 384. **Acetone** and **Aceto-acetic acid** (often called diacetic acid) are present together in the urine in cases of ketosis. *Small* amounts are detected by Rothera's test and *large* amounts by Gerhardt's test.

Rothera's Test.—Add to 5 ml. urine a small crystal of sodium nitro-prusside and a few drops of liq. ammon. fort., shaking well: a permanganate colour appears and gradually deepens. The sensitiveness of the reaction is greatly increased by saturation of the urine with crystals of ammonium sulphate.

The *Acetest* tablet also contains sodium nitro-prusside and gives a permanganate colour in the presence of acetone.

Gerhardt's Test is performed by adding a few drops of a strong aqueous solution of ferric chloride, until in excess of the amount required to precipitate the phosphates, when a Burgundy-red colour appears. This same colour is given by salicylates. When urine gives a positive Gerhardt's test, Rothera's reaction develops very quickly due to the large amount of ketone bodies present.

Diacetic acid and acetone have long been known to be present in the urine in many cases of diabetes mellitus. One or both are also present in starvation and inanition, prolonged vomiting and gastro-intestinal diseases which prevent assimilation, severe acute diseases of the liver (such as acute yellow atrophy, delayed chloroform poisoning and eclampsia), in febrile states, in cases with an ill-balanced diet with a large excess of fat and insufficient sugar, and also in sea-sickness and cyclical vomiting in children (§ 271), even before the vomiting commences. In ketosis there is a deficiency in the utilisation of carbohydrates; the subsequent incomplete oxidation of fats leads to the formation of oxybutyric acid, aceto-acetic acid and acetone.

In the normal person the ratio of acid to base in the blood and tissues is maintained at a steady level by the intake of bases with the food, by the neutralisation of acid by ammonia, and by the elimination of acid radicles by the kidneys and of H_2CO_3 by the lungs.

Acidæmia indicates that these compensatory mechanisms have failed and so the H-ion concentration in the blood and tissues rises above normal and the pH is below 7·4. (The pH may fall as low as 7·0.) Three varieties occur:—(1) It may be exogenous, the result of taking by mouth large quantities of acids (as in aspirin poisoning, when taking HCl, sodium acid phosphate or ammonium chloride, which is converted into urea and HCl.) (2) Metabolic causes arise in renal failure, when acids (especially NaH_2PO_4) cannot be sufficiently excreted; and in diabetes mellitus when diacetic acid accumulates. (3) In advanced pulmonary disease (severe emphysema and chronic bronchitis) H_2CO_3 cannot be excreted in sufficient amounts through the lungs. In the first two of these types (the exogenous and metabolic) the plasma sodium bicarbonate falls as the acid radicles accumulate, but in the third variety (the respiratory type) it rises to try and keep pace with the rising H_2CO_3 in the blood.

The clinical *symptoms* are—(1) an increase in the depth and to some extent the rate of respiration (air-hunger) sometimes with a hissing sound. If it is due to ketosis, there is (2) an ethereal odour to the breadth and (3) ketone bodies will be found in the urine.

Treatment of Acidæmia and Ketosis.—When exogenous and metabolic causes are in operation, sodium bicarbonate is given orally or as an isotonic solution (B.P.) intravenously (5·0 per cent.); or sodium lactate (one-sixth molar) may be used intravenously instead. For ketosis, the most rapid results are given by intravenous injection of 250 ml. of sodium bicarbonate (4 per cent.), and dextrose (5 per cent.) and should be used with insulin. When the ketosis occurs with diabetes mellitus, see §§ 423, 424.

Alkalæmia is the reverse of acidæmia. It is the condition when the H-ion concentration in the blood and tissues is below normal, and the pH rises. If it occurs slowly, it is compensated by a retention of acids, especially H_2CO_3; if rapidly, the blood actually becomes more alkaline. The usual *symptoms* are headache, nausea, vomiting, abdominal pain, thirst, mental irritability; in severe cases, symptoms of tetany ensue (§ 1030), ushered in with tingling of the fingers and toes: coma may lead to a fatal issue. On examination the patient looks ill, usually has a flushed dehydrated face, a furred tongue and suffused conjunctivæ; the urine may contain a trace of albumen and in severe cases acetone occurs. *Causes.*—(1) After excessive vomiting, as with pyloric and high intestinal obstruction; (2) after excessive doses of alkalies by mouth, especially $NaHCO_3$; (3) with hyperpnœa due to mountain climbing, forced breathing at rest or exposure to a hot, moist climate, with excessive loss of CO_2, and therefore of H_2CO_3 from the blood.

Treatment.—The cause must be removed, vomiting allayed, the lack of chlorides compensated by large doses of normal saline solutions by mouth, per rectum, or intravenously, and acid administered in the form of ammonium chloride (3–6 G.) or dilute hydrochloric acid by mouth, or calcium chloride (1–2 G.) intravenously.

§ 385. **Pus** in the urine is detected by the microscope: chemical tests should not be used, as they only show the presence of large amounts of pus. The presence of one or two leucocytes in the deposit of a fresh specimen of urine is normal. Up to 10 cells per c.mm. is normal (Dukes). When pus comes from the *kidney*, the urine is, at any rate when first passed, acid, and the pus is uniformly disseminated through the urine, and remains so for some time. When it comes from the *bladder*, the urine is usually alkaline or neutral, and the pus soon collects into a creamy layer at the bottom of the glass.

When in *very considerable quantity*, pus may be detected by the addition of a few drops of tinct. guaiaci, when a greenish-blue colour appears. *In small quantities* it is essential to examine the deposit microscopically for pus cells.

§ 386. **Other constituents** met in urine are albumoses, homogentesic acid, melanin, indican, amino-acids and steroids.

Albumosuria occurs in many different conditions, *e.g.*, with abscess formation, during the resolution of pneumonia, with acute yellow atrophy of the liver, with asthma and with some cases of nephritis. It is only clinically significant in the form of *Bence-Jones' protein* as a globulin, which is present in about 50 per cent. of the cases of multiple myeloma or Kahler's disease.

Tests.—Slightly acidify 50 ml. urine with 33 per cent. acetic acid. To 5 ml. urine in each of 3 test-tubes, add 0, 1 and 2 drops of 33 per cent. acetic acid and place in a water-bath with a thermometer. When Bence-Jones' protein is present, the urine suddenly becomes turbid at a temperature between 40–55° C. On boiling, in at least one tube the protein redissolves. Bradshaw's test depends on a dense white ring forming at the junction of urine and concentrated HCl in a test-tube. (Other proteins when in large quantities give a faint white ring.) *Electrophoresis* of the urine (and of the serum) in myelomatosis with Bence-Jones' protein reveals a dense band of a globulin in the $\beta\gamma$ range or rarely is an α_2 globulin; such findings are especially significant when albumen is absent.

Alcaptonuria is a condition where the urine darkens from the surface downwards on standing exposed to the air or on addition of alkalies, due to the presence of *homogentesic acid*. It is due to an inborn error of metabolism, and has no known clinical significance. Its only importance lies in the fact that it reduces Fehling's solution and simulates glycosuria. (See § 766.)

Melanuria occurs when there are extensive deposits of melanotic sarcoma. Fresh urine is usually colourless (melanogen) but becomes dark on standing (melanin).

Test.—To 5 ml. of urine add 3–4 drops of freshly prepared sodium nitro-prusside solution, and 10–12 drops of 40 per cent. caustic soda and shake. Then add sufficient 33 per cent. acetic acid to acidify, when a Prussian-blue colour develops.

Amino-aciduria is detected by *paper chromatography* and has been the subject of intense study in recent years. Among the amino-acids excreted are cystine, lysine arginine and ornithine. Two types occur: (*a*) when amino-acids are in excess in the blood plasma and (*b*) when the plasma content is normal but there is a failure of absorption in the distal convoluted tubules of the kidneys. The presence of amino-acids assumes considerable importance in congenital cystinuria (with cystine stone formation in the renal passages), cystinosis, severe liver damage including hepato-lenticular degeneration (Wilson's disease), the Fanconi syndrome (§ 422), galactosæmia of infants and other forms of mental disease. Urine containing *phenylpyruvic acid* (Phenylketonuria) gives a well-marked green colour with ferric chloride solution— a colour which fades in a few minutes. It is found in certain conditions of low-grade mental deficiency. Diets low in phenylalanine help in treatment.

Paper Chromatography.—A paper chromatogram is prepared by placing near one end of a piece of filter paper a small drop of the urine or other fluid under investigation. The spot so formed is dried and the end of the filter paper nearest to the spot is placed in a solvent reservoir. Paper and reservoir are enclosed in an air-tight vessel. Solvent is added to the reservoir and passes by capillarity along the length of the paper. As the solvent moves it takes with it at different rates the various components which are present in the spot. After the solvent has travelled a suitable distance the paper is removed from the vessel, dried and treated with a reagent which will produce coloured compounds with some of the components of the original mixture. These coloured areas, distributed at different distances along the length of the paper, show by their position the identity of the compounds originally present. The quantity of the different materials is indicated by the size or intensity of the coloured area. Of the *urinary sugars* fructose, lactose and pentose can readily be distinguished from glucose by this method. Unfortunately the separation of glucose from galactose is much more difficult. For the detection of *amino-acidurias* paper chromatography is the method of choice. In phenylketonuria there is an abnormal excretion of phenyl-pyruvic acid and phenylalanine. Abnormal quantities of cystine, lysine, arginine, ornithine are excreted in cystinuria. The generalised amino-aciduria of Wilson's disease and the Fanconi syndrome can readily be detected.

Steroids of many different varieties are found in urine: these include 17-ketosteroids, 17-hydroxycorticosteroids and aldosterone. Twenty-four-hour bulk specimens are required for their quantitative estimation.

Normal Constituents of the Urine.

Normally the urine consists of water containing about 4 per cent. of solids by weight, of which urea comprises from 2·5 to 3 per cent. of the total urine, amounting to about 30 G. per diem.

§ 387. Urea.—A healthy male adult, weighing, say 140 pounds, excretes daily an average of 1,200 to 1,500 ml. urine (42 to 53 fl. oz.), containing 30 G. of urea. These figures vary widely in health, and are much less for a lighter person taking less food. If the kidneys are acting well, the urea output is dependent on the intake of nitrogenous food, but it is considerably diminished after vomiting or diarrhœa. A specimen for estimation should be taken from the urine of twenty-four hours, mixed and measured (§ 378). Deficient elimination of urea (with a rise in blood urea) occurs sooner or later in nearly all renal diseases (see Uræmia, § 370), in certain hepatic diseases, in myxœdema, Addison's disease and melancholia. (See Kidney Efficiency Tests, § 389.)

Estimation of Urea.—For accurate results it is necessary to determine the *total nitrogen* in the urine; but since the greater proportion is in the form of urea, it is most convenient to estimate the urea excretion.

The apparatus usually employed is Gerrard's Ureameter or some modification of it. It is fitted up as shown in Fig. 117. 25 ml. of freshly prepared solution of sodium hypobromite are placed in the wide-mouthed jar (A). Then a small tube containing

5 ml. of urine (B) is carefully introduced so that it stands up against the side of the wide glass jar, which is tightly stoppered. Next, the reservoir (C) is filled with water: the stopcock (E) of the cylinder (D) is opened and the reservoir raised till the water in the cylinder is at zero and level with that in the reservoir; the stopcock (E) is closed. Then the jar (A) is tilted so that the urine mixes with the hypobromite. Effervescence occurs as the liberated nitrogen enters the cylinder and displaces water, driving it into the reservoir. After allowing to cool for ten minutes, the reservoir is moved until the water in it and the cylinder are level; then the amount of gas is read. The cylinder is graduated in percentage of urea.

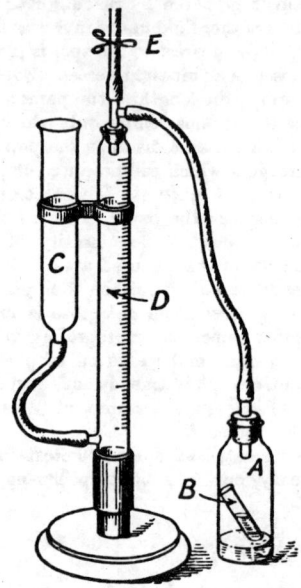

§ 388. **Uric acid,** either free or combined in the form of urates, is normally present in a sample from a day's collection of urine to the extent of 0·7 G. per diem. Uric acid and urates separate out as a cloudiness or deposit (§§ 390 and 393) when there is high acidity. This dissolves on warming or with alkali. Their chemical quantitative estimation is difficult.

CHLORIDES.—The chlorides found in the urine are principally salts of sodium, and vary in *health*, according to the food taken, from about 11 to 15 G. daily. In *disease*, the chlorides are increased during convalescence from fevers, during the absorption of œdema or other forms of serous exudations and in diabetes insipidus. Except in malaria, they are diminished in acute fevers, especially in pneumonia (reappearing 2 or 3 days after the crisis), in diabetic coma, in renal diseases with œdema, during vomiting and diarrhœa.

FIG. 117.—GERRARD'S UREAMETER.

The *Fantus test* is a useful bedside method of indicating the amount of chloride present. The test-tube and the pipette used must previously be rinsed with distilled water and washed each time before containing a fresh solution. Into the test-tube 10 drops of urine and one drop of potassium chromate (20 per cent.) are measured; silver nitrate (2·9 per cent.) is added from the same pipette until a brick-red colour of silver chromate develops. The number of drops of silver nitrate solution needed indicates the number of grammes of sodium chloride per litre in the urine.

PHOSPHATES (§ 393) occur in two groups: the alkaline phosphates, salts of potassium, sodium and ammonium; and the earthy phosphates, salts of calcium and magnesium. The former are readily soluble; the latter are readily deposited when the urine is neutral or alkaline, especially when heated.

Tests.—In an *alkaline* or neutral urine, the earthy phosphates form a cloudy precipitate, which is increased on boiling, but disappears on adding weak acetic acid. Microscopic examination is indispensable when, as often happens, both are present.

CALCIUM excretion in the urine is an approximate measure of the serum calcium. *Test.*—Equal parts of Sulkowitch's reagent and of a 24-hour specimen of urine are mixed in a test-tube. If no precipitate occurs the serum calcium is probably below 7·5 mg. per cent.; a fine milky cloud indicates a normal amount and a milky precipitate means a high serum calcium content. The results are often low in osteomalacia and osteoporosis.

§ 389. **Kidney Efficiency Tests.**—Certain tests yield invaluable evidence as to the condition of the kidneys. These have usurped the position of the older tests for the amount of urea in the urine, which was formerly regarded as the chief source of information. Several of these tests should be confided to the skilled laboratory worker. This is true especially of the examination of the blood for protein and non-protein nitrogen.

1. *Estimation of Blood Urea.*—The most accurate method is by means of urease in the soya bean, but for practical purposes a much more rapid method is by means of sodium hypobromite. *Ambard's Method.*—Into a 25 ml. measuring flask deliver approximately 10 ml. of 20 per cent. trichloracetic acid. To this add 10 ml. of blood, and make up to the 25 ml. mark with water. Filter off the coagulated protein, and take a measured quantity (10–15 ml.) of the clear filtrate. Pour this into the urea apparatus by squeezing some air out of the rubber bag, filling the cup with the solution, and introducing this into the apparatus by releasing the pressure on the rubber. Add a few drops of phenolphthalein and sufficient strong caustic soda to

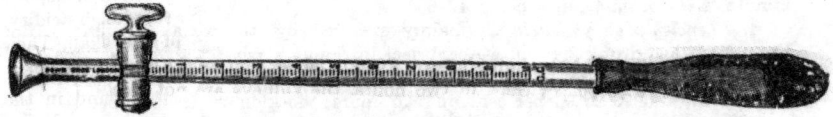

FIG. 118.—AMBARD'S APPARATUS FOR ESTIMATING BLOOD UREA. (¼ scale.)

make the contents alkaline. By pressing on the rubber bag, drive all the air from the apparatus to the top of the tap. Then fill the cup to the level of the neck with sodium hypobromite, and release this into the apparatus, taking care that no air enters. Invert the apparatus several times till all the nitrogen has been evolved, and measure the quantity of this by releasing the bag from the apparatus in a cylinder of water, and measuring the quantity of gas when the levels of fluid are the same inside and outside the apparatus. Suppose 13 ml. of filtrate were used, and evolved 0·8 ml. of nitrogen. This amount of filtrate was derived from $\dfrac{13 \times 10}{25}$ ml. of blood. Knowing that 1 G. of urea liberates 354 ml. nitrogen at N.T.P., the amount of urea present in the blood is readily calculated. Normally the blood has 20 to 50 mg. of urea per 100 ml. In renal diseases it rises considerably higher; about 100 mg. per 100 ml. blood may be taken as definitely pathological. A high blood urea may occasionally occur without renal disease (§§ 372 and 387); then the prognosis varies with the cause. In doubtful cases the urea excretion should be measured. The urea concentration test and the urea clearance test will help to decide whether the condition is due to disease of the kidney. Usually there is urea retention in the blood with chronic interstitial nephritis but not with subacute parenchymatous nephritis.

2. *The Urea Concentration Test* introduced by Maclean is a valuable guide to the function of the kidney. The bladder is emptied, and the patient drinks 15 G. urea solved in 100 ml. water. The urine passed at the end of 1, 2 and 3 hours is separately collected, measured and the urea percentage in each specimen estimated. The volume in the first hour may be increased by the diuretic effect of urea, and if it exceeds 120 ml. the result should be discarded. The second sample is often the more important because of this diuresis. Above 2·5 per cent. urea in any sample means normal concentration. In chronic interstitial nephritis there is less; serious cases show a concentration of only 1·0 to 1·5 per cent. urea. The fallacy of this test is that it may not show even severe grades of renal insufficiency in certain cases, particularly in subacute parenchymatous nephritis, because the urea is concentrated, owing to the small output of fluid. This is partly overcome by estimating the total urea excretion in each hour. In at least one period, 10 per cent. of the ingested dose of urea is secreted by the normal kidneys. More accurate estimation is by the urea clearance tests.

3. *Van Slyke's Method for Determining Urea Clearance.*—The test is best performed between breakfast and lunch. Before the test, vigorous exercise must be avoided, and the previous meal must have been moderate and without coffee. Just prior to the test, and again 1 hour later, a glass of water is given. At a noted time, the bladder is emptied; at the end of the first hour a sample of blood is taken for blood urea estimation; at about the end of the first hour, urine is passed, the time recorded, and the whole specimen put into a labelled bottle. At the end of a second hour urine is again passed, and the whole specimen put into another labelled bottle.

For persons over 16 years, and of average build, the following methods are used to calculate the results (in others, correction factors have to be applied).

$$\text{The Maximum Clearance} = \frac{\text{per cent. urea in urine (U)}}{\text{per cent. urea in blood (B)}} \times \frac{\text{Vol. of urine in ml.}}{\text{per minute (V)}}$$

is used where the output exceeds 2 ml. per minute, the normal values being 64–99.

The Standard Clearance $= \frac{U}{B}\sqrt{V}$ is used where the output is less than 2 ml. per minute, the normal values being 40–68.

4. *Phenolsulphonophthalein* is mainly excreted by the renal tubules. After the patient has drunk 300 ml. water, inject intramuscularly 6 mg. of the dye, and examine the urine 70 and 130 minutes after. If 40 to 50 per cent. of the dye is excreted in an hour, and 70 to 90 per cent. in two hours, the kidneys are not diseased.

(c) The Urinary Deposit.

§ 390. Cloudiness of the Urine (naked-eye examination).—In healthy urine there is no deposit, but many of the normal constituents, and some abnormal substances, may become evident as a sediment or turbidity after the urine has cooled.

(1) A bulky pinkish turbidity and deposit in an acid urine, which form when the urine cools, indicates the presence of *urates*. It is the commonest of urinary deposits. (2) *Uric Acid* is evident to the naked eye as a sandy deposit resembling red cayenne pepper. (3) A white flocculent turbidity in an alkaline or neutral urine indicates the presence of *phosphates*, which are cleared at once by the addition of a few drops of 2 per cent. acetic acid. (4) *Calcium oxalate* gives a typical " powdered-wig " deposit of fine white points seen on the surface of a mucous cloud. (5) A fine cloud of *vesical mucus* is normally present in the urine, although it is only visible when the entangled débris and epithelial cells are sufficiently plentiful. (6) *Pus* forms a deposit which resembles phosphates to the naked eye, but it is readily distinguished under the microscope. (7) *Prostatic threads* (" floaters ") are elongated fine white threads which float in the urine and indicate chronic prostatitis. (8) Urine is sometimes cloudy from the presence of *bacteria*, and this cloudiness cannot be cleared by boiling or the addition of acids.

§ 391. Specimens of the deposit must always be examined **microscopically** in cases of **suspected** renal disease. The urinary deposit is best examined after the urine has stood for some hours in a conical glass, or after the specimen has been centrifugalised. Examine the deposit first under a $\frac{1}{4}$ or $\frac{1}{2}$ inch objective, then under a $\frac{1}{6}$ or higher. It normally contains foreign substances, such as cotton and woollen fibres, etc., and a few bladder (and in women nearly always a few vaginal) epithelial cells, which are recognised by their large and nucleated appearance. Inquiry should always be made as to the sex of the patient, and in women if any leucorrhœa is present.   If so, it may be necessary to obtain a mid-stream or a catheter specimen of urine.

The urinary deposit may contain ORGANISED SUBSTANCES (§ 392), or CRYSTALLINE and inorganic substances (§ 393).

§ 392. The **Organised Constituents** of the urinary sediment are of far more serious import than the crystalline .substances.   They comprise TUBE-CASTS (which are the most important), EPITHELIAL CELLS, PUS CELLS, BLOOD CELLS, spermatozoa, and certain rarer structures such as bacteria.

Tube-casts and renal **Epithelial Cells** are present in all renal diseases attended by shedding or destruction of the renal epithelium.   The casts are composed of blood cells or renal epithelial cells moulded together in the convoluted tubules during the absorption of water.   When tube-casts are abundant in the urine, microscopic examination of the sediment permits of their ready detection.   But if, on the other hand, they are present only in small numbers, they may be easily overlooked, especially when, as in chronic interstitial nephritis and in amyloid disease, the urine is abundant and of low specific gravity, so that any suspended matter is deposited only slowly and incompletely.   Moreover, in these instances, the casts are apt to be of the hyaline variety, and their almost transparent character renders them inconspicuous objects in the microscopic field. To detect the presence of casts *a fresh specimen of urine is often essential*, as they rapidly disappear in alkaline or decomposing urine.

THE SEARCH FOR TUBE-CASTS must be conducted with great care if the risk of a false conclusion is to be avoided.   One of the best methods, after settlement or centrifugalisation of the deposit, is to examine it with a moderately low power of the microscope, using a narrow diaphragm and shading the light so as to have the field only feebly illuminated.   Any suspicious-looking object can be brought into the centre of the field and examined with a stronger lens.   In this way casts may be detected which in a strong light would readily be missed, and if several slides have been prepared and examined in this manner the detection of any casts present in the urine is rendered fairly certain.   But the examination *of a fresh specimen* should be repeated on several occasions in any urine containing albumen before a negative conclusion is finally arrived at.   The addition of a few drops of methylene blue to the urine before centrifugalisation is of assistance.   The casts do not stain at first, but in those containing cells the nuclei stain; and the casts stand out against the pale blue background of the fluid.

The clinical importance of tube-casts in the urine is that, with but few exceptions, they indicate disease of the renal epithelium.   Thus, when found in a urine containing albumen, they indicate that the albuminuria is a result of some structural change in the kidney.   Similarly in cases of pyuria and hæmaturia the detection of tube-casts not only suggests that the pus and blood are of renal origin, but that the kidney is affected. It must be remembered that more than one part of the urinary tract may be diseased at one and the same time.   In the urine of patients who are jaundiced, tube-casts may often be found without, either at the time or subsequently, any evidence of renal disease.

In general terms, *epithelial casts* and *blood casts* are indicative cf the earlier and more acute stages of nephritis.   *Waxy casts* are not peculiar to lardaceous kidney, but occur in other forms of long-standing renal disease. These and *fatty casts* indicate that the inflammatory process is passing to a degenerative stage. *Granular casts* are more abundant in chronic renal disease. *Hyaline casts*, which must not be confused with waxy casts, occur in all forms of nephritis, both acute and chronic.

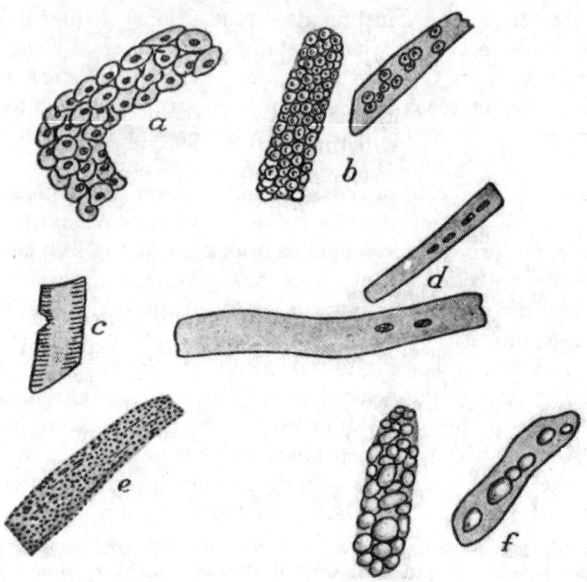

Fig. 119.—RENAL TUBE-CASTS.—*a*, epithelial casts; *b*, blood casts; *c*, waxy cast; *d*, hyaline casts; *e*, granular cast; *f*, fatty casts.

The relative proportion of epithelial, granular, and hyaline casts (Fig. 119) is affected by the condition of the urine. In highly acid and in alkaline urine the casts tend to be hyaline; in acid urine, granular. Tube-casts in abundance always form a serious symptom, but one or two hyaline casts occur in normal urine. They are more abundant in the acute than the chronic forms of renal disease. Their *absence* does not count for very much, as they may be easily missed or undergo disintegration in the urine. The continued presence of hyaline and granular casts is more serious than the temporary appearance of other types.

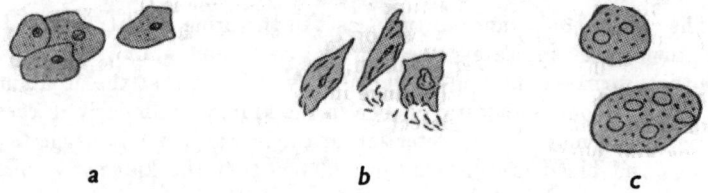

Fig. 120.—RENAL EPITHELIUM—*a*, normal; *b*, disintegrating; *c*, fatty.

Renal Epithelial Cells (Fig. 120) in a urinary deposit have much the same significance as the presence of tube-casts. The cells are *spherical* and rather smaller than bladder or vaginal epithelium. They may be seen isolated or in small groups. In acute nephritis they may be found in an unaltered condition, but in chronic disease they become degenerate, and may thus appear crowded with fat globules. BLADDER or VAGINAL EPITHELIUM (Fig. 121) is met with as collections of squamous cells; transitional, spindle-shaped and other forms of epithelium may also be derived from the bladder. TAILED EPITHELIUM may be derived from the pelvis

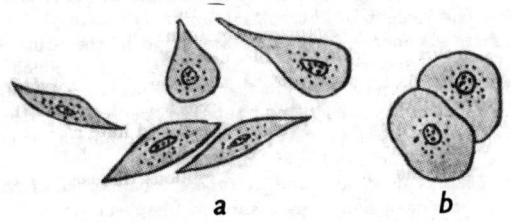

FIG. 121.—TAILED EPITHELIUM (*a*) from the pelvis of the kidney; and BLADDER EPITHELIAL CELLS (*b*).

of the kidney: the male urethra and the prostate gland yield epithelium practically identical with this.

Pus Cells, under the microscope, are of globular form with a diameter about one-third larger than that of a red blood cell: they are opaque and granular, but when treated with acetic acid they clear, and a nucleus is seen (Fig. 122, *d* and *e*). Pus cells may or may not accompany bacilli in the urine.

Red Blood Cells.—When only in small numbers, they may be seen microscopically, but do not give the chemical reactions (§ 382). In most fresh urines they are readily distinguished, as they retain their bi-concave form and the outline shows a double contour (Fig. 122, *a*). But sometimes

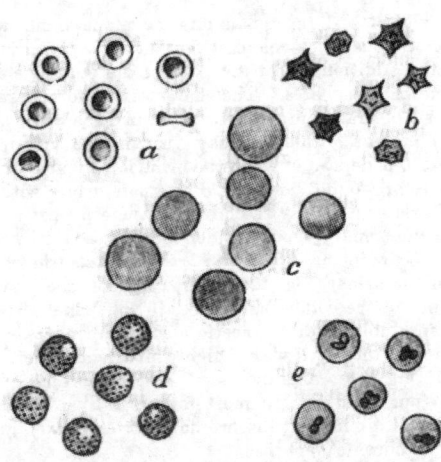

FIG. 122.—Various appearances of RED BLOOD CORPUSCLES and PUS CELLS in the URINE.—*a*, normal red blood corpuscles; *b*, crenated; *c*, in hypotonic solution; *d*, pus cells; *e*, pus cells + acetic acid. In very pale, watery urine the red corpuscles may be so pale as to escape detection (*c*). They may then be revealed by adding a solution of iodine in potassium iodide.

the cells become much changed. Thus in a very dilute urine they are apt to become distended by imbibition, and then are seen as circles having sharp delicate outlines (c). In other instances they become crenated, shrunken, and deformed (b).

Spermatozoa may occasionally be found in the urine. Each has a minute oval or pear-shaped head, from the larger extremity of which there passes a long and delicate tail. The total measurement of the spermatozoon is about $\frac{1}{600}$ inch in length.

Micro-organisms.—Numerous organisms are found in the urine, especially when decomposition has occurred within the bladder. *E. coli* is much the commonest (§ 416); other organisms found are *B. proteus*, *B. pyocyaneus*, *B. subtilis*, streptococci, staphylococci, occasionally gonococci, and tubercle bacilli (see § 419). The *Typhoid bacillus* may be abundant in cases of typhoid fever, and long after health is restored it may remain a potent source of infection to others.

The *Tubercle bacillus* may be found in tuberculous disease of the bladder or of the kidney, and is therefore a sign of great value. In appearance under the microscope it resembles the smegma bacillus. Its presence should always be suspected when pus cells are abundant and yet the urine remains sterile on culture. Its special staining reaction is given in § 1202. It is difficult to find in the urine early in the disease and the deposit of a 24-hours specimen should be examined. In obscure cases a guinea pig should be inoculated or a culture made (§ 1203).

§ 393. **Crystalline and Inorganic Deposits** in urine are usually of less serious import than the organised substances above noted.

In ACID URINES we meet chiefly urates, uric acid, oxalates and, more rarely, stellar phosphates, cystine, xanthine, hippuric acid, tyrosine and leucin.

In neutral or ALKALINE URINES we meet chiefly triple phosphates (occasionally ammonium urate and calcium carbonate).

In urines of EITHER REACTION amorphous deposits of potassium or ammonium urate and phosphates and carbonates of the alkaline earths may be met.

1. URATES, chiefly of sodium, potassium or ammonium, when in excess are deposited as an amorphous brick-coloured deposit after the urine has become cold. On heating or on the addition of caustic potash, the deposit clears, both tests distinguishing urates from phosphates. The characteristic forms are shown in Fig. 123. An occasional deposit of urates in a concentrated urine is of no importance. When they are *constantly* present a calculus may form in the kidney or bladder.

2. FREE URIC ACID is deposited when the urine is very acid or poor in salts and in pigment, and is therefore found chiefly in dilute pale urines with deficiency of salts. The red deposit of uric acid closely resembles cayenne pepper to the naked eye. It may be detected in the urinary deposit under the microscope by the *colour* and *shape* of the crystals. It occurs in the form of *red-brown crystals* (the only coloured crystals commonly found in the urine) (Fig. 124). Uric acid assumes many different shapes, owing to the presence of the colloid substances in the urine. This deposit is soluble in caustic potash, insoluble in dilute acetic acid, the converse of phosphates.

In health, uric acid is increased with a highly nitrogenous diet, after much exercise, after meals, and during the " alkaline tide " of the morning. It is also increased after any excess of purine intake, in most fevers, in liver diseases, and during and after acute gout. It is diminished in chronic gout, especially just before the acute exacerbations and in chronic nephritis.

3. PHOSPHATES occur as a white deposit or flocculent turbidity in FEEBLY ACID, NEUTRAL or ALKALINE urine, in three different forms, which in order of frequency are (1) *Amorphous phosphates of calcium* form the thick white deposit that is apt to

be mistaken for pus, but which is more readily shaken up in the urine. These and all other phosphates are soluble in acetic acid (which distinguishes the deposit from pus). (2) *Triple phosphate* of ammonium and magnesium (Fig. 125) is found in urine which has undergone alkaline fermentation. In markedly ammoniacal urine " feathery phosphates " are found. (3) *Basic magnesium phosphate* occurs in large rhombic

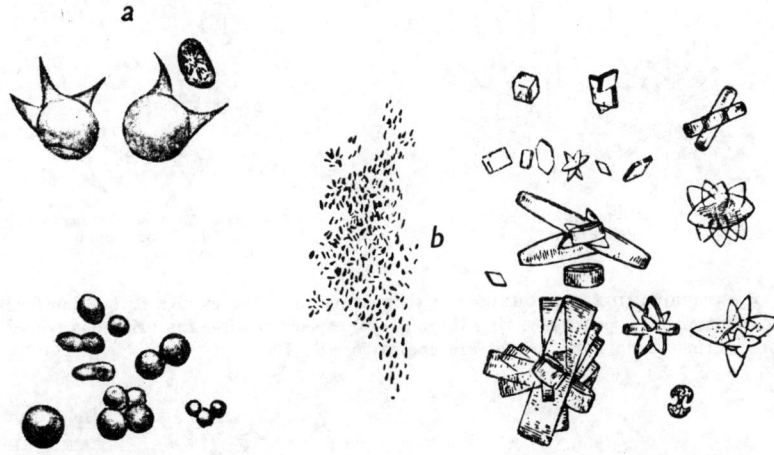

FIG. 123.—URATES.—*a*, " Hedgehog " crystals of sodium urate; *b*, amorphous urates; *c*, ammonium urate crystals (found in alkaline urine).

FIG. 124.—URIC ACID crystals (red-brown).—The two top rows show, from left to right, the evolution in a colloid medium of the "lozenge-shaped" crystal from the primary rhombic prism. In the lower right-hand corner is the "dumb-bell" form occasionally met.

plates, not grouped, but scattered. (4) *Neutral or dicalcium phosphate* occurs in neutral or alkaline urine as " stellar phosphates " (Fig. 126). They decompose on the addition of ammonia. The constant presence of phosphate deposits may be

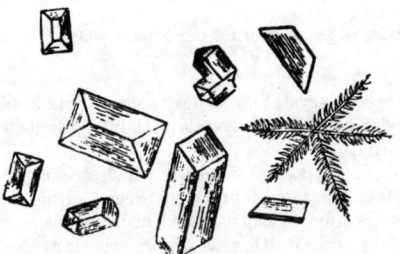

FIG. 125.—TRIPLE PHOSPHATE—" house-top " and " feathery " crystals.

associated with symptoms of phosphaturia (§ 431), and usually does not indicate excess eliminated, but only alkalinity of the urine. *Monocalcium phosphate* occurs chiefly in acid urines.

4. OXALATES are chiefly met as *calcium oxalate* (Fig. 127). They are soluble in hydrochloric acid, insoluble in acetic acid or caustic potash. The presence of crystals

of calcium oxalate is not necessarily indicative of an excess (OXALURIA, § 431); their presence may suggest the nature of a calculus.

5. *Calcium Carbonate* is a rare deposit, consisting of tiny spheres and dumb-bells, or of amorphous granules, effervescing and dissolving in acetic acid. The *Carbonates of the Alkaline Earths* are rarely found.

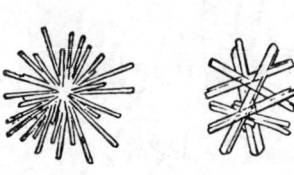

FIG. 126.—NEUTRAL OR "STELLAR" PHOSPHATE.

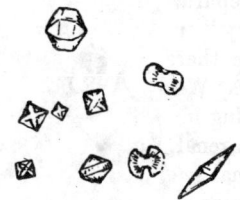

FIG. 127.—CALCIUM OXALATE— " envelope " and " dumb- bell " crystals.

6. SULPHONAMIDE COMPOUNDS and their acetyl derivatives in a crystalline form are common in patients receiving these drugs, especially after the urine has cooled. Some forms which may be met are shown in Fig. 128.

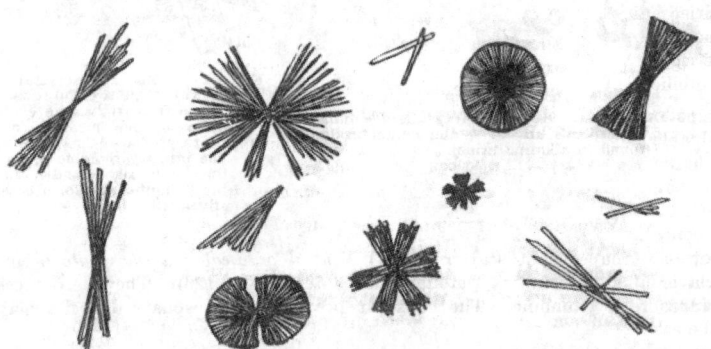

FIG. 128.—CRYSTALS OF SULPHONAMIDE COMPOUNDS which may be found in urine (Prof. R. J. Harrison).

When a patient is taking crystalline drugs, such as potassium acetate and sodium phosphate, or even liquor ammoniæ, crystals without pathological significance some-times appear in the urine.

7. *Certain rare and less important deposits*, which occur only in acid urines, are as follows: *Hippuric Acid* occurs as four-sided prisms, either scattered or in groups. It is present after the ingestion of benzoic acid in large doses, cranberries, and other fruits. *Calcium Sulphate* occurs either as amorphous granules, or, very rarely, as long colourless needles or elongated tables with truncated ends. It is detected by being insoluble in ammonia and acids. *Cholesterol* (Fig. 113) is rare among urinary deposits. It forms laminated plates with longitudinal striæ, and a notch at one end. *Cystine* occurs as hexagonal plates soluble in ammonia in large amount in congenital cystinuria.

PHYSICAL EXAMINATION OF THE KIDNEYS

§ 394. A dull " sickening " pain is usually felt on firmly compressing the kidney with both hands, but there is no tenderness in a healthy organ. Tenderness may be elicited in cases of calculus and other forms of pyelitis, perinephric inflammation, abscess, or tumour of the organ, and in " dropped kidney " in neurotic subjects. Kidney tumours tend to grow forwards, where there is least resistance, pushing the resonant colon *in front* of them. When, therefore, the palpating hand encounters resistance and swelling in the lumbar region *posteriorly*, it is probably due to a peri- or extra-renal, rather than to a renal condition (see Fig. 50). The diagnosis of renal swellings from other abdominal tumours has been given in § 263. An extra-renal tumour may press the kidney backwards, so that the apex of the tumour may be due to the displaced kidney.

In the majority of renal disorders the physical examination of the kidney is of secondary importance to the examination of the urine. The kidneys are situated on either side of the spine, about 3 inches from the middle line; the right is slightly lower than the left, owing to the position of the liver just above it. The upper end of the right kidney reaches to the *lower* edge of the eleventh rib; the left kidney reaches as high as the *upper* edge of the eleventh rib. The kidneys lie partly in the hypochondriac and partly in the lumbar regions, and are therefore much higher than is commonly supposed, in relation to the anterior abdominal wall. The lower end of the right kidney is 1 inch and that of the left kidney 1½ inches *above* the level of the umbilicus.

Palpation.—Even in normal conditions the lower border of the right kidney may be palpable in thin people. In those whose abdominal walls are lax—in women who have borne children, for instance—it is surprising how frequently the right kidney can be palpated. The patient should lie on the back, with the abdominal muscles relaxed. The physician, standing on the right of the patient, should place his left hand beneath the patient's back, close under the ribs, just external to the quadratus lumborum. The right hand is laid flat over the anterior surface of the abdomen, in the mid-clavicular line, with the fingers pointing upwards, just below the liver. Pressure backwards, as if to meet the left hand, is made by the right hand. The patient should then be asked to draw a deep breath, and as he does so the rounded lower edge of the kidney is felt to slip between the opposing hands. When the ligaments of the kidney are relaxed—*movable kidney*—the fingers of the right hand may be able to palpate the upper border of the organ, and to retain it during expiration. A kidney is said to be " *floating* " when it can not only be readily palpated, but can be pushed below the umbilicus or freely moved about in the abdominal cavity.

Percussion does not enable us to define the margins of the kidney, for the organ is too deeply seated. The feature of primary importance in this connection is its relation to the colon, which is pushed forward by enlargement or tumour of the kidney. Consequently the anterior surface of such growths is always resonant, there being dullness at the side which is continuous with that at the back; whereas with enlargements of the spleen or gall-bladder there is dullness anteriorly and resonance at the side.

Radiography is often of great help. In cases of doubtful renal calculus a *radiogram* usually settles the diagnosis. By *pyelography* an outline of the pelves of the kidneys, and of the ureters can be obtained. In retrograde pyelography, a 10–15 per cent. solution of potassium iodide is injected through a ureteric catheter, and on X-ray examination an opaque shadow is thrown where the solution has penetrated (Fig. 131). With *excretion urography* diodone B.P. (35, 50 or 70 per cent.) or sodium diatrizoate (Hypaque) are injected intravenously in doses of 20 ml. and X-ray

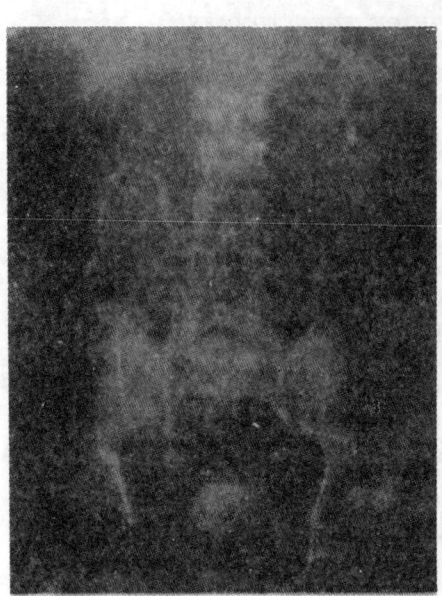

FIG. 129.—NORMAL RETROGRADE PYELOGRAPHY

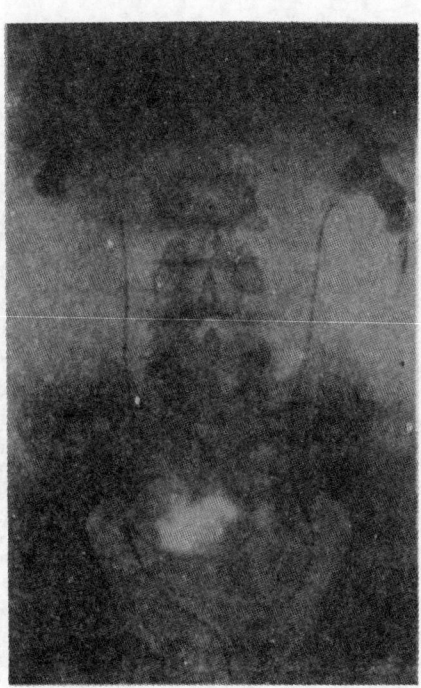

FIG. 130.—LARGE BILATERAL BRANCHED RENAL CALCULI (" coral calculi "), with ureteric catheters in position.

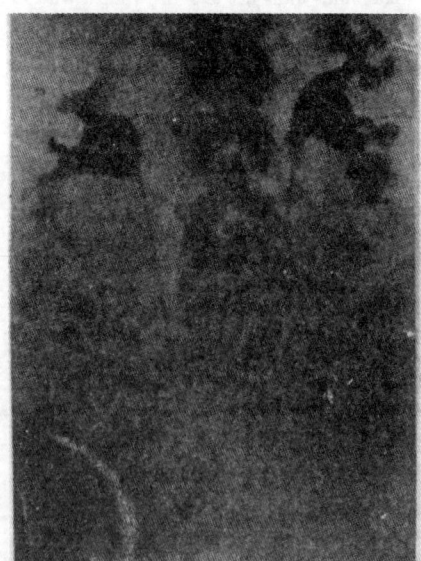

FIG. 131.—BILATERAL POLYCYSTIC KIDNEYS, demonstrated by retrograde pyelography. (X-Rays kindly supplied by Dr. J. Russell-Reynolds.)

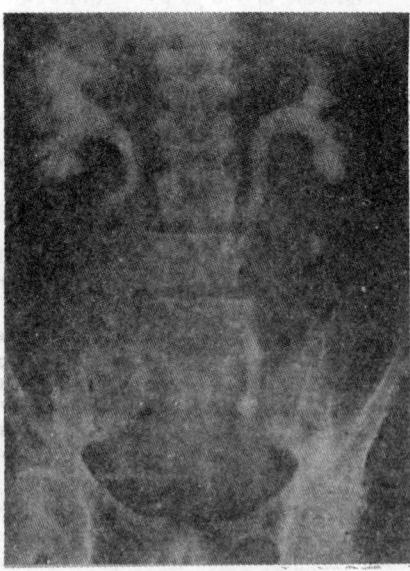

FIG. 132.—BILATERAL HYDRONEPHROSIS in a child, with demonstration of renal pelves with iodoxylum (excretion urography).

examination 5, 10, 30 and 50 minutes later gives information as to the secreting power of the kidneys and a picture of the outline of the whole renal tract (Fig. 129). Care must be taken that no drop enters the tissues around the vein.

Cystoscopy reveals the condition of the bladder and of the ureteric orifices: the orifices may be the seat of congestion or ulceration. The previous injection of indigo-carmine or methylene blue may make the differences of the flow from the orifices more obvious (*chromo-cystoscopy*). Through the cystoscope the ureters may be catheterised and a separate specimen of urine obtained from each kidney.

Perirenal Insufflation of the kidneys and suprarenals is performed by inserting a needle through the sacro-coccygeal foramen into the pre-sacral fascia. One litre of oxygen is slowly injected; about 30 minutes later it has ascended to the perirenal fascia when plain or tomographic X-rays will reveal the kidneys and suprarenals.

Aortography is performed by injecting diodone into the aorta via a needle or via a catheter inserted into the femoral artery. The renal arteries and their branches are clearly seen in serial films. The method is not without danger.

Renal Biopsy under a local anæsthetic permits a small portion of kidney substance to be obtained through a needle, for subsequent histological examination. An intra-venous pyelogram helps to locate the exact position of the kidney beforehand.

PART C.   *URINARY DISORDERS, THEIR DIAGNOSIS, PROGNOSIS AND TREATMENT*

§ 395. Routine Procedure and Classification.—*First*, having ascertained that the patient's LEADING SYMPTOM refers to the kidneys or renal passages; and, *secondly*, the data of his ILLNESS, particularly as to whether it is of an ACUTE or CHRONIC nature; we proceed, *thirdly*, to examine the urine. The ROUTINE EXAMINATION of the URINE in everyday practice consists of Inspection, Reaction, Specific Gravity, Tests for Albumen and for Sugar. The subsequent more detailed examination depends upon circumstances. As stated, the examination of the urine stands, in relation to renal disease, as the local signs do to diseases of other organs. Few diseases, certainly no common disorders of the kidneys, are unattended by some change in the urine. On the other hand, the LOCAL EXAMINATION of the kidney, by palpation, percussion and by radiography, is more difficult, but should never be omitted in any case which is at all obscure.

Classification.—We will deal with urinary disorders under their respective cardinal symptoms as follows:

§ 396. Albuminuria (proteinuria) occurs especially when a greatly increased amount of albumen is filtered through diseased glomeruli or when there is a rise in the renal venous pressure.

Protein passes through the normal glomerular membrane in amounts up to 200 mg. per 100 ml.; this is completely absorbed in the normal proximal convoluted tubules after being broken down by the tubular cells to amino-acids.

The causes come under these groups:

A. The ALBUMEN is ASSOCIATED with BLOOD and CASTS and the disease is **acute**: Acute nephritis (§ 397).

There is marked ALBUMINURIA and SUPPRESSION OF URINE; the disease may be Acute Tubular Necrosis (§ 428).

B. The ALBUMEN is PERSISTENT and is ASSOCIATED with CASTS; BLOOD is present microscopically, and ŒDEMA may be marked; the disease is **subacute**: Subacute parenchymatous nephritis: § 398.

(a) With marked œdema.
(b) Without marked œdema.

C. The ALBUMEN is ASSOCIATED with CASTS; BLOOD is USUALLY ABSENT and the disease is **chronic**: § 399.

D. The ALBUMEN is NOT USUALLY ASSOCIATED with CASTS or BLOOD; it may be INTERMITTENT, and the condition is usually **chronic**— I. physiological; II. orthostatic; III. kyphotic; IV. toxæmic; V. pregnancy; VI. drugs; VII. endogenous poisons; VIII. mild renal congestion; IX. chronic gout and arteriosclerosis; X. urinary calculi and crystals; XI. leaky kidney or residual albuminuria; XII. anæmia; XIII. obscure causes (§ 410).

E. The ALBUMEN is ASSOCIATED with BLOOD, and CASTS are SCANTY or ABSENT—Hæmaturia (§§ 411–412).

F. The ALBUMEN is ASSOCIATED with PUS—Pyuria (§ 416).

A. *The illness came on recently and is* **acute**; *the urine contains a considerable quantity of* ALBUMEN *and* TUBE-CASTS: *it is or has been* " SMOKY " *from the presence of blood.   The disease is* ACUTE NEPHRITIS.

§ 397. Acute Nephritis (Synonym: Acute glomerulo-tubular nephritis; formerly called Acute Bright's Disease).—In this disease the inflammation begins and predominates in the glomeruli and to a less extent in the tubules (the parenchyma) of the organ. The condition usually lasts five or six weeks, and may terminate in recovery or pass into a subacute condition. The disease exists in two forms: (*a*) acute diffuse glomerulo-tubular nephritis; (*b*) acute focal glomerulo-tubular nephritis.

(*a*) **Acute diffuse glomerulo-tubular nephritis** (Ellis type I) is due to an intoxication of the kidney, usually one to three weeks after an acute hæmolytic streptococcal infection. The diffuse involvement causes temporary renal failure.

Symptoms.—(1) The albumen is often in considerable quantity, and the urine may even " go solid " on boiling. (2) The other characters of the urine are: (i.) It is scanty, sometimes only 10 or 20 fl. oz. a day, or less. Consequently, the specific gravity is high, although the diurnal quantity of urea is diminished. (ii.) It varies from a turbid or " smoky " to a dark brown hue from the presence of blood. (iii.) Epithelial, red cell and granular casts, free renal epithelium, and red and white blood-corpuscles are present. (3) Œdema is usually moderate in extent and severity, and is first noticed in the loose areolar tissue below the eyes, in the legs and back and in the genitals. There may be collections of œdematous fluid in the serous cavities. (4) There is a waxy pallor of the skin. (5) A degree of malaise, with discomfort and even pain in the loins or abdomen, may be present, but there is only a slight elevation of temperature for about four or five days: mild anæmia is common. (6) Uræmic symptoms may come on early—*e.g.*, (i.) occasional vomiting, (ii.) headache, (iii.) drowsiness, (iv.) some shortness of breath, (v.) the blood urea is often raised. (7) In the course of a few days the blood pressure may become high, and the second aortic sound accentuated.

Etiology.—(1) Acute infection is the commonest cause. The microorganism is usually the streptococcus hæmolyticus, commonly found in the tonsils, rarely in the respiratory passages, nasal sinuses or middle ear, or in the skin (*e.g.*, erysipelas). This explains its common occurrence with scarlet fever. Other acute infections are influenza, typhoid, malaria, cerebro-spinal fever, staphylococcal infection and trench fever. (2) Hidden foci of sepsis, cholecystitis, empyema, etc. (3) Sudden chill may predispose. (4) A family tendency is common.

No organisms are found in the renal lesions; the condition is thought to be due to a chemical substance released by the hæmolytic streptococci causing an antigen-antibody reaction in the glomeruli.

Prognosis.—Acute nephritis will terminate (1) usually in complete recovery in a few weeks, when treatment and hygienic surroundings are good (80 per cent. of cases). This is usual with children; with adults complete recovery is not so common, unless the original focus of infection rapidly subsides. (2) Partial recovery. If the disease lasts longer than two months, it develops into the condition known as large white kidney (Subacute Parenchymatous Nephritis, § 398). (3) Death may occur from uræmia, from œdema into the serous cavities, or from other complications. The chief *complications* are: (a) Uræmia; (b) hypertensive encephalopathy; (c) inflammations of the *serous* membranes, such as pleurisy, pericarditis, or peritonitis, which are usually latent—*i.e.*, attended by little or no pain; and (d) infections of the *mucous* membranes, such as bronchitis, bronchopneumonia, gastro-enteritis; (e) œdema of the lungs or of the glottis; (f) cardiac dilatation and left ventricular failure with pulmonary œdema; (g) erysipelas, cellulitis and various other *skin diseases* are very prone to attack patients with acute nephritis. The prognosis, therefore, of acute nephritis is grave in proportion to (i.) the persistence of œdema, oliguria, gross albuminuria, and hypertension beyond two weeks; (ii.) the development of uræmic symptoms; and (iii.) the nature and severity of the complications.

Treatment.—The indications are to relieve the kidney by giving it as little to do as possible during the acute stage; a chart of the fluid intake and output each twenty-four hours should be kept and the blood pressure recorded regularly. (i.) The diet should be salt-free, low in its protein content, and consist at first of 1½–2 pints of fluid daily, with added glucose (see diet in § 296, VII, Stage I) unless the blood urea is over 100 mg. per cent., when more fluid is essential. After 3–4 days the hæmaturia has often diminished, the blood pressure fallen, and the volume of urine increased (" critical diuresis "), when further quantities of fluid and more carbohydrate may be added (Stage II). About the 10th–14th day it is usually possible to give a still more liberal diet (Stage III). It is unwise to restrict the diet for too long a period as this undermines the patient's resistance. (ii.) Penicillin is required to combat the infection, initially by injection and then in a suitable form by further injections or orally. (iii.) To obviate the danger from exposure to cold, the patient must be kept strictly confined to bed till all red blood cells have disappeared from the urine. Cases of scarlet fever should be kept in bed during convalescence, because they are so apt to develop this disease. Mild purgatives are useful when there is much œdema. Diuretics are contra-indicated in the early stage and mersalyl should certainly be used with caution. Alkalies such as sodium or potassium bicarbonate or citrate may be given to prevent an acid urine still further damaging the inflamed renal epithelium. (iv.) Local counter-irritation over the kidneys, with kaolin poultices is indicated when the volume of urine is low. Digitalis can be given if the heart is feeble. During *convalescence*, tonics, especially iron, must be given. For the treatment of Uræmia, see § 372.

In scarlet fever albuminuria frequently comes on between the sixteenth and twenty-sixth day, at which time also acute nephritis may supervene. To avoid this risk, scarlet fever patients should be kept in bed a month, and the urine kept alkaline (Osman).

(b) **Acute focal glomerulo-tubular nephritis** arises during the height of the acute stage of an infection, again usually due to streptococcus hæmolyticus. Only a certain number of the glomeruli are involved; probably the micro-organisms produce minute emboli in them, and so signs of renal failure are usually absent.

Symptoms.—(1) The condition is commonest in children. (2) Hæmaturia and cylinduria are present; the bleeding may be profuse; the amount of albumen is such as can be accounted for by the bleeding, or little in excess of this. (3) Dull aching in the loins is common. (4) There is no renal failure; symptoms and signs of uræmia are absent, there is no œdema, no rise in the blood urea or blood-pressure. (5) Relapse may occur with recurrence of the original infection. The *prognosis* is usually excellent; chronic nephritis ensues rarely. The *treatment* is as for the diffuse variety, except that there is no need for restriction of fluids, and not so much need to restrict the protein.

B. *The* ALBUMEN *is* PERSISTENT *and is* ASSOCIATED WITH CASTS; BLOOD *is present microscopically* and ŒDEMA MAY BE PRESENT; *the disease is* Subacute parenchymatous Nephritis.

§ 398. When the symptoms and signs of acute nephritis do not subside within 6–8 weeks, the disease has entered the subacute phase. A large number of patients are first seen at this stage, occasionally because they have neglected to obtain advice, or more usually because there is no initial acute infection and the disease has been insidious from the commencement. There are two extremes of this clinical condition: (*a*) In the usual variety œdema is the most prominent feature; (*b*) in rare cases œdema may be largely absent: intermediate cases are often seen. In either case, if the disease persists, it usually passes into the stage of secondary contracted kidney (§ 400).

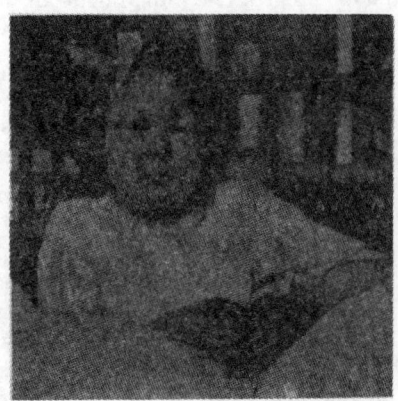

FIG. 133.—A case of Subacute Nephritis with Anasarca.

(*a*) *The illness has been present for two or more months, and the general symptoms of renal disease pronounced;* GENERALISED ŒDEMA IS MARKED, *the* URINE SCANTY, *and* ALBUMEN *and* CASTS ARE ABUNDANT. *The disease is* SUBACUTE PARENCHYMATOUS NEPHRITIS (nephrotic type).

Subacute Parenchymatous Nephritis (synonyms: Large White Kidney, Subacute Glomerulo-tubular nephritis, Ellis type II, formerly called Chronic Parenchymatous Nephritis) usually develops insidiously.

Symptoms.—(1) The albuminuria is considerable, and often reaches 2·0–3·0 G. per cent.: the daily loss may be 20–30 G. (2) The other characters of the urine are: (i.) the diurnal quantity is diminished, (ii.) the specific gravity tends to be high, (iii.) it is often turbid with urates, (iv.) all forms of casts are met (§ 392), (v.) blood is rarely absent but is usually only detected microscopically: relapses temporarily increase the amount of blood. (3) Generalised œdema is *the* prominent clinical feature. At first it is most marked in the face, giving a general puffiness: soon it appears in all the loose cellular tissues of the body, and the serous cavities become involved, causing a generalised collection of tissue-fluid (anasarca). The amount of œdema varies at different times, so that the patient may lose or gain many pounds in weight in the course of a few weeks. (4) A marked degree of anæmia is present sooner or later, the hæmoglobin falling to ½–¼ the usual values. (5) Lassitude and digestive disorders are common. (6) The blood pressure and the blood urea are normal or very little raised. (7) The plasma albumen is markedly lowered (to 1·0–2·0 G. per cent.) while the plasma globulin is raised, giving an albumen/globulin ratio around or below 1·0 : 1·0; the blood cholesterol is high. (8) After many months the œdema may subside. It is rare for the condition to be cured: more often the blood pressure and the blood urea are found to increase simultaneously with the disappearance of the œdema, renal function tests show progressive impairment of function, and the condition becomes chronic (secondary contracted kidney).

(b) *The illness is subacute, the urine containing* ALBUMEN, TUBE CASTS *and* RED CELLS: *the patient is* PALE, *shows occasional* PUFFINESS OF THE FACE, *and renal function tests show* PROGRESSIVE IMPAIRMENT OF RENAL FUNCTION. *The disease is* SUBACUTE NEPHRITIS WITHOUT MARKED ŒDEMA.

This variety is more commonly overlooked than the nephrotic variety, on account of the slight degree of œdema. The *symptoms* are: (1) The urine invariably contains a small quantity of albumen, and hyaline and granular casts. Microscopically, red cells are almost invariably present, indicating that the inflammatory process is still active. (2) Periodically, slight œdema may appear, especially in the face. (3) Symptoms of general debility, lassitude, anæmia, and headaches are present. (4) The blood pressure is raised, the systolic pressure being commonly 20–50 mm. above normal. (5) The blood urea is raised and kidney efficiency tests give a poor result. (6) The nephrotic type may supervene later.

Etiology of Subacute Nephritis.—The cause is usually not known. However carefully a septic focus is sought, according to Ellis it is rarely found. The insidious onset over a period of weeks or months makes the search more difficult. The average age of onset is later than in the acute varieties. Occasionally tertiary syphilis is causal.

Several factors cause œdema. The glomerular damage allows an increased amount of albumen to filter through the glomeruli, resulting in hypoproteinæmia. Due to loss of osmotic pressure in the plasma more fluid then passes into the tissue-spaces. Sodium retention also follows the glomerular damage and is accentuated by the increased reabsorption in the distal convoluted tubules under the influence of the adrenal cortical hormones (especially aldosterone).

Diagnosis of Subacute Nephritis.—When the insidious form occurs in young women it is often mistaken for *simple anæmia*; in all such cases, examine the urine for albumen and tube casts. In the later stages it may be mistaken for *chronic interstitial nephritis*; but in that disease the patient is usually older, and see Table XXIII (p. 567). In certain cases which present *both renal and cardiac symptoms*, it may be very difficult to say *which condition is the primary* one.[1]   In such cases it is important to note the following points: (i.) If there is a *history* of rheumatic fever and previous attacks of œdema, it is probable that the cardiac condition is primary. (ii.) The presence of *other than mitral* systolic murmurs points to cardiac disease; a mitral regurgitation murmur *alone* might be due to the cardiac failure following renal disease.   (iii.) The *urine*, when there is any difficulty in diagnosis, is in both cases scanty and albuminous.   Many tube-casts, and an appreciably raised blood urea, point to renal disease; the rapid clearing up of the œdema and improvement of the urine after a short period of rest in bed points to heart disease.   (iv.) A *hard pulse* favours kidney disease, but an irregular soft pulse is found with cardiac failure secondary both to renal and to cardiac disease.   Widespread œdema in undernourished children in the tropics is caused by kwashiorkor (§ 29).

Prognosis.—It is rare for the disease to be arrested, but the prognosis is better in the non-œdematous variety and has been improved by modern methods of treatment.   It is not uncommon for acute relapses to occur. A useful guide to the prognosis is furnished by successive renal function tests every six months.   Death occurs with complications of uræmia, or as with acute nephritis.   The prognosis is grave in proportion to (1) the amount of œdema and albuminuria; (2) diminution of urine and of nitrogen excretion; (3) the height of the blood pressure.   When this rises progressively the outlook is grave, whereas if the pressure remains the same or falls, the prognosis improves correspondingly.   (4) Uræmic symptoms. *Complications* such as infections, pleural effusions and pulmonary œdema add to the gravity of the case.   When the stage of contraction sets in, life may be prolonged with care.

Treatment.—So long as subacute inflammation is present, the patient should be confined to bed, and this is essential when œdema is present. The main objects are to reduce or abolish œdema, to relieve the kidneys as far as possible and to prevent complications.   (i.) *Œdema* is best controlled by tab. prednisolone in full doses.   For the first 10 days the adult dose is 40 mg. a day, followed for the next 10 days by 20 mg. a day, after which the dose should be reduced to 5–10 mg. a day for a period of months. On this regime it is usual (but not invariable) to obtain a marked diuresis which commences on the 10th–14th day, and with this the amount of protein lost in the urine is greatly reduced.   The loss of œdema fluid causes the loss of many pounds in weight but as the body tissues are replenished in protein and fat a gradual gain in weight then occurs.   During this intensive steroid therapy the plasma potassium often falls; this must be checked by periodic plasma estimations and by giving potassium chloride in a capsule t.d.s.   In the place of prednisolone some prefer corresponding doses of a long-acting, ACTH preparation by injection.   (ii.) *Penicillin*

---

[1] It is well to bear in mind that when both cardiac and renal disease are present, they may be associated in three ways: (a) Cardiac disease may produce renal disease (§ 410. VIII).   (b) Renal disease may produce cardiac disease, as when acute or chronic nephritis lead to cardiac hypertrophy and failure.   (c) They may both be the result of a common cause—*e.g.*, gout.

or some other antibiotic should be given each day to prevent and to control infections which are much more likely to occur when giving these large doses of steroids. Septic foci must be searched for and carefully removed. The author has had encouraging results from penicillin therapy alone, even when a definite focus of infection cannot be found: but the penicillin must be given within 2 weeks of the onset of clinical symptoms. (iii.) *Diet.* When oedema is present, the kidneys find it difficult to secrete sodium chloride and water, and an enormous amount of albumen (often 10–25 G. daily) is lost in the urine. The rational line of therapy is to limit the amount of fluid ingested to that which the kidneys can secrete per day, and to avoid salt as far as possible. A salt-substitute (such as Neoselarom) may be used instead. Once the gross oedema has been overcome the protein intake should be of a high order, and this is of additional value for the urea so produced is a valuable diuretic (Maclean). · A diet meeting these needs is given (§ 296, VII B). If benefit is to be obtained with such a diet it should show itself in 6–8 weeks, and it is useless to continue it otherwise. In this case an ordinary diet can be resumed, with some restriction of total fluid and salt intake. It is unwise to use a high-protein diet if the blood urea is already raised, and in any case weekly blood urea estimations are desirable: in these circumstances the Karell diet is often used (§ 296, VII. B). When there is little or no oedema, these strict diets are unnecessary and may be harmful by lowering the patient's resistance. The Stage III diet of acute nephritis is then useful. (iv.) Pleural effusions and acute pulmonary oedema should be watched for and the usual remedies given. (v.) In cases which do not respond to the steroids, hydrochlorothiazide in full doses (50 mg. once or twice a day) together with potassium chloride, or chlorthalidone (Hygroton) may aid diuresis and do not produce toxic effects on the kidneys. Thyroid gr. 3–5 a day may help to reduce oedema. If fluid-retention still persists, in the more chronic stages, intramuscular injections of mersalyl are now used more freely than was once thought possible; the toxic effects on the renal tubules are usually transitory, but need careful watching. This drug must never be given intravenously in nephritis, for in cases with a low plasma albumen sudden myocardial failure may occur. (vi.) To prevent further renal damage, chill and exposure must be avoided, the bowels regulated, and all alcohol forbidden. (vii.) Although concentrated plasma transfusions are usually disappointing in that the transfused protein is rapidly eliminated, when anæmia is severe a blood transfusion is often helpful.

Nephrosis is a term used to describe a special type of parenchymatous nephritis. The essential lesion is a lipoid degeneration of the kidney tubules, without any signs of inflammation. Thus, in addition to marked oedema and albuminuria, there is hypercholesteræmia and hypothyroidism: but there are no cardio-vascular changes nor is there any nitrogen retention. At autopsy, the masses of lipoid in the tubules form the so-called " myelin " deposits.

C. *The* ALBUMEN *is* ASSOCIATED WITH CASTS. BLOOD *is usually* ABSENT *and the condition is* CHRONIC. *The disease is* CHRONIC NEPHRITIS.

§ 399. There are three common and two less common varieties of chronic renal disease attended with more or less albuminuria, which, when occurring in their typical forms, present well-marked clinical distinctions, as shown in tabular form on p. 567. (I.) In the condition of SECONDARY CONTRACTED KIDNEY, we are dealing with the end result of progressive acute and subacute nephritis with gradual destruction of the kidneys and replacement by fibrous tissue. (II.) In CHRONIC INTERSTITIAL NEPHRITIS there is no such history of previous acute or subacute nephritis; the onset is usually insidious, hypertension and arterial disease are often marked, and pathologically there is found considerable increase in the interstitial tissue of the kidneys and hyperplasia of the middle coats of the arteries. (III) CHRONIC PYELONEPHRITIS is often difficult to distinguish clinically from chronic interstitial nephritis but it is a common cause of renal failure. Hypertension may or may not be present but anæmia is common. The two less common varieties are (IV.) DIABETIC NEPHRITIS which arises in long-standing diabetics who develop a considerable degree of albuminuria in association with arteriosclerotic changes elsewhere in the body. (V.) In the AMYLOID (Waxy) Kidney the vessels are primarily involved, the lardaceous degeneration beginning in the middle coat. Pathologists make many sub-divisions, but these represent the five clinically recognisable groups of chronic renal changes attended by albuminuria.

Following an attack of ACUTE *or* SUBACUTE NEPHRITIS *the patient complains of the symptoms of* INCIPIENT URÆMIA. *There is a small quantity of* ALBUMEN, POLYURIA *is present,* ŒDEMA *is slight or absent. The condition is one of* SECONDARY CONTRACTED KIDNEY.

§ 400. I. Secondary Contracted Kidney (Synonym: Chronic Diffuse Nephritis). *Symptoms:* (1) Urinary changes: (i.) diminution of the large amount of albumen which was present in the early stage; (ii.) the volume of the urine rises; (iii.) the specific gravity falls, and the urea content is considerably reduced. (2) The œdema disappears as the diurnal quantity of the urine increases. (3) The blood urea and the blood pressure rise progressively, and the left ventricle hypertrophies. (4) In the terminal stage of renal failure the urinary volume falls and uræmic symptoms ensue. In children a condition of renal rickets may accompany this form of nephritis. The treatment is as for chronic interstitial nephritis.

§ 401. II. Chronic Interstitial Nephritis used to be regarded as a single clinical entity, but now different varieties are becoming recognised. It is convenient to reserve this term for a composite group of cases distinguished by *persistent albuminuria* and *cylindruria*, often with hypertension, in which the progressive renal destruction is not due to a previous attack of acute or subacute nephritis. In one variety the primary cause is arterial disease associated with hypertension, benign or malignant, and recent experimental and clinical evidence regards the chronic renal destruction as being due to the diminution of blood supply to the kidneys. In another variety the kidneys are primarily at fault, due to congenital or acquired lesions: here the renal destruction often causes the liberation of a pressor substance which produces hypertension, the resultant arterial disease causing a " vicious circle." The clinical symptoms produced in these different types are influenced in part by the age of the patient, as when chronic nephritis causes renal rickets and renal dwarfism. A classification which includes most of these forms of chronic interstitial nephritis is:—

Chronic Nephritis develops in a *middle-aged* or *elderly patient* suffering from *hypertension* (hypertensive nephritis).

(a) Benign hypertension (Benign Nephrosclerosis).

(b) Malignant hypertension (Malignant Nephrosclerosis).

Chronic Nephritis occurs in a *young person*, previously in good health, and *may* or *may not* be associated with *hypertension*. It is probably due to some congenital abnormality in the kidneys (renal dysbiotrophy).

(c) Chronic type.

(d) Rose Bradford type with acute symptoms.

or Chronic Nephritis occurs in a *young or middle-aged person* as a result of a *congenital cystic defect* (Congenital Cystic Kidneys). § 432, V.

(e) Chronic Nephritis occurs as a result of renal destruction by other causes, *e.g.*, renal calculus, hydronephrosis, an enlarged prostate.

The patient is MIDDLE-AGED OR ELDERLY *and has suffered from* BENIGN HYPERTENSION *for years. The* DIURNAL QUANTITY OF URINE *increases, and* ALBUMINURIA *and* CASTS *appear: later signs of* INCIPIENT URÆMIA *develop. The disease is* CHRONIC NEPHRITIS *with* BENIGN HYPERTENSION.

§ 402. II(a). **Benign Nephrosclerosis.**—BENIGN HYPERTENSION is a condition which for long periods is non-progressive, or very slowly progressive, and associated in the majority of cases with no renal changes and no albuminuria (§ 96). In a small number of cases, albuminuria and casts appear later, due probably to renal arteriosclerosis.

Symptoms.—(1) The symptoms of benign hypertension are fully described in § 96. When impairment of kidney function follows (i.) the albuminuria is small in amount, and many samples of urine may be examined without finding any. In cold weather, however, when there is deficient skin action, there is generally a trace, especially after a chill or any cause which produces renal congestion. The other characters of the urine are: (ii.) The diurnal quantity is increased (perhaps to 100 fl. oz.). The patient has to get up at night several times to pass large quantities of water. (iii.) The specific gravity is low (1002 to 1010), owing chiefly to the increased quantity of urine. (iv.) The urine is clear, pale, and contains but few casts, and these are chiefly hyaline or granular (Fig. 119). (2) Œdema is usually absent, when it occurs it is due to secondary cardiac failure. (3) The patient may look robust, but sometimes he has a greyish pallor. (4) The pulse indicates persistent high blood pressure, associated with hypertrophy of the left ventricle, and with a thickened condition of all the arteries. (5) There develops a condition of chronic or incipient uræmia (§ 371), due to the deficient elimination of nitrogenous and other substances.

Diagnosis.—Often the patient has been known to have hypertension for many years. Although degenerative retinal changes associated with retinal arteriosclerosis are found, *papillœdema is not present.*

Prognosis.—The disease is very slowly progressive, even when renal damage is present. The older the patient the better the outlook, and he is more likely to die of heart failure or apoplexy than of uræmia, even when renal disease is well established. With proper care and treatment, the patient may live for five or ten years. The amount of albumen is no criterion as regards prognosis in chronic interstitial, as it is in parenchymatous, nephritis.

The patient has suffered from HEADACHE *and other symptoms of* HYPERTENSION *for months or years.* VOMITING, PRECORDIAL PAIN *and* ALBUMINURIA *develop, with* PAPILLŒDEMA. *The disease is* CHRONIC NEPHRITIS *with* MALIGNANT HYPERTENSION (MALIGNANT NEPHROSCLEROSIS).

§ 403. II(*b*). Malignant Nephrosclerosis (Syn. Chronic Focal Glomerular Nephritis) is accompanied by widespread cardio-vascular changes. There is no history of antecedent acute or subacute nephritis; often the patient has been in normal health and not known to have hypertension before symptoms arise. In other cases there has been benign hypertension for years, the condition developing into malignant hypertension in the course of a few months (see § 96).

Symptoms.—(i.) Headache, especially on waking, with vomiting, is associated with attacks of precordial pain, breathlessness and nocturnal paroxysmal dyspnœa. An epileptiform convulsion may be the first symptom. (ii.) The blood pressure is very high, with figures of 240 mm. (systolic) and 130 mm. (diastolic) or more. A figure of 290/180 is not unusual in association with hypertensive cerebral attacks (§ 97). (iii.) The left ventricle is hypertrophied, the brachial and radial arteries contracted and hardened, and in the late stages stress and failure of the left ventricle are shown by attacks of œdema of the lungs, by tachycardia, premature beats, pulsus alternans and gallop rhythm. (iv.) Failing vision is due to changes in the fundus oculi: the fundi show papillœdema, contracted silver-wired arteries and patches of retinal degeneration, especially at the maculæ (§ 1132) and Plate XXI. Whereas in the early stages of malignant hypertension there is little evidence of renal damage, later this becomes a prominent feature; when this occurs, (v.) the specific gravity of the urine becomes more and more fixed around 1012, albuminuria is marked, and the urinary deposit contains some red and white blood cells, and a number of hyaline and granular casts; (vi.) the blood urea may be normal when the patient is first seen, but later rises to 300 mg. per cent. or more in spite of treatment; (vii.) symptoms of incipient uræmia become more marked, with loss of appetite and considerable loss of weight, thirst, impairment of mental and physical vigour, and tremor and twitchings of the muscles; hiccup is often very troublesome.

The *Diagnosis* depends on the very high blood pressure, the retinal changes (and especially the papillœdema), the moderate or considerable albuminuria and the absence of a previous history of nephritis. Hypersecretion of aldersterone may be confused with malignant nephrosclerosis.

Etiology.—(i.) The disease may occur at any age, but most often between 30 and 50 years of age. (ii.) A family history of hypertension is very common. The condition may be the result of a pheochromocytoma (§ 97).

Structural Pathology. (See § 95.) The kidneys are a little smaller than normal. There is fibrinoid necrosis especially of the afferent glomerular arterioles, with acute focal degeneration of the glomeruli, and severe degenerative changes in the tubules.

Prognosis.—The course of the disease is relatively rapid once the kidneys are involved; patients rarely live more than 1–2 years after diagnosis. The greater the degree of hypertension, of albuminuria and especially of papillœdema when first seen, the worse is the prognosis.

The patient, who is UNDER 30 YEARS OF AGE, *is found to have* ALBUMINURIA. *There is no previous history of acute or subacute nephritis.* HYPERTENSION *may or may not be present.* ANÆMIA *is common. The course of the disease is slow, but* URÆMIA *supervenes after a period of years. The disease is* CHRONIC NEPHRITIS *probably due to a* CONGENITAL DEFECT *in the kidneys.*

§ 404. II(c). Congenital Renal Defects with Nephritis.—This little-understood group has recently been separated from the heterogeneous group of chronic interstitial nephritis, and merits a separate description.

Symptoms.—(i.) The patient, who is usually 15–20 years of age, is found on routine examination to have chronic albuminuria. The amount of albumen is never large. The urine contains some red cells, and occasional granular and hyaline casts. (ii.) For months or years the patient may otherwise appear to be in perfect health, but sooner or later lassitude, attacks of pallor, and occasional headaches make their appearance. (iii.) A moderate or severe refractory anæmia may be the presenting symptom. (iv.) From the time the patient is first seen there is often polyuria, the renal function tests give a poor result, with deficient urea concentration and urea clearance, and often a blood urea raised above the normal. (v.) In some the blood pressure is raised, but it may be normal throughout. (vi.) In cases before puberty, signs of renal infantilism or of renal rickets (§ 608) may be present. (vii.) Secondary hyperparathyroidism sometimes occurs later.

Diagnosis.—In the earlier stages it may be difficult to distinguish postural or orthostatic albuminuria, especially as the amount of albumen in both cases is reduced by rest in bed. Impaired renal function tests prove the kidneys to be diseased. Sometimes only one kidney is affected —this becomes very shrunken, the opposite kidney being hypertrophied and healthy. This state of affairs is best revealed by intravenous or by ascending pyelography, or by renal biopsy.

Etiology.—These cases are believed to be due to an inborn tendency to renal degeneration (dysbiotrophy); rarely they are familial, and at autopsy it is not unusual to find such congenital abnormalities as double ureters. Chronic pyelonephritis is apt to be superimposed.

Prognosis.—The course is very slowly progressive, and it is common to find the patient living 5 to 10 years after the disease is discovered. It is often surprising how long a young person will live with a blood urea persistently raised at a level of 100 mg. per cent. or more. The rapidity of the renal failure is best judged by periodic renal function tests. When only one kidney is diseased, removal may effect a cure.

§ 405. II(d). *The patient is commonly* 15–26 YEARS OF AGE, *and has not previously suffered from acute or subacute nephritis.* He may be SUDDENLY TAKEN ILL *with* URÆMIA, *and is found to have a* VERY HIGH BLOOD PRESSURE. *The disease is probably* CHRONIC NEPHRITIS *(Rose Bradford type) with* SMALL WHITE KIDNEYS.

The cause is unknown, but it does not follow acute or subacute nephritis. It may be the result of unrecognised pyelonephritis in utero or in infancy. Often the first symptom is an attack of uræmia in an apparently healthy person. There is no œdema, the blood pressure is very high, the respiration assumes a hissing quality, and the urine is normal in quantity, of low specific gravity, with a few casts and more albumen than is met in the cases with red granular kidney.

§ 406. II(e). *A patient with* HYPERTENSION *and* ALBUMINURIA *also has symptoms of a* RENAL CALCULUS, HYDRONEPHROSIS, *or* OTHER DISEASE OF THE KIDNEYS. *The disease may be* CHRONIC NEPHRITIS *associated with a* SURGICAL KIDNEY LESION.

As already discussed in §§ 88, 95, any lesion of a kidney which produces chronic renal destruction may cause the liberation of a pressor substance which produces hypertension and subsequent chronic nephritis in the sound kidney. Such lesions are renal tuberculosis, renal calculus, hydronephrosis, or a renal tumour. When unilateral lesions are present, the progressive hypertension and the chronic nephritic lesions in the sound kidney may be controlled by surgical removal of the diseased kidney, and in certain cases the blood pressure may return to normal. In future it will therefore be necessary to investigate for these several conditions (*q.v.*) as part of the routine investigation of cases of hypertension and chronic nephritis.

A patient develops symptoms of INCIPIENT URÆMIA *and* HYPERTENSION *is sometimes a prominent feature; there may be a previous history of* PYELONEPHRITIS. *The disease is likely to be* CHRONIC PYELONEPHRITIS.

§ 407. III. Chronic Pyelonephritis is a common cause of renal disease, with a marked variation in the degree of renal failure from month to month. It occurs in younger women who may or may not give a history of recurrent pyelitis, especially with pregnancy, or in older men who have prostatic retention. When it occurs in children or adolescents a congenital renal defect may already exist. The disease affects one or both kidneys; the discovery of unilateral disease is usually made during the investigation of the cause of severe hypertension.

Symptoms vary considerably in different cases. They may be (i.) those of severe hypertension (§§ 96, 97); (ii.) those of unexplained anæmia which does not respond to the usual methods of treatment; (iii.) a history of previous attacks of pyelitis; (iv.) a tendency to puffiness of the face; (v.) polyuria and frequency of micturition are common. (vi.) Albuminuria is slight or absent and only becomes marked in the later stages, the urine may contain no casts or abnormal cells and be sterile on culture. (vii.) Terminal uræmia is usual.

Unusual symptoms are (viii.) renal rickets and renal infantilism: (ix.) episodic weakness or paralysis of the limbs due to excessive potassium loss (hypokalæmia): (x.) " salt-losing " nephritis with a low serum sodium content and a very low blood pressure (even pigmentation) which may closely mimic Addison's disease. (xi.) Nephro-calcinosis is sometimes found.

Diagnosis is by finding a raised blood urea or a defect in renal efficiency tests. In the earlier stages an intravenous pyelogram will reveal disease on one or both sides: the X-rays may show that one kidney is almost functionless while the opposite kidney is enlarged and secretes freely; or that the calyces of one part of a kidney are distorted and slightly hydro-nephrotic—this latter change may best be shown with a retrograde pyelogram. A renal biopsy is especially useful in confirming the diagnosis.

Etiology.—The cause is a recurrent infection of the kidney substance usually with *E. coli* but sometimes following other infections such as subacute bacterial endocarditis. The disease progresses insidiously months or years after the infection has disappeared. Apart from the cases of recurrent pyelitis in women, any cause of ascending infection in either sex may be causal, whether this be due to an enlarged prostate or uterus, diverticulitis or a neurogenic condition (and see § 419).

Structural Pathology.—The affected kidneys are greatly reduced in size by scarring. They show triangular areas of fibrosis with the bases attached to the renal capsule and the apices tapering to the renal medulla and pelvis. Confined to the fibrotic areas there is infiltration with plasma cells and lymphocytes. Intrarenal obstruction causes cyst-like distension of some of the renal tubules, which may resemble a miniature condition of hydronephrosis.

Prognosis.—The condition may exist for years but tends slowly to progress. The best results are obtained by removing a unilaterally diseased kidney, discovered in the course of investigation of severe hypertension, but even in these cases a complete cure is unusual. When hypertension co-exists the progress of renal failure is usually more rapid.

A patient who has had DIABETES *for years develops* ALBUMINURIA *which gradually becomes more severe, accompanied by* HYPERTENSION *and later* DIABETIC RETINOPATHY. *The disease is* DIABETIC RENAL DISEASE.

§ 408. IV. **Diabetic Renal Disease** (Kimmelstiel–Wilson syndrome) is becoming more common since diabetic patients live so much longer than a few decades ago: it is found equally in mild or in severe cases of diabetes of ten or more years' standing. The progressively severe albuminuria and hypertension result in uræmia, cardiac infarction or a cerebro-vascular catastrophy. In some there is in addition a chronic urinary infection.

Treatment of Chronic Nephritis.—The first aim is to discover the cause whenever possible. General measures include the avoidance of excessive mental or physical exertion and of exposure to cold or to infection. When the blood urea is raised a suitable dietary needs to be given (§ 296, VII C) and alcohol must be allowed in extreme moderation. Pregnancy is not permissible, as it increases the renal damage, and abortions or a macerated foetus usually result. It is generally agreed that severe hypertension aggravates the renal damage, so that if the blood pressure can be lowered before renal impairment is marked, life may be considerably prolonged. Therefore hypotensive drugs are valuable (§ 96). Infections in the urine (§ 419), as well as septic foci should be eliminated, and drugs which damage the kidneys (*e.g.*, phenol, cantharides, mercurial salts) avoided. The sulpha-drugs and the antibiotics (other than penicillin) must be given in smaller doses than usual if renal impairment is marked. When unilateral renal disease is present, such as chronic pyelonephritis or a calculus, considera-

TABLE XXIII.—CHRONIC ALBUMINURIA OF RENAL ORIGIN.

	Quantity of Albumen.	Tendency to Uræmia.	Quantity of Urine.	Tendency to Œdema.
Subacute Parenchymatous Nephritis.	Large.	Moderate.	Diminished or normal.	Great.
Secondary Contracted Kidney.	Moderate.	Great.	Increased.	Slight.
Chronic Interstitial Nephritis.	Varies with the cause.	Great.	Increased.	Very slight.
Chronic Pyelonephritis.	Small at first.	Great.	Increased.	Slight.
Diabetic Renal Disease.	Large.	Great.	Increased.	Very slight.
Amyloid Kidney.	Very great.	Slight.	Greatly increased.	Slight.

tions of nephrectomy arise. Otherwise the treatment is that of the main complications: (i.) Left ventricular failure will need rest in bed, the relief of hypertension and of insomnia (§ 62). (ii.) Anæmia does not necessarily respond to iron salts, and these may be injurious by leading to constipation: in certain cases transfusion of concentrated red cells and small doses of ACTH may stimulate a hypoplasic bone marrow. (iv.) Treatment often resolves itself into the treatment of uræmia (§ 372).

There is abundant albumen with the passage of LARGE QUANTITIES of urine, but little tendency to œdema and uræmia; the patient is anæmic; there is a history of prolonged SUPPURATION, RHEUMATOID DISEASE or of SYPHILIS; and there may be evidences of lardaceous disease elsewhere. The disease is AMYLOID KIDNEY.

§ 409. V. Amyloid Kidney (Waxy or Lardaceous Kidney) is generally part of a widespread lardaceous disease. With more efficient modern surgical methods, amyloid degeneration is becoming a rare condition.

Symptoms.—(1) The albumen, though it may be small in quantity in the early stage, is marked when the condition is established. (i.) The diurnal quantity is greatly increased, even to 150 fl. oz.; (ii.) the specific gravity is very low, but the urea is not diminished till the later stages; (iii.) the colour is pale and clear; (iv.) all varieties of casts may be found, including amyloid and fatty casts. (2) There is great pallor of the surface and anæmia, but there may be no œdema, till near the end. In cases with great cachexia œdema *may* occur early (§ 29). (3) Other evidence of lardaceous disease is present—enlargement of the liver and spleen; consequently hæmorrhages may occur from different parts. Amyloid disease of the bowel causes intractable diarrhœa,. and when it involves the suprarenals the blood pressure is low.

For the *Diagnosis, Prognosis* and *Treatment* of Amyloid disease see § 346.

D. *The* ALBUMEN *is* NOT *usually* ASSOCIATED *with* CASTS *or* BLOOD; *the condition is often* INTERMITTENT *and tends to be chronic.*

§ 410. The chief causes to be reviewed are:

I. PHYSIOLOGICAL.—Albumen occurs regularly in the urine of new-born infants in the first week of life, apparently due to the kidney not having gained its normal semi-permeability. Albumen is also present for some hours after any severe exercise, such as running or rowing. Probably the albuminuria is due to a temporary vaso-constriction of the renal vessels during exercise.

II. ORTHOSTATIC or FUNCTIONAL albuminuria occurs in the adolescent, as a result of the upright position. It therefore disappears at night, when asleep and in the horizontal position; occasionally it continues to be excreted for the first hour after lying down. It is commonest (i.) in young people; (ii.) it shows a familial tendency; (iii.) it occurs in tall people, during the periods of most active growth and does not occur after the age of 25; it is associated with (iv.) a tendency to attacks of pallor, faintness and fatigue states; and (v.) a low systolic blood pressure and often a low pulse pressure. *Diagnosis:* casts and other evidences of renal failure are absent, renal efficiency tests give normal findings and, if the patient voids urine an hour after going to bed, the early morning specimen is free of albumen. The albuminuria often disappears with full doses of calcium salts. Mild cases of nephritis also may show albuminuria when the patient stands upright for long, but other evidences of renal disease are present.

III. KYPHOTIC albuminuria is due to a kyphotic stance causing pressure on the left renal vein. It disappears on correcting the cause.

IV. Any form of TOXÆMIA may produce albuminuria. The milder cases probably recover completely, with no permanent renal damage; more severe cases tend to progress to acute or chronic nephritis. In hyperpyrexia albuminuria is invariably present. A small quantity of albumen is common in febrile conditions, *e.g.*, in pneumonia, typhoid, diphtheria, diarrhœa and vomiting of infants, the reaction stage of cholera, secondary syphilis, tuberculosis, streptococcal infections and in any septicæmia. The albumen may be accompanied by some casts in the severe forms, but it disappears completely within 2 or 3 weeks of the subsidence of the fever.

V. PREGNANCY.—The cause of the albuminuria is almost certainly a toxæmia, although mechanical pressure may play a part. The condition is more common in primiparæ. *Mild cases* occur after the sixth month; the first sign is sudden œdema due to salt and water retention, so that the patient gains more than 2 lb. in weight in one week. The blood pressure is slightly raised (systolic up to 150 mm.). Albuminuria (up to 0·2 per cent.) follows with an excess of renal epithelial cells and occasionally of casts, but there are no signs of renal failure, such as retinitis or urea retention. The condition rapidly disappears in the puerperium, but may recur in subsequent pregnancies. *Severe cases* may begin as mild cases, or they may start suddenly, often with eclampsia. The blood pressure is considerable (up to 230–240 mm.), and there is usually evidence of hepatic or renal failure with oliguria or anuria, retinitis, headaches, drowsiness, muscular twitchings, epigastric pain and a raised blood urea. The condition may respond to medical treatment or may need artificial termination of pregnancy. It sometimes passes into chronic nephritis, and tends to recur in subsequent pregnancies.

Prophylaxis is by ensuring that no woman gains more than 3 lb. in weight in one week, or more than 2 stone during the whole pregnancy.

VI. DRUGS and POISONS are closely allied to the previous group. Common causes are mercury, arsenic, phosphorus, phenol, salicylic acid, quinine, lead, gold, cantharides, turpentine, alcoholism, and vegetable or animal poisons such as mushroom or fish poisoning. This cause is recognised by: (i.) the presence of the drug in the urine; (ii.) there may be a history of the administration of the drug; and (iii.) the albuminuria usually disappears when the drug is stopped.

VII. ENDOGENOUS POISONS such as jaundice, diabetes and acute gout may all cause temporary albuminuria.

VIII. Mild RENAL CONGESTION causes albuminuria in: (i.) right-sided heart failure; (ii.) rapid catheterisation of a distended bladder (and see Hæmaturia, § 411); (iii.) after epileptic fits.

IX. Chronic GOUT and ARTERIOSCLEROSIS lead to an ischæmia of focal areas in the kidneys. The urine is copious, of low specific gravity and contains at times a trace of albumen. The blood pressure is raised, but there is no tendency to uræmia (see § 93).

X. URINARY CALCULI and CRYSTALS, especially oxalates, and CYSTITIS may give rise to albuminuria, but other signs are usually present (§ 413).

XI. "LEAKY KIDNEY" or "RESIDUAL ALBUMINURIA" is a name given to a condition of albuminuria which follows a past attack of nephritis, and is due to albumen leaking through the healed scars. It is known by: (i.) the absence of signs of renal failure, and the renal function tests are normal: (ii.) absence of casts: (iii.) normal blood pressure; (iv.) the condition is not associated with progressive renal disease.

XII. ANÆMIA.—Severe anæmia may be accompanied by a trace of albumen.

XIII. OBSCURE CAUSES, *e.g.*, when albumen appears for unknown reasons, as (1) after burns and other causes of severe shock. (2) In exophthalmic goitre the albuminuria is usually temporary, though it may last for months. It may vary in amount at different times on the same day, which tends to show that it is of vaso-motor origin. The urine in other respects is healthy. (3) Excessive study or other cause of nervous strain has been reported to have occasioned albuminuria. (4) Certain cases of cerebral tumour, and other conditions in which there is increased intracranial pressure, have been attended by albuminuria.

The *Prognosis* of albuminuria in the above groups is that of its cause. Before giving a prognosis it is important to examine thoroughly and repeatedly the urine, for casts in particular, so as to be satisfied that the kidneys are structurally healthy. Young subjects with functional albuminuria are not necessarily predisposed to kidney troubles, but they are often below par; the albuminuria will disappear as the general condition improves. The prognosis as to life is excellent.

Treatment.—The treatment must be directed to the cause. Rest in bed will do a good deal for the renal complication of cardiac disease. In the *albuminuria of pregnancy* careful investigations should be made, and the amount of urea watched. If (1) there is a clear history of renal disease prior to pregnancy, or (2) puerperal eclampsia has occurred in previous pregnancies, or (3) the renal disease, no matter of what kind it may be, is distinctly *progressive in its nature*, then termination of pregnancy or induction of premature labour should be advised. For the treatment of functional albuminuria general hygienic and dietetic rules must be followed. The administration of calcium lactate and alkalies temporarily stops the albuminuria.

E. *The* ALBUMEN *is* ASSOCIATED WITH BLOOD, *and* CASTS *are scanty or absent*—HÆMATURIA. When the condition is associated with severe abdominal pain, see renal colic, § 413.

§ 411. Hæmaturia.—When the patient is " passing blood " in the urine, an endeavour should be made to ascertain if the blood comes chiefly at the beginning of micturition, chiefly at the end, or whether it is intimately mixed with the urine and gives to it a " smoky " tint. For the tests for blood in the urine and the methods of distinguishing it from hæmoglobinuria, see § 382. The *fallacy* of menstrual blood must be avoided.

1. *If the blood is bright crimson and comes chiefly* AT THE COMMENCEMENT *of micturition, it is probably of* URETHRAL *or* PROSTATIC *origin.*

In these circumstances, which are mainly of surgical interest, there will probably be a history of injury or gonorrhœa. Enlargement of the prostate is sometimes causal; when the gland is congested or contains an abscess there is local pain or tenderness and rectal irritation. Urethral angioma and excessive sexual indulgence in the male and urethral caruncle in the female may lead to hæmaturia.

2. *If the blood comes most freely* AT THE END *of micturition, and especially if in clots, it is probably of* VESICAL *origin.*

The COMMONEST CAUSES of vesical hæmorrhage are:

I. ACUTE CYSTITIS, chiefly at its onset (see § 418). The bleeding is usually slight.

II. CALCULUS, or stone, in the bladder. Here the hæmorrhage is worse after exercise, moderate in amount, and there is pain, which, like the bleeding, is worse at the end of micturition and after exercise or jolting, and is frequently referred to the point of the penis. The ensuing cystitis may complicate the symptoms and render the diagnosis of stone difficult, but its detection by X-ray, the sound or cystoscope is conclusive.

III. TUMOURS of the bladder.—The hæmorrhage here, especially in *papillomata*, is usually great in amount. Shreds of the growth may be passed, and cystitis may develop. In *cancerous* tumours the hæmorrhage is more or less intermittent and resists treatment; there are pain and cachexia, and sometimes the growth may be palpable above the pubes or per rectum. Extension of tumours of neighbouring organs, or even spread of inflammation or congestion, as in appendicitis or dysenteric ulcers, may cause hæmaturia. The cystoscope is the best means we have of recognising the condition of the bladder.

IV. An enlarged PROSTATE may produce hæmaturia either from congestion or from the rupture of enlarged veins near the neck of the bladder.

V. Some of the LESS COMMON CAUSES of vesical hæmaturia are TUBERCULOUS DISEASE of the bladder, VESICAL VARIX, certain constitutional diseases such as SCURVY and PURPURA, and SCHISTOSOMA HÆMATOBIUM.

VI. § 412. Schistosomiasis (Syn.; *Bilharziasis*).—The endemic hæmaturia of the Middle East and Africa results from the depositions of schistosomal eggs in the bladder by the adult female worm—*Schistosoma hæmatobium*—which lives in the portal system (§ 315, (3)) and pelvic plexuses of veins. Ova occur chiefly in the liver, bladder, lungs, prostate, lower third of the ureter, and in the pelvic viscera of the female; occasionally they are deposited in the pancreas, spleen and colon. Carcinoma of the bladder or penis may occur.

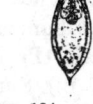

FIG. 134. — EGG of *Schistosoma hæmatobium*, magnified about 120.

Symptoms: Urticarial eruptions, terminal hæmaturia, frequency, perineal, penile and suprapubic pain and aching in the lumbar region. The blood is bright red, occurs at the end of micturition and is increased by exercise. Cystoscopic examination in the early stages shows round, yellowish-white, pseudo-tubercles and ulcers; later, papillomata and sandy patches may develop. Schistosomal complement fixation reactions and intradermal tests are generally positive, and eosinophilia may be present, especially in the early stages. In the majority of cases terminal spined eggs are readily demonstrable in the urine. As the disease progresses the clinical picture may be modified by complications. Ureteric involvement may lead to back pressure on the kidney with hydronephrosis and chronic nephritis. Secondary bacterial infection of the genito-urinary tract is common leading to septic cystitis, pyelonephritis and pyonephrosis; urethral fistulæ and vesical calculi may occur.

Etiology.—After the eggs in the excreta come in contact with water, motile miracidia are set free, enter certain fresh-water snails of the *Bulinus* species and develop in the liver into sporocysts and later cercariæ; these in turn escape into water, penetrate the skin of man during bathing, or invade the mucous membrane of the mouth and the œsophagus during drinking.

Treatment.—Antimony is specific, and the treatment of uncomplicated cases is highly satisfactory. The details of treatment are the same as in schistosomal dysentery (see § 315, (3) (a)). The presence of hepatic cirrhosis, splenomegaly, septic cystitis and renal involvement render effective treatment difficult; surgery may be required for complications.

3. *If the blood is* INTIMATELY MIXED *with the urine, causing it to assume a " smoky " tint, it is probably of* RENAL *origin. In these cases also the tests for blood should be carefully applied, and fallacies avoided* (§ 382).

Symptoms and signs pointing to the kidney will usually be detected on examination.

The CAUSES of RENAL HÆMORRHAGE may for convenience be grouped under these headings: (I) Inflammation; (II) Severe congestion; (III) Nephroptosis; (IV) Blood conditions; (V) Renal calculus and crystals; (VI) Drugs; (VII) New growths; (VIII) Essential hæmaturia; (IX) Paroxysmal hæmoglobinuria; (X) Injury; (XI) Porphyrinuria and Porphyria resemble hæmaturia (§ 415).

I. INFLAMMATION: (i.) In acute nephritis the urine also contains casts (§ 397); (ii.) in subacute and chronic nephritis and in congenital cystic kidneys bleeding may occur during an acute exacerbation, or as a consequence of high blood pressure, in the same way that bleeding may occur from the nose (epistaxis) or into the brain; (iii.) Acute pyelitis (§ 419); (iv.) Infarction, due to subacute bacterial endocarditis (§ 50a); (v.) Tuberculous disease of the kidney (§ 419); (vi.) Parasites, *e.g.*, *Schistosoma hæmatobia* (see above). The *Microfilaria sanguinis hominis* usually causes chyluria, but hæmaturia may also occur.

II. SEVERE CONGESTION.—Mild congestion causes albuminuria, but marked congestion causes hæmaturia also. (i.) The commonest cause is right-sided heart failure (§ 55). The scanty, highly-coloured urine contains at first albumen only, but later a large quantity of albumen, accompanied by blood. Particularly in long-standing cases, there is an excess of hyaline casts. (ii.) Sudden congestion occurs after rapid catheterisation of a distended bladder, probably as a result of sudden relief of a bilateral hydronephrosis. Suppression of the urine may also ensue. It can be avoided by emptying the bladder gradually. (iii.) Thrombosis of the renal vein causes acute congestion. It occurs chiefly with streptococcal infections, and rarely in cachectic states—sudden hæmaturia with rapid enlargement of a tender kidney is very suggestive. (iv.) Sudden congestion may occur with a patient who has been bedridden for many months, as with a fractured femur (Wilson), usually on the second day of walking. There is colic, hæmaturia, and pain in the loin, which disappear when the patient returns to bed for a few days.

III. NEPHROPTOSIS, with or without aberrant renal vessels, may produce intermittent attacks of hæmaturia, probably congestive in origin.

IV. BLOOD CONDITIONS, especially purpura, scurvy and malaria.

V. Renal CALCULI and CRYSTALS, particularly oxalates, produce renal colic and hæmaturia (§ 413).

VI. DRUGS, particularly phenindione B.P. (Dindevan), dicoumarol, sulphathiazole and other sulpha-drugs, salicylates, phenol and its derivatives, and hexamine, can cause hæmaturia.

VII. NEW GROWTHS of the kidney (carcinoma, sarcoma, hypernephroma and polycystic disease), or of the renal pelvis (papilloma, carcinoma) (§ 432). The hæmaturia is often painless, and either intermittent or continuous.

VIII. ESSENTIAL HÆMATURIA (nephritis dolorosa hæmorrhagica) is a name given to a group of cases in young adults in which either slight or severe unilateral hæmorrhage is accompanied by paroxysmal colic or dull renal pain. The cause is probably a patchy nephritis; bleeding usually ceases dramatically after nephrotomy; nephrectomy should not be performed.

IX. PAROXYSMAL HÆMOGLOBINURIA is not, strictly speaking, hæmaturia. Free hæmoglobin is plentiful in the urine (§ 414), but blood discs are absent.

X. **Injury of the Kidney,** laceration or rupture, is usually caused by a fall on the back of the loin, or in " buffer accidents " on the railway, or in street accidents. There may be no bruising or external signs, but a laceration of the kidney may be inferred from (1) the history of such an accident; (2) a tense swelling (due to extravasated blood) with increased area of dullness in the region of the kidney; and (3) copious hæmaturia. In a few cases there is no hæmaturia, and the other two evidences have to be relied on. Immediate operation is sometimes necessary, the collapse being treated by blood transfusion or saline injections.

§ **413. Renal Calculus and Renal Colic.**—Calculi may form either in the pelvis of the kidney (Fig. 130), or more rarely in its substance. Two stones occur in acid urines. The commonest form, dark brown in colour, consists of *calcium oxalate*, and gives rise to more acute symptoms, for each bristles with sharp-pointed crystals which cause bleeding and colour the calculus. Another form consists of *uric acid* and urates mixed in varying proportions (§§ 388, 393). These form light brown stones, round or branching, and are the commonest stones in gouty subjects, and those whose highly acid urine habitually deposits urates. Calculi are often multiple. Compound stones consist of an oxalate or organic nucleus, or alternate layers. In an *alkaline* urine phosphate stones are sometimes found, usually when infection is present. Cystine and xanthin are rarely met with renal calculi. Various *events* may happen. (1) A large calculus may remain in the renal pelvis for years without causing pain but sooner or later chronic pyelonephritis occurs (§ 419 and Fig. 130); or (2) by its movement produce acute symptoms, RENAL COLIC. (3) It may obstruct the ureter and lead to hydro- or pyo-nephrosis (§ 432). (4) If the other kidney is not healthy sudden blocking may lead to obstructive suppression (§ 428). (5) It may pass into the bladder and result in cystitis. (6) Small stones may be voided through the urethra as " gravel." (7) In rare cases small calculi become encysted and quiescent. (8) Hypertension may develop (§§ 88, 406). The clinical history of renal calculus consists of (a) *attacks of renal colic*, separated by (b) *intervals* in which the symptoms are those of calculous pyelitis.

The *Symptoms of Renal Colic* consist of severe paroxysms of lancinating pain, starting in one loin, shooting down to the front of the thigh or testicle or vulva on that side. This is associated with retraction of the testicle and with frequency of micturition, and is attended by vomiting, shivering, sweating, pallor, and a certain amount of collapse. These symptoms are in most cases followed by hæmaturia, the urine containing blood and pus cells, but usually no casts. Crystals may be present, and reveal the nature of the stone. Most blood and pain occur with an oxalate calculus.

The *Diagnosis* of renal from other forms of colic is given in Table XIV, § 247. Cystoscopic examination may reveal blood issuing from one ureteral orifice or even an impacted calculus. A plain X-ray film is of assistance except in the case of uric acid and cystine stones; these are more likely to be seen by X-ray pyelography. All the symptoms of renal colic may arise simply from the irritation of *fine crystals*. They may also be produced without alteration in the urine by *movable kidney*; or by the passage of *clots* of blood or *caseous material* down the ureter. *Malignant* disease of the kidney may be mistaken for calculus, but in that case the blood is more copious and more constant, and the pain is less severe, but more continuous.

Etiology.—Known predisposing causes to the formation of renal calculi are metabolic peculiarities, anatomical abnormalities, high concentration of the urine, infections and obstruction in the urinary passages. A monotonous and unsatisfactory diet in the poor is contributory in India and the Far East.

Treatment.—(1) Of the colic and (2) during the intervals. 1. The treatment of an attack of *renal colic* consists mainly in the relief of the symptoms—pain, vomiting, and collapse. Usually nothing avails except injections of morphia, papaverine, ephedrine, Trasentin or atropine. Locally, hot applications relieve. After the painful attacks the patient must rest to allow the inflammation to subside. 2. The treatment in the intervals resolves itself into the removal of the stone, and treatment directed to the pyelitis. The urine in all cases should be kept diluted by drinking plenty of fluid. Dietetic treatment is of use in some cases. If oxalates are being passed, any dyspepsia should be carefully treated; for diet, see § 296, XIV; if the urine is kept strongly acid with sodium acid phosphate or with ammonium chloride, the crystals are kept in solution. In uric acid cases a purin-free diet is given and in cystinuria a largely vegetarian diet and an alkaline urine are helpful. The alkaline waters are very useful here, such as those of Vichy, Ems and Contrexéville. With a uric acid or cystine calculus give a vegetarian diet. Large doses of alkaline salts are certainly useful, especially the citrate and the acid tartrate of potassium. Begin with potassium citrate gr. 50 in 4 fl. oz. of water every 4 hours until the urine is alkaline, and then give an effervescing drink, consisting of sodium bicarbonate gr. 60, and citric acid gr. 40 in 4 oz. of water, t.i.d. This treatment should not be continued if the urine is or has become ammoniacal. For pyelitis, see § 419. Operative treatment is called for if the stone is of large size or becomes impacted in the lower end of the ureter; small stones are often passed spontaneously. Before operation the function of the other kidney must be investigated.

Hyperparathyroidism due to an adenoma can occur with minimal bone changes: any patient with a renal calculus (especially if multiple) and a serum calcium over 12 mg. per cent. should be suspect.

§ 414. In **Paroxysmal hæmoglobinuria** porter-coloured urine is passed at intervals. An attack commences abruptly with (1) a rigor and temperature to 104°, nausea, headache and malaise. (2) Abdominal cramp, aching pains in the back and legs: severe shock may follow. (3) An hour or so later the patient passes dark, highly albuminous urine, showing the spectroscopic bands of methæmoglobin, oxyhæmoglobin and hæmatin, containing no red cells, but albumen, red cell casts and amorphous hæmosiderin may be present. Anuria is a dangerous sequela. (4) In severe cases, a hæmolytic anæmia is present which may endanger life. Thrombosis and infarcts are common. Free hæmoglobin can often be detected in the plasma as well as in the urine. Each attack lasts a few hours, passes off suddenly only to recur later.

The types are—(1) In 90 per cent. of the cases (Roberts) the attacks are connected with chill to the surface. In this type attacks are induced by immersing a hand in ice-cold water for 10–20 minutes. A hæmolysin is present in the serum which unites with the red cells when the temperature is lowered and lyses them when the temperature rises again (Donath-Landsteiner reaction). The cause is usually syphilitic as in most cases stigmata of acquired or congenital syphilis are present, the Wassermann reaction is positive, and the disease is cured by antisyphilitic measures.

(2) March hæmoglobinuria. In the second decade hæmoglobinuria may follow severe exertion, and especially running on a metalled road. Muscle pains and hæmoglobinæmia are usually absent, and it has been suggested the hæmolysis occurs locally in the renal vessels (Witts). It is often accompanied by lordosis, and treatment to overcome this helps. Patients are spontaneously cured in a year or so.

(3) Recurrent hæmoglobinuria, usually occurring at night with a hæmolytic anæmia (Marchiafava-Micheli syndrome), is often associated with splenomegaly, some bronzing of the skin and a constant reticulocytosis. Sooner or later the severe anæmia and hæmolysis endanger life, but splenectomy and transfusions are unavailing. The cause is associated with an altered pH in the blood at night. Death usually occurs in three to five years.

(4) Massive toxæmia with *Cl. Welchii* or with the Bartonella of Oroya fever, and the hyperacute form of Lederer's anæmia, are occasional causes.

(5) Favism following ingestion of the sensitised portion of the bean *Vicia fava*, grown in Mediterranean areas and especially in Sardinia.

(6) In paralytic myoglobinuria the pigment is myoglobin and is associated with muscle pains, cramp, weakness and paralysis of skeletal muscles. Attacks may be spontaneous or brought on by exertion. The urinary pigment is distinguished by the spectroscope.

The *Diagnosis* depends on the precipitating cause. Only in the form due to exposure to cold is syphilis a factor.

The *Treatment* consists of rest in bed during the attacks, with warmth.

Hæmoglobinuria and Methæmoglobinuria occasionally accompany severe burns and acute infective diseases, especially malaria. The blood contains an excess of bilirubin and the urine an excess of urobilin. It may be produced by toxic doses of potassium chlorate, nitrites, phenacetin, phenazone, acetanilide, arseniuretted hydrogen, and quinine in those who have had malaria. Blackwater fever, see § 513. Hæmoglobinuria also occurs after incompatible blood transfusions (§ 547).

Epidemic Hæmoglobinuria is seen in the new-born, with jaundice and nervous symptoms.

§ 415. XI. **Porphyrinuria and Porphyria** indicate an excess of porphyrins in the urine. When in large amounts these may give a red or " port wine " reddish-brown colour to the urine when freshly passed or after standing, and they give a pink fluorescence in ultraviolet light. In adults the daily excretion of porphyrins in urine is up to 0·1 mg. and in fæces up to 0·4 mg.; in disease the urine may contain even 100 mg. a day.

In the synthesis of hæmoglobin porphobilinogen forms porphyrins which with added iron produce hæm; this links with globin to form hæmoglobin.

Secondary Porphyrinuria is not familial. The excess of porphyrins (chiefly coproporphyrin III) is not enough to colour the urine for the amount is usually less than 5 mg. a day. It is consistently found in infections, hæmolytic and pernicious anæmia, in liver disease (especially cirrhosis) and is an important early sign of poisoning with benzol, lead and other heavy metals. No symptoms arise from its presence.

Primary Porphyria is due to an inborn error of metabolism. The urine and fæces contain a considerable amount of one or more porphyrins, often sufficient to colour the urine. The varieties are recognised are I. *Congenital*, II. *Hepatic*.

I *Congenital Porphyria* is familial but very rare. *Symptoms.*—The chief feature is the red coloured urine at birth or in infancy. The normoblasts of the bone marrow, the plasma, urine and fæces contain high concentrations of porphyrins (especially uroporphyrin I and coproporphyrin I) which stain the teeth red (erythrodontia), and cause the skin to be photosensitive. In the spring and summer the exposed parts develop a bulbous eruption (hydroa æstivale, § 678). There may be a hæmolytic anæmia, enlargement of the liver and spleen, loss of digits and hypertrichosis. The *Prognosis* is poor. *Treatment* is by protection from direct sunlight even through window panes; splenectomy may help hæmolytic cases.

II. *Hepatic Porphyria* may be produced by increased porphyrin synthesis in the liver; there is no excess of porphyrins in the bone marrow. The liver is damaged to a greater or lesser extent and cirrhosis may follow. The condition usually first shows itself between 20–40 years of age. There is frequently a family history and many cases have been traced to a single Swedish ancestor (Swedish and N. European type) or to a South African forbear. Four types with different groups of symptoms are recognised, but there is often overlapping.

(a) *Intermittent Acute Porphyria* is much the most common.

Symptoms.—Attacks of severe burning or colicky pain, vomiting and constipation suggest an acute abdominal emergency and operation has often been performed in error. There is no abdominal rigidity or rebound tenderness and often no leucocytosis. In attacks the urine is usually normal in colour and darkens on standing; this is due to porphobilinogen (a colourless chromogen in amounts even up to 50 mg. a day) being slowly converted to uroporphyrin III. Uroporphyrin I and coproporphyrin I which stain the urine red and cause photosensitivity are rarely present. However with Ehrlich's aldehyde reagent porphobilinogen gives a red colour which is not extracted by chloroform (as is urobilinogen). Attacks, which appear to be severe in proportion to the plasma porphobilinogen content, are often precipitated or aggravated by barbiturates (such as thiopentone intravenously), by alcohol, sulphonal, trional or by infections. Neurological symptoms often occur sooner or later with hysteria or other psychological disturbances, delirium, coma, convulsions, optic atrophy, neuritic pain, flaccid paralysis of one or more extremities, and even bulbar palsy and respiratory failure. Paroxysmal hypertension or jaundice are met; the skin can become brown independent of photosensitivity. During remissions the urine may or may not contain porphobilinogen.

The *Prognosis* is good unless irreversible neurological disease has already occurred.

Treatment of the acute attacks is with chlorpromazine which gives prompt relief from abdominal pain and recent neurological symptoms. Abdominal pain and hypertension are also relieved by injections of ganglionic blocking drugs. *Prophylaxis* is by strict avoidance of all drugs (especially barbiturates) which precipitate attacks.

(b) *Porphyria Cutanea Tarda* (Syn. Chronic Porphyria) is more common in men. Excess uroporphyrin I in the plasma causes photosensitisation and bullæ (hydroa æstivale), or urticarial and eczematous reactions. The skin is often brownish in colour; there may be hirsutism. The urine and fæces contain excess of porphyrins.

The *Prognosis* is good in uncomplicated cases.

Treatment is by avoiding direct sunlight (§§ 628, 678).

(c) A *mixed type of Porphyria* with a combination of the Intermittent Acute Symptoms (abdominal and neurological) and those of chronic porphyria occurs in the South African variety but not in the Swedish type. In the former the skin may show symptoms years before others occur.

(d) A *Latent Variety* is found in relatives of those affected by overt disease. It is most easily recognised by a screening test by which an excess of protoporphyrin and coproporphyrin in the stools causes fluorescence in ultraviolet light.

F. The patient complains of LASSITUDE **and ill-health, which may be associated with fever; the urine is found to contain** PUS **(§ 392)—i.e., there is** PYURIA. **With few exceptions, when the pus comes from the** BLADDER **the urine is** ALKALINE, **and the pus remains diffused through the urine; but when it comes from the** KIDNEYS **or any other part of the urinary passages, the urine is** ACID, **and the pus settles at the bottom. Pus cells are often accompanied by a trace of albumen in the urine.**

§ 416. Pyuria.—If we except the rupture of an abscess into the urinary passages, there are three sources of pus in the urine:

1. From the **Urethra** (*e.g.*, gonorrhœal or *B. coli* infection).
2. From the **Bladder** (cystitis).
3. From the **Kidney** (pyelitis).—The chief forms are due to *B. coli* INFECTION, or to ASCENDING, CALCULOUS or TUBERCULOUS PYELITIS.

Abscesses bursting into the Urinary Tract.—The abscesses most liable to burst into the urinary tract are those due to diverticulitis, or of the prostate (below), pelvis, perineum, liver, psoas sheath or perinephric tissues. (i.) The urine is usually acid; (ii.) the pus is in large quantity and settles at the bottom; (iii.) there is a clinical history of abscess prior to the appearance of pus in the urine; and (iv.) localising signs of the abscess may be present.

In health a few leucocytes may be passed. For accuracy a cell count is necessary; Dukes found 0–10 pus cells per c.mm. in normal people. A properly collected catheter specimen is necessary to exclude pus cells from the generative organs. A number of leucocytes are present in acute and subacute nephritis. Special precautions may have to be taken in women to exclude pus mixing with the urine as it is passed (false pyuria). When the presence of pus is suspected, the reaction should be tested immediately after it is passed, before decomposition makes the urine ammoniacal.

1. The **pus** *comes chiefly at the* BEGINNING OF MICTURITION, *and the urine is* ACID; *there is* PAIN IN THE URETHRA *during micturition.* The pus comes from the URETHRA, and is usually caused by one of three conditions:

I. URETHRITIS.—There is pain, swelling, and redness of the meatus, scalding during micturition, and a discharge of pus or muco-pus especially in the early morning. Two main types exist, both of venereal origin, Gonococcal and Non-specific urethritis.

The patient, who may be either sex, complains of a SUDDEN BURNING PAIN *and* DISCHARGE FROM THE URETHRA *and also (in a woman)* FROM THE VAGINA. *The disease may be* ACUTE GONORRHŒA.

§ 417. Acute Gonorrhœa is caused by sexual contact with an infected person.

Symptoms occur within two to six days. There is an acute purulent discharge from the urethra in both sexes and also from the cervix uteri and vagina of the female, with enlarged inguinal glands. In *men* there may be a *local* spread to the littré glands, prostate, seminal vesicles and epididymi, and in *women* to Bartholin's glands, Skene's tubules, the racemose glands of the cervical canal or to the Fallopian tubes. In association with a secondary infection pelvic peritonitis may arise. When the conjunctiva is accidentally inoculated with the discharge a grave ophthalmia occurs. *Chronic Gonorrhœa* may ensue from these foci, and bacterial exotoxins cause metastatic complications in the synovial membranes or periarticular tissues of joints, in the eyes and the skin.

Diagnosis and Etiology.—The causal organism is the *N. gonorrhœa*. This may be identified as a gram-negative intracellular diplococcus in pus obtained from the urethra, the cervix uteri, or by prostatic massage; it may be seen in freshly stained films or from cultures on suitable media.

Treatment.—The infection usually responds to two daily injections of procaine penicillin 600,000 units. Resistant cases need inj. streptomycin 1·0 G. daily for two days, concurrently with sulphathiazole 1·5 G. eight-hourly by day and by night for five days. The male urethral discharge may also be cleared with irrigations of potass. permanganate (1 in 10,000 solution) and in females by dry swabbing of the vagina and fornices. Complications call for more intensive and prolonged treatment with penicillin, the tetracyclines and erythromycin, drainage of the genito-urinary foci, warm douches or short-wave diathermy.

Non-specific (abacterial) cases are due to an unknown organism. The amount of purulent or muco-purulent discharge is much less and may be overlooked unless an early-morning specimen of urine is examined for pus cells. In men there may also be prostatitis and in women cervicitis and proctitis. Especially in men a blood-stream spread is liable to cause a high temperature, polyarthritis, conjunctivitis and iritis (Reiter's syndrome). *Treatment.*—For non-specific urethritis give each day inject. streptomycin sulph. 1 G. with tab. trisulphonamide (N.F.) 5·0 G., or otherwise caps. oxytetracycline (B.P.) 0·5 G. q.d.s., or tab. spiramycin 1·0 G. q.d.s., all in five-day courses.

II. Prostatic abscess is known by: (1) pain in the perineum, which is worse at the end of micturition; (2) the finger in the rectum detects a tender, fluctuating swelling; (3) the symptoms closely resemble those of vesical calculus with concurrent cystitis. It may be distinguished from this, however, by: (i.) a history of gonorrhœa, which is a common cause of prostatic abscess; (ii.) the signs on examination per rectum; (iii.) a discharge occurring in the intervals between micturition, and (iv.) examining the urine after prostatic massage. Some cases are due to *E. coli.*

III. Perineal Abscess is detected by the local signs.

2. *The* pus *comes chiefly at the* END OF MICTURITION, *or is intimately mixed with the urine. There is* SUPRAPUBIC PAIN *or* DISCOMFORT *and frequency of micturition.*[1] The pus comes from the BLADDER, and is indicative of CYSTITIS.

§ 418. Cystitis, or inflammation of the bladder, occurs in two well-recognised forms—acute and chronic.

(*a*) ACUTE CYSTITIS.—(1) In this condition the pus is in small amount, and in severe cases there may be considerable hæmaturia at the onset. At first the urine is acid, but it soon becomes alkaline, and ropy with pus and mucus. (2) There are pain and tenderness in the hypogastrium. (3) Micturition is frequent and painful (" scalding "). There is a constant desire to pass water immediately after micturition (strangury); this relieves the pain for a short time, unless the cystitis is due to stone in the bladder, when the pain is severe *after* micturition, because the inflamed walls of the emptied bladder come into contact with the stone. (4) Hæmaturia may be the chief symptom. (5) There is generally constitutional disturbance with pyrexia.

(*b*) In CHRONIC CYSTITIS (which may supervene upon the acute form, or may be chronic from the onset), there is (1) a larger amount of pus. (2) The urine is alkaline directly it is passed and contains a large amount of ropy mucus.[1] (3) The pain and other symptoms are less severe than in acute cystitis.

---

[1] The urine may be acid—(i.) at the onset of acute cystitis; (ii.) in the stage of recovery from chronic cystitis; (iii.) in the early stage of tubercle and new growths of the bladder; (iv.) in cystitis due to *E. coli.* In all other conditions in which the urine contains pus derived from the bladder the reaction is alkaline.

Etiology.—Infection of the bladder is rarely primary in origin. Predisposing causes are: (i.) the presence of residual urine. This occurs with prostatic enlargement, urethral stricture, atony of the bladder in old age, and various nervous diseases producing paralysis and retention (§ 429). (ii.) Stone or foreign body; (iii.) papilloma, carcinoma and other tumours; (iv.) diverticulum of the bladder; (v.) following surgical operations on the bladder or other pelvic organs. Infection spreads to the bladder: (i.) in most cases in the stream of urine from the renal pelvis, as in *E. coli* and tuberculous pyelonephritis; (ii.) from adjacent organs, especially cervicitis, diverticulitis or growths of the colon and rectum (forming a fistula), pelvic cellulitis or pelvic peritonitis; (iii.) via the urethra, as after the passage of infected instruments or foreign bodies introduced by the patient, by extension of urethritis, and possibly via the wide urethra of women, especially when there is infection of Bartholin's glands or Skene's ducts, or a perianal crack or fissure. Almost any variety of organism may be found, but the most common are (*a*) in acid urine *E. coli*, tubercle bacilli and gonococci, (*b*) in neutral urine *E. coli* and streptococci, (*c*) in alkaline urine staphylococci and *B. proteus.* For schistosomiasis, see § 412.

Differentiations.—(1) Cystitis due to VESICAL CALCULUS.—In addition to the symptoms of simple cystitis, there are (i.) very severe pain at the end of micturition lasting for some time after, shooting down the urethra; pain is often much worse after jolting, as on a bus ride. (ii.) Hæmaturia is common, though in some cases it may be so slight that it is detected only by the microscope; (iii.) sometimes there is a preceding history of renal colic (§ 413); (iv.) the stone may be detected by the sound, the cystoscope or by radiography.

(2) Cystitis due to NEW GROWTH IN THE BLADDER, or ULCERATION, is characterised by (i.) continuous suprapubic pain, with paroxysms of lancinating pain, quite independent of micturition and movement; (ii.) copious hæmorrhage at intervals; (iii.) the urine may contain cancer cells or tubercle bacilli; a tumour may be felt per rectum or through the abdominal wall. (iv.) Cystoscopic examination or radiography may settle the diagnosis. The cancerous ulcer is often covered by a fine deposit of calcium phosphate which gives a characteristic X-ray appearance.

(3) ABACTERIAL PYURIA causes the symptoms and signs of cystitis and urethritis, but organisms cannot be cultured from the urine and tubercle bacilli cannot be found. The amount of pus from the bladder and urethra may be considerable and cystoscopy reveals generalised cystitis. *Treatment:* the disease fails to respond to the usual urinary antiseptics but disappears rapidly after 1 or 2 small doses of neoarsphenamine. Relapse may occur unless septic foci are treated.

Prognosis.—Cystitis is not dangerous to life unless the inflammation spreads upwards from the bladder to the kidneys and produces pyelonephritis; but, on the other hand, it is a very troublesome, painful complaint, and has a special liability to recur. When the cause is not removable—*e.g.*, in cystitis due to tumours of the bladder—the prognosis is grave. When it is due to retention of urine, and when it is due to gonorrhœa, it tends to cause ascending pyelitis and pyelonephritis. When there is pre-existing hydronephrosis (§ 432) and acute cystitis develops, the inflammation is almost certain to extend upwards to the kidney, and so lead to pyonephrosis.

Treatment.—The cause must be sought, and, if possible, removed. A catheter or " mid-stream " specimen of urine must be bacteriologically examined and sensitivity tests performed. (*a*) Otherwise, in the *acute* form absolute rest in bed with milk diet is necessary. Copious libations of water, barley-water and other bland fluids are called for. The drug chosen will depend on the infecting micro-organism (see Table XXIV).

TABLE XXIV. DRUGS USED IN TREATMENT OF CYSTITIS
AND RECURRENT PYELONEPHRITIS.

Infecting Organism.	Drugs and Doses most effective (in order of choice).	Comments.
E. coli	A sulphonamide. Initial dose 2 G., then 1 G. q.d.s. for 7 days.	Tab. trisulphonamide (N.F.) preferable, with alkaline mixture.
	Nitrofurantoin (Furadantin) 100 mg. t.d.s. for 10 days.	
	Sulphafurazole (Gantrisin) 1 G. 4-hourly for 7 days.	Nausea, vomiting and rashes may occur.
	Tetracycline (B.P.) or chloramphenicol (B.P.) 0·5 G. t.d.s. for 5 days.	Only effective in acid urine.
	Sulphamethizole (Urolucosil) 200 mg. six-hourly for 7 days.	Fluid intake should not be increased.
	Inj. streptomycin sulphate (B.P.) 1 G. b.d. for 5 days.	Much more effective in alkaline urine. Older patients need smaller doses.
B. proteus Ps. pyocyanea	Inj. benzyl-penicillin 250,000 units b.d. for 7 days. Inj. streptomycin sulph. (B.P.) (as above). Chloramphenicol (B.P.) 0·5 G. t.d.s. for 5 days. Nitrofurantoin (as above).	A sulphonamide is sometimes effective and may be combined with inj. penicillin or inj. streptomycin.
Strep. fæcalis	Inj. benzyl-penicillin (B.P.) (as above). Tetracycline (B.P.) or chloramphenicol (B.P.) (as above). Inj. streptomycin sulph. (as above).	
Staphylococci	Benzyl-penicillin (B.P.) (as above). Tetracycline (B.P.) or chloramphenicol (B.P.) (as above).	

B. proteus and *Ps. pyocyaneus* infections are most obstinate and may also need lavage with acriflavine (1 in 8,000). Bladder pain and discomfort are best relieved by dicyclomine hydrochlor. (Wyovin) 10 mg. t.d.s., or tab. Pyridium 200 mg. t.d.s. before meals. (*b*) For the *chronic* and *subacute* forms, apart from the drugs just mentioned, it may be necessary to wash out the bladder with acriflavine, or mercury oxycyanide ($\frac{1}{4000}$ - $\frac{1}{8000}$), followed by normal saline to prevent mercurialism. *Prophylactically* penicillin injections are very valuable in those with a paralysed bladder, *e.g.*, in paraplegia.

3. *The* **pus** *is present in urine which is usually* ACID *when freshly passed* (**acid pyuria**), *the pus cells are at first disseminated through the urine, but later they form a* SEDIMENT, *and there is* PAIN, *perhaps* SWELLING *of the kidney, and* PYREXIA; the pus comes from the kidney—the disease is PYELONEPHRITIS.[1]

§ 419. Pyelonephritis is indicated by the symptoms just mentioned. The condition was formerly termed pyelitis, but it is now believed that the kidney substance is always involved in the presence of infection of the renal pelvis. The urine, which is acid unless there be concurrent cystitis, contains, in addition to pus cells (Fig. 122), epithelial cells from the renal mucosa and often red blood cells; but unless the renal parenchyma is severely involved, the number of casts and the amount of albumen is slight; nor is there any renal œdema. There is increased frequency of micturition. Renal pain and tenderness are nearly always present, but vary widely in degree and character in the three varieties about to be mentioned. *The kidney should always be carefully examined* (§ 394), because, in addition to the renal congestion, all forms of pyelitis are liable to result in partial or complete obstruction of the infundibula, and the gradual supervention of pyonephrosis. A few pus cells in the urine may be found in acute nephritis and with typhoid and other fevers. Apart from these there are four well-marked varieties of acid pyuria.

(I) PRIMARY INFECTIVE PYELONEPHRITIS.—This is the commonest group, and in the majority of cases the kidney is primarily infected from the blood-stream by the bacillus coli. The disease occurs chiefly in females, either children or adults, and especially during pregnancy. The right kidney is most commonly involved, but both kidneys or only the left may be affected. The disease may be acute or chronic. (*a*) ACUTE PYELO-NEPHRITIS. *Symptoms:* (i.) *Constitutional:* sudden onset, with headache, languor, anorexia, shivering, sweating, dry furred tongue and pyrexia of swinging type, up to 103 or 104° F. In adults, one or more rigors, and in children convulsions may occur. (ii.) *Urinary:* The first symptoms are often due to bladder irritation—frequency of micturition, perhaps every 15 to 20 minutes, sometimes associated with strangury. Later, a dull ache in the loin is felt, and local tenderness and rigidity develop. Sometimes acute abdominal pain may simulate appendicitis. The urine is concentrated, and contains a trace of albumen, pus cells, bacilli, occasionally a considerable amount of blood. In the earlier stages the amount of pus

---

[1] In obscure or resistant cases it may be necessary to collect a specimen of urine from each kidney by ureteric catheterisation. This will confirm that pus cells and organisms are derived from the *kidney*, and will decide whether from one or both sides. This procedure should never be undertaken if the bladder is extensively septic, lest ascending pyelonephritis be induced.

and bacilli may be microscopic, but later the urine is uniformly turbid, gives a shimmering appearance when rotated in a glass, and has an unmistakable fishy odour, due to the presence of sulphides. (*b*) SUBACUTE or CHRONIC PYELONEPHRITIS, or BACILLURIA. *Symptoms:* (i.) *Constitutional:* general ill-health, headache, periodic low-grade pyrexia; (ii) *Urinary:* frequency of micturition, enuresis in children, pain in the loins or hypogastrium. The urine shows a trace of albumen, pus, bacilli and occasional hæmaturia, as in the acute form. After a period of years, chronic nephritis and uræmia may ensue (§ 407).

Etiology.—(i.) The *Bacillus coli* is the common infecting agent and usually comes (*a*) from the blood-stream; it may arrive (*b*) from the colon, and (*c*) from the pelvic organs by the lymphatics. (ii.) When other organisms are present, such as staphylococci, streptococci, *B. pyocyaneus*, *B. proteus* or *B. subtilis*, the infection is often secondary to some other disease of (*a*) the kidneys, such as hydronephrosis, tuberculosis, or to some congenital abnormality, such as double ureters: or (*b*) disease of the bladder, prostate, cervix uteri, Bartholin's glands or Skene's crypts.

II. ASCENDING PYELITIS OR PYELONEPHRITIS arises from: (*a*) *extension of primary infective pyelitis*; (*b*) *obstruction of the urinary passages* below the kidney. The resulting retention and decomposition of the urine causes infection to arise, which may go on to pyonephrosis. (*c*) *Extension of cystitis* without obstruction, and thus the numerous causes of the latter disease (§ 418) are brought into operation. *Symptoms:* (i.) A high swinging temperature, often with repeated rigors. (ii.) Pain, tenderness, rigidity, and often a considerable enlargement of the kidney may be felt in the loin. (iii.) There may be a history of the cause, *e.g.*, enlarged prostate, renal calculus. (iv.) Often both kidneys are involved, with gradual diminution of the urinary output and symptoms of uræmia. *Treatment:* Surgical aid should be sought early. Special investigations as to the cause and the functional condition of the kidneys should be undertaken.

III. CALCULOUS PYELITIS is due to the irritation and obstruction set up by the presence of a stone. The *Differential Symptoms* are: (i.) A history of renal colic (§ 413) is often obtainable; with a large " stag-horn " calculus this is absent. (ii.) Pain on the diseased side, which varies with exercise; and (iii.) hæmaturia, also varying with exercise. (iv.) The quantity of pus often varies from day to day, and the patient may feel easier after its discharge, as the retained pus causes pain and sometimes swelling. (v.) Attacks of intermittent pyrexia and sometimes rigors. (vi.) Crystals in the urine aid the diagnosis of the cause.

IV. TUBERCULOUS PYELONEPHRITIS.—Tuberculous disease of the kidney may be primary or secondary to tubercle elsewhere, and is often associated with tuberculous infection of the genital system. Sometimes both kidneys are diseased. This condition may be difficult to diagnose from Calculous Pyelitis. *Differential Symptoms:* (i.) Increased frequency of micturition, and perhaps strangury, is the commonest early symptom; (ii.) hæmaturia occurs in 75 per cent. of cases; (iii.) dull pain in the loins, liable to colicy exacerbations from the passage of caseous masses; (iv.) *pyrexia of a regularly intermitting type*; (v.) the urine is acid, contains some albumen, pus and often red blood cells. Tubercle bacilli may be demonstrated in the deposit of a 24-hours' specimen, by culture, or by guinea-pig inoculations; other organisms are absent unless secondary infection has occurred. A sterile pyuria is often tuberculous or due to abacterial pyuria; (vi.) the cystoscope may show the presence of swelling or ulceration at the mouth of one ureter. Pyelography shows distortion of the structure of the affected area.

Renal tuberculosis may produce a small acute lesion or a larger chronic caseous area in the renal substance, or it may ulcerate one or more renal papillæ. Concomitant fibrosis produces obstruction to the flow of urine. Therefore the tuberculous focus may or may not be constantly in connection with the bladder (the " open " and the " closed " types). In the latter, many specimens of urine may have to be searched before tubercle bacilli are found.

Prognosis.—With modern methods of treatment, uncomplicated coli pyelitis usually clears up within 3–4 weeks, and provided the urine has been rendered sterile, as shown by examination of catheter specimens, relapse is unlikely. The course of ascending pyelitis depends very much upon the cause, the possibility of its removal, the age of the patient and the general condition: it used to be the common mode of death after fracture of the spine or transverse myelitis. Calculous pyelitis may last for years, but after surgical removal it may be possible to sterilise the urine with modern drugs. In the tuberculous form the prognosis depends on whether one or both kidneys are involved, the results of successful medical or surgical treatment and the presence of lesions elsewhere. Pyonephrosis (§ 432) may follow all the chronic forms of pyelonephritis.

Treatment.—In all forms of pyelonephritis fluid diet and warm drinks, rest in bed and warmth, are essential. (1.) The most common form is that due to *E. coli* infection. When there is fever, the best treatment is by a combination of sulphonamides (trisulphonamide N.F.) combined with equal parts of potassium citrate and sodium bicarbonate (gr. 30 of each): these latter must be given four-, three- or two-hourly (even at night) until every specimen of urine is alkaline to litmus paper. At the same time copious drinks of fluid must be given (4 to 6 pints daily); with this the temperature should settle in 3 to 4 days and the urine be sterile in 7 to 10 days. If the infection does not respond to this treatment, perhaps because the *E. coli* are sulphonamide-resistant, sensitivity tests should be performed and other drugs used (Table XXIV, page 580). Inject. streptomycin sulph. often proves effective when other remedies have failed. A rotating course of a sulphonamide, tetracycline, nitrofurantoin and sulphamethizole, giving each for a week at a time, is helpful in resistant or relapsing cases. Whichever method of treatment is used, it must be continued until two successive specimens of urine at an interval of 7 days are sterile. If the urine remains infected or relapse occurs X-ray examination, cystoscopy and urethroscopy are often necessary. *General measures.*—Apart from a high fluid intake and a light diet until the temperature has settled, the bowels must be regulated by mild aperients, such as paraffin, petroleum agar, senna, etc., so that the stools are neither constipated nor loose. (2.) When the infecting pyogenic organism is other than *E. coli* the appropriate drugs should be used (Table XXIV). (3.) Some cases call for nephrectomy or other surgical measures. Before operation it is necessary to determine which kidney is diseased and the state of activity of the healthy kidney. This is seen by the cystoscope, the ureteral catheter and sometimes by X-ray. In cases of *calculous pyelonephritis*, large doses of potassium citrate and bicarbonate may be employed for uric acid calculi; for oxalates, see Oxaluria (§ 431); and nephrolithotomy is needed in nearly all cases. (4.) In cases of *tuberculous pyelonephritis* the outlook has been greatly improved by chemotherapy. At least two of the three drugs inject. streptomycin sulph. 1 G., P.A.S. 16-20 G. and isoniazid 300 mg. should be given daily for 12-18 months, choosing the drugs to which the tubercle bacilli are most sensitive by laboratory tests (p. 230). Streptomycin is especially indicated when secondary infection is present but is better avoided in extensive tuberculous cystitis as it causes more fibrosis. If the urine can be rendered permanently free of tubercle bacilli surgery is not necessary. Operative measures are required after 3-4 months' chemotherapy if tubercle bacilli persist in the urine or recur later; this is most likely to happen when one kidney is extensively involved and in ulcero-cavernous lesions. Then, after renal function tests, nephrectomy with ureterectomy, or in some cases local resection of part of a kidney, are required.

A **diminution in the specific gravity,** *when marked and continuous, even in the absence of albumen, is suggestive of* CHRONIC INTERSTITIAL NEPHRITIS, *or more rarely* DIABETES INSIPIDUS. **A marked increase** *in the specific gravity is suggestive of* DIABETES MELLITUS.

§ 420. The other **causes of altered specific gravity** are relatively less important, because they are identified mainly by other means. Nevertheless, the specific gravity of the urine is an extremely important feature, because, in the absence of sugar, it is a MEASURE OF THE UREA and SODIUM CHLORIDE EXCRETION, the specific gravity being higher in direct proportion to the amounts contained in a given sample of urine. Therefore, it is a very fair measure of the power of concentration of the two kidneys taken together (and see § 376). For this purpose an early-morning specimen is essential, to avoid the effect of food and drink consumed during the day.

The specific gravity is DIMINISHED in—

1. Increased intake of fluid.
2. When the kidney reserve is called upon (see introduction to this section), as in Chronic Interstitial Nephritis, Secondary Contracted Kidney, etc.
3. Polyuria, and all the diseases mentioned below under that heading, excepting Diabetes Mellitus.
4. Myxœdema and other conditions with lowered nitrogenous metabolism.

The specific gravity is INCREASED in—

1. Diabetes Mellitus (owing to the sugar).
2. Some renal diseases where the quantity of water is considerably diminished, such as Acute Nephritis, Subacute Parenchymatous Nephritis, or the Cardiac Kidney.
3. Febrile and other conditions where the nitrogenous disintegration is excessive.
4. Whenever the urine becomes concentrated by profuse sweating, vomiting, diarrhœa, or diminished intake of fluid.

An **increase in the quantity of urine** (POLYURIA) *is complained of by the patient in several important diseases.*

§ 421. In **Polyuria** it is necessary to measure the total diurnal quantity, since patients are very apt to mistake increased frequency for increased quantity, and *vice versa*. It must be remembered that *in old age*, there is normally some increase in the diurnal excretion due to loss of concentrating power in the renal tubules.

Otherwise there is INCREASED QUANTITY of urine secreted in—

1. *Diabetes mellitus*, which is known by the high specific gravity of the urine and persistent glycosuria.
2. *Diabetes insipidus*—low specific gravity and malaise, but no sugar.
3. *Chronic interstitial nephritis*, which is known by the persistent low specific gravity of the urine, slight albuminuria, etc. (§ 401).
4. *Amyloid kidney*, which is known by the low specific gravity of the urine and great albuminuria (§ 409).
5. *Dietl's crises* are known by a dull pain in the loin which becomes more severe, associated with an enlarged tender, and often mobile, kidney. As the pain subsides, polyuria occurs for a few hours, with decreasing tenderness and swelling of the affected kidney: recurrences are common. The condition is not due to hydronephrosis but to temporary engorgement of a mobile kidney which becomes twisted on its pedicle: the polyuria is a reaction to the establishment of a normal blood flow as the attack subsides.
6. *Convalescence* after fevers.
7. *Temporary polyuria* occurs in Dietl's crises, alcoholism, following an attack of paroxysmal tachycardia or of asthma, hysteria, nervous excitement, and any condition giving rise to a reactionary or paralytic condition of the abdominal sympathetic. Cerebral tumours may be accompanied by polyuria.
8. During the administration of *diuretics*.
9. During the *absorption of exudations*, such as generalised œdema (anasarca).

The patient complains of **polyuria**; *the urine is of* HIGH SPECIFIC GRAVITY, *and* CONSTANTLY *contains* GLUCOSE (**glycosuria**); *there are also fatigue, thirst, and, in spite of a voracious appetite, gradual loss of flesh.* The disease is DIABETES MELLITUS. (See § 381 for Fallacies.)

§ 422. Temporary Glycosuria may arise in many conditions in which the carbohydrate metabolism is deranged; often it is of little or no consequence. (1) There may be a temporary diminution of sugar tolerance, particularly with septic infections (boils, etc.) in the elderly. (2) Chronic alcoholism. (3) Graves' disease. (4) Pregnancy and suckling (lactosuria). (5) Conditions, such as head injuries, meningitis or tumour affecting the brain, especially the pituitary or the fourth ventricle. (6) Dietetic errors, as after a heavy meal, especially in the obese. (7) During the paroxysms of ague and collapse of cholera. (8) After acute fevers, such as mumps. (9) At times of sudden emotion (as at a medical examination) or physical stress (*e.g.*, asphyxial conditions) due to excess of adrenalin in the blood. (10) After epileptic fits.

(11) **Lag glycosuria** is a condition where the blood sugar rises rapidly after a meal to a value above the renal threshold; the fasting value is normal and the blood sugar returns to normal at the usual rate. It is believed to be due to a delay in the action of insulin, and also occurs after gastro-enterostomy. Its presence can only be satisfactorily determined by a sugar tolerance curve, and it has no clinical significance.

(12) **Renal glycosuria** (Diabetes innocens, renal diabetes). When a small quantity of sugar is excreted in the urine, and yet the blood sugar is not above normal (§ 423), the condition is one of renal glycosuria. Glucose is normally present in the glomerular

filtrate and renal glycosuria is caused by a deficient reabsorption in the proximal convoluted tubules. The condition may be found accidentally whilst the urine is being examined. The sugar excretion in this condition is not much affected by increasing the carbohydrate in the diet; in the true diabetic the contrary is true. A sugar tolerance test and a study of the blood-sugar curve is required before diagnosing the glycosuria as renal (Fig. 135 (3)).   No treatment is required for this condition.

(13) The **Fanconi Syndrome** is a rare hereditary disease due to impaired tubular reabsorption of glucose (renal diabetes), amino-acids and phosphorus; the latter causes osteomalacia. *Symptoms* occur in infants and young children and occasionally in

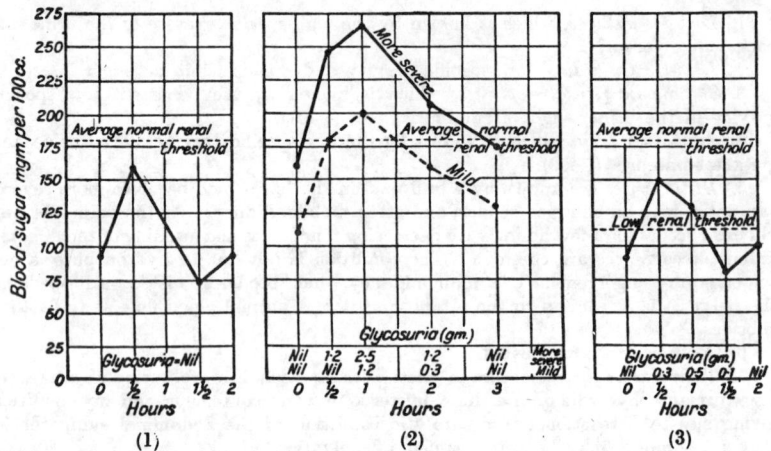

FIG. 135.—SUGAR TOLERANCE CURVES after 50 grammes glucose, with corresponding urinary sugars. (1) Normal. (2) Curves of mild and more severe diabetics. (3) Renal glycosuria showing lowered renal threshold.

adults. They are (1) Glycosuria with polyuria and polydipsia; (2) those of rickets with infantilism; deformities of long bones and fractures are common; (3) uræmia and liver cirrhosis may follow.

The *Diagnosis* is made by the family history, the X-ray changes in the bones, the abnormally low blood-phosphate levels, and finding glucose and large quantities of amino-acids (by paper chromatography) in the urine.

Treatment is unsatisfactory: large doses of calciferol, a high intake of calcium and phosphorus and combating the low alkali reserve of the serum may help.

§ 423. Diabetes Mellitus is a very common constitutional disease, characterised by the passage of large quantities of urine containing glucose. It is estimated that there are a quarter of a million persons with this disease in Great Britain at the present time.

Symptoms.—The patient may first complain of the symptoms of the disease itself, or of one of its complications (*e.g.*, cataract, gangrene). The primary symptoms are: (i.) The urine is abundant (polyuria), and may amount to 6–15 pints a day; clear, pale, but of high specific gravity, 1030–1050—raised beyond that which would be expected from the concentration as judged by the amount of pigment present. Sugar may vary from 1 to 9 per cent., is often accompanied by ketone bodies, and a trace of albumen may be present. If the urine drops on the boot, a crystalline deposit may be noticed by the patient. (ii.) Excessive thirst (polydipsia) and a dry tongue, which may become raw and cracked. (iii.) Cramps in the legs are common. (iv.) Loss of weight may be extreme, and is a gauge of the severity of the condition. (v.) The appetite is normal or excessive (especially in relation to the weight), unless ketosis or other complications are present, when it usually fails. (vi.) General symptoms such as lassitude, progressive weakness and ready fatigue. (vii.) The skin may lose its elasticity and become dry: it often acquires a yellow tint, especially on the hands and face, by which the disease may be suspected. This is due to an excess of a yellow pigment (carotene) circulating in the blood and staining the tissues. (viii.) The blood sugar is above the normal. This may be determined by estimating the fasting value (normally 70–100 mg. per cent.) or by a sugar tolerance estimation. In this test, after determining the fasting value, 50 grammes of glucose are administered and the blood-sugar value determined each ½ hour for 1½–2 hours. Typical curves are shown (Fig. 135).

Varieties.—There are two well-marked varieties: (a) A mild form met in grossly obese middle-aged people, where there are few symptoms, little or no ketosis and often no weight loss due to the disease. Removal of the excess weight removes the sugar from the urine and often causes the previous diabetic type of glucose tolerance curve to revert to normal. In this group the main cause is the consumption of food far above the bodily requirements: the plasma insulin level is almost within the normal range. (b) The variety with more severe symptoms, marked ketosis and considerable weight loss occurs in acute and chronic forms. In both of these the plasma insulin is markedly deficient. Whereas the acute form usually occurs in children or young adults, and occasionally after head injuries, the chronic form occurs in later life and sometimes follows temporary glycosuria (§ 422).

Complications are numerous: (1) *Occlusive vascular disease* is by far the most common. (a) Especially in obese subjects in their later years simple atheroma and /or hypertensive arteriolar disease are very frequent. Occlusive vascular disease in the legs is forty times more common in diabetics, causing intermittent claudication; gangrene readily supervenes in the toes and feet, usually of the dry variety; secondary infections readily arise in corns, ulcers, etc., and may produce a moist gangrene. Gangrene is due to ischæmia, and/or sepsis and /or neuropathy—or to all three. Symptoms due to coronary and cerebral atheroma are also frequent. (b) Renal lesions of vascular origin are often found. Glomerulo-sclerosis of the renal capillaries causes albuminuria: where this is advanced, copious albuminuria with hypertension and œdema are associated with a rising blood urea (Kimmelstiel–Wilson syndrome) (§ 408). Pyelonephritis is also common. (c) Capillary lesions often co-exist with the glomerular sclerosis; they are best seen in the unsupported capillaries of the retina as red dots which represent micro-aneurysms. (2) *Ketosis* and *coma* are due to defective fat metabolism. The excessive fat utilisation is shown by the excess of fat in the blood (lipæmia): in the absence of sufficient glucose utilisation, the end products of fat metabolism cannot be converted to CO_2 and water, and accumulate in the blood as β oxybutyric and aceto-acetic acids. The former is comparatively harmless but the latter stimulates respiration and depresses the brain, producing drowsiness and finally coma. In the more usual form of diabetic coma these ketone acids are secreted by the lungs and kidneys, and by losing CO_2 are partly converted to acetone, giving a sweet-smelling breath and the ferric chloride and Rothera's tests in the urine (§ 384). A rarer and more fatal variety is that in which the kidneys are unable to secrete these ketone bodies (anuric form), the urine being scanty or absent, containing albumen and abundant casts, and with a corresponding rise in blood urea. THE SYMPTOMS OF KETOSIS are (i.) in the *earlier stages*, loss of appetite, abdominal pain, nausea and vomiting; drowsiness is usually present but occasionally may be replaced by undue restlessness, irritability and giddiness. In the *later stages* coma develops. This is accompanied by slow deep breathing (" air hunger "), a sweet-smelling breath, diminution in the urinary volume which may be extreme in the anuric form, and usually the presence of acetone and aceto-acetic acid in the urine, with a lowered intraocular tension of the eyeballs. (3) *Infections,* especially staphylococcal and tuberculous, are liable to arise. The former may give rise to skin infections— pruritus vulvæ, boils, carbuncles and deep-seated abscesses; the latter commonly causes pulmonary tuberculosis. It is essential to examine the urine in all cases of pruritus vulvæ, boils and carbuncles, and of acute infections, especially in elderly subjects with pneumonia, who are not responding satisfactorily to treatment. In young persons yearly routine chest X-rays are highly desirable. (4) Ocular changes may be transient or permanent. The former is due to dehydration of the lens with temporary blurring of vision. Permanent damage results from retinopathy (§ 1133), cataract and sometimes retinitis proliferans. (5) Polyneuritis (§ 980) is common and cerebral changes (depression or restlessness, mania and melancholia) make satisfactory treatment difficult. Diarrhœa at night is associated with a raised protein in the C.S.F. (6) Pregnancy markedly increases the need for insulin: the fœtal mortality in the last month of pregnancy is 20–25 per cent. so Cæsarean section at the 36th week is highly desirable.

Diagnosis.—In any of the conditions mentioned under *Complications* the urine should be examined. This is the key to the diagnosis. In *diabetes insipidus, granular kidney, amyloid kidney,* and with excessive fluid intake (as in beer-drinkers) the quantity of urine is excessive, but in none of these conditions is sugar present. Three golden rules will enable us to identify a case of diabetes which otherwise might be overlooked: Always examine the urine of a patient suffering from (1) boils or eczema of the genitals, (2) apparently causeless wasting, and (3) in any case of coma. Other causes of glycosuria are discussed in § 422.

Etiology.—(1) A deficient production of insulin occurs when the β cells of the islets of Langerhans are diseased. The α cells of the islets secrete an anti-insulin substance (glucagon) which converts liver glycogen into glucose. Deficient insulin secretion may be due to (a) an inherited tendency. The disease often runs in families, especially in the Jewish race; in successive generations it tends to occur at an earlier age, with corresponding increase in severity of the disease. (b) Infections: A *generalised infection* (i.) calls for a greater output of insulin, which may not be forthcoming, and (ii.) may damage the pancreatic cells. With *acute infections* (boils, carbuncles, pneumonia) the disease may first manifest itself, the condition being temporary or permanent. (c) Progressive fibrosis of the pancreas occurs in hæmochromatosis and sometimes in tertiary syphilis. (d) A gradual obliteration of blood supply is met in arteriosclerosis of the cœliac axis and pancreatic arteries. (2) Overaction of the thyroid gland, especially primary thyrotoxicosis, causes a rise in blood-sugar level which the pancreas tries to correct. When thyrotoxicosis and diabetes occur together, wasting is rapid and often extreme. In some cases of thyrotoxicosis the blood-sugar level is not raised, but glycosuria occurs due to a lowering of the renal threshold (renal diabetes). (3) The pituitary secretes a diabetogenic hormone which not only stimulates the production of glucose from glycogen and from non-carbohydrate sources but also prevents the metabolism of sugar by the tissues. Oversecretion of the pituitary (as in tumour or acromegaly) may produce glycosuria. (4) Hypersecretion of the suprarenal cortex (Cushing's syndrome) is a rare cause. (5) Temporary glycosuria from overaction of the suprarenals occurs in times of sudden stress and emotion (§ 422).

Prognosis.—This depends on the age of the patient and, particularly in younger persons, the care taken over the diet and the use of insulin. Before the discovery of insulin, if the disease was established in a young adult, life rarely lasted more than two years. Since the discovery of insulin the outlook has much improved and most patients *with proper treatment and control of the disease* lead an almost normal life to the expected age. The middle-aged or elderly overweight diabetic is often readily controlled by simple weight reduction, which causes the blood sugar to return to normal levels; and provided weight is not put on again the diabetes remains in abeyance. *Mild cases* who are of average weight, after the age of 40 years are often rendered sugar-free by simple reduction of the carbohydrate intake to 120-160 G. a day without the use of insulin. More *severe diabetics*, *i.e.*, those of a younger age, those with ketosis or who are underweight, always require the injection of insulin, and the younger the patient the larger the dose. Once the condition has been adequately controlled, the amount of insulin required may often be reduced for a period of months or even years, although later on it usually has to be increased again up to a dose (usually 50-75 units a day) which need not be further increased. The presence of *complications* adds to the gravity of the disease when there is pulmonary tuberculosis, a septic infection or gangrene, but with modern methods, including the use of antibiotics, these

are now much more readily controlled. Unless neglected or badly managed, **most** patients with diabetic coma survive. Other complications, especially **those** due to arterial disease and those occurring in the eye (cataract, **retinitis,** etc.) are much more likely to occur and to be progressive when the **patient** is careless with the control of the diabetes, with prolonged periods **of** hyperglycæmia.

In *Treatment* certain objects should be achieved: (i.) sufficient calories must be given to maintain normal nutrition; (ii.) the diet taken must prevent ketosis; (iii.) as much variety as possible should be allowed; (iv.) the blood sugar should be maintained within normal limits.

Middle-aged or elderly *obese* diabetics should be given a 1,000-calorie diet (§ 296. VI) with considerable restriction of bread, sugar and other carbohydrates until their weight is reduced to that which existed before obesity set in. To calculate the calories necessary for a *young* diabetic and especially in a patient who has lost a considerable amount of weight, it is necessary to give a diet in proportion to the normal weight before the disease set in, and if this weight is not known it can be estimated from tables (see Table at end of book). In adults the values per kilo of the normal weight are: (*a*) sedentary workers, 30–35 calories (15 calories per 1 lb.), (*b*) for those doing moderate muscular work 35–45 calories, and (*c*) for heavy manual workers 45–60 calories. Diabetics can live a healthy life consuming rather fewer calories than the average man or woman, and the guide as to whether the diet is sufficient is by regular weighing: under no conditions should a diabetic patient (especially when treated with insulin) become overweight. The amount to be given as protein is about $\frac{2}{3}$ gram per kilo, the amount of fat is just under 1 gram per kilo and the remaining calories are made up with carbohydrate. In practice it is rarely considered necessary nowadays to weigh the protein and the fat-containing foods — patients are allowed average small helpings of fish, meat, bird, cheese, bacon and eggs: these amount to 60–90 G. of protein and 70–110 G. of fat a day. On the other hand the amount of carbohydrate prescribed must be strictly adhered to.[1] The present tendency is to give more carbohydrate than formerly, with amounts in different patients between 100 and 220 G. a day. The advantages of this higher carbohydrate and rather low fat diet are (i.) it is more palatable and more closely resembles the normal diet, (ii.) it is cheaper, (iii.) the sugar tolerance increases in proportion to the carbohydrate value of the diet, (iv.) insulin requirements are not greater than on a high-fat, low-carbohydrate diet, (v.) the patient feels better, (vi.) ketosis and complications such as arteriosclerosis and infective disorders are less common, (vii.) the heart muscle keeps in better condition. There are several convenient methods of giving as much variety as possible. Lawrence's " Line ration " scheme is easy to follow and is arranged to save

---

[1] Many of the advertised starch-free breads are by no means what they claim to be; the careful physician should examine them for starch with the iodine test, and for sugar by boiling them with dilute sulphuric acid, neutralising with caustic potash and adding Fehling's solution. Soluble saccharin B.P. is taken in place of sugar.

trouble in calculating. A " black line " contains 10 G. of carbohydrate (41 calories). The carbohydrate in one line can be replaced by the corresponding number of grammes in another line. Diets worked out on the Lawrence Scheme are set out in § 296. VIII. In children, extra calories and protein must be allowed for growth.

INSULIN is now manufactured in seven different varieties which have shorter or longer durations of action. The object of giving insulin is to supplement the patient's own supply, when by dieting alone the sugar in the urine cannot be controlled and when the blood sugar remains above 180-200 mg. per cent. It is essential in all young diabetics and in the presence of ketosis. (a) *Insulin B.P.*, better known as *soluble insulin* (S.I.), is a clear acid solution which begins to act within ½ hour of injection. It is useful to stabilise the severe diabetic as it can be given 3-4 times a day to get the disease under control. It should be started immediately the patient is seen if the amount of ketosis in the urine is sufficient to give a positive ferric chloride test. During stabilisation the urine must be tested four-hourly, and the insulin administered once, twice or three times daily according to the severity of the case, 15-20 minutes before the principal meals. The dose should be increased by 6 units daily until the urine is sugar-free, and then it is wise to perform blood-sugar estimations to make sure the values are within normal limits. For severe cases, double and quadruple strengths of insulin are available.

(b) Once the patient's blood sugars are stabilised and ketosis has disappeared, most patients can change from the shorter-acting S.I. to longer acting preparations, so that only one, or occasionally two, doses need to be given each 24 hours. The prolonged actions are due to insulin being combined with protamine or with globin, which in the presence of traces of zinc have a still more prolonged effect. (*Protamine zinc insulin (P.Z.I.) and globin zinc insulin.*)

(c) More recently insulin has been joined with zinc without a foreign protein, but the suspension has to be in an acetate buffer. Three varieties of this *insulin zinc suspension* (I.Z.S.) exist: (i.) Ultra-lente (crystalline) which is very long acting, (ii.) Semi-lente (amorphous) which is relatively short acting, and (iii.) Lente which is a combination of the first two (7 parts of crystalline and 3 parts of amorphous zinc insulin). Lente insulin is in common use, for it gives a fairly uniform action over a period of 24 hours. A similar effect to that of lente insulin is produced by a mixture of P.Z.I. with a small dose of S.I. measured into the same syringe and given as a single injection (Table XXV). (The S.I. must be measured into the syringe before the P.Z.I. is added to avoid precipitation of the rest of the S.I. in the bottle by any P.Z.I. accidentally introduced.) Isophane insulin (N.P.H.) is now rarely used. The amount of carbohydrate portions must be increased at the meals corresponding to the times when the particular insulin preparation has the strongest action: thus lunch and tea must be fairly large when using globin insulin with zinc because of the liability to hypoglycæmia in the late afternoon: and when P.Z.I. or lente insulin are given, a bedtime meal of 10–20 G. of carbohydrate are also essential to prevent insidious hypoglycæmia during the sleeping hours. In severe cases which cannot be stabilised with a single dose of P.Z.I. with S.I., or by lente insulin, 12-hourly injections of globin insulin with zinc may prove helpful. Urticarial reactions to the

TABLE XXV. TIMES AT WHICH THE DIFFERENT TYPES OF INSULIN PRODUCE THEIR EFFECTS ON THE BLOOD SUGAR.

Type of insulin.	Maximum effect after injection (overdose causes hypoglycæmia): in hours.	Total duration of action after injection: in hours.	Comments.
I. Quick-acting Soluble insulin.	small doses 2–4 large doses 6–8	6 9–12	Clear solution: may be combined with P.Z.I. but not with I.Z.S.
II. Longer acting Globin insulin with Zn. I.Z.S. amorphous (semi-lente).	small doses 5–8 large doses 8–12	8 16	Cloudy suspensions.
III. Very long acting P.Z. insulin. I.Z.S. crystalline (ultra-lente).	small doses 5–8 large doses 18–24	12 24–30	Useful in smaller doses: undesirable in doses above 40 units because of varying rates of absorption from day to day.
IV. Combination of above P.Z.I. with S.I. I.Z.S. (lente insulin) composed of 7 parts ultra-lente and 3 parts semi-lente.	4–8 and again 12–24	4–30	Both in common use for moderate and severe diabetes.

Of these longer-acting insulins (i) P.Z. Insulin either alone or with Sol. Insulin and (ii) I.Z.S. (lente insulin) are the most often employed.

insulins combined with protein may be avoided by using lente insulin. After stabilisation with any of these preparations the dose of insulin may have to be varied from time to time as the disease gets more or less severe; and the patient should not only be instructed how to ward off hypoglycæmic reactions but also how to give his own insulin and test the urine regularly for sugar and acetone.

Ketosis is usually effectively controlled by the combination of insulin with increased carbohydrate and diminished fat in the diet. In pyrexial disorders, there is an increased need of insulin, whereas in pregnancy the dose must be immediately reduced by one half directly after childbirth.

Tolbutamide and certain other oral preparations, when given in tablet form, lower the blood sugar in mild cases of diabetes. They can replace injections of insulin in patients who do not need more than 30 units a day, but they are not effective in children or in those under 40 years of age and they cannot replace insulin when ketonuria is present. *Tolbutamide* in doses of 0·50 G. two or three times a day has a short-lived action, the effect of each dose lasting about 3 hours. *Chlorpropamide* is more effective than tolbutamide. Given with breakfast in an initial dose of 500 mg., often reduced later to 200 mg., it has a hypoglycæmic effect lasting 24 hours or more; it may produce drug rashes, gastro-intestinal upsets and occasionally jaundice. *Metahexamide* also acts for 24 hours or more. In initial doses of 300 mg. at breakfast, reduced later to 200 mg., 100 mg., or even 50 mg. after a few days when a satisfactory hypoglycæmic effect has been attained, it is well tolerated; jaundice is rarely seen after its use. *Phenethyldiguanide* 75 mg. per dose needs to be given twice a day and is liable to produce nausea and vomiting. A combination of chlorpropamide or metahexamide with phenethyldiguanide may be more effective than using one drug only.

§ 424. Treatment of Severe Diabetic Ketosis (Precoma) and of Diabetic Coma. Diabetic precoma is present when the patient is very drowsy, has air-hunger, severe ketosis (and a strongly positive reaction in the urine to the ferric chloride test), sometimes vomiting, but during which he can still swallow fluids. The patient should immediately be given N/2 saline by mouth. With this Lawrence advises an injection of soluble insulin 40 units, the dose to be repeated after 4 hours if the amount of sugar in the urine produces a red or yellow precipitate with Benedict's solution; but only 20 units are needed if the precipitate is green and no insulin is needed if the test is blue.

In diabetic coma the main indications are to combat the dehydration, the ketosis and the circulatory collapse. At this stage the patient is relatively resistant to insulin and 50–100 units of *soluble* insulin should be given immediately (one half being administered intravenously); 2 litres of N-saline needs to be given via an intravenous drip in the first 3 hours. (In severe cases the first litre of saline should be of twice normal strength and 0·5–1·0 litres of blood plasma or dextran also given.) Stimulants such as noradenaline, metaraminol or hydrocortisone can be administered via the intravenous tube. If *consciousness returns*, 500 G. of glucose should be dissolved in 2,500 ml. of half-normal saline, and 100 ml. administered by mouth each hour, with 10 units of insulin hourly, until the blood sugar level falls to 300 mg. per cent. If the *patient is still unconscious*, 50 G. of glucose in 0·5–1·0 litres of normal saline are given (preferably) into a vein or by a duodenal tube, with 30–50 units of insulin intramusc. each 4 hours until consciousness returns. Then the intravenous medication may be replaced by the half-normal saline and glucose by mouth, until with the control of the ketosis, milk, Benger's food, etc., may be commenced. In the "anuric" variety still larger doses of intravenous saline ($1\frac{1}{2}$–2 litres in the first hour) with 100–200 units of insulin must be given at once: subsequently further intravenous dextrose-saline (0·5–1·0 litres) with saline per rectum must be combined with 4-hourly insulin until the urine is passed in adequate quantities. When an infection has precipitated coma, often there is no pyrexia, but leucocytosis gives valuable confirmation and penicillin is often necessary. The doses of insulin may then have to be very large, even 500–600 units in 24 hours, but regular blood sugar analyses are essential when using such doses. At the commencement of treatment the stomach should be washed out, throughout the patient should be kept warm and in bed for 3–4 days. Potassium deficiency of the plasma may occur a few hours after commencing treatment due to the insulin and sodium chloride given in large doses causing potassium to pass into the intracellular fluids: this may cause death from cardiac failure unless potassium chloride is given (2 G. of potassium chloride by mout⸍ t.d.s. for 2 days only).

Estimation of the Blood Sugar. Folin-Wu Method.—Blood is obtained from a finger prick, and 0·2 ml. is measured accurately into 1·6 ml. of sodium tungstate solution in a centrifuge tube. Then 0·2 ml. of 2/3N sulphuric acid is added, and the whole is shaken. By this means the blood is diluted ten times, and the protein coagulated. The protein precipitate is centrifuged off, or allowed to settle, and 0·75 ml. of the supernatant fluid is pipetted into the special hard-glass boiling-tube. From two standard solutions containing respectively 0·01 per cent. and 0·02 per cent. glucose, 0·75 ml. of each are placed in similar hard-glass tubes. To each of these three, 0·75 ml. of the copper solution is added, and the solutions shaken together. The tubes are boiled for exactly six minutes in a boiling water-bath, and after cooling in a cold water-bath for three to five minutes, 0·75 ml. of the sodium molybdate solution is added, and each tube has distilled water added to the 9 ml. mark. The relative depths of the colour of the blue solutions are compared in a colorimeter or in Nessler tubes, the amount of sugar present in each being proportional to the depth of the colour. Suppose a depth of 50 mm. of the unknown sugar solution matches a depth of 40 mm. of the 0·02 per cent. standard sugar solution, the unknown solution contains $\frac{40}{50} \times 0·02$ per cent. sugar. Allowing for the dilution of the blood × 10, the blood sugar value is $\frac{40}{50} \times 0·02 \times 10$ per cent. = 0·16 per cent. The normal fasting blood sugar is 0·08 to 0·10 per cent. After a meal it may rise to 170 mg. per cent. Values above 200 mg. per cent. are abnormally high. The blood sugar becomes too low after an overdose of insulin, and may fall to 30–50 mg. per cent.

The *glucose-oxidase test* is specific for blood glucose but gives rather lower figures.

Congenital Galactosæmia is becoming more frequently recognised. It is a familial condition in which the infant is unable to convert galactose (derived from lactose) into glucose.

Symptoms commence in the early weeks or months of life. Wasting, dehydration, lethargy and often vomiting are usual and the urine strongly reduces Benedict's solution; there is often albuminuria, and amino-aciduria is always present. The liver soon enlarges, jaundice is present in two-thirds of the cases, intercurrent infections often occur and unless the condition is treated early, cataract and mental retardation follow.

The *Diagnosis* is by finding sugar in the urine which is non-fermentable: the blood galactose content is high and the urinary sugar is identified as galactose by paper chromatography.

The *Prognosis* is good only if it is recognised early. Death may occur in the early weeks or months of life from intercurrent infection. Complete recovery is possible. *Treatment* is by excluding milk and milk products (such as butter) from the diet. Milk substitutes such as Nutramigen, or Casilan with arachis oil and coconut oil with vitamins should be given. Within a few days the galactosuria disappears and the liver decreases in size.

§ 425. Hypoglycæmia and Hypoglycæmic Coma are due to a rapid fall in the blood sugar to a low level. This may be due to an overdose of insulin or to endogenous causes.

Symptoms.—Early symptoms are believed to be due to the sudden release of adrenalin: these are a sense of weakness, " sinking feelings," anxiety, sweating, tremors, palpitation, pallor, hunger-pains, nausea, vomiting and headache. Numbness of the lips, hemiparesis and occasionally diplopia may occur. Difficulty of waking in the mornings may be complained of (Garland). *Later symptoms* are due to the effects on cerebral function: they take many different forms and tend to be repetitive in the same patient. These include (i.) amnesia with automatism lasting seconds, minutes or hours during which the behaviour is normal. There is permanent loss of memory during this time: (ii.) attacks of unusual behaviour during which the patient may be confused, noisy, even violent, dysarthric or ataxic: (iii.) involvement of the special senses may cause diplopia, visual hallucinations, macropsia or micropsia, olfactory hallucinations, vestibular symptoms with rotary vertigo—but without tinnitus or deafness: (iv.) transient or prolonged coma may occur (§ 855): (v.) major epileptic convulsions are met but such patients never develop status epilepticus.

The *diagnosis* is made by the symptoms. It is confirmed by special tests:—(i.) by finding a blood sugar value under 60 mg. per cent.: a value below 50 mg. per cent. is diagnostic. (ii.) In spontaneous cases (*i.e.*, not due to insulin injections) typical attacks are often induced when a patient in a fasting condition is injected with 5–10 units of insulin. (iii.) A prolonged glucose tolerance test carried out for 5 or 6 hours shows a fall of blood sugar below 50 mg. per cent. after the first 2 or 3 hours. (iv.) Following inject. adrenalin 1 ml. subcut. in a starving person, the blood sugar taken at $\frac{1}{4}$-hour intervals for 1 hour rises by at least 35 mg. per cent.: this rise fails to occur in the presence of hypoglycæmia. (v.) An electro-encephalogram shows a depressed cortical function and later disappearance of the alpha rhythm during the hypoglycæmic period. (vi.) When in doubt as to whether the symptoms present are due to hypoglycæmia a diagnostic procedure is to give 1 oz. of glucose by mouth or 10 ml. of a 20 per cent. solution intravenously: unless the patient is in deep or prolonged coma the immediate symptoms are dramatically relieved and the E.E.G. signs disappear.

Etiology.—Although a low blood sugar value is important, the rapidity of fall of the blood sugar in a short space of time is probably of even greater importance. Attacks are therefore often induced by vigorous exercise before meals. The only *exogenous* cause is an overdose of injected insulin. When symptoms occur at the same time on succeeding days, the dose injected is too large. Coma is usually due to carelessness on the part of the patient, as when the usual dose of insulin is taken without being followed by a meal, or in the presence of vomiting. *Endogenous* causes are (i.) the over-production of insulin (hyper-insulinism) by islet cell tumours of the pancreas. There may be a single adenoma, multiple adenomata, multiple microscopic adenomatosis of the pancreas or an islet-cell carcinoma. (ii.) Especially since partial gastrectomy has been so frequently performed for the treatment of peptic ulcer a high carbohydrate meal passing rapidly into the small intestine may cause a temporary high blood sugar and then a rapid fall due to overstimulating the insulin-producing mechanism, and therefore hypoglycæmic symptoms. (iii.) A functional hypoglycæmia occurs for a similar reason in some individuals with an unstable personality and a rapidly emptying stomach, in the absence of a gastric operation. (iv.) Anterior pituitary deficiency may cause hypoglycæmia and coma. The low blood sugars of Von Gierke's disease (§ 345), liver failure and Addison's disease do not cause symptoms.

Prognosis.—In the milder types of hypoglycæmia rapid recovery occurs on giving glucose. After a large overdose of insulin, administered accidentally or for purposes of suicide, resulting in prolonged coma and a very low blood sugar value, irreversible changes may occur in the brain cells which causes permanent loss of the higher faculties or prolonged coma and death. To prevent this, any patient with coma due to an undiagnosed cause should be given intravenous dextrose *immediately* unless the blood sugar can be rapidly estimated.

Treatment.—Following an overdose of insulin, administer 1 oz. of sugar by mouth; if the patient is unconscious 10 ml. of 20 per cent. dextrose should be given intravenously or sugar given via a stomach-tube. The blood sugar is also raised by an injection of adrenalin (Ⅲ 10–15) or of posterior pituitary extract (0·5–1·0 ml.). In spontaneous hyperinsulinism the same immediate measures should be used and then a high carbohydrate diet prescribed: small doses of thyroid (gr. 1–2) may help. If these measures are insufficient, surgical removal of the adenoma or carcinoma will be curative, or if a local tumour is not located, total pancreatectomy or removal of the tail of the pancreas will reduce the amount of insulin secreted. In those cases following gastric operation or due to rapid gastric emptying, a low-carbohydrate high-fat and high-protein diet is of help.

The patient complains of polyuria *and many of the other symptoms of* Diabetes Mellitus, *but the* SPECIFIC GRAVITY OF THE URINE IS LOW, *and there is* NO SUGAR. The disease is DIABETES INSIPIDUS.

§ 426. Diabetes Insipidus is characterised by great and persistent increase in the quantity of the urine, without glycosuria and albuminuria, attended by distressing thirst; in severe cases loss of weight is marked.

Symptoms.—(1) The amount of urine may be very great, from 5 to 10 litres per day. It is pale in colour, so that it resembles clear water. The specific gravity averages 1002 to 1005. The diurnal amount of solid constituents is as a rule not very much increased, and no other abnormality is usually found. Occasionally traces of albumen and sugar appear towards the end. (2) In the mild form of the disease polyuria and thirst are the only symptoms; but in the more severe variety nearly all the symptoms mentioned under Diabetes Mellitus are also present—dry skin, emaciation, large appetite, and alternating constipation and diarrhœa. Indeed, it is distinguished from that condition only by the absence of glycosuria. Intercurrent attacks of pyrexia have been observed. (3) Nervous symptoms are common in this disease—irritability of temper, disturbed sleep, occipital headache, neuralgic pains in the lumbar region, diminished reflexes and muscular twitchings.

Diagnosis.—The disease is apt in its early stages to be mistaken for *chronic interstitial nephritis*, but the greater age of the patient, the presence of traces of albumen, and of cardio-vascular symptoms, and the absence of thirst and voracious appetite distinguish the latter condition. With *amyloid kidney* there is albumen, and with both *hydronephrosis* and *polycystic kidney* a tumour is generally palpable in the region of the kidney. In *Diabetes Mellitus* there is glycosuria. In the majority of cases the diagnosis can be confirmed by the relief of symptoms following an injection of posterior pituitary extract.

Etiology.—The cause is a deficient secretion of the anti-diuretic hormone of the posterior lobe of the pituitary. This normally acts on the thin segment of Henle's loop in the renal tubules and promotes absorption of water (not of sodium chloride) after the glomerular filtrate has in large part been absorbed in the proximal convoluted tubules. Affection of the sub-thalamic area is more common than is involvement of the post-pituitary itself; complete removal of the pituitary body does not cause this condition, suggesting that the anterior lobe produces an antagonist to the anti-diuretic hormone. Men are more commonly affected than women, especially in early middle age or in childhood. Some cases are hereditary or familial. Other causal factors are: head injury involving the hypothalamus or the post-pituitary, a primary tumour or secondary metastases, syphilis, meningitis, encephalitis, xanthoma in Hand-Schüller-Christian disease or hyperparathyroidism.

Prognosis.—The milder varieties may last for many years, and exist mainly as an inconvenience. In the severe forms, especially those due to intracranial tumours, the course may be rapid. When setting in acutely after head injury (which may be attended by some glycosuria at first) recovery may ensue after a year or so. In general terms, acute cases are more hopeful than those which start insidiously; hereditary and familial cases respond poorly to post. pituitary compounds, perhaps because the primary defect is in the renal tubules. Death takes place from exhaustion, drowsiness passing into coma with or without convulsions, or from complications such as phthisis or pneumonia.

Treatment.—Substances which increase diuresis, such as tea, coffee, alcohol and salt, should be avoided, but the amount of fluid taken should not be reduced below that which the patient can comfortably manage. The active principle in the pituitary is supplied by giving injections of posterior pituitary extract, or better still pitressin tannate in oil (5 units per ml. each 24–72 hours), both of which contain the antidiuretic factor. In some cases the missing factor can be given by painting pituitary extract on the nasal mucosa or by inhaling piton snuff. However these are given, the extracts tend to lose their efficacy after a time. Anti-syphilitic treatment is given when there is a positive Wassermann.

A **decrease in the quantity of urine** (OLIGURIA) occurs in two distinct conditions:—

    A. Retention of Urine in the Bladder (§ 427).

    B. Suppression of Urine which may be Obstructive or Non-obstructive (§ 428).

The patient complains that he **cannot pass water**, *and a* DISTENDED BLADDER *can be made out by palpation and percussion above the pubes, or by the passage of a catheter.* The condition is RETENTION OF URINE.

§ 427. A. The Causes of **Retention of Urine** come mainly within the province of the surgeon. Those of *sudden* onset are often due to urethral spasm or congestion; those of *gradual* onset are more numerous. The age and sex of the patient may aid us.

Thus, in *childhood* we may suspect impacted calculus or foreign body, a congenital valve of the urethra, phimosis, or a ligature round the penis; in *women*, tumours pressing on the neck of the bladder (*e.g.*, fibroid or retroverted enlarged uterus), hysteria, or reflex irritation after parturition; in young or middle-aged *adults*, urethral stricture, gonorrhœa with congested mucous membrane, spasm after exposure to cold or a drinking bout, or tabes dorsalis; in *old men*, prostatic enlargement or atony of the bladder. At all ages there may be a calculus or tumour blocking the neck of the bladder, paralysis of the bladder from diseased or injured spinal cord or brain, or reflex spasm after operations around the perineum. Hydronephrosis commonly results.

The *Treatment* is mainly surgical. Before undertaking any operation the blood urea (§ 389) should be estimated. If this is high, over 75 mg. per cent., there is interference with the kidney function and operation may be dangerous; drainage of the bladder improves the condition and operation may be safe later on. In cases of spasm a hot bath or hot fomentations to the abdomen give relief. Hysterical and other nervous affections are referred to elsewhere. Atony and simple vesical paralysis may be treated by an injection of carbacholum. B.P. (doryl) or a mixture containing nux vomica and belladonna.

The patient complains that he has not passed any water for some time, but there are NO EVIDENCES *of a* DISTENDED BLADDER, *and on passing a catheter it is found to be empty, or nearly so.* The condition is SUPPRESSION OF URINE.

§ 428. B. **Suppression of Urine** (Syn., Oliguria or Anuria) is a very grave condition. A catheter should always be passed before the diagnosis of suppression is made. There are two kinds: I. OBSTRUCTIVE suppression, which is due to some obstruction to the flow of urine through the ureters; and II. NON-OBSTRUCTIVE suppression, which is due to the non-secretion of urine by the kidneys. The latter form is sometimes spoken of as true suppression.

I. OBSTRUCTIVE SUPPRESSION is due to blocking of both ureters (the kidneys being healthy) by (i.) renal calculi: (ii.) a renal calculus blocking one ureter may cause reflex suppression in the other kidney; (iii.) blocking of both ureters by sulphonamide crystals (especially after sulphathiazole and sulphadiazine); (iv.) tumour at the base of the bladder; (v.) malformation of the ureters, *e.g.*, aberrant renal vessels, periureteritis fibrosa. When only one ureter is blocked, the urine that passes is clear, of low specific gravity, and non-albuminous; but, provided the other kidney is healthy, there is no renal inadequacy, the healthy kidney undergoing compensatory hypertrophy (see also Hydronephrosis, § 432). When both ureters are blocked, a condition known as " *latent uræmia* " arises.

The *Symptoms* are: the patient passes no urine for several days, and may complain of nothing except slight drowsiness, but after eight or ten days he becomes restless, with contracted pupils, subnormal temperature, dry brown tongue, and muscular twitchings. In other cases vomiting may be so severe as to suggest the presence of intestinal obstruction. Death is usually sudden, after ten to fourteen days, the mind remaining clear to the end.

II. NON-OBSTRUCTIVE SUPPRESSION is the result of severe renal failure due to Acute or Chronic causes:

1. Acute Nephritis (§ 397).
2. Acute Tubular Necrosis (see below).
3. Subacute Nephritis (§ 398).
4. The final stages of Chronic Interstitial Nephritis (§ 401), Malignant Nephrosclerosis (§ 403), Chronic Pyelonephritis (§ 419), and of Secondary Contracted Kidney (§ 400).
5. The Cardiac Kidney and some other Renal Congestions, including thrombosis of the inferior vena cava.
6. Febrile States including Heat Stroke.
∴ Diabetic Coma in its Anuric form (§ 423).

8. Polyarteritis Nodosa (§ 98).
9. Whenever there is profound collapse and shock, profuse vomiting, diarrhœa, perspiration or when little fluid is taken.
10. Embolism or thrombosis of both renal arteries (very rare). This may follow aortography.

The *Symptoms* are:—(1) any urine passed is highly coloured and concentrated (high specific gravity), and may contain albumen and casts (indicating that the suppression is due to renal disease); (2) there may be urgent vomiting, diarrhœa and sweating. The other symptoms are those of acute uræmia (§ 372) and those of the cause.

Acute Tubular Necrosis (Syn., Lower Nephron Necrosis) occurs in the distal convoluted tubules and is usually the result of a prolonged fall in blood pressure or of toxic damage to the tubules. It was first recognised during World War II following crush injuries, but is now known to follow many other causes.

CRUSH INJURIES follow severe crushing of a limb under débris. The urinary output due to the initial shock falls further, with marked albuminuria, myohæmoglobinuria and dark-brown granular casts. Complete suppression often follows with incessant vomiting and thirst. At an early stage due to the muscle trauma, severe hyperpotassæmia (hyperkalæmia) results, the blood urea reaching a maximum on the sixth to ninth days. If some urinary secretion persists recovery may ensue.

Etiology.—The cause may be due to a reflex from the injured limb causing the blood flow in the kidneys to by-pass the renal glomeruli via the vasa recta (" renal shunt ") giving rise to anoxia, or the tissue trauma may produce an endogenous, chemical toxin which affects the renal tubules.

Other causes of Acute Tubular Necrosis are (i.) the prolonged application of a tourniquet to a limb; (ii.) after severe abdominal operations or injuries; (iii.) especially after operation on cases of severe obstructive jaundice; (iv.) severe burns; (v.) obstetric shock; (vi.) concealed accidental uterine hæmorrhage; (vii.) incompatible blood transfusions; (viii.) with hæmolytic anæmias; (ix.) following acute poisoning with salts of mercury, lead, phenol, phosphorus, carbon tetrachloride, potassium bichromate, turpentine or with certain sulphonamide drugs; (x.) with prolonged circulatory collapse after overdose of ganglion-blocking drugs; (xi.) after passage of a catheter, cystoscopy, ascending pyelography or other instrumentation.

Prognosis of Suppression.—Suppression is a very serious condition, though the gravity depends somewhat upon the cause. Of the *obstructive* forms, calculus blocking one ureter, the kidney of the opposite side being healthy, is perhaps the most favourable. If the obstruction affects both ureters and is not removed, death will occur in about eleven days after the obstruction began. In the *non-obstructive* forms death or partial recovery takes place in a few days.

Treatment.—In acute *non-obstructive suppression* the treatment is that of acute uræmia (§ 372). In crush injuries intravenous calcium gluconate will antagonise the effects of hyperpotassæmia. When a sulphonamide drug is causal, lavage through a ureteric catheter by 2·5 per cent. sodium bicarbonate will remove crystals from the ureters: otherwise bilateral nephrostomy may be required. In some cases good results have been obtained from blocking the sympathetic vaso-constrictor fibres to the kidneys with either a spinal anæsthetic, or a bilateral paravertebral block with procaine. Decapsulation of the kidneys may relieve, for the kidneys are often in a state of " cloudy swelling," and when given space to expand recover their function.

For the treatment of *obstructive suppression* a surgeon should be consulted at once.

The patient has **lost the power of controlling the flow of urine** *and the clothes or bed-clothes are soaked with it—the condition is* INCONTINENCE OF URINE.

§ 429.· **Incontinence of Urine** may be *true* or *false incontinence*.

(a) TRUE INCONTINENCE occurs when the urine dribbles away involuntarily as fast as it is formed. The bladder fails to retain urine, either temporarily or permanently. It is common in old people, especially when bed-ridden during acute illnesses or with cerebral arteriosclerosis. Incontinence of fæces may co-exist. Other causes are vesico-vaginal fistula, paralysis or dilatation of the sphincter after the operation of lithotrity, or paralysis of the sphincter associated with neurological diseases (§ 806).

(b) FALSE INCONTINENCE is due to the overflow from a distended bladder in *retention* of urine. It is recognised by the signs of a full bladder and by the relief afforded by a catheter (see § 971).

Treatment of true incontinence is essential as otherwise bed-sores are soon likely to arise. The bedpan should be used two-hourly and any infection of the bladder remedied. As a temporary measure during acute illness, an indwelling catheter may be used in combination with a urinary antiseptic. Special bedpans, and for permanently bed-ridden women, special beds have been devised (and see § 858). False incontinence must be remedied by catheterisation and by treatment of the cause.

NOCTURNAL INCONTINENCE (enuresis) in children is a troublesome and frequent condition; if untreated it may persist into adult life. Usually the child has gained proper control of the urine by the age of 2-2½ years, and nocturnal incontinence shows itself later. When complete continence has never been attained, lesions such as spina bifida, a congenital valve in or imperfect development of the urethra must be looked for. In all cases it is important to exclude lesions such as stone in the bladder, cystitis or pyelitis, renal tuberculosis, polycystic kidney or polyuria with chronic nephritis. Reflex causes such as threadworms, a local vulvitis, and, according to some, phimosis or naso-pharyngeal adenoids may be contributory. Having excluded organic diseases, the children having nocturnal incontinence come usually under three types: (i.) In the largest group the condition is the result of an anxiety neurosis; such children are intensely worried about their trouble, are made worse by punishment or the jibes of their brothers and sisters, and so long as their parents continue to regard the condition as a fault, it remains incurable. (ii.) In a small proportion, carelessness and laziness of habit is causal. These children are usually obese and mentally sluggish. (iii.) In a few, mental deficiency is present, making training in their earlier years impossible. In such, diurnal incontinence of urine, and often of fæces, results.

Both *Prognosis* and *Treatment* turn almost entirely upon the cause, and are hopeful in proportion as this is removable. The power of retention of the urine is a habit which can be cultivated in early life, and the relative frequency in different individuals varies with habits engendered in infancy and childhood. Local lesions and reflex causes must be removed when possible. Where there is an anxiety state, it is well to explain the condition to the child, in kindly fashion; stop punishments and scoldings, and adopt a confident attitude that the condition will ultimately be curable.

Fluids towards the end of the day should be strictly limited, and the bladder emptied at bedtime. A simple expedient is to let the child keep a calendar which he marks himself, crossing out the nights on which enuresis has occurred; a suitable reward for gradual improvement often works wonders. Most drugs probably act by suggestion, but bromides, belladonna and ephedrine are helpful. Operative measures are not necessary or justified unless organic disease is present. In the sluggish, lazy child, thyroid is useful.

The patient has **repeated calls to pass urine** but INCONTINENCE IS UNUSUAL *and only amounts to a little dribbling—the condition is* INCREASED FREQUENCY OF MICTURITION.

§ 430. Increased Frequency of Micturition is a very common complaint.

The patient can hold his water, but the calls to urinate are too frequent, and sometimes so urgent that a few drops dribble away before arrangements can be made. " Stress incontinence " indicates that any sudden strain, *e.g.*, emotion, laughing, crying, coughing, will cause dribbling. The normal time during which the urine can be retained varies in different individuals, and also according to the amount of fluid taken; but 4 or 5 hours is a fair average. It is longer in the female than the male; some women can retain the urine for 10 or 12 hours. The habit is injurious, and is said to lead to abnormal flexions of the uterus.

Etiology.—The first point to determine is whether there is any marked increase in the diurnal quantity, as in diabetes mellitus, diabetes insipidus or chronic nephritis, because any of the causes of polyuria (§ 421) may be a cause of increased frequency of micturition. In young adults diabetes is the commonest, but in advancing years chronic nephritis and enlarged prostate are the most common causes. Our attention is often first drawn to the latter condition because the patient develops a habit of rising several times at night to pass urine. It is not always easy to decide whether the quantity is increased or not, as the patient is apt to think that, because he passes urine too often, he passes too much: it may be necessary to measure the diurnal volume (§ 378). There remains three groups of causes of increased frequency to consider: 1. Some cause of *local irritation* is undoubtedly the most frequent. *Bacilluria* may for long cause no symptom except increased frequency of micturition; this is a common symptom in coli bacilluria. The *bladder* may be irritable, owing to an enlarged prostate (the usual cause of abnormal frequency after middle-age), chronic cystitis, ulceration, tumour, stone, oxaluria, or pressure upon the viscus by a displaced or enlarged uterus. Or the irritation may be in the *kidneys* from the presence of stone, tubercle or other cause of pyelonephritis (§ 419). Or the irritation may be *reflex*, from disease in the vicinity of the bladder, worms, phimosis, fissure, piles, prolapse or polypus of the rectum, vascular urethral caruncle (a cause frequently overlooked in women), pelvic inflammation or varicocele. 2. *Constitutional* causes are occasionally associated with this condition, such as anxiety states, hysteria or sexual excesses.   3. The *sphincter* may be incompetent, especially with cystocele.   And see § 458.   *A congenital* want of development of the sphincter is sometimes present.   True congenital cases are rare, and defective action of the sphincter is more frequently due, especially in women and children, to some of the reflex causes above mentioned, the habit persisting after the cause has been removed.

Treatment is that of the cause.   The irritability of the bladder may be reduced by giving small doses of barbiturates or bromides, or by tab. dicyclomine hydrochlor. 10 mg. t.i.d.

§ 431.   *The urine presents a* cloudiness, *due to some* CRYSTALLINE *or* OTHER DEPOSIT; it may be URATES, URIC ACID, PHOSPHATES, OXALATES or FAT, unless it be pus (§ 416), blood (§ 411), or bacteria (§ 392).

With excess of URATES *the urine,* CLEAR *when first passed, becomes cloudy, with a pinkish* AMORPHOUS DEPOSIT *when it gets cold; the deposit dissolving again when heated in a tube.*   This condition is still believed by many to be due to functional derangement of the liver.   Various other conditions with which excess of urates and uric acid in the urine may be associated, as a more or less subordinate symptom, have already been referred to in § 393.

The clinical significance of uric acid and urates is still a subject of debate.   The deposit may be physiological when occurring after a heavy meal or undue exercise.

In *Multiple Myeloma* the urine may be cloudy on standing or even passing, due to the presence of the Bence-Jones protein (§§ 386, 613).

Phosphaturia *is usually indicated by cloudiness in a neutral or alkaline urine* (§§ 390 and 393).   It signifies decreased acidity of the urine rather than increased excretion of phosphates.   Phosphates frequently occur in the urine in such quantity as to cause a turbidity even when *first passed.*   They appear especially towards the end of micturition and may alarm the patient unnecessarily.   Phosphates may be especially abundant in the " alkaline tide " of the early morning or after dinner, after taking antacid drugs, and may cause an iridescent " scum " on the surface of the water. There may be no symptoms, even when phosphates are passed in large quantities; but phosphaturia may be accompanied by depression and anxiety.   Phosphates in *excess* occur with hyperchlorhydria, wasting disease and after a diet rich in fruit and vegetable.   Phosphates are *diminished* in pregnancy and in convalescence after fevers. *A deposit of triple phosphates* in freshly passed urine indicates decomposition in the bladder.

The *treatment* is based on the cause.   Usually all that is necessary is reassurance that no organic disease is present.   When cystitis is present it needs appropriate treatment (§ 418).

Oxaluria *is generally indicated by a " powdered wig " deposit on the top of the mucus which settles at the bottom* (§ 393).   Transient oxaluria has no clinical significance except as indicating the *nature* of a stone, which has revealed its *presence* by other symptoms.   It is also found after a diet of rhubarb, sorrel, spinach, tea and coffee, or cocoa.   But oxaluria is also connected with other clinical conditions.   (1) Renal colic, hæmaturia and albuminuria are due to irritation of the renal tract by the very hard crystals.   (2) Pancreatic disease: they are said to be abundant in the early stages of chronic pancreatitis.   (3) Other observers have connected certain nervous symptoms, such as mental depression; it is probable that these symptoms are connected with the concurrent dyspepsia.   (4) Oxaluria is associated with abnormal fermentation of sugar in the intestine.   Urates are generally precipitated in the urine at the same time.   (5) Oxalates occur in large excess in paroxysmal hæmoglobinuria (§ 414).

Treatment consists in avoiding foods which contain oxalates and those which allow excessive carbohydrate fermentation in the intestine. See Diet (§ 296. XIV). The formation of crystals is prevented by the ingestion of magnesia. Calculi of oxalates are reduced by rendering the urine strongly acid with acid sodium phosphate or ammonium chloride.

Fat may occur in the urine in subacute parenchymatous nephritis attended by much fatty degeneration of the epithelium, and after fractures of the bones. It is found in great abundance in **Chyluria.** The presence of chyle in the urine gives a milky white appearance and the power of coagulating: it is only visible under the microscope with a $\frac{1}{12}$-in. objective and with dark ground illumination. *In this country* enlarged glands or new growths are the principal causes. The back pressure on the lymphatic vessels of the kidneys and bladder causes some of them to rupture into the urinary tract. *In the tropics* chyluria is due to the filaria sanguinis hominis producing obstruction of the thoracic duct. The urine passed at night is the more completely white; that passed by day may be mixed with blood. Embryos are to be found in the urine with a few red and white blood-cells, albumen, fat and shreds of fibrin. Chyluria may follow trauma, and may accompany leukæmia in rare cases.

Prognosis.—The patient may live twenty years with but little impairment of health. In other cases, however, great debility and mental depression may be present.

Treatment.—Prevent the disease by boiling the drinking-water. To meet the loss of weight give plenty of nourishing food.

In *Pseudo-Chyluria* the milky appearance of the urine is due to the presence of the same material that occurs in pseudo-chylous ascites.

§ 432. Renal Tumours may be of six kinds: (I.) HYDRONEPHROSIS; (II.) PYONEPHROSIS; (III.) PERINEPHRIC ABSCESS; (IV.) MALIGNANT DISEASE; (V.) POLYCYSTIC DISEASE; and (VI.) MOVABLE KIDNEY. The

last-named is described under Abdominal Pain (§ 254), which is the symptom for which advice is sought. Extravasation of blood after injury to the kidney may simulate a tumour.

The *Physical Signs* common to all tumours of the kidney and their diagnosis from other ABDOMINAL TUMOURS are given in §§ 263 and 394.

I. **Hydronephrosis** is a term indicating a cystic tumour of one or both kidneys, caused by the gradual or intermittent obstruction of the urinary passages, and the consequent dilatation of the pelvis of the kidney. It is always present with normal pregnancy.

The *Symptoms* by which this tumour is recognised are: (1) Intermittent attacks of renal pain, often with vomiting. (2) If large, a renal tumour develops. (3) Local pressure symptoms may arise, causing pain or disturbance of function of the neighbouring organs. (4) Constitutional and general symptoms are absent, unless the stagnant urine becomes infected. (5) It may be discovered on investigating for the cause of pyelitis, the condition having been unrecognised previously.

Etiology.—The causes of obstruction to the outflow of the urine may be (i.) *congenital* (narrowed ureters, aberrant renal vessels, a valve in the urethra); (ii.) *acquired* causes, which may occur (a) in the *urethra*, such as stricture or enlarged prostate; (b) in the *ureter*, such as occur from stone or blood-clot; pressure by pelvic or other tumours; contraction after operation, injury or disease of the ureter; kinking, as in movable kidney (often associated with aberrant renal vessels). These acquired causes give rise to a *gradual obstruction* (Fig. 132), and when the obstruction is intermittent the tumour may become very large, when it is liable to be mistaken for an ovarian cyst, or even for ascites. In such cases a trocar introduced at operation will reveal fluid free of the albumen which is always present in an ascitic fluid. *Complete obstruction* of a ureter causes atrophy of the kidney, not hydronephrosis.

Prognosis.—If the condition is unilateral and intermittent it may cause little trouble, and may disappear after a duration of years. On the other hand, a double hydronephrosis is very serious, as it leads to uræmia. A surgeon should be consulted early. The complications are rupture into the peritoneum or pleura; suppuration in the pelvis of the kidney (pyonephrosis); or uræmia, due to atrophy of the substance of both kidneys.

Treatment.—In all cases the cause must be ascertained and, if possible, treated. Surgical treatment is usually advisable.

II. **Pyonephrosis** is a cystic tumour of the kidney due to distension of the pelvis and calyces by fluid containing pus. It is consequent on obstruction to the free outlet of the urine in septic cases of pyelitis, or sepsis supervening on hydronephrosis.

The *Symptoms* are: (1) The tumour is tender to palpation; (2) symptoms of pyelonephritis are present—pyuria, intermittent pyrexia, sometimes rigors, a toxic appearance, and dull pain in the loin; (3) at intervals, when the obstruction is removed or diminished, the tumour may subside, coincident with the passage of a large quantity of pus in the urine.

The *Causes* are: (1) pyelonephritis (§ 419), with blocking, partial or complete, of the ureter; or (2) hydronephrosis (*vide* Causes of this above) becoming septic—*e.g.*, from extension upwards of cystitis.

Diagnosis.—(1) From *hydronephrosis*, which has no tenderness or fever; (2) from *perinephric abscess*, which has greater tenderness in the loin and a more superficial swelling, with local signs of abscess sooner or later.

Prognosis.—The condition is serious. A tuberculous pyonephrosis may undergo cure by fibrosis. The structure of the kidney is largely destroyed, and in bilateral cases, uræmia will result. A fatal issue is rapidly brought about by the tumour bursting into the abdomen or chest.

Treatment is surgical and nephrectomy is usually indicated. Lavage through a ureteric catheter may temporarily relieve.

III. **Perinephric Abscess** is fairly common. It may arise by (i.) a blood-stream infection often associated with boils; (ii.) extension from kidney disease (pyelonephritis pyonephrosis or tuberculosis); (iii.) extension from a perityphlitic abscess; (iv.) extension from other organs—*e.g.*, abscess of the liver, empyema or spinal caries; (v.) after an injury. The *Symptoms* are: (1) dull, aching pain in the loin, sometimes radiating down the leg; (2) deep-seated resistance of the erector spinæ, tenderness on pressure in the post-renal angle, or in the hypochondrium in front; (3) the temperature is continuous, or pyæmic in acute cases with sudden onset, or intermittent in insidious cases; (4) the leg on the same side is kept flexed and the patient stoops when walking; (5) swelling, with œdema of the skin, which appears late in the disorder, is felt between the iliac crest and the last rib, and it may be fluctuant; (6) the urine may or may not be altered according to the cause, but traces of albumen are common; (7) marked leucocytosis; (8) collapse of the base of the lung and sometimes a small pleural effusion. The *Diagnosis* is difficult in the early stage when pain alone is present, when it may readily be mistaken for *lumbago, appendicitis* or *spinal disease,* but there is no fever in the first of these. Later it may be mistaken for a *renal tumour,* but in a simple tumour fever is absent, and the leg would not be held constantly flexed; the aspirating needle may be used. In *pyonephrosis* there is not such acute pain or tenderness. *Prognosis.*—The abscess tends to open or to burrow its way in various directions, into the alimentary or urinary canals, peritoneum, or pleura. It may point in the lumbar region or various other directions, and burrow for a considerable distance. *Treatment.*—In the early stages, before the diagnosis can be certain, give penicillin, hot fomentations and opium for the pain; as soon as pus is recognised operative procedure is necessary.

IV. **Malignant Disease starting in the Kidney** is a rare condition. It affects children under nine (in whom *sarcoma* chiefly occurs), and adults over forty (in whom usually it is *carcinoma*), there being a remarkable immunity between these age periods. RENAL SARCOMA is the commonest abdominal growth in children (Wilms' tumour). It is met in the first five years of life and grows to an enormous size. Between the ages of 10 and 30, malignant disease is rare; it is, however, common in people between 50 and 60. The commonest form of CARCINOMA in adults is a *hypernephroma*. It may lie latent for years and then assume great malignancy: metastases occur in the opposite kidney, grow along the renal veins and produce early deposits in bones. A carcinoma of glandular type or a malignant papilloma of the renal pelvis are much rarer.

The *Symptoms* are: (1) The tumour is rapidly growing, usually of firm consistence, but if of very rapid growth it may appear fluctuating; (2) hæmaturia, frequent, intermittent, and of moderate amount; (3) progressive emaciation; (4) the pain is variable, sometimes it is very severe, owing to pressure upon or infiltration of the neighbouring organs. Sometimes pain is entirely absent, and the tumour may have attained a very large size before any symptoms occur; (4) in left-sided hypernephroma left varicocele occurs, and is a valuable early diagnostic sign. (5) In hypernephroma, a spontaneous fracture of bone or an unexplained pyrexia may be the first symptom.

Diagnosis.—When a tumour occurs in a movable kidney it is apt to be mistaken for *ovarian tumour* or *fibroid*, and vaginal examination is necessary (see § 263 for diagnostic points). *Tuberculous* kidney in a child may present difficulty, but the pain is less, and pyuria is present rather than hæmaturia. *Pyonephrosis* is accompanied by fever, the swelling is fluctuant, and there is a history of pyuria. *Retroperitoneal* and *renal sarcoma* are the chief causes of enormous abdominal tumours in children. The diagnosis of malignant tumours is not usually difficult.

The *Prognosis* is very grave. If untreated, death occurs in six to twelve months after detection of the growth, the cancer of adults being of somewhat slower growth. *Treatment* is usually too late; early excision gives the only chance of life.

Benign Tumours affecting the kidney are fibromata, lipomata, angiomata or adenomata.

V. **Polycystic Disease of the Kidneys** is a rare condition, usually of congenital origin and often familial, in which both kidneys contain cysts of varying size and number.

Symptoms.—(1) There is complaint of a dull dragging pain in one or both loins. (2) With this there is a tumour in one or both loins, but usually larger on one side; the surface is irregular and feels cystic, although the kidneys feel very firm otherwise. (3) The other symptoms are those of chronic interstitial nephritis (§ 401), the urine is abundant, pale, of low specific gravity, containing traces of albumen, and occasionally blood and casts. The heart becomes hypertrophied, and the pulse indicates high blood pressure. (4) Polycystic disease may co-exist in the liver, spleen, ovaries and pancreas. The patient may have excellent health for many years, or may develop symptoms of chronic uræmia. It may give rise to an enormous tumour in the fœtus and obstruct delivery. In children, symptoms may be associated with renal rickets.

The *Diagnosis* may be difficult. When symptoms of granular kidney occur, together with a tumour in both renal regions, the condition may be diagnosed as polycystic kidney. The tumours have to be diagnosed from other abdominal tumours (§ 263). Pyelography reveals a large kidney with elongated calyces (Fig. 131).

Etiology.—The disease is usually familial. In the majority, the patients are middle-aged.

Prognosis.—The younger the patient the worse the prognosis. In those diagnosed in middle age, it is common for them to survive 20–30 years.

Treatment is similar to that of nephritis. Death may occur from uræmia or the same complications as those of interstitial nephritis. Operation must not be performed as the condition is bilateral. A surgical support may be of value when the weight of the tumour is producing symptoms.

Hydatid cyst may occur in the kidney, and may be difficult to differentiate from other cysts unless it opens into the pelvis of the organ, when the characteristic hooklets (**Fig. 112**) are found in the urine. The passage of vesicles may cause renal colic. The condition may be suspected if (i.) the tumour has the " hydatid thrill " on palpation; (ii.) there is evidence of cysts elsewhere; and (iii.) there is a history of residence in infected countries. (iv.) Eosinophilia may be present. The complement fixation test and the Casoni reaction aid diagnosis (§ 347).

The *Prognosis* is generally not grave. The cyst may last for years with no symptoms, or it may burst into the pelvis of the kidney. It may open into the stomach or bowel, with temporary recovery; or into the chest, which is a serious complication. It may become very large and give rise to pressure signs.

Treatment is surgical.

CHAPTER XIV

DISEASES OF THE FEMALE REPRODUCTIVE ORGANS

DISEASES and disorders of the genito-urinary tract have a wide influence upon the physiological welfare of the individual as a whole. General diseases also may have a marked influence upon reproductive functions. The physician must, therefore, take into consideration the reproductive system when investigating the condition of the patient and especially when there is evidence of endocrine imbalance. In a volume on Clinical Medicine it is essential to give some consideration to the methods of investigation and the general treatment of disorders of the pelvic organs of women. The aim of the gynæcologist is to restore and preserve the reproductive function whenever possible, reserving radical surgical treatment for those cases where no alternative exists. The present chapter deals with gynæcological problems along general medical lines, merely indicating the lines of treatment to be adopted when surgery becomes essential.

§ 433. The Physiology of the Reproductive System.—Research into the hormones of the ovary and pituitary has thrown much light upon reproductive function and has assisted in the evaluation of various gynæcological disorders. Before discussing the diseases affecting the pelvic organs a brief account of these hormones is necessary in order to understand how their functions affect the reproductive system as a whole.

Ovarian Hormones.—Before *puberty*, the secretion of the *granulosa cells* of the primordial follicles in the ovary is associated with the early development and growth of the genital organs. At puberty a striking change occurs in the ovary; the first development and rupture of Graäfian follicles begins and œstrogens are produced in larger amounts from the granulosa cells which line the follicles. The œstrogenic (or follicular) hormone has been described as the "hormone of preparation" since its function is to prepare the body as a whole for the function of reproduction. Thus it causes growth of the vagina with thickening of its lining epithelium and secretion of glycogen by the epithelial cells: it stimulates growth of the uterine muscle so that the uterus reaches its adult size with proliferation of the uterine mucosa or endometrium; it is responsible for growth of the breasts by proliferation of their glandular system and for the appearance of the other secondary sexual characteristics. A Graäfian follicle develops and ripens in each menstrual cycle and about mid cycle *ovulation* occurs with extrusion of the ovum. The Graäfian follicle collapses and its lining cells form the *corpus luteum* which secretes the hormone known as progesterone. Progesterone has been described as the "hormone of pregnancy" since it is found mainly in the premenstrual stage of the menstrual cycle when the body is prepared for pregnancy, and during pregnancy itself. It is responsible for secretory changes in the endometrium and in the breasts. When the secretion of œstrogen is deficient, the development of the genital organs is arrested, the secondary sex characteristics fail to appear, menstruation does not occur and sterility results. Substitution therapy with œstrogenic hormones may cause some development of the genital organs.

When oöphorectomy is performed in adults, atrophic changes may occur in the uterus and other genital organs. These changes may be partially arrested and some degree of normal function may be restored in the uterus and other pelvic organs by administration of œstrogens. Injection of œstrogenic hormone in castrated rats and mice is followed by desquamative changes in the superficial cells of the vagina similar to those seen in œstrus in the normal animal. Œstrogen also causes some mammary activity. It arrests the reduction of the granular cells in the anterior pituitary which appears after castration.

Menopausal changes follow diminishing œstrogen secretion. Symptoms arising from these may be relieved by giving preparations of œstrogenic hormones or their synthetic substitutes such as stilbœstrol.

Menstruation.—At puberty menstruation begins. The menstrual cycle is generally reckoned from the first day of menstruation and has two main phases: (i.) the proliferative or follicular phase, which is brought about by secretion of œstrogen; the uterine mucosa gradually proliferates during this phase which lasts until ovulation. (ii.) The secretory or progestational phase follows, the corpus luteum producing œstrogen and progesterone which together cause secretory changes in the endometrium.

Ovulation takes place about 14 days before the next menstrual period is expected. If the ovum is not fertilised, the corpus luteum degenerates, the superficial layers of the uterine mucosa are cast off, hæmorrhage occurs and a fresh menstrual cycle begins. The process is initiated by withdrawal of œstrogen and of progesterone; the latter modifies the effect of œstrogen on the endometrium. The degenerate corpus luteum becomes converted first into a waxy body, the *corpus albicans* and later into scar tissue. If fertilisation does occur, the corpus luteum develops further and its secretion of œstrogen and progesterone is increased. The corpus luteum of pregnancy persists for the first three or four months of pregnancy, its functions of producing œstrogens and progesterone being gradually taken over by the placenta. The persistence of the corpus luteum in early pregnancy is brought about by the secretion of chorionic gonadotrophins by the fœtal chorionic tissues. *The menstrual flow* consists at first of desquamated epithelium from the uterus, fluid blood, which does not normally clot, serum and some white blood cells. Towards the end of the period the loss is scanty and brownish in colour. The total amount lost varies considerably in individual normal women but has been estimated as between 2 and 8 fl. ozs. The length of the cycle, that is the interval from one period to the next, also shows considerable individual variation but is usually about 28 to 31 days. When examining specimens of the uterine mucosa after endometrial biopsy or by curettage it is important to note the length of the cycle and the exact date of the last menstrual period so that the histological findings can be correlated with the phase of the menstrual cycle.

Temperature variations in the menstrual cycle.—Basal body temperature varies during the cycle; immediately after menstruation it is at a relatively low level. At the time of ovulation a slight drop occurs and this is followed by a rise of two-tenths to three-tenths of a degree, corresponding to the progestational phase. About two days before menstruation the temperature falls again to its original level, unless pregnancy has occurred, in which case the temperature rise is maintained. This temperature curve can be used as a means of determining the date of ovulation and as a means of diagnosing early pregnancy; the temperature readings must be taken under truly basal conditions (immediately on waking) for any activity, including eating, drinking or smoking, will give fallacious results.

§ **434. The Anterior lobe of the Pituitary** is closely associated with ovarian function. It produces three gonadotrophic hormones: œstrogen inhibits the production of these hormones, so that when there is ovarian deficiency (after castration or at the menopause) excess of gonadotrophins is found. (1) *The follicle-stimulating hormone* is produced in both sexes; in females it acts on the ovary to cause ripening of the ovum, growth of the follicle and production of œstrogenic hormone. (2) *The luteinising hormone* is also found in both sexes; it acts with follicle-stimulating hormone in the female to produce ovulation and luteinisation of the Graäfian follicle. (3) *The luteotrophic hormone* stimulates the luteinised follicle to produce progesterone. It is probably identical with *prolactin* which is stored in the anterior pituitary during pregnancy and released after delivery of the placenta to cause secretion of milk.

These hormones of the anterior pituitary have no direct action on the uterus and are effective only through intact and functioning ovaries. In practice, treatment with anterior pituitary hormones has proved disappointing and it is rarely possible to reproduce clinically the effects seen in experimental animals. They must be used with caution as anterior pituitary hormones are complex proteins. Their administration, which must be by injection, may cause the production of anti-hormones which will not only neutralise the effect of further treatment, but may also neutralise the natural hormones produced by the patient's own pituitary.

The **Posterior lobe of the Pituitary** produces at least two hormones. One of these is the *anti-diuretic hormone*; when given in large doses it causes general contraction of all smooth muscle including that of the uterus and the blood vessels, thus causing a rise of blood pressure. The other hormone, *oxytocin*, acts on the uterus in the human subject only in the later weeks of pregnancy and the early days of the puerperium. Towards the end of pregnancy the human uterus becomes progressively more sensitive to oxytocin and this is in some way connected with the onset of labour.

The **Chorionic Villi of the Placenta** produce a hormone which resembles those of the anterior pituitary in some respects and is generally known as *chorionic gonadotrophin*. It may be demonstrated in blood and urine early in pregnancy, as early as the 35th day after the last menstrual period and is the basis of most of the tests for pregnancy in common use. It is also produced in some pathological conditions, as in hydatidiform mole, chorion epithelioma and teratoma. Tests for pregnancy (§ 1211) are based on the presence in the urine of chorionic gonadotrophin and the following are in current use: the Aschheim-Zondek test uses immature female mice; the Friedmann test uses a female rabbit; for the Hogben or " toad " test, the female *Xenopus lævis*, or South African clawed toad is used. Female rats are used for the " two-hour " rat test. A recently developed pregnancy test employs male frogs or toads; in these chorionic gonadotrophin induces spermatogenesis.

The **Thyroid gland** is concerned with reproduction, though its role in this respect is still obscure. Excess of thyroid secretion may result in menstrual disturbances such as amenorrhœa while cretins and those with myxœdema are often sterile. In severe thyroid deficiency, ovulation often fails to occur and the result may be anovulatory cycles with episodes of prolonged bleeding. (See §§ 444, 575.) This may be reversed by giving thyroid extract.

§ 435. Hormone Therapy is now a recognised part of gynæcological practice, though knowledge is still incomplete regarding the mode of action of the hormones of the anterior pituitary and the gonads and of the controlling effects they have on each other. The discovery of reliable synthetic substitutes for the ovarian hormones has permitted great advances in treatment.

Œstrogenic (follicular) hormones.—Naturally occurring œstrogens may be given by injection, by implantation of fused pellets and also as ointments and vaginal pessaries. They are relatively ineffective when given by mouth. The two most commonly used are œstrone and œstradiol. A dosage of 1 to 2 mg. on alternate days by injection for three weeks will be followed by withdrawal bleeding in castrated women. Synthetic œstrogens have the advantage that they are active when given by mouth; they may also be given by injection, inunction or as vaginal pessaries. The three most commonly used are stilbœstrol, dienœstrol and hexœstrol. Of these the most active is stilbœstrol, which is four times more active than dienœstrol and eighteen times more active than hexœstrol. A dosage of 2 mg. of stilbœstrol a day for 21 days will cause withdrawal bleeding in castrated women when treatment is stopped. There is a tendency for nausea and vomiting to occur in non-pregnant women given stilbœstrol, but this is uncommon when the dosage is 2 mg. a day or less. Ethinyl œstradiol is a powerful and relatively non-toxic synthetic œstrogen; 0·05 mg. of ethinyl œstradiol is roughly equivalent in its effects to 1 mg. of stilbœstrol.

Progestagens.—The naturally occurring hormone progesterone may be given by injection or by implantation of fused pellets. The synthetic equivalent *ethisterone* B.P. may be given by mouth, though to obtain a similar effect the dosage must be

C.M.—X

ten to twenty times that of the natural hormone given by injection. New powerful synthetic progestagens include norethisterone (Primolut N), norethisterone acetate (Primodos, Anovlar), norethynodrel (Enavid); these commercial preparations contain ethinylœstradiol. They are used clinically to replace the action of progesterone; as they inhibit ovulation they are also used as oral contraceptives.

Androgens are used in the treatment of various gynæcological disorders either alone or combined with œstrogens. The male hormone testosterone may be administered by injection, by inunction or by implantation of fused pellets. Methyl testosterone is active by mouth and the amount absorbed can be increased by giving it through the buccal mucosa.

PART A. SYMPTOMATOLOGY

§ 436. Diseases of the pelvic organs have both Local and General symptoms. LOCAL SYMPTOMS are: Irritation or swelling around the vaginal orifice, vaginal discharge, including leucorrhœa, painful menstruation (dysmenorrhœa), excessive menstruation (menorrhagia), deficient menstruation (amenorrhœa or oligomenorrhœa), pain in the region of the organs, acute and chronic; backache, various disorders of function (such as dysuria, dyspareunia and infertility); tumours and swellings.

GENERAL SYMPTOMS consist of: (1) Malaise and general ill-health. The condition of chronic invalidism caused by pelvic disorders may be altogether out of proportion to the amount of local trouble. Such chronic ill-health frequently dates from pregnancy and childbirth. (2) Disorders of the abdominal or pelvic viscera often cause symptoms of dyspepsia. (3) Anæmia, due to excessive uterine hæmorrhage, toxæmia from degenerating tumours or as a result of pregnancy. (4) Obscure pains with a general hypersensitiveness of the nervous system may follow derangements of the reproductive system. (5) The premenstrual Syndrome.

THE PREMENSTRUAL SYNDROME (Syn. Premenstrual Tension) is a condition where profound depression, irritability, emotional outbursts and sometimes insomnia occur during the 7 to 10 days before menstruation. These may be accompanied by a bloated feeling and even an actual gain in weight; pain in the breasts (mastalgia) is common. This syndrome is common after the age of 30 and is rare in younger women. *Treatment* is largely empirical. Restriction of fluid and of the salt intake with the administration of diuretics have been recommended. Hormone treatment may take the form of inject. progesterone, 10 mg. on alternate days for 10 days before menstruation. Tab. ethisterone B.P. 25 mg. or tab. methyl testosterone B.P. (10 mg. sublingually) may be given for 10 days commencing on the 15th day of the cycle. A tranquilliser such as meprobamate 200 mg. t.d.s. may help.

Case-taking in diseases of women differs somewhat from that given in Chapter I. The following summary will form a guide to the principal questions to be answered as a matter of routine:

1. What is the leading symptom complained of by the patient, its periodicity and its duration?
2. History—name, age, married or single.
   (a) If married, how long? How many children and dates of birth of each? Character of pregnancies, confinements and puerperia? Any complications after childbirth? Any miscarriages?
   (b) Menstruation—age at which it commenced? (1) Regular? How often does it occur? How many days does it last? (2) Is it profuse and does the flow contain

clots? Has there been any recent change in the character of the flow? (3) Is pain present, before onset or during period? Has pain always been present? If not, when did it begin? Where is the pain? In back, legs or one or other side of lower abdomen? What relation has pain to the flow? Is it continuous?

(c) Is there any intermenstrual discharge—duration, quantity, white, yellow, clear, thin or thick? Offensive? With blood?

(d) Micturition—painful, frequent during day or night? Any incontinence? Condition of bowels, regular? Are purgatives taken as a rule? Is there pain on defæcation?

(e) If married, is there dyspareunia? Are contraceptives used? If so what? If infertility, voluntary or involuntary? For how long?

(f) Other symptoms and history of past illnesses and operations.

PART B. PHYSICAL EXAMINATION

§ 437. An abdominal examination is a matter of routine in all gynæcological cases.

(a) *An External Examination* of the abdomen by inspection, palpation, percussion and auscultation (§ 240). For a thorough examination of the pelvic organs the patient should lie on her back with knees flexed and shoulders raised; this relaxes the abdominal muscles. The degree of rigidity or contraction of the abdominal muscles can be ascertained. Is rigidity due to the cold hands of the examiner or to clumsy methods of palpation ? Or is it a guard to prevent the examining hand from touching a deep-seated lesion ? Is the rigidity due to nervousness, and will it pass off when the patient is more at ease ? Place the warmed hand, cup-shaped, on the abdominal wall, very lightly at first. If the patient is encouraged to talk, her attention will be diverted from tender areas which may be more or less due to a condition of hypersensitiveness. If the normal areas are palpated first, the painful regions may be found to be less resistant as the examination proceeds. If there is tenderness in a particular area, is it local or referred from a deep organ ? If so, the pathological lesion may be in the intestine or the parietal peritoneum may be involved. Is there any abdominal tumour or enlargement of any viscus ? Is free fluid present ?

(b) *Pelvic Examination.*—There need be no unnecessary exposure of the patient during the vulvo-vaginal examination. A light blanket or a sheet is thrown over the knees and lower abdomen. This examination is mainly undertaken in the case of a married woman or one who has borne a child. Virgins should only be examined per vaginam in exceptional circumstances and the examination is generally best made under anæsthesia; if a pelvic examination is necessary it may be performed per rectum, the patient lying on her left side. A satisfactory bimanual examination of the pelvic organs may be made by this route though, in excessively nervous women, spasm of the muscles often makes this examination of little value. To perform a *vaginal examination* one finger of either hand is covered with a rubber glove or finger stall, lubricated with liquid soap, glycerine jelly or obstetric cream, and gently introduced into the vaginal opening, care being taken not to touch with the thumb the sensitive anterior portion of the vulva which includes the clitoris. The skin should not be soiled with the lubricant. The *vulva* is first inspected for any local soreness or inflammation or for the presence of a swelling. The condition of the *vaginal walls* should be noted—dry or moist, a normal pink or fiery red, as a whole or in patches, atrophic or swollen; the position and condition of the cervix, patulous or soft as in pregnancy, conical, firm, granular, scarred or friable. Bleeding or discharge should be noted.

(c) *The Bimanual Examination* is next made by placing the finger in the anterior vaginal fornix and palpating the uterus with the external hand pressed firmly above the symphysis pubis. The size, shape, position and mobility of the uterus can be felt between the two hands. The examination may also aid in defining whether a painful area is low down or high up in the pelvic cavity. As a rule the uterus itself is not painful on palpation; pain on examination indicates congestion, adhesions, inflammatory conditions of the peritoneum or ovarian lesions. Palpation of the ovary sometimes gives a sensation of sickness—a valuable aid in localising its position. By shifting the finger into the lateral vaginal fornix and following it with the external hand it is possible to feel tubal or ovarian tumours. A tumour in the pouch of Douglas behind the uterus may be felt through the posterior vaginal fornix. The bladder and the rectum must be empty.

Difficulties in examination may be overcome by giving an *anæsthetic*. This produces relaxation of the abdomen, so that palpation of the pelvic organs is easy on bimanual examination. The disadvantage of an anæsthetic is that areas of tenderness are not then ascertained and deep palpation may even cause damage as in cases of ectopic pregnancy or pyosalpinx.

X-ray examinations are useful in localising appendix complications, and will reveal the presence of a calculus, a calcified fibroid or bony tumours; a hystero-salpingogram (after the injection into the uterus of iodised fluid) will reveal the outline of the uterine cavity and the condition of the Fallopian tubes. X-rays also show the position and condition of the spine, the vertebræ and the joints, also any spinal or pelvic deformity and pregnancy after the sixteenth week.

Instruments employed in the examination of the pelvic organs.

1. *Vaginal Specula.*—The Ferguson speculum is a tube; the bivalve (Cusco or Brewer) consists of two limbs jointed together; the duckbill (Sims) is a retractor of the perineum. The first gives good exposure of the cervix; the second is best for the examination of the vaginal walls; the third for operative measures. Note the condition of the mucous membrane and the character of any discharge. In passing the speculum, do not forget that the vaginal canal is directed upwards and backwards; less pain is produced by quick movements in the right direction than by slow bungling. If it is necessary, apply treatment to the vagina or cervix by means of a probe covered with cotton-wool or by a pledglet of cotton-wool held in a sponge forceps; do this before withdrawing the speculum.

2. The *Volsellum* is a form of hooked forceps used for drawing down the cervix. It is contra-indicated in those conditions in which the sound is contra-indicated and in tubal pregnancy. Owing to its painful effect upon the cervix it should rarely be used in the unanæsthetised patient.

3. The use of the *Uterine Sound* often yields valuable information. The uses of the sound are to discover (1) the length of the uterus, which is normally about

3½ inches from the external os to the fundus, and the thickness of its wall prior to dilatation and curettage; (2) the position of the uterine cavity; (3) the state of the external and internal os of the cervix; (4) the presence of tumours in the uterine cavity. The sound should not be passed in pregnancy and if there is a septic lesion of the vagina or cervix there is a danger of carrying infection to the upper part of the genital tract. Great care must be exercised in cases where cancer is suspected owing to the risk of perforating the uterus. It must be passed with due aseptic and antiseptic precautions so that its use in the consulting room or out-patient department is to be deprecated. It is generally used in the anæsthetised patient, but it may be used gently without an anæsthetic, especially as a preliminary to such procedures as tubal insufflation, endometrial biopsy or hystero-salpingography. A bimanual examination must always be made before the sound is passed.

EXAMINATION OF A VAGINAL DISCHARGE gives valuable information (see § 440). A little discharge is removed with a sterile swab, or with a glass pipette with a rubber

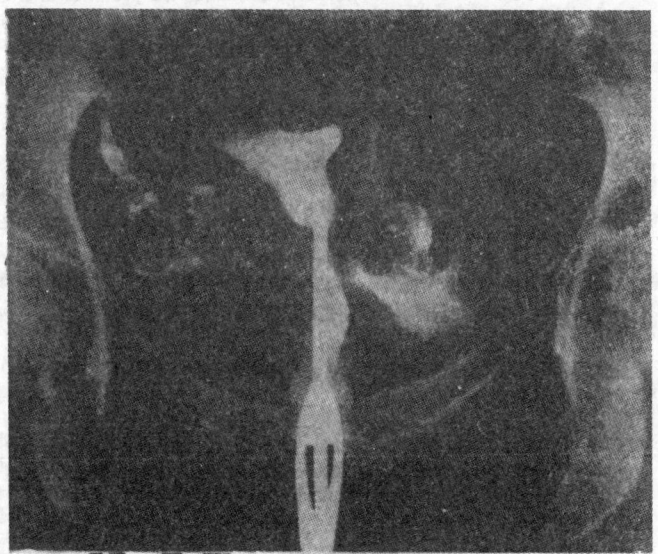

FIG. 136.—Normal Hysterosalpingogram showing the outline of the Uterus and a spill of the iodised fluid into the peritoneum.

nozzle attached. The discharge may be examined directly under the microscope in a drop of normal saline. Culture tubes should also be inoculated for bacteriological examination. Swabs may be transported in a special " transport medium " if they have to wait some time before reaching a bacteriological laboratory.

The aspiration pipette may also be used to obtain a sample of vaginal secretion for the purpose of making a vaginal smear. A thin film is made on a glass slide and this is fixed and stained by the method of Papanicolaou. When seen under the microscope the epithelial cells of the vagina are large, flat with irregular faint outlines; the nuclei stain deeply. When these cells are numerous there is healthy tissue in the vaginal wall with normal secretion of œstrogen. Variations are seen at different phases of the menstrual cycle. In the follicular phase the vaginal smear shows leucopenia and cornified squamous cells with small pyknotic nuclei; in the post-menopausal phase of non-cornified squamous cells with large nuclei or compact cells with larger nuclei from the deeper layers of the vaginal epithelium. Administration of œstrogens will produce a temporary change from the second phase to the first.

In cases of cancer of the uterus, malignant cells may be detected in the vagina smear before clinical evidence of the disease is apparent (see § 1213). Cancer of the cervix may be diagnosed by Ayre's method of taking a smear from the area surrounding the external os with a small wooden spatula. The diagnosis of cancer is never made on examination of smears alone but must always be confirmed by biopsy.

DILATATION OF THE CERVIX may be performed by the (1) *Slow Method* (seldom employed); laminaria tents are inserted and left *in situ* for some hours, or by (2) the *Rapid Method* with dilators (Hégar's, Fenton's or Heywood Smith's), metal or vulcanite instruments of graduated sizes. General anæsthesia is necessary. First a bimanual examination is made. Then insert the posterior vaginal speculum, fix the anterior lip of the cervix with a volsellum or ring forceps, draw well down, measure the length of the uterus with a sound, and insert dilators gradually one after the other until the cervix is dilated. The uterine cavity should then be explored with a ring forceps or intra-uterine forceps; the curette is then used. Curettings must always be submitted to histological examination, or vital information, including the presence of a growth, may be missed. Dilatation of the cervix is contra-indicated in pregnancy and must be performed with great caution in the presence of cancer. Care is also needed when the tissues are softened by recent pregnancy.

PART C. DISEASES OF WOMEN: THEIR DIAGNOSIS, PROGNOSIS AND TREATMENT

§ 438. Routine Procedure and Classification.—Having ascertained the patient's principal or *Leading Symptom*, and the leading facts as to the *History* according to the scheme given in Part B., proceed, unless the nature of the case is not already apparent, to the *Physical Examination* (subject to the reservations mentioned in Part B.).

The diseases are considered under the various cardinal symptoms to which they give rise—viz.:

(A) Morbid alterations of the vulva and external parts .. .. .. § 439
(B) Leucorrhœa and other causes of discharge .. .. .. § 440
(C) Pain connected with menstruation (dysmenorrhœa) .. .. § 441
  Endometriosis .. .. § 442
(D) Hæmorrhage .. .. §§ 443–450
(E) Amenorrhœa .. .. § 451
(F) Pain in the lower abdomen, not necessarily connected with menstruation (pelvic pain), Cellulitis, Salpingitis and Tuberculosis; Uterine displacements .. .. §§ 452–456
(G) Pelvic tumours .. .. §§ 457–459
(H) Disorders of micturition and defæcation, pain on sitting, dyspareunia .. .. § 460
(I) Backache, chronic .. .. § 461
(J) Sterility .. .. § 462

§ 439. (A) Morbid Alterations of the Vulva.—A few of the common alterations are enumerated here.

VULVITIS in children may be caused by the migration of threadworms, streptococcal, coli and other bacterial infections, uncleanliness, gonorrhœa or masturbation. In adults it may be secondary to vaginitis.

PRURITUS AND ECZEMA VULVÆ may be very obstinate conditions. Inquire for : allergic cause such as use of detergents (including those used for washing underwear), antiseptics or strong soaps. Careful examination must always be made for pediculi or irritating discharges from the uterus, vagina, urethra or from the minute ducts near the vaginal orifice. Diabetes and glycosuria with associated fungus or yeast infection of the mucous membrane are not uncommon causes.

A CARUNCLE is a minute, red, irritable tumour situated usually just within the urethral orifice, and is a frequent cause of painful micturition, painful sitting and dyspareunia. Two main types are seen—a granuloma and a papilloma. The latter are often painless but both may bleed. Slight prolapse of the urethral mucous membrane may give rise to a red swelling which may be mistaken for a caruncle, especially in the aged.

ABSCESS of the vulva may be associated with boils; often it follows inflammation with suppuration in Bartholin's gland. HERPES is an eruption of a small group of vesicles. They readily rupture, leaving round, superficial ulcers which may become secondarily infected.

NOMA (GANGRENE OF THE VULVA), DIPHTHERIA, AGRANULOCYTOSIS, CHANCRES, CONDYLOMATA, INFECTIVE WARTS, ULCERS (simple or malignant) and TUBERCULOSIS (§ 455) may also affect the part. For LEUCOPLAKIA and KRAUROSIS see §§ 746, 752; LICHEN SIMPLEX and LICHEN SCLEROSUS § 752.

CARCINOMA OF THE VULVA most often takes the form of ulceration on the inner surface of the labium minus; it may affect the clitoris, or rarely, Bartholin's gland: it is a highly malignant and almost entirely radio-resistant growth. Early diagnosis is essential if radical surgery, which is the only satisfactory treatment, is to be successful.

In the *Treatment of vulval* conditions cleanliness is essential and on the whole the lack of this is one of the most frequent causes of vulvitis. Use of harsh soaps or disinfectants should however be forbidden. *Urethral caruncle* is treated by cauterisation, diathermy fulguration or by operation. *Abscesses* require surgical treatment. The treatment of *pruritus vulvæ* may tax every therapeutic resource. Severe cases should remain in bed. All scratching is forbidden and to ensure this sedatives in the form of adequate doses of barbiturates may be needed during the acute stage. Every effort should be made to determine the *cause* and it must be remembered that many conditions belonging to the realm of dermatology such as lichen planus, epidermophytosis and seborrhœic eczema may affect the vulva. The opinion of a dermatologist may be invaluable. Investigation includes examination of several specimens of urine to exclude glycosuria and bacteriological investigation of a vaginal and urethral swab to exclude pathogenic organisms. Vaginal discharge if present should be treated. The question of an allergic sensitisation of the vulva must be considered and it must be remembered that symptoms may continue after the cause has been removed. In post-menopausal women, atrophic changes may be treated by application of ointments containing œstrogens, such as ung. stilbœstrol 0·05 per cent. Hydrocortisone ointment (2·5 per cent.) may be tried. A warm alkaline bath before retiring to bed often gives temporary relief and may be taken as a preliminary to applying local remedies. In cases where no cause is found treatment is symptomatic. Relief is often given by the use of cremor calaminæ to which is added phenol 1 per cent., by cremor zinci with liq. carb. deterg., 0·5 to 1 per cent. In cases where there is an allergic cause, oral or local use of antihistamines may prove helpful. In intractable cases, local application of Grenz rays, deep X-ray therapy or even vulvectomy may become necessary.

(a) *There is a white* NON-PURULENT DISCHARGE *from the* VULVAL ORIFICE; *the condition is* LEUCORRHŒA.

§ **440.** (B) **Leucorrhœa** is a discharge colloquially known as " the whites "; a small amount of secretion is healthy and this tends to increase at the time of ovulation and before the onset of menstruation in normal women. Leucorrhœa is usually a simple increase of the normal secretion of the genital tract, a non-infective type of discharge, not to be confused with the purulent discharge associated with inflammatory conditions of the vagina, cervix, uterus or tubes.

Diagnosis.—While a complete investigation may be undesirable in the case of young girls, much may be discovered from examination of the discharge alone. The normal vaginal secretion is acid, due to lactic acid formed by Döderlein's bacilli: the pH of about 4·4 deters the growth of other organisms. When the discharge gives a pH of 5·6 or over, this is suggestive of local infection. A smear shows whether epithelial or pus cells predominate and the presence and type of micro-organisms may be determined by microscopical examination and by culture. A thin discharge is usually of vaginal, a tenacious glairy mucus of cervical or uterine origin. A foul-smelling discharge, worse after the period, usually indicates infection of the vagina, cervix or uterine body.

Etiology.—Leucorrhœa is common (1) at puberty, (2) at the time of ovulation and before menstruation, (3) with sexual excitement, (4) in pregnancy; and may accompany (5) local congestion due to undue exertion, constipation, gastro-intestinal disorders and other causes of pelvic congestion, (6) debility, anæmia and malnutrition. (7) A congenital erosion of the cervix is a common cause in girls and young women. (8) During treatment with œstrogens, increased secretion in the form of leucorrhœa is not uncommon.

Treatment.—Remove any local cause; improve health with exercise, fresh air and general tonic treatment. Provided the discharge is no more than a slight excess of normal secretion, explanation and reassurance will suffice. Douches are usually unnecessary; the best is lactic acid ℳ 60 to Ō i, or vinegar ℳ 60 to Ō i. Freshly prepared lactic acid pessaries may be of benefit.

(b) *There is a* PURULENT DISCHARGE which comes from the VAGINA; *the condition is* **vaginitis, acute** *or* **chronic.**

In ACUTE VAGINITIS the discharge is profuse, yellow or greenish, sometimes blood-stained, attended by dysuria and local signs of inflammation. The chief *Causes* are: (1) Trauma, due to pins, other foreign bodies and worms in children, or in the adult an irritant pessary, a foreign body (tampons, contraceptive appliances, etc.), too strong douches or excessive coitus; (2) infection with *E. coli*, streptococci, staphylococci, other micro-organisms and fungi of various kinds; (3) gonorrhœa, which is hard to diagnose from other infections of the vagina except by bacteriological examination of the discharge; (4) extension from adjacent parts, such as the urethra or Bartholin's glands; (5) a diphtheritic form; and (6) agranulo-cytosis (§ 155). Acute vaginitis of gonorrhœal origin (§ 417) is dangerous because of the liability of the infection to extend to the uterus, tubes and peritoneum and to the bladder and the kidney.

Diagnosis.—Find the cause; in children examination under anæsthesia may be necessary to exclude a foreign body. A vaginal swab should be taken and examined directly under the microscope and cultured. The sensitivity to antibiotics of any pathogenic organisms isolated should be determined.

Treatment.—Remove foreign body if present and treat residual vaginitis by douches of lactic acid, ℥ 60 to Ō i. A thorough vaginal toilet is carried out with a speculum; hydrogen peroxide is useful for removing pus and cleansing the vagina; in children and virgins the first treatment should be carried out under general anæsthesia. Antibiotics may be given orally, by injection or in the form of vaginal pessaries according to the sensitivity of the infecting organism. Painting the vagina with an aqueous solution of gentian violet, 1 per cent., is often effective.

Acute gonorrhœal vaginitis res-ponds rapidly to penicillin given by intramuscular injection. A single injection of 300,000 units is gener-ally sufficient to cure the infection but further treatment may be re-quired if relapse occurs. Care must be taken that this does not mask a coincident syphilitic infection (§ 417).

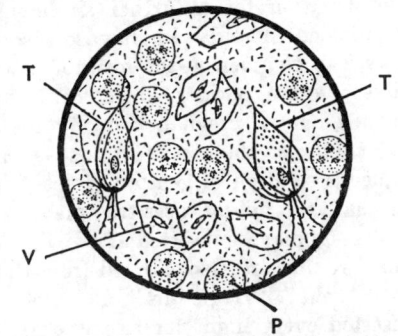

FIG. 137.—A Diagram drawn from a Microscopic Specimen of Vaginal Secretion. It shows Trichomonas Vaginalis Organisms (T) with Flagellæ; also Pus Cells (P) and Vaginal Epithelial Cells (V).

In CHRONIC VAGINITIS there is a thick, continuous, opaque discharge, usually with local signs of inflam-mation. The *Causes* are: (1) antecedent acute vaginitis; (2) various con-stitutional conditions, such as general debility, vitamin deficiency, diabetes, old age, alcoholism, anæmia and convalescence from fevers; (3) new growths of the vagina or cervix; (4) irritant foreign bodies and other causes mentioned under Acute Vaginitis.

Trichomonas Vaginitis due to a flagellated protozoon is common (Fig. 137). It may cause intense prurigo, intertrigo, dyspareunia and acute pain on urination. The vagina is red and tender, the vault filled with a thin, yellow or greyish-yellow purulent fluid, frothy, offensive, often acid in reaction. The origin of the parasite is unknown: a similar organism is found in the large bowel, while it may be found also in the bladder. It may be harboured in the male urethra without causing symptoms and in an inactive form so that reinfection may follow coitus; many cases are complicated by infection with other organisms. Relapse after each period is common; the trichomonas does not ascend to the upper genital tract and is never found above the external os of the cervix.

Vaginal Thrush is due to a yeast-like organism, known variously as *Monilia, Oidium Albicans* or *Candida Albicans* (Fig. 86). It causes a thick white curdy discharge, often with external irritation and varying evidence of vaginal inflammation. It is common in pregnant women and in women with glycosuria or diabetes: occasionally it occurs in normal, non-pregnant women.

Treatment.—(1) Treat any constitutional disease and remove foreign bodies or new growths. (2) Deal with any primary cause originating in the cervix or body of the uterus. (3) For *trichomonas vaginitis* first cleanse the vagina thoroughly with hydrogen peroxide and treat with one of the many preparations now available. Acetarsol vaginal tablets give satisfactory results: two should be inserted high in the vagina each night for a week; then they should be used on alternate nights for a further two or three weeks. Treatment should be continued during the week following menstruation for a further six months to prevent relapse. Acetarsol vaginal compound with flavazole sometimes gives better results. This may also be given in the form of powder for vaginal insufflation, as may silver picrate powder, 1 per cent. Vaginal insufflation must *never* be carried out in pregnancy owing to the risk of air embolism. (4) For *vaginal thrush* the best treatment is painting the vagina with a 1 per cent. aqueous solution of gentian violet. In severe cases this must be carried out daily; in milder cases treatment two or three times a week will suffice; a tampon may be inserted after painting to prevent staining of underwear. Good results are also claimed from the use of fungicide preparations such as " Mycil," " Dequadin " or " Nystatin " pessaries; one or two may be inserted every night for two weeks. When *vaginitis continually relapses* seek and treat any source of reinfection in the cervix.

SENILE VAGINITIS may occur in elderly women and with the menopause. The vaginal lining shows atrophy and red patches, sometimes with submucous hæmorrhages; the discharge may be blood-stained and adhesive bands may form near the cervix. The glycogen content of the vaginal epithelium is diminished; the normal acid reaction is lost and the normal vaginal flora disappears, often being replaced by pathogenic bacteria. The cervix and urethra may be involved. Senile vaginitis often responds to œstrogens either by injection, orally or locally in the form of pessaries; very small doses are sufficient, such as 0·5 mg. of stilbœstrol by mouth daily. Lactic acid pessaries may be given in addition.

VULVO-VAGINITIS IN CHILDREN should be investigated by excluding a foreign body or other local lesion and by taking a swab for bacteriological examination including the sensitivity to antibiotics of any organisms present. *Treatment* is best given by oral administration of the appropriate chemotherapy or antibiotic; if the organism is sensitive to penicillin this can be given by injection. Local treatment is best avoided or restricted to sitz baths and local irrigation of the vagina through a fine catheter.

DISCHARGE OF Uterine Origin may be due to cervicitis, endometritis (including tuberculosis), cancer (see Hæmorrhage) or salpingitis (§ 454).

I. In Cervicitis, or inflammation of the cervix or cervical erosion, the discharge is more or less constant and usually consists of *glairy material* like white of egg but it may be muco-purulent.

Symptoms, in addition to discharge may include backache, pelvic or lower abdominal pain, dyspareunia, infertility, frequency of micturition, general malaise and other signs of a septic focus. Erosion of the cervix may cause slight bleeding in pregnant women but in the non-pregnant bleeding is suspicious of malignant change.

Diagnosis depends on feeling a raised velvety area on the vaginal portion of the cervix; examination with a speculum reveals a raised bright red area around the external os. Retention cysts may be seen, usually around the edge. Cervicitis must be diagnosed from other lesions of the cervix. These include a cervical polyp, which is often seen in association with erosion; ectropion, when the lips of the torn cervix evert, exposing the cervical canal; and cancer of the cervix. Here the age is not much guide, as cancer may appear in a young patient. Cancer is hard to the touch and friable, readily breaking down and bleeding when touched, and there is usually a blood-stained discharge. Histological examination of a thorough biopsy of the cervix will determine the diagnosis and this should always be performed in doubtful cases. When fixity of the uterus and cachexia have appeared the diagnosis is simple. There is reason to believe that chronic cervicitis may be a premalignant lesion.

Etiology.—Erosion of the cervix may be congenital due to persistence of columnar epithelium on the *portio vaginalis*; some cases accompany chronic infection of the cervix, as in chronic gonorrhœa; many cases are acquired as a result of childbearing.

Treatment is most satisfactorily carried out by electro-cauterisation of the cervix; this simple procedure can be carried out in the consulting room or the out-patient department and no anæsthetic is necessary. The cervix is exposed and the external os wiped dry with cotton-wool. The point of a nasal cautery, heated to red heat, is inserted into the cervical canal and three to four radial incisions are made on the anterior and posterior lips of the cervix. The eroded area sloughs and healing occurs by regrowth of squamous epithelium in 8 to 10 weeks. The patient should be warned to expect a little bleeding during the 14 days following cauterisation and to refrain from coitus during this time. Slight discharge may persist until healing is complete.

ECTROPION of the cervix occurs mainly in parous women in whom the cervix has been bilaterally torn at childbirth; rarely it may follow instrumentation of the cervix. *Symptoms* are similar to those of cervicitis, a thick, mucopurulent discharge being the outstanding symptom. *Diagnosis* depends on examination with a speculum. *Treatment* is surgical, repair of the cervix or trachelorrhaphy in women of childbearing age or amputation of the cervix in post-menopausal women.

II. **Endometritis** may be acute or chronic and both may give rise to leucorrhœa. *Acute Endometritis* occurs in acute gonorrhœa and in puerperal infection of the uterus which may follow abortion (often criminal abortion) or childbirth. The symptoms are usually those of an acute pelvic infection (§ 453) and the treatment is that of this condition.

Chronic Endometritis is relatively uncommon in adult women. It may cause a persistent leucorrhœa, accompanied by menorrhagia, pelvic pain and backache. Diagnosis is made by microscopical examination of curettings. *Treatment* is unsatisfactory; some cases are improved by curettage alone; every effort must be made to improve the patient's general health, but in intractable cases hysterectomy may be required.

SENILE ENDOMETRITIS occurs in post-menopausal women and is characterised by a persistent, watery, sometimes blood-stained discharge from the uterus. Curettage is essential to exclude cancer, and release of retained discharge by dilatation of the cervix in the uterus is often sufficient to cure the condition.

TUBERCULOUS ENDOMETRITIS is found most commonly in women aged between 20 and 40; it is usually associated with a tuberculous salpingitis (see § 455). Infertility may be the only complaint, but in some cases there is a persistent white discharge from the uterus and in advanced cases, with destruction and caseation of the endometrium, amenorrhœa may occur. *Diagnosis* depends on histological examination, culture and guinea-pig inoculation of material obtained by endometrial biopsy or curettage. The *treatment* is that of pelvic tuberculosis (§ 455):

Pyometra is a collection of pus, or of blood and pus, in the uterus.

Symptoms.—There may be a corresponding discharge from the uterus, accompanied by pelvic pain. Examination may reveal a slightly enlarged uterus, with pus exuding from the cervix.

Etiology.—Causes include congenital atresia of the vagina or cervix, retention of lochia with puerperal endometritis, stenosis of the cervix following operation or radiotherapy, tuberculosis or senile endometritis, and cancer of the cervix or of the body of the uterus.

Treatment consists of evacuation of the pus by gentle dilatation of the cervix, followed later by treating the underlying cause. Appropriate antibiotics should be given after the organisms have been cultured.

§ 441. (C) **Dysmenorrhœa** is pain during or associated with the menstrual period. Three main types are described: (1) SPASMODIC, Intrinsic or Primary, due to muscular ischæmia of the uterus on account of strong muscular contraction during menstruation; (2) CONGESTIVE, Pre-menstrual or Secondary due to chronic pelvic sepsis or pelvic endometriosis; (3)

MEMBRANOUS, due to the passage of the endometrium shed at menstruation as a cast from the uterine cavity.

The patient is BETWEEN 16 AND 30 *years of age and complains of* SEVERE PAIN AT THE ONSET OF MENSTRUATION. *The condition is probably* SPASMODIC DYSMENORRHŒA.

(1) **Spasmodic Dysmenorrhœa** accounts for the majority of cases in young women. Few, if any, women do not experience some discomfort at the onset of menstruation but in those who suffer from spasmodic dysmenorrhœa, severe pain is felt, usually during the first hours or days of the menstrual flow; it may be a continuous ache or may resemble colic or spasm; the pain may be accompanied by vomiting, headache and general malaise. The pain may be felt in the lower abdomen or pelvis and may be referred to the sacral region or down the legs. It is most frequent in young, single women or in married women in association with sterility; it often disappears spontaneously after the age of 30. It does not as a rule begin at the onset of menstruation, but two or three years later and sometimes not until the age of 18 or older. It is frequently associated with a sedentary occupation, such as office work, and with deficient exercise and open air; it also occurs where there is overstrain or lack of occupation or interests. There is good reason to believe that young women with this type of dysmenorrhœa have a lowered threshold for pain; this may be brought about by emotional disturbance and is often greatly improved when an active life is taken up in the country. It is rare to find any evidence of pathological change in the pelvic organs, and findings such as that of congenital retroversion of the uterus are almost certainly coincidental. Nor is there any evidence to associate it with underdevelopment of the uterus, in fact in these cases the uterine muscle is unusually well developed; it is believed that pain is caused by ischæmia due to powerful uterine contractions which occur during the early days of menstruation. Childbirth often cures such cases, probably because the parous uterus is more vascular and less liable to become ischæmic.

Treatment.—In the case of unmarried women vaginal examination is not necessary unless some pathological condition is suspected; rectal examination is sufficient to exclude any gross lesion such as a pelvic tumour. Vaginal examination should be made under general anæsthesia; if local treatment such as dilatation and curettage is indicated it is carried out at the same time. *General* treatment such as good diet, vitamins, avoidance of constipation, attention to anæmia and dental sepsis, open-air games or exercise should be advised; dancing, or attendance at an evening gymnastic class are useful substitutes for those whose occupation precludes much exercise in the open air. Hot baths often relieve the pain if taken before and at the onset of the period and also throughout its duration. Considerable success is achieved in dealing with girls of all classes when interesting occupation is found and activity encouraged; the practice of staying in bed at the time of menstruation should be forbidden. In some cases, however, these simple hygienic measures are insufficient and, owing to the severity of the pain, the girl is incapacitated; special treatment is then required.

Remedial treatment at the time of the period consists of a hot drink and a short rest with a hot-water bottle, carefully protected to avoid burning the skin, on the lower abdomen. Simple analgesics such as aspirin, phenacetin and codein are often successful; a combination of aspirin, phenacetin with dextroamphetamine (" Edrisal ") gives relief in many cases. Alcohol and drugs of addiction such as morphine and pethidine should never be given. It is important to reassure the girl (and her mother) that the presence of pain at menstruation does not necessarily indicate pelvic disease or sterility. Administration of œstrogens has proved valuable; some believe that their effect is to inhibit ovulation and thus cause painless withdrawal bleeding. If this view is held they should be given from the 5th day of the cycle for 21 days: stilbœstrol in a dose of 1 mg. twice a day, by mouth, is often effective or, if it is not well tolerated, ethinyl œstradiol 0·05 mg. may be given twice daily. This treatment is so often successful that it is always worth a trial. Treatment should be continued for 3 or 4 cycles and then a month's rest from treatment given to prevent permanent inhibition of the pituitary. There is no evidence that treatment with œstrogens properly given in this way ever causes permanent harmful effects and the dysmenorrhœa is often relieved completely after 3 or 4 months' treatment. Other authorities claim equally good results from administration of œstrogens in the second half of the cycle, *i.e.*, stilbœstrol 1 mg. twice a day for 14 days, commencing on the 15th day of the cycle (counting from the first day of the menstrual flow). Progestational steroids which inhibit ovulation (§ 435) may give dramatic relief; give one tablet of Conovid-E or of Anovlar nightly for 20 nights in each cycle, beginning on the fifth day of menstruation. Administration is most effective when the tablet is allowed to dissolve slowly under the tongue. Dilatation of the cervix is worth a trial when hormone treatment is unsuccessful; under a general anæsthetic the cervix is slowly dilated as far as possible. Sometimes the relief following this procedure is only temporary, lasting a few months, in which case it is well worth repeating it, as a second dilatation often gives more permanent relief. In intractable cases, pelvic sympathectomy may be undertaken but this should be reserved for cases where all other means of treatment have proved unsuccessful; in practice it is rarely required.

The patient is BETWEEN 30 AND 40 *years of age and complains of* PAIN (*sometimes severe*) *which begins* SEVERAL DAYS BEFORE MENSTRUATION. *The condition may be* CONGESTIVE DYSMENORRHŒA.

(2) **Congestive, Secondary or Acquired Dysmenorrhœa** tends to occur in older women and is rare before the age of 25 and uncommon before 30.

Symptoms.—The pain usually begins three or four days, or up to a week, before menstruation and may be relieved or aggravated at its onset. The pain is continuous and felt either in the pelvis or as a low backache. Exercise and movement aggravate while rest improves this type of dysmenorrhœa; other symptoms such as menorrhagia, infertility and dyspareunia are often associated with it.

Diagnosis.—In chronic salpingitis (§ 454) there is usually, but not invariably, a history of an acute pelvic infection such as gonorrhœa, puerperal sepsis following childbirth or abortion, or appendicitis with pelvic peritonitis.

Etiology.—The two principal causes of congestive dysmenorrhœa are chronic salpingitis and pelvic endometriosis but it may occur with fibroids or acquired retroversion of the uterus with prolapsed ovaries.

Treatment consists in using simple analgesics and the application of heat to the pelvis; this is most effectively given by pelvic short-wave diathermy. Surgical treatment may be required in intractable cases.

§ **442. Endometriosis** is now recognised as a common and important disease of the female pelvic organs. It may cause congestive dysmenorrhœa. The growth closely resembles endometrium in its histological characteristics and in its tendency to periodic bleeding. It thus takes on menstrual changes during the period with congestion, swelling and hæmorrhage. The ovaries are most often affected, but the growth may be found in the uterine muscle and in other sites such as the recto-vaginal septum, pelvic peritoneum, bowel, bladder, umbilicus and perineum.

Symptoms.—Pain due to pelvic endometriosis occurs before the onset of the menstrual flow and is relieved thereby; sterility is usual and there may be dyspareunia and other symptoms such as hæmaturia, depending on the situation of the growth. Fibroids are present in the uterus in about one-third of the cases and menorrhagia is a frequent associated symptom. Endometriosis occurs mainly in women aged 30 to 40; it is rare in those who have borne children and is believed to be cured by childbearing in the rare cases where conception occurs.

Treatment is generally surgical, conservative operation in younger women and radical removal of the pelvic organs in older women who do not wish for children. In minor cases androgens (methyl testosterone 5 mg. sublingually for 100 days) may prove successful; this may be repeated after one month's rest from treatment. Progestational steroids (up to 100 mg. daily for 6–9 months) cure some cases.

The woman between the AGES OF 15 AND 45 *complains of* VERY INTENSE PAIN AT THE ONSET OF MENSTRUATION *which is* RELIEVED BY THE PASSAGE OF A CAST. *The condition is* MEMBRANOUS DYSMENORRHŒA.

(3) **Membranous Dysmenorrhœa** is uncommon. *Symptoms.*—Severe **pain is** associated with the passage of portions of or a complete cast of the uterus; this may occur at every menstruation or at occasional cycles. The pain is similar to that of labour pains and is due to the contractions of the uterus in its efforts to evacuate the cast. It is believed that minor degrees of this condition with passage of large fragments of endometrium, but not a complete cast, may be responsible for **some cases**

of so-called spasmodic dysmenorrhœa. In true membranous dysmenorrhœa, there is slight bleeding; at first the pain is not severe but increases and reaches its height, resembling in severity that associated with an acute abdominal emergency, as the membrane is being passed. The cast may be solid or may be hollow and triangular in shape like the cavity of the uterus. In some cases the openings of the Fallopian tubes and the internal os may be recognisable. Under the microscope fibrin is seen with leucocytes, red blood corpuscles and remnants of uterine glands and vessels. The cast is distinguished from extrusions from the uterus in cases of ectopic pregnancy or uterine abortion by the absence of decidual cells or chorionic villi. There may be a history of recurrent attacks unassociated with early symptoms of pregnancy.

Treatment sometimes proves difficult; the best results are obtained with œstrogens given orally in the form of stilbœstrol, 1 mg. twice daily or ethinyl œstradiol 0·05 mg. twice daily for 21 days commencing on the 5th day of the cycle. Dilatation and curettage, which may need to be repeated, cures some cases. Intractable cases in older women, especially if there is an associated pelvic pathology such as a uterine fibroid, are best treated by hysterectomy.

Mittelschmerz.—This pain occurs midway between the periods and is unusual before 20 years of age. It is associated with ovulation and many women notice a slight twinge of pain on one or other side of the pelvis at about this time. More severe pain is likely to be associated with a lesion such as chronic sepsis, endometriosis, sclero-cystic disease of the ovary or acquired retroversion of the uterus with prolapsed ovaries. The appropriate *treatment* for these pathological lesions should be carried out. Cases with no evident pathology may respond to analgesics; hormones, either œstrogens or androgens given in small doses from the end of one period to the beginning of the next may be helpful, possibly by inhibiting ovulation.

§ 443. (D) Hæmorrhage.—*Menorrhagia* indicates an excessive flow at the monthly period; *Metrorrhagia* indicates irregular hæmorrhage from the uterus, irrespective of the period. It may be difficult to separate these, as their causes are more or less identical, and they often occur together. Hæmorrhage from the *vulva or vagina* is usually slight in quantity, and its cause readily discovered by inspection. Hæmorrhage from the *cervix* is usually due to polypi, cervical erosion or malignant disease; rarely, it is due to ulceration, syphilitic or tuberculous, or to injury by a pessary. All these are made out on inspection with a vaginal speculum. Hæmorrhage after coitus is suggestive at all ages, but especially in older women, of malignant disease or a polypus hanging from the cervix.

Local causes of hæmorrhage from the *uterus* are: Endometritis, fibrosis or metritis, fibroids, polypi of the uterus, endometrioma of the uterus (often called adenomyoma), inflammation of the adnexa and in the pelvis, abortion, extra-uterine fœtation, malignant disease, incarcerated retroverted uterus, œstrogen-secreting ovarian tumours (occasionally) and chronic inversion of the uterus. Displacements and malposition of the uterus rarely cause symptoms unless accompanied by pelvic inflammation, pelvic endometriosis or adhesions. *Constitutional* or *functional* causes are considered in § 444.

In women *over 35* any of the above causes may give rise to hæmorrhage, but malignant disease must be excluded; it must be remembered that cancer of the uterus does occur, though rarely, in much younger women. The sudden supervention of *hæmorrhage* with *acute pain* suggests a miscarriage or an extra-uterine fœtation (§§ 445, 446). In women *past the menopause* some lesion of the uterus, especially cancer or uterine polypus, is nearly always present.

Many of the above-mentioned causes of uterine hæmorrhage are dealt with elsewhere. The following are considered here:

(I) Certain Constitutional or Functional Conditions (§ 444);

(II) Abortion, Ectopic Gestation and Hydatidiform Mole (§§ 445, 446);

(III) Uterine Fibroid or Polypus (§ 447);

(IV) Chronic Subinvolution (§ 448);

(V) Uterine Endometriosis or Adenomyosis (§ 449); and

(VI) Malignant Disease (§ 450).

§ **444.** I. Certain CONSTITUTIONAL or FUNCTIONAL conditions may cause hæmorrhage. (1) Some women have too profuse periods all their lives, and it must be remembered that the pattern of normal menstruation varies greatly from one woman to another; those with profuse periods may be of plethoric build, usually with florid countenances and they tend to excessive flow on trivial exciting-causes. (2) Excessive loss at menstruation may be associated with hypertension; (3) too many and too frequent pregnancies and prolonged lactation; (4) residence in tropical climates; (5) acute specific fevers, sepsis, purpura and other blood conditions; (6) strong emotion may cause a single heavy hæmorrhage, probably through the hypothalamus and its effect on the pituitary. (7) Congestion, as with heart or liver disease; also after sudden change of temperature or over-exertion. (8) Endocrine imbalance, as at the onset of puberty, when it is due to unovulatory bleeding with excess secretion of œstrogens. The flow may occur every two or three weeks and be prolonged, though the amount may not be increased, and it may be readily excited by a hot bath or a day of unusual exercise. Other endocrine causes are a deficiency of thyroid and unbalanced production of pituitary and ovarian hormones. This may result in metropathia hæmorrhagica.

Metropathia hæmorrhagica is due to excessive œstrogen stimulation and absence of luteal influence, leading to cystic hyperplasia of the endometrium. With this follicular cysts of the ovary occur.

Symptoms.—There is a loss of menstrual rhythm, often with a preliminary period of amenorrhœa followed by profuse and lengthy bleeding. There are no abnormal physical signs in the uterus.

Treatment may be medical or surgical. Anæmia should be corrected and in severe cases blood transfusion may be required. Hormone treatment consists in injecting progesterone daily in 10 mg. doses for 10 days; ethisterone 50 mg. daily by mouth may be given instead. After stopping treatment, withdrawal bleeding will temporarily occur in the form of a " medical curettage "; 15 days after the first day of the withdrawal bleeding the treatment should be repeated. Alternatively, œstrogens may be used to stop metropathic bleeding. Stilbœstrol in large doses up to 20 mg. or more daily (or ethinyl œstradiol up to 1 mg. daily) may be required initially.   The dose should be gradually reduced to maintain the patient free of bleeding for three weeks: then withdrawal bleeding is permitted.   During the last 10 days of œstrogen treatment it is advisable to give progesterone or ethisterone, as above.   *Curettage* of the uterus is essential to establish the diagnosis of metropathia and is at least temporarily curative, in a proportion of cases.   In some, especially those under 30, spontaneous cure may occur.   In women over 40, hysterectomy is the treatment of choice.   Metropathia must be regarded as a premalignant condition.

§ 445. II. **Abortion** (Syn. Miscarriage) may be threatened, inevitable, missed, incomplete, complete or septic.   There may be a history of interference either by the patient herself or by some other person.   In *threatened abortion* bleeding is usually slight and pain is absent; it may occur at any time before the 28th week of pregnancy.   The cervix is closed and the uterus is enlarged to correspond with the period of amenorrhœa preceding the bleeding.   In *inevitable abortion* bleeding is more profuse and accompanied by cramp-like pains, similar to those of labour.   The cervix is open and a portion of the products of conception can be felt in the cervical canal: abortion usually takes place in a matter of hours.   In *missed abortion* there is a persistent brownish discharge from the uterus, sometimes preceded by slight bleeding; the symptoms and signs of pregnancy regress and growth of the uterus ceases.   The biological tests for pregnancy (such as the Aschheim-Zondek test) become negative 7 to 14 days after the death of the embryo.   In *incomplete abortion* part of the products of conception is passed, while the retained products give rise to intermittent bleeding which may be profuse; the uterus is slightly enlarged and the cervix is patulous.   In *complete abortion*, the products of conception have been passed complete; the cervix is almost closed and the uterus of normal size or only slightly enlarged.   Bleeding is usually slight and ceases within a week; if bleeding continues beyond this time, retention of some of the products of conception must be suspected.   *Septic abortion*, often criminal in origin, is a form of puerperal sepsis.   The symptoms and signs are those of uterine infection, often with evidence of spread beyond the uterus, such as salpingitis, pelvic venous thrombosis, pelvic peritonitis, septicæmia or pyæmia.

§ 446. **Extra-uterine Pregnancy** (or Ectopic Gestation) is the term applied to a condition where pregnancy takes place outside the uterus, usually in the Fallopian tube but rarely in the ovary.   Tubal pregnancy may terminate in one of four ways; the fœtus may die and be retained in the tube, forming a tubal mole; the pregnancy may be aborted through the abdominal ostium of the tube with a varying amount of bleeding into the peritoneal cavity, forming a pelvic hæmatocœle; the tube may rupture, on account of erosion of its wall by the trophoblast, with invasion of a blood-vessel causing diffuse intraperitoneal hæmorrhage; rarely, the embryo is extruded from the tube and continues to grow and develop in the peritoneal cavity, forming a secondary abdominal pregnancy.

Symptoms.—(1) There are symptoms of early pregnancy—amenorrhœa and sometimes morning sickness; (2) in many cases paroxysmal pains are experienced in one iliac fossa; (3) slight bleeding from the uterus occurs, sometimes accompanied by the discharge of a membrane or cast from the uterus; (4) on bimanual examination the cervix is soft as in early pregnancy the uterus appears soft and slightly enlarged and there is a tender pulsatile swelling in one vaginal fornix.   (5) In many cases, however, none of the above symptoms is noticed by the patient and advice is not sought until tubal abortion or rupture of the tube has occurred.   Tubal abortion is accompanied by the formation of a pelvic hæmatocœle; intraperitoneal rupture by the symptoms and signs of diffuse intraperitoneal hæmorrhage (§ 245).   Prognosis and treatment of haematocœle is discussed in § 452.

Hydatidiform or vesicular mole is a disease of the chorion which undergoes hydropic degeneration so that the chorionic villi are converted into tiny vesicles, the size of currants.   The fœtus is usually absorbed in an early stage but may persist. *Symptoms.*—Signs of pregnancy appear with amenorrhœa, breast changes and morning sickness, which is often severe.   The uterus may enlarge rapidly and eventually, though sometimes not for 12 or 16 weeks, bleeding occurs due to separation of the abnormal chorion.   Vesicles may be present in the discharge.   *Diagnosis* depends on finding a large uterus of " doughy " consistency from which fœtal parts are absent to palpation: an X-ray confirms the absence of fœtal bones.   Biological tests for pregnancy such as the Aschheim-Zondek are positive in urine diluted one in a hundred or even one in five hundred times (and see Chorion Epithelioma, § 450).

§ 447. III. A uterine fibroid may cause hæmorrhage.

The *symptoms* vary with the position of the tumour.   These tumours may be *submucous*, *interstitial* or *subserous*.   When the fibroid is submucous or interstitial the symptoms are (1) menorrhagia and metrorrhagia; (2) discharge and sometimes dysmenorrhœa.   (3) On examination with the sound the uterine cavity is found to be enlarged; and (4) on bimanual examination enlargement of the uterus, which is usually hard and bossed from the presence of more than one fibroid, can be detected.   The submucous variety tends to become polypoid, remaining attached to the uterine wall by a pedicle. The *subserous* fibroid may present no symptoms for many years and may even then be discovered by accident; rarely a subserous fibroid becomes pedunculated and the stalk of the fibroid undergoes acute torsion, so that the patient presents with symptoms and signs of an acute abdomen.   With subserous fibroids menorrhagia does not usually occur and pressure symptoms may be the earliest indication of its presence.   In uterine fibroids of all kinds the rate of growth, though it varies somewhat, is nearly always slow; but as the tumour increases it may be felt by the patient herself and there will be symptoms of pressure upon the surrounding organs, such as frequency of micturition, varicose veins, backache and pain in the legs.   Fibroids, especially when very large, tend to undergo degenerative changes which give rise to pain and symptoms of toxæmia.

Uterine polypus.   The most common forms are fibroid polypi and mucous polypi of the endometrium or cervical mucosa.   Placental polypi occur, arising after labour or abortion from retained products of conception.

Adenomyomatous polypi may occur in uterine adenomyosis (endometrioma). Carcinomatous or sarcomatous polypi also occur; these may be primary or may result from malignant changes in a benign polypus. *Symptoms.*—Polypus of the uterus causes at first a discharge which may be offensive; bleeding, at first slight in amount and intermittent but later profuse and continuous, may follow. A small polypus can be made out with certainty only by dilating the cervix and exploring the uterine cavity. When a polypus is larger or springs from the cervix, examination with a speculum reveals it hanging from the os into the vagina; such a polypus may be easily removed by seizing it with forceps and twisting the pedicle till it drops off. Every polypus, however removed, should *always* be submitted to histological examination owing to the relative frequency of malignant change.

§ 448. IV. **Chronic Subinvolution,** or the non-return of the uterus to its normal size after labour or abortion, may be a cause of menorrhagia. After confinement the uterus begins to diminish in size, resuming its normal non-pregnant size in about two months. When the process of involution is incomplete the uterus remains large and bulky with an excess of fibrous tissue in its walls; the condition is sometimes referred to as FIBROSIS UTERI or MYOHYPERPLASIA. In cases of subinvolution we find (1) on bimanual examination that the uterus is enlarged; (2) it may be retroverted and lower than normal; (3) the patient complains mainly of profuse periods but also may complain of backache, bearing-down pain and discharge; and (4) lassitude, weakness, general malaise and anæmia.

Etiology.—(1) Retained products of conception. (2) Puerperal sepsis, often leading to chronic pelvic inflammation. (3) Numerous pregnancies, often in rapid succession.

§ 449. V. **Endometriosis or Adenomyosis of the uterus** occurs mainly in nulliparous women, aged between 30 and 40. The uterine muscle is invaded by endometrium: the invasion, which is localised to the uterus, may be diffuse, or there may be a single localised deposit, in which case this is referred to as an adenomyoma or endometrioma. The endometrium may remain inactive or may undergo the typical changes of the menstrual cycle. The chief *Symptom* is profuse menorrhagia; there is often a feeling of weight with premenstrual dysmenorrhœa and the uterus is felt to be enlarged and firm (and see § 442).

§ 450. VI. **Malignant Disease** of the uterus is met in four forms: (a) Cancer of the cervix, chiefly in multiparæ; (b) cancer of the body, seen equally in nulliparæ and multiparæ mainly between the ages of 55 and 65; (c) sarcoma of the uterus is rare and generally arises from malignant degeneration in uterine fibroids; and (d) chorionepithelioma, a very rare form following abortion, parturition or hydatidiform mole.

(a) CANCER OF THE CERVIX runs a variable course but its progress is usually more rapid in younger women.

Symptoms.—(1) On digital examination at an early stage, the os feels hard, friable, and granular; it is so characteristic that this feature and the blood-stained discharge upon the finger are alone, in experienced hands, sufficient to diagnose the disease. (2) At a later stage examination reveals a mushroom-like growth (" cauliflower excrescence ") or crater-like depression, readily breaking down and readily bleeding. It spreads to the vaginal wall, to the uterosacral ligaments, broad ligaments and body of the uterus, leading to fixation of the uterus and a hardness which is easily made out on palpation. (3) Metrorrhagia and menorrhagia are present. (4) In the intervals between the marked hæmorrhages, and indeed in the early stages, there is a continuous watery discharge, often pinkish-brown in colour, often with a very offensive odour. In the early stages, slight bleeding may follow coitus or exertion. (5) Local pain is usually a late symptom, but like the wasting and cachexia, is sure to supervene sooner or later. Pain points to invasion of the cellular tissue by the growth.

Less commonly cancer of the cervix may arise, by *malignant degeneration in a cervical mucous polypus*; another variety arises within the cervical canal, the *endocervical carcinoma*. This latter is a dangerous and insidious growth which tends to spread beyond the uterus at an early stage, while the appearance of typical symptoms and signs may be delayed.

Early *Diagnosis* offers the best hope of cure. Every case of discharge and bleeding, especially in women over 40, demands the most complete investigation; suspicious ulceration of the cervix must be fully examined by biopsy and polypi removed from the cervix must always be submitted to histological examination.

(*b*) CANCER OF THE BODY OF THE UTERUS is met mainly in women over 50 years of age. Bleeding occurs at a later stage than in cancer of the cervix.

Symptoms.—(1) A watery discharge, usually coming in gushes; (2) metrorrhagia, and in the intervals a pinkish or blood-stained discharge; (3) the uterus may appear to be enlarged on bimanual examination but this is not always the case; (4) fixation of the uterus, due to spread to the broad ligaments or peritoneum, occurs in advanced cases; (5) cachexia, pain and other general symptoms resemble those of cancer elsewhere.

The *Diagnosis* can only be made by histological examination of curettings; a thorough diagnostic curettage must be carried out in *all* cases of menopausal or post-menopausal bleeding.

Cancer of the uterus may sometimes be diagnosed by examination of vaginal smears stained by the method of Papanicolaou (§ 1213); this method is chiefly of value for " screening " clinically normal women for the purpose of diagnosing cancer at the earliest possible stage. The results of a vaginal smear should never be accepted as diagnostic but must always be confirmed by curettage or biopsy of the cervix.

(*c*) SARCOMA OF THE UTERUS is relatively rare. It occurs mainly in post-menopausal women and may arise from malignant degeneration in a fibroid. The *Symptoms* may consist of post-menopausal bleeding, rapid enlargement of a pelvic tumour, pelvic pain and ascites. The growth spreads rapidly and metastasises early.

(*d*) CHORION EPITHELIOMA is a very rare malignant tumour of the uterus which follows hydatidiform mole, abortion or confinement. *Symptoms.*—Bleeding may occur but in some cases metastases are widespread before there is any bleeding from the uterus.   *Diagnosis.*—The Aschheim-Zondek test and other biological tests for pregnancy are positive from urine diluted 100 or even 500 times.   Curettage may reveal the diagnosis but when the growth is deep in the uterine muscle it may escape the curette.   The ovaries contain thecalutein cysts.   *Treatment* consists in early removal of the uterus.   In a few cases the metastases clear up when the primary growth is removed.   A cytotoxic agent, tab. methotrexate, is giving good results.

The *Diagnosis of Hæmorrhage.*—Every effort should be made to find the cause.   In adult women all cases of intermenstrual bleeding and most cases of menorrhagia will require examination under anæsthesia with curettage of the uterus and histological examination of the curettings.   At the same time a polypus may be removed and biopsies should be taken from any doubtful ulceration of the cervix.   Before carrying out this examination it is advisable to assess the patient's general condition.   An estimation of hæmoglobin should be carried out in every case; where blood dyscrasia is suspected, a full blood count with estimation of platelets, bleeding time and clotting time should be performed.

The *Prognosis of Hæmorrhage* depends upon the cause.   Uterine bleeding is of itself not fatal to life, but some forms are very intractable and lead to anæmia, debility, discomfort and inability to fulfil the duties of life. Some of the causes of hæmorrhage interfere seriously with the normal reproductive capacity.   (1) Functional bleeding at the MENOPAUSE or of SUBINVOLUTION may undergo spontaneous recovery; that due to some constitutional conditions may be amenable to treatment; with chronic inflammation, metropathia and adenomyosis the outlook is not favourable. (2) The prognosis in a case of FIBROID depends on the age of the patient and the position of the fibroids; in younger women they can often be removed by myomectomy and the reproductive function left intact.   Small subserous fibroids may be present for many years without causing symptoms and such symptoms as arise are those due to pressure.   (3) Cancer is the most serious of all causes of hæmorrhage.   The chance of recovery depends upon the diagnosis of the disease and its treatment *at an early stage.*   It is a wise rule to regard every menopausal or post-menopausal woman who complains of irregular bleeding as a potential sufferer from cancer until a full investigation, including a curettage, has excluded it.   Improved results with modern treatment, surgery, radium and X-rays, depend upon treating the disease in its early stages.

Treatment of Hæmorrhage—(i.) Unless there is uncontrollable bleeding, anæmia should be treated and the level of hæmoglobin raised to 70 per cent. (10 G. per 100 ml.) before any operative procedure, including curettage, is carried out.   (ii.) An exception to this rule may be made in the case of puberty bleeding occurring in girls under the age of 18.   Here, a satisfactory response is almost invariably obtained to hormone treatment.   This is best given as follows:

On the 5th day of an episode of bleeding, commence treatment with tab. stilbœstrol 1 mg. twice daily for 21 days; should bleeding commence again during treatment, stop for five days and recommence with double the dose.   Continue until treatment has produced 21 days free from bleeding.   On the 5th day of the next episode of bleeding, repeat œstrogen treatment as before for 21 days. After three regular cycles have thus been produced proceed as follows: 4th month, stilbœstrol as before for 21 days. For the last 10 days of treatment add tab. ethisterone, 20 mg. daily; 5th month, halve the dosage of stilbœstrol, increase ethisterone to 30 mg. daily; 6th month, quarter the dose of stilbœstrol, increase ethisterone to 40 mg. daily. Then stop all treatment and in most cases regular normal menstruation will ensue. Where stilbœstrol is not well tolerated, ethinyl œstradiol may be used, with 0·05 mg. in the place of 1 mg. of stilbœstrol.

(iii.) In adult women remedial treatment is directed to the cause.   (iv.) Functional uterine hæmorrhage, that is bleeding without evident pelvic pathology, may prove difficult. Methyl testosterone helps some cases; good results may sometimes be obtained by combining this with ethisterone during the second half of the menstrual cycle. Other cases of functional bleeding, including those due to metropathia hæmorrhagica, irregular shedding of the endometrium or hyperplasia of the endometrium are cured by curettage alone. Cases of metropathia may respond to administration of progesterone, ethisterone or the new synthetic progestagens (§ 435), dosage being planned so that "progestagen withdrawal" bleedings are produced cyclically at intervals of about 28 days (§ 435). Emergency treatment of acute, profuse functional hæmorrhage consists in administration of large doses of œstrogens, say tab. stilbœstrol 10 mg. every two hours, till bleeding is controlled. A single large dose of testosterone, 100 mg. by injection, may also be effective. In cases of intractable bleeding, hysterectomy may be the only treatment. In women at or near the menopause, artificial menopause may be induced by radium or X-rays, provided careful investigation, including a full curettage, has excluded malignant disease. (v.) Bleeding due to retained products of conception after childbirth, uterine abortion or hydatidiform mole requires careful and thorough evacuation of the uterus. Bleeding may be severe and steps must be taken to combat this. Hydatidiform mole is occasionally dealt with by hysterotomy, but in women near the menopause, who already have a number of children, hysterectomy is the treatment of choice. When the uterus is not removed, serial biological tests for pregnancy must be performed, every three months for the first year and every six months for the second year; a positive test leads immediately to a suspicion of chorionepithelioma, though it may be due to normal pregnancy. Further investigation, including biological tests with urine diluted 1/200 and 1/500, is demanded.   (vi.) Fibroids may be treated by hysterectomy or myomectomy, the choice resting with the surgeon. An artificial menopause can be carried out when the patient is unfit for major surgery.

§ **451.** (E) **Amenorrhœa** is that condition in which menstruation is absent. The term oligomenorrhœa is applied to those cases where menstruation is deficient or where the periods occur at abnormally long intervals. *Physiological* amenorrhœa is the cessation of the menses which occurs in menopause, pregnancy and during lactation. The term *primary* amenorrhœa is applied to the condition where menstruation never occurs, as in rare cases where there is a congenital absence of the organs concerned, and also in cases of infantile uterus and undeveloped ovaries. *Apparent* amenorrhœa or cryptomenorrhœa is that form in which there are symptoms of menstruation such as a feeling of fullness in the breasts and abdominal pain every month, but the menstrual flow is retained behind an imperforate hymen, an occluded os or vagina. In *secondary* amenorrhœa, the flow, after having been once established, ceases for a time.

The Menopause, or climacteric, is the epoch at which the reproductive activity of the female undergoes involution and the menses, which are the sign of that activity, cease. This may take place in three ways: (*a*) the menses may cease gradually, appearing at gradually lengthening intervals until finally they stop altogether; (*b*) they may cease quite suddenly; (*c*) there may be a series of hæmorrhages.

Symptoms.—When menstruation ceases at the normal age of the menopause, the patient should be reassured that the occurrence is physiological and reminded that in a healthy woman this process takes place with no disturbance of her normal life. Sexual intercourse can of course continue normally. Attendant phenomena of the menopause may be as follows: (1) The age varies considerably, between 35 and 55, the average being between 45 and 50. (2) " Hot flushes, " a generalised vaso-motor disturbance, felt as a wave of heat spreading up over the face and head and sometimes accompanied by sweating. (3) Nervous phenomena may appear at this time—insomnia, irritability, restlessness and depression. (4) At and after the menopause, atrophic changes occur throughout the genital organs; the uterus shrinks and its muscle wall becomes thin. The vaginal folds become smooth and there may be some contraction of the introitus, leading to dyspareunia. The extent of this change may be estimated by microscopical examination of vaginal smears. (5) Fibroids and other pelvic lesions such as endometriosis tend to involute at this time, but must be carefully watched.

Diagnosis.—Menorrhagia and in particular irregular uterine bleeding require most careful investigation at this age when cancer is especially liable to develop. Irregular uterine bleeding must *always* be investigated by a careful and thorough curettage of the uterus, followed by histological examination of the curettings; any ulceration of the cervix must be investigated by biopsy. Such irregular bleeding must never be lightly dismissed as " simply due to the Change."

Treatment is necessary for constitutional symptoms such as hot flushes. They are believed to be due to excess of pituitary secretion, released by the failure of ovarian function; they can be relieved by giving sex hormones, œstrogens, progesterone or testosterone. Œstrogens may be given by mouth: daily doses are œstrone 2 mg., stilbœstrol 0·5 to 1 mg., dienœstrol 0·3 to 1 mg., or ethinyl œstradiol 0·01 to 0·05 mg. If œstrogens are used the dosage should be kept to a minimum and treatment should never be continuous; it is best given for three weeks at a time with a week's rest and every effort should be made to discontinue treatment as soon as symptoms are relieved. Methyl testosterone 5 mg. daily relieves some who do not respond to œstrogens.

ARTIFICIAL MENOPAUSE following surgical removal of the ovaries or after a radium menopause may cause severe symptoms. Hot flushes, sweating, irritability and depression are common. When the uterus is removed but the ovaries conserved symptoms are generally less severe. Marital disturbance may occur, due to fear of coitus or to dyspareunia. There is a tendency to gain weight, which is partly due to water retention. Substitution therapy with hormones should be given as in the menopausal syndrome. Obesity is treated by a low-sodium, high-protein reducing diet with restricted fluid intake. Small doses of thyroid, gr. 1 a day, help some patients.

Pregnancy is the chief physiological cause of amenorrhœa before the menopause. The *General Symptoms* are as follows: (1) Morning sickness is usually one of the earliest, coming on from about the 6th week and ceasing by 16 weeks; frequent micturition is also a symptom. (2) The breasts feel tense, tender and full and become enlarged. Montgomery's tubercles, which are the enlarged pouting mouths of sebaceous glands, appear on the areola of the nipple. The nipples themselves may become pigmented and a dark area or " secondary areola " may surround them. Dilated veins, coursing over the surface of the breast, become apparent by the 12th week. After this time, the breasts may contain colostrum. *Local Signs.* The *earlier signs* are: (1) On digital examination, there is a softening of the cervix which is unmistakable to the educated finger; the vagina feels warm and moist due to increased secretion; (2) a gradual increase in the size of the uterus becomes apparent; this is associated with a change in shape so that the uterus feels globular instead of pear-shaped. Hégar's sign is due to softening and thinning of the lower segment of the uterus so that, on bimanual examination, the fingers appear to meet in the anterior vaginal fornix; this sign is observed from the 6th to the 10th week. Piscacek's sign, present about this time, is also elicited on bimanual examination; the uterine fundus appears to be separate from the cervix, owing to softening and thinning of the lower uterine segment. Palmer's sign consists of regular, rhythmic contractions of the uterus, elicited on bimanual examination. From the 12th week, the uterus becomes palpable per abdomen and unmistakable *later signs* appear—viz., (3) about the 18th to the 22nd week, fœtal movements can be felt by the patient and by the physician, and (4) the fœtal heart sounds (at the rate of 120 to 140 per minute) may be heard on auscultation, usually midway between the umbilicus and one or other anterior superior spine; and (5) external ballottement of fœtal parts can be made out after the 20th week. (6) X-ray examination will demonstrate the fœtal skeleton after the 16th week of pregnancy.

The *diagnosis* of pregnancy occasionally presents difficulty. The accuracy of diagnosis has been enhanced by the introduction of biological tests such as the Aschheim-Zondek and other tests which depend on the presence of chorionic, anterior pituitary-like gonadotrophins in the urine (§ 1211). It must be remembered that a negative test is often obtained after the 14th week in normal pregnancy, as a sharp fall in gonadotrophin excretion occurs at this time.

The *Causes* of SECONDARY AMENORRHŒA may be divided into constitutional and local causes. (*a*) *Constitutional* causes are the most frequent. Endocrine imbalance as a cause of primary amenorrhœa is considered in the introductory paragraph to this chapter (§ 433); to this may be ascribed the amenorrhœa following a sudden change of abode or mode of life, anxiety, stress or mental shock. Such amenorrhœa is common in young women who leave home between the ages of 18 and 22. It also occurs with pulmonary tuberculosis, anæmia, after severe illness or prolonged lactation, in chronic alcoholism and chronic poisoning with cocaine or opium, and sometimes with pyrexia. Certain tumours of the anterior pituitary or adrenal cortex are also causes. (*b*) The most important *local* cause is pelvic tuberculosis which may lead to total destruction, with caseation, of the endometrium. Certain ovarian tumours, especially the masculinising tumour called the arrhenoblastoma, may be associated with amenorrhœa.

Treatment of constitutional causes consists of general measures to improve health; causes associated with disease such as pulmonary tuberculosis must be investigated and treated. In cases where no serious disease exists, spontaneous recovery with return of the menses is the rule. Treatment with œstrogens alone, or combined with progestogens (*vide* § 450) is successful in provoking cyclical bleeding except in cases where the uterus is too small and underdeveloped to respond. In cases of functional amenorrhœa, the production of artificial cycles by means of hormone treatment may be followed by a return of normal spontaneous menstruation.

§ 452. (F) Pelvic Pain.—Pain in and about the pelvis is one of the commonest symptoms of disorder of the female reproductive organs. " Bearing down " is often spoken of; and " backache ", or pain over the sacrum, is so constant a feature of pelvic disorders that it has come to have that association in the minds of the laity. The position and character of the pain vary with different diseases but its degree is largely influenced by the temperament of the patient. Reference has already been made to painful menstruation (dysmenorrhœa), but the causes of continuous pain (without reference to the menstrual period) are usually due to inflammatory lesions of the reproductive organs, to pelvic endometriosis or malignant disease. Referred pain is frequently present in acute gynæcological lesions because the parietal peritoneum is involved.

CLINICAL INVESTIGATION OF **Acute Pelvic Pain.**—To ascertain the significance of pain in a given case attention must be paid to the general mental or nervous condition of the patient. The method of procedure in the investigation of abdominal pain in § 242 should be studied here.

(1) The HISTORY of the ONSET and the AREA of PAIN give valuable indications as to the nature of the lesion. If the pain begins at the umbilicus and later extends

to the right iliac fossa suspect appendicitis. If the pain starts in the lower abdomen and later settles into one or both iliac fossæ, suspect tubal disease, which is often associated with pelvic inflammation (§ 453 *et seq.*).

(2) TENDERNESS is present either in the skin (hyperæsthesia) or in the deep structures (deep tenderness) in association with congestion or inflammation of underlying organs. In appendicitis there is usually deep tenderness over MacBurney's point, but if the appendix is in the pelvis, tenderness may be much more marked on vaginal or rectal examination. If the maximum tenderness is close to the anterior superior spine, the appendix is to the outer side of the normally situated cæcum; but if the maximum tenderness is on the lower part of the right rectus abdominis, close to the middle line, the appendix is hanging over the brim of the pelvis. Any other inflamed organ in the pelvis may cause much more tenderness by vaginal or rectal examination than by abdominal palpation. And see § 248.

(3) RIGIDITY is generally associated with deep-seated tenderness and usually indicates an acute inflammatory condition.

(4) Inquire as to MENSTRUAL IRREGULARITY, which gives an important indication as to pregnancy or abortion.

(5) VAGINAL DISCHARGE, if acute or severe, may point to extension upwards of gonorrhœal or other sepsis.

(6) RECTAL OR VAGINAL EXAMINATION must never be omitted, as it detects tenderness, swelling, discharge or displacement.

The CAUSES OF PELVIC PAIN are many. Pain may arise in the organs of reproduction or in the other organs lying in the pelvis. *Diagnosis* as to the cause may be difficult: particular attention should be given to the SUDDENNESS OF ONSET, the SEVERITY AND TYPE of pain, whether it is ATTENDED BY COLLAPSE or UTERINE BLEEDING, and whether there are CONSTITUTIONAL SIGNS and LOCAL SIGNS OF PELVIC INFLAMMATION (pyrexia and the signs discussed in § 244). The diseases can be classified as follows:

I. ACUTE PELVIC PAIN *came on* VERY SUDDENLY *accompanied by* FAINT-NESS *or* COLLAPSE *and often* UTERINE BLEEDING. The cause is probably ABORTION (§ 445). Less commonly there is a RUPTURED OR LEAKING ECTOPIC PREGNANCY (§ 446), and rarely HÆMORRHAGE FROM THE OVARY, both of which produce a PELVIC HÆMATOCŒLE.

Pelvic Hæmatocœle is an effusion of blood either into the peritoneal cavity (intraperitoneal) or into the connective tissues of the broad ligament (extraperitoneal) due to the above-mentioned causes. There is a *sudden onset* of (1) severe pain, starting in one iliac fossa and soon spreading over the lower part of the abdomen; occasionally it is referred to the shoulder. The pain is accompanied by (2) faintness, perhaps collapse with (3) nausea and in some cases vomiting. (4) There may be some uterine bleeding with discharge of a cast of the interior of the uterus. (5) On examination, the uterus in the intraperitoneal variety of pelvic hæmatocœle is found pushed forwards behind the pubes, while in the extraperitoneal variety the swelling is smaller and causes lateral displacement of the uterus as in pelvic cellulitis. The intraperitoneal variety, if large, forms a lump which can be felt on bimanual examination, both in Douglas' pouch and above the pubes, and the abdomen is tense and distended. After 48 hours, adhesions form and the uterus is fixed; signs of pelvic inflammation may ensue. The temperature rises 24 hours after the onset of pain when pelvic peritonitis commences.

Diagnosis.—If the bleeding is (*a*) rapid and intraperitoneal it may become excessive; in addition to the symptoms of abdominal pain and collapse, there are symptoms caused by hæmorrhage, viz. pallor, restlessness and air hunger. The diagnosis from a ruptured viscus (§ 243) may be difficult at first. (*b*) When extraperitoneal, bleeding is usually slow, limited in amount and tends to become encysted. At first there may be acute pain and collapse but the symptoms may subside after a few hours, and attacks of pain may recur at intervals for days. The local signs resemble *pelvic cellulitis* from which it may be diagnosed by a history pointing to extra-uterine pregnancy, and by the fact that pyrexia is absent at the onset.

Prognosis.—Death has been known to occur in about an hour from massive hæmorrhage. In smaller hæmorrhages adhesions form and the exudation may be (i.) entirely absorbed or (ii.) may go on to suppuration with a danger of peritonitis or pelvic cellulitis. In rare cases, where secondary rupture occurs into the peritoneum, the fœtus may live till term, when the patient goes through a spurious labour. In undiagnosed cases the fœtus may become mummified, forming a *lithopædion.*

Treatment is operative in all cases once the diagnosis is firmly established. If there is difficulty in diagnosis between a tubal lesion and acute appendicitis it is safest to operate.

II. *The* PELVIC PAIN *came on* ACUTELY *and* RECENTLY, *accompanied by more or less* CONSTITUTIONAL DISTURBANCE. · The condition may be

(*a*) *Infection* of the pelvic organs—the uterus, Fallopian tubes (salpingitis), the pelvic cellular tissues (pelvic cellulitis) or pelvic veins. As *pelvic peritonitis* is always secondary to some other infection it is not separately described here.

(*b*) *Torsion* of the pedicle of an ovarian cyst (§ 246) or of a pedunculated subperitoneal uterine fibroid (§ 447), a tender tumour, which is firm and separate from the uterus is felt on palpation.

(*c*) *Uterine pain* may arise during pregnancy, with abortion (§ 445), with spasmodic and membranous dysmenorrhœa (§§ 441, 442), with degenerating fibroids (§ 447), with uterine endometriosis (adenomyosis) (§ 449) and with tuberculous pyometra (§ 455). It may be associated with alterations in menstruation and may be spasmodic in character, due to irregular uterine contractions.

(*d*) *Tubal gestation* (§ 446) which may rupture, causes spasmodic pain in the pelvis. When intra-abdominal bleeding is slight, collapse and shock are largely absent.

(*e*) *Other causes* are acute appendicitis (§ 248), acute pyelitis (§ 419), renal colic (§ 413), diverticulitis (§ 328).

§ 453. **Acute Infection of the Pelvic Organs** is a frequent cause of acute pelvic or lower abdominal pain. Infection may reach the pelvic organs in various ways and there is usually a history or evidence of the mode of infection. (1) Infection may spread upwards through the genital tract, involving the cervix, endometrium, Fallopian tubes and ovaries, as in *gonorrhœa*. (2) After childbirth or abortion the placental site in the uterus may become infected, causing *puerperal sepsis*; septic abortion, which in most cases has been criminally induced, is a frequent cause. Infection may spread to other parts of the genital tract or more widely. (3) The pelvic organs may become infected through the pelvic peritoneum as in peritonitis due to acute appendicitis, and occasionally after pelvic operations. (4) Rarely, infection takes place through the blood-stream in cases of septicæmia. (5) Infected tears of the cervix or vagina such as may follow childbirth or operations may cause spread of infection to the cellular tissue in the pelvis, causing *pelvic cellulitis*. (6) Septic thrombi may form in the pelvic veins in certain puerperal infections or after pelvic operations, leading to a condition of pelvic thrombo-phlebitis. Tuberculous infection is discussed in § 455.

Acute Salpingitis is the commonest result of acute pelvic infection.

Symptoms.—(1) Severe pain across the lower abdomen; (2) on examination, distension, tenderness and rigidity of the lower abdomen and (3) a tender swelling may be felt. (4) The legs are flexed; the patient lies on her back. (5) The temperature is high and the pulse quick, indicating the severity of the condition. (6) On bimanual examination there is great tenderness and pain on moving the cervix. (7) A swelling may be felt to either side of, or behind the uterus, pushing it forward; the uterus becomes fixed owing to adhesions. (8) There is usually bleeding or a muco-purulent discharge from the cervix.

Varieties.—The common types are (1) pyosalpinx where the tube is closed and tensely distended with pus. (2) When the Fallopian tube is infected; the ovary is generally involved to a varying degree, and in advanced infections a *tubo-ovarian abscess* forms. (3) The pelvic peritoneum is usually involved and pus may collect, leading to the development of a *pelvic abscess*. This may point into the vagina or rectum, upwards in the direction of Poupart's ligament, or very rarely pus may track along the ureter and point in the region of the kidney. Femoral thrombophlebitis is a frequent complication.

In **Acute Pelvic Cellulitis** there is likewise a great variation in the severity of the infection.

Symptoms.—Pain may be referred to one leg (which may be drawn up to relieve the pain) and on examination the swelling of the pelvis may be limited to one side with displacement of the uterus, or may surround the cervix in a circle of induration and tenderness. (2) Backache may be marked. (3) Dragging pain is a feature when there are posterior peritoneal adhesions. (4) Pus may form in acute or subacute septic conditions of the cellular tissue, again resulting in a pelvic abscess.

Pelvic Thrombophlebitis follows puerperal sepsis (especially with an anærobic streptococcus) and pelvic operations, especially those that involve deep dissection of the parametrium.

Symptoms.—There is a persistent low-grade fever with acute exacerbations when small septic emboli lodge in the lungs. The patient complains of feeling generally unwell. Examination of the pelvis shows no local physical signs of disease. Femoral thrombophlebitis often follows.

Prognosis of Acute Pelvic Infections.—Prompt treatment with the appropriate antibiotic will usually cause rapid subsidence of the symptoms and signs and complete recovery is the rule. In severe acute infections abscess formation may take place before treatment becomes effective; the abscess may point and evacuate itself spontaneously or surgical intervention may become necessary. In neglected cases, widespread adhesions form and the condition progresses to chronic pelvic peritonitis; the patient will probably have chronic pelvic pain, menorrhagia, discharge and dysmenorrhœa all her life, resulting in chronic invalidism and nervous symptoms. Sterility is the rule and dyspareunia may be present. Relapses with acute pain and fever may occur, especially following a chill or over-exertion.

Treatment of Acute Pelvic Infections.—The principles to be adopted are (1) absolute rest in bed; (2) application of warmth. Local heat in the form of hot-water bottles, an electric pad or a hot cradle may be helpful; care must be taken to avoid burning the skin. Pelvic diathermy is of value in pelvic sepsis when the acute stage has passed. (3) Pain is relieved by analgesics as indicated in Chapter IX. Aspirin or tab. codein co., or a mixture of aspirin and phenacetin may be sufficient. Morphine, pethidine and amidone B.P. (Physeptone) are used only in severe conditions, and when the diagnosis has been established, as they tend to mask symptoms and thus to delay proper surgical treatment. (4) Every attempt is made to discover the infecting organism and to determine its sensitivities. In all cases a cervical swab should be taken. In severe infections treatment should be begun before the result of bacteriological tests is available. A sulphonamide, such as sulphadimidine, 1 G. every six hours, and penicillin 500,000 units every six hours are given. In most cases there is a dramatic response to treatment, the symptoms and signs subsiding within 48 hours. If there is no response during this time, a change is made to one of the tetracyclines such as chlortetracycline B.P. (Aureomycin) or oxytetracycline B.P. (Terramycin). Acute salpingitis is best treated medically except when the diagnosis is uncertain or when abscess formation occurs. Surgical treatment is not indicated in acute pelvic infections, except in two circumstances. If the diagnosis is in doubt as between an acute pelvic infection and acute appendicitis it is safer to perform laparotomy. An abscess must be drained, preferably by the vaginal route.

III. *The* PELVIC PAIN *is of a* CHRONIC *nature and* RECURS FREQUENTLY.

(a) WHEN IT IS ACCOMPANIED BY A LOW-GRADE TEMPERATURE *it may be due to* CHRONIC SALPINGITIS, CHRONIC PELVIC CELLULITIS, SCLEROCYSTIC DISEASE OF THE OVARY, TUBERCULOSIS *of the pelvic organs,* TUBERCULOUS

GLANDS (§ 573), CHRONIC PYELITIS (§ 419) *or to* CROHN'S DISEASE *of the ileum* (§ 312, *c*).

(*b*) *When there is* NO ACCOMPANYING PYREXIA *almost any of the different diseases mentioned in this chapter may be suspected. Examination may reveal* ENDOMETRIOSIS (§ 442), ENDOCERVICITIS (§ 440), CHRONIC PELVIC CELLULITIS or UTERINE DISPLACEMENT; *or careful bimanual examination may reveal a* PROLAPSED OVARY *or an* INFLAMED TUBE (§ 454).

§ **454. Chronic Salpingitis** may or may not follow the acute form.

Symptoms.—(1) Pain in the lower abdomen, in one of both iliac regions. (2) Backache is usual, the pain is constant, bearing down and is much worse at the menstrual period; it frequently takes the form of premenstrual or congestive dysmenorrhœa, pain beginning 3 or 4 days or even a week before the flow which may relieve it.   (3) Menorrhagia or heavy irregular uterine bleeding may occur.   (4) Dyspareunia may be caused by pus tubes bound down by adhesions to the posterior wall of the uterus and pelvic peritoneum.   (5) Sterility is the rule as the tubes are closed by infection. (6) The general health is poor, the woman exhibiting signs of the " chronic pelvic woman " and often becoming wrongly labelled neurotic.   (7) Exacerbations of the disease may occur, in a subacute form, giving a picture similar to that of acute salpingitis, but with less severe symptoms and signs. (8) On bimanual examination the uterus is found to be retroverted and fixed by adhesions, posteriorly or to one or other side, and (9) there is tenderness due to adhesions, especially in the ovarian region.

Hydrosalpinx occurs when the infection is slight and the closed tube distended with clear fluid and *chronic interstitial salpingitis* when the tube is only slightly enlarged but its wall is greatly thickened and its lumen partly or completely obliterated.   For tuberculous salpingitis, see § 455.

In **Chronic Pelvic Cellulitis** (1) there is a deep aching pelvic pain with deep dyspareunia.   (2) Backache may be troublesome.   (3) On examination of the pelvis the swelling may be on one side only, displacing the uterus to the opposite side, or the cervix may be surrounded by a tender induration.   Pus may form after a period of some weeks: the swelling felt in one lateral fornix becomes larger, pushing the uterus to one side and presenting as a firm lump which may extend to the iliac fossa and become palpable above Poupart's ligament. (See pelvic abscess, § 453.)   (4) Instead of pus, adhesions with fibrous tissue may form: these do not interfere with pregnancy and may be slowly absorbed.

Treatment of Chronic Salpingitis and Chronic Pelvic Cellulitis.—If there is evidence of active infection, this should be treated as described in acute pelvic infections.   Otherwise medical treatment is mainly with pelvic short-wave diathermy; remarkable improvement is often seen.   When this fails, the patient can be saved from chronic invalidism and disability only by radical surgery, which should include at least removal of the uterus and Fallopian tubes.

Sclerocystic disease of the ovary may be a manifestation of chronic infection or may arise from endocrine causes. Both ovaries are enlarged and filled with small retention cysts; the outer coat is thickened. The patient complains of chronic pelvic pain, irregular bleeding and sterility. *Treatment* is surgical and consists in the excision of a wedge from each ovary.

§ **455. Tuberculosis of the Pelvic Organs** is mainly active during the reproductive period, most cases occurring between 15 and 35. It has been estimated that pelvic tuberculosis is found at routine autopsy in 1 per cent. of all women, but in 5 per cent. of women suffering from tuberculosis elsewhere; 10 per cent. of all cases of chronic salpingitis are believed to be tuberculous.

General Symptoms.—Many cases remain dormant for years and may only be discovered in the course of investigations for sterility, at laparotomy or at autopsy. The pelvic organs are affected in the following order of frequency: Fallopian tubes, uterus, ovaries, cervix, vulva and vagina.

Tuberculosis of the Fallopian tubes is the most frequent of all the tuberculous lesions of the female genitalia. (*a*) In the ulcero-caseous variety the tube is closed and distended with tuberculous (caseous) pus. Dense adhesions often form to the surrounding peritoneum. (*b*) In the *interstitial* variety or nodular salpingitis, the wall of the tube is generally thickened though the abdominal ostium remains patent.

Tuberculosis of the uterus affects chiefly the endometrium; in most cases it is secondary to disease of the Fallopian tubes. The most common type is the *caseous variety*; slow caseation affects the endometrium which is gradually destroyed so that eventually amenorrhœa results. In the *chronic diffuse variety*, minute tubercles are scattered throughout the endometrium and the underlying muscular layer. A third variety, *miliary* tuberculosis, is occasionally found in women dying from generalised miliary disease. *Symptoms* may be absent; sterility or persistent leucorrhœa may be complained of. Menorrhagia may occur, but amenorrhœa results when the disease has totally destroyed the endometrium. Pain may occur with a tuberculous *pyometra*.

Tuberculosis of the ovaries may be secondary to tuberculous salpingitis or to tuberculous peritonitis. In the early stages giant-cell systems are found in the ovaries; later, caseation with the formation of a cold abscess may occur. The tube and ovary may form one abscess cavity—a tuberculous tubo-ovarian abscess.

Tuberculosis of the cervix generally occurs in association with tuberculosis of the endometrium. It occurs in two varieties: (*a*) the ulcerative form may resemble cervical erosion; (*b*) The proliferative form may closely resemble squamous epithelioma of the cervix. Both forms give rise to blood-stained, often offensive, vaginal discharge. *Diagnosis* is made by biopsy of the cervix.

Tuberculosis of the vulva exists in two forms: (*a*) In the ulcerative form, the vulva is covered with multiple small indolent ulcers which may fuse to form a serpiginous ulcer. These have a yellowish base and purple œdematous edges. (*b*) The proliferative form is less common and leads to elephantiasis of the vulva, with enormous swelling of the labia. Painful micturition, pruritus and pain are the most frequent symptoms. *Diagnosis* may be made on clinical appearances and often confirmed by biopsy, though in proliferative cases with much fibrosis it may be difficult to find the typical giant-cell systems.

Tuberculosis of the vagina is rarely primary, but usually secondary to tuberculosis of the cervix; the ulcerative form is the commonest but a miliary form exists.

Tuberculosis of the pelvic peritoneum occurs in three forms. In the *miliary* variety, which is often associated with generalised peritoneal tuberculosis, the peritoneum is studded with tubercles. Ascites may eventually occur, but the condition may remain dormant for some time (and see § 573). In the *ulcero-caseous* variety, masses of tuberculous granulation tissue form and these may break down to form a tuberculous pelvic abscess. Fistulae may develop. In the *fibroplastic* variety, adhesions form with encysted collections of free fluid.

Diagnosis.—Tuberculous salpingitis and oöphoritis should be suspected when salpingitis occurs with no history of appendicitis or of other cause for pelvic infection. The presence of tuberculous disease elsewhere, of nocturnal pyrexia or a raised sedimentation rate may strengthen the suspicion. Confirmation depends on finding the tubercle bacillus, or at least the typical histological features of tuberculosis. Since in most cases of tuberculous salpingitis the endometrium is involved, biopsy is the most important preliminary investigation: the endometrium should be submitted to histological examination, culture for tubercle bacilli and inoculation of a guinea-pig. The disease is sometimes diagnosed when laparotomy is carried out for an obscure pelvic mass or for pelvic pain.

Etiology.—The blood-stream is the most frequent route of infection, but tubercle bacilli may reach the Fallopian tubes from the bowel or mesenteric glands. In generalised tuberculous peritonitis, the pelvic peritoneum will become involved; in cases of generalised miliary tuberculosis, the pelvic organs may be affected as a part of the disease. Tuberculosis of the vulva is often secondary to tuberculous infection of the bowel.

Treatment should be conservative in most cases and should consist initially of streptomycin, 1 G. 3 to 6 times weekly for 12 weeks with para-amino-salicylic acid 12 to 20 G. daily for 12 weeks. Isoniazid, 100 mg. thrice daily, may be given in addition. This treatment should be carried out under sanatorium conditions. Progress is observed by serial endometrial biopsies and by sedimentation rates. *Surgery* is indicated in those cases which fail to respond, or relapse in spite of adequate medical treatment; also in cases where there are large caseous pelvic masses. Operation should always be carried out under a cover of streptomycin and PAS and the danger of fistula formation in cases with multiple adhesions must be borne in mind. Surgery should be radical and should always consist of a pelvic clearance. Some cases will be found to be inoperable in view of extensive adhesions or involvement of the bladder or rectum. Deep X-ray therapy may be successful in the treatment of inoperable disease.

The **pain** *is of a* **chronic** *character, is of considerable duration, and is* UNATTENDED *by* PYREXIA. Almost any of the different diseases mentioned in this chapter may be suspected. Examination may reveal METRITIS, ENDOCERVICITIS, CHRONIC PELVIC INFLAMMATION (§ 454) or a UTERINE DISPLACEMENT; or careful bimanual examination may reveal a PROLAPSED OVARY, or an INFLAMED TUBE. UTERINE DISPLACEMENTS AND PELVIC TUMOURS alone remain to be considered. PROLAPSE OF THE UTERUS is a cause of dragging pain, in its early stages.

§ 456. **Uterine Displacements.**—The normal position of the uterus is one of anteversion, with slight anterior flexion. The uterus undergoes physiological displacements according to the fullness of the bladder and rectum. In itself a displacement leads to no symptom; the symptoms so often associated with displacements are due to inflammatory processes or to endometriosis in or near the uterus which have caused the displacement. Tumours and inflammatory exudation in the pelvis may cause LATERAL or UPWARD DISPLACEMENTS of the uterus.

FORWARD DISPLACEMENTS (ANTEFLEXION).—On bimanual examination the os is found to be high up and the fundus is felt unduly far forward. In nulliparæ, stenosis of the os or an elongated cervix may accompany a forward displacement of congenital origin. As above stated, *Symptoms* may be entirely absent and attention is first drawn to the condition when other mischief such as pelvic inflammation, endometriosis, parametritis or a history of dysmenorrhœa, sterility or recurrent abortions is present.

Etiology.—(1) A congenitally ill-developed uterus is often displaced forwards. Forward displacement, which is uncommon, is diagnosed as pathological, rather than physiological, when there is lessened mobility of the uterus, and pain on attempting to move it. Forward displacements are found in association with (2) pelvic peritonitis with adhesions and (3) cellulitis affecting the utero-sacral ligaments.

Treatment.—Slow dilatation of the cervix with graduated metal dilators is the best treatment for congenital cases; this may have to be repeated more than once. In cases associated with chronic sepsis, short-wave diathermy offers the best hope of improvement.

BACKWARD UTERINE DISPLACEMENTS consist of RETROVERSION AND RETROFLEXION. In a backward displacement there is some degree of descent of the uterus. Retro-displacements in themselves cause no symptoms; the majority are congenital in origin. On examination the finger detects the forward displacement of the cervix which is often somewhat lower than normal. The uterus is not palpable in the anterior fornix, whereas a lump is felt in the posterior fornix which is recognised as the body of the uterus because it is movable with the cervix and can be felt to be continuous with the cervix.

Symptoms arise when pelvic adhesions are present, or when the displaced organ interferes with other organs in the vicinity. In such conditions, a retroverted uterus gives rise to (1) pain in the back and the lower abdomen of a bearing-down, dull aching character; (2) deep dyspareunia, due to pressure on prolapsed ovaries; (3) constipation and painful defæcation, especially if associated with endometriosis. (4) After the 14th week of pregnancy, an incarcerated retroverted gravid uterus may cause retention with dribbling of urine.

Diagnosis.—The diagnosis of a backward displacement is not difficult, but the diagnosis of the cause may be obscure. It is important first of all to determine whether the uterus is freely movable or not, as the prognosis and treatment differ.

Etiology.—(i.) Congenital; (ii.) the dragging of adhesions consequent on pelvic peritonitis or pelvic endometriosis; (iii.) changes in the uterus such as subinvolution or tumours; (iv.) relaxation of the ligaments as in incipient prolapse; (v.) displacement by pelvic tumours such as those of the ovary; (vi.) very rarely, a sudden fall or strain. (vii.) An over distended bladder, as in the puerperal woman. Several of these causes may act in combination; thus subinvolution together with relaxation of the ligaments causes a retroversion with a certain amount of downward displacement of the uterus, as pointed out in Prolapse (§ 459).

Prognosis.—(1) So long as the uterus is freely movable and not enlarged there may be no symptoms referable to the displacement. In women of neurotic disposition, it is unwise to suggest that the uterus is displaced. (2) Some retro-displacements are apt to lead to congestion and enlargement of the uterine body with prolapse of the ovaries. Adhesions may form when there is chronic inflammation or endometriosis affecting the tubes or ovaries. (3) Where the uterus is bound by adhesions there may be a condition which, according to Playfair, is " not fatal, but tends to life-long discomfort."

Treatment.—If the displacement is giving rise to no symptoms, no treatment is required. If there is pain, such as backache or dyspareunia, the uterus should be replaced and a Smith-Hodge pessary inserted. This may be possible without anæsthesia, but often it is necessary to give an anæsthetic before the uterus can be replaced. A fixed retroversion which cannot be replaced under anæsthesia suggests major pelvic disease and laparotomy followed by the appropriate treatment is advisable. Retroversion of the gravid uterus persisting after 12 weeks should be treated by rest in bed, preferably in the semi-prone position. Bimanual replacement of the gravid uterus may be possible, but if a gentle attempt fails, a rubber ring pessary, of the largest size which can be tolerated without discomfort, is inserted. The pressure of the pessary, combined with muscular movements of the patient, is almost always successful in causing the uterus to rise up out of the pelvis; the pessary is removed at the 16th week of pregnancy. Retention of urine is dealt with by catheterisation; the bladder should be emptied gradually and infection of the urinary tract prevented, or treated if present. Ventrosuspension of the uterus by Gilliam's method, or by one of the other operations devised for this purpose, is successful in non-pregnant women when it has been proved that the retroversion is causing symptoms. A "pessary test" is advisable; a Smith-Hodge pessary is inserted, after replacing the retroverted uterus, and left in position for at least 4 weeks. If the symptoms are relieved, but recur with recurrence of the retroversion after removing the pessary, then operation is justified.

§ 457. (G) The following are some of the more important **Pelvic Tumours and Vaginal Swellings:**—

(a) *Internal Tumours.*

(i.) Uterine Fibroid (§ 447).

(ii.) Cervical or Uterine Polyp (§ 447).

(iii.) Cervical or Uterine Cancer (§ 450).

(iv.) Retroverted Uterus (§ 456).

(v.) Pelvic Cellulitis (§§ 453, 454).

(vi.) Ovarian Tumour (§ 261).

(vii.) Pyosalpinx (§§ 453, 455).

(viii.) Appendix Abscess (§ 248).

(ix.) Pelvic Hæmatocœle (§ 452).

(x.) Hydatid of Pelvis.

(b) *External Swellings* or *Swelling about the Vulva* may be due to:—

(i.) Prolapse of the uterus.

(ii.) Prolapse of the vaginal walls (cystocœle and rectocœle).

(iii.) Abscesses, cysts or tumours of Bartholin's gland.

(iv.) Uterine polypus with a long pedicle.

(v.) Local conditions of the vulva such as abscess, hæmatoma, sebaceous cyst or carcinoma.

(vi.) Cysts of the vaginal wall, usually found on the anterior wall, about the size of an egg and painless.

(vii.) Inguinal hernia.

Most of these various conditions have already been referred to, but three conditions which may appear as external swellings remain to be described—PROLAPSE OF THE VAGINAL WALLS, PROLAPSE OF THE UTERUS and INVERSION OF THE UTERUS.

§ 458. **Prolapse of the Vaginal Walls** is most common in women who have borne children. Cystocœle is a herniation of the bladder into the anterior vaginal wall; this may be felt by the patient as a lump in the vagina and in extreme cases may project beyond the vulva. Prolapse of the posterior wall also occurs, and when the rectum is prolapsed it is named rectocœle; the pouch of Douglas may also herniate into the posterior vaginal wall, producing the condition known as enterocœle (because small or large intestine may occupy the swelling) or pouch of Douglas hernia.

CYSTOCŒLE may cause a variety of *Symptoms* associated with micturition (see also § 460); this may include frequency, precipitancy, urgency, stress incontinence or difficulty in emptying the bladder until the prolapsed part is pushed up. A very large cystocœle may pull the base of the bladder down to such a degree that the lower ends of the ureters are kinked; ureteric obstruction leading to hydronephrosis and ultimately to renal failure sometimes results. The urethra may be prolapsed or displaced with the bladder; occasionally prolapse of the urethra or *urethrocœle* is found with little or no cystocœle (§ 439). The *diagnosis* of cystocœle from a cyst of the vagina is made by passing a sound per urethram and with one finger in the vagina feeling the point of the instrument in the bladder.

RECTOCŒLE also causes a lump which is felt in the vagina; a large rectocœle will also cause constipation. The desire to defæcate is felt, but the rectum cannot be completely emptied. Rectocœle is often associated with a deficient perineum following injury at childbirth. For the *Treatment* of prolapse of the vagina see below.

§ 459. **Prolapse of the Uterus** is its displacement downwards. Three degrees of displacement are described: (i.) The organ may occupy a position somewhat lower than normal; (ii.) it may have partly passed through the vaginal orifice (procidentia); and (iii.) in complete procidentia it lies entirely outside the vulva, the body lying in the inverted vaginal wall.

In slighter cases the vaginal wall is seen coming down on asking the patient to strain or cough. In more severe degrees the cervix is seen outside the vulva and the body of the uterus can be felt. The other *Symptoms* of prolapse of the uterus are as follows: (i.) the uterus is elongated, the cervix is frequently hypertrophic and there may be accompanying endocervicitis or endometritis; (ii.) in early cases there may be incontinent, urgent or frequent micturition; later there is difficulty in passing water until the prolapsed organ is pushed up. (iii.) Sometimes there is a feeling of weight or a bearing-down feeling in the pelvis, but more often no pain is complained of, only the discomfort of the lump during walking or sitting. In the early stages, however, a dragging backache may be a prominent feature. (iv.) The uterus is usually retroflexed. (v.) Leucorrhœa is usually troublesome. Ulceration of the prolapsed parts, called decubitus ulcer, is apt to supervene on procidentia.

Etiology.—Prolapse occurs mainly in parous women, and most cases must be held to arise directly or indirectly as a result of childbirth. Congenital weakness of the supports of the uterus and vagina must be a factor, as evidenced by the occasional occurrence of prolapse in nulliparæ and by the fact that a woman may bear several children without sustaining prolapse. It is mainly a disease of working-class women, and laborious occupations involving muscular strain contribute to its causation. It may come on immediately after childbirth, or more often, in later life, at or near the menopause. Exciting causes are (i.) increased abdominal pressure, such as occurs with muscular strain, sagging of enlarged viscera or undue deposit of abdominal fat. (ii.) Weakness or relaxation of the supporting muscles and ligaments such as occurs after childbirth, in menopausal and in post-menopausal women. (iii.) Increased weight of the pelvic organs as in chronic subinvolution of the uterus or tumours of the uterus or ovaries.

Treatment.—Preventive treatment is most important. This includes proper management of labour and careful suture of lacerations sustained at childbirth: in the puerperium, early ambulation and physiotherapy in the form of abdominal massage and exercises to improve the tone of the abdominal and pelvic muscles. Many cases of incipient prolapse can be cured by weight reduction where necessary and faradism and exercises to the pelvic floor under trained supervision. Where there is visceroptosis, a well-fitting belt to support the abdominal organs and prevent downward pressure on the pelvis is very beneficial.

For established prolapse, the best results are obtained with operative repair. Pessaries may be used where operation is contra-indicated owing to the patient's age or general condition, but their effect is mainly palliative.

Inversion of the Uterus.—Sudden inversion may occur in the third stage of labour, but here we are concerned only with the chronic form of inversion, a very rare condition. It may be the sequel to acute inversion if the patient survives the initial shock, or to the dragging of a tumour. The fundus alone may be inverted through the os, or the whole uterus may be inverted. (1) The swelling is red, bleeds readily and is tender. (2) The uterine sound cannot be passed the normal distance if at all. (3) Bimanually the fundus is found to be missing: and if a sound is placed in the bladder in the middle line and the finger in the rectum these can be made to meet without any uterus being felt. (4) There may be symptoms of bearing down, menorrhagia and leucorrhœa. (5) The orifices of the Fallopian tubes can sometimes be distinguished. A *Diagnosis* may have to be made from a fibroid polyp, in which the fundus is present in its normal position.

Prognosis.—There is no tendency to spontaneous cure. Treatment is operative in most cases. Where the uterus is normal it can occasionally be replaced with Aveling's repositor. For details of operative treatment, the reader should consult a textbook on Gynæcology.

§ **460.** (H) It is proposed to discuss briefly the causes of the following symptoms for which the physician may be consulted: (a) DISORDERED MICTURITION (Retention, Unduly Frequent, Painful or Difficult Micturition and Incontinence); (b) PAINFUL DEFÆCATION; (c) PAIN ON SITTING; and (d) DYSPAREUNIA.

(a) **Disordered Micturition** is dealt with more fully in kidney diseases (§§ 416 to 421); here only a few of those special to the female will be mentioned.

I. RETENTION OF URINE.—The *Causes* peculiar to women are impacted fibroids and ovarian tumours, malignant disease of the cervix, involving the vagina, tumours of the vagina, retroverted gravid uterus (especially about the 14th week of pregnancy) and other conditions causing obstruction to the urinary passage consequent on pressure over the mouth of the bladder. The condition also occurs after operations on the pelvic organs, after childbirth (especially after difficult or instrumental delivery or Cæsarean section). Retention of urine in women may be due to hysteria or may occasionally occur when the bladder has been allowed to become overfilled.

II. FREQUENT MICTURITION may be caused in women by (i.) pressure on the bladder in early or late pregnancy; an enlarged anteflexed uterus or a pelvic tumour; (ii.) a vascular caruncle of the urethra; (iii.) acute cystitis; (iv) cystocœle or urethrocœle; (v.) pelvic inflammation, especially during the early stages; (vi.) calculi, crystals or foreign bodies in the bladder; and (vii.) various nervous conditions.

III. PAINFUL MICTURITION is found especially in connection with urethral caruncle, cystitis, after childbirth or operation, in cervicitis and in the early stages of pelvic inflammation.

IV. DIFFICULT MICTURITION is found (i.) after labour, when the parts are swollen and bruised; (ii.) after operations on the pelvic organs; (iii.) in severe degrees of uterine prolapse, in which case the symptom may be relieved by pressing up the prolapsed parts; (iv.) all causes of incomplete obstruction.

V. INCONTINENCE OF URINE is found in fistula between the urinary tract and the genital tract, e.g. vesico-vaginal, vesico-uterine or uretero-vaginal. STRESS INCONTINENCE is a common disorder in which incontinence occurs on effort, such as coughing or sneezing; it is due to weakness of the support of the bladder neck and is usually though not always associated with cystocœle or urethrocœle. URGE INCONTINENCE is a condition in which incontinence of urine occurs when the bladder is full and the urge to micturate cannot be immediately satisfied. It also tends to occur with prolapse of the bladder or urethra.

(b) **Painful Defæcation** may be due to (i.) a retroverted and retroflexed uterus, especially when bound down by adhesions; (ii.) an incarcerated retroverted pregnant uterus; (iii.) acute pelvic infection; (iv.) endometriosis, especially affecting the recto-vaginal septum; (v.) a pelvic tumour pressing upon the rectum and (vi.) rectal disease, e.g., hæmorrhoids, proctitis, fissure, fistula-in-ano or ischio-rectal abscess.

(c) **Pain on Sitting and Coccydynia** may be associated with painful defæcation. (1) The commoner *external* causes of painful sitting are (i.) a vascular caruncle of the urethra;(ii.) vulvitis and all other acute conditions of the vulva;(iii.)hæmorrhoids; fissure of the anus, fistula -in-ano or ischio-rectal abscess. (2) The *internal* causes of painful sitting may depend upon (i.) an increased pressure within the pelvis—*e.g.*, pelvic inflammation, or any tumour within the pelvis; (ii.) injury or inflammation affecting the sacro-sciatic or sacro-coccygeal ligaments; (iii.) undue mobility of the sacro-iliac joints after parturition; or (iv.) arthritis, rheumatism or tuberculosis affecting the same joint; (v.) dislocation or un-united fracture, inflammation or "neuralgia" of the coccyx.

The *Diagnosis* of pelvic inflammation is discussed elsewhere. *Neuralgia* of the coccyx is recognised by the fact that the coccyx is tender to touch. There may be associated constipation or disorder of the rectum. Injury of the sacro-sciatic or sacro-coccygeal ligaments is known by: (i.) the history of pain often dates from childbirth or from the injury which produced it; (ii.) pain is produced by pressure on the ligaments which tightens them; and (iii.) there is no swelling or dislocation of the bone. *Dislocation of the coccyx* consists in most cases of backward displacement and is then rarely a cause of pain or tenderness. When the coccyx is dislocated forwards a much more painful condition results, so that the patient usually sits on one ischial tuberosity, *i.e.*, sits sideways. *Undue mobility* of the joints or *sacro-iliac strain* may occur during late pregnancy or may result from labour, including instrumental delivery, or there may be a history of accident or sudden strain. Slight cases are difficult to diagnose but the condition may be apparent on X-ray, especially if the pictures are taken with the patient standing in different positions. X-rays will also reveal disease of the joints or the surrounding bone. *Rheumatism* is known by the absence of other local signs and by the shifting character of the pain, and perhaps the fact that the patient has other manifestations of rheumatism.

Prognosis and Treatment.—Vulvitis and pelvic inflammations are discussed elsewhere. Neuralgia of the coccyx may be cured by hot baths, analgesics, infra-red radiation or short-wave diathermy. Dislocation of the coccyx if backward may cause no great inconvenience; if recent it may be reduced at the time but if long-standing it is best left alone. A forward dislocation, on the other hand, may be much more troublesome and may be curable only by removal of the coccyx. Sacro-iliac strain tends to spontaneous recovery. A few cases are helped by manipulation of the joints. In other cases a period of rest is advised, followed by the wearing of a sacro-iliac support when walking is resumed.

(d) **Dyspareunia** (painful coitus) arises from a variety of causes. (1) The most frequent is a functional spasm of the vaginal musculature (vaginismus), often occurring in neurotic patients. Fear of coitus, or a conscious or subconscious fear of pregnancy and childbirth, may be contributing factors. In these circumstances the attempt to pass a finger into the vagina or to insert a speculum may elicit violent spasm, affecting not only the vaginal muscles and even a state of general spasm with opisthotonos. (2) Painful coitus may result from a rigid perineum, or an abnormally thick or imperfectly dilated hymen. (3) Other local conditions should be carefully looked for, such as a vascular caruncle of the urethra, vulvitis or vaginitis (§ 440). Fissures or small ulcers of the vulva or anus may be causes of discomfort and may remain undiscovered for months or perhaps years. Prolapse may cause pain and difficulty through mechanical obstruction. (4) A prolapsed ovary, generally associated with retroversion of the uterus, or pelvic endometriosis may cause pain on deep penetration. (5) Chronic pelvic inflammation, including endocervicitis, salpingitis and pelvic peritonitis may also cause deep pain. (6) In elderly women kraurosis vulvæ may lead to shrinking of the vulva and vagina to a point where coitus is impossible without agonising pain. (7) Occasionally, though this is rare, there may be disproportion between the individuals concerned. (8) After childbirth, and especially if the perineum has been torn and has either been sewn up too tightly or has been slow to heal, pain and tenderness may persist for many months and in a few cases may require surgical treatment.

Prognosis and Treatment.—Dyspareunia leads to considerable discomfort and distress, not only to the individuals concerned but to home life in general, and may have far-reaching consequences. Many women are naturally disinclined to discuss this symptom but are usually glad to be given the opportunity of doing so; tactful encouragement will generally lead the most shy and reluctant patient to give a full history. The problem should always be discussed frankly and without embarrassment. Examination should begin with a very careful and minute examination of the vulva in a good light. Spasmodic contraction on touching the parts may give the diagnosis of vaginismus. Vaginal examination will reveal a rigid hymen or a tight introitus. Causes of deep dyspareunia may be elicited on bimanual examination, while examination with a speculum reveals cervicitis or vaginitis. *Treatment* will depend on the cause. Vaginismus may be treated by manual dilatation under anæsthesia, followed by insertion of vaginal dilators. The patient must be taught to insert gradually increasing sizes for herself. Psychotherapeutic treatment and adjustment of marital relationships may be required when there is underlying neurosis. The use of a lubricant or of a cocaine ointment, and the fitting of a reliable contraceptive may all prove helpful. Where there is mechanical obstruction at the introitus, perineotomy should be performed; during the healing process the patient must learn to pass graduated vaginal dilators.

§ 461. (I) **Backache.**—Pain in the back may accompany many diseases, *e.g.*, those of the chest; for these see § 103. We are here concerned with pain in the lumbar region which is so frequently complained of, especially in women. Chronic backache was often, in the past, attributed to some abnormal condition of the reproductive organs, and patients came under the care of the gynæcologist: a common condition, cervicitis, may have pain referred to the back. Since backache has been studied as an orthopœdic problem, it is found to be due most frequently to strain of the sacro-iliac, lumbo-sacral and other joints. The condition frequently follows pregnancy and labour. Badly balanced conditions of the spine contribute to the symptoms, which may be confused with gynæcological lesions. These cases improve with orthopædic treatment.

PHYSICAL EXAMINATION.—When the patient complains of backache, the physician should make a thorough examination of the region over which the pain is felt. For the adequate performance of this examination it is essential that the patient should be stripped. If the clothes are only removed so far as the waist, important physical phenomena may be overlooked. Note first whether there is any curvature of the spine, displacement, tumour or redness. By palpation endeavour to make out the presence of any tenderness or swelling. Examine next the precise position of the pain; whether it is unilateral or bilateral; whether it is accompanied by tenderness or not; whether it is aggravated by the movements of certain muscles or joints or is accompanied by muscle spasm; whether it radiates along the course of any nerve. Examine the lumbo-sacral and sacro-iliac joints and the costo-vertebral joints and ascertain whether pressure over these joints elicits pain. An examination should be made next of the viscera; visceroptosis, associated with weakness of the muscles of the abdominal wall and back may be present. Vaginal and rectal examinations help to reveal disorders in these regions. The urine may reveal kidney disease. In the absence of such causes, X-ray examination should be made. The history of the onset of pain, and of the concomitant symptoms at the time of the onset, may give important clues in the diagnosis.

CAUSES OF BACKACHE.—Sometimes the case belongs to the province of the gynæcologist, as in *Pressure pain* and *Bearing-down pain.*

(1) *Pressure pain* may occur as a result of *displacement of the uterus,* although this is infrequent unless some other complication is present. *Pelvic tumours* may also give rise to pain.

(2) *Bearing-down pain* may indicate uterine enlargement and displacement (§§ 456, 457), *e.g.*, retroflexion, retroversion and prolapse, endometriosis or tumours pressing on the rectum. It is also frequent with inflammatory lesions in or near the uterus. Constipation is a frequent cause. Pain of this type is present in advanced malignant conditions of the uterus or ovaries.

(3) Backache occurs in many *acute diseases,* such as acute pyelitis, and at the onset of many acute specific fevers, notably influenza, acute anterior poliomyelitis and small-pox, and its cause is then recognised by pyrexia and other general symptoms.

(4) *Functional Causes.*—In nervous individuals, whose general health is below par, FATIGUE is often evidenced by backache. It is frequently

met after childbirth, after febrile illnesses, after operations and in association with constipation. The treatment consists of rehabilitation, with graduated exercise, good diet, vitamins and adequate rest. A corset with a back brace may be necessary.

(5) **Lumbago** is the term applied to a variety of causes of backache, but in its most familiar form it represents a condition of fibrositis affecting the lumbar musculature. The clinical features are: (i.) a history of sudden onset, usually while stooping; (ii.) the pain is increased by movement of the lumbar muscles, and is relieved by local warmth; (iii.) tender nodules are palpable near the origin and insertion of the muscles affected. *Treatment* consists of the application of heat and massage to the affected muscles. Intramuscular injection into painful nodules of local analgesics, such as procaine 1 or 2 per cent. or lignocaine 1 or 2 per cent. often gives immediate relief (and see § 604).

(6) DEFORMITY OF THE SPINE, whether it be due to Pott's disease or to simple lateral curvature (scoliosis), is a cause of backache. The later stages of Pott's disease (tuberculosis of the vertebræ) show an angular curvature and come chiefly under the notice of the orthopædic surgeon. The early stages may be overlooked, as no symptom may be present except pain. X-ray reveals the cause. Prolonged rest, with general and special medical treatment as in other forms of tuberculosis, and a surgical support are required. The slighter forms of lateral curvature are a frequent cause of backache, especially on standing; in the early stages this cause of pain may be missed unless care is taken to examine the patient completely stripped.

(7) SECONDARY DEPOSITS, MYELOMATOSIS and a SPINAL TUMOUR give intractable backache. X-ray examination is essential.

(8) **Sacro-iliac strain** or **subluxation** may be caused by a jerk, as when stepping from a kerb, or when stooping to lift a heavy object. It often occurs without apparent cause in the later weeks of pregnancy or soon after delivery. Pain is felt intermittently for a time, then is continuous and spreads over the buttock and leg. *Symptoms.*—(i.) Pain and tenderness over the joint is made out on palpation, or when the ilium is pressed inwards by the physician; (ii) pain is elicited by flexing the thigh on the abdomen while the knee is fully flexed; (iii.) the patient may complain of pain along the course of one sciatic nerve, made worse by standing on one leg; (iv.) there is usually a history of strain, except in pregnancy. *Diagnosis.*— Especially in the early stages this may be very difficult. Many cases later reveal themselves as being due to an intervertebral disc lesion or to spondylitis deformans. *Treatment.*—When a recent strain is the cause, rest the back and strap the joint for support; otherwise heat, massage, exercises and manipulation are necessary.

(9) **Sacro-iliac tuberculosis,** usually in young women, is usually unilateral and causes chronic pain over the affected joint. X-ray examination greatly aids diagnosis.

(10) **Osteo-arthritis** gives constant pain, made worse by even slight exertion. The condition is diagnosed by X-ray.

(11) A DISPLACED INTERVERTEBRAL DISC (§ 1020) is recognised as a frequent cause of backache, usually of sudden onset.

(12) Backache may be due to disease connected with the KIDNEYS such as pyelonephritis, hydronephrosis, pyonephrosis, polycystic kidneys, tumour and stone. Examination of the urine may first lead to the suspicion that the kidneys are diseased but it must be remembered that some renal diseases lead to no abnormality in the urine itself and a full investigation including pyelography may be necessary to establish the diagnosis.

(13) ABDOMINAL TUMOURS such as cancer of the stomach or rectum, tumours of the spine, retro-peritoneal sarcoma and aneurysm may cause backache.

(14) GALL-STONES and a GASTRIC or DUODENAL ULCER may also give rise to pain in the back rather than to the more typical pain in the front of the abdomen; CHRONIC PANCREATITIS and CANCER OF THE PANCREAS also cause backache.

(15) **Spondylitis** or inflammation of the vertebral joints must be mentioned as a cause of backache. In its most usual form it is a manifestion of osteo-arthritis of the spine, but tends to affect individuals in a younger age group, *e.g.*, 30 to 40, than osteo-arthritis of other joints: rarely it follows typhoid fever or syphilis. The "*typhoid spine*" appears a variable time after typhoid fever. There is pain and tenderness, sometimes starting pains along the nerves, occasionally paresis and wasting. The diagnosis from *polyneuritis* and tuberculous *disease of the vertebræ* is made by a positive Widal reaction. X-rays show osteo-periostitis. Kyphosis may result if the condition is not treated by rest.

(16) *Spondylitis deformans*, although much less common in women than in men (§ 601), is becoming recognised with increased frequency as a cause of persistent low backache in women. *Symptoms* include pain distributed over the sacrum and buttocks associated with stiffness, especially in the morning. A high E.S.R., anæmia and the X-ray appearances aid diagnosis.

(17) RECTAL disease including hæmorrhoids presents in some cases as low backache.

Treatment.—Appropriate treatment can be carried out when the cause is known. When no obvious lesion is found, and especially in women who have borne children, a well-fitting belt or elastic corset is beneficial and should be worn continually; it should be kept in position by suspenders and shoulder-straps and should not end at the waist-line. Backache is one of the commonest symptoms complained of by women; a gynæcological cause should always be carefully excluded but when none is found orthopædic advice should be sought.

§ 462.   (J) **Sterility** is that condition of a woman who under ordinary circumstances of reproduction does not bring forth a living child. Natural sterility may be either *absolute* or *relative*. In absolute sterility conception cannot take place without treatment; in relative, sometimes called " one-child sterility," a fœtus is cast off before viable or one child only is born. Whether a woman will be sterile or not is practically decided within three years of marriage; only 7 per cent. bear children after that time.

Etiology.—(1) In 25 per cent. of cases a single absolute cause will be found. Any condition causing dyspareunia or vaginismus, any deformity, mal-development, inflammatory condition, new growth, displacement or obstruction to coitus may result in failure to conceive. (2) 75 per cent. of infertile marriages are due to a totality of multiple infertility factors, which, in themselves, may be of little importance. If a fertile couple be investigated, one or two of these infertility factors will be found, but in an infertile couple the number varies between two and eight factors; investigation and treatment is thus directed to removing as many as possible of these, so that the fertility level of the sterile couple may be raised well above the threshold of conception. In an ordinary case with four or five infertility factors, the removal of two or three may result in conception occurring. Thus it follows that any one of several therapeutic measures may be successful.

FEMALE INFERTILITY FACTORS.—*Local* genital factors are the more common, such as (1) minor degrees of genital hypoplasia indicated by a relatively long cervix and a small firm uterine body; (2) hostile viscosity of the endo-cervical mucus; (3) tubal blockage; (4) absence of or mechanical impediments to ovulation such as small cystic ovaries; (5) uterine displacements. Retro-displacements reduce fertility, anteflexions generally form part of an endocrine factor. (6) Important *general* causes are endocrine deficiencies of the thyroid, anterior pituitary and ovary; (7) chronic intoxications, particularly focal, such as appendicitis and chronic cholecystitis; (8) dietetic errors such as insufficient protein and absence of fresh foods; (9) general debility and anæmia. (10) Obesity due to other than endocrine causes.

Investigation.—(1) First inquire into the *medical history*:—(i.) General questions concerning age, duration of marriage, any history of past abdominal inflammation such as appendicitis, salpingitis or septic abortion. (ii.) Any discharge requires careful investigation. (iii.) Whether menstruation is normal, whether it started late, whether it is infrequent, excessive or small in amount. (iv.) Frequency of coitus.

(2) Next *examine* the wife, preferably at about the time of ovulation: (i.) Look for any evidence of endocrine disturbance suggesting thyroid deficiency or virilism, and note the general development. (ii.) Examine the vaginal mucosa; if it is thick, rugose and pink, ovulation is probably taking place; when it has more the appearance of a vaginal mucosa at the menopause, then fertility is reduced, as ovulation is less likely. (iii.) Examine the vaginal discharge; if it shows a semi-solid ground rice appearance it is indicative of hyper-acidity. Frank pus may be present, the result of inflammation, most probably due to the *Trichomonas*. (iv.) Note the position and accessibility of the external os, and, if at the expected time of ovulation, whether the cervical mucus is clear and extensile, and with a pH in the region of 7·5. Turbid mucus at this time indicates impaired fertility. The cervix may show an erosion. (v.) Bi-manual examination may reveal gross abnormalities of the uterus but more likely a disturbance of the utero-cervical index only. If the examination is being carried out in the week preceding the period, a diagnostic scrape may be taken from the uterine cavity which will indicate the presence or absence of ovulation in that particular month. An isolated negative finding indicates the absence of ovulation that month only and is not proof of permanent absence of ovulation. Any tubal swelling would suggest tubal occlusion.

(3) If nothing abnormal is detected the husband should be tested.

MALE INFERTILITY FACTORS are most often constitutional states producing relative deficiencies in the semen, such as general infective and toxic states, dietetic errors, obesity, endocrine disturbances and drug abuse. Local causes are less common. In an infertile marriage it will be found that 8 per cent. of the males are absolutely sterile, 60 per cent. are distinctly sub-fertile, and only 25 per cent. are normally fertile; the remainder are borderline. Apart from constitutional states, the faults in the male are due either to faulty delivery of the semen, the result of premature ejaculation, to failure of erection or normal erection with failure of ejaculation. The presence of a varicocœle or the constant wearing of a suspensory bandage may, by raising the testicular temperature, impair spermatogenesis.

Investigation.—Two tests are necessary. (1) After four days' abstention a fresh specimen of semen is examined and should show in the region of one hundred million motile sperms per ml., with less than 20 per cent. of abnormal heads. Less than sixty million or more than 20 per cent. abnormal heads indicates male infertility, but cases of pregnancy have occurred with much lower counts. (2) The post-coital test of Huhner. If live and active spermatozoa are found penetrating the cervical mucus, it is reasonable to exclude the husband.

Treatment.—(1). If both parties, as a result of these investigations, appear to be normal and are under thirty, and if a reasonable time for conception to occur has not elapsed, give them some general advice and ask them to report in six months. (i.) Advise as to the best days for coitus relative to ovulation time, and as to the most favourable positions to be adopted in abnormal positions of the cervix. (ii.) Calculate the most likely dates for ovulation to take place. (iii.) Advise rest at the expected time of the next period, and if this does not arrive, to continue resting throughout the normal duration of the expected period. (iv.) Should the period not arrive, advise against further coitus.

(2) Assuming the husband to be normal, a post-coital test at the time of ovulation should be performed. It is as well to remember that high fertility in one partner may well outweigh the low fertility in the other. Thus, the presence of a favourable cervical plug of mucus may allow the penetration of feeble spermatozoa, and vice versa. Hence the great importance of the post-coital test. About the time of ovulation the cervical plug of mucus should be clear, colourless and like glycerine in consistency; it does not dry quickly, is very extensile and contains few leucocytes and cervical cells. It is probable that the normal cervical plug as seen in the fertile woman is a response to œstrin stimulation, and does not necessarily mean that ovulation has occurred. If the post-coital test shows that the normal plug is absent, treatment consists in giving 0·1 mg. of stilbœstrol during the first ten days of the menstrual cycle. If this has no effect, then double the dose in the next cycle. Larger doses should not be given, as ovulation may be suppressed. *If the penetration of the cervical plug by spermatozoa is normal, then the cause of the infertility must be sought elsewhere.*

(3) The wife may have to be treated for:—(i.) Failure of ovulation. This is likely if the basal temperature chart does not show the two- or three-fifths of a degree rise at the time of ovulation. This test is of great use if the following conditions are fulfilled:—the thermometer must be held in the mouth for 5 minutes and the temperature is to be taken first thing in the morning, before any movement has taken place (§ 433). A diagnostic curettage, with a special curette, taken during the week before the expected period, or better still, on the first day of the period, does not show the typical secretory glands, with crenated margins and fern-like tufts projecting down into their lumens. In 5 per cent. of such cases evidence of a tuberculous infection will be found in the endometrium. In some cases of failure of ovulation, graduated stimulating doses of X-rays to the ovaries have proved successful. Pelvic diathermy has also been used. In the absence of menstruation, cycle regulation may be attempted as follows:—(a) give stilbœstrol 2 mg. daily for 20 days, during the last 6 days of which give in addition ethisterone 10 mg. daily. Oestrin withdrawal bleeding will follow, this treatment some days later. (b) On the fifth day of this bleeding repeat the course of treatment, but increase the ethisterone to 20 mg. on the last 6 days. (c) On the fifth day of this œstrin withdrawal bleeding start a further course, but reduce the stilbœstrol to 1 mg. daily and increase the ethisterone to 30 mg. (d) Give a final course, reducing the stilbœstrol to 0·5 mg. and increasing the ethisterone to 40 mg. (ii.) Failure of the ovum to imbed. This is most likely if the endometrium is inadequately prepared. In such cases the endometrium should be prepared for nidation as follows:—dienœstrol 3 mg. by mouth, together with ethisterone 5 mg. dissolved under the tongue should be taken daily, starting 3 days before the calculated date of ovulation and continuing either until the onset of the next period, or until amenorrhœa due to pregnancy has been present for four months, by which time the placenta will be formed. This form of treatment is very useful in cases of repeated miscarriage, and is prescribed not so much as a replacement therapy, but to

make up for a deficiency. (iii.) Obstruction to the entry of the ovum to the tubes and uterus. (a) Tubal occlusion. Try repeated insufflations. Lipiodol injections will indicate the site of occlusion. (This should not be carried out during the week following the period.) (b) Uterine hypoplasia. Little can be done to develop an undersized uterus once the urge to development has ceased: pregnancy has occasionally followed curettage in some of these cases. (c) Endocrine disturbances, as indicated by obesity and amenorrhœa. Thyroid deficiency, indicated by a low basal metabolic rate must be dealt with. Thyroid given to the limit of tolerance if successful in reducing the weight and producing normal menstruation, is often followed by conception. (iv.) Any organic cause must be removed. In the vagina, vaginitis due to *Trichomonas* infestation is a frequent cause. Cervical infection with erosion and cervicitis, does not favour conception; in these cases adequate treatment with sulphonamides and antibiotics may be successful, but frequently dilatation and linear cauterisation may be necessary.

Artificial Insemination is indicated where coitus is impossible due to male deformity or where the cervical discharge is proved to be persistently lethal to the sperms. Careful attention to the health and hygiene of adolescents, with a view to preventing genital hypoplasia, the correct teaching of sex hygiene to avoid pelvic congestion, the eradication of venereal disease will help to reduce considerably the number of infertile marriages.

CHAPTER XV

PYREXIA AND THE INFECTIVE DISEASES

WHEN a patient is suffering from some general or constitutional derangement, he complains of a vague " feeling of illness " (*i.e.*, malaise), or of " weakness " (debility, asthenia). He feels " generally " ill, and perhaps looks ill, but may be unable to mention any localising symptom, such as pain in the side or palpitation. Now, the first thing to do in such circumstances is to ascertain whether he is feverish or not, because all such conditions may be divided into two large clinical groups: A. **Debility with pyrexia,** which includes the Acute Specific Fevers and disorders in which there exists some localised inflammation; and B. **Debility without pyrexia,** which includes the different forms of Anæmia and various toxic and nutritional disorders. The latter will be dealt with in Chapter XVI. In this chapter we are concerned solely with the various conditions attended by elevation of the body temperature.

§ 465. **Definitions.**—The term **Acute Specific Fever** (or Specific Febrile Disease) has been applied to those fevers which are due to a specific or special agent, introduced into the body from without, and which run a definite course. If the infection was contracted from a previous case, but without contact with the patient, it was said to be an *Infectious* disease (*e.g.*, scarlatina); if the disease was produced only by physical contact with a person suffering from the malady, it was called *Contagious* (*e.g.*, syphilis); but these terms have always been used somewhat loosely and indifferently, and it would be better not to attempt any such distinction but to speak of them collectively as *Infective*. There is direct or inferential proof in all the acute specific fevers that they are of bacterial or parasitic origin. At first the organisms themselves were supposed to be the active agents of these diseases, but now in most cases the *causa vera* of the pyrexia and other symptoms is known to be a toxin or toxins which are produced by the infecting agent. This branch of knowledge has made enormous advances during the last three-quarters of a century (*cf.* §§ 523 *et seq.*).

Bacteriology is dealt with in Chapter XXII. The chief clinical characteristics which cause us to suspect a disease of being **bacterial in origin** are:

1. The occurrence of the disease in question in an *epidemic* form—*i.e.*, in the form of an outbreak, or as a series of cases which suggest that the patients contracted the disease either from one another or from a common source, the infection being conveyed to them through the air, the water or other ingesta, or by the bite of an insect.

2. Two features are common to all infective diseases: (i.) *Pyrexia* is present at some time during the course; [1] and (ii.) in many cases the disease runs a more or less *definite course*—definite onset, gradual increase (fastigium) to an acme, gradual or sudden defervescence, followed by complete restoration to health, or death.

3. The constant presence in the blood, tissues or excretions of the patient of a *bacterium* or *protozoon*, which is not there normally.

The *pathological proof* that a particular organism is causally related to the disease consists in applying certain experimental tests (see § 474).

---

[1] Some diseases have become so attenuated (*e.g.*, rubella and chicken-pox) that pyrexia may at times be absent, although most of the other clinical features are present.

4. The fact that the attack is more or less protective against subsequent infection.

Epidemic, Endemic, and Sporadic are terms by which it is usual to express the relative prevalence of infectious diseases. A disease is said to be *Epidemic* when a large number of cases arise by infection from a common source or from one another at one time, followed by an interval in which relatively few arise. Thus epidemics of measles, scarlet fever and diphtheria arise from time to time. A disease is said to be *Sporadic* when it occurs only in isolated cases. Thus we speak of a sporadic case of mumps when no other cases of it have been known to occur about the same time and in the same district. An *Endemic* disease is one which is constantly present in a certain district. Thus measles is endemic in London, malaria in Central Africa and cholera in India.

PART A. SYMPTOMATOLOGY

§ 466. Pyrexia and Symptoms which may attend it.—Pyrexia may in some instances be unattended by any symptoms, but in nearly all cases the patient whose temperature is elevated complains of feeling " chilly," or he may have shivering or rigors; or perhaps he feels " burning hot." Headache, restlessness and vague pains in the limbs and back are also common symptoms, in addition to the malaise or weakness. His skin is hot and dry to the touch, his pulse and respiration are rapid, his appetite is poor, tongue furred and bowels constipated, his urine scanty and highly coloured: in young children vomiting and convulsions may herald a pyrexial illness. In severe cases of fever there is great prostration, considerable mental dullness, and there may be delirium, or the " typhoid state." By these symptoms we suspect the presence of pyrexia, and the suspicion is confirmed and the degree of fever ascertained, by the clinical thermometer (see below). Infective diseases pass through various STAGES which have many features in common: in severe cases, and often in association with high temperatures, RIGORS, DELIRIUM and PROFOUND TOXÆMIA (the " TYPHOID STATE ") may occur.

§ 467. Incubation and other Stages of Acute Specific Fevers.—Particularly in epidemics, the infective or specific fevers conform to a common pattern and run a *definite course* (*e.g.*, measles). However, it must be remembered that the same organism may at times give rise to dissimilar diseases: *e.g.*, the same strain of hæmolytic streptococci may produce acute tonsillitis, scarlet fever or puerperal fever in three different individuals.

It is a curious fact that a person does not develop the disease directly after he has been exposed to infection. The interval is called the stage of *incubation*. The patient is usually quite well during this stage, but there may be transient fever (" illness of infection ") for a few hours after exposure. The incubation period varies in different diseases (Table XXVI). During at least part of this time a healthy person who has been exposed to infection needs to be isolated (" placed in quarantine "), to see if he will develop the disease. A glance at the first column in the table will show that a period of THREE WEEKS will cover the incubation of all the eruptive fevers. The actual *invasion* or development of the symptoms of the disease is usually more or less abrupt, except in typhoid fever,

TABLE XXVI.—SHOWING INCUBATION, DATE OF THE RASH, AND DURA-
TION OF INFECTION OF THE PRINCIPAL INFECTIVE DISORDERS

DISEASE.	INCUBATION PERIOD.	DAY OF DISEASE ON WHICH RASH APPEARS.	INFECTIOUS PERIOD, or period during which the *patient* need be isolated.
Varicella.	10 to 21 days, average 14.	The rash is usually the 1st symptom noticed.	Till all scabs have separated, or 14 days, whichever is the shorter.
Scarlet Fever.	2 to 4 days, average 2¼.	1st or 2nd.	From commencement of illness for 14 days in mild cases or those given specific treatment, provided clinical evidence of infection has gone. Rhinorrhœa, and possibly otorrhœa, may retain infection for 6 months or more.
Small-pox.	12 days.	3rd.	From commencement till not a trace left of scabs and the last seed has been removed. Most virulent during vesiculation, pustulation, and scabbing. 3 to 8 weeks.
Measles.	7 to 14 days, average 10.	4th.	*Great* in early period *before* rash out. Till rash has faded, usually 1 week after rash appears.
Rubella.	14 to 19 days.	1st to 4th.	5 to 6 days from commencement.
Typhus.	12 to 14 days.	4th or 5th.	Probably 3 to 4 weeks.
Typhoid and Paratyphoid.	8 to 21 days, usually 10 to 14.	Average 2nd week.	When three consecutive weekly stool and urine specimens fail to grow the bacilli. In typhoid the Vi agglutination should also be negative. "Carriers" may retain their infection for many years.
Dengue.	2 to 6 days.	Initial rash 1st day. Terminal rash 4th.	
Diphtheria.	1 to 6 days, usually 2 to 4.	None.	Until 3 consecutive swabs from nose and throat, and any ear discharge, fail to grow the organism.

The period of incubation of the other infective disorders so far as we know is given approximately below. This is important, as the duration of quarantine depends on the period of incubation. In cases with a relatively long incubation period, such as mumps, chicken-pox, measles and rubella, it is not necessary to isolate contacts for the first week after exposure.

Malaria, 12 hours and upwards.
Erysipelas, 1 to 7 days.
Cerebro-spinal fever, 1 to 3 days.
Influenza, 1 to 3 days.
Pneumonia, 1 to 3 days.
Anthrax, 2 or 3 days.
Gonorrhœa, 2 or 3 days.
Plague, 3 to 7 days.
Glanders, 3 to 18 days.
Tetanus, usually 3 to 21 days.
Mumps, 3 to 28 days (average 17).

Relapsing fever, 4 to 10 days.
Glandular fever, 5 to 12 days.
Whooping-cough, 7 to 14 days.
Malta fever, about 9 days.
Cholera, 1 to 5 days.
Yellow fever, 3 to 6 days.
Syphilis, 15 to 25 days.
Hydrophobia, 35 to 70 days.
Tuberculosis, probably some weeks.
Infective Hepatitis, 17 to 35 days.
Undulant Fever (Brucellosis), 2 to 4 weeks.

whooping-cough and sometimes measles. *Prodromal symptoms* at the
onset of the disease proper may indicate that a disease is commencing,
but not permit an exact diagnosis. An *eruption* appears upon the skin
within the next four days (except in typhoid fever) in those diseases which
develop a rash, and which are called on that account the EXANTHEMATA.
(Enanthemata are the lesions seen on the mucous membranes.) The
fever and other symptoms go on increasing until the *acme* is reached.
Remissions indicate temporary diminution of symptoms, and *recrudescences*
aggravation of the disease. Finally, the last stage—the stage of *defervescence* supervenes, and gradually the patient convalesces unless a *relapse*
occurs.

§ 468. Rigors often indicate the sudden onset of pyrexia. A rigor is an
attack of shivering attended by elevation of temperature and great
acceleration of pulse rate, rapidly followed (usually) by sweating and a fall
in the temperature. Such an attack may vary widely in severity from a
simple feeling of " chilliness down the back," to a shaking of the whole
body, so that the patient shakes the bed beneath him. Severe rigors
occur typically and *regularly* in the course of malaria, also at frequent but
irregular intervals throughout the course of septicæmia and pyæmia. In
childhood, rigors are often replaced by convulsions.

1. First, ascertain that the shivering is not of purely nervous origin,
because a trembling much resembling a rigor may occur solely as the result
of fright or from slighter causes in nervous people.

2. Procure, if possible, a series of temperature records, because rigors
occur in association with several conditions which can only be differentiated in this way.

Causes.—The causes of rigors are very numerous, but they are best
approached in a general way as follows:

(*a*) Coming on in a person *previously healthy*, one should always suspect
the advent of some acute illness. In children the eruptive fevers are
sometimes ushered in with either convulsions or rigors. In adults,
pyelonephritis, septicæmia, pneumonia, pyæmia, peritonitis, the eruptive
fevers, malaria or influenza may be suspected.

(*b*) *Septic Infection.*—When rigors *supervene in the course of an illness*
of any kind, abscess or pent-up pus in some position should always be
the first thing thought of. *Before the days of the thermometer the doctor
used to rely upon shivering and sweating as an infallible indication of the
formation of pus.* For instance, in a case of pleurisy with an effusion,
which has hitherto been serous, the occurrence of shivering indicates that
the contents of the chest have become purulent (empyema). Similarly, a
rigor occurring with otitis media suggests extension to the mastoid cells,
or may point to lateral sinus thrombosis. Rigors occurring in a case of
cardio-valvular disease indicate the occurrence of infected emboli, or the
supervention of bacterial endocarditis. Shiverings and sweatings may
occur during the course of tuberculosis and many other conditions mentioned under the Causes of Intermitting Pyrexia (§ 511). If no obvious

cause for an attack of shivering appears, we may suspect some internal suppuration, such as appendicitis, or ulceration in some part of the urinary, biliary or alimentary canals. If the rigor is due to a collection of pus, a definite leucocytosis will be found.

(c) The *passing of a catheter* is often followed by a severe rigor, and sometimes the temperature goes suddenly up to 105° or 106° F, and as suddenly falls again. Sudden obstruction in the biliary or renal passages is often attended by rigors, followed by a feeling of heat and sweating, and the temperature may go up to 105° F; these examples are probably due to bacterial invasion through minute abrasions. A rigor, too, may be set up by the intravenous injection of some chemical substance (*e.g.*, neoarsphenamine) or a therapeutic serum, such as diphtheria antitoxin, or after blood transfusion. Therapeutic use has been made of this by injecting T.A.B. vaccine, sulphur and foreign proteins to produce pyrexia.

(d) *Neurasthenic* and *hysterical* patients often have shivering attacks, without pyrexia. An attack of shivering may also constitute a symptom of *vaso-motor disorder*. Thus it is a symptom of the reaction which follows, and often forms part of the " flush-storms " chiefly met with at the climacteric, without elevation of temperature.

(e) *Cholecystitis* may cause short attacks of shivering without pyrexia. It cannot be too strongly emphasised that the presence of pus, even in large quantities (e.g., in a subphrenic abscess), may fail to evoke rigors or even a rise of temperature if large doses of antibiotics are being given.

The *Prognosis* and *Treatment* belong to the several causal conditions, but in any case the patient should be kept warm in bed with a hot-water bottle to his feet: aspirin, a barbiturate or morphia will soothe the nervous system.

§ 469. **Delirium,** or incoherence of thought, is another symptom which frequently accompanies pyrexia. The older authors used to describe three varieties of delirium: (1) Delirium ferox, in which the patient is very violent and maniacal; (2) typhoid delirium, in which the patient lies on his back muttering, with subsultus tendinum; (3) delirium tremens, in which there is great sleeplessness, hallucinations and tremors, not necessarily due to alcohol. The nature of the delirium is not always constant in any given disease. For clinical purposes, the *causes of delirium* may be divided into two groups—FEBRILE and NON-FEBRILE. It is important, therefore, to take the temperature at once in every case of delirium. Alcoholic subjects and children, especially if neurotic, are predisposed to delirium when attacked with only slight fever.

a. Febrile Delirium may arise under four circumstances:

1. ACUTE LOCAL INFLAMMATION in some part of the body, such as pneumonia. It is advisable, therefore, to examine all the organs.

2. DISEASES OF THE BRAIN (Encephalitis), or OF THE MENINGES, such as tuberculous meningitis. The latter is accompanied by headache, vomiting, retraction of the head, intolerance of light, and paralysis of cranial nerves.

3. All the ACUTE SPECIFIC FEVERS are liable to be accompanied by delirium. The tendency, however, varies considerably, though it is usually directly related to the height of the temperature and the nervous stability of the individual. It is important to bear this in mind, because, as a prognostic indication, delirium occurring in a disease like measles or acute rheumatism, in which it is rare, has a much more serious meaning than when it occurs in pneumonia, where it is more usual (see Table XXVII).

4. Certain cases of DELIRIUM TREMENS of a SEVERE KIND are accompanied by an elevation of temperature. Indeed, the prognosis in this affection may largely depend upon the temperature. We must be careful to exclude local inflammations in such cases, for they are apt to come on very insidiously. In the worst cases of ACUTE DELIRIOUS MANIA also the temperature may be considerably elevated (see b 6, below).

TABLE XXVII.—SHOWING THE RELATIVE FREQUENCY OF DELIRIUM IN THE VARIOUS INFECTIVE FEVERS

Frequent in—	Occasional in—	Rare in—
Confluent Small-pox	Remittent Fever	Influenza
Typhus	Yellow Fever	Mumps
Lobar Pneumonia	Small-pox (modified)	Dysentery
Typhoid Fever (after 1st week)	Measles	Cholera
Meningitis	Relapsing Fever	Acute Rheumatism
Encephalitis	Scarlet Fever	Diphtheria
Erysipelas	Malaria	Rubella
Plague		Varicella
Malignant Endocarditis		
Septicæmia		

b. Non-febrile Delirium may arise under six conditions:

1. DELIRIUM TREMENS (Delirium à Potu) is, as just mentioned, usually unattended by a rise of temperature, and is undoubtedly the commonest cause of non-febrile delirium. It is recognised by the history, the muscular tremors, sleeplessness and the characteristic hallucinations.

2. CHRONIC RENAL DISEASE, and especially chronic interstitial nephritis, gives rise in its advanced stages to a muttering delirium or incoherence, which thus becomes a symptom of the gravest import, and generally heralds coma and death. The delirium is due to uræmia, and occurs in other renal diseases.

3. POST-FEBRILE DELIRIUM (Post-Febrile Mania).—During the convalescence of pneumonia and other exhausting diseases, especially such as run a protracted course, and have been attended with a high degree of pyrexia, mental symptoms may develop. These symptoms, which usually make their appearance without any warning, give great uneasiness to the friends. Nevertheless, by means of good food and nursing care, and fresh air, such mental symptoms will entirely disappear. Before

venturing on a prognosis, however, inquiry should always be made for any family history of mental disease, for a hereditary tendency greatly lessens the chance of recovery. The condition is recognised by the history of the previous condition. Sometimes the mental derangement consists simply of loss of memory, especially for the names of persons and things, but more often the mind " wanders " and there are delusions.

4. REFLEX DELIRIUM.—Trousseau mentioned cases of children with intestinal worms who had delirium, and described several cases which were caused by tickling the soles of the feet. The transient delirium connected with the severe pain of childbirth is possibly of the same nature.

5. DELIRIANT DRUGS should always be suspected when delirium develops suddenly in a person in health, especially children in the country, in the absence of any of the foregoing causes. The most important are belladonna, hyoscyamus, hyoscine, cannabis indica, stramonium and others of the solanaceæ, d-amphetamine, antipyrin, camphor in rare cases, œnanthe crocata, cocculus indicus (with which beer used to be adulterated), poisonous fungi and sometimes in bromism and with salicylic acid and its salts when given in large doses. Delirium may ensue when a patient is recovering from the effects of poisonous gases. Morphia in some people invariably produces delirium.

6. ACUTE MANIA sometimes comes on very suddenly, and only differs from " delirium ferox " or maniacal delirium in not being referable to some bodily disease or toxæmia. Delirium occurs in the advanced stage. of many mental diseases. We identify these conditions by (1) the temperature is not as a rule elevated; (2) it affects a person previously in good health; and (3) the exclusion of any organic lesion by a careful examination of the nervous and other systems. As regards the temperature there is an exception in the rare and serious condition known as " acute delirious mania," in which marked pyrexia is present (and see § 1178).

Prognosis.—Febrile delirium is not necessarily a grave symptom when it is associated with a *disease in which its occurrence is usual*—*e.g.*, meningitis—and especially when the cause is only temporary; but its presence adds considerably to the gravity of a case if the occurrence of delirium is unusual (see Table XXVII), for it indicates a very severe attack, or the occurrence of complications, or both. *Non-febrile* delirium is a grave symptom in chronic renal disease. The prognosis is serious as regards mental recovery in all patients who have a hereditary tendency to mental disorder. In acute mania the prognosis is grave.

Treatment.—It is necessary to provide a nurse or attendant, and restraint may be called for. *Remedial Treatment.*—An ice-bag to the head for an intracranial inflammation; good nourishing food for mania and post-febrile delirium. *Symptomatic treatment* consists of the administration of sedatives, such as Somnifaine, sod. pentobarbitone (Nembutal), chloral, Calcibronat, the bromides and paraldehyde (injected) (Table LI). Opium and morphia require caution, especially if there is liver disease; in delirium tremens they are most helpful in some cases by procuring sleep, but in others they only aggravate the maniacal condition. Periodical sponging with cold or ice-cold water often has a steadying effect. In post-febrile delirium and other conditions where the brain is suffering from malnutrition, opium in small doses is a valuable remedy, and may be given without fear if the liver and kidneys are healthy.

§ 470. **Profound Toxæmia of Infective Origin** (Synonym: THE TYPHOID STATE) may be described as a condition of semi-consciousness or unconsciousness (coma) attended by elevation of temperature and muttering delirium, due to toxæmia. The name of this condition was derived from its frequent association with typhus, but it is met in many other fevers. With reference to the question of pyrexia, it should be stated that the comatose condition, due to renal disease (uræmia), advanced liver disease (cholæmia) and various poisons (particularly opium), has sometimes been described as the typhoid state, but these are apyrexial conditions, and it is preferable to include only those with pyrexia. In short, the typhoid state corresponds clinically to a state of coma *plus* pyrexia and muttering delirium.

Symptoms.—The typhoid state is always secondary to some febrile condition, in the course of which it arises: the height of the temperature and its persistence depend chiefly upon the nature of the primary disease. The first *mental symptom* usually noticed is sleeplessness with delirium, generally of the muttering variety, but by and by stupor supervenes, which gradually deepens. The mental faculties are obscured, but the unconsciousness is not always so complete as one would imagine. The profound disturbance of the nervous system is evidenced by prostration, restlessness, subsultus tendinum (muscular twitchings), floccitatio or carphology (picking at the bedclothes), unconscious evacuation of bladder and bowels, and in extreme cases, convulsions. The *physical condition* is indicated by the pale and often cyanosed colour: the tongue is dry, brown, furred and tremulous: and sordes collects upon the lips and teeth. The pulse is rapid, feeble and irregular, and the heart-sounds distant. The respiration is usually rapid, but shallow. The pupils are dilated, but the patient does not see. Nevertheless, he looks about at imaginary objects— " coma vigil." Dysphagia, diarrhœa and stertorous breathing are very serious indications of profound stupor.

Diagnosis.—(1) The " *typhoid state,*" as above mentioned, may be distinguished from *coma* by the presence of pyrexia, and the absence of evidences of renal or liver disease, apoplexy, or other cause of the coma. (2) Certain acute *inflammations of the brain and meninges* are attended by pyrexia, and offer considerable difficulty—particularly with tuberculous meningitis (§ 886). The presence of papillœdema, head retraction, paralysis of the cranial nerves on the one hand, and the signs of the primary disease which has produced the typhoid condition on the other, are evidences upon which we can rely in many instances.

Causes.—Patients with an alcoholic history or with chronic nephritis are predisposed to the development of the typhoid state.

1. The ACUTE INFECTIOUS FEVERS are the commonest causes, and particularly typhoid and typhus fevers. The Typhoid State occurs as an ordinary symptom of a grave attack in the course of these two diseases and in some others (see Table XXVIII). In another group of diseases it occurs only occasionally, and in others it is rare. If it arises in either of these latter groups, it indicates either (1) a very severe variety of the disease, or (2) some serious complications; and, in any case, that the patient is likely to die.

2. Certain other INFLAMMATORY or INFECTIVE DISORDERS with local manifestations may be attended by the typhoid state, such as acute lobar pneumonia, acute pulmonary tuberculosis, infective endocarditis, acute meningitis and encephalitis lethargica.

3. Certain acute IDIOPATHIC DISEASES may, in rare instances, be attended by the typhoid state, such as acute gout and very intense forms of delirium tremens. It is extremely rare in acute rheumatism, unless accompanied by peri- or endo-carditis.

TABLE XXVIII.—RELATIVE FREQUENCY OF THE TYPHOID STATE IN DIFFERENT DISEASES. ALCOHOLIC SUBJECTS AND PATIENTS WITH CHRONIC NEPHRITIS ARE PREDISPOSED TO THE TYPHOID STATE

Frequently met with, especially towards the end, in—	*Occasionally met with in—*	*Rare in—*
Typhoid (Enteric) Fever	Scarlet Fever	Cholera
Typhus	Measles with broncho-	Variola (modified)
Confluent Small-pox (unmodified)	pneumonia	Dysentery
Erysipelas (severe)	Cerebro-Spinal Fever	Malaria
Septicæmia (including Bacterial Endocarditis and Osteomyelitis)	Anthrax (Internal)	Relapsing Fever
Meningitis—especially tuberculous	Remittent Fever	Acute Rheumatism
Encephalitis	Undulant Fever	
Lobar Pneumonia	(Brucellosis)	
Acute Miliary Tuberculosis		
Acute Glanders		
Acute Anthrax		
Remittent Fever		
Cerebral and Hæmorrhagic Malaria		
Yellow Fever		
Plague		

Diagnosis of the Cause.—The clinical investigation should be conducted on the same lines as in cases of pyrexia. Is it due to *local* or *generalised* inflammation ? First, every organ in the body should be thoroughly examined so as to exclude local disorders. Secondly, we proceed to the diagnosis of the general fevers from one another, and, if possible, obtain a series of temperature records. In cases where the cause of the typhoid condition is obscure, septicæmia, especially with endocardial involvement, should always be suspected, and its origin carefully sought.

Prognosis.—The typhoid state, like delirium, has a less serious import in diseases such as typhoid fever, in which it is frequently met with. But it is always a grave condition, and indicates profound cerebral and general toxæmia. Occurring in the course of scarlet fever, erysipelas or measles, it often indicates pulmonary or cardiac complications and is proportionately serious. As regards symptoms, the profundity of the stupor is a measure of the intensity of the toxæmia, and dysphagia, uncontrolled diarrhœa, stertor or convulsions are generally lethal signs.

The Treatment of a condition such as this arising in the course of so many diseases must necessarily vary, and our first duty is *to ascertain what disease is in operation*. The toxæmia is partly bacterial and partly the result of disordered metabolism and elimination. The indications are (1) to destroy the causal organism, *e.g.*, by the appropriate antibiotic; (2) to support the patient's strength by nutriment and stimulants; and (3) to counteract and eliminate the toxins. The use of alcohol in the treatment of fevers as in other branches of medicine has of late years considerably declined. As regards symptomatic treatment, if the delirium be very violent, sedatives such as inject. paraldehyde 4–10 ml. intramusc. or large doses of chloral and bromide, even up to 40 grains of each, are indicated. Opium should be avoided, as it prevents the elimination of the poison. For the treatment of Hyperpyrexia, see § 528.

PART B. PHYSICAL EXAMINATION

The clinical investigation of pyrexial disorders consists of (1) CLINICAL THERMOMETRY; (2) AN EXAMINATION OF THE ORGANS; and (3) BACTERIOLOGICAL INVESTIGATION.

§ 471. Clinical Thermometry and Types of Pyrexia.—The temperature is ascertained by means of the clinical thermometer: readings are usually taken in the mouth or the axilla. Mouth temperatures must be taken before meals, for food, drinks or mouth breathing cause false readings: a half-minute thermometer must be kept in the mouth for at least one minute, and in the axilla for ten minutes, to give accurate records. The temperature may also be taken in the rectum, where it is $\frac{1}{2}°$ to 1° higher than in the mouth. In children the thermometer may be held in the groin, the thigh being flexed to the abdomen for the purpose. The normal temperature of the body varies between about 97·8° and 99° F; average 98·4° F. It is lowest about 4 A.M. and highest about 8 P.M. It tends to be *lower* in old age and *higher* in hot weather and in infancy, especially after an attack of crying. The temperature is often subnormal after a loss of blood, during convalescence, in cardiac failure and in all states of collapse. The latter is sometimes the direct result of toxæmia.

A temperature of 100° is regarded as slight fever.
„   „   „ 102° „   „   „ moderate fever.
„   „   „ 104° „   „   „ high fever.
„   „   „ 105° and upwards is regarded as hyperpyrexia.

THE TEMPERATURE CHART.—*Very little information can be derived from a single observation of a patient's temperature, and in all cases of pyrexia one must know the course which it runs from day to day and hour to hour.* In most cases of fever it is hardly possible to come to any conclusion without seeing a "chart" of the case—*i.e.*, a series of records. In all cases of pyrexia the temperature should be **taken and recorded morning and evening;** and in all acute cases it should be taken 4-hourly. The pulse, respiration and blood pressure should also be observed, especially in abdominal inflammation, extensive broncho-pneumonia, and with severe attacks of diphtheria, where the temperature alone does not give

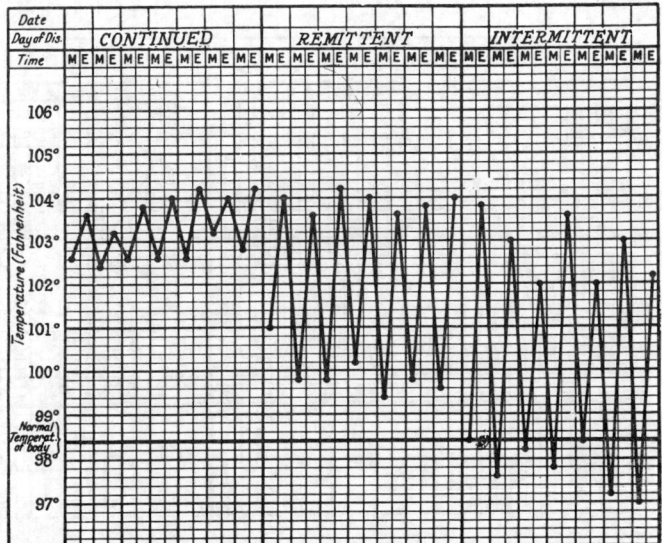

FIG. 138.—TYPES OF PYREXIA.—Continued pyrexia showing only the normal variations in th morning and evening. Remittent pyrexia showing a drop of several degrees each day. Inter nittent pyrexia where the temperature comes down to normal at some time every day.

us a true idea of the amount of mischief which is going on. In brcncho-pneumonia the rapidity of respiration is often the most reliable indication. The onset of pyrexia may be gradual, as in typhoid fever or diphtheria, but more often it is sudden and may be accompanied by a rigor, as is sometimes seen in pneumonia cr small-pox. Remember that the *onset is apt to be very sudden* in scarlet fever, erysipelas and small-pox; it is *gradual* (taking perhaps two or three days) in measles, typhoid fever and pertussis. During the next few days the temperature generally increases until the *acme* is reached. The termination may be gradual, when it is said to terminate by *lysis* as in typhoid; or pyrexia may terminate suddenly by *crisis*, as in some cases of lobar pneumonia (Fig. 56, § 121) and relapsing fever.

Types of Pyrexia.—In the absence of any eruption, the COURSE OF THE

TEMPERATURE is our best, and may be our only, guide. It is usual to describe three types of pyrexia, according to the course which the temperature pursues from day to day (Fig. 138); (i.) *Continued Fever*, where the temperature remains elevated for a considerable period, and where the *diurnal variation often does not exceed the normal diurnal variation*— viz., one, or at most one and a half degrees; (ii.) *Remittent Fever*, when the diurnal variation is greater than the normal diurnal variation, but where the temperature never comes down quite to normal; (iii.) *Intermittent Fever*, where the temperature at some time of the day is normal or subnormal, and at another time of the day, usually in the evening, it is raised one, two or more degrees. But for clinical purposes the two latter may

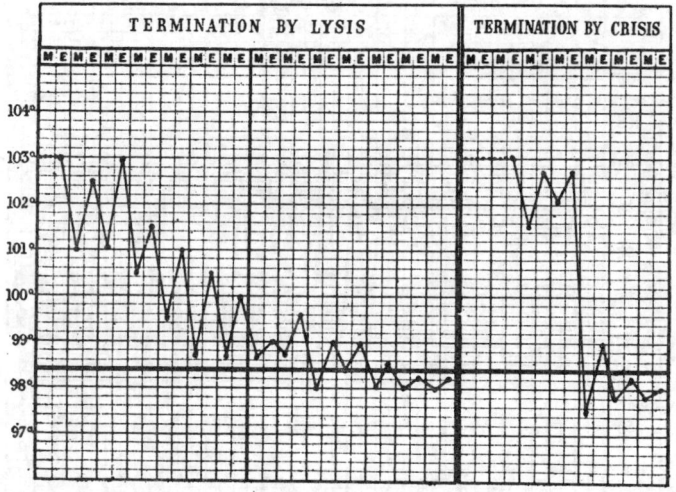

FIG. 139.—TERMINATION OF PYREXIA BY LYSIS AND CRISIS.

be grouped together, and thus we have TWO GROUPS of fevers—one in which the pyrexia is practically CONTINUOUS, and another in which there is a remission, or INTERMISSION, once or more often during the twenty-four hours, usually in the morning.

The following are useful facts to remember regarding temperatures: (i.) The sudden advent of high fever in a previously healthy person without other symptoms indicates, in England, Influenza, Tonsillitis, Scarlet Fever, Pneumonia or Erysipelas. A very gradual advent is suggestive of Tuberculosis and sometimes of Typhoid Fever. (ii.) A fresh rise after the temperature has begun to fall indicates a complication or a relapse. (iii.) A sudden fall in the course of a fever (especially Typhoid Fever) may indicate internal hæmorrhage, perforation of one of the viscera, or profuse diarrhœa. (iv.) A considerable rise in diseases usually non-febrile, such as tetanus, delirium tremens, cancer, epilepsy, apoplexy, cholera, etc., generally indicates a fatal termination.

§ 472. Subnormal Temperature.—The temperature of the surface of the body, as indicated in the mouth or axilla, is rarely more than one or two degrees below normal. When it is below 96° the condition usually amounts to collapse. Subnormal temperature is not so important, for purposes of diagnosis, as elevation of temperature; but in the first four instances given below it may aid us in their differentiation. Subnormal temperature adds to the gravity of the prognosis in most wasting disorders. With regard to treatment. temperature readings below the normal are indications for the application of external warmth, nourishment, and the administration of stimulants.

Causes.—1. Subnormal temperature as an indication of *lowered vitality* occurs in normal circumstances in the aged, in whom the temperature is habitually several fractions of a degree below normal.

2. The temperature drops suddenly in *internal hæmorrhage* and in *abdominal rupture* or *perforation*: rupture of an abdominal cyst, traumatic rupture of the liver, spleen or kidney, or perforation of a peptic ulcer or of an ulcer of the bowel are usually attended by other and more distinctive signs (§ 243). In typhoid fever this sudden fall may be the only indication of these serious complications.

3. In all severe *abdominal inflammations* prostration and collapse are marked features, and the temperature may in some cases be subnormal, although there may be considerable constitutional disturbance, as shown by the prostration, and the rapid pulse (§ 239).

4. Subnormal temperature occurs in several other disorders in which it is not of much diagnostic significance, because we depend upon other signs for their identification. Thus, the temperature of the body is lowered (i.) when there is an excessive withdrawal of heat from the body, as in cases of inanition or exposure combined with privation, or with extensive weeping skin eruptions; (ii.) with dehydration *e.g.*, when large quantities of fluid are evacuated, as in severe diarrhœa, or in cholera (when the temperature may be 90° in axilla, though 105° in rectum); (iii.) in states of inanition or cachexia—*e.g.*, during convalescence from fevers, Addison's disease, cancer (especially of the alimentary canal), diabetes and chronic mental disorders; (iv.) when there is deficient oxygenation, as in cases of congenital heart disease, cardiac failure, alcoholism, jaundice, uræmia and myxœdema; (v.) in some diseases of the central nervous system, such as cerebral hæmorrhage or cerebral tumour; and (vi.) in poisoning by phosphorus, morphia, phenol and other drugs.

5. In all states of COLLAPSE the temperature is considerably lowered (2° or more). Indeed, this is one of the chief means by which it may be distinguished from syncope.

§ 473. Examination of Organs.—All the viscera must be carefully examined in accordance with the Scheme of Case-taking, pp. 6 and 7, so that local causes for the pyrexia may be excluded. Examination of the urine or the stools may reveal an unsuspected cause of pyrexia. For *clinical* purposes there are two large groups of causes of pyrexia: (*a*) **local inflammation:** such as pleurisy, appendicitis, abscess of the liver, etc., and (*b*) **general bacteræmic or toxæmic conditions,** like scarlet fever, rheumatic fever, and streptococcal or coli infection.

If any local inflammation is found, turn to the chapter dealing with the disease of that part. But it must still be remembered that some constitutional disease (*e.g.*, some specific fever) *may* be present, of which the local disease is a complication. Thus pneumonia, which would be discovered in the course of our examination, is a frequent complication of typhoid fever; and endocarditis of rheumatic fever. There are two features which may lead us to suspect a combination of disorders such as this: (1) The signs and symptoms of the local disorder may be of an aberrant type (*e.g., see Atypical Acute Pneumonia,* § 123); and (2) the constitutional disturbance presented by the patient would be greater in degree or different in kind than would accompany the local disease if it were the only disease present.

§ 474. **The Examination of the Blood** often affords most valuable information, and it may be useful to make a complete blood-count or stain a film (§§ 541 and 542), to take blood for the purpose of culture or to determine the Widal and Wassermann reactions (§§ 1208 and 1207). In certain cases the erythrocyte sedimentation rate (§ 1210) is also useful.

PART C. THE DIAGNOSIS, PROGNOSIS AND TREATMENT OF PYREXIAL DISORDERS

§ 475. **Routine Procedure and Classification.**—In cases of pyrexia we must investigate, as in other cases, three points:

First, THE LEADING SYMPTOM complained of by the patient will be one or more of those mentioned in § 466.

Secondly, THE HISTORY OF THE ILLNESS. The *date* when the symptoms commenced—*i.e.*, the PRECISE DURATION OF THE ILLNESS—is a most important matter. A few of the fevers—*e.g.*, typhoid fever and diphtheria—commence insidiously; but the majority are ushered in suddenly, very often with an attack of shivering (a rigor). Throughout the entire course of every case of fever the physician should have constantly in mind the " day of the disease," [1] so that he may know what events to expect at that particular period of the case. In typhoid fever, for instance, on the fourteenth day, or a little later, the diurnal range of the temperature should commence to be more marked, and during the next few days special care should be exercised to avoid hæmorrhage or perforation.

Thirdly, THE EXAMINATION OF THE PATIENT comprises three important matters: (1) Physical examination; (2) is there, or has there been, a rash ? and (3) the temperature and its course.

(1) EVERY ORGAN must be systematically examined (Scheme of Case-taking, pp. 6 and 7), and as carefully and thoroughly as the patient's condition will allow, in order that we may DETECT or EXCLUDE ANY LOCAL DISEASE. This is important, because all cases of pyrexia are associated with or due to some **local inflammatory disease**, or some **generalised febrile disorder** (*e.g.*, typhoid fever), or both.

(2) WHETHER THERE IS OR HAS BEEN ANY RASH is the next question. The first of the groups (*vide infra*) into which all fevers may be divided comprises those in which a rash distinctive of the disease appears within the first 4 days (with one exception) after the illness. The day on which it appears in each disease should always be in mind (Table XXVI).

(3) THE TEMPERATURE **and its course** is the next point to investigate; and it is of the greatest importance to obtain a CHART or succession of readings, after the manner described in § 471. The DURATION of the fever

---

[1] The fourth day of a disease is the third day *after* its commencement. Thus the rash of measles appears on the fourth day, and, supposing the patient were taken ill on a Monday, the rash would appear on Thursday.

is of assistance in diagnosis, especially when it has lasted longer than 2 or 3 weeks.[1]

The **classification** of pyrexial disorders may conveniently be based upon the results of our examination—namely, the eruption, if present, and the course of the temperature.

GROUP I.—ACUTE EXANTHEMATA or ERUPTIVE FEVERS—*i.e.*, fevers which are characterised by AN ERUPTION (*i.e.*, a RASH) distinctive of each disease appearing on one of the first 4 days of the illness (§§ 476 *et seq.*).

GROUP II.—CONTINUED FEVERS—*i.e.*, fevers in which the temperature runs a more or less continuous course, and which present NO ERUPTION during the first 4 days (§ 492).

GROUP III.—INTERMITTENT FEVERS—*i.e.*, fevers in which the temperature runs an intermittent (or remittent) course, and which present NO ERUPTION (§ 511).

If the physical examination reveals signs of disease of some particular organ, reference should be made to § 473, and to the chapter on diseases of that organ.

GROUP I. THE ACUTE EXANTHEMATA OR ERUPTIVE FEVERS

In all the diseases in this group the onset of the pyrexia is more or less abrupt, and in the majority a well-marked GENERAL ERUPTION appears during the *first four days* of the illness.[2] The course of the pyrexia varies considerably in the disorders in this group.

Common.		*Rare.*	
I. Chicken-pox (first day) ..	§ 476	VIII. Dengue (first day) ..	§ 483
II. Scarlet Fever (second day)	§ 477	IX. Classical Typhus (fourth or	
III. Erysipelas (second day) and		fifth day)	§ 484
Erysipeloid	§ 478	X. Rocky Mountain Fever	§ 485
IV. Small-pox (third day) ..	§ 479	XI. Scrub Typhus (rash fifth to	
V. Measles (fourth day) ..	§ 481	seventh day)	§ 486
VI. Rubella (first to fourth day)	§ 482	XII. Q Fever	§ 487
VII. Typhoid Fever (usually eighth to		XIII. Trench Fever	§ 488
tenth day), influenza, cerebro-		XIV. Rickettsial Pox	§ 489
spinal meningitis, plague, and		XV. Anthrax	§ 490
other members of Group II, occa-		XVI. Acute Glanders	§ 491
sionally present early rashes. § 492			

In each of the acute exanthemata the ERUPTION has special and DISTINCTIVE CHARACTERS, which, together with the DAY OF THE DISEASE on which the eruption appears, may enable one to differentiate the members of this group from one another. SCARLET FEVER may be regarded as the type, but it will be convenient to take them in the order in which the eruption appears. In England TYPHUS is hardly ever seen, and DENGUE is not met. ANTHRAX and GLANDERS are, like hydrophobia, derived from animals.

---

[1] Excluding diphtheria and the exanthemata, it is found that the majority of short fevers, of a few days' duration, are due to " common colds,' " rheumatism," " constipation " and " influenza."

[2] Incomplete forms (formes frustes), in which the rash or other characteristic symptoms are absent, may occur especially during an epidemic.

Some DRUGS IN COMMON USE may give rashes and pyrexia ("drug fever "): common examples are the sulphonamides and the barbiturates which at times can mimic the eruptive fevers closely.

§ 476. I. Varicella (Synonym: **Chicken-Pox**) may be defined as an acute infectious disease, manifested by an eruption of successive crops of limpid vesicles, usually accompanied by slight exacerbations of fever. It is in most cases a trivial disorder of childhood. It was differentiated from small-pox by Heberden in 1767, but its autonomy was disputed for nearly a hundred years later.

Symptoms.—Especially in young- children the characteristic rash is generally the first sign noticed. In older children and in adults *prodromal symptoms* precede this rash for the first 12 to 24 hours and give rise to a temperature even to 101–102°, malaise, headache, backache and sometimes a prodromal scarlatiniform, morbilliform or urticarial rash. In any case within 24 hours the *characteristic eruption* appears: this consists of dark pink, slightly raised, ovoid, or somewhat pyramidal papules, which in the course of a few hours become vesicular. The typical vesicle is at first a thin-walled, translucent, unilocular, glistening bleb, which contains a clear fluid in the most superficial layer of the skin: some of the lesions are ovoid and in the direction of the folds of the skin. After a day or so the fluid is invaded by staphylococci, causing the fluid to become turbid: the vesicle meanwhile loses its tension and dries into a scab which within 10 to 14 days separates, leaving a pigmented scab but rarely extensive scarring. Some of the papules do not proceed to vesiculation at all, but dry up. The essential feature of this eruption is that it *comes out in successive crops*, and so we see different stages of the rash on the same area of skin: this process rarely exceeds 4 days and is often less. The earliest lesions often appear on the mucous membranes of the palate and cheeks, which should always be inspected: on the skin, first the back, and then the front of the chest and abdomen are invaded: soon the whole body is affected, including the face and limbs, but as the lesions spread away from the centre, so they become much less numerous. Hence the density of the lesions is much less on the forearms and hands than on the upper arms; is less on the lower legs and feet than on the thighs, and is less on the upper face and scalp than on the lower face and neck. On the arms and legs, the *flexor* rather than the *extensor* surfaces are affected. The number of lesions can be very variable: in some the whole body seems to be covered, in others only isolated vesicles are to be seen.

The whole disease seldom lasts longer than 10 days, and may be so trivial as to pass unnoticed by the patient. The temperature rarely exceeds 103° F, and mild cases may be afebrile throughout. A case ceases to be infectious after the primary scabs have separated. The incubation period is usually about a fortnight, with limits from 10 to 21 days (see Table XXVI). A *quarantine period* is unnecessary, but child-contacts should be kept under regular observation for 21 days.

Varieties.—A *non-eruptive form* (varicella sine varicellis) may occur,

but abortive lesions may have been missed in some of these cases.
Varicella bullosa and *V. ulcerosa* occur most commonly in children with a
concomitant infection with virulent streptococci as in those who have
simultaneous impetigo contagiosa or scarlet fever. *V. gangrenosa* occurs
when the lesions are infected by hæmolytic streptococci or by C. diphtheriæ. *V. hæmorrhagica* in which bleeding occurs into and between the
vesicles, and from the mucous membranes, is very rare but usually fatal.

Diagnosis.—*Modified Variola* is the chief disease from which it has to
be differentiated, although this should not be difficult, because in small-
pox (i.) the rash comes out definitely on the third day; (ii.) it does not

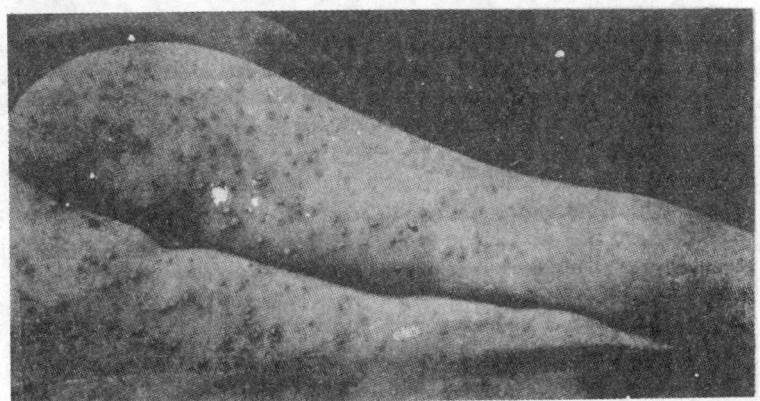

Fig. 140.—Chicken-pox eruption showing some papules, the superficial pearly vesicles and the varying
size of the pocks on the fourth day of the eruption.

appear in successive crops; (iii.) its favourite situations are the distal
extremities; (iv.) the evolution of the pock is much less rapid; and (v.) the
constitutional symptoms are very definite and characteristic ; and see
p. 681. *Herpes zoster* is distinguished by the limited area, and grouping
of the vesicles (§§ 676, 1021). *Pemphigus* is identified by the size and
chronic character of the blebs, but a bullous or pemphigoid form of varicella
may occur. *Dermatitis Herpetiformis* is very chronic, its vesicles occur in
groups, and irritation is severe. In *Scabies* the chest and abdomen are
not the most affected areas, and oral lesions are never seen.

Etiology.—Varicella is essentially a disease of childhood, but adults
are not exempt; even elderly persons may be attacked. It occurs in
epidemics, for the most part of limited extent, though it is endemic in
London. One attack usually confers immunity, but there are many
reported cases of second and even third attacks. Other infectious fevers
predispose to it; attacks following scarlet fever are apt to be severe.
The disease is transmitted mainly by droplet infection, but can be carried
by feeding utensils and by the hands and clothing of contacts. The
disease can be inoculated, though not so constantly as small-pox. The
vesicle fluid has been found by C. R. Amies and others to contain elemen-

tary bodies which are much smaller than those of small-pox and which are agglutinated by the serum of patients convalescent from varicella.

There is a close relationship between the virus of chicken-pox and of herpes zoster, and the elementary bodies of the two appear identical (Amies). A patient with herpes zoster can cause contacts to develop chicken-pox after the usual incubation period, and more rarely the reverse occurs. Yet an individual who has had chicken-pox is not protected against herpes zoster. Rake and his colleagues (1948) demonstrated with the electron microscope that the virus particles of the two diseases were identical in size and appearance; and that the virus from a case of herpes zoster is clumped by convalescent serum from that patient or from another suffering from chicken-pox.

Prognosis.—An attack is usually over in a week or 10 days, but it is apt, particularly in adults, to be followed by weakness which indeed may be more troublesome than the disease itself. Death is very rare apart from the hæmorrhagic form and secondary infection (see *varieties*). Rare *complications* include encephalitis, meningitis, myelitis, neuritis, pneumonia, arthritis and fibrositis, from all of which recovery is usual.

Treatment.—The itching is generally the chief trouble. The child should be prevented from scratching the pocks. The early application to each crop of papules or vesicles of 2–3 coats of a paint (cresol 0·5, tannic acid 12·5, collodion flexile 100) decreases the amount of pustulation and subsequent scarring (Mitman). The oral lesions need frequent mouth washes. When the lesions are infected by hæmolytic streptococci or by C. diphtheriæ, give full doses of penicillin and diphtheria antitoxin. Chemotherapeutic and antibiotic drugs should not be used locally because of the risk of skin sensitisation. Isolation need not be maintained for more than 14 days from the first appearance of the eruption.

§ 477. II. **Scarlet Fever** (Synonym: Scarlatina) used to be one of the most serious, and one of the commonest, of the eruptive fevers. It is still very prevalent, especially in those under ten years of age, though its severity has undergone remarkable mitigation in this country during recent years. It may be defined as an infective febrile disease due to a hæmolytic streptococcus, attended by inflammation of the tonsils, a punctiform eruption on the skin, and usually followed by pinhole desquamation. There are six characteristic *Symptoms*. (1) After a period of incubation which varies from 1 to 7 days, though usually 2 to 4, there is a *sudden advent of high fever* to 100–103°, reaching a maximum on the second or third day (Fig. 141). As with other hæmolytic streptococcal infections, the pulse is rapid, 120 or over: headache and muscular pains are usual. *Vomiting* with the initial rise of temperature occurs in 80 per cent. of cases. In the absence of complications, the temperature gradually subsides to normal about the fifth or sixth day. It does not, as in small-pox, subside when the rash comes out. (2) A *sore throat*, with enlarged lymph glands at the angles of the jaw, is complained of or seen on the first day. The tonsils are inflamed and often develop a follicular exudate on both sides, which can be removed without causing bleeding: the fauces become uniformly red or scarlet in colour, whereas the palate shows a punctate redness. Sore throat occurs with several of the exanthemata. In scarlet fever it is the tonsils and pharynx that are affected (rarely the larynx); in measles the larynx is chiefly affected; in small-pox both the larynx and pharynx are involved. The inflammation may become very severe, and is always attended with more or less glandular swelling. (3) The *eruption* is the next symptom and is remarkably regular in its appearance, 24 to 36 hours after the advent of the pyrexia. It has two elements—a generalised red blush, disappearing on pressure, and a number of minute points

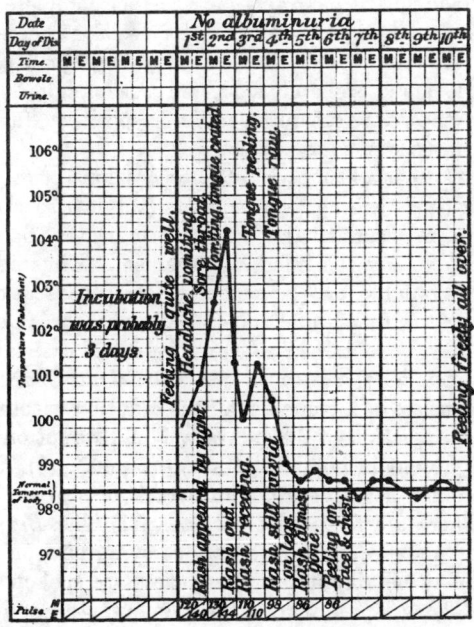

FIG. 141.—SCARLET FEVER.—Arthur M——, æt. 5. A typical mild case, especially as regards the initial symptoms, the rash, the tongue and the desquamation. The various incidents are shown on the chart.

(punctate erythema) slightly raised and redder than the surrounding skin. The flush is first seen on the face, and is rapidly followed by the punctate rash which starts on the neck and quickly spreads to the chest, trunk and upper arms. The forearms and hands and the legs are not affected at first, but within the first 24 hours the whole body is covered. There are certain special points to notice: (a) the face is flushed, but has no punctiform rash. (b) In contrast to measles and German measles, the face in scarlet fever usually shows a *circumoral pallor*. (c) Punctate hæmorrhages may be seen, especially in the flexures of the elbows (Pastia's sign). (d) Miliary sudamina may occur if the rash is severe. The rash continues to be well marked until the fourth or fifth day of the disease, but disappears earlier if antitoxin or penicillin have been given: slight staining may remain. (4) In the early stages the *tongue* becomes reddened along the edges, and covered with a thick white fur—" Strawberry and cream tongue." Soon the brilliant red papillæ show through, and as the fur separates leaves a bright red denuded surface resembling a ripe rasp-berry. Some confusion has arisen from the term " strawberry tongue " having been applied to both these conditions. (5) *Desquamation* (" peel-ing ") is apt to occur with any severe skin inflammation, but it is more characteristic in this than in any other fever. It begins about the fourth day, and continues for 4 to 6, or 8 weeks—first on the face, and, following the order of the rash, *last on the palms and soles*, the complete desquamation of which may be very tedious. In the latter position the flakes are large; elsewhere they are small and shreddy. (6) The *blood* shows a poly-morphonuclear leucocytosis and moderate eosinophilia. According to some observers, the Wassermann reaction is positive during the acute stage, though this is denied by others.

The primary cause is a hæmolytic streptococcal infection, usually of the throat, and sometimes arising from wounds (surgical scarlatina) or from the uterus (puerperal scarlatina). The rash indicates the production of an erythrogenic toxin by the infecting organism. Thus additional signs of the disease are available for (7) a hæmolytic streptococcus can be isolated from the primary source of infection (usually the throat and nose). A positive result may be obtained in non-scarlatinal cases, but a reliable negative report excludes the disease. (8) The *Schultz-Charlton* reaction or *Extinction Sign* consists of a blanching of the eruption within 8 to 24 hours of intracutaneous injection of 0·2 ml. of a 1 in 10 dilution of scarlatinal antitoxin. It is absent in non-scarlatinal eruptions. (9) A *positive Dick test* (p. 656) becomes negative after an attack of scarlet fever.

Varieties.—There are four chief varieties: (1) The *Benign*, simple or ordinary type as above described. Various symptoms—*e.g.*, rash, fever or sore throat—may be absent and these cases are spoken of as *latent* or *formes frustes*. (2) *Modified* scarlet fever follows the administration of penicillin or scarlatinal antitoxin within the first 1 to 2 days. Within 48 hours the temperature settles to normal, the intensity of the sore throat and rash is considerably lessened and desquamation may not occur. (3) In *Septic Scarlet Fever*, Scarlatina Ulcerosa or Anginosa, the ordinary symptoms are aggravated by a septic infection of the throat, with an exudate which may spread beyond the tonsils and may produce local ulceration even of the fauces and palate. From this focus septic material is absorbed, the upper cervical glands may suppurate and the middle ears become involved. The rash is often faint, but a blotchy or gyrate eruption frequently appears on the face and limbs in the second or third week. (4) In the *Toxic* form the patient is seized with high fever, delirium, and marked cardio-vascular weakness; the vomiting per-sists, the rash is very intense, but the throat symptoms often ill-marked, and the patient dies during the first week. Toxic scarlet fever of such intensity as to deserve the name *Malignant*, with low muttering delirium, usually a marked rash, and death without complications in a few days, is a very rare variety.

Diagnosis.—The diagnosis of scarlatina is not difficult in typical cases. The abrupt advent of high fever, accompanied by vomiting and sore throat in a child who has not had the disease, is always extremely suggestive, and if the disease is prevalent the diagnosis is almost certain. During the first few days the greatest difficulty is sometimes experienced in the diagnosis from *tonsillitis*, and especially that variety due to other strains of hæmolytic streptococci. Vomiting is more common in scarlatinal cases, and a careful watch must be kept for the rash and for subsequent desquamation. *Diphtheria* has no punctate rash, though a flush may be seen on the chest and arms, but the characteristic membrane appears on the throat and the tongue remains coated. In doubtful cases it is best to act as if the graver disease were present (see Table X, § 157). *Measles* is associated with marked catarrhal symptoms in the eyes, nose and bronchi, and Koplik's spots are usually present. The characteristic differences between the rashes of the two diseases are best seen on the limbs. *Dengue* (§ 483) is accompanied by severe articular pains and a morbilliform eruption on the fourth day; the diagnosis is easier when the eruption is present. The scarlatinal rash is distinguished from the diffuse prodromal erythema of *small-pox* by the fact that the latter starts in the groins or axillæ, and invades the oral circle if the rash is diffuse; and lumbar pain is usually complained of. *Enema rashes* and *Epidemic Exfoliative Dermatitis* are sometimes mistaken for scarlatina. A *septic rash* may be scarlatiniform, but is distinguished by fever of a pyæmic type, the presence of a septic focus, and the absence of characteristic punctation. The erythema of *belladonna poisoning* is accompanied by great thirst, dryness of the fauces and dilatation of the pupils. *Sulphonamide* and other *drug rashes* may be a source of confusion.

Etiology.—The disease is highly infectious, especially at the onset and during the early stages. It is due to a hæmolytic streptococcal infection with an organism belonging to Lancefield's group A, and capable of producing a toxin which causes the characteristic skin rash. The infection is propagated through the air for short distances as a droplet-infection from other cases, from healthy carriers, or from an infection derived from a case recently discharged from hospital (" return cases "). More rarely the organisms are conveyed by dust or by direct contact with an infected spoon, fork or the nurse's fingers: outbreaks due to infected milk have been recorded.

The patient used to be regarded as infectious until desquamation had ceased, a period averaging 4 to 6 weeks, or even longer. There is no evidence that the desquamation of scarlet fever is ever infectious, traditional belief notwithstanding. On the other hand, the infection may survive in the mucous discharges from the throat and nose, and possibly the ears, for many weeks, long after the peeling has completely finished.

One attack usually gives immunity for life. *Relapses* or second attacks are believed to arise in those who have developed a poor immunity from the first attack (shown by a persistently positive Dick test), and who are infected by a different serological type of hæmolytic streptococcus.

A hæmolytic streptococcus (Lancefield group A) has been proved to be the causal organism, on the following grounds: (1) inoculation of an apparently pure culture has produced scarlet fever in volunteers; (2) intracutaneous injection of a filtrate of the culture gives a strongly positive reaction in susceptible subjects (Dick test); (3) preparation of a serum by immunisation of a horse with the scarlatinal type of *Streptococcus hæmolyticus* has a curative effect. The presence or absence of a rash depends on the susceptibility of the individual and the capacity of the organism to produce a highly active erythrogenic toxin.

The *Dick Test* is performed by injecting intradermally one skin test dose of scarlatinal exotoxin, contained in 0·2 ml. of fluid. In 8 to 12 hours, there appears a small circular erythematous area which reaches its maximum in 18 hours after injection, then rapidly fades. To avoid pseudo-positive reactions, a control test should be carried out simultaneously. A true positive result is found in 70 to 100 per cent. of cases of scarlet fever in the first three days of the disease, as well as in susceptible persons. The test possesses some diagnostic value: conversion of a positive reaction in the acute stage into a negative reaction at the end of the week or fortnight indicates that the disease is scarlet fever.

Prognosis.—The disease has become very much milder in Great Britain; whereas in 1870 the death-rate per million living was 1,446, now it is 0·5; even so over 50,000 cases are notified annually. It still remains serious in other parts of the world. The danger is greater in those under five years: untoward symptoms arise when the throat infection is severe, the temperature above 105°, when cardio-vascular toxæmia is marked and with persistent vomiting. Delirium at night is more or less usual in severe cases, but violent delirium or stupor is a bad sign. The septic, toxic, malignant and hæmorrhagic forms always cause anxiety. *Complications* and *Sequelæ* are now rare when penicillin or another suitable antibiotic is given early. They are: (1) Some degree of upper cervical adenitis is usual: abscess formation is now very rare. (2) Otitis media and mastoiditis. (3) Acute nephritis is seen in untreated cases at the end of the third week, very rarely after the fourth. It usually shows itself by slight pyrexia, albuminuria and the presence of casts. This may soon clear up or may proceed to more severe acute nephritis: chronic nephritis may follow. (4) Scarlatinal rheumatism occurs in the third week, and is due to supervening acute rheumatic fever, often with carditis. (5) Acute sinusitis, ulcerative stomatitis and broncho-pneumonia are relatively rare. Among the *sequelæ* subacute rheumatism and chorea are occasionally found.

Treatment.—With the milder cases now prevailing, it is no longer necessary to insist on treatment in an infectious diseases hospital, so long as the patient can be isolated and nursed at home (*Hygienic* treatment is considered in §§ 526 *et seq.*). Strict bed rest for a week is necessary even in the mildest cases, to prevent complications: a well-ventilated room is essential. Aspirin is useful as a gargle and to swallow in the initial stages: kaolin poultices form a useful application to the cervical glands. *Specific treatment* is with chemotherapy and antibiotics against the organism, and streptococcal antitoxin against the toxin. The routine use of antitoxin is no longer necessary, but for severe cases the dose is 10,000 units intramusc. and 20,000 or 40,000 units intravenously. (A unit of streptococcal antitoxin is the quantity required to neutralise 50 skin-test doses of scarlet fever toxin.) Penicillin alone is very effective in most cases; sulphonamides alone do not give such good results. The best results are obtained when the two drugs are combined. For *mild cases* administer procaine penicillin intramusc. 600,000 units once daily for 5 days; or give an initial dose of procaine penicillin and follow this by oral tablets of penicillin 4-hourly, half an hour before meals—phenoxymethylpenicillin 125–250 mg. or phenethicillin (Broxil) are commonly used. *Severe cases* need crystalline penicillin 0·5–1·0 million units 6-hourly with sulphonamides and antitoxin if necessary. *Isolation.*—After treatment with antibiotics the mild and uncomplicated case may be discharged home when clinically free from infection (*i.e.*, no nasal or ear discharge, a healthy throat, no enlarged cervical glands) in 12–14 days. " Release swabs " need not be taken. Children should be able to return to school after a further week. *Complications* indicate the need for sensitivity tests on the organism and a change of the specific remedy being used. If an abscess forms in the neck, or in the middle ear, incision will be necessary. For the treatment of acute nephritis or acute rheumatism, see §§ 397, 592. The occurrence of return cases, *i.e.*, cases of scarlet fever arising in the same family within a month of the patient (primary case) being sent back home should not take place nowadays.

Prophylaxis can be promoted by: (1) Oral penicillin, giving tab. phenoxymethylpenicillin 125 mg. or tab. phenethicillin (Broxil) (Table XXXV) half an hour before meals 12-hourly for 10 days or a daily dose of sulphadiazine (1 G.) for 12 days. (2) 3,000 units of antitoxin (intramusc.) produces temporary immunity for 10 to 14 days. (3) *Active immunisation* with graduated doses of scarlatinal toxin is no longer considered necessary in Great Britain.

§ 478. III. **Erysipelas** may be defined as an acute febrile infectious disease, characterised by a progressive marginated redness and tumefaction of the skin, usually attacking the face, or the neighbourhood of wounds. (1) *The Stage of Invasion.*—After an incubation period of 1 to 7 days the advent is abrupt, as in scarlet fever and small-pox. The temperature on the evening of the same day may be 103° to 104° F, or more. Vomiting is very common, and so also are muscular pains, especially pain in the back, like that of small-pox. (2) The *Rash* begins about 24 to 36 hours after the advent of fever, as a tense red spot on the face (facial erysipelas) or at the site of an abrasion (which may be microscopic). It often commences just within the external nares on one side at the junction of the skin and mucous membrane. It enlarges, spreads, becomes bright red and tender: where the skin is loose as in the eyelids or the scrotum, œdema is well marked. Thin-walled bullæ may form in the centre of the inflammatory area. The advancing edge is sharply defined and raised, the receding edge indefinite. The rash may vary in duration from 3 to 4 days to a fortnight: it is materially shortened by chemotherapy. Delirium at night is not unusual in elderly people. Convalescence becomes established, and desquamation occurs in the course of 1 to 3 weeks. During this last stage albumen may appear in the urine, if it has not appeared before.

Diagnosis.—Erysipelas is to be diagnosed from *erythema* complicated by cellulitis, in which the margin is less raised, and there is less fever. *Cavernous sinus thrombosis,* often arising from a nasal furuncle, causes a unilateral fan of cyanotic skin from the nose to the eye. In *herpes* of the first division of the fifth nerve vesicles occur in groups, are limited to one side of the face, and are unattended by fever.

Varieties.—(i.) Although erysipelas and cellulitis are often classified as separate diseases, spread of the infection from the skin to the subcutaneous tissues may give a combination of both (erysipelo-cellulitis). (ii.) Phlegmonous erysipelas or gangrenous erysipelas are severe varieties with suppuration or extensive sloughing. (iii.) Erysipelas neonatorum can be a fatal variety; death may be due to peritonitis by inflammation spreading along the umbilical cord.

Etiology.—It is a highly contagious malady due to a local infection with a hæmolytic streptococcus. Persons are predisposed to it, especially alcoholics, by wounds and unhygienic conditions. Infants and persons over forty are most liable. In so-called idiopathic cases the organism is probably introduced through a minute and hardly visible scratch. The presence of a wound is the strongest predisposing cause and it spreads amongst surgical patients with great rapidity. One attack gives no immunity; on the contrary, it predisposes, and some elderly people are liable to an attack of facial erysipelas every year.

Prognosis.—The usual course is favourable, but the disease is more dangerous in infancy or old persons, alcoholic or plethoric patients, and those affected with chronic diseases, especially nephritis. The death-rate in England and Wales is now virtually nil. Hyperpyrexia, persistent vomiting, lividity of the rash, and typhoid delirium are untoward symptoms. *Complications* include cellulitis with residual abscesses, septicæmia, broncho-pneumonia and acute nephritis. Death may occur by coma or syncope.

Treatment (Hygienic Treatment, see §§ 526 *et seq.*). The treatment of erysipelas has been revolutionised by the administration of either penicillin or a sulphonamide, which have a remarkably favourable effect on the duration of the spread of the local lesion, the length of primary pyrexia and of the toxæmia. The drug of choice is inject. benzylpenicillin, and in young children and in all severe cases it is prudent to administer a sulphonamide as well. Local applications are unnecessary, but on the face and eyelids local bathing gives relief.

Erysipeloid is a common disease which affects the fingers, hands and wrists. It is usually occupational in origin in those preparing food or handling whales, seals, fish, meat and sometimes poultry.

Symptoms.—There is usually a history of a cut, scratch or puncture, often by a meat or fish bone, fish skin or butcher's knife up to 2 weeks previously. At the site of inoculation there is a central bluish-red spot with a reddened margin; lymphangitis and lymphadenitis follow but suppuration does not occur.

Etiology.—The cause is a saphrophytic organism *Erysipelothrix rhusiopathiæ.*

Treatment.—Without drug therapy the disease disappears within 1 to 4 weeks, but injections of penicillin or capsules of one of the tetracyclines shorten its duration. The sulphonamides are ineffective. *Prophylaxis* in those especially exposed to infection is by wearing rubber gloves and frequent washing of the hands.

§ **479.** IV. **Small-pox** (Variola) is a highly infectious eruptive fever, the eruption passing through the stages of papule, vesicle, pustule and scab with subsequent scarring. It essentially exists in THREE FORMS. (A) A virulent or classical Eastern form—Variola Major. (B) A mild form in the unvaccinated, a type originating in America and the W. Indies —Variola Minor or Alastrim. These two types breed true and are caused by different strains of the same virus. (C) Small-pox modified by previous vaccination—Modified Small-pox.

(A) VARIOLA MAJOR. The *Symptoms* fall into two groups: (1) *Prodromal.* After a definite incubation period of 12 days, characteristic constitutional symptoms appear—viz., sudden advent of shivering and high fever (101–104° F), with severe headache and *pain in the back.* The most noticeable features of this primary fever are the severity of the pain in the back (which is present even in the mildest cases), and the frequent occurrence of vomiting: cough and bronchitis are common. *Prostration is marked,* the face becomes grey in colour, the conjunctivæ suffused and the tongue furred. The mind may be active and the patient sleepless, or a toxic delirium with mental confusion may be present. During the stage of primary fever there is, as a rule, no eruption, but in some cases a prodromal rash makes its appearance on the second day. This may be (i.) erythematous, generally found in the groins or other folds, occasionally it covers the whole body, in which case the outlook is grave; (ii.) morbilliform, usually occupying the apron area, but also occasionally diffuse; or (iii.) a profuse hæmorrhagic eruption sometimes appears on the anterior surface of the abdomen and thighs and indicates a very severe attack. After 2 or 2½ days, these initial symptoms disappear, the temperature drops, and on the third day the true small-pox eruption appears. (2) During the *Eruptive stage,* the temperature at first remains much lower—the patient, indeed, may feel comparatively well. The earliest lesions are often visible in the mouth and involvement of the larynx and pharynx causes a sore throat. On the skin, for the first few hours (of the third day) there is a macular eruption which rapidly gives place to a crop of papules of *shotty hardness* which can be felt even more readily than they can be seen, like small shot beneath the skin (Plate XVA): each papule is surrounded by a pink areola. They are of centrifugal distribution and first appear on the forehead and on the fronts of the wrists. Then the eruption travels over the whole body, the chest, abdomen, groins and legs being least affected; lesions on the trunk are mainly on the back, the axillæ being comparatively free. This papular stage is complete in 48 hours, and the papules then more or less simultaneously become vesicular (on the fifth or sixth days). The eruption *comes out in one crop* and is never multiform in any given area of skin as in varicella. Some of the

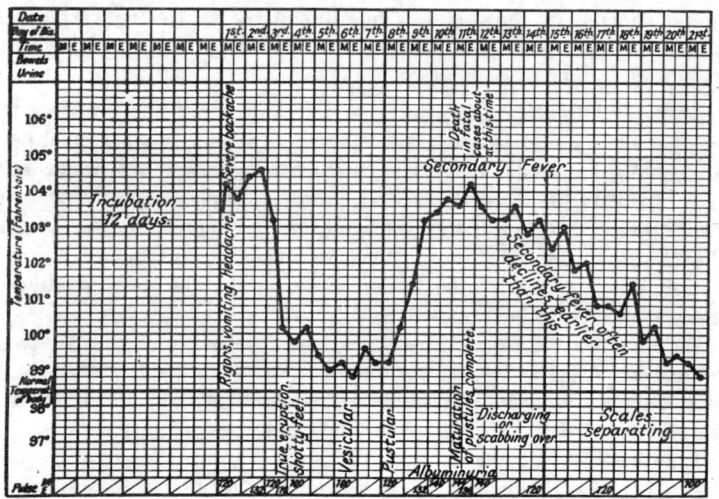

FIG. 142.—UNMODIFIED SMALL-POX.—Severe confluent case, unvaccinated, terminating in recovery. The various incidents are shown in the chart.

papules, however, may abort and not proceed to vesiculation. Each vesicle enlarges, and by the seventh or eighth day has become pustular: with this a secondary suppurative fever develops, which may last 6 to 8 days and be attended by rigors (Fig. 142). In typical cases, unmodified by vaccination, each vesicle presents a depressed centre which is held down by a bridle (umbilication). The next day (eighth day) the bridle ruptures, and each pustule becomes hemispherical, about as large as a split pea, with an inflamed and indurated base, and at this time considerable œdema of the skin is present. These pustules gradually dry into scabs, which separate about the fifteenth to the twentieth day, though in some situations, such as the scalp, forehead and sides of the nose, considerably later, leaving patches of congested skin, and in severe cases a pitted cicatrix. The extent of the eruption and the amount of inflammatory induration varies considerably. Sometimes only the face and wrists

PLATE XV (A)

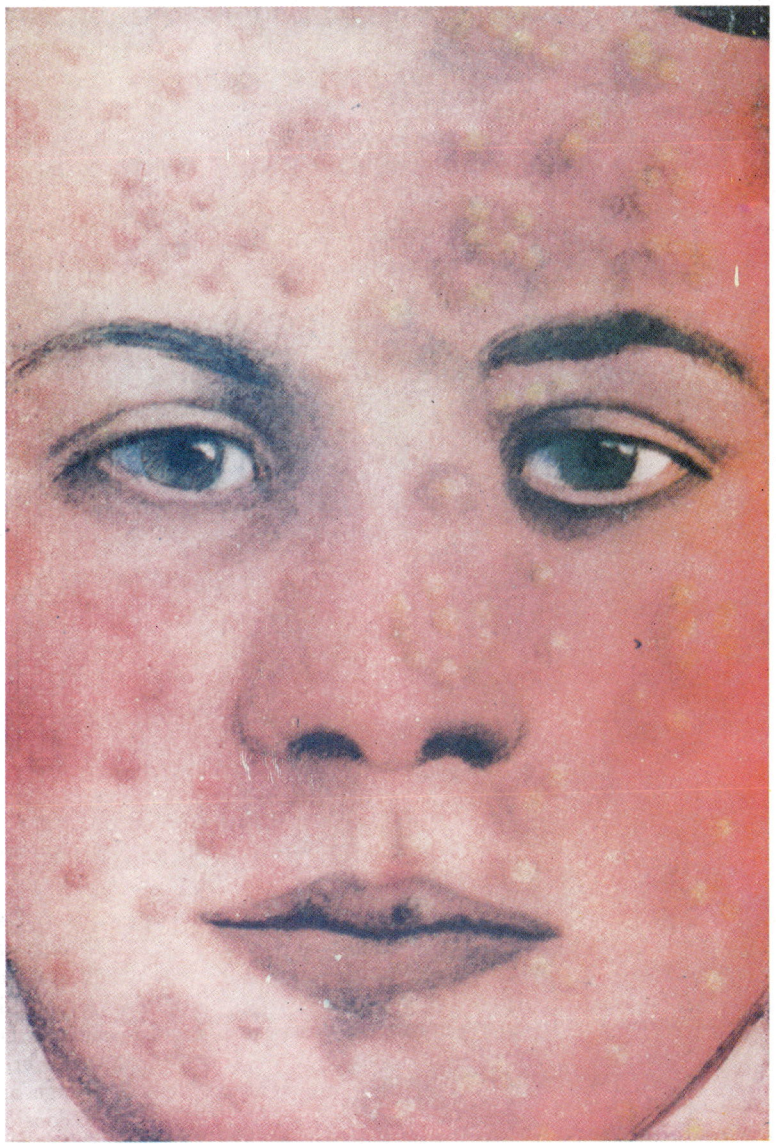

SMALL-POX.

Right side of face (left of observer) represents the papules of the second day of the eruption. The other, pustular, side represents the sixth day of the eruption; a few of the pustules show commencing umbllication.

Drawn from nature by Miss Mabel Green.

PLATE XV (B)

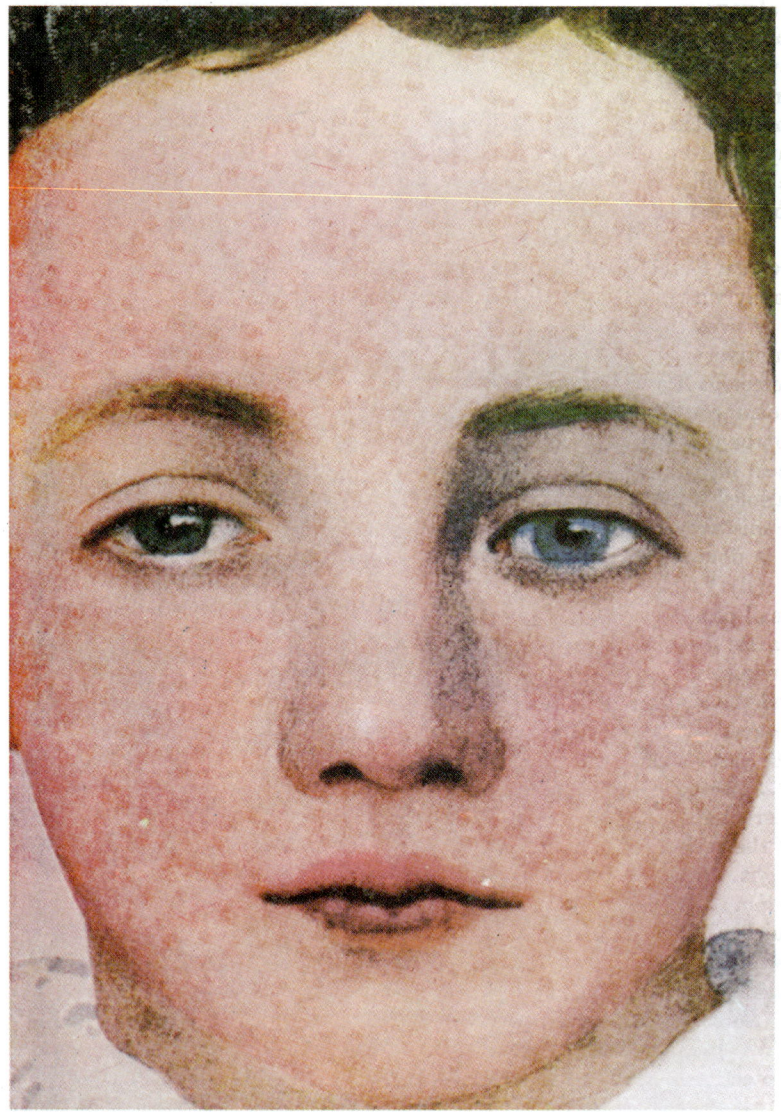

MEASLES.

The eruption, which is very plentiful, is eighteen hours old (second day of rash). Note the evidence of coryza in the eyes and nose.

Drawn from nature by Miss Mabel Green.

present a few spots; sometimes the whole body is covered.   The eruption is always most profuse where the skin has been irritated by any cause. The eruption on the legs always presents a proportionate retardation of development, since it appears last in this situation.   Consequently, before certifying a patient as free from infection, the soles of the feet should be carefully examined, and should the thick epidermis be found to harbour any dried-up remnants of obsolescent pocks (or " seeds "), these should be carefully dug out and removed before the case can be regarded as free from possible infection.

Varieties.—It is sufficient to describe four varieties according to the severity of the disease, the severity of the symptoms corresponding very closely with the character and extent of the eruption on the face: (1) *Mild or Discrete*, (2) *Confluent* and (3) *Malignant or Hæmorrhagic*.   During the eruptive stage, a hæmorrhagic prodromal rash may be associated with hæmorrhages within and beneath the skin, and from most, if not all, of the mucous membranes.   Death ensues early, even before the vesicles appear (Fig. 144).   In a second variety, which is less fatal, hæmorrhages occur into and between the pustules.   (4) A *non-eruptive form* (variola sine variolis) has been described as in the other acute exanthemata, and may be mistaken for influenza.   It occurs among contacts recently vaccinated; it is doubtful whether it is infective to others.

(B) Variola Minor (Synonym: Alastrim) is the term applied to true small-pox occurring in an unvaccinated person in which the severity of the disease has been considerably lessened (as compared with *V. major*) due to diminished toxicity of the organisms: the typical lesions tend to abort and the secondary fever is relatively slight.   In Great Britain during the 25-year period up to Dec. 1961 there have been 281 cases of *V. major* and 146 cases of *V. minor*.

Symptoms.—(1) The incubation period is often prolonged beyond the characteristic 12-day period of *V. major*: 15 to 17 days to the appearance of the rash is quite common.   (2) The prodromal symptoms are usually slight.   (3) The distribution of the typical lesions is the same as in *V. major*.   (4) The papules appear more slowly, but the lesions mature more quickly.   This may give a deceptive appearance of crops of lesions such as are met in chicken-pox.   (5) A considerable number of papules and vesicles abort, and so secondary infection and its associated fever is slight.

Etiology.—The fact that the virus of *V. minor* is the same as the virus of *V. major* (of ordinary small-pox) is shown by (1) vaccination is equally protective against both; (2) the distribution of the eruption is the same; (3) the sera derived from patients with *V. minor* and *V. major* give the same agglutination reactions with virus obtained from the lesions of *V. minor* and *V. major*.

(C) Modified Small-pox (Synonym: Varioloid) is the disease which arises when a previously vaccinated person develops *V. major*: immunity is only partial, and may be the result either of unsatisfactory vaccination, or of vaccination many years previously.

Symptoms.—(1) The primary fever and early symptoms are often indistinguishable from *V. major*, and the eruption appears on the fourteenth day. (2) Certain portions of the eruption abort and do not pass through all stages. (3) As a consequence several stages of the eruption may occasionally be seen on the same portion of skin. (4) The general eruption may be very scanty, and may consist of not more than a dozen papules, which may not even undergo vesiculation. (5) There is little, if any, secondary (suppurative) fever (Fig. 143).

TABLE XXIX.—DIFFERENTIATION BETWEEN

	CHICKEN-POX	SMALL-POX
Age	Especially children.	Any age.
Degree of illness	Slight.	More severe, often with prostration.
Prodromal symptons	Usually slight in children; more severe in adults. No symptoms before the rash.	Severe for 2–3 days before the rash: high temp., headache, backache, vomiting.
Prodromal rash	Uncommon: most on chest and arms.	More common: especially groins.
Main Eruption:—		
Temperature of eruption	On *First day.* Rises as rash appears.	On *third or fourth* days. Settles as rash appears.
Typical rash	Evolves quickly: *successive crops* for 4 days: several stages on one portion of skin.	Evolves slowly: *one crop only.*
Earliest and most profuse skin lesions	Chest and abdomen: fewer on face and limbs. Centripetal distribution.	Forehead, wrists and forearms: less on the trunk. Centrifugal distribution; the axillæ, groins and pressure areas on back relatively free.
On limbs	Flexor surfaces especially.	Extensor surfaces especially.
Early stage	Superficial papules becoming vesicular in a few hours.	Deep shotty papules becoming vesicular in 2 days.
Umbilication of vesicles	Absent.	Present.
Shape of vesicles	May be oval.	Circular.
Pustulation of vesicles	Within 4 days.	Seventh or eighth day of illness.
Scars	Absent or slight.	Marked.
Secondary Fever	Absent or slight.	Marked.
Vaccination against small-pox	Ineffective.	Successful vaccination prevents the disease.

Diagnosis of Small-pox.—There are three important diagnostic features: (i.) Sudden advent of high fever, often with a rigor; (ii.) headache, *backache*, and vomiting at onset of the disease, of which there should always be a history, even in the mildest cases; (iii.) the distribution of the papules and vesicles; (iv.) the most important single factor is the *distribution* of the rash; difficulty may occur when chicken-pox in the adult causes severe constitutional symptoms or a profuse rash on the face. The main diagnostic points and the differentiation from *varicella* are set out in Table XXIX. *Measles* is the disease which is most often mistaken for variola in the early stages of the case, and therefore two plates of these diseases are presented side by side (Plates XVA and B). Measles is distinguished by the redness of and the running from the eyes, with other signs of catarrh, and the presence of Koplik's spots (§ 481) on the buccal mucous membrane. The rash, too, is macular rather than papular, and the individual spots as they increase in size spread out in patchy coalescence. In febrile *roseola* or lichen, the fever lasts only 24 hours, the efflorescence appears all over

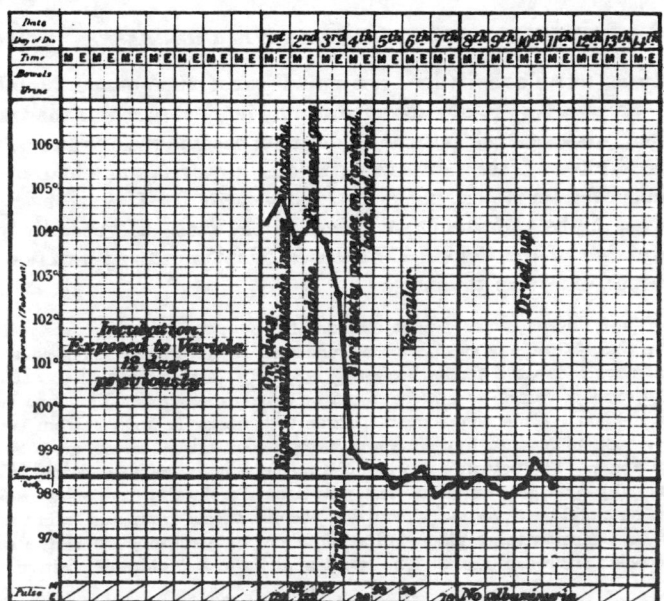

FIG. 143.—A mild case of MODIFIED VARIOLA occurring in a young woman, æt. 22, who had been vaccinated two years previously and who presented three visible cicatrices of the primary vaccination. Initial symptoms severe. No secondary fever.

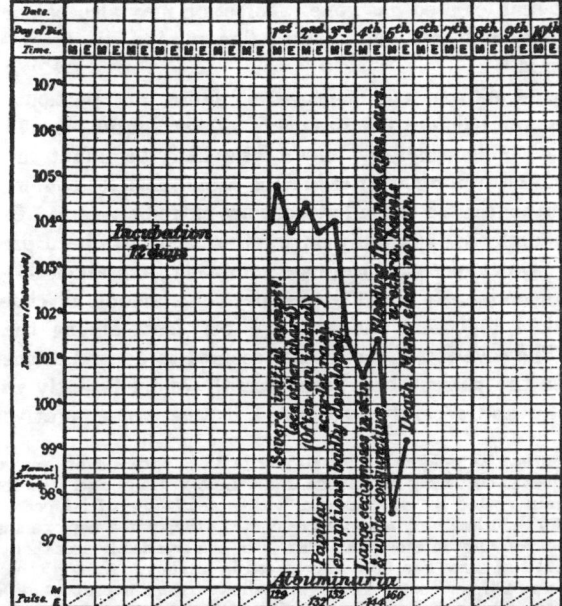

FIG. 144.—A case of MALIGNANT HÆMORRHAGIC SMALL-POX (as distinct from those cases of confluent small-pox with hæmorrhages in the pustules).—Patient unvaccinated. Death occurred on the 5th day. The various incidents are shown on the chart.

the body at once, and it does not go to any further stage. *Syphilitic papules* and *pustules* are not accompanied by marked pyrexia: they remain unchanged, while in small-pox the lesions soon become vesicles and pustules (and see § 705). *Lichen urticatus* (papular urticaria) in children may be mistaken for small-pox, but is distinguished by the (1) rash being profuse on the limbs and absent or sparse on the face, (2) generally superficial situation of the lesions, (3) absence of inflammatory reaction, and (4) presence of severe itching.

Pathological investigations are of considerable assistance in diagnosis. (1) The virus from vesicular fluid or specimen scrapings is readily grown on the chorio-allantois of the 10 days incubated fertile hen's egg. After 3 further days' incubation, the plaques of virus of variola and vaccinia can be clearly distinguished. Varicella does not grow thereon. (2) A complement fixation test, using the antigen from vesicular fluid or scrapings against hyperimmune antivaccinal rabbit serum gives a result within 24 hours. The patient's vaccinal history must be taken into account in interpretation. (3) Agar-gel diffusion test. Antigen, preferably vesicular fluid, is incubated on a slide with anti-sera from the vaccinia-variola group and from varicella, separately. Diffusion takes place and a white precipitate forms where the antigen and its specific antiserum meet. The result is given in 2–5 hours if positive.

Etiology.—Guarnieri described what were first regarded as protozoa in the epithelial cells of the small-pox vesiclé, but were subsequently proved by Paschen to be the elementary bodies or virus of the disease. The patient is highly infectious from the first skin or mouth blemish until the last scab or seed has gone. Infection may also be conveyed by feeding utensils, clothing and infected fingers, and via crusts from the skin of patients.

Prognosis.—Children, and especially infants, are particularly prone to the disease, and before the discovery of vaccination in 1796 (§ 480), it was a cause of considerably more than half the infant mortality in Great Britain and other countries.[1] One attack usually confers complete immunity: authenticated second attacks are extremely rare. In *V. major* the prognosis depends (1) mainly on whether there has been prophylactic vaccination. Until recently, the case mortality was about 37 per cent. among the *unvaccinated*; about 5 or 6 per cent. among all classes of the *vaccinated* taken together; and about ½ per cent. among the *properly vaccinated*. The severity of the disease seemed to depend almost entirely upon whether the patient had been recently and efficiently *vaccinated*.[2] In the healthy and recently vaccinated it was a comparatively trivial

[1] Warrington had an epidemic of small-pox in 1773, with a death-rate of 26·5 per 1,000, all the deaths occurring in persons under nine years of age. In 1892–3 Warrington was again visited by an epidemic, with a death-rate of 1·1 per 1,000 of the inhabitants, who then had only about 1 per cent. unvaccinated persons among them.

[2] During the Warrington epidemic, 1892–3, in the *infected* houses there were 2,535 persons, and 2,223 of these had been vaccinated in infancy. Among these latter the case-mortality was 5·2 per cent. The figures showed that in proportion as the vaccination had been more efficient, the severity of the disease was less. Of the 667 cases which occurred in this epidemic, not one had been vaccinated or revaccinated within seven years of the attack.—Appendix to the Report of the Roy. Com. on Vaccination, 1894.

disorder, but in the unvaccinated, especially in infancy, it was one of the gravest diseases. Even so, it must be realised that vaccination is not an absolute safeguard against even virulent small-pox. (2) The second factor is the question of *age*: the official records of the outbreak in Warrington in 1773 showed that of 211 fatal cases, 166 were under three years of age. (3) Alcohol and plethora add to the gravity of the disease. As regards the *varieties*, the confluent, in which the rash may come out on the second day and is very abundant, is much more dangerous than the discrete form. In the former the fever does not subside on the third day, and there is a great tendency to hyperpyrexia and complications. Speaking generally, the more copious the rash, the greater the danger. True hæmorrhagic small-pox is invariably fatal, but if hæmorrhage occurs *into* the vesicular or pustular rash, there is a chance of recovery. As regards *untoward symptoms*, the more severe the primary fever in the unvaccinated, the more severe will be the disease, but this is not necessarily so in the vaccinated; profuse salivation is a bad symptom; the case is grave if there be no swelling of the skin at about the ninth day, and still graver if the swelling goes suddenly away. The case fatality of variola minor in recent epidemics is about 0·2 per cent.

Complications.—(1) Bronchitis is common in the more severe cases. Pneumonia, empyema and rarely œdema glottidis are often fatal. (2) A toxic myocarditis occurs in the toxic and hæmorrhagic cases, and with a severe secondary fever. Endocarditis and pericarditis are rare. (3) Nervous complications include encephalitis with delirium and convulsions, hemiplegia or acute ataxia: post-febrile psychosis may occur. (4) Some degree of conjunctivitis is not unusual: painless corneal ulcers may produce a panophthalmia and destruction of the eye. (5) Erysipelas and cutaneous abscesses are common during the secondary fever.

Treatment.—Prophylaxis. It should be remembered that vaccination is capable of modifying the disease even after exposure to infection, because the incubation period of variola is 12 days and that of vaccinia only 8 days. Vaccination may, therefore, be performed with efficacy during the first 3 or 4 days after exposure; and every member of an infected household should be vaccinated immediately the disease breaks out therein. For its efficiency in the prevention and modification of small-pox, see pp. 684 and 687. Treatment *of an attack* demands immediate notification and transfer to a special small-pox hospital. The patient should be nursed on a special mattress and kept as quiet as possible; the heart muscle should be carefully guarded by skilful nursing. Headache and pains in the neck and limbs in the earlier stages require aspirin and even the use of morphia or heroin: restlessness and delirium in the secondary toxic stage need full doses of sedatives and narcotics. The eyes should be examined in a good light each day. To protect the skin, the whole body may be painted daily with potassium permanganate solution (5 per cent.) from the early papular stage: a weak dettol solution is comforting and acts as a deodorant. Finsen reported that the exclusion of all except red rays from the sickroom was beneficial, but this has not proved very helpful in this country. The Variola virus is not sensitive to any antibiotic. In the control of the secondary infection and secondary fever, sulphonamides have, on the whole, been disappointing; but the use of penicillin or other antibiotics from the start of vesiculation is the treatment of choice. Hyperimmune anti-variola gamma-globulin, prepared from blood taken from a recently vaccinated subject, is available in Great Britain through the Public Health Laboratory Service: it may prove of value to small-pox contacts. *Hygienic Treatment* is given in §§ 526 *et seq.*

§ 480. **Vaccinia.**—VACCINATION is the production in a person of the disease called vaccinia, by inoculating him with lymph containing attenuated living vaccinia virus; this is taken from the vesicles on the skin of healthy calves or sheep which are suffering from vaccinia as a result of previous inoculation with the virus.

It was noticed in 1769 by a German that people engaged in the milking of cows were exempt from small-pox. Jenner, in 1796, placed the subject on a scientific basis, and ascertained that the inoculation of a human being with the lymph taken from the unbroken vesicles on the udder of a calf suffering from vaccinia protected that person from small-pox. He was also the first to inoculate this disease (vaccinia) from person to person by taking the lymph from the vesicle on the arm which had matured on the eighth day after inoculation. Vaccination was made compulsory in 1853. In 1897 this law was repealed in response to an outcry among the public that syphilis and (?) other diseases could be conveyed from person to person in this way. Syphilis certainly has, in rare instances, been conveyed by arm to arm vaccination; but by using calf-lymph or sheep-lymph this is entirely avoided. Compulsory vaccination has been abolished by the National Health Act (1946). All " Government " lymph issued in Great Britain today is sheep-lymph which has been diluted 1 in 5 with glycerol-saline, together with a preservative. A dried vaccine (Lister Institute) is more suitable for tropical conditions on account of its greater stability. Goodpasteur has perfected a method by which the virus is grown on the chorio-allantoic membrane of chick embryos.

Rules for vaccination.—The older method of four areas of vaccination has now been superseded. The area of skin to be vaccinated may be over the deltoid, on the abdomen, or over the outer side of the calf: this is washed with soap and water and allowed to dry thoroughly. Two methods of insertion may be used: (1) A scratch not more than ¼ inch long is made by a sterile round-pointed needle, which should not draw blood: the lymph is ejected from the capillary tube over this prepared area, or alternatively the scratch may be made through the lymph. (2) The multiple-pressure method has largely superseded the scratch method as it produces a higher immunity and also more " takes " in re-vaccinations. A drop of lymph is placed on the skin and the point of a Hagedorn needle is applied through the lymph; then pressure is applied on the side of the shaft of the needle so as to indent the skin but not to draw blood. Twenty pressures are made (*i.e.*, the skin is indented 20 times) over an area not greater than ⅛ inch diameter. For primary vaccination this is done with one drop of lymph, for re-vaccination with two drops of lymph and in a small-pox contact with three drops of lymph. A sterile (not antiseptic) dressing is then applied. *Primary vaccination* is safest and best performed in the third–sixth month of life. *Re-vaccination* is necessary each 5 to 7 years, if immunity is to be maintained. Skin disease, especially unhealed eczema or an open wound, a poor general state of health or anæmia, the first 3 months of pregnancy and recent exposure to other acute specific fevers, are the only indications to postpone vaccination. Contact cases with eczema, or in early pregnancy, should be given 20 ml. of convalescent serum instead of being vaccinated.

The Phenomena of Vaccination.—The primary reaction (vaccinia) occurs with a successful vaccination in a person vaccinated for the first time or after a very long interval (*i.e.*, in someone who possesses little or no immunity). On the second or third day a slight pimple, on the fourth day a definite papule and on the fifth day a bluish-white cupped vesicle appears. On the eighth day (the same day of the week as that on which the operation was performed) the vesicle *becomes pustular* and the areola increases during the next 2 days: at the same time the axillary or groin glands draining the area become swollen and painful. After the tenth day the pustule dries up; the scab falls on the fourteenth or fifteenth day, leaving a pitted cicatrix. Successful *re-vaccination* occurs earlier and the vesicle appears sooner because there is already a partial immunity. This accelerated reaction is known as *vaccinoid*. Following re-vaccination, the immediate reaction should be regarded as a sensitivity reaction; then a red itchy papule develops in 12 hours and fades within 3 days—although this may indicate that the person is completely immune to vaccinia and to small-pox it is dangerous to assume this; the only criterion of success is vesiculation.

It is now generally accepted that (1) efficient primary vaccination offers absolute protection against *infection* for the ensuing 5 or 6 years, and relative protection (gradually diminishing) for a considerable time; (2) primary vaccination lessens the *severity of the attack* of small-pox if contracted during the ensuing 20 or 30 years; (3) re-vaccination affords absolute *immunity from attack* during the ensuing 5 or 6 years, and relative protection for the rest of life; and (4) if everybody were vaccinated in infancy and again at twelve and twenty-one, small-pox would be exterminated.

Complications of Vaccination.—*Generalised vaccinia* is a rare condition found almost exclusively in children following the first vaccination. It generally occurs between the ninth and fourteenth days after vaccination and may be later still. It usually appears as a single crop of papules which mature into vesicles and pustules and later crust: occasionally there are separate crops for 5 to 6 weeks. The distribution of the lesions is not that of small-pox and there is greater variation in size of the lesions. Toxæmia is likely to be severe, but is only likely to be serious and even fatal when it supervenes on a pre-existing skin disease, especially eczema, seborrhœic dermatitis or impetigo. *Accidental vaccinia.*—Persons in charge of recently vaccinated children have frequently been inoculated by lymph from the child's arm, in various parts of the body, especially on the face, lips and eyes, and occasionally on the mouth, throat and genitals.

Various transient *rashes* of a scarlatiniform or morbilliform type, urticaria, erythema multiforme, and hæmorrhagic eruptions occur. *Secondary infections* such as impetigo, furunculosis, erysipelas, cellulitis and gangrene have become rare since the introduction of calf-lymph.

Post-vaccinal encephalitis, and less frequently other nervous manifestations such as meningitis, myelitis or polyneuritis develop 9 to 15 days after vaccination. *Symptoms.*—There is a sudden onset with pyrexia, headache and vomiting, which may be followed by delirium, convulsions or coma. Residual damage is rare, for cases usually end in coma and death, or in complete recovery. These sequelæ occur practically only in connection with primary vaccination, and the great majority have been found in children of school age; only 7·2 per cent. of 509 cases of post-vaccinal encephalitis occurred in the first year of life (McNair Scott). The best *treatment* of these nervous sequelæ is by intravenous injection of 5–10 ml. of the serum of a person recently successfully vaccinated with the same lymph (and see § 895).

§ 481. V. **Measles** (Synonym: Morbilli) may be defined as an infectious febrile disease attended by catarrh of the ocular, nasal and respiratory mucous membranes, and by an eruption of minute elevated papules which, as they enlarge, become aggregated into irregular and often crescentic groups. It is still very common, and in England and Wales over 750,000 cases were notified in 1961.

Symptoms commence after an incubation period of 7 to 14 days, usually 10 or 11. At the commencement of the incubation period and a few hours after infection, there may be a transient febrile catarrh and a fleeting rash; this may occur in 10 per cent. of cases and is known as the " illness of infection." Then the typical attack commences at the end of the incubation period. (1) *Prodromal symptoms* occur in the first 4 days until the typical rash appears: (i.) Pyrexia comes on abruptly, though not as suddenly as in scarlet fever, rising to 102–103° F on the evening of the first day. During the next 2 days it usually declines a little (Fig. 146). (ii.) Catarrhal symptoms arise, often with some sneezing and redness of the conjunctivæ. During the next 3 days these increase, with profuse lacrymation, redness and œdema of the conjunctivæ, a running nose, faucial injection, and a short dry cough with catarrh of the larynx and bronchi—indeed, if the temperature is not very high the case may be mistaken for coryza. The tonsils are inflamed and may present an exudation. (iii.) Koplik has described spots, which appear on the second or third day of the prodromal period, on the buccal mucous membrane opposite the bicuspid or molar teeth, and especially around and in front of the parotid duct. They are better seen in daylight than in artificial light and are often more numerous on one cheek than on the other: the typical lesions are *minute* white spots of pin-point dimensions surrounded by a red flush (§ 211). At times discrete and few in number, they may on occasion be very numerous, when they give an appearance of a white stippling on a slightly raised reddened base. They may be confused with

the much larger patches of thrush, but Koplik's spots are ⸱   away
only with difficulty. As they occur in at least 90 per cent. ⸱⸱ ⸱⸱ cases,
their diagnostic significance, before the typical rash appears, cannot be
over-estimated. (iv.) The tongue is at first furred, but gradually clears,
so that as the rash appears the tongue may come to resemble the strawberry tongue of scarlet fever. (v.) Transient prodromal rashes of macular
or scarlatiniform type are rare. (vi.) During the whole of this first phase
the child looks and is "a picture of misery." Photophobia is usual.

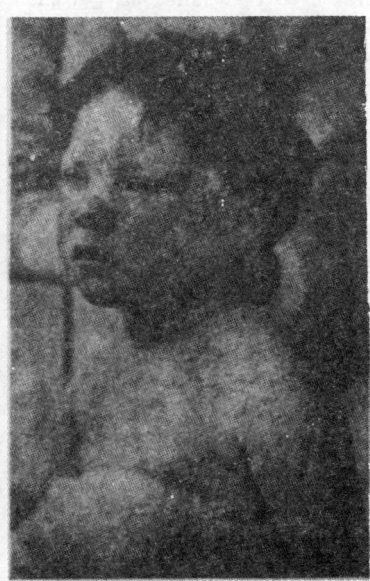

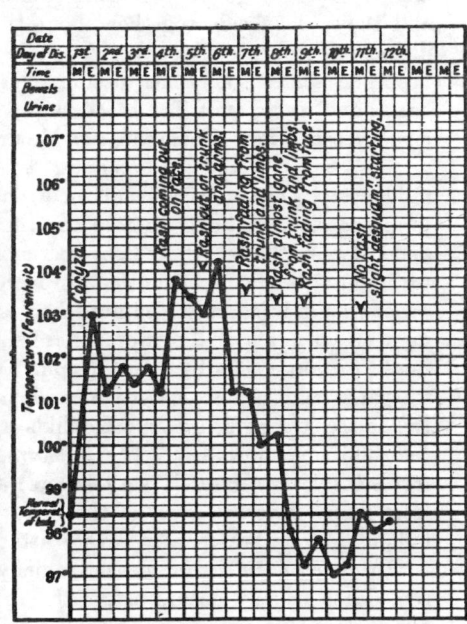

FIG. 145.—Measles—showing the catarrhal signs of conjunctivitis and nasal discharge, with the dusky macular rash coalescing into crescentic forms, with sub-cuticular œdema.

FIG. 146.—MEASLES.—Ethel H——, æt. 5. The various incidents are shown upon the chart.

Stage of Eruption. (i.) The typical rash appears on the third or more
usually on the fourth day (Coloured Plate II). It commences behind the
ears and along the hair margin of the forehead, temples and neck. Within
a few hours the whole face is involved (including the circum-oral region)
and then the whole body is affected: even so the rash is always more
marked on the face and trunk than on the more distant areas of the body.
At first there is a reddish-brown erythema, which develops into a *macular
rash* the colour of which may darken even to a maroon colour. Initially
the individual lesions are discrete, but as they become more numerous
they tend in the course of the next 2 days to coalesce into regularly shaped
blotchy patches. These are soft and velvety to the touch and the colour
fades on pressure, thus differing from the early stage of small-pox papules.

Soon the lesions begin to recede, and at the end of 48 hours to fade: within 4 to 5 days of its appearance (the ninth day of the disease) the rash has completely disappeared, except that a brownish mottling of the skin ("measles staining") remains for some time. (ii.) Occasionally the macules become petechial. (iii.) The temperature rises somewhat as the rash appears, remains up for the 2 days of its development (until the sixth day), and then falls by crisis (Fig. 146). (iv.) The constitutional symptoms (malaise, headache, insomnia, etc.) and the catarrhal symptoms (especially the cough) go on increasing during the development of the rash, and they all subside together about the sixth to the eighth day of the illness, as convalescence begins. (v.) Slight desquamation of minute bran-like scales sometimes occurs over the whole body, including the hands and feet. (vi.) The blood shows a leucopenia which is replaced by leucocytosis when a complication occurs.

Varieties.—Modified, Attenuated or Abortive Measles indicates a very mild attack, either as a result of a natural immunity or of the use of prophylactic measures. Before the third month of life, measles is rare, and between the fourth and seventh months attacks are usually modified by immune bodies transmitted through the placenta. In later life, the prophylactic injection of immune bodies (*vide infra*) may result in a very mild attack: catarrhal symptoms are slight, the temperature may not be raised for more than 24 hours, Koplik's spots may be absent and the rash is sparse and pale coloured: complications do not arise. Occasionally the initial temperature and Koplik's spots are not followed by a rash (morbilli sine morbillis). The *hæmorrhagic* or malignant variety (toxic), fortunately now rare, is very severe, and is attended by hæmorrhages from many different areas of the body: it is usually fatal. Occasionally bullous lesions are seen in severe attacks (Morbilli bullosa).

In *toxic or suffocative* measles, chiefly of rachitic and avitamised children, death usually occurs before the fourth day from cardio-respiratory failure (pulmonary œdema, cyanosis and coma). *Congenital* measles is a rare and mild form in which the mother and the child, which is often born prematurely, both have the rash at the same stage.

The *Diagnosis* from a severe common cold in the absence of Koplik's spots, is very difficult until the eruption appears. *Rubella* tends to occur at a later age than measles. The catarrhal symptoms and the temperature are much less marked although in adults and even in adolescents, rubella can produce severe catarrhal and constitutional symptoms. Enlarged sub-occipital glands are characteristic of rubella, while Koplik's spots are conclusive proof of measles. *Variola* often presents a difficulty; bronchial catarrh is common to both, but watering of the eyes and nose favours measles, while the presence of pain in the back and vomiting aid us considerably in diagnosing variola. The differences between the rashes are referred to on p. 682. *Erythema Multiforme* is somewhat like measles, but is recognised by the absence of catarrh, pyrexia and of Koplik's spots. The rash due to *sulphonamide drugs* is often morbilliform. A *serum rash* is especially suggestive and may lead to temporary confusion. The paramount importance of recognising Koplik's spots in the early diagnosis of measles can hardly be exaggerated.

Etiology.—Measles is especially a disease of childhood, and few escape. It is endemic in England, and two-yearly epidemics occur, especially in the spring and winter. The essential cause is a filter-passing virus which has been identified in the nasal secretions, the blood and in the brain when encephalitis occurs: the organism can be cultured on the chorioallantoic membrane of hen's eggs. It is spread by droplet infection from the nasal and bronchial secretions. Measles is most infectious before the eruption has appeared, and its infectivity disappears rapidly so that most cases are not infectious a week after the rash has appeared. Secondary infections by hæmolytic streptococci and by pneumococci are responsible for many of the complications. One attack confers relative immunity: the majority of so-called second attacks are probably rubella.

Prognosis.—Measles is not a serious disease in itself, except in infancy. It has become much milder in type in the last 30 to 40 years, and the death-rate in England and Wales is now 0·2 per thousand cases, but in children under 1 year it may rise to 3·0 per thousand. In countries where it has not previously been endemic, sudden epidemics may occur; in Greenland in 1951 99·9 per cent. of the population were affected with a death-rate of 18 per thousand cases. The most important determining factors otherwise are poverty and overcrowding, and the proportion of very young children. Children up to the age of 5 months are often immune and those up to the age of 9 months relatively immune (*vide supra*): after this age, and especially in the poorer classes, secondary infections are very prone to cause pneumonia, but even then much of the terror of this complication has been removed by modern chemotherapy and antibiotics. In middle-class children, the maximum incidence of measles is during the school age, when *complications* are fewer. (1) The most important and most common complication is broncho-pneumonia: even when recovery occurs, some residual pulmonary fibrosis and even bronchiectasis may ensue. (2) Catarrhal laryngitis, laryngismus or laryngeal diphtheria also occur. (3) In all cases of measles with sudden aggravation of fever for no apparent cause, acute otitis media should be suspected: this is usually caused by a hæmolytic streptococcal infection, especially before the age of 3 years, and often results in residual damage and even total deafness with deaf-mutism. (4) Conjunctivitis is a normal phenomena, but corneal ulceration which may proceed to perforation and panophthalmitis is dangerous. (5) Cancrum oris is rare nowadays; it is usually due to infection by Vincent's organisms, and begins as an ulcer on the inner surface of the cheek, surrounded by intense inflammation: soon a black slough appears, perhaps followed by perforation. (6) Acute enteritis in children before the age of 2 years may occur alone or with broncho-pneumonia. (7) Encephalitis occurs more frequently with measles than in any other acute exanthem: about the eighth day when the temperature has returned to normal, it is ushered in by drowsiness or convulsions: focal symptoms such as aphasia, hemiplegia and weakness of the external ocular muscles may result. The mortality rate of these complications is 20 per cent.; 40 per cent. make a complete recovery and the remainder have persistent defects, especially problems of behaviour and a decrease of mental capacity. A recognised *sequela* is tuberculosis, especially of the bronchial glands: it follows measles and whooping-cough more frequently than any other febrile disease, though measles does not rouse dormant tuberculosis into activity nor aggravate active disease so frequently as was formerly supposed.

Prophylaxis.—The·best and most effective remedy now used is gamma-globulin prepared from normal adult plasma and obtainable through the Public Health Laboratory Service: it gives minimal reactions and no case of jaundice following its use has been recorded. The dose given, dissolved in 3 ml. of sterile water, is shown in Table XXX. No permanent immunity results if this is used to prevent an attack developing—such immunity only follows an attenuated attack.

TABLE XXX.—MEASLES PROPHYLAXIS

with Gamma-globulin (intramusc.) and Convalescent serum (intramusc.)

Preparation used.	Age.	Doses for		Days after exposure to be given.
		Complete protection.	Attenuation.	
Gamma-globulin	Under 1 year 1–2 years 3 years and over	250 mg. 500 mg. 750 mg.	At all ages give 250 mg.	For protection 0–5 For attenuation 5–9
Convalescent serum	Up to 3 years Over 5 years	Age in years × 2 ml. 10 ml.	Age in years × 1 ml. Age in years × 2 ml. 5 ml.	0–5 5–9 5–9

Convalescent serum from a patient on the fourteenth day after the start of an attack is less effective but has a high antibody content; if prepared from one donor the risk of homologous serum jaundice is minimal. Prevention of an attack results if it is given before the fifth day of exposure to infection and attenuation if it is given before the ninth day. Adult serum and whole blood have a lower antibody content; for this reason and because of the risk of the young patient contracting jaundice (§ 334), which is of greater severity than in adults, these are now rarely given. Placental extract (immune globulin) tends to give severe local and general reactions and is rarely used.

Contacts who have not had measles should be closely watched from the end of the first week until 17 days after exposure and isolated immediately suspicious symptoms arise. Preventive measures are necessary in weakly children, in those in hospital or in bad environmental conditions. Exclusion from school may be desirable if the child is not entirely fit.

Treatment.—The patient is put into a shaded room, with plenty of fresh air. Admission to a fever hospital is better avoided if adequate isolation and nursing can be given at home, for cross-infection with hæmolytic streptococci and other organisms is thus avoided. Bronchitis is treated by a mixture containing ipecacuanha. (General treatment, see §§ 526 *et seq.*) For broncho-pneumonia and other complications, penicillin and/or the sulphonamides (§ 122) are of great value: the oxygen tent may be invaluable in small children. Particular attention must be paid to the ears, and to the hygiene of the eyes, the mouth and the nose.

§ 482. VI. **Rubella**, or German Measles (Synonym: Röteln), may be defined as an acute infectious disease, characterised by a polymorphous eruption, frequent enlargement of the lymphatic glands, little or no constitutional disturbance and almost invariably runs a mild course.

The *Symptoms* vary somewhat in different epidemics. (1) After a period of incubation varying between 14 and 19 days, and more often 17 or 18 days, the temperature rises to 99–101°. This is accompanied in adults by headache, pains in the limbs, and soon after by *slight* conjunctivitis and catarrhal symptoms. Usually the glands are swollen, the most characteristic being the upper cervical and occipital groups. Tender swelling of the posterior cervical glands is sometimes present several days before the rash appears, the patient often complaining of "stiff neck," which he usually ascribes to having sat in a draught, or some such reasonable explanation. Occasionally the glands in other areas enlarge. Especially in children, the rash may be the first symptom of the disease, and the constitutional symptoms and primary fever are slight or absent. (2) The rash usually occurs within 24 hours of the first symptoms: rarely it is delayed until the third or fourth day. It consists of minute round or oval rose-red spots, varying in size from a pin's head to a pea, very slightly raised, never papular. The rash at the outset appears behind the ears and on the forehead and face, and it is like that of early measles. In a day or two it becomes confluent, or nearly so, on the trunk, but on the limbs the rash is always discrete and sparse. In adults, itching may be troublesome. The rash usually lasts 2 to 3 days, and the severity of the attack is in direct relation to the severity and duration of the eruption. It is sometimes followed by slight desquamation and transient brownish staining. The blood shows a characteristic excess of Türk cells and often of plasma cells.

Diagnosis.—The characteristic features of rubella are the relative absence of catarrhal symptoms, the early appearance of the rash, and the cervical adenitis. In *measles*, the rash appears later in the disease, the temperature is usually higher and remains up for about 6 days: the child is miserable, catarrhal symptoms are marked and Koplik's spots can be identified. *Scarlet fever* shows an abrupt onset, with high fever and a high pulse-rate: the sore throat is marked with possibly a tonsillar exudate: headache and vomiting are usual. The rash appears on the *neck* and spreads downwards and is punctate in type, sparing the circumoral region: petechiæ occur in the flexures (Pastia's sign) and the Schultz-Charlton test is positive. *Glandular fever* is identified by the more widespread enlargement of the glands and by the blood picture: rashes are rare in this disease, but sore throat with an exudation on the tonsils is common. In *secondary Syphilis*, the rash is not irritable and the roseola spares the face (§ 705). Some *drug* and *serum rashes* may have to be considered.

Etiology.—It is mainly a disease of late childhood, or of young adults. It is not so infectious as either measles or scarlet fever. One attack confers immunity. It is caused by a virus which can be obtained from pharyngeal-saline washings at the height of the rash.

Prognosis.—It is a much more trivial disease than measles. *Complications* are rare: polyarthritis and severe rheumatic manifestations, purpura hæmorrhagica and encephalitis have been recorded. The chief *sequelæ* are in mothers who contract the disease in the first 4 months of pregnancy —the danger is much greater in the first and second months. Abortions and stillbirths are then more likely to occur, and 10 to 25 per cent. of the children are likely not to survive their second birthday or to be born with congenital defects, especially cataract, deaf-mutism, mental changes and congenital heart disease. These do not occur when the disease is contracted in later pregnancy.

Treatment is purely symptomatic. Isolation is necessary for 5 to 6 days. *Prophylaxis.*—When contact has occurred in a pregnant woman who has not had previous rubella, no action need be taken after the fourth month; within the first 4 months of pregnancy, such a patient should immediately receive gamma-globulin (prepared from rubella convalescent serum) 1·5 G. and white cell counts performed on her blood between 14 and 24 days after contact, for subclinical attacks still produce large numbers of Türk cells and plasma cells.

VI*a.* The term " **fourth disease,** " was suggested by Clement Dukes in 1900 as a provisional name for an acute exanthem which he regarded as distinct from scarlet fever, measles and rubella. The great majority of experts, however, do not recognise its autonomy, and are of opinion that most of the cases so described were examples of mild scarlet fever or rubella.

VI*b.* Erythema infectiosum, or " **fifth disease,** " is an acute exanthem appearing in epidemic or sporadic form in children between 5 and 12 years of age. It is characterised by its typical localisation on the cheeks and extremities, and almost complete absence of constitutional disturbance, complications and sequelæ. On the face, where it first appears as rose-red macules, it assumes the form of a butterfly's wings on both cheeks, which are hot and swollen; a few patches are also found on the forehead and chin. The rash next involves the extremities, especially the extensor surfaces where it develops a circinate appearance. On the trunk, which often escapes, the rash is usually morbilliform and lasts about 9 days. It is not followed by pigmentation or desquamation. The infectivity is very slight; it is uncommon to find several cases in a family or institution. The *prognosis* is excellent. No *treatment* is required.

VI*c.* **Exanthemum subitum, Roseola infantum** or " **sixth disease,** " is the name given in 1921 to an acute exanthem which occurs in children under 2 years of age. It usually runs a mild course without any symptoms beyond a 3-day fever and a morbilliform rash, which appears on the fourth day, simultaneously with the fall of the temperature. It fades without leaving pigmentation or desquamation. Cases have been reported mainly in the United States, in Europe and Japan, but only a few in Great Britain.

VII. TYPHOID and some fevers rare with a rash after the fourth day are described in Group II.

§ 483. VIII. Dengue (Break-bone fever: Dandy fever).—This is a specific fever lasting not more than 7 days and mainly confined to tropical climates. After an incubation period of 3 to 7 days there is sudden onset, with chilly feelings or a rigor followed by headache, aching eyeballs and rapid rise of temperature (100–105° F). Excruciating backache and joint pains follow; the joints are involved with peri-articular swelling and redness. The tongue is furred and the conjunctivæ injected. Often within 1 to 2 days the skin over the face, neck and chest becomes flushed and reddened (primary rash). Anorexia, vomiting, restlessness and insomnia may ensue. The pulse, which is at first rapid, now slows, and by the third or fourth day the temperature falls to 100° F or lower, with sweating and perhaps diarrhœa. The patient temporarily feels better, but after a few hours to 3 days the temperature again rises, the fever lasting 2 to 3 days, and a typical saddle-back chart results. The pain returns and a measly or scarlatiniform eruption (secondary rash) appears, which implicates the limbs and perhaps the trunk and lasts a few hours to 3 days. Desquamation and itching follow. A leucopenia with relative lymphocytosis is characteristic.

Etiology.—The disease, which may occur in big epidemics, is due to a filterable virus, transmitted by aëdine mosquitoes. All ages and both sexes are susceptible and the virus is demonstrable in the blood for the first 3 days. One attack does not invariably confer immunity. The mortality rate is 0·1 to 0·5 per cent.

The *Diagnosis* is easy during an epidemic, but sporadic cases have to be differentiated from typhus, yellow fever and sand-fly fever.

Treatment.—Prevention depends on anti-mosquito measures. Medicinal therapy is symptomatic.

THE RICKETTSIAL DISEASES (Table XXXI). CLASSICAL or EXANTHEMATIC TYPHUS is transmitted from man to man by lice, and occurs in *epidemic* form (Brill's disease is a sporadic recrudescence of this infection). MURINE TYPHUS is serologically closely related, and is fundamentally a disease of rodents: it is transmitted from animal to animal and to man by fleas: in man the disease resembles classical typhus but is milder and occurs in *endemic* form. ROCKY MOUNTAIN SPOTTED FEVER and certain other forms of Tick Typhus are transmitted from animal reservoirs to man by various ticks. SCRUB TYPHUS is an epizootic (*i.e.*, endemic) disease of rodents which is transmitted from animal to animal and to man by the bites of the larvæ of various species of mites. Q FEVER is also a rickettsial disease of man, transmitted from animal reservoirs by ticks, but it differs serologically and clinically from the other tick typhuses. TRENCH FEVER is a rickettsial disease of man transmitted by lice. RICKETTSIAL POX is transmitted from mice by a mite.

The Weil-Felix reaction is of value in recognising certain of these fevers, since in some of the infections the sera of patients will agglutinate special strains of *B. proteus*. Three strains are used—*B. proteus* OX19, OX2 and OXK. Sera from patients with classical or with murine typhus agglutinate OX19 and usually OX2; sera from tick typhus cases may sometimes agglutinate them, but weakly. Strain OXK is strongly agglutinated by sera from cases of scrub typhus. Agglutinins appear early in the second week of disease and may rise as high as 1 in 30,000 during convalescence. In the field a slide technique may be used as a rough guide. Specific complement-fixation tests are now also used.

§ 484. IX. Classical or Louse Typhus (Syn., Typhus exanthematicus, Hospital and Gaol Fever) is no longer found in England; its disappearance is a triumph of hygiene. As lice do not survive excessive heat, typhus appears in epidemics and may occur at any time of the year in Europe, but only during the cool weather in countries like Egypt and Palestine. Lice become infected some 5 to 10 days after feeding on infected human blood and remain infective for life. The causative agent, *Rickettsia prowazeki*, is found in the epithelial cells lining the gut of the louse and in its excreta; man acquires the disease by infected excreta entering through abrasions and not by the actual bite of the louse. Typhus is associated with overcrowding and personal squalor and is common in times of war, siege and famine. Both sexes are equally susceptible.

Symptoms.—(i.) The period of incubation varies from 5 to 20 days, but is usually about a fortnight. (ii.) There may be prodromal symptoms in the form of malaise,

TABLE XXXI.—THE TYPHUS GROUP OF FEVERS

	Disease.	Vector.	Rickettsia Organism.	Reservoir.	Weil-Felix Reaction.	Remarks.
The Typhus Fevers	CLASSICAL or EPIDEMIC TYPHUS—usually severe BRILL'S DISEASE (mild late manifestation)	Lice	R. prowazeki	Man	OX19+++ OX2 ++ OXK −	May be differentiated by using specific suspensions of rickettsias in agglutination and complement fixation reactions.
	MURINE or ENDEMIC TYPHUS — widespread and usually benign. Ship typhus (Toulon), Urban Shop typhus (Malaya, etc.)	Rat fleas	R. mooseri	Rats and mice	OX19+++ OX2 ++ OXK −	
	TICK TYPHUS:— (a) ROCKY MOUNTAIN SPOTTED FEVER	Ticks	R. rickettsii	Wild rodents and ticks	OX19+ OX2 + OXK + (Variable low titres)	
	With local lesions:— (b) FIÈVRE BOUTONNEUSE (Mediterranean), TICK TYPHUS	,,	R. conori (R. pijperi)	Dog, rodents and ticks	OX19+ OX2 +	
	SCRUB TYPHUS (Tsutsugamushi fever)	Larval Trombiculid mites	R. orientalis (R. tsutsugamushi)	Field rodents and mites	OX19− OX2 − OXK+++	
	Q FEVER	Tick faeces Dust borne. Milk	R. burneti (R. diasporica)	? Cattle		Complement fixation test is positive.
	TRENCH FEVER . . .	Lice	R. quintana	Man		
	RICKETTSIAL POX . .	Mouse mites	R. akari	House mice		

but the onset is usually abrupt with shivering, rise of temperature to 103° or 104° F, and sometimes vomiting. The face and eyes are congested, the tongue coated, the breath foul, and there is persistent headache, bronchitis, and a characteristic drunken or stuporose appearance. In rare fulminating cases there may be fits and delirium. After a week of great prostration delirium develops, sometimes drowsiness and coma. The temperature remains high for 12 to 14 days, with slight morning remissions; then falls by rapid lysis as a rule, less frequently by crisis. (iii.) The spleen may be palpable, but the abdomen is not distended. (iv.) The rash appears on the fourth or fifth day, first on the abdomen and axillæ, and spreads to the chest, back and trunk: the face is rarely involved. It has two elements: a dusky subcuticular mottling.

and purple roseolar macules, which may become petechial. (v.) There is no definite blood picture, but a leucocytosis of 12,000 to 15,000 is common.

Diagnosis.—The Weil-Felix reaction (*i.e.*, agglutination of *B. proteus* OX19 by the serum of typhus cases in dilutions of 1–100 to 1–2,000 or higher) is a very valuable reaction, but is not obtained until the end of the first week. (1) *Typhoid fever* was originally confused with typhus, but differs in its insidious onset, type of temperature, leucopenia, rash, bacteriology and serology. (2) In *measles* the eruption resembles the typhus spots, and appears at the same date, but in typhus it does not involve the face, it is never preceded by catarrh, is never papular, and becomes petechial. (3) Some *malarial* fevers occasionally present difficulty, but they have no eruption. (4) *Uræmia* and other causes of coma may be mistaken for it. (5) Apical *pneumonia*, *meningitis*, and other causes of the *typhoid state* may be confused with typhus. The cerebro-spinal fluid may be increased in pressure and contain an excess of lymphocytes in typhus. The bubonic swellings in *plague* occur earlier, during the first week.

Prognosis.—Case-mortality, 20–40 per cent.: between the age of 15 and 25, 4 per cent.; over 50, 50 per cent. or more. Thus the mortality is greatly influenced by the age of the patient, and by previous preventive inoculation. One attack usually confers immunity. Typhus is always a serious disease, especially in the plethoric and alcoholic. It terminates fatally in three ways : (i.) Toxic myocarditis is a very common accompaniment; (ii.) coma from toxæmia; or (iii.) pneumonia. Untoward symptoms are (i.) a weak, irregular or intermittent pulse, or other indications of cardiac weakness; (ii.) an abundant rash, with high fever; (iii.) early and protracted cerebral signs or protracted hiccough; (iv.) all complications, especially pulmonary. Of the *complications* and *sequelæ*, (i.) the pulmonary are the worst, especially broncho-pneumonia and hypostatic congestion of the lungs; œdema glottidis and pleurisy are less common. Other complications are (ii.) hyperpyrexia and meningitis; (iii) femoral and other thromboses; (iv.) gangrene of the extremities from embolism, bed-sores and pyæmic abscesses (v.) cardiac weakness, which may remain for a long time, on account of the granular degeneration of the muscle ; (vi.) post-febrile mania ; and (vii.) paralysis of various parts.

Brill's disease is a mild form of typhus found in the United States of America. It occurs sporadically among immigrants from eastern Europe and is now considered to be due to exacerbations of latent louse-borne infections. *Symptoms.*—The onset is generally rapid; the fever, which is of continuous type, terminates by crisis about the fourteenth day. Frontal headache, mental apathy and profound prostration are notable features. The eruption, which is maculo-papular and rarely petechial in type, appears about the fifth day. The mortality is low and does not exceed 2 per cent.

Murine Typhus is world-wide, but occurs especially in Mexico, U.S.A., Palestine, N. Africa, Egypt and Abyssinia. It is similar to but milder than louse-borne typhus; it is transmitted by fleas from infected rats. Unlike the virus of louse-borne typhus, the murine virus produces a characteristic reaction in the tunica vaginalis of male guinea-pigs. Protective measures include anti-rat campaigns, destroying fleas by dusting rat runs and floors with 5–10 per cent. DDT, and protective vaccination of individuals.

§ 485. X. **Rocky Mountain Spotted Fever.**—*Symptoms:* During the incubation period of 4 to 12 days irritation and pain may be experienced in the tick-bites. The fever often commences with a slight rigor, and the temperature rapidly rises to 103°, and later to 105° or even 107° F; the maximum is reached by the fifth to the twelfth day. About the third day the eruption appears in the form of macules on the wrists and ankles; these rapidly spread all over the body, including the face, and may become hæmorrhagic. The spleen is palpable and tender. There may be slight bronchitis and sore throat. Epistaxis and jaundice are not infrequent. Pneumonia is a common complication. Gangrene of the fingers, genitals, etc., may occur. The temperature in favourable cases falls by lysis; if it remains high the patient lapses into a typhoid state and does not recover. Early albuminuria and a leucocytosis with an increase in monocytes are found.

Etiology.—It is due to *Rickettsia rickettsii*, spread by ticks of the genus *Dermacentor* which live on certain domesticated animals and rodents harbouring the infective agent. It occurs not only in the Western States of the United States of America but also in certain Eastern States and in Columbia.

Diagnosis.—The disease resembles typhoid and louse typhus. From the former it is differentiated by the eruption, but it cannot always be distinguished from typhus. Exposure to infection by residence in an infected region may be taken into account.

The *prognosis* varies in different localities. The Western form has a mortality as high as 90 per cent.: the Eastern form is milder and the mortality is only 5–10 per cent.

Prophylaxis consists in the avoidance of the places which are tick-infested and by destroying the ticks by the application of ammonia, turpentine, etc. The bite may be cauterised with pure phenol. Vaccination by injection of formolised suspensions of triturated infected ticks gives good protection.

Other forms of Tick Typhus occur in the Mediterranean basin (fièvre boutonneuse, transmitted from dogs by the dog tick); also in Africa, India, S. America and elsewhere. The illness is seldom severe.

§ 486. XI. Scrub Typhus (Syn., Japanese River Fever, Tsutsugamushi Fever, tropical typhus, mite typhus—Sumatra, Australia, India, Burma, etc., rural scrub typhus—Malaya).—A typhus-like disease occurring in scattered areas throughout the Far East and Australia.

Symptoms.—Some 5 to 14 days after being bitten by mites the patient develops a shiver, headache, giddiness and fever lasting 2 to 3 weeks. This is at first continuous and later remittent in type. Locally there is a small ulcer or ulcers associated with a dark areola and redness, with lymphangitis and enlargement of the regional lymph glands. On the fifth to seventh day a papular and red macular eruption appears involving the face and trunk, limbs, hands and feet. The spleen may be enlarged. When the scab separates it may leave a punched-out ulcer in the second week which may take weeks to heal. The Weil-Felix reaction is strongly positive to *B. Proteus* OXK, and there is a leucopenia associated with a decrease in the neutrophils.

Etiology.—The disease is due to *R. orientalis*, transmitted by the bites of various species of larval *Trombicula* mite, the animal reservoirs of infection being various field rodents. The larva bores into the skin and causes local necrosis and ulceration followed by lymphangitis and adenitis.

Prognosis.—The mortality varies from 5 to 60 per cent.: it is better in the young and in a subsequent than in the first attack.

Prophylaxis.—Excellent protection against mites is given by impregnating clothing and bedding with dimethyl phthalate.

§ 487. XII. Q Fever occurs widely throughout the world as a disease primarily of cattle; it is sometimes transmitted to man and 11 outbreaks have been recorded in Great Britain in the last 10 years. Adults handling livestock or working in slaughter-houses are primarily affected and children are rarely involved.

Symptoms.—The onset is sudden after an uncertain period of incubation. There is high fever often swinging to 103°, usually a severe retro-orbital headache, delirium, occasionally nausea and vomiting. Pain in the back and chest is accompanied in the first few days by drenching sweats and a dry cough: most cases develop an atypical pneumonia (§ 123), with slight physical signs; X-ray examination shows diffuse patchy consolidation in both lung fields. The illness usually lasts 1–4 weeks and deaths are rare.

Diagnosis is by a positive complement-fixation reaction after the first week, by blood culture, or by intraperitoneal injection of blood or urine into guinea-pigs.

Etiology.—The organism, *Rickettsia burneti*, is inhaled from the dried fæces of various ticks which are chiefly carried by domestic ruminants, sheep and cattle; the infecting agent is then transmitted to man by inhalation of dried dust or in milk. The ticks may also infect domestic and wild birds, rats, the shrew mouse, dormice and mountain rabbits. Outbreaks from these sources usually occur in the spring and autumn, particularly from parturient animals, but arise from human respiratory cross-infection at any time of the year. *R. burneti* can persist in the human being for years; relapses, cases with a chronic illness and subacute infective endocarditis are recorded.

§ 488. XIII. Trench Fever (Syn., Weigl's disease and similar fevers of Russia and Poland) is characterised by fever of a relapsing type and frequently but by no means invariably, by pains in the shins. It only occurs in times of war.

Symptoms.—In the acute type there is high fever for 5 to 8 days, and after an afebrile period there are relapses recurring at 5-day intervals. A macular rash, chiefly affecting the thorax and abdomen, is found in about 80 per cent. at the onset or during a relapse. Slight and transient nephritis is frequent. In the chronic type the onset shows only a lengthy period of increasing incapacity. In both types the febrile wave is accompanied by severe headache, tenderness of the loin and calf muscles and pains in the shins with nocturnal exacerbations. The spleen is sometimes enlarged. *Etiology.*—The cause is probably *Rickettsia quintana*, transmitted in the excreta of lice. *Prognosis.*—Trench fever may run a protracted course, and the patient develop a neurasthenic condition. *Treatment* is symptomatic.

§ 489. XIV. Rickettsial Pox has recently been described in New York as being carried by a blood-sucking mouse mite, which transmits *R. akari*.

Symptoms.—Initially there is a deep-seated single papule which enlarges to form a vesicle: in 1-2 weeks a scab forms which leaves a small scar. A week after the initial lesion there is sudden fever to 103-104°, gradually declining over the next 7 days. Frontal headache, photophobia and backache may be associated with nausea, vomiting and transient splenic enlargement. Within the first 4 days of fever a maculo-papular rash appears which vesiculates and gives black crusts.

The *Prognosis* is excellent.

TREATMENT OF THE TYPHUS FEVERS.—Caps. chloramphenicol B.P. or chlortetracycline (Aureomycin) are extremely effective and one of these should be given as soon as possible. The initial dose is 3·0 G., followed by 0·25 G. 3-hourly for 24 hours and then by smaller doses for another 6 days. The maintenance of the fluid and electrolyte balance is important and careful nursing is required. For Q fever give 0·5 G. every 4 hours until the temperature has been normal for 3 days. *Prophylaxis.*—In an epidemic of classical typhus prompt delousing of the whole surrounding population with dicophane (DDT) powder dusted on to skin, hair and clothes must be undertaken at once; it remains lethal to lice for several weeks. All clothing and bedding needs steam disinfection. Medical and nursing personnel and others at special risk should wear protective clothing impregnated with an insect repellent. *Prophylactic vaccines*, which are fairly effective, are available against the louse- and flea-borne diseases, but not against the tick- or mite-borne fevers.

§ 490. XV. Anthrax (Syn., Malignant Pustule) is due to infection with the *Bacillus anthracis*. The lesion is almost always situated on exposed parts, the dorsum of the hand, arm or face; 82 per cent. of the cases show the pustule on the head or neck. It affects woolsorters, furriers, feltmakers, ragsorters and others who come in contact with animals or their hides, fur or bonemeal; 40 per cent. of the cases in British leather-workers are due to handling Chinese or East Indian goods. No case has been traced to wet salted hides.

Symptoms.—The incubation period is 24 to 72 hours. First a papule forms at the seat of inoculation, which rapidly enlarges, and becomes on the second day a vesicle, with serous or hæmorrhagic contents and with considerable local œdema. On the third day this bursts, leaving a raw exuding surface, which, on the fourth day, turns to a dry black slough, surrounded by a zone of intense inflammation slightly raised above the surface. Upon this inflammatory zone there appears, also on the fourth day, a characteristic ring of small red vesicles. The œdema extends around, and the lymphatics and the glands inflame. The pain is usually very slight, and no pus forms until about the tenth day, when the slough begins to separate. The constitutional symptoms bear no proportion to the local mischief. The pyrexia may be so slight as not to interfere with the patient's ordinary work, and it may not come on until some days after the local signs. Usually, however, it is severe, comes on early, soon assumes a typhoid character, and there is a positive blood culture. *Intestinal* and *Pulmonary* types are also described, according to the method of infection. In the former intense vomiting and diarrhœa occur, with great prostration and cramps, with, in some cases, cyanosis and dyspnœa, and towards the end convulsions and spasms. The spleen is enlarged. In the pulmonary type, due to inhalation of diseased wool or hair (*woolsorters' disease*), there are urgent dyspnœa, and pain in the chest of sudden onset. The temperature rises to 102° to 103° F, and death may occur with profound collapse in 24 hours. Sometimes delirium and convulsions, or diarrhœa and vomiting, occur.

Diagnosis.—It may have to be diagnosed in the first place from the sting of an insect, from various conditions which lead to solitary vesicles or bullæ on the second day, from erysipelas (if on the face), lymphangitis and other causes of œdema. The occupation of the patient assists, but a diagnosis may be made by examining the serum or secretion of the sore, stained by Gram's method (§ 1202), under the microscope; the *Bacillus anthracis* is thus readily discovered.

Prognosis.—The mortality varies with the position of the primary lesion, being 40 per cent. when this is on the neck or face, and 12 per cent. when situated elsewhere. In the gastro-intestinal, pulmonary and meningitic forms it is over 90 per cent.

Treatment with penicillin and streptomycin is not always successful and has now been superseded by caps. chloramphenicol or otherwise by one of the tetracyclines in doses of 0·5 G. 4-hourly for 3 days. Anti-anthrax serum 200–500 ml. each 12–24 hours is only occasionally used. Surgical procedures may spread the disease. Mild antiseptics such as a dilute solution of formalin can be applied to the lesion.

§ 491. XVI. Glanders (Syn., Equinia) may be defined as an infectious febrile disease attended by a discharge from the nostrils, and sometimes an eruption on the skin, due to the inoculation of the *Bacillus mallei*, in a person attending to HORSES affected with the disease. The eruption, which only occurs in ACUTE GLANDERS, consists of a general erythema, on which a crop of pustules of hemispherical shape appear in the course of a few days or hours. They vary in size between a lentil and a florin. There are also nodules of granulomatous material in the subcutaneous tissue and muscles, which usually suppurate, leaving large foul ulcers. The other symptoms are (i.) a copious discharge of viscid, semipurulent matter from the nostrils; (ii.) pains in the limbs and joints; and (iii.) high fever, with rigors and prostration, passing on to the typhoid state.

In CHRONIC GLANDERS (Farcy) the pyrexia and constitutional symptoms are absent, also the cutaneous eruptions (erythema, pustules and nodules which leave ulcers and sinuses). The discharge from the nose may be the only sign.

Diagnosis.—The pustules of acute glanders resemble those of variola, but they are larger, are not umbilicated, and the temperature in glanders does not fall with the rash in those cases which present a generalised pustular eruption. The pain and swelling of the joints and limbs bear some resemblance to acute rheumatism, and still more to pyæmia. The reaction to mallein may assist.

Treatment.—At present the disease is extremely fatal. Specific serum and vaccine treatment have been unsuccessful. Sulphadiazine in full doses for 3 weeks has been reported upon as curative, and inj. streptomycin has given good results. In FARCY or CHRONIC GLANDERS the death-rate is 40 or 50 per cent.

GROUP II. CONTINUED PYREXIA

§ **492.** In this group the pyrexia tends to assume a CONTINUED TYPE —*i.e.*, it runs a continuous course except for the slight normal diurnal variation (§ 471). This group is distinguished from Group I by the absence of an eruption during the first four days of the illness. It is distinguished from Group III mainly by the course of the pyrexia, though aberrant types of one group are found in the other.

Some of the fevers rare in this country have an eruption which develops usually after the fourth day.

TYPHOID FEVER, which may be taken as a type, may in exceptional cases present no other symptoms than *the characteristic pyrexia*. The rash, when present, may be ill-marked, and does not appear till the second week of the disease. In DIPHTHERIA there is the characteristic *throat lesion*; in INFLUENZA there are *pains in the limbs* and a more sudden advent; in PERTUSSIS the *characteristic cough*; and in MUMPS the *parotitis*. Various PATHOLOGICAL TESTS may aid diagnosis. CHOLERA (§ 311) and DYSENTERY (§ 308) might also be included in this group, but the pyrexial disturbance is quite a subordinate feature compared with the intestinal manifestations.

Long-continued fevers which cause difficulty in diagnosis are usually due to tuberculosis, malignant disease (especially of the kidney or bronchus), typhoid or paratyphoid fever, sepsis, subacute bacterial endocarditis, urinary infection, malaria, glandular fever, brucellosis, syphilis, reticulosis, Hodgkin's disease, polyarteritis nodosa or disseminated lupus erythematosus.

Under " sepsis " are included all abscesses such as originate in the appendix, gall-bladder, genito-urinary tract, or alimentary canal or empyema (§§ 499 and 517).

<table>
<tr><td colspan="2">*Common*</td><td colspan="2">*Rare in Britain*</td></tr>
<tr><td>I. Influenza .. .. ..</td><td>§ 493</td><td>IX. Plague .. .. ..</td><td>§ 501</td></tr>
<tr><td>II. Whooping-cough.. ..</td><td>§ 494</td><td>X. Undulant fever.. ..</td><td>§ 502</td></tr>
<tr><td>III. Mumps .. .. ..</td><td>§ 495</td><td>XI. Yellow fever .. ..</td><td>§ 503</td></tr>
<tr><td>IV. The Enteric Fevers (Typhoid</td><td></td><td>XII. Cerebro-spinal fever ..</td><td>§ 504</td></tr>
<tr><td>and Paratyphoid) ..</td><td>§ 496</td><td>XIII. Relapsing fever ..</td><td>§ 505</td></tr>
<tr><td>V. Diphtheria .. ..</td><td>§ 497</td><td>XIV. Other fevers, rare or un-</td><td></td></tr>
<tr><td>VI. Glandular fever .. ..</td><td>§ 498</td><td>known in this country,</td><td></td></tr>
<tr><td>VII. Rheumatic fever, pneu-</td><td></td><td>transmitted by ticks,</td><td></td></tr>
<tr><td>monia, and various other</td><td></td><td>sand-flies, etc.; Tular-</td><td></td></tr>
<tr><td>inflammatory disorders,</td><td></td><td>æmia, Kala-azar, Phle-</td><td></td></tr>
<tr><td>usually attended by local</td><td></td><td>botomus fever, Rat-</td><td></td></tr>
<tr><td>signs .. .. ..</td><td>§ 499</td><td>bite fever .. ..</td><td>§ 506</td></tr>
<tr><td>VIII. Syphilis .. .. ..</td><td>§ 500</td><td>XV. Psittacosis .. ..</td><td>§ 507</td></tr>
<tr><td></td><td></td><td>XVI. Cat-scratch fever ..</td><td>§ 508</td></tr>
<tr><td></td><td></td><td>XVII. Bornholm Disease ..</td><td>§ 509</td></tr>
<tr><td></td><td></td><td>XVIII. Toxoplasmosis .. ..</td><td>§ 509a</td></tr>
<tr><td></td><td></td><td>XIX. Heat stroke .. ..</td><td>§ 510</td></tr>
<tr><td></td><td></td><td>XX. Weil's Disease .. ..</td><td>§ 334b</td></tr>
</table>

§ **493.** I. **Influenza** is an acute fever which, although endemic in the winter and spring months, is liable to break out in widespread epidemics affecting even 30–70 per cent. of the population. It has been known for at least five centuries, and certain of the great pandemics have been

attended by a considerable mortality: that of 1918–19 produced nearly 20 million deaths.

Symptoms.—(1) After an incubation period of 1 to 3 days, the patient's temperature rises in a few hours to 102–104°. The onset is frequently attended by severe headache, pain behind the eyes, shivering, anorexia, and pains in the limbs and back which form such a characteristic feature of influenza. (2) The pulse rate is often relatively slowed in proportion to the temperature, and a true bradycardia may occur. (3) The constitutional symptoms, malaise and prostration are out of all proportion to the pyrexia and to the local signs. (4) Catarrh usually accompanies the fever—*i.e.*, there is some redness and watering of the eyes, nasal catarrh, sore throat and a dry cough. (5) The face is flushed and the tongue heavily coated. (6) *Eruptions* of erythematous or urticarial type occur. (7) Some cases present only the above symptoms and signs: but *types of the disease* occur in which different systems of the body are attacked. Some of the symptoms thus presented are of the nature of complications: (i.) The *respiratory tract* is very frequently involved, and laryngitis, tracheitis, bronchitis and pneumonia may arise. *Fulminating influenza* follows the usual initial symptoms with dyspnœa, retro-sternal pain, cyanosis, frothy hæmorrhagic sputum which causes death from widespread tracheo-bronchitis and lung hæmorrhages within 2–3 days. (ii.) The *heart* may be affected by myocarditis. (iii.) Involvement of the *alimentary* tract may be evidenced by gastro-enteritis, diarrhœa, vomiting, etc. (" gastric influenza "). (iv., The *nervous system* may possibly be attacked, and encephalomyelitis occur. Cases of disseminated sclerosis and encephalitis lethargica have been attributed to this disease. Influenzal meningitis is due to Pfeiffer's bacillus and not to true influenza.

Diagnosis.—The term " influenza " is often improperly applied to what is really febrile catarrh. In addition to the absence of the influenza virus in febrile catarrh, this clinical distinction is drawn by C. H. Stuart Harris: (1) Premonitory symptoms, such as coryza, sore throat or cough, are uncommon in influenza, in which the onset is sudden, whereas febrile catarrh starts insidiously with a " cold " and fever. (2) The first symptoms of influenza are constitutional rather than respiratory. (3) The cough in influenza is short and dry; in febrile catarrh it is paroxysmal, painful and often productive. (4) Sore throat is constant in febrile catarrh, but is not a feature of influenza. (5) Laryngitis is rarely severe in influenza, but a very hoarse voice is common in febrile catarrh. (6) Bronchiolitis and pneumonia are the characteristic complications of influenza, and basal bronchitis and broncho-pneumonia of febrile catarrh. Leucopenia is usual in uncomplicated cases.

Etiology.—The agent responsible is a virus, of which three varieties, A, B and C, have so far been identified. Virus A in particular consists of many strains with different antigenic activities; Asiatic virus A is antigenically different from the viruses met in recent epidemic years. Wilson-Smith, Andrewes and Laidlaw have reproduced influenza in ferrets by intranasal installation of filtrates of throat and nose washings containing the virus from influenza patients, and have found that mice are susceptible to the virus of human and swine influenza, and that this virus can be retransmitted to man. The virus can be grown on the developing chick embryo, and the serum of human convalescents contains specific virus-neutralising antibodies. Virus A is mainly responsible for major outbreaks and epidemics; virus B is essentially endemic and can cause epidemics; virus C is widespread and produces milder symptoms than virus A and virus B, often in the form of subclinical influenza. Pfeiffer's bacillus is not causal, but this organism, hæmolytic streptococci or *Staphylococcus aureus* are responsible for many of the complications. One attack confers no immunity: old and young, rich and poor are attacked alike.

Prognosis.—The case-mortality is about 1 per cent. among the old and young together. In middle-aged and elderly people the respiratory type is very apt to end fatally with pneumonia, and undoubtedly many cases presumed to be primary pneumonia are really secondary to influenza. Usually it is fatal only through its complications—chiefly respiratory in type and often accompanied by a penicillin-resistant staphylococcal infection which results in profound toxæmia and circulatory collapse. The disease itself is usually trivial, and the patient soon recovers.

Complications are chiefly respiratory, and include sinusitis, otitis media and mastoiditis, bronchitis and broncho-pneumonia. These are caused almost entirely by the associated secondary infections. Relapses are common. The *sequelæ* are often more troublesome than the disease itself: (i.) There is a neuro-vascular asthenia, causing weakness in the legs, tachycardia or bradycardia, palpitation, flushings, faintings, perspiration, dyspnœa and the like. (ii.) Anxiety states, depression, neurasthenia, neuritis and neuralgia may be very persistent. Insomnia can be very troublesome.

Treatment.—There is no specific treatment. During the attack, and for several days after the temperature has become normal, the patient should be kept in bed in view of the sequelæ: aspirin, sodium salicylate and codein will reduce the fever and lessen the pains in the limbs. For the complicating infections, the sulphonamides and /or penicillin are most useful. In severe cases where a penicillin-resistant staphylococcus may be present, methicillin (Celbenin) should be injected in doses of 1 G. each 4 hours; otherwise give benzylpenicillin with either inject. streptomycin 1 G. each 8–12 hours or with oral erythromycin 1 G. 6-hourly. In these cases the oxygen tent is essential, and hydrocortisone 25 mg. 2-hourly (intravenously) has been favourably reported on. *Prophylaxis.*—It is well to keep elderly people away from infection during an epidemic. A patient is not infectious to others 48 hours from the onset, unless pneumonia ensues, when infection can be transmitted up to 6 days. The prophylactic value of a vaccine, prepared by virus culture on embryonic hen's egg, with two doses at a 4-weekly interval, is giving good results in 30–40 per cent. of cases.

§ 494. II. Whooping-Cough (Pertussis) is an acute specific infectious disease of world-wide distribution characterised by an initial catarrh, and usually followed by paroxysmal attacks of coughing, succeeded by a long noisy inspiration (or whoop) and usually vomiting. The condition is the most serious of the infectious diseases of children in Great Britain at the present time. It is most common in those under 5 years of age, but adults are not exempt. The patients are highly infectious before the nature of the illness can be diagnosed.

Symptoms.—Following an incubation period of 7–14 days there is (1) a preliminary *Catarrhal Stage* which is apt to be overlooked unless inquired for. Running from the nose and sometimes from the eyes is attended by malaise and a low-grade temperature. Soon a short dry cough develops and becomes more persistent, and the individual coughs become grouped together. This catarrhal state lasts up to a week or more, and is followed by (2) *Paroxysms of Coughing* for weeks or months. (i.) These are more noticeable at night and vary considerably in severity. In milder cases there are a series of explosive coughs in rapid succession, followed by a long-drawn inspiration. In typical cases the explosive coughs follow one another until the child has largely emptied the lungs of expired air, and this is succeeded by a loud inspiratory crow or *whoop*, through the narrowed chink of the half-closed glottis. One attack may succeed another, punctuated by a series of whoops, until the child manages to dislodge and cough up a small piece of tenacious mucus, often with *vomiting*. In the process, the face and eyes become more and more congested, and the lips cyanosed, and when the attack is over there is temporary exhaustion. (ii.) The onset of an attack is often recognised by the child who runs to his mother for comfort: attacks are made more frequent by food and by any excitement. (iii.) As a result of the straining cough, the face remains somewhat swollen between the attacks; and subconjunctival hæmorrhages, epistaxis and a blood-streaked sputum may occur. (iv.) The number and severity of the paroxysms increases to a maximum which is maintained for a week or more, and then starts to decrease. The whoop gradually disappears, but the paroxysmal cough persists for weeks or months after the acute phase has passed. (v.) The temperature is lower than in the catarrhal phase, unless complications ensue, but usually there is some tachycardia: in milder cases the child is apparently quite well between the attacks of coughing, although a puffiness of the face may persist. (vi.) There are no characteristic physical signs in the lungs, and bronchitic signs are generally not as numerous as the severity of the cough would suggest. (vii.) The disturbed sleep and the difficulties of feeding cause considerable exhaustion even for weeks or months. (viii.) There is a tendency for the whoop to return on taking a fresh cold, for months or years, without any return of the original infection.

The clinical *varieties* are: (1) The disease passes through the catarrhal stage to that of the paroxysmal cough, but whooping never eventuates: even in the absence of whooping, repeated paroxysms of coughing succeeded by vomiting, render the diagnosis almost certain. (2) In some adults, and when broncho-pneumonia supervenes in the catarrhal stage in children, the cough may be spasmodic without being paroxysmal. (3) In one atypical form in infants, attacks of sneezing or hiccough replace the paroxysmal cough.

The *Diagnosis* is usually simple during an epidemic, but otherwise the early catarrhal symptoms may be mistaken for *coryza*. Tuberculosis or other causes of *enlargement of the tracheo-bronchial glands* gives rise to a paroxysmal cough, but the whoop is absent. In the first stage of the disease there is a leucopenia, but during the second stage there is a leucocytosis usually ranging from 15,000 even up to 27,000, with 70–80 per cent. of lymphocytes. The erythrocyte sedimentation rate is slightly retarded or normal in uncomplicated cases, but rises with any complication. Isolation of *H. pertussis*, either by the cough plate method, or by inoculating a plate of Bordet-Gengou-penicillin or diamidine-fluoride penicillin medium from a per-nasal swab, is the most certain means of diagnosis early in the disease, and is of particular value in atypical and abortive cases.

Etiology.—Bordet and Gengou found that the causal organism is a cocco-bacillus (*Hæmophilus pertussis*) which is most abundant in the respiratory mucus in the catarrhal stage. The less common *H. parapertussis* produces a milder disease; it differs from *H. pertussis* culturally, serologically and in its antigenic properties.

Prognosis.—With the decrease of virulence of diphtheria, scarlet fever and measles, whooping-cough has become one of the most serious of the specific diseases of childhood, and as such is now compulsorily notifiable in England and Wales. The incidence of the disease is not materially lessening, but deaths from the disease have dropped from 4,000–6,000 a year 35 years ago to 27 in 1961. The immediate prognosis depends particularly on the age of the child, as it is much more likely to be fatal under one year especially in the first 6 months of life: otherwise on the severity of the attack, and especially on the occurrence of secondary infections with a hæmolytic streptococcus, pneumococcus or *H. influenzæ*: then a serious *complication* is broncho-pneumonia, the importance of which has lessened with the advent of chemotherapy. Convulsions in infancy are more liable to occur if there is a tendency to infantile tetany. Spasm of the glottis may be the cause of sudden death. Other complications include cerebral or retro-bulbar hæmorrhages, otitis media, right-sided cardiac dilatation; an ulcer under the frenum of the tongue is due to the forced protrusion against the teeth in the act of coughing. Among the *sequelæ* there is a particular tendency for broncho-pneumonia to be followed by fibroid lung and bronchiectasis; whooping-cough may reactivate a dormant tuberculous infection in the chest: and herniæ or prolapse of the rectum are seen. Recurrence is very unusual.

Treatment.—The child should be nursed in an airy room, with considerable bed spacing from other children to prevent secondary infections being spread from the one to the other. Food should be in small quantities at short intervals, and if a feed is vomited, another immediately after is less likely to set up a paroxysm of coughing. Belladonna is the most useful drug: children will stand ℳ 10–15 of tinct. belladonnæ if the dose is increased gradually: it may be usefully combined with small doses of chloral and of bromide. Antipyrin, ephedrine and phenobarbitone (gr. $\frac{1}{12}$ at 3 months, gr. $\frac{1}{8}$ at one year t.i.d.) have been advocated. Small doses of potassium iodide in the third week may help expectoration. Penicillin, streptomycin and the sulphonamides are of no use against the disease itself but are of great value for the secondary infections which cause broncho-pneumonia later in the disease. Chloramphenicol and chlortetracycline (Aureomycin) 25 mg./kilo a day in 6-hourly doses are of limited value in reducing the severity of the infection if given in the first week of the disease. Collapse of the lung is treated with antibiotics and posturo-percussion drainage: penicillin is the first choice for chest and ear complications. For convulsions sodium phenobarbitone or chloral hydrate are most successful: chloroform inhalation may be needed. In uncomplicated cases high-flying at 12,000 feet, or an equivalent low pressure in a decompression chamber for one hour, helps in 30–40 per cent. of cases, especially in lessening the tendency to vomit. A period of *isolation* of 4 weeks from the onset of the whoop is sufficient, but infectivity does not necessarily last as long as this, and many cases can be proved to be no longer infectious after 3 weeks—by taking per-nasal swabs at intervals of 1 to 2 days. The value of vaccines in treatment is not proven, but 10–20 ml. of convalescent serum is of distinct value in the initial catarrhal stages. In *prophylaxis* hyper-immune human gamma-globulin has been favourably reported on. Although useless in treatment, vaccines help to prevent the disease occurring: preferably starting at the age of 2–3 months a typical course consists of 3 doses of 20,000 million Phase 1 organisms at monthly intervals with a similar " boosting " dose before entering school-life. In Great Britain it is now common to give a vaccine composed of *H. pertussis*, tetanus and diphtheria toxoids before the age of 6 months.

§ 495. III. **Mumps (Acute Epidemic Parotitis)** is an acute febrile infectious disorder characterised by inflammatory swelling of one or both parotid glands. The period of incubation is usually 17–18 days, and in exceptional cases up to 4 weeks.

The *Symptoms* usually commence with (1) moderate fever (102° F). This usually commences insidiously, but may start with a rigor. The pulse is often slowed. (2) There are constitutional symptoms with headache, malaise, anorexia and constipation. (3) Attention may be drawn to the neck by a complaint of sore throat and stiffness in the neck. (4) When looked for, and especially in an epidemic, there is at an early stage, redness around the mouth of the parotid duct on one or both sides. *Characteristic symptoms* appear on the first to the fourth day with (5) pain and swelling of one or both parotid glands. Usually one side is first affected, followed by the other in a day or two: both may be affected together, or one side may escape altogether. The glands are acutely tender, the skin over them is stretched, and trismus may be so marked as to prevent the mouth being opened more than a quarter of an inch. (6) The secretion of saliva is usually suppressed, the mouth becomes dry and the tongue remains furred. (7) Local pain and the deficiency of saliva make swallowing a very painful process. (8) The blood shows a leucocytosis chiefly due to an increase of lymphocytes. The temperature subsides in 3 or 4 days to a week, constipation becomes less troublesome, and the glandular swellings slowly subside, unless complications ensue.

Varieties.—Particularly in epidemics, the submaxillary and even the sublingual glands are also affected. Sometimes the parotid glands escape, and one or more of the other salivary glands are alone involved. Meningo-encephalitis without parotitis, due to the virus, has been described.

Diagnosis.—Enlargement of a *pre-auricular lymph gland* is unilateral due to some local source of sepsis, and does not involve the deep part of the gland. *Simple and suppurative parotitis* (§ 9) are associated with oral sepsis such as occurs in typhoid and typhus fever, and in abdominal and cachectic states; mumps is almost always bilateral and very rarely suppurates. Care must always be taken to exclude " the bull-neck " of *toxic diphtheria*; *Mikulicz' Syndrome* is usually mistaken for mumps (§ 9). In the *uveo-parotid syndrome* the parotitis is harder and less obvious, and only the pre-auricular part of the gland is involved. Most cases show a rise in serum amylase commencing on the first or second day of the salivary gland swelling.

Etiology.—It is almost entirely confined to children and the young between 5 and 25. It is rare in the very young and very old, but is often epidemic and runs through a school. The infective agent is a filterable virus spread by droplet-infection from the nasal secretions and saliva of patients: the disease can be reproduced from these sources in monkeys, and is most infectious at the end of the incubation period. Death is very rare. The chief *complications* are (1) orchitis, and much less often, oophoritis. Orchitis is very rare before puberty and is most frequent in young adults who are sexually active. It usually follows about 7–10 days from the commencement, when the parotitis and fever have settled. There is sudden pyrexia, with enlargement of one testicle, which becomes very tender and possibly fluctuant; the inflammation settles slowly in a week or 10 days. Subsequent sterility is rare but subfertility may occur when both testicles are involved. Anxiety about this may cause impotence of psychogenic origin. In some epidemics there may be a swelling of a mammary gland or of a testicle, preceding or accompanying that of the parotids, and cases occur in which there is no parotitis. (2) Meningo-encephalitis is not uncommon in the presence of orchitis: most cases recover. Other complications are (3) albuminuria, most liable to occur in severe attacks and in adults; (4) pancreatitis (§ 358); (5) meningitis, usually ill-developed, but sometimes typical; (6) encephalitis; (7) neuritis; (8) otitis interna of the organ of Corti, which usually causes permanent deafness; (9) œdema of the larynx secondary to submaxillary localisation of mumps; (10) joint symptoms, usually arthralgia, but sometimes serous or suppurative arthritis. Diabetes mellitus is an occasional sequel.

Treatment.—Antibiotics are valueless. Rest in bed is essential until the glands have subsided and the temperature is normal: and the patient is isolated for at least a fortnight. Infectious precautions with all feeding utensils and handkerchiefs are necessary. A kaolin poultice to the neck is comforting. Feeding may of necessity be through a straw, and rarely nutrient enemata are required. Orchitis and the other complications are less likely to occur if the patient is kept in bed and the bowels freely opened: sexual stimulation of any kind should be avoided.

Orchitis and severe encephalitis may be controlled by tab. prednisolone 10–15 mg. 6-hourly or by inject. corticotrophin (gel) 100 mg. daily for 1–2 doses. *Prophylaxis:* injection of convalescent serum 20 ml. within 5 days of contact gives passive immunity for 2 weeks.

The ENTERIC FEVERS include Typhoid and the Paratyphoid Fevers. In young children the clinical picture differs from that in adults, and commonly manifests itself as gastro-enteritis or broncho-pneumonia.

§ 496. IV. **Typhoid Fever** is an acute specific fever of about 4 or 5 weeks' duration, and is due to the ingestion of typhoid bacilli. In contrast to the fevers in Group I, the onset is insidious but profound toxæmia develops, often attended by successive crops of rose-coloured spots and characteristic ulceration of the Peyer's patches of the small intestine.

Symptoms.—The period of incubation is 10 to 14 days, but may be shorter or longer. There is a stage of increasing illness and bacteræmia (first week), followed by a continued high temperature and profound prostration (second and third weeks): in cases that recover there follows a slow decline in fever (fourth and fifth weeks) before convalescence is established.

First week.—(i.) The most important early symptom is severe frontal headache: otherwise there are simple malaise and lassitude, some degree of bronchial cough, epistaxis and disturbed nights. (ii.) Anorexia and nausea are associated with abdominal discomfort, flatulence and indefinite pain in the right iliac fossa. The bowels are irregular with constipation or temporary looseness of action. (iii.) The tongue is always heavily coated with a white fur. (iv.) The temperature is characteristic (Fig. 147), tending to rise in step-ladder fashion, being higher in the evening than in the morning. Yet the pulse rate is often slowed in proportion to the temperature, and rather soft. (v.) The bacteræmic nature of the symptoms in this first week is demonstrated by the frequency with which a positive blood culture can be obtained. A polymorph leucopenia is almost invariable.

During the *second and third weeks* the condition of the patient deteriorates. The *three characteristic features* in this stage are: (i.) The temperature remains up (continued pyrexia) at 103° to 105° F, the diurnal remissions often being no more than are met with in health (Fig. 147). The pulse, slow in proportion to the temperature, is soft and often dicrotic in character and the blood pressure lowered. (ii.) The rash generally appears about the seventh to twelfth day (average, tenth) in successive crops [1] of small rose-coloured lenticular spots, slightly elevated, soft and disappearing on pressure. Each spot lasts about 3 or 4 days. They are never petechial. They are chiefly seen on the abdomen, sometimes on the rest of the trunk, very rarely on the face or limbs. The number of these spots varies considerably, but they are seldom abundant. They may be very small, and thus be overlooked or mistaken for flea-bites. (iii.) The spleen is generally enlarged during this period. It is seldom large, it may be tender and the lower edge is rather soft, which makes it more difficult to feel. Otherwise, (iv.) Lethargy becomes very marked and gives rise to an aspect which is fairly characteristic (*facies typhosa*): the drowsiness deepens to semi-coma and in severe cases the typhoid state eventually supervenes (§ 470). (v.) Some diarrhœa is usually present after the first week—at least in cases of moderate severity—and the stools are of a characteristic pea-soup or yellow ochre colour—this feature is of less value as a means of diagnosis if the patient is wholly on a milk diet. The number of stools passed in 24 hours is very variable, but tends to decrease in the third week. In more than half the cases there is no diarrhœa throughout, but these include the large proportion of mild attacks: complete absence of diarrhœa is exceptional in cases of any severity. (vi.) Tympanitic distension of the abdomen (meteorism) is common (especially if the patient be injudiciously fed), and there is pain and gurgling in the right iliac fossa, though great care should be used to elicit this symptom, as the intestinal wall is thinned by disease. (vii.) The mouth becomes dry and sordes collect on the teeth and lips. The tongue at first develops a brown fur, but in the second week this clears, and the tongue becomes glazed and dry or red and smooth: shallow transverse fissures are often seen on it. (viii.) A toxic albuminuria is usual.

The *fourth and fifth weeks* are characterised by a gradual improvement in the patient's condition. (i.) The temperature gradually falls in a stepladder fashion, the reverse of the initial rise (Fig. 147). (ii.) The extreme mental and physical apathy give place to a slowly renewed interest. With increasing appetite weight is gradually regained. (iii.) The stools become more formed and constipation often follows. Prolonged *convalescence* is necessary, for energy is slow in returning. After an apyrexial period, relapse may occur, with a recrudescence of the symptomatology, although such is rarely as severe as the original attack. It is particularly during the third and fourth weeks that the dreaded complications of perforation or hæmorrhage of the ulcerated Peyer's patches are most liable to occur.

The *varieties* of typhoid fever are legion. It is a safe rule to remember that continued fever of any kind may be due to typhoid, whatever symptoms are presented. The predominant symptoms may be those of bronchopneumonia or of meningitis. In the *septicæmic variety*, the disease com-

---

[1] This fact may be revealed by enclosing each of the spots which appear on one day by a circle, next day by a triangle, and so on, by a skin pencil or aniline ink.

mences suddenly with a rapid rise of temperature, vomiting and rigors: intestinal symptoms are usually absent. In the *ambulatory form* the patient keeps about, and perforative peritonitis or intestinal hæmorrhage may be the first manifestation.

Diagnosis.—The chief clinical features are the insidious onset and prolonged course of the illness, the profound prostration, the temperature chart and slowed pulse rate, the rash and the enlarged spleen. By cultural methods the organism may be found in the blood (especially in the first week), in the stools (first to third weeks) or in the urine (third week). A blood count which shows a polymorph leucopenia in the presence of a high temperature is highly suggestive of uncomplicated typhoid. The Widal reaction is rarely positive before the tenth to fourteenth days, and may be negative throughout: however, a positive reaction is diagnostic. Difficulty may arise in previously inoculated persons: even so in the acute stage the " O " (somatic) antigen titre rises, while the " H " (flagellar) antigen titre remains low throughout. Undoubtedly many slight cases of typhoid are overlooked and regarded as *Febricula.* Slight cases may also be mistaken for *influenza,* which except for the more sudden advent and brief duration, much resembles mild typhoid. The other *specific fevers* in this group may also have to be excluded. In most cases of typhoid a mild *bronchitis* and *hypostatic congestion* of the lungs occurs, and it is common to confuse this with the early stages of typhoid fever. Early headache and delirium may suggest *tuberculous meningitis,* but the latter is recognised (apart from examination of the cerebro-spinal fluid) by (i.) the retracted abdomen: (ii.) the headache persists longer, and may concur instead of alternating with delirium: (iii.) signs of increased intracranial pressure and local cranial palsies supervene. (It must be remembered that true meningitis and also pneumonia occur due to typhoid bacilli.) *Typhus Fever* has a sudden onset with high fever, a greater tendency to delirium in the early stages, conjunctival injection, a rash on the fourth day which is dark red in colour and does not invade the face, and the Weil-Felix reaction is positive. *Acute Pulmonary* or *Miliary Tuberculosis* sometimes closely resembles typhoid. The positive signs of typhoid are wanting, and the presence of tuberculosis is suggested by (i.) the intermittent character of the temperature and its prolonged course; (ii.) the lung symptoms are much more marked; (iii.) the rapidity of breathing is out of proportion to the other signs of illness; and (iv.) the result of a chest X-ray. *Malignant endocarditis* is recognised by (i.) the intermittent character of the temperature (usually), often with rigors, (ii.) the cardiac signs, and (iii.) the positive blood culture. Pyæmia is differentiated by the wide range and irregularity of the pyrexia.

Undulant fever (§ 502) resembles typhoid in its insidious onset, high fever and enlargement of the spleen, but is distinguished by the patient's serum agglutinating *Brucella abortus* and having no effect on the organisms of the typhoid group. *Tularæmia,* which, like undulant fever, may attack laboratory workers and cause a prolonged fever, is also distinguished by an agglutination test.

Etiology.—Typhoid fever is due to the *Salmonella typhi* (the Eberth-Gaffky bacillus). Most epidemics are due to contamination of the water supply by sewage: especially in rural areas this is more common after a dry summer when leakage from cesspools and drains permits contamination

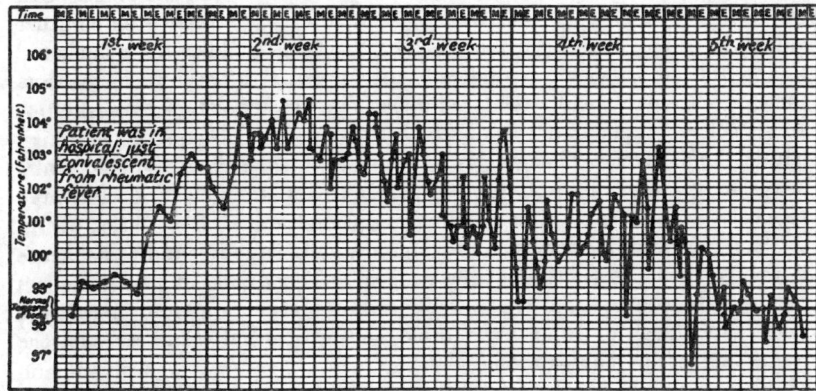

FIG. 147.—TYPHOID FEVER (typical chart), Henry H——, æt. 22, was in hospital when he developed typhoid fever, which was not treated by antibiotics. There was an apathetic mental condition, feeling of profound illness and headache, watery pea-soup stools, and bronchial catarrh. The chart shows the continued character of the pyrexia in the second and third weeks, with gradually increasing remissions in the fourth and fifth weeks.

of shallow wells. Infection has also been traced from sewage-contaminated waters to oysters and other shell-fish, to ice-creams and to the milk supply. In a patient, *all discharges from the stomach, bowels, bladder and lungs* are

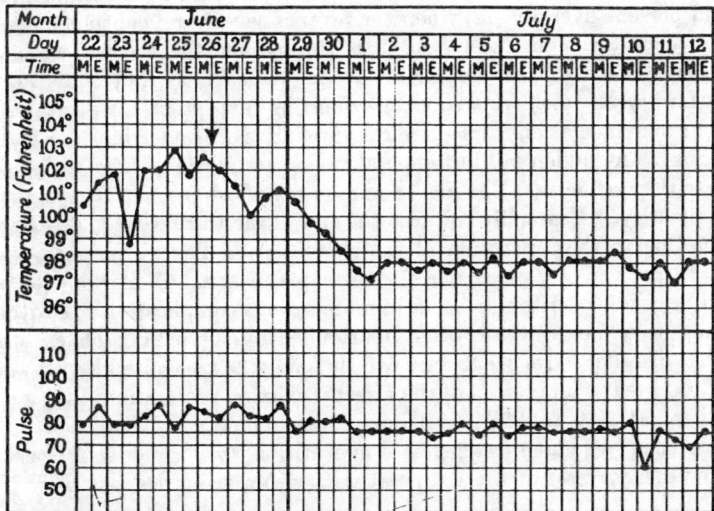

FIG. 148.—TYPHOID FEVER treated with Chloramphenicol (started as marked by arrow). Note rapid subsidence of temperature (cf. Fig. 147).

infective: thus nurses and friends of patients contract the disease by handling bed-pans, sheets, and other articles contaminated by these excreta: the discharges become more virulent after standing for 12 to 24 hours. The urine and fæces may contain typhoid bacilli long after restoration to health: " typhoid carriers " [1] are persons whose stools have been shown to carry bacilli many years after an attack—the original nature may not have been recognised. The gall-bladder often harbours the organisms which are periodically discharged into the bowel and thus the stools are periodically rendered infective. Second attacks are rare but an attack of typhoid does not protect against a subsequent attack of paratyphoid fever. The greatly diminished incidence of typhoid fever in recent years has been attributed partly to the immunisation of a large proportion of the susceptible population during the two Great Wars, partly to the more careful supervision of water and milk supplies, and to chlorination of any water which may be suspect. The toxins of typhoid seem particularly prone to produce weakness of muscular action: hence the extreme asthenia of voluntary muscle, the myocardial weakness, and the hypotonia of involuntary muscle.

Prognosis.—The case mortality varies in different epidemics from 5 to 20 per cent. It is always a serious disease on account of the numerous complications, prolonged course and its exhausting nature. The usual duration is 4 or 5 weeks, though it can vary from 10 days to 6 weeks even without relapses which are by no means infrequent. Many fatal issues would be avoided if it were remembered that slight attacks require just as much care as severe ones, being liable to hæmorrhage or perforation if the patient does not remain at rest. The prognosis is more favourable between 5 and 10 years of age. It is more serious (i.) in children under 3 and persons over 60: (ii.) when the fever is severe and continued, especially when it remains above 104° F throughout the second week and especially if the diurnal remissions do not increase, as they should do, in the third week: (iii.) when there is vomiting (except at an early stage), urgent diarrhœa at any time, severe tympanites or hæmorrhage, or marked delirium. A sudden fall in temperature suggests hæmorrhage, or perforation with peritonitis. The most common *complications* are: (1) Pneumonia and pleurisy. Especially towards the end of the third week. (2) Hæmorrhage due to the separation of the sloughs from Peyer's patches, occurs in 8–10 per cent. of cases, and for the same reason. (3) Perforation with local or general peritonitis is a still more serious complication. Peritonitis arising in typhoid fever is often unattended by the pain so characteristic of that disorder. Its occurrence can then only be recognised by (i.) vomiting; (ii.) great aggravation of the already existing prostration; (iii.) a small rapid pulse (120 to 140); (iv.) immobility followed by distension of the abdomen; (v.) sudden frequency of micturition; (vi.) a sudden fall, usually followed by a rise, of the temperature; (vii.) a rising leucocytosis; (viii.)

---

[1] The best example was " Typhoid Mary," who during her employment as cook in different households and institutions initiated 10 outbreaks with 51 cases.

the *facies Hippocratica*. (4) Myocarditis is present to some extent in every case: it can be severe and associated with a general circulatory failure of toxæmic origin, which may prove fatal. (5) Other complications are thrombosis of the femoral or popliteal vein, local suppuration and inflammation, such as parotitis, periostitis, cholecystitis, cancrum oris and laryngeal ulceration; and, rarely, arthritis leading to dislocation, typhoid spine due to spondylitis (§§ 461, 15) and rupture of the rectus abdominis, simulating intestinal perforation. As *sequelæ* multiple abscesses, various psychoses, polyneuritis, phthisis and miliary tuberculosis may occur.

The temperature may rise again after convalescence has begun. Such *recrudesence* may be due to too liberal a diet, excitement, or constipation; or it may be due to a *relapse*, which occurs in about 10 to 15 per cent. of all cases. There is usually an apyrexial interval of about 5 to 10 days, but sometimes the temperature has never dropped satisfactorily. The second attack is usually less severe and shorter than the first, but there may be fatal relapses. As many as five relapses may occur, though more than two are rare in this country.

Treatment.—Specific treatment is with chloramphenicol. The sooner this is started the better, but often the diagnosis is not made until the disease is in the second or third week and then toxæmia is already marked. Give caps. chloramphenicol 2·0 G. initially and then 0·5 G. each 6 hours for 5 days; 0·5 G. 8-hourly should then be continued for another 2 weeks. When oral administration is difficult adults can have 1·0 G. each 8–12 hours intramusc. In severely ill patients some give smaller doses at first due to the fear of sensitivity reactions; but in cases with marked prostration the chloramphenicol may be combined with tab. prednisolone 5–10 mg. each 4 hours, the dose being reduced gradually over a period of 4–7 days as recovery ensues. The temperature usually falls to normal within 7–10 days of starting this treatment and toxæmia rapidly abates. Ampicillin (Penbritin), one of the new semi-synthetic penicillin compounds, is not proving as effective against organisms of the typhoid group as was first thought. For adults the dose is 750 mg. 8-hourly for the first 4–5 days, with decreasing doses subsequently. The high concentration of the drug in the bile and the urine may be advantageous. T.A.B. vaccine 0·1 ml. 2–3 times a week for 2 weeks is sometimes used to boost active immunity. The *other indications* are (*a*) to conserve the energy of the patient and to prevent hæmorrhage or perforation by skilled nursing; (*b*) to give a high-calorie low-residue diet and to avoid meteorism; (*c*) to correct electrolyte imbalance; (*d*) to use such drugs as will reduce diarrhœa and flatulence; and (*e*) to use barrier nursing in its strictest sense. (*a*) *Bed rest* is of the highest importance, and as the patient will probably be in bed for at least 6 weeks, a sorbo type of mattress is most comfortable. During the third and fourth weeks when (in those not having an antibiotic at an early stage) the dangers of hæmorrhage and perforation are greatest, the patient should not be allowed to turn himself in bed: perforation may occur if a patient is allowed to raise himself as in changing a draw-sheet.

It is a great mistake, however, to keep the patient continually on the flat of his back, as this tends to induce congestion of the lung bases and also the formation of bed sores—he should be carefully turned every 2 hours by day. Especial attention should be paid to the care of the skin and of the mouth. (b) The *diet* now given is of higher nutritive value than used to be the custom, and this undoubtedly supports the patient's strength. Milk in quantities of 2–3 pints a day is the staple diet; it should be sufficiently diluted and barley water, lime-water or sodium citrate (2 gr. to 1 fl. oz.) added to prevent the formation of curds. Custards, junkets, jellies, eggs, chicken broths, clear soup, beef tea, chocolate and cocoa are nutritious and non-putrefactive: Complan and Farex are useful high-calorie additions. Toast, cereals, plain biscuits, and boiled or steamed pounded fish are added if the patient can digest them. Predigested foods such as Benger's are an aid to promote assimilation, especially if the tongue is heavily furred, and pepsin is said to be of service. (c) *Salt depletion* is particularly common in hot countries and where diarrhœa is profuse: this condition may be overlooked when toxæmia is profound. It should be suspected when drowsiness and apathy are marked, with a rapid feeble pulse, low blood pressure and syncope; and confirmed by the Fantus test of the urine (§ 388) and by electrolyte studies of the serum. It will necessitate the prompt use of intravenous saline. (d) *Diarrhœa*, if profuse, must be checked by enemata of starch and opium (℥ 30 of tinct. opii to 3 fl. oz. of mucilage of starch); or liq. morphinæ ℥ 20, with dilute sulphuric acid ℥ 10, every 3 or 4 hours. If these fail, give bismuth salicylate. Constipation should never be treated by purgatives, but by glycerin suppositories, liquid paraffin by mouth, aided by cautious small enemata. If the abdomen is tympanitic, reduce the amount of food and of milk and give it peptonised or more diluted: a flatus tube or a small turpentine enema may help. Hæmorrhage should be checked by the administration of opium, absolute rest must be enjoined, and the amount of the diet temporarily reduced. For perforation, immediate laparotomy and suture of the bowel is usually necessary. (e) *Barrier-nursing*. Typhoid patients have been treated in a general hospital ward, but are often better dealt with in an infectious diseases hospital. Doctors and nurses should already have been protected by T.A.B. vaccine. They must wear gowns and rubber gloves when handling bedpans and urinals. The hands must be washed after doing anything for the patient. The stools must be immersed in and stirred with liq. cresol sap. (Lysol) 10 per cent. which is left in contact for 12 hours: the urine and other excreta, personal and bed linen, crockery, bedpans and the separate thermometer must be disinfected for several hours with 5 per cent. phenol.

Typhoid relapses need treatment on the same lines as the original attack.

Typhoid carriers arise in those persons who harbour the bacilli and excrete them at regular or at irregular intervals. There may previously have been a recognised attack of typhoid, or such may not have occurred, the disease having been mistaken for influenza, etc. Such persons are most dangerous when they handle food, milk or water supplies. The carrier state may be temporary or permanent: for its detection bacteriological testing of the stools and urine is necessary. If the Vi (Virulence) agglutinins are present, and particularly if with tests at 3-monthly intervals the titre is rising, a carrier state must be strongly suspected, and a considerable number of specimens of stool and urine examined. Urinary carriers may respond to sulphonamides or to ampicillin. Fæcal carriers are more obstinate and the organisms may be shown by laboratory tests to be resistant to chloramphenicol. Treatment will depend on the results of sensitivity tests and may be (i.) a second course of chloramphenicol; (ii.) oral neomycin or ampicillin may be effective; (iii.) procaine penicillin (intramusc.) 3-hourly for 7 days with tab. probenecid which inhibits the tubular excretion of penicillin by the kidneys. Cholecystectomy does not always cure and is not to be lightly undertaken. When cured the Vi agglutinins should disappear with the *S. typhi*.

Prophylactic Treatment is based on a knowledge of the origin of the disease and its mode of introduction into the system via the mouth. The incidence of typhoid in a community is a fair index of the purity of its water supply: when any doubt arises, and especially in rural areas, the water should be boiled or chlorinated. General measures necessitate a careful search for carriers, their proper supervision and control; all carriers and suspected cases must maintain a high standard of personal hygiene (washing hands, etc.) and must not handle food, water or milk consumed by the public. Preventive vaccination subcut. or intramusc., originally introduced by the late Sir Almroth Wright, has proved an established success, as was well exemplified in the fighting forces during the last two Great Wars (for the method, see § 525). Felix has prepared a particularly efficacious vaccine containing Vi and O antigens. Vaccine therapy is not effective in the treatment of typhoid fever.

Paratyphoid Fever is due to infection by *B. paratyphosus* A, B or C. Paratyphoid A is almost unknown in England and Holland, and is uncommon in Germany, but is common in France, Italy, the Balkan countries, Soviet Russia and the tropics. Paratyphoid B is now more common than typhoid fever in this country. Paratyphoid C, which is much less frequent, is prevalent in the Middle East and Mediterranean. Paratyphoid has assumed such prominence that inoculation against the A and B paratyphoid fevers has to be carried out as carefully as against typhoid fever. A mixed vaccine (T.A.B.) is usually employed (§ 525).

Symptoms.—On clinical grounds, differentiation from typhoid fever in any individual case is at the best uncertain. It is best distinguished by cultural examinations and the Widal test. However, in paratyphoid infection, the disease tends to be rather less severe, and to run a shorter course: in fact, the temperature may return to normal within 2–3 weeks. It has often been remarked that paratyphoid infection tends to give a much greater profusion of the eruption on the trunk, and that the spots tend to be more obvious as they are darker in colour: but often no rash is visible at any stage of an attack.   Intestinal symptoms and complications are not so frequent, in consequence of which the mortality rate in some epidemics is only 1–2 per cent.   Even so, it is most unwise to presume on this.

Treatment is as for typhoid fever and care to guard against intestinal hæmorrhage and perforation must be just as strict.   Mixed infections of two or more of the varieties of enteric fever are not uncommon.

Enteric Fever in Infants and Young Children usually does not conform to the clinical picture presented above.   Whether the cases occur sporadically or in epidemics, it is often necessary at first to make a tentative diagnosis of " pyrexia of uncertain origin."   The onset is often sudden, and in infants the presenting symptom is that of gastro-enteritis: in slightly older children, the symptoms and signs are those of bronchopneumonia, of meningitis or of appendicitis, the origin of which is only established by careful bacteriological study.   Even in children dying of the disease, intestinal hæmorrhage and perforation are rare.   Relapses are more frequent than in adults.

§ **497. V. Diphtheria** is an infectious fever due to the Klebs-Loeffler or diphtheria bacillus (§ 1202).   Since 1940 when prophylactic immunisation was introduced into Great Britain the death-rate from diphtheria has dropped from an average of 3,000 persons a year to under 30 a year. It most commonly involves the throat, but may start on or spread to the nose or larynx, and more rarely the ear, the conjunctiva, the vagina or a wound of the skin.   The organisms rarely penetrate the surface, but multiply and cause the formation of a surface coagulum (" the membrane ").   Dangers arise chiefly from the absorbed exotoxins which attack especially the myocardium and the peripheral nerves: in the narrow laryngeal passages of children, obstruction to respiration is serious.

Symptoms of Faucial Diphtheria.—The incubation period is variable, but it is often 2 to 4 days.   (1) The onset is usually gradual (extending over a day or two), but in some cases is more sudden.   (2) There is general listlessness, *pallor*, and often headache and vomiting.   A trace of albumen in the urine is common.   (3) The temperature is low in proportion to the appearance of illness, and temperatures above 100° F are unusual: in many of the worst cases the patient is apyrexial.   The pulse is soft and rapid.   (4) Sore throat and dysphagia, though usual, are not always complained of by young children.   For the first few hours the throat may only be congested.   Within 24 hours one or both tonsils shows a characteristic patch of creamy-white, wash-leather-like membrane situated on an obviously congested surface, and if forcibly removed this leaves bleeding-points.   The patches tend to run together, and to spread beyond the tonsils on to the fauces, soft palate, uvula and pharyngeal wall.   The presence of membrane on these parts is a diagnostic feature of great value from simple tonsillitis.   The size and rapidity of spread of the membrane and the amount of œdema present, are an index of the

severity of the case.   (5) The membrane spreads to the larynx and bronchi
in certain cases, and it may spread upwards to the nose (especially in
children).   An ichorous discharge from the nostrils in a child lying prostrate and fretful in bed is very characteristic of severe diphtheria.   (6) The
glands at the angles of the jaws are enlarged even in mild cases, and the
patient may complain that the neck feels stiff.   When the membrane inside the throat is extensive, the glands become much more swollen, and

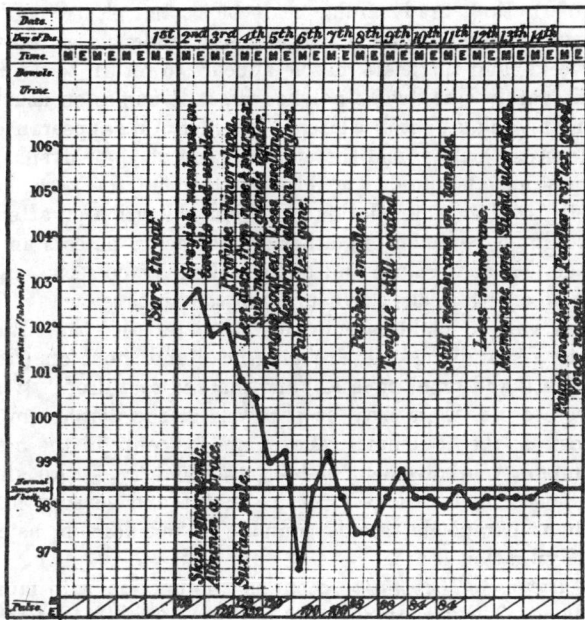

FIG. 149.—DIPHTHERIA.—Male, æt. 9.   An ordinary case of faucial diphtheria without implication
of larynx.   The palate was still anæsthetic one month later.   Not followed by paralysis.   The
different events are indicated on the chart.

these and the surrounding œdema may give an appearance of " a bull-
neck."   (7) There is often a diagnostic odour to the breath: recognition
of this is most valuable, but depends a great deal on the observer's acuity
of smell.   In mild cases and particularly in those energetically treated by
antitoxin at a very early stage, the disease aborts in a few days and the
membrane separates.   In moderate and in severe cases, and especially in
those who are not given antitoxin until later, the toxin may have become
fixed in the tissues, and the patient's condition then undergoes a change
for the worse.   Even when the case appears to be mild, and is treated
early, these toxic effects may arise, and so every case must be treated by
strict bed rest.   The three major specific effects of the toxæmia are: (8)
In the first week, and in virulent cases, general toxæmia gives rise to death
by the seventh day.   (9) From the end of the first week and progressively

during the second week, myocardial damage and failure occur. Slight cases show a rise of pulse rate, a fall in systemic blood pressure and some enlargement of the heart to the left: in more severe cases, tachycardia is marked (up to 140 per minute), the heart sounds become feeble, the blood pressure may fall to very low levels: and the resulting failure of the cerebral circulation leads to restlessness, drowsiness and coma, while failure of the right heart causes symptoms or signs of this disease (§ 55): vomiting, progressive liver engorgement and suppression of urine occur in fatal cases. Disorders of rhythm, bradycardia, heart block and electro-cardiographic changes have all been recorded. There is a tendency to recovery in a period of weeks, and the heart muscle appears to return to normal. (10) Diphtheritic paralysis is due to polyneuritis. It comes on usually in the third or fourth week, sometimes later. In order of its appearance we find: (i.) it starts in the palate, and therefore a nasal voice or dysphagia is the earliest symptom, and fluids are returned through the nose. (ii.) Next we may get loss of accommodation, with blurred vision on attempting to read. A squint is common but other cranial nerve pareses are unusual. At this stage loss of the knee and ankle jerks may be seen. (iii.) About the seventh to eighth weeks polyneuritis of the limbs is seen (§ 975). The attitude and gait in children may be characteristic, the little patient walking with a shambling gait, drooping head and shoulders (from weakness of the neck and trunk muscles) and marked foot-drop. (iv.) Especially in severe cases, there may be paralysis of the diaphragm, pharynx and intercostals: the abdominal reflexes are lost only in the most severe cases. Temporary involvement of the pyramidal tract with an extensor plantar response, and various forms of motor and sensory impairment occur, such as paraplegia, ataxia, numbness, formication, astereognosis and loss of vibration sense.

Other Varieties of Diphtheria occur in conjunction with faucial diphtheria or alone. The varieties are: (1) Laryngeal diphtheria (membranous croup). Symptoms.—The patient is usually under 5 years of age and (i.) there is a croupy cough with a hoarse cry: (ii.) there is inspiratory stridor, followed soon by (iii.) symptoms of laryngeal obstruction. These may be continuous, or intermittent, with inspiratory recession of the ribs and of the suprasternal notch accentuated by the use of the accessory muscles of respiration, and some cyanosis. (iv.) The child is pale and ill, with a low grade temperature and other signs of diphtheritic toxaemia. (2) Nasal diphtheria, when it occurs alone, is a mild disease of young children (§ 179. V). (3) The auditory meatus, the conjunctiva, the vagina and wounds of the surface may harbour diphtheria bacilli. Care must be taken to prove these organisms are pathogenic, and not diphtheroids which are normal inhabitants of mucous membranes and of the skin.

The Diagnosis of diphtheria is made by finding the C. diphtheriæ (Klebs-Loeffler bacillus) in swabbings from a characteristic membranous lesion. In cases of doubt a virulence test must be performed. The diagnosis of the sore throat caused by tonsillitis, scarlet fever, and diphtheria presents certain difficulties, and is given in Table X, § 157. *Follicular tonsillitis* is distinguished by the absence of the definite wash-leather-like patches on the fauces, nasal, or laryngeal passages, and usually the presence of higher fever. There may also be a history of previous attacks, though an inference based on this may be very misleading. Albuminuria, too, is much less common. *Scarlet fever* is distinguished by its abrupt onset, higher fever, rash, strawberry tongue, and generally the absence of membrane from the throat. Simple " *croup* " (catarrhal laryngitis) is distinguished by the history of previous attacks and the absence of patches in the throat, but this is often the case in true diphtheria, in which case an appeal must be made to bacteriology. *Membranous croup* is always diphtheritic. *Vincent's Angina* is distinguished by the bacteriological examination (§ 155e), and the fact that the patch is usually depressed instead of being raised above the surface. For differentiating *agranulocytic angina* and the anginose variety of *glandular fever*, see § 155f, d.

Etiology.—The disease is due to the diphtheria bacillus (*Corynebacterium diphtheriæ*), of which three strains are now recognised, *gravis*, *intermedius* and *mitis*: generally speaking, the gravis strains are the most virulent and produce most toxin, whereas some mitis strains are avirulent to man. The infection is spread by droplet infection and by fomites—cups, spoons, etc.: occasionally it is conveyed by milk. Diphtheria carriers may be the cause of local epidemics.

Prognosis.—The case-mortality varied widely in different epidemics, and used to be 25 to 50 per cent.; since the introduction of serum therapy it has fallen to 3 or 4 per cent. Faucial cases in adults are usually mild. During the first week, the disease in little children is often fatal, by the spread of membrane to the larynx. The prognosis is greatly improved when adequate doses of serum are given in the first 24 hours: every few hours' delay, especially in virulent cases, increases the risk of complications and lessens the recovery rate. *Untoward Symptoms.*—The prognosis is unfavourable in severe cases, especially when (i.) fœtor of the breath is marked; (ii.) periglandular œdema forming a " bull-neck " is present; (iii.) in the presence of hæmorrhage or epistaxis, purpuric cases being almost invariably fatal; (iv.) marked albuminuria is a bad sign. Other unfavourable symptoms are (v.) a low temperature with severe local lesions; (vi.) when the membrane is extensive, thick and persistent, especially in young patients; (vii.) rapid extension of the membrane to the larynx, leading to croupy cough, dyspnœa and cyanosis. *Complications.*—Apart from toxic myocarditis and polyneuritis (*vide supra*), these are: (1) Bronchopneumonia, formerly so frequent in laryngeal cases, now attacks only 4 per cent. since modern treatment is available. (2) Nephritis during convalescence is very infrequent, and permanent lesions of the kidney are rare. (3) Otitis media is not uncommon. (4) Embolism secondary to cardiac thrombosis may occur and give rise to hemiplegia or gangrene of a limb from blocking of a main artery.

Treatment.—The indications are (*a*) to neutralise the toxin; (*b*) to keep the patient at rest in order to diminish the effects of myocarditis and polyneuritis; (c) to inhibit the local process and (d) to treat complications. (1) *Antitoxin* will neutralise diphtheria toxin only if it has not become fixed in the tissues. It is therefore vitally important to administer a sufficient dose immediately the condition is suspected or diagnosed, without waiting for bacteriological confirmation. The dose depends on the degree of toxæmia and the day of the disease (the fourth day being a late stage). It varies from 30,000 units (intramusc.) in a mild case with membrane on one tonsil, to 80,000 units intravenously in a moderate case with membrane on both tonsils and slight periadenitis. In severe faucial diphtheria with a " bull-neck " give 200,000 units intravenously with due precautions for allergic reactions. (2) *Penicillin* should be injected; it helps to clear *C. diphtheria* from the site of the lesion and controls secondary infection. The dose is 500,000 units (intramusc.) 12-hourly. (3) *Heart failure* is liable to occur about the tenth to the fourteenth day in severe cases. From the commencement of the disease, therefore, the patient must be kept lying down and at *strict rest in bed*—one pillow at the most being allowed for comfort: during this time he must be fed and washed. This position is maintained even in mild cases for 2 weeks, and for longer in more severe cases, and any subsequent activity will be curtailed immediately evidence of myocarditis shows itself. In a severe case, when myocarditis is likely to be followed by polyneuritis, it is not unusual for the patient to have to remain in bed for 2-3 months. Extra activity is only allowed very gradually. Glucose should be freely given by mouth; in severe or malignant cases, and in the presence of vomiting, 50 ml. of 50 per cent. dextrose should be given intravenously once or twice daily. Restlessness must be combated by sedatives and even by small doses of morphia. (4) An *oxygen* tent with at least 50 per cent. oxygen is indicated in critical cases to reduce the strain on the circulation. (5) The *diet* should contain adequate protein and carbohydrate and be increased gradually. Palatal paralysis necessitates semi-solids, whilst pharyngeal paralysis requires nasal feeding and postural drainage (to prevent inhalation of saliva, etc.). Failing this, dextrose-saline or plasma intravenously or rectal fluids are administered pending a return of swallowing. (6) Antitoxin has rendered *local* treatment by syringing, spraying or swabbing unnecessary. (7) In *costo-phrenic paralysis* a cabinet respirator, *e.g.*, Drinker or Alligator machine, is essential. Patients may be gradually removed from the respirator by using the Cuirass or the Bragg-Paul apparatus or the Rocking bed.

When THE LARYNX is involved, the dose of antitoxin for cases of primary laryngeal diphtheria is 40,000-80,000 units intramusc., but when the disease is secondary to the throat give 200,000 units intravenously. Steam inhalations, antihistamines and chlortetracycline (Aureomycin) in the place of penicillin are indicated: give chlortetracycline 6-hourly (15-20 mg./kilo for children and 1·5-2·0 G. a day for adults during 24 hours). Direct laryngoscopy with suction of the membrane is helpful. Laryngeal

intubation has proved successful in some hands but the tube is liable to
be coughed out.   High tracheostomy through the second and third tracheal
rings is vital in urgent cases and when there is œdema or ulceration; it
should be carried out early and all laryngeal cases should be watched for
inspiratory epigastric recession.   Sterile instruments must be available
for immediate use and oxygen may be helpful.

   Freedom from infection is proved by three negative cultures for *C. diphtheriæ*, taken from the nose and the throat at not less than 2-day intervals.
Prophylaxis.—A carrier of virulent *C. diphtheriæ* may be (1) a person who
has just recovered from an attack (convalescent carrier), or (2) one who
is innocently harbouring the infection.   Especially in the latter the virulence of the organism must be proved.   When a carrier state is persistent,
any local contributory cause should be treated: it will often respond to
systemic penicillin, or in faucial cases to tonsillectomy.

   The question of susceptibility to diphtheria is settled by the Schick test.   This is
described, together with the method of prophylactic immunisation, in § 525, p. 775.
Although diphtheria may sometimes occur in the immunised, the attack in the great
majority of such cases is mild and fatalities are very rare.

   § **498. VI. Glandular Fever** (Syn., Infectious mononucleosis) is an
infectious fever occurring in sporadic or epidemic form, in children and
adults (especially young adults), probably due to a virus.   After an incubation period of 5 to 12 days the disease shows itself in one of three fairly
well-defined clinical syndromes, but overlapping between these syndromes
is often seen.

   The GLANDULAR TYPE is the commonest, and occurs chiefly in children
and young adults.   *Symptoms* are: (i.) Sudden onset with fever of 101° to
103° F, often with vomiting; (ii.) transient sore throat or mild tonsillitis;
(iii.) severe frontal headache and limb pains; (iv.) sweating may be profuse; (v.) on the second or third day painful enlargement of the upper
cervical glands, which remain discrete and tender.   Sometimes they reach
a considerable size, and are followed by enlargement of the axillary, inguinal and epitrochlear glands.   (vi.) Abdominal pain and tenderness,
with pyrexia and vomiting, indicate enlargement of abdominal glands, and
may precede cervical adenitis—then appendicitis is often diagnosed.   (vii.)
Some enlargement of the liver and spleen is common; (viii.) a painful cough
may indicate enlarged mediastinal glands.   (ix.) At the junction of the
hard and soft palate multiple pin-point petechiæ occur 3–14 days after
the onset.

   In the ANGINOSE VARIETY a membrane is present on the tonsils and
surrounding œdema is severe—simulating diphtheria.   Vincent's bacilli
and spirochætes are often present in the membrane (§ 155*d*, *e*).

   The FEBRILE FORM is most common in adults.   *Symptoms.*—(i.) There
is a sudden onset, with sore throat, headache and even a rigor.   (ii.)
Macular, papular or urticarial rashes appear particularly on the trunk,
towards the end of the first week.   (iii.) Glandular enlargement is relatively late—even in the third week.   (iv.) Fever may be prolonged for

3 or even 4 weeks; at first remittent, it later becomes intermittent. (v.)
Splenomegaly is rare.

In all three clinical forms, the course of the disease may be prolonged.
In the glandular variety the glands begin to decrease in 5–7 days without
suppuration, but may still be palpable months afterwards: the fever often
takes 2 to 3 weeks to settle and leaves considerable exhaustion. The
Wassermann reaction may be completely or incompletely positive.
Shortly after the commencement, the blood shows a leucocytosis between
6,000 and 40,000 per c.mm.: the differential count reveals a large number
of mature and immature mononuclear cells, which may constitute 60–
75 per cent. of the total: sometimes cells of the lymphocytic variety
predominate.

Diagnosis.—Owing to the difference in prognosis the diagnosis from
leukæmia is very important. In glandular fever the onset is usually sudden, sweating is marked, the cervical glands are usually first involved,
and purpura is very rare. In *acute leukæmia* there is often previous
malaise, the glands in different areas enlarge simultaneously, anæmia and
purpura are common, and the patient progressively deteriorates. An
agglutination test (*Paul-Bunnell test*) shows the presence of heterophile
agglutinins for sheep cells in the serum: it is positive in about 70 per cent.
of cases of glandular fever after the end of the first week, in a dilution
of at least 1 in 64 (§ 1209). The serum glutamic pyruvic transaminase
is often high.

The *prognosis* is excellent but convalescence is often protracted.
Complications.—A relapse, hæmorrhagic nephritis, hepatitis or a ruptured
spleen may occur.

Treatment is symptomatic and convalescence should be reasonably prolonged. Antibiotics help to control secondary infection but do not affect
the primary disease.

§ 499. VII. **Rheumatic Fever, Pneumonia and other Inflammatory
Conditions** which usually present well-marked **local manifestations.**—The
three groups of fevers just described are those commonly met in England,
in which the pyrexia may run a continued course, and which have no
eruption during the first 4 days. But it must not be forgotten that
certain inflammatory disorders may give rise to pyrexia of a continuous
type, and that the usual local signs of these disorders may be absent,
at the time when the patient is first seen. It will be well, therefore, to
mention those which might be mistaken for an acute specific fever.

(*a*) OBSCURE (so-called) LOCAL[1] INFLAMMATORY DISEASES are mostly
met as complications secondary to fevers. They can usually be detected
by a thorough examination of all the organs in the body (§ 473). Nevertheless, certain cases of (1) *pericarditis* or *infective endocarditis,* or
(2) *pneumonia, pleurisy* or *empyema,* may be latent—*i.e.,* the usual
physical signs may occasionally be wanting or overlooked. (3) Various

---

[1] The word " local " is here used in a qualified sense. Many of these diseases with
local manifestations are now known to be due to a general infection.

affections in or around the *throat, nose and ear*; (4) some *abdominal* disorders, such as cholecystitis, pyelitis, deep-seated abscesses (hepatic, subphrenic, perinephric, tubal), inflammation of the mesenteric glands or pancreas, etc.; (5) cases of *sarcoma* and *carcinoma*, especially of the kidney, liver, lung and stomach and when metastases are present; or (6) inflammation of the *meninges*, tuberculous or epidemic, may also give rise to an elevation of temperature sometimes unattended by marked local symptoms; (7) *parasitic infections*, trichinosis, actinomycosis. In obscure cases of long-continued fever the causes to be suspected are pulmonary tuberculosis, pyelonephritis, infective endocarditis, typhoid and undulant fever, deep-seated abdominal abscesses, malignant and Hodgkin's disease (cf. §§ 517–519).

(*b*) Certain GENERAL DISORDERS are attended by pyrexia, which may similarly give rise to difficulties in diagnosis. (1) In *rheumatic fever* and *acute gout* the pyrexia is nearly always continuous. The joint lesions are the cardinal feature in these cases; but it must not be forgotten that acute rheumatism may commence with inflammation of the pericardium (the structure of which very much resembles that of a joint), and that the joint lesions may not be apparent for several days. (2) There are several conditions special to infancy, childhood and adolescence which are attended by continued pyrexia: (i.) *Acute anterior poliomyelitis* is attended at its outset by a considerable rise in temperature, which may last for several days, and be accompanied by restlessness, peevishness, etc.; (ii.) *meningitis*, tuberculous or epidemic. (3) Septicæmia, and see § 516. (4) Certain blood diseases, especially acute leukæmia and pernicious anæmia, may for a time be overlooked. (5) Examination of the urine may reveal bacilluria, an unsuspected cause of pyrexia. (6) *Constipation* also may cause fever. (7) *Drug fever* is increasingly being recognised during the use of the sulphonamides, barbiturates, penicillin and a number of other preparations. (8) *A nervous or hysterical pyrexia* has been described, and the temperature may go up in an erratic manner, at odd times, in nervous subjects. But while admitting that the nervous system plays a very important part in the production of fever it is difficult to prove that there is not a compound cause in operation in such cases. Only a thorough *bacteriological* and *post-mortem* examination would enable us to be certain that none of the many obscure foci of inflammation above mentioned were present.

§ **500.** VIII. **Syphilis** resembles the specific fevers in having a period of incubation followed by a characteristic eruption. One attack renders a person immune to a second attack, except in cases where the first was cured by treatment. It differs from other specific fevers in the extreme length of its course, which may last many years, in the long intervals which may separate its various manifestations, and above all in its liability to recur without fresh infection. It is caused by infection with *Treponema pallidum* (*Spirochæta pallida*) and is of especial importance in medicine by reason of its protean manifestations. If not recognised and treated early, it is liable to break out anew during the whole lifetime of the individual, even after many years of quiescence: in its later stages it may produce serious inflammatory and degenerative lesions in many different parts of the body, particularly in the cardio-vascular and central nervous systems. There are two chief forms: (A) Acquired, and (B) Congenital Syphilis.

(A) ACQUIRED SYPHILIS. *Symptoms.*—When no history of primary syphilis is obtainable and no physical signs discovered, the disease may be latent and unsuspected. For convenience the symptoms of syphilis are divided into four stages. There is a *period of incubation* which generally lasts about 3 weeks but which may vary between 10 and 90 days. *Primary Stage.*—(i.) At the end of the incubation period there generally appears at the site of inoculation a primary chancre. The initial manifestation is a flat, elevated, painless papule which slowly enlarges and later breaks down to form an indurated ulcer with a slight serous discharge (the hard or Hunterian chancre). It is usually single, and since the infection is commonly conveyed by sexual intercourse, it is likely to be found most commonly on the prepuce or glans penis of the male, and the vulva or cervix of the female. An extra-genital primary chancre may occur, particularly on the lip, finger or anus—in the latter site it may be mistaken for a fissure or a pile. Occasionally the initial papule desquamates without ulceration: and when the primary lesion occurs on the cervix or vagina it will often be entirely overlooked. (ii.) Within 1 to 2 weeks the lymphatic glands draining the primary focus become enlarged and hardened—especially in the groin. (iii.) The lesion after a time cicatrises and may leave behind a scar, or some slight coloration, but it often heals without leaving any mark. The disease is a generalised infection long before the chancre develops at the site of entry.

The *Secondary* symptoms are later reactions to this and make their appearance about 3 to 6 weeks after the first appearance of the chancre (4 to 12 weeks after inoculation). They comprise a rash, sore throat, "mucous patches," enlargement of the lymph glands, condylomata, pyrexia and other constitutional symptoms. (i.) The early *rash* appears chiefly on the chest and abdomen as a faint generalised dusky macular eruption which takes about 3 weeks to mature and 3 weeks to decline (it may be brought out more clearly by a warm bath) (§ 625). Subsequently there are rashes of many different kinds—macular, papular, scaly, pustular and tubercular, but never eczematous or vesicular. They are generalised and symmetrical in distribution, with a preference for the forehead and flexor surfaces, and characteristically *reddish-brown* in colour, *polymorphic* in type, and *never irritate* (§ 705). (ii.) The *sore throat* may be slight, but on the other hand pain on swallowing may be marked and the voice may be husky. The accompanying erythema is described in § 162. (iii.) " *Mucous patches* " (or " snail-tracks ") are seen on the lips, tonsils, pillars of the fauces, soft palate and uvula, and tend to be symmetrical (§ 162): similar lesions may also occur at the corners of the

mouth and at other mucous orifices, and their secretions are all highly
infectious. (iv.) The *lymph glands* near the primary focus become
involved and as a secondary manifestation generalised lymphadenopathy
may develop and persist for months or years: the hardness of the glands
aids diagnosis. (v.) Condylomata are warty masses which occur on moist
warm parts of the skin and abound with *treponemata*. (vi.) A low-grade
pyrexia is often overlooked (§ 520), and may be accompanied by pain in
the limbs. (vii.) There is loss of appetite, general malaise and some loss
of weight. The hair may fall out and the nail-beds become affected by
an indolent inflammation. The liver, spleen and thyroid may enlarge:
the eyes may become affected by iritis or choroido-retinitis: the joints
with synovitis and the bones with periostitis in which the pain is worse
at night. Any of these symptoms may recur again and again in the
ensuing months or years.

The *Tertiary* stage is the result of a syphilitic invasion of the various
organs of the body early in the disease and indicates that the patient
has not been adequately treated in the primary or secondary stages.
The organisms may lie dormant for many years before producing noticeable clinical disease. As may be seen by studying the preceding and
succeeding pages, almost any organ may be affected. Some of the principal results are as follows: (i.) All the *skin* symptoms noted in the secondary
stage may recur, but they are much less profuse and are apt to be asymmetrical in distribution, serpiginous in outline, lenticular or nodular in
shape, with a greater tendency to deep ulceration, suppuration or scarring,
and to be followed by more loss of tissue. (ii.) Nodular or infiltrating
gummatous deposits are followed by scarring and perhaps by ulceration.
These may involve the mucous membranes (especially in the mouth and
naso-pharynx): the liver, spleen and other abdominal organs: the lungs
and mediastinum, the heart, brain and other vital structures. The
bones are often attacked by gummatous periosteal deposits, leading
in the hard palate and nasal septum to perforation, and in the other flat
bones and the long bones to a diffuse periostitis or to more localised
" nodes." (iii.) In the cardio-vascular system, the wall of the thoracic
aorta and the aortic valves are infiltrated and weakened (§ 80) so that an
aneurysm may occur: the smaller arteries (especially of the brain) show
an endarteritis and may become thrombosed (§ 99). (iv.) The *lymphatic
glands* may remain enlarged. (v.) Intermitting *pyrexia* may accompany
the formation of gummata (Fig. 156). (vi.) *Lardaceous disease* of the
liver, spleen, kidneys or intestine may ensue. (vii.) The principal result
of the invasion of the *central nervous system* is often the production 10–20
years later of tabes dorsalis (§ 1022), general paralysis of the insane (§ 1190),
or both (tabo-paresis). (viii.) In a few untreated or malignant cases of
syphilis there is cachexia which may be fatal.

Varieties.—In practice, it is convenient to recognise two main types of
syphilis. Civilised communities are now more resistant to the disease than
a hundred or more years ago and most cases assume a benign type: in such

the influence of adequate treatment during the primary and secondary stages will prevent any tertiary stage developing. In others, and particularly in primitive races not previously exposed to the disease, a more virulent form ensues: this may be enhanced by a debilitated state of the individual, and by inadequate treatment in the earlier stages causing the organisms to develop a resistance to subsequent remedies.

(B) CONGENITAL or " HEREDITARY " SYPHILIS is now rare. Syphilis is no longer regarded as a cause of abortion for this is not more frequent in syphilitic than in normal women. On the other hand, it does cause the child to die within the uterus (Still-birth), or, being born alive to die of marasmus within the first 12 or 18 months. Even so, the greater proportion of syphilitic children pass through infancy with few characteristic clinical lesions. There is no primary chancre in a congenital syphilitic child, and if symptoms arise they conform more or less to the secondary symptoms above described. In the small number of infants who do develop symptoms early in life, at the age of a few weeks " snuffles " occurs, and this so interferes with feeding that it contributes to marasmus. In these there is often a ham-coloured eruption on the buttocks, flexures, palms or soles: the general condition deteriorates, the cry is hoarse, the bones are tender and a fatal gastro-enteritis, bronchitis or pneumonia terminates the picture. Epiphysitis may cause pseudo-paralysis, but in a large number of children, a symptomless epiphysitis or periostitis, demonstrated only by X-ray examination, is valuable evidence of active disease. About the sixth year the permanent incisors appear, and frequently present a " screw-driver " shape and a notched border described by Sir Jonathan Hutchinson (Fig. 4). At any later date, and even in early adult life, interstitial keratitis, periostitis, synovitis, or *sudden* eighth nerve deafness in one ear rapidly followed by similar deafness in the other ear, may appear. More rarely the skin, viscera and the nervous system are attacked (with the development of juvenile tabes or G.P.I.) —Table XXXII. Even without symptoms the C.S.F. is often pathological. The residual lesions of congenital syphilis persist throughout life as hall-marks (stigmata) of the disease, and are summarised in Table XXXIII.

The *Diagnosis* of the Hunterian chancre has to be made from herpes genitalis which usually occurs as a group of vesicles, from scabies in which the characteristic signs is also found in other sites and from epithelioma. Also from the non-Hunterian chancre or soft sore: in the latter pain is a marked feature, the ulceration is deeper, and the edges are softer and less deeply infiltrated. Pityriasis rosea and drug rashes may be confused with the eruption of the secondary stage, but the concomitant lesions present in syphilis and the positive serology will indicate the diagnosis. Identification of the *Treponema pallidum* under the dark-ground illumination of the microscope will settle the diagnosis (Fig. 150). The Wassermann, Kahn and other tests for syphilis (§ 1207) are very helpful: they usually become positive about 10 days after the appearance of the chancre and are always positive in the secondary stage. Even in

TABLE XXXII.—HEREDITARY SYPHILIS

A. MANIFESTATIONS IN INFANTS (3 weeks to 12 months).

Stillbirths are common. When born alive are usually healthy. Soon a small number of infants develop symptoms resembling the secondary stage of acquired syphilis. The lesions are:

I. Mucous membranes { Snuffles and hoarse cry.
                      Condylomata around anus or mouth.

II. Marasmus, leading to wizened appearance: very marked wasting, often fatal.

III. Skin { Papular
           Scaly
           Pustular
           Bullous
           Polymorphic } Always symmetrical, transitory, ham-coloured, becoming deep-brown; on buttocks because of urine and fæces; in flexures because of perspiration. Patches of peeling erythema about the palms and soles, nates, etc. Circum-oral eczema produces rhagades on healing.

IV. Epiphysitis and Periostitis—Tenderness of bones, abscesses, or caries of long bones.
Skull: cranio-tabes, *i.e.*, thinning in one place, thickening in another (rare).
In many, symptomless periostitis or epiphysitis can be demonstrated radio-graphically.

V. Large cirrhotic liver.

VI. " White " (interstitial) pneumonia—usually found only at autopsy.

B. MANIFESTATIONS IN CHILDREN AND YOUNG ADULTS—
rare before 5 years of age.

I. Interstitial Keratitis—an acute painful inflammation first of one cornea, then the other. As it resolves appears like ground-glass. Between the tenth and twentieth year. Clears up very slowly with treatment, but some scarring remains.

II. Deafness, often in association with interstitial keratitis. Characteristically comes on suddenly with noises in the ears, without pain or otorrhœa. Usually causes complete deafness within 24 hours, and within a week the opposite ear is similarly affected. Treatment has no effect.

III. Periostitis of long bones (rarely of the skull)—generally causes thickening (sabre-tibia), or nodes, occasionally suppuration.

IV. Synovitis is painless and persistent—knees or other large joints (Clutton's joints).

V. Skin, mucous membranes and viscera fairly often affected at this stage, with lesions of tertiary type.

VI. Nervous system rarely involved (juvenile tabes and G.P.I.). C.S.F. much more frequently gives positive W.R.

the presence of active disease, negative results may be met in the tertiary stage, especially in those who have had incomplete treatment earlier. In this case a positive result by examination of the cerebro-spinal fluid denoting neuro-syphilis may be helpful (§ 1204). It must not be forgotten that " false positive " results of the Wassermann reaction may be met, especially in and following such conditions as benign tertian malaria, infectious mononucleosis, some of the collagen diseases, mumps, measles and other specific fevers of childhood, after the injection of tetanus toxoid and inoculation for small-pox. In most of these cases positive findings sooner or later revert to negative results without treatment. In any obscure clinical condition, the possibility of a syphilitic cause should be borne in mind: and in the absence of confirmation by examination of the

TABLE XXXIII.—HALL-MARKS OF PREVIOUS LESIONS OF CONGENITAL
SYPHILIS

NOTE.—Only a few of these may be present in any individual case. Signs may also
be present in brothers and sisters.

I. *Tegumentary System.*	*Skin*—Peribuccal cicatrices radiating from mouth (rhagades). *Eruptions* (rare)—Lupoid ulceration, gradually spreading. *Mucous membranes*—Cicatrices of the throat and palate. Hole in nasal septum or palate.
II. *Bones and Joints.*	*Cranial malformations*—prominent frontal eminences, natiform cranium, asymmetry, hydrocephalus. *Nasal malformations*—"saddle nose," depressed septum. *Tibial deformities*—"sabre-blade" or nodular tibia. *Joint lesions*—Chronic painless effusions (Clutton's joints).
III. *Hutchinson's Triad.*	1. Eye—{ The remnants of interstitial keratitis (striæ in cornea), old iritis, or choroidal atrophy. 2. Ear—Total nerve deafness. 3. Teeth—Microdontism, "screw-driver" incisor teeth (Fig. 4), with central notch in the cutting edge.
IV. *Constitutional Effects.*	Infantile build. Retardation of growth and mental development, of dentition and of puberty.

blood or C.S.F., a careful therapeutic trial can be made with anti-syphilitic
remedies.

Etiology.—The specific organism is a feebly staining spirochæte, *Treponema pallidum (Spiro-
chæta pallida).* It can be
obtained not only from
the primary sore, but in
abundance from condylo-
mata, and with more difficulty from the viscera in
secondary, tertiary and
congenital syphilis. The
organism has a corkscrew
shape with from eight to
twelve curves (Fig. 150).
With the dark-field microscope it is differentiated
from a commonly occur-
ring spirillum, the *Treponema refringens,* in that
the latter has fewer and
less delicate curves and
more active movement.

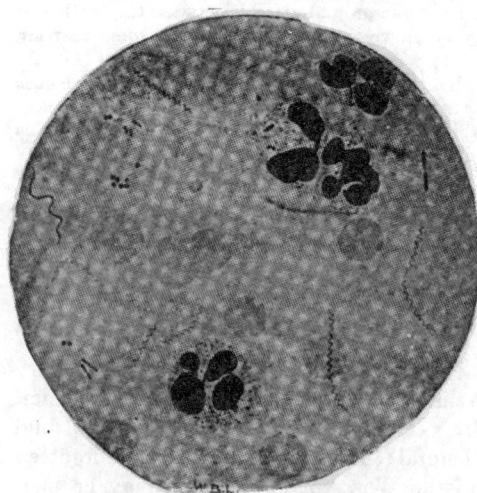

FIG. 150.--TREPONEMA PALLIDUM (SPIROCHÆTA PALLIDA) of
SYPHILIS, magnified about 500 diameters. The organism
is of a spiral form like a long corkscrew. The wavy
organism on the left is the *Treponema refringens.*

Inoculation can only take place through a minor abrasion of the skin
or mucous membrane, and may occur in three ways: (*a*) Usually it is by
direct contact with an infected person, generally during sexual intercourse;
and in some cases by suckling (as in wet nurses), kissing, and (in doctors

and midwives) as a result of examining diseased persons; (*b*) contaminated articles—*e.g.*, spoons, cups, pipes, towels or surgical instruments have sometimes been suspected. In the first two stages the blood and the moist exudations of all the lesions are certainly infectious. In the later stages some difference of opinion exists as to the infectivity of the blood and secretions, but generally speaking infection is rare after 5 years from the onset of the disease. (*c*) In bygone days the use of human vaccine lymph, even when free from blood, for vaccination purposes from arm to arm was the occasional means of propagating syphilis, but the frequency of this was certainly exaggerated.

In the young pregnant woman suffering from early syphilis, the chance of transmission to the child is high (approx. 90 per cent.). When she has had syphilis for 5 years or more, the infection is attenuated and transmission is much less frequent. It is probably true to say that a father never transmits the infection directly to the offspring and only does so by first infecting the mother who later develops a positive Wassermann reaction. When a pregnant woman with latent syphilis is found to have a repeatedly positive Wassermann test, it is imperative that she should be treated throughout pregnancy, thus ensuring that the child will be born healthy.

Prognosis.—The toxæmia of syphilis is particularly virulent in the fœtus: in infancy it may cause fatal marasmus. Following the secondary stage, untreated adults fall into four groups: (*a*) one-third remain symptomless throughout life, with a persistent positive W.R.; (*b*) one-third are likewise symptomless, with a W.R. which ultimately becomes negative; (*c*) one-sixth develop early tertiary symptoms which abort spontaneously, and (*d*) one-sixth develop and suffer from disease afflicting many different systems of the body. The first two groups are termed *latent syphilis.* Unfortunately it is not possible to know beforehand whether the disease will remain latent, or whether it will cause future complications in some vital part. In general, when serial blood reactions become weaker and finally negative, such complications are very unlikely. The severity and duration of an attack of syphilis are influenced by many circumstances, and particularly by the habits and mode of life (especially intemperance), age, occupation, exposure, privation and pre-existing disease (such as tuberculosis and nephritis). The factor which influences the prognosis of syphilis most is adequate and continuous treatment during its earlier stages.

Treatment is of two kinds, prophylactic and curative. *Prophylaxis* is best carried out within half an hour of exposure by thoroughly rubbing in to the exposed site calomel ointment (33 per cent.) which must be left *in situ* for 48 hours. There is no evidence that prophylactic penicillin is of value: on the contrary, it must not be used for it can mask infection and result in latent or tertiary syphilis. If the disease does occur subsequently it can be successfully treated. *Curative treatment* should be begun as soon as possible after diagnosis is made. The most successful results are obtained when treatment is commenced before the secondary symptoms appear and while the serological tests are still negative.   Because of the social aspects (contact tracing and the prolonged surveillance necessary before cure can be assumed), treatment is best carried out in a Special Clinic.   The clinical signs of infection rapidly clear but considerably more treatment is necessary to prevent relapses and to cure the disease, which is a generalised systemic infection long before the primary chancre appears.

Whereas in the earlier part of this century the standard treatment was by the injection of arsenicals and of bismuth for periods of 1 year or more, for over 15 years routine treatment has been with penicillin; except in refractory cases and those patients allergic to penicillin, this has largely superseded treatment with the organic arsenicals and bismuth.   Adverse reactions are infrequent and treatment is completed in a shorter time. At first, it was common practice to give an 8-day course of penicillin, followed by one 10-week course of organic arsenic combined with bismuth injections, and there is no doubt that this procedure was more consistently curative than the present standard treatments; but patients have become increasingly intolerant of the arsenical injections and most venereologists now content themselves with a longer course of penicillin alone, or with penicillin followed by a 10-week course of bismuth.   In either case, close surveillance is necessary for at least 2 years after completing treatment and clinical or serological relapse must be treated by more intensive methods.

Early Disease.—(Primary, Secondary and Latent Syphilis in the first 3 years from the date of infection.)   Early syphilis usually responds to large daily doses of penicillin sustaining a constant demonstrable blood titre for 2 weeks.   To achieve this, benzylpenicillin B.P. 1 mega-unit has to be injected at 8-hourly intervals and calls for in-patient treatment; alternatively inject. procaine penicillin B.P. 900,000 units at 24-hourly intervals is adequate in out-patients attending daily; the diffusibility is increased if combined with benzylpenicillin 300,000 units (*i.e.*, inject. fortified procaine benzylpenicillin B.P.) and achieves a higher rate of cure (a total combined course of 16·8 mega-units in 14 days).   Inject. benzathine penicillin B.P. and inject. benethamine penicillin B.P. maintain a recognisable penicillin titre for 3 days, and it is claimed that cure can be achieved with a dose of 900,000 units twice weekly for several weeks. Attempts have been made to combine these penicillins into a long-acting reservoir of antibiotics but this is still experimental and not yet suitable for general adoption.   If clinical or serological tests do not give satisfactory results a further course of penicillin, often followed by a course of bismuth (*vide infra*), should be given within 4–6 weeks.   In all cases of apparent cure, blood tests are performed every month for the first 3 months and then every 3 months for 2 years; also the cerebro-spinal fluid must be found free of reaction during the second year before treatment is finally passed as satisfactory.

An increasing number of patients are becoming allergic to penicillin, and inquiry should always be made as to whether they have received the antibiotic previously and if they experienced any adverse reactions. Penicillin sensitivity with a drug rash develops immediately after the first injection or about the twelfth day from the start of treatment. It can be relieved by daily intravenous injections of calcium gluconate (10 per cent.), by antihistamines, or in severe cases by prednisolone 5 mg. q.d.s. for a few days. In patients known to be allergic to penicillin, a broad-spectrum antibiotic should be used: e.g., chloramphenicol B.P. or erythromycin B.P. 500 mg. at strict 6-hourly intervals, by day and night, for 10 days (total 20 G.).

Late Disease.—It is wise to avoid intensive treatment at the onset. In late latent and tertiary syphilis it is more important to treat the patient than the disease and due regard must be paid to the condition of the heart, brain, liver, lungs and kidneys; much harm may be done by injudicious intensive treatment. Commence with a course of potassium iodide (vide infra) and then give inject. procaine penicillin in small initial doses of 50,000 units: this is doubled each day if no untoward reactions occur until the full dose of procaine penicillin 900,000 units and benzylpenicillin 300,000 units (fortified benzylpenicillin B.P. 1·2 mega-units) can be safely given daily for 14 days. This should be followed by a 10-week course of bismuth (vide infra); later a further 14-day course of penicillin may be deemed necessary. Active neuro-syphilis, as indicated by positive C.S.F. findings, needs more intensive treatment: benzylpenicillin is more easily diffusible into the nervous system and one mega-unit should be given every 8 hours for 20 days (total 60 mega-units). Fever therapy with artificially induced malaria or the Kettering Hypertherm, is not now considered necessary except for refractory cases. In late syphilis, it is the progress of the disease that we aim to control and damage already suffered by specialised tissues may persist. The positive serological tests of latent and tertiary syphilis will seldom be reversed and are not an indication for treatment, in the absence of special clinical indications, after adequate measures have been employed. Tertiary lesions, particularly of the heart and central nervous system, often persist after full treatment and, in the absence of physical signs of active disease and persisting activity in the C.S.F., do not call for further specific treatment.

Other Drug treatment.—In the past potassium iodide, mercury, bismuth and organic arsenical compounds were used. Potassium iodide has no lethal effect on treponemata and is only of value in the tertiary stages: it prepares the way for safe intensive treatment of late lesions by dissolving gummatous material, and it is particularly valuable in the absorption and healing of gummata in organs such as the skin, liver, spleen or bones. Start with potassium iodide gr. 5 t.i.d. and increase daily by gr. 5 in the total daily dose until a total of gr. 90 a day is taken. Mercury was originally used for syphilis but was superseded by bismuth and the arsphenamines: it is rarely used except occasionally in superficial glossitis. Bismuth intramusc. is often given after the course of treatment of early syphilis with penicillin, particularly in severe or refractory cases. Ten weekly doses of 0·2 G. of the insoluble metallic suspension (inject. bismuthi B.P.) or the oxychloride are injected into the upper and outer quadrant of the buttock: to avoid the danger of accidental intravenous injections, always insert the needle first and make certain that no blood flows, then attach the charged syringe and gently withdraw the piston to ensure that a vein has not been entered; after slowly injecting the dose massage the area for 30 seconds to disseminate the bismuth along the tissue planes. Before bismuth therapy make sure the gums are healthy and that decayed teeth are removed; in an infected mouth a blue line of bismuth sulphide will occur along the gum margin causing salivation and stomatitis and even ulceration of the gums and buccal mucosa; this is treated by the administration of sulphonamides and a mouthwash containing sulphurated potash (B.P.C.) 0·5 per cent. in peppermint water. Albuminuria and loss of weight call for termination of bismuth therapy.

The organic arsenical compounds were introduced by Ehrlich in 1910, when he discovered Salvarsan or " 606 " (arsphenamine B.P.). This trivalent arsenical substance was toxic to the treponema and to the patient and, with Experiment 914, he produced the better tolerated neoarsphenamine B.P. (N.A.B.—" 914 "). These and related compounds are not directly bactericidal to the treponemata but are stored, chiefly in the liver; in the presence of oxygen they slowly liberate arsenoxides which are the lethal agents. After a smaller initial dose neoarsphenamine 0·6 G. is made into solution with sterile distilled water 6 ml. and the freshly made solution is injected intravenously once a week for 10 weeks, often with a concomitant course of bismuth. Administered only by the intravenous route great care must be taken that none of the solution enters the perivenous tissues, as it causes severe pain and produces chemical cellulitis and necrosis: this accident can, to some extent, be alleviated by the immediate infiltration of sodium thiosulphate (5 ml. of 10 per cent. solution). Do not inject neoarsphenamine after a heavy meal, if the patient is hungry or has recently taken alcohol. It is not well tolerated by elderly or debilitated subjects and special care is needed if it is administered to patients with liver, kidney or cardio-vascular disease. Occasional untoward reactions to treatment must be mentioned: (1) Symptoms resembling anaphylaxis (nitritoid crisis) may occur during or immediately after injection: inject. adrenaline ♏ 10 subcut. controls the condition. (2) The Jarisch-Herxheimer reaction is due to sudden liberation of toxins at the site of the treponemata in the blood-vessels; a few hours after the injection there is a transient fever or rigors, and the local œdema and inflammation may narrow the lumen of the blood-vessels causing obstruction, *e.g.*, of the coronary arteries. In early syphilis it is incidental but in the tertiary stage with coronary or cerebro-vascular disease, the reaction may be fatal; it can be avoided by preliminary gradual treatment with iodides or very small repeated doses of penicillin. When a patient is being treated for gonorrhœa by penicillin, the occurrence of such a Herxheimer reaction with general symptoms, should be regarded as suggestive of an incubating syphilitic infection. (3) Arsenical hepatitis may be allergic in the second week of treatment and later on toxic from accumulation of the drug in the liver, but it is more often due to a virus-transmitted hepatitis (§ 334). (4) Other toxic effects are arsenical dermatitis, acute encephalopathy, purpura and aplastic anæmia. When allergic complications occur, treat with antihistamines or steroids; toxic complications respond to inject. dimercaprol B.P. (B.A.L.) 2 ml. intramuscularly, 6-hourly on the first day and 8-hourly on the second and third days. *Tryparsamide* (a pentavalent arsenical compound) has greater permeability into the central nervous tissue and is preferable for late syphilis of this type, if adjuvant methods are required. Oxophenarsine B.P., the active substance which destroys the treponemata, was more recently used but it is rapidly excreted and needs several injections in 1 week; it is not free from untoward reactions and it is not much used in this country.

Marriage should be deferred until the minimum of 2 years' surveillance has been completed with no clinical relapse, completely negative serology and satisfactory C.S.F. findings. A patient is then considered cured but a woman should always be advised to have one full course of penicillin during pregnancy to prevent the risk of unsuspected dormant infection involving the fœtus.

Congenital syphilis is now rare as a result of the performance of routine serological tests in antenatal clinics and the efficacy of penicillin given to those mothers who are found to have positive blood tests. The blood in the umbilical cord reflects the state of the mother's blood and, if the strength of the reaction in the child decreases during the next few months to become negative by the sixth month, active treatment is not required. If, however, the reaction remains positive or becomes increasingly so, or if symptoms of infection are present, treatment is immediately needed. Inject. benzylpenicillin is recommended: in infancy give 6,000 units per lb. bodyweight at 8-hourly intervals for 15 days; alternatively procaine penicillin 300,000 units each 24 hours for 15 days is used, but this tends to give painful local swellings in the limited tissue available. The absorption of oral penicillin is unreliable and should not be used in congenital syphilis.

Many authorities augment penicillin treatment with one or more courses of appropriate doses of bismuth or arsenic. Owing to the difficulty of intravenous treatment, neoarsphenamine is replaced by intramusc. injections of sulpharsphenamine (B.P.) which is well tolerated by children. The dosage is calculated on the weight rather than on the age: Table XXXIV shows the maximum weekly doses at different ages but allowance must be made for a child above or below the average weight. A quarter of the maximum dose is given for the first injection, a half dose for the second injection and this is followed by 8 weekly injections. Alternatively 10 weekly doses of inject. bismuthi (B.P.) into the buttocks may be given alone or concurrently with the arsenical; a rest period of 4 weeks is allowed before undertaking a further course.

TABLE XXXIV. TREATMENT OF CONGENITAL SYPHILIS WITH
SULPHARSPHENAMINE AND BISMUTH

(Maximum weekly dosage for children of average weight)

Age	*Sulpharsphenamine*	*Bismuth*
Birth . . .	0·025 Gramme	0·025 Gramme
3 Months . .	0·05 ,,	0·025 ,,
1 Year . . .	0·10 ,,	0·05 ,,
5 Years . .	0·30 ,,	0·10 ,,
10 Years . .	0·45 ,,	0·15 ,,

The C.S.F. should be examined if the serological tests of the blood are still positive after two such courses of further treatment, and in all cases regular clinical and serological examinations are needed until after puberty. In late childhood and adolescence intravenous neoarsphenamine is tolerated better than sulpharsphenamine and in adults with late congenital syphilis treatment follows the pattern advocated for latent and tertiary syphilis.

The remaining fevers in this group are PLAGUE, UNDULANT FEVER, YELLOW FEVER, *which are met abroad;* CEREBRO-SPINAL FEVER, *which until recent years has for a long time been rare in this country; and* RELAPSING FEVER, *met in epidemic form only in times of famine. In* HAY FEVER, DYSENTERY *and* CHOLERA, *there is some disturbance of the temperature.* WEIL'S DISEASE *is described in* § 334*b*.

§ **501. IX. Plague** (Bubonic Plague, Typhus Bubonicus, Oriental Plague, the Black Death) may be defined as a highly infectious and fatal fever, characterised by inflammatory glandular and periglandular swellings, hæmorrhages beneath the skin and from the mucous membranes.   The last great epidemic in London was in 1666; the disease disappeared from this country at the end of the seventeenth century, probably because of the destruction of the black rat by the Norwegian brown rat.   Its chief epidemic centres at the present day are Northern India, China, Mongolia and Uganda. Since 1894 there has been a pandemic over most of the civilised world, and our present knowledge of the disease has therefore greatly increased.

Symptoms.—(1) The incubation period from is 2 to 10 days.   (2) There is often a prodromal stage, with depression and pains, but usually the onset is sudden, with shivering, and fever rising to 103° or even 107° F.   Mental aberration is not uncommon.   Prostration is marked, and may be accompanied by vertigo, staggering gait and lethargy, soon passing into the typhoid state.   The spleen and liver may be enlarged.   In some cases the speech is halting and staccato, the expression vacant, and the eyes congested; the condition is sometimes mistaken for acute alcoholism. A small vesicle, corresponding to a flea bite, is occasionally observed in the early stages of the disease; and examination of the fluid contents may reveal plague bacilli. (3) On the second or third day a tender swelling of the lymph glands (bubo) appears, the affected group, dependent on the site of the infecting flea bite, being inguinal and femoral in 70 per cent., axillary in 20 per cent. and cervical and submaxillary in 10 per cent. of the patients.   The glands rapidly enlarge, pain is intense and suppuration generally supervenes from the seventh to the twelfth day, if the patient survives. (4) Petechiæ and subcutaneous hæmorrhages are not uncommon.   A distinctive rash is rare, but when present it resembles typhus.   There are six principal *varieties*, which prevail in different epidemics: (i.) The *bubonic* variety is the commonest, glandular swellings occurring in quite 70 per cent. of all the cases.   The causal organism is frequently recovered on blood culture. (ii.) The *septicæmic* type is very fatal: the glands enlarge slightly, but they do not suppurate; (iii.) a *fulminant* form, with high fever, little glandular enlargement, vomiting of blood, and death within a few hours; (iv.) a *pneumonic* form, which may be mistaken for bronchitis, influenzal pneumonia or broncho-pneumonia, attended by intense prostration, no glandular enlargement, and death usually on the third to the fifth day; herpes is absent and the pulse-respiration ratio not so much altered as in true pneumonia; (v.) an *abortive* form, in which there are buboes without much fever, subsiding in 14 days; and (vi.) an *ambulant* or mild form, with chronic glandular enlargement, great anæmia and weakness.   Intestinal, cerebral and cellulo-cutaneous types are also encountered.

Diagnosis.—Early in an epidemic bubonic plague may have to be distinguished from filarial adenitis, lymphogranuloma venereum, soft sore or syphilitic bubo, tularæmia and rat-bite fever.   Gland puncture reveals plague bacilli in both smears and culture of the gland juice, and in most of the severe cases of bubonic plague *Pasteurella pestis* can be cultured from the peripheral blood at some stage of the disease.   In pneumonic plague the sputum is watery and sanguineous, never viscid and rusty as in pneumonia; the bipolar plague bacilli are present in great numbers in smears of the sputum and this particular form is directly transmitted from individual to individual by droplet infection.   Septicæmic plague is diagnosed by positive blood cultures.

Etiology.—Plague is due to the *Pasteurella pestis*.   Outbreaks of plague were often preceded by a large mortality among rats and other rodents, and it is now known that the bubonic form of the disease is spread by them.   The fleas infesting rats convey the infection to man.   The alimentary tract of the flea becomes blocked by a mass of bacilli, the result of growth from infected blood previously imbibed; some of these bacilli are voided during attempts to suck blood and so pass to a fresh victim, being enabled to enter through the puncture made by the flea. Filth and overcrowding predispose to plague. The pneumonic form is directly conveyed from man to man by droplet infection. Age and sex have little influence.

Prognosis.—The case-mortality in the early periods of epidemics is generally 50 per cent. in untreated cases. In the usual course of bubonic plague death occurs before the sixth day; or, if the patient is to recover, convalescence starts between the sixth and tenth day. The pneumonic variety was so fatal before treatment with streptomycin was introduced that of 43,000 cases in Manchuria only three recovered. Prolonged suppuration of the glands may delay convalescence considerably. The course of the disease is very difficult to forecast. Hæmorrhages usually herald death. The *sequelæ* include boils, pneumonia, dropsy, partial paralysis and mental disorder.

Treatment.—Bed rest, careful nursing and a fluid diet are essential. Isolation is advisable in all cases and imperative in pneumonic cases. The attendants on these latter patients should wear protective clothing and masks and may be given prophylactic streptomycin 0·5–1·0 G. daily for short periods. Streptomycin intramusc. is the most effective antibiotic and should be administered with a sulphonamide, preferably sulphadiazine. Streptomycin 1 G. is given immediately, then 0·5 G. 4-hourly until the temperature has been normal for 2 days. Concurrently sulphadiazine is given orally, 4 G. immediately, 1 G. 4-hourly until the temperature has been normal for 2 days, then 0·5 G. 4-hourly for a further 10 days: these large doses must be combined with a copious fluid intake and measures to render the urine alkaline. The tetracyclines and chloramphenicol are also very valuable especially in the pneumonic form. The buboes should be treated with hot fomentations, a kaolin poultice or glycerin of belladonna paste, and incised when suppuration occurs. Morphia may be necessary for the pain. *Prophylaxis.*—General measures consist of rat control and the use of 10 per cent. DDT powder on rat runs to kill the fleas. Contacts of known cases should be given prophylactic courses of sulphadiazine or sulphamerazine 6 G. a day for 3–7 days. Prophylactic vaccines are of some value.

§ 502. X. Undulant Fever. There are two main types: (1) Malta Fever, found particularly in those countries which border on the Mediterranean, in S. Africa, in the southern portions of the U.S.A., and the Punjab, due to *Brucella melitensis.* All ages and both sexes are liable to contract the disease. It is conveyed to man by the milk of infected goats which need not show any signs of ill health. (2) Abortus fever, contracted from cattle or swine suffering from contagious abortion due to *Brucella abortus* (an organism closely related to *Brucella melitensis*). It is prevalent on the continent of Europe, especially Denmark, in North Africa and the United States. In England many cases are being reported and the disease is by no means uncommon. The disease is conveyed by drinking raw milk, handling the carcases or hides, removing the animal's placenta or slaughtering pigs. Porcine strains of *Brucella* (*B. suis*) are also known.

Symptoms.—The incubation period is 14 days, though exceptionally it appears to be very much longer; the prodromata include malaise, muscular pains and dyspepsia. Soon increasing headache, fever and muscular pains cause the patient to seek advice. The temperature keeps high (102–104° F) for about 14 days, and may then drop for a few days, only to rise again. After several such undulations the temperature becomes intermittent, with a marked rise at night. The general health of the patient suffers in many ways, the chief symptoms being gastro-intestinal. There are muscular and joint pains, which may be accompanied by considerable swelling, sore throat, sweating, anæmia, enlarged painful spleen and bronchitis. There are three varieties of the disease. The *malignant* is of acute onset, and runs a rapid course to a fatal termination, preceded by the typhoid state and hyperpyrexia. The *intermittent* variety is of very slow onset, and runs a long course, with sudden elevation of the temperature each evening often with a rigor. The patient does not as a rule make any complaint of specific symptoms until his general health begins to be affected. The *ambulatory* type includes the not infrequent cases in which the *Brucella melitensis* is found in the blood of persons who are in no respect ill. A *chronic* form is described which is often very difficult to confirm bacteriologically. The symptoms commonly complained of are long-standing night sweats and rheumatic pains; the findings are occasional enlargement of the liver, spleen and lymph glands, with little loss of weight, a relatively normal blood count and erythrocyte sedimentation rate.

The *Diagnosis* is suggested by the clinical signs and often by the patient's occupation. The differential diagnosis includes the enteric fevers, chronic malaria, rheumatic fever, kala-azar, subacute bacterial endocarditis, tuberculosis and the reticuloses. The organism can be cultured from the blood, urine or sternal marrow. (*Br. abortus* grows better in an atmosphere containing 10 per cent. CO_2.) After a few weeks the agglutinin reaction of the blood usually becomes positive at titres of 1/100 to 1/500 or higher (a wide range of dilutions should be tried as zones of inhibition are common in the lower dilutions). Later the complement-fixation test, which is only group specific, becomes positive. A positive intradermal test, using a killed culture, is often obtained. In doubtful cases blood can be inoculated into the peritoneal cavity of a guinea pig.

Prognosis.—In the common type the mortality is about 3 per cent. Complications are arthritis, osteitis, neuritis, orchitis, parotitis, mammitis, bronchitis, pneumonia, cardiac failure and hyperpyrexia, the latter being the usual cause of death. The disease may last 2 years or longer; the average is 3 to 6 months. *Brucella melitensis* infections are usually much more severe than infections by *Brucella abortus.*

Treatment.—Careful nursing and a nourishing diet adequate in vitamins is important. When the temperature exceeds 103° F tepid sponging should be instituted. Chlortetracycline (Aureomycin) 0·5 G. 6-hourly for 10 days will arrest the fever but relapses are common. Then intensive treatment must be instituted and some authorities prefer this from the commencement. This consists of chlortetracycline 0·5 G. 6-hourly, inject. streptomycin 0·75 G. 12-hourly and tab. trisulphonamide 1·0 G. 6-hourly for 3 weeks. This combination is bactericidal whereas each drug given alone is mainly bacteriostatic. Penicillin is useless. *Prophylaxis* consists in avoiding the milk, cheese and carcases of infected goats and cows. Milk is rendered safe by boiling or pasteurisation. Laboratory workers must handle *Brucella* cultures with great care. S19 vaccine administered to young animals has greatly reduced the incidence of the infection.

§ 503. XI. **Yellow Fever** is an acute infectious disease endemic in a large part of tropical Africa and South America; in severe cases it is accompanied by jaundice, black vomitus and other evidences of hæmorrhage into the mucous membranes or skin.

Symptoms.—The incubation period in man is from 3 to 5 days in mosquito-transmitted infections, and up to 10 days in laboratory workers who have contracted infection from contact with blood containing the virus. Mild, ordinary and fulminating clinical types of the disease are encountered. (*a*) In the *mild* or larval infections there is headache, vomiting and fever of short duration, lasting a few days. Albuminuria is generally demonstrable, but jaundice, if it develops, is mild. (*b*) In the *ordinary* type three stages are recognised, the *sthenic*, the *remission* and the *asthenic* stage. (i.) The onset is generally sudden with chilly sensations or a rigor, the temperature rising to 103° or 104° F on the first day. Frontal headache, backache, pains in the limbs and photophobia are characteristic, the face is flushed, the conjunctivæ injected and the tongue furred with bright red edges. Albuminuria appears about the second day and rapidly increases and the urine soon contains casts; bile salts and pigments are found later. At first the pulse is rapid and bounding, but later it slows and by the third day equals only 60 to 70 per minute despite the elevated temperature. (ii.) About the third or fourth day the temperature drops considerably or falls to normal. (iii.) After the short remission the fever usually returns for 2 or 3 days. In this stage the liver is enlarged and tender, epigastric discomfort is marked, and hiccough and jaundice with hyperbilirubinæmia and a biphasic van den Bergh reaction are common. There is no splenic enlargement. Petechiæ, melæna and black vomit may appear, while oliguria and anuria with nitrogenous retention and acidosis are the rule in fatal cases. Hypotension and bradycardia, due to involvement of the A-V bundle, are characteristic. Death may occur from the fifth to the twelfth day. Leucocytes vary from 5,000 to 15,000 per c.mm.

(c) *Fulminating* cases develop high fever, purpuric skin rashes, oozing from the gums, early black vomitus and melæna. Jaundice is intense. Hiccough, tremor, delirium and coma due to cholæmia, and uræmia with anurla develop. Death occurs on the third or fourth day.

Etiology.—Yellow fever is due to a filterable virus. Although clinically indistinguishable, three types of yellow fever are recognised, namely, urban, rural and jungle. The first two are transmitted normally by the tiger-banded mosquito, *Aëdes ægypti* (*Stegomyia fasciata*); the third is transmitted by various forest mosquitoes from various animal reservoirs. The blood of man is infective during the first 3 days of fever, but never the excreta. One attack confers immunity and convalescent human serum protects the susceptible monkey, *Macacus rhesus*, when exposed to the virus. The virus may traverse the intact skin in either man or monkey; and in this way many research workers have contracted fatal infections.

Diagnosis.—Important points in diagnosis from other tropical fevers are the severe prostration, early albuminuria, slow pulse, jaundice and the absence of splenic enlargement. In mild cases, intracerebral inoculation into mice of the patient's blood in the early days of the disease produces an encephalitis. Later, and in recovered cases, immune bodies in the patient's blood may be demonstrated by the mouse protection test: mice whose brains have been previously traumatised by injected starch solution are inoculated intraperitoneally with mixtures of virus and suspected serum. If the serum contains no immune bodies, encephalitis results: whereas if immune bodies are present (due to previous infection of the patient), the mice remain well. *Leptospirosis* closely simulates yellow fever, but there is extreme muscular tenderness, neutrophil leucocytosis and a history of a recent immersion accident or an occupational relationship to rats; see § 334. *Malaria* complicated by jaundice is recognised by the splenomegaly and parasites in the blood, and *blackwater fever* by the hæmoglobinuria. *Infective hepatitis, toxic hepatitis* and *acute yellow atrophy* all have a more gradual onset and no stage of remission. In *relapsing fever* with jaundice there is enlargement of the spleen and spirochætes are readily demonstrable in the blood.

Prognosis.—In the average case the mortality is about 20 per cent. Intense and early jaundice, severe nervous disturbances, intractable hiccough, widespread hæmorrhages into the skin and from mucous membranes and anuria are of bad omen.

Treatment.—(a) *Curative* treatment is unsatisfactory. Careful nursing and abundant fluids during the acute phases of the illness are imperative and a chart of the fluid intake and output must be kept. Glucose and sodium bicarbonate should be added to all drinks, and 1 to 2 pints of 5 per cent. dextrose may be given intravenously each 24 hours. The development of shock calls for immediate plasma transfusion. Tepid sponging and sedatives are good for the insomnia but antipyretics must not be given. Gradual increase of food is allowed after the temperature has been normal several days. (b) *Prophylactic* treatment includes all measures for the destruction of the mosquito vector, *Aëdes ægypti*, a domestic mosquito which may bite during both day and night. Prophylactic inoculation with chick-embryo cultures of low virulence pantropic virus is protective for 6 years; human serum is no longer used in preparing the vaccine. Rubber gloves should be worn when collecting blood for laboratory purposes, and infected patients should be screened during the first 4 days of fever.

§ **504. XII. Cerebro-Spinal Fever** (Syn., Meningococcal Fever, Meningoccocal Meningitis, Spotted Fever) is due to the meningococcus invading the blood stream from the naso-pharynx, and later reaching the meninges. In some cases two separate stages are evident, with symptoms of septicæmia followed by those of meningitis, but the stages often overlap. *Principal Symptoms:* (i.) In the initial stages there may be nasopharyngeal catarrh: (ii.) fever, accompanied by fleeting joint pains, headache, vomiting and later, skin rashes. The temperature is often irregular at the onset and even subsides to normal for a day or so, before rising again. It is rarely over 102–104° F except for a terminal hyperpyrexia. These septicæmic symptoms are accompanied or succeeded by (iii.) symptoms of irritative intracranial inflammation, such as very severe headache, vomiting, photophobia, restlessness, drowsiness and delirium. There is always retraction of the head, and sometimes opisthotonus, owing to the rigidity of the muscles of the back. Hyperæsthesia, especially along the spine, neck stiffness, and severe pain in the back, may be so great that all movement is intolerable. Kernig's and Brudzinski's signs are usually present. Compression symptoms may supervene later. (iv.) A prominent feature is the presence of an eruption, often symmetrical. Herpes simplex is frequent except in infants, and may have unusual localisation. Urticaria and erythema may occur. On the second day or later a purpuric rash sometimes appears, and may cover the body (" spotted fever "); its frequency varies considerably in different epidemics; in some it has been rare. (v.) Polymorphonuclear leucocytosis appears early. Unusual *Varieties* are: (i.) The fulminating type is associated with the Waterhouse-Friderichsen Syndrome (§ 245); in this, septicæmia and often hyperpyrexia are associated with acute circulatory collapse and anuria, cyanosis, purpura and often death within 24 hours. With this (ii.) an acute encephalitis may co-exist or the latter may occur alone. The brain involvement gives deep coma and stertorous breathing, sometimes with convulsions: meningitis is not necessarily present. (iii) Abortive forms occur with moderately severe headache, fever and neck stiffness; the C.S.F. shows polymorph cells, but meningococci may be very difficult to demonstrate. (iv.) Chronic septicæmic cases show moderate fever, occasional rigors, muscle and joint pains, headache and rose-red spots, sometimes resembling erythema nodosum: a positive blood culture is obtained, but the meninges may or may not be involved later. (v.) Posterior basic meningitis of infants.

POSTERIOR BASIC MENINGITIS is a subacute form of this disease occurring in infants from 3 to 12 months old, characterised by (i.) an acute onset with convulsions and gastro-enteritis, or a gradual onset with drowsiness, vomiting and a meningitic cry. (ii.) A few days later there is the gradual onset of the retraction of the head which may amount to opisthotonos with flexor and extensor spasms in the limbs; (iii.) staring of the eyes, with blindness, appearing quite early in the disease, unassociated with changes in the optic nerves, and due to involvement of the occipital cortex; strabismus is common; (iv.) rigidity of the limbs, which may be localised or confined to one extremity; (v.) paroxysms of high fever lasting a day or two at a time. The onset of *Hydrocephalus* is heralded by *vomiting* and *wasting*, with enlargement of the skull in infants, bulging of the fontanelles and opening of the sutures between the bones. A resonant or " cracked pot " note is present on percussion over the anterior horn of the lateral ventricle in infants in whom the fontanelles are closed.

Diagnosis.—If the patient is seen in the septicæmic stage a post-nasal swab and blood culture will show meningococci. Usually the patient is first seen in the meningitic stage and then a diagnostic lumbar puncture is essential—it will reveal a turbid fluid with pus cells and often intra- or extra-cellular Gram-negative diplococci. In tuberculous meningitis the onset is more insidious, there is no eruption and the C.S.F. findings are characteristic (Table LXVI). Care should be taken to exclude anterior poliomyelitis, in which a stage of cerebral irritation lasting even 7 to 10 days is not uncommon. During an epidemic of cerebro-spinal fever the diagnosis is much easier.

Etiology of Cerebro-spinal fever.—It occurs sporadically and in epidemics, usually in persons under 20; some epidemics have occurred chiefly among infants, and males more than females. It is most frequent in winter and spring. Although becoming rare in this country it is still common in other parts of the world. It is undoubtedly infectious, although much less so than the acute exanthemata. " Carriers " play the chief part in its spread, overcrowding, especially of sleeping quarters, greatly increasing the danger of transmission which occurs as the result of the droplets of secretion being sprayed around during coughing and sneezing. It is due to the *Neisseria meningitidis* (*Diplococcus intracellularis meningitidis* of Weichselbaum), which is Gram-negative and best grown on tryp-agar or ascitic fluid.

Prognosis.—The overall fatality rate in Great Britain is about 7·5 per cent., but for those under 1 year and over 65 years the figure rises to 25–30 per cent. These figures show the need for early and adequate treatment. Amongst the unfavourable signs are the occurrence of hyperpyrexia, purpura, broncho-pneumonia or circulatory collapse or encephalitis (see above): an unduly prolonged period of illness. The other common complications are acute arthritis, acute sinusitis and optic neuritis. Amongst the sequelæ may be mentioned deafness, iridochoroiditis, panophthalmitis, subacute arthritis, orchitis, chronic hydrocephalus, and transient paralysis of the limbs, aphasia and dementia.

Treatment consists in isolating the patient and nursing him in a darkened room: all attendants must wear masks and gowns. When the initial diagnostic lumbar puncture is done, 20,000 units of sterile benzylpenicillin in 10 ml. should be inserted into the cerebro-spinal fluid. The results have been revolutionised by the use of tabs. sulphathiazole and sulphadiazine; sulphamethazine is not quite so effective. (For dosage see Table XXXV.) *These sulpha drugs must never be given intrathecally.* Intramusc. injections of soluble salts of these drugs have been given up because their solutions are very irritant owing to their strongly alkaline reaction. The neutral preparation Soluthiazole can be given in an initial dose of 2·0 G. by intramuscular medication or via a continuous drip into a vein. Later oral preparations can be substituted. These large doses always demand a copious fluid intake and simultaneous administration of alkalies. Penicillin is not so effective as the sulphonamides and does not easily pass the blood-brain barrier but it may be given in addition. Fulminant cases with circulatory collapse may respond to intravenous hydrocortisone 100 mg. 12-hourly or to a nor-adrenaline drip (§ 52) together with 600 ml. of human plasma and then 600 ml. 5 per cent. dextrose in half-normal saline, in addition to Soluthiazole and penicillin intravenously. Apart from the initial diagnostic puncture, lumbar puncture is usually unnecessary. Frequent doses of chloral hydrate and potass. bromide āā 20 gr., injections of paraldehyde and caps. sodium amylobarbitone may be given with advantage. Retention of urine should be looked for, dehydration corrected, nasal feeding used where necessary and the use of an oxygen tent is sometimes required. *Prophylaxis.*—Even as small a dose of sulphadiazine as 2 G. has cleared meningococci from the noses of carriers.

§ 505. XIII. Relapsing Fever (Syn., Famine Fever, Spirillum Fever) embraces a group of infectious fevers due to *Spirochæta recurrentis* found in the blood, spread either by lice (widespread form) or by ticks (Central African, Peruvian and American forms). The incubation period varies from 5 to 9 days. The primary fever lasts generally from 5 to 7 days, and short febrile relapses are common.

LOUSE-BORNE RELAPSING FEVER. *Symptoms.*—(1) The fever has a sudden onset, with rigor, headache, backache and pains in the limbs. The face is flushed, the eyes injected and photophobia is common. Often there is an initial erythematous rash and later roseolar macules or petechiæ. The temperature rapidly rises and after remaining elevated for 6 or 7 days, returns to normal by crisis. The fall is preceded and attended by profuse perspiration or diarrhœa, or both. This is followed by an interval of about a week, during which the patient feels exhausted, and the pulse and temperature are subnormal. At the end of this time a relapse occurs which is similar to the first attack, but shorter, lasting 3 or 4 days. In rare cases there is a second and even a third relapse. (2) Abdominal pain and tenderness, and definite enlargement of the spleen and liver, are present in most cases. Jaundice and epistaxis are not uncommon in severe cases; sometimes there is vomiting of blood. Delirium is very rare, but if present is of the noisy kind, and occurs at the crisis. Convalescence is slow. (3) Spirochætes are found in the blood during the pyrexial period. A neutrophil leucocytosis accompanies the fever and a leucopenia the afebrile period.

TICK-BORNE RELAPSING FEVER is endemic in Central Africa, sporadic in the Middle East, and never assumes the epidemic proportions of the lice-borne fevers. It differs from the louse-borne form in the shorter duration of the initial fever, in the greater number of relapses and the paucity of spirochætes in the peripheral blood. Epistaxis, hæmaturia and jaundice may occur and the central nervous system may be involved with paresis of the cranial nerves and coma; the C.S.F. may show increased pressure and lymphocytosis. Complications are pneumonia, parotitis and iritis. It is often more resistant to treatment, e.g., with organic arsenic, than the louse-borne form.

The *Diagnosis of Relapsing Fever* depends on demonstration of the organism in the blood. Intraperitoneal injection of patient's blood into young white mice or rats may help diagnosis, as spirochætes may appear in the animal's blood in 24–48 hours.

Prognosis.—The case-mortality averages about 5 per cent., but may be very high in the African form. Age has not much influence, but dissipation and debility are unfavourable. One attack does not confer immunity from a second. Death, which occurs generally at the height of the first attack, is usually due to syncope, from hæmorrhage or from myocardial degeneration. When occurring later, it may be due to complications. Untoward symptoms include hæmorrhage, suppression of urine, the typhoid state, cerebral symptoms, or indications of a weak heart. A rapid pulse, a high temperature, and even jaundice, are not necessarily unfavourable.

Treatment.—Neoarsphenamine 0·45 G. should be given intravenously very slowly, as early as possible, preferably when the temperature is rising; if given when a natural crisis is imminent grave collapse may occur. In the louse-borne disease one dose is usually effective; in the tick-borne disease relapses may occur and the dose is then repeated. Although penicillin cuts short the fever it does not permanently prevent relapses but terramycin is often completely successful in a dose of 0·5 G. 6-hourly. *Prophylaxis* is by delousing, using the methods detailed for epidemic typhus (§ 484).

§ **506.** XIV. Apart from the relapsing fever above described, there are several forms of fever transmitted by ticks, sand-flies and animals. The best known of these are: Tularæmia, Kala-azar, Phlebotomus and Rat-bite Fevers.

Tularæmia (Syn., Deer-fly Fever, Pahvant Valley Fever, Ohara's Disease). A rodent disease, due to *Pasteurella tularense*, transmissible to man and prevalent in the United States of America, Russia, Europe and Japan; many accidental infections have occurred among laboratory workers.

Symptoms.—Two principal forms of the disease have been described—ulcero-glandular and typhoid. The glandular form is characterised by fever, rigors, gener-alised pain, headache, the formation of a papule which ulcerates, and enlargement of the regional lymphatic glands. It is the type common in butchers, poultry-men and trappers. In the typhoid type there is a fever of varying degree which lasts a considerable time. There are no localising symptoms; it is the type generally found in laboratory workers. The *diagnosis* is made by agglutination of *P. tularense* by the patient's serum or by culture of the organism from the local lesions or glands.

Etiology.—(1) The organism *P. tularense* is introduced by the bite of a horse-fly or of a wood-tick. (2) Also by contamination of hands or the conjunctival sac with internal organs or body fluids of rabbits, hares, squirrels, water-rats or other animals infected with *P. tularense* and (3) the ingestion of their uncooked flesh.

Prognosis.—Convalescence is slow, but recovery usually occurs without sequelæ. The chief complications are broncho-pneumonia, pleural effusion, abscesses in the lungs, liver and spleen, peritonitis and meningitis. The mortality rate is very low.

Treatment.—Streptomycin intramusc. 0·5 G. 8-hourly to a total of 4·0 G. combined with a course of a sulphonamide will cure the glandular form. In the typhoid form the drugs should be continued until the patient is afebrile. The tetracyclines are not quite so efficacious but can be used when streptomycin is contra-indicated.

Kala-azar.—A disease found in China, India, Africa and S. America associated with enlargement of the spleen and liver, anæmia and leucopenia, some wasting and irregular fever of long duration. It is caused by *Leishmania donovani*, which are found in monocytes in the peripheral blood and in the reticulo-endothelium of the viscera and bone marrow. An infantile form of the disease occurs throughout the Mediterranean littoral. Transmission is by sand-flies.

Symptoms.—The incubation period varies from 1 to 12 months and the onset is occasionally sudden with fever; usually it is more insidious. When established there are (1) irregular remittent or intermittent pyrexia, the temperature charts sometimes showing a double daily rise in the afternoon and evening; (2) increased pigmentation of the skin; (3) anæmia of secondary type associated with marked leucopenia (1,000–5,000 cells per cubic millimetre): there is a relative increase in lymphocytes and monocytes, a decrease in neutrophils with disappearance of the eosinophils; (4) loss of weight, and cachexia; (5) splenomegaly, the spleen being first soft and doughy but not tender, and later enlarging and becoming very hard. Diarrhœa, enlargement of the liver, night sweats, asthenia and low blood pressure may develop. Cancrum oris associated with agranulocytosis, otitis media, hæmorrhage from mucous membranes, purpura and secondary infections like influenza, pneumonia and tuberculosis may cause death. Hepatitis and cirrhosis, and post kala-azar dermal leishmanoid may follow the disease.

Diagnosis.—Kala-azar has to be distinguished from leukæmia, Banti's disease, the reticuloses, schistosomiasis, chronic malaria, undulant fever, relapsing fever and typhoid fever. The diagnosis is made by finding the parasites in material aspirated from the spleen, liver, bone marrow or lymph gland. The formol-gel test is usually positive after 2 to 5 months: the serum added to a drop of commercial formalin becomes opalescent within 1 or 2 minutes and coagulates solid like boiled egg white in 20 minutes. A positive reaction, associated with leucopenia, is valuable evidence of kala-azar. Sometimes the parasites are demonstrable in blood smears and they may be cultured on rabbit blood agar medium at 22° C.

Treatment.—Antimony compounds are generally curative, although refractory cases are encountered especially in the Mediterranean. Trivalent antimony compounds have now been replaced by the less toxic pentavalent compounds. Sodium stibogluconate, 0·6 G. in 6 ml. fluid intravenously daily for 7 days, the course being repeated after a week's rest, gives very good results. Other pentavalent antimonial compounds are also used. Ascites and nephritis are indications for care in the use of antimony, and if pneumonia or jaundice supervenes the injections may have to be suspended until these complications are cured. Children tolerate a relatively larger dose than adults. In antimony-resistant cases, pentamidine isothionate (B.P.C.) (0·2 to 0·3 G. daily for 10 to 14 days) may be used. Cure is indicated by decrease in the size of the spleen, an absence of pyrexia and clinical symptoms extending over a period of 6 months, a negative formol-gel test and a permanent disappearance of parasites. Where agranulocytosis occurs penicillin injections will help to prevent secondary infections. Injections of pentnucleotide should be given without delay.

Phlebotomus Fever (Syn., Sand-fly Fever, Papataci Fever, Three Days' Fever) is a fever affecting new-comers in the summer months in the Balkans, Malta, Crete, Mesopotamia, Egypt, India and other parts of the tropics and subtropics.

Symptoms.—After an incubation period of 2 to 7 days the patient has a rigor, followed by severe headache, fever and severe pain in the eyeballs and brow, back and calves of the legs. The eyes are congested, the face flushed, the tongue foul. The fever lasts from 1 to 5 days, most often 72 hours. Vomiting, bradycardia and leucopenia with relative lymphocytosis may occur. The disease is never fatal. Recurrence is most unusual.

Etiology.—The disease is due to a filterable virus transmitted to man by the bite of a sand-fly (*Phlebotomus* species). The virus is present in the peripheral blood during the first 2 days and can be transmitted by direct inoculation. The *diagnosis* lies between influenza, malaria and dengue, the latter showing secondary rises of temperature and a rash not observed in sand-fly fever.

Treatment.—Medical treatment consists of aspirin, phenacetin and caffeine citrate or even opium for the pain; cold sponging is beneficial when the fever is high. The disease is best prevented by the application of an insecticide to the sand-flies' breeding places and the use of special small meshed nets at night (they can pass through the meshes of an ordinary mosquito net and only bite at night). Repellents, such as dimethyl phthalate, are useful.

Rat-bite Fever (Syn., Sodoku) has long been described in Japan as occurring after the bites of rats and cats. Cases are also met in Europe and America. There are two varieties: (1) The first is due to *Spirillum minus*, and the *symptoms* are: (i.) There is a history of a rat-bite which is followed by local pain, swelling and a purple-red discoloration; (ii.) this develops into a chancre-like ulcer 1–3 weeks after the bite, with lymphangitis and lymphadenitis; (iii.) there is fever even to 105° F, which recurs at intervals of about 6 days. It may last a day or a week and assume an intermittent type; (iv.) the fever is accompanied in most cases by a large macular or papular rash; (v.) the blood shows a moderate leucocytosis, but blood cultures are negative: the Kahn reaction may be positive but the Wassermann reaction is negative. (2) The second is caused by *Streptobacillus moniliformis*. *Symptoms:* (i.) After the rat-bite the wound heals quickly: but (ii.) within 2–5 days there is high fever, severe arthritis, and sometimes painful nodules in the muscles: (iii.) there is often secondary anæmia and polymorph leucocytosis.

Treatment.—The disease caused by *Spirillum minus* responds to neoarsphenamine and to penicillin (given for 7–10 days): that due to the *Streptobacillus* to penicillin or to the tetracyclines.

§ 507. XV. Psittacosis is a disease of parrots due to a filterable virus. The infection is contracted by inhalation of excreta from infected birds, including the green Amazonian parrot, grey parrots and budgerigars.

Symptoms.—The incubation period varies from 7 to 12 days and the onset is acute or gradual, usually acute. Headache is marked, the patient becomes dull and apathetic and a typhoid-like condition may develop; occasionally epistaxis occurs. The spleen is not generally palpable; small rose spots may appear, somewhat resembling those of typhoid fever. Pulmonary symptoms are frequent and may be present from the onset, or develop some days later (§ 123). There is not much expectoration as a rule, but cough is troublesome. The pulse respiration ratio is low. Physical signs vary, but are not infrequently those of massive consolidation with woody dullness on percussion. The disease may terminate in recovery after 2 or 3 weeks. The death rate is about 15 per cent. Recrudescence during convalescence is sometimes observed.

Diagnosis.—The diagnosis is made from a history of contact with a sick bird by a patient who is affected with an obscure fever resembling typhoid or pneumonia. Agglutination and complement fixation tests are helpful in diagnosis.

Treatment.—Prophylaxis consists of forbidding the importation of infected birds and strict quarantine. Sick parrots should be immediately destroyed and cages treated with antiseptics. *Treatment* is with chloramphenicol or a tetracycline.

§ 508. XVI. Cat-scratch Fever is a benign condition with case reports from many parts of the world.

Symptoms.—In over 50 per cent. of cases there is a history of a scratch or close contact with a domestic cat. Other almost identical cases follow pricks by thorns, splinters, meat-bones and insect bites. *Local symptoms.*—At the site of injury, in half the cases there develops a red papule, vesicle or pustule followed by regional lymphadenitis usually of the epitrochlear and axillary glands, sometimes of the inguinal glands. These attain a large size, may suppurate and produce a sinus, the pus being sterile. The glands remain enlarged for weeks or months but ultimately subside completely. *General symptoms* are not severe and comprise low grade fever, headache and malaise. Unilateral granular or ulcerative conjunctivitis has been described.

Diagnosis.—The condition may be mistaken for tuberculosis, Hodgkin's disease or other forms of reticulosis. The blood shows a leucopenia with a relative lymphocytosis. A specific diagnostic test is with heated pus from affected lymph nodes, intradermal injection of which causes in 48 hours a tuberculin-type of papule or erythema.

Etiology.—A virus of the psittacosis-lymphogranuloma venereum group is suspected but the causal organism has not been identified. Even the cat has not been conclusively proved to be the vector as suspected cats give a negative intradermal test.

Prognosis.—All cases ultimately recover. Encephalitis, encephalomyelitis and radiculitis occasionally occur.

Treatment is symptomatic. Suppurating glands need aspiration. Chlortetracycline (Aureomycin) and terramycin may help to shorten the course of the disease.

§ 509. XVII. **Bornholm Disease** (Syn., Epidemic pleurodynia, epidemic myalgia, devil's grip) is an acute febrile illness which produces widespread outbreaks in the early autumn in Great Britain and occurs in many other parts of the world. More than one member of a family is often affected, especially children under 15 years of age.

Symptoms.—After an incubation period of 3–5 days, the onset is usually very sudden and even dramatic, with acute spasmodic myalgic pain especially at the lower rib margin or in the upper abdomen on one or both sides. Acute local tenderness in one spot may occur, the pain is aggravated by deep breathing, coughing or sneezing, and when the diaphragm is affected there may be board-like rigidity of the muscles which simulates an acute upper abdominal emergency. In an epidemic other cases show a less severe pain and some only slight pain in the muscles. The temperature rises rapidly to 102–104° F, with a frontal headache, nausea, sweating is often profuse and there may be a general myalgia. Occasionally there is initially a sore throat, with anorexia and a rigor shortly before the pain commences. A loud pleural rub is sometimes heard. The temperature is intermittent and finally settles in 3–4 days. Although X-ray signs in the lungs are usually absent, pneumonitis has been described. One or two relapses may occur.

Diagnosis is from a perforated peptic ulcer or other acute upper abdominal condition, and from other causes of diaphragmatic pleurisy.

Etiology.—A member of the Cocksackie virus B group is probably responsible and has been isolated from the stools in a considerable proportion of cases.

Prognosis.—All cases recover in a few days: occasional complications are meningism, meningo-encephalitis, and acute orchitis at the end of the first week of the illness.

Treatment is symptomatic with bed rest and the use of analgesics.

§ 509a. XVIII. **Toxoplasmosis** is an unusual disease of man and animals due to a small protozoan parasite *Toxoplasma gondii.* It occurs in most parts of the world, including Great Britain. Infants and small children are much more severely affected than adults.

Symptoms.—Two main types exist. (i.) *Congenital* infection takes place through the placenta and is the most commonly recognised variety; the mother is free of symptoms and only one child of each mother is affected. When acquired early in pregnancy abortion or stillbirth are usual, infection in later infancy or at birth causes in the first 3 months of life hydrocephalus, chorio-retinitis or encephalomyelitis with muscular twitchings and convulsions; the majority of such infants die in the first few weeks of life, and the few that survive often show calcified granulomata in the brain, microphthalmia with hydrocephalus, a greater or lesser degree of blindness and mental deficiency. Those affected late in pregnancy may also show the primary signs of the infection with a fluctuating temperature, jaundice, enlargement of the liver and spleen (in 50 per cent. of cases) and sometimes purpura or a maculopapular rash. (ii.) *Acquired* disease in young children is much more serious than in adults in whom the diagnosis is more benign and often missed. Active infection gives rise to: (*a*) Adults most commonly show enlargement of lymph glands in one or more areas with a marked or low fever, headache, muscle pains, often anæmia and slight leucocytosis with a predominance of lymphocytes. Recovery occurs slowly over a period of weeks or months during which time the glands remain palpable. (*b*) The rare acute exanthematous form causes sudden fever, often ushered in by a rigor, a widespread maculo-papular rash and the principal local feature is a diffuse interstitial pneumonia resembling virus pneumonia; myocarditis and meningo-encephalitis may occur. (*c*) Children have fever, headache, delirium and convulsions due to meningo-encephalitis—the C.S.F. shows a leucocytosis, increased protein and often xanthochromia.

Diagnosis.—In infants the condition is more easily recognised. In young adults the clinical and blood pictures resemble *infectious mononucleosis*, but the Paul-Bunnell reaction is negative. Confusion with *polioencephalitis* and *typhus fever* may occur. With glandular enlargement a lymph node biopsy, or otherwise examination of the C.S.F., muscle biopsy or bone marrow smears may reveal the organism which can be grown on the chorio-atlantoic membrane of developing chick embryos. Laboratory mice are susceptible. In acute infections the complement fixation test (to a titre above 1 in 10) and the cytoplasmin-modifying (dye) test (titre above 1 in 250) become positive in 1–2 weeks. The toxoplasmin skin sensitivity test becomes slowly positive over a period of many months.

Etiology.—Although the causal organism is known the method of transmission to man is very uncertain: domestic animals (dogs, cats and rabbits) are suspected. Entry to human beings can be gained via the placenta, the mother's milk, by inhalation, ingestion or through shaven skin.

Prognosis.—The disease is most lethal when the infant acquires it during pregnancy or in the first few weeks of life. In adults the rare acute exanthematous type can be rapidly fatal.

Treatment is by pyrimethamine (Daraprim) combined with sulphadiazine. The former is given with an initial loading dose of 50 mg. and continued in doses of 25–50 mg. daily for 10–14 days; the daily dose of sulphadiazine is 1 G. q.d.s. for a similar period.

§ 510. XIX. Disturbances of Heat Regulation.

—In the tropics or where atmospheric temperature and humidity become unduly high, breakdown may occur of the physiological control of the body temperature and of water-electrolyte balance.

(i.) **Heat Hyperpyrexia** (Syn., Heat-stroke) is due to exposure to continuous excessive heat (not necessarily sunlight), especially in unacclimatised individuals and in the elderly.

Symptoms.—There may be premonitory restlessness, irritability, headache, giddiness, drowsiness or gastro-intestinal upsets. In others the onset is sudden with fever, convulsions, delirium and coma with a rectal temperature of 110° F or more, a rapid pulse and fast shallow respirations. The skin is hot and dry due to inhibition of sweating, the face and conjunctivæ congested, the pupils dilated and later cyanosis appears. There is incontinence of urine and fæces; the urine contains albumen and perhaps ketone bodies. In the stage of coma, unless appropriate treatment be rapidly started, death may quickly follow from respiratory failure or shock. Gastro-intestinal features with severe vomiting and diarrhœa are sometimes prominent. As recovery ensues the temperature remains at 101–103° F for a few days with headache and a dry skin.

Diagnosis.—*Cerebral malaria* with coma may be mistaken for heat-stroke, and *vice versa*. Splenomegaly and the presence of parasites in the blood films should prevent confusion, though in any case of doubt 10 grains of quinine dihydrochloride in 10 ml. of distilled water should be injected slowly intravenously. *Cerebral hæmorrhage* into the pons is associated with coma and hyperpyrexia, but the pupils are pin-point in size and lumbar puncture may reveal blood-stained cerebro-spinal fluid.

Etiology.—Predisposing factors include excessive clothing (especially of the conventional European type), lack of air movement and especially a high humidity which limit heat loss by preventing evaporation of sweat, excessive exercise with over-production of heat (such as troops carrying heavy packs), intemperance and patients with fever such as is due to pneumonia or malaria.

Prognosis.—This largely depends on the rapidity with which treatment is instituted. In the choleraic type and in comatose patients with temperatures over 109° F the outlook is grave.

Treatment.—The patient is nursed in a cool room, is covered only by a moist sheet and is fanned vigorously. Ice is applied to the head and neck. Dehydration and shock require intravenous normal saline, dextrose-saline or plasma; saline enemate are also helpful. When the rectal temperature falls to 102° F active treatment is stopped, the temperature usually continues to fall and natural sweating is re-established. *Prophylaxis* is by avoiding the conditions which precipitated the condition, with adequate sleep and a sufficient intake of sodium chloride and of water. Those particularly susceptible must live in a cooler climate or otherwise reside in dwellings made of non-conducting materials (and never in tents) and must wear suitable loose-fitting clothes (and see § 528).

(ii.) **Thermogenic Anhidrosis** usually occurs after long exposure to high temperatures and there is often a previous history of extensive " prickly heat."

The *Symptoms*, which are worst during the hottest part of the day, consist of exhaustion, headache, anorexia, dyspnœa and palpitation after exercise. Sweating is diminished or absent on the trunk and limbs but normal on the face and neck. The salt content of the sweat is high. The skin eruption, which is characteristic, is composed of tiny greyish papules, about 1 mm. in diameter, surmounted usually by clear vesicles. It occurs in patches on the trunk and limbs and does not itch. *Treatment* is by rest in a cool environment for about 2 weeks.

(iii.) **Heat Exhaustion** is due to copious sweating of salt and water without adequate replacement. It occurs in natives and visitors to hot moist tropical climates who undertake heavy manual work or who suffer from febrile illnesses.

Symptoms usually come on over several days. There is a complaint of headache, anorexia, nausea, giddiness, tinnitus and visual disturbances. Vomiting always occurs in serious cases and may be severe; muscular cramps often follow. The patient is exhausted and anxious. The rectal temperature may reach 102° F—not higher; the pulse rate is usually fast and the blood pressure low. Sweating is normal and the skin pale, cold and moist. The volume of urine is 500 ml. or less per day and it may contain albumen and casts; the chloride content is low or absent. In severe cases a condition of shock with suppression of urine leads to acute uræmia which is often fatal. The blood volume is reduced causing a corresponding hæmoconcentration.

Treatment.—The water electrolyte balance is restored by mouth if possible, otherwise by intravenous fluids. By mouth 5–6 pints of fluid with sodium chloride 25–40 G. are given in the first 24 hours. In severe shock an initial bottle of plasma is given intravenously; with severe dehydration 2 pints of normal saline are given intravenously in the first hour followed by 1 pint each 4 hours (maximum 6 pints in all in the first 24 hours). Subsequent parenteral treatment is seldom necessary. The urinary chloride concentration is watched and hypotonic saline given by mouth when it begins to rise. In all cases an intake-output fluid chart must be kept. Recovery is usually rapid. The possible presence of a concomitant malarial infection must not be forgotten.

(iv.) **Heat Cramps** without appreciable rise of temperature are also due to loss of chloride through excessive sweating. They occur in miners, stokers, engineers, ship's firemen and furnacemen a few hours after starting heavy manual shift-work.

Symptoms.—The muscle spasms in the calves later spreading to the arms and the abdominal muscles, and even giving rise to intestinal cramps are most painful and may last several hours.

Treatment is by giving normal saline by mouth or in severe cases intravenously, combined with the use of morphia for pain. *Prophylaxis* is by giving salt containing foods, effervescing drinks containing sodium chloride tablets and even salted beer.

HAY FEVER (Hay Asthma), especially the constitutional variety, DYSENTERY and CHOLERA, give rise to a certain amount of pyrexia of a continued type. Hay Fever (§ 179) is recognised by the violent attacks of sneezing. Dysentery (§ 309).—Acute dysenteries may be attended at the onset by some degree of pyrexia, but much the most important symptom is diarrhœa. In Cholera (§ 311) the abdominal cramps, collapse and diarrhœa are the leading symptoms. During the collapse stage the temperature may be as high as 105° F in the rectum, although in the axilla and mouth it is subnormal. In the reaction stage, if the patient lives, there is usually a degree or so of pyrexia lasting from a week to a fortnight.

Finally, there are several diseases which in their typical forms belong to Group III or, belonging to Group I, are seen perhaps before or after the eruption comes out, which may present pyrexia of a continued type. It is well in all cases of difficulty or doubt to remember this, and to pass in review the members of all three groups.

§ 511. In this group of diseases the pyrexia is of an INTERMITTENT (or remittent) type—*i.e.*, the temperature drops at regular or irregular intervals to normal (or nearly to normal). This group is distinguished from Group I by the complete absence of eruption. It is distinguished from Group II mainly by the wide variations of the temperature.

Common		*Rare*	
I. Malaria	§ 512	Amœbiasis	§ 519
II. Latent tuberculosis ..	§ 514	Visceral syphilis	§ 520
III. Acute miliary tuberculosis	§ 515	Infective endocarditis ..	§§ 50, 520
IV. Acute septicæmia and pyæmia	§ 516	Hodgkin's disease	§ 584
		Pernicious anæmia	§ 548
V. Subacute septic conditions (abscesses, ulceration, etc.)	§ 517	Leukæmia	§ 554
		Polyarteritis nodosa	§ 98
VI. Malignant disease	§ 518	Systemic lupus erythematosus	§ 602
VII. Typhoid and paratyphoid fever (some cases) and occasionally influenza ..	§ 496	Opium habit	§ 1185
		Trypanosomiasis	§ 521
		Filariasis bancrofti	§ 522
		Trichinosis	§ 606

The clinical investigation of these diseases is often attended by considerable difficulty. MALARIA, which may be regarded as the type of this group, is essentially a *paroxysmal pyrexia*, each paroxysm having three stages (cold, hot and sweating), and each paroxysm being typically *separated by one or more days' interval of apyrexia*, except in certain subtertian fevers. TUBERCULOSIS has a daily rise and fall, and is a good example of *regular diurnally* intermitting pyrexia. ACUTE SEPTICÆMIA, on the other hand, is noted for the *irregular* character and wide range of its temperature and the severity of the rigors. CHRONIC SEPTIC CONDITIONS occupy a position midway between these two types—regular and irregular intermitting pyrexia. In a given case of intermitting pyrexia which has arisen in a tropical or subtropical climate, malaria, undulant fever, amœbiasis or tropical liver abscess, or filariasis are probable, but in England the commonest cause is probably a latent focus of infection, malignant disease or tuberculosis. Tubercle as a cause of this type of fever is nearly as common in the tropics as elsewhere. The SERUM REACTIONS aid us to some extent in the diagnosis of this group.

Turning to the rarer diseases, which must always be kept in mind, INFECTIVE ENDOCARDITIS is chiefly remarkable for the *long course* it may run. In HODGKIN'S DISEASE we usually find the enlarged *glands*; and in PERNICIOUS ANÆMIA the skin is very sallow, and the blood picture is characteristic.

It follows therefore that if we have a patient's temperature chart before us, and it shows definite intermissions or remissions, the disease will belong to one of three sub-groups:

A. REGULAR INTERMITTENT PYREXIA, with one or two days' INTERVAL, which contains only one disease—Malaria   ..   ..   ..   § 512
B. REGULAR INTERMITTENT PYREXIA occurring DAILY, such as Tuberculosis ..   ..   §§ 514 *et seq.*
C. IRREGULAR INTERMITTENT PYREXIA, such as Septicæmia, and other pyogenic processes   ..   ..   §§ 516 *et seq.*

§ 512. I. **Malaria** (Syn., Ague, Intermittent Fever, Remittent Fever, Jungle Fever).—Malaria is a non-contagious disease caused by four different parasites which infect the red blood corpuscles of man and give rise to periodic paroxysms of fever, enlargement of the spleen and anæmia: transmission is by anopheline mosquitoes.

Symptoms.—The incubation period varies from 10 to 20 days as a rule, but may be delayed for months. At onset the initial fever may be continuous or remittent in type. Some time elapses before the typical periodic fever, commencing frequently about mid-day with headache and aches and pains in the limbs and joints, develops. The ague paroxysm has three characteristic phases. First, the *cold* stage, lasting ¼ to 2 hours, in which the patient, who lies curled up in bed covered with blankets, feels and looks cold, and shivers or has a rigor despite the fact that the internal temperature is rising; the skin may be livid and the nails blue. This is followed by a *hot* stage in which blankets are discarded. The face is flushed, the skin dry and hot, and nausea, a high temperature (103° to 106°) and perhaps vomiting and delirium may ensue; this generally lasts 4 to 5 hours. Then begins the *sweating* stage, which lasts 1 to 2 hours and is accompanied by a critical fall in temperature and profuse perspiration which soaks the bedclothes. An apyrexial interval follows, its duration being determined by the species of infecting parasite. In *malignant tertian* the cold, hot and sweating stages are less pronounced and the temperature is rarely so high, but the fever generally lasts at least 12 hours and may continue for days. Examination of the patient during the fever generally reveals a tender and palpable enlargement of the spleen, parasites are to be found in the blood and secondary anæmia is frequent. Herpes is commonly seen on the lips.

VARIETIES OF MALARIA.—There are three common species of malarial parasites, the so-called benign tertian (*Plasmodium vivax*), the quartan (*Plasmodium malariæ*) and the malignant tertian (*Plasmodium falciparum*). A fourth species, *Plasmodium ovale*, is found in some districts: its effects are similar to those of *P. vivax*. There are several types of periodicity (Fig. 151): (1) TERTIAN fever with febrile attacks every alternate day (*P. vivax* or *P. ovale* infection): (2) QUARTAN fever, with attacks every fourth day, and a 2-day apyrexial interval (*P. malariæ*): (3) an IRREGULAR or CONTINUOUS fever with a tendency to tertian periodicity (*P. falci-*

parum): (4) DAILY OR OTHER PHASIC FEVERS are due to double infec ion
by one or more species. Uncomplicated cases of the benign forms of
malaria (*i.e.*, *P. vivax*, *P. malariæ* and *P. ovale*) are rarely fatal.

Malignant Tertian malaria (*P. falciparum*) carries a worse prognosi.
and is much more difficult to diagnose: the infected corpuscles adhere to
one another and to the walls of the capillaries producing local tissue anoxia,
and the symptoms vary according to the organs chiefly involved. *Pernicious complications* can develop without warning at any stage and may
end fatally unless promptly treated. (i.) *Cerebral malaria* causes delirium,
stupor and coma, and may give rise to an epileptiform attack, various
pareses and hemiplegia. Meningitis may be simulated. (ii.) *Hyper-*

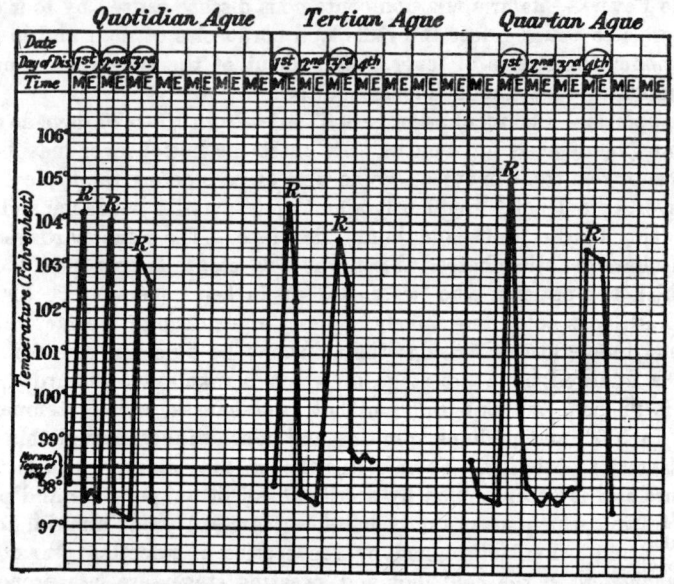

FIG. 151.—TYPES OF MALARIA.—Quotidian (daily) due to two cycles of vivax parasites; Tertian (every
other day); and Quartan (every third day). " R " indicates the rigor which ushers in the cold
stage.

pyrexia causes an internal temperature of 107–111° F, but the skin may
be cold. (iii.) *Algid malaria* is a condition of medical shock resembling
acute adrenal insufficiency. (iv.) *Abdominal malaria*, by affecting the
blood supply to the alimentary tract, may produce epigastric pain, vomiting of blood-stained material, purging, and even the passage of blood and
mucus (choleraic malaria). (v.) " *Bilious* " *remittent fever* may show
hæmolytic jaundice alone, or toxic jaundice with a biphasic van den Bergh
reaction and bile salts and bile pigments in the urine. Bilious vomiting,
dark fæces and urobilinuria occur in both varieties, and in some cases
very severe hæmolytic anæmia may ensue.

Diagnosis.—The spleen is always enlarged in malaria, though at the
onset or when a patient has been taking an antimalarial drug, it may

not be palpable. In chronic cases in hyperendemic areas great enlargement ensues and the spleen often extends below the umbilicus or even
into the pelvis. Not infrequently the liver is enlarged and tender. Malaria, especially during the primary fever, may be mistaken for other
tropical febrile diseases such as typhoid, paratyphoid, relapsing fever and
kala-azar: later, periodic fever commencing about mid-day, splenomegaly,
anæmia and the response to specific remedies suggest the diagnosis. In
all cases of tropical fever, every effort should be made to demonstrate
parasites in the blood (Plate XVIII) by taking blood films before treatment
is commenced. After full doses of a schizonticidal drug the fever should
fall in 72 nours provided the drug is being absorbed. In the apyrexial
periods, urobilinuria, leucopenia and a monocytosis of 12 to 15 per cent.
are suggestive of malaria, while hyperbilirubinæmia is not infrequent.
Where secondary anæmia is present, polychromasia, anisocytosis and
poikilocytosis are frequent findings.

Etiology.—Malaria has a widespread geographical distribution. In the
tropics malignant tertian preponderates, causing a high infant and child
mortality and at times dangerous epidemics; in colder climates benign
tertian is met, manifesting a definite seasonal prevalence. In Europe,
malaria does not occur above the 3,000-ft. level. All races and both sexes
are susceptible and children surviving in hyperendemic areas gradually
acquire a relative immunity or tolerance; there is a progressive decrease
in the parasitic and spleen rate as age advances.

Life Cycle of Malarial Parasites (see § 542).—(1) Sporozoites are inoculated with
the saliva of infected anopheline mosquitoes during the act of biting. (2) Soon
after inoculation the parasites enter tissue cells (they have recently been demonstrated
the polygonal cells of the human liver) where they undergo a non-pigmented cycle
of asexual development (the pre-erythrocytic phase). During this phase they are
relatively insusceptible to schizonticidal drugs, but *P. falciparum* is killed by proguanil
hydrochlor. (Paludrine) and pyrimethamine (Daraprim) in prophylactic doses.
(3) Merozoites are liberated at the end of the pre-erythrocytic phase and the majority
infect the red blood cells thus starting the cycle of schizogony. Here the parasites
can be killed by schizonticidal drugs. The young parasite appears as unpigmented
rings of cytoplasm with one or more dots of chromatin (the trophozoite). It becomes
amœboid (the schizont) and develops a brown pigment. The chromatin then divides
and becomes distributed peripherally with its surrounding cytoplasm, forming spores
(merozoites). These then rupture the corpuscle, causing the patient's rigor, and
re-enter other corpuscles, so renewing this asexual cycle. (4) In the case of *P. vivax*,
P. ovale and *P. malariæ* parasites, it is believed that some of the pre-erythrocytic
merozoites re-enter tissue cells and there persist (the exo-erythrocytic phase). From
time to time they release merozoites into the blood-stream to re-establish the asexual
cycle and thus bring about the *relapses*. This tissue phase is also relatively resistant
to schizonticidal drugs but is eradicated by 8-amino-quinolines (such as pamaquin).
P. falciparum has no exo-erythrocytic phase; relapses in this case arise from persistence
of red cell infection. (5) From time to time sexual forms (gametocytes) appear in the
peripheral blood and when these are sucked up by a suitable anopheline mosquito
fertilisation ensues in the stomach of the mosquito. The stomach wall is penetrated,
and after a series of local developmental changes the mature oöcyst ruptures and
sporozoites are liberated into the body cavity and reach the salivary gland and saliva.
Under satisfactory temperature conditions the mosquito phase of the life cycle takes
about 10 days.

Prognosis.—In the tropics malaria is a major cause of death, and cases of malignant tertian with pernicious manifestations frequently succumb rapidly if untreated. The benign infections are not so often fatal in the absence of complications. The chronic, repeatedly infected malaria case is liable to develop cachexia, pigmented skin, anæmia and " ague-cake " spleen and may die of intercurrent diseases like sepsis, pleurisy, pneumonia and dysentery, or in the presence of certain conditioned deficiencies of hæmopoïetic substances develop a hæmolytic nutritional macrocytic anæmia which is often fatal, especially in pregnancy. Blackwater fever may supervene in chronic infections with *P. falciparum*. Rupture of the spleen may follow slight trauma. Nephritis with œdema is not infrequent in quartan malaria. Other complications include neuralgia, iritis, corneal ulceration and retinal hæmorrhages, amnesia, while certain psychoses may follow cerebral malaria. Abortion often occurs. After a patient has left an endemic area, relapses can occur up to 2 years with malignant tertian fever; up to 3 years and exceptionally considerably longer with benign tertian; and up to 7 years with quartan fever.

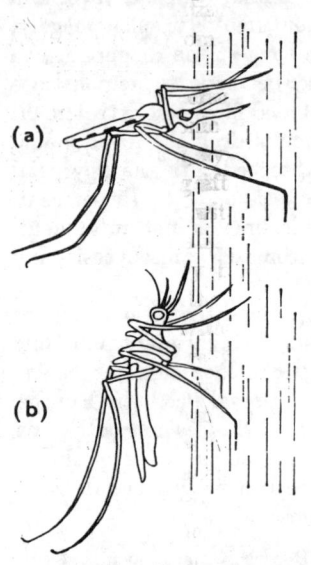

FIG. 152.—MOSQUITOES settling on a wall. There are two chief types of mosquitoes—Anopheline and Culicine—easily differentiated by their attitudes when resting upon a wall. Anopheles (*a*) is the more dangerous one, and is recognised by its spotted wings and its tilted attitude: Culex (*b*) rests parallel to the surface. Anopheline larvæ lie flat on the surface of puddles, whereas Culicine larvæ lie more perpendicularly, and if disturbed rush to the bottom of the pool. Anopheline larvæ are found in puddles which contain algæ and which are too large to be dried up in a week (time needed for the mature insect to be hatched). They are not found in pools which contain minnows, nor in shallow rain pools that are easily dried up. In certain districts they may be found even in rapid streams.

Prophylaxis.—In order to get rid of the mosquito larvæ, marshy tracts and swamps must be drained and cisterns and wells screened. In potential breeding places which cannot be drained or screened, dicophane (DDT) 5 per cent. in kerosene oil (♏ 60 to a pool of 1 sq. yard) kills all larvæ in 6 hours. Protection against mosquitoes is by residual spraying of DDT, or of DDT and pyrethrum, in a suitable solvent; these leave a fine powder of insecticide on the inside walls of dwellings, which is effective for about 6 weeks. Houses should be made mosquito proof where possible. *Individual protection* is by using mosquito nets at night, suitable clothing and mosquito boots by day, and by the application of repellents such as dimethyl phthalate as a cream or lotion to exposed parts. Drug treatment is by the regular use of proguanil hydrochlor. (Paludrine) 100 mg. daily or pyrimethamine (Daraprim) 50 mg. weekly; these are true causal prophylactics against *P. falciparum* and suppress clinical manifestations in all other types of malaria by antagonising folinic acid which is necessary for nuclear division of the schizonts. Chloroquine (base) 300 mg. weekly and mepacrine hydrochlor. 100 mg. daily are also good suppressive drugs. Each of these should be started 2 weeks before reaching, and continued for 4 weeks after leaving, an endemic area.

Treatment.—The *ordinary attack* is treated by oral schizonticidal drugs (which act on the asexual blood parasites). Preferably give the 4-amino-quinoline drug chloroquine (base) 600 mg. immediately, 300 mg. 6 hours later and then 300 mg. daily for 2 days; otherwise mepacrine hydrochlor. 300 mg. t.d.s. on the first day, then 200 mg. for 2 days followed by 100 mg. t.i.d. for 5 days; or a quinine compound 10 gr. t.d.s. for 7 to 10 days. This latter is much less used nowadays and if taken repeatedly it carries some risk of inducing blackwater fever in *P. falciparum* infections. Proguanil hydrochlor. (Paludrine) and pyrimethamine are also schizonticides but in non-immune patients they act too slowly and are best reserved for prophylaxis and suppression. When *vomiting* or *pernicious complications* of falciparum malaria are present or are threatened, give at once a rapidly acting schizonticide as irreversible changes in vital organs may otherwise occur; intravenous chloroquine sulphate 200 mg. or quinine dihydrochlor. 10 gr. dissolved in 20 ml. normal saline and injected very slowly over a period of 10 minutes, are best for emergencies; intramusc. chloroquine hydrochlor. 300 mg. or mepacrine hydrochlor. 300 mg. act effectively but rather more slowly. *Never give mepacrine intravenously.* Serious symptoms are usually controlled by one or two parenteral injections at a 6-hour interval after which oral therapy can be started. CHILDREN should be given doses strictly in accordance with body weight, but intramusc. mepacrine should not be given to infants as it is liable to cause convulsions. When a patient is in coma lumbar puncture with removal of cerebro-spinal fluid may help recovery. In dehydrated and unconscious patients intravenous dextrose solution is of value and hyperpyrexia needs tepid sponging. *Relapses* in benign tertian (*P. vivax* and *P. ovale*) and quartan (*P. malariæ*) cases are prevented by giving an 8-amino-quinoline drug after the schizonticidal course; of these primaquine phosphate 7·5 mg. t.d.s. for 2 weeks is less toxic than pamaquin.

Toxic effects from antimalarial drugs are rare. Proguanil hydrochlor. and pyrimethamine in ordinary doses are not harmful. Chloroquine may cause transient and unimportant difficulty in visual accommodation; mepacrine stains the skin yellow and may cause dermatitis or psychotic behaviour necessitating change to another drug. Quinine in therapeutic doses can be expected to cause tinnitus and deafness and should be replaced if rashes, hæmoglobinuria or amblyopia occur; it should not be used routinely in hyperendemic areas with *P. falciparum* as it fails to suppress certain strains of this organism. Primaquine phosphate and pamaquin cause unimportant methæmoglobinæmia but must be stopped if methæmoglobinuria or severe gastro-intestinal symptoms appear; they may produce severe hæmolysis in those of the Negro race possibly due to a genetic pre-disposition to these drugs.

§ 513. " Blackwater Fever " (Syn., Hæmoglobinuric Fever), so named from the colour of the urine, is an acute illness developing in patients infected with latent or demonstrable malignant tertian malaria: clinically, it is characterised by the rapid destruction of red blood corpuscles, resulting in hæmoglobinæmia, hæmoglobinuria, fever, vomiting, jaundice and anæmia.

Symptoms.—The onset cannot be foretold. It generally comes on suddenly with chill, fever and loin pain, followed by epigastric discomfort, bilious vomiting and the passage of red urine which in severe cases soon becomes porter-coloured, due to the presence of the blood pigments, oxyhæmoglobin (in alkaline urine) and methæmoglobin (in acid urine). Hæmolytic jaundice follows a few hours after onset and anæmia rapidly develops but may be masked by hæmoconcentration; 50 per cent. of the corpuscles may be destroyed overnight. Low blood pressure, pallor, restlessness and cold extremities are characteristic of the early stage. Hiccough and Cheyne-Stokes' breathing often develop in severe cases. The spleen and liver are enlarged and tender and the urine shows albumen, blood pigments, urobilin and a characteristic brown granular sediment containing granular casts; red corpuscles are scanty or absent. Blood chemistry shows a hyperbilirubinæmia and increased blood urea; the plasma contains oxyhæmoglobin and a pigment, methæmalbumin, which had previously been regarded as methæmoglobin. In severe cases anuria and acidosis due to renal failure may supervene. Malarial parasites are sometimes found before and during the first few hours of an attack, but generally soon disappear. The fever generally declines in 3 to 4 days, the vomiting lessens and the urine clears; a post hæmoglobinuric fever sometimes persists. Different clinical types include (1) Transient mild hæmo-globinuria. (2) Fulminating cases, often dying in 48 hours. (3) Anuric cases in which oliguria and anuria culminate in death some 7 to 10 days later with uræmia. (4) Intermittent hæmoglobinuria lasting 8 days or longer. (5) Hyperpyrexia followed by death.

Mechanism of Hæmolysis and Anuria.—The hæmolytic agent acts intravascularly on the corpuscles, liberating oxyhæmoglobin, and possibly originates from the reticulo-endothelium hypertrophied as a result of chronic malaria. The liberated blood pigment is dealt with by the liver and kidneys. Hyperbilirubinæmia, hæmolytic jaundice and pleocholia with bilious vomiting and dark brown stools result, and absorption of the excess of stercobilin produces urobilinuria. Some of the circulating hæmoglobin is secreted by the kidney as oxyhæmoglobin, and if the urine be acid is converted into methæmoglobin and acid hæmatin. It is now considered that intra-renal vascular changes producing anoxæmia of the kidney are chiefly responsible for the failure of renal function and anuria.

Diagnosis.—The disease must be distinguished from relapsing fever, leptospirosis and yellow fever by the spectroscopic demonstration of oxyhæmoglobin and methæ-moglobin in the urine. The history of residence in malarial countries and of malarial infection is important.

Etiology.—It occurs in various hyperendemic areas of malignant tertian malaria in Africa, India, America and the Balkan peninsula, and generally affects the patient who has been taking quinine irregularly. The exact cause of the hæmolysis is not known, but it generally follows the administration of quinine. With efficient pro-phylaxis of malignant tertian (*P. falciparum*) malaria, as by the use of paludrine, blackwater fever is becoming rarer.

Prognosis.—The case mortality is about 25 per cent. and death results from sudden heart failure, anæmia or anuria. One attack predisposes to another; even if the patient returns to Europe attacks may recur unless the malarial infection be eradicated.

Treatment.—Blackwater fever is best prevented by the eradication of malignant tertian malaria. The patient must be carefully nursed in a recumbent position. A schizonticidal drug (*not quinine*) should be given at once by injection, whether parasites can be found or not. A transfusion of carefully cross-matched blood should always be ready and given if the red cell count falls below 1·5 million; this may save the patient's life if further hæmolysis occurs. Intravenous plasma followed by saline or dextrose infusions are often needed to restore blood volume and to replace lost fluid and salt, but excess is dangerous. When renal failure has occurred alkalis and diuretics do not help, but spinal anæsthesia or " an artificial kidney " should theoretically be useful. Cortisone serves to prevent further hæmolyses. It must not be forgotten that a full course of the schizonticide must be completed orally. During convalescence iron and liver therapy should be instituted.

§ **514.** II. **Latent Tuberculosis.**—Tuberculosis is often said to be latent in the absence of the obvious signs or local manifestations. In all cases of unexplained pyrexia in this country, one of the possible causes to be suspected is tuberculosis in some part of the body. Although occasionally the extension of a tuberculous lesion in the lung may be entirely symptomless and unattended by any appreciable rise of temperature, it is a good clinical axiom that active tuberculosis in any part of the body is usually associated with a daily intermitting pyrexia; and the degree of fever is a fair indication of the degree of activity of the process. Fig. 153 is a chart recorded from a case with active tuberculosis: the temperature drops each morning to (about) normal, and rises each evening one, two or more degrees, occasionally *vice versa* (§ 515). The patient may seek advice on account of weakness, dyspepsia, loss of weight and other vague symptoms. Such a condition may persist for weeks without any local manifestations, as in the cases referred to under Tuberculous Meningitis (§ 886). The lungs, peritoneum, kidneys and various other organs may be affected. (1) The commonest locality in adult life is the *lungs*. In this case X-ray evidence of disease often precedes physical signs: when these appear they may resemble bronchitis or simple pulmonary congestion (§§ 117, 131). (2) Apart from the lungs, the *meninges, peritoneum* and other *serous membranes* are perhaps the commonest positions in childhood in which tuberculosis may be present without definite signs. (3) In the *kidney*, tuberculous pyelonephritis may be readily overlooked, and in suspicious cases the urine should be carefully examined for pus and tubercle bacilli (§ 419). (4) Tuberculosis may also be latent in other situations, such as the Fallopian tubes, uterus (§ 455) and other viscera; and, finally, the tuberculous process may be generalised, and give rise to *Acute Miliary Tuberculosis.*

§ **515.** III. **Acute Miliary Tuberculosis** may be of the meningeal type, usually known as tuberculous meningitis (§ 886); of the pulmonary type or " acute phthisis " (§ 117); or of the generalised type, with which we are now concerned. It is characterised by intermitting pyrexia, prostration, and a tendency to profound toxæmia—due to a generalised spread of the tubercle bacilli.

Symptoms.—(1) The onset is insidious and for some time there are no localising symptoms or signs. The patient is often a child or young adult who complains of lethargy, which is found to be associated with an evening rise of temperature and a rapid pulse. The inverse type—*i.e.*, a lower temperature in the evening than in the morning—is said to be more common in this than in any other form of tuberculosis. (2) The lassitude increases, the daily rise of temperature becomes more marked (Fig. 153), and with this increase of toxæmia there is headache, loss of appetite and of weight, often a dry tongue and insomnia. In the course of a few weeks profound toxæmia develops, with wandering of the mind, a muttering delirium (especially at night) and progressive cachexia. (3) By now, localising signs have often shown themselves in one or more organs, with an especial tendency to signs of tuberculous meningitis. In others, there are signs of generalised bronchitis, with numerous fine râles scattered over the lungs; sometimes the involvement of the peritoneum is shown by general tumidity, with occasionally a palpable spleen. (4) X-ray examination of the lungs is essential as it may reveal the typical " snow-storm " appearance of the lung fields (Fig. 54). (5) Investigation of the cerebro-spinal fluid may be valuable.

Diagnosis.—(1) Cases of acute miliary tuberculosis in the early stage are sometimes admitted to hospital as bronchitis, in the later stages as typhoid fever. The

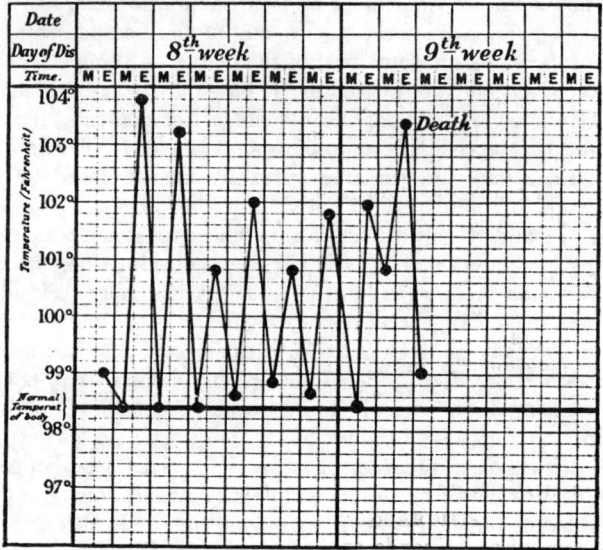

FIG. 153.— ACUTE MILIARY TUBERCULOSIS.— Geo. W——, æt. 49. Seven weeks' history of vague illness before admission, during which time there was profuse hæmoptysis on one occasion; the signs in the chest were very indefinite. After death the lungs were found to be sparsely studded with miliary tuberculosis. The liver and peritoneum were also dotted with tiny tubercles hardly visible to the naked eye.

possibility of miliary tuberculosis should be remembered in all cases of " *bronchitis* " attended by an intermitting pyrexia, especially in young adults. The presence of tubercle bacilli in the sputum is unusual; the sputum is usually small in amount, and indeed cough and sputum may be absent. Choroidal tubercles are sometimes visible on ophthalmoscopic examination, and settle the diagnosis (§ 1137). (2) The course of the disease may closely resemble the *typhoid fevers*: the slowed pulse, rose-red spots and a palpable spleen favour one of these. A positive blood culture and later a positive Widal reaction are found in typhoid and paratyphoid.

Etiology.—The disease is due to dissemination via the blood-stream (bacteræmia) of tubercle bacilli throughout the body. The usual cause is rupture into a vein of a subacute or chronic focus (often a caseating gland), in a person with a low resistance.

Prognosis.—Until modern therapy was instituted the disease was almost uniformly fatal within 4–8 weeks. Now with early adequate treatment 80–90 per cent. of patients recover completely, although a few are left with some mental impairment.

Treatment.—(1) Isoniazid is the most important drug as this is rapidly absorbed and quickly diffuses into the body tissues, including the cerebro-spinal fluid: its effect is mainly bacteriostatic and it must be combined with intramusc. injections of streptomycin and/or with caps. sodium aminosalicylate (PAS) by mouth. In such a serious condition it is probably best to commence with all 3 drugs. To *adults* give (i.) tab. isoniazid 75 mg. 6-hourly with (ii.) inject. streptomycin 0·50–0·75 G. 12-hourly and (iii.) PAS 4 G. 6-hourly. *Children* require (i.) inject. streptomycin 10 mg. 12-hourly for each 1 lb. body weight (max. 1·0 G. a day), (ii.) isoniazid 8 mg./lb. for two initial doses and then 1·0–1·25 mg./lb. 6-hourly with (iii.) PAS 25·0–37·5 mg./lb. 6-hourly. PAS can be given intravenously at first. When meningitis is present many authorities give on alternate days, for 4 doses, intrathecal streptomycin 50–100 mg. (20 mg. for infants) with or without isoniazid 20 mg.; some also give a short course of inject. corticotrophin (ACTH) gel 25 mg. each 12 hours. The isoniazid, streptomycin and PAS must be given for many weeks and until the C.S.F. sugar has risen to 50 mg. per cent. A continuation course of isoniazid and inject. streptomycin is essential for at least 6 (often 12) months to prevent relapse. These large doses of isoniazid may produce polyneuritis and a burning sensation in the limbs which is in part prevented by tab. pyridoxine 50 mg. t.d.s. (2) Feeding via a nasal catheter or with a spoon with as high a calorie diet as possible is most important. (3) A 4-hourly temperature chart, regular chest X-rays and examination of the ocular fundi are routine measures.

§ 516. IV. **Acute Septicæmia** and **Acute Pyæmia**[1] are diseases characterised by a wide range of temperature, accompanied by rigors and sweating, due to the direct infection of the blood by a micro-organism, usually through some breach of surface in the skin or mucous membrane.

The *Symptoms* are (1) pyrexia, which runs a very characteristic course, and is distinguished from all other diseases not of septic origin by a wide and *very irregular* range of the temperature (Fig. 154). The remissions may occur several times a day, and have not the diurnal regularity which marks the two preceding classes of disease (§§ 514 and 520). There may be as much as 6° or 7° difference between the temperature in the course of a few hours: when it rises suddenly the temperature is often accompanied by a rigor (§ 468), followed by very profuse perspiration and a rapid fall. The pulse is rapid and compressible. (2) Toxic symptoms include prostration, headache, anorexia, nausea, a dry furred tongue, often constipation, and aches and pains in the muscles: the skin is sallow, and anæmia may develop. The mind is clear at first, and remains so for a considerable time, but towards the end there is a tendency to the typhoid state (§ 470). (3) Later on in the disease emboli may occur in different parts of the body: in the lungs they give rise to a generalised congestion and patches of pneumonic consolidation or abscess (as in the case given in Fig. 154). (4) In PYÆMIA the emboli occur primarily in the arteries of the lungs, and from the very beginning they suppurate and form abscesses, which constitute centres of secondary infection elsewhere. (5) The spleen may become palpable: and deposits of pus may occur in or around the joints or in other

---

[1] In *Bacteræmia*, living organisms are present in the blood-stream but do not produce clinical symptoms and signs. *Septicæmia* is a clinical rather than a pathological conception. A bacteræmia is present, and in addition the patient exhibits signs and symptoms of infection of the blood-stream. *Pyæmia* is a condition of metastatic abscess formation due to the presence of infected thrombi in the blood-stream.

parts of the body. The serous cavities may contain pus, constituting empyema or pyo-pericarditis. The leucocytosis and other changes in the

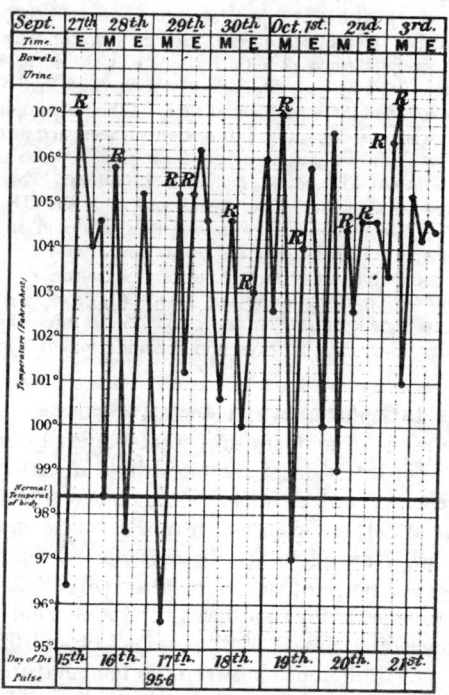

FIG. 154.—ACUTE PYÆMIA (typical of an irregularly intermitting pyrexia).—Catherine W——, æt. 6. She was taken ill somewhat suddenly 14 days previously with shivering and vomiting. On admission to hospital she was seriously ill. There were no physical signs excepting a systolic bruit over the whole cardiac area and slight enlargement of the spleen. Three days later, there was rusty sputum with streaks of blood: dullness and crepitations over the back of the right lung. She was delirious from time to time, and died 6 days later. At autopsy pus was found in the mastoid cells; there was sinus thrombosis secondary to long-standing middle ear disease (of which a history was now obtained) with infarcts in the kidney, and pyo-pneumothorax secondary to rupture of one of the gangrenous-looking abscesses of the lung.

blood may aid diagnosis; *a positive blood culture clinches the diagnosis*, and should always be performed when a *local* cause for pyrexia cannot be found.

Portal Pyæmia (Syn., Portal pylephlebitis) is a condition where the primary focus is in the alimentary tract, the veins of which drain into the portal vein. Appendicitis is the commonest cause and the abscesses are usually confined to the liver. A high leucocytosis with a negative blood culture aids the diagnosis.

Acute Osteomyelitis (Acute Periostitis) is an infective process which may set in very suddenly, usually after an injury to one of the superficial bones, generally the tibia (§ 607). If untreated it may be succeeded by pyæmia. In children there may be no history of injury. The diagnosis is easy when the tissues round the diseased bone are swollen, but during the first day or two pain is often complained of near a joint, and may lead one to diagnose rheumatic fever.

Diagnosis.—Whenever septicæmia or pyæmia is at all likely, one or more blood cultures must be taken at the height of the fever, for a positive blood culture confirms the diagnosis and identifies the responsible organism. The diagnosis is suggested when there is an external wound or abrasion, perhaps accompanied by lymphangitis; and it should never be difficult when there is a wide variation of the temperature, coupled with the rigors and the sweats. The chart of a typical acute case is characteristic. When due to some internal cause, it may resemble infective endocarditis, acute rheumatism, typhoid fever, coli bacilluria, pneumonia, malaria and remittent fever. But when carefully recorded temperatures of several days are available, and a thorough examination of the organs is made, the diagnosis should not be difficult. *Streptococcal* septicæmia is marked by high fever, rapid pulse (over 120/min.), joint pains, skin rashes, rapidly developing anæmia, hæmaturia and often diarrhœa. *Staphylococcal* septicæmia is often associated with a previous history of boils or carbuncles, an initial slow pulse and a tendency to form abscesses in the renal cortex, bones and joints. With *pneumococcal* infections there is no primary focus, a hot dry skin, herpes labialis and a considerable rise in the respiration rate even in the absence of lung signs.

Etiology.—The principal cause is the introduction of a virulent organism either through the *skin* or through a *mucous membrane*. In addition, there is often a lowered resistance of the patient. (1) A mere prick or scratch of the skin may permit the entrance of micro-organisms: cases have been caused by doctors and nurses becoming infected by an accidental prick or cut during a surgical operation or while dressing an infected wound. In recent years there has been an intensive study of the spread of virulent organisms of two varieties. (*a*) Cross infection with hæmolytic streptococci still sometimes occurs in maternity units. After recent parturition, the surface of the uterus resembles an open wound, and offers a large surface for the passage of organisms directly into the venous sinuses, by introduction of an infected glove or instrument: here again the original source may be a droplet infection from the nose or throat of a doctor or midwife. The disease is then called PUERPERAL FEVER, or Puerperal septicæmia: when the infection is derived from a previous case of puerperal septicæmia it is especially virulent due to the phenomenon of *passage*. *Also when a young woman is admitted with septicæmia, a recent abortion, perhaps criminally induced, should always be borne in mind.* Such an infection readily responds to treatment with penicillin, a sulphonamide or one of the tetracyclines for hæmolytic streptococci do not develop drug-resistance. (*b*) In the last few years cross-infection with staphylococci has become a much greater menace, particularly in hospital practice. A very large number of different strains of this organism have been identified by phage-typing and some strains are particularly virulent. Staphylococci may be transmitted from carriers, for about 40 per cent. of newly admitted patients harbour these organisms, particularly in their clothes and in their skin (especially around the perineum). Droplet infection from the nose is not now regarded as of such importance as it was a few years ago: dust, woollen blankets and bedding, soiled instruments and

fingers are believed to be of much greater importance. The ability to
infect wounds and to invade mucous membranes (especially of the lungs)
depends not only on the phage-type of the staphylococcus but on its concentration in the immediate, environment of the patient. Unlike hæmolytic streptococci, staphylococci develop a resistance to penicillin, by
virtue of producing a penicillinase, and to the sulphonamides and the tetracyclines and so are able to produce epidemics which have*become much
more serious since the introduction of these chemotherapeutic and antibiotic substances. These resistant strains are still mainly susceptible to
neomycin, bacitracin and to the newer penicillin methicillin (Celbenin) in
therapeutic concentrations. In this manner a variety of bacteria and
viruses can enter the blood-stream through the tonsils, naso-pharynx,
bronchial mucosa, mastoid cells and the intestinal biliary and urinary
passages. (2) The ability to invade the human body also depends on the
innate resistance of the individual. A lowered resistance may be due to
hygienic causes—overcrowding, lack of fresh air and sunlight, and to
poverty: or to special *predisposing causes*—diabetes mellitus, alcoholism,
hyperthyroidism, chronic nephritis, agranulocytosis, agammaglobulinæmia,
or a recent surgical operation as well as to ill health due to bad teeth or
infected tonsils.

The *Prognosis* has been remarkably altered by modern treatment.
Whereas cases of virulent infection from a wound or from parturition
used to run a rapid and fatal course in 10 to 12 days, nowadays the
majority respond to a sulpha-drug, to one of the penicillins, streptomycin
or to some other antibiotics when given early and in adequate doses.
There still remains a small proportion of cases in which the disease is so
fulminant that treatment has no time to be effective; or the responsible
organism may be resistant to all chemotherapeutic and antibiotic agents at
present available. Not all cases are of this extreme virulence, and there
are a number in which small quantities of infected material are constantly
leaking into the general circulation from some *internal* source over many
weeks or months, especially when there is an untreated or undrained
primary focus (as in the patient referred to in Fig. 154). There is, in
fact, no hard-and-fast line to be drawn between the *acute* septicæmia now
under consideration and the *subacute* and *chronic* septicæmia due to pent-
up pus or ulceration described later (§ 517). Acute pyæmia is just as
serious and, if untreated, often fatal. Death may occur either by the
intensity of the infection, asthenia, or complications. The *untoward
symptoms* are a very high temperature, frequent rigors, or cerebral symptoms. The most frequent *complications* are (1) broncho-pneumonia, which
invariably occurs in severe cases; (2) pericarditis, peritonitis or pleurisy,
which usually becomes purulent; and (3) suppurative inflammation of
the lungs, liver, spleen, brain and other organs, consequent on the infected
emboli; (4) acute infective endocarditis. Among the sequelæ in certain
less acute cases which recover is a destructive form of arthritis.

Treatment.—The indications are (1) to find the cause and to identify the invading organism; (2) whenever possible to administer chemotherapeutic drugs which will lead to the destruction of the causal bacteria; (3) to relieve the symptoms and support the strength of the patient. (1) The *source of the infection* must first be identified. Subsequently drainage of any infected material may be necessary, *e.g.*, surgical drainage of an abscess. (2) The term *Chemotherapy* means the use of drugs which are without serious detriment to the patient but which inhibit the multiplication of susceptible organisms (bacteriostasis) thus allowing the defensive mechanisms of the body to destroy them. In practice, the commonest of these in use is the sulphonamide group of drugs—the " sulpha-compounds." Antibiotics are substances derived from fungi or bacteria which exert a bacteriostatic and /or bactericidal effect in low concentrations on different classes of micro-organisms, not only on bacteria but on the rickettsiæ, some protozoa and even the larger viruses. The *sulphonamides* in common use at the present time for systemic infections are sulphadimidine, sulphamerazine, sulphadiazine and sulphamethoxypyridazine (Midicel); these have largely replaced sulphanilamide, sulphapyridine and sulphathiazole as they are more effective and less toxic. These sulpha-drugs are much cheaper than the antibiotics, are readily absorbed when given by mouth and rapidly penetrate most of the body tissues; they are still the drugs of choice in meningococcal meningitis and in combination with inject. streptomycin in meningitis due to *H. influenzæ, E. coli* and *K. pneumoniæ* (Friedlander); they are also of great value in treatment of acute bacillary dysentery, in some urinary infections and in patients who develop an untoward reaction with the antibiotics. For blood-stream infections a blood concentration of 5–10 mg. (and sometimes 10–15 mg.) per cent. is necessary; these are readily obtained by standard doses given each 4–6 hours by mouth. It is usual to give the half-gramme tablets in a high initial dose and then to continue with 4-hourly doses subsequently. (For the uses and dosage see Tables XXXV and XXXVI.) During their administration plenty of fluid and an alkaline mixture must be prescribed, as otherwise the drugs or their acetyl derivatives may crystallise out and produce blockage of the renal tubules. Other toxic effects include nausea, mental depression, skin rashes and drug fever: it is advisable to discontinue administration after a week, unless the blood is watched for leucopenia and agranulocytosis. In certain cases it is helpful to determine the sensitivity of the organism to the particular sulphonamide beforehand, to ensure an adequate therapeutic effect. The *antibiotics* have become popular in recent years. It is customary to speak of them as " broad-spectrum " antibiotics when they are effective against a wide variety of organisms and " narrow-spectrum " antibiotics when they are active against a relatively small number of different organisms. *Penicillin* was the first antibiotic to be discovered and its use has revolutionised medical and surgical treatment. It is now mainly derived from the mould *P. chrysogenum* and is bacteriostatic and bactericidal on a number of organisms; now that the penicillin " nucleus " (6-aminopenicillanic acid) has been

TABLE XXXV.—EFFECT OF SULPHONAMIDES AND OF ANTIBIOTICS ON ORGANISMS

	Uses	Toxic effects may be	Used against	Sometimes used against
Sulphonamides (oral) Sulphadimidine Sulphamerazine Sulphadiazine	Most valuable against all forms of acute purulent meningitis. Usually well tolerated and slowly excreted: need to be given with plenty of fluid and alkali for maximum of 7–10 days. Sometimes used for synergism with an antibiotic.	R. she Fever Drowsiness Jaundice Agranulocytosis (rare)	E. coli Pf. mallei (glanders) N. meningitidis Past. pestis Past. tularense Pneumococci Str. pyogenes	Dysentery bacilli N. gonorrhœa Proteus vulgaris Staphylococci
Sulphamethoxypyridazine (Midicel)	Very slowly excreted: single daily dose gives continuous high blood level.			
Sulphacetamide Sulphafurazole (Gantrisin)	Rapidly excreted and give high concentration for urinary infection.			
Succinyl-sulphathiazole Phthalyl-sulphathiazole	Little absorbed from intestine and used as intestinal antiseptics in large doses.			
Sulphaguanidine	More absorbed than the other two and more liable to give toxic effects.			
Soluthiazole (by injection)	A neutral solution; can be given intravenously or intramusc. when speed is essential.			
Nitrofurantoin (Furadantin)	In urinary infections.	Nausea, vomiting Diarrhœa	E. coli Proteus Ps. pyocyaneus	
Penicillin				
Benzylpenicillin	*Preparations to be given by subcut. or intramusc. injection* Rapidly gives high blood level but rapidly excreted. Many organisms are resistant.	Severe allergic reactions Skin rashes Glossitis Fever	B. anthracis C. diphtheriæ Lepto. ictero-hæmorrhagiæ N. gonorrhœa N. meningitidis Pneumococci Spirillum minus Str. fæcalis (in urine) Str. pyogenes Str. viridans Trep. pallidum Trep. pertenue (Yaws) Vincent's organisms	Actinomyces Proteus Staphylococci
Procaine penicillin	Low solubility and slowly excreted: each dose lasts 24 hours.			
Fortified procaine penicillin Methicillin (Celbenin)	Contains benzylpenicillin and procaine penicillin. Resistant to penicillinase and should be reserved for penicillin-resistant staphylococci. Less effective against other organisms.	Painful injection		
Phenoxymethyl-penicillin (penicillin V) Phenethicillin: Phenoxyethyl penicillin (Broxil) Propicillin: Phenoxypropyl penicillin (Brocillin) Phenbenicillin: Phenoxybenzyl penicillin (Penspek) Ampicillin (Penbritin)	*Preparations to be given orally, ½ hour before meals* Probably more effective than penicillin V. Wide spectrum: useless against penicillinase forming staphs. and coli.	Reactions less common than with injected Penicillins.		Generally speaking acts against above organisms but less rapid in action and less effective than injected penicillins.
Benzylpenicillin also used as lozenge or ointment				

TABLE XXXV (*continued*)

	Uses	*Toxic effects may be*	*Used against*	*Sometimes used against*
Streptomycin sulphate (by injection)	Not absorbed by mouth. Short courses by injection are valuable but organisms readily develop resistance. In tuberculosis must be combined with PAS or INAH. In other infections often given with penicillin.	On 8th cranial nerve Contact dermatitis	*B. anthracis* *E. coli* Friedlander's bacilli *M. tuberculosis* *Past. pestis* (plague) *Past. tularense* Pneumococci Pneumobacilli Streptococci	*Bact. ærogenes* *B. mallei* (glanders) *B. pyocyaneus* Brucella Dysentery bacilli *H. influenzæ* Proteus *S. typhi* Salmonellæ Staphylococci
Chloramphenicol (oral)	Rapidly absorbed. Drug-resistance unusual.	Diarrhœa Vomiting Agranulocytosis *Staph.* enterocolitis	*Bact. ærogenes* *B. anthracis* *E. coli* *H. influenzæ* Pneumobacilli Pneumococci Rickettsia (typhus) Salmonellæ *S. typhi* Streptococci Larger viruses (psittacosis and lymphogranuloma venereum)	Actinomyces *Brucella abortus* Dysentery bacilli *E. histolytica* *H. pertussis* Proteus *Ps. pyocyaneus* Staphylococci
Tetracyclines (oral) (Intravenous and intramusc. occasionally) Chlortetracycline (Aureomycin) Oxytetracycline (Terramycin) Tetracycline (Achromycin) Demethylchlortetracycline (Ledermycin) Also used as ointments	Readily absorbed, especially tetracycline. Passes into all body tissues (C.S.F. not freely). Drug resistance unusual.	Diarrhœa Vomiting Stomatitis *Staph.* enterocolitis Liver damage (rare)	Brucella *C. diphtheriæ* *Ducrey's bacilli* (chancroid) Friedlander's bacilli *H. influenzæ* Pneumococci *Spirchæta recurrentis* (relapsing fever) Viruses of pneumonia	*B. anthracis* Cat-scratch fever *Cl. Welchii* Dysentery bacilli *E. coli* *Past. tularense* Proteus *Ps. pyocyaneus* Rickettsia (typhus) Salmonellæ Staphyococci Larger viruses
Bacitracin (intramusc. occasionally) Main use is locally	As solution or ointment to skin and eyes where penicillin-resistant organism present.	Albuminuria Anorexia (Painful injection)		Staphylococci Streptococci
Erythromycin (oral) Occasionally used as ointment	Main use against Gram-positive cocci especially when penicillin-resistant or patient sensitive to penicillin. Organisms rapidly develop resistance. Valuable in *Staph. entero-colitis.*	Occasional diarrhœa	*C. diphtheriæ* *H. influenzæ* Neisseria Staphylococci Streptococci	*E. histolytica* Pneumococci
Polymyxin B (intramusc.)	Only used when severe infection refractory to other drugs. Main effect on Gram-negative bacilli especially in urine. Intrathecal for *Ps.pyocyaneus* meningitis.	Albuminuria Oliguria Dizziness Fever (painful injection)	*Ps. pyocyanea*	*E. coli* (in urine)
Spiramycin (oral)	Low toxicity. Chief use against penicillin-resistant staphylococci and patients sensitive to penicillin. Valuable in *Staph. entero-colitis.*		Staphylococci *Str. fæcalis*	

761

TABLE XXXV (continued)

	Uses	Toxic effects may be	Used against	Sometimes used against
Vancomycin (intravenous or intramusc.)	Main use against penicillin-resistant staphylococci.	Thrombophlebitis Fever Deafness (occasionally)	Staphylococci	
Gramicidin (Syn. Tyrothricin) Local use only in skin and mouth	Dangerous when injected. Acts on Gram-positive cocci and some bacilli. Action enhanced by penicillin and neomycin.		Staphylococci Streptococci	Proteus Ps. pyocyaneus
Neomycin (intramusc. occasionally) Main use is locally	Resembles streptomycin; not absorbed by mouth. Rarely used intramusc. against organisms resistant to streptomycin (including tubercle bacilli).	Albuminuria On 8th cranial nerve Candida infection	Gram-positive and negative infections of skin and mucous membranes	Tubercle bacilli
Neostatin (oral)	Little is absorbed. Antifungicidal action in mouth and intestine.		Candida albicans	

isolated a number of semi-synthetic penicillin derivatives of therapeutic importance are being produced for administration by intramuscular injection and by mouth.   Penicillin is largely free of undesirable side-effects and even considerable over-dosage produces no toxic effects on the patient (unless given in large doses intrathecally).   It does not readily diffuse into the cerebro-spinal fluid.   The dose is measured in Oxford Standard units (Table XXXVI).   Drug fever, urticaria and penicillin-resistance of certain organisms is met especially with repeated and prolonged courses of penicillin.   It can also be used locally by injection into abscesses, empyemata and into the cerebro-spinal canal, as well as locally into wounds, as pastilles in the mouth, and by inhalation as an aerosol.   Streptomycin is derived from the soil organism Actinomyces griseus, and differs from penicillin in being effective against such gram-negative organisms as those of the coli-typhoid group, and against the tubercle bacillus (Table XXXV).   It is not appreciably absorbed when given by mouth and for systemic use has to be injected intramuscularly each 12–24 hours.   Not only do organisms develop resistance to its use rather rapidly but it is liable to produce undesirable side-effects on the eighth cranial nerve as well as contact dermatitis in nurses and others handling it.   Chloramphenicol (Chloromycetin) was originally obtained from Streptomyces venezuelæ and is now prepared synthetically. It has a very wide antibacterial spectrum and is useful in a large variety of diseases; but especially in children and when given for any length of time it can produce agranulocytosis.   It has an almost specific effect against the typhoid-paratyphoid organisms.   The tetracyclines include chlor-

TABLE XXXVI.—DOSES OF SULPHONAMIDES AND PRINCIPAL ANTIBIOTICS RECOMMENDED

	Severe Infections	*Milder Infections*	*Remarks*
	Initial and Subsequent Doses in Grammes		
Sulphonamides *Adults*	2: 2: then 1 4-hourly for 3 days: then 1 8-hourly for 4–6 days	2: 1 4-hourly for 36 hours: then 1 6-hourly for 2 days: then 1 8-hourly for 2 days	Intravenous Soluthiazole can be given initially. Give fluids and alkalis freely. Continue treatment until temperature normal for 3 days.
Children 0–2 years	1: then ½ 4-hourly for 3 days	¼–½: then ⅛–¼ 4-hourly for 3 days	
3–5 years	1½: then ¾ 4-hourly for 3 days	¾: then ¼–½ 4-hourly for 3 days	
5–15 years	2–2½: then ¾–1 4-hourly for 3 days	1: then ½ 4-hourly for 3 days	
Penicillin	*Inject. in Mega Units* (1,000,000 units)		
Adults Benzylpenicillin	1: then ½ 8- or 12-hourly	¼–½ 12-hourly	Continue treatment until temperature normal for 3 days. Children require rather smaller doses by injection.
Procaine penicillin	0·6 12-hourly	0·3 12-hourly	
Methicillin (Celbenin)	1 Gramme 4-hourly injected		Especially useful against penicillin-resistant staphylococci.
	Doses in Milligrammes by mouth, ½ hour before meals		
Phenoxymethyl-penicillin (penicillin-V)	500 mg. 4- to 6-hourly	125–250 mg. (400,000 units) 4-hourly	
Phenethicillin (Broxil)	”	”	
Propicillin (Brocillin)	”	”	
Phenbenicillin (Penspek)	”	125–250 mg. 6-hourly	
Ampicillin	”	”	
Children Phenoxymethyl penicillin Children 0–2 years	60 mg. (100,000 units) 4-hourly	30 mg. 4-hourly	Initial doses of benzylpenicillin desirable. Doses continued until temperature normal for 3 days.
3–15 years	125 mg. 4-hourly	60 mg. 4-hourly	
Phenethicillin Propicillin Phenbenicillin 0–2 years	30 mg. 4-hourly	20 mg. 4-hourly	
3–15 years	60 mg. 4-hourly	30 mg. 4-hourly	
Empyema	After pus removed by aspiration inject. 100,000–500,000 units of benzylpenicillin into cavity in 5–10 ml. on alternate days.		
Arthritis (pyogenic)	After pus removed inject. 50,000–100,000 units of benzylpenicillin in 3 ml. into joint on alternate days.		
Streptomycin (intramusc.) Adults	0·50–0·75 G. 12-hourly	1·0 G. each 24 hours	Potentiates the effect of penicillin.
Children	10 mg./lb. body weight 12-hourly	5 mg./lb. body weight 12-hourly	
Adults (intrathecal)	100 mg. alt. days for 4 doses		For use in meningitis.
Children (intrathecal)	20–50 mg. alt. days for 4 doses		”
Chloramphenicol and Tetracyclines Adults	1 G.: then 0·5 G. each 4 hours for 2 days: then 0·5 G. each 6 hours	0·5 G.: then 0·25 G. each 4 hours for 2 days: then 0·25 G. each 6 hours	If vomiting, initial slow intravenous inj. 1·0 G. 12-hourly: then intramusc. 0·25 G. 12-hourly.
Children	3–5 mg./lb. body weight each 6 hours	1–2 mgm./lb. body weight each 6 hours	The oral dose of Ledermycin is rather less.

tetracycline (Aureomycin), oxytetracycline (Terramycin) and tetracycline (Achromycin). These three broad-spectrum antibiotics are bacteriostatic and bactericidal and are effective even against some of the viruses. They have slightly different effects against different species of bacteria but possess the great advantage that they can be administered orally in capsules, and rarely produce drug fever or drug eruptions. After 4–5 days they are very liable to produce severe entero-colitis, and they are still very expensive. Other antibiotics which are sometimes used include bacitracin, erythromycin, polymyxin B, spiramycin, and for local use gramicidin, neomycin and nystatin. Whenever an antibiotic is given (especially with penicillin and streptomycin) full doses must be used as otherwise drug-resistance of the infecting organism is likely to occur. As the temperature falls smaller doses may be given (except in tuberculosis) but these doses must be maintained until the patient has been afebrile for 72 hours. If the temperature fails to respond the organism is probably already of a resistant type. (3) The patient's general resistance is encouraged by a free supply of fresh air, at least 5 pints of fluid daily, with sugar as the principal food, restful sleep and especially in anæmic cases by blood transfusion.

§ **517. V. Subacute and Chronic Septic Conditions** (*e.g.*, **Abscess, Ulceration, etc.**) also give rise to intermitting pyrexia. The various clinical conditions met under this heading are due to the absorption of some septic or toxic material into the circulation. The possible sources of the sepsis are numerous, and may be grouped into two divisions—(*a*) ABSCESS and (*b*) SIMPLE INFLAMMATION often with ULCERATION (internal or external). Clinically, the former is more acute than the latter.

(*a*) ABSCESS (PENT-UP PUS).—Pus never forms in any part of the body —*e.g.*, in the pleura (empyema), in the liver (hepatic abscess) or elsewhere—without an intermitting or remitting pyrexia: this may be accompanied by "chills," "shivers" or "rigors." Before the clinical thermometer was invented, these shiverings (sometimes followed by sweatings) were the chief symptoms by which the formation of pus was identified. It must however be remembered that chemotherapy (especially with the sulpha-drugs) and occasionally the antibiotics may allow pus to develop— sometimes in considerable amounts—while the patient remains apyrexial: it is thus easy to mask the presence of a dangerous infection in a hidden area, *e.g.*, in the mastoid air-cells, or in a subphrenic abscess. In the presence of an abscess, there are marked constitutional effects such as lassitude, debility, pallor (though with a hectic flush on the cheeks) and loss of weight. The blood should always be examined for a leucocytosis; an increase in the polymorphonuclear cells will afford strong confirmation that pus is present.

Etiology.—Abscess or pent-up pus in any position may produce these symptoms, and careful search should be made for abscess of the liver, gall-bladder, pelvic cellulitis or abscess, appendicitis (Figs. 154, 155), caries of the spine, mastoiditis, sinusitis, a dental apical abscess, intracranial abscess, empyema, pyonephrosis, subphrenic and perinephric abscess, etc. Pain is the chief localising symptom, but it may be absent, especially in children. On giving free exit to the pus the pyrexia should rapidly subside.

(*b*) SIMPLE INFLAMMATION, with or without ULCERATION of an INTERNAL or EXTERNAL surface, is always attended by some degree of intermitting pyrexia, running a more chronic course than the foregoing. This fever also differs from the last in the usual absence of definite rigors. Sometimes the shivering may not amount to more than " chills down the spine "— perhaps thought to be " malaria "—and sweating which is hardly noticed. The morning temperature is normal, or almost normal, and it is raised one or two degrees some time during the day. Anæmia and failing health are always present, and some degree of leucocytosis is usual. This kind of fever, due to prolonged suppuration and attended by chronic wasting, was

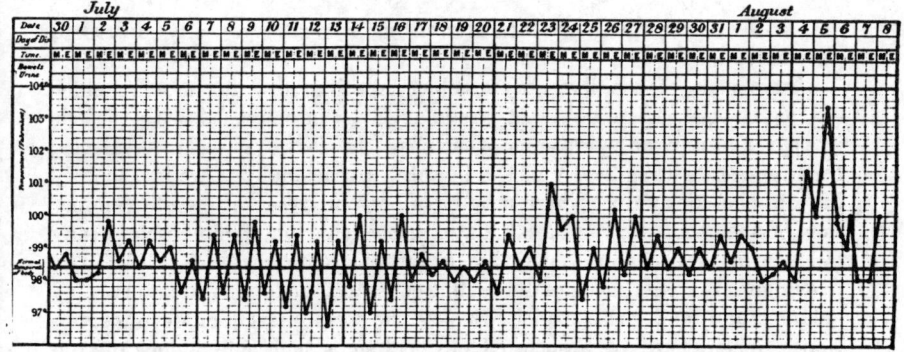

FIG. 155.— CHRONIC PYÆMIA.— Frank T——, æt. 31, had had an attack of gonorrhœal rheumatism 2 years before, from which he had recovered. The present illness had come on gradually a month or so before admission. Stiffness and pain in the joints were the chief symptoms, and the urethra being *absolutely normal*, it was regarded as a case of chronic rheumatism, though none of the usual remedies had any effect. The joints became progressively worse, and though he complained of abdominal pain from time to time attention was not directed to that cavity. He died some two months later suddenly from perforation of the appendix. A review of the case pointed to a chronic septic process having its origin in the appendix, and especially affecting joints which had been previously diseased.

formerly known as *Hectic Fever* (Greek, ἑπτιπός " habitual "). When due to a discharging sinus—for instance, connected with caries, or necrosis of a bone, or a bed-sore—the cause is obvious. But the condition may also be set up by inflammation or ulceration of any of the mucous membranes or internal passages—*e.g.*, ulcerative colitis, appendicitis (Fig. 155). It is called *Urinary Fever* when it arises from chronic infection of some part of the urinary passages—*e.g.*, with a stone impacted in the ureter, or a urethral stricture, or chronic pyelonephritis. This cause may be suspected if there be a history of renal colic. Similarly, *Acute Cholangitis* (infection of the biliary passages) may be suspected if there be a history of biliary colic. When the infection, due to gall-stones, is situated in the *gall-bladder*, colic and jaundice may be absent and the patient complains only of the " chills."

§ 518. VI. Malignant Disease as a cause of obscure pyrexia is becoming more common in an ageing population.

Symptoms.—The temperature may rise in an irregular manner to 99·5–100° F., but in some can mount in the evening to 103–104° F. Accompanying this are the symptoms and signs of malignancy (§ 571).

Diagnosis.—Apart from careful clinical examination of the chest and abdomen in particular, there is very commonly a high erythrocyte sedimentation rate, usually anæmia and sometimes a polymorph leucocytosis of 20,000–35,000 per c.mm.

Etiology.—The cause may be malignant disease associated with an infection as in carcinoma of the bronchus (§ 138) or colon. Other cases show no evidence of infection. Although carcinoma or sarcoma in any part of the body may be the cause, hypernephroma of a kidney or deposits in the liver should be especially suspect.

§ 519. The **rarer causes of Intermitting Pyrexia** are fully described elsewhere.

Amœbiasis of the liver or amœbic hepatitis may for months show few signs other than bouts of irregular fever interspersed with periods of apyrexia, and no symptoms other than those of dyspepsia, flatulence, constipation or irregularity of the bowels. Occasionally there is a history of right shoulder pain. There may have been no dysentery, and examination of the stools and of fæcal material collected on sigmoidoscopy may fail to reveal cysts or vegetative forms of *Entamœba histolytica*. The liver signs are sometimes indefinite, but generally the organ is demonstrably enlarged and tenderness is elicited below the costal margin on deep inspiration. When there are associated physical signs such as evidence of consolidation or fluid at the base of the right lung, or when X-ray reveals upward bulging or " splinting " of the diaphragm, an abscess of the liver is almost certainly present. There is a mild polymorphonuclear neutrophil leucocytosis, but even when the condition of hepatitis has gone on to abscess formation a neutrophilia not exceeding 80 per cent. and a total count not exceeding 15,000 per c.mm. are common findings. Amœbiasis should be suspected in obscure cases of fever when the patient has lived in the tropics. Within 48–72 hours, the temperature responds to emetine. Such patients show marked improvement in health when the parasites are eradicated. It is among the amœbic carriers that many cases of hepatitis and liver abscess are found, as infection often persists unsuspected for long periods. Also refer to Abscess of the Liver (§ 336) and Amœbiasis (§ 315).

§ 520. Visceral Syphilis.—There are two different stages of syphilis in which intermitting pyrexia may occur. (*a*) At the first development of the primary roseolar eruption there may be some fever. This is generally overlooked, but at other times it may be accompanied by thirst, loss of appetite, and shivering. It always occurs within 65 days of the date of the infection, and is only present if no early treatment be given. (*b*) In the later secondary and tertiary stages of the disease intermitting pyrexia may occur in connection with syphilitic periostitis, or gummata of the internal organs. Syphilitic lesions of this kind should be considered in cases of prolonged intermitting pyrexia, especially when attended by anæmia. The morning temperature is normal, but in the evening it goes up one, two or more degrees (Fig. 156). There may also be rigors, nocturnal sweating, and paroxysms of pain in the joints; these symptoms speedily subside when iodide is given. In obscure cases careful investigation should be made of the eyes, liver, ribs, clavicles and other bones; the Wassermann reaction should be tested. In rare instances the fever may be continued and simulate typhoid. When the diagnosis has been confirmed a full course of anti-syphilitic treatment must be given.

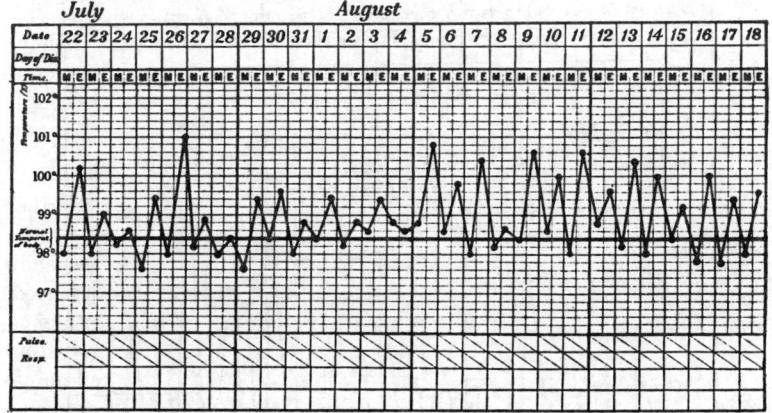

FIG. 156.—VISCERAL SYPHILIS.—Annie L——, æt. 66. The temperature subsided under iodide in large doses, but she ultimately died of exhaustion and hypostatic pneumonia. Autopsy— Gummata of liver and bones, hypertrophic cirrhosis, widespread fibrosis of organs.

INFLUENZA, TYPHOID and PARATYPHOID fever, especially when modified by previous inoculation, and other diseases described in Groups I and II may be attended by pyrexia of an intermitting type.

TYPHOID FEVER during the first 2 weeks of its course is attended by typically continued pyrexia, but in the concluding stage of the disease the temperature gradually drops each morning to normal, and the case may be seen for the first time in this stage. Under certain other circumstances also the temperature may be intermitting —viz.: (i.) In rare instances it may commence with symptoms of ague (see *Varieties*, p. 709); (ii.) in very mild cases; (iii.) after lasting a few days, the fever sometimes aborts and takes on an intermitting type.

KALA-AZAR has usually intermittent fever after the first period, during which there is fever of a remittent type (§ 506).

Various LOCAL INFLAMMATORY DISEASES, other than the septic conditions previously mentioned, may at times be attended by intermittent pyrexia. In cirrhosis of the liver, for instance, a prolonged fever with daily oscillations is occasionally observed.

INFECTIVE ENDOCARDITIS (Multiple Systemic Embolism) (§ 50) is always attended by pyrexia of an irregularly intermitting type, sometimes with rigors and sweatings, very much resembling the chart of septicæmia, though the temperature is usually a little more diurnally regular, and rigors are not usually so frequent (compare charts, Figs. 157 and 154). Infective Endocarditis is favoured by (i.) a loud cardiac murmur detected quite early in the case; (ii.) a history of acute rheumatism; (iii.) the secondary emboli in this disease are more frequently found in the systemic arteries, such as those of the spleen, liver and kidneys, and they do not result in abscesses.

HODGKIN'S DISEASE is recognised by the enlargement of the lymphatic glands and pyrexia of a remitting or intermitting type (§ 584). Sometimes a periodic temperature occurs with glandular enlargement confined to the mediastinal or retroperitoneal glands (Pel-Ebstein Syndrome).

In PERNICIOUS ANÆMIA the temperature is sometimes subnormal, but it is often attended by exacerbations of slight fever of an intermitting type. The disease is also identified by the intense sallowness of the skin and the condition of the blood.

In ACUTE LYMPHATIC LEUKÆMIA the temperature is high and irregular, somewhat resembling that of septicæmia. It can be diagnosed by the examination of the blood, when there is found to be an increase in lymphocytes (§ 554).

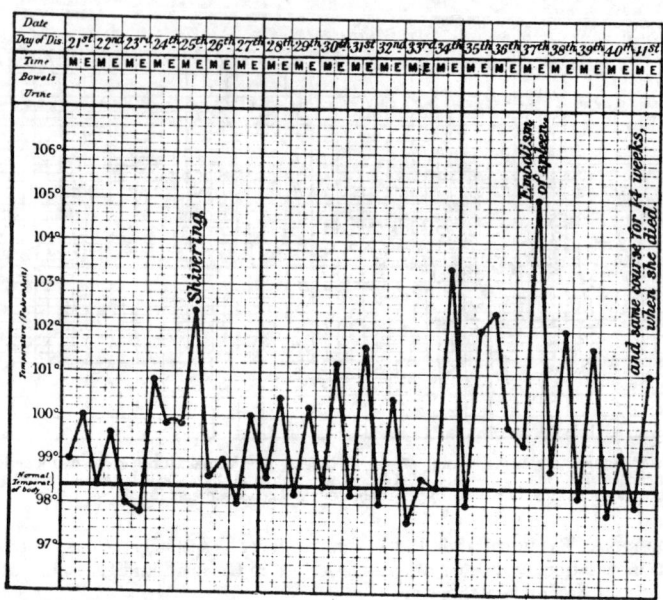

FIG. 157.—INFECTIVE ENDOCARDITIS in a woman, æt. 42. The 3 weeks shown illustrate the course of the temperature which lasted 17 weeks, when she died.

The OPIUM OR MORPHIA HABIT (§ 1185) is attended from time to time by attacks of intermittent pyrexia, during the reaction stage, in which there are cold, hot and sweating stages. Cases are recorded where no cause could be found, but the attack ceased on giving opium.

§ 521. African Trypanosomiasis (Syn., Sleeping Sickness), a disease confined to tropical Africa, is characterised by enlargement of the glands, fleeting intermittent erythematous rashes, irregular pyrexia, excessive sleepiness and mental degeneration.

Symptoms.—The incubation period following the bite of infected tsetse flies varies from 1 to 3 weeks. Two stages are recognised: (1) In the *first* trypanosomes are demonstrable in the blood and lymphatic gland juice. There may be a history of a papule at the site of the bite—the " trypanosomal chancre." Irregular, remittent or intermittent fever with periods of apyrexia may last for some months. The pulse is rapid, the respirations accelerated. Patches of circinate erythema appear, mainly on the trunk, and localised puffiness may implicate the feet, legs and face. Polyadenitis with painless enlargement of the posterior cervical glands is common; sometimes the epitrochlear, supraclavicular and axillary or femoral glands may be the group affected. The spleen is generally palpable at this stage and deep hyperæsthesia, especially over bones like the tibia, is characteristic; there is often a definite latent period after pressure before pain appears. This stage is well marked in Europeans, but may not be so evident in natives. Many months may elapse before the second stage, due to trypanosomes invading the central nervous system, occurs. (2) Here the cerebro-spinal fluid contains an excess of lymphocytes and globulin: trypanosomes are sometimes difficult to find. The patient develops lack of concentration, headache, insomnia, loss of weight and slight tremor of the tongue associated with polyadenitis. Later, the countenance becomes apathetic and morose, emotional instability and laziness increase, and the patient drops off to sleep even when eating. The gait is shuffling, the speech mumbled and slow, and fibrillary tremors develop in the lips and hands. Ataxia is marked and the reflexes increased. Finally, owing to muscular weakness, the patient takes to bed; bed-sores and flexure contractures develop, and coma or convulsions terminate the picture.

Diagnosis.—This can only be made with certainty on finding the parasite by gland puncture, in the blood or in the cerebro-spinal fluid. Where C.N.S. involvement is doubtful lumbar puncture should not be done until treatment with antrypol or pentamidine has been started. Otherwise there is a risk of the needle infecting the C.S.F. from the blood. Guinea-pigs or rats should be inoculated in unproven cases.

Etiology.—The trypanosome is introduced into the body by the bite of a tsetse fly. There are two varieties of trypanosomiasis: (i.) a chronic form, lasting months to years, due to *Trypanosoma gambiense* and occurring more in the western half of tropical Africa. This is transmitted by *Glossina palpalis* and allied species; these tsetse flies require shade and proximity to water. (ii.) An acute form, lasting weeks or months, due to *T. rhodesiense*, occurs especially in Rhodesia, Tanganyika and Nyasaland. It is carried by *G. morsitans* and related species which breed in more open orchard bush.

Prognosis.—With treatment many patients infected with *T. gambiense* and, in the early stages, with *T. rhodesiense* recover, but in the later stages of rhodesiense infections the outlook is grave.

Treatment.—First-stage infections of either type respond to suramin (1 G. weekly) intravenously for 10 doses: albuminuria, nephritis and rarely dermatitis may follow its administration. Pentamidine is also effective in this stage; 2–3 mg./kilo is given intramusc. daily or on alternate days for up to 10 injections. Neither of these drugs penetrate the central nervous system. Therefore in all second-stage *T. gambiense* cases tryparsamide, which does penetrate the C.N.S., must also be used in doses of 2–4 G. weekly intravenously for 10 weeks. The drug must have been recently manufactured and freshly dissolved for each injection. Optic atrophy may occur, especially with old tryparsamide, so the patient's visual acuity must be tested before each injection, and inquiry made into the presence of unusual optic phenomena. *T. rhodesiense* and some strains of *T. gambiense* are always resistant to tryparsamide; these resistant cases, previously fatal, may respond to a new drug Melarsoprol (Mel B) in doses of 3·6 mg./kilo intravenously daily for 3 days, with second and third courses at 10-day intervals when necessary. Melarsoprol is very liable to produce encephalopathy but the risk is lessened if suramin is given first. *Prophylaxis.*—Pentamidine 250 mg. intramusc. will protect a man at risk for 3 to 6 months in *T. gambiense* regions of Africa. There is no drug prophylaxis against *T. rhodesiense*.

Chaga's disease in S. America is due to a trypanosome carried by certain bugs. There is a first stage, usually in children, of fever, which, if survived, may lead to a chronic stage characterised by signs of myocardial damage. **Trichinosis** (§ 606) is usually accompanied by intermittent fever. **Rat-bite** fever may show a temperature of an intermittent type (§ 506).

§ 522. Filariasis bancrofti is widespread in tropical countries. It is the result of infection with *Wüchereria bancrofti* which invade the lymph vessels and lymph glands; it produces embryos (microfilariæ) which also invade the blood-stream.

Symptoms.—After an incubation period of up to 2 years, *early symptoms* comprise (1) recurrent attacks of fever and often rigors associated with acute lymphadenitis and lymphangitis. A distinguishing feature is that the lymphangitis starts at the enlarged lymph glands and spreads down the limb (*i.e.*, it is usually centrifugal); (2) the primary site is usually in the legs with painful and tender enlargement of the inguinal glands. Recurrent funiculitis and epididymo-orchitis are also common with acute tenderness of the spermatic cords, scrotum and testicles. The arms are less commonly involved with enlargement of the epitrochlear and axillary glands; sometimes the breasts are affected; (3) the skin in the area of the blocked lymphatics becomes dull red and œdematous and nodules may be present in the lymph vessels at the site of an adult worm; (4) attacks of abdominal pain indicate enlargement of the retro-peritoneal lymphatics; (5) secondary infection of the affected part is usually streptococcal and causes further rises of temperature and inflammation of the lymphatics. *Late symptoms* are due to intermittent and finally permanent obstruction of the lymph drainage; (6) the lymph glands affected earlier remain permanently enlarged; (7) elephantiasis of the legs may result in such gross enlargement that walking becomes impossible and similar changes in the scrotum and testicles produces elephantiasis of these organs with hydrocœle (§ 580); (8) chylous ascties and chyluria are due to rupture of the enlarged lymph vessels into the peritoneum, the pelvis of the kidney or into the bladder; (9) the skin remains coarse and thickened, and indolent ulcers or abscesses may form.

Diagnosis is made on the characteristic history. When lymphatic nodules are present, excision and microscopy may reveal an adult worm, and embryos (microfilariæ) can be found in the blood at night (§ 542). Eosinophilia is almost invariably present. The lymphœdema of Milroy's disease occurs in those who have not resided in tropical areas and is often accompanied by a family history of the condition (§ 580).

Prognosis.—Although grossly incapacitated by the size and weight of the lymphœdematous areas the disease does not materially shorten life unless intercurrent infection supervenes.

Treatment.—In the acute stages bed-rest is essential and the affected limb must be elevated. When secondary infection occurs, inject. benzylpenicillin or another suitable antibiotic is necessary. Once the acute phase has subsided tab. diethylcarbamazine citrate B.P. (Banocide) should be given; at first use small doses and slowly increase to 2 mg./kilo body weight t.d.s. for 3 weeks. This causes rapid disappearance of microfilariæ from the blood but adult worms are affected much more slowly. The drug should be repeated each 6 months so long as active infection persists. Plastic surgery of the genitals and breasts give good results but it is not so successful when attempted on the limbs.

Remedial treatment has, for the most part, been given under each disease, but there are some important matters relating to all infections in common which must now be referred to—viz., **Immunisation, Serum Therapy, Antibiotic and Chemotherapy** (and see § 516), **Notification** and **Isolation, Disinfection, Diet,** and the treatment of **Pyrexia** and **Hyperpyrexia.**

§ 523. **Infection and Immunity.**—Man lives in constant contact with germs; these may be large as with the protozoa, small as with the different types of bacteria or ultra-microscopic as with the viruses. The healthy person possesses a certain natural immunity against these various organisms, but this varies greatly in different individuals and in different races; thus tuberculosis is much more serious in negroes than in the white-skinned population. Some of the mechanisms by which infections are resisted are known, but there are many unknown factors, discovery of which may provide the information necessary to prevent infection by deliberate immunisation.

To produce disease bacteria almost invariably have to enter the body. Intact skin is an efficient protection against organisms and its normal resident population of bacteria is killed by drying or through the action of substances excreted in the sweat. The mucous membranes also possess inherent powers of resistance which may be lessened by previous damage such as may be produced by chemical substances; thus the smoke-filled atmosphere of industrial cities damages the mucous membrane of the bronchi and encourages a subsequent infection. Bacteria in the eye may be killed by lysozyme or will be washed away in the tears via the naso-lachrymal duct to the nose. Many air-borne bacteria are deposited on the lining mucous membrane of the nose and of the pharynx, and together with those from the eye and those ingested in the food are carried down into the stomach. Here the majority are killed by acid or by the gastric ferments, this being one reason why in an outbreak of a disease such as typhoid fever only some of those at risk contact the disease. Resistance to invasion of the wall of the gut by *Entamœba histolytica* is dependent on the concentration of the proteolytic enzymes; if these are inhibited (as by the presence of serum) invasion by the parasites is much more likely to occur. When an organism has overcome these primary barriers in the skin or the mucous membranes it (*a*) may remain on the surface and pro-duce exotoxins. These are relatively stable substances which are absorbed into the blood-stream and paralyse the activity of certain tissues. Thus in diphtheria and tetanus powerful toxins are produced which have a great affinity for nervous tissue. (*b*) Otherwise the organism invades the tissues and may cause a local infection (such as an abscess) or it passes into the blood-stream (bacteræmia or septicæmia). Some organisms, *e.g.*, those responsible for gas gangrene, both invade the tissues and produce an exo-toxin. On entering the body bacteria are met by phagocytes and anti-bodies, and by substances in the blood such as the recently discovered properdin.

Agranulocytosis is a condition occurring for no known reason, or secondarily to poisoning by a drug, in which there is an extreme lack of white cells. It is often accompanied by ulceration of the throat and perhaps of other tissue (§§ 155(*f*), 541).

The organisms may enter the red blood cells, as with protozoal infec-tions such as malaria, and this susceptibility of the erythrocytes is limited to certain groups of animals, where the concentration of potassium is high and of sodium is low. The various bacteria which gain entrance to the body likewise seem to have a selective affinity for certain tissues—thus the pneumococcus attacks the areas lined by endothelial cells as in the lungs, the meninges, the peritoneum or the joints. The viruses also pro-duce a preliminary viræmia and then may succeed in establishing them-selves in particular tissue cells: thus abortive cases of acute anterior polio-myelitis are those in which the virus grows in living cells of the gut and a viræmia occurs; if the virus once establishes itself in the cells of the central nervous system paralytic phenomena ensue. Once a virus has established itself intracellularly it is relatively resistant to the immunological processes of the body.

Antibodies are substances present in body fluids whose formation is stimulated by antigens. Antigens can be derived from many substances and not only from protozoa, bacteria and viruses. The principal requirement is that the molecule should be large, and probably for this reason the majority of antigens are proteins. Antibodies also possess a large molecule and are contained in the globulin portion of the blood. In general, antibodies react only against the antigen which stimulates their formation. Different types are made, including those which will agglutinate, precipitate or lyse bacteria. Because of the specificity of the antigen–antibody reaction it can be used as the basis of diagnostic tests.

Agammaglobulinæmia or hypoglobulinæmia is a rare condition mainly of children but sometimes met in adults where there is a failure to produce antibodies in response to an infection and so recurring infections are met; yet the patient recovers from an infection in a normal manner. The condition is congenital and sometimes hereditary in origin, but often disappears in adult life.

Resistance to the attacks of various organisms may be (i.) *Inherited*. Some races and certain families possess a much higher immunity to particular organisms than do others. But this is only relative and a sufficiently large dose will cause them to succumb. Infants who are breast-fed derive antibodies to a large number of diseases from the mother's milk. Recent work has suggested that malaria in breast-fed infants is suppressed because the mother's milk is deficient in *p*-aminobenzoic acid; if this is added to the mother's milk a malarial infection is much more readily established in a breast-fed infant. (ii.) *Active acquired immunity* to many diseases is developed as a patient recovers from them and antibodies can usually be demonstrated in the blood. Thus the blood of patients recovering spontaneously from diphtheria or tetanus contains antitoxin which will neutralise the exotoxin responsible for the infection. It is not always possible to demonstrate such antibodies and in some diseases antibodies in the tissues, or some other mechanism, may be responsible for the acquired immunity. Virus infections may also, as with small-pox, measles and mumps, produce an immunity which lasts many years; but others such as the virus of the common cold, give a very short-lived immunity after infection. (iii.) *Artificial acquired immunity* is similar to (ii.) above. Vaccine therapy is based on the principle of producing immunity by the administration of one or more doses of dead or of living but harmless organisms. The earliest example was Jenner's use of living cowpox vaccine to protect against small-pox. Now protection can be offered against many diseases and the use of B.C.G. vaccine to Mantoux-negative children and adults has played a notable part in decreasing the ravages of tuberculosis. In general, where it has been possible to use a living vaccine such as an attenuated strain of yellow fever virus, or a single toxin as in the case of tetanus and diphtheria, protection is more certain than if the vaccine has to be made of killed organisms—as in the prevention of typhoid fever. (iv.) In *passive immunity* protection is provided by serum containing antibodies produced in other people or animals and administered by injection. The patient plays no active part therefore in the process: usually in about 3 weeks the donated antibodies are excreted and destroyed. This occurs naturally in that the placenta allows the passage of antibodies, and the new-born baby starts life with circulating antibodies derived from its mother. Passive immunity may be employed artificially for either treatment or protection. In the past it was used extensively in the treatment of infections, but except for a few and notably for diphtheria, tetanus and botulism, it has been replaced by chemotherapy. Examples of prophylaxis in passive immunity are the use of diphtheria antitoxin, of tetanus antitoxin, and of convalescent measles serum (or gamma-globulin containing measles antibody) for the temporary protection of individuals exposed to these infections. For diphtheria and tetanus, prevention by active immunisation before exposure is a much preferable policy. (v.) *Chemotherapy and the antibiotics* are also used in certain diseases to protect the patient from infections. Thus the prophylaxis of rheumatic fever now consists of the daily administration of penicillin (usually penicillin-V by mouth) to prevent re-infection of the throat with hæmolytic streptococci. The incidence of malaria has been greatly reduced by the regular use of drugs such as proguanil hydrochlor. (Paludrin) or pyrimethamine (Daraprim) (§ 512). Unlike the protection afforded by active immunisation the protection afforded by any of these chemical compounds rapidly disappears when the drugs are stopped.

§ 524. **Serum Therapy.**—Serum may be given by three routes: (1) Intravenous. This is the method of choice when immediate immunisation is required, for the antitoxin is thus instantly available. It is also the best way when doses have to be large, or frequently repeated, or when its use has been unduly delayed. On the other hand, the immunity is less lasting. (2) Intramuscular. The gluteus maximus and the vastus lateralis are the most convenient muscles. This method is less rapid in its effects, the maximum concentration of antitoxin not being present till 24 hours after the injection. It is much safer, and requires a less elaborate technique. (3) The subcutaneous method is the slowest and the easiest. The maximum concentration is not reached till 72 hours after injection. This route may be of great value as a reserve in support of the intravenous, the antitoxin being maintained in the circulation by slow absorption. The intrathecal method of administration is no longer used.

Serum Reactions.—Antisera made in horses will contain some horse protein and a proportion of patients can be expected to react. Anaphylactic shock is the most serious reaction and may be fatal within minutes. Serum sickness of the delayed type occurs 7 to 12 days after the infection, and in the accelerated type seen in those who have had previous injections, 3 to 4 days after the injection. Both types are characterised by fever, rashes, œdema and joint pains. Patients should always be kept under observation for 30 minutes after the administration of antiserum, and *antiserum should never be given unless a syringe and inject. adrenalin B.P. is immediately available.* Adrenalin intramuscularly 0·5 to 1 ml. repeated if necessary in 15 minutes, with an intramuscular antihistamine will usually bring about rapid recovery from anaphylactic shock.

Before antiserum is given inquiry should be made as to previous injections of horse serum and for any history of allergic conditions such as asthma or infantile eczema. If there is no history of allergy a trial dose of 0·2 ml. of undiluted antiserum should be given subcutaneously, and in the absence of general symptoms in 30 minutes, can be followed with the full intramuscular dose. If there is a history of allergy the trial dose should be of 0·2 ml. of a 1 in 10 dilution of antiserum followed by a second trial dose of 0·2 ml. of undiluted serum 30 minutes later. If there is no general reaction the full dose may then be given. Following a general reaction and its treatment it is necessary to wait until the blood pressure has returned to normal and rashes have subsided (usually 6 to 12 hours) before the next trial dose of 0·2 ml. of undiluted toxin is given: if there is no reaction to this the full dose may be injected 30 minutes later.

§ 525. **The Treatment of Infections** has been revolutionised by the use of chemotherapeutic and antibiotic drugs. The specific treatment of individual diseases has been discussed in the appropriate sections of this book. There are certain general principles which apply to all treatment. Before treatment is begun, the doctor should ask himself if it is necessary. Antibiotics are frequently prescribed for no clear reason, and indiscriminate use may carry the risk of sensitisation to the drug, toxic reactions and replacement of sensitive bacteria by resistant strains. Not all infections can be treated by chemotherapy alone. In some infections, *e.g.*, chronic osteomyelitis, the drug will be unable to reach bacteria in sufficient concentration to destroy them, or may not be able to destroy them because the bacteria are not multiplying fast enough to render them susceptible to the drug's action. For successful treatment chemotherapy may have to be accompanied by surgery. Urinary infections also provide an example of the inability of chemotherapy by itself to cure patients: while acute infections in otherwise normal patients will respond well, the prospects of keeping the urine sterile in patients with obstructive lesions of the urinary tract are poor.

Antibiotics should be used to which the infecting organism is likely to be sensitive, and if there is doubt, laboratory sensitivity tests should be carried out. In most cases they will give a reliable guide, although for some infections, *e.g.*, typhoid fever, they can be misleading and in others, *e.g.*, subacute bacterial endocarditis, the most promising drug or combination of drugs can sometimes only be chosen after relatively complicated tests. Some antibiotics are more likely to produce resistant bacteria than others and this should be borne in mind. When treatment has to be prolonged, *e.g.*, in tuberculosis, combinations of drugs have been shown to reduce greatly the likelihood of resistant strains appearing. Patients may become sensitive to almost any drug and the reactions can be serious. Before treatment is begun an inquiry should be made as to any history of sensitisation, and a watch should be kept for its development during treatment.

Finally, if the response is poor, what should be done? If it is certain that the response is poor the case should be reviewed in its entirety. In some instances the original diagnosis may have been wrong, in others conditions may have changed, *e.g.*, through the development of an abscess. Considerable clinical acumen may be needed to weigh the many factors involved; but the main principle, that antibiotics should be prescribed in adequate doses and for a stated period only, should be kept in mind. Continued use of an antibiotic which is obviously ineffective will do the patient no good, and may subject him and perhaps other patients to unnecessary risks.

SERUM AND VACCINE THERAPY

DIPHTHERIA.—An antitoxic serum has been on the market since 1895. When given early enough and in large enough doses, antitoxin has been found to be of the greatest value for patients suffering from the disease (see further details in § 497).

Prophylaxis.—By means of the Schick test we can find out who is susceptible to diphtheria and who immune. Technique: By means of a very fine needle Schick Test Toxin (B.P.) 0·2 ml. is injected into the skin of the flexor aspect of one forearm, while into the skin of the other forearm, as a control, is injected a similar quantity of Schick Test Control (B.P.) consisting of heated (inactivated) toxin. The results of the reaction come under four heads: 1. *Negative:* complete absence of any reaction in either arm indicates that the patient is immune to diphtheria. 2. *Positive:* complete absence of reaction in the control arm. The test arm shows after 24–36 hours a red circumscribed flush which reaches its maximum on the fourth day, when it may be 1 to 2 cm. in diameter. After this it fades till by the seventh day a brown desquamating stain is left, which may remain for some weeks. Interpretation: the patient is susceptible to diphtheria. 3. *Negative and Pseudo:* by the end of 24 hours a diffuse red flush which is equal in both arms has developed. By the fourth day this will have faded to a brownish stain, equal in both arms. Interpretation: the patient is immune. The reaction is the non-specific result of a foreign protein. 4. *Positive and Pseudo:* at 24 hours the reaction is as in 3, a diffuse red flush equal on both arms, but by the fourth day the flush on the control arm has faded, while that on the test arm has developed to the circumscribed red area seen in 2, which in its turn fades by the seventh day. Interpretation: the patient is susceptible. If possible the patient should be seen daily till the seventh day; if only a single visit is possible, it should be on the fourth day.

The Schick test allows us to separate the immune from the non-immune. It now remains to immunise the non-immune. Two methods are available: 1. In cases, particularly children, who have been exposed to diphtheria and who have not been previously actively immunised it is wise to confer *passive immunity* by injecting 500–2,000 units of diphtheria antitoxin intramuscularly. This will afford protection for 3 weeks, but may not be successful if the child is already incubating diphtheria. 2. *Active immunisation* can be carried out with toxoid-antitoxin floccules (T.A.F.), alum precipitated toxoid (A.P.T.) or formol toxoid (F.T.). A.P.T. is the best immunising agent. It consists of a suspension of the washed precipitate produced by adding a small amount of alum to diphtheria toxoid. For children under 8 years the dose is 0·3 ml. with a further dose of 0·5 ml. a month later. It has two drawbacks. In adults it may cause local and general reactions, and at all ages it has been accused of producing poliomyelitis in patients who would otherwise have had only a non-paralytic attack of the disease. In countries where there is a risk of poliomyelitis F.T. may be used for immunising children. This preparation consists of purified toxin rendered atoxic with formalin and is given in two doses of 1 ml. separated by at least 4 weeks. The immunity should be reinforced by a single dose of 0·5 ml. of F.T. on first going to school and again at the age of 8. Adults are probably best immunised with T.A.F. Consisting of a suspension of floccules formed when toxoid and antitoxin are mixed, T.A.F. normally causes no reaction, although the trace of horse serum in the antitoxin may give rise to trouble in patients very sensitive to horse proteins. Three doses of 1 ml. are given at 3-weekly intervals.

A combined diphtheria, tetanus and whooping-cough preparation is now being widely used for the primary immunisation of children, and poliomyelitis vaccine may shortly be included in it.

TETANUS.—*Passive immunisation* with tetanus antitoxin is effective as a prophylactic measure: 3,000 international units should be given subcutaneously or intramuscularly after any deep injury which may be contaminated with soil or dirt. The precautions to be taken in administering the serum are outlined in § 524. As immunity from a single dose lasts only about 10 days a second dose should be given after this period if the wound has not healed and conditions suitable for the growth of *Cl. tetani* are still present. Antitoxin should also be given to patients about to undergo operation on old sites of injury in which spores may lurk, dormant but alive; but it is preferable to immunise the patient actively with tetanus toxoid previously.

Active immunisation.—Tetanus toxoid (the toxin rendered atoxic by formalin) is used to produce a high degree of immunity in those persons who may be exposed to tetanus. In countries where umbilical tetanus of infants is common the disease has been prevented by active immunisation of mothers during pregnancy. The dose is 1 ml. followed by 1 ml. 1 month later and a third dose of 1 ml. after a year. There are virtually no undesirable reactions. If an actively immunised person is injured a boosting dose of 1 ml. should be given; tetanus antitoxin is then unnecessary. This regime resulted in only 11 cases and 4 deaths among the 10·7 million men in the U.S.A. armed forces in World War II.

TUBERCULOSIS.—In *diagnosis* Koch's " old Tuberculin " is used. It is prepared by evaporating a 6-week old culture of tubercle bacilli in glycerol broth, sterilising by heat and then filtering. Some use the purified protein derivative (P.P.D.) of this tuberculin instead of the whole tuberculin. The diagnostic application depends on the fact that the tissues of a patient with tuberculosis become hypersensitive to tuberculin. In man the *Mantoux test* is commonly employed: it may be performed by (i.) injecting intradermally 0·1 ml. of the appropriate dilution of old Tuberculin. In the full test 1 tuberculin unit (T.U.) is injected: if this is negative at 72 hours it is followed by 10 units and again if negative by 100 units. (1 T.U. in 0·1 ml. corresponds to 1 in 10,000 dilution, 10 T.U. in 0·1 ml. to 1 in 1,000 and 100 T.U. in 0·1 ml. to 1 in 100.) A positive test consists of a raised indurated area with a diameter of at least 6 mm. appearing within 72 hours; erythema without induration is disregarded. (ii.) Heaf's multiple puncture method is with a small " gun " by which 6 needles are stabbed through an end plate: the stabs carry some of the contents of one drop of tuberculin P.P.D. (equivalent to 100,000 units of P.P.D. tuberculin in 1 ml.): Protoderm (Allen & Hanburys) is a convenient preparation of this. When the result is read between the fourth and seventh days a minimal positive reaction is indicated by palpable induration around at least four punctures. A *positive* reaction by either of these methods does not indicate more than that the patient has been infected by tuberculosis and does not indicate whether the infection is healed or active, although in young children it may often be regarded as an indication of recent infection. A *negative* reaction usually excludes active disease although between one and two per thousand adults give a negative reaction even when tubercle bacilli are present in the sputum. *False negative* reactions also occur when the infection has so recently occurred that there has been no time for antibodies to form, in labour and in the puerperium as well as in very acute (*e.g.*, miliary) tuberculosis. A positive reaction without clinical evidence of active disease indicates a certain degree of immunity, and negative reactors are much more susceptible to infection and to contract clinical tuberculosis.

Prophylactic Vaccination against Tuberculosis.—The object is to give a harmless primary infection with avirulent tubercle bacilli, which will confer immunity against a later virulent infection. Plainly only those who have not yet been infected should be immunised and vaccination is therefore always preceded by Mantoux testing. It is advocated especially in children of tuberculous parents, in medical students and in nurses who are Mantoux-negative. For vaccination B.C.G. (Bacille Calmette-Guérin) is used. This is a living vaccine of an attenuated strain of tubercle bacilli, given as a single intradermal injection of 0·1 ml. The normal reaction develops as a painless papule which is greatest in size between 3 and 6 weeks and which may break down to form a shallow ulcer. Complications consisting of regional adenitis and delayed healing of the ulcer are rare. In Great Britain B.C.G. confers substantial protection (approximately 80 per cent.) against tuberculosis for at least 5 years and probably for 6 years or more. There is virtually no risk that progressive tuberculosis will occur as a result of the inoculation—only three cases have been seen in over 100 million vaccinated persons, and fewer fatalities have been caused by B.C.G. than with any other prophylactic immunisation. Following successful vaccination a previously Mantoux-negative person becomes Mantoux-positive after 8 to 12 weeks.

POLIOMYELITIS VACCINATION.—Active immunity may be produced against poliomyelitis with dead or living vaccines of the three types of poliomyelitis virus. When given intramuscularly, two injections a month apart are followed by a third 9 months later. Live vaccines consist of living attenuated strains of virus, which can be given by mouth. Evidence is increasing that substantial protection is afforded by both methods.

WHOOPING-COUGH.—A good vaccine of killed *H. pertussis* will protect children against infection or modify the illness when protection is not complete. It should be given before the sixth month of life and may be combined with diphtheria and tetanus prophylactics.

ANTI-CATARRHAL VACCINES consist of mixtures of organisms which may infect or may be found in the air passages. Although in use for many years, it is not universally agreed that they are of value.

TYPHOID AND PARATYPHOID INFECTION.—*Prophylactic* inoculation with dead typhoid and paratyphoid bacilli protects against enteric fever, although the protection is probably not as certain as was once thought. The usual T.A.B. vaccine consists of typhoid and paratyphoid A and B bacilli either killed by heat and preserved with phenol, or alcohol killed. Two subcutaneous doses are given at least 10 days apart: with the heat-killed vaccine the first dose is 0·50 ml. and the second 1·0 ml. With the alcohol-treated vaccine half these doses are used. Other vaccines incorporate also paratyphoid C or tetanus toxoid. Avoidance of active exercise and alcohol for 24 hours after the inoculation will reduce the risk of a general reaction.

CHOLERA.—Vaccines made of killed suspensions of *V. choleræ* are used in the prevention of cholera. The usual course consists of two injections at weekly intervals, the first containing 4,000 million and the second 8,000 million organisms. The protection afforded is less than that given by T.A.B., and has not yet been completely assessed.

PLAGUE.—Haffkine vaccine, consisting of two doses of heat-killed *Past. pestis*, provides some protection for a short period—stated to be 2 to 20 months. Severe general reactions may be produced. Recently animals have been successfully immunised with a non-toxic mixture of antigenic fractions, and there are hopes that this method will be applicable to human beings.

YELLOW FEVER.—The prophylactic vaccine consists of an attenuated living yellow fever virus, and only one dose is needed. The immunity is virtually complete, and lasts for at least 6 years.

SMALL-POX.—See §§ 479, 480.

SNAKE BITE.—The adder is the only poisonous snake occurring in Britain and its bite is rarely fatal. The majority of adults and children over 10 will recover with rest and administration of an antihistamine. In severe cases and in young children antivenin should be given—2 ml. through the fang marks and 8 ml. intravenously. As there is a considerable likelihood of a reaction, it is wise to give an antihistamine beforehand. Polyvalent antivenins prepared against the venoms of several snakes or antivenins prepared against single snakes are available in many countries. They should be given as soon as possible.

GAS GANGRENE.—Immunisation against gas gangrene is impracticable and surgical removal of dead tissue and dirt from a wound is the most important prophylactic measure. It is doubtful if anti-gas gangrene serum is of value in the treatment of the established infection, and it is certain that its use entails a considerable risk of acute or delayed reaction. Clostridia are moderately sensitive to penicillin, and this antibiotic should be given in substantial doses (500,000 units 6-hourly) for prophylaxis, e.g., after high thigh amputation, and in large doses in treatment (1 million units 2-hourly).

RABIES (Syn., Hydrophobia).—Anti-rabies treatment should not be given to persons who have only had a minimal exposure to infection, as the chances of neuroparalytic accidents may be greater than the risk of contracting rabies. Patients bitten by a rabid dog or, in appropriate countries, by a wolf, jackal, fox, bat or other wild animal, should be immunised at once. To do this hyperimmune serum is given immediately, and a course of injections begun with Semple type vaccine, consisting of infected brain tissue treated with phenol to kill the virus. When the patient has been licked or bitten by an apparently normal dog, the dog should be observed for 10 days. If during this time rabies develops, the patient should be immunised. If at the end of the period the dog has remained healthy immunisation is not required.

§ 526. Notification and Isolation.—Two duties are laid upon the medical practitioner in cases of the commoner infectious diseases: (1) NOTIFICATION of the case to the medical officer of health of the district in which the case arises. The notifiable complaints in most districts are Anthrax: Cholera: Diphtheria (including Membranous croup): Dysentery, amœbic or bacillary: Acute encephalitis, infective or post-infectious: Enteric fevers (typhoid and paratyphoid): Erysipelas: Farcy: Food poisoning (Foods and Drugs Act, 1938): Malaria: Measles: Meningococcal infection: Ophthalmia neonatorum: Plague: Pneumonia, acute primary and acute influenzal: Acute poliomyelitis, paralytic or non-paralytic: Puerperal pyrexia: Relapsing fever: Scarlet fever: Small-pox: Tuberculosis (all forms): Typhus fever: Whooping-cough. Any infectious disease may at any time be added to the list at the option of the Sanitary Authority. A medical practitioner is bound, under a penalty of forty shillings, to notify any of the diseases named " immediately on becoming aware " of its existence. (2) IMMEDIATE REMOVAL of the patient to an infectious diseases hospital is compulsory for the more dangerous infectious diseases; otherwise the parents or guardians must make proper and adequate arrangements for the isolation of the case at home. In some places the removal is superintended by the medical officer of health.

For ISOLATION at HOME, carpets, curtains and superfluous furniture should have been previously removed. Books and articles in use must be such as can be afterwards burned. The nurse in charge of an infectious case should wear a washable dress when on duty, and should hold no communication with others, nor should she go out of doors without having first changed her wearing apparel, and, if possible, taken a bath. An airy, quiet room at the top of the house, having cubic space of about 12 × 12 × 10 feet, is desirable. The air in this space required to be changed three or four times in every hour. The bedstead should be so placed as to be accessible on both sides. The temperature, read on a thermometer suspended near the bed, and away from draughts, should be 60° F.

VENTILATION must be ample in fever cases, because of the danger of mixed infections. Many of these cases are due to droplet infection from one patient to another, and that is why mixed infections are more apt to arise when there is not free ventilation and sufficient cubic space. This partly explains the higher death-rate from infectious diseases when overcrowding occurred in former days. The direction of the wind should be constantly noted, and to avoid draught, the windows or ventilators opened on the side of the room away from the wind. A " sash-board " is an excellent contrivance for avoiding draught. It should be about 6 to 8 inches broad, and fit across the bottom of the window, so that the lower sash can be raised without a visible opening, and then ventilation takes place behind the sash-board, and also in the middle of the window, the air in both cases being directed upwards. The chief principle in ventilation is that the current of air always takes place from a colder to a hotter medium—usually, therefore, from outside to the inside of a room. The chimney, when the fire is alight, is the only reliable exit. Make the window your inlet in preference to the door.

§ 527. Disinfection and Prevention.—Before discussing the means employed for disinfection, it is necessary to consider how infection is conveyed. There are three principal ways: through the *air*, by *water* or other ingesta, and by *direct contact* or inoculation.

(a) As regards the *air-borne* group, their infectivity varies, also the distance to which the infection in an active state may be carried. For instance, erysipelas and typhus probably do not spread beyond a few feet, but small-pox and chicken-pox may spread a considerable distance. A frequent mode of spread of bacteria and viruses from the mouth and throat of an infected person is by *droplet infection*. Minute drops of saliva or nasal discharge, with adhering organisms, are dispersed for some distance into the surrounding air during talking, coughing or sneezing. These organisms usually enter *via* the respiratory tract (nose, throat, tonsils or lungs); occasionally milk or other foods are contaminated and may be the source of the infection. Streptococci, tubercle and other bacilli can remain virulent in dust for several weeks.

(b) Fevers conveyed *by water, milk* or *other ingesta* are typhoid, paratyphoid, cholera, dysentery, undulant fever, and rarely scarlet fever and diphtheria. Two facts form the basis of the propagation and prevention of these diseases:—(1) All matters coming from the patient's bowel and stomach are infective, in typhoid the urine also; (2) to produce the disease the organism must be introduced by the mouth into the alimentary canal. Acute poliomyelitis is now known to be carried in the fæces.

(c) In the third group the infection is introduced into the blood or tissues of the body by means of a *wound* or a *scratch*, or by the *bite of an insect*. Our profession pays a penalty every year to this group of disorders—a pathologist receives a scratch during post-mortem work, or a surgeon pricks his finger during an operation on a septic appendix. Some of these diseases were formerly considered to depend upon climatic influence, e.g., malaria, which is now known to be introduced into the body by the bite of a mosquito. Tetanus enters through a wound or scratch contaminated with soil; plague is conveyed by rat fleas; typhus by lice. Others in this group are the fevers due to tick bites, glanders, anthrax, leptospirosis and hydrophobia.

The procedure for disinfection differs somewhat according to which of the above three groups the fever belongs. There is now an increasing tendency to concentrate chiefly upon current disinfection during the illness. Formerly much stress was laid on fumigation and spraying the patient's room after the illness. With careful current disinfection it is unnecessary to have terminal disinfection after measles, scarlet fever and diphtheria.

Current disinfection, i.e., that carried out during the illness in the sickroom. All unnecessary furniture and furnishings such as curtains and carpets should be removed. Hæmolytic streptococci can be conveyed by books, but as a general rule infection (except with small-pox and typhoid fever) is rarely conveyed by bedding and other inanimate objects. Before being washed, the *bed-linen*, blankets and clothes must be soaked in 1 per cent. solution of " white fluid " or in Cyllin 1 in 160 (1 fl. oz. to the gallon). Food and drinking *utensils* should be boiled for 5 minutes; they must also be protected from flies. *Thermometers* are kept in 5 per cent. phenol. The nurse should remove gross contamination from her hands by washing and should then immerse the hands in stabilised hypochlorite solution (1 per cent.) or in cetrimide solution (1 per cent.). *Sputum* and nasal discharge should be collected in gauze or paper handkerchiefs and burned. Allow no *dust* to accumulate.

With fevers conveyed by water and other ingesta, in addition to the above precautions, it is essential that the excreta are covered and mixed with an equal quantity of a general disinfectant (black or white fluid) and allowed to stand for 2 hours before being emptied down the drain pipe or buried in earth. *Prophylaxis.*—All drinking water should be boiled if there is the slightest suspicion of its being contaminated by leakage, soakage (however small) from cesspools, drains, or the reckless casting of slops, and by flies. Food utensils must be disinfected carefully by boiling, and flies must be prevented from access to food and to excreta. All handlers of food or every individual where large groups of men are crowded together, as in armies, should be examined and treated if found to be " carriers," *i.e.*, apparently healthy persons in whose excreta the cysts of the amœba of dysentery or typhoid, paratyphoid or cholera bacilli abound.

List of *common disinfectants* for use in the sick room: Extreme heat (200° F or more, and preferably moist); fumes of burning sulphur (SO_2); chlorinated lime, 1 to 5 per cent.; phenol, 5 per cent.; dettol; formalin, 2 to 10 per cent.; lysol, 1 per cent. (or liq. cres. sap. fort., 1½ oz. to 1 gallon water); corrosive sublimate, gr. 10 to 1 gallon (as well as those mentioned above).

Terminal Disinfection.—Burn as many articles of clothing as possible; boil others. Mattresses and blankets, books and all clothing which cannot be boiled, should be sent to be disinfected by steam. Boots and shoes can be washed over with lysol. Furniture should be moved from walls, and drawers, cupboards, etc., disinfected with a liquid spray. Wallpapers in some cases are stripped and the walls treated with hot lime. Doors and windows are closed, crevices are stopped, and the whole room is kept closed for 6 hours after being thoroughly sprayed with formalin by means of a hand-worked pump. Formalin 8 oz., glycerin 8 oz., water 1 gallon, is the disinfectant most often employed. Then the windows are opened and all is washed down with hot water and soap, and the room is well aired.

Disinfection and the PREVENTION OF DISEASES caused by scratches, bites, etc., differ in each individual case. Thus septicæmia and tetanus almost ceased in surgical cases with the introduction of cleanliness and asepsis. Various tropical fevers are conveyed to man by the bites of mosquitoes, flies, fleas and bugs. The prophylaxis of these conditions includes measures directed to the extermination of the insect responsible and avoidance of places in which they are known to be present. Insecticides and repellents such as DDT and dimethylphthalate play a large part in preventing disease. Where plague is endemic rats must be destroyed and DDT powder (10 per cent.) put in their runs; where bugs infected with disease are found it may be necessary to burn the huts, etc., in which eggs are likely to have been deposited. With many of these insect pests knowledge of their life-history is the necessary preliminary to effective steps for their destruction.

§ 528. The **Treatment of pyrexia and hyperpyrexia** comprises six indications:

(1) *Heat production can be diminished and heat loss increased* to some extent by means of *drugs*, known as antipyretics, such as aspirin and phenacetin. Quinine in full doses (say 5 grains every 3 or 4 hours) may be given until the temperature comes down or toxic symptoms are produced (ringing in the ears, deafness, headache, etc.). Salicylates, especially in rheumatic affections, and aconite are also useful. Among the mild diaphoretics are liquor ammoniæ acetatis, potassium nitrate, spiritus ætheris nitrosi, and camphor: also lemon drinks, dilute acids and salines.

The Graduated Bath.—Place the patient in a bath one-third full of water at 90° or 95° F. Every 5 minutes reduce the temperature 5° until 60° F is reached. If the fever be not then reduced to 100° F or lower, continue for further quarter of an hour. The pulse must be closely watched and stimulants given if necessary.

The Wet Pack.—Take off the night-shirt and superfluous bedclothes and place the patient on a blanket. Moderately wring a sheet out of ice-cold water and lay it along his side. Gently roll him over on to it, and completely envelop him in it, head and all, except the face, so that it is next to his skin, without creases or air, between the legs and beneath the arms. Cover these latter with wet towels. Then put two cradles over the patient, and blankets over all. Leave him thus packed for 20 to 40 minutes, until his temperature, taken in the mouth, is reduced to the required extent.

Tepid Sponging.—Lay the patient in a blanket and sponge him gradually all over with tepid water (about 75°). Do half the body at a time, the other half being covered up. Continue the process for 20 to 40 minutes, until the fever is reduced.

(2) *The application of ice* in large ice-bags for the head, chest and abdomen has been used when other means are not available, but the weight of the bags and their localised application are objections to their use.

(3) *Diminish the work done by the internal organs* by diet (§ 296. XVIII), and by promoting the action of the skin and bowels, in order to relieve the kidneys.

(4) In all fevers it is necessary *to watch the heart* and blood pressure carefully, and, if necessary, administer suitable stimulants, such as nikethamide B.P. (Coramine) or metaraminol.   The pulse should be recorded several times a day in all fever cases.

(5) *Symptomatic treatment* has been dealt with in the preceding pages.

(6) *Watch for and treat complications* as they arise.   The chief of these are (i.) cardiovascular (*vide supra*), and (ii.) delirium and insomnia.   If the delirium be of the *raving* kind, chloral and bromides should be given in full doses; if of the *muttering* or typhoid variety, stimulants.   Insomnia may be relieved by the same treatment. (iii.) Pulmonary complications, (iv.) suppression or retention of urine, and (v.) collapse, are all dealt with elsewhere (and see § 510).

CHAPTER XVI

GENERAL DEBILITY, PALLOR, EMACIATION

A FEELING of general weakness and lassitude is a symptom common to many diseases, but we are now concerned with those in which this is the only obvious, or at least the most prominent, symptom for which the patient seeks relief. Diseases in which debility is the chief symptom may be classified clinically into two great groups according to whether they come on acutely and are attended by pyrexia, or not. Debility coming on acutely and attended by pyrexia was fully dealt with in the preceding chapter. There still remains a large group of diseases in which the weakness is of gradual onset, runs a chronic and indefinite course, and is unattended for the most part by any notable elevation of temperature; and these diseases may be attended by pallor or by emaciation. Here we shall often meet with the beginnings of disease, beginnings which may, however, lead to a serious and fatal issue. It is, therefore, of the highest importance that an exact diagnosis should be made and treatment adopted as early as possible.

Many of the debilitating conditions mentioned in this chapter may be unattended by any other symptom, or only by the pallor of anæmia or the wasting of malnutrition, and many give rise to no characteristic anatomical changes: even their pathology may be obscure.

PART A. SYMPTOMATOLOGY

§ 535. General Debility.—Malaise, lassitude, inability to complete a day's work, are some of the terms used to describe the symptom under consideration, which is essentially chronic in its course. The weakness is generalised, and it may affect the mind as well as the body, for there is not only a disinclination to take muscular exercise, but an inability to concentrate the attention or accomplish mental work. The weakness may vary in kind and degree from very slight malaise to a total incapacity to move. Many diseases in this category are apt to be overlooked in their earlier and more curable phases. The patient may attribute his ailment to " slight indigestion," or think he has " been working too hard," or " wants a change," and perhaps he calls on his doctor " as he was passing " just to confirm his own diagnosis and " give him a tonic." These cases may tax the young practitioner's skill and tact in several ways. Fresh from studying instances of marked diseases in hospitals, he may regard these cases as trivial and " uninteresting "; and even if he detects the beginning of some insidious condition the patient may meet

782

his suggestion of serious ailment not only with surprise, but even with resentment and distrust. Some tact, therefore, is required, and the practitioner may find it wise to confide in some discreet relative or friend.

Fallacies.—The distinction of general debility from *paralysis* is not usually difficult, though patients with polyneuritis, early paraplegia, general paralysis of the insane, bulbar paralysis, and various other forms of paresis, often complain simply of weakness. Patients who are overworked, sleepless or suffering from a *chronic anxiety state* or *neurasthenia* often complain of " feeling below par," of physical or mental exhaustion and may lose weight. Cases of *malingering* offer far more difficulty in diagnosis, for we are almost entirely dependent upon the patient's own statements. The question of motive should be considered and an exhaustive examination made by the most up-to-date methods, but even then we may in justice be compelled for awhile to give the patient the benefit of the doubt. In many cases it is only by keeping the patient under daily observation, and with the aid of intelligent, experienced and well-trained nurses, that a correct conclusion can be gained. The *Causes* of debility are discussed in §§ 545 and 573.

Pallor of the Skin—*i.e.*, deficiency of its normal colour—is a frequent accompaniment of cases in which debility is complained of by the patient. The causes are discussed in §§ 545 *et seq.*

Fallacies.—Slight *jaundice* may resemble some forms of pallor. In *town-dwellers and those who habitually remain indoors* pallor of the face is common. In certain " delicate " families a pale face is more or less normal. Europeans who have lived long in the *tropics* are usually pale and " anæmic " looking, but the blood may not confirm anæmia. On the other hand, patients with dyspepsia may have a flushed face even in the presence of anæmia. *Nervous* conditions may cause transient constriction of the vessels and pallor which may be mistaken for anæmia. Many patients who " go white " with nervous emotion are mistakenly supposed to be anæmic; in anæmia the pallor has a waxy or yellow tinge, which is absent in pallor of vaso-motor origin. With a glance at the colour of the lips, conjunctivæ and mucous membranes one can usually distinguish the conditions.

Emaciation, or loss of flesh, may also be associated with general debility, and its presence adds considerably to the gravity of a case, for it may indicate either serious organic disease such as cancer or tubercle, or definite defect in the alimentation or metabolism of the body, such as is produced by a digestive derangement or chronic nephritis. It is manifested to the patient by his clothes becoming looser, or his face becoming thinner, and to the physician by pinching up a fold of skin between the finger and thumb. But the only reliable test is a definite loss of weight, and it is advisable at the outset to record the weight of all patients who come to us complaining of debility. When possible *note the exact weight*; the patient should be weighed in a dressing gown, of which the weight is known. A reliable weighing machine should be in every consulting room. The causes of emaciation are discussed in §§ 569 *et seq.*

Fallacies.—A normal loss of adipose tissue may occur about the climacteric, but the reverse is quite as usual. Amyotrophy, unless generalised, is not to be confused with emaciation; it is usually localised. The diet a person has been taking will, within certain limits, influence his weight considerably, and one who has been taking only nitrogenous food may be many pounds under his normal weight.

PART B. PHYSICAL EXAMINATION

§ 536. The physical examination of cases of general debility, pallor or emaciation, comprise (1) EXAMINATION OF THE VISCERA; (2) OBSERVATIONS ON THE WEIGHT, and in some cases on the TEMPERATURE; and (3) AN EXAMINATION OF THE BLOOD.

1. An examination of the VISCERA AND EXCRETA should be systematically conducted (see Scheme, pp. 6 and 7), because we may be dealing with some incipient disease, the signs of which are obscure. Inquiries should be especially directed to the food intake and the state of the digestive organs.

2. The WEIGHT of the patient should be noted, and, if possible, compared with previous records. It is a wise precaution to take the patient's TEMPERATURE, and to obtain a series of records (§ 471).

3. An examination of the BLOOD is necessary. This consists of (1) estimation of hæmoglobin; (2) blood counts of the red and white corpuscles; (3) examination of blood films. In most cases these three will be sufficient for a routine examination; but in other cases it is necessary to make (4) an examination for parasites and other abnormal constituents; (5) certain physical and chemical properties of the blood, and (6) biopsy of bone marrow.

EXAMINATION OF THE BLOOD

§ 537. **Apparatus and Methods.**—APPARATUS REQUIRED.—A hæmoglobinometer of Haldane's or Sahli's type or a colorimeter incorporating a photo-electric cell; a counting chamber (hæmocytometer) of the Neubauer or Thoma type; a sharp Hagedorn needle or other sterile lancet; Hayem's solution; Toison's fluid; Leishman's, Wright's or Giemsa's stain; distilled water. For *counting cells* in the hæmocytometer chamber certain diluting fluids are necessary. For red cells normal saline or Hayem's solution (sod. chloride 1 G., sod. sulphate 5 G., mercury perchloride 0·5 G., distilled water to 200 ml.) are used as diluting fluids. For white cells use either a 0·3 per cent. solution of acetic acid containing a few drops of methylene blue: or Toison's fluid (methyl violet 0·025 G., neutral glycerin 30 ml., distilled water 80 ml. to which is added a solution of sodium chloride 1 G. and sodium sulphate 8 G. in 80 ml. of distilled water; the solution is filtered before use). Blood pipettes are best cleaned as soon as possible after their use first with water, then with alcohol and then ether until they are dry.

METHOD OF OBTAINING BLOOD.—Reliable results are only obtained if standard conditions are observed as much as possible, in order to avoid physiological variations in the blood after meals, after exercise or with the time of day. In most cases 10 a.m. and 2 p.m. are the most suitable times for blood collection. The lobe of the ear is less painful and out of sight of the patient and therefore is preferable to the finger, but if the finger must be used the puncture should be made at the side and not on the ball.

After gentle cleaning, a sufficiently deep puncture is made with the needle (which is best mounted on a cork acting also as a stopper for the bottle of alcohol), to obtain blood without squeezing. As an alternative 5 ml. of blood from a venepuncture may be put into a tube containing 4 mg. solid potassium oxalate and 6 mg. ammonium

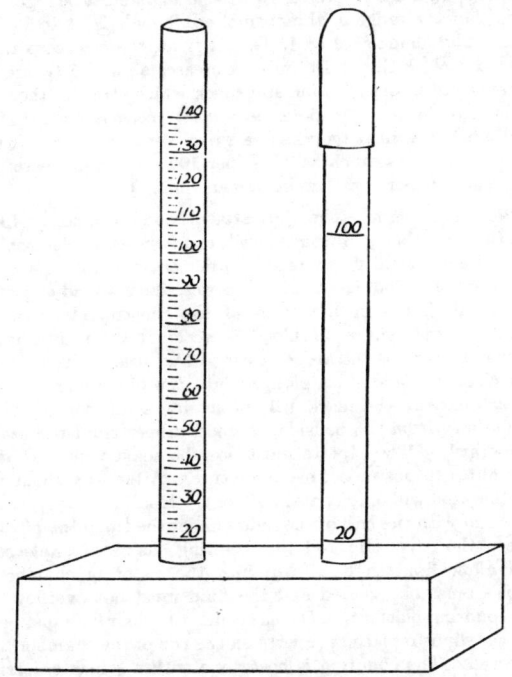

FIG. 158.—HALDANE HÆMOGLOBINOMETER. The right-hand tube is the standard (100% = 14·8 G. hæmoglobin per 100 ml.)

oxalate, or into a bottle containing sequestrin and gently shaken. This will provide an isotonic solution suitable for many blood tests.

§ 538. The Hæmoglobin Estimation is the most useful and most frequent blood test. With *Haldane's method*, 20 c.mm. of blood are sucked up in a straight capillary pipette and quickly blown into a small quantity of distilled water in the comparator tube. A stream of coal gas is gently played on the surface through a glass pipette for a minute or so and then the mixture is gradually diluted with distilled water until the depth of pink matches the standard tube. The percentage figure is read off the upper level of the fluid. The comparison should be made in daylight. When coal gas is not available *Sahli's method* can be used which involves the use of N/10 hydrochloric acid as a diluent. With this method it is necessary to wait about 10 minutes for the solution to turn brown so that it matches the standard. *Tallquist's scales* may be used as a rough screening method. A drop of blood is allowed to dry on a special piece of blotting paper and as soon as dry the depth of colour is compared with a printed chart. This must be done in full daylight. *Colorimeter methods* involving the use of photoelectric cells are probably more reliable than the methods described, but can only be used in the laboratory.

The amount of hæmoglobin is often expressed in terms of per cent. of the normal. Owing to the confusion caused by different standards (in Sahli's method 100 per cent. corresponds to 17·4 G. per 100 ml. and in Haldane's method to 14·8 G. per 100 ml.)

the most useful way is to express the amount of hæmoglobin in G. per 100 ml. of blood. The normal average for both sexes has now been accepted as 14·8 G. of hæmoglobin per 100 ml. of blood and this has been provisionally agreed to as 100 per cent. (see Table XXXVII).

The Significance of Increase or Decrease of Hæmoglobin must be regarded in the light of the knowledge that the range of the normal adult male is 14 to 17 G. per 100 ml. and of the normal adult female 12 to 15 G. It is for these reasons that the normal average is regarded as 14·8 G. per 100 ml. Increases above 17 G. are abnormal. A *temporary increase* occurs in dehydration and shock which is due to the reduced volume of plasma in the circulation. A more *permanent increase* occurs after prolonged residence at high altitudes, in polycythæmia rubra vera and in erythrocytosis where the level may be raised to as much as 21 G. per 100 ml. A decrease of hæmoglobin below 12 G. (approx. 80 per cent.) indicates anæmia.

§ 539. **Red Blood Cell Count.**—The apparatus needed is a mixing pipette, Hayem's fluid and a counting chamber. Automatic cell counters using electronic devices may in the future become sufficiently accurate in order to supersede the more traditional methods. The drop of blood is obtained as described already (§ 537). Blood is sucked up to the mark 0·5 in the stem of the pipette. It is necessary to be very accurate in this manœuvre; if blood is accidentally sucked into the mixing chamber, the pipette must be discarded, cleaned and dried. The tip of the pipette is wiped with a clean rag and then plunged into the diluent from which enough is sucked up to reach exactly the mark 101, producing a dilution of 1 in 200. If the laboratory is some way from the bedside, a broad rubber band will seal both ends of the pipette temporarily. The pipette must now be shaken in more than one plane for at least 3 minutes to ensure an even mixture. After this about four drops are discarded, since the stem will only contain diluent. Holding the pipette obliquely and sealing the upper end with the ball of the index finger the tip of the pipette is placed in the space between the cover slip and the counting chamber. Release of the index finger will then allow fluid to be drawn into the counting chamber by capillary traction. Bubbles must be avoided and the fluid must not overflow into the ditch surrounding the counting platform. If this occurs, the chamber must be cleaned again and when the cover slip is replaced properly on the rim of the chamber, Newton's rings should show up well. The counting is best done with a $\frac{2}{3}$ inch objective and a high ($\times$ 15) eyepiece. The ruling on the platform varies in different types of counting chambers, but the Neubauer and Thoma types (Fig. 159) are generally most useful. The small squares have an area of $\frac{1}{400}$ sq. mm. and a depth of $\frac{1}{10}$ mm. (capacity $\frac{1}{4000}$ c.mm.). When corpuscles lie on dividing lines, only those over the upper and the left-hand lines are counted, those on the lower and the right-hand lines are ignored. *Calculation of number of red cells in 1 c.mm. of blood.* If, for example, 80 squares contain 500 cells, since the blood has been diluted 200 times, 1 c.mm. of blood contains

$$\frac{500}{80} \times 4{,}000 \times 200 \text{ cells} = 5{,}000{,}000 \text{ cells.}$$

The *Significance of Increase or Decrease of the Number of Red Cells.*—Since the red cell count is a laborious and difficult laboratory procedure even in skilled hands, it is wise to restrict requesting a red cell count to those cases where a count can be expected to provide useful information or in conjunction with the estimation of the mean corpuscular volume. The average number of red cells per c.mm. of blood in health is about 5 million (Table XXXVII). *Physiological variations.* Fasting, sweating and residence at high altitudes cause increases to about 6 million. In the newborn infant 7 to 8 million red cells per c.mm. is a normal figure during the first week or so. During the later weeks of pregnancy the number of red cells usually decreases to about 4 million. *In Disease* the number of red cells is increased (i.) in chronic pulmonary conditions when the blood in the pulmonary circulation is insufficiently oxygenated; (ii.) in congenital valvular disease and in septal defects of the heart when arterial and venous blood is mixed, the red cells may number up to 10 million per c.mm.; (iii.) with hæmo-concentration following attacks of diarrhœa or water loss for other causes, after vomiting and after severe burns; (iv.) in the crises of Addison's disease; (v.) in poly-cythæmia rubra vera (§ 31). Cyanosis does not in itself cause an increase of red cells. A *decreased number* of red cells occurs after hæmorrhage and in anæmia, whether primary or secondary. The decrease may be very marked in pernicious anæmia, but usually less marked in iron deficiency anæmia.

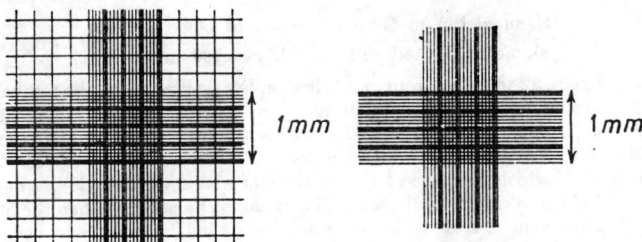

FIG. 159.—Types of ruling for counting chambers.

THE MORPHOLOGICAL CHARACTERISTICS OF RED CELLS are estimated by a number of indices, sometimes referred to as absolute values:

1. The *Colour Index* approximately indicates the amount of hæmoglobin in each red cell. Because for the calculation of the colour index the figure of 5 million red cells per c.mm. is considered to be the normal and because only the percentage figures for hæmoglobin are taken, the colour index is not as useful in hæmatological diagnosis as are other values. It is, however, still widely used, and is calculated as follows:—

$$\frac{\text{Hæmoglobin (expressed as per cent. of normal using Haldane's method)}}{\text{Number of red cells per c.mm., divided by } 5{,}000{,}000}$$

Normally the colour index ranges from 0·85 to 1·10. In anæmia it may be lower or higher than normal or within the normal ranges, again showing that the usefulness of the colour index is restricted. Usually anæmias characterised by large red cells, such as pernicious anæmia, have a high colour index, and anæmias with a deficiency of hæmoglobin which is greater than the deficiency of the cells have a low colour index.

2. The *Mean Corpuscular Diameter* indicates the *size of the red cells*, but only uses two dimensions for a three-dimensional particle. It is estimated accurately by the laborious Price-Jones curve in which 1,000 stained red cells are measured microscopically at a known magnification, remembering that staining causes slight shrinkage of the cells. Less accurately, but more usefully, the mean cell diameter is estimated by a halometer using an unstained film. The normal range is 6·9 to 7·7μ with an average of 7·2μ. In macrocytic anæmias such as pernicious anæmia, cells may measure 8·5 to 9·0μ.

3. The *Mean Corpuscular Volume* is obtained by the relationship between the red cell count and the hæmatocrit. Wintrobe's hæmatocrit tube, a graduated glass tube 11 cm. long and with a 2·5 mm. bore, is filled with oxalated blood to the mark 10 and then centrifuged at a speed of 3,000 revolutions per minute for half an hour. The red cells are thus collected into a compact mass (packed cell volume) and its percentage volume is read from the calibration on the glass tube; normally this is 45 per cent. The mean corpuscular volume is calculated as follows:—

$$\frac{\text{Volume of packed cells in ml. per } 1{,}000 \text{ ml. of blood}}{\text{Red cells in millions per c.mm.}}$$

It is expressed in cubic microns. The normal range is 78 to 94 c.μ. Higher figures than these indicate macrocytosis; lower figures, which are found more rarely, indicate microcytosis. Cases in which macrocytosis is found should be investigated most carefully, because many of them will require treatment with the specific hæmatinics such as cyanocobalamin (vitamin B_{12}).

4. *The Mean Corpuscular Hæmoglobin Concentration* of red cells is the most useful index in order to detect iron-deficiency. Since it relies on relatively simple and therefore relatively accurate methods, *i.e.*, the estimation of hæmoglobin and the packed cell volume, it is also sensitive and accurate. It indicates the amount of hæmoglobin per unit volume of red cells and therefore is an index of saturation. It is calculated as follows:—

$$\frac{\text{Hæmoglobin in G. per 100 ml. of blood}}{\text{Volume of packed cells in ml. per 100 ml.}} \times 100$$

Its normal range is 32 to 38 per cent. and this implies saturation of the red cells with hæmoglobin. When such values are obtained in cases of anæmia, this is termed normochromic. Increases of the M.C.H.C. above 38 per cent. rarely if ever occur, because the red cell cannot be over-saturated. Therefore the older term " hyperchromic anæmia " which is derived from an anæmia with a colour index of more than unity, has strictly speaking no real basis and should not be used. When the M.C.H.C. is less than 32 per cent. a state of hypochromia exists indicating a deficiency of iron.

5. *The Mean Corpuscular Hæmoglobin* indicates the average hæmoglobin content of an average single red cell in micromicrograms ($\gamma\gamma$). It is calculated as follows:

$$\frac{\text{Hæmoglobin in G. per 1,000 ml. of blood}}{\text{Red cells in millions per c.mm.}}$$

Normally it ranges 27 to 32 $\gamma\gamma$. In most cases red cells contain an average amount of hæmoglobin of about 30 $\gamma\gamma$. If higher figures are obtained, it indicates that there is more hæmoglobin per cell and since over-saturation is not possible, it means that the average red cell in such a case must be either larger in size (macrocytic as in pernicious anæmia) or in volume (spherocytic as in hæmolytic anæmia), or both.

6. Normal red cells are circular, bi-concave, non-nucleated discs measuring 6·7 to 7·7μ in diameter ($\frac{1}{3200}$ inch) and 86 c.μ in volume.

TABLE XXXVII—NORMAL HÆMOGLOBIN AND NUMBERS OF RED AND WHITE CELLS

	Average	Range
Hæmoglobin	14·8 G. per 100 ml. (= 100%)	
„ (men)	15·8 „ „ „ „	14–17 G.
„ (women).	13·7 „ „ „ „	12–15 G.
Red Cells	5 million per c.mm.	
„ (men)	5·5 „ „ „	5 – 6 million
„ (women)	4·8 „ „ „	4·2-5·5 million
Colour Index	1·0	0·85-1·1
Mean Cell Diameter	7·2 μ	6·9-7·7 μ
Packed Cell Volume	Adult males 47 per cent.	40-54 per cent.
	adult females 42 „ „	37–47 „ „
Mean Cell Volume	86 c.μ	78–94 c.μ
Mean Corpuscular Hæmoglobin Concentration	34 per cent.	32-38 per cent.
Mean Corpuscular Hæmoglobin	30 $\gamma\gamma$	27-32 $\gamma\gamma$
Reticulocytes	1 per 100 red cells	

White Cells (Leucocytes) normal range: 3,000–12,000 per c.mm.

	Absolute Numbers per c.mm.	Percentage
Neutrophil polymorphs	1,600–7,500	33–75
Eosinophils	400	up to 6
Basophils	200	up to 2
Lymphocytes	1,000–4,500	15–60
Monocytes	800	up to 10

§ 540. **White Blood Cell (Leucocyte) Count.**—The technique of white cell counts is very similar to that of the red cell count. In the stem of the special pipette, blood from a prick in the lobe of the ear is taken up to the mark 0·5.   The pipette is then filled to the mark 11 with Thoma's or Toison's fluid.   The pipette is shaken for 2 to 3 minutes.   The contents of the stem are discharged and a small drop from the pipette is introduced into the counting chamber.

In the Neubauer hæmocytometer counting chamber the contents of the two large squares (that is 2 sq. mm.) are counted.   Since the depth of the chamber is $\frac{1}{10}$ mm. the cubic capacity of the two chambers is 0·2 c.mm.: with the dilution 1 in 20, it is only necessary to add 00 to the figure obtained.   Normally leucocytes number 3,000 to 12,000 per c.mm. (see Table XXXVII).

§ 541. **Microscopical Examination of the Blood.**   Fresh blood may be examined by placing a small drop of blood on a slide, covering it with a cover slip and ringing it with Vaseline or paraffin in order to avoid evaporation.   Abnormalities of red cells and abnormal structures such as pigment or microfilariæ may be readily observed by this method.   Rouleaux formation of red cells is easily seen, excess of white cells can be noted.   Freshly made unstained blood smears may reveal alteration in the shape or size of blood cells.   Such examinations must be made with a partially closed substage iris diaphragm or with a phase contrast microscope.   It is necessary to use a high dry objective ($\frac{1}{4}$ in.) and a ×7 or ×10 eyepiece.   Detailed and repeated examination of stained preparations can only be made with a $\frac{1}{12}$-inch oil-immersion lens.

A blood *smear* or *film* is made on a cover slip or, a little easier, on a slide.   Clean slides, free of grease, are kept in absolute alcohol.   They only require wiping before use.   A slide from which a corner has been broken off is used as a spreader.   This has the result that the smear is narrower than the slide on which it is made, a useful fact, because the blunt-nosed objective cannot satisfactorily travel to the edge of the slide. With the spreader a small drop of blood is picked up without touching the skin and transferred to the slide.   The drop is allowed to spread along the edge of the spreader which is held at 45° and the blood is pulled along in the acute angle between spreader and slide.   Increasing the angle between spreader and slide and pulling the spreader along more rapidly will produce thicker films.   The finger should not touch the film once it is made and the slide should be waved rapidly to dry it.   The more rapid the drying, the better the preparation.   If it is necessary to keep the film for several days before staining, dip it in absolute alcohol and allow it to drain.

Staining is one of the few arts left in the modern laboratory, but standardised methods make good films possible even under adverse conditions.   Most nuclei take up basic dyes such as hæmatoxylin or methylene blue; the cytoplasm of red cells takes up acid dyes only.   A composite stain such as Leishman's or Wright's is therefore used to allow for the various affinities of parts of the cells to be displayed tinctorially.   *Method.*—The dry film placed on the staining rack is flooded with Leishman's stain and left covered for $\frac{1}{2}$ to 1 minute.   An equal part of buffered distilled water is added and the mixture is left 8 to 10 minutes.   The slide is then washed with ordinary tap water and its under surface is wiped clean.   It is left to drain the excess water for a few minutes; drying by blotting tends to spoil films.

Variations of the Morphology of the Red Cells in Disease take several forms: (1) poikilocytosis; (2) anisocytosis; (3) polychromasia; (4) central pallor; (5) punctate basophilia; (6) reticulocytes; (7) nucleated red cells.

(1) *Poikilocytosis* is variation in shape of the red cells.   They may resemble flasks or pears.   Poikilocytosis is seen in almost all cases of severe anæmia, but most marked in pernicious anæmia in relapse.

(2) *Anisocytosis* is variation in the size of red cells.   Its most marked degrees are seen in pernicious anæmia, but during the phase of regeneration after blood loss it is also often present.   When large cells predominate, macrocytic or megalocytic anæmia is present, but these terms merely indicate that cells are large.   In microcytic anæmia anisocytosis is not usually a striking feature.

(3) *Polychromasia* (polychromatophilia) is variation in colour of red cells when stained with polychrome stains.   Normally red cells stain an even bright pink with Leishman's stain, but in the centre the staining is lighter due to the smaller amount

of cytoplasm there. In many cases of severe anæmia, particularly during phases of regeneration, many red cells stain with a bluish hue, and sometimes bluish hues and pinkish areas are seen within one cell. The bluish colour is due to the retention in the cell of the remnants of reticular material and polychromatic cells are therefore younger red cells.

(4) *Central pallor.* Normally the central area of the red cell can just be appreciated. In iron-deficiency this is increased and often referred to as central pallor. It rarely appears in other anæmias.

(5) *Punctate basophilia* or basophilic " stippling " refers to the presence of blue dots in the pink cytoplasm of the red cells. They consist of reticular matter and in most cases the number of polychromatic cells and of stippled cells is roughly equivalent to the number of reticulocytes. Punctate basophilia is particularly marked in anæmia due to lead poisoning, but also occurs in other types of severe anæmia. Howell-Jolly bodies occur in many red cells in severe anæmia and after splenectomy; they are present as one or two larger bluish or purple bodies.

(6) *Reticulocytes* are young red blood corpuscles, showing a network of reticular matter when stained supravitally. Their number indicates approximately the rate of the production of new red cells. In ordinary films stained with Leishman's method, cells which would be reticulocytes appear as polychromatic or stippled cells. Normally reticulocytes number 0·1 to 1·0 per 100 red cells. *Supra-vital staining of reticulocytes.*— A drop of 0·1 per cent. alcoholic solution of brilliant cresyl blue is placed on a slide and allowed to evaporate. With the spreader a small drop of blood is placed on the area marked by the dried-up cresyl blue. The spreader is held at 45° and supported at such an angle so as to form a moist chamber to allow reticulocytes to take up the stain. After a minute the spreader is used in the usual way, a film is spread and allowed to dry. The film is counterstained with Leishman's stain. Reticulocytes show a network or granules of bluish material in their cytoplasm.

(7) *Nucleated Red Cells* (erythroblastosis) must be regarded as a danger signal. They must be carefully distinguished from lymphocytes, which they resemble in size and shape, but not as regards their nuclei. There are two distinct lines of development of the red cells, the normoblastic and the megaloblastic. They are both derived from the *proerythroblast*, the earliest cell that can be identified as erythroid. It is a large cell with deep blue cytoplasm and a regular chromatin nuclear network (Plate XVI). Normally a series of normoblasts are derived from the proerythroblast: (1) the *early basophilic normoblast* has a deeply basophilic cytoplasm and a nucleus similar to the proerythroblast, but no nucleoli; (2) the *intermediate normoblast* has a polychromatic cytoplasm and a condensed nucleus; (3) the *late normoblast* has a hæmoglobinised acidophilic (orthochromatic) pink-staining cytoplasm and a dense small nucleus. This cell may easily be confused with a lymphocyte. In fœtal life and in pernicious anæmia the proerythroblast produces *megaloblasts*, although a number of cells develop normally on normoblastic lines. Megaloblasts are generally larger than normoblasts and their nuclei have a fine lace-work type of pattern of their chromatin structure. Megaloblasts show hæmoglobinisation earlier than normoblasts, and sometimes this occurs in small patches. Megaloblasts are rarely seen in the peripheral blood, even in pernicious anæmia, but this diagnosis may be made from the appearance of megalocytes (macrocytes) and certain changes in leucocytes and platelets.

Variations of the Leucocytes occur in their absolute numbers (Table XXXVII) and their structural characteristics. It must be remembered that the relative numbers of cells obtained by the differential count are only of value in order to obtain the absolute numbers. It is necessary to stain a blood film in order to perform a differential count. There are several kinds of leucocytes and the predominating variety may give valuable clues to the diagnosis. Apart from the standard method of staining a blood film, two other important methods of investigating the white cells are:—(1) The *Oxidase Reaction* helps to distinguish the earlier cells of the myeloid series from those of the lymphatic series. The granules of the myeloid cells contain oxidases, but the earliest myeloid cells do not have granules in their cytoplasm and therefore are

PLATE XVI

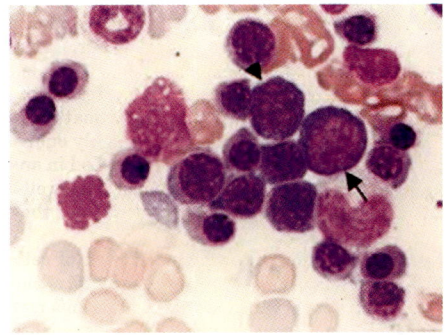

(a) Precursors of normal red cells in the bone marrow

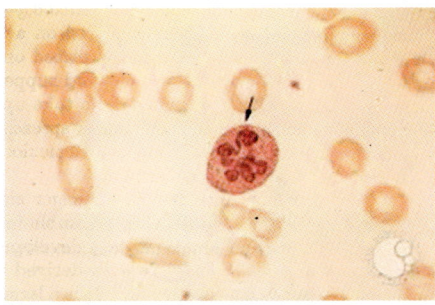

(b) Pernicious anaemia

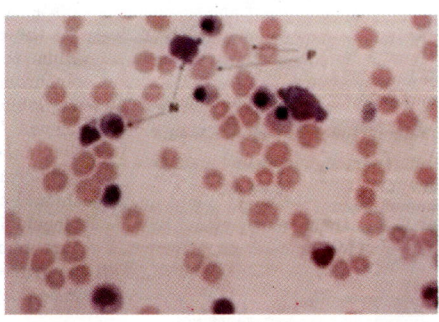

(c) Haemolytic diseases of the newborn

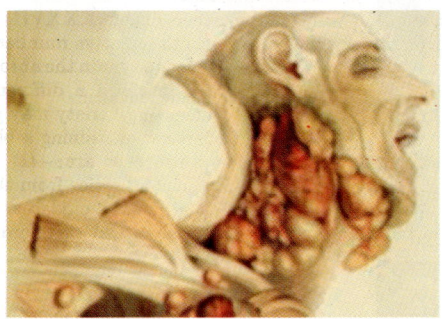

(d) Hodgkin's disease

PLATE XVII

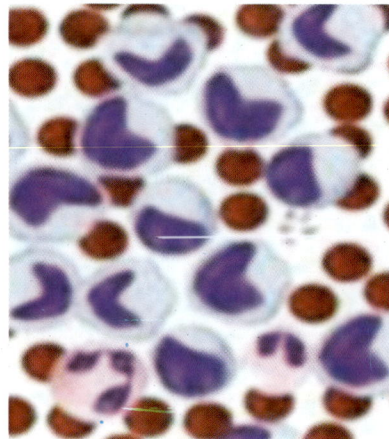

(a) Acute myeloid leukaemia

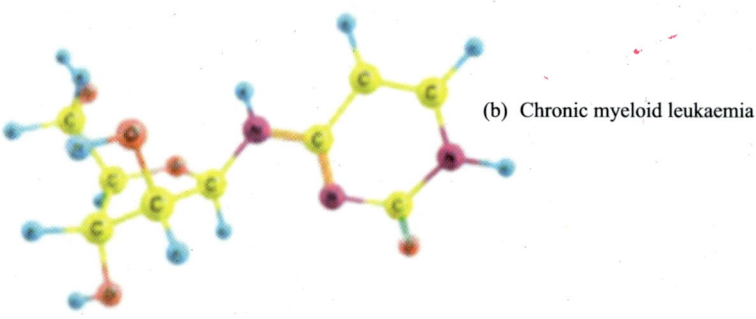

(b) Chronic myeloid leukaemia

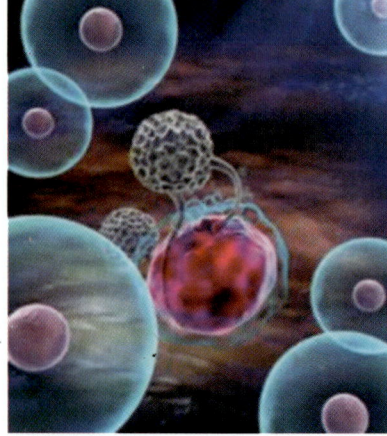

(c) Chronic lymphatic leukaemia

oxidase-negative, just as are the cells of the lymphatic series. In Washburn's method a solution of benzidine in ethyl alcohol containing also sodium nitroprusside is dropped on the slide and after two minutes a weak solution of hydrogen peroxide is added. After 5 minutes the slide is washed, dried and counterstained with Leishman's stain. The oxidase-positive granules show up golden brown. (2) *Supravital preparations* with Janus green and neutral red are used to observe the active movements of the cells and their mitochondria. The myeloid cells show more active movements than lymphocytes and monocytes.

The *normal ranges of leucocytes* are given in Table XXXVII. The types of cells are as follows:—

(1) *Neutrophil polymorphonuclear cells* comprise 33 to 75 per cent. of all white cells in the blood. They are about twice the size of red cells (*i.e.*, 15μ in diameter) and have in their faintly grey cytoplasm fine slightly red-staining small granules which are termed neutrophil, but are in reality slightly acidophilic. Their nuclei are elongated and usually lobed, similar to a string of sausages. In the female the neutrophils have a drumstick-like appendage of the nucleus, present in about 1 in 5 cells, but absent in cells from males. The number of lobes varies from 2 to 5 and generally the younger cells have 2 lobes. In some conditions cells with more than 3 or 4 lobes predominate; for example in pernicious anæmia cells with 6 or 8 lobes are common. A numerical assay of the distribution of the lobes sometimes helps diagnosis, and such Arneth counts may distinguish degenerative and regenerative conditions. In the Pelger-Huët nuclear familial anomaly no cells have more than 2 lobes. Where there is a severely toxic state the neutrophils show " toxic " granulation, which is a much heavier and often darker type of granulation than normal.

The neutrophil is derived from the bone marrow cells, is actively phagocytic and amœboid. Its immediate precursor is the myelocyte which has a similar cytoplasm, but a single oval nucleus. This is descended from the myeloblast with a basophilic non-granular cytoplasm and a dense nucleus which contains nucleoli.

(2) *Eosinophil cells* contain coarse bright red staining granules in their cytoplasm and otherwise have the same characteristics as neutrophils, but rarely have more than 3 lobes to their nuclei. They are not phagocytic but are amœboid and are also derived from the bone marrow.

(3) *Basophils* or *mast cells* have coarse, dark-blue staining granules in the cytoplasm and usually only 1 or 2 lobes to their nuclei. Like the eosinophils they are derived from the bone marrow through the stages of the myelocytes.

(4) *Lymphocytes* comprise about 15 to 60 per cent. of the total number of white cells. They have a single solid nucleus with dense chromatin. Their cytoplasm is usually light blue and clear, but occasionally contains a few azure granules which are small, irregular and stain red. The large lymphocyte has much cytoplasm and the small lymphocyte has only a rim of cytoplasm. Lymphocytes are derived from the spleen, lymph glands and other centres of lymphoid tissue, their precursor being the lymphoblast. They are not phagocytic and are only sluggishly amœboid.

(5) *Monocytes* are sometimes called " large hyaline " or " transitional " leucocytes. They have a large, usually somewhat irregular nucleus with a fine chromatin structure and a light blue, slightly cloudy cytoplasm which occasionally contains small vacuoles and a few fine red granules. They are sluggishly amœboid. Some monocytes are derived from the bone marrow, but their precise origin and their function is not known.

(6) *Plasma cells* are occasionally seen in peripheral blood films. They have an oval shape and dark-blue cytoplasm. Their nucleus is situated eccentrically in the cytoplasm and its chromatin network gives it a cart-wheel appearance.

Leucocytosis and Leucopenia.—Increases in the white cells above 12,000 per c.mm. and figures below 3,000 per c.mm. are usually abnormal.

(1) PHYSIOLOGICAL LEUCOCYTOSIS is an increase of the number of neutrophils due to natural causes. In the newborn infant white cells usually number 15,000 to 20,000 per c.mm. and most of them are neutrophils. The number slowly decreases until at the age of 7 years the normal figures are stabilised. In the later stages of pregnancy

and during the earlier parts of the puerperium, even without sepsis, there is usually a moderate leucocytosis. After meals, after exercise and after a cold bath there is usually a transient rise of leucocytes.

(2) PATHOLOGICAL LEUCOCYTOSIS.—(a) *Neutrophil polymorph leucocytosis* occurs in septic states. It is found in (i.) Acute infections, such as septicæmia, pneumonia, acute appendicitis, peritonitis, meningitis, scarlet fever, acute poliomyelitis and diphtheria. (ii.) It is less marked in chronic infections such as syphilis and tuberculosis, except where an abscess has formed or where there is much necrosis of tissue. When pus is under pressure, the number of leucocytes rises to very high figures, even to 50,000 per c.mm. as in empyema, appendix abscess, subphrenic abscess. In acute abscesses the pus consists largely of pus cells which are degenerate neutrophil polymorph cells. A very high leucocyte count indicates an unfavourable prognosis, as also does failure to develop leucocytosis in infection and leucopenia. In pneumonia after the crisis and after satisfactory drainage of an abscess the leucocytosis soon disappears. Leucocytosis also develops (iii.) after hæmorrhage, acute hæmolysis, in extensive bruising and after blood transfusions, (iv.) after operations, particularly if they involve much laceration, (v.) in acute poisoning and acute gout, (vi.) in advanced malignant disease when there is much tissue breakdown of the tumour or when there is widespread metastasis in the bone marrow or liver. (vii.) Leucocytosis is marked in certain blood dyscrasias, such as polycythæmia and myeloid leukæmia and in the terminal stages of certain types of reticulosis such as Hodgkin's disease. Artificially produced leucocytosis following the injection of blood, milk or nucleic acid preparations in an effort to overcome leucopenia or aplastic marrow conditions is usually a therapeutic failure.

With infections younger cells with fewer lobes to their nuclei predominate and become very numerous. Metamyelocytes and myelocytes appear—these have only a single round or oval nucleus. When this occurs, it is called " shift to the left " in the nuclear index of the Arneth or Schilling counts. A moderate shift to the left occurs in infection, a marked shift involving many myelocytes (of about 30 to 50 per cent. of all leucocytes present) suggests chronic myeloid leukæmia and extreme shift to the left involving myeloblasts suggests acute myeloid leukæmia or an acute relapse in a chronic case.

(b) *Lymphocytosis*, an increase in the number of lymphocytes, occurs (i.) in the more chronic infections, such as tuberculosis and secondary syphilis, but not when tissue breakdown is marked such as in tuberculous cavities, nor in widespread miliary tuberculosis or in tuberculous meningitis; (ii.) in pertussis and in glandular fever and other virus infections; (iii.) during the recovery from infectious or toxic states; (iv.) in lymphatic leukæmia and (v.) in the subacute infective conditions of infancy and childhood.

(c) *Eosinophilia*, an increase of eosinophils, occurs (i.) in infestation with certain parasites, particularly hydatid disease, trichinosis, filariasis, ankylostomiasis and bilharzia; (ii.) in certain skin conditions, particularly psoriasis, pruritus and dermatitis herpetiformis; (iii.) in asthmatic and other allergic disorders such as hay fever and rhinitis; (iv.) in Lœffler's syndrome which consists of spasmodic bronchitis, leucocytosis and eosinophilia; (v.) in tropical eosinophilia, perhaps an allergic condition; (vi.) in familial eosinophilia where the number of eosinophils is increased in several members of a family without any discoverable cause; (vii.) during the recovery from infective or toxic states and during the absorption of a hæmorrhagic pleural effusion; (viii.) after taking certain drugs, particularly sulphonamides and after injections with tuberculin. (ix.) Some patients with Hodgkin's disease have bouts or longer periods of eosinophilia. (x.) In myeloid leukæmia and in polycythæmia the eosinophils are often increased.

LOCAL ACCUMULATIONS of eosinophil cells occur in (i.) the nasal secretion and in the nasal mucosa in allergic rhinitis, (ii.) certain cases of conjunctivitis, (iii.) the bronchial secretion of some cases of asthma, (iv.) pleural effusions following pneumonia, and (v.) the majority of cases of Hodgkin's disease in the spleen or lymph glands.

(d) *Monocytes* are increased in number in glandular fever, occasionally in tuberculosis, Boeck's sarcoidosis and syphilis, and transiently during recovery from infectious states before the polymorph neutrophils show any changes. They are also increased in monocytic leukæmia.

(e) *Immature leucocytes* are present in the peripheral blood whenever there is an increase of leucocytes, but only a few may be present. In carcinomatosis of the skeletal system when there are many deposits of carcinoma in the bone marrow, immature myeloid cells, usually myelocytes, are present as well as normoblasts (leuco-erythroblastic reaction). This may also occur in myelosclerosis and syphilis (§ 551). Myelocytes in significant numbers occur in chronic myeloid leukæmia and myeloblasts in the acute form. Lymphoblasts occur in acute lymphatic leukæmia.

(f) *Other leucocytes* such as plasma cells occur occasionally in the peripheral blood. Very rarely nuclei of megakaryocytes or cells from malignant tumours are seen.

Leucopenia is the decrease in the number of leucocytes in the peripheral blood. When this occurs, it is necessary to remember that the percentage figures obtained by the differential count do not reflect the actual state of the blood, but the absolute figures will indicate whether all leucocytes are decreased in number (leucopenia), or only the neutrophils (neutropenia) or the lymphocytes (lymphopenia). In a patient with neutropenia the percentage figures can show a relative lymphocytosis while the absolute figures will indicate normal or subnormal figures for the lymphocytes.

Neutropenia and Agranulocytosis. Neutropenia may not be recognised as such clinically, but especially when there is a coincident rise of temperature, the low neutrophil count can give a useful clue to diagnosis. The most severe form is agranulocytosis (malignant neutropenia) which is twice as common in women as in men, and in this variety there is severe illness. *Symptoms*—(1) There is fever, exhaustion and often slight jaundice, as many of the causal agents are toxic to the liver. Rigors and delirium are of serious significance. (2) Necrotic ulceration (agranulocytic angina) occurs in the mouth, pharynx and around the anal and vaginal orifices due to bacterial invasion; septicæmia often co-exists. (3) The blood count shows a deficiency and even complete absence of neutrophil leucocytes. Any reduction of the neutrophils below 1,000 per c.mm. is of serious significance.

Etiology.—(1) *Infections* which show leucopenia and a moderate or high pyrexia are measles, German measles, typhoid and paratyphoid fever, abortus fever, psittacosis, infective hepatitis, small-pox (in the first four days), miliary tuberculosis, some chronic cases of malaria, kala-azar and in many forms of septicæmia (especially staphylococcal). Leucopenia also occurs in infective conditions which normally produce a neutrophil leucocytosis when the infection is overwhelming in its severity. (2) *Drugs* and *industrial poisons* which may be causal in susceptible individuals are amidopyrin, thiouracil derivatives, chloramphenicol, phenylbutazone, tridione and preparations of arsenic, bismuth and gold. Less frequent causes are the barbiturates, sulphonamides, diparcol, pyribenzamine, benzol, mercury, antimony and lead. With amidopyrin and the barbiturates a hæmo-agglutinin may develop. (3) *Diseases of the bone marrow* which may be responsible are those which produce hypoplasia or aplasia (as in aplastic anæmia and some cases of leuco-erythroblastic anæmia) or those in which there is a maturation arrest as in leukæmia and agranulocytic angina. (4) In some *blood dyscrasias* the other portions of the bone marrow may depress or suppress the myeloid system as in pernicious anæmia, primary splenic neutropenia, splenic anæmia, disseminated lupus erythematosus and Gaucher's disease. (5) *Ionising irradiations* and the use of radio-mimetic drugs (such as nitrogen mustard) are occasionally responsible.

Prognosis.—In agranulocytosis when the bone marrow shows abundance of myelocytes and few mature neutrophils (maturation arrest) the prognosis is fair. When the marrow shows almost complete absence of myeloid and neutrophil cells, sometimes accompanied by hypoplasia of the erythroid and megakaryocytic cells (aplastic type) the prognosis is grave.

Treatment must include treatment of the cause, the immediate cessation of any drug which may have played a part and prevention of secondary infection by barrier nursing and injection of penicillin 500,000 units 8-hourly. Other antibiotics may be used but never chloramphenicol. A large fluid intake should be coupled with a full diet; folic acid and pyridoxine (Vitamin B_6) 150-200 mg. intravenously or by mouth daily are advisable. Regular toilet of the mouth, the corticosteroids and transfusion of fresh blood may help. In cyclical and in primary splenic neutropenia splenectomy offers a reasonable prospect of cure.

Melanæmia indicates the presence in the peripheral blood of isolated masses or clumps of black pigment, either in the cells or in the plasma. It occurs in malaria, relapsing fever, in widespread malignant melanomatosis and in melanosis.

Lipæmia occurs when *fresh* plasma or serum has a pale-pinkish fatty appearance. After standing for several hours plasma often becomes opalescent but this is not true lipæmia. A milky appearance due to a considerable amount of fat in suspension occurs in health after a meal rich in fats, and in some cases of diabetes mellitus, of nephrosis and of xanthomatosis.

Platelets are small (3 to 5μ) irregular bodies which in blood films tend to occur in groups. As their disintegration results in the production of thromboplastin they are concerned with coagulation and hæmostasis. Normally they number 150,000 to 400,000 per c.mm. For *counting platelets* place a drop of 3·8 per cent. sodium citrate on the clean finger, prick with a needle through the drop of fluid and let some blood ooze into it. A smear is made from the diluted blood and is stained with Leishman's method. The platelets are counted against the red cells and when the number of red cells is known, the number of platelets can be calculated.

Thrombocythæmia.—The number of platelets is increased after (i.) hæmorrhage, (ii.) a blood transfusion, (iii.) splenectomy; (iv.) in chronic myeloid leukæmia and (v.) polycythæmia rubra vera. In thrombocythæmia, whether primary or secondary, thromboses and hæmorrhages may occur and the platelets may number as many as 1 to 2 million per c.mm.

Thrombocytopenia.—The number of platelets is reduced in (i.) idiopathic thrombocytopenic purpura, (ii.) pernicious anæmia, (iii.) Gaucher's disease, (iv.) scurvy, (v.) acute myeloid leukæmia or the late stages of chronic myeloid leukæmia, (vi.) aplastic anæmia and (vii.) other induced types of bone marrow aplasia due to benzol or other drugs, such as gold or phenylbutazone, and (viii.) after exposure to X-rays, radium or atomic irradiation.

§ 542. **Parasites found in the Blood.**—The detection of micro-organisms of clinical importance found in the blood is dealt with in Chapter XXII. *Bartonella baçilliformis* infects the red corpuscles of patients in Peru suffering from Oroya Fever. Certain pathogenic protozoa such as *malarial* parasites, *trypanosomes* and *Leishman-Donovan bodies* as well as filarial embryos, may be found in tropical patients; those of *Wuchereria bancrofti* are nocturnal, being found in the blood at night; those of *Loa loa*, from West Africa, which causes Calabar swellings, are found in the day time. In the relapsing fevers spirochætes may be found during the pyrexial periods.

Staining.—Thick blood films are " dehæmoglobinised " and stained with Field's stain. Parasites seen in these are then specifically identified in thin films stained by Leishman's method.

The PARASITE OF MALARIAL FEVER is a protozoon, inhabiting the red corpuscles which it destroys, but if schizonticidal drugs are being taken, only sexual forms (gametocytes) are likely to be found (and see Plate XVIII).

Varieties.—The life history of the protozoa is described in § 512. Each of the four species is identified in the blood by its characteristic asexual intracorpuscular phase and by its gametocytes. *Plasmodium vivax*, the benign tertian parasite, is first seen within the corpuscle as a small, clear, ovoid body about 2μ in diameter, possessing active amœboid movement. It gradually increases in size, becomes vacuolated, and after the lapse of a few hours becomes ring-shaped (stage 1), with a peripheral chromatin dot. After about 6 hours the larger amœboid form develops (stage 2), containing one or two refractile granules of brown pigment, while the erythrocytes show enlargement, pallor and fine granules known as Schüffner's dots, staining red with Romanowsky stains. At the stage of full growth the parasite occupies more of the enlarged corpuscle

PLATE XVIII

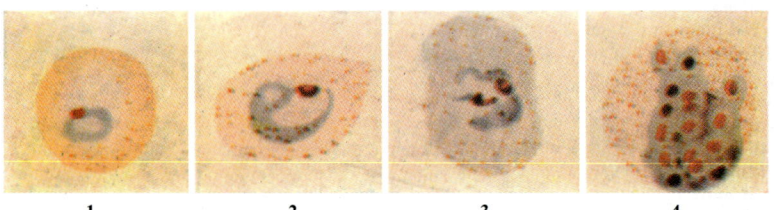

| 1 | 2 | 3 | 4 |

PARASITE OF MALARIAL FEVER SEEN IN PERIPHERAL BLOOD SMEARS.

1–4. STAGE OF BENIGN TERTIAN (P. VIVAX). (1) *Parasite with vacuole in centre and chromatin nucleus.* (2) *Parasite developing into amoeboid trophozoite: red cell enlarging and Schüffner's dots beginning to appear.* (3) *Trophozoite still increasing in size and beginning to divide (schizogony): Schüffner's dots more visible.* (4) *Divided schizont (forming merozoites) before rupture of red cell.*

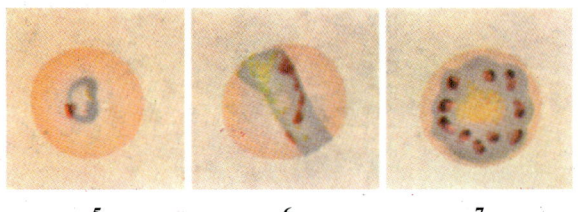

| 5 | 6 | 7 |

5–7. STAGES OF QUARTAN MALARIA (P. MALARIAE). *Similar stage to 1–4, but parasite remains more compact (sometimes assuming bond forms—see 6): red cells do not enlarge and Schüffner's dots are absent.*

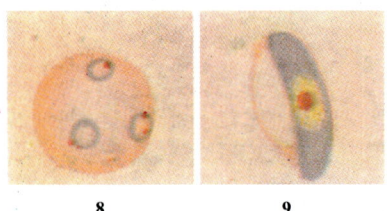

| 8 | 9 |

8–9. STAGES OF MALIGNANT TERTIAN (P. FALCIPARUM): (8) *Ring forms. The growing trophozoites and schizonts are not seen in the peripheral blood except in very severe infections.* (9) *The crescent is the gametocyte.*

(Reproduced by permission from *The Microscopic Diagnosis of Tropical Diseases.*

Farbenfabriken Bayer A.G.)

(stage 3). Now the pigment gathers in the centre of the parasite and chromatin divides, and the protoplasm is arranged around these masses so that rosettes of from 15 to 20 segments are formed (stage 4); these are set free as merozoites by the rupture of the red blood corpuscles containing them, and masses of insoluble pigment enter the bloodstream; this is subsequently taken up by the reticulo-endothelial cells in the liver, spleen and bone marrow. This phase of " segmentation " is complete in about 48 hours, and corresponds clinically to a fresh paroxysm of the fever. These merozoites enter fresh red blood corpuscles and the cycle is repeated. Some of the rings develop into the *sexual* gametocytes if the patient is not treated early.

Plasmodium malariæ, the quartan parasite, first appears as a small, round, clear mass of cytoplasm which becomes vacuolated to form a ring difficult to distinguish from *P. vivax* (stage 5). It has feeble amœboid movement, develops slowly, and takes 72 hours to complete its cycle. After a few hours, coarse dark pigment granules appear; as growth develops the organism tends to be stretched as a band across the corpuscle (stage 6). By the third day pigment, coarser and blacker than that of the tertian form, gathers round its periphery. On the fourth day segmentation takes place, the pigment flows in towards the centre, and here forms the radiating lines which produce the beautiful " daisy rosette " so characteristic of the quartan parasite (stage 7). It breaks up eventually into 8 to 10 spores, and these with the insoluble pigment becomes free in the blood-stream. The development of the gametocyte resembles that of the benign tertian variety. There is no enlargement of the red corpuscle.

Plasmodium falciparum, the parasite of the *malignant tertian* fever, is first seen in the red blood-cells as a tiny, unpigmented, hyaline body, 48 hours being needed for its development. At first it exhibits energetic amœboid movements, but ultimately settles into a bright, colourless, ring-like form, with one or two chromatin dots (stage 8). There is frequently multiple infection of a single corpuscle. Often the parasite seems adherent to the outside of the corpuscle. The rosette or sporulating stage is rarely seen in the peripheral blood. In about a week (during the period of remission) characteristic crescent bodies, containing masses of coarse pigment granules, begin to appear, and increase in number rapidly. They are incapable of sporulation, and represent the sexual form—the gametocyte—(stage 9), of which there are male and female forms. They ultimately degenerate if not taken up by the mosquito.

Plasmodium ovale causes a mild type of tertian fever. It is found in oval-shaped red cells with Schüffner's dots. It resembles *P. vivax* but the schizont has only 6 to 12 merozoites and has a central mass of pigment. The parasite occupies only three-quarters of a red cell.

Filariasis is caused in tropical climates by various nematode worms (round worms) invading the tissues of human beings: their embryos (micro-filariæ) can be found in the blood. Four varieties of worms are recognised. (i.) *Wuchereria bancrofti* and the related *Brugia malayi*; (ii.) the filarial worm *loa loa*; (iii.) *Tetrapetalonema perstans* and (iv.) *Onchocerca volvulus*.

Wuchereria bancrofti (Syn. *Filaria bancrofti*) and *Brugia malayi* (Syn. *F. malayi*) are transmitted by various species of anopheline, culicine or aëdine mosquitoes in which the embryos, sucked up with the blood, take 10 to 40 days to develop. The microfilariæ are readily seen in a fresh drop of blood in a cover-glass preparation examined under the low or medium power of the microscope; the detailed morphology may be studied in a thick film dehæmoglobinised and stained with hæmalum. The embryos may be found in 20 per cent. of apparently healthy residents in certain tropical countries. The embryos come into the peripheral blood at night (from 6 p.m. to 10 a.m.) and disappear during the day; the maximum number is usually found about midnight. It may be necessary to make repeated examinations at intervals of 2 hours to find them. Should a victim of the parasite alter his usual habits, and sleep during the day, the microfilarial periodicity is reversed. The adult filariæ inhabit the lymphatics, where they give birth to immense numbers of embryos, many of which are destroyed. In the Pacific Islands the mosquito transmitter is *Aëdes variegatus* which bites in the daytime.

No periodicity exists and the worm causing filariasis there is not identical with *W. bancrofti*. Adult parasites after their death may cause lymphangitis, various forms of elephantiasis, lymph-scrotum, hæmatochyluria, chylous diarrhœa and ascites, usually related to their blocking of the lymphatic circulation (§ 522).

Loa loa is a filarial worm transmitted by certain species of mango-fly (Chrysops). The adult worms cause " calabar swellings " in the subcutaneous tissues and when they cross the conjunctiva there is local conjunctivitis. After some months typical sheathed embryos (micro-filariæ) occur in the blood during the daytime with a diurnal periodicity (Fig. 160). (For *Symptoms* and *Diagnosis* see § 657.)

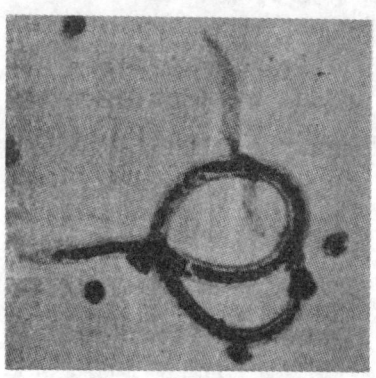

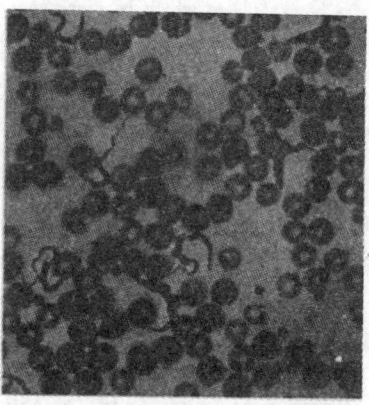

FIG. 160.—Thick dehæmoglobinised blood film showing microfilariæ of *Loa loa*; note sheath and the irregular and diffusely staining column of nuclei which extend almost to tip of tail. (× 400).

FIG. 161.—*Trypanosoma rhodesiense* in blood film. (× 480).

Tetrapetalonema perstans is a harmless filarial worm whose unsheathed embryos are often found in the blood of people from Africa.

Onchocerca volvulus is a filarial worm carried by a species of Simulium flies. It produces subcutaneous nodules and severe eye lesions which often cause blindness (§ 724). The micro-filariæ (larvæ) can be demonstrated in skin shavings and may be found in the blood.

Trypanosoma.—The parasite of TRYPANOSOMIASIS (§ 521) is a flagellated protozoon. It is usually obtained by gland puncture, and can also be demonstrated in the blood and cerebro-spinal fluid. It is found free in the blood. One end of the parasite is drawn out into a whip-like process, the flagellum; the other end is bluntly conical; the body itself is short and thick, and its substance granular. It contains a trophonucleus and a kinetonucleus. Attached to one side is a transparent, flange-like process, the undulating membrane. The length of the parasite, including the flagellum, is about 18μ to 25μ. It is best stained by Leishman's or Giemsa's stain (Fig. 161).

LEISHMANIA.—The protozoa of KALA-AZAR are found in the spleen, liver, bone marrow, the blood and in the lymphatic glands. The commonest form found is a small ovoid body longer than it is broad, less than 2μ in diameter, measuring about one-fifth of a red corpuscle in its longest axis. Stained with Leishman's stain the parasite shows two nuclei: one is small, rod-shaped, and stains deeply; the other is larger, rounded, and stains less deeply. Similar bodies are found in Oriental sore and in Espundia. Leishmania in culture elongate and develop a flagellum.

RELAPSING FEVERS.—The spirochætes causing these fevers can be stained by the Leishman method in blood smears. Fine focussing is requisite, and the morphology varies considerably. In fresh blood their active motility renders them conspicuous against dark ground illumination.   The spirochætes are found in the blood during the pyrexial periods only.

§ 543. **Chemical and Physical Properties of the Blood.**—In Table XXXVIII are shown the substances which can be readily detected in the blood, and the findings in the normal subject.   Individual sections should be consulted for variations from the normal, see Table at end of book.

The FRAGILITY of red cells is tested by placing a drop of blood in salt solutions of strength varying by 0·05 per cent. and extending from 0·30 to 0·70 per cent.   When

TABLE XXXVIII.—BLOOD CHEMISTRY

Substance.	Plasma or Serum content in mg. per 100 ml. (unless otherwise stated).	m.Eq./litre.
Alkali reserve as CO_2	53–77 vols. per cent.	23–34
Amylase, diastase	3–10 (Wohlgemuth) units per 1 ml.	
Bilirubin	0·1–0·5	
Calcium	9–11	4·5–5·5
Chlorides (as Sodium Chloride)	560–620	96–106
Cholesterol (total)	150–260	
Creatinine	1–2	
Iron (as Fe)		
Male	80–150 micrograms per 100 ml.	
Female	60–120 „ „ „	
Phosphatase		
acid	1–3 King-Armstrong units	
alkaline	3–13 „ „ „	
Phosphate as (inorganic phosphorus)		
Adult	2–4	
Child	4–6	
Potassium	15–22	3·9–5·6
Proteins total	5·6–8·5 G. per 100 ml.	
Albumin	4·0–6·7 „ „	
Globulin	1·2–2·9 „ „	
Fibrinogen (plasma)	0·2–0·4 „ „	
Pseudocholinesterase	55–120 units	
Sodium	315–350	137–152
Sugar (fasting)	80–120	
Thymol turbidity	1–4 units	
Transaminases		
-serum glutamic oxalacetic transaminase (S.G.O.T.)	Up to 40 Sigma-Frankel units per ml.	
-serum glutamic pyruvic transaminase (S.G.P.T.)	„	
Urea	15–40	
Uric acid	1–5 (Folin's method)	
Zinc sulphate turbidity	4–8 units	

the red cells have settled, a slight red tinge is seen above them in some tubes, whilst in others the red cells have completely hæmolysed.   Hæmolysis is said to start in the tube in which the first red tinge is seen and to be complete in that in which the red cells are all hæmolysed.   It is customary to test a normal person in a second set of tubes for comparison.   Normally, hæmolysis commences in the 0·45 tube and is complete in the 0·30 tube.   The fragility of the red cells is a diagnostic point in acholuric jaundice (§ 331).   *Quantitative estimation* of hæmolysis gives more information than the simple qualitative test described, because it detects fragility of a small number of corpuscles in a sample in which most of the cells exhibit normal saline fragility.   It is carried out by red cell counts on the different samples.

SPECTROSCOPIC EXAMINATION of the blood.—The instrument chiefly used for clinical purposes is Browning's spectroscope.   It is used by holding up a glass containing a very dilute solution of blood, and looking through it at the daylight, or at a white cloud, with a spectroscope placed between the blood solution and the eyes.   Carboxyhæmoglobin is found in poisoning from coal gas, stoves, petrol fumes (§ 577). Methæmoglobinæmia and sulphæmoglobinæmia are occasional complications of therapy with sulphonamide drugs. Methæmoglobin is also formed in nitro-benzol and potassium chlorate poisoning and in other conditions (§§ 32, 382, 414). Hæmatoporphyrin has been found in the urine in sulphonal poisoning.

ELECTROPHORESIS.—The different serum proteins carry electrical charges of differing magnitudes, which cause them to migrate at different rates under the influence of an electric field.

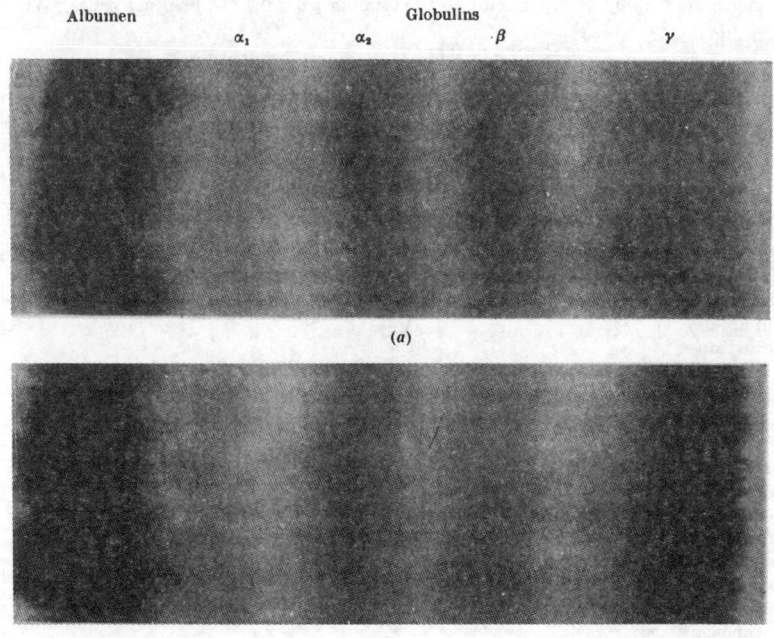

FIG. 162.—ELECTROPHORETIC PATTERNS. (a) Normal pattern. (b) Increased γ-globulin in a case of Hodgkin's disease.

Technique.—A piece of filter paper soaked in a buffer solution is used to connect two reservoirs of the buffer. The reservoirs are joined to the positive and negative poles of a battery. A thin line of the protein solution under investigation is placed on the wet paper and a current passed through the paper. After a suitable time the paper is removed and the protein fixed to the paper by drying at an elevated temperature. The protein bands are made visible by dipping in a dye which stains the protein but not the paper. The albumen fraction moves furthest from the site of application of the protein, then follow the α_1, α_2, β and γ globulins.

The relative proportions of each component vary widely in disease. In myelomatosis an abnormal band is often found in the region of the β or γ globulins. Nephrosis is associated with a decrease in albumen and high β or γ globulins. In cirrhosis all the globulin fractions may be increased. In agammaglobulinæmia the γ globulin is missing. In most diseases the changes which occur in the plasma protein pattern tend to be non-specific and in only a few instances, such as nephrosis, is it possible to associate electrophoretic patterns with disease states. The large amount of γ globulin shown in the illustration was present in the serum of a patient suffering from Hodgkin's disease (Fig. 162). A similar picture could equally well have been produced from a case of cirrhosis or multiple myelomatosis.

BLOOD COAGULATION is now known to be a complex process. The four stages in which it is known to occur are :—

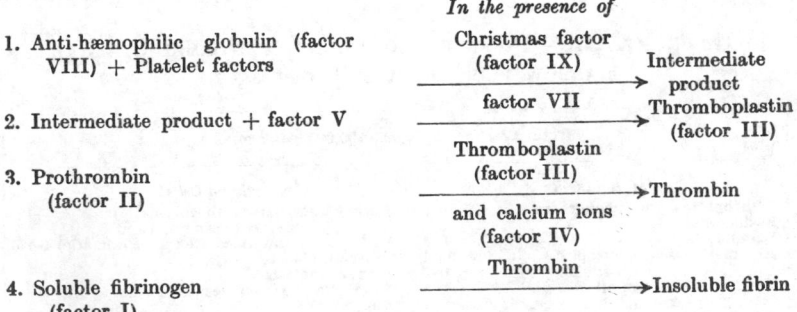

In the presence of

1. Anti-hæmophilic globulin (factor VIII) + Platelet factors

Christmas factor (factor IX)
→ Intermediate product

2. Intermediate product + factor V

factor VII
→ Thromboplastin (factor III)

3. Prothrombin (factor II)

Thromboplastin (factor III)
→ Thrombin
and calcium ions (factor IV)

4. Soluble fibrinogen (factor I)

Thrombin
→ Insoluble fibrin

Technique.—The CLOTTING TIME is estimated by Lee and White's method. With dry needle and syringe 4 ml. of blood is obtained by a clean venepuncture and 1 ml. is placed in each of 4 small test-tubes. As soon as the blood enters the barrel of the syringe the stop-watch is started. The test-tubes are placed in a water bath at 37° C and are fully inverted every 30 seconds, until a firm clot is formed and the tube can be turned upside down without the blood moving. Normally the clotting time is 4 to 9 minutes. The clotting time is *prolonged* in most cases of hæmophilia and Christmas disease (often to more than 2 hours), to a lesser extent in obstructive jaundice and liver failure, in leukæmia and in aplastic anæmia of whatever etiology. The clotting time is slightly *shortened* after hæmorrhage, splenectomy, blood transfusions, a general anæsthetic and in some fevers. The prolongation of the clotting time caused by heparin given for therapeutic reasons can be corrected by the use of vitamin K_1.

Anti-hæmophilic globulin. Factor V and Factor VII are estimated by specialised procedures. These and the thromboplastin generation test of Biggs and Macfarlane help in the accurate diagnosis of the hæmorrhagic diseases.

The PROTHROMBIN TIME is a useful test in certain hæmorrhagic states, in obstructive jaundice, in hæmorrhagic disease of the newborn and during the administration of anti-coagulants for thrombotic diseases. *Technique.*—In Quick's method 0·1 ml. of the patient's plasma is added to 0·1 ml. of thromboplastin and when 0·1 ml. of calcium chloride is added to the mixture, in the water bath at 37° C, the stop-watch is started. The small test tube is tilted backwards and forwards until the sample clots. The normal prothrombin time is 13 to 15 seconds. A normal control should always be tested at the same time and this should be recorded with the result. The estimation of a prothrombin index or of the prothrombin content is not a reliable way to assess the amount of prothrombin. In anti-coagulant treatment for thrombotic states it is desirable to maintain the prothrombin time at a level of 2 to 3 times the normal.

The BLEEDING TIME does not bear any close relationship to blood coagulation, but is roughly in proportion to the number of blood platelets and is also a measure of the retractility of blood-vessels. *Technique.*—After puncturing the finger with a Hagedorn needle or an automatic lancet, the finger is placed in water at 37° C and the issue of blood from the puncture wound is observed. After a minute or so it slows down and normally stops in 2 minutes. In thrombocytopenia the bleeding time is prolonged, sometimes to more than half an hour. In hæmophilia the bleeding time is normal.

§ 544. **Bone Marrow Biopsy** is a valuable method of investigation when examination of the peripheral blood has shown that we are dealing with a disorder of hæmopoiesis. The technique is described in § 1201. From the material obtained the number of nucleated cells (normally 20,000–100,000 per c.mm.) is estimated in the usual counting chamber; also smears are made on glass slides and stained with Leishman's or with other special stains; the rest is allowed to clot, fixed and histological sections are cut. After scanning 2 or 3 smears, paying attention to larger cells like megakaryocytes or to clumps of cells, at least 500 cells are classified in a differential count (Table XXXIX).

TABLE XXXIX.—DIFFERENTIAL COUNT OF NORMAL STERNAL MARROW FROM SMEARS (Percentages)

Total Cell Count 20,000–100,000 per c.mm.

Myeloid Cells		*Erythroid Cells*	
Neutrophil polymorphonuclears	20–50	Normoblasts : late (orthochromatic)	7–19
Eosinophils	0–4	,, early (basophilic) and	
Basophils	0–1	intermediate (polychromatic)	4–15
Metamyelocytes : neutrophil	2·5–10	Proerythroblasts	0–4
,, eosinophil	0–2·5	Hæmocytoblasts	0–1
Myelocytes : neutrophil	2–8	Megaloblasts are not seen in normal adult	
,, eosinophil	0–1	marrow.	
Promyelocytes	0·5–5·0		
Myeloblasts	0–2·5		

Myeloid–Erythroid ratio 8 1 to 2 : 1

Other Cells			
Lymphocytes	5–20	Reticulum cells	0–1
Monocytes	0–5	Megakaryocytes	0·2–1
Plasma cells	0–1		

In DIAGNOSIS the results are of value : (i.) With pernicious anæmia typical megaloblasts are found during a relapse, but these disappear within two days of treatment with specific hæmatinics; (ii.) a doubtful case of subacute combined degeneration when anæmia is slight, and (iii.) leukæmia (especially in atypical or aleukæmic forms) may be confirmed. It is also useful in (iv.) other blood diseases such as erythræmic myelosis, thrombocytopenia; (v.) malignant diseases, especially myelomatosis, secondary carcinomatosis or sarcomatosis of the bone marrow; (vi.) disseminated lupus erythematosus (when L.E. cells are found), the reticuloses, Gaucher's disease and allied disorders; (vii.) infections such as malaria, kala-azar, trypanosomiasis. (viii.) In brucellosis a positive culture may be obtained. An unsuccessful marrow puncture may suggest aplastic anæmia and an increased bony resistance is met in myelosclerosis. In *Prognosis*, serial marrow examinations in cases of leukæmia furnish the best information in controlling treatment by steroids or chemotherapy; recognition of a remission rests primarily on the reversion of the marrow to an almost normal state. In conditions such as myelosclerosis the difficulty of obtaining marrow tissue by needle puncture and its extremely hypoplastic nature serves as a warning against splenectomy. In prolonged radiotherapy it gives an assessment of the amount of marrow damage.

Hæmophilia and related coagulation defects are the only conditions contra-indicating marrow biopsy. In hæmolytic and iron-deficiency anæmias it is of little value.

APLASIA OF THE BONE MARROW may concern only the red cells (aplastic anæmia, § 552), only the leucocytes (leucopenia, agranulocytosis, §§ 155f, 541), only the platelets (thrombocytopenia) or any combination of these. In most cases the severity of the disease varies in different cell systems and the most prominent lesion is reflected in the name given.

*PART C.   DISEASES WHICH GIVE RISE TO GENERAL DEBILITY, WITH
OR WITHOUT ANÆMIA AND EMACIATION: THEIR DIAGNOSIS,
PROGNOSIS AND TREATMENT.*

§ 545. Routine Procedure and Classification.—Here, as elsewhere, we
have three points to investigate:

First, the LEADING and perhaps the only SYMPTOM complained of by
the patient will be debility, or pallor of the skin, or loss of flesh.

Secondly, the HISTORY OF THE ILLNESS, its date, mode of onset and
mode of evolution.   Often these data are vague, but special inquiries
should be directed to the condition of the digestion in times past and
to any other points relating to nutrition.

Thirdly, the PHYSICAL EXAMINATION of the patient, commencing with
that physiological system to which the results of our previous inquiries
have directed attention, and then going through all the systems seriatim.
An examination of the blood should be made in all anæmic or doubtful
cases—viz., hæmoglobin, cell counts, red cell indices and blood smears.

Classification.—If there is PALLOR OF THE SKIN and ANÆMIA is suspected, turn first to Group I, BELOW.

If LOSS OF WEIGHT is most prominent, turn to Group II, § 569.

If GENERAL DEBILITY (without obvious pallor or loss of weight) is most
prominent, turn to Group III, § 574.

GROUP I.   PALLOR OF THE SKIN AND ANÆMIC DISORDERS

PALLOR OF THE SKIN may be due to:

(A) ANÆMIA.—The degree of pallor is approximately in proportion to
the degree of hæmoglobin deficiency; the lack of red colour in a drop of
blood is confirmatory.   Although the deficiency of hæmoglobin in the
capillaries causes them to be pale, an even more important factor is the
associated vaso-constriction.   In every case where anæmia is suspected
the amount of hæmoglobin must be estimated; when a lowered value is
obtained it is essential to proceed to estimate the red cell count, the red
cell indices and to examine a blood smear (§§ 539–541).   In other cases
(B) the anæmia is slight and the pallor of the skin is due to a variety of
causes, *e.g.*, syphilis, renal or hepatic disease.

The pallor presents to the experienced observer a difference in kind and degree
in the several affections (and see § 10).   Thus, the lemon-yellow of pernicious anæmia,
the earthy tint of carcinoma, the sallowness of aortic disease and interstitial nephritis,
the pasty white of parenchymatous nephritis, and the transparent waxy look of
lardaceous disease are very suggestive to the careful observer.   The age of the patient
often gives a valuable clue.   The microscopic examination of the blood also reveals
differences which are mentioned below.   For Fallacies, see § 535.

A. *The patient complains of* LACK OF ENERGY, SHORTNESS OF BREATH
ON EXERTION *and the other symptoms of anæmia.*   PALLOR *is marked and*
THE BLOOD IS MARKEDLY DEFICIENT IN HÆMOGLOBIN.   *The condition is
one of* ANÆMIA.

C.M.—D D

Symptoms Common to all **Anæmias** are (1) failing strength for physical and mental work accompanied by pallor of the surface. The pallor is marked in the nail-beds, the palms of the hands, the lips, the tongue and conjunctivæ (as may be observed by pulling down the lower lid), and the sclerotics have a bluish colour. (2) Cardio-vascular symptoms, such as dyspnœa on slight exertion, palpitation, giddiness and fainting. The heart is dilated in many cases, with precordial discomfort. Hæmic murmurs are heard, especially over the pulmonary area. In marked cases the " bruit de diable " is present—a continuous hum heard when the stethoscope is gently placed over the jugular vein in the neck. Œdema of the ankles at night is common; venous thrombosis is rare. **Hæmic or Anæmic Murmurs** (§ 42) are usually soft and blowing, but may be loud and rasping; loudest in the pulmonary area, but may be heard all over the precordium, rarely in the axilla; often louder when the patient is lying down or has rested, and apt to vary from day to day. (3) Disturbances of digestion— deficient or capricious appetite, discomfort or even vomiting after food: gastric atony and gastroptosis. Constipation is often present. (4) Symptoms referable to the nervous system—faintness or actual fainting, vertigo, headache, tinnitus, defective attention, nervousness, irritability or depression of spirits, spots before the eyes. Vaso-motor signs are frequent such as a tendency to " dead fingers." (5) Amenorrhœa is usual, dysmenorrhœa not infrequent; menorrhagia may lead to anæmia.

Synthesis and Breakdown of Hæmoglobin.—There is a constant synthesis and breakdown of hæmoglobin to the extent of 8 G. a day in the healthy adult. The hæmoglobin molecule consists of an iron-containing portion (hæm) loosely combined with a series of polypeptide chains (globins). Hæm is a ferrous protoporphyrin (protoporphyrin III) and for its formation a sufficiency of iron is essential. The iron is absorbed in the ferrous form mainly in the duodenum (§ 549); it is then oxidised to the ferric state and linked in the mucosal cells with an iron-free protein (apoferritin) to form ferritin. When the cells have become saturated with iron, the " mucosal block " prevents further absorption until iron has been transferred to the blood. The amount of iron ultimately absorbed is governed by the amount already stored in the body. Ferritin is conveyed through the blood as transferrin to be stored as ferritin in the liver, spleen, bone marrow and other tissues. From these sources it is taken to the bone marrow to be synthesised in the erythroid cells into hæm and ultimately into hæmoglobin. After an average life of about 120 days the red cells are broken down by hæmolysis, but the greater part of the hæmoglobin set free is not lost to the body for it joins with haptoglobin to form a combination which is not excreted by the kidneys; then it is conserved as hæmosiderin in the cells of the marrow and of the reticulo-endothelial system. Such hæmoglobin as is not conjugated in this way is converted by cells of the reticulo-endothelial system into bilirubin.

The CAUSES OF ANÆMIA may be:
(*a*) Hæmorrhage, either manifest or occult.
(*b*) Deficient formation of red blood cells.
(*c*) Excessive breakdown (hæmolysis) of red blood cells.

(*a*) § **546. Hæmorrhage** is the commonest cause of pallor and anæmia and so is considered first. A patient rarely complains of symptoms until the hæmoglobin has fallen below 70 per cent. of normal, and many maintain fair health with much lower values. A sudden drop in hæmoglobin produces symptoms early; a slow drop is much less noticed by the patient.

Manifest hæmorrhage occurs with hæmatemesis, hæmoptysis, hæmaturia, epistaxis, menorrhagia, bleeding piles or melæna, or with surgical injuries. The history reveals the nature of the hæmorrhage, although in unobservant patients or in women with menorrhagia leading questions as to abnormal bleeding may be necessary. If the hæmorrhage is acute and severe, giddiness, sudden faintness or even collapse is present during the period of blood loss.

Occult hæmorrhage may be in such small repeated quantities as to be unnoticed, as when it occurs from a peptic ulcer or carcinoma of the stomach, when blood oozes in small amounts almost continuously. Small amounts of blood may also be lost in cases with internal piles or with ankylostomiasis; in these cases, the blood may be demonstrated by occult blood tests of the stools (§ 303). Sometimes hæmorrhage may remain hidden, when it occurs into the internal organs or serous cavities, *e.g.*, in a ruptured ectopic gestation or with suprarenal hæmorrhage in infants.

The hæmorrhage may be contributed to by an abnormal tendency to bleeding, such as occurs in the hæmorrhagic diseases: hæmophilia (§ 561), severe purpura, including thrombocytopenic purpura and Henoch's purpura (§ 595), in certain liver diseases (§ 333) and with hereditary capillary telangiectasis (§ 769). In infants, scurvy and hæmorrhagic disease of the newborn must be considered.

The *type of anæmia* resulting from hæmorrhage depends on whether the blood loss was sudden and large or frequent and small. In the first case the anæmia is usually normocytic and normochromic; in the second, as the iron stores in the body have probably been depleted by the long continued loss of blood, the blood picture is usually indistinguishable from that of a simple iron deficiency anæmia (§ 549) and the red cells are normocytic or microcytic and hypochromic.

Treatment must deal with the underlying cause. Blood transfusions may be necessary and the administration of iron will help to overcome iron deficiency and stimulate hæmopoiesis.

§ 547. **Blood Transfusion** is carried out for three main purposes: (1) when it is necessary to restore the *volume* of the circulating blood—after a sudden severe hæmorrhage or in shock; (2) to *replenish missing elements*, as in chronic anæmia where the deficiency of red cells leads to anoxia or in hæmophilia where the deficiency of antihæmophilic globulin leads to hæmorrhage; (3) when it is essential to *remove or dilute foreign antibodies* which destroy the red cells as in hæmolytic disease of the newborn. For the maximum benefit the *correct fluid* must be chosen for the various indications and the *right amount* should be given at the *right rate of flow* according to the condition of the patient.

INDICATIONS.—(1) Anæmia following a severe *brisk hæmorrhage* is corrected by a transfusion of fresh blood. This has a hæmostatic effect, overcomes the circulatory failure and the reduction of the oxygen-carrying capacity, and shortens the period of recovery. (2) Anæmia due to *chronic blood loss* must be corrected when the hæmoglobin reaches a level dangerous to life (40 per cent. of normal), but the rate of administration must be carefully adjusted because the myocardium is often in poor condition due to fatty change.   Major surgical operations should not be undertaken until the hæmoglobin has been restored to at least 70 per cent.   In the presence of anæmia convalescence is prolonged and post-operative wound repair is delayed.   (3) *In shock* the circulating blood becomes concentrated (hæmoconcentration) and the increased viscosity embarrasses the circulation.   Transfusion should restore the blood volume and maintain the systolic blood pressure at a level of at least 100 mm. Hg.   Surgical operations below such a pressure increase the risk to life.   (4) When a severe acute or chronic *infection* or *toxæmia* is accompanied by anæmia with a hæmoglobin of 70 per cent. or less, transfusion corrects the anæmia at least temporarily, helps the patient's resistance and supplies non-specific protective elements such as complement. Examples of this are septicæmia, ulcerative colitis and rheumatoid arthritis.   (5) *Hæmorrhagic states* and blood disorders : (*a*) in a severe relapse of pernicious anæmia cardiac failure threatens life and transfusion will overcome the delay of the onset of remission until specific treatment such as with vitamin B$_{12}$ takes effect.   (*b*) In other anæmias transfusions should be given with caution, and only when the type of disorder has been established and after the blood to be transfused has been most carefully matched.   (*c*) In thrombocytopenia transfusion temporarily increases the numbers of platelets in the circulation to a level at which the danger of hæmorrhage is reduced. (*d*) Transfusion of fresh blood remains the best treatment in hæmophilia and is a specific, although temporary, remedy.   When the coagulation time is prolonged and an acute hæmophilic hæmorrhage has occurred, fresh blood provides enough anti-hæmophilic globulin (Factor VIII) and therefore has a hæmostatic effect.   (*e*) When the bone marrow is aplastic, either primarily as in aplast· ; anæmia or secondarily as in the suppression of erythropoiesis by leukæmia, Hodgkin's disease or radiotherapy, blood transfusion supplies enough red cells to prolong life and may provide time gained for other more specific methods of treatment.   (6) In *hæmolytic disease of the newborn* blood transfusion may be curative.   (7) In *carbon monoxide poisoning* from coal gas or other substances interfering with the formation of oxyhæmoglobin, venesection followed by a transfusion of a large amount of blood may be life saving.

Relative Merits of Fresh and Stored Blood.—Blood collected with sterile precautions by the method described later and kept refrigerated at 2–4° C for not more than three weeks raises the level of hæmoglobin and restores the blood volume.   Because in stored blood there is a rapid loss of leucocytes, platelets, other coagulation factors and non-specific protective elements, fresh blood (less than 24 hours old) is preferable for patients with a disorder of the blood (when it is desirable that transfused red cells should survive as long as possible), or for a hæmorrhagic state (when coagulation factors are needed). In anæmia complicated by sepsis fresh blood is more valuable than stored blood.

Blood Grouping.—The agglutination reactions observed in mixtures of red cells and serum (or plasma) led Landsteiner in 1901 to divide human beings into 3 and later

TABLE XL.—BLOOD GROUPS AND BLOOD GROUP SUBSTANCES

Blood Group			Blood Group Substances		Transfusion		
International Classification	Moss Numbering	Jansky Numbering	Agglutinogen in Red Cells	Agglutinin in Serum	Donor can give blood to Groups	Recipient can receive blood from Groups	Incidence in Europeans (Per cent.)
AB . . .	1	4	A and B	none	AB only	AB, A, B, O (Universal recipient)	4
A . . .	2	2	A	β (anti-B)	A and AB	A and O	42
B . . .	3	3	B	α (anti-A)	B and AB	B and O	9
O . . .	4	1	none	α and β	All groups (Universal donor)	O only	45

4 blood groups. A numerical classification was first used but an International nomenclature based on the agglutinogens is now almost universally adopted. The four blood groups depend on the presence or absence of two agglutinogens (A and B) in the red cells and two agglutinins (α or anti-A, and β or anti-B) in the serum or plasma. Reaction between an agglutinogen and its corresponding agglutinin (e.g., group A cells and α-agglutinins) causes clumping of red cells (or agglutination) and later lysis. An agglutinogen and its corresponding agglutinin cannot therefore exist together in one and the same blood. Table XL and Fig. 163 show the classification of blood groups, their blood group substances, their incidence in Europeans and the possibilities of compatible transfusions.

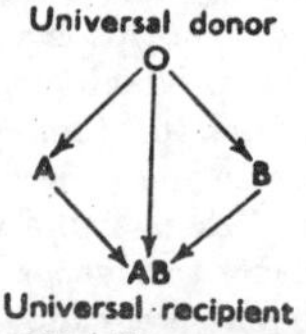

When blood of group O is transfused to a person other than from group O, the α- and β-agglutinins in the transfused blood are diluted in the recipient's blood to such an extent that their concentration is usually too weak to cause any significant reaction; a reaction after transfusing group O blood can very rarely occur when the titres of α- and β-agglutinins are unusually high.

Universal donor

Universal recipient

FIG. 163.—BLOOD GROUPS
AND TRANSFUSIONS.

The arrows indicate the likelihood of a compatible blood transfusion.

Technique of Blood Grouping.—A small drop of a stock A-serum (containing β-agglutinin) is placed on a microscope slide marked A and a small drop of a stock B-serum (containing α-agglutinins) is placed on another slide marked B, using separate pipettes. These stock sera must have high titres of agglutinins. A small quantity of the blood to be grouped is diluted with N-saline to produce an approximately 5 per cent. suspension of red cells; capillary or oxalated blood from a fresh sample is suitable. A small drop of this suspension is placed alongside the stock sera on the slides, which are then gently rocked to mix the red cell suspension and sera; these mixtures are allowed to stand for 10 to 15 minutes. The slides are then rocked more strongly and examined. Agglutination is " positive " when the homogeneous red mixture shows a fine or coarse granular appearance which can be easily seen by the naked eye. The preparation should be examined with the microscope; in cases of doubt protect the preparation with a cover slip, put them in a Petri dish with a piece of moist filter paper, leave them in the incubator at 37° C for about 20 minutes, and then re-examine them microscopically. The possible reactions with the test sera are shown in Table XLI. Ideally and as a check on the results obtained, the serum of the blood being examined should be tested for agglutinins with suspensions of known group A and group B red cells using the same technique.

TABLE XLI.—DETERMINATION OF BLOOD GROUPS

Group A serum (containing β-agglutinin)	Group B serum (containing α-agglutinin)	Group of Blood tested
mixed with a suspension of red cells from the blood under examination:		
+	+	AB
0	+	A
+	0	B
0	0	O

(+ = agglutination; 0 = no agglutination)

The Rhesus Antigen was discovered in 1940 by Landsteiner and Wiener, who found that red cells from 85 per cent. of American white people were agglutinated by the serum of a rabbit which had been injected with red cells from a rhesus monkey. Persons whose blood gives this reaction have a blood group factor called rhesus antigen and they are Rh-positive. In the other 15 per cent. the blood does not give this reaction as it lacks the rhesus antigen; they are Rh-negative and therefore may develop a rhesus antibody if the rhesus antigen should be introduced into their circulation. This may occur by transfusion or during pregnancy. (*a*) If a Rh-negative person is transfused with Rh-positive blood the rhesus antibody resulting from this may agglutinate the red cells of any subsequent Rh-positive blood which may be transfused, setting up a hæmolytic reaction. (*b*) When a Rh-negative woman becomes pregnant with a fœtus whose red cells are Rh-positive like those of its father, she produces rhesus antibody: this is a danger to the fœtus for it crosses the placenta into the fœtal circulation producing agglutination with subsequent hæmolysis of the fœtal red cells and damage to other fœtal tissue cells. This may lead to death *in utero*, to hydrops fœtalis or to hæmolytic disease of the newborn (icterus gravis neonatorum, § 330*a*). The risk is slight with the first pregnancy (unless the Rh-negative mother has previously received a transfusion of Rh-positive blood), but it increases with each subsequent pregnancy, just as it does in men or women of all ages with each transfusion, of Rh-positive blood. The risk becomes greater as the titre of the Rh-antibodies rises.

Rhesus Grouping must be carried out as a routine measure before any blood is transfused, for about 50 per cent. of Rh-negative recipients develop antibodies if given transfusions of Rh-positive blood. The Rh-grouping is particularly important before transfusions to (1) all young women, (2) all mothers who have had repeated stillbirths or whose newborn babies were jaundiced or anæmic, (3) any patient who may require further transfusions or who has already had a transfusion. The test serum for the Rh-antigen is usually derived from Rh-negative mothers sensitised against a Rh-positive fœtus. *Method.*—Add to one drop of such test serum in a small tube a similar-sized drop of a weak saline-suspension of red cells. The mixture is incubated for 2 hours at 37° C. The red cell sediment is then transferred to a slide with a pipette and examined with the low power of the microscope. If agglutination is present (that is if the cells clump together) the cells are Rh-positive; if absent, Rh-negative.

The rapid advances made during the last 20 years in immuno-hæmatology have made present-day knowledge a complex subject. Special textbooks should be consulted. Fisher's theory, which is now almost universally accepted, suggests that each chromosome concerned with the Rh-system carries three antigens of the three allelomorphic pairs, C and c, D and d, E and e. Combinations of these may produce eight allelomorphic genes CDe, CDE, CdE, Cde, cde, cdE, cDE, cDe. Each cell has two chromosomes, receiving one from each parent; a common genotype being CDe/CDe. The most important rhesus antigen is D, which is present in 85 per cent. of Europeans. The corresponding antigen is anti-D. The principal selection of cells for transfusion is made with pure anti-D sera. Red cells agglutinated by it are called Rhesus-positive; those not agglutinated are called Rhesus-negative and have a genotype containing -d-/-d-. Because of the unreliability of some anti-D sera this simple agglutination test should always be supplemented by *a direct cross-matching test before transfusion*.

CHOICE OF DONOR.—The blood donor should be a healthy person of either sex whose veins are readily felt in the cubital fossa. Age does not matter within wide limits. A fatty meal is best avoided before a blood donation. Certain *precautions* are necessary: (1) Syphilis, malaria and infective hepatitis are transmissible diseases which should be excluded in the donor. Syphilis is usually detected by the Wassermann reaction or a similar serological test, but these tests are occasionally negative or only doubtfully positive in the late primary or early secondary stages when the disease is most infectious. Storage in the blood bank for 6 days or more at 2–4° C will usually kill all spirochætes. It is safe to use a donor with a past history of malaria so long as he has (in the absence of treatment) had no febrile bout attributable to malaria for three years, nor resided in a malarial district during this period. Malarial plasmodia survive storage. In an emergency when no other blood is available, malarial blood may be used provided the recipient is treated with quinine immediately after the transfusion. Those who have had infective hepatitis or jaundice during the previous 18 months and those with allergic tendencies should not give blood. The processing and production of serum and plasma eliminates spirochætes and plasmodia during the filtration and subsequent drying, but the virus of infective hepatitis survives such procedures. (2) A husband should not give blood to his wife during the child-bearing period because of the risk that she may become sensitised to an agglutinogen which may be contained in the blood group of future children, who may then suffer from hæmolytic disease. (3) For deliberate transfusion the donor should be of the same ABO blood group as the patient, rather than a convenient Group O " universal donor," because of the risk of damage to the recipient's red cells by the presence of agglutinins particularly when large volumes of blood are transfused.

A direct matching test for compatibility between the patient's serum and a weak suspension of the donor's red cells in saline should always be made before any transfusion. The technique used will reveal compatibility within the ABO blood groups (Table XLI) but will not reveal Rh-incompatibility. So long as the recipient is Rh-positive (85 per cent. of white people) the Rh-group plays no part in the choice of donor. Sensitisation of these Rh-positive recipients is highly unlikely. Other red cell antigens such as the M and N factors, the Lutheran antibody, the Kell-Cellano agglutinogen, the Lewis antibody and the Duffy antigen do not play an important part in the selection of a donor—they only assume importance in some patients requiring repeated transfusions.

Indications for Rh-negative Blood.—It is highly desirable and may be essential that Rh-negative patients should only be transfused with Rh-negative blood, after ascertaining that their ABO groups are compatible. Since only 15 per cent. of donors are Rh-negative, this recommendation cannot always be met. However Rh-negative blood only, of the appropriate ABO groups, should be transfused to (1) Rh-negative young women. Transfusion of Rh-positive blood may sensitise a Rh-negative woman and may cause hæmolytic disease even in her first child, should she marry a Rh-positive husband. (2) Mothers of children with hæmolytic disease of the newborn or with a history of stillbirths. In 90 per cent. of such cases the child is Rh-positive and the mother Rh-negative with a Rh-antibody in her blood. (3) Rh-negative patients of either sex who may require further transfusions or who have had any previous transfusions. If a Rh-negative person is repeatedly transfused with Rh-positive blood, he may become sensitised with formation of an Rh-antibody and this may cause an incompatible transfusion reaction. (4) Infants with hæmolytic disease are usually Rh-positive. They may have a high content of Rh-antibody in their blood derived from their mother. Because of this, transfused Rh-negative blood is much less likely to be hæmolysed. Although the mother is probably Rh-negative, her blood is unsuitable because it contains Rh-antibody.

COLLECTION AND ADMINISTRATION OF BLOOD.—The equipment used in Great Britain in the National Blood Transfusion Service was developed and well tried before and during World War II. Transfusion equipment and technique in other countries is essentially similar in design with only slight variations. The bottle (Fig. 164) marked at 180 ml. and at 540 ml. is slightly waisted for ease of holding and is closed with a rubber wad set in an aluminium screw-cap; it is provided with a metal band and a loop at the base for hanging when inverted. As anticoagulant it contains 2 per cent. disodium citrate (100 ml.) and 15 per cent. glucose solution (20 ml.), made with freshly distilled water. This mixture ensures good keeping qualities for 420 ml. blood for about three weeks. *All equipment for blood transfusion is fully sterilised and all procedures should be carried out with an aseptic technique.*

Collecting Blood from the Donor.—The donor should be told that he will not feel anything unpleasant and that a small amount of local anæsthetic will be injected near the selected vein. He should lie comfortably on a couch and the elbow should rest on a firm cushion. The upper arm is compressed and a suitable vein is chosen. A sphygmomanometer cuff is placed on the upper arm and when all is ready this is inflated to about 40 mm. The skin in the bend of the elbow is cleansed with a swab soaked in ether, 80 per cent. methyl alcohol or other suitable solution. With a fine needle about 0·5 ml. of local anæsthetic (2 per cent. procaine hydrochlor.) is injected into the skin and subcutaneous tissue near or over the selected vein. After 2 or 3 minutes the needle of the taking set, with the bevel pointing downwards, is pushed gently and firmly in a slightly oblique path into the vein and then secured with adhesive plaster. As soon as the blood flow starts the bottle, which is held well below the patient's arm, should be gently and continuously shaken to produce an even mixture, as far as possible free of blood clots. The donor may be encouraged to open and close his fingers over a bandage or round a piece of wood without bending the wrist or elbow. When the 540 ml. mark has been reached (*i.e.*, 420 ml. of blood has been donated) the pressure in the sphygmomanometer cuff is released, the needle is gently withdrawn and the blood running in the rubber tubing is collected for purposes of testing in a small pilot test-tube or into a special receiving tube incorporated in the neck of the bottle. The main bottle containing the blood and (in the first of these arrangements) the pilot test-tube must be immediately labelled with the patient's name, the date, etc. A small dressing is applied over the venepuncture mark and kept in position for

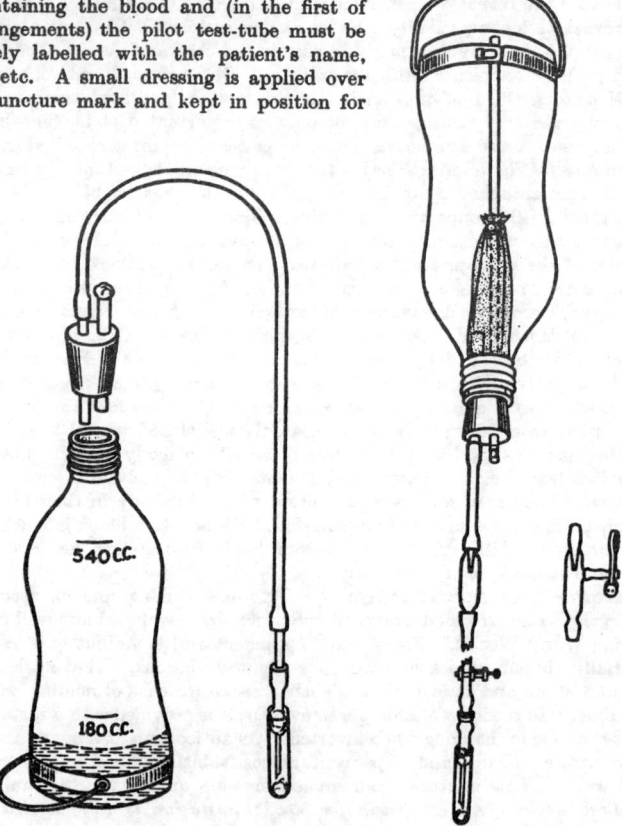

A   B

FIG. 164.—Standard Set for A. Blood Collection (" Taking set ").
B. Blood Administration ("Giving set").

24 hours. The donor should be allowed to rest for 10–15 minutes after the donation and should then be given some refreshment such as a cup of tea.

Administering Blood to the Patient.—Before giving a bottle of stored blood to the patient, when it is removed from the refrigerator make sure that (1) the details on the label tally with those of the laboratory report of the cross-matching test, and (2) there is no evidence of hæmolysis as shown by a pink zone just above the sedimented red cells, or of infection as shown by colour changes or turbidity. Blood showing such changes must be discarded. The bottle is then gently inverted a few times to secure an even mixture of the contents. If time permits the bottle should be placed for 20–30 minutes in water at 37° C but overheating must be avoided as it causes hæmolysis.

After removing the screw cap from the bottle, the rubber bung of the giving set is inserted firmly into the bottle. The long tube, which measures 25 cm., reaches almost to the bottom of the bottle to serve as an air inlet once the bottle is inverted (Fig. 164B). The inner opening of the shorter tube (6·5 cm. long) is encased in a gas mantle or fine-mesh metal filter so that blood clots cannot enter the drip-feed tube; the outer end of this same tube is connected by rubber tubing to a drip-feed glass bulb and then by about 90 cm. of rubber tubing to an adaptor and a sharp narrow-bore needle; a short distance above the adaptor there is a screw-clip with which to regulate the rate of flow. Having made sure the clip is screwed tightly on the rubber tubing and inserted the rubber bung, suspend the bottle on a hook near the patient. The two pieces of the adaptor are disconnected and the distal end with its short piece of tubing and needle are temporarily laid aside on a sterile towel. The small cork from the air inlet tube of the bottle is removed and the screw clip temporarily released to feed the system with blood.

Then select a suitable vein of the patient (see below) and after preparing the vein insert the needle; as soon as the blood flows freely the pressure around the upper arm is released and the male adaptor on the bottle side of the giving set is joined to the female adaptor near the needle. The screw-clip is slightly released, and the rate of flow of the blood adjusted to that deemed necessary, after which the needle is secured to the patient's skin by adhesive strapping. If the patient is restless the limb used for the transfusion may have to be bandaged to a back splint. To give subsequent bottles of blood the same administering unit is used again, and only the bottle containing the blood needs changing. A careful record must be kept of the details of the bottles of blood and other fluids given, the rate of flow and the time taken, with a 4-hourly temperature and pulse chart. It is desirable to record the blood pressure levels each hour. The site of infusion needs to be inspected regularly and the rate of flow checked. Occasionally a sample of blood is required for estimation of the blood electrolytes; this is obtained by temporarily disconnecting at the adaptor. Injection of fluids through the rubber tubing carries with it the risk of introducing air with subsequent air embolism.

Choice of Vein.—For the patient's comfort a vein in the forearm is preferable and allows greater freedom of movement of the elbow; in an emergency a vein in the cubital fossa is normally more prominent and less likely to be collapsed. When a " cut-down " on to a vein cannot be avoided, a short incision is made parallel to the vein selected and the vein dissected free; a cannula may then be inserted through an oblique cut in the vein and secured by a ligature. In children and in some adults who are to continue infusions for some time the internal saphenous vein in front of the internal malleolus is recommended; in infants one of the scalp veins and a small needle (such as a No. 14 record needle) may be used.

Dosage and Rate of Flow.—The amount of blood transfused must be decided for each case; one bottle of blood may be expected to raise the hæmoglobin value by 5–7 per cent. (0·7–1·0 G. per 100 ml.). After an acute hæmorrhage the amount transfused should be about the same as the amount lost; in shock one bottle of blood should raise the blood pressure about 10 mm. Hg. When the transfusion is to replace the loss of red cells the volume transfused is reduced by the use of red cell concentrates. The *rate of flow* varies according to circumstances. After an acute hæmorrhage the first two bottles should be given rapidly (one bottle in half an hour), but with larger volumes and after the blood pressure has returned to normal the rate of flow is usually 40–60 drops per minute through the drip bulb (approximately one bottle in 4 hours). Too fast a rate embarrasses the heart, distends the neck veins and may cause a rigor. *Children* require a higher proportion to body weight than adults, and usually need 20 ml. of whole blood per 1 Kg. (2¼ lb.) of body weight.

CONCENTRATED RED CELL SUSPENSIONS (" PACKED CELLS ") are prepared by syphoning off the supernatant plasma from two bottles of well-matched blood after the maximum sedimentation of red cells has occurred. The plasma can be used for other purposes and should not be discarded. Because of the slight risk of infection during preparation and because the removal of the plasma and of the glucose (which is a part of the anti-coagulant mixture) makes the red cells less stable, the suspension must be used within 24 hours. Such red cell suspensions should be pooled and administered slowly. The blood volume is only slightly increased by such suspensions and in shock whole blood is usually preferable. Packed cells are most useful in the treatment of anæmia (a) prior to operation, (b) in the presence of myocardial degeneration or heart failure, (c) in the anæmia associated with nephritis and (d) in aplastic anæmia, whether primary or secondary.

Exchange Transfusion.—Premature and full-term infants with hæmolytic disease of the newborn whose cord blood hæmoglobin is less than 11 G. per 100 ml. are treated by exchange transfusion made with a 20-ml. syringe and a three-way stop-cock which permits alternating withdrawal and transfusion; about 500-ml. of well-matched and slightly warmed blood may be given in exchange at one operation during the first two. days of life. Usually no further treatment is necessary (§ 330a).

Intramedullary infusion of blood or saline may be given where no surface veins are available, *e.g.,* in extensive burns or scalds. In adults and in children over two years the blood or saline is given through a bone marrow biopsy needle firmly set in the first part of the body of the sternum just below the sternal angle: after removal of the stilette connect the needle with the male adaptor of the transfusion set prepared as for an ordinary intravenous transfusion. In children under two years old the upper part of the tibia may be similarly used, approaching the bone from the upper and inner aspect. A slow steady flow into the marrow is achieved by gravity alone, the rate of flow tending gradually to increase in rate; pressure must be avoided.

BLOOD SUBSTITUTES.—For the treatment of shock whole blood, plasma and serum are about equally effective, but the red cells of whole blood begin to hæmolyse after storage for 3 weeks. *Fluid plasma* keeps in the dark at room temperature for about 2 years but after filtration it sometimes clots. This does not occur with serum, which is easier to prepare and keeps well for 2 years.

Dried Human Plasma and Serum remains well preserved, when prepared by approved methods, for 10 years; it does not need to be stored in a refrigerator but should be kept in a dark cool atmosphere. Plasma is obtained from citrated blood and serum from clotted blood. After reconstitution plasma contains about 5 per cent. of protein, including fibrinogen; owing to the diluent it contains less protein than serum—the latter has no fibrinogen but possesses about 7 per cent. of protein. During their preparation the plasma or serum from various blood groups is pooled. The resulting low agglutinin content makes it possible to ignore the blood groups during infusion.

For *Reconstitution,* to the dried solids from 400 ml. of plasma or serum contained in the usual bottle add an equivalent amount of sterile pyrogen-free distilled water (supplied in another bottle) just before use. To aid solution the mixture should be shaken and warmed to 37° C and the reconstituted fluid then has an opalescent appearance. The protein content may be raised by using less distilled water but then transfusion reactions are more frequent.

Indications.—The main use of plasma or serum is in the treatment of shock, the high protein content causing the blood volume to be restored and maintained much more effectively than by normal saline, but they should not be used when anæmia is present which makes it necessary to replace red cells. When the hæmoglobin level is less than 7 G. per 100 ml. (50 per cent.) *and* there is shock a whole blood transfusion must be given until the hæmoglobin has reached 11 G. per 100 ml. (75 per cent.) and the red cells are 3·7 million per c.mm. In shock without much hæmorrhage hæmo-concentration is frequently present, particularly following multiple injuries, crush injuries, extensive surgical operations and with burns and scalds, and under these conditions the shock can be effectively combated and the fall of blood pressure corrected and effectively maintained by the infusion of the proteins of plasma or serum. To avoid hæmo-concentration being overcorrected, with resulting hæmo-dilution, after the transfusion of two bottles of plasma or serum one bottle of whole blood should be given, the hæmoglobin and the blood pressure levels both needing to be checked periodically. Hypoproteinæmia in patients with nephrosis or chronic nephritis can be temporarily checked by plasma or serum infusions. They may also be given to patients requiring whole blood, pending the availability of the whole blood and its cross-matching and Rh-grouping.

Solutions of Various Inorganic Salts usually isotonic with the blood are given intravenously and by other routes for a variety of purposes. *Normal Saline Solution* (inject. sodium chloride B.P.) is 0·9 per cent. NaCl in distilled water. *Dextrose-saline* is also isotonic with the blood plasma and usually consists of 4 per cent. dextrose with 0·18 per cent. sodium chloride (one part of N saline to four parts of 5 per cent. dextrose in distilled water). *Ringer-Locke* solution (B.P.C.) is an isotonic solution with a more balanced electrolyte content as it contains sodium chloride, potassium chloride, calcium chloride, sodium bicarbonate and dextrose. These three solutions are useful in water or sodium chloride depletion but may be dangerous in shock, for the reduction of plasma proteins makes it impossible to retain the water in the circulation; they also increase the risk of pulmonary œdema.

Indications for intravenous saline solutions include: (i.) when no other fluid can be taken by mouth, about 5-6 pints must be given in 24 hours by slow continuous drip ;(ii.) severe diarrhœa; (iii.) the crises of Addison's disease and of severe anterior pituitary deficiency; (iv.) uræmia, diabetic coma; and (v.) in poisoning from aspirin, carbolic acid or strychnine. As with blood transfusions a regular check must be kept on the blood pressure, the filling of the neck veins, the pulse and temperature. Regular hæmoglobin estimations help to prevent hæmo-dilution and hæmo-concentration. Blood electrolyte analyses (sodium, potassium, chloride and bicarbonate) make it possible to achieve electrolyte balance by promptly varying the constitution of the fluids being given. A wise precaution is to add 5 ml. of 20 per cent. calcium chloride to the intravenous drip for every bottle of blood administered.

Rectal saline may be given as a half-strength solution (0·45 per cent. sodium chloride) with a slow continuous drip of about 60 drops per minute through a rubber catheter. This is particularly suitable in dehydration and for the first 24–48 hours after abdominal operations.

Subcutaneous saline (0·9 per cent. sodium chloride) is given into the loose areolar tissue of the thigh or abdominal wall at a rate of about 250 ml. in 4–6 hours.

Dextran is a polymerised polysaccharide compound of glucose units. Its administration helps to restore the blood pressure when blood products are not available but it does not overcome the danger of dilution of plasma proteins and of red cells.

Fractionated Blood Proteins are available as dry powders. (i.) Albumen helps to restore blood volume. (ii.) Immune globulins prevent or attenuate measles (§ 481). (iii.) Fibrinogen is used as a hæmostatic. (iv.) Antihæmophilic globulin, which also contains fibrinogen, is specific for the treatment of acute bleeding in hæmophilia. The human preparation can be given repeatedly but antihæmophilic globulin prepared from beef or pork can only be given once because of sensitisation to the foreign protein.

TRANSFUSION REACTIONS AND COMPLICATIONS may be classified as follows:—

(1) *Simple febrile reactions* occur in 2–5 per cent. of all transfusions. They are due to foreign protein, dead bacteria, inadequately prepared distilled water or the transfusion of over-age blood. These reactions usually develop towards the end or shortly after a transfusion and may be accompanied by rigors. *Treatment* is by reducing the rate of flow or stopping the transfusion of blood, keeping the patient warm and giving brandy. If more severe, a hypodermic injection of morphia (gr. ⅓–½) and inject. adrenaline B.P.(ℳ 10–15) are given. The remainder of the blood being transfused should be bacteriologically investigated and if necessary the appropriate antibiotic should be given. Transient mild jaundice and renal complications occasionally develop following the transfusion of over-age blood.

(2) *Reactions due to transfusion of incompatible blood* should be prevented by careful blood grouping, a direct cross-matching test and by realising that a clerical error may be dangerous to life.   As little as 50 ml. of incompatible blood may cause rapid death from circulatory collapse, but larger quantities are sometimes tolerated with little or no reaction.

Symptoms include violent pain in the back or loins, rigors, respiratory embarrassment, circulatory collapse, hæmoglobinuria or oliguria, jaundice, urticaria and focal symptoms due to small hæmorrhages or emboli in the brain, mesentery and myocardium.   If the patient survives the immediate symptoms, uræmia and renal failure may follow.   Incompatibility in the ABO group is more likely to cause severe reaction than incompatibility in the Rh-group, although the latter may cause jaundice some hours after the transfusion.   The renal damage following an incompatible transfusion is due to arterial spasm and ischæmia and not due to blocking of the renal tubules by the products of hæmolysed red cells as was once believed ; at autopsy acute tubular necrosis is a common finding (§ 428).

Treatment.—(a) In the first phase of shock and peripheral circulatory failure, plasma should be given if dehydration is present, but compatible blood must be given if much blood has been lost.   These measures must be prompt and continued for about 12 hours.   (b) In the second stage of renal failure which may become evident in 24 hours and which lasts for a few days up to 3 weeks, the danger is mainly one of electrolyte imbalance.   The intake and loss of water should be balanced; and potassium intoxication and water retention overcome by peritoneal dialysis or with the artificial kidney.   (c) In the third stage of diuresis as the danger of renal failure diminishes, the control of water and of salt balance become more important.   Frequent blood electrolyte estimations must guide the decision to increase or decrease sodium, potassium, chloride and water.   (d) In convalescence which may last 1-9 months the treatment is similar to that of chronic nephritis; it needs to be continued until the renal function is back to normal.

(3) *Mild allergic manifestations.*—e.g., urticaria or localised œdema—are sometimes caused by hypersensitivity to plasma proteins; they respond to inject. adrenaline or to the anti-histamines.   Grossly infected blood may produce a clinical condition resembling severe protein shock.

COMPLICATIONS OF TRANSFUSIONS are (1) Circulatory with cardiac failure and pulmonary œdema.   The circulation may easily be overloaded, particularly in an anæmic patient whose heart may suffer from fatty changes in the myocardium.   The type of fluid given, its volume and the rate of transfusion must be carefully judged to prevent this.   (2) Transmission of disease by way of a transfusion is rare except with homologous serum hepatitis (§ 334 and page 806).   The virus of hepatitis may be transmitted from apparently healthy donors, and because the incubation period is so long the association between jaundice and the previous transfusion may be overlooked.   In most cases the disease is mild but occasionally it can lead to acute yellow atrophy and death (§ 334a).

§ 547a.   SERUM ELECTROLYTE CONCENTRATIONS AND IMBALANCES.—Flame photometry provides a ready method of estimating the serum sodium and potassium concentrations; these are supplemented by measuring the serum content of chloride and of bicarbonate.   The serum electrolytes are in dynamic equilibrium with the same electrolytes in the extra-cellular fluids and in the cells but they are not necessarily in proportion to one another.   Thus potassium, which is normally in a high concentration in the cells, passes into the serum to make up for loss of extra-cellular fluid and of sodium chloride in severe diarrhœa and/or vomiting: this causes a lowered intracellular content of potassium with a raised serum potassium value.

The serum sodium values are important chiefly because they give an index of the osmotic pressure of the body-fluids; they do not necessarily reflect the total amount of fluid or salt present in the body for they can be low in states of dehydration, and also in states of over-hydration when the body tissues are œdematous and contain an excess of sodium.   The clinical states associated with low and with high potassium serum concentrations are much more clearly defined than those associated with corresponding changes in the values of the sodium. In clinical practice it is rare to find a pathological variation of a single substance in the serum—usually several are involved.

Hyponatræmia (low serum-sodium values) occurs with water intoxication (cellular over-hydration), in patients on a low sodium diet and in those who are vigorously treated with diuretics. The *Symptoms* are mental apathy, disorientation and later convulsions and coma. The voluntary muscles may show loss of tone and of tendon reflexes, and cramp is common; nausea and vomiting may be produced. *Treatment* is by infusion of hypertonic NaCl, or in states of deficiency of blood bicarbonate by the addition of intravenous sodium bicarbonate or sodium lactate.

Hypernatræmia (high serum-sodium values) is usually due to a deficient water intake when the patient is already apathetic or in coma. It is well illustrated by the condition of shipwrecked sailors who are short of water, and is produced in those who voluntarily abstain from drinking water, after the infusion of excess of hypertonic saline and in aldosteronism. The *symptoms* are excessive thirst and mental imbalance leading to coma. *Treatment* is by giving intravenous 5 per cent. dextrose or water by mouth.

Hypokalæmia (low serum-potassium values—below 3 mEq./litre) occurs after the use of diuretics (especially the chlorothiazides), in potassium-losing nephritis, in familial periodic paralysis, in severe diarrhœa and vomiting, in the treatment of diabetic coma by N-saline and insulin and in Conn's syndrome. The *Symptoms* are (i.) weakness of the voluntary muscles, hypotonia and loss of the tendon reflexes; (ii.) tachycardia, various arrhythmias and an increased susceptibility to digitalis, accompanied by electrocardiographic changes with a decreased QRS amplitude, prolonged and often depressed ST segment, flattening or inversion of the T waves and the appearance of U waves; (iii.) cardiac failure and myocardial necrosis; (iv.) polyuria and thirst and (v.) mental disturbances and paralytic ileus. *Treatment* is by giving potassium chloride 5–10 G. a day, or intravenously at a concentration not above 2 G. per litre.

Hyperkalæmia (high serum-potassium values) also notably affects the skeletal and the cardiac muscles. It follows excessive doses of potassium salts and may be found in chronic nephritis. *Symptoms.*—(i.) There may be widespread muscle weakness or paralysis (including the diaphragm). (ii.) The electrocardiogram shows a peaked T wave, distortion of the QRS complex with intraventricular block and when it reaches 7 mEq./litre the heart action becomes irregular and may become arrested in diastole; (iii.) paræsthesiæ may occur. *Treatment* is by giving glucose and insulin; intravenous calcium salts help.

(b) *The patient is* ANÆMIC, *but* HÆMORRHAGE HAS BEEN EXCLUDED *as the cause of the anæmia.* *There is often a* PRIMARY DISEASE OF THE BLOOD FORMING ORGANS *with* DEFICIENT FORMATION OR EXCESSIVE DESTRUCTION *of the hæmoglobin and red blood cells.* The causes are:—

Common.

I. Pernicious anæmia (§ 548).

II. Iron-deficiency anæmia (§ 549).

III. *Associated with Acute or Chronic Infection or Toxic Processes* (§ 550).
   Acute: especially
      Septicæmia(§ 516).
      Subacute bacterial endocarditis (§ 50a).
      Acute rheumatic carditis (§ 592).

   Chronic: especially
      Focal sepsis and
      Suppuration (§ 517).

Common (contd.)

Renal disease (§ 371).
Tuberculosis (§ 131).
Amyloid disease (§ 409).
IV. *With marked emaciation.*
      Carcinomatosis (§ 551).
      Leuco-erythroblastic anæmia (§ 551).

Rarer.

I. Aplastic anæmia (§ 552).
II. Acquired hæmolytic anæmia (§ 553).

Rarer (contd.)

With enlarged spleen and/or lymph glands.
- III. Acute leukæmia (§ 554).
- IV. Acute erythræmic myelosis (§ 555).
- V. Chronic myeloid leukæmia (§ 556).
- VI. Chronic lymphatic leukæmia (§ 557).
- VII. Leukæmoid blood states (§ 558).
- VIII. Hodgkin's disease (§ 584).
- IX. Acholuric jaundice (§ 331).
- X. Splenic anæmia (§ 559).
- XI. Myelomatosis (§§ 559 and 613).
- XII. Osteosclerosis and myelofibrosis (§ 559).
- XIII. Gaucher's disease (§ 559).

Rarer (contd.)

With spongy gums, tender limbs and hæmorrhages.
- XIV. Scurvy (§ 560).

With recurrent bleeding after trivial injuries.
- XV. Hæmophilia (§ 561).

With hæmoglobin in the urine.
- XVI. Paroxysmal or nocturnal hæmoglobinuria (§ 414).

With residence in the tropics.
- XVII. Malaria (§ 512).
- XVIII. Ankylostomiasis (§ 563).
- XIX. Sickle-cell anæmia (§ 564).

With destruction of red cells or marrow.
- XX. Hæmolytic anæmia (§ 565).
- XXI. After exposure to ionising radiation or industrial poisons (§ 566).

For the Anæmias in Infancy and Childhood see § 567.

The patient is **markedly anæmic** *and there is* NO EVIDENCE OF MANIFEST OR OCCULT HÆMORRHAGE OR OTHER OBVIOUS ORGANIC LESION. *The patient is at or past middle-age, may show a* LEMON-YELLOW COLOUR IN THE SKIN AND COMPLAIN OF A SORE TONGUE AND OF PARÆSTHESIÆ IN THE FINGERS OR TOES. *The disease is probably* PERNICIOUS ANÆMIA.

§ 548. I. Pernicious Anæmia (Syn. Addisonian Anæmia) is met in persons of both sexes and its course shows remissions and relapses. It is characterised by large red cells in the blood due to the formation of megaloblasts in the bone marrow and is caused by the lack of Castle's gastric intrinsic factor.

Symptoms include general debility, loss of weight, pallor and those of anæmia *per se* (§ 545) but even in advanced cases dyspnœa may not be marked. The symptoms peculiar to the disease comprise: (1) The general appearance, a lemon-yellow tint in the skin with a distinct malar flush occurs in a severe relapse. Almost all patients have silver-grey hair or the hair has become prematurely grey. They often look well-nourished in spite of some loss of weight. A low-grade fever may occur even in the absence of infection. (2) The tongue is sore, red and raw, smooth and denuded of papillæ in 50 per cent. of cases. The soreness disappears spontaneously and also with specific treatment. (3) Anorexia, nausea, vomiting and diarrhœa are the result of gastro-intestinal disturbances, which may cause colicky pain. A fractional test meal shows achylia gastrica so that no acid or pepsin is secreted even after an injection of histamine. The presence of free hydrochloric acid in the gastric juice of a patient suspected of pernicious anæmia should make one question the diagnosis. The achylia usually persists even when the anæmia is fully

rectified.   Following the loss of hydrochloric acid and of pepsin the loss of
the gastric intrinsic factor is slowly progressive.   (4) The spleen is slightly
enlarged in a few cases.   (5) Neurological symptoms are common.   Tingling
and numbness of the fingers and of the toes are due to peripheral neuritis.
This condition and the symptoms and signs of subacute combined degeneration of the cord (§ 950) may precede obvious anæmia and cause difficulty
in diagnosis.   The cranial nerves are not usually affected but optic neuritis
may be an early symptom.   Euphoria is fairly common; depression and
lack of mental energy are unusual.   (6) Hæmorrhages into the retina, ear
or sometimes into other organs are rare.

   Blood changes (Fig. 165): (1) *Red cells.*   (a) The red cell deficiency is

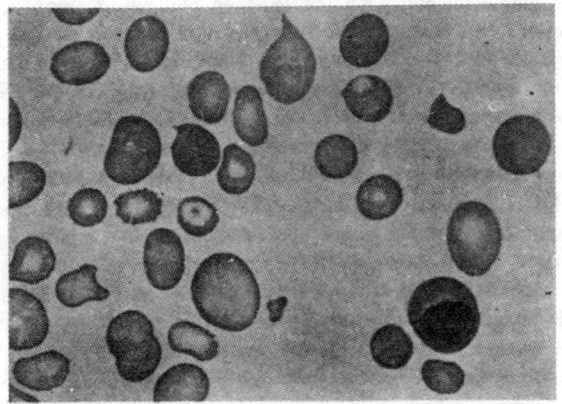

FIG. 165.—Blood film of patient in a relapse of Pernicious Anæmia.

much more marked than is the hæmoglobin deficiency.   The hæmoglobin
is often around 20–40 per cent. (3·0–6·0 G. per 100 ml.).   (b) The colour
index is above 1·0, for the larger red cells contain more hæmoglobin than
cells of normal size; even so the mean corpuscular hæmoglobin concentration is within the normal range unless there is also an iron deficiency
(" dimorphic anæmia ").   (c) The mean corpuscular diameter is often 8 to
9μ (normal average 7·3 μ); and the mean corpuscular volume is about
120 cu. microns (normal average 86 cu. μ).   (d) There is marked anisocytosis with many large cells (megalocytes) but also many small cells
(microcytes).   The frequency distribution (Price-Jones) curve shows a
depressed and broadened peak which is shifted to the right.   Poikilocytosis
is marked; nucleated red cells, some with small pyknotic nuclei and others
with a typical megaloblastic appearance are seen in the blood of patients
with a severe relapse.   (2) *White cells.*   In a well marked case there is a
leucopenia, the neutrophils numbering 2,000 per c.mm. or less; some of
these have 5 or 6 lobes to their nuclei.   Myelocytes also occur.   (3) *Platelets.*
In about 25 per cent. of cases these are reduced to 40,000–80,000 per c.mm.

(4) The *indirect Van den Bergh reaction* (§ 333) shows an excess of serum bilirubin (approx. 1·0 mg. per 100 ml.). The urine contains an excess of urobilinogen (§ 383). (5) The *bone marrow* in a typical case shows many megaloblasts (§ 541) even when the blood is not markedly anæmic. The normal myeloid–erythroid ratio in the blood is 8 : 1 or 2 : 1 (Table XXXIX) but in pernicious anæmia this may be altered to 1 : 10. Giant forms of neutrophils and myelocytes are common. Within 24 hours of a single dose of cyanocobalamin (B₁₂) most megaloblasts are transformed into normoblasts, the effects lasting 6 months or more. (6) Gastric biopsy specimens show atrophy of all the coats of the stomach. (7) The serum B₁₂ level is low and the Schilling test (§ 1216) is of great value.

Diagnosis.—The age and appearance of the patient, the insidious onset, raw tongue, paræsthesiæ, with the low red cell count, high colour index, raised mean red-cell diameter and corpuscular volume, and especially the achylia gastrica and the megaloblastic bone marrow make the diagnosis easy in most cases. A most important diagnostic feature is the high reticulocyte response (even up to 20 per cent.) which follows 8–10 days after specific therapy has been started. The distinction from other megaloblastic anæmias is made on the history and the results of investigations (p. 819). Anæmia with large cells (macrocytes) and nucleated red cells can occur during rapid blood regeneration as after a large hæmorrhage, after prolonged severe exercise, after splenectomy and in diseases of the liver involving destruction of the liver parenchyma. In *acholuric jaundice* the osmotic fragility is altered. *Iron-deficiency anæmia* is much more common in women; the skin is not lemon-yellow in colour, the serum bilirubin value is normal and koilonychia is common. The blood shows a low mean corpuscular hæmoglobin concentration. *Dimorphic anæmia* is occasionally seen when pernicious anæmia and iron-deficiency anæmia co-exist, especially when there is rapid regeneration of red cells induced by vitamin B₁₂ injections. *Carcinoma of the stomach* with hæmatogenous spread to the bone marrow may cause a similar type of anæmia. *Aplastic anæmia* and aleukæmic leukæmia are excluded by examination of the blood and of the bone marrow.

Etiology.—Pernicious anæmia is met chiefly after the age of 40; it affects the white races in particular and is rarely seen in Negroes and Asiatics. Several members of a family are affected in 10 per cent. of cases. Chronic gastritis leading to atrophy of the gastric mucous membrane may be a common factor. The specific defect in pernicious anæmia is the absence from the gastric juice of Castle's intrinsic factor, without which cyanocobalamin cannot be properly absorbed.

Cyanocobalamin (B.P.), otherwise known as Vitamin B₁₂, is regarded as identical with the extrinsic factor, present in the ordinary diet. It is present in the media on which *Streptomyces griseus* has been cultured, as well as in liver; it contains cobalt and can be crystallised as small red needles. The intrinsic factor (hæmopoietin) is contained in normal gastric juice and in man is secreted in a higher concentration from the cardiac portion of the

TABLE XLII.—THE ETIOLOGY OF THE MACROCYTIC ANÆMIAS

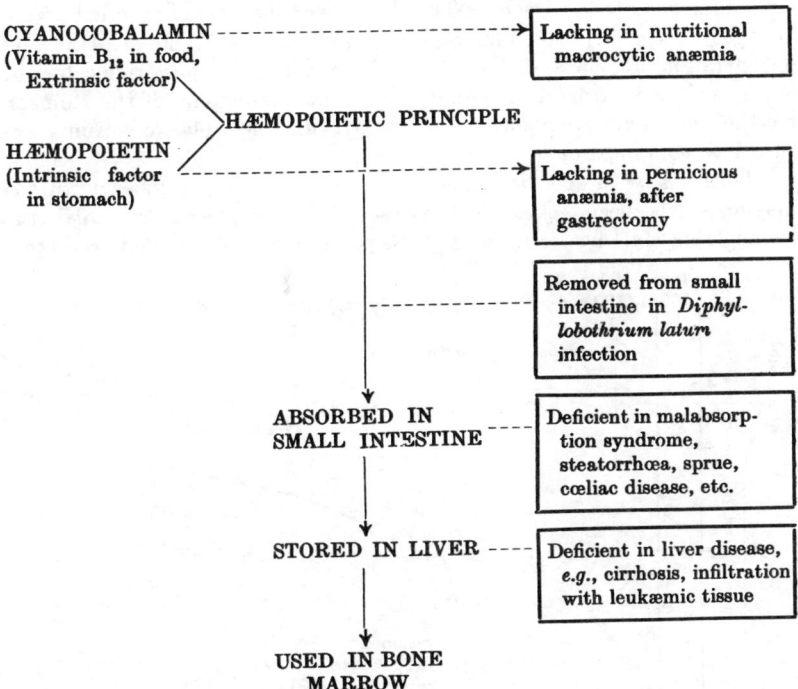

CYANOCOBALAMIN - → | Lacking in nutritional macrocytic anæmia
(Vitamin B$_{12}$ in food, Extrinsic factor)

HÆMOPOIETIC PRINCIPLE

HÆMOPOIETIN - → | Lacking in pernicious anæmia, after gastrectomy
(Intrinsic factor in stomach)

- - - - - - - - - - - - | Removed from small intestine in *Diphyllobothrium latum* infection

ABSORBED IN SMALL INTESTINE - - - - | Deficient in malabsorption syndrome, steatorrhœa, sprue, cœliac disease, etc.

STORED IN LIVER - - - - | Deficient in liver disease, *e.g.*, cirrhosis, infiltration with leukæmic tissue

USED IN BONE MARROW

stomach—in certain animals more is obtained from the pyloric end. Cyanocobalamin can only be absorbed in the presence of the intrinsic factor, in the duodenum and upper part of the small intestine; it is then stored particularly in the liver. A deficient absorption of vitamin B$_{12}$ can be corrected by injecting it parenterally or as an injection of liver concentrate, or by feeding the intrinsic factor in the form of desiccated hog's stomach. In the absence of a sufficiency of intrinsic factor or of extrinsic factor, or when their absorption or storage is faulty, the red bone marrow fails to produce an orderly series of normoblasts and the earliest red cell precursors (the proerythroblasts) produce instead a series of megaloblasts which may outnumber the other cells in the marrow. These are stored in the bone marrow and produce a megalocytic anæmia, as well as causing disturbances of the myeloid cells and the megakaryocytes—thus producing the blood picture previously described. Adequate treatment usually corrects these changes.

Prognosis.—Before the discovery of the specific effect of liver therapy, pernicious anæmia was slowly progressive and almost always fatal. Following efficient regular treatment with inject. cyanocobalamin or with liver extracts no patient need now die from the disease. Although modern treatment no longer makes the disease " pernicious " or fatal, the name pernicious anæmia retains its usefulness. If *complications* occur this is a sign of inadequate treatment. The chief are cardiac weakness due to fatty changes in the myocardium, vomiting and diarrhœa, polyneuritis and degeneration of the spinal cord chiefly affecting the posterior columns. With modern treatment of pernicious anæmia, carcinoma of the stomach has become more frequent. Chronic arthritis and aplastic anæmia are rare late complications.

Treatment with specific remedies should not be commenced until the diagnosis has been established. Rest in bed is necessary until the hæmoglobin level has returned to 9 G. per 100 ml. (60 per cent. Haldane)

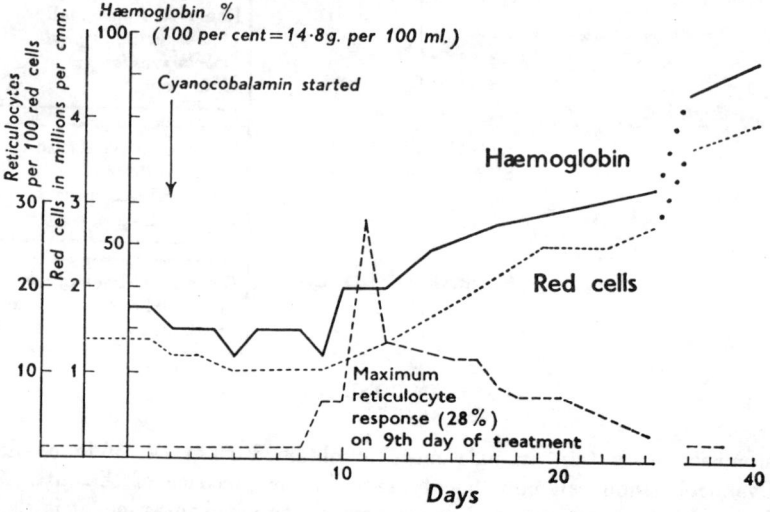

FIG. 166.—Hæmatological response of patient with severe Pernicious Anæmia to administration of cyanocobalamin. (In this patient it was given with the intrinsic factor, by mouth.)

because of the damage due to fatty changes in the myocardium. Transfusion of well-matched blood helps seriously ill patients and when sepsis is present, until specific measures have had time to act. A *relapse* is easily and most economically treated by intramusc. injections of cyanocobalamin (B.P.) in daily doses of 100 μg. until recovery is complete (Fig. 166); larger doses are necessary in the presence of sepsis or arteriosclerosis. Allergic reactions to vitamin B_{12} are very rare. Often the patient has a sense of well-being after one or two doses, but treatment *must* be continued; very few patients with typical Addisonian anæmia do not respond to this. Hydroxycobalamin (Neocytamen) in similar doses is probably rather more effective than cyanocobalamin. Alternatively, carefully standardised preparations of liver extract may be injected intramusc.—with an initial dose of 15 (U.S.P.) units, then 10 units daily for a week, followed by 10 units once a week and thereafter 10–15 units each 2–3 weeks for the rest of the patient's life. Raw or undercooked liver, proteolysed liver and desiccated stomach extracts are now rarely given. In addition to

specific therapy iron preparations may be needed to overcome the shortage of iron in the tissues resulting from the rapid production of red cells;
the indication for iron is when the mean corpuscular hæmoglobin concentration falls below 32 per cent. *Maintenance treatment* must never
stop and must be adjusted to the individual patient's needs, so as to maintain the red cell count above 5,000,000 per c.mm. The danger of subacute combined degeneration of the cord increases when this level is not
maintained. The patient should be told that his feeling of well-being is not
an index of satisfactory treatment. Monthly clinical and hæmatological
examinations can be combined with monthly injections of cyanocobalamin.
The dose must be increased during an acute infection: sometimes it is
necessary to change the preparation used to effect a satisfactory hæmatological response. A combination of oral vitamin B_{12} with the intrinsic
factor may be taken by mouth (Fig. 166) but the response is not always
satisfactory. Folic acid (5–20 mg. daily) by mouth induces a satisfactory
response in the blood but gives no protection against neurological complications; it can be used in *pernicious anæmia of pregnancy* which in any case
resolves during the puerperium. A few cases fail to respond to vitamin B_{12}
due to hypothyroidism, but do so when given small doses of thyroid.

Other Megaloblastic Anæmias resemble pernicious anæmia in many
ways but they tend to be less severe clinically and pathologically.

(1) MEGALOCYTIC TROPICAL ANÆMIA (§ 562), which is widespread in
the thickly populated areas of Asia and Africa, is due to deficiency of the
extrinsic factor in the diet. It becomes more obvious with malnutrition
and a very poor protein intake.

(2) PARTIAL GASTRECTOMY and CARCINOMA OF THE STOMACH cause a
failure in production of the intrinsic factor. A certain number of such
patients develop macrocytic anæmia.

(3) The MALABSORPTION SYNDROME causes a failure of absorption of
the hæmopoietic principle in the small intestine (§ 316). This occurs in
idiopathic steatorrhœa, cœliac disease, sprue and more rarely in chronic
diarrhœa and in intestinal hurry. With gastro-colic fistulæ, blind loops
of the ileum and after gastro-enterostomy the formed hæmopoietic factor
may be destroyed in the gut by the altered bacterial flora.

(4) The DIPHYLLOBOTHRIUM LATUM worm (§ 304), the fish tapeworm,
causes anæmia indistinguishable clinically and hæmatologically from pernicious anæmia. The worm has a peculiar avidity for vitamin B_{12} and
may assimilate large quantities. *Treatment* with the vitamin is therefore
unsuccessful until the worm has been expelled.

(5) SEVERE LIVER DISEASE such as cirrhosis and heavy infiltration with
leukæmic tissue may cause macrocytic anæmia, sometimes with a megaloblastic marrow, because the liver cannot store the hæmopoietic principle.

(6) *Achrestic Anæmia* was regarded as a type of megaloblastic anæmia due to
failure of the bone marrow to utilise the hæmopoietic principle present in the liver.
Its existence is now in doubt for there are a number of cases of anæmia resembling
pernicious anæmia which are refractory to accepted lines of treatment but which may
respond to one or more of proteolysed liver, folic acid or fresh liver.

Whatever the cause of megaloblastic anæmia, one of the most important diagnostic features of this group is the reticulocyte response (up to 15–20 per cent.) which follows 8 to 10 days after administration of the specific hæmatinic and the disappearance of the megaloblastic bone marrow (normoblastic transformation) 3 to 4 days after commencing treatment, with a clinical and hæmatological remission.

The patient is a woman of middle-age with **anæmia** *who is in poor health;* the SPLEEN MAY BE PALPABLE, the FINGER-NAILS ARE SPOON-SHAPED and THE BLOOD *shows the red cells to be smaller than normal, pale and with a low mean corpuscular hæmoglobin concentration.* *The disease is probably* IRON-DEFICIENCY ANÆMIA.

§ 549. II. **Iron-Deficiency Anæmia** (Syn. Simple Hypochromic Anæmia) is insidious in onset and chiefly affects women over the age of 35. Less severe forms are common in infancy and childhood. It responds to adequate doses of iron but may recur later. It is more marked following menorrhagia and during pregnancy.

Symptoms comprise those due to anæmia *per se* (§ 545) and those belonging to the disease itself. The latter are: (1) poor health with weakness, lassitude, headaches, loss of appetite, indigestion, chronic abdominal pain and constipation. (2) The skin and mucous membranes are pale although the tongue may be red and usually painless. (3) Dysphagia, glossitis and anæmia characterise the Plummer-Vinson syndrome (§ 226); this may be associated with post-cricoid or œsophageal webs which need cutting through an œsophagoscope. (4) In most cases there is a low acid content of the gastric juice or achlorhydria. (5) The spleen may be moderately enlarged. (6) Spoon-shaped, thin brittle nails (koilonychia) are common (Fig. 168).

Blood changes. There is a deficiency of hæmoglobin which is greater than the deficiency of red cells; thus the hæmoglobin may be 30 to 50 per cent. (5·0–7·5 G. per 100 ml.) and the red cells 3·5 to 4·5 million per c.mm.: this causes a low colour index (0·4–0·6), pallor of the red cells (hypochromia) and a low mean corpuscular hæmoglobin concentration (23–29 per cent.). The red cells are usually smaller than normal (mean cell diameter 6·5–6·8 μ), and the mean corpuscular volume 60–70 cu.μ (normal 78–94 cu.μ). When stained the cells show marked anisocytosis and poikilocytosis and sometimes consist merely of a ring of cytoplasm ("pessary forms"); when anæmia is severe normoblasts may be seen. The leucocytes and platelets are usually normal or a little reduced in numbers. The plasma is usually pale due to a reduction of iron compounds down to half the usual amount (normal 100–120 μg. per 100 ml.). *The bone marrow* shows normoblastic hyperplasia, the red cell precursors making up half the number of red cells.

Diagnosis.—Because of the vague symptoms, patients may be diagnosed as having a neurosis; a careful clinical and hæmatological examination will disclose an iron-deficiency anæmia. *Pernicious anæmia* is distinguished by the symptoms and the characteristic blood and bone marrow findings. *Aplastic anæmia* causes neutropenia and thrombocytopenia as well. Other conditions which cause an iron-deficiency anæmia and a similar blood picture are recurrent hæmorrhage as from the gastro-intestinal tract, from hæmorrhoids or from uterine fibroids; chronic infections such as from tuberculosis or dental sepsis; ankylostomiasis or other helminth infestation, carcinomatosis and myxœdema. If the patient fails to respond to iron therapy the diagnosis must be reviewed but in favourable cases the hæmoglobin does not rise more quickly than 1 per cent. a day. SECONDARY ANÆMIA which often has the characters of an iron-deficiency anæmia, is more common than a PRIMARY ANÆMIA—that is

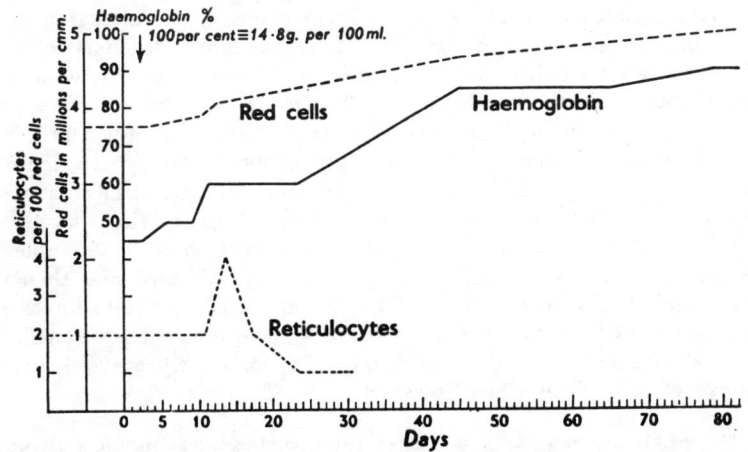

FIG. 167.—A woman of 50 years with severe Iron-deficiency Anæmia. Before treatment mean-cell diameter 6·8 μ and mean hæmoglobin concentration 23 per cent. Treatment started on day 1 with 215 mg. of oral iron daily and was continued throughout the whole period.

anæmia in the course of a disorder of erythropoiesis. Until the underlying cause has been treated successfully, iron therapy will not help.

Etiology.—The immediate cause is unknown but a diet lacking in animal protein and an insufficiency of iron in the diet, linked with inadequate absorption due to hypochlorhydria are important factors, especially when combined with excessive blood loss. Multiple pregnancies are a frequent cause. *Premature infants* are especially liable to suffer from iron-deficiency.

Iron Metabolism. Only a small proportion of iron in the diet is available for the synthesis of hæmoglobin (§ 545). Inorganic iron is readily absorbed (ferrous iron more so than ferric iron), but iron in organic combination must first be broken down. Because iron salts are poorly dissociated in neutral or alkaline solutions, most of the absorption occurs in the stomach and upper part of the small intestine within 4–8 hours of ingestion. The normal serum iron is 100 μg. per 100 ml., the unsaturated iron-binding capacity 200 μg., making the total iron saturation capacity 300 μg. per 100 ml. of serum. The ordinary diet must supply 5 mg. of iron daily for a normal man, but 15 mg. is needed daily by a woman or a growing child.

Prognosis.—The disease is never fatal by itself, but it is a common cause of prolonged ill-health and a liability to infections. No woman should be allowed to undertake childbirth unless the hæmoglobin has been checked and iron-deficiency corrected.

Treatment.—Iron therapy is specific in this disease and it is better to give too much than only just enough. Suitable preparations are ferrous sulphate 0·5 G. t.i.d., iron and ammonium citrate 2 G. in chloroform water, Blaud's pill (ferrous carbonate) 1 G. t.i.d. or ferrous gluconate 0·6 G. t.i.d. The patient should be warned that during treatment the stools will be black; and if these doses cause headache, nausea, attacks of diarrhœa and sometimes constipation, they may have to be reduced. Iron and ammonium citrate solution taken in milk and ferrous gluconate are much less likely to produce these side-effects. Intravenous saccharated iron oxide (such as Ferrivenin) or intramusc. iron–dextran complex (such as Imferon) are useful when oral iron preparations are poorly tolerated. Occasionally ascorbic acid assists the absorption of iron. When there is dyspepsia, acid hydrochlor. dil. $\mathfrak{M}$ 60 in water t.i.d. is of value. Adjustment of the diet alone seldom achieves a good response but a good wholesome diet should be supplemented by liver, brown bread and oatmeal. In many instances the plasma proteins are low and then a high protein diet is necessary. About a week after commencing treatment there is a temporary increase of reticulocytes (up to 10 per cent. of red cells) and then the hæmoglobin begins to rise slowly. Treatment must be continued until the hæmoglobin is back to normal; as relapses are common the hæmoglobin value should be estimated each 3 to 6 months for a few years and further courses of iron given when necessary.

Chlorosis is now very rare. It is a peculiar type of iron-deficiency anæmia which occurs in young women at or soon after puberty. The *symptoms* are those of anæmia and the name was derived from the unusual greenish-yellow colour of the complexion. There is also scanty menstruation or amenorrhœa and a perverted appetite. The blood volume is usually increased. *Treatment* with iron preparations must be continued for a long time and measures taken to ensure plenty of fresh air and outdoor exercise.

The patient is PALE *and* ANÆMIC, *there is* RECURRING PYREXIA *and careful search reveals an* ACUTE *or* CHRONIC *infection.*

§ 550. III. Infection causes anæmia by preventing proper utilisation of essential erythropoietic substances or by a toxic effect on the bone marrow, or it may destroy red cells by hæmolysis.

Symptoms.—The anæmia produced is of varying severity; the red cells are usually of normal size but eventually tend to resemble a mild iron-deficiency anæmia; occasionally acute or chronic aplastic episodes occur. Infection is usually accompanied by intermittent pyrexia (§ 471) and by weakness and wasting (§ 569). A full blood examination is of value. Most pyogenic infections cause a neutrophil leucocytosis of 10,000–20,000 per c.mm.; when the figure reaches 60,000–80,000 per c.mm., an abscess or peritonitis must be looked for. Severe infections may cause myelocytes to appear with excessive " toxic " granulation in the neutrophils. In many

virus infections the leucocytes are normal or there is a temporary increase
in the lymphocytes and monocytes.

Etiology.—Septicæmia, bacterial endocarditis, the acute fevers including rheumatic fever, staphylococcal infections (such as osteomyelitis,
perinephric abscess and staphylococcal pneumonia), hæmolytic streptococcal infections (such as scarlet fever and puerperal sepsis), ulcerative
colitis, tropical protozoal diseases (such as malaria and kala-azar) and
most forms of chronic suppuration all cause anæmia of varying degree.
Hæmolytic anæmias may occur in gas gangrene (due to *Cl. Welchii* infection), septicæmia with *Strep. hæmolyticus*, malaria and in some virus
infections.

Treatment is that of the underlying condition. To ensure a sufficiency
of the erythropoietic factors the diet should be as full and varied as possible. When there is evidence of iron-deficiency, iron salts should be
administered. When anæmia is severe, a transfusion of fresh blood
compensates for the deficiency of red cells, and supplies fresh complement
and other immune bodies which may be lacking. Some antibiotics used in
treatment can cause anæmia and neutropenia; weekly blood counts are
then desirable. When antibiotics or other drugs known to produce
agranulocytosis are being given (§ 541), patients should be told to report
a sore throat as soon as possible as this may precede neutropenia; all
treatment likely to damage the bone marrow must be stopped and a
transfusion of fresh blood given.

The patient is PALE *and* ANÆMIC *and loss of weight is marked. The
symptoms, physical examination and special investigations by X-rays,
pathological tests etc. reveal* MALIGNANT DISEASE.

§ 551. IV. **Carcinoma, Sarcoma** and other malignant diseases are
often accompanied by anæmia, pallor, weakness and loss of weight, the
characteristics of malignant cachexia. The hæmoglobin deficiency may
be one of the most pronounced clinical symptoms. The type of anæmia
often suggests iron-deficiency but does not respond to iron salts in large
doses; this is partly due to the release of toxic substances when a malignant
tumour undergoes necrosis. An intermittent pyrexia with a neutrophil
leucocytosis may suggest the anæmia of infection rather than of malignant
disease. Occasionally carcinoma of the stomach is associated with
pernicious anæmia.

Leuco-erythroblastic Anæmia indicates a blood condition in which
anæmia is accompanied by immature leucocytes (usually myelocytes) and
nucleated red-cell precursors (usually late normoblasts). It is due to
irritation or replacement of the bone marrow by (i.) *secondary* deposits of
growth (metastases) in the marrow; (ii.) multiple foci of *Hodgkin's disease*,
myelomatosis or sarcoidosis, (iii.) *myelofibrosis, myelosclerosis* and *erythræmic
myelosis*; (iv.) *syphilitic disease*. These conditions are revealed by X-ray
examination of the ribs, spine, skull and long bones (which may also reveal
pathological fractures) and by bone marrow biopsy (§§ 544, 1201).

Rarer Causes of Anæmia

§ 552. I. **Aplastic Anæmia** is a severe disease in which the bone marrow loses its power of producing all forms of blood cells. Most cases occur in young adults and both sexes are equally affected. The *primary* or idiopathic form is of unknown origin and is much rarer than the *secondary* form which may be due to: (i.) certain poisons, especially the aromatic hydrocarbons (benzol, benzene, trinitrotoluene); arsenic, mercury, gold and lead preparations; tridione; chloramphenicol; sulphonamide and thiouracil derivatives; (ii.) the action of ionising radiations; (iii.) advanced renal disease.

The *symptoms* are (1) those of profound anæmia with breathlessness at rest and a raised jugular venous pressure. (2) Hæmorrhages occur into the skin as purpura, from any of the mucous membranes, in the retina and even as subarachnoid hæmorrhage, largely due to the thrombocytopenia. (3) Sore throat, stomatitis, aphthous ulcers and diarrhœa are mainly the result of severe neutropenia and therefore deficiency of phagocytes. (4) The blood shows severe anæmia with a reduction of red cells (1-2 million per c.mm.) but with a normal colour index and a normal or increased mean cell diameter; evidence of regeneration in the bone marrow, *i.e.*, reticulocytes, and nucleated red cells, is absent. The leucopenia is mainly due to lack of neutrophil polymorphs (less than 1,500 per c.mm.); although a differential count may show a relative lymphocytosis of 95 per cent. the absolute figures often show a deficiency of lymphocytes. The platelets are frequently less than 50,000 per c.mm.

The *Diagnosis* can only be made by a careful examination of the blood and especially by bone marrow biopsy (§§ 544, 1201). The latter helps to distinguish the two chief types: (1) the complete aplasia or severe hypoplasia with a jelly-like or a fatty marrow containing few cells (usually of idiopathic origin), and (2) the form due to a maturation defect with a cellular marrow but with no mature cells; most of those seen are intermediate normoblasts, myelocytes and immature megakaryocytes. This is more common in the secondary type of the disease.

The *Prognosis* with complete aplasia is bad and the disease is rapidly fatal; regular weekly or monthly blood transfusions may keep the patient with partial aplasia alive until the bone marrow starts to produce cells once more.

Treatment by transfusions of fresh blood from a donor in whom a leucocytosis has been artificially induced, and the administration of proteolysed liver and of pyridoxin by mouth are occasionally helpful. Treatment otherwise is as described for agranulocytosis (§ 541) by stopping all drugs potentially causative, barrier nursing, penicillin injections, prednisolone or injection of ACTH. *Prophylaxis* is by the regular supervision of industrial workers exposed to substances which may cause this condition. In the maturation type of aplastic anæmia splenectomy has sometimes been carried out with good results and with a return to normal health with almost normal blood counts; the operation has been done on the assumption that the spleen inhibits proper maturation of the marrow cells. The term *hypersplenism* has been used to describe this phenomenon. The hypoplastic anæmia often met with chronic renal disease only improves when the kidney lesions have been overcome.

§ 553. II. **Acute Acquired Hæmolytic Anæmia** (Syn. Lederer's Anæmia) is a rare disease of young adults who develop acute hæmolytic anæmia with fever, headache, abdominal pain and anorexia with slight jaundice. The blood may show a leucoerythroblastic reaction which makes it difficult to distinguish from acute leukæmia but there is a marked reticuloœytosis.

A *Chronic form of Acquired Hæmolytic Anæmia* is more commonly seen in older persons. The symptoms and blood findings are similar to those of the acute variety but there is commonly enlargement of the liver and spleen with a tendency to relapses and remissions.

The *diagnosis* is usually suggested by a positive Coombs' test for the presence of hæmolysins, and the favourable response to blood transfusion or splenectomy.

Prognosis.—Many cases rapidly end fatally or the temperature may fall and recovery occur in a few weeks.

Treatment by the corticosteroids or ACTH combined with blood transfusions may be successful.   If these are not effective splenectomy should be advised.

The patient is PALE.   The SPLEEN *or the* LYMPH GLANDS *or both are* ENLARGED.   EXAMINATION OF THE BLOOD *may show typical changes*.   The disease is probably LEUKÆMIA, HODGKIN'S DISEASE, LYMPHOSARCOMA, ACHOLURIC JAUNDICE, SPLENIC ANÆMIA, a Sequela of MALARIA, OSTEO-SCLEROSIS, MYELOFIBROSIS or GAUCHER'S DISEASE.

Leukæmia is a disease characterised by progressive anæmia and the appearance in the blood stream of abnormal leucocytes, often in large numbers progressing to a fatal termination.   There is usually enlargement of the spleen and/or of the lymph glands and of the liver.   The three chief varieties are: (1) *myeloid*, affecting the myeloid or granular cells of the bone marrow; (2) *lymphatic*, primarily involving the lymphocytes and lymphatic tissue; and (3) the rarer monocytic form, involving changes in the monocytes and reticulo-endothelial tissues.   There are also a number of *atypical forms* of leukæmia with distinct clinical and hæmatological characteristics. Practically every case shows infiltration with leukæmic tissue of the bone marrow, spleen, lymph glands, liver and other organs.   Should the total leucocyte count be normal or below normal, the disease is termed *aleukæmic* leukæmia.   The different types may be grouped into acute and chronic leukæmia.

§ 554. III. Acute Leukæmia is more common in children and young adults.   It may be myeloid, lymphatic or monocytic with a white cell count of 50,000-100,000 per c.mm.   A few cases show 500,000 cells per c.mm.; about a third of the cases are aleukæmic.   Many primitive forms of leucocyte are usually to be found.   As many patients die within a few days or weeks of the diagnosis, it is not always easy to identify whether one is dealing with acute leukæmia, a very acute exacerbation of chronic leukæmia or the terminal phase of chronic leukæmia.   *Symptoms* usually suggest a sudden severe disease.   (1) The first is often extreme weakness out of proportion to the other early symptoms.   (2) Fever is sometimes very high, swinging and with rigors but with no discoverable cause; and blood cultures are sterile.   (3) Aching pains in the limbs simulate acute rheumatic fever.   (4) Severe anæmia is present. (5) Bleeding from the mucous membranes, oozing from swollen gums, purpura in the skin and hæmorrhages into the retina, the joints, serous cavities and the br in are partly due to reduction of the blood platelets.   (6) There is often stomatitis, ulc ration of the gums, fauces and palate with enlargement of the tonsils and salivary lands. (7) The spleen is only moderately enlarged.   (8) The lymph glands are enlarged in the lymphatic type, those in the neck are often further enlarged by infection in the mouth or throat.   (9) Other infections, especially in the respiratory tract, tend to cai se still higher temperatures.   (10) Raised pink nodules in the skin due to leukæmic d posits may appear in increasing numbers.

IN CHILDREN tumours occur usually in relation to bones which are the eat of excessive hæmopoietic activity, such as the skull, the spine and the sternum.   In acute myeloid leukæmia these are termed *chloroma* for they have a greenish tinge when freshly cut.   In acute lymphatic leukæmia similar grey tumours are termed *lymphoma*.

Diagnosis is made by blood examination in the majority of cases.   The blood and bone marrow show large numbers of primitive cells.   In acute myeloid leukæmia myeloblasts in the blood may show mitotic figures and may contain Auer bodies; in acute lymphatic leukæmia the lymphoblasts have only 1–2 nucleoli and do not contain oxidase-positive granules: in the acute monocytic form monocyte-like forms may resemble paramyeloblasts and have vacuoles in the cytoplasm.   Sternal puncture must be done with great care for the cortex of the bone is thinned in proportion as the medullary cavity is expanded by the leukæmic tissue.

Etiology.—The cause is not known but in the last few years attention has been drawn to the increase in survivors of atom-bomb explosions, in radiologists and in those who have had large doses of diagnostic or therapeutic X-ray exposures. Even so these probably explain the incidence of only 5–10 per cent. of cases.

Treatment consists in attempts to convert acute leukæmia into a chronic form, or to induce a temporary remission. Blood transfusion, folic acid antagonists (such as aminopterin 1·0 mg. daily by mouth), corticotrophin (5 mg. q.d.s. intramusc.), corticosteroids by mouth and other anti-mitotic and anti-metabolite substances are more effective in children than in adults. No possibility of cure exists at present. Antibiotics must be used with care as the phagocytic power of the leucocytes is diminished, and radiotherapy is contra-indicated.

- § 555. IV. Acute Erythræmic Myelosis (Syn. Erythromyelosis, di Guglielmo's disease) is regarded as the red cell counterpart of acute leukæmia. *Symptoms.*—From the onset there is severe anæmia, irregular fever and moderate enlargement of the spleen and liver. The blood and bone marrow show large numbers of red cell precursors, many of which are atypical and resemble megaloblasts. *Treatment* has no effect and the condition is usually fatal in a few weeks.

Chronic forms of this disease are even rarer. Cases showing the features of myeloid leukæmia and erythræmic myelosis are called erythroleukæmia. Their *diagnosis* may be very difficult.

§ 556. V. Chronic Myeloid Leukæmia (Syn. Leukæmic myelosis, Splenomedullary leukæmia).

Symptoms.—(1) Abdominal swelling and a feeling of a dragging weight due to the greatly enlarged spleen is often the first complaint. (2) The symptoms of anæmia (§ 545) and (3) lassitude and loss of weight are common. (4) Infarction may cause pain and a friction rub over the spleen. Spontaneous venous thromboses occur, such as in the corpora cavernosa causing priapism without libido. (5) Tenderness on pressure over the sternum is due to the thinned cortex of bone resulting from the hyperplasia of the myeloid cells in the bone marrow. (6) Fever and pruritus occur in the later stages of the disease. (7) Hæmorrhages from the nose, the gastro-intestinal tract, in the retinæ or into the skin appear in the terminal stages when thrombocytopenia has developed.

Diagnosis.—The most important sign is the great enlargement of the spleen which may reach the pelvis; the splenic notches can still be felt. The liver is also enlarged, sometimes greatly. The lymph glands may be slightly enlarged. Blood changes are usually characteristic. Although at first there may be polycythæmia, anæmia soon appears and becomes progressive. There are numerous polychromatic red cells and reticulocytes, and nucleated red cell precursors may number 30,000 per c.mm.; where early and intermediate normoblasts are frequent, a mistaken diagnosis of pernicious anæmia may be made. The platelets may be increased to 1 million at first but in the late stages can fall even to 10,000 per c.mm. The white cell count is normal in a few cases, but usually is very high—even 300,000 to 1,000,000 per c.mm.; the neutrophil polymorphs account for 30–70 per cent., myelocytes 15–50 per cent. and myeloblasts 2–5 per cent. Eosinophils and basophils are increased and when in large numbers justify the terms eosinophilic or basophilic leukæmia. In more acute phases the myeloblasts increase to 20–30 per cent., just before death they may increase further with a resemblance to acute myeloid leukæmia.

Etiology.—The disease is most common between 30 and 65 years of age, equally in men and women. It is regarded as a malignant tumour-like formation arising from the myeloid tissue, akin to sarcoma; this extraordinary overgrowth invades all the organs of the body and produces in the marrow a grey-green sheen within a thin cortex of bone. The ultimate cause is unknown; a similar disease in mice, rats and fowls can be transmitted by cell-free filtrates of tissues, but this is always specific to each species. The human disease has not been transmitted; but familial and hereditary factors and ionising radiations play a part.

Prognosis.—The disease is incurable and ultimately fatal. The average duration of life after diagnosis is about 3 years but a few patients survive 25 years. It is uncommon to observe more than three major remissions in any one patient. Marked increases of myelocytes and especially of myeloblasts suggest a more rapidly fatal course. Death occurs from exhaustion, intercurrent infection or hæmorrhage, frequently in the brain.

Treatment does not materially prolong life; but it relieves symptoms and keeps patients comfortable, happy and at work. When there is evidence of iron-deficiency, iron is given but inject. cyanocobalamin may accelerate the course of the disease; blood transfusions are very helpful when anæmia is marked. If there is evidence of hæmolysis, splenectomy is considered justifiable by some, in spite of the risk of operation. Infections must be avoided as they produce a marked deterioration of health. X-ray therapy is the treatment of choice, either to the spleen, to the bones or to the whole body; it reduces the size of the spleen and the number of white cells in the blood and often causes a rise in the hæmoglobin value, with a feeling of improved health. Of the drugs which help to arrest mitosis of the abnormal cells, myleran 4 mg. daily by mouth is the best, although intravenous radio-active phosphorus (P^{32}) 1–2 millicuries twice a week is helpful. An alternative is to use a drug which blocks nucleic acid synthesis; 6-mercaptopurin 150–200 mg. a day is less effective but is the best. All forms of treatment must be controlled by regular blood counts, including platelet counts; the doses must be reduced as soon as a significant drop in the number of leucocytes occurs and stopped when the figure falls to about 15,000 per c.mm.

TABLE XLIII. DIFFERENTIAL DIAGNOSIS OF CHRONIC LEUKÆMIA AND OTHER CAUSES OF SPLENOMEGALY.

	Enlargement of Spleen	Enlargement of Lymph Glands	Leucocytes per c.mm.	Other Features
Chronic Myeloid Leukæmia	Gross; may reach pelvis	May be slightly enlarged	Usually 50,000 to 500,000; 30 per cent. myelocytes	Progressive anæmia; enlargement of liver
Chronic Lymphatic Leukæmia	Moderate; rarely gross	Moderate, soft enlargement	30,000 to 200,000; 90 per cent. lymphocytes	Slowly progressive anæmia
Hodgkin's Disease	Usually slight; may be massive	Marked and usually firm	Normal or slight increase (20,000)	Anæmia in late stages; occasional eosinophilia; intermittent fever
Splenic Anæmia	Large	None	Neutropenia (1,500)	Portal hypertension; œsophageal varices cause hæmorrhage; cirrhosis of liver later
Gaucher's Disease	Massive	None	Neutropenia (1,500)	Familial: moderate anæmia; brown pigmentation of skin; pingueculæ
Acholuric Jaundice (Hereditary Spherocytosis)	Large	None	Normal or slight increase (20,000)	Familial; crises of anæmia; reticulocytosis; increased osmotic fragility of red cells

§ 557. VI. Chronic Lymphatic Leukæmia. *Symptoms.*—(1) Insidious but progressive enlargement of the lymph glands. (2) General symptoms with lassitude, weakness and loss of weight often precede the glands. (3) The symptoms of anæmia (§ 545). (4) In some cases the spleen is markedly enlarged and so causes a dragging pain in the left hypochondrium, but this is not so striking as in myeloid leukæmia. (5) The liver is uniformly enlarged. (6) Nodules in the skin and (7) intense pruritus with a general redness of the skin (erythroderma) are more common in lymphatic leukæmia. (8) Purpura may occur. (9) Enlarged mediastinal glands may cause dyspnœa or dysphagia. (10) The lachrymal and salivary glands may enlarge and give rise to Mikulicz' syndrome (§ 9). (11) The blood shows little anæmia in the earlier stages before the bone marrow is extensively involved. The leucocytes may number up to 200,000 per c.mm. and more than 90 per cent. are lymphocytes, usually of the small type. Lymphoblasts with nucleoli in the nuclei and with a more basophilic cytoplasm than usual are seen in the more acute cases and in exacerbations. In the very early stages the bone marrow may show no abnormality, but later a predominantly lymphatic picture develops, and nucleated red cell precursors appear in the blood. (12) Occasionally hæmolytic episodes occur even before the spleen is markedly enlarged.

Diagnosis.—This is usually made from the general enlargement of the lymph glands, the moderate enlargement of the spleen and the typical blood picture. Biopsy of the spleen or of a lymph gland shows disappearance of the normal architecture and replacement by a uniform mass of lymphocytes. In *aleukæmic* cases with a normal total white cell count, diagnosis may be difficult; it is established by a high percentage of lymphocytes in the blood, an increased number in the marrow and by a lymph gland biopsy. *Pertussis* and *glandular fever* may show a marked lymphocytosis; in the former the lymph glands are not enlarged and in the latter a positive Paul-Bunnell test will be distinctive. *Lymphosarcoma* shows an identical microscopic appearance in the lymph glands but no changes in the white blood count.

Etiology.—The incidence is during middle and later life, and men are more often affected than women. The cause is not known. A similar disease occurs in mice, and in the lymphomatosis of cattle and dogs. Although there are points in favour of an infective etiology in animals, lymphatic leukæmia in man is at present regarded as a malignant tumour-like condition of the lymphatic series of cells.

Prognosis.—There is no cure but the outlook as regards life is rather better than in chronic myeloid leukæmia. The more chronic forms seen in old age have a comparatively low malignancy and patients may live 10 to 20 years after the diagnosis.

Treatment has no real influence on the progress and duration of the disease but helps to relieve symptoms. Patients with few or no symptoms may not require any treatment for a long time. X-ray therapy to areas where enlarged lymphatic tissue is causing pressure effects gives relief. Corticosteroids benefit a few patients, especially when there are hæmolytic episodes—otherwise these may be treated by splenectomy. Nitrogen mustard and its derivative triethylene melamine (TEM) and radio-active phosphorus (P^{32}) are useful. Blood transfusions which raise the hæmoglobin to over 80 per cent. are of considerable value and may produce a sustained remission. Treatment must be controlled by the clinical condition of the patient and by regular blood counts.

§ **558.** VII. **Leukæmoid blood pictures:** Certain diseases are sometimes accompanied by blood changes which, if divorced from the clinical picture, may suggest leukæmia. Measles, pertussis and glandular fever may simulate lymphatic leukæmia because of a high lymphocytosis. Acute infections, generalised or miliary tuberculosis and sarcoidosis simulate myeloid leukæmia, because of the high neutrophil count and the appearance of myelocytes or even myeloblasts. Proper correlation with the clinical condition, bone marrow biopsy and other laboratory tests, and repeated blood counts usually solve the diagnostic problem. The absence of leukæmic infiltration in the organs excludes leukæmia.

VIII. HODGKIN'S DISEASE (§ 584) and Reticulum cell Sarcoma cause enlargement of groups of lymph glands. In the later stages splenomegaly and anæmia occur.

IX. ACHOLURIC JAUNDICE (Syn. Congenital Hæmolytic Jaundice) causes anæmia, enlargement of the spleen and recurrent attacks of jaundice. It is often found in other members of the family (§ 331).

§ **559.** X. **Splenic Anæmia** (Banti's disease) is a rare chronic condition.

Symptoms.—(1) These are enlargement of the spleen and sometimes of the liver, but not of the lymph glands; (2) slowly progressive anæmia which may have features of a hæmorrhagic or an iron-deficiency anæmia, but rarely of a macrocytic anæmia; (3) a neutropenia and sometimes a thrombocytopenia. Later (4) hæmorrhages take place from gastro-œsophageal varices and (5) the liver is cirrhotic with ascites mainly due to portal hypertension. In the *first stage* of the disease the spleen enlarges and anæmia of an iron-deficiency type develops and progresses slowly for 3–10 years. In the *second stage*, which lasts up to 2 years, there are attacks of pain over the splenic area when the spleen enlarges still further due to congestion or thrombosis of the spiculae vascular area; the spleen otherwise becomes smaller because of fibrotic changes but the liver enlarges further due to hyperplasia of the liver lobules and proliferation of the bile ducts. Attacks of mild jaundice occur especially if there is intra-hepatic block of the portal system: and in the active stages of the disease attacks of fever occur. The portal hypertension causes recurrent hæmatemeses and dyspepsia with loss of weight. The anæmia becomes more severe, the leucocytes and the platelets become reduced in number and there may be evidence to suggest hæmolytic changes to complete the picture of hypersplenism. The *third and final* stage is characterised by periportal cirrhosis of the liver, hæmatemeses or melæna, ascites, cachexia and eventually hepatic failure and death.

The *Diagnosis* depends chiefly on the insidious onset of gross splenomegaly and anæmia. The spleen reaches as far as or below the umbilical level. Other conditions causing marked splenic enlargement usually show other features:—In *leukæmia* there are the typical leucocytic changes; in *Hodgkin's disease* and *lymphosarcoma* the lymph glands are enlarged; in *Gaucher's disease* there are areas of pigmentation, changes in the bones and the finding of typical cells; in *pernicious anæmia* the spleen is rarely large and the megaloblastic anæmia responds to cyanocobalamin injections. In *acholuric jaundice* (§ 331) the osmotic fragility of the red cells is increased, while in thalassæmia (Cooley's anæmia) there is usually leucocytosis and the blood often contains fœtal hæmoglobin (§ 567). In *kala-azar* there is a history of residence abroad and the parasite is found by liver or sternal puncture. In *Felty's syndrome*, apart from the enlarged liver and spleen with leucopenia, there are the signs of rheumatoid arthritis with accompanying pyrexia. Distinction from *cirrhosis of the liver* is at times very difficult; the earlier history and changes in the blood preceding the later symptoms are most helpful.

Etiology.—The primary cause is unknown. Men are more often affected than women but the disease may occur at any age.

Prognosis.—The disease is slowly progressive, but chronic ill-health may be interrupted by irregular remissions lasting years. Treatment has little effect on the over-all prognosis but tends to prevent complications such as thrombosis. Once cirrhosis has developed the prognosis depends on the state of the liver rather than of the spleen. Hæmorrhages and sudden death occur even years after splenectomy.

Treatment must be adjusted to the individual case and is largely symptomatic. In mild chronic cases without hæmorrhage large doses of iron may help the anæmia. If œsophageal varices cause repeated or severe hæmorrhages, they may require transsection of the affected area. Splenectomy in the earlier stages, with or without portocaval anastomosis, may relieve portal hypertension. Before splenectomy it is necessary to demonstrate by bone marrow biopsy that the spleen is not the only area of hæmopoiesis. At operation it is helpful to remove a small portion of liver for biopsy; after operation the rise in the platelets which occurs after splenectomy is particularly dangerous as it predisposes to thrombosis; this can be avoided by anticoagulant therapy.

XI. MYELOMATOSIS occurs in middle or later life with the formation of multiple tumours in the bone marrow; the cells forming these resemble plasma cells. The early symptom is pain in the bones, especially of the vertebral column, ribs and pelvis (§ 613). Anæmia is a relatively late symptom; Bence-Jones' protein may be found in the urine.

XII. Osteosclerosis and Myelofibrosis are two disorders which cannot always be distinguished from one another. In most cases they run a chronic course but with remissions. In the different phases of development, varying diagnostic features may be found, but leuco-erythroblastic anæmia (§ 551) of varying severity and splenomegaly are common. Since the bone marrow is largely replaced by dense bone or by fibrous tissue, hæmopoiesis takes place in the spleen, lymph glands, liver and other organs (extramedullary hæmopoiesis, myeloid metaplasia). In *Osteosclerosis* (Marble-bone disease of Albers-Schönberg, § 617) the marrow cavity is reduced by the thickened cortex of the bones. *Symptoms* usually commence in childhood, but the solid bone is more brittle than normal and may fracture with trivial injury. Sternal puncture may be impossible, and even trephining may be difficult because of the hard bone. In *Myelofibrosis* the marrow is replaced by fibrous tissue. The blood contains many myelocytes and even myeloblasts, and early normoblasts. It may be regarded as a benign scirrhous form of myeloid leukæmia; occasionally a frankly leukæmic picture develops, particularly after irradiation of the spleen or splenectomy.

Megakaryocytic leukæmia (Syn. Giant-cell reticulosis) is a condition in which megakaryocytes or cells resembling them are found in many organs, and they or their fragments may even appear in the blood. The symptoms comprise a leuco-erythroblastic anæmia with a large spleen and liver.

Diagnosis of these three disorders requires prolonged clinical and hæmatological observation. X-ray examination of the bones helps to differentiate osteosclerosis from myelofibrosis. The *prognosis* is that of a slowly progressive disease lasting 2 to 5 years or even 20 years. When thrombocytopenia is present the danger of hæmorrhage will shorten life. *Treatment* does not affect the ultimate issue. Repeated transfusions help; occasionally specific hæmatinics are useful but they may apparently cause rapid deterioration and even leukæmic transformation in some cases. Splenectomy is sometimes necessary when the large spleen embarrasses other abdominal viscera, but it should only be considered when it is established that hæmopoiesis is satisfactorily carried on in other sites. Instead of splenectomy some advocate deep X-ray therapy to the spleen.

XIII. **Gaucher's Disease** is a rare, congenital and familial condition found most commonly in the Jewish race, due to a disturbance of lipoid metabolism.

Symptoms.—The yellowish-brown pigmentation of the face and hands, with triangular pigmented areas in the scleræ (pingueculæ) becomes more marked as the disease progresses. The liver and spleen become enlarged; these organs together with the bone marrow and lymph glands contain many nests of Gaucher cells, which have a small pyknotic nucleus and much cytoplasm containing a network of fine fibrils. The blood shows anæmia and neutropenia.

Diagnosis rests on finding Gaucher cells in the bone marrow or spleen.

Etiology.—The material in the Gaucher cells is the lipoid kerasin, a cerebroside containing galactose, lactose and sometimes glucose.

Prognosis.—The disease is ultimately fatal but may be so chronic that death does not occur until middle age.

Treatment.—If there are signs of hypersplenism or if the weight of the spleen causes symptoms, splenectomy should be considered, but this has no effect on the course of the disease.

An *Infantile form* is rapidly fatal.

Niemann-Pick's disease has similar symptoms. The infantile form is always fatal before the age of 2 but the adult form is more chronic. The cells have a foamy cytoplasm containing lecithin.

Hand-Schüller-Christian disease is a disorder principally of infants and children in which the main cells contain a great excess of cholesterol or of its esters. *Symptoms* comprise (1) exophthalmos, (2) diabetes insipidus, (3) bony defects of the skull and of the long bones, but the pituitary fossa is radiographically normal. In ea. 'y life the condition is rapidly fatal, but in older children and adults may go on for years. *Treatment* is that of diabetes insipidus (§ 426); X-ray therapy to the masses in the skull and long bones may be helpful.

The patient is very pale and anæmic, and there are or have been SPONGINESS *of the* GUMS, PURPURIC SPOTS, *and brawny indurations of the legs. This disease is probably* SCURVY.

§ 560 XIV. **Scurvy** is a " deficiency disease " due to a too long continued diet lacking in vitamin C. Scurvy is attended by extreme debility, anæmia, sponginess of the gums, and hæmorrhages.

The disease may occur in adults, or in infants especially between 6 and 18 months of life. Certain *symptoms* are common to both. (i.) Pains in the back and limbs occur early, and in infants the associated tenderness causes them to scream when touched. (ii.) The gums become swollen, spongy and bleed easily. If untreated sloughing may follow, the teeth become loosened and the breath offensive. When there are no teeth these changes are absent. (iii.) Hæmorrhages occur. In adults capillary bleeding occurs around hyperkeratotic hair follicles especially on the outer aspect of the upper arms. There is a marked tendency to bruising, and purpuric spots and subcutaneous ecchymoses are common about the flexures of the joints especially in the popliteal space. Swellings due to hæmorrhages into the skin are purple but if beneath the skin the colour may be pale. Subperiosteal ecchymoses are more usual in adults than in children; at all ages hæmaturia is common, and epistaxis and melæna may occur. In infancy, hæmaturia may be the first sign. Hæmorrhages under the periosteum of the orbit causes proptosis, and occasionally intracranial hæmorrhage produces cerebral symptoms. (iv.) A marked anæmia causes pallor; there is a deficient maturation of the red cells, and although the bone marrow is hyper-cellular the blood shows a normochromic normocytic anæmia with very scanty platelets. (v.) There is profound bodily weakness and prostration with loss of appetite and usually a histamine-fast achylia gastrica. This weakness and the pains in the legs made it impossible for sailors afflicted during the Middle Ages to secure fruit and vegetables even when they reached the shores of desert islands. (vi.) Often there are striking psychological changes of resentment and depression. (vii.) Constipation, albuminuria and microscopic hæmaturia are often met. (viii.) Death may ensue suddenly without an adequate cause being found at autopsy; but hæmorrhages into the brain, the meninges or the pericardium may be causal. (ix.) Infections such as pneumonia are common; and wounds heal slowly.

IN INFANCY (Barlow's disease) the symptoms are those already enumerated, the special features being (i.) the child is very still when at rest (pseudo-paralysis) but cries when washed or dressed and screams if the limbs are touched. (ii.) Sponginess of the gums around erupted teeth is common. (iii.) Emaciation is often absent but muscular weakness, pallor and anæmia are usual. (iv.) The temperature may be raised to 100–102° F due to large and recent hæmorrhages or to infective complications. (v.) The anterior ends of the ribs at the costo-chondral junctions become expanded almost to twice the normal size, with backward displacement of the sternum and costal cartilages. (vi.) X-ray examination shows a loss of differentiation in the cancellous bone leading to a " ground-glass " appearance and the cortex is thinned. In acute cases there is a narrow line of dense bone (the Trümmerfeld zone or " the white line of scurvy ") at the ends of the diaphysis as calcification proceeds while the growth of the soft tissues ceases. In more chronic cases there is a wide zone of translucency on the diaphysial side of the " white line " through which fracture and even dislocation may occur.

Diagnosis.—The diagnosis of scurvy from other causes of purpuric eruptions is afforded by the condition of the gums, the hard brawny swellings which are peculiar to scurvy and by the marked tenderness of the limbs. Slighter cases are, however, sometimes difficult to diagnose at first as similar symptoms may be seen with purpura. The capillary resistance test is usually positive. A blood count should at once distinguish scurvy from *acute leukæmia*, which is also accompanied by stomatitis and hæmorrhage of the gums. *Acute rheumatism* does not occur under 3 years of age and it affects the joints, which are free in scurvy. *Infantile paralysis* is also associated with a temperature, tender limbs and paralysis, but is not accompanied by spongy gums, swellings of the legs or hæmorrhages; moreover the tendon reflexes are not lost in scurvy. *Acute osteomyelitis* usually causes pain and tenderness in one or two bones only. *Syphilitic pseudo-paralysis* occurs at a younger age (under 6 months), and crepitation with pain on moving the limb may be found, due to the separation of the epiphysis from the diaphysis. An acute swelling of the bone may raise the suspicion of *sarcoma*. When doubt exists the therapeutic test of administering an adequate dose of ascorbic acid greatly helps diagnosis, for in cases of scurvy the symptoms and signs subside in a very few days.

Etiology.—Scurvy is due to the absence of vitamin C (Ascorbic Acid). It used to be the scourge of the British Navy, until the introduction of lemon juice as a prophylactic. It is occasionally seen when prolonged strict dieting has been practised for the treatment of peptic ulcers, and in those who never eat fresh vegetables and fruit.

Breast-fed infants are less liable to develop scurvy as they derive some vitamin C from their mother's milk; the content of fresh cow's milk is low and such vitamin as is present is largely destroyed when cow's milk is pasteurised, dried or condensed. The average daily requirement of vitamin C for an adult is 60–70 mg. and for an infant 25–50 mg.; these amounts are higher during pregnancy, lactation and during the post-operative period when a wound is healing.

Prognosis.—Under vigorous treatment symptoms rapidly subside in the course of a week. Unfavourable symptoms are severe dyspnœa, syncope, scanty urine and high temperatures.

Treatment.—Prophylaxis consists in giving vitamin C daily to infants in the form of one teaspoonful of orange juice or rose-hip syrup at the age of 2 months, increased to the juice of one whole orange at 6 months. Concentrated orange juice is distributed by Infant Welfare Clinics in the United Kingdom. Vitamin C is also contained in large amount in the juice of fresh lemons, oranges, and in fresh green vegetables; in moderate amount in roots, such as swedes and potatoes; and in small amount in milk and fresh meat. Prolonged boiling and alkalies destroy the vitamin; soda should not be used in cooking vegetables. *Curative treatment* is by giving ascorbic acid in tablet form; initially infants need at least 100 mg. and adults 600 mg. a day. When vomiting or diarrhœa are present sodium ascorbate should be given intravenously. After symptoms have subsided this should be replaced by the regular consumption of orange, lemon, fresh tomato or swede juice with potato pulp and raw-meat juice. *Local* treatment consists in wrapping the limb in cotton wool and preventing injury.

The patient is a YOUNG MAN *who complains of* RECURRENT SEVERE BLEEDING *after minor injuries and of* INVOLVEMENT OF JOINTS. *The disease is probably* HÆMOPHILIA.

§ 561. XV. Hæmophilia (Syn. Classical Hæmophilia, Hæmophilia A) is a rare hereditary disease affecting males but transmitted by females, characterised by a life-long tendency to excessive hæmorrhage. Spontaneous cases also occur.

The *symptoms* are due to the hæmorrhagic tendency: (1) Bleeding from the skin or mucous membranes usually appears first after the age of 2 years when the boy becomes more active: it does not occur from the umbilical cord at birth. Scratches and knocks which normally heal readily can cause *prolonged* bleeding which is not always *severe.* Circumcision or the extraction of a tooth cause almost uncontrollable bleeding and capillary oozing lasting several days. Epistaxes, hæmatemesis and hæmaturia occur. The blood clots slowly and large hæmatomata form which compress the adjacent structures. (2) Hæmorrhages into and around joints may affect any joint but particularly the knees and elbows. They cause (i.) the acute onset of an effusion into the joint which becomes hot and tender; followed by synovitis and pariarticular swelling; (ii.) pyrexia; (iii.) after repeated attacks or when recovery is slow there is loss of joint cartilage, lipping of the surfaces, fibrosis and osteo-arthritis; ankylosis may develop. This leads to crippling, gaps in education and a much reduced income.

Diagnosis.—A single severe hæmorrhage does not suggest hæmophilia, but recurrent hæmorrhages after trivial causes are characteristic. There is often a family history of a bleeding tendency in the males. The joint affections must not be confused with other causes of acute or chronic arthritis (§§ 592, 596). The blood will show normal bleeding and prothrombin times but the clotting time (§ 543) is greatly prolonged. The thromboplastin generation test (Biggs and Douglas) and the assay of the anti-hæmophilic globulin show the typical patterns of hæmophilia. *Thrombocytopenia* must be excluded by a platelet count. Other hæmorrhagic conditions which cause diagnostic difficulties include *purpura simplex* with its increased capillary fragility (Hess's test), *Henoch-Schönlein purpura, hereditary hæmorrhagic telangiectasia, constitutional thrombopathy* (von Willebrand's disease) which shows a normal platelet count but prolonged bleeding time, and congenital and acquired deficiency of fibrinogen where the prothrombin time is greatly prolonged.

Etiology.—The condition is due to a deficiency or absence of anti-hæmophilic globulin in the plasma (§ 543) which remains throughout life. Symptoms are severe when under 5 per cent. of the globulin is present and usually mild when over 10 per cent. is present. It occurs in families over many generations, and is transmitted by the female who is unaffected and whose blood shows no abnormality. The tendency is transmitted as a Mendelian sex-linked recessive character. If a carrier marries a healthy male, half the sons are hæmophilic (the other half being normal) and half the daughters are carriers (the other half not being carriers). If a hæmophilic man marries a healthy woman all their sons are normal and all their daughters are carriers. Normal children in hæmophilic families do not pass on the hæmophilic trait. About half the cases of hæmophilia are sporadic and without a family history, possibly due to a spontaneous mutation; their sons and daughters transmit the condition in the classical manner.

Treatment.—Hæmophilic patients should be protected as far as possible from injury; gymnastics and competitive sports must not be undertaken but ordinary swimming is a useful exercise. When bleeding occurs, rest is essential and local treatment is adopted aimed at stopping bleeding and promoting rapid wound healing. Gentle pressure should not be applied beyond 5 minutes as necrosis may ensue; cold packs may help. Dressings or fibrin-foam soaked in thrombin or Russell's viper venom (1 in 10,000 solution) should be applied and left in position as long as possible. Epistaxis and bleeding after dental extraction should be treated similarly. With massive hæmorrhages into muscles or into the deeper tissues of the limbs and trunk attempts at draining the extravasated blood are useless. Hæmorrhage affecting the neck may cause asphyxia due to hæmorrhage and œdema extending into and around the pharynx and larynx; this may require tracheostomy. The missing blood fraction is supplied by the prompt transfusion of fresh blood or of freeze-dried plasma; these may have to be repeated at 24-hourly intervals. In an emergency, bovine or porcine antihæmophilic globulin may be given but this cannot be repeated owing to the development of allergy. Only operations essential to life should be undertaken, and the patient must be protected by transfusions of *fresh* blood or freeze-dried plasma before, during and afterwards; a litre of *fresh* human plasma usually raises the level of antihæmophilic globulin to a level which makes operation safe.

Hæmophilia-like diseases. Two varieties are recognised:—

(i.) *Christmas disease* (Syn. Hæmophilia B, plasma thromboplastin component deficiency) is named after the patient first discovered to show this. It resembles hæmophilia as a sex-linked recessive condition but is only 10–20 per cent. as common as classical hæmophilia. The *symptoms* are the same as in hæmophilia A but the bleeding tendency is less severe.

Etiology.—The deficient Christmas factor is in the β-globulin fraction of plasma, in contrast to antihæmophilic globulin which is in the fibrinogen fraction. Hæmophilic plasma does not lack Christmas factor, and Christmas-disease plasma does not lack antihæmophilic globulin; the addition of the one plasma to the other will shorten the clotting time in each case. When antihæmophilic globulin is added to hæmophilic plasma it shortens the clotting time, but does not do so when added to Christmas disease plasma.

Treatment.—The Christmas factor is more stable than the antihæmophilic factor and when hæmorrhage occurs in a patient with this condition, apart from the use of fresh blood and freeze-dried plasma, stored blood may be transfused.

(ii.) *Parahæmophilia* resembles hæmophilia but is due to a congenital or familial deficiency of factor V or factor VII.

C.M.—E E

XVI. Paroxysmal or Nocturnal Hæmoglobinuria occurs when intra-vascular hæmolysis raises the level of the free hæmoglobin above the renal threshold (§ 414). *There is pallor of the skin and the patient has* BEEN IN THE TROPICS. Inquiry should be made for MALARIA, CHRONIC DYSENTERY, WORMS and other PARASITES, or other TROPICAL DISEASES.

§ 562. XVII.—Various **Tropical Diseases** and **Parasitic** conditions rarely seen in England, but very common in tropical and subtropical areas, are attended by intense anæmia. There are three groups:

(1) *Microcytic Tropical Anæmia* is by far the most common. It is usually due to insufficient iron in the diet or to hæmorrhage; occasionally there is failure to absorb sufficient iron. The blood shows the changes described in § 549, and such anæmias are particularly common in breast-fed infants, in pregnancy and in association with hookworm infestation.

(2) *Normocytic Tropical Anæmia* occurs when the average diameter of the red cell is within normal limits and the colour index is usually between 0·8 to 1·0. Most cases are due to *parasitic* diseases such as malaria (where it may be associated with blackwater fever), kala-azar, trypanosomiasis, amœbiasis (especially with a liver abscess) or schistosomiasis. Chronic *bacterial* diseases such as leprosy and brucellosis are also causal.

(3) *Macrocytic Tropical Anæmia* is usually due to various forms of a conditioned malabsorption syndrome (§ 316). The classical example is tropical sprue (§ 318) in which anæmia is sometimes absent in the earlier stages, but in which macrocytic anæmia develops later and then the blood picture may be indistinguishable from that of pernicious anæmia. However, the histamine test meal shows acid in 70 per cent. of sprue cases, which with the characteristic stools, intestinal flatulence, great loss of weight an·' absence of spinal cord involvement distinguish it from pernicious anæmia. Lesser ·f intestinal malabsorption produce macrocytic megaloblastic anæmia quite commonly in pregnant women, and in peasant people living on a low-protein high-carbohydrate diet (nutritional macrocytic anæmia). These anæmias usually respond well to high doses of folic acid by mouth (5 mg. t.i.d.), Marmite (1 drachm thrice daily) but sometimes parenteral cyanocobalamin (Vitamin B_{12}) is also needed.

Oroya Fever of the Andes, due to *Bartonella bacilliformis* which is located in the red cells, is associated with a severe hæmolytic macrocytic anæmia with a megaloblastic bone marrow closely resembling pernicious anæmia. Hyperbilirubinæmia is present, but there is a leucocytosis of some 20,000 per c.mm. with the neutrophils forming 60–70 per cent. There is no response to cyanocobalamin therapy but chloramphenicol will effect a cure if given early in the disease.

DIPHYLLOBOTHRIUM LATUM infestation (§ 548) is sometimes associated with anæmia indistinguishable from pernicious anæmia. It responds to inject. cyanocobalamin therapy and is permanently cured by the successful removal of the tape-worm.

§ 563. XVIII. Ankylostome Worms may produce no symptoms, but heavy infections in the badly nourished result in anæmia (of the microcytic hypochromic type), asthenia and debility. In severe cases the skin becomes yellow and dry, the mucous membranes pale, and dyspnœa, palpitation, pulsating cervical veins, hæmic murmurs, retinal hæmorrhages, œdema of the feet and serous effusions may be found. Epigastric tenderness, enlarged liver, dyspepsia, mental and physical lethargy are characteristic. Occult blood may occur in the stools, but melæna is rare. The two species affecting man are *Ankylostoma duodenale* and *Necator americanus*; their ova are voided in the fæces. In warm, moist earth rhabditiform larvæ subsequently develop, and infect man by boring through the skin, invading the blood-vessels, passing to the right heart and finally the lungs, whence they proceed *via* the trachea, œsophagus and stomach to their adult habitat—the duodenum and jejunum. Although infrequently fatal, ankylostomiasis predisposes to intercurrent diseases like pneumonia and dysentery. Ankylostome dermatitis may result from invasion of the skin by the larvæ, and later anæmia with a low colour index (0·5) and eosinophilia may be found.

The *Diagnosis* is made by finding the eggs in the fæces either in ordinary smears or by a flotation concentration method. Anæmia associated with eosinophilia in miners or people from the tropics should arouse suspicion.

Treatment.—Prevention includes the wearing of good shoes and boots, the proper disposal of night soil and the treatment of carriers. In miners proper sanitary arrangements are essential. Medical treatment consists in the administration of tetrachlorethylene 4 ml., after preliminary light diet and saline purgation. A further purge should be given an hour after the drug. Tetrachlorethylene is contra-indicated in cases of liver or renal disease. Hexyl resorcinol 1·0 G. in gelatin capsules is a good substitute (§ 323). Iron should be prescribed as for hypochromic anæmia (§ 549), and a well-balanced diet given, adequate in proteins and vitamins.

§ 564. XIX. Sickle-cell Disease and Anæmia.—The sickle-cell trait is a hereditary Mendelian dominant characteristic which appears in individuals of African and some Mediterranean and Asiatic races: the trait is heterozygous because it is inherited from only one parent. A proportion of the red cells become elongated and sickle-shaped in low oxygen tensions; this is due to the presence of an abnormal hæmoglobin (Sickle-hæmoglobin or Hb.S) which makes up about 40 per cent. of the total hæmoglobin. Those with the trait have among their red cells in venous blood about 1 per cent. of sickle cells. Most subjects are symptomless throughout life and may possess an actual advantage in areas where falciparum malaria has a high mortality.

Sickle-cells are demonstrated *in vitro* (1) by placing a drop of freshly drawn blood on a slide and sealing with a cover slip and a ring of paraffin; on standing for several hours a number of the red cells become sickle-shaped. (2) A wet film treated with a reducing agent such as sodium metabisulphite brings out the changes much more rapidly.

Sickle-cell Anæmia occurs when the inheritance of the change is homozygous, *i.e.*, inherited from both parents. The children therefore have a very high proportion of Hb.S in their cells and the venous blood shows 30-50 per cent. of the red cells to have this change.

Symptoms date from childhood. When sickling occurs *in vivo* in these large numbers of red cells (1) there are irregular " crises " of hæmolysis and anæmia with paroxysms of temperature to 103°-104° F; (2) jaundice and sometimes hæmoglobinuria follow the attacks; (3) there are pains in the bones and joints, and abdominal pain; (4) the liver becomes enlarged and there is splenic pain but rarely sphenomegaly; (5) intravascular thrombosis followed by infarction accounts for a number of these symptoms and for the frequent occurrence of ulcers on the legs. (6) The blood shows a moderate or high leucocytosis (up to 40,000 per c.mm.) but the coagulation time, the number of platelets and the red cell fragility are normal. (7) Osteoporosis and other bone changes are found.

Diagnosis is by demonstrating the large proportion of sickle-cells in the blood (*vide supra*), and from Cooley's anæmia.

Prognosis.—Once symptoms have developed the ultimate prognosis is bad and many die before the age of 40. Sudden death may occur, or cardiac failure and coma appear more gradually.

Treatment.—*Prophylaxis* is by avoiding anoxia during anæsthesia or high-flying. In a crisis blood transfusion is the only hopeful measure. Splenectomy, liver extracts and iron are of no value.

OTHER ABNORMAL HÆMOGLOBINS. In those of West African descent, Hb.C is comparatively common and may cause a milder type of hæmolytic anæmia in homozygous individuals. Mixed types of these abnormal forms of hæmoglobin such as Hb.S-C disease, produce a similar anæmia especially in pregnancy. A hypochromic anæmia which fails to respond to treatment with iron salts, and in which the iron-binding capacity of the serum is low, may be due to the thalassæmia trait (Cooley's anæmia).

§ 565. XX. Excessive Breakdown of Red Cells (Hæmolysis) also causes anæmia. There are many causes of this, a number of which have been described elsewhere but it is convenient to collect them into a group. Many cases of anæmia are due chiefly to a deficient formation of red cells in the marrow (hæmopoiesis), but even in these some premature destruction of the red cells (hæmolysis) occurs so that the life span of the average cell is below the normal 120 days. A mild degree of hæmolysis should be suspected when the hæmoglobin level of the blood progressively falls, and when this is accompanied by an excess of serum bilirubin (van den Bergh reaction, § 333) and of urobilin in the urine, with a raised reticulocyte percentage; normoblasts may be seen in the blood. Rapid hæmolysis produces the same results in an intensified degree, and gives rise to hæmolytic jaundice (§ 330) and even hæmoglobinuria. Confirmation that the red cells are destroyed prematurely is also obtained by incubating the patient's red cells with radio-active chromium (Cr^{51}), re-infusing them and measuring the radio-activity by monitoring over the liver, spleen, heart and spine.

Causes —(1) *Infections* such as septicæmia and virus diseases produce anæmia chiefly by depressing hæmopoiesis. However, *Cl. Welchii* infections may produce hæmolytic changes. Malarial parasites enter the red cells and cause their premature destruction, and malignant tertian malaria (*P. falciparum*) can cause rapid hæmolysis. Oroya fever with its intracorpuscular parasite acts similarly. (2) *Poisoning* by certain chemical substances, especially in industry, may be responsible. Arsene, phenylhydrazine, para-aminophenol, dinitrobenzene, naphthalene and snake venom are particularly dangerous. The sulphonamides have in rare instances produced acute hæmolytic anæmia. Severe burns may also be a cause. Favism follows the ingestion of the horse bean *Vicia fava* in sensitised persons. (3) *Hæmolysins* play an important part in incompatible blood transfusions (p. 812), hæmolytic disease of the newborn (§ 567), acute acquired (Lederer's) anæmia (§ 553), paroxysmal hæmoglobinuria (§ 414); and sometimes in conjunction with malignant disease, chronic lymphatic leukæmia, Hodgkin's disease, sarcoidosis and other reticuloses. (4) *Hereditary defects of red cells* are responsible in acholuric jaundice (hereditary spherocytosis, § 331), hereditary elliptosis (see below); and *hereditary defects of hæmoglobins* in thalassæmia (Cooley's anæmia) and in sickle-cell anæmia and allied disorders (§ 564).

Hereditary Elliptocytosis may exist merely as a harmless, symptomless trait; its inheritance follows the Mendelian dominant pattern. *Symptoms* arise when increased hæmolysis occurs, after an intercurrent infection. This may lead to mild jaundice, anæmia, gall stones and ulcers on the legs. *Treatment* in the severely anæmic patient is with transfusion which is a useful palliative measure. Splenectomy is often beneficial.

There is a history of exposure to IONISING RADIATION, or to INDUSTRIAL or other CHEMICAL POISONS.

§ 566. XXI. Ionising Radiations produce different effects on the human body depending on the dose used, the method of application and the sensitivity of the individual. They may be applied externally or internally. *External irradiation* is either hard and penetrating (X- or γ-rays) or soft and superficial (X- or β-rays). Very high energies are sometimes used to produce beams of great penetration (fast and slow neutrons, β-rays, X-rays and electrons). *Internal irradiation* can be given with radium and some other isotopes such as cobalt[60], gold[198], tantalum[182]; these are applied in containers such as needles or tubes for interstitial or intracavitary implantation, *e.g.*, in the treatment of carcinomata of the tongue, uterine cervix or bladder. Another method of internal irradiation is with radio-active isotopes given by mouth or by intravenous injection when a local action is needed on structures such as the bone marrow or the thyroid gland (β- or γ-rays).

(1) PENETRATING RADIATIONS given for the purpose of radiotherapy may produce nausea especially when applied to the chest or abdomen and on rare occasions in particularly sensitive individuals this may go on to the acute disease.

(a) *Acute Disease* (Acute Radiation Sickness). Patients lose their appetite, develop nausea and often vomit. There is general malaise, headache and often a low-grade temperature. It is essential to perform blood counts during and after radiotherapy; they may show leucopenia or thrombocytopenia, and if treatment is continued after this stage permanent damage to the blood-forming organs may ensue. The effects of a single very large dose of α-, β- and γ-radiation were demonstrated by the atom bomb explosions over Hiroshima and Nagasaki in 1945 when about 165,000 persons lost their lives, and also by accidents in atomic energy plants. Here also individual susceptibility was very variable. In the most severe cases vomiting, diarrhœa and fever were followed by dehydration, toxæmia and rapid death. In the first few days pharyngeal lesions and gross infection were due partly to a local effect but also to agranulocytosis with leucocyte counts of only 200 per c.mm.; death followed within 3 weeks. In less severe cases hæmorrhages occurred from the nose, stomach, renal pelves and in the brain and meninges within 3–5 weeks, due to thrombocytopenia. Others developed aplastic anæmia within 5–7 weeks, with red cell counts falling to 1 million per c.mm.; the bone marrow showed either aplasia or ineffective hyperplasia. Total epilation was usual.

Prognosis.—In those exposed to atomic radiation recovery is rare when the leucocyte count falls below 600 per c.mm. In those less severely affected, marrow regeneration commences during the second week.

Treatment of those receiving radiotherapy. Nausea and vomiting are reduced by giving pyridoxine hydrochlor. with hydrochloric acid orally, or by intravenous pyridoxine (100–200 mg.). Chlorpromazine or the antihistamines also help. After atomic explosions the only hope is by free administration of intravenous fluids, blood transfusions and the use of large doses of inject. benzylpenicillin or other antibiotics.

(b) *Chronic Disease* can occur in those exposed to small doses of ionising radiation over long periods. Modern methods of protection have made this a rarity in radiologists and radiographers, those working in radio-active isotope departments or with radium or strontium, and in those exposed to the fall-out of radio-active dusts. Others liable to exposure are workers with luminous watches and clocks, television sets, X-ray fluoroscopy for shoe fitting and those treated by radio-therapy for chronic diseases such as ankylosing spondylitis.

Symptoms depend on the total dosage and on the frequency, site and extent of the body exposed. GENERAL EFFECTS are: (i.) the blood shows a reduction in the lymphocytes and later in the neutrophils. A total white cell count of 2,000 per c.mm. or less is a definite danger signal, as is a rise in the absolute numbers of monocytes. A reduction in the number of platelets is also dangerous. Anæmia of the normocytic or iron-deficiency type may occur, and later still aplastic anæmia ensues. *Leukæmia* can develop; between 1929 and 1948 there were nine times as many deaths in American radiologists from leukæmia as among other American doctors. (ii.) Degenerative changes take place in the testes and ovaries. After moderate exposure fertility returns in 1–3 years. (iii.) Genetic effects may occur. In pregnancy the fœtus must be screened and the mother given as little exposure as possible, especially in the first three months of pregnancy. (iv.) LOCAL EFFECTS on the skin include erythema, epilation, pigmentation and even telangiectasia. Surgical operations on an area of skin previously exposed to irradiation even several years previously usually makes healing difficult. The effect on the skin and the degenerative changes in the smaller blood vessels have in the past led to necrosis and dry gangrene of the fingers of radiologists.

Treatment is almost entirely prophylactic. Radiologists, radiographers and others exposed in the course of their work to the cumulative effects of scattered irradiation must wear lead and rubber gloves and aprons and other shielding devices. Personnel and premises need to be checked by monitoring with small photographic films or capacity condensers. Working in dark or poorly ventilated rooms should be reduced to a minimum. Examination of the blood needs to be carried out every three months as long as the occupational risks continue. If the lymphocytes fall below 1,500 per c.mm. or the neutrophils below 3,000 per c.mm. or if anæmia is present, a few weeks' holiday is advisable. Anæmia may be rectified by adequate doses of iron. Any person showing even a slight degree of susceptibility to the effects of irradiation, whether in medicine or in industry, must be permanently excluded from contact.

(2) NON-PENETRATING RADIATIONS with β-particles are used for surface applications where treatment to a depth of not more than a few millimetres is required. Radio-active phosphorus (P^{32}) and strontium[90] plaques are mostly used, the latter for treating diseases of the cornea while ensuring that the lens of the eye receives no ionisation. *Internal* radio-active isotopes are being increasingly used in diagnosis and in the treatment of medical conditions. Thus iodine[131] and iodine[132] are used most commonly for estimation of the degree of thyroid activity and I^{131} is also used for treatment of hyperthyroidism (§ 186) and of iodine-concentrating thyroid carcinoma. Isotopes used in the detection of various diseases are sodium[24], chromium[51], tritium[3], cobalt[58], iron[59] and arsenic[76] but special precautions in well-equipped departments are necessary when using these as they are highly dangerous.

INDUSTRIAL AND OTHER CHEMICAL POISONS may cause anæmia. Lead poisoning is dealt with in § 568. *Benzol, benzene* and their derivatives are widely used in the leather, rubber, paint, cleaning, photographic and motor industries. *Symptoms* of chronic poisoning by benzene, toluene, xylol and trinitrotoluene are lassitude, giddiness, indigestion and nausea; in severe cases agranulocytosis or aplastic anæmia may occur.

§ 567. Anæmia in Infancy and Childhood.

—In children the hæmo-poietic system, like all other parts of the body, is more sensitive to outside influences and reacts more vigorously to them. Its activity is complicated by the development and growth of the child, and the necessity to acquire immunity. The normal values in children are shown in Table XLIV. Features which are especially prominent in children are: (*a*) Since all the bones contain active red marrow there is no fatty yellow marrow which can be transformed into red marrow under stress; therefore anæmia occurs at an earlier stage of a disease than in adults and tends to be more severe. Reticulocytes and nucleated red cell precursors appear early. (*b*) The spleen, lymph glands and other centres of lymphoid tissue such as the tonsils, adenoids, Peyer's patches in the ileum and the appendix become much more readily enlarged in children and may give rise to a variety of symptoms. This hyperplasia is often continued long after an infection has subsided, and when it is unduly prolonged in " lymphatic " children chronic ill-health may result. Marked enlargement of the spleen occurs in splenic anæmia, Hodgkin's disease and leukæmia. (*c*) Leucocytosis and particularly lymphocytosis reach higher figures in childhood and myelocytes appear more readily.

TABLE XLIV.—BLOOD COUNTS OF NORMAL INFANTS AND CHILDREN AT DIFFERENT AGES

	At birth	2 days old	14 days old	3 months	12 months	12 years	Remarks
Hæmoglobin per 100 ml. (in Grammes and Haldane percentages).	20 G. (140%)	19 G. (130%)	17·8 G. (120%)	11·0 G. (75%)	13·3 G. (90%)	14·85 G. (100%)	
Red cells per c.mm.	7·0 million	6·5 million	5·5 million	5·4 million	5·2 million	5·2 million	At birth late normoblasts fairly numerous
Reticulocytes as per cent. of red cells	5–10%			←————Under 1·0 per cent.————→			
Leucocytes per c.mm. Absolute values : Neutrophils Lymphocytes	18,000 12,000 3,000	14,000 8,000 3,000	17,000 10,000	Slowly fall to adult values at 12 years Adult values after 7 days old Slowly fall to adult values at 10 years			
Platelets per c.mm.	←— — — — —·— — — —250,000–500,000— — — — — — — — →						

Fœtal hæmoglobin (Hb.F) accounts for 60–90 per cent. of the total Hb. at birth ; it disappears by the twelfth month.
In artificially fed babies the above figures are lower.
In premature babies, the above figures may be 25 per cent. lower and the milestones are reached at later stages.

All forms of anæmia, described above in adults, occur in children, but true pernicious anæmia is extremely rare. Generally speaking the causes are the same as in adults although some forms are peculiar to children.

Anæmia in Infancy.

I. Nutritional Anæmia.
II. Anæmia due to Infection.
III. Infantile Scurvy (§ 560).
IV. Hæmolytic Anæmia of the New Born.
V. Hæmorrhagic Disease of the New Born.

Anæmia in later Infancy and Childhood.

I. Nutritional Anæmia.
II. Anæmia due to Infection.
III. Parasitic diseases, especially malaria (§ 512) and Leishmaniasis (§ 506).

Anæmia in later Infancy and Childhood (contd.).

IV. Acholuric Jaundice (Hereditary Spherocytosis) (§ 331).
V. Chronic Hæmolytic Anæmia.
VI. Acute Acquired Hæmolytic Anæmia (Lederer's Anæmia) (§ 553).
VII. Sickle-cell Anæmia (§ 564).
VIII. Thalassæmia (Cooley's Anæmia).
IX. Aplastic and Hypoplastic Anæmia (§ 552).
X. Hæmophilia (§ 561).
XI. Idiopathic Pulmonary Hæmosiderosis.

I. **Nutritional Anæmia of Infancy and Childhood.**—Anæmia in *infancy* is almost always of the iron-deficiency type.

Symptoms.—The infant or child will appear unduly pale and listless. Anæmia may also be suspected when recurrent infections occur, for anæmic children are much more prone to these. The *diagnosis* will be confirmed by blood examination.

Etiology.—(1) Neonatal iron-deficiency anæmia and (2) the nutritional anæmia of later infancy may be avoided by (*a*) ensuring an adequate supply of iron to the mother during the last 3 months of pregnancy as two-thirds of the fœtal iron is stored during this time; and (*b*) not permitting breast-feeding from an anæmic mother for too long a period without supple-·· nting with iron-containing foods. Cow's milk or dried milk products ·····.···· even less iron than human milk. (3) In anæmia of prematurity whu·h is most marked when the hæmoglobin reaches its physiological lowe··t level at 3 months, the infant has not had the opportunity to acquire an adequate store of iron and the bone marrow does not respond well. (4) The anæmia of multiple births is also due to exhaustion of the mother's iron reserves.

In *later infancy and childhood* alimentary anæmia may develop when the foods with a high iron-content, such as meat and vegetables, are not provided in sufficient quantity due to poverty. Chronic diarrhœa (§ 312), intestinal hurry and cœliac disease (§ 317) also cause deficient iron absorption.

II. **Anæmia due to Infection.**—Any acute or chronic infection leads to anæmia especially during periods of rapid growth, by depressing the erythropoietic function of the bone marrow. The hæmoglobin may fall to 7 G. per 100 ml. (50 per cent.). Infections with pyogenic organisms, in ·· ····ulosis and malaria, to a lesser extent with the acute specific fevers and the toxæmia of nephritis are common causes. *Treatment* with iron and a full diet tends to be ineffective until the underlying cause has been eradicated.

III. INFANTILE SCURVY is described in § 560.

IV. **Hæmolytic Anæmia of the New Born** (Syn. Congenital Hæmolytic Anæmia) occurs in some Rhesus-positive babies of Rh-negative mothers. Hæmolytic antibodies developed by the mother pass through the placenta and cause destruction of the red cells and therefore anæmia in the *fœtus* with gross œdema (hydrops fœtalis) and in the *new-born* jaundice (icterus neonatorum, § 330*a*) or hæmolytic anæmia. To over-come the loss of red cells by hæmolysis, increased erythropoiesis continues in the liver, spleen and other organs where normally it ceases after birth. The hæmoglobin falls to levels sometimes as low as 4 G. per 100 ml. (30 per cent.) and the blood smears show many late and intermediate normoblasts. If the parents differ in their Rh-groups the mother's blood should be tested for antibodies and if their titre rises appropriate steps can be prepared (and see § 547).

Treatment.—When the cord blood contains more than 14·8 G. per 100 ml. (100 per cent.) no treatment is necessary and the infant usually thrives normally. When there is moderate anæmia a simple small blood transfusion frequently suffices. Babies who are severely anæmic, premature or show a serum bilirubin value above 5 mg. per cent. require an exchange transfusion (§ 330*a* and p. 810). The red cell and blood groups of the mother and baby indicate the type of blood to be given and a *direct compatibility test must be performed.*

V. **Hæmorrhagic Disease of the New Born** (Syn. Melæna neonatorum) occurs during the first five days of life causing melæna or hæmatemesis, or more rarely hæmorrhage from the umbilicus, mucous or serous membranes, into the skin or internal organs, or following circumcision. It is due to a shortage of vitamin K, producing deficiency of plasma prothrombin which is normally at a low level during the first few days of life. *Treatment* is by intramusc. injection of synthetic vitamin K (menaphthone) or one of its analogues of which 1–2 mg. may have to be repeated daily. Particularly if much blood has been lost 20 ml. of whole blood may have to be transfused to supply prothrombin rapidly. Once the prothrombin deficiency has been overcome iron therapy will be needed.

OTHER ANÆMIAS OCCURRING IN LATER INFANCY AND CHILDHOOD :—

Acholuric Jaundice (Syn. Hereditary Spherocytosis) is described in § 331.

Chronic Hæmolytic Anæmia in childhood is nearly always symptomatic and may present features of hypersplenism (and see §§ 552, 565).

VI. *Acute Acquired Hæmolytic Anæmia* (Lederer's Anæmia) may first appear in children.

VII. *Sickle-cell Anæmia* is described in § 564.

VIII. **Thalassæmia** (Syn. Cooley's Anæmia) is predominantly but not exclusively found in children of Mediterranean people. It is a rare familial condition in which the osmotic resistance of the red cells to hypotonic saline and their mechanical fragility are increased, but survival of the cells when measured by labelling them with Cr^{51} is usually reduced. The full disease (thalassæmia major) is the homozygous expression of the Mendelian dominant. The trait (thalassæmia minor) and the almost symptomless form (thalassæmia minima) arise from heterozygous inheritance.

Symptoms are most marked in thalassæmia major. (1) There is hæmolytic anæmia; (2) the spleen may be enlarged, in some cases to an enormous size; (3) the liver is also enlarged; (4) the Mongolian face is due to the bones of the vault of the skull, the zygoma and the maxilla being filled with red bone marrow in an attempt to compensate for the continued blood loss by hæmolysis. The other bones of the skeleton are similarly affected and their thinned cortex and widened diploë may lead to pathological fractures. (5) The blood shows a constant high reticulocytosis (30 per cent.) and severe erythroblastosis which, particularly in the presence of a high leucocytosis with many myelocytes may suggest acute erythræmic myelosis or even leukæmia. Although the blood shows the changes of iron-deficiency, such as microcytosis and hypochromia, the serum iron and the iron-binding capacity are normal and there may even be hæmosiderosis. The red cells are often mis-shapen with target cells. The amount of fœtal hæmoglobin present may be 40–90 per cent.

Prognosis.—The full disease leads to death before puberty.

Treatment.—The anæmia is entirely refractory to iron therapy. The less severe forms may benefit by splenectomy, at least by a reduced need for blood transfusion.

IX. **Aplastic and Hypoplastic Anæmias** are rare. Symptomatic cases occur in nephritis and in malignant conditions. A familial type of hypoplastic anæmia, with neutropenia and thrombocytopenia in children, has been described by Fanconi; it is associated with brown pigmentation of the skin and with skeletal abnormalities such as microcephaly and mal-development of the extremities, or with urogenital defects such as a solitary or a horse-shoe kidney. Transfusions may prolong life but splenectomy is useless.

X. **Hæmophilia** is described in § 561.

XI. **Idiopathic Pulmonary Hæmosiderosis** is a rare condition in children and young adults causing anæmia, often of a severe nature, cyanosis, hæmoptysis, fever and later jaundice. X-ray shows diffuse infiltration of both lungs, almost miliary in type. *Diagnosis* is added by aspiration lung puncture which shows siderocytes on microscopic examination. *Etiology.*—The condition is not generalised as in transfusion siderosis. The decrease in the elastic fibres in the pulmonary interstitial tissue reduces the distensibility of the lungs, and promotes capillary stasis, hæmorrhages and brown induration in the lungs. No effective *treatment* is known.

B. PALLOR OF THE SKIN IS MARKED, *but* ANÆMIA IS SLIGHT, *the drop in the hæmoglobin content of the blood relatively small, and is* NOT READILY AMENABLE TO IRON ADMINISTRATION. The common causes are:—

I. Acute and chronic renal diseases.
II. Chronic hepatic disease.
III. Latent tuberculosis.
IV. Gastro-intestinal conditions.
V. Cardio-vascular conditions.
VI. Syphilis (§ 500).
VII. Lead poisoning (§ 568).
VIII. Addison's disease, myxædema and other diseases of Groups II and III.

I. **Acute and Chronic Renal Diseases** are usually accompanied by a pallor which may readily be mistaken for **primary anæmia**. This is especially the case in parenchymatous nephritis (§ 398), which is apt to affect young people. The pallor is of **an ivory whiteness**, is usually accompanied by a certain amount of œdema, and the urine reveals albumen and tube casts. Chronic interstitial nephritis (§ 401) usually occurs in older people; it is generally attended by sallowness, but progressive asthenia is its more constant and striking symptom.

II. **Chronic Liver Disease,** and especially cirrhosis of the liver, may be attended by an anæmic pallor; but it is usually attended also by a very characteristic dilatation of the venous capillaries in the face (§ 342).

III. **Latent Tuberculosis** is generally attended by pallor, weakness, and loss of weight (§ 131). The pallor may be marked and gives rise to a diagnosis of anæmia which is not supported by the blood examination. If pallor and general debility in a young patient do not respond to iron and general tonic measures, tuberculosis should be suspected. The disease may be latent in the sense that there are no obvious clinical manifestations, *e.g.*, no abnormal physical signs to be found in the lungs or elsewhere. The condition is described more fully in § 514.

IV. **Gastro-intestinal conditions** and especially simple dyspepsia, constipation, colitis and other disorders of the alimentary canal are frequently associated with pallor and often with secondary hypochromic anæmia. Indeed, these conditions and confinement indoors are perhaps the commonest causes of pallor among town-dwellers. Focal sepsis as with septic tonsils, dental abscesses, nasal sinus disease and pyorrhœa alveolaris may cause marked pallor and some anæmia. A dietetic deficiency, particularly of meat, may also act in a lesser degree. In colitis and other intestinal conditions pallor may be noticeable; the skin loses its lustre and there are dark rings under the eyes. In some of these patients the cæcum is loaded and abnormal intestinal organisms are found.

V. Certain **Cardio-Vascular conditions.** Infective endocarditis produces a toxic pallor associated with anæmia. Pallor also occurs in one type of hyperpieses (§ 88), in acute pericarditis (§ 46) and endocarditis (§ 49) and in aortic valvular disease.

VI. **Syphilis** leads to a degree of pallor which may simulate simple anæmia closely; it may be accompanied by a moderate degree of anæmia, even quite late in the disease. The condition is described fully in § 500.

§ 568. VII. Plumbism (Syn. Chronic Lead Poisoning, Saturnism). Chronic ill-health, usually associated with a number of other symptoms, results from the slow absorption of lead into the system. Acute lead poisoning is rare.

Symptoms.—(1) Pallor is very marked, due to vascular spasm rather than to anæmia. The pale pasty appearance of lead workers who are insufficiently protected is well known : with this, general asthenia and loss of weight are usual. (2) Attacks of severe intestinal colic are accompanied by obstinate constipation. An acute attack of colic may be associated with general malaise, a rise of temperature and some degree of abdominal tenderness and rigidity : during the attacks the pulse is slowed. The presence of recurrent attacks of colic is of diagnostic aid. (3) Nervous symptoms: lead has a special tendency to attack the peripheral nerves, and especially the motor cells and fibres; the musculo-spiral nerves are most commonly affected, leading to bilateral wrist-drop, but the supinator longus muscles escape (Fig. 247). Sometimes the paralysis is generalised. Otherwise the brain cells may be involved (saturnine encephalopathy); neurasthenia is common and in typical cases severe headache, acute mania, and convulsions occur (p. 1151). The mental condition may deteriorate until the patient is unable to look after himself. In others, optic neuritis and various degrees of amblyopia may occur : tremor is often present without paralysis, especially if the lead has entered the system by inhalation, as in glass-blowers. (4) Chronic renal changes may ensue, leading to chronic nephritis and uræmia. With this, an advanced degree of arteriosclerosis may be met, leading to fainting fits, and even hemiplegia. (5) In those with teeth, the gums show a punctate " blue line " close to the gum margin; this is much more marked when dental sepsis is present, permitting the formation of hydrogen sulphide, with the deposition of lead sulphide; a hand lens is of help in identifying this. A similar line is met in those receiving bismuth injections; in copper poisoning the line is brighter and more greenish. (6) Punctate basophilia (§ 541) in the red cells is present in anyone in contact with lead; when the number of red cells showing this stippling shows a sharp and persistent rise, toxic symptoms are likely to ensue. (7) In chronic cases, and particularly in women, marked secondary anæmia, and a relative lymphocytosis of the white cells, may be found. (8) Coproporphyrins are found in the urine in considerable quantities by the spectroscope.

Diagnosis.—Vague ill-health, pallor, the blue line, recurring colic and nervous symptoms occurring in a lead worker are diagnostic. In industry a falling hæmoglobin value and basophilic stippling of the red cells are the best guides to plumbism. Lead poisoning can occur at any age, *e.g.*, in babies and small children it has occurred due to the use of lead nipple shields, lead applications to the nipples and lead paint on toys or cot sides. Estimation of the urinary excretion over a 3-day period may be valuable in diagnosis. Other causes of abdominal pain, constipation and anæmia such as *carcinoma coli* must not be overlooked.

Etiology.—Some appear to be immune; women are more susceptible than men. Lead may enter the system by the mouth, the lungs or the skin. (1) Epidemics have been caused by water contaminated with lead, when stored in lead cisterns; soft water and slightly acid water has dissolved some of the lead carbonate found inside leaden pipes. Poisoning has occurred with food contaminated with lead, when stored in lead-lined or pewter vessels, and with drink, such as beer or cider which has lain several hours in a pewter or leaden pipe. Other causes are lead used for abortion, sucking paint off toys, sleeping in newly painted rooms, hair dyes, grease paint and face powders containing lead. (2) Lead is still more poisonous when its dust or fumes are inhaled, as occurs with those manufacturing lead accumulators or brass alloys, compositors, painters, pewterers and those exposed to fumes of melted lead, and lead glaze workers. A subacute form of poisoning occurs in those engaged in ship-breaking with oxyacetylene flames and has followed the use of old lead battery cases as a source of cheap fuel. (3) Lead can be absorbed through the skin; possibly some of the cases due to face powders and grease paint acquire it by this route.

Prognosis.—In spite of modern methods of protection in those working with lead cases still occur. Chronic ill-health results with a case-mortality of 10 per cent.

Treatment.—The first indication is the avoidance of the cause. Those who are exposed to the poison by reason of their occupation must observe the greatest personal cleanliness; the face, hands and teeth should be cleansed before meals. Adequate ventilation of the workroom is essential and a respirator worn if the air contains much dust. When pain is present give rest in bed, warm local applications, magnesium sulphate and inject antispasmodics such as pethidine or hyoscine hydrobromide. Intravenous calcium gluconate (10 ml. of 20 per cent. solution) repeated in 3 and in 6 hours will arrest severe lead colic. Older methods of treatment with inject. para-thormone and ammonium chloride have now been replaced by administration of sodium calciumedetate (B.P.C.) intravenously; this substance exchanges its calcium for lead ions to form a water-soluble lead compound which is non-ionisable and which is rapidly secreted in the urine. The dose in 500 mg. per 30 lb. body weight 12-hourly, each dose being given in at least 600 ml. of N-saline or dextrose solution over a period of 3 hours. These doses must not be given more than 5 days each week for 2 weeks; after a 10-day rest period a second course of treatment may be given.

Acute and Subacute Lead Poisoning may result accidentally from swallowing lead compounds or inhaling lead fumes in high concentration. The *symptoms* after swallowing lead salts are a sense of constriction in the gullet with acute gastro-enteritis, prostration and collapse. A blue line on the gums does not occur for some weeks. *Treatment* is with stomach lavage, followed by well-diluted magnesium sulphate and by sodium calciumedetate (*vide supra*).

Tetra-ethyl Lead Poisoning occurs when unprotected persons handle this heavy oily substance or clean out storage tanks which have held ethyl petrol. It is readily absorbed through the lungs and the skin. The *Symptoms* are (i.) anorexia, nausea, loss of weight; (ii.) muscular weakness, " rheumatic " pains and a coarse tremor; (iii.) mental symptoms with delusions, hallucinations and motor restlessness. Punctate basophilia does not occur. *Treatment* is with small repeated doses of barbiturates, intravenous dextrose solution and in severe cases intravenous magnesium sulphate up to a maximum of 4·0 G. as a 2·0 per cent. solution.

VIII. Finally, in various conditions referred to in Group II (Emaciation), or Group III (Debility) (p. 855), Pallor may be the symptom which first attracts our notice. ADDISON'S DISEASE is one of these; another is early MYXŒDEMA (§ 575) and the puffiness of the eyes, the failing memory, loss of hair and bodily weakness may for a time escape observation, or be attributed to other causes. MYELO-MATOSIS (§ 613) also may first come under notice for anæmia.

GROUP II. EMACIATION

When loss of weight is complained of or noticed by the physician it must be verified on a reliable pair of scales; and routine subsequent weighings each 1–2 weeks insisted on. WASTING is a common sequence of nearly all acute and many chronic diseases, but when it is the leading or only symptom the following conditions should be borne in mind; for fallacies see § 535.

Marasmus in children may be caused by defective feeding, diarrhœa, constipation, persistent vomiting, hereditary syphilis, rickets, certain nervous states, tuberculosis of the lungs, lymphatic glands or of the peritoneum. These are discussed in §§ 572 *et seq.*

§ **569.** I. TUBERCULOSIS is often first evidenced by an apparently cause-less loss of weight. In latent tuberculosis (§ 514) the trunk and limbs may be wasted although the face is plump and rosy. There is a daily rise in temperature, tendency to night sweats, and careful search will usually reveal an active focus in the lungs (§ 131), peritoneum (§ 573), Fallopian tubes (§ 455), or in the lymphatic glands (§ 581).

II. DIABETES MELLITUS in the young may even impress the patient by the inconsistency of the ravenous appetite and constant thirst with the loss of weight. On the other hand, some middle-aged patients with diabetes are well-nourished and even obese (§ 423).

III. HYPERTHYROIDISM is usually recognised in the young when we meet the combination of exophthalmos, restlessness and nervousness, tachycardia and full thyroid; but in elderly and latent cases the diagnosis may be much more difficult (§ 186).

IV. DEFECTIVE FEEDING and DIGESTIVE DISORDERS constitute one of the largest groups of conditions causing loss of flesh. *Vomiting* and/or *diarrhœa* of any origin cause rapid wasting and dehydration, especially in children. Careful questioning may elicit the fact that the food intake is insufficient in *quantity*; many who live very busy lives regularly miss one or more meals a day, and those who live alone " may not bother " to cook satisfactory meals for themselves. In others the diet is defective in *quality*—perhaps consisting mainly of meat, fruit, vegetables and salads, all of which have a relatively low calorie value. Young women may affect a purposeful reduction in weight by eating insufficient and non-nutritious food. Although rare in this country, a deficiency of vitamins may be causal—especially those of the vitamin B group; thus in pellagra anorexia and loss of weight are early symptoms. Those who oversmoke or consume large quantities of alcoholic spirits often have no inclination to take proper meals.

Digestive Disorders.—Defective teeth and ill-fitting dentures make proper mastication difficult; these or the loss of taste and smell contribute to a poor appetite. Most derangements of the STOMACH cause wasting—gastritis, peptic ulceration, carcinoma and particularly pyloric obstruction with its associated vomiting. Various INTESTINAL DISORDERS may also be causal, such as colitis (especially ulcerative colitis), chronic constipation, intestinal worms and amœbiasis which may be long overlooked. Among the rarer causes, the malabsorption syndrome and especially the various causes of steatorrhœa (§ 316) car lead to considerable loss of weight and of energy.

V. CHRONIC INFECTION may cause emaciation due to long-continued absorption of toxins from defective teeth, tonsils or other hidden foci, or by producing periodic blood-stream infections causing bacteræmia or septicæmia.

VI. DISEASES of the NERVOUS SYSTEM may start with or present generalised wasting, as in bulbar paralysis and paralysis agitans. Wasting due to disappearance of muscular tissue alone, at first localised and later generalised, occurs in *motor-neurone disease* and in *myopathy*.

VII. PSYCHONEUROSES AND PSYCHOTIC STATES form an extremely varied and common cause of loss of weight. Before making this diagnosis it is most important to exclude physical disease and to remember that wasting in a patient with a psychoneurotic condition may be aggravated by a physical cause such as pulmonary tuberculosis. An *anxiety neurosis* is usually associated with progressive loss of weight amounting even to several stones; it is well known that sudden grief as with the loss of a husband or wife and other prolonged emotional stresses are causal. Such causes, especially in young women, have to be differentiated from hyperthyroidism; in both there is emotional instability and tachycardia, but in anxiety states the sleeping pulse rate is not above normal, excessive sweating is usually confined to the hands and the axillæ, and the basal metabolic rate is not raised. *Refusal of food* and consequent starvation is a symptom of hysteria and various psychoses. A variety of this condition is *selective food faddism*, where the patient believes herself incapable of digesting certain foods which are consequently eliminated from the diet. One such patient, troubled with flatulence, lived for years only on preserved ginger and peppermint creams, until scurvy developed. Loss of weight may also be a symptom of an oncoming psychosis such as *schizophrenia*. Some of the cases develop pulmonary tuberculosis. In the variety of manic-depressive psychosis known as *cyclothymia* the patient may lose weight during the periods of excitement, whilst in the alternating depressed phases menstruation is abolished and the patient's weight increases. Profound restlessness especially at night, anxiety and other psychoneurotic manifestations may occur in patients with inexplicable upper abdominal pain due to carcinoma of the pancreas or of the prepyloric area of the stomach. *Anorexia nervosa* is an extreme condition of loss of appetite and loss of weight.

Anorexia Nervosa occurs almost entirely in adolescent and young women—99·5 per cent. of cases are females (see also §§ 273, 1273).

Symptoms.—There is a gradual but progressive loss of appetite so that less and less food is taken until all food is refused. A small meal is associated with a feeling of great fullness and often by vomiting shortly afterwards—this may be hidden from the parents and the doctor. Abdominal pain is strikingly absent. Loss of weight becomes extreme down to 5 stone or less, constipation is severe and amenorrhœa invariable from an early stage. The temperature and pulse rate become subnormal and the body and legs are covered with a fine downy hair. In spite of the extreme weight loss the mental and physical energy is excessive until a late stage when apathy and drowsiness complicated by bed-sores develop. The urine contains no albumen or sugar, but ketone bodies may be present due to starvation.

Diagnosis is from *pituitary cachexia* which usually starts at a later age, is associated with signs of premature senility and with lack of axillary and pubic hair. *Tuberculosis* causes pyrexia, a raised erythrocyte sedimentation rate and often a positive result on a chest X-ray. *Drugs* such as thyroid and amphetamine which reduce weight must be excluded. *Carcinoma of the stomach* is more common in men after 40 years of age.

Etiology.—The condition is believed to be purely psychogenic in origin; no causal physical disease has been found. It may come on as a result of a hidden fear or worry, and may follow deliberate dieting for weight reduction in an overweight girl.

Prognosis.—Patients will sometimes succumb unless energetic treatment is given. Even when weight loss is corrected, relapse may occur. Amenorrhœa often persists for years afterwards.

Treatment can only be undertaken by removing the patient to hospital away from over-anxious parents. The condition must be explained to the patient, and at a later stage psychotherapy is often helpful. A doctor or nurse must sit with the patient until the whole of each moderate sized meal has been consumed. In severe cases temporary feeding via a stomach tube may be needed. In the earlier stages tab. meprobamate 400 mg. twice daily helps; ethyl-nortestosterone (Nilevar) 10 mg. t.i.d. or 25 mg. intramusc. on alternate days helps to produce a large gain in weight and nitrogen retention.

RARER CAUSES

§ 570. **VIII. Pituitary Cachexia** (Syn. Simmond's disease) is caused by destruction or atrophy and sometimes by lack of development of the anterior lobe of the pituitary. This leads to deficiency of hormones necessary for nutrition and growth, and of the adrenocorticotrophic (ACTH), thyrotrophic (TSH) and gonadotrophic hormones. The excretion of these may not be impaired to the same degree so that varying clinical pictures of deficiency of the adrenal cortex, the thyroid and the gonadal functions are met. The condition is much more common in women than in men.

Symptoms.—In *adults*: (1) there is extreme emaciation with a wizened appearance, little subcutaneous fat, a dry wrinkled skin and asthenia; (2) deficiency of ACTH causes hypotension, low blood sugar values and a flat glucose tolerance curve—this may lead to *coma* with marked hypoglycæmia, dehydration with a low serum sodium chloride and hypothermia; (3) deficiency of the thyroid-stimulating hormone causes a slow pulse rate, a low metabolic rate, constipation and also mental slowness which is not usually so marked as in primary myxœdema; (4) lack of gonadotrophic hormone causes amenorrhœa, loss of secondary sexual characteristics, of the pubic and axillary hair and atrophy of the ovaries and uterus. In men there is loss of hair on the face and impotence. (5) Anæmia is usually of the normocytic variety but may be microcytic or macrocytic. (6) Achlorhydria is common. In *children* the findings are similar to those of adults but puberty is much delayed or absent, growth in height is slow or ceases (dwarfism) and epiphyseal union is delayed. *Progeria* is an extreme condition of Simmonds' disease occurring in a child or young adult, associated with premature arteriosclerosis and loss of hair, teeth and nails. After several years death usually occurs, with lethargy and coma.

Diagnosis.—In women the typical signs are the wizened look and wasting, the signs of myxœdema and the obstinate amenorrhœa. In myxœdema due to primary thyroid deficiency, in striking contrast to these pituitary cases, there is a considerable gain in weight, and menorrhagia unless the patient is past the menopause. Anterior pituitary coma must be differentiated from other causes of loss of consciousness (§ 850). The 24-hour urine shows a very low output of 17-ketosteroids and of the follicle-stimulating hormone, and the blood a low content of protein-bound iodine; there is a marked increase of tolerance to insulin.

Etiology.—By far the commonest cause of destruction of the cells of the anterior pituitary is infarction following thrombosis of the pituitary veins after a severe post-partum hæmorrhage. More rarely it is the result of pressure or destruction by a cranio-pharyngioma, suprasellar cyst or chromophobe adenoma, or by deliberate surgical destruction in the treatment of metastasising carcinoma of the breast or ovary. Rarely a granuloma due to tuberculosis, syphilis or sarcoidosis is found. There is atrophy not only of the anterior lobe of the pituitary but also of the suprarenal cortex, thyroid, ovaries, uterus and testes.

Treatment.—A remarkable improvement is usually affected by regular injections of a long-acting preparation of corticotrophin (ACTH) in doses of 20–40 units once daily. It is usually more convenient and just as effective, to give instead oral corticone acetate (12·5–40 mg. in divided doses daily); this rapidly relieves the symptoms, including the mental and physical inertia and the intolerance of cold. In either case thyroid gr. $\frac{1}{2}$–$1\frac{1}{2}$ a day further improves the metabolism. Even with the addition of stilbœstrol it is rare to overcome amenorrhœa, but should pregnancy be achieved there is often a spontaneous recovery—unless a post-partum hæmorrhage recurs. Anterior pituitary coma requires immediate treatment with a rapid intravenous N/2 saline infusion with 5 per cent. dextrose, and with hydrocortisone acetate 100 mg. added to the drip; this must be supplemented by ACTH gel 40 units or hydrocortisone acetate 100 units intramusc.

IX. DRUGS may act by depressing the mental or physical faculties or by impairing digestion. Drug addicts (*e.g.*, morphia, heroin, cocaine) are almost invariably emaciated. Drug addiction to thyroid and amphetamine have been recorded. The later stages of chronic alcoholism may produce marked loss of weight.

X. Other rare causes such as DIABETES INSIPIDUS, PANCREATIC DISEASES, PERNICIOUS ANÆMIA, HODGKIN'S DISEASE, CIRRHOSIS of the liver and SYPHILIS, are described in their respective paragraphs.

Localised absence of fat occurs in the rare condition called PROGRESSIVE LIPODYSTROPHY. Fat disappears from the face, arms and upper body and accumulates over the lower trunk, hips and lower extremities (§ 16).

In ELDERLY SUBJECTS, although any of the above causes may be in operation, suspect especially:—

§ 571. XI. **Malignant Disease** (Carcinoma and Sarcoma) is one of the commonest causes of loss of weight and of strength, leading to emaciation. Carcinoma must always be considered when these symptoms arise in a patient at or past middle age; it is much more common than sarcoma which is the commonest form of malignant disease in children and young adults. A rare third variety is a malignant teratoma derived from embryonic tissue. The essential features of a malignant tumour are the tendency to invade neighbouring parts, to recur after removal and to metastasise in distant areas. *Carcinomata* may arise from any epithelial or mucous surface; common primary sites are the bronchus, stomach, colon, rectum, breast, uterus, tongue, œsophagus and skin. The primary source of the growth may be latent when it arises in the stomach, colon, pancreas, thyroid, breast or prostate. *Sarcomata* arise from connective tissue of mesodermal origin, especially from lymph glands, bones, cartilage, fibrous tissue, brain, spinal cord, retina and in the kidney in children (Wilm's tumour). Malignant growths vary considerably in their rate of growth and dissemination : with carcinomata, those with an abundant hard stroma (scirrhous types) are relatively slow growing as compared with the tumours which consist almost entirely of malignant cells and which are soft (like brain tissue—encephaloid types). Among sarcomata the melanotic and round-celled forms are very malignant, whereas fibro-sarcomata are the slowest growing.

In England and Wales in 1959 malignant disease accounted for 18 per cent. of all deaths. The commonest site of origin was the bronchus and lung (14 per cent.) and if those cases are included which were not specified as to whether the bronchus and lung were primary or secondary, this figure rises to 21 per cent. Other common primary sites were stomach (14 per cent.), breast (9 per cent.), rectum (6 per cent.) and the pancreas, prostate and uterus (each 4 per cent.).

Early Symptoms.—(1) The initial symptoms may depend on the *primary site of the disease.* Thus the patient may first seek advice for (i.) a lump (as in the breast); (ii.) pain (from local invasion); (iii.) a repeated blood-stained secretion (*e.g.*, from the bronchus) or a continuous blood-stained discharge (*e.g.*, from the uterus or rectum); or (iv.) symptoms and signs of obstruction (*e.g.*, of the colon or pylorus). The diagnosis of these has been considered already (the abdomen, § 263; the chest, §§ 81, 138). (2) In other cases the first evidence of the disorder may be from the *disorganisation produced by metastases.* Carcinomata usually spread *via* the lymphatic system (with certain notable exceptions, *e.g.*, hypernephroma of a kidney which spreads *via* the blood-stream). They tend to invade (i.) neighbouring glands; (ii.) the liver, often with hard, tender nodules and producing obstructive jaundice; (iii.) adjacent structures to which they become adherent; (iv.) the serous sacs by a spread through their serous covering, producing effusions (often blood-stained) in the peritoneum or pleura; when they gravitate into the pelvis as from a carcinoma of the stomach there is often secondary involvement of the ovaries or deposits in the other pelvic organs; (v.) the bones. Cancer of the breast, bronchus, kidney, thyroid, prostate or ovary also invades the blood-vessels and may be recognised by a constant pain in the back from metastases in the vertebræ, by a spontaneous fracture or by X-ray evidence of a metastasis in the lung. Carcinoma of a bronchus often first declares itself by the occurrence of a cerebral metastasis. Sarcomata usually spread by the blood-stream, with metastases in the lungs, liver, bones or skin; but a lymphosarcoma tends to spread via the lymphatic channels. (3) The patient may first seek advice for the symptoms of general debility. Especially prominent are (i.) loss of general energy and

strength, (ii.) loss of appetite, (iii.) loss of weight. *Late Symptoms.*—
Cancerous cachexia occurs: the patient looks ill, becomes anæmic and the
skin assumes a yellowish, earthy or sallow hue and becomes inelastic. An
irregular temperature arises, especially when the growth ulcerates through
to the surface of the skin or mucous membrane, or when the liver is involved.

Diagnosis.—Malignant disease may have to be diagnosed from all the
other conditions which give rise to emaciation. (1) A thorough clinical
examination must be carried out in every case, including the rectum and
pelvic organs. (2) When malignancy is suspected a careful X-ray examination of the possible primary sites is essential. X-ray examination of the
lungs may reveal metastases. (3) Any obscure cause of anæmia in a
middle-aged or elderly person can be due to carcinoma; occult blood tests
of the stool may reveal persistent bleeding into the digestive tract. (4) In
any case of doubt, especially when persistent pain is accompanied by progressive weight loss and anæmia, surgical exploration or a biopsy must
be carried out to ensure early diagnosis and treatment.

Etiology.—The cause of cancer in human beings is not known. It is
generally agreed that whereas the cells of normal tissues multiply and grow
in a controlled manner to the benefit of the host, cancerous tumours are
composed of tissue cells whose growth is unrestrained: they are of a primitive
type, with an exuberant rate of growth and multiplication, and a histological pattern which may bear little or no resemblance to the cell proto-
type which gave rise to them; ultimately they destroy the host which
harbours them. One of the earliest phases in cancer research was the
recognition of the striking resemblance between the appearances and
behaviour of cancer cells and of embryonic cells. It is possible that the
cancer cell is a somatic mutant by loss, or inactivation of key proteins or
enzyme-proteins, necessary in the normal cell for the physiological regulation of growth and division (A. Haddow). The most important factors
now recognised as being contributory or causal are: (1) Carcinogenic
chemical agents. For years cancer of the scrotum in chimney sweeps has
been recognised as being the result of contamination of the skin by soot.
Later it was agreed that cancer of the skin due to impregnation by mineral
lubricating oils occurred in shale-oil operatives and in coal and tar workers
due to dibenzanthracene, and that cancer of the bladder can be the result
of working in the dye industries with α- or β-naphthylamine, benzidine,
auramine or fuchsin. Now hundreds of chemical carcinogens are known.
Lung cancer which today forms the largest group of cancerous growths in
the human being, is commonly believed to be due to carcinogenic factors in
tobacco smoke (§ 138). (2) An entirely different group of potential chemical
carcinogens is that of the naturally occurring and synthetic sex-hormones
(steroids). Malignant growths appear on occasions when these are administered in large amounts, withdrawn or imbalanced. During the child-
bearing period, cancer of the breast may remit to a remarkable degree if
naturally-occurring œstrogens are " neutralised " by testosterone; and
synthetic œstrogens may act similarly when the disease occurs after

menopause. Similarly cancer of the male breast may remit after orchi-dectomy and cancer of the prostate often responds to large doses of a synthetic œstrogen. Cases of extensive metastases from cancer of the breast in woman remit for an average of two years after complete elimina-tion of œstrogen production by bilateral oophorectomy combined with removal of both suprarenals (with replacement by corticosteroids). (3) Irradiation with high total doses of X-rays in cases of lupus vulgaris and in thyrotoxicosis can produce carcinomata and new powerful penetrating rays may produce fibrosarcoma. Likewise exposure to ionising radiations may produce leukæmic effects. (4) Although specific viruses or virus-like agents will produce the growth and transference of tumours such as the Rous sarcoma of chicken, the Shope papilloma of rabbits and mammary cancer in mice, there is as yet no evidence that viral agents produce malignant tumours in man. (5) Heredity and blood groups do on occasions cause an increased susceptibility to certain types of cancer in human beings. (6) There is evidence that some persons affected by cancer are able to build up a resistance to the disease.

The *Prognosis* in untreated cases is always grave, the course rarely lasting more than one, or, at the outside, two years. A few cases of undoubted malignant disease have undergone spontaneous involution. The prognosis depends largely on whether the disease is detected at an early stage so that it may be removed or arrested.

In 1957 the Registrar-General gave the 5-year survival rates for early disease treated radically as follows (the survival rates for all cases being given in brackets): cancer of the female breast 67 per cent. (37 per cent.); cervix uteri 50 per cent. (35 per cent.); stomach 28 per cent. (5 per cent.); intestine 45 per cent. (17 per cent.); lung 14 per cent. (2 per cent.).

The prognosis also depends on (1) the position and accessibility of the growth, how far vital structures are involved, and whether it is on or near the surface; (2) the structure of the tumour (*vide supra*); and (3) the age of the patient, for growth is more rapid in the young. When the primary growth has been removed, seedling growths may cause local recurrences or distant metastases even 10 to 20 years afterwards.

Treatment can be considered under that of (*a*) the disease itself and (*b*) symptomatic measures. (*a*) The PRIMARY DISEASE and its secondary deposits are treated by four main methods: (i.) *Radical surgery* with removal of the primary growth, of the local lesions produced by direct spread and of the regional lymph glands which may be involved, is still much the most satisfactory procedure; but this is useless when detectable visceral metastases have formed. (ii.) *Endocrine therapy* is particularly useful in cancer of the breast and prostate. In women with cancer of the breast, androgens (such as subcutaneous implantation of testosterone 1,000 mg.) often combined with ovariectomy are used before menopause; after the age of 60 synthetic œstrogens may be given. In favourable cases there is decrease in the size of the regional lymph glands, relief of pain and recalci-fication of areas of deposits in bones, but such benefits rarely last more than 1 to 2 years. Cancer of the male breast often remits after orchidectomy. With cancer of the prostate, œstrogens in full doses combine with curettage of the testicular cells often cause retrogression of the primary growth as well as of secondary metastases in bones. (iii.) *Chemical agents* are chiefly of value in the leukæmias (§§ 556, 557), but are also used in patients with Hodgkin's disease, chorion epithelioma (§ 450) and various reticuloses. (iv.) *Radiotherapy* aims at decreasing the rate of growth and sometimes destroying a radio-sensitive tumour: it has been estimated that about 10 per cent. of tumours are totally radio-resistant. Modern X-ray apparatuses such as the 2-million electron volt generator, the 4-million electron volt linear accelerator, the betatron and the large cobalt units have largely replaced older machines and have greatly altered the clinical aspects and results of irradiation. In some cases radio-active isotopes are valuable (§ 190). SYMPTOMATIC measures for the relief of pain and of emotional distress include skilled nursing care, the administration of analgesics and more recently of chlorpromazine.

A **Carcinoid tumour** is of low malignancy arising typically from argentaffin cells in the small intestine, and metastasising later in the liver. Rarely similar symptoms are produced by an oat-celled carcinoma or a "metastasising adenoma" of the bronchus. The argentaffin cells produce excessive amounts of serotonin (5-hydroxy-tryptamine, 5 H.T.) which is excreted in the urine as 5-hydroxy-indole acetic acid, thus confirming the diagnosis.

Symptoms are of three types. (1) The malabsorption syndrome with diarrhœa partly due to the effect of 5 H.T. in stimulating intestinal muscle; later (2) attacks of bright flushing of the face superimposed on a dark purplish suffused facies; (3) a thick deposit on the inner wall of the right heart causing the signs of tricuspid or pulmonary stenosis and later right-sided heart failure.

Treatment is by removal of the primary tumour; and temporary relief of symptoms may be achieved by removal of a single large deposit in the liver.

XII. SENILE DECAY AND GENERAL ARTERIOSCLEROSIS. Many people lose weight in their later years, especially as their mental and physical faculties decline. Some gain weight as a result of enforced idleness and immoderate appetite (and see § 574).

XIII. CHRONIC NEPHRITIS and Chronic Pyelonephritis may be an unsuspected cause in an older person until the urine is examined (§ 399). The associated nausea and vomiting of the later stages add to the wasting, and the rapidity of the loss of weight is a fair guide to the prognosis.

§ 572. **Marasmus in Children.**—Infants and children emaciate with almost any disorder and with surprising rapidity. An attack of diarrhœa may give rise to loss of much weight in 24 hours. The principal causes are:

(*a*) Those which occur chiefly under two years of age: Defective or improper food or feeding; those associated with diarrhœa or constipation; those associated with persistent vomiting; hereditary syphilis; and rickets.

(*b*) Those which are met with chiefly after two years of age: Nervous causes, certain constitutional conditions, and tuberculosis of the lungs, peritoneum, or lymphatic glands.

I. DEFECTIVE FEEDING is a common cause of emaciation. Such children are always fretful, underweight, late in sitting up and teething, with poor muscular tone and often anæmia. The bowels are irregular, constipation often alternating with diarrhœa is common, and the stools furnish a good index as to the chief defect in assimilation present—undigested " curds " of protein, greasy masses of soaps and fats, or green and explosive stools due to excess of carbohydrate. Breast milk may be too plentiful or too little, or when breast feeding is continued beyond the ninth month iron and other deficiencies occur. About the third-fourth months it is usual to commence mixed feeding to supplement breast or artificial milk foods. For further information special books on the feeding of infants must be consulted. In older children the diet is often unbalanced: thus the poorer child usually has too much sugar, white bread and biscuits and too little milk. The wealthy child has often too much fat (butter, milk and cream) and too little carbohydrate.

II. DIARRHŒA and CONSTIPATION are potent causes of wasting in infancy and childhood; they are due to dietetic errors or defective cleanliness in the nursery and may be associated with intestinal worms. Infantile diarrhœa is discussed in § 310. Chronic constipation undoubtedly causes marasmus. In a family two children died of marasmus associated with obstinate constipation; the third child who, the mother stated, exactly resembled the others in all particulars, was following the same fatal course until systematic treatment by an aperient mixture restored the health.

III. PERSISTENT VOMITING may be due to errors of diet, especially too frequent or over-feeding, or to gastro-intestinal catarrh. Careful dieting cures most cases. The reflex and other causes of vomiting (§ 271) must be considered when simple treatment is unavailing. In intractable cases feeding by a nasal catheter has been resorted to. Hypertrophic stenosis of the pylorus is a rare cause of vomiting in infants (§ 271).

IV. HEREDITARY SYPHILIS is recognised by snuffles and other signs which appear generally during the first six months (see § 500).

V. RICKETS (§ 608) may be accompanied by wasting, but is more common in children who are overweight. It appears between the sixth and the eighteenth month of life; rarely after two years of age, unless associated with renal or cœliac disease (§ 608).

In *older children*, in addition to the above-mentioned causes which may continue to operate, wasting is due to VI. NERVOUS CAUSES. A child in an unhappy environment, or who inherits a nervous disposition, is usually thin, restless, and subject to gastro-intestinal attacks. Dr. Cameron has drawn attention to a well-known type—the child full of energy, soon exhausted, and subject to attacks of prostration with pallor, irritability, even vomiting and fever. These children apparently have a defective fat metabolism and are in better health when the fat in their diet is reduced and the sugar increased. Cyclical vomiting is a closely allied condition (§ 271).

VII. CONSTITUTIONAL CONDITIONS such as asthma (§ 127), cœliac disease (§ 317), recurrent bronchitis and congenital abnormalities often cause wasting.

VIII. PULMONARY TUBERCULOSIS is usually insidious in onset as in adults. It more commonly affects the bases than the apices and causes a chronic cough, persistent pyrexia and wasting. Tubercle bacilli can usually be detected in sputum, from stomach washings or in the stools.

§ 573. IX. **Tuberculous Peritonitis** is a wasting disorder occurring for the most part in children of two years and upwards, due to tuberculosis of the peritoneum and the mesenteric glands. This form was formerly known as tabes mesenterica.

Symptoms.—The onset is very insidious, and may extend over many months. Gradually the limbs and face become shrunken, and there are anæmia, listlessness, attacks of pyrexia, and sometimes abdominal cramps. The leading physical sign is the enlarged abdomen, which is generally tympanitic on percussion. There are three main types: (i.) the ascitic, (ii.) the fibro-caseous adhesive, and (iii.) the loculated type, which is a combination of the first two. (i.) In the ascitic variety, the patient complains of little pain; gastro-intestinal symptoms may be absent, but ascites is present. Ascites unaccompanied by general œdema in a young adult is usually due to tuberculous peritonitis. A sample of fluid shows an excess of protein and of lymphocytes, and guinea-pig inoculations often confirm the diagnosis. (ii.) In the adhesive variety, there is matting together of the peritoneum and intestines; this may be localised or generalised. Attacks of diarrhœa or constipation occur, perhaps with signs of intestinal obstruction. Pain and tenderness may be marked features, and localised thickenings and masses with a doughy feeling can be palpated. The rolled-up omentum often forms a tumour stretching across the upper abdomen below the edge of the liver. (iii.) In the loculated variety matting occurs, with encysted fluid in the centre. The hectic fever so common in tuberculosis may be present, and sometimes the disease runs a more acute course with pyrexia, resembling typhoid fever. (iv.) Tuberculosis of the ileo-caecal group of lymph glands causes general ill-health, and may cause local pain and swelling often confused with appendicitis.

Diagnosis.—In addition to the diseases just mentioned, tuberculous peritonitis may have to be distinguished from the distension of the bowels due to improper feeding, in which there is generally no pyrexia, no resistant masses, and disappearance on regulating the diet. X-rays may reveal calcification of the tuberculous masses in chronic cases. The Mantoux test is strongly positive. *Rickets* (§ 608) may show a distended abdomen, but the characteristic rachitic changes in the skeleton differentiate it. In *Hirschsprung's disease* large enemata bring away the masses palpable through the abdominal wall (§ 324). *Cœliac disease* (see § 317).

Etiology.—Tuberculosis of the mesenteric glands is usually due to the ingestion of infected milk: it may occur at almost any age, but is rare under two. Males are affected more than females. If the mucous membrane of the alimentary canal is diseased, the risk of infection is greater. The miliary type with ascites may be of systemic origin. Other varieties arise by extension from tuberculous enteritis, salpingitis, ileo-cæcal or mesenteric gland tuberculosis.

Prognosis.—Before the introduction of modern methods of treatment, the course of the disease was apt to show intervals of apparent recovery interrupted by relapses. The ascitic cases usually made the best recovery. Untoward symptoms were acute local pain and tenderness due to peritonitis, persistent diarrhœa and evidence of tuberculosis elsewhere. *Complications* included miliary tuberculosis, abscesses bursting in various situations such as into the peritoneum or forming a chronic fistula on the surface as at the umbilicus. Intestinal obstruction sometimes followed the forma-tion of bands of adhesions. Adequate and prolonged treatment with modern methods usually causes the disease to resolve without such complications.

Treatment is by a period of bed rest, specific antibiotic and chemotherapy (§ 131) and a full diet. Only when there is obstruction of the lacteals with steatorrhœa need the fat intake be restricted. Although open operation and swabbing out the fluid was often curative in the past, this is now rarely necessary. Prophylactic measures consist in sterilising or pasteurising cow's milk, and regulating the supply whence it is obtained. The disease is now much less common in Britain than formerly, since pasteurisation of milk has been generally adopted.

GROUP III. DEBILITY ONLY (ASTHENIA)

The causes of debility not necessarily accompanied either by pallor or by emaciation are as numerous as those of the two preceding groups, and it must be remembered that all the disorders in both of those groups may commence with weakness only; in short, the majority of chronic disorders begin with debility. After any acute illness debility is present; this is usual after fevers, and is especially marked after influenza. The fallacies (§ 535) and methods of examination have already been given.

It should be remembered that profound fatigue may be complained of for a few days to a week before the onset of any acute disease. The same symptom may be complained of, before any sign is evident, in cases of tonsillitis or even of the " common cold."

COMMONER CAUSES

I.   Senile decay and arterial disease.
II.   Disease of the Nervous System, functional or organic.
III.   Chronic infections. Focal infection and tuberculosis.
IV.   Chronic dyspepsia and many other abdominal diseases.
V.   Chronic nephritis.
VI.   Myxœdema.
VII.   Conditions referred to in Groups I and II, and especially the early stages of Diabetes Mellitus, Hyperthyroidism, Anæmia of any origin (especially Pernicious Anæmia) and Leukæmia.
VIII.   After shock or operation, or after the specific fevers.

RARER CAUSES

IX.   Addison's disease.
X.   Hæmochromatosis.
XI.   Diseases of the Pancreas, Acromegaly, Myelomatosis, Beri-beri, Pellagra, Alkalosis, Hypoglycæmia.
XII.   Carbon monoxide poisoning.

When a patient is suffering from debility or loss of vigour of mind and body without any very marked pallor or obvious loss of flesh, and without any marked physical signs or other evidence of disease, in the *first half* of life one would suspect neurasthenia, chronic dyspepsia or gastro-intestinal disorders, incipient or latent tuberculosis, diabetes mellitus or diabetes insipidus.

In the *second half* of life one would suspect senile decay, chronic nephritis, focal infection, cardiac valvular or aortic disease, diabetes, myxœdema, Addison's disease; and failing these, some of the conditions previously mentioned among the anæmic or wasting disorders (Groups I and II).

§ 574. I. Senile Decay and Arterial Disease.—As we advance in years the power both of body and mind notably declines. This should not be very obvious under sixty, but the age at which it appears differs considerably in different persons, and still more in different families, for the onset of decay in human beings, as in plants and animals, is largely a question of heredity plus the previous habits of the individual. It is also contributed to by chronic alcoholism, gout, hypertension, syphilis, hypothyroidism, chronic nephritis, focal infection and occasionally by chronic lead poisoning. Structurally there is a general tendency to degeneration or atrophy of the parenchyma or functionally active tissues, and slight increase in the tissues, such as fibrous and supporting tissues, in all the organs and structures of the body. This is seen particularly in the cardio-vascular system, where the deeper layers of the intima first show signs of senile degeneration (§ 93).

Symptoms.—Consequent on the changes above mentioned there is a universal lowering of vitality and nutrition, and the general enfeeblement of thought, word and act which results in the mumbling, fumbling and stumbling of old age. Physical weakness comes on so slowly that the patient may be hardly aware of it. In the second half of life, and especially in those with an alcoholic history, widespread arteriosclerosis, often with accompanying myocardial degeneration, may produce no other symptom than lack of mental and physical energy. It is not sufficiently recognised that widespread disease of the arteries alone is the commonest cause of progressive mental and bodily enfeeblement in the elderly and can occur even at the age of 50 years.

The following case illustrates this: Jessie T—— (æt. 49) first began to complain of muscular and mental weakness four years previously. This gradually increased, so that at the time of admission she could only walk by pushing a chair before her, and she resembled a person with paraplegia. There were no physical signs in any organ, no evidence of disease in the nervous system at any time, and the urine was always normal. She became progressively more and more enfeebled in body and mind, gradually took to bed, and died, ten years after admission, of progressive asthenia. At autopsy all the organs were normal, both macro- and microscopically, with the exception of atrophy; but there was extreme and widespread disease of all the arteries of the body and of the brain, the main change being brown atrophy of the heart muscle and narrowing and thickening of the arteries.

The symptoms affect different systems of the body in different individuals. *Cerebral arteriosclerosis* causes slowing of the mental processes, deficient powers of concentration and a gradually failing memory, especially for recent events. Vertigo is frequent and a series of small strokes may occur. Senile dementia is sometimes seen in the later stages (§ 1187). In others the symptoms associated with carotid or basilar artery insufficiency may show themselves (§ 904). A large number of other cerebral vascular symptoms may be experienced, and even syncope may occur (§§ 35, 833). Thrombosis, hæmorrhage and aneurysmal formation are complications which may develop in many different areas. *Cardiac ischæmia* gives rise to shortness of breath on exertion and the symptoms of angina pectoris. It is very common in later life to hear a systolic murmur at the mitral or aortic areas due to hardening of the valve cusps. *Disease of the peripheral arteries* causes a sense of weakness in the legs, intermittent claudication and even senile gangrene (§§ 586, 587). A poor blood supply via the splanchnic vessels produces flatulence, a diminished appetite and sometimes diarrhœa which contribute to the loss of weight so commonly seen in the aged. There is a *reduced resistance to infection* in different parts of the body and bronchitis, pneumonia and chronic pyelonephritis are common and often determine the end. The urine should be examined each few months for albumen which may indicate chronic nephritis, and also for sugar as diabetes in the elderly is usually of a mild type and produces few symptoms.

The *Prognosis* depends on the rate of progress of the arteriosclerotic changes and to a greater extent on the degree and type of changes in the various tissues resulting from this. When mental and physical stress are diminished so that the demands on the circulation are lessened, the prognosis is correspondingly improved. Any chronic infection, however slight, is poorly tolerated; chronic constipation which is particularly liable to lead to fæcal impaction of the rectum in patients who are largely bedridden, can cause serious deterioration in health until it is remedied.

Treatment.—It is most important that elderly people should be given an occupation or interests in life which lie within their capacity. Nothing produces more rapid deterioration than forcing an ageing man or woman to discard his or her everyday pursuits so that he or she spends most of the day either in a chair or lying in bed. A business man may be greatly helped by going to his office for a shortened day three or four times a week and a housewife should be encouraged to carry on her less arduous househol l duties as long as possible. The food should be light, nutritious and ea il y assimilable but small in quantity; it is remarkable how small a quantit y the aged require. A daily supplement of vitamins (especially of the vitan iin B group) is often helpful. A little whisky or a similar stimulant at be lt ne is often called for. Regular exercise and a daily walk in the fresh air v. in the weather allows is essential. Elderly people do not need so iai h sleep as in their younger years but a long night's rest in bed and an aft r-noon " nap " are necessary. Remember to keep them warm, do not ovt r-feed them and keep them away from relatives and friends who may briig a respiratory infection into their homes.

II. DISEASES OF THE NERVOUS SYSTEM, FUNCTIONAL OR ORGANIC. In various *functional and degenerative conditions of the nervous system* general weakness may be the chief complaint. *Sleeplessness, worry and mental strain* are potent causes in modern life. This is especially true of functional disorders, such as neurasthenia and hysteria, where the weakness may amount to complete prostration. Such cases are usually seen in the first half of life or middle age. *Toxic* or *infective* causes may be present, such as addiction to alcohol, tobacco or morphine, and bromide intoxication. *Polyneuritis* is often described by the patient as causing general weakness, in which the limbs are especially involved. Among the gross lesions which may develop insidiously, with weakness, are *paralysis agitans, bulbar paralysis*, and frontal *cerebral tumour*—diseases more often met in the second half of life. *Myasthenia gravis* is a rare condition, usually evidenced by local and generalised weakness (§ 988).

III. FOCAL INFECTION should be looked for in long-continued debility without any definite cause. Fleeting or constant " rheumatic " pains and low-grade pyrexia may also be present. Pus in the antrum, sinuses or tonsil is often unsuspected. A dead tooth, with a granuloma at its root not always shown on X-ray, may in time cause serious illness. Uterine or cervical discharge may be overlooked. EARLY TUBERCULOSIS of the lungs and other areas should always be remembered in cases of unexplained general debility, especially in younger persons.

IV. CHRONIC DYSPEPSIA, gastritis, visceroptosis, and other obscure DISEASES WITHIN THE ABDOMEN may be attended for long by debility only. Gastro-intestinal troubles produce debility by causing toxæmia and mal-assimilation of food. In *E. coli* infections, before the development of urinary signs, there is often a history of many months of readily induced fatigue. In women there is often, but not always, a concurrent history of frequent micturition; in children this may be absent. *Mucous colitis* may be especially mentioned, also *chronic appendicitis, abdominal cancer*, and many of the other conditions mentioned in Chapter IX.

V. CHRONIC INTERSTITIAL NEPHRITIS (§ 401) AND CHRONIC PYELO-NEPHRITIS (§ 407) cause progressive enfeeblement coming on at or past middle life. Chronic nephritis is apt to be mistaken for senility; failing vigour is the leading symptom for which the patient seeks advice in a large proportion of both these conditions. Sometimes this weakness is accompanied by general muscular wasting, but quite as often there is none. The complexion is generally sallow, but there is no definite pallor till late in the disease. Hypertension is often present. Headache is common, chronic interstitial nephritis being one of the commonest causes of headache coming on after middle life.

§ 575. VI. **Myxœdema** ($\mu \acute{v} \xi a$, mucus; $o \acute{\iota} \delta \eta \mu a$, swelling) is in most cases an insidious disease which often remains undiagnosed for many months. It is characterised by weakness, lethargy, and other manifestations of deficiency in the metabolic processes of the body, due to diminished thyroid function. It was first described by Sir William Gull (1874), so named by Dr. Ord (1878) who at first believed it constituted a new and till then undescribed form of generalised œdema. Extracellular mucoid material develops in many of the organs and tissues of the body, particularly in the skin round the hair follicles, sweat and sebaceous gland, in the subcutaneous tissues and in the tongue; this does not allow pitting on pressure.

Symptoms.—(1) The weakness is associated with a characteristic slowness of action, thought and speech. It usually comes on very gradually, but occasionally is of acute onset and is much more common in women at the menopause, in whom the milder degrees are often overlooked. (2) The aspect is so characteristic that when the doctor has once seen a case he recognises it again directly (Fig. 1). The skin has a yellow tint which contrasts with a flush on the cheeks. The face is smooth and expressionless, is slightly puffy especially around the eyes, the eyebrows are thin especially in the outer parts, and the hair of the scalp is coarse, dry, sparse and unruly. (3) There is a deposit of connective tissue in the skin as a whole, often with pads above the clavicles, back of the neck and over the deltoids. The hands become puffy and spade-like. The skin is dry and inelastic, and rarely sweats: it looks œdematous but does not pit on pressure except around the ankles. (4) The tongue is broad and flabby. (5) The mental processes are dulled, the speech is slowed and often husky, and at times wandering of thought and action may give rise to hallucinations or to mild dementia, " myxœdema madness." In some, sudden coma sets in. (6) The knee and ankle jerks are sluggish but are maintained for longer than usual. Occasionally the limb muscles ache, fatigue readily, are stiff and a little swollen (Hoffman's syndrome). The temperature is subnormal, the hands and feet cold and blue and intolerance of cold weather is usual. (7) The pulse rate is slowed to 45–60 per minute, but myocardial degeneration often ensues with a dilated heart, poor heart sounds, and even a rapid pulse rate. Angina pectoris due to coronary disease is often complained of and the blood-vessels as a whole become prematurely sclerotic, often with a raised blood pressure. (8) Digestive processes are slowed and obstinate constipation with a dilated colon is the rule. (9) Menorrhagia is usual unless the patient has passed the menopause. The 24-hour urinary excretion of 17-ketosteroids is low. (10) Anæmia may be of the iron-deficiency type, may be normochromic or rarely megaloblastic; hypoplasia of the bone marrow is sometimes present. (11) Albuminuria in small amounts is often found. (12) The basal metabolic rate is lowered, and a considerable gain in weight is usual. (13) The thyroid gland is commonly diminished in size, but may be larger than normal. In rare instances the condition is not primarily due to under-action of the thyroid gland but to diminution of the *thyrotropic hormone of the pituitary*, when amenorrhœa, *loss* of weight, and other evidences of anterior pituitary deficiency accompany the myxœdema (§ 570).

Diagnosis.—The cardinal symptoms are loss of energy, extreme intolerance of cold weather, a dry skin and falling hair, pads above the clavicles, constipation, bradycardia and gain in weight. Myxœdema may be mistaken in its earlier stages for *anæmia* and the other disorders mentioned in Group I, and also for the other various causes of *debility*. It may be diagnosed from chronic nephritis and other forms of renal disease by the absence of generalised *pitting* œdema, and by examination of the blood and urine.

Special Investigations.—(1) A lowered basal metabolic rate, even as low as minus 30–40 per cent., is diagnostic (§ 1214). (2) The radio-iodine uptake of the thyroid gland is much below normal but the patient must not have been given iodine-containing drugs or thiouracil preparations beforehand. (3) The protein-bound iodine in the blood is liable to similar fallacies, but otherwise is a good measure of the amount of circulating thyroid hormone; values below 4 μg./100 ml. indicate hypothyroidism. (4) The electro-cardiogram shows a low voltage in all the leads and often flattened or inverted T-waves in the limb leads. (5) The blood cholesterol may be high from the commencement or only rise to high levels late in the disease (and see § 184).

Etiology.—The disease is due to a deficiency of thyroid function and is much more common in women around or after the menopause. It often runs in families, some members of which may be hyperthyroid. The gland is usually small and fibrotic but can be of normal dimensions. The cause of the thyroid atrophy is not established but many cases are believed to be due to destruction of the gland by an auto-immunological process whereby anti-bodies develop to destroy thyroglobulin as it is formed in the gland. Occasionally myxœdema may be post-operative or the result of treatment with thiouracil preparations or radio-iodine. The extracellular material in the skin and other tissues is a muco-polysaccharide in combination with protein. For juvenile myxœdema see § 192.

Prognosis.—Before the introduction of the thyroid treatment advanced cases rarely lived more than a few years, dying usually of cardio-vascular changes or some intercurrent disease. Cardio-vascular complications still occur unless patients are treated early and continue treatment for the rest of their lives.

Treatment by the oral administration of thyroid is so efficacious that this may be used as a means of diagnosis. Thyroid (B.P.) is best given once a day commencing with gr. ¼ to prevent reactions, but the dose needs to be increased to a maximum of gr. 2, 3 or even gr. 5 daily until symptoms are controlled. The drug must be given very cautiously in the presence of angina, tachycardia or other signs of myocardial degeneration and must never be pushed to the point of *producing* tachycardia. Many prefer l-thyroxine sodium (B.P.C.) starting with 0·05 mg. and increasing to 0·2, 0·3 or 0·5 mg. daily because of its greater stability. Complete recovery should follow after a few weeks or months of treatment but the patient must continue the preparation indefinitely: for the effect of treatment see Fig. 1. In cases of urgency, as in myxœdemic mania or coma, intra-venous l-triiodothyronine sodium (20–60 μg. daily) produces an even more rapid response, but for maintenance l-thyroxine or thyroid is preferable.

LOCALISED MYXŒDEMA occurs in the presence of hyper- or hypo-thyroidism and consists of a thickened plaque of skin, usually over both shins.

RARER CAUSES OF DEBILITY

§ 576. IX. **Addison's Disease** is a rare condition, described by Dr. Addison in 1855, characterised by progressive loss of strength and weight, general pigmentation of the skin and hypotension due to disease of the cortex of the suprarenal glands.

The *Symptoms* come under five categories: (1) Progressive *physical weakness* is its most marked feature and may appear long before any other symptom. It is unaccompanied, as a rule, either by anæmia or marked emaciation until perhaps at a late stage. Uncomplicated cases present a subnormal temperature throughout, but in those of tuberculous origin a low-grade temperature is common. (2) *Pigmentation* of the skin ensues sooner or later in most people, but may be slight or absent in the very fair skinned. The colour begins with a yellowish tint, which gradually deepens into a bronze mahogany colour in those of dark complexion. The localities most affected are the exposed parts (the face, neck and hands), those where pigmentation is normally present, such as the axillæ and nipples, and sites of pressure (*e.g.*, the waist); the palms are scarcely affected but the creases of the hands and fingers show the pigmentation. The edge of a patch of colour shades gradually into the healthy skin around, which makes it difficult to discover such a patch in its early stage. The mucous membranes of the cheeks, soft and hard palate, gums, lips and the sides of the tongue frequently show pigmented patches. (3) *Gastric* symptoms generally occur at some time, such as nausea, vomiting, hiccough, and pain in the upper abdomen and loins. Loss of weight is usual. Pains in the limbs may also be complained of. There is often constipation, but sometimes there is intractable diarrhœa, which may be fatal. (4) *Cardiovascular symptoms* may be present—palpitation, dyspnœa, sighing, yawning, a poor peripheral circulation, and later a tendency to collapse. A marked feature is the low systolic and diastolic pressure (*e.g.*, 70S–50D). (5) *Nervous symptoms* are less common, but may consist of headache, vertigo and nervousness. The mind is clear, except towards the end, when delirium, convulsions, or coma may set in. (6) *Crises* in the symptoms and signs are precipitated by infection, even minor operations, over-excitement and cessation of treatment: in them there is collapse, dehydration and hypoglycæmia, a subnormal temperature with a rapid feeble pulse, a very low blood pressure, vomiting and diarrhœa with oliguria or anuria: irritability or stupor may precede death. (7) The *blood* shows mild anæmia except in the crises when dehydration tends to produce polycythæmia. The blood sugar is normal or subnormal but the blood urea a little raised (up to 80 mg. per cent.). The sodium and chloride content of the plasma are usually low (below 300 and 330 mg. per cent. respectively), whereas the potassium is usually high. These groups of symptoms vary in their predominance, but asthenia and a low blood pressure are always present, and pigmentation nearly always. An acute variety may occur.

The *Diagnosis* is often difficult in the early stages on account of the vagueness of the symptoms, but should be suspected when the systolic pressure is under 100 mm. and especially when under 90 mm.; some patients have a low blood pressure for most of their lives without Addison's disease appearing. The pigmentation resembles that of other cachectic states but the latter rarely show pigmentation of the mucous membranes. The low serum values of the sodium and chloride are distinctive. *Cancer of the pylorus* is accompanied by sallowness, which is often mistaken for the pigmentation of Addison's disease. Both, moreover, are accompanied by enfeeblement, gastric pain and vomiting. Other *pigmentary conditions* are mentioned under pigmentation (§ 754); slight jaundice, the pigmentation of malaria, chloasma and arsenical pigmentation are the chief causes of error in diagnosis. *Chronic nephritis*, neurasthenia, and other conditions attended by asthenia have been mistaken for the disease.

Special Investigations to confirm the diagnosis.—(1) The *Kepler test* measures the rate of secretion of water after giving a water-load of 9 ml./lb. (20 ml./kg.) body weight. The test is carried out in the morning before the physiological increased secretion of anti-diuretic hormone occurs later in the day. The normal person secretes at least 80 per cent. of the quantity ingested within 4 hours, but in Addison's disease the quantity falls much below this level (even to 4 per cent. of the quantity given), although diuresis occurs later. This test may produce mild symptoms of an adrenal crisis. When it is repeated after giving inject. adrenocorticotrophin (ACTH) 25 mg. 6-hourly for 3 days, the result on the third day still shows the same deficiency, as there is no adrenal cortex to respond to ACTH, but when it is repeated after giving cortisone acetate 100 mg. or prednisolone acetate 20 mg. 4 hours beforehand the result reverts to normal. (2) The 24-hour output of urinary 17-ketogenic steroids and of 17-keto-steroids is well below normal and is unaffected when the estimation is repeated on the third day of a 3-day course of inject. ACTH. (3) In those with tuberculous supra-renals calcification in the glands may be seen by X-ray tomography.

Etiology.—Patients are usually 20–40 years old and the disease affects men and women equally. It is due to deficiency of the various suprarenal cortical hormones and at least 75 per cent. must be destroyed before symptoms occur. The destruction of the suprarenal cortex is a result of : (i.) tuberculosis is still the commonest cause but rarely affects the medulla of the gland; (ii.) slow progressive atrophy of the cortex is of unknown origin—in a few cases the glands have been normal at autopsy but their nerve supply has been destroyed; (iii.) rarely infarction, hæmorrhage, carcinomatous deposits, amyloid or hæmochromatosis are causal; (iv.) the glands may have been surgically removed for treatment of carcinomatosis. *Secondary adrenal cortical insufficiency* is due to destruction of the anterior lobe of the pituitary (§ 570); this causes the adrenal glands to diminish in size and to secrete less of their hormones; but they resume normal function after injecting ACTH; patients with anterior pituitary deficiency do not pigment as do those with Addison's disease. The melanin pigment in the deeper layers of the skin of Addison's disease is thought to be due to an excessive secretion of melanocyte-secreting hormone from the anterior pituitary in response to reduced cortical function.

The gluco-corticoids from the suprarenal cortex (mainly hydrocortisone) not only cause increased glucose production from tissue protein with increased storage of glycogen in the liver, but help to maintain the blood pressure and to ensure a normal glomerular filtration in the kidneys; therefore absence of these steroids decreases water secretion and allows the blood urea to rise. The mineralocorticoids of the suprarenal cortex (mainly aldosterone) greatly aid the absorption of water, sodium and chloride in the convoluted tubules of the kidneys so that a deficiency of these causes excessive loss of sodium chloride in the urine and retention of potassium. The resulting hyper-kalæmia causes weakness of voluntary and of cardiac muscle with corresponding electrocardiographic changes (p. 813).

Prognosis.—Without treatment the disease lasts a few months or years. With adequate treatment the patient may be restored to normal health and pigmentation often lessens, but relapses are liable to occur. Unless carefully watched for and quickly dealt with, a comparatively mild infection may still be a frequent cause of death.

Treatment of mild cases is with a glucocorticoid, using either cortisone or predniso-lone. As the suprarenal cortex in health produces approx. 15 mg. of hydrocortisone a day, the dose required by mouth of cortisone is 12·5 mg., or prednisolone 2·5 mg., twice or three times daily. These preparations have some sodium chloride retaining properties but sodium chloride 1 G. t.d.s. on food or in capsules may also be needed. This regime rectifies the muscular weakness, mental apathy, low blood pressure and liability to infections. More severe cases require a mineralocorticoid as well, either as deoxycortone acetate (DCA) B.P. 2–5 mg. in oil intramusc. two or three times a week, or as 100–300 mg. pellets implanted each 6–9 months (a 100-mg. pellet releases 0·3–0·45 mg. daily). Many prefer to give instead tab. fludrocortisone acetate 0·1 to 0·3 mg. orally in divided doses daily, as this has a glucocorticoid and a still stronger mineralocorticoid effect. When an *adrenal crisis* occurs, as with an infection, double-strength intravenous dextrose-saline must be given combined with hydrocortisone 100 mg. in the first hour and another 200 mg. in the next 12–24 hours; cortisone by mouth in similar doses is rapidly absorbed and can be used instead. Patients with tuberculosis also require anti-tuberculous measures. *Prophylactic* treatment consists in avoiding cold, infections and over-exertion.

§ 577. X. Hæmochromatosis (Bronzed Diabetes) is a rare disease, often showing a hereditary tendency, almost confined to the male sex. It depends on an abnormal metabolism of iron, whereby the iron-containing pigment hæmosiderin and iron-free hæmofuscin are retained in excessive amounts in the tissues; the iron-binding capacity of the serum is almost saturated and the body contains up to ten times its normal complement of iron. The liver, pancreas, skin and suprarenals suffer most and the cardinal *symptoms* of the disease depend on this. They are : (1) cirrhosis of the liver, with ascites; (2) glycosuria, usually permanent and leading to coma, but in some cases appearing late as a subsidiary feature; (3) pigmentation of the skin, giving rise to a slaty colour, occurring chiefly on exposed areas and not on the oral mucous membrane; (4) those of Addison's disease; (5) genital hypoplasia is usual.

Diagnosis can be confirmed by biopsy of the skin and of the liver.

The *Prognosis* depends mainly on efficient treatment and life may then be prolonged for a number of years.

Treatment is (1) of the diabetes and the prevention of diabetic coma; (2) the excess of iron in the body can be removed by regular venesection. In this disease blood depletion is very rapidly corrected by blood regeneration. Daily venesection of 500 ml. removes 250 mg. of iron and is carried out until the red cell count falls to 3·0–3·5 million per mm., subsequently 500 ml. are removed weekly for 6–24 months, with regular hæmoglobin and red cell estimations. Liver biopsy confirms the marked loss of hæmosiderin from the liver cells that ensues.

XI. **Disease of the Pancreas, acromegaly, myelomatosis, beri-beri, pellagra, alkalosis and other conditions mentioned in Groups I and II** (*q.v.*), may come on with debility only, or the patient may seek relief for debility. *Hypoglycæmia* (§ 425) is often overlooked; the exhaustion in such cases is relieved by taking food.

XII. **Carbon monoxide poisoning** should be borne in mind when lassitude, slight giddiness or headache are often present. Other symptoms are nausea, vomiting, palpitation, inability to move the limbs. The onset, however, is often sudden with collapse and loss of consciousness. Slight gas leaks, imperceptible to smell, can cause malaise. Petrol fumes in closed cars, escape of noxious coal and anthracite fumes from ill-ventilated chimneys or through overheated metal stove casings, are often unsuspected causes of poor health. In large doses this gas causes collapse or coma without any warning. (See § 856.) The *diagnosis* is made by removing 10 ml. of blood from a vein and examining its spectrum.

Treatment is by artificial respiration applied even for several hours when breathing has stopped, combined with the inhalation of 95 per cent. oxygen with 5 per cent. carbon dioxide.

CHAPTER XVII

THE EXTREMITIES

IN the preceding pages we have seen on several occasions that so-called local diseases, such as pneumonia and endocarditis, have by scientific research been shown to be only local manifestations of a general bacterial infection. This principle will here again be illustrated, for a gouty joint is only the local evidence of disordered metabolism, and acute rheumatism is probably initiated by bacteria. Probably all joint diseases (other than traumatic) are local manifestations of some toxic, septic or other inflammatory condition. In conformity, however, with the scheme of this work, whereby all diseases are approached from a symptomatic stand-point, certain diseases, the symptoms and physical signs of which are referable mainly or entirely to the upper or lower extremities, will now be considered.

PART A. SYMPTOMATOLOGY

The CARDINAL SYMPTOM referable to the extremities is **pain** (or painful sensations of some kind), which may or may not be accompanied by some **physical change.**

§ 578. **Pain in the Limbs** should be investigated, like **pain** in other situations, as to its *position, character, degree, constancy* and *duration.* Its position may be localised to the skin, or to a joint or some other structure, or be generalised, as in sheer exhaustion; its character may be sharp and shooting (as in tabes) or dull and heavy (as in vascular lesions), or like " pins and needles " (as in nerve and neuro-vascular lesions). The skin, subcutaneous tissues, nerves, muscles and vessels must be examined for a local cause; but it must be remembered that pains in the limbs, especially in the legs, may be due to a generalised infection which may not be evident for some time after the onset of the pain. So also disease of the brain, spinal cord, chest or abdomen may be the causal condition; hence a thorough examination, including investigation of the urine, blood and even lumbar puncture, may be necessary in obscure cases. Pain in the limbs may come on *acutely* or *insidiously.*

(a) *Acute pain in the limbs* coming on more or less SUDDENLY may herald influenza, tonsillitis, typhoid fever, malignant endocarditis, variola, scarlatina or some other specific fever. In many cases of influenza this pain and pyrexia are the only symptoms. *Acute rheumatism* and *Gout* also come on rapidly with pain referable to the muscles, bones or joints, and so does *Dengue* (" break-bone " fever). In *Trench fever* there is great pain and tenderness in the legs, especially in the shins. *Trichinosis* is attended by excruciating muscular pain in the second stage of the disease, when the parasite begins to migrate. *Scurvy, osteomyelitis* and *epiphysitis*

864

are other causes of pain in the limbs associated with pyrexia. A sudden severe pain in the limb is felt when *embolism* of an artery occurs: so also in *thrombosis* of a vein. In either case pyrexia may be absent.

(*b*) *Subacute and chronic pains in the limbs* coming on more or less *insidiously* may be due to (1) affections of the *nerves*, of central or local origin and especially to sciatica and polyneuritis. Carcinoma of the prostate may produce pains in the legs with demonstrable deposits in the pelvic bones. Polyneuritis may be due to many different causes (§ 974). Similar pains may occur in neurasthenia. Other causes of *nerve* origin are tabes dorsalis, cervical rib, cerebral tumour and meningitis, disease of the vertebræ or spinal cord, neuralgia and acroparæsthesia. Severe pain in the foot should lead us to suspect flat foot or metatarsalgia. Metatarsalgia (Morton's disease) is a neuralgia of the foot due to lateral displacement of the heads of the metatarsal bones which press upon the nerves, and may also produce a corn (for which, indeed, the patient may seek advice). (2) Pains in the *joints* or *muscles* are characteristic of chronic rheumatism, rheumatoid arthritis, osteoarthritis, gout and all forms of *synovitis*. (3) *Vascular* affections are such as intermittent claudication, thrombosis, embolism, erythromelalgia, aneurysm, varicose veins, phlegmasia alba dolens, Raynaud's disease, periarteritis nodosa and gangrene. "Numbness" and tingling are characteristic of vascular affections, and may indicate a vasomotor disorder, or may be due to a *neurological* cause such as neuritis, the incipient stage of tabes, disseminated sclerosis or other organic nerve disease. (4) Certain *skin* diseases are accompanied by pains in the limbs. (5) *Growing pains* (so-called) in children may be of serious import, as the first evidence of subacute rheumatism, which may produce endocarditis with permanent damage unless the condition is recognised and dealt with early. (6) Pains in the legs may be due to orthopædic and postural defects of the feet and spine. (7) Various diseases of the *bones* (§ 607) begin insidiously, with indefinite, vague pain in the limb or limbs. This must be especially remembered in children. Acute or chronic inflammation may arise, and unless the bone be superficial there may be no surface indications. Osteomyelitis is very serious, and requires prompt recognition. Syphilis can cause pain in the bones, worse at night. Other causes are Paget's disease, multiple myeloma, osteomalacia, osteoporosis, acromegaly, Cushing's syndrome, eunuchoidism, rickets, blood diseases and tumours. (8) A *muscular* strain or rupture of muscular fibres may leave a chronic pain and partial loss of function unattended by any physical sign. Other causes of muscle pain are acute myositis, rheumatic fibrositis, trichinosis, tumours and myositis ossificans. (9) *Local injury* or pressure due to injury from a crutch, or sleeping in a cramped position, or lymphatic glands or other tumours in the axilla, neck or pelvis can be causal. Heavy rings may cause ulnar neuralgia. Shooting pains down the arms, especially the left, occur in aneurysm of the aorta and angina (see also § 1004). (10) A careful examination of the *chest* should be made, for pain down the arm may indicate disease in that region; *e.g.*, apical pleurisy, cardiac disease, aneurysm or other mediastinal tumour. (11) Disease of the *pelvis*, vertebræ and hip joint are frequently overlooked causes of pain in the legs.

PART B. PHYSICAL EXAMINATION

The physical signs referable to the extremities consist mainly of some visible or tangible alteration in the skin and general contour of the limbs, the joints, the muscles, the bones, or the vessels and nerves.

§ 578a. Inspection of the Limb may reveal generalised redness or alteration of colour, œdema, varicose veins, or some other diffuse or localised swelling. Skin rashes are dealt with in Chapters XV and XVIII and œdema of both legs in § 29.

Inspection of the hands, when carefully performed, tells a great deal concerning the temperament, habits and diseases of a patient. The long, thin, dextrous *fingers*, perpetually on the move, almost surely indicate a nervous temperament and imaginative disposition, just as the short, thick, almost clumsy fingers and hands of another

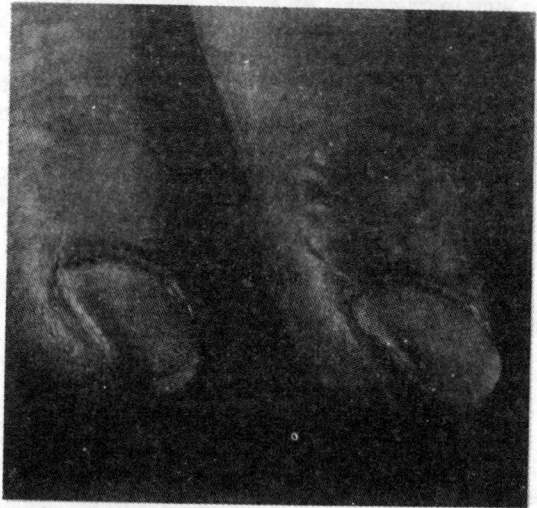

FIG. 168.—KOILONYCHIA occurring in a woman with Iron deficiency Anæmia.

bespeak slowness, deliberation and doggedness. The occupation of a patient may often be learned from a glance at the palms. Some people habitually have cold, damp, clammy hands; they often suffer from alcoholic habits, hyperthyroidism, rheumatoid arthritis or some other condition causing a defective vaso-motor tone. Fibrous nodules over the proximal finger joints occur with rheumatic or other chronic diseases. The *nails* and nail-beds afford information. They are dusky with impaired circulation and pale in anæmia; compression on the tip of the nail should not completely empty the capillaries as it does in anæmia. In aortic regurgitation compression of the nail tip reveals capillary pulsation. A transverse ridge or white mark in the nails indicates injury or arrested growth, and may mark the date of an illness a few months previously. It is useful to remember that the nail takes five to six months to grow from root to tip. Atrophic and hollowed nails (Koilonychia, Spoon nails) may be congenital; when acquired, iron deficiency anæmia is usually present (Fig. 168). Various distortions of the nail occur in Raynaud's disease, neuritis and injury, as with manicuring.   Pitted, dark and discoloured nails may be due to eczema, psoriasis, ringworm or monilial (thrush) infection.   *Clubbed fingers*—i.e., fingers with a bulbous end and great convexity of the nails (filbert-shaped nails)—occur in (i.) cardiac disease, especially congenital disorders associated with cyanosis, valvular disease acquired in early life and subacute bacterial endocarditis; (ii.) pulmonary disease with fibroid lung, bronchiectasis, lung abscess, empyema and carcinoma of the bronchus; (iii.) other causes include cirrhosis of the liver, steatorrhœa and poly- cythæmia rubra vera; (iv.) it can occur in those in good health, and as a family char- acteristic.   Hypertrophic osteo-arthropathy is a more advanced condition in which in addition to clubbing of the fingers and toes there is general enlargement of the bones and soft tissues of the hands and feet.   *Glossy fingers* (fingers with smooth, thin ʳkin) are the result of a neuritic atrophy, and are associated with destructive and paralytic lesions of the nerve trunks; they also occur in scleroderma.   *Dactylitis* is a thickening of one phalanx due to disease of the bone, with infiltration of the tissues of the fingers, resulting in a deformity known as the "champagne bottle finger." It is met with chiefly in tuberculous and sometimes in syphilitic children.   Heberden's nodes, lipping and distortion of the terminal phalangeal joints, are in reality osteo- arthritis of the fingers.   Gouty nodules of urate of soda form white masses near the joints, just beneath the skin, and have a superficial resemblance to Heberden's nodes. Scars may be due to painless injuries, as in syringomyelia or tabes, to previous sinuses as in gout, and to tertiary ulcers of the leg.   The bone ends of the wrists are enlarged in rickets, syphilis and pulmonary osteo-arthropathy.   Erythema of the palms is seen in pregnancy and in liver cirrhosis, and in the latter there is often an irregular "flapping tremor" when the fingers and hands are extended.   "Spade-shaped" hands with thickened tissues, suggest myxœdema; large flat hands with osseous enlargement occur in acromegaly and pulmonary osteoarthropathy.   The "claw- hand" (*main en griffe*) occurs as the result of injury or neuritis of the ulnar and median nerves; it is also seen in progressive muscular atrophy, syringomyelia and cervical pachymeningitis.   Wrist-drop is characteristic of musculo-spiral nerve paralysis.

§ 579. **Varicose veins** consist of dilatation and tortuosity of the super- ficial veins, and occur chiefly in the legs, where their tortuous elevations are characteristic.

Symptoms may be absent.   The most common complaints are an aching pain and a sense of tiredness in the legs, or irritation and discoloration of the skin over a distended vein.   Œdema around the ankle at the end of the day is common.   In the varices thrombophlebitis may occur, varicose eczema or ulceration can develop in the lower legs, and severe hæmorrhage may ensue if they rupture.

Etiology.—Varicose veins are caused by incompetent valves at the sapheno-femoral or sapheno-popliteal junctions, or when the valves of the communicating veins joining the superficial and deep veins are deficient so that blood drains from the deep veins into the superficial vessels.   They are much more likely to occur in those with a strong family history of the disorder, when thrombophlebitis has obstructed the deep veins, or when the valves in the superficial veins have been damaged by direct trauma or by phlebitis; once these defects are present the varicosity is aggravated by obesity, pregnancy, in those who stand a great deal and by tight garters.

Treatment.—Three methods are available.   (1) Support with suitable elastic stockings is most helpful in the elderly and in pregnancy.   "One-way stretch " stockings should be ordered when support is only needed below the knee, but " two-way stretch " stockings are necessary when a full-length stocking is required.   (2) When the long or short saphenous veins are dilated for a considerable distance or when symptoms arise or complications occur, ligature at the site of incompetence may be combined with stripping the superficial veins from the legs.   (3) Local injections are best reserved for localised varices with only slight incompetence of the valves, in patients in whom localised varices persist or recur after surgical removal of the main superficial veins, or when it is necessary to remove the varices for cosmetic reasons.   There is a marked tendency for varices treated by this method to recur, but in suitable cases considerable relief of symptoms is obtained and the procedure can be repeated later.

Technique.—To be most effective the sclerosing solution must be injected into an empty vein.   After slightly distending the vessel with a lightly-applied tourniquet the vein is entered with a short-bevelled number 15 or 16 needle attached to a Record syringe; the tourniquet is then removed, the leg elevated to empty the vein and 0·5 to 2·0 ml. of the sclerosing solution is injected, depending on the size of the vein; after resting quietly in the same position for 10 minutes to allow the sclerosing solution to act the patient can become ambulant and resume his or her normal occupation.   Inject very slowly and begin with the lower veins; the solutions used are ethanolamine oleate B.P. (ethamolin) or sodium morrhuate, both in a 5 per cent. solution.

§ **580. Œdema of one limb** (localised dropsy) is a swelling which pits on pressure.   There are three main varieties which present different clinical characteristics:

(1) LOCALISED ŒDEMA in *one area* of a limb indicates a local cause, usually inflammatory œdema (*e.g.*, cellulitis), local thrombosis, angioneurotic œdema or osteomyelitis.

(2) GENERALISED ŒDEMA of the greater part or whole of a limb which *readily pits on pressure* points to *obstruction of the main vein, by thrombosis* within or *by pressure* from without.

(*a*) *Simple venous thrombosis* indicates primary clotting within a vein with or without secondary inflammation in the wall of the vein subsequently; *thrombophlebitis* indicates a primary inflammatory reaction in the vein wall followed by clot formation.   These two types are difficult to differentiate clinically.

Symptoms depend on the importance of the vein to the flow of blood from the limb, *i.e.*, whether a superficial or a deep vein is involved or whether the main vein (*e.g.*, the common femoral vein) is affected.   In the majority of cases there is local pain, tenderness and often swelling at the seat of obstruction, with some irregular fever and general malaise. A *thrombosed superficial vein* can be easily seen and felt as a linear, tender bluish-red swelling lying just under the skin, whereas a thrombosed vein lying more deeply in the subcutaneous tissues may be more difficult to identify.   These two types produce local œdema adjacent to their course but no generalised œdema.   *Deep vein thrombosis* is still more difficult to identify and may involve one of the smaller vessels, especially in the calf, or the main popliteal, the deep or the common femoral vein or the external iliac vein, or in the arm the brachial or axillary vein. In these cases there may be little or no pain or tenderness but a main vein thrombosis always causes extensive œdema below the site of obstruction. The calf is a common site of a clot, in which case there is œdema around the ankle, local tenderness of the calf muscle and pain which is increased by dorsi-flexing the foot (Homan's sign); the skin below the level of the clot may be a little congested and the superficial veins distended. In a proportion of cases the first evidence of a pre-existing deep vein thrombosis is a sudden pulmonary embolism (§ 105), especially about the tenth day after an operation. *Phlegmasia alba dolens* (white leg) often follows pregnancy and is caused by thrombosis of the main femoral and even the external iliac vein. The whole leg rapidly becomes greatly swollen even to twice the normal size, painful and pale in colour, the femoral vein is tender and may be felt to contain a clot. In *thrombosis migrans*, thrombosis occurs in several arteries and veins in various parts of the body at different times. A femoral, coronary, pulmonary and cerebral thrombosis may all occur in the same individual; a carcinoma (especially of the pancreas) or a septic focus is believed to be causal in many cases: the prognosis is often grave.

Etiology.—Thrombophlebitis is much more common in the veins of the legs than in the arms and in those over 40 to 50 years of age. Usually there are two or more factors present in any given case. Those recognised are (i.) an increased coagulability of the blood which may depend on changes in a micro-film of fluid inside the vessel wall, on an increased amount of silver-staining cement substance between the endothelial cells and on factors which allow the blood platelets to adhere to the endothelial wall; (ii.) stasis of the blood is important, especially with confinement to bed and pressure on the calf veins such as occurs in right heart failure or when lying anæsthetised on a hard operating table, or with pillows behind the knees: varicose veins also predispose; (iii.) increased intra-abdominal pressure slows the return of venous blood as in obstetric cases and in obesity; (iv.) parturition and all surgical operations increase the number of circulating platelets; operations on the pelvis or on an inguinal hernia (adjacent to the femoral vein) also particularly dispose to thrombosis; (v.) focal sepsis (especially apical infection of the teeth) or tinea tarsi; (vi.) Buerger's disease of the arteries is often preceded by venous thrombosis suggesting that similar changes in the walls of the veins are operative; (vii.) direct trauma and intravenous therapy are well-recognised causes; (viii.) growths may compress the veins from outside. Carcinoma of the stomach, of the lung, of the thyroid or of the pancreas may first manifest itself by unexplained single or multiple thromboses. With a pancreatic cancer thrombosis of the veins and even of the smaller arteries may be due to an excess of circulating trypsin.

Prognosis.—Venous thromboses all tend to be recanalised and those of smaller vessels clear completely. Clots in larger deep veins produce more severe venous insufficiency with œdema for several weeks or even permanently, and varicose veins may ensue. The most serious complication is pulmonary embolism.

Treatment.—When thrombosis is confined to a *superficial* vein, especially one that is varicose, a firm bandage is applied and the patient may then become ambulant. But when a *deep vein* is involved, when œdema is present or the vein is of larger size and above the knee, bed rest is

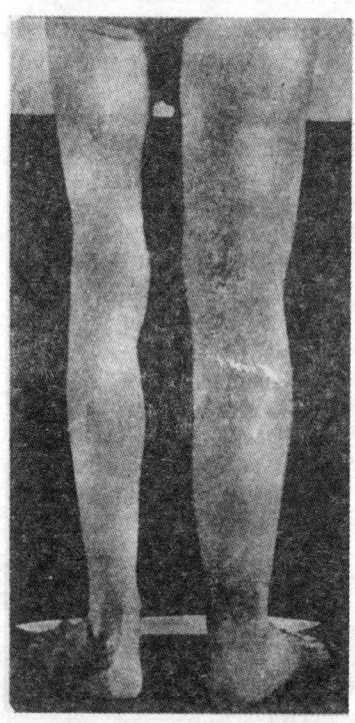

essential, with the foot of the bed raised 12–18 inches, the leg being made comfortable on *soft* pillows. Anticoagulant treatment prevents the spread of the clot and hastens its resolution. Heparin acts rapidly and is given intravenously in doses of 12,500–15,000 units regularly each 6 hours, or by intravenous drip (20–30 units per minute) combined with phenindione (Dindevan) by mouth, the heparin being discontinued once the phenindione comes into full action after 24 to 36 hours; Bauer combines this with active movements of the limb on the first day. These anticoagulant measures should only be used in hospital where the prothrombin time can be estimated, the object being to keep the value at 2–2½ times of the control. The diet should be low in fats but with plenty of fluid especially during the first week. When a focus of infection is thought to be operative, antibiotics are indicated, but their routine use is of little or no value. Ligature of the common femoral or iliac veins is rarely performed today. *Prophylaxis* demands, after childbirth or after any operation and especially those on the abdomen, early movements of the legs followed by early ambulation, breathing exercises and raising the calves from the operating table; in coronary occlusion immediate anticoagulant therapy greatly decreases the chance of venous thrombosis in the legs.

FIG. 169.—LYMPHŒDEMA in a man about 40 years of age who had never been abroad.

(b) *Pressure upon a vein* by a tumour can cause œdema. This occurs with enlarged glands in the axilla or elsewhere, aneurysm, or other intrathoracic growth pressing upon the veins coming from the arm; pelvic cellulitis, carcinoma of the prostate, bladder, ovary or uterus, bands of adhesion, or other intrapelvic growths pressing on the veins from the leg.

(3) GENERALISED ŒDEMA of the thigh or of the whole of a limb which *does not easily pit on pressure* is due to lymphatic obstruction (Lymphœdema, Elephantiasis Lymphangiectodes); and see Fig. 169.

Lymphœdema is more solid than that of venous obstruction as the fluid is under greater tension in smaller tissue spaces and may result in fibrosis or overgrowth of adipose tissue.   It occurs (1) after blockage of the lymphatics by carcinoma, removal of a tumour (especially of the breast), or deep X-ray therapy; (2) after recurrent lymphangitis.   Lymphœdema of one or both thighs and of the vulva occurs with carcinoma of the pelvic organs or tissues.   (3) It is met chiefly in tropical countries in persons whose blood contains filarial embryos (either *F. bancrofti* or *F. malayi*). The adult worms block the lymphatics.   (4) **Milroy's Hereditary Œdema** starts at birth or up to the age of puberty and affects several members of a family. The œdema usually starts around the feet and ankles and later ascends to the knees and rarely to the thighs; it has an abrupt line of demarcation at the level of the hip, knee or ankle.   There may be a history of attacks of fever with increase of swelling. The *cause* is unknown.   The *diagnosis* rests on the history, and similar œdema in other members of the family.   *Treatment* consists in adequate support for the limbs. the use of diuretics and sometimes operative measures such as excision of sheets of double fascia (Kondoléon's operation) have been tried.   Steroid therapy has occasionally been of service.

§ 581. **Swelling of the Lymph Glands** in the neck, axillæ, groins or elsewhere on the surface of the body or limbs may be due to: I. injury, septic or infective processes; II. tuberculosis; III. cancer; IV. lymphosarcoma; V. syphilis; VI. lymphogranuloma inguinale; VII. chancroid; VIII. acute specific fevers; IX. leukæmia; X. Hodgkin's disease; XI. glandular fever, § 498; XII. sarcoidosis, § 141; XIII. cat-scratch fever, § 508; XIV. plague, § 501; XV. trypanosomiasis, § 521; XVI. scrub typhus, § 486; XVII. toxoplasmosis, § 509a.   In I, II, III, VII and XVI the glands enlarge adjacent to some focus of disease, and the glandular swelling usually remains localised; in the remainder all the lymph glands tend to become affected.

I. *Local* injuries, septic sores, infected tonsillar crypts and abscesses give rise to enlargement of the neighbouring lymphatic glands.   Pain and enlargement of the glands in the groin, for instance, may be due to direct injury to those glands; but more usually to a sore on the foot or around the toe-nails, through which infection has occurred.   *Post-mortem scratches* or inoculation from septicæmic cases are of a much more virulent nature. Red streaks along the course of the lymphatics indicate lymphangitis. The glands at the elbow and axilla become acutely painful and tender, and may rapidly suppurate.   In the absence of antibiotic therapy general septicæmia and death ensue in a day or two.

II. *Tuberculous disease* occurs most often in children.   (a) The commoner type affects the upper cervical glands, causing tenderness and enlargement, usually on one side only in the earlier stages.   At first discrete, the capsules of the glands are later broken through by caseous material, causing matting together and finally a sinus to the skin.   (b) A rare form (endothelial tuberculosis) is more common in adults: there is general enlargement of the lymphatic glands and often splenic enlargement. The glands rarely mat together and constitutional disturbance is slight.

Treatment is with isoniazid 100 mg.b.d., combined with sodium amino-salicylate (P.A.S.) 5 G. t.i.d. or with inject. streptomycin sulphate 1·0 G. four times a week for 12 to 18 months. When an abscess forms it may be aspirated and a buffered solution containing streptomycin sulphate 0·25 G. injected locally on one or two occasions.

III. *Cancer* gives rise first to enlargement of the adjacent glands (§ 571). These glands are known by their hardness and their tendency to invade and become fixed to adjacent tissues.

IV. *Lymphosarcoma* is a growth starting in the lymph glands, or in the lymphoid tissue of structures such as the thymus. Usually commencing at a later age than Hodgkin's disease the enlarged glands may for a long time be localised in one area, or may involve most of the lymph glands simultaneously. *Symptoms* depend on the site and the extent of the disease and the larger masses seen in the neck or the medias-tinum produce marked pressure effects (§ 81). The *diagnosis* may be possible only after excision and examination of a gland, and *treatment* is on the lines of that of Hodgkin's disease.

Reticulum cell sarcoma closely resembles lymphosarcoma, and is differentiated only by careful histological examination of a gland.

V. *Syphilis* first affects the lymphatic glands in the neighbourhood of the chancre (and therefore usually in the groin). They are small, hard (shotty), painless and only perceptible on palpation. In the secondary stage these become larger but do not suppurate as with a soft chancre; at the same time there is universal lymphadenitis, and careful palpation for many years afterwards may still reveal this (§ 500).

§ 582. VI. **Lymphogranuloma inguinale** (Syn. L. venereum, Climatic or Tropical Bubo) is a venereal disease caused by a filterable virus which is common in Oriental countries and America and is now appearing in Europe.

Symptoms.—The incubation period varies from a few days to 3 weeks. The *Primary* lesion consists of small herpetiform ulcers on the penis. The *Secondary* phase shows swelling of the medial group of inguinal glands between 1 to 6 weeks later. Both sides may be involved. Discomfort, tenderness and groin pain accompanied by fever may first suggest the condition. The glands at first are hard to the touch and somewhat tender; the surrounding skin becomes red, then bluish-violet. Sub-sequently they remain indolent, or fluctuation occurs and sinuses form in about half the cases. Generally the iliac glands are palpable as a hard mass above Poupart's ligament. General features include fever of remittent type which may last 7–10 days or many weeks, anorexia and loss of weight. In women a chronic elephantoid condition of the vulva may ensue, also stricture of the rectum.

Diagnosis.—Herpes genitalis resembles the primary lesion, while filarial involve-ment of the lymph glands, septic and tuberculous adenitis, venereal buboes due to chancroid, gonorrhœa and syphilis, and buboes due to plague, rat-bite fever, cat-scratch fever and tularæmia may need differentiation. A history of cohabitation with native women is an important aid to diagnosis. This is confirmed by Frei's intradermal test, which is performed with sterilised diluted pus or mouse-brain virus. A reddish, infiltrated papule of from 7·5–20 mm. diameter appearing within 48 hours is evidence of infection with the virus of climatic bubo.

Prognosis.—The disease is rarely fatal, but enlarged glands, sinuses or ulcers in the groin may take 18 months to heal.

Treatment.—The patient is put to bed on a nutritious diet and chlortetracycline (Aureomycin) or chloramphenicol given for 10 days in doses of 0·5 G. 6-hourly. Sulph-onamides are sometimes effective. Pus should be aspirated under aseptic con-ditions, the needle being inserted through healthy skin some distance from the bubo; incision of the glands should not be undertaken.

§ 583. VII. **Chancroid** is a venereal disease due to Ducrey's bacillus (*Hæmophilus* *ducreyi*) and usually causes inguinal adenitis and suppuration. Although primarily a tropical disease it is now seen in most countries throughout the world and sometimes in Great Britain.

Symptoms occur after an incubation period of 3 to 5 days in the form of a painful red papule on the genitalia, which soon becomes a pustule and then a very painful ulcer which is *not indurated*; lesions are often multiple. The inguinal glands become swollen, tender, may suppurate and ulcerate, with painful lymphangitis.

Diagnosis is suggested by the frequent multiple character of the ulcers and the lack of induration of the papules. It is confirmed when the bacillus is identified by direct smear or by culture, but a co-existing *Treponema pallidum* infection should be looked for and recognised by dark-ground examination.

Treatment is with a sulphonamide in doses of 5·0 G. daily for 10 days. Those allergic to sulphonamides should be given chlortetracycline or chloramphenicol 0·5 G. t.i.d. for a week. In response to such treatment the ulcers heal in 7 to 10 days, but the patient should be kept under observation and serological tests for syphilis performed for the next 6 months.

VIII. In most of the *acute specific fevers* there is, as in syphilis, a slight generalised glandular enlargement. After *Whooping cough* isolated glandular enlargements are not uncommon. In those fevers which have a local manifestation—the throat in scarlet fever and diphtheria, for instance—the adjacent glands are first and chiefly affected. In *German measles* the occipital glands are especially noticeable. In bubonic plague the enlargement is great; in milder cases of *plague* only slight glandular swelling and fever occur (pestis minor). *Rheumatoid arthritis* is accompanied by enlargement of the glands and spleen, especially in children.

IX. In *Leukæmia* there is a generalised enlargement, and the blood changes are characteristic (§§ 554, 557).

§ 584. X. Hodgkin's disease (Syn. Lymphadenoma) is characterised by progressive enlargement of the lymph glands; enlargement of the spleen; and later progressive anæmia without other important blood changes.

Symptoms.—(1) Enlargement of lymph glands. Those in the neck are often first affected, but in other cases the primary glandular enlargement may occur in the mediastinal, abdominal or groin glands. Although at first the glands vary in size and may even disappear for a while, sooner or later other groups are affected, until widespread adenopathy is present. The glands are sometimes painful and tender: are freely movable over each other and over adjacent structures; of rubbery consistency; without a tendency to break down. (2) Enlargement of mediastinal and mesenteric glands may produce special symptoms, due to pressure upon important structures, such as the veins in the thorax and abdomen, the trachea and bronchi, and the œsophagus. (3) A peribronchial invasion produces the symptoms and signs of a mediastinal tumour. (4) Enlargement of the spleen occurs later, and is sometimes very marked. (5) Fever is present, either as a low irregular fever, or occasionally as an undulating fever, the waves varying in length from a week or 10 days to a month or more. This undulating fever in lymphadenoma is known as the Pel-Ebstein syndrome and may be present even for months before the glands become palpable. (6) Symptoms of anæmia are slight at first, but later become more severe. The blood changes are not characteristic, apart from the anæmia, though there is often a high polymorph leucocytosis, and an eosinophilia in 15 per cent. of cases (Plate XVI). (7) General pruritus, sometimes severe, and various eruptions occur, including herpes zoster. (8) Bronzing of the skin may be seen. (9) Spinal deposits cause spinal compression. (10) Deposits in bone cause persistent pain especially in the lumbar spine. (11) The blood sedimentation rate sooner or later reaches very high figures.

Diagnosis.—The disease must be distinguished from others giving rise to enlarged lymph glands. It is distinguished from *lymphatic leukæmia* by the absence of the blood changes of that disease; from *glandular fever, secondary syphilis, rubella,* secondary deposits of *malignant disease,* etc., by the size, consistency and distribution of the glands, together with the progress of the case, and the absence of evidence of the other diseases. Occasionally it may be difficult to distinguish between Hodgkin's disease affecting only one set of glands and some other diseases, especially *lympho-sarcoma* and *tuberculosis*; it may be necessary to excise a gland, under local anæsthesia, to establish the diagnosis by histological examination. Mervyn Gordon has established a biological test; after the intracerebral inoculation of an emulsion of a fresh gland into a rabbit, encephalitis with ataxia and spasticity of the hind limbs, and convulsions, may prove fatal. A similar encephalitogenic agent is present also in normal bone marrow and spleen and is believed by some to be a reaction to eosinophils.

Etiology.—Males are more frequently affected than females, and most often about middle age. The cause is undecided: although many of the features are those of a neoplasm, others much more closely resemble those of an infection. Mervyn Gordon has described certain " elementary bodies " as being possibly causal. The histological changes are those of a granulomatous process which causes enlargement of the lymphatic structures, but in which almost all the organs are involved. At autopsy the most striking feature is enlargement of the lymph glands, the spleen and the liver, but changes occur in almost all the organs of the body, including the bones and the bone marrow.

The *prognosis* is bad. The patient becomes progressively weaker and more anæmic, and pressure upon important structures by the enlarged glands may hasten the end. The more chronic cases may live for 10 years after the diagnosis is made; febrile cases usually die within a year.

Treatment.—When there is only a single small group of glands in one region, complete excision followed by radiotherapy is the treatment of choice. When more widespread, deep X-ray therapy is preferable; many prefer to combine this with a cytotoxic agent and especially one of the nitrogen-mustard group such as mustine hydrochlor. (B.P.C.) 0·1 mg./Kg. body weight intravenously twice a week. The total dose for each course should not exceed 0·6 mg./Kg. General measures must be taken to correct anæmia and to improve the health and strength. Unfortunately the disease sooner or later becomes resistant to all forms of treatment.

§ **584a.** The JOINTS, MUSCLES, BONES, VESSELS, NERVES and CONSTITU-TIONAL SYMPTOMS should be next investigated.

The **joints** may need investigation for pain, tenderness, heat, swelling or redness, and for loss of function or range of movement. The affected and the unaffected sides should be carefully compared. Slight degrees of fluid in a joint are often difficult to detect. The active movements (those which the patient can make) and the passive movements (those made by the doctor) should, with due consideration and caution, be tested. Among the *fallacies*, paralysis, or muscular weakness is often simulated by chronic joint diseases, and *vice versa*, and pain in the limbs from various causes will often simulate a stiffness of the joint. Disease near a joint may be mistaken for disease in a joint. Pain may be referred, *e.g.*, in hip-joint disease pain is often complained of in the knee. In neuritis pain may be referred to the joint supplied by the affected nerve. X-rays may help diagnosis. In acute joint disease the fallacies of epiphysitis and acute osteomyelitis must be avoided. The presence of associated symptoms may aid; for example, tophi suggest gout; subcutaneous nodules, rheumatism.

The **muscles** may be investigated for tenderness, stiffness, swelling or wasting. The investigation of paralysis, tonic or clonic spasm, or wasting, is given under diseases of the nervous system (Chapter XIX). We are here concerned only with pain, tenderness, or swelling localised in the muscles and fasciæ (§ 604); the presence of these localised symptoms helps to differentiate muscular diseases from paralysis and other diseases of the nervous system. To decide that the lesion is not in the bones or ligaments may be difficult; if it be in the muscle, the pain is greater during active than passive movement of the affected muscle; if in the ligaments or joints, the pain is about equal.

Disease situated in the **bones** may be evidenced by pain, tenderness, swelling or deformity. The physician may be first consulted when pain is the only symptom, and the diagnosis presents considerable difficulty. X-ray examination is of great value.

In the diagnosis of SWELLINGS CONNECTED WITH BONES it is well to remember the following data. Symptoms come on *acutely* with trauma, periostitis and osteomyelitis; slowly and *chronically* with caries, necrosis, chronic periostitis and osteitis, rickets, syphilis and tumour. In regard to physical signs the *diaphysis* is mainly affected in acute and chronic inflammation, in sarcomatous and other tumours; the *epiphysis* in rickets, syphilis and central sarcoma. The consistency of the swelling is *soft* in abscess and vascular sarcomata, *hard* in chronic inflammation. As regards the mode and rate of growth, the swelling *progressively enlarges* in inflammatory and malignant tumours, and is *relatively slow* or *stationary* in chronic inflammation and benign tumours; *receding* swellings are always inflammatory.

The **vessels** and **nerves** need examination when any of the symptoms indicate their implication, as in erythromelalgia and some other conditions in Group I below. Pressure along their course may elicit tenderness, indicative of inflammation. For symptoms of peripheral neuritis see §§ 974 *et seq.*; thrombosis of a vein, § 580, embolism of an artery, § 99 and § 587, and periarteritis, § 98.

The **viscera** should be examined, particularly in acute joint diseases which are almost always the product of some systemic disorder—*e.g.*, the heart must always be examined in rheumatic conditions, the kidneys and the urine in gout.

Pyrexia and **Constitutional Symptoms** are present in a considerable number of diseases of the extremities, particularly in the acute joint and bone disorders, and they may be investigated on the lines laid down in Chapter XV. Rigors and sweating indicate a pyogenic process. Characteristic blood changes are found in several diseases, notably glandular and septic diseases.

The **mental state** should be investigated when organic disease has been excluded or when the symptoms far outweigh the organic signs. The term psychosomatic rheumatism has been applied to these cases (§ 605).

PART C. DIAGNOSIS, PROGNOSIS AND TREATMENT OF DISEASES CAUSING SYMPTOMS REFERABLE TO THE EXTREMITIES

Routine Examination and Classification.—As a matter of routine, as in other cases, investigate—

First, the LEADING SYMPTOM, which in this instance is very often as visible or palpable to the patient as to the physician.

Secondly, the HISTORY of the case, its mode of onset (acute or chronic), and evolution in chronological order.

Thirdly, examine the AFFECTED LIMB or limbs, their colour and contour, the joints, muscles, bones, vessels or nerves, as may be indicated; and, finally, examine the VISCERA and the TEMPERATURE. The movements, reflexes and sensation should be tested in cases where neurological disease is suspected. An X-ray examination is often essential.

If there is any visible abnormality in the COLOUR of the hands or limbs, turn to Group I, below.

If the symptoms point to JOINT disease, acute or chronic, turn to Group II, § 592 (Acute), or § 596 (Chronic).

If the symptoms point to disease of the MUSCLES (rare), turn to § 604.

If the symptoms point to disease of the BONES, turn to § 607.

If the symptoms point to disease of the NERVOUS SYSTEM, turn to § 790.

GROUP I. ALTERATIONS IN COLOUR OF THE EXTREMITIES

This group comprises the following medical conditions. Other alterations in colour or contour, such as œdema of one limb, clubbed fingers and varicose veins, have been referred to in §§ 578 to 580. Pigment alterations are described in § 754. There remain—

I. Cyanosis, § 585.
II. Intermittent claudication, § 586.
III. Gangrene, § 587.

IV. Trench-foot and Frost-bite, § 588.
V. Raynaud's disease and Dead hands, § 589.
VI. Erythromelalgia, Nutritional Erythromelalgia and Acroteric Scleroderma, § 590.
VII. Pink Disease, § 591.

The HANDS *and/or the* FEET *present a uniformly* DEEP PURPLE COLOUR *often with a feeling of coldness, especially* IN COLD WEATHER. *The condition is* CYANOSIS OF THE EXTREMITIES.

§ 585. I. **Cyanosis** (Blueness) of the extremities.—Blueness and redness of the extremities appear to be due to a vaso-motor condition, to arteriosclerotic narrowing of the arteries by old age, or to polycythæmia (§ 31). After infantile paralysis the affected limbs are blue and cold, with defective circulation. In ACROCYANOSIS all the fingers, both hands and wrists, even the forearms, are cold, blue and swollen. Attacks are much worse in the cold weather but unlike erythromelalgia there is little or no pain. The condition may affect the feet to a less extent and is almost confined to young women. ERYTHROCYANOSIS CRURUM PUELLARUM is a similar condition affecting the lower legs and ankles in girls (§ 627). The feet usually escape but chilblains are often present and the ankles swollen. Occasionally the blueness extends on to the thighs and the poorly nourished skin of the lower legs may ulcerate. Bazin's disease is a separate entity (§ 707) but may accompany the blue state of the legs. These patients are often stout and take little exercise; in some, thyroid insufficiency is present. *Treatment* consists in wearing warm underclothes, woollen stockings and bootees. Outdoor exercise is essential and thyroid in small doses should be combined with tab. calcium with vitamin D (B.P.C.)—two tablets to be taken regularly before breakfast.

A patient, USUALLY A MAN OVER 50 YEARS *of age, complains of* CRAMP IN THE CALF *of one or both legs* AFTER WALKING *several hundred yards; the pain ceases on resting. The condition is probably* INTERMITTENT CLAUDICATION.

§ 586. II. **Intermittent Claudication** (Syn. Angina cruris, Intermittent limping) is a painful condition of the muscles due to the blood supply being insufficient to meet the demands of exercise. There are two varieties: (A) The arteriosclerotic form is common in later life, but (B) thromboangiitis obliterans occurs as a much rarer condition in younger persons.

(A) ARTERIOSCLEROSIS first produces rigidity and narrowing of the main arteries of the legs, especially in the femoral and popliteal vessels; later occlusion by thrombosis on one or both sides is common. Men are much more frequently affected than women (see also § 574).

Symptoms.—Three stages are described: (1) After walking a certain distance, especially up-hill, a cramp-like pain is felt in one or both calves but this slowly disappears if the pace of walking is reduced. (2) Later the pain is more severe and causes the patient to stop; the pain then disappears but recurs after walking a similar distance. The legs feel weak and may go cold and numb. Arterial pulsation in the popliteal and especially in the dorsal pedal and posterior tibial arteries is greatly reduced and disappears when an arterial thrombus has formed. At this stage, when the patient lies flat on a couch and the legs are raised, the skin of the feet goes dead white, in contrast to the extreme congestion and purple colour which occurs on standing. (3) In the third stage the pain on walking 20–30 yards is intolerable. Also *rest pain* is present at night when the patient is in bed and relief is only obtained by hanging the feet over the side of the bed or by sleeping in a chair. Gangrene may supervene. Because the femoral arteries in Hunter's canal or the popliteal arteries are commonly at fault the pain is usually confined to the calf muscles, but occlusions of the anterior tibial arteries produce pain in the anterior tibial muscles; and when on occasions the gluteal arteries are affected the pain occurs on the outer side of the hips. The poor nutrition of the feet causes wasting of the fatty pads of the toes, changes in the nails and infection.

(B) THROMBO-ANGIITIS OBLITERANS (Buerger's disease) is the result of an inflammatory condition of the intima and media of the larger and medium-sized arteries, especially in the legs. It occurs in localised patches and also affects the veins so that the two may be matted together. It causes symptoms of arterial occlusion in the twenties and thirties at an age when arteriosclerotic symptoms are very rare; but it is no longer believed to show a predilection for those of the Jewish or Russian races.

Symptoms.—There is often a history of attacks of venous thrombosis before the symptoms of arterial insufficiency and occlusion arise, or the two may coincide. The symptoms and signs in the legs are otherwise the same as those described in arteriosclerosis (A above); disease in the vessels of the arms, in the coronary, cerebral and abdominal arteries also give rise to corresponding symptoms. Gangrene of the toes and feet in young men is almost invariably due to Buerger's disease.

Diagnosis of Intermittent Claudication.—The characteristic pain in the calves and the colour changes in the feet and toes with posture are usually diagnostic. Unless the patient is very fat pulsation in the femoral, popliteal, posterior tibial and dorsal pedal arteries should be felt when the legs and feet are warm, although the arterial pulsation of the dorsal pedal arteries is occasionally very small; therefore absent pulsation is of great diagnostic value and may be confirmed by an oscillometer. *Arthritis of the hip or knee* and *fasciitis* of the ilio-tibial tract may have to be differentiated. *X-ray examination* with a rapid series of films immediately after injecting diodone (B.P.) into the femoral artery or the abdominal aorta (Arteriography) will demonstrate narrowing or occlusion of the main vessels and the extent of a collateral circulation (Fig. 170).

Etiology.—The symptoms are due to an accumulation of lactic acid and other metabolites as a result of exercise combined with anoxia of the muscles (especially the gastrocnemius and soleus). Arteriosclerotic

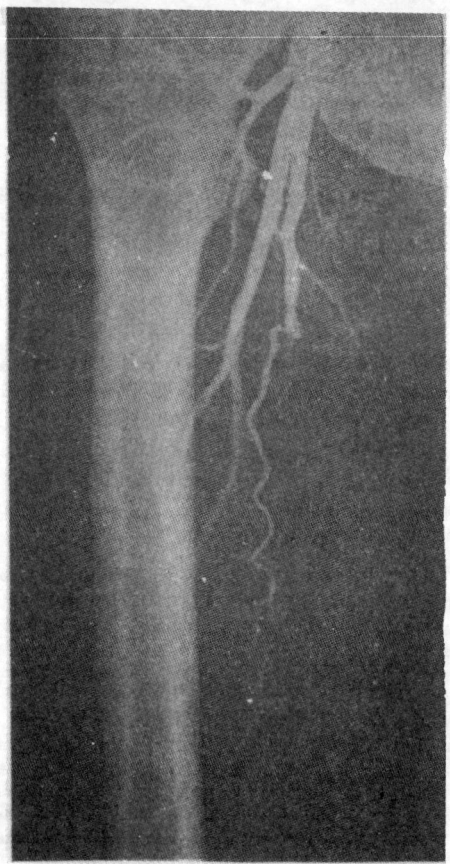

FIG. 170.—ARTERIOGRAPHY; following the injection of diodone into the right common femoral artery occlusion of the superficial and deep femoral arteries and a partial collateral circulation is shown.

patients may show other evidences of arterial damage such as hypertension or coronary artery disease. Diabetes greatly aggravates the condition. Thrombo-angiitis obliterans is very rare in non-smokers.

Prognosis.—With arteriosclerosis the symptoms may slowly disappear in a period of a year or so as collateral arteries open up to make good the deficiency, but in Buerger's disease the condition is likely to be progressive and sooner or later results in amputation of one or both legs.

Treatment aims at reducing the intensity of work of the muscles and improving the arterial circulation. Walking should be at a slower pace and is more comfortably undertaken on soft turf than on hard ground, with the heels of the shoes raised by rubber pads. In both varieties smoking must be given up and obesity corrected. A long course of short-wave diathermy over a period of 6 to 8 months applied to the lower pelvis and thighs helps to open up new blood vessels, and in some, prolonged anticoagulant therapy undoubtedly helps. Tolazine hydrochlor. (Priscol) occasionally aids and aspirin or a tot of whisky at bedtime may relieve nocturnal rest pain. *Surgical measures* in young and middle-aged patients include lumbar sympathectomy, arterial grafting (with homografts or plastic materials) when the femoral, popliteal and subclavian arteries are occluded; and when the internal iliac arteries are blocked endarterectomy with removal of the diseased inner layers can avoid the necessity of amputation.

One or more fingers or toes and perhaps part of a hand or foot, become COLD, PURPLE, PERHAPS SHRIVELLED *and evoke a characteristic odour; all sensation is lost but severe pain is present in the adjacent living tissues, often with secondary infection.*—GANGRENE *is present.*

§ 587. III. **Gangrene** indicates death of the tissues with necrosis. It may be localised (*e.g.*, due to persistent pressure on the heel or malleolus of a bed-ridden patient) or more extensive and cause death of the periphery of a limb. The feet and legs are much more commonly involved than the hands and arms, partly due to the less effective collateral circulation in the former. Three types are described but there is often a combination of these. They are:

(*a*) DRY GANGRENE is the most common and is almost invariably due to an arterial block. The extremity becomes white, cold and anæsthetic; soon it becomes painful, dark as the blood pigment changes in colour and then shrunken as the fluid evaporates. Gradually the part becomes dry and mummified. As thrombosis slowly extends up the limb the gangrene spreads until a line of demarcation forms where an adequate blood supply is reached (Fig. 177*b*).

Etiology.—The commonest type is senile gangrene due to arteriosclerosis of the leg vessels; in Rob's series of cases of gangrene of the feet 86 per cent. were due to this while 8 per cent. were due to thrombo-angiitis obliterans. Other causes are sudden embolic blocking of an artery, trauma to a main artery, Mönckeberg's sclerosis with intimal damage, Raynaud's disease (usually in the fingers), a tight plaster cast, frost-bite, ergot poisoning and the accidental intra-arterial injection of sodium thiopentone. An enfeebled heart action aggravates the condition. When an artery suddenly becomes occluded, reflex spasm above the block frequently follows. The artery is tender at the seat of embolism and ceases to pulsate below.

(*b*) MOIST GANGRENE occurs when the part is engorged with blood and is aggravated when there is arterial combined with venous occlusion, the result of thrombosis, pressure, injury or inflammation; it is commonly seen on the toes or feet of diabetics or of the elderly following local trauma and infection. The part involved becomes cold, purple or mottled, blebs then form on the surface and a bright red line separates the dead from the living tissue. The dead part may ultimately slough off and leave an ulcer.

Treatment of both these varieties by modern methods has greatly improved the prognosis. *Medical measures* entail keeping the patient flat in bed; the foot should not be raised and the nutritional needs of the affected part lowered by cold air from a fan or by surrounding the part

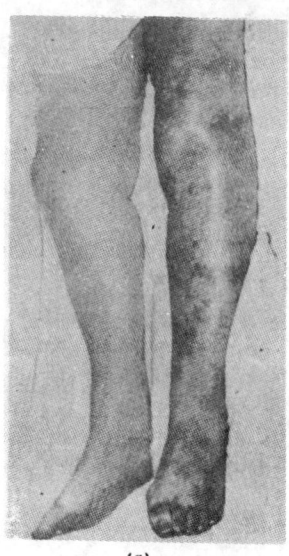 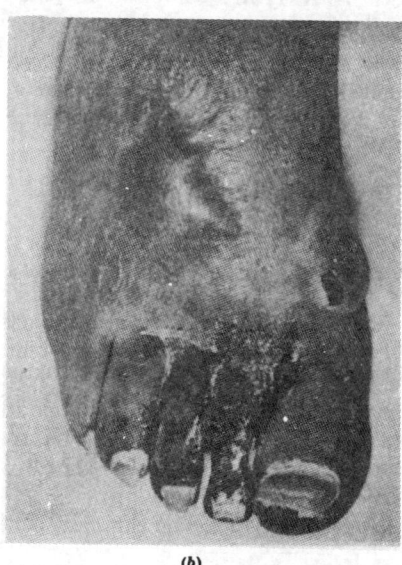

(a) (b)

FIG. 171.—(*a*) Leg of woman aged 83 with embolus in left common iliac artery due to auricular fibrillation; the whole leg was cold and discoloured prior to commencement of gangrene. (*b*) Dry gangrene affecting chiefly the second and third toes of a diabetic man, aged 70.

with ice. Infection is controlled by systemic antibiotics and by the local application of a powder containing penicillin (1,000 units) in sterile sulphanilamide (1·0 G.). Nicotinic acid (25 mg. each 1–2 hours) and alcohol by mouth improve the circulation by dilating the arterioles, and anticoagulants (especially intravenous heparin) aid resolution of blood clot. Especially in Buerger's disease tobacco smoking is better avoided altogether. *Surgical treatment* may involve lumbar sympathectomy to denervate the collateral circulation around an arterial block and to lessen arterial spasm. When large vessels are involved removal of an arterial embolus or thrombus may be necessary; in other cases a homologous arterial transplant or an autogenous venous graft is inserted to by-pass the blocked vessel. Later on, amputation may be required to remove the gangrenous tissues. *Prophylaxis* is by avoiding ill-fitting shoes or other sources of trauma, the use of careful chiropody in the elderly, keeping the feet dry and clean and taking care to avoid tinea infection.

(c) GAS GANGRENE is due to infection and necrosis of muscles, by spore-forming anærobic organisms such as *Cl. welchii*, *Cl. œdematiens* and *Cl. septicum*, with which streptococci and staphylococci are often associated. If untreated the infection spreads with local thrombosis and the production of toxins. There is local swelling with crepitations and a dark brown discoloration from which, on incision, bubbles of gas escape with a musty odour. Toxæmia is usually profound.

Treatment.—The condition usually responds to mixed gas-gangrene antitoxin B.P. combined with full doses of one of the tetracycline drugs; but as these drugs do not penetrate devitalised tissues, drainage and surgical excision of the devitalised tissue and sometimes amputation of a limb are still of major importance.

§ 588. IV. Trench Foot occurs when blood stasis is present as a result of standing for long periods in cold wet trenches at temperatures a little above freezing point. It was common in World War I and on the Russian front in World War II.

Symptoms.—(1) There is numbness and later great pain with hyperæsthesia, confined as a rule to the feet, but sometimes also affecting the hands; later (2) œdema of the feet with blebs, ulcers or other cutaneous lesions occur; (3) these minor injuries may lead to moist gangrene.

Treatment is by slowly warming the feet, keeping them elevated and dry with an antiseptic dusting powder. Rubbing should be avoided.

Frost-bite is the result of exposure to temperatures below freezing point, especially at a high altitude and in a high wind. The fingers, toes or the ears actually freeze, ice crystals form in the tissues and the circulation ceases.

Symptoms.—(1) The onset is often sudden, with loss of sensation including that of cold. The skin becomes waxy pale and the affected joints are stiffened. (2) When the whole thickness of skin is involved it becomes necrotic, the nails may be lost and some permanent anæsthesia may remain. (3) Destruction of the whole part causes dry or moist gangrene. Recurrences are common on re-exposure.

Treatment.—The feet must be kept at rest and rapidly warmed with warm air or water until the temperature is approximately normal. The application of heat must then be stopped. Massage is useful during this period. Hot drinks and sleep are essential, but alcohol is better avoided. In the absence of infection, amputation of a gangrenous area should be delayed until there is a clear line of demarcation between the living and dead tissues. Prophylaxis consists in wearing loose warm dry clothing, with Balaclava helmets and warm gloves: two pairs of socks should be worn in well-fitting boots: all clothing must be windproof.

A YOUNG WOMAN *complains that* ONE OR MORE FINGERS SUDDENLY BECOME DEAD *for an hour or more, and this occurs* SYMMETRICALLY *on the two sides especially in cold weather; in long-standing cases* ULCERS MAY FORM *on the finger-tips—the condition is* RAYNAUD'S DISEASE.

§ 589. V. Raynaud's Disease (Syn. Raynaud's Phenomenon, Local Asphyxia of the Extremities) was first described in 1862 by Raynaud. It is characterised by local recurrent attacks of occlusion of the digital arteries in one or more of the fingers, for the most part symmetrically on the two hands. In severe long-standing cases this may ultimately result in gangrene. Occasionally the toes are involved. Two varieties of the disease have been described—a syncopal type due to generalised vascular spasm, and an asphyxial type due to spasm of the arterioles and dilatation of the capillaries.

Symptoms.—(1) First there is sudden pallor (*local syncope*), coldness and numbness of the distal parts of one or more of the fingers or toes, usually the corresponding finger or toe on both sides, coming on in attacks, lasting up to an hour or more. This pale stage, due to occlusion of the arteries, arterioles and capillaries, is generally followed by (2) coldness and local asphyxia, with cyanosis when the capillaries dilate. (3) In the third or reactionary stage, as the blood flow recommences the affected parts become bright red or dark purple, there is considerable pain and swelling with paræsthesiæ. Sometimes the pale stage is very definite, sometimes it is absent or so transient as to be unobserved. Occasionally the entire hands are involved. (4) In the more severe cases and after frequent attacks the nails become impoverished or lost, local ulcers and *gangrene* occur in the area affected; the dead area becomes separated from the living part and the ulcer that is left heals normally, but slowly. Occasional cases have been recorded of extensive multiple gangrene. X-ray reveals atrophic changes in the bones. The attacks described may be the only symptom, but in most cases other symptoms of considerable clinical interest may be observed. In some there is a generalised scleroderma, the skin appearing to be stretched and smooth, or sometimes cracked; in such cases all the fingers are pale and dead-looking, their entire substance becomes wasted and the nails may be lost. In other cases erythematous blotches occur from time to time in different parts of the body, leaving bruise-like stains. Transient attacks of hemiplegia and aphasia have been observed, also of paroxysmal hæmoglobinuria. Effusion into the phalangeal and other joints may supervene, which can result in ankylosis.

The *Diagnosis* is usually simple. The earlier stages are allied to *erythromelalgia, sclerodactyly* (§ 751), and to " dead hands," but these affections are not so localised to the fingers' *ends*, are less severe, and never go on to gangrene. Local vaso-motor symptoms, affecting usually only one arm, may be due to a *cervical rib.*

Etiology.—The disease is much more common in women and may be familial. It usually starts between the ages of 15 and 30, especially in those with a nervous temperament. Attacks are brought on most often by exposure to cold; they are more frequent at the menopause, after childbirth or surgical operations and under mental stress. In susceptible persons idiosyncrasy to smoking and to phenobarbitone plays a part. Mechanical factors are also important, especially partial occlusion of the subclavian artery by a cervical rib or by hyperabduction of the arms above the head during sleep or at work. The use of vibrating tools may be causal. The condition is at first due to vaso-motor spasm, but later permanent narrowing occurs, making treatment less successful.

Prognosis.—The disease runs a prolonged course of many years. The attacks become more prolonged and frequent, and the patient gradually becomes more and more helpless. There are many degrees of severity, ranging from a small localised syncope or asphyxia to gangrene of the entire segment of a limb. It is a curious circumstance that, in most cases, once a finger has become gangrenous the stump does not become similarly affected later on.   The subjects of this malady in a marked form rarely reach old age, but usually die of some intercurrent disease.

Treatment.—The affected limbs must be kept warm and the patient protected from exposure to cold. Warm underclothing which should cover the upper arms and the thighs, and lined gloves and bootees, should be worn. It is wise to stop smoking permanently in those who benefit from temporary abstention. Thyroid is beneficial and nitroglycerin has been used. Tablets of tolazine hydrochlor. (Priscol) 25 mg. and of dibenyline 20 mg. up to four times daily produce still better vaso-dilatation. Intense pain may occasionally need inject. pethidine hydrochlor. Removal of the sympathetic chain below Th. 1 ganglion to below Th. 3 ganglion removes a large number of the sympathetic nerve fibres to the upper limb (they extend from Th. 1 to Th. 10), but leaves the outflow to the eye (Th. 1) unaffected and so prevents Horner's syndrome. Some surgeons prefer stellate ganglionectomy with the associated Horner's syndrome as being more effective. These operations and lumbar sympathectomy are performed in severe cases with complete relief of symptoms. Operations must be done early, before the vessels become permanently narrowed, the most suitable cases being those which, before operation, show good vaso-dilatation and a rise in skin temperature in response to an artificial rise in body temperature or when the vaso-motor nerves are paralysed by a spinal anæsthetic.

Dead Hands (Pallor of the Fingers).—Many patients—but particularly those who present other evidences of an inherent vaso-motor instability—complain that the hands or finger-tips " go dead," or white, like those of a corpse, and feel numb and cold. These attacks, which rarely last very long, may happen in warm summer weather, without any obvious cause. This vascular disorder resembles the early phase of Raynaud's disease. These attacks are not as a rule serious. Treatment is similar to that of Raynaud's disease.

Raynaud's Syndrome with cold sensitivity of the fingers, superficial ulcers, and localised purpura which can be reproduced by applying ice to the fingers, is seen in **Cryoglobulinæmia.** The blood plasma contains cryoglobulins which are precipitated by cold and redissolved at body temperature; 50 per cent. of these cases have myelomatosis, and others have liver cirrhosis, chronic lymphatic leukæmia, lupus erythematosus, etc.

§ 590. VI. **Erythromelalgia** is a painful burning sensation accompanied by redness and swelling, symmetrically affecting the hands and sometimes the feet: it may spread to the arms and legs. Attacks occur in paroxysms, and although one side may be more affected than the other, both sides are affected simultaneously. Paroxysms often commence when the limbs hang down, are worse after strenuous exercise and after placing them in very hot or very cold water. They are particularly trouble-

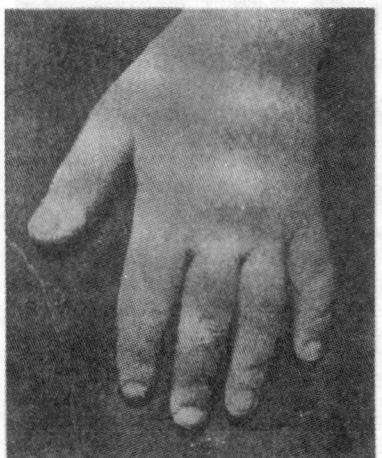

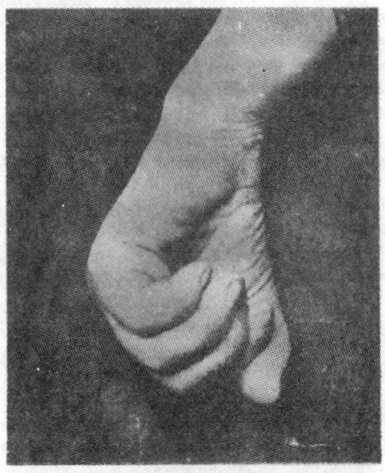

FIG. 172*a*.—ERYTHROMELALGIA in a woman aged about 30.

FIG. 172*b*.—ERYTHROMELALGIA, showing maximum closure of the hand.

some when lying in bed and produce insomnia. An attack starts with tingling and numbness in the fingers or toes (*acroparæsthesia*), spreads to the hands or feet and later on a painful redness supervenes. There is no paralysis but the fingers cannot be fully flexed as they become swollen; the pain and swelling are lessened by holding the hands over the head, or by raising the feet.

Diagnosis.—The swelling and redness affect the whole hand (Figs. 172*a* and *b*) —not in patches as in chilblains, lupus or erythema. In the cyanotic form of *Raynaud's disease* the symptoms start and prevail in one or two finger-tips and the fingers are intensely cold; in erythromelalgia all the fingers and both hands are equally involved and the hands are warm. It is a prolonged and painful condition, never fatal.

Etiology.—Women are more prone to the disease, in a proportion of 20 to 1, between 18 and 25 and chiefly at the climacteric. It is believed to be neurogenic in origin due to a sympathetic-parasympathetic imbalance—the symptoms resembling those of cholinergic overactivity. Several cases have exhibited, concurrently with a severe paroxysm of the erythromelalgic symptoms, erythematous blotches on other parts of the body, and severe " rheumatic " pains in the limbs.

Treatment is by attention to the general health and avoiding factors which cause the attacks. Antihistamines or aspirin are of considerable help and barbiturates may be needed to ensure sleep.

Nutritional Erythromelalgia (Syn. the Burning-feet syndrome) is seen in the grossly undernourished and sometimes in severe alcoholics (and see § 983).

Symptoms.—There is an intense burning in the feet with some aches and pains in the legs, and in severe cases there may be burning in the fingers and hands. The pain is excruciating and prevents sleep at night and there is great difficulty in walking. Examination shows only slight redness of the feet, sometimes combined with evidence of other vitamin deficiencies such as glossitis or cheilosis. Autopsy reveals changes in the arteries and arterioles of the feet.

Treatment is by the administration of a full diet and vitamin B complex; pantothenic acid and yeast have been reported to give good results.

Acroteric Scleroderma (Hutchinson) or **Sclerodactyly** is a scleroderma affecting the hands and feet, and sometimes the nose, in which the skin is bluish and thickened at first, white and atrophic afterwards (§ 751).

§ 591. VII. Pink Disease (Syn. Erythrœdema) is a rare disease which runs a course of several months, with characteristic swelling and redness of the hands and feet, affecting children under 4 years of age.

Symptoms: (i.) There is often a preliminary stage with fever (100° to 102° F), malaise, muscular weakness and loss of weight. For about a month irritability and sleeplessness, bouts of profuse sweating and severe itching of the skin are prominent. (ii.) Then the hands and feet swell, become bright pink or cyanosed and cold. Photophobia is marked, there is almost invariably a rapid pulse; coryza, stomatitis and often vesicles with staphylococcal complications, are common. (iii.) There is poor muscle tone with reduction or absence of the tendon reflexes. (iv.) Recovery is slow and it is many months before the child becomes normal.

Diagnosis.—*Infantile paralysis* is usually suspected and the condition may not be recognised until the development of pink swelling of the extremities.

Etiology.—The disease affects children under 3½ years old, the majority being between 6 and 24 months. The cause is almost certainly due to hypersensitivity to mercurial salts contained in " teething powders " and used for treatment of congenital syphilis; the disease has become very rare since these salts were omitted.

Prognosis.—There are no sequelæ and an attack does not recur. Children nursed at home usually recover, but in hospital there is great risk of infection, such as bronchopneumonia and gastro-enteritis. Secondary infections of the skin such as pustules and onychia are common.

Treatment.—Nursing in the open air with light clothing is recommended. Talc should be dusted over the extremities; painting with spirit prevents the development of pustules. For mouth lesions, the child may chew a swab soaked in hydrogen peroxide 1 in 4; a string ensures that this is not swallowed. The diet must have an adequate vitamin content, and all mercurial salts are avoided.

GROUP II. JOINT DISEASES

The methods of examination and exclusion of fallacies have already been described. Arthritic disorders may conveniently be grouped into acute, subacute and chronic (see § 596).

(a) *Acute Joint Diseases*

Acute joint diseases come on more or less abruptly, and as a rule are attended by the local and general signs of inflammation. Acute rheumatism is essentially an erratic polyarthritis from the commencement; acute gout usually affects a single joint; most of the other causes start in one joint, but (excepting VIII, IX and X) tend to a progressive involvement of others. It is worth noting that all the acute joint disorders (traumatism being excluded) are due either to some infective process or to some other systemic disorder. These facts emphasise the necessity of investigating the constitutional symptoms, the viscera and the blood.

A CHILD OR YOUNG ADULT *complains of* ACUTE PAIN *and often* SWELLING IN SEVERAL JOINTS; *as the inflammation subsides in these joints others are affected. The patient has a* HIGH TEMPERATURE *and there may be cardiac involvement, especially* ENDOCARDITIS. *The disease is* ACUTE RHEUMATISM.

§ 582. I. Acute Rheumatism (Rheumatic Fever) is mainly a disease of temperate climates. In Great Britain it has become progressively less severe and less frequent over the last 50–60 years, but some 4,000 children still fall victims each year. It is rare before 4 years of age and first attacks are very unusual after 25. Especially in children, second, third or more attacks are common, particularly in the winter months. Acute rheumatism is capable of many manifestations with inflammation in a number of organs, especially in the serous membranes of the joints, the endocardium and the pericardium (all of which resemble one another histologically). The chief types of disease are: (A) Acute Rheumatic Polyarthritis; (B) Subacute rheumatism which is largely confined to children. Both types are often accompanied by cardiac disease. (C) Rheumatic carditis may occur alone with no other evidence of acute rheumatism.

(A) ACUTE RHEUMATIC POLYARTHRITIS (Syn. Acute Rheumatic Fever) is the common variety met in young adults, but can occur in children.

Symptoms.—(1) There is usually a history of *tonsillitis* due to the *β-hæmolytic streptococcus* (Lancefield Group A) 1 to 3 weeks previously. (2) The fever of the attack of acute rheumatism comes on in the course of 24 hours, setting in before or at the same time as the joints are inflamed. It is of a continued type (Fig. 173), usually remaining about 102° or 103° F for some days. The onset of any inflammatory complication in the endocardium, pericardium or elsewhere is marked by renewed higher fever, pain but rarely delirium. The usual accompaniments of pyrexia are present—viz., the urine is scanty and highly coloured, the tongue coated, the pulse quick and bounding usually over 100. Hyperpyrexia

occasionally occurs.   (3) In adults there is a *profuse perspiration* which
has a sour disagreeable odour and an acid reaction, but in children this
is unusual; later on sudaminal vesicles are frequently seen.   Erythematous, purpuric and other *rashes* occasionally appear.   (4) The two distinguishing features of the *joint lesions* of acute rheumatism are their
wandering or metastatic character, and the absence of suppuration.   First
one joint is affected, but within a day or so another is involved, the first
joint having almost recovered; finally several may be affected together.
The knees, ankles, wrists and elbows are those most commonly affected;
occasionally only one joint is involved.   Such joints are acutely painful
on the slightest movement; they are warm, not particularly tender to

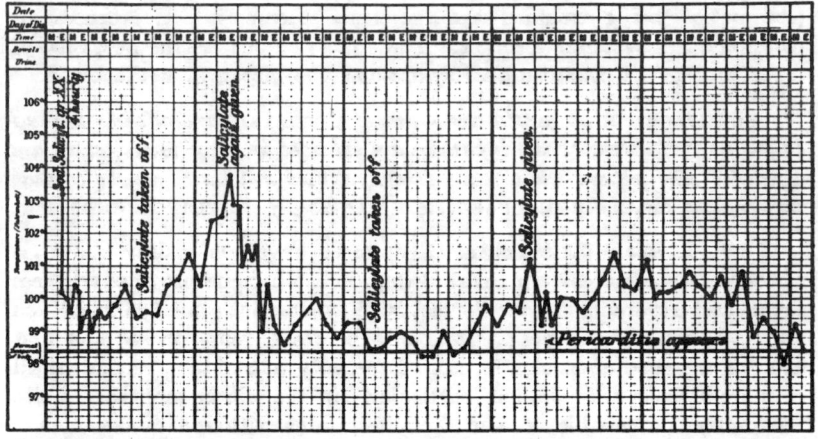

FIG. 173.—RHEUMATIC FEVER.—Henry H——, æt. 22; the chart shows the efficacy of sod. salicylate
in reducing the temperature until pericarditis appears; then it has little effect.

touch and are more likely to show an effusion in an adult.   The skin over
the joints is either unaltered in colour or shows a faint flush.   (5) *Cardiac
involvement* is the most important feature of acute rheumatism because
it is much less amenable to treatment and may leave considerable permanent damage in the heart.   It is much more frequent in children; the
earliest sign is usually that of *mitral endocarditis* with a soft apical systolic
murmur which soon acquires a harsher quality (§ 49); a mitral diastolic
murmur may also be heard.   The aortic valve is rarely affected until
after the age of puberty.   Myocarditis is commonly present with some
dilatation of the heart.   A *pericardial rub* is always evidence of serious
cardiac damage and may be accompanied by a pericardial effusion (§ 46).
(6) *Rheumatic nodules* occasionally occur.   They are small movable bodies,
usually fibrinous, but may become fibrous.   They are generally symmetrically placed on opposite sides of the body and appear on bony
prominences and prominent tendons.   The commonest places to find them
are about the elbows, knees, malleoli, occipital curved lines, posterior

spinous processes of the vertebræ, and knuckles. (7) *Chorea* may be the
first and only sign of rheumatism, but is frequently followed by arthritis
and endocarditis. (8) Pneumonia, pleurisy and peritonitis, all occur rarely.
(9) In untreated cases the fever and local inflammation will last 4 to
6 weeks, but it is characteristic of the disease that the pain and swelling
of the joints and the fever rapidly subside with adequate doses of sodium
salicylate; on the other hand this drug has little effect on the temperature
and the course of inflammation involving the heart. (10) Anæmia develops
rapidly in many cases, especially in those with active carditis and may be
moderately intense in convalescence. (11) Relapses are common even in
the convalescent stage.

The *Diagnosis* of rheumatic fever in the adult is not as a rule difficult,
and there may be a history of previous attacks. In children and in adults
by the time symptoms arise there is a considerable rise in the serum titre
of streptococcal anti-hæmolysins (normal upper limit 200 unit per ml.)
even though the preceding hæmolytic streptococcal sore throat is not
clinically recognisable; but this organism may still be found in culture
of a throat swab. *Acute gout* is distinguished by the features mentioned
in Table XLV. *Acute rheumatoid arthritis* affects chiefly the larger joints
or the fingers (§ 594); the swelling is fusiform, and does not subside
under treatment by salicylates. *Septicæmia*, especially streptococcal, and
pyæmia may closely resemble rheumatic fever. In these pyrexia shows a
marked diurnal variation, often with rigors and delirium, and the leucocytosis is often higher than in rheumatic fever (in which it rarely exceeds
15,000). In any doubtful case, blood culture must be performed early.
Osteomyelitis starting near an epiphysis may be mistaken for rheumatic
fever. *Meningococcal septicæmia* causes confusion at first, as in the septicæmic stage flitting pains in the joints and muscles occur. The presence
of marked headache, facial herpes and purpura help to distinguish this
condition, and a post-nasal culture usually grows meningococci. *Acute
poliomyelitis* in children causes pains in the limbs before paralysis sets in,
pains in the neck with some stiffness and a lymphocytic response in the
C.S.F. *Lymphatic leukæmia* may be difficult to distinguish until a blood
count is performed. *Henoch-Schönlein purpura* may cause joint swelling
in addition to urticaria and gastro-intestinal symptoms. *Polyarteritis
nodosa* and *disseminated lupus erythematosus* do not often occur before
20 years of age. *Gonorrhœal arthritis* usually affects the knees or the
small tarsal or carpal joints (see § 594. III and § 598); the condition is
more chronic, and there is a history of gleet. Among the other diseases
which sometimes have to be differentiated are *dengue*, which has a characteristic eruption; *trichinosis*, in which the pain and swelling are referable
rather to the muscles; in *infective endocarditis* the temperature is intermittent, salicylates are of little use, and a positive blood culture is often
obtained. The secondary arthritis of *cerebro-spinal fever* and *dysentery*
must be borne in mind. *Infantile scurvy* and *syphilitic epiphysitis* rarely
occur after the age of 2, whereas acute rheumatism is rare before 3.

(B) SUBACUTE RHEUMATISM has now become much more common than is the florid type of acute rheumatism just described. Principally a disease of children over the age of 4, it seldom produces acute arthritis but it is very prone to cause unrecognised cardiac disease because the constitutional symptoms are so much less obvious.

Symptoms.—(1) The child complains of " growing-pains." These are fairly severe, enough to cause crying; they occur by day or by night, are present in the arms as well as in the legs and even are present in the intercostal and abdominal muscles. Sometimes pain with or without swelling is present in the joints, or in the structures around the joints. (2) There is a great tendency to sore throats with enlarged cervical glands and a Lancefield group A hæmolytic streptococcus in a throat swab. (3) Usually a low grade fever to 100° F is present. (4) Evidence of cardiac disease is shown by the presence of murmurs at the mitral orifice, with cardiac enlargement, a persistently raised sleeping pulse rate and sometimes pericarditis. (5) Rheumatic nodules are rare.

The *Diagnosis* is from the other disorders mentioned in (A) above. " Growing-pains " must not be regarded as necessarily of rheumatic origin; they occur in many states of general debility, or with postural defects, anæmia or " nervous exhaustion " in children. In these conditions they are present as fatigue pains after exercise, they are much more marked at the end of the day, they tend to disappear in bed at night and they are not usually accompanied by pyrexia. In these debilitated children extracardiac or functional murmurs are often present and require to be distinguished from organic valvular conditions (§ 42). A raised erythrocyte sedimentation rate and a high or rising anti-streptolysin titre is strong confirmatory evidence of a true rheumatic infection; a titre less than 50 units per ml. virtually excludes this diagnosis.

(C) RHEUMATIC CARDITIS is found in some 4 per cent. of those with established mitral stenosis, in whom no previous history of acute or subacute rheumatism can be elicited. The value of periodic routine medical examination in school children in identifying these children at an earlier stage is obvious.

Etiology.—Hereditary and familial factors are important, and the disease is much more prevalent among the poor and the artisan classes; girls are rather more prone to attacks than are boys. Exposure to cold or chill, fatigue and a state of " prerheumatic debility " with loss of weight and of appetite all play a part. The immediate cause is not known; the most important single etiological agent so far identified is the β-hæmolytic streptococcus (Lancefield group A) which usually resides in the throat. Approximately 3 weeks after invasion acute rheumatism occurs. The general consensus of opinion is that during this period a state of hyperimmunity is being developed so that the affected person has more antibodies to hæmolytic streptococci in his blood than do normal people. Then an allergic reaction occurs in the tissues between the antibodies and the bacterial allergens which gave rise to them so that acute rheumatism results. Re-infections with these hæmolytic streptococci cause recurrences of acute rheumatism. Even so routine tonsillectomy does not act as a preventive; diabetics are less liable to acute rheumatism than others. Attempts to incriminate an infecting agent in the heart valves and elsewhere have not survived critical examination or

the proofs required by Koch's postulates. In 1900 F. J. Poynton and Alexander
Paine isolated a diplococcus from the blood exudates, and cardiac valves of rheumatic
cases, which answered the tests of specificity. This has been corroborated by others
but still awaits general acceptance.

The possibility that the hæmolytic streptococcus enables a virus to act as the
primary infecting agent must not be overlooked. The occurrence of localised outbreaks of acute rheumatism in those living and sleeping in confined conditions, and
especially following an epidemic oi acute streptococcal sore throat, strongly support
the view of its being a specific infective disease.

Prognosis of Acute and Subacute Rheumatism.—The disease is not
dangerous to life when it attacks the joints only, but when the heart is
severely affected the prognosis is more grave. One attack predisposes to
future attacks. Other untoward symptoms are hyperpyrexia and cerebral
symptoms. The younger the patient the more likely is relapse to occur.
An attack is grave in proportion to the height of the temperature, the
involvement of the heart, the presence of pericarditis and of rheumatic
nodules; a pericardial effusion with a considerably enlarged area of cardiac
dullness, signs at the left lung base and a raised venous pressure carries a
much worse prognosis than does dry pericarditis.

Treatment.—Absolute rest in bed is essential: the patient should be
between blankets to absorb perspiration, and allowed one pillow if it adds
to his comfort. If severe carditis supervenes, the Fowler position may
be the only one possible. Copious fluids must be taken as for pyrexia
(§ 296, XVIII). Sodium salicylate combined with at least an equal amount
of sodium bicarbonate will relieve the joint pains and cause the temperature
to fall almost to normal within 72 hours, provided large doses are administered to give a plasma concentration of 30–35 mg. per cent.; usual doses
for an adult are 20 gr. every 2 hours during the first 2 days (maximum
200 gr. in 24 hours), then smaller maintenance doses till the temperature
is normal or toxic symptoms of the drug ensue—viz., headache, deafness
and buzzing in the ears, vomiting, albuminuria or delirium. Children
under 12 years of age require half these doses. When salicylates fail to
control the fever, either the diagnosis is incorrect or severe carditis (often
with pericarditis) is present (Fig. 173). Instead of sodium salicylate with
sodium bicarbonate some authorities prefer to avoid this large intake of
sodium and use aspirin 1 gr./lb. body weight per day (maximum 140 gr.
a day) in divided doses 4-hourly for 6 or more weeks. The place of
corticotrophin (ACTH) and of the steroids in therapy has not been
settled but there is considerable evidence that when given in large doses
within the first 2 or 3 weeks of the onset of acute rheumatism there is a
reduction in the number of patients left with residual cardiac murmurs;
the best results seem to have been produced by inject. ACTH 1 mg./lb.
body weight or oral cortisone 3 mg./lb. body weight daily in divided doses
for 4, 6 or 8 weeks. Penicillin should be given at the same time, especially
when a hæmolytic streptococcus persists in the throat. Local remedies
to relieve pain consist of wrapping the joints in cotton-wool, or applying
lead and opium lotion, oil of wintergreen or compound liniment of menthol

(B.P.C.).   To relieve the pain of pericarditis a leech, or a blister with liq. iodi fort. over the precordium is of service.   With hyperpyrexia a graduated hot bath or an ice pack may be required.   Once the acute phase has subsided, before allowing extra activity it is important that there is no evidence of active carditis.   The best guides are the absence of pyrexia or tachycardia, the heart should be normal in size and the murmurs at a stationary stage, the patient should be gaining ½–1 lb. in weight each week and the blood sedimentation rate should have returned to normal. Then slowly graduated extra activity is allowed; in severe cases 6–9 months in bed may be necessary.   As *prophylaxis* to avoid relapses and second attacks, and to prevent streptococcal throats arising, oral penicillin should be given as phenoxymethylpenicillin B.P. 120 mg. b.d. or as benzyl-penicillin 300,000 units b.d. during school age or for 5 years after an attack, whichever is the longer.   Such measures cut down the likelihood of a relapse to one quarter.   When in spite of these measures a streptococcal throat occurs, give an immediate single injection of fortified pro-caine penicillin 3 ml. (1·2 mega-units) followed by oral phenoxymethyl-penicillin 120 mg. t.i.d.   A sulphonamide in a dose of 0·5 G. b.d. is given instead of penicillin in those sensitive to this drug.   When school children suffer with " growing-pains " or tonsillitis, a strict watch should be kept on them, and rest in bed ordered if the heart shows any suspicious signs.

A MAN OVER 40 YEARS *of age wakes in the early hours with sudden severe pain in a* BIG TOE JOINT, *which soon becomes* ACUTELY SWOLLEN, TENDER AND RED.   *The symptoms persist for a few days with a low grade pyrexia after which they spontaneously subside—the disease is* ACUTE GOUT.

§ 593.   II.   **Acute Gout** is due to a disordered metabolism with an excess of uric acid in the blood and tissues.   It is characterised by recurrent attacks of acute inflammation of one or more joints with deposition of sodium biurate crystals in the cartilages of the joints and other skeletal tissues.   Gout is one of the oldest known diseases, is fairly common in temperate climates and is easily overlooked in its earlier stages.   It occurs in acute and in chronic forms (§ 600) and is a cause of fibrositis (§ 604).

Symptoms of an acute attack are often preceded by dyspepsia, aching in the limbs or a mild catarrhal illness.   The onset of an attack is usually sudden, often in the middle of the night.   It most likely affects one of the smaller joints and especially the metatarso-phalangeal joint of a big toe.   (1) In the *earlier attacks* the joint becomes very painful, throbs, burns and is stiff; the temperature rises to 101–102° F and after a bout of sweating the patient may fall asleep for a few hours.   On waking he finds the joint is hot, swollen, shining and bluish-red in colour with exquisite tenderness so that he may not bear the touch of the bed-clothes on the joint.   Suppuration never occurs.   The pain eases in the day-time but becomes worse the following night; after a few days the inflammation subsides and leaves no residual signs.   During the bout there is a polymorph leucocytosis of 20,000 or more and the blood uric acid is raised; the urine is concentrated and contains a trace of albumen but less uric acid than before the attack. Glycosuria may be present. (2) After an interval of 12 months or more a second attack occurs in the same or in another joint, usually a toe or finger, foot or hand, ankle, wrist or knee. In the absence of prolonged treatment, (3) *subsequent attacks* come at shorter intervals, even every few months, and may affect more than one joint at a time, but the inflammation does not flit from one joint to another as in acute rheumatism; (4) then the affected joints never completely settle down in the intervening periods, the disease becomes chronic and permanent changes take place in the joints. For *chronic gout* and its associated symptoms see § 600.

Varieties.—(1) In *subacute gout* the attack is milder and there are wandering pains resembling fibrositis with little or no joint involvement. (2) So-called *irregular gout* is a misnomer, but gouty patients are particularly liable to develop eczema and other skin rashes, headaches, gastrointestinal, cardio-vascular or catarrhal symptoms.

The *Diagnosis* is not difficult except from *acute rheumatism* and *acute rheumatoid arthritis*. In all these conditions the erythrocyte sedimentation rate is raised; but in gout there is an increase of the blood uric acid to 6–9 mg. per cent., especially just before and during an acute attack. It should be remembered that the uric acid content is also high in chronic nephritis and in certain blood diseases, especially in the leukæmias, polycythæmia and myelosclerosis.

TABLE XLV.—DIAGNOSIS BETWEEN ACUTE GOUT AND ACUTE RHEUMATISM

Acute Gout.	*Acute Rheumatism.*
In typical cases:	In typical cases:
Middle age; male sex.	Youth; either sex.
Preference for smaller joints; never wandering from joint to joint.	Preference for larger joints; usually wandering from joint to joint.
Swelling is usually red, tense, pitting on pressure, acutely tender. Pain persists during rest.	Swelling is hot, but pale; pain only on pressure or movement of joint.
Ears may show tophi.	No tophi.
Fever may be slight or transient.	Fever always marked and continuous.

Etiology.—The most important factor is a hereditary tendency which occurs in 50–75 per cent. of cases; men are more liable than women in a proportion of between five and ten to one. The disease is rare under 30 and it is uncommon to see it start after 50; when it occurs in women it is almost invariably after the menopause. The predisposition is transmitted mainly through the male line; but rarely it may be transmitted by an unaffected female and reappears in the sons. Attacks are more frequent in the changeable weather of spring and autumn. Plumbism has now become a very rare cause.

The height of the blood uric acid is not the sole cause of attacks; in gouty families many men show a raised blood uric acid with no symptoms of gout and in the various blood diseases accompanied by a rapid break-down of red cells the blood uric acid may be as high as 10 mg. per cent. and yet no symptoms of this arise. Uric acid is derived from *exogenous* sources, especially cellular protein foods such as liver, sweetbread, kidneys, fish roe; and from *endogenous* sources of which one of the most important is nucleic acid. The normal man excretes uric acid and urates through the renal glomeruli but reabsorbs 90 per cent. in the tubules; there is no evidence in the early stages of the disease of any impairment of renal function although this does occur later when secondary renal damage occurs in the renal vessels so that glomerular filtration becomes inefficient.

Precipitating causes of attacks of gout include (1) alcohol, especially forms containing a high percentage of sugar and alcohol such as port wine, brown sherry, Madeira, sweet red or white wines and beer. Gout is very rare among Scottish artisans; a possible explanation is that the beverage of the Scottish artisan is whisky while that of the English working-man is beer which contains over one grain per pint of purine bodies. (2) Obesity and (3) severe mental or physical fatigue are important factors. (4) A local injury may determine the joint affected. (5) Attacks often follow an infection such as pneumonia or even a simple catarrh of the nose and throat.

The excess uric acid in the blood is deposited as sodium biurate first in the cartilages of the joints and of the ears (later producing characteristic tophi). As the disease progresses similar deposits are found in the ends of the bones (with X-ray changes), in the ligaments and other periarticular tissues, as well as in tendon sheaths, bursæ and in the blood vessels pro-ducing arteriosclerosis and the " gouty kidney."

Prognosis.—An attack is never fatal and in the earlier stages of the disease the patient soon makes a complete recovery. Recurrent attacks tend to recur in the same joint. Many patients can remain free of all attacks and of the secondary complications of gout if they are willing to take uricosuric drugs for the rest of their lives so that the blood uric acid remains at a normal level. But when the disease starts in early life some young adults develop chronic gout and tophaceous deposits in spite of early and conscientious treatment; and these die before the age of 50. Gout tends to shorten life mainly because of the cardio-vascular changes and the resulting kidney disease with hypertension (§ 410). Arteriosclerotic changes in the coronary arteries and in the cardiac valves are common.

Treatment during an attack.—(1) When a joint of the foot or leg is involved the patient will have to rest in bed for a few days. (2) A low diet of milk and farinaceous food and complete abstinence from alcohol should be enjoined. (3) Alkaline carbonates and citrates of potassium, lithium and sodium with additional fluid by mouth promote the solution of uric acid. Three drugs are available to relieve the pain of acute gout and to promote a quicker excretion of uric acid: (4) Phenylbutazone B.P.

(Butazolidin) often results in complete relief of symptoms in 48 hours with a rapid lowering of the blood uric acid and an increased renal excretion. The dose is 800 mg. on the first day, 400-600 mg. on the second day and 200 mg. for a further 2 or 3 days. When given for only this short period toxic symptoms of the drug are uncommon. (5) Colchichine with an initial dose of 1·0 mg. followed by 0·5 mg. 2-hourly for 6-10 doses rapidly gives relief and should then be given in doses of 0·5 mg. for another 7 days; nausea, vomiting and diarrhœa are not infrequent with these doses but can usually be controlled by tincture of opium. (6) Sodium salicylate 20 gr. 5 times a day combined with sodium bicarbonate, or alternatively aspirin 15 gr. q.d.s. is also very effective. Cinchophen B.P. (Atophan) is no longer used because it may prove fatal by producing acute liver necrosis. (7) *Local* treatment consists of applying lotio plumbi cum opio (B.P.) or a spirit lotion, before wrapping the joint in cotton-wool.

Treatment between attacks—i.e., preventive treatment—resolves itself into (1) a question of diet. When the patient is overweight a lower calorie diet should be combined with one containing a low content of purines and of oxalate forming foods (§ 296. XV). (2) Mental and physical fatigue must be prevented and (3) regular outdoor exercise is necessary. (4) To promote uric acid excretion a combination of tab. probenecid (0·5 G.) once, twice or thrice a day should be combined with tab. colchichine 0·5 mg. once or twice a day with the aim of keeping the blood uric acid within normal limits. Probenecid 0·5 G q.i.d. has been shown to increase the excretion of uric acid between 33 and 200 per cent. but the effect is neutralised by salicylate in any form. Sulphinpyrazone (Anturan), a pyrazolidine compound allied to phenylbutazone, is said to be even more effective as a uricosuric drug than probenecid or the salicylates but it may cause gastro-intestinal symptoms: the dose is 100 mg. two or three times a day. It should not be used for acute attacks. (5) Visits to spas such as Bath, Harrogate, Buxton, Strathpeffer, Carlsbad, Royat and Aix-les-Bains help by reason of the mental rest, physiotherapy and dietetic measures used and the waters consumed. Mineral waters (Carlsbad, Vichy, Hunyadi Janos, Friedrichshall) can be freely taken.

Soon after a DISCHARGE FROM THE URETHRA OR VAGINA *there is* ACUTE ARTHRITIS *of one or more joints which* DOES NOT RESPOND TO SALICYLATES —*the disease may be* GONOCOCCAL ARTHRITIS.

§ **594.** III. **Acute Gonococcal Arthritis** is due to infection from the uro-genital organs during the acute stage of gonorrhœa (§ 417). It is more common in men than in women, and is particularly apt to supervene when the prostatic portion of the urethra is involved. The disease commences soon after the acute uro-genital infection (often about the fourth or fifth week). The commonest finding is a synovitis of the joint, but more severe attacks involve the cartilage, bone and periosteum in and around the joints.

Symptoms.—There may still be a discharge from the urethra of the male or from the cervix and vagina of the female, but when the joints become affected the gleet sometimes disappears, a circumstance which can cause an error in diagnosis. A single joint may be affected but it is more common to find several joints involved; the symmetrical joint involvement seen in acute rheumatoid arthritis is unusual, the commonest joints being a knee, wrist or ankle. These become swollen with fluid, hot and tender, and the joints first affected do not get better as others become involved; also the intermittent temperature and the inflamed joints show no response to salicylates. A gonococcal cause is particularly suggested when there is involvement of a sterno-clavicular, temporomandibular or other unusual joint. Although there is rarely suppuration, untreated cases or those resistant to treatment may result in extensive destruction of the joints, deformities and even ankylosis. The disease can occur in children.

Diagnosis is by the history of infection, a positive smear or culture of the gonococcus from the primary sites and a positive complement-fixation reaction in the blood serum or in the fluid removed from a joint. The gonococcus can only be found in the synovial fluid of about 15 per cent. of cases.

Treatment is by bed rest and giving full doses of procaine penicillin; although many cases may be cured by a single dose of 600,000 units intramusc., others need repeated doses even for a month. A small number of cases of proven gonococcal arthritis are penicillin resistant, in which case inject. streptomycin, chloramphenicol, the tetracyclines or the sulpha drugs should be tried, alone or in combination. Short-wave diathermy to the joints may be helpful for the gonococcus cannot exist at the temperature to which the joint is raised; some prefer artificial fever therapy as by T.A.B. intravenously. Secondary infection in the prostate or the cervix can be removed by prostatic massage with local diathermy. The patient should avoid any possibility of a fresh attack of gonorrhœa.

Reiter's disease (Syn. Reiter's syndrome) is especially common in young men and may be independent of sexual contact.

Symptoms.—There is an acute polyarthritis affecting especially the joints of the legs (knees and ankles) and less commonly the wrists, shoulders, spine and occasionally the hips; this is accompanied by a non-specific urethritis with a discharge which may be copious or scanty, purulent or mucoid. Conjunctivitis or iritis often precede the polyarthritis and there may be nausea, vomiting, cough, slight fever and skin lesions. The cause is unknown but a virus is suspected; the condition is often confused with gonococcal arthritis. Many cases clear up spontaneously in 3 or 4 months, but some develop a condition resembling chronic rheumatoid disease.

Treatment.—Penicillin, tetracyclines and the sulphonamides are useless. Some appear to benefit from chloramphenicol or corticosteroids in large doses. Bed rest, splinting severely affected joints, aspirin for pain and artificial fever therapy with intravenous T.A.B. vaccine are the most hopeful lines of treatment.

IV. **Acute Rheumatoid Arthritis** may start in a manner indistinguishable from acute rheumatism, but the joint swellings persist and become more typically those of rheumatoid arthritis later (§ 597).

V. Acute Suppurative Arthritis. *Septicæmia* and *Pyæmia* have been described in § 516. In some cases of acute general infection the joints are not involved, but in others there is a marked tendency to inflammation in and around the joints. This may occur with pneumococcal, staphylococcal or streptococcal septicæmia, with typhoid fever and rarely with infective endocarditis. It is differentiated from other joint lesions by: (1) the swelling does not shift its position, as it does in acute rheumatism; (2) the joint may be red and show evidences of suppuration; (3) the constitutional symptoms are characteristic, especially the wide and irregular temperature, often rigors and sweatings, and the leucocytosis is usually above 15,000; (4) a cause may be revealed in the shape of an internal or external pyogenic focus.

VI. Other **acute specific diseases** may lead to arthritis. The joint disease can be identified only by the presence or history of the disease which it complicates. In *adults* with dengue fever joint swelling is often part of the disease; in cerebro-spinal meningitis and in brucellosis the joints are often affected. In *children* the joints may be affected in the early stages of acute poliomyelitis: measles, typhoid, mumps and influenza are rarer causes. Synovitis sometimes follows the administration of antitoxins, *i.e.*, serum reactions (§ 524) and of penicillin.

VII. There are four remaining generalised disorders associated with joint trouble —viz., Henoch-Schönlein Purpura, Scurvy, Hæmophilia and Leukæmia.

§ 595. Henoch-Schönlein Purpura (Syn. Henoch-Schönlein Syndrome, Anaphylactoid Purpura, Peliosis Rheumatica) is more frequent in male children between 3 and 12 years of age but can occur in adults up to 30. Relapse is common. *Schönlein's disease* produces pain in and around the joints not due to rheumatic fever, associated with a skin eruption (§ 767); *Henoch's purpura* produces acute abdominal pain with bleeding into the coats of the intestine.

Symptoms.—(1) There is an initial pyrexia, rarely above 100°, which may follow a hæmolytic streptococcal throat infection. (2) The eruption is often the first symptom; it presents most often as a macular rash with surrounding erythema on the extensor surfaces of the elbows and forearms or of the lower legs and may affect the buttocks. It is roughly symmetrical, itching at first and may leave brown staining. Scanty or more profuse patches of purpura may be seen, and occasionally ecchymoses or even necrosis with bulla or ulcer formation can occur. (3) Within the first 7 days joint pains, tenderness and swelling occur; the amount of effusion into a joint is never great and the swelling tends to be periarticular rather than intra-articular. (4) Henoch's purpura may co-exist and give acute abdominal symptoms. (5) Acute nephritis, often hæmorrhagic, is common and may lead to subacute or chronic nephritis. (6) Hess's capillary fragility test may be positive, and bleeding can occur into other areas such as the brain or eyeball. (7) The blood may show an increase in polymorphs and/or eosinophils, but unlike purpura hæmorrhagica, the blood platelets, the bleeding and clotting times are normal. A mild anæmia may be produced.

Etiology.—There is an aseptic inflammation of the capillaries which allows blood plasma and red cells to escape. The condition is regarded as a sensitisation to foreign protein. Many cases follow a hæmolytic streptococcal throat infection, but allergy to foods is sometimes responsible and the condition clears when the offending article is removed from the diet.

Prognosis.—This is usually good unless the kidneys are severely involved, in which case chronic nephritis and uræmia may develop.

Treatment is by bed rest and treating a streptococcal throat. Once the condition is established penicillin, the sulphonamides and salicylates seem to be valueless The antihistamines have been used with good results, and otherwise the corticosteroids have been favourably reported on when used in full doses such as tab. prednisolone 5-10 mg. t.i.d. for 4 weeks, followed by smaller doses for the next 1 to 2 months. A course of iron may be needed for anæmia.

HENOCH'S PURPURA ABDOMINALIS is another variety of anaphylactoid purpura, and all or any of the symptoms recorded above may be present. The *chief symptom* is severe colic, occurring independently of diet, associated with constipation or diarrhœa and the passage of blood or blood-stained stools. Vomiting may be severe, with or without blood and a tumour due to hæmorrhage into the submucous coats of the intestine may occur—especially in the lower ileum. The condition is apt to be mistaken for intussusception—this complication or sometimes perforation may occur. The *diagnosis* is aided by finding a few spots of purpura or other skin rashes, or red cells in the urine. Attacks may recur at intervals for years. *Treatment* is on the lines of Schönlein's purpura, but small doses of opium may be needed when colic is severe.

In SCURVY (§ 560) tender non-suppurative swellings occur beneath the periosteum near the joints, but the joints themselves are not often affected. The disease is recognised by the spongy bleeding gums, anæmia and other symptoms of scurvy.

In HÆMOPHILIA (§ 561) the larger joints are usually affected. The joint lesion is due to the extravasation of blood into the joint cavities, and usually supervenes suddenly after a slight blow. It frequently recurs, and may ultimately lead to ankylosis. *Diagnosis* is mainly by the history of hæmorrhages in the patient and by the family history; the onset is usually between the ages of 7 and 14 and only affects males.

In ACUTE LEUKÆMIA joint symptoms may predominate in the earlier stages. Swelling is usually slight, but there is considerable pain, with limitation of movement and some pyrexia, which make the distinction from acute rheumatism difficult. The pain may be due to small purpuric hæmorrhages into the joints. Sooner or later purpuric retinitis, generalised purpura, enlargement of lymphatic glands and of the spleen aid diagnosis. The ends of the bones may present a frosted glass appearance on X-ray examination, and a blood count is usually diagnostic.

VIII. **Acute Traumatic Synovitis** is recognised by the history of an injury, though one must bear in mind (1) that many constitutional processes, especially gout, are lighted up by a very slight injury, and (2) that in childhood the history of trauma may be wanting.

IX. **Intermittent Hydrarthrosis** possibly comes under this heading. In adult life the knee joints swell at periodic intervals, which the patient can foretell almost to a day. There is no fever and no local redness or warmth over the joint. Nothing accurate is known of its etiology. It has been ascribed to allergy, but some cases later develop rheumatoid disease. *Treatment* is symptomatic.

Palindromic Rheumatism resembles intermittent hydrarthrosis in that there are short recurrent attacks of acute pain and swelling in one or more joints. The differentiation is by the complete irregularity of occurrence of the attacks, pain and warmth in the joints are more marked and any joint may be affected. A causal relationship to giant urticaria has been suspected. Even after multiple attacks in the same joint chronic damage never develops. *Treatment* is again symptomatic; no method of cure is known.

X. **Extension** from epiphysitis or osteomyelitis (§ 607) or other bone disease in childhood—set up very likely by injury—may produce acute inflammation in a joint, and the serious nature of the condition may be overlooked unless the correct meaning of the pyrexia and constitutional disturbance is appreciated.

(b) Subacute and Chronic Joint Diseases

These joint disorders come under the following headings:—

I. Osteo-arthritis, § 596.
II. Rheumatoid arthritis, § 597.
III. Chronic gonococcal arthritis, § 598.
IV. Chronic infective arthritis, § 599.
V. Chronic gout, § 600.
VI. Ankylosing spondylitis, § 601.
VII. Systemic lupus erythematosis, § 602.

VIII. Polyarteritis nodosa, § 98.
IX. Tuberculous joint disease, § 603.
X. Syphilitic arthritis.
XI. Hysterical joint affections.
XII. Neuropathic arthritis (e.g., Tabes, Syringomyelia and Raynaud's disease).

Clinically some of these joint diseases resemble one another in their physical signs and their history, and many cases are met which it is almost impossible to place definitely under one or other classification.

A middle-aged or elderly patient complains of PROGRESSIVE PAIN *in* ONE OR SEVERAL JOINTS; STIFFNESS AND GRATING *are felt on movement but there are no constitutional symptoms.* *The disease is likely to be* OSTEO-ARTHRITIS.

§ 596. I. **Osteo-arthritis** is a chronic degenerative disease of joints, progressive in character and occurring in middle and later life. It may affect one or several joints and can affect any joint in the body. The condition is seen radiographically in most people after the age of 40 but only a small proportion develop symptoms; thus in one large series X-ray changes were found in 90 per cent., but symptoms were only present in 5 per cent. Therefore it is most important to be sure that the symptoms complained of are due to osteo-arthritis and not to some other cause.

Symptoms.—(1) Pain is present especially during and after use; thus there may be little pain in a knee until the patient walks. The severity varies from a slight dull ache to a severe sharp pain; this may be localised to the joint, may spread to the adjacent muscles or be referred through nerve roots or trunks to distant areas. (2) Stiffness is felt after resting or when first getting out of bed. (3) Scrunching and grating are audible and may be felt by the patient or by the examining fingers with active and passive movements. (4) Swelling, warmth and tenderness may occur. Distension of a joint is due to a thickened synovial membrane and to the occurrence of an acute effusion; and there may be encysted collections of fluid near a large joint, lying in spaces bounded by muscles and connective tissue. (5) Lipping and osteophytes may be felt at the margins of larger joints, especially the knees. Lipping is due to hypertrophied cartilaginous fringes at the articular margins and when these calcify they produce the osteophytes. (6) Limitation of movement develops as the disease advances, largely due to muscle spasm or to periarticular adhesions and sometimes to the mechanical changes produced. (7) Considerable deformity may result from the weakness of the muscles and ligaments, and from the absorption of the ends of the bones so that displacement and even shortening occurs. There is no constitutional disturbance in

C.M.—G G

this disease; the patient often looks robust. Muscular atrophy is less marked than in rheumatoid arthritis, but muscle spasm around a painful joint causes further limitation of movement. Contractures and ankylosis do not develop. A patient with arthritic hips and knees tends with advancing age to become more immobile and therefore often puts on a good deal of weight.

The symptoms produced vary with the position and type of the joints affected.

1. *The Knees* are most commonly affected in women, especially domestic workers at and past middle age; excessive weight is an important aggravating factor. Pain and stiffness are noticed on walking and going downstairs and the knees may give way suddenly. Because they are easily accessible, the swelling warmth and lipping are readily detected. X-ray examination shows narrowing of the joint space and calcification in the cruciate ligaments and the patellar ligament—the changes are often more marked in the patello-femoral area than elsewhere. Menopausal arthritis is a special variety of this (see below).

2. *The Hip-Joint* is more commonly involved in men over 50 and leads to considerable crippling. Osteo-arthritis may be unilateral or bilateral, and is often independent of arthritis elsewhere. It may be the result of repeated small traumata (especially falls off a horse), Perthé's disease, coxa vara, old infective or tuberculous disease, or epiphysitis. Pain is felt most severely in the groin but may radiate down the outer side of the thigh to the knee; the condition is distinguished from sciatica, with which it is often confused, by the position of the pain and the fixity of the joint. The earliest limitation of movement is of rotation; later all movements become difficult and painful, the thigh becomes adducted and externally rotated and while walking the patient leans over to the affected side when he puts weight on the diseased hip joint. Wasting is limited to the buttock and thigh muscles; the limb may be shortened.

3. *The Metatarso-phalangeal Joint* of one or both *big toes* is affected after an injury or recurrent attacks of gout and produces hallux rigidus.

4. *The Carpo-metacarpal Joint* of one or both *thumbs* are painful, loose and grate and the bones can be felt to be lipped.

5. *Cervical Osteo-arthritis* (*Spondylosis*) is usually due to postero-lateral disc protrusion and sometimes to changes in the articular surfaces. The result is a narrowing of the intervertebral foramina by osteophytes, between cervical 3–7 vertebræ, especially in C 5–6 and C 6–7 areas. At first there is complaint of stiffness, and limitation of movement is found; in a proportion of cases this develops into a painful condition in which, as a result of adhesions to and compression of the cervical nerve roots, there is a dull aching or burning pain in the occipital area, or in the lower neck or arm associated with paræsthesiæ and even loss of motor function (§ 1004).

6. *Dorsal Osteo-arthritis* is radiographically present in the majority of elderly persons, especially between D 7–10 vertebræ; the bodies of the

vertebræ later may become wedge-shaped with the production of kyphosis and when disc protrusions occur they give rise to pain in the distribution of the lower dorsal nerve roots.

7. *Lumbar Osteo-arthritis* is a similar condition, most marked between L 3–5 vertebræ. It produces a low backache and sciatic pain (§§ 604, 1019).

8. *The Generalised Form.*—In this condition most of the joints in the body may be attacked, including those of the spine. In the hands, the distal interphalangeal joints and the carpo-metacarpal joints of the thumbs are usually selected, and show the characteristic grating and lipping, not the fusiform swelling of rheumatoid arthritis.

Other Varieties are:—

Heberden's Nodes. These are the commonest and best known variety of osteo-arthritis. They occur independently of osteo-arthritis in other areas. In women, in whom there is often an inherited tendency, they are very frequent, but they are rare in men. The nodes form bony outgrowths which occur in symmetrical fashion at the sides of the distal interphalangeal joints of the hands. They are usually painless, but may be painful, and produce numbness and tingling in the fingers. Little bursal swellings occasionally accompany them. In advanced cases the terminal phalanges are bent acutely toward the radial side.

Menopausal Arthritis (Syn. Climacteric Arthritis) occurs in women between 40 and 55 years of age and involves principally the knees, and to a lesser extent the wrists and fingers. In the early stage there is swelling, due to synovitis, and pain; in the knee this is usually on the inner side. Later, osteo-arthritic change may supervene. Obesity and panniculitis are usually present, with signs of hypothyroidism.

Diagnosis is from other varieties of monarticular and multiple arthritis and from the diseases around joints which affect the soft tissues (§ 604). Arthritis of a joint produces limitation of movement in *all* directions whereas disease of the soft tissues limits movement in one or several directions. Other varieties of polyarthritis, and especially rheumatoid arthritis and gout, often give rise to osteo-arthritis later. The erythrocyte sedimentation rate and the sheep cell agglutination test give normal results in purely degenerative disease. *X-ray examination* is often of help in confirming the diagnosis (Fig. 175c); the joint space in osteo-arthritis is narrowed and calcified osteophytes are usually well seen. Later the large joints show wearing away of the subchondral bone which then undergoes sclerosis in an attempt at repair. Especially in vertebral disease, in addition to antero-posterior and lateral views, oblique views are essential to demonstrate narrowing of the intervertebral foramina.

Etiology.—Osteo-arthritis is essentially a degenerative condition, sometimes named " degenerative arthritis." It is partly the result of ageing of the joints, the process being aggravated by major or repeated minor traumatic factors which accounts for its localisation in certain joints in men doing manual work. In the lumbar spine, hip- and knee-joints the condition is certainly aggravated by obesity and by abnormal strains due to faulty posture. Fatigue, overwork, sleeplessness and toxic influences may induce symptoms because they aggravate such postural deformities.

The primary change is in the cartilage of a joint, which even in the twenties may show softening (chondromalacia); small portions may flake off and cause a knee-joint to "catch." In the next stage the cartilage develops grooves in the direction of the main movement of a joint, and later it wears through where the weight-bearing and other pressures are greatest. The subchondral bone becomes more vascular and undergoes osteosclerosis where it forms part of a joint—as it becomes polished it is said to be eburnated. Meanwhile the edges of the articular cartilage hypertrophy and later calcify to produce osteophytes. The synovial membrane hypertrophies and produces villi with some excess of joint fluid; later it undergoes fibrosis. In certain vascular areas, especially in the head of the femur, cysts may form which communicate with the joint. Small loose foreign bodies or "joint mice" are believed to originate from calcified villi which separate from the synovial membrane.

Prognosis.—If treated early, temporary improvement may occur, but speaking broadly, the disease is progressive. The form occurring in the hip-joint of old men is very intractable, but that in the knees of women at the menopause more remediable. The crippling is not great, but patients with the joints of the lower extremities affected will often be afraid to get about, because of the fear of the knees giving way. Relieving abnormal strains as by the correction of obesity, of bad postures and improving the general health often cause relief of symptoms even though the joint changes remain.

Treatment.—*General* measures consist in attention to the general health. Pain and the progress of the disease are often greatly lessened by the loss of even a few pounds of excess weight. In menopausal arthritis this can be aided by regular small doses of thyroid. *Local* measures include (1) local applications such as Scott's dressing, a kaolin poultice and liniments containing menthol, camphor and methyl salicylate may be used. Heat is very welcome, and may be given as radiant heat, diathermy, paraffin wax baths or infra-red rays. (2) *Abnormal strains* must be corrected as far as possible. Remedial exercises to correct faulty posture and wasting of muscles are valuable. Particularly in osteo-arthritis of the knees and lumbar spine, correction of flat foot, genu valgum and other orthopædic deformities are necessary. (3) A period of *bed-rest* or with splinting will help the acute phase to subside when a joint suddenly becomes painful. (4) *Local injections* into joints such as sterile procaine hydrochlor. (2·0 per cent.) 5 ml. are useful but hydrocortisone or prednisolone should not be added more than once or twice at the outside. (5) *Deep X-ray* is useful in selected cases for the relief of pain. (6) *Analgesics* with the use of aspirin or aspirin compounds, phenylbutazone and sometimes chloroquine are used as described in § 597. The oral administration of corticosteroids is seldom justified. (7) *Surgical measures* are helpful especially in advanced osteo-arthritis of the hip where various forms of arthroplasty have now become established practice. When a single joint is grossly diseased and the cause of much pain which does not respond to other measures, arthrodesis is often justified.

A WOMAN *complains of* STIFFNESS, *and later* PAIN AND SWELLING, IN THE JOINTS OF THE FINGERS; *larger joints are soon affected. The condition progresses and is associated with* CONSTITUTIONAL SYMPTOMS *and some pyrexia; she probably has* RHEUMATOID DISEASE.

§ 597. II. Rheumatoid Disease (Syn. Rheumatoid Arthritis) is a systemic condition which produces intra-articular and periarticular inflammation. Although the principal symptoms relate to the joints, it is now regarded as a disease of mesenchymal connective tissue which affects many organs—skeletal tissues including bones, muscles, tendons, fascia, synovia and bursæ; the lungs and pleura; the heart and pericardium and sometimes

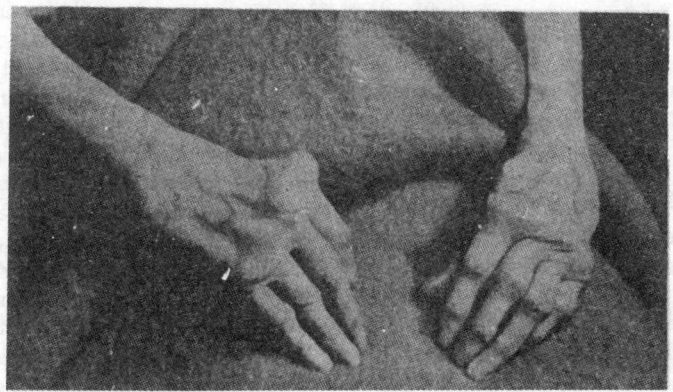

FIG. 174.—RHEUMATOID ARTHRITIS in a woman, showing deformity of wrists and fingers.

the spleen and the eye. It affects women more frequently than men in the proportion of five to one. The classical type affecting women between 20 and 45 years of age is now tending to give place to a disease in which first attacks occur in young, middle-aged and even elderly adults alike. The disease is common in Great Britain at the present time; a recent survey showed 4 per 1,000 adults to be affected.

The onset may be acute, subacute or chronic. In the acute form (§ 594) the condition closely resembles acute rheumatism but the joints remain swollen, prove intractable to the administration of salicylates and later assume the typical characters. A subacute onset is much the commonest. Sometimes the condition is chronic throughout so that over a period of years a gradual deformity of the fingers develops leading to joint and bone destruction, without pain ever being complained of.

Symptoms.—(1) *Prodromal* symptoms are often the first manifestation, so that for months the patient complains of anorexia, excessive fatigue, transient muscle and joint pains and progressive loss of weight. In others there may be a recent history of metatarsalgia, tenosynovitis, bursitis, capsulitis of the shoulder or a painful heel. (2) Then the *arthritic* symptoms commence in one of several different ways: (i.) they usually affect the second and third fingers of the proximal row of interphalangeal joints of the fingers; soon other interphalangeal joints and the metacarpo-phalangeal joints are involved, the lesions being more or less bilaterally symmetrical. (ii.) In others the corresponding joints of the feet are first complained of. In both these types the disease may remain confined to the hands or feet: in others the wrists, tarsal joints, ankles, knees and elbows soon become involved, followed by the shoulders and last of all the hips, so that the progression of the joint disease is from the periphery. Yet the distal interphalangeal joints are usually spared, although the intervertebral joints can be affected. (iii.) In another group one of the larger joints is the first to be affected—a wrist, knee or ankle, followed some weeks, months or even years later by a number of other joints. During the ACTIVE STAGE the joints are first felt to be stiff during the first few hours after rising. Soon they become painful on movement and swollen, as well as tender to pressure and warmer than the surrounding parts; gradually movement of the joints becomes limited. The swelling is fusiform in shape because the lesion is a combination of synovitis and peri-arthritis; a polymorphonuclear viscid fluid collects in the joint cavity and so no grating can be elicited. The periarticular tissues are softened and weakened so that deformities arise, the most common being an ulnar deviation of the fingers. There is considerable muscle wasting above and below the affected joints, to a much greater extent than can be explained by disuse. If the active stage is severe and of long duration, very marked limitation of movement occurs, due to the formation of adhesions around and in the joints as well as to secondary contracture of muscles, so that partial dislocation (subluxation) or ankylosis may be found. (3) Even in the early stages the peripheral circulation is poor, the *skin* of the hands and feet is cold and sweaty. Later the skin becomes glossy, atrophied and often parchment-like. Pigmentation is common as circumscribed spots like freckles, or as diffuse spreading patches especially on the face and neck and on the back of the wrists and forearms, but it may be general. (4) *Subcutaneous nodules* are often present usually in the form of flat masses in bursæ, especially in the olecranon bursæ, but they may be present as large and sometimes tender masses in the subcutaneous tissues, especially of the forearms or the fingers. (5) Enlargement of the epitrochlear, axillary and inguinal *glands* draining the affected joints is common. (6) *Constitutional* symptoms are present especially during the active stage. The temperature is usually above normal in the evening and may reach 102–103° F; the pulse is quickened often out of proportion to the temperature; the anorexia and loss of weight of the prodromal period continues; anæmia with a hæmoglobin value of 60–80 per cent. (Haldane) develops. *Less frequent symptoms* and signs include: (7) the lungs may show a chronic interstitial pneumonia with fibrosis, or bronchiolitis or a

honeycomb lung, or wet or dry pleurisy; (8) the heart muscle is weakened
by myocarditis, and sometimes endocarditis or pericarditis are present;
(9) the *mental state* often becomes one of depression which is aggravated
by the sleeplessness caused by the painful joints. After many months
of active disease, the acute phase tends to die out, but recurrences can
occur months or years later.

In the CHRONIC STAGE there is residual limitation of movement and
deformity of the previously affected joints, so that the knees cannot be
fully extended or fully flexed, the fingers assume a permanent flexion with
ulnar deviation, and the feet become flattened with the toes hyperextended at the metatarso-phalangeal joints so that the ball of the foot
is formed by the heads of the metatarsal bones over which corns develop.
In the advanced stages, contractures of the tendons and joint capsules,
secondary osteo-arthritis or a fibrous or bony ankylosis are frequently seen.

Diagnosis.—In the typical case this is relatively easy, as when it commences in a woman with involvement of the proximal interphalangeal
or the metacarpo-phalangeal joints and soon involves other areas producing
a spindle-shaped swelling of the joints, lymphatic gland enlargement and

TABLE XLVI.—TABLE OF DIAGNOSIS.

Infective Arthritis.	Chronic Gout.	Rheumatoid Arthritis.	Osteo-arthritis.
Either sex; middle life or over.	Generally male sex; over 40.	Chiefly female sex; often 20 to 45.	Either sex; the hips in men, the knees in women; 40 to 60.
Poor and debilitated. Insidious onset.	Family tendency usual. History of sudden onset and acute attacks with severe pain. Skin over joints red, swollen and œdematous.	Inherited tendency is common. Onset acute, subacute or insidious. Constitutional symptoms present with pyrexia, anæmia, loss of weight.	Onset insidious; course, progressive. No constitutional symptoms.
Tends to affect the larger joints; hips, knees, wrists, elbows and shoulders.	Only one joint affected at first; usually the metatarso-phalangeal of the great toe. Usually asymmetrical.	Generally polyarticular. Temporo-maxillary joint may be affected. Spreads from the smaller joints to the larger; proximal interphalangeal joints usually affected. Usually symmetrical.	Polyarticular or mono-articular. Temporo-maxillary joint rarely, if ever, affected.
Thickening of synovial membrane; marked rarefaction of bones and irregular overgrowth around the joints.	Deposits of urate of soda round the joints. Tophi may be present in cartilages of ears. Blood uric acid increased.	Spindle-shaped enlargement with ulnar deviation and later some fixation. No lipping or osteophytes in early stages.	Radial deviation of terminal phalanges. Lipping and osteophytes marked. Cartilage and bone absorbed.

constitutional symptoms. When however it commenced in one of the
larger joints early diagnosis is not so easy. The sheep-cell agglutination
test of Rose-Waaler or the recent simple modification as the latex test of
Singer and Plotz gives positive results in 85–90 per cent. of those with true

rheumatoid disease; this test gives positive results in lower titres in other collagen diseases as well as in liver cirrhosis, ulcerative colitis, myelomatosis and certain febrile diseases. A positive test appears to be due to a macroglobulin in the blood which by electrophoresis follows the rapidly migrating gammaglobulin (§ 543); the highest titre at which the test is positive and the height of the erythrocyte sedimentation rate are usually directly proportional to the activity of the rheumatoid process, although on rare occasions the E.S.R. can be normal in the presence of advanced disease. *Gouty arthritis* is much more common in men, gives rise to acute attacks especially in a big toe with a red and very painful swelling which subsides in a few days. *Osteo-arthritis* comes on insidiously, usually in a knee- or hip-joint and tends to occur at a later age. *Gonococcal* and other forms of *infective arthritis* should be considered in any case of acute arthritis with atypical features. *Disseminated lupus erythematosus* can easily be confused with acute and subacute rheumatoid disease, especially when marked constitutional changes are present. In both there is polyarthritis which does not respond to salicylates but which does respond to corticosteroids. When the patient already shows signs of localised lupus erythematosis the diagnosis is certain, but this is unusual; a certain diagnosis between the two conditions may be impossible for some while, especially as there is a high erythrocyte sedimentation rate in both and the presence of the " L.E." phenomenon in the blood has been reported in 15 to 25 per cent. of cases of advanced rheumatoid disease. However, permanent joint changes are uncommon in lupus erythematosus and leucopenia is usual, contrasting with the mild polymorphonuclear leucocytosis of rheumatoid disease. *Polyarteritis nodosa* also commences on occasions with acute polyarthritis but soon other symptoms of this disease of the smaller blood-vessels will arise. *X-ray examination* of the joints may show no change at first; soon there is osteoporosis of the ends of the bones adjacent to the joints and then diminution in the joint space becomes demonstrable.

Etiology.—The immediate cause is not known but certain predisposing factors are established: (1) a hereditary tendency occurs in 17 per cent. of cases and 20 per cent. of their relations give a positive Rose-Waaler test (as compared with 2 to 3 per cent. of adults in non-rheumatoid families); (2) there is a previous history of true rheumatic fever in 10 per cent. of cases; (3) overwork and psychological stress not only appear to cause first attacks but to cause relapses; (4) endocrine factors play a part, so that 20 to 25 per cent. of cases occur within a year of the menopause— the maximal incidence of new cases is now in the 45-54 age group; (5) a lowered resistance frequently precedes an attack; apical abscesses, pyorrhœa alveolaris, septic conditions of the nose, antrum, sinuses, ears and throat, tonsils, gall-bladder or digestive tract, chronic cervicitis, cystitis, colitis, and ulcerating piles may act as contributory causes, but that they are not the real cause is shown by the fact that dealing with such does not necessarily bring about lasting improvement.

The primary damage in a joint is in the periarticular tissues, the capsule of the joint and the synovial membrane; granulation tissue (pannus) spreads inwards from the junction of the synovial membrane with the articular cartilage until the latter is entirely replaced by granulation tissue. The underlying bone simultaneously becomes more vascular and osteoporotic.

Prognosis.—The younger the patient at the onset, the more crippled does she become as age advances. Those who have efficient treatment within the first year have a much better outlook than those who remain untreated for several years. Rheumatoid disease tends to be self-limiting and in a proportion of cases the active disease dies out without leaving any permanent joint disorganisation or appreciable incapacity. Others progress in spite of continuous and active treatment so that ultimately they become severely crippled and some 10 per cent. become bedridden. Steroid therapy frequently relieves pain and may make the difference between working and not working, or between being bed-ridden and being able to get around the house with the help of furniture (Kersley); but it makes no difference to the progressive degeneration shown by serial X-rays of the joints, and the X-ray and pathological changes may be aggravated because relief of pain encourages the patient to overwork the diseased joints. A remission may be spontaneous, but is usual during pregnancy and may be permanent following an attack of jaundice. A well-recognised *complication* is amyloid disease which should be suspected when persistent albuminuria develops—it may be confirmed by the congo-red test or by renal biopsy. Some degree of osteo-arthritis always develops and is often severe.

Treatment.—In the acute stages and in relapse (*a*) *bed-rest* is essential and a period of some weeks in hospital is often of great help. The skin must be kept active by light clothing and regular baths; treatment on an open-air balcony or in a special hut is often most useful. (*b*) *Pain* is best relieved by bed-rest and by one or more of the analgesic drugs; aspirin in the form of calcium aspirin or aspirin-glycine (Paynocil) may be prescribed with other analgesics as in tab. codein. co. (B.P.) or with phenacetin and aspirin. Paracetamol (Panadol) is helpful to some who are intolerant of aspirin. (*c*) The *diet* needs to be abundant and nourishing to combat the wasting; thus a 10-stone person will need 2,500 calories with large quantities of fats, milk, eggs, fruit and green vegetables. As the appetite is often poor and the glucose-tolerance reduced, insulin injections (6 to 10 units before meals twice a day) may be given. (*d*) *Prevention of deformities* is accomplished by suitable splints worn at night or for the whole 24 hours; a short period of complete rest in a plaster-of-Paris jacket for 10 to 14 days often aids a very painful swollen joint. The upper arms should be at a right angle; the elbow at a little less than a right angle; the wrist supinated and dorsiflexed; the fingers nearly extended. The hips and knees should be extended, the feet dorsiflexed. When pain has diminished, massage and small doses of galvanism are indicated to prevent wasting and fixation. (*e*) *An infective focus* must be sought and removed, surgical measures being conducted under an antibiotic cover as with penicillin. (*f*) *Gold salts* (sodium aurothiomalate B.P., Myocrisin) are widely used as they frequently cause a remission of the disease, especially if it has been present for less than 12 months; but infective foci should first be attended to. Doses at weekly intervals are increased from 10 to 100 mg. until a total of 1·0 G. has been given. Second or third courses are often required after an interval of 6 to 12 months, especially when the blood sedimentation rate remains high. The patient's condition is aggravated if a fresh dose is given before the reaction due to the preceding one has subsided: before each dose toxic phenomena such as stomatitis, skin rashes, albuminuria and symptoms of agranulocytosis should be looked for; if such effects are produced the course must be stopped immediately. In those who are intolerant to these larger weekly doses, subsequent courses may be cautiously administered giving calcium aurothiomalate B.P. as this is less toxic, and the weekly dose should not exceed 50 mg.—often a weekly dose of 5 to 10 mg. may be best tolerated up to a total dose of 1·0 G. (*g*) *Phenylbutazone* B.P. (Butazolidin) is a valuable analgesic which undoubtedly suppresses active disease in the joints in daily doses of 200–400 mg., but toxic effects may arise even with these doses. (*h*) The *corticosteroids* and inject. corticotrophin (ACTH) have been in frequent use since Hench and his colleagues at the Mayo Clinic first described their use in 1949. There is no evidence of suprarenal inadequacy in rheumatoid disease and these drugs act solely by suppressing the inflammatory reaction in the joints and elsewhere. After a few days the pain, swelling and even the stiffness of the joints is markedly reduced and in some may disappear completely; at the same time the pyrexia and sweating may cease, the erythrocyte sedimentation rate falls and the appetite and the anæmia improve so that euphoria takes the place of depression. Prednisone and prednisolone acetates by mouth are four times more powerful than the corresponding doses of cortisone acetate and the doses used must be the smallest which will afford adequate relief of symptoms. Larger doses are always necessary in the more severe cases but divided doses of prednisolone above 15 mg. a day will almost certainly produce unpleasant and even intolerable side-effects. Their use cannot be a substitute for the measures already described. Once a patient has embarked on a course of treatment with steroids, it cannot suddenly be stopped because of the serious results of sudden withdrawal. In many cases the steroids will have to be withdrawn gradually because of the side-effects, the occurrence of complications of the therapy or the failure of treatment to justify their continued use. Some have found a combination of gold injections with corticosteroid therapy more helpful than either given separately. Medical Research Council trials with an average dose of cortisone acetate 75 mg. a day to one series of patients, and aspirin, 4·5 G. a day to a comparable series, have revealed little difference in the relief of their symptoms or in the X-ray films of their hands and feet, E.S.R. and hæmoglobin levels at the end of one, two or three years; although aspirin compounds are so much cheaper a considerable number of patients (estimated at 25 per cent.) are unable to tolerate these large doses of aspirin.   Aspiration of a joint and then injection of intra-articular hydrocortisone or prednisolone have given good results, but if a joint is treated in this way on more than one or two occasions, X-ray examination reveals considerable increase in the rate of joint damage.   (*i*) *Chloroquine phosphate* B.P. 250 mg. b.d. or the rather less toxic hydroxychloroquine sulphate 400 mg. b.d. produce no benefit for the first 3 weeks, but prolonged administration produces a suppression of symptoms in rather more than half the cases treated, with a complete remission in a quarter.   Toxic effects include nausea, headache, pruritus and blurring of vision due to corneal changes.   (*j*) The *anæmia* of rheumatoid disease does not respond to oral iron therapy; blood transfusions give temporary benefit but the cells tend to be rapidly destroyed.   Injected iron preparations give the best response.   (*k*) *Physiotherapy* with local heat or wax baths and active and passive movements help to relieve pain, lessen muscle wasting and prevent contractures.   After the active stage has passed, mobilisation of the joints by gradual exercises and movement in slings, correction of contractures and deformities by manipulation under anæsthesia, followed by vigorous exercises and methods of general rehabilitation help to restore good health.

Rheumatoid Disease and Psoriasis (Syn. Psoriatic Arthritis) is well known. Changes in the skin and nails often precede the arthritis by many years, but the two may occur together.   The joint changes closely resemble those of the usual forms of rheumatoid disease, but the metatarso-phalangeal joints are often severely involved and the ends of the small bones largely destroyed.   The Rose-Waaler test gives consistently negative results.   *Treatment* is as for rheumatoid disease; although the joints respond well to corticosteroids the skin does not improve.

Felty's Syndrome is a rare condition of adults (usually women of 40–50 years of age) in which the joint symptoms of rheumatoid disease are combined with pyrexia, splenomegaly, anæmia, leucopenia and sometimes generalised lymph gland enlargement.   *Treatment* with steroid therapy suppresses the joint disease and splenectomy often helps the anæmia.

In *Children* a juvenile form of rheumatoid disease resembles the lesions of adults. The multiple arthritis described by Dr. G. F. Still (Still's disease), associated with pallor, fever, wasting and enlargement of the lymphatic glands and spleen, differs from the description given above only in the frequency of affection of the glands and the splenic enlargement; a rash with small macular lesions is present on the limbs and trunk in 25 per cent. of cases, and eye lesions are much more common than in adults. *Treatment* is as for the disease of adults and prednisolone given over a long period is of great symptomatic value.

A young or middle-aged MAN *has* PAINFUL SWELLING *of one or more of* the LARGER JOINTS *and sometimes of an* UNUSUAL SMALL JOINT; *there may be a history of previous urethral discharge and the* GONOCOCCAL COMPLEMENT-FIXATION TEST *is* STRONGLY POSITIVE.   *The condition is probably* CHRONIC GONOCOCCAL ARTHRITIS.

§ **598. III. Chronic Gonococcal Arthritis.**—Since the advent of effective treatment for acute gonorrhœa, this has become much less common.   It may follow months or years after acquiring the infection, and is due to a chronic focus in the prostatic urethra or prostate of the male, or in the cervix uteri of the female. It resembles other cases of infective arthritis but the cause may be overlooked if it is not borne in mind.

Symptoms are more likely in men than women. There is often no history of a previous uro-genital discharge. The disease may be mon-articular or polyarticular but in the latter there is not the same tendency to a bilateral symmetry of the joints affected as in rheumatoid disease. The more common joints to give symptoms are one or both knees, ankles, wrists, elbows or shoulders, but the sacro-iliac, mandibular and sterno-clavicular joints may be diseased. The affected joints are painful, hot, swollen and tender due to synovitis, but in severe cases the articular cartilage, periosteum and ligaments may be destroyed leading to X-ray changes with narrowing of the joint space, decalcification of the ends of the bones and ultimately to osteo-arthritis: in the spine ankylosis may ensue. The temperature is raised, sometimes to 102° F. Other symptoms which particularly suggest a gonococcal origin are (i.) involvement of tendon sheaths, particularly those of the flexor tendons above the wrists, or (ii.) of fibrous tissues especially the plantar fascia. (iii.) The tendo achillis is sometimes painful, (iv.) periostitis of the os calcis may be found and (v.) irido-cyclitis may occur at the same time as the joints are diseased.

Diagnosis is especially helped by a strongly positive complement-fixation reaction of the blood serum or of the synovial fluid. It is often difficult to demonstrate the intra-cellular gram-negative organisms in pus cells from the primary site.

Treatment is as for the acute variety. In some cases the effect of even a single dose of penicillin is dramatic, a bed-ridden patient with polyarthritis being apparently cured in 3 or 4 days. It is however not unusual to encounter penicillin-resistant organisms which need prolonged treatment with chemotherapy, and the other measures described in § 594. Diathermy to the prostate and cervix is helpful in removing secondary infection.

There is ACUTE PAIN *and* SWELLING *in one or more of the* LARGER JOINTS, *and* *rheumatoid disease, gonococcal arthritis and gout have been excluded·* *Search reveals a* FOCUS OF INFECTION—*the disease is likely to be* CHRONIC INFECTIVE ARTHRITIS.

§ 599. IV. Chronic Infective Arthritis is distinct from suppurative arthritis (§ 594) in that it is rare to be able to culture organisms from the joint and the condition is usually subacute or chronic. Apart from chronic gonococcal arthritis (§ 598) a variety of other organisms are causal.

Symptoms.—The arthritis is usually an affection of the larger joints and occurs equally in men and women who are often at or past middle age. It may present as one or more acute attacks or come on insidiously from the beginning. Usually one joint is first affected and others are involved later. In the acute phases there is an acute or subacute synovitis, the joint becoming more or less swollen, tender and painful on movement; there is often a mild degree of pyrexia and sometimes other evidence of toxæmia such as anæmia. In advanced cases osteo-arthritic changes supervene. A focus of infection also accentuates rheumatoid disease and may precipitate an attack of gout.

The *diagnosis* from *chronic gout* may be difficult, but there are no tophi, the blood uric acid is not raised and there are no constitutional evidences of gout. *Osteo-arthritis* is more chronic and shows lipping and other characteristic bony changes. In *rheumatoid arthritis* there is a greater tendency for multiple involvement of the smaller joints and the changes are also periarticular. In infective arthritis X-ray examination shows a general absorption of calcium salts in the ends of the bones adjoining the affected joints.

Etiology.—Apart from gonococcal cases and Reiter's disease, the cause may reside in a hidden focus of infection, often due to a streptococcus, on the apex of one or more teeth, in the tonsils or nasal sinuses and sometimes in the appendix or the female pelvic organs. Other causes are chronic ulcerative colitis (with which a staphylococcus may be associated), acute bacillary dysentery, brucellosis, tuberculosis and syphilis.

Treatment must primarily be directed to the identification and elimination of the cause, with antibiotic therapy where indicated.

§ **600. V. Chronic Gout** usually supervenes upon a succession of acute attacks (§ 593); rarely it is subacute or chronic from the beginning. Several joints which have previously been involved in the acute attacks are involved; they are stiff, painful on movement and may be the subject of renewed acute attacks. Sometimes sodium biurate ("chalk stones") can be seen under the skin and may discharge through it, leaving chronic scars or sinuses which usually heal rapidly. Secondary osteo-arthritis commonly ensues. The patient, usually a man over middle age, suffers from frequent acute or subacute exacerbations of joint trouble, with early generalised arteriosclerosis (especially of the coronary and cerebral vessels), hypertension, sometimes dyspepsia and phlebitis, and a lowered resistance to catarrhal and other infections. Gouty tophi are often present; they consist of aggregations of sodium biurate analogous to the deposits in and around the joints, and are commonly situated in the cartilages of the ears near the helix and in bursal sacs. The urine contains albumen from time to time which becomes more persistent as chronic renal disease develops.

The *Diagnosis* from other forms of chronic arthritis is not always easy. In general terms chronic gout occurs in those who have a family history of the disease, it occurs much more commonly in men, is associated with a history of paroxysms of acute gout and with a blood uric acid above 4 mg. per cent. (see also table, § 597). Gouty tophi in the cartilages of the ears and the presence of healed sinuses over the joints are diagnostic. X-ray films, especially of the fingers and toes, show a general rarefaction of the bones near the joints with small translucent areas where

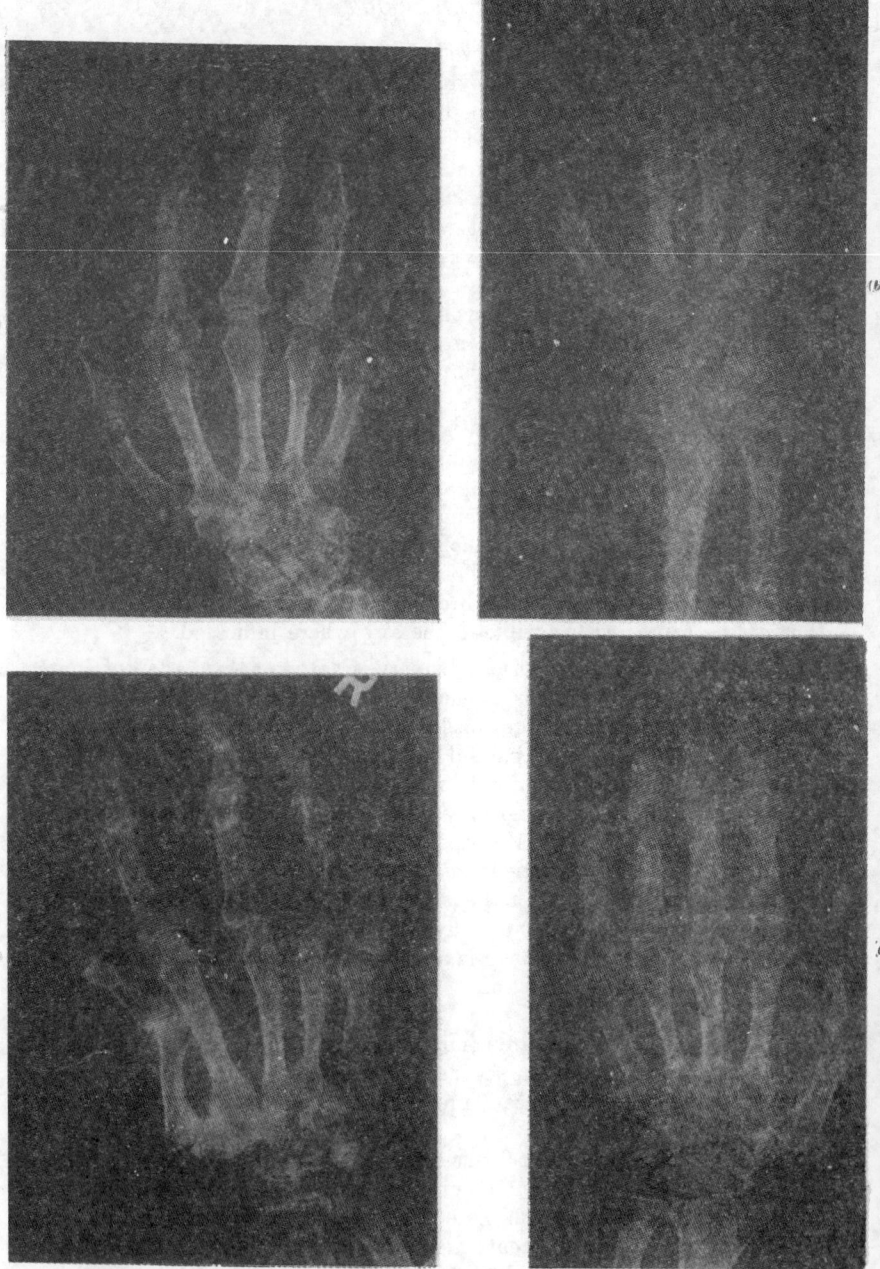

FIG. 175(a).—ADVANCED GOUT, with large areas of decalcification at the ends of the metacarpals and phalanges. Note the soft tissue swelling of the fingers. (b) GONORRHŒAL ARTHRITIS of wrist and carpal joints. Decalcification and loss of definition of the joint surfaces are well seen. Note the new periosteal bone on the shaft of the radius. (c) OSTEO-ARTHRITIS, especially between the interphalangeal joints, and at the base of the first metacarpal. (d) Typical RHEUMATOID (atrophic) ARTHRITIS showing decalcification of the bones; the outlines of the joints are as yet unaffected.

the bone is replaced by urate crystals.   Later osteo-arthritic changes are added (Fig. 175a).

The *Prognosis* in patients first seen in an advanced stage, who do not persevere with treatment for the rest of their lives or who are resistant to treatment (§ 593), is serious.   It mainly depends on three factors: (i.) the condition of the kidneys and the presence of signs of renal failure; (ii.) the degree of hypertension and (iii.) the presence of angina pectoris, coronary ischæmia or myocardial failure.   The patient may die with uræmia, pericarditis, pleurisy or cerebral hæmorrhage.

Treatment is described under Acute Gout.   The efficacy of modern methods in a large proportion of cases is seen not only by the prevention of acute attacks and of the complications which otherwise arise but also by the gradual absorption of gouty deposits in the skin, the bones and the cartilages of the ears.

A YOUNG MAN *complains that for weeks or months he has had* PAIN AND STIFFNESS *in the* LOWER BACK *or possibly in the* NECK; *the* SPINE *shows* MARKED LOSS OF MOBILITY *and there are* SYMPTOMS OF GENERAL ILL-HEALTH *—the condition may prove to be* ANKYLOSING SPONDYLITIS.

§ 601. VI. Ankylosing Spondylitis (Syn. Spondylitis Deformans) was formerly classified under rheumatoid arthritis, but is now recognised as a separate entity. It affects the invertebral and costo-vertebral joints and especially the sacro-iliac joints; it may also involve the shoulder- and hip-joints and sometimes other large joints of the arms or legs, but rarely the joints of the fingers and toes.   It is relatively common, produces considerable disablement but rarely leads to chronic invalidism.

Symptoms.—The age of onset is usually in the twenties, and men are affected ten times more often than women.   (1) Initially there is a complaint of transient pains or stiffness in the back or limbs for some weeks or months; at this stage there may be a swollen joint such as a knee or ankle.   (2) In the second stage there is great pain and stiffness in the back; the usual type is in the lumbo-sacral spine, and with this there may be pain in the buttocks or in the distribution of the sciatic nerves. A less common variety is where the symptoms are chiefly related to the cervical spine. Sooner or later all the spinal joints are involved and pain may radiate along the intercostal nerves to the chest or abdomen, simulating pleurisy or an abdominal complaint.   With this, constitutional symptoms are marked, the patient looks pale and ill and often has a low-grade evening pyrexia; there is appreciable loss of weight and of appetite and moderate anæmia.   Examination of the spine shows great lack of mobility, pain on movement, spasm of the para-vertebral muscles and often local tenderness over the spinous processes.   One or more of the larger peripheral joints is often swollen and painful.   (3) After a period of years the spine becomes more and more fixed in an attitude of flexion to which the name " poker back " is aptly applied; he is compelled to stand and to walk with his face pointing to his feet; with this fixed kyphosis the breathing becomes mainly or entirely abdominal due to fixation of the costo-vertebral joints.   A similar change in the hips or shoulders will produce partial or complete fixation of these joints also.   The X-ray changes are best seen in the sacro-iliac joints at an early stage—there is initially osteoporosis and later reossification with obliteration of the joint spaces: similar changes take place in the vertebral joints with calcification of the edges of the intervertebral discs and of the spinal ligaments.   The erythrocyte sedimentation rate is very high from the commencement of the disease.

Diagnosis in the earlier stages is from " fibrositis," recurrent lumbago, lower back strain and from intervertebral disc lesions.   The X-ray changes in the sacro-iliac joints and the high E.S.R. are characteristic. *Sacro-iliac osteosclerosis* is solely confined to women (see below and § 461).

Etiology.—The condition is no longer regarded as venereal; a certain number of cases occur in Reiter's disease, and iritis and non-specific urethritis are fairly common. The initial changes in the joints are in the synovial membranes, with a later spread to the capsules of the joints which become fibrosed and later calcified. There is a family tendency to rheumatoid disease in a number of cases; but ankylosing spondylitis is a separate entity because it is very frequent in young *men*, the small joints of the hands and feet are rarely affected, there are no subcutaneous nodules or enlarged lymph glands, the histological appearances are different and the Rose-Waaler sheep-cell test is seldom positive unless there is also peripheral rheumatoid arthritis, in which event 100 per cent. of positive results are obtained.

Prognosis.—The condition is disabling and liable to exacerbations and relapses over a period of years; finally the active disease dies out. Throughout, patients are able to undertake light occupations. When the costo-vertebral joints are fused and chest breathing becomes impossible there is a considerable tendency to bronchitis and broncho-pneumonia.

Treatment.—Repeated doses of aspirin are of great help. Oral prednisolone and injections of corticotrophin (gel) produce great symptomatic relief and can be continued for a period of years in the smallest doses required to control symptoms. Phenylbutazone B.P. may be used as for rheumatoid disease. Local deep X-ray therapy gives relief for several years and is still used in spite of the slight danger of producing leukæmia.

Sacro-iliac Osteosclerosis (Syn. Osteitis Condensans Ilii) only occurs in young women, frequently after pregnancy. The principal *symptom* is a low backache which may come and go. Other joints of the vertebral column are not involved and X-ray examination shows at an early stage dense sclerosis in the iliac border of the sacro-iliac joints with a normal joint space. *Treatment* is by local heat, avoiding faulty postures and lifting heavy objects while the lumbo-sacral spine is flexed.

§ 602. VII. Systemic Lupus Erythematosus (Syn. Disseminated Lupus Erythematosus) in recent years has come to be recognised as a relatively common disease, especially in women of middle and later age. Although it may follow discoid and other local skin lesions (§ 631) it much more commonly starts as a generalised disease. The manifestations in the different organs are numerous.

Symptoms vary in different cases.—(1) Pain in the joints is the first to be complained of in 90 per cent. of patients. There may be a general aching of the joints and muscles (resembling fibrositis), a migratory form of polyarthritis or a chronic form hardly distinguishable from rheumatoid disease. (2) A severe constitutional disturbance follows, with a high evening temperature, profuse sweating, loss of appetite and loss of weight. (3) Anæmia is usually noticed and this is accompanied by a polymorph leucopenia; sometimes a severe hæmolytic anæmia arises. (4) Skin changes are of several different types and tend to occur late; purpura, petechiæ, ulcers in the mouth and less commonly rashes which resemble lichen planus or psoriasis. Alopecia areata may be found. (5) Enlarged and sometimes tender superficial lymph glands are sometimes associated with enlargement of the liver and spleen. (6) Pleurisy often occurs but large effusions are rare; pulmonary infiltration and consolidation may give rise to severe dyspnœa. (7) The heart and blood-vessels may show a variety of changes; myocardial damage gives rise to enlargement and failure, and pericarditis or endocarditis can be found. Vascular occlusion of the vessels of the fingers gives rise to the Raynaud phenomena and on occasion local gangrene occurs. (8) Renal involvement causes albuminuria, microscopic hæmaturia and renal casts; œdema and later uræmia are always of serious significance. (9) Epileptiform convulsions, hemiplegia and psychoneurosis are mainly the result of vascular damage to the brain. (10) Abdominal pain, nausea and vomiting may be met.

Diagnosis is often extremely difficult in the earlier stages. Joint symptoms with high fever, a sterile blood culture, leucopenia and an erythrocyte sedimentation rate above 100 mm. in the first hour (Westergren) are highly suggestive. (This high E.S.R. is associated with a considerable amount of an abnormal gamma-globulin in the plasma.) The presence of lupus erythematosus cells in the blood (in 80 to 90 per cent. of cases) is very helpful and newer methods are giving an even higher percentage of positive results—but positive findings are encountered in other diseases (§ 1212). Histological examination, as of a lymph-node, may reveal a small artery showing fibrinoid necrosis of the arterial wall and a narrowed lumen—highly suggestive features of the disease. A false-positive Wassermann reaction is misleading.

Etiology.—This is not known for certain. The present view is that auto-antibodies are formed to an antigen which is frequently the patient's own connective tissue (comparable to Hashimoto's thyroiditis, § 187), but on occasions it may be the result of drug administration. Sulphonamides are not so commonly suspected as formerly; hydralazine (Apresoline) can probably give rise to this disease.

Prognosis.—The natural course is subject to spontaneous remissions. Death may occur in a matter of weeks or the patient may survive a number of years; some live 10 years or more. The prognosis is much worse in the presence of renal disease and is usually fatal from uræmia or from an intercurrent infection.

Treatment.—In the absence of symptoms no treatment is called for; but bed-rest is necessary in the acute phases. The use of inject. corticotrophin B.P. (ACTH) and of the corticosteroids in full doses by mouth almost invariably produce a remission, but these drugs need to be given for long periods and to be resumed when a relapse occurs. More recently chloroquine phosphate, hydroxychloroquine sulphate and mepacrine hydrochlor. (300 mg. or more a day) have given good results and a combination of these drugs with the steroids has been advocated.

VIII. POLYARTERITIS NODOSA has a close clinical resemblance to systemic lupus erythematosus and may give rise to subacute polyarthritis (§ 98).

Sjogren's Syndrome is a rare cause of a rheumatoid type of polyarthritis mainly in middle-aged women, accompanied by a dry mouth, dysphagia, conjunctivitis with keratitis, and rhinitis sicca. The *cause* is unknown and *treatment* is disappointing.

§ 603. Tuberculosis, Syphilis, Hysteria, Tabes Dorsalis and nervous disorders also affect the joints.

IX. **Tuberculous Joint Disease.**—Tuberculosis affects chiefly the synovial membrane, but it may commence in the articular ends of the bones. This is *par excellence* the monoarticular joint disease of children.

Symptoms.—The onset is insidious, though not infrequently the symptoms date from an injury. Generally the disease is in the knee, though sometimes it is in the hip, although the pain may still be referred to the knee through the obturator nerve; any joint may be affected. The child may complain of slight pain which gives rise to limping, weeks or months before anything else is apparent. The affected joint swells; it is pale, and has a pulpy or doughy feel beneath the finger, and fluctuation may be felt. If untreated, an abscess develops. The constitutional symptoms consist of an intermitting pyrexia and general debility which are present from the very beginning.

The *Cause* is usually infection with bovine tuberculosis. In a chronic synovitis in adults tubercle bacilli can often be identified in aspirated joint fluid. The disease is now much rarer in children in Great Britain since milk has been pasteurised; in advanced life a more destructive form may occur. If neglected, extensive destruction of the joint follows, and frequently tuberculous disease in other organs.

Treatment is by the prolonged administration of specific antituberculous drugs (§ 131) combined with complete rest of the affected joint in a plaster jacket. A good diet, sunlight and fresh air are essential.

X. **Syphilitic Joint Disease.**—In the secondary stage of syphilis there may be (i.) a subacute arthritis with redness and pain, or (ii.) an indolent hydrarthrosis with little pain. In the tertiary stage the differential features are: (1) One or several joints may be affected. The synovial membrane may be attacked, leading to a doughy swelling; or the ligaments or cartilage. (2) The joint manifests no signs of acute inflammation, but there is occasionally some effusion. (3) The pain is moderate during the day, but subject to nocturnal exacerbations. (4) Other evidences of syphilis are generally present. (5) The condition responds to large doses of penicillin. It may occur in children (§ 500).

A PSEUDO-PARALYSIS OF SYPHILITIC ORIGIN occurs in infants due to epiphysitis and later a separation of the cartilage from the diaphysis may occur, and be mistaken for joint disease or for infantile paralysis. The affected part is acutely tender. The condition may be readily recognised by X-ray examination—indeed similar changes may be seen in the epiphyses with periostitis even in the absence of symptoms.

XI. **Hysterical Joint Disorder** is often a muscular stiffening and immobility. It usually affects the hip or the knee, and often dates from some trifling injury. The joint is fixed, tender (often more tender to light touches than to deep pressure), sometimes swollen, and the local temperature may be raised. Sometimes there are no physical signs referable to the joint at all. The loss of function may be entirely due to muscular rigidity and in the case of the hip-joint the condition may very precisely mimic tuberculous disease of this joint. This *Diagnosis*, which is often difficult, rests mainly on (1) the absence of evidence of serious disease in the affected joint when examined under anæsthesia; (2) the disproportionate loss of function; (3) absence of X-ray changes. For *Treatment* see § 1173.

XII. **Neuropathic Arthritis** (Syn. Neuro-Arthropathy, Tabetic Arthropathy).— Two diseases of the spinal cord are sometimes, though comparatively rarely, attended with chronic disease in the joints—viz., *Tabes Dorsalis* and *Syringomyelia*. In both arthritis may occur in an early stage of the disease, when nervous symptoms are few, and extensive disintegration of the joint may take place, without pain, heat, or redness, and without giving rise to much inconvenience. X-rays shows gross destruction of the bone, and even dislocation. In *tabes dorsalis* the associated joint lesion is known as tabetic arthropathy, or **Charcot's joint disease** (see § 1022), which especially occurs in the lower limbs. Occupation chiefly determines which joints are involved; thus in a blacksmith the arms, and in a soldier the legs are affected (Fig. 254). This lesion may occur without the patient suffering any pain; it may go on to extensive disorganisation with increased mobility and new bony formations before the patient seeks advice. In all such cases the pupils and ankle- and knee-jerks should be examined.

Syringomyelia is characterised by muscular atrophy and dissociated anæsthesia. The arthritis is limited almost entirely to the upper limbs (§ 1005).

In *Raynaud's Disease* (§ 589) subacute or chronic synovitis sometimes occurs, associated with an atrophic condition of the bones.

In *Diabetes Mellitus* with polyneuritis and a spread of infection from the soft tissues (*e.g.*, a perforating ulcer), a condition resembling Charcot's joints occurs especially in the areas of the tarsal and metatarsal bones, and sometimes in the ankle- and knee-joints.

GROUP III. *NON-ARTICULAR RHEUMATISM AND PRIMARY DISEASES OF MUSCLES*

Here we are concerned with lesions in the skeletal tissues other than the joints. They do not give rise to pain and swelling of a joint but to pain outside a joint especially in muscles, tendons, ligaments, synovia, bursæ, aponeuroses and other mesodermal tissues. The causes of pain in the limbs were discussed in § 578, and those of primary neurological origin will be dealt with in Chapter XIX.

I. Non-articular rheumatism, § 604.
II. Psychosomatic rheumatism, § 605.
III. Tumours, § 605.
IV. Trichinosis, § 606.
V. Idiopathic myositis, § 606.

§ 604. I. Non-articular Rheumatism is still often known as fibrositis, but with increasing knowledge we now realise that many different conditions can be differentiated, for inflammation of the fibrous tissue *per se* is relatively rare. However, the cause of pain in the limbs and trunk is often obscure and the term *fibrositis* is a convenient label for these. Diseases in this category are extremely common in Great Britain, can be very incapacitating and prone to recur. Symptoms may occur in those who are in perfect health, but certain constitutional conditions have often been present for weeks or months beforehand, especially in women with chronic fatigue, insomnia, constipation and at menopause.

The GENERAL SYMPTOMS are: (1) Pain may be a persistent dull ache or can come on so suddenly that the patient is unable to straighten up after bending. (2) Stiffness is often present. Pain and stiffness are usually relieved by rest but are much more marked when movements are recommenced, *e.g.*, on first getting out of bed. (3) The pain may be fairly widely distributed and removed from the site of the lesion. Acute tenderness is often present on deep pressure at the point of origin of the pain. (4) Tender nodules are sometimes present. These can be due to local areas of muscle spasm (F. Elliott) or to protrusion of fatty lobules which become œdematous as they herniate through a thin fascial covering in the paravertebral muscles (Copeman). (5) Occasionally attacks occur in epidemic form associated with slight pyrexia. One variety of this is Bornholm disease (§ 509).

LOCAL SYMPTOMS referable to various areas of the body are:—

(A) **Lumbo-sacral back pain** is much the commonest. Often described as **lumbago,** the pain may be present in the lumbo-sacral area of the back, on one or both sides of the sacrum, in the iliac crest or down the outer side of the thigh. Intra-abdominal and pelvic conditions which cause backache must be excluded—such as chronic peptic ulcer, renal and pancreatic disease, salpingitis and malignant conditions in the pelvis (§ 461).

(1) *The pain is dull or nagging* and liable to *acute exacerbations* after sitting in a flexed position in a chair, or when straightening the back with the knees straight especially when lifting a heavy object. This occurs in healthy men and women, or in tired overworked housewives who are gaining weight too quickly and whose spine assumes a faulty posture—only in severe or neurasthenic cases does the patient take to bed.

The *Diagnosis* is from an *intervertebral disc* lesion which causes sudden crippling pain often spreading into one or both sciatic nerves. *Osteo-*

arthritis of the lumbar spine, which also may produce sciatic pain, can be, demonstrated by X-ray.

Etiology.—Two varieties are distinguishable. (i.) Especially in young women there may be a sudden *sprain* due to tearing some of the fibres of the interspinous, lumbo-sacral or sacro-iliac ligaments—the so-called " sprung back." This occurs after a sudden fall, blow or severe sprain when lifting a heavy object. There is very marked local tenderness to deep pressure at the site of the lesion when the spine is flexed (trigger areas) with reproduction of the pain complained of; and there is temporary relief immediately after injecting procaine hydrochlor. (2·0 per cent.) at the most tender point—this is usually in the ligament between lumbar 4–5 or lumbar 5–sacral 1 spines. (ii.) Usually at an older age there is a *postural strain* of the back when the intervertebral ligaments are submitted to extra tension especially with gain in weight at menopause or when they have been recently softened by childbirth. Men complain of this after unaccustomed work or exercise. Such a person assumes a faulty posture in the lumbo-sacral region; and the condition may be aggravated by anxiety and by focal sepsis.

Treatment is by correcting obesity, bad postures and other aggravating factors. The patient must avoid lifting and carrying heavy weights and must be shown how to rise from a stooping position with the knees flexed. Analgesic drugs and local heat help to relieve pain and repeated injections of procaine hydrochlor. into painful areas often aid. In obstinate cases a supporting corset must be worn for a time.

(2) *The pain is sudden and severe usually in the lower lumbar and sacral region* and may come on during a particular movement such as with a twisting strain or lifting a heavy weight. Commonly there is a previous history of a dull backache, due in many cases to intervertebral disc degeneration. In the acute attack it may be impossible to straighten the flexed spine; the erector spinæ muscles go into spasm and the pain may radiate into one or both sciatic nerves, especially on sneezing or coughing, producing the motor and sensory signs of sciatic neuritis. The cause is protrusion of the nucleus pulposus of an intervertebral disc into the spinal canal, usually between lumbar 5–sacral 1 vertebræ but often between L 4–L 5 and sometimes higher up. This condition is liable to recur (§ 1020).

(3) *Sudden severe pain not necessarily localised to the lower lumbar and sacral region* also accompanies collapse of a vertebral body as in carcinomatosis, myelomatosis, tuberculous caries and osteoporosis.

(4) *A more chronic pain* also occurs in osteo-arthritis, ankylosing spondylitis and spondylolisthesis (§ 461).

After a careful history, physical and X-ray examinations have excluded the above conditions:—

(5) *Sudden severe pain* or *more usually a persistent intolerable ache* in the mid-lumbar or lumbo-sacral areas appears to be due to primary disease of the fascial covering of the lumbar muscles. This is to be regarded as true **lumbago** and here again the pain may extend into a sciatic nerve.

In the more severe attacks the patient has to take to his bed for there
is marked spasm of the lumbar muscles. These are the cases in which
tender nodules can be palpated (*vide supra*) and injection of these followed
by radiant heat and deep massage affords great relief. Otherwise relief
from pain is secured with analgesic drugs—aspirin, tab. codein co. or full
doses of sodium salicylate. Locally counter-irritants and cataplasma
kaolini should be used. Sometimes an attack may be aborted by a
Turkish bath. For more *chronic cases*, radiant heat, infra-red rays and
diathermy allay pain. In cases of recurring lumbago, *B. acidophilus*
taken over a long period has proved useful (and see § 461).

(B) **Cervical and upper dorsal pain** and stiffness is usually due to cervical osteo-arthritis (spondylosis) as described in §§ 596, 1004. It is probable that some painful conditions of the upper neck and suboccipital
muscles are due to fibrositis and muscle tension comparable to those of
lumbago. The pain can be referred to the occipital and even to the vertical
areas of the skull. *Panniculitis* occurs in middle-aged and elderly subjects,
especially overweight women who complain of pain across the back of
the lower neck and between the shoulders where there is a diffuse thickening of the subcutaneous tissues. Tender areas are easily made out on
pressure and the skin dimples on being picked up. Similar tenderness is
made out in the adipose tissue of the inner sides of the knees and along the
outer sides of the thighs, with signs of mild hypothyroidism (and see § 824).

(C) **Persistent pain around the shoulder girdle** on one or both sides can
be due to a number of causes. (1) The commonest is cervical spondylosis
(§ 1004) or an intervertebral disc lesion of the mid cervical spine (§ 1018).
Other causes include tuberculosis of the vertebræ, acute and chronic
osteomyelitis or caries of the clavicle, scapula or head of the humerus and
referred pain from apical pleurisy, carcinoma of an apical bronchus and
myocardial ischæmia. (2) *Pain in the shoulder girdle which also radiates
into the arm, forearm and hand* is usually due to an intervertebral disc lesion
in cervical 5-6-7 areas or to compression of the lower cervical nerves by
a cervical rib as in the rib pressure syndrome (and see §§ 999, 1018), as
well as to the chest diseases just enumerated. (3) *Pain at the shoulder tip
extends down to the deltoid insertion*; the most likely cause is inflammation
of the subacromial bursa and of the underlying supraspinatus tendon close
to its insertion into the greater tuberosity of the humerus. This is present
in middle age and produces pain when the arm is actively raised to a right
angle at the shoulder and when it is lowered. Passive movement of the
arm through the same range and actively moving the arm above a right
angle are painless. The condition may follow an injury such as a fall on
to the elbow or hand and is very persistent for a period of months but
there is no muscle wasting. Calcification in the tendon is sometimes seen
by X-ray. (4) A *frozen shoulder* is due to the same inflammation spreading to the entire capsule of the joint (pericapsulitis) and to the long head
of biceps and its accompanying tendon sheath in the bicipital groove.
Severe pain in the shoulder area spreading down to the deltoid insertion

is accompanied by gradual fixation, so the joint is immobile in all directions. Pain is worse at night, seriously interferes with sleep and with dressing and feeding. *Treatment* of frozen shoulder is by resting the arm in a sling combined with short-wave diathermy and prolonged administration of small doses of prednisolone by mouth. A local injection of a steroid may be helpful and analgesics must be used freely. The condition always clears up in 12 to 18 months and this period may be shortened by operative measures.

(D) " **Tennis elbow.**" *Pain on the outer side of the elbow* is accompanied by *marked local tenderness* in the tendons of origin of the extensor muscles. The pain spreads into the forearm when the muscles actively contract against resistance. This form of tendinitis heals slowly and is aided by a local injection of procaine hydrochlor. with hydrocortisone. "*Golfer's elbow*" is a similar condition in the tendons of origin of the flexor muscles from the internal condyle.

(E) **A painful heel** may be the result of achillis tendinitis which is often associated with a subachillis bursitis. Young adults who stand for long periods develop this as a result of the pressure of the heel of a tight shoe. Pain may also be present under the heel after a long period in bed; this is helped by avoiding soft slippers and wearing shoes with firm soles.

(F) **Plantar fasciitis** is a most troublesome condition in middle-aged men of heavy build. There is pain and tenderness over a localised area in front of the medial tuberosity of the calcaneus. The pain disappears as soon as the patient sits or lies down but recurs immediately he stands or walks. It is a self-limiting disease which persists for months; it may be helped by rubber heels and sorbo-rubber pads in the heels of the shoes.

§ 605. II. Psychosomatic Rheumatism (Syn. Tension pain) is a musculo-skeletal expression of a psychoneurotic or " functional " disorder: it is a common condition especially in women.

Symptoms.—The patient often describes a burning or aching sensation or a pain, the distribution of which does not conform to that of a known organic lesion; it is frequently distributed widely over the body and may be bilaterally symmetrical. As with other types of functional disorder the pain is constant day and night for weeks or months with no inter-mission, and is worse when the patient is tired or anxious. Other symptoms of emotional tension are present with insomnia, excessive fatigue, irritability and depression. Loss of weight is usual and mild anæmia may be found. Physical examination reveals no organic disease which can explain the symptoms complained of, or the mild degree of arthritis is such as would normally be symptomless.

Diagnosis.—Organic disease must be excluded by a complete physical examination, X-ray of the area complained of and by a full blood count and erythrocyte sedimentation rate. Conditions which are especially liable to be overlooked are ankylosing spondylitis, myelomatosis, unsuspected carcinomatosis and primary bone tumours.

Treatment.—It is most unwise to tell the patient that she has mild arthritis as this will be regarded as incurable. Reassurance, adequate rest and sleep and correction of anæmia are of service. For the treatment of psychoneurosis see § 1172.

III. **Tumours** in the substance of the muscles may give rise to pain and tenderness usually associated with swelling. The pain and tenderness are at first strictly localised to the seat of the disease, and there is a thickening or tumour discoverable on careful palpation. In some cases—*e.g.*, syphilitic and malignant growths—the lymphatic glands in the neighbourhood are enlarged. The chief tumours affecting muscles are (*a*) innocent—syphilitic gumma; abscess, which may arise from a gumma, or be of inflammatory origin, especially after typhoid and influenza; innocent neoplasms such as fibroma, lipoma, angioma, hydatid cysts and hæmatoma. (*b*) Malignant growths, sarcoma, and carcinoma (by extension). First determine whether the swelling is inflammatory or non-inflammatory, malignant (and rapidly growing) or non-malignant, by an investigation of the swelling, the glands, the history and the concurrent symptoms. The diagnosis and treatment is mainly surgical.

§ 606. IV. Trichinosis (Syn. Trichiniasis) is in Great Britain a comparatively rare disease; but several localised outbreaks have been recorded in recent years. It is due to a nematode worm (*Trichinella spiralis*) which is conveyed to man by " measly " pork or pork sausages, insufficiently cooked. Bear, seal and walrus meat may also convey the infection. The capsules of the worm are digested in the human stomach and the embryos set free; they multiply and breed in the intestinal canal in the ensuing week, each female producing several hundred embryos which develop rapidly. After mating, the female worm penetrates the walls of the intestine and deposits small larvæ which reach the blood-stream; they are small enough to pass through the capillaries of the lung to reach the muscles where, after 2–3 weeks, they become encysted. They have been found alive and capable of developing 10 years after their entrance.

Symptoms are now much milder than in years gone by; only in severe cases are there the three typical stages. The *first* stage is now rarely seen. In it there is sometimes diarrhœa, but abdominal pain, vomiting and urticaria are rare. The *second* stage starts about 2 weeks after infestation, and lasts 2–3 weeks; this coincides with the migration of the embryos. The most constant feature is œdema of the eyelids which is almost invariable; there is usually headache with pain behind the eyelids, photophobia, and stiffness and aching in the limbs. On occasions there are hæmoptyses and pneumonia, hæmorrhages under the finger-nails, mental symptoms with lethargy and confusion, melancholia, meningitic or encephalitic symptoms; monoplegia, cerebellar signs, oculogyric crises and extensor plantar responses are met. The wandering of the embryos in the muscles produces shortening and rigidity especially of the biceps, and in severe cases chewing, swallowing, or moving the eyeballs aggravate the pain. Pyrexia may be present to 102–103° F with sweating, and later there may be loss of weight. In the *third* stage as the larvæ settle in the muscles 4–6 weeks after infestation the patient gradually recovers, the temperature subsides and the larvæ become encysted, but the aching of the muscles may continue for several months. The severity of the muscle pain varies in proportion to the number of larvæ present.

Diagnosis.—In slight cases the distinction from muscular rheumatism may be difficult, though the puffiness of the eyelids, the muscular pains, the headache and the widespread muscular tenderness should aid us, especially when this occurs in a family or other local epidemic. Cases may be mistaken for rheumatic fever or for typhoid fever. In trichinosis there is a marked leucocytosis, even reaching 30,000 per c.mm. or more, with a great increase in the eosinophil cells which may amount to 40 per cent. of all leucocytes; the absolute eosinophil count varies between 1,000 and 5,000 per c.mm. The stools after a large dose of calomel may be searched for adult worms; the female adult measures about ⅛ inch, the male rather less; the characteristic feature is the " cell body " at the anterior end of the intestine of the parasite. A skin test is not positive early in the disease; later a positive result will show as an erythema one hour after injecting an extract of trichinellæ. The embryos may be found in the blood in the third week and later a biopsy of the affected deltoid muscle may reveal encysting larvæ. In after years X-ray examination may reveal calcified cysts. Very mild infestation is common in Germany; in the U.S.A. 20 per cent. of routine autopsies have shown evidence of larvæ in the muscle of the diaphragm.

Etiology.—Human beings, pigs and rats all harbour the parasite, in each of which there is an identical life cycle; there is no primary stage in one host and secondary stage in another. The pig is infected by eating pig offal or an infected rat. The pork consumed by human beings shows trichinosis when it looks " measly " to the naked eye or when examined by a hand lens. The larvæ (Fig. 176) or muscle trichinæ consist of an ovoid capsule (translucent or infiltrated by lime salts) containing two or more embryos coiled up within it. The embryos are 0·6 to 1·0 mm. long, with a pointed head and rounded tail. Cold storage of pork at minus 15° C for 3 weeks destroys the larvæ, and this is often used in prophylaxis. Otherwise thorough cooking kills the parasite, but in larger joints the temperature may not kill the organisms in the interior; therefore sausages and pork should be thoroughly cooked.

Prognosis.—The disease can end fatally between the second and sixth week; the intensity and duration of the symptoms indicating the severity of the attack—these are diarrhœa, hæmoptysis or pneumonia, the involvement of respiratory muscles and exhaustion. Health may not be restored for several months.

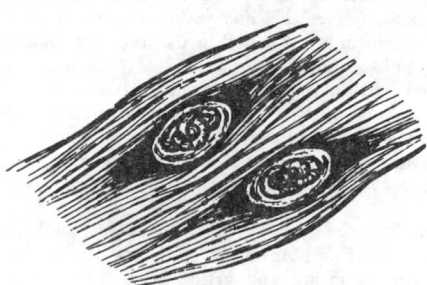

Fig. 176.—Larvæ of the Trichina Spiralis encysted in muscle.

Treatment.—If the patient is seen within 2 or 3 hours after eating infected meat an emetic should be given. If the disease is discovered within 24 or 30 hours the gastro-intestinal tract must be thoroughly cleared out. Glycerin in large doses has been recommended in the first stage as its hygroscopic properties destroy the nematode. Piperazine citrate, tetrachlorethylene, santonin and thymol are also recommended. If, however, the second stage is reached, and the embryos are migrating, the treatment must be symptomatic, because nothing will destroy them. For the pain and tenderness, opium and other anodynes may be required. Prednisolone helps to support strength and lessen muscle pain in severe cases.

V. **Myositis,** or inflammation and swelling of the voluntary muscles, is a rare condition. Four forms are recognised.

(*a*) *Localised,* in which pain, tenderness, swelling and impaired movement are localised to one muscle or group of muscles; this occurs in pyæmia; in typhoid fever it is especially prone to involve the muscles of the abdominal wall when it may simulate an intra-abdominal catastrophe.

(*b*) *Acute generalised myositis* is usually due to Trichinosis.

(*c*) *Progressive generalised ossifying myositis* is rare; it usually commences in children and goes on to produce ossification in muscles, tendons, aponeuroses and ligaments with a hard wooden feeling to the limbs and back. It is well seen on X-ray and either leads to the patient becoming bed-ridden and dying from intercurrent infection or to spontaneous recovery over a period of months or years.

(*d*) *Dermatomyositis* may follow an acute throat infection; it is sometimes associated with a reticulosis or neoplasm and the disease disappears when these have been successfully treated. The *symptoms* are those of a severe illness with a general and symmetrical weakness and aching in the muscles, some pyrexia and an erythematous rash which may be followed by scleroderma; the muscles of speech and of swallowing are often affected. Severe muscular wasting ensues and pneumonia often follows. The erythrocyte sedimentation rate is high and the blood also shows anæmia and a polymorph leucocytosis. *Treatment* is by a prolonged course of corticosteroids or with sodium para-aminobenzoate 12–16 G. daily. When the acute stage is over, physiotherapy is needed to overcome the stiffness and contractures.

GROUP IV. BONE DISEASES

The acute diseases of bone are of especial interest to the surgeon: the chronic diseases are, in the main, of medical interest. Nevertheless, all bone diseases are frequently seen by the physician, especially in their early stages. Pain and deep-seated tenderness are often their chief and sometimes their only symptoms. Pyrexia and constitutional derangement may be present. Deep-seated swelling and deformity may appear later and, if the bone is superficial, œdema and redness of the skin.

Acute Bone Diseases

I. Acute osteomyelitis .. .. § 607   III. Acute epiphysitis .. .. § 607
II. Acute localised periostitis   § 607

§ 607. I. Acute Osteomyelitis (Syn. Acute Necrosis of Bone) is due to an acute infection usually affecting only one bone, accompanied by severe constitutional disturbances. It occurs principally in children between 2 and 18 years of age and is rare in adults. The disease is primarily an infection of the metaphysis near the end of a long bone, very often the tibia or the lower end of the femur. It is the only really acute disease of bone although acute symptoms resembling those of osteomyelitis may arise with LOCAL PERIOSTITIS following trauma.

Symptoms often follow a local injury and comprise (1) severe pain and extreme local tenderness coming on in the course of a few hours, starting near the end of a long bone. (2) In a day or so, as the pus makes its way to the surface under the periosteum, there is local swelling, redness and heat. (3) Constitutional symptoms develop shortly and (in the absence of treatment) become very marked; the temperature is 102–104° F, there may be rigors and prostration. A blood culture is positive in 50 per cent. of cases.

The *Diagnosis* is from acute rheumatism which it may at first resemble because of the pain near a joint; but in rheumatism there is early involvement of other joints, cardiac signs may be present and sweating is marked, whereas in osteomyelitis some movement of the joint is possible and the leucocyte count is usually higher (up to 30,000 per c.mm.).

Etiology.—Acute osteomyelitis is usually due to a coagulase-positive staphylococcus arising from a focus on the skin, in the tonsils or from a wound; occasionally pneumococci and *H. influenzæ* are causal. Infection is due to bacteræmia, the organisms settling in a small traumatised area in the cancellous bone of the metaphysis. A small abscess forms which usually makes its way towards the surface under the periosteum, or occasionally into the medulla of the bone. Unless promptly treated, acute necrosis of the bone ensues as its blood supply is cut off by thrombosis of the nutrient artery and by pus stripping up the periosteum which provides the only alternative blood supply.

Prognosis.—This has been revolutionised by penicillin which often prevents abscess formation if given in the first 1–2 days. Penicillin-resistant staphylococci are becoming more common and blood cultures to isolate the organism and test its sensitivity to penicillin and to other antibiotics are essential.

Treatment.—As soon as it is suspected, intensive penicillin therapy must be started with 1 mega-unit of inject. benzylpenicillin in divided doses each day; then injections of fortified procaine penicillin B.P. may be substituted and given daily for 3 weeks. When pus is suspected drill holes should be made to drain the abscess.. In any case the limb must be completely immobilised till healing is complete.

II. Acute Localised Periostitis may arise from trauma, and if not infected it soon subsides. If infected either from a wound or from the blood, suppuration and necrosis take place, and the condition becomes chronic (§ 612).

III. Acute Epiphysitis is inflammation beginning in the growing line, which in early life separates the epiphysis from the shaft of the long bone. The *acute* form is met in very early infancy and is usually due to injury associated with a staphylococcal infection. It may resemble acute osteomyelitis, but the profound constitutional disturbance is lacking. It is distinguished from acute rheumatism by the age of the patient, and by the excellent response of most cases to adequate doses of penicillin. Other varieties are due to infantile scurvy (§ 560) and congenital syphilis (§ 500). In the *chronic* form the process is much slower, and differs from rickets in being localised to one joint. It is generally due to syphilis or tuberculosis.

Chronic Bone Diseases and Deformities

The bones are live and active tissues undergoing a constant process of bone destruction and of new bone formation comparable to the changes in most other organs of the body. Throughout life bone destruction takes place in one stage, through the medium of osteoclasts. In contrast to this new bone is formed in two stages, first by the formation of a protein matrix (osteoid tissue) and then by its calcification, these processes being the function of the osteoblasts. In health there is an equilibrium between the formation and destruction of bone so that it remains the same, both histologically and chemically.

When this equilibrium is upset the bone density may be (1) DE-CREASED in osteomalacia, osteoporosis, osteitis deformans, myelomatosis and by new growth in bone. *Osteomalacia* occurs when there is a defect of calcification of the osteoid tissue so that true bone cannot be formed. The commonest cause is rickets (including late rickets, cœliac and renal rickets), in which there is usually a deficiency of vitamin D, and sometimes of calcium or of inorganic phosphate. *Osteoporosis* occurs when the protein matrix (osteoid) is deficient. This is usually of endocrine origin (especially with disease of the parathyroids or of the suprarenal cortex). In osteitis deformans there is overactivity of the osteoclasts due to an unknown cause. (2) INCREASED bone density (*Osteosclerosis*) is much rarer. It occurs in *marble bone disease*, the inhalation or ingestion of excessive amounts of fluorides (*fluorosis*) and with some sclerosing types of metastasing *carcinomatosis*.

§ 608. I. Rickets is a general metabolic disorder of childhood due to lack of vitamin D; this leads to deficient calcification of bone with epiphy-

seal enlargement and the production of various deformities of the skeleton.
First described in 1675 by Glisson it used to be extremely common, but
during the last 50 years it has become rare in Great Britain.

Symptoms.—The earliest for which we are consulted, coming on between
the sixth and twelfth month of life, are delay in sitting up or standing,
gastro-intestinal disorders, respiratory catarrh, sweating about the head
or the symptoms of infantile tetany. The bone changes are painless.
The *earliest signs* are in the bones. (i.) The rib-ends are enlarged at the
junctions with their costal cartilages and thus produce an appearance of
" beading "—the " rickety rosary." (ii.) The head shows the anterior
fontanelle to be larger than normal and to close late so that instead of
being closed by the fifteenth to the sixteenth month it may remain open
even in the third year. Calcification in the frontal and parietal bones
is largely centred around the frontal and parietal eminences which become
prominent; and there may be thinning of the skull bones (craniotabes)
especially in the occipital region. Rather *later skeletal changes* are:—
(iii.) A chest deformity due to sinking in at the costo-chondral junctions,
so that the sternum and cartilages stand out prominently in front (" pigeon-
breast "), and are united to the ribs along a deep lateral groove. Harrison's
sulcus is another groove which runs transversely across the chest just
above the lower costal margin. (iv.) The enlarged epiphyses at the ends
of the long bones are often best seen and felt at the wrists: they show
diagnostic X-ray changes. (v.) The spine has a general backward curvature when the child sits up (kyphosis) due to muscular weakness. Scoliosis
may ensue later. (vi.) The pelvis becomes deformed and in later life this
causes difficulty in childbirth. (vii.) The pull of the muscles on the softened
bones causes bowing of the arms when the child crawls, and of the legs
which curve forwards and outwards. *Non-skeletal changes* include: (viii.) A
poor muscle tone of the whole body, which materially contributes to the
delay in sitting, standing and walking. (ix.) The poor tone in the
abdominal wall together with the gaseous distension due to too much
carbohydrate in the diet produces " a pot-belly." (x.) In advanced cases
the liver and spleen are both enlarged. (xi.) The milk teeth are late in
appearing. (xii.) Iron deficiency anæmia is common. (xiii.) Symptoms
of infantile tetany arise giving laryngismus stridulus, carpo-pedal spasm
and even generalised convulsions.

Diagnosis.—In rickets the important points are its more frequent
occurrence in artificially fed children, the lack of pain and tenderness in
the epiphyses, the onset after the fourth and usually the sixth month,
the beading of the ribs, the large anterior fontanelle and the late appearance of the first teeth. X-ray examination of a wrist shows a characteristic
picture, with a broadened concave end to the diaphysis and a fluffy indistinct outline to the ends of the bones. There is also a general osteoporosis.
In *hereditary syphilis* the epiphysitis occurs in the first few months of life,
is painful and usually occurs only in one bone, with other undoubted signs
of syphilis (§ 500). *Infantile scurvy* causes acutely painful and tender

swellings under the periosteum of the shafts of the long bones (§ 560). *Achondroplasia* is a rare condition (§ 616).

TABLE XLVII.—DIFFERENTIAL DIAGNOSIS OF RICKETS, CONGENITAL SYPHILIS AND HYDROCEPHALUS.

	Rickets.	*Congenital Syphilis.*	*Hydrocephalus.*
I. History.	Gastro-intestinal irritation, sweating about head. Improper feeding.	Snuffles and rash. Possibly condylomata.	Congenital, or acquired after meningeal inflammation, or due to tumour pressing on veins.
II. Age of patient.	Rarely commences before 6 months or after the second year.	Symptoms first appear third week to the third month.	Congenital or acquired.
III. Shape of head.	Often compressed antero - posteriorly. Frontal eminences marked.	Irregular prominence on frontal and parietal bones. Skull termed natiform. Depressed bridge of nose.	Bulges in all directions. General tendency to assume a globular form.
IV. Fontanelles.	Close late.	Appear to be depressed in the hollow between the four prominences.	Bulging, separation of the bones at the sutures.
V. Other peculiarities.	Epiphyseal enlargements, delayed dentition, etc.	Pegged and notched permanent teeth. Scars about mouth.	Stunted growth, sometimes mental deficiency.

Etiology.—The lack of vitamin D affects both sexes equally, and the disease is more frequent in cities and during the dark months of the year. This vitamin is essential for the absorption of calcium and to a less extent of phosphorus from the small intestine. At least ten different substances of similar chemical composition are known which will prevent or cure rickets: the term vitamin D is usually taken to include irradiated ergosterol (otherwise known as calciferol or vitamin D_2) and irradiated 7-dehydrocholesterol (vitamin D_3). Vitamin D_2 is synthetic and derived from ergosterol found in yeast, plants and fungi. Vitamin D_3 is formed by the action of ultra-violet radiation or of natural sunlight on the precursors found in the skin and is the natural form occurring in cod liver and halibut liver oils. Therefore exposure of the skin to natural sunlight and to ultra-violet rays from lamps can prevent and cure rickets. In vitamin D deficiency the blood plasma is usually deficient in inorganic phosphate or more rarely in calcium.

Prognosis.—When the disease is treated before osseous changes are marked it readily responds; otherwise permanent deformities of the limbs, spine, chest and pelvis result, and the growth is stunted. Genu valgum (knock-knee), genu varum (bow-leg) and flat foot often occur. Rickets contributes to death because of a lowered resistance to bronchitis, pneumonia or gastro-intestinal disorders, or due to the convulsions of tetany.

Other complications include a liability to green-stick fractures and a delayed second dentition with crowded teeth due to defective growth of the jaws.

Treatment.—The first essential is to give vitamin D by mouth in a dose of 2,000 I.U. daily; this is contained in 0·25 ml. of liq. vitamin D conc. (B.P.) or 15 drops of halibut liver oil. It is wise to correct the unbalanced diet which often accompanies rickets by reducing starches and giving fresh milk, butter, cream and fresh fruit. Exposure of the body to ultra-violet rays, such as are found in natural sunlight or from U.V. lamps, is also curative. *Prophylaxis* is by giving a child of 6 months 600–800 I.U. daily, contained in cod liver oil (B.P.) 2 teaspoonsful (8 ml.) or in halibut-liver oil, 5 drops. Calciferol and irradiated ergosterol in large doses are dangerous. Only in severe cases are splints necessary for two to three weeks to prevent the patient walking.

Other Varieties of Rickets include:—

(1) *Late Rickets* may be seen up to the age of puberty when animal fats and dairy produce are in very short supply for a long period, as during World War I. Rickets in the child is the counterpart of osteomalacia of the adult, except for the effects on the growth of bone of the former; and girls and young women who live under the Purdah system in India and who veil themselves out-of-doors are liable to similar skeletal abnormalities.

(2) *Cœliac Rickets* occurs in severe cases of cœliac disease in children (§ 317); the bone changes resemble those of severe ordinary rickets and improve when treatment becomes effective. It is caused by deficient absorption of calcium and vitamin D, but does not usually show itself until the child begins to grow, with the corresponding increase in the demand for these substances. The ultimate prognosis is good; liq. vitamin D. conc. (B.P.) 0·3–0·5 ml. daily is necessary.

(3) *Renal Rickets* is the result of chronic renal disease. It usually starts about the age of seven, but may date from birth or occur at puberty. The chief features of the rickets are the stunted growth (" renal dwarfism ") and genu valgum (knock-knee), but on careful examination other signs of rickets such as enlarged epiphyses are found. The renal symptoms include polyuria, polydipsia with an excessive volume of urine of low specific gravity and usually a little albuminuria (§ 404). The blood shows retention of nitrogen bodies and of phosphate with a very low alkali reserve (renal acidosis). The bony deformities are due to the kidney being unable to excrete phosphate, leading to a relative insufficiency of calcium (Parsons).

The *Fanconi syndrome*, with its defect of tubular reabsorption (especially of phosphate), is a special variety of this (§ 422). The ultimate prognosis is bad and most cases die in the second decade.

Treatment.—The ricketic symptoms are best treated by the administration of alkali, calcium gluconate and vitamin D in a daily dose of 20,000 I.U., but this does not affect the underlying renal disease. Exposure of the body to the ultra-violet rays of natural sunlight or of artificial lamps, although curative in ordinary rickets, aggravates renal rickets (Parsons).

(4) *Hypophosphatasia* is sometimes met. Phosphatase is necessary for the deposition of calcium phosphate in bone; and a lack of this ferment is general in all tissues. Deficiency is best shown in the serum. The symptoms of rickets are accompanied by early loss of teeth, osteoporosis and sometimes there is papillœdema with blindness.

§ **609.** II. **Osteomalacia** in adults (Syn. Mollities ossium) is the counterpart of rickets in children. It is a chronic disorder usually commencing at 20 to 30 years of age, especially in women in India, China, Japan and other Far-Eastern countries; it is rare in Great Britain. There is a reduced calcification of newly formed osteoid tissue which leads to a general decrease in the bone density of the skeleton ("decalcification"). The bones become soft and fragile.

Symptoms.—(1) There is an aching pain in the back and thighs, which is worse at night; this is accompanied by weakness of the muscles of the limbs. The bones are often *tender*. (2) In the course of a few months *bending* of the weight-bearing bones occurs with bowing of the legs; the spine becomes deformed with a diminished stature, the pelvis flattens leading to difficulty in childbirth and coxa vara may occur. (3) Stress fractures are common but they heal readily. (4) Tetany is common. The condition is aggravated by puberty (late rickets), during pregnancy and lactation. It is often associated with iron-deficiency anæmia.

Diagnosis.—The deformities are characteristic. X-ray examination in the earlier stages shows increased bone trabeculation due to increased growth of uncalcified matrix. In the late stages there is general lack of calcification of the bones, which acquire a frosted or ground glass appearance.

Etiology.—The mineral content of the bones is decreased by (i.) lack of vitamin D and sometimes of calcium in the diet as a result of famine or extreme poverty. (ii.) In Great Britain the commonest cause is failure of absorption of calcium and/or vitamin D from the small intestine in any condition which gives rise to chronic steatorrhœa (§ 316). (iii.) Chronic renal disease, especially renal tubular absorption defects, is a rare cause.

Treatment is by remedying the cause and giving calciferol in doses of 50,000 I.U. daily. Ultra-violet rays are helpful except in renal disease.

§ 610. III. Osteoporosis is much more frequent in Great Britain than is osteomalacia; it occurs in women after the menopause and in very elderly men. The primary cause is a deficiency of bone matrix (osteoid) which may occur as a result of the inadequate replacement or the excessive breakdown of this protein substance.

Symptoms are caused by the softening and collapse of the bodies of the middle and lower dorsal and especially of the lumbar vertebræ; later on the long bones may be affected. There is a low back pain which is occasionally more severe after a minor fall if sudden vertebral collapse takes place. Fractures occur especially in the vertebræ and in the long bones. Although at first the general nutrition is good, loss of weight occurs later.

Diagnosis.—The condition should be suspected when a woman past middle age complains of the above symptoms. X-ray examination with lateral views of the lower dorsal and lumbar vertebræ shows normal intervertebral disc spaces but irregular collapse of the vertebral bodies with loss of the normal reticulation of the bones; the skull usually escapes these changes. For the blood findings see Table XLVIII.

Etiology.—The *rebuilding* of the protein-matrix of bones depends on (1) an adequate amount of body protein—this is deficient with a grossly

TABLE XLVIII.—BIOCHEMICAL CHANGES IN SERUM IN BONE DISEASES.

	Calcium.	Inorganic Phosphate.	Alkaline Phosphatase.
Osteomalacia.	Normal or lowered.	Normal or usually low.	Raised or high.
Osteoporosis.	Normal.	Normal or raised.	Normal.
Hyperparathyroidism.	Raised.	Low.	Raised.
Osteitis Deformans.	Normal.	Normal.	Raised.

deficient protein diet or with prolonged protein loss; (2) a sufficiency of œstrogens, androgens and to a less extent of thyroid hormone; (3) the daily use of bones, so that prolonged bed-rest is harmful. Increased *destruction* of the protein-matrix (osteoclasis) occurs with the prolonged administration of large doses of corticosteroids and of corticotrophin (ACTH) as in the treatment of disseminated lupus erythematosus or advanced rheumatoid disease, as well as with Cushing's syndrome and prolonged hyperthyroidism.

Prognosis.—The condition is usually far advanced before symptoms arise; it has been found that over 60 per cent. of the vertebræ has been absorbed before X-ray changes are evident. In the absence of treatment the condition is progressive. Repeated pregnancies aggravate the disease.

Treatment is by removing the cause such as the use of large doses of corticosteroid drugs. The production of osteoid is encouraged by the prolonged administration over a period of one or more years of œstrogens and of androgens. In post-menopausal osteoporosis give tab. stilbœstrol 0·5 mg. t.i.d. or tab. ethinyl œstradiol 0·02 mg. t.i.d. together with tab. methyl-testosterone 5 mg. t.d.s. In elderly men only the androgen is required. If these are poorly tolerated and the androgens produce unpleasant virilising effects they should be replaced by tab. norethandrolone (Nilevar) 10 mg. t.d.s. or inject. nandrolone (Durabolin) 25 mg. once a week, as these have much weaker androgenic side-effects. All these preparations also aid the retention of calcium salts. Fluid retention has to be rectified by diuretics.

§ **611. IV. Osteitis Deformans** (Syn. Paget's disease of bone) is fairly frequent in those over 40 years of age, and is rather more common in men than women. There is a very chronic enlargement of the diameter of the bones accompanied by a rarefying osteitis with enlargement of the Haversian spaces. Paget's disease may be found in one bone or in several, and gradually extends but never involves the whole skeleton. The bones most frequently affected are the pelvis, lower vertebræ, tibia, femur, vault of the skull and clavicle.

Symptoms.—(1) In many cases there are no symptoms or they may occur only after 10 years or more, the condition being an incidental finding during X-ray examination for some other purpose. The general health is rarely affected. When symptoms are present they depend a good deal on the bone or bones involved. (2) Pain is the most frequent symptom and varies from a dull ache to a severe burning or shooting pain. When the bone is superficial there is considerable warmth over it due to the increased blood supply through the affected area. Involvement of the skull commonly produces a headache. (3) Deformity is most obvious in the tibia which becomes broadened and bowed. When the femur or tibia of one or both sides is extensively affected this is very noticeable and the knees become widely separated. (4) The patient may complain of a very slow increase in the size of the vault of the skull necessitating a larger size in hats, but the face is not involved. (5) Progressive deafness and tinnitus are due to the changes in the petrous temporal bones or to compression of the auditory nerves. Less frequently loss of vision results from compression of the optic nerve at the optic foramen. (6) Root pain due to compression of the spinal nerve roots is unusual and spinal cord compression is very rare. (7) In an advanced stage the head is projected forwards by the kyphosis and both legs are bowed outward and forward. (8) Osteo-arthritis in the hips, knees, ankles or spine is due to the abnormal stresses which result from the bone deformities.

Diagnosis is from *carcinomatous deposits* in bone, especially from the prostate. The X-ray appearances of the spine and pelvic bones can on occasions be similar. In *osteitis deformans* the absorption of the cortex makes it resemble the medulla, the trabeculæ are more marked and more widely separated; the broadening and bowing of this disease is never seen in carcinoma and discovery of a mottled appearance in the thickened bones of the skull is also characteristic. Whereas in osteitis deformans the serum alkaline phosphatase is raised, in carcinoma of the prostate the serum acid phosphatase is high. Unlike *hyperparathyroidism*, in Paget's disease the serum calcium and phosphate are normal. *Syphilitic osteitis* may have to be considered when only one bone is affected.

Etiology.—The cause is unknown but a metabolic disturbance of bone is suspected. The bone is full of osteoclasts and osteoblasts; the former cause reabsorption especially of the cortical bone whereas the latter lay down new bone under the periosteum. The vascularity of the affected bones is greatly increased and the decalcified areas represent a considerable arterio-venous shunt which can give rise to heart failure.

Prognosis.—Patients are usually able to continue their normal life with this disease. Osteo-arthritis may involve the neighbouring joints, especially in the lumbar spine and the legs. Pathological fractures occur but heal readily. On occasions there is circulatory failure. Osteogenic sarcoma, especially in the pelvic bones, is rare.

Treatment does not affect the course of the disease. Pain is relieved by analgesics, by the regular administration of prednisolone or by local deep X-ray therapy. Some, having obtained success by modifying the calcium phosphorus ratio in certain osteoporotic diseases in animals, report favourably on the effects of a diet rich in calcium and poor in phosphorus, and advocate a high consumption of milk, with calcium sodium lactate and calciferol.

§ 612. V. Chronic Periostitis and Osteitis includes a number of tuberculous, syphilitic, and other conditions leading to caries, necrosis, and other anatomical changes in the bone. Periostitis and osteitis are dealt with together, for although the disease may start in the bone or the periosteum, it soon spreads to the other.

The *Symptoms* of periostitis and osteitis may begin with pain, redness and swelling. Usually they are more insidious, with pain still a prominent feature (especially at night) and with enlargement of the bone; this may be followed by softening (caries) or death of a portion of the bone (necrosis) with signs of abscess formation.

Causes and their differentiation: (1) *Trauma* alone, without sepsis or toxæmia of some kind, is a rare cause of chronic periostitis or osteitis. It is recognised by the history and only one bone is affected. (2) The favourite seat of *tuberculosis* is the epiphysis, where it induces a chronic epiphysitis, especially in the neighbourhood of the hip or knee. Sometimes it gives rise to osteitis, as in the fingers where it results in a characteristic thickening of the metacarpals and phalanges known as tuberculous dactylitis. In any position it may go on to caries or necrosis. Tuberculosis of the bones is recognised by (i.) the younger age of the patient; (ii.) a tuberculous family history; (iii.) the characteristic intermitting pyrexia; (iv.) signs of tuberculosis in the lungs and elsewhere; (v.) the chronicity of the process; and (vi.) the frequent limitation to one bone. (3) *Syphilis* of the bones is common both in the acquired and the hereditary disease. (*a*) *Acquired syphilis* may take the form of a chronic diffuse or localised periostitis (nodes), or on the other hand, a diffuse or a gummatous (localised) osteitis. It is recognised by (i.) the nocturnal pains in the bones, which are such a frequent manifestation of syphilis; (ii.) other evidence of syphilis; and (iii.) positive serological tests. (*b*) *Hereditary syphilis* may give rise in childhood and early life to the same lesions as the acquired disease. In infancy (in addition to the foregoing) chronic epiphysitis may be mistaken for rickets. One or several bones may be affected, but it never presents the same symmetry as rickets. The deformities resulting from hereditary lesions (§ 500) and the physiognomy are characteristic— the bosses on the frontal and parietal bones (Parrot's nodes), the depressed bridge of the nose, scars about the angle of the mouth, Hutchinson's teeth, and perhaps keratitis (Tables XXXII and XXXIII). (4) *Gout* may give rise to chronic periosteal thickening. (5) *Osteogenic sarcoma* usually produces considerable pain and often causes new bone to be laid down under the periosteum.

For *Diagnosis* X-ray examination of the bones is essential.

For the adequate *Treatment* of most of these different conditions, rest and surgical aid are necessary. The treatment of tuberculosis, syphilis and gout have already been dealt with.

VI. Tumours of Bones may produce no symptoms until the swelling is noticed. This applies chiefly to INNOCENT tumours which may have been present for many years before they are discovered. *Exostoses* may occur on almost any bone, and *Enchondromata* are most common on the metacarpals and phalanges. Both are usually multiple. A *fibroma* or *angioma* is rare. A *giant-cell tumour* (osteoclastoma, focal osteitis fibrosa) usually starts in early adult life before the epiphysis closes. It produces a gradual cyst-like expansion of the end of one or more bones and may produce a pathological fracture; unless malignant change is occurring treatment is by curettage or deep X-ray. MALIGNANT tumours grow ı ʰh more quickly and are liable to produce pain, swelling or fractures. *Sarcomata* can be of varying malignancy. An *osteogenic sarcoma* is the most frequent and the most malignant; it is usually seen at the distal end of the femur or the proximal end of the tibia or humerus, and readily produces metastases in the lungs. Other varieties of sarcoma are fibrosarcoma, chondrosarcoma, angiosarcoma and malignant giant-cell tumours. *Carcinoma* starting in any part of the body may produce bone metastases, but many fail to do so. When a metastasis in bone does occur, the primary source is usually in the breast, prostate, kidney, bronchus or thyroid. The common symptoms are pain or a pathological fracture: as they usually start in the medulla of a bone the complaint of a swelling occurs late.

C.M.—H H

Certain rare forms of chronic bone disease must be described.

§ 613. VII. Multiple Myeloma (Syn. Myelomatosis, Kahler's disease) is a condition in which " myeloma " cells, arising from plasma cells or their precursors in the bone marrow, undergo a malignant type of growth. They invade the bones producing multiple tumours and anæmia. The disease is more common in men than women and is rare before 40.

Symptoms.—The onset is insidious. In the *early stages* there is pain in the dorso-lumbar spine, ribs and sternum. The pain in the back extends to the chest and abdomen, is aggravated by sneezing, coughing and by exertion, and unlike metastatic carcinoma usually goes during sleep. The affected bones are sometimes extremely tender and often fracture without apparent cause. There is considerable loss of energy and loss of weight, and usually a low-grade fever. The blood shows anæmia with a normal or low leucocyte count, although a leuco-erythroblastic or a myeloid-leukæmoid reaction is occasionally met (§§ 551, 558): the peripheral blood may show myeloma cells. Bence-Jones' protein is found in the urine in about half the cases and nephritis with a raised blood urea but without hypertension is common. In the *later stages* the patient becomes more bed-ridden and anæmic. The dorso-lumbar vertebræ collapse causing kyphosis and extension of the disease into the spinal canal may cause sciatic pain or spinal cord compression. Sooner or later the long bones and the skull become affected. Palpable masses may be felt in the scalp or around the pelvic or shoulder girdles.

T'ie *Diagnosis* should be suspected when there is vertebra pain and tenderness, especially in the presence of anæmia and a very high erythrocyte sedimentation rate (§ 1210). By serum electrophoresis two types are recognised; the first (usually in older patients) shows a sharp band in the γ-globulin region, and the second a band in the β-2a globulin range. X-ray examination of the vertebræ, ribs and often of the skull shows small focal areas of rarefaction accompanied by collapse of the vertebral bodies and pathological fractures; there is also considerable general osteoporosis. Confirmation of the disease is by finding a considerable excess of " plasma cells " by examination of the bone marrow or biopsy of a rib. The serum calcium and phosphate are usually normal, but in the active stages of the disease they may be raised: the serum alkaline phosphatase is normal.

Prognosis.—The disease is invariably fatal within 2 to 3 years of the onset, usually from uræmia and sometimes from amyloidosis.

Treatment is disappointing. Analgesic drugs are needed for pain. Prednisolone helps some and deep X-ray therapy often gives relief from local symptoms. A cyclophosphamide in the form of Endoxan 200 mg. daily (a total dose of 4·0 G.) intravenously often produces a remission, but must be stopped when the leucocytes fall to 2,000 per c.mm.: it often produces hair fall. In those with β-2a globulin as shown by serum electrophoresis Melphalan is useful.

§ 614. VIII. Hyperparathyroidism (Syn. Osteitis fibrosa cystica) is a rare disease of the parathyroids due to a local adenoma, carcinoma or to diffuse hypertrophy of the glands. The effects resemble those of prolonged administration of an active extract of parathyroid, such as parathormone (Collip). There is increased breakdown of the bone matrix due to excessive osteoclast activity. The bones become decalcified, with loss of calcium and phosphate, which are excreted in the urine and may form renal calculi. The bones become progressively rarefied, with cyst formation, which may form large tender tumours. At the same time spontaneous fractures and bending of the bones cause progressive loss of stature. Gastro-intestinal disturbances with attacks of headache and vomiting are common. Polyuria and polydipsia commonly occur. The muscles become hypotonic. The *diagnosis* is confirmed by the blood findings, as the calcium is raised to perhaps 15–16 mg. per cent., the phosphorus is below normal and the alkaline phosphatase high. X-ray examination shows the decalcification and cyst formation; at an early stage subperiosteal erosions are seen, particularly in the bones of the fingers. After successful removal of the parathyroid tumour, and large doses of calcium and calciferol, the bones slowly recalcify, and the headaches and gastro-intestinal symptoms are lost, with a return of the blood to normal (and see § 413).

Other Varieties of Hyperparathyroidism:—

(1) *Recurrent renal calculi* can occur due to parathyroid hyperplasia or tumour even when the serum calcium and phosphate values are normal. In addition the daily urinary output of calcium may be within normal limits. The *Diagnosis* of the hyperparathyroid state in these cases is difficult: the serum calcium may be temporarily raised and then return to normal. A raised ionised calcium value in the serum (above 6·2 mg. per cent.) may prove helpful. Some postulate that another parathyroid hormone other than parathormone may be responsible.

(2) *Secondary hyperparathyroidism* can occur in response to long-standing renal failure, especially when due to chronic pyelonephritis. In this condition the bones become osteoporotic.

§ 615. IX. Acromegaly is a rare disease of the anterior pituitary gland, with overgrowth in the skeletal tissues. The onset is often so gradual that patients may not be aware of the changes.

Symptoms.—(1) Headache is often a marked feature and tends to be bitemporal. (2) The bones and the cutaneous and subcutaneous tissues of the face and of the hands and feet enlarge, producing a characteristic appearance (Fig. 7). In the *face* the features are coarsened by considerable enlargement of the supra-orbital ridges, the nose and the cheek bones; the lower jaw is especially enlarged and may project beyond the upper jaw (prognathism) so that the teeth no longer meet. These bony changes are aggravated by the thickening of the soft tissues of the face, with hypertrophy of the eyelids, nose, lips, ears and the tongue. The skull bones also enlarge but to a much less extent. The broadening of the *hands and feet* is recognised by the patient requiring a larger size in gloves and shoes. Later in the disease there may be a similar enlargement of the bones of the thorax and kyphosis of the spine. (3) Hypertrophy of the general musculature leads to excessive strength for a while, but later muscular weakness occurs. (4) The voice may deepen due to enlargement of the larynx. (5) Pains in the joints are due to changes in the articular cartilages and softening of ligaments, which produce a degenerative type of arthritis with instability and even recurring effusions in the joints. (6) When due to a *tumour*, the headache is associated sooner or later with bitemporal hemianopia, and/or with gradual optic atrophy (§ 1046). (7) As the basophile cells of the pituitary are encroached upon and the production of the gonadotropic hormones lessens, amenorrhœa and sexual impotence occur and a goitre may form. Glycosuria is sometimes seen in the earlier stages.

Diagnosis.—*Osteitis deformans* causes enlargement of the vault of the skull whereas acromegaly produces hypertrophy of the facial bones. *Myxœdema* resembles acromegaly, but is known by the dry skin, the sluggish mentality and the absence of all bony enlargement. In acromegaly due to a tumour X-ray is likely to show an enlarged sella turcica. The serum phosphate is usually high and there may be a diminished glucose tolerance. The visual fields should be regularly charted whenever there is a suspicion of a tumour (Fig. 261). For hypertrophic osteo-arthropathy see below.

Etiology.—The primary change is an increased secretion of the growth hormone of the eosinophil cells in the anterior lobe of the pituitary gland. This may be due to hypertrophy or to an adenoma of these cells; when this takes place at a young age it produces gigantism (§ 805), and after the epiphyses have united acromegaly. The latter usually starts before 40 years of age, about the twenty-fifth year, and is a little more frequent in women.

Prognosis.—Acromegaly runs a prolonged course over many years, but 80 per cent. of cases die of cardio-vascular disease before the age of 60.

Treatment.—Extract of thyroid may help in the early stages. X-ray therapy is the best treatment of patients with simple hypertrophy of the eosinophil cells. An adenoma calls for surgical treatment when there is progressive loss of the visual fields or of central vision.

§ 616. X. Achondroplasia (Syn. Chondrodystrophia Fœtalis) is a rare condition which dates from fœtal life and may occur in successive generations.

Symptoms.—The striking feature is the dwarfism, so that the adult is between 4 feet and 4 feet 6 inches in height. This is due to considerable shortening of the bones of the limbs, in contrast to which the trunk is little affected. The shortened arms cause the hands only to reach to the hips when standing, instead of half-way down the thighs. The epiphyses are considerably thickened (producing enlargement of the

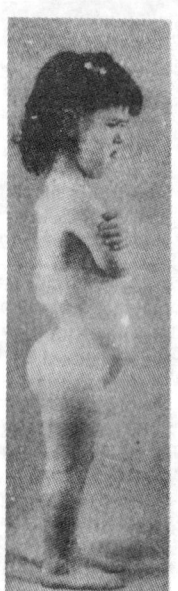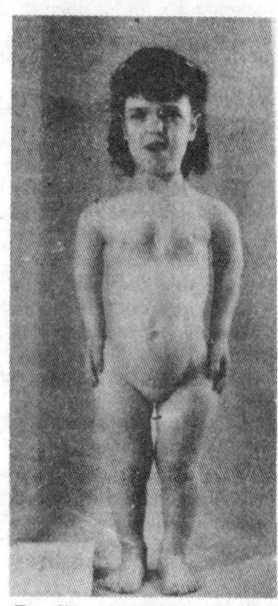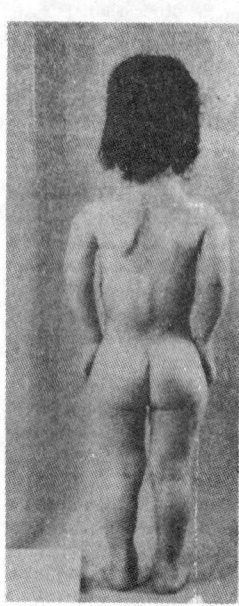

FIG. 177.—A case of ACHONDROPLASIA.

articulations) which give rise to the former misleading name " fœtal rickets." The fingers and toes are shortened, taper and are abducted from one another. The cranium is enlarged, with a bulging forehead which causes a resemblance to hydrocephalus; the face is small and the bridge of the nose depressed. On standing the limbs are seem to be rather bowed, there is a pronounced lumbar lordosis, and a characteristic waddling gait (Fig. 177). The muscular, sexual and the mental development are normal; there is a sharp distinction from the mental deficiency, facial aspect, and the changes in the hair and skin characteristic of cretinism. X-ray of the limbs shows no signs of rickets, but the epiphyseal centres are closer to the shafts than normal.

Prognosis.—Many are still-born. The disease does not shorten life, except that the pelvic deformity causes difficulty in childbirth so that Cæsarian section is usually required. No *treatment* is known.

§ 617. XI. Hypertrophic Osteo-arthropathy (Syn. Pulmonary osteo-arthropathy) is a chronic condition of hyperplasia associated with chronic pulmonary disorders. There is symmetrical enlargement of the bones of the hands and feet and of the lower ends of the long bones of the forearms and lower legs, but the face and head are not enlarged. The fingers show marked clubbing and the nails are curved over the terminal phalanges (" filbert nails "). The finger- and toe-joints may be swollen, and in about a third of the cases the wrists, knees and ankles are swollen.

Etiology.—There are a variety of causes, which include diseases of the lungs such as bronchiectasis, lung abscess, empyema or carcinoma; sometimes no cause can be found.

Treatment is that of the cause. The changes rapidly regress when the original disease has been eliminated.

XII. **Leontiasis Ossea** is the term given to a rare condition of early adult life in which there are symmetrical hyperostoses of the facial bones and skull, which encroach upon the cranial cavity, and so may lead to death.

XIII. **Fragilitis ossium** and **osteogenesis imperfecta** are terms now used almost synonymously for a condition of abnormal bone fragility due to a very thin cortex of bone; the long bones and the ribs break very easily after trivial injuries. It is usually hereditary. There are two varieties—(*a*) ante-natal, in which multiple fractures are found at birth; (*b*) in the early years of life fractures occur with slight injury or even from a sudden muscular pull. The fractures heal well and the general health may not be interfered with, but gross deformities and diminution of stature occur. Blue sclerotics are more common in this second variety.

XIV. **Cleido-cranio-dysostosis** is a congenital defect. There is absence of bone at the outer third of the clavicle, with persistence of the acromio-clavicular ligament, and deficient ossification of the cranial bones.

XV. **Marble bones** (Syn. Infantile osteosclerosis, Albers-Schönberg's disease) are very rare and occur in children and young adults, showing (i.) undue fragility of the bones associated with dense osteosclerosis throughout the body, which obliterates the marrow cavities; (ii.) severe anæmia (often with nucleated red cells, myeloblasts, and myelocytes in a blood film (§ 541); and (iii.) enlargement of the spleen and liver, proptosis and optic atrophy may appear. The X-ray appearances are characteristic.

XVI. **Perthés' disease** (pseudo-coxalgia) is a rare disease which causes fragmentation of the epiphysis of the head of the femur. It occurs in children under 12, and is evidenced first by a limp and limited abduction; later there is shortening and muscular wasting. X-ray decides the diagnosis. There is usually spontaneous recovery in a few years.

CHAPTER XVIII

THE SKIN

THE skin is a large and vital organ with numerous complex functions indispensable to the health and survival of the individual. An intact and healthy skin provides protection against physical and chemical trauma and against infective agents. It plays a large part in the regulation of body temperature and has important excretory functions. It has nervous functions, as a sense organ for the perception of local sensation and as an organ of emotional expression. The reticulo-endothelial system in the skin has immunological functions and is one site of antibody formation. Under the influence of ultraviolet light vitamin D_3 is formed in the skin from ergosterol.

Extensive structural or functional disorders of the skin can give rise to serious systemic disturbances. Thus gross reduction of thermoregulatory sweating is the cause of tropical anhidrotic asthenia, and severe persistent pruritus, destroying peace of mind and rendering sleep almost impossible, may produce loss of weight and distressing psychological symptoms. Conversely many systemic disorders and some psychological states are associated with modifications of skin structure or function.

Skin lesions may parallel those in other organs less readily accessible to direct clinical examination, as in sarcoidosis and polyarteritis nodosa. Here also the superficial vascular networks are exposed directly to view; circulating micro-organisms, toxins and chemical substances may be trapped in the capillary loops or may injure some component of the network giving rise to visible skin lesions. Many disturbances of endocrine function produce skin changes, and the patient's emotional state is often reflected in his skin. Dietary deficiencies or excesses may produce lesions of distinctive character or may significantly modify skin reactions. Finally this organ is of particular importance as an indicator of allergic and immunological reactions by means of its spontaneous eruptions, or through the results of special tests carefully applied and critically interpreted.

The interplay of external and of internal factors, both physical and emotional, concerned in the production of skin eruptions is highly complex and infinitely variable. Accuracy in diagnosis and success in therapy are unlikely to be achieved if the patient's general physical state, his personality and his social background are ignored. The present chapter emphasises the symptomatic and morphological aspects of skin disorders. The logical analysis of symptoms and signs in terms of the physiopathological changes which produce them provides the only rational approach to diagnosis; the importance of careful assessment of the patient as a person must not be overlooked.

PART A. SYMPTOMATOLOGY

The patient usually seeks advice because he has become aware of the presence of visible changes such as an ERUPTION or of a functional disturbance such as excessive sweating. The lesions may or may not be accompanied by subjective sensations. Although pain, paræsthesiæ and other symptoms are occasionally present in skin disorders the common and characteristic symptom is pruritus.

§ 620. **Pruritus,** or itching, is mediated by pain receptors and is independent of touch and the temperature senses. Impulses conveying pruritus ascend the spinal cord in the anterolateral tract. There may be an itching centre in the hypothalamus and a reflex scratch centre in the medulla.

The symptom of itching should never be disregarded. Although on investigation it may prove to be a manifestation of some trivial condition it is always acutely distressing to the sufferer and may occasionally be a presenting symptom of serious organic disease. Analysis of this symptom, the factors that appear to determine its exacerbations and remissions, disturbance of sleep and intrusion on daytime activities and the imagery employed by the patient to describe it, often provide useful information. The *causes* of pruritus can conveniently be classified in three groups:—

(*a*) Pruritus *secondary* to visible skin lesions. In general acute eruptions are irritable and chronic eruptions less so, but there are many exceptions. Dermatitis herpetiformis and scabies almost invariably produce itching; eczema, urticaria and lichen planus usually are accompanied by it, whilst syphilis and psoriasis commonly give rise to no subjective symptoms. Itching is inconstant in pityriasis rosea and seborrhœic dermatitis.

(*b*) *Localised* pruritus without visible skin lesions other than those produced by rubbing and scratching. More than one site may be involved. This wide group includes (i.) pediculosis capitis and pediculosis pubis, (ii.) lichen simplex (localised neurodermatitis) which includes many cases of anogenital pruritus; (iii.) onchocerciasis, due to a parasitic worm, occurs in tropical climates (§ 724).

(*c*) *Generalised* pruritus without visible skin changes. Among the more important causes are:—(1) Parasitic infestations, especially pediculosis corporis. (2) Diabetes, without relation to the severity of the disease. Some patients show a diabetic type of glucose tolerance curve even in the absence of clinical diabetes. (3) Pregnancy during the last month. It tends to recur with successive pregnancies. (4) Reticuloses, leukæmia and as an early manifestation of Hodgkin's disease. (5) Some cases of carcinoma. (6) Liver disease. Especially with jaundice; it may develop before jaundice is detected and is more frequent and more severe in obstructive than in infective jaundice. (7) Endocrine disorders, especially hypothyroidism. (8) Uræmia in which it is of serious prognostic significance. (9) Drug sensitivity. (10) Asteatosis—excessive degreasing of the skin—in old age, especially in winter. (11) SENILE PRURITUS; this diagnosis should never be accepted until all other causes have been excluded. Degenerative changes in the skin are believed to be responsible for true senile pruritus. Dryness of the skin, anæmia, cardiac insufficiency, hypertension and emotional factors may be contributory. (12) Psychogenic pruritus, a generalised pruritus of psychogenic origin without visible skin changes, is uncommon. In younger patients it may herald a schizophrenic state. In elderly women there may be delusions of infestation.

Complications accompanying persistent pruritus. Any prolonged and extensive inflammatory disease of the skin accompanied by persistent pruritus may give rise to a benign hyperplasia of the lymph nodes draining the affected areas of skin. The skin may become pigmented. This condition has been described as *lipomelanic reticulosis*: it is benign but those not familiar with the distinctive histological changes are liable to misinterpret their significance.

Nervous tension and anxiety may accentuate pruritus of organic origin. For *treatment* see § 1172.

PART B. PHYSICAL EXAMINATION

A complete examination of the patient is sometimes necessary and routine testing of the urine for albumen and sugar can seldom be omitted. The skin should be examined in a good light, and preferably in daylight.

Very little APPARATUS is necessary—a hand lens is useful, a torch and a tongue-depressor are frequently required and a microscope is essential. An ordinary glass microscope slide is adequate for diascopy; where the blood is expelled from a lesion by firm pressure characteristic features may be revealed, as in lupus vulgaris. A pair of forceps, preferably of Whitfield's pattern, is needed for the removal of hairs and a scalpel for the preparation of scrapings from lesions suspected of being of mycotic origin. Hairs or skin scrapings from suspected ringworm infections should be soaked in 10 per cent. potassium hydroxide, warmed gently and examined for mycelium under the lower power of the microscope. In a large school clinic or in an outpatient department Wood's Light—ultraviolet light passed through a nickel-glass filter—is a great asset in the rapid diagnosis of certain types of scalp ringworm. The indications for special bacteriological, mycological and biochemical investigations will be mentioned in later sections.

HISTOLOGICAL EXAMINATION (biopsy) is often essential when the clinical diagnosis is in doubt, particularly when malignancy is possible. An elliptical specimen of full skin thickness should be removed under local anæsthesia. A common fault is to excise too small a fragment.

PATCH TESTING is described in § 671.

The CLINICAL EXAMINATION of the skin should be conducted by Inspection and by Palpation.

§ 621. **Inspection.**—The whole skin surface must be examined in any extensive eruption. Lesions of diagnostic appearance may be present in some sites, whilst those in others are fading, or are so modified by secondary infection or by overtreatment as to be unrecognisable. The buccal mucous membrane should also be examined.

(1) Note first the *distribution* of the lesions: it is often of assistance in

diagnosis as many eruptions tend to favour certain sites. The *generalised* or *symmetrical* eruption of *rapid* onset is more likely to have an internal cause, infective or toxic; an *asymmetrical* eruption confined to a single site is often of exogenous origin; but there are many exceptions. The distribution of the eruption may sometimes give an obvious indication of the factor which has provoked it or has determined its site (*e.g.*, venous hypostasis in the leg), but it often aids diagnosis merely by its conformation to a well-recognised pattern, as in lichen planus, psoriasis or pityriasis rosea. If the morphological characteristics are in favour of a particular diagnosis this should not be abandoned because the distribution is unusual, but it must be critically reviewed.

(2) Then examine closely the *individual* lesions paying special attention to those which are in different stages of their evolution and those which have apparently been modified by treatment or by scratching. Try to differentiate the primary lesions from such secondary changes.

(3) The development of new lesions in scratch marks (the Kœbner isomorphic phenomenon) is a feature of lichen planus, psoriasis, plane warts and molluscum contagiosum.

(4) The irregular clustering of insect bites and of their complications, the result of the biting habits of the insects responsible, are always helpful in diagnosis. An annular configuration is common in granuloma annulare and erythema annulare, and is sometimes seen in psoriasis and in lichen planus (especially on the forehead and on the penis).

Palpation of the lesions will determine their consistency, their depth in the skin and the presence of tenderness.

§ **622. The terms employed** in describing the lesions and the histological changes present, must be understood before considering their classification, diagnosis and treatment. If the visible changes are constantly considered in terms of the pathological changes which produce them the accuracy with which they are interpreted will increase rapidly with practice. Any attempt to rely solely on visual memory—an aircraft spotter's technique—will lead to many errors which can be avoided by a logical approach to each case.

1. A *macule* is a small circumscribed area of altered colour. It is not felt by the finger and is of normal texture. Histologically there may be simple vaso-dilatation or pigmentary changes as described below.

2. A *papule* is a circumscribed solid lesion, easily palpable. A *wheal* is a soft papule, usually lasting only a few hours, produced by transient œdema of the dermis.

Papules are commonly produced by any of the following pathological changes, singly or in combination. (*a*) Hyperkeratosis—thickening of the horny layer. (*b*) Acanthosis—thickening of the rete mucosum of the epidermis—as in chronic eczema. (*c*) Parakeratosis—production of abnormal horn cells as in psoriasis. (*d*) Spongiosis—intercellular œdema of the rete mucosum—the essential change of eczema. (*e*) Malignant or premalignant proliferation of the epidermis. (*f*) Localised œdema of the dermis as in urticaria. (*g*) Inflammatory cellular infiltration of the

dermis as in lupus vulgaris. (*h*) Abnormalities of connective tissue elements.
(*i*) Local reticulo-endothelial hyperplasia. (*j*) Abnormal metabolic deposits—
xanthomatosis. (*k*) Miscellaneous abnormalities of developmental origin such as
cellular and vascular nævi.

Although dermal and epidermal changes are usually associated it is often possible
to decide whether the papule is predominantly of epidermal origin—as for example
a wart, or a dermal lesion beneath an intact epidermis as in granuloma annulare.

3. *A nodule* is essentially an enlarged papule although nodules often
lie more deeply in the skin or are hypodermal.

The same combinations of pathological changes which give rise to papules can
produce nodules, but the epidermis is less commonly involved and certain changes
in the hypoderm may be conspicuous: (*a*) Perivascular inflammatory changes surrounding hypodermal arterioles and venules as in Bazin's disease or in nodular vasculitis. (*b*) Localised degenerative and inflammatory changes in the subcutaneous fat
—panniculitis.

4. *Erythema* is a diffuse area of redness, either universal or of limited
extent. It is produced by vaso-dilation in the dermis and if at all persistent
is usually accompanied or followed by epidermal changes.

5. *Vesicles* and *bullæ* are collections of clear fluid within or beneath
the epidermis. Bullæ are for practical purposes merely large vesicles.

Vesicles may be formed as the result of spongiosis (a combination of intercellular
and intracellular œdema of the epidermis) as in eczema, or by dissolution of the
intercellular bridges (acantholysis) with distinctive cytological abnormalities as in
such virus infections as herpes simplex and herpes zoster. The bullæ of impetigo
are formed by separation of the horny layer alone. In dermatitis herpetiformis
they form at the dermo-epidermal junction whilst in pemphigus they are usually
formed by acantholysis and lie within the epidermis.

6. *Pustules* are localised collections of pus. It is helpful to determine
whether pustular lesions are follicular in distribution and whether they were
pustular on their first appearance or have developed from vesicles or other
lesions.

7. A *scale* is formed of horn, either normal or abnormal.

Normal horn separates in scales after such inflammatory processes as scarlatina.
The scales of psoriasis consist of abnormal parakeratotic horn and owe their silvery
appearance to the air trapped between the horn cells.

8. *Crusts* are formed of dried serum, pus or blood.

9. *Atrophy* may develop as the sequel to severe inflammation which
has destroyed the hair follicles and connective tissue or it may arise as
a primary change. Atrophic skin is smooth and featureless: hair follicles
are absent. There may be scars in the popular sense of the term, or the
affected skin may be soft and finely wrinkled, in which case fixed dilatation
of small vessels in the dermis which have lost their normal support from
the surrounding connective tissue may be a conspicuous feature
(telangiectasia).

10. *Pigmentary changes.*—The colour of normal skin depends on the
thickness of the horny layer, on the circulation and the volume of reduced

and oxyhæmoglobin in the superficial vessels and on the presence of other pigments in the skin and subcutaneous tissues. The most important are melanin and its disintegration product melanoid. A *yellowish-brown* coloration is produced by melanin granules in the upper dermis, while a *blue-black* tinge occurs when the pigment is in the lower dermis. Racial and constitutional differences in skin pigmentation depend on the quantity of melanin present. An *orange-yellow* colour may be imparted to the skin by carotene, a pigment in the subcutaneous fat and in the horny layer of the epidermis. In various pathological states melanin or carotene may be present in excessive quantity or in abnormal sites but many pigments not found in normal skin may also be encountered. Thus a reddish-brown staining is produced by hæmosiderin (a break-down product of hæmoglobin) in the lower legs in the presence of venous insufficiency. A *yellow* colour occurs when the skin is stained by the bile pigments in jaundice. Some drugs stain the skin, especially mepacrine, which also gives a yellow colour. A *purple-grey* and *slate-grey* pigmentation occur after prolonged overdosage with gold and silver compounds respectively.

11. *Excoriations* are usually (i.) secondary lesions and are inflicted by the patient in his efforts to relieve the intense irritation of many pruritic skin disorders including those of psychogenic origin. There are deep and vigorous linear markings in parasitic infestations, often leading to secondary infection: these are in striking contrast to the usual absence of scratch marks in senile pruritus, in urticaria and in lichen planus. Excoriations, sometimes punctiform, may be conspicuous in eczema. In lichen simplex and in atopic eczema (§ 671(2)) rubbing gives rise to thickening, pigmentation and an increase of the normal skin markings—lichenification. The former occurs frequently on the nape of the neck in women or on the outer aspect of the lower leg in men, and is common in anogenital pruritus. It may complicate a pre-existing skin lesion, or pruritus of psychogenic origin. (ii.) Excoriations are the only significant objective lesions present in acne excorié (§ 635) of the face in adolescent girls and neurotic excoriations of the neck and shoulders are sometimes seen in nervous women. (iii.) Excoriations, which may be numerous and deep, are sometimes a feature of parasitophobia in elderly women and are also seen in some forms of dermatitis artefacta.

§ 623. **Dermatitis Artefacta** occurs in the psychologically abnormal individual, the gross hysteric or the psychotic. The *clinical forms* are as variable as the ingenious methods employed to produce them. The bizarre nature and distribution of the lesions, sometimes conforming to the patient's concept of the disease she hopes to simulate, usually makes diagnosis obvious. Blisters, burns or ulcers may be produced with caustics, disinfectants or lighted cigarettes, friction with abrasives or even the application of fæces to produce infection. Some patients seem to be unconscious of the fact that they are themselves inflicting the lesions. From their presence they obtain either direct pecuniary benefit or, much more commonly, direct or indirect emotional advantage. At times a pre-existing lesion, often trivial, is perpetuated but commonly the entire lesion is self-inflicted. *Treatment* is a psychiatric problem.

THE ETIOLOGY OF SKIN DISORDERS

A large number of the commonest skin disorders strikingly demonstrate the impossibility of attributing many pathological conditions to any single cause. For example a patient with an industrial dermatitis caused primarily by detergents may have an underlying inherited skin defect and the course of the dermatitis may be unduly prolonged by emotional instability. The cause of any particular skin condition may often fall into more than one of the following groups: 1. Skin disorders genetically determined (genodermatoses). 2. Developmental defects of the skin (nævi). 3. Age changes. 4. Reactions to physical and chemical agents. 5. Allergic disorders. 6. Parasitic infestations. 7. Infections with bacteria, viruses or fungi. 8. Nutritional, metabolic or endocrine disorders. 9. Vascular disturbances. 10. Psychogenic illness. 11. Benign and malignant neoplasms. 12. Disorders of unknown origin.

PART C. DIAGNOSIS, PROGNOSIS AND TREATMENT OF SKIN DISORDERS

Routine Procedure and Classification. A detailed and careful HISTORY is essential. Special attention should be paid to a family or personal history of skin disorders (especially eczema, asthma or hay fever), to the past and present occupation and to any hobbies. Residence in the tropics or subtropics will increase the diagnostic possibilities. It is essential to know whether the patient was taking any medicines at the time of onset of the skin eruption and inquiry must always be made concerning recent local applications which may have produced secondary skin lesions.

Knowledge of the *duration* of the lesions may allow the differentiation of those of very similar morphological appearance. Any coincidence of remissions and exacerbations with environmental and occupational changes should be noted. The site of onset should be related to possible exposure to external irritants. Subjective symptoms should be carefully analysed. Finally any apparent relationship between emotional stress and exacerbations of the eruption should be inquired into.

In the following classification skin disorders are classified according to their most conspicuous features.

GROUP   I. If the lesions are DRY and consist of:

    (a) *macules* or erythema, turn to .. .. § 624
    (b) *papules*, turn to .. .. § 635
    (c) *wheals*, turn to .. .. § 652
If (d) *scales* are a conspicuous feature turn to .. .. § 658

GROUP   II. If the lesions are MOIST and exudative with vesicles, bullæ or
                crusts, turn first to .. .. § 670
GROUP III. If the lesions are *pustular* turn first to .. .. .. § 687
GROUP IV. If the lesions are *multiform* .. .. § 705
GROUP V. If the lesions are *nodular* .. .. § 706
GROUP VI. If there is *ulceration* .. .. § 735
GROUP VII. If the lesions are *horny* or *warty* .. .. § 741

GROUP I. LESIONS USUALLY DRY

(a) *Eruptions which consist predominately of diffuse or localised Erythema*

Generalised	*Localised*
I. Exanthemata (§ 476).	I. Erythema pernio (chilblains) (§ 627); chronic perniosis; erythrocyanosis; acrocyanosis; livido reticularis.
II. Dermatitis medicamentosa (drug eruptions) (§ 624).	
III. Roseola syphilitica (§ 625).	II. Erythema solare (light eruptions) (§ 628).
IV. Erythema scarlatiniforme (§ 626).	III. Erythema intertrigo and gluteale (including napkin eruptions) (§ 629).
	IV. Rosacea (§ 630).
	V. Lupus erythematosus (§ 631).
	VI. Erysipelas and erysipeloid (§ 632).
	VII. Pellagra (§ 633).
	VIII. Other forms of erythema (§ 634).

Erythema, the visible manifestation of cutaneous vaso-dilatation, may occur at an early stage of many skin eruptions including the eczema-dermatitis group, but in the conditions listed above erythema is a conspicuous feature at all stages although it may be accompanied or followed by other changes.

I. The **Exanthemata** or eruptive fevers are fully described in Chapter XV, where they form Group I of the acute specific fevers.

§ 624. II. Dermatitis medicamentosa.—Drug eruptions are of great importance. They may give early warning of an acquired sensitivity to a drug, continued administration of which could have serious or even fatal consequences. Moreover, they may simulate a wide variety of other conditions. It is important to differentiate between drug eruptions which are the result of the direct toxic action of the drug and which may disappear if the dosage is reduced, and the very much more common eruptions which depend on one of several types of acquired allergic sensitivity and which are likely to recur when the drug, or related drugs, are administered even in minute doses. In other cases the eruption is the result of interference by the drug with the natural balance of bacterial or yeast flora. Few drug eruptions are specific but many drugs produce eruptions of certain well-defined types and it is therefore often possible to suspect that an eruption in a patient receiving many drugs is due to one rather than to another—often a matter of considerable importance. Eruptions caused by drugs in frequent use are listed below. Many drugs may provoke any one of a variety of different eruptions.

Erythema, which may be scarlatiniform: arsphenamine, atropine, belladonna, chloral hydrate, para-aminosalicylic acid, quinine.

Macules or *maculopapules*, often morbilliform: antipyrin, barbiturates, chloramphenicol, chlorpromazine, codeine, salts of gold and mercury, para-aminosalicylic acid, penicillin, phenylbutazone, streptomycin, sulphonamides, tetracyclines, thiouracil. A *morbilliform*, *scarlatiniform* or *eczematous* eruption may progress into an exfoliative dermatitis, if the drug is continued.

Urticaria: arsphenamine, gold salts, insulin, liver extracts, penicillin, salicylates and aspirin, foreign serum.

Erythema multiforme: barbiturates, phenylbutazone, salicylates.

Eczematous reactions: arsphenamine (often flexural at onset), salts of gold and mercury, penicillin, sulphonamides (favour light-exposed areas).

Bullæ: barbiturates (may simulate erythema multiforme exudativum), bromides, iodides.

Purpura: carbromal, iodides, meprobamate, quinidine, quinine, sedormid.

Anogenital pruritus and *dermatitis:* chloramphenicol, gold salts, tetracyclines.

Exfoliative dermatitis: arsphenamine, barbiturates, salts of gold and mercury, para-aminosalicylic acid, phenylbutazone.

Pigmentation: inorganic arsenic, salts of gold and silver, phenolphthalein.

Acneiform pustules: bromides, iodides.

Lichenoid papules: gold salts, mepacrine.

Keratoses: inorganic arsenical compounds.

Granulomatous nodules and *plaques:* bromides, iodides.

Fixed eruption: This is a sharply circumscribed round or oval plaque, red and œdematous, becoming dusky and violaceous. The œdema may be sufficiently intense to induce the formation of a large bulla on the plaque. When the reaction subsides brown pigmentation remains and persists for some weeks. The eruption recurs in the identical site whenever the drug responsible is ingested: antipyrin, phenytoin (Epanutin), phenacetin, phenolphthalein (in many proprietary laxatives), sulphonamides.

§ 625. III. Roseola syphilitica is the traditional term applied to the early macular eruption of secondary syphilis. It may develop within a week of the appearance of the chancre or as long as 6 or 8 weeks after. The roseola consists of pink or dull red macules from a few millimetres to over a centimetre in diameter. The sites of predilection are the abdomen and flanks, the back, shoulders and upper arms. The eruption may remain inconspicuous and fade in a few days or may become papular, when extension to the face, palms and soles often occurs.

Diagnosis is assisted by the presence of constitutional symptoms, generalised lymphadenopathy and mucosal erosions. The healing chancre may still be palpable. The Wassermann reaction is positive in 98·5 per cent. of cases; it is important to ask about recent treatment with antibiotics which may have modified the course of the disease. Differential diagnosis must exclude acute exanthemata, drug eruptions and pityriasis rosea.

§ 626. IV. Erythema Scarlatiniforme, as its name implies, closely resembles scarlet fever, but the onset may be subacute and fever and constitutional symptoms may be mild. There is no strawberry tongue, *Strep. hæmolyticus* cannot be isolated from the throat and recurrent attacks are not uncommon. If " surgical scarlatina " and drug eruptions are excluded many cases remain for which no cause can be discovered. Occasionally a scarlatiniform or morbilliform erythema occurs in association with food poisoning or after small-pox vaccination.

Erythema of more or less LOCALISED distribution

§ 627. I. Erythema pernio (Perniosis—Chilblains).—(i.) The common form affects mainly the toes, heels and fingers of children and young

women. They result from an abnormal response of the small vessels of
the skin to cold and damp; cold is not the only factor as they are relatively
uncommon outside England and Western Europe. Patches of erythema
are transformed into firm swellings by serous exudation. In severe cases
there may be blister formation and ulceration.

Treatment is often unsatisfactory. Warm clothing and sufficient
physical exercise are important. Nicotinic acid 25–50 mg. two or three
times daily is sometimes useful. Some find the following ointment helpful
—phenol 1, camphor 6, balsam of Peru 2, paraff. moll. 2·5, paraff. durum
7·5, anhydrous lanolin to 100.

(ii.) CHRONIC PERNIOSIS is often misdiagnosed as erythema induratum.
Young women are usually affected but these lesions also occur in either
sex at any age on limbs paralysed by poliomyelitis. Dull bluish-red
nodules develop on the lower calves and may ulcerate. They persist
throughout the colder months of the year and in severe cases may not
disappear completely even in the summer.

(iii.) ERYTHROCYANOSIS affects young women aged 12–25 (§ 585).
The lower legs are often fat with prominent follicles. A symmetrical
cyanotic erythema with a sharp lower margin just above the malleoli
extends six or nine inches up the posterior and lateral aspects of the legs.
The affected areas feel diffusely infiltrated. The changes are most marked
in the cold weather when nodular perniosis may develop but the disability
is largely cosmetic. The condition improves as the patient gets older.
Massage, surging sinusoidal baths, exercises and bandaging are useful;
warm stockings and fur-lined boots should be worn.

(iv.) In ACROCYANOSIS the hands are cold, blue and slightly puffy.
There are no episodes of blanching and no trophic changes. Women with
vaso-motor instability are usually affected (§ 585).

(v.) LIVEDO RETICULARIS presents as a dull red or slightly cyanotic
reticular mottling of the skin of the extremities. The changes are
accentuated by exposure to cold.

§ 628. II. **Erythema solare** (Sunburn) is the normal response of the
skin to exposure to ultraviolet light in the wavelength range 2,900–
3,300 Å. Erythema begins within an hour of exposure. If the dose
has been larger there is also œdema which reaches its maximum on the
second day when a secondary erythema may develop. Blistering, fever
and collapse occur in severe cases. Desquamation follows after several
days. Existing pigment begins to darken immediately after exposure and
new pigment is formed after a few days. Increased tolerance to sunlight
after repeated exposures is largely due to thickening of the horny layer.

Treatment.—Reasonably good protection against sunburn is provided
by para-aminobenzoic acid 10 per cent. in a vanishing cream base. If
sunburn is severe, and particularly if constitutional symptoms are present,
the patient should be put to bed and an antihistamine such as promethazine
hydrochlor. (Phenergan) 25 mg. t.d.s. prescribed. Bland local applications are indicated.

Other skin reactions caused by Sunlight include: (i.) *Eczema solare:* an eczematous reaction to sunlight. Even brief exposure may provoke erythema and œdema followed by exudation and crusting. It develops as the result of the photosensitising action of certain substances either ingested or in external contact with the skin. It may occur in the absence of any discoverable cause particularly after severe sunburn. Among the drugs the sulphonamides and chlorpromazine are the most common offenders; tar and some of its products, certain plants and vegetable oils are the most usual external sensitisers.

Treatment.—The cause must be determined and further contact avoided, but the light-sensitivity may be very persistent and treatment long and tedious.

(ii.) *Polymorphic light eruptions* (including Hutchinson's summer eruption and prurigo æstivalis) depend on an inborn or acquired sensitivity to sunlight. The lesions consist of irritable œdematous papules or dull red or pink plaques, and must be differentiated from lupus erythematosus. Light screens may be helpful but chloroquin in the doses used in lupus erythematosus is more effective.

(iii.) *Urticaria solaris* is rare: sensitisation to certain specific wavelengths of light results in the development of urticarial wheals in light-exposed areas.

(iv.) *Porphyria* is a rare defect of pigment metabolism. The congenital form starts in early infancy. Blisters may develop on light-exposed skin; the teeth and bones are stained red and the urine, which is characteristically pink, red or black, contains uroporphyrin I. In the acute form, which affects mainly adult women, there is no photosensitivity and abdominal and neurological symptoms predominate. A chronic type—porphyria cutanea tarda—affects both sexes, but most often men, usually after the age of 40. The exposed skin is pigmented, scarred and thickened and blisters develop from light or trauma (and see § 415).

(v.) *Hydroa æstivale* and *Xeroderma pigmentosum* are two rare inherited defects occurring in childhood. In the former blisters appear on light-exposed areas: they may leave vacciniform scars. Spontaneous recovery may take place at puberty. *Xeroderma pigmentosum* is a serious condition in which freckle-like pigmentation, atrophic scarring, telangiectasia and keratoses appear on light-exposed skin. The keratoses develop into epitheliomata and unless patients are kept under regular careful supervision the expectation of life is poor.

§ 629. III. Erythema intertrigo (Intertrigo) and erythema gluteale (Napkin Rash).

Symptoms.—Intertrigo affects those parts of the body where two skin surfaces are in close apposition, viz.: beneath the breasts, the axillæ, the upper and inner thighs, the genito-crural flexures, the natal cleft, and in infants the deep folds of the neck. At first there is a simple traumatic erythema strictly limited to the surfaces actually in contact, but friction and sweating often result in secondary infection and overtreatment may produce an eczematous dermatitis. The condition is more common in hot weather and in those who are overweight. Poor hygiene is an important contributory factor. One form is a manifestation of seborrhœic dermatitis.

Diagnosis.—*Tinea cruris* extends down the inner thighs as an inflammatory plaque with a vesicular margin. *Moniliasis* may show a festooned outline beyond which are the characteristic small flat pustules. *Psoriasis* in the older patient may involve the anogenital region; unless there are typical lesions elsewhere on the body differentiation may be difficult.

Treatment.—First examine the urine for sugar. Give the patient a low carbohydrate diet if she is overweight. In severe cases bed rest is an advantage. Bathe the affected surfaces with potassium permanganate

1/5,000, apply lotio calaminæ oleosa and then separate them with strips of gauze. After a few days substitute a simple dusting powder.

Erythema gluteale. *Symptoms.*—This common napkin eruption of infants must be differentiated from intertrigo. It spares the flexures and favours the convex surfaces, the buttocks, the genitalia, the backs of the calves, sometimes the lower abdominal wall and the heels. Initially a diffuse dull erythema, it may present as red eroded papules.

Diagnosis.—In congenital syphilis other stigmata of the disease are present.

Etiology.—The skin is irritated by ammonia produced by bacteria from urea. Secondary infection produces the later lesions.

Treatment.—The highest possible standard of hygiene is necessary and napkins should be frequently changed. The skin can be protected with soft paraffin B.P., ung. aquosum or a silicone barrier cream. When the napkins are thoroughly boiled and well rinsed they should require no further preparation but as an additional precaution they can be soaked in mercury perchloride solution (1 in 4,000) before the final rinse.

§ **630.** IV. **Rosacea** occurs in three stages: (1) The earliest consists of a recurrent congestive erythema of the nose and cheeks, and sometimes also of the forehead and chin. At first there are intervals of freedom but the erythema gradually becomes more persistent. (2) Later permanent dilatation of the small blood-vessels (telangiectasia) develops and further disfigurement is caused by papules and pustules in the congested areas. (3) In severe cases sebaceous hyperplasia may be marked and there may be gross enlargement of the nose (rhinophyma). An irregular dyspepsia may be associated with rosacea. Many patients notice that fatigue, anxiety, heat and exposure to sunlight aggravate the condition. Premenstrual exacerbations are common.

Mild blepharitis and conjunctivitis are often associated with rosacea but are non-specific. The most important associated ocular lesion is corneal vascularisation which can proceed to keratitis and corneal ulceration. The incidence of keratitis is not related to the severity of the rosacea and although the skin and ocular changes may develop simultaneously either may precede the other by many years.

Diagnosis is usually not difficult. In lupus erythematosus, atrophic scarring and horny follicular plugs are distinctive features. In acne, comedones are often present and congestive erythema is absent.

Etiology.—Rosacea is seen in patients of both sexes and at all ages from puberty onwards, but more often in women than men. In women it is common between 30 and 50 and in men between 50 and 65. The basic cause is vaso-motor instability due to emotional stress. It seems probable that endocrine and other factors which have been previously incriminated merely play a contributory role by increasing vaso-motor instability. Gastroscopic investigations suggest that changes in the gastric mucosa may parallel those in the skin, both having a common origin.

Treatment.—The patient must reduce his commitments and obtain sufficient relaxation. Tea, coffee, alcohol and other articles of diet causing flushing must be restricted. Mild sedation with phenobarbitone is often helpful. Although there is now known to be no constant association with achlorhydria, acid hydrochloric dil. ℥. 30 diluted and taken with the main meals is often useful. In women with menopausal symptoms œstrogens should be prescribed to control them. During the early congestive phase bland soothing local applications are required. Later lotio calaminæ with 2 per cent. sulphur can be applied by day and ichthammol 2 per cent. in zinc cream B.P. at night. Chloroquin 0·25 G. daily is valuable in light-sensitive cases. When there is papule and pustule formation or sebaceous hyperplasia zinc paste containing 2–4 per cent. sulphur should be used. Cryotherapy with a soft slush prepared from carbon dioxide snow, acetone and sulphur is valuable where there is disfiguring early rhinophyma or gross telangiectasia—weekly treatments over a period of two or three months can greatly improve the cosmetic appearance. In severe rhinophyma plastic surgery is indicated.

§ 631. V. **Lupus Erythematosus** has been intensively investigated in recent years and new diagnostic techniques have caused many cases to be recognised which previously masqueraded under other diagnoses.

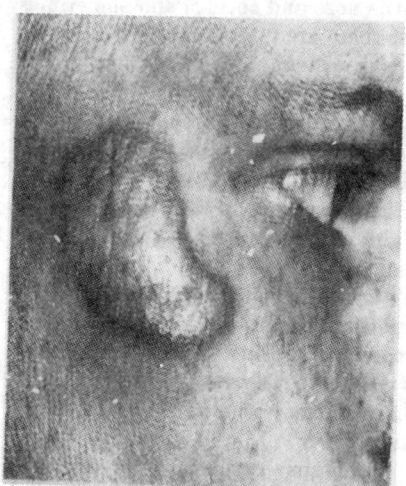

FIG. 178.—LUPUS ERYTHEMATOSUS. A sharply defined plaque of fixed erythema. The telangiectasia and the prominent plugged follicles can be distinguished.

Symptoms. — These may be local and limited to the skin, or generalised with marked systemic involvement. No sharp line can be drawn between the different types.

(A) The *localised* variety occurs in three forms: (i.) The *chronic discoid* type is the commonest variety. It especially affects women around 40 years of age. Lesions occur most frequently on the face where they assume a butterfly distribution or persist as discrete discoid patches. The scalp may be involved. A sharply defined plaque of congestive erythema is covered by scales, underneath which small plugs extend into the enlarged hair follicles. As congestion subsides atrophic scarring and telangiectasia become evident. Slow or rapid centrifugal extension may occur. (ii.) In the *acute localised œdematous* type the lesions are circumscribed œdematous plaques, which may completely disappear or may develop into chronic discoid lesions. (iii.) In the *chronic disseminated type,* numerous extensive lesions of the chronic discoid type are present but systemic symptoms are slight or absent and L.E. cells (see below) are not found.

(B) The *systemic* form is described in § 602. Skin lesions may be limited to transitory erythema and in many cases are entirely absent. Erythematous, purpuric or bullous eruptions are found in association with high fever, systemic symptoms and a positive test for L.E. cells in the acute disseminated variety. Active œdematous skin lesions with low-grade fever and milder systemic effects are present in the subacute disseminated disease—in which the L.E. test may be positive or negative.

Diagnosis.—In the localised varieties, diagnosis may be confirmed by histological examination. In the systemic types the skin changes, if present, may show no distinctive features. Laboratory procedures which help to establish a diagnosis are a raised erythrocyte sedimentation rate, leucopenia, hyperglobulinæmia and especially the finding of L.E. cells in the peripheral blood (§ 1212), or bone marrow (Plate XVII).

Etiology.—The cause is unknown. Many factors previously incriminated in individual cases are probably provocative rather than causative. Light sensitivity is frequent and exposure to sunlight may produce exacerbations. Hypersensitivity reactions to drugs, especially sulphonamides, are manifestations of progressive disturbance of immune responses which result in the persistence of harmful autoantibody to white and red blood cells and various tissue components.

Prognosis.—Chronic discoid lesions may in a few months regress to leave permanent scarring or may become active and periodically extend for many years before becoming permanently inactive. Some long-standing cases of the chronic discoid type develop into the acute systemic variety; this is most likely to occur in young women and seldom occurs in older women or in men. A large proportion of the acute generalised type are acute from the onset.

Treatment.—For the treatment of systemic disease see § 602. When the skin lesions are of the chronic discoid type and without systemic symptoms outpatient treatment is satisfactory. The antimalarial drugs are now the treatment of choice. Chloroquine, hydroxychloroquine and mepacrine are suitable: if one fails or is poorly tolerated the others should be tried. Treatment must be continued for several months. Chloroquine sulphate 0·2–0·6 G. daily or hydroxychloroquine sulphate 0·4–0·8 G. daily may cause slight nausea but side effects are few. Mepacrine 0·1 G. twice or thrice daily is an alternative, but produces yellow staining of the skin and rarely has caused aplastic anæmia. All drugs give best results in early cases. To prevent relapse a smaller maintenance dose is sometimes desirable after maximum improvement has been achieved. Cosmetic disfigurement by residual scarring can often be reduced by applications of carbon dioxide snow. Young women who are affected should avoid direct sunlight and can be provided with a light-screen (see § 628).

§ 632. VI. Erysipelas and **Erysipeloid** are described in § 478.

Symptoms of Erysipeloid.—The usual localised form develops after an incubation period of 2–3 days as a sharply marginated area of dusky erythema, at the border of which vesicles may be seen. Spontaneous cure occurs in about 3 weeks. A systemic form of the infection is very rare. *Treatment* with parenteral penicillin is rapidly effective.

§ **633.** VII. **Pellagra** is a deficiency disease of a complex origin.

Symptoms.—The classical triad of dermatitis, diarrhœa and dementia is encountered only in severe cases. *Prodromal symptoms* are anorexia, dyspepsia, loss of weight, asthenia, insomnia, depression and confusion. (i.) The *skin* lesions appear symmetrically on those parts of the body exposed to light—the face, neck, backs of hands and wrists and sometimes the lower legs, feet and ankles. Patchy or diffuse areas of erythema resembling severe sunburn soon becomes pigmented. Later these become scaly, thickened and cracked; they are sharply demarcated, often with a pigmented border. Hyperkeratosis, fissuring and pigmentation develop at sites of friction or pressure. Pigmentation and excoriation of the anogenital skin are often conspicuous. In the milder cases, such as are seen in Britain, there may be no skin lesions or only erythema and pigmentation. (ii.) The *gastro-intestinal* tract may be involved early, the patient complaining of burning and soreness of the tongue, mouth and throat and of excessive salivation (ptyalism). Nausea, vomiting, abdominal distension and pain after food are frequently present and severe persistent diarrhœa is characteristic of the later stages. The tongue is smooth, red and swollen and an aphthous stomatitis may develop. Achylia gastrica may be present, and some cases have anæmia, occasionally of megalocytic type. Vaginitis and proctitis may occur. (iii.) *Nervous symptoms* include in the early stages depression, apprehension, increased irritability, insomnia, headache and burning sensation in the extremities. Later tremor, jerky movements, altered reflexes and a spastic or ataxic gait occur. Many patients die in mental hospitals of a paranoid or delusional psychosis.

Etiology.—Pellagra occurs at any age and in any race, more commonly in women. It is endemic in the Southern United States, in some countries of Southern Europe and in the Middle East. The essential cause is deficiency of nicotinic acid, resulting from an inadequate intake of the vitamin, or its poor assimilation and utilisation or the ingestion of an antivitamin. Tryptophane, an essential amino-acid, present in most proteins, can partly replace nicotinic acid in the diet. Maize contains a negligible quantity of this amino-acid and also contains an antivitamin. Hence the high incidence of pellagra where maize forms the staple diet. Most victims of the disease also suffer from protein and other dietary deficiencies. The cases met in Britain usually occur in chronic alcoholics who substitute alcohol for food, in the elderly, indigent and eccentric and in patients with extensive disease of the gastro-intestinal tract or liver, when assimilation of food is impaired.

Prognosis.—The disease runs a chronic course and is subject to partial remissions which may be seasonal but, untreated, it is ultimately fatal in from 3 to 15 years.

Treatment.—It is doubtful whether the administration of nicotinic acid alone will prevent or cure pellagra if the diet is also deficient in protein and in the other water-soluble vitamins. The patient should be treated in bed on a diet high in calories, low in carbohydrate and rich in protein, with ample fresh milk, lean meat, marmite and fresh vegetables. Whole vitamin B complex should be given, and if specific signs of B_1 deficiency are present this vitamin should be administered parenterally in large doses. Nicotinamide is necessary orally in a daily dose of 500 mg. for 7–10 days and then in a small maintenance dose. In severe cases 200 mg. daily should be given parenterally. Iron and ascorbic acid are usually also required.

§ **634.** VIII. **Other forms of erythema:** (i.) Erythema may be produced by the action of *primary irritants* and may proceed to eczema. The *diagnosis* should be established by the distribution and the history. (ii.) Erythema occurs together with scaling in *exfoliative dermatitis* (§ 665). (iii.) In *dermatomyositis*, erythema especially of the face, and associated

with swelling of the eyelids, is a frequent early manifestation (§ 606).
(iv.) In *pregnancy* until after delivery and in *hepatic cirrhosis* there is
often erythema of the palms and of the soles of the feet. (v.) *Leprosy*
may present as dull red macules or plaques (§ 715). (vi.) *Annular
erythema.* Annular lesions may occur in Urticaria. The other forms of
annular erythema are uncommon. *E. annulare centrifugum* occurs on the
trunk, thighs or upper arms and slowly enlarging infiltrated rings may
persist for months or longer before undergoing spontaneous involution.
E. chronica migrans is probably a reaction to the bite of certain insects.
E. annulare rheumaticum consists of a patchy broken network of small
rings, is transitory, and is frequently associated with rheumatic fever.

(b) *Eruptions which in their typical forms are predominantly papular*

Common.		Rare.
I. Acne vulgaris (§ 635).	VIII.	Granuloma annulare (§ 644).
II. Prurigo (§ 636).	IX.	Papular syphilide (§ 645).
III. Lichen planus (§ 637).	X.	Tuberculides (§ 646).
IV. Plane warts (§ 638).	XI.	Keratosis pilaris (§ 647).
V. Molluscum contagiosum (§ 639).	XII.	Keratosis follicularis (Darier's
VI. Scabies (§ 640): other Mite infes-		Disease) (§ 648).
tations (§ 641) including Pedi-	XIII.	Adenoma sebaceum (§ 649).
culosis Corporis and P. Pubis	XIV.	Fox-Fordyce Disease (§ 650).
(§ 642).	XV.	Eruptions which may occur in
VII. Erythema multiforme (§ 643).		papular forms or may pass
		through a papular stage (§ 651).

§ 635. I. **Acne Vulgaris** in its mildest form afflicts the majority of
adolescents. In at least 10 per cent. it is of sufficient severity to induce
the patient to seek treatment.

Symptoms.—The characteristic lesion is the comedo, a blackened horny
follicular plug. In most cases the eruption is polymorphic and consists
of varying combinations of comedones, papules, pustules, indurated
nodules and cysts. The sites of predilection are the face, the back and
shoulders, the chest and the back of the neck. Many patients with acne
have a greasy, coarse, thickened skin with prominent follicular orifices.
The scalp is often greasy or scaly.

Acne usually appears at puberty but may develop considerably later.
Some forms of facial acne in women may first appear in the middle twenties
and acne of the back or of the neck in men often develops after the age of
25. The maximum incidence is between 17 and 19 after which it declines
but severe cases persisting for many years are by no means rare.

Diagnosis seldom presents difficulty. If halogen eruptions are excluded only papular *syphilides*, certain papular *tuberculides* and *adenoma
sebaceum* require consideration.

Etiology.—Both the basic seborrhœic state and the tendency to acne
itself may be familial. Androgenic stimulation of the pilosebaceous
follicles and thickening of the horny layer take place at puberty: acne is
unknown in castrates. In some older patients the ratio of androgenic to

œstrogenic substances may be abnormal but in the great majority an increased susceptibility of the follicles to normal levels of androgen must be postulated. The pilosebaceous follicle functions as a unit for the formation of both hair and sebum and when much sebum is formed the hair is too small to maintain the patency of the follicular orifice. The various types of acne lesion then arise from the retention of sebum and the reaction of the tissues to its presence. A contributory role in its development and persistence is played by numerous factors which may stimulate sebaceous secretion, interfere with the free escape of sebum from the follicles or increase the secondary inflammatory changes. These include (i.) fatigue and emotional stress, (ii.) certain foods, particularly chocolate, (iii.) lack of open-air exercise, (iv.) the habit of squeezing the lesions or of sitting for long periods with the hands to the face. (v.) " Tonics " and other medicines containing iodides or bromides can cause acute pustular exacerbations, as do (vi.) the *Corticosteroids*.

Special Varieties.—(1) *Occupational acne* may be caused by (a) *mineral oils* which also provoke follicular pustulation on the forearms and thighs. (b) *Tar* or *pitch*, when pigmentation and light-sensitivity are often associated with small acneiform papules of the face, arms and thighs. (c) *Chlorinated naphthalene* and related substances which cause a widespread eruption of large comedones on the face and trunk and sometimes on the genitalia. (2) *Acne excorié* occurs in young women. The underlying lesions of acne vulgaris may be trivial but the excoriations may be disfiguring. Psychiatric treatment is sometimes required. (3) *Acne varioliformis* is uncommon. Indolent papules along the frontal hair-margin and on the temples heal to leave pitted scars.

Treatment.—It is never justifiable to inform a young person that he will " grow out " of his acne. A great many will do so, but in others the persistence of disfiguring lesions, perhaps leaving permanent scars, can have important psychological consequences at a shy and self-conscious age. All cases, however mild, need vigorous and sympathetic treatment. First attend to the contributory factors mentioned above. The patient must have sufficient sleep, a well-balanced diet and open-air exercise. Affected regions should be washed twice daily with hot water and soap. If there are many comedones they should be removed with a comedo expressor after steaming the face. Local applications are designed to produce peeling; in the mildest cases lotio calaminæ (B.P.) with 2 per cent. precipitated sulphur may suffice. More commonly lotio sulphuris co. (N.F.) or lotio potass. sulphurata c. zinco (N.F.) will be prescribed. In the average case one of these lotions should be applied each morning and sulphur 6 per cent. in zinc paste or Pasta resorcin et sulph. (N.F.) each night. The strength of the application can be progressively increased.

Vitamin A (50,000 units twice daily) may be of value, especially in cases with much comedo formation. The use of œstrogens appears logical but since they are only effective in high doses which produce undesirable side effects, it is doubtful whether in males they should be given even to the most severe cases. Broad spectrum antibiotics administered for long

PLATE XIX

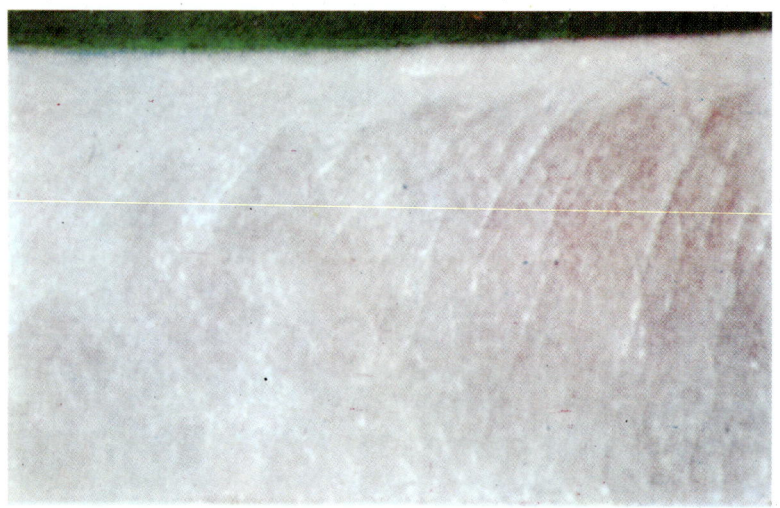

Fig. 179.—LICHEN PLANUS OF THE FLEXOR ASPECT OF THE FOREARM.

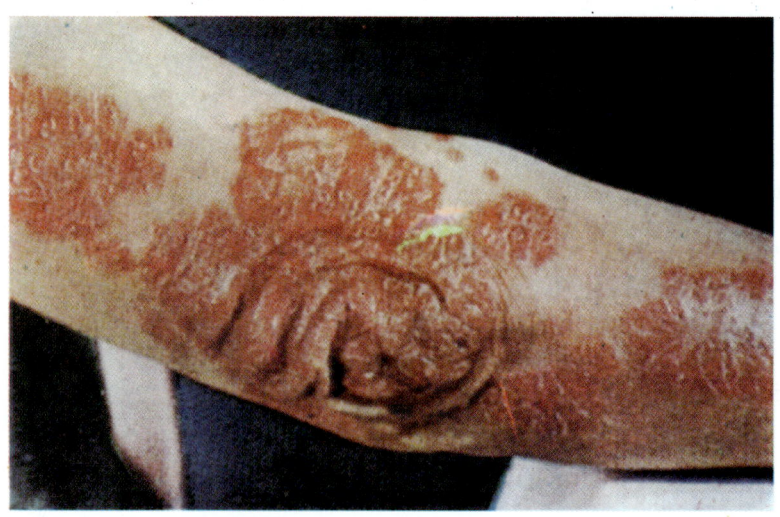

Fig. 183.—PSORIASIS OF THE ELBOW REGION.

periods often control pustular and cystic lesions and are justifiable in acute exacerbations or where serious scarring would result. Chlortetracycline or triacetyloleandomycin (Evramycin) is given in a dose of 125–250 mg. daily after initial control with a higher dose for a few days. Staphylococcal toxoid or vaccines are of questionable value but may be given intradermally rather than subcutaneously in pustular acne. Ultraviolet light is valuable. Superficial X-ray therapy is seldom necessary. Acne scarring may be improved by applications of carbon dioxide snow or by dermabrasion.

§ **636. II. Prurigo.**—Barber defined as prurigo a condition in which itching is the first and essential symptom, but in which certain skin changes are present either primarily or as the result of scratching. Dermatological text-books formerly devoted much space to this condition but the majority of the diseases so classified are now more logically considered under other headings. The term is still employed in a descriptive sense and for the rare disorders, prurigo nodularis and prurigo of Hebra.

Prurigo of Besnier—the later form of infantile eczema; see § 671(2).

Prurigo simplex—Papular urticaria; see § 656.

§ **637. III. Lichen planus** is of unknown origin: nervous factors seem frequently to play an important role. It is rare in childhood and is usually seen in middle life, affecting women rather more often than men.

Symptoms.—On the *skin* the characteristic lesion is a shining flat-topped, polygonal papule, dull pink or violaceous in colour. This is usually irritable, especially at the onset: irritation may be very severe. The sites of predilection are the flexor surfaces of the wrists and forearms, around the waist, the inner surfaces of the thighs and the lower legs. Other sites may be involved and the eruption may either be widespread or limited to a single site. New papules

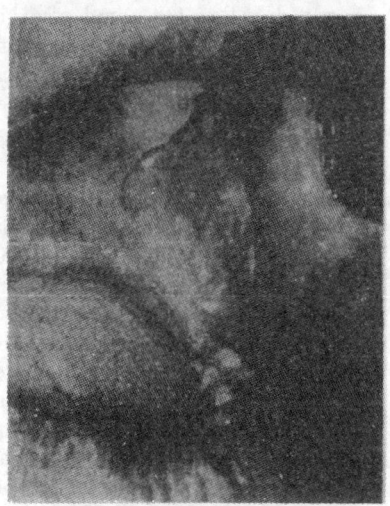

FIG. 180.—LICHEN PLANUS on the mucous membrane of the mouth. The lacey milk-white patches may confirm the diagnosis of suspected skin lesions. If only the mucous membrane is involved confusion with leucoplakia is possible. A tongue depressor is seen on the top right-hand corner of the photograph.

tend to appear in scratch marks. In severe cases of acute onset the papules may be light pink in colour and slightly œdematous. On the lower legs they are often hypertrophic, large and horny. Annular lesions may occur especially on the glans penis and on the forehead. The *oral mucous membrane* may be involved, either alone, or with an eruption elsewhere. The lesions appear as milky-white papules or as irregularly reticulate chalky streaks, which are often confused with leucoplakia. On the *scalp* a cicatricial alopecia is produced.

Diagnosis.—The lichenoid drug eruptions occasionally provoked by mepacrine, and by gold and bismuth salts must be considered.

Prognosis.—It runs a variable course. Some cases clear in a month or two but others persist for many months or even years. The papules are usually followed by marked pigmentation.

Treatment.—Acute cases benefit from rest in bed and if very severe may be treated with the corticosteroids which in small doses may be rapidly curative. Sedation is usually required to lessen the irritation. Preparations of bismuth or mercury have recently fallen into disrepute as controlled studies suggest the heavy metals do not affect the course of the disease. Calamine lotion or other bland antipruritic applications may help. In hypertrophic lichen planus salicylic acid ointment (5 per cent.) or occlusive tar paste bandages (such as Coltapaste) are useful. An intralesional injection of triamcinolone cures a localised hypertrophic plaque.

§ **638.** IV. **Plane warts** are caused by the same virus as common warts (§ 741) especially in children and young women. They are skin-coloured or greyish-yellow flat papules varying from a pin's head to 5 mm. or more in diameter, and often in very large numbers. They particularly occur on the backs of the hands and the face. New warts tend to appear in scratch marks. For *Treatment* see § 741.

§ **639.** V. **Molluscum Contagiosum** is a relatively uncommon virus infection.

Symptoms.—The lesions develop in the course of a few weeks as domed shining white papules, often umbilicated and traditionally compared with pearl buttons. There may be a solitary lesion or many hundreds. They are frequently irregularly grouped in one region of the body—the face including the eyelids, the trunk, the thighs and genitalia. They may persist unchanged for many months or may, sometimes after trauma, become acutely inflamed and undergo spontaneous cure.

Etiology.—Hired or borrowed towels at swimming or Turkish baths may transmit the infection, but frequently its source cannot be ascertained.

Treatment is simple. The lesions may be removed with a sharp curette using an ethyl chloride spray to provide local analgesia or pure trichloracetic acid may be applied to the centre of each papule on a sharpened wooden probe.

§ **640.** VI. **Scabies and other Mite infestations.**—The reaction of the host to infestation by ectoparasites, and hence the nature of the skin lesions, may be modified by the development of an allergic sensitivity either to substances injected in biting or to the parasite itself, its excreta and débris. Scratching and secondary infection may partially conceal the original lesions.

The *primary* lesions of scabies are burrows, vesicles and papules. The burrows are $\frac{1}{4}$–$\frac{1}{2}$ inch long and may be curved or S-shaped: they are usually situated between the fingers, on the ulnar border of the hand, on the anterior axillary folds, around the nipples or on the penis, and in infants on the palms or soles.   The vesicles may occur at the inner end of burrows, or independently of burrows, especially at the sides of the fingers.   The papules are small and numerous and are seen mainly on the thighs, buttocks and abdominal wall.   The *secordary* lesions are scratch marks, pustules and impetigo—the presence of impetigo on the buttocks or in other unusual sites should always suggest the possibility of scabies.   Irritation is often severe, especially at night, but may be mild in those of low intelligence.

Etiology.—Scabies is caused by *Sarcoptus* (*Acarus*) *scabiei*.   The fertilised adult female burrows into the skin, extending the small " moulting pocket " in which she was previously maturing, to form a tunnel in which eggs are laid.   The disease is transmitted by close contact: spread by fomites is uncommon.   In most parts of Britain scabies is now rare but the incidence may possibly be increasing.   It was extremely common during World War II, but war conditions cannot be solely responsible as a steady increase was noted in many countries for 3-4 years before the War.

The *Diagnosis* is usually suggested by the distribution of the eruption but the burrows should always be sought—with a little practice the acarus can be lifted out of a burrow on the point of a needle.

Treatment must be a family affair.   Unless close contacts of the patient are examined and treated constant reinfection will occur.   Sulphur ointment has been largely replaced by more effective remedies, which include emulsion of benzyl benzoate (25 per cent.), tetraethylthiuram monosulphide (Tetmosol) and crotamiton ointment (Eurax).   Whichever preparation is employed the following routine should be closely followed:— the patient must take a hot bath, apply the remedy to the entire skin surface except the face and neck, and then resume his previous day and night clothing.   Repeat this procedure after 48 hours, when the underclothing and bedding must be changed.   Normal washing provides adequate disinfection of clothing and bedding.   When treatment has been properly carried out failures are few: treatment should not be repeated within a fortnight and never without a further careful medical examination.

Other forms of Scabies.—*Norwegian scabies* produces thick crusted lesions in the usual distribution of scabies, but in addition the nails may be grossly thickened. Mental defectives, especially Mongols, are commonly affected, but it can occur in malnourished patients of normal intelligence.   It is an abnormal host reaction to the *Sarcoptus scabiei*.   The usual *treatment* is employed.

Animal scabies may occasionally occur in man.   Horse, camel and cat scabies have been reported.   The eruption is papular or papulovesicular but there are no burrows.

§ **641. Other Mite infestations** are uncommon, but many are certainly overlooked. *Grain itch*, caused by *Pediculoides ventricosus*, affects farm labourers handling straw or dockers unloading cargoes of grain.   *Copra* and *cheese mites*, *rat mites* and the *mites of domestic birds*, poultry or small cage-birds, may at times give rise to eruptions of papules, wheals and papulovesicles.   The distribution of the lesions depends on the mode of exposure to the mite.   There are no burrows.

§ 642. **Pediculosis corporis** must be remembered as a cause of generalised pruritus, especially in the elderly and indigent. Primary lesions are rarely seen but excoriations, secondary infection and pigmentation are often conspicuous. The ova or nits are found in the creases of the clothing, and occasionally on the body hairs.

Pediculosis pubis is caused by the crab-louse, *Phthirius pubis*, and is often transmitted by venereal contact.

Symptoms.—There is pruritus of the pubic region; there may be bluish macular stains on the lower abdominal wall. Constitutional symptoms such as headache and malaise can accompany heavy infestation.

Treatment.—Both forms of pediculosis readily respond to local applications of DDT powder.

OTHER INSECT BITES are due to *bed bugs* and *fleas*, human and animal. *Mosquitoes, gnats, harvest mites* and other insects can cause urticarial wheals, more persistent papules or bullæ according to the victim's sensitivity to the injected substances. The *diagnosis* is usually suggested by the asymmetrical distribution in irregular groups on exposed parts or around constrictions in the clothing but varies according to the biting habits of the individual species. *Treatment.*—Dimethyl phthalate is a useful repellent. The relationship of papular urticaria to insect bites is discussed in § 656.

§ 643. VII. Erythema Multiforme.

Symptoms.—In the usual form crops of dull or bluish-red, œdematous papules are symmetrically distributed on the back of the hands, the forearms, the backs of the feet, the buccal and other mucous membranes and

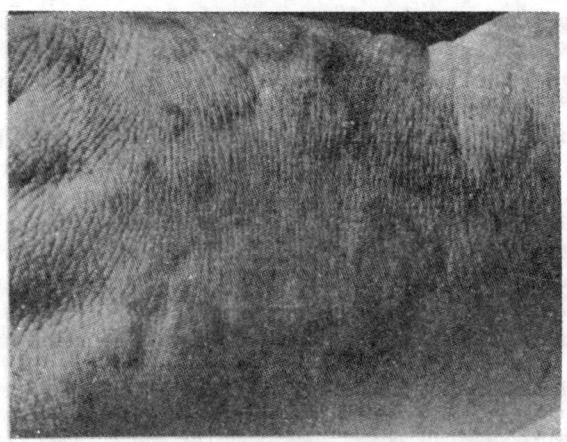

FIG. 181.—ERYTHEMA MULTIFORME. The back of the hand is a common site. Note the "target" appearance of individual lesions.

the face and neck. Lesions may also occur on the palms and the soles. In the mildest cases only the hands are involved but in serious cases the eruption may be generalised. There may be a preceding sore throat and some constitutional symptoms but these are often absent. The lesions take two or three weeks to clear, but recurrent attacks, which may be seasonal, are not uncommon. *Variations.* In the *Iris* type of E. multiforme the lesions show three zones, a central bulla, which may be hæmorrhagic, a cyanotic zone and a red periphery. Other clinical forms show varying combinations of wheals, bullæ and purpura. The severe bullous variant (*E. multiforme exudativum*) is described in § 682.

Diagnosis is based on the distribution and the characteristic appearance of the lesions. The histological changes differentiate clinically similar eruptions.

Etiology.—The term *E. multiforme* was formerly applied rather indiscriminately to a variety of eruptions of polymorphic character but is now restricted to (i.) a benign and often recurrent eruption, of unknown origin, (ii.) morphologically similar eruptions provoked by various recognisable causes:—drugs, especially phenobarbitone; systemic bacterial infections; herpes simplex, which may be associated with recurrent attacks, often of the *iris* type; malignant disease; deep X-ray therapy.

Treatment is rarely necessary in the common idiopathic type. In the symptomatic type the cause should be sought and eliminated.

§ **644.** VIII. **Granuloma annulare** is relatively uncommon: it usually occurs in children or young adults.

Symptoms.—The lesions are firm skin-coloured papules which are frequently but

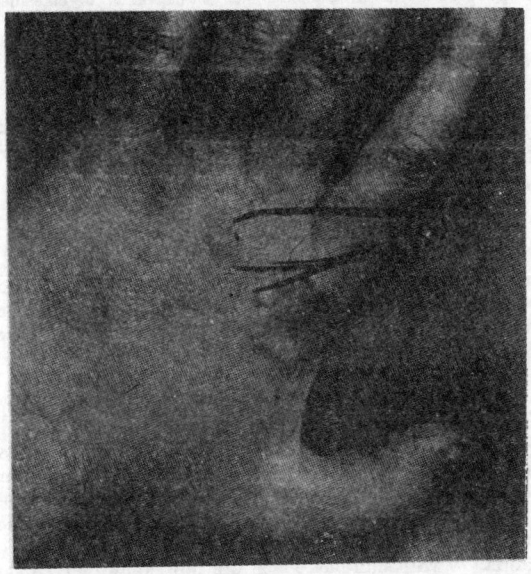

FIG. 182.—GRANULOMA ANNULARE.

not always in rings. They occur typically on the backs of the hands, on the feet or on the extensor surfaces of the arms and legs. They may persist for months or years, but ultimately disappear spontaneously.

Etiology.—The cause is unknown.

Treatment.—Some have claimed good results from vitamin E (α-tocopherol) 300 mg. daily. The lesions sometimes disappear when traumatised accidentally or after a biopsy, and in areas such as the fingers under Elastoplast occlusion. Unsightly lesions may be effectively treated by infiltration with cortisone acetate suspension.

§ **645. IX. Papular Syphilide.**—The papule is the distinctive lesion of secondary syphilis and usually occurs within six months after infection, but occasionally much later, especially in relapses after inadequate treatment.

Symptoms.—The papules may be the earliest skin lesion or may follow a macular eruption. They are indurated, copper-coloured and occur most commonly on the face, arms, palms, soles, abdomen and anogenital region, but may be generalised. There is often wide variation in the size of the papules: in general in the earlier stages they are numerous, small and symmetrically distributed, and in the later stage fewer, larger (lenticular) and often grouped. Special terms are used to describe numerous morphological variants—*corymbose, lichenoid, follicular,* etc. Itching is usually absent. Constitutional symptoms may be present; the patient looks and feels ill. Generalised enlargement of lymphatic glands is usual. In the anogenital region and sometimes in other areas where the skin is macerated by sweating and friction *condylomata* occur. These are moist papules, bathed in highly infective secretions; they may become hypertrophic.

§ **646. X. Tuberculosis of the skin** is now relatively uncommon in Britain as the result of more effective methods of treatment, improved living conditions and public health measures which reduce the opportunities for spread of infection. The clinical manifestations depend on the route by which the organism reaches the skin and the patient's immunological state.

The more important forms of *cutaneous tuberculosis* may be classified in two main groups:

A. **Progressive tuberculosis of the skin**

1. The Primary complex (§ 738).
2. Lupus vulgaris (§ 709).
3. Tuberculosis verrucosa (§ 744).
4. Scrofuloderma (§ 738).
5. Tuberculous ulcers in advanced disease (§ 738).

B. **The Tuberculides**

1. Erythema induratum (§ 707).
2. Papulonecrotic tuberculides.
3. Lichen scrofulosorum.

The TUBERCULIDES are the result of hæmatogenous dissemination of tubercle bacilli in those who have developed some degree of allergy and immunity to the infection. The *papulonecrotic tuberculide* occurs in children and young adults. Crops of dusky red firm papules appear on the backs of the hands and feet, the knees and the elbows, and occasionally on other sites. The papules break down to form small indolent ulcers, and heal in a few weeks, leaving depressed scars. Crops may appear at irregular intervals for months. *Acnitis* or *acne agminata* is a papulonecrotic tuberculide presenting as groups of brownish-red papules on the cheeks, the upper lip, forehead and chin, leaving small scars. *Lichen scrofulosorum* is now very rare. The eruption consists of discoid or oval groups of small skin-coloured follicular papules on the trunk of children: it gradually involutes over a period of months.

Many conditions were formerly regarded as tuberculides solely on inadequate histological criteria. Two conditions which are now known to be non-tuberculous are conveniently considered here. (i.) *Lupus miliaris facei* is seen in adults as an eruption of small discrete brownish-red papules, often grouped around the eyelids, on the cheeks and around the angles of the mouth. (ii.) The so-called *rosaceous tuberculide* usually occurs in women who, on a rosaceous background of erythema and telangiectasia, develop crops of yellowish-brown papules on the forehead, the sides of the cheeks and the chin. Both conditions are of unknown origin and are benign.

§ **647. XI. Keratosis Pilaris** occurs mainly in children and young adults as skin-coloured horny follicular papules on the extensor surfaces of the limbs. It is often associated with ichthyosis and may occur in vitamin A and vitamin C deficiencies. *Treatment.*—An ointment of salicylic acid (5 per cent.) will remove the lesions and vitamins should be prescribed when indicated.

§ **648.** XII. **Keratosis Follicularis** (Darier's Disease) is rare. The eruption consists of skin-coloured or brownish firm spherical follicular papules with a rather greasy surface. They may become confluent and in intertriginous areas may be moist, crusted and vegetating. The distribution is variable, but is usually symmetrical and often involves the face, neck, chest and back and later the limbs and inguinal region. The nail plates are often thickened. The cause is unknown. Familial cases have been reported. *Diagnosis* is confirmed by biopsy as the histological changes are distinctive. *Treatment* with high doses of vitamin A is sometimes successful. Local measures include keratolytic ointments and, for limited areas, X-ray therapy.

§ **649.** XIII. **Adenoma Sebaceum** is one of the cutaneous manifestations of the rare congenital neurocutaneous syndrome known as Tuberous Sclerosis or Epiloia (§§ 1049, 1194 (c)). Small hemispherical teleangiectatic papules appear on the nose and cheeks, often in a " butterfly " distribution, in childhood or occasionally at or after puberty. The other manifestations of the syndrome should be sought. Cosmetic *treatment* of the skin lesions may be undertaken with the diathermy.

§ **650.** XIV. **Fox-Fordyce Disease** is rare. Most patients are women. Numerous intensely irritating small smooth skin-coloured or pink papules occur in the axillæ, the pubic region and on the areolæ of the nipples. *Treatment* is difficult, but X-ray therapy or thorium-X may be helpful.

§ **651.** XV. *Eruptions which occur in papular forms or pass through a papular stage.* Mild or early eczematous eruptions may be papular but the development of the groups of typical papulovesicles usually rapidly establishes the diagnosis. Some *drug eruptions* are papular (§ 624). The *guttate form of psoriasis* may present as an extensive papular eruption. Horny papules on the backs of the fingers are a feature of pityriasis rubra pilaris (§ 668).

C. Wheals

The varieties are:

I. Evanescent spontaneous whealing
   Urticaria: Angioneurotic œdema (§ 652).
   Cholinergic urticaria (§ 653).
II. Whealing provoked by friction
   On normal skin—Dermographism (§ 654).
   On pigmented macules or nodules—Urticaria pigmentosa (§ 764).
III. Wheals succeeded by papules
   Insect bites (§ 655).
   Papular urticaria (§ 656).
IV. Wheals and large painless swellings
   Loiasis (§ 657).

§ **652.** I. **Urticaria** (Nettle-rash, Hives). *Symptoms.*—There is a localised or widespread eruption of wheals preceded and accompanied by severe itching. The individual wheal is evanescent, often fading after a few minutes, and seldom persisting longer than a few hours. Often therefore no lesions are present at the time of examination and a diagnosis must be made on the history. The wheals are frequently about 1 cm. in diameter, firm pink or white papules surrounded by a red flare, but the size and shape are very variable and annular and gyrate configurations are not uncommon.

Urticaria is rare before 10 or after 60 years of age; women are more often affected than men. Acute and chronic forms occur. Acute attacks may be ushered in by mild gastro-intestinal or other constitutional symptoms and fever and may last for a few hours or for several days. In the chronic forms constitutional symptoms are rare. ` It may recur at short intervals, sometimes at the same hour each day, for months or years.

In GIANT URTICARIA (Angioneurotic œdema: Quincke's disease) the wheals are very large and involve the subcutaneous tissue producing firm circumscribed swellings. Characteristically the lips, eyelids and genitalia are swollen but the giant wheals may involve the limbs or trunk or the tongue and the glottis, possibly with fatal results. Men are affected slightly more often than women and there may be a familial tendency. Giant urticaria is present in over 10 per cent. of cases of common urticaria.

Pathogenesis of the Wheal.—The urticarial wheal is analogous to the " triple response " of Lewis after the introduction of histamine into the skin. This and allied substances act directly on the minute vessels of the skin and also initiate an axon-reflex. Because the release of histamine with the production of whealing can result from antigen–antibody reactions it must not be assumed that all cases necessarily have an allergic basis. Many different mechanisms are probably concerned.

Etiology.—In acute urticaria the cause can frequently be established but in chronic and recurrent urticaria the cause often remains unknown even after the most careful investigation. In general, investigation by skin tests is not of value and elimination diets and trial exposure to the suspected cause must be employed. Common causes are: (i.) Food allergy. Shell-fish and crustacea are the commonest of a wide variety of foods which have been incriminated. Gastro-intestinal symptoms are often also present. (ii.) Drug allergy (see § 624). Some drugs, notably penicillin, give rise either to simple urticaria or to a reaction of serum sickness type in which fever, joint pain and swelling are associated with urticaria. (iii.) Inhalant allergy is not a common cause of urticaria although it may occasionally accompany attacks of hay fever. (iv.) Parasites: intestinal worms, hydatid disease, amœbiasis. (v.) Bacterial infection was formerly believed to be a frequent cause and alleged " septic foci " were eradicated. Proven cases are very uncommon. Mild cases of anaphylactoid purpura (§ 767) may present as a purely urticarial reaction mainly on the extensor surface of the limbs and buttocks. The purpuric element may fail to develop. (vi.) Physical factors. Urticaria may be provoked by light, cold, heat or exertion. The diagnosis can usually be established if the possibility is recognised. Cold urticaria is of particular importance as sudden immersion in cold water may provoke an intense reaction with collapse from histaminic shock and a real risk of death from drowning. (vii.) Psychogenic factors are of the greatest importance. Fatigue and

overwork predispose and frustration and resentment are more lrectly
provocative. In many cases more than one factor is oncerned.
Endocrine and metabolic disturbances may play a contributo role. In
angioneurotic œdema the same complex of factors requires investigation
and the same two groups are distinguished: the acute cases are often
caused by drug and food allergy and the chronic cases are often of emotional
but sometimes of unknown origin.

Treatment.—If specific allergic sensitivity is conclusively established
the food or drug responsible should be avoided. If this is impracticable
desensitisation can be considered but the treatment may be hazardous and
the result uncertain. In urticaria of emotional origin the patient is often
helped greatly if she discusses her problems with her doctor. Psychiatric
advice may be required. Local applications are not of great value but
lotio calaminæ B.P. to which is added phenol 1 per cent. may give slight
relief. In an acute attack of angioneurotic œdema inject. adrenalin
hydrochlor. B.P. ℳ 1–10 subcutaneously is usually effective. Ephedrine
gr. $\frac{1}{4}$–$\frac{1}{2}$ twice daily may be useful. The antihistamines are less effective
than in urticaria. These drugs may be safely administered over prolonged
periods but care should be taken in the choice of drug and its dose. The
anti-whealing effect varies considerably from one individual to another and
the character and severity of the side effects are even more variable.
Promezathine hydrochloride (Phenergan) 25 mg. b.d. or .t.d.s. and
chlorcyclizine hydrochloride (Histantin) 75 mg. t.d.s. have a powerful
anti-whealing effect. Both cause less drowsiness than diphenhydramine
hydrochloride (Benadryl). Many other antihistamines are available. It
is often useful to combine Phenergan or Histantin by day with Benadryl
at night.

In some cases a period of rest and hypnotics to ensure sound sleep prove
of greater value. Any probably contributory or predisposing factors
should be treated. In some resistant cases of unknown cause a course of
autohæmotherapy or intramuscular injections of a crude liver extract may
quite empirically prove helpful.

It is important to differentiate true urticaria including giant urticaria ·
in which the symptoms consist solely of wheals arising spontaneously, from
dermographism and from the conditions in which the urticarial wheal
represents but one phase of an eruption of different character—papular
urticaria and urticaria pigmentosa.

§ 653. In **Cholinogenic Urticaria** the eruption is profuse and consists of very
small rounded wheals of uniform size surrounded by irregular flares, and occurs
especially in young adults or in children. Attacks are provoked by warmth, exertion,
excitement or by injections of cholinergic drugs. The attacks may be suppressed by
antihistamines in larger doses than are required in histaminic urticarias.

§ **654.** II. **Dermographism** (Factitious urticaria) was found by Lewis
in 5 per cent. of healthy subjects. A wheal results from firm pressure on
the skin with a blunt point. Dermographism is not more common in
patients with urticaria: the cause is not known but there is no evidence

that it is allergic.　Dermographism is often a coincidental finding but it is sometimes of clinical significance: the patient complains of generalised irritation and may have noticed wheals at sites of friction or after scratching.　This condition has been called dermographic prurigo and may be of psychogenic origin.

§ 655. III. Insect bites, nettle stings, jelly-fish stings, etc., may induce simple wheal formation by the introduction of a foreign substance.　With many insect bites an acquired sensitivity to the injected substance modifies and prolongs the tissue response—see papular urticaria.

§ 656. Papular Urticaria (Strophulus, Lichen urticatus, Prurigo simplex) occurs most frequently in children between 1 and 5: infants and adults may be affected.　The essential lesion is an evanescent wheal replaced by a small firm papule which may persist for up to a week: a pigmented macule may follow.　The papules may be surmounted by small vesicles: on the legs they may be bullous.　New lesions characteristically develop in irregular groups at intervals over a period of weeks or months.　They are most numerous on the legs, thighs and buttocks but can occur anywhere, even on the palms and soles, and in some reported series have been numerous on the face and neck.　The condition is much commoner in warm weather and may clear in the winter only to recur the following summer.　It invariably ceases immediately a child is admitted to hospital irrespective of his diet.

Etiology.—In newborn babies and other persons not previously bitten by a particular insect species there may be no perceptible reaction.　After repeated bites an allergic sensitivity may be acquired and, depending on the degree of sensitivity, a wheal, followed by a papule or bulla results. Further bites may produce desensitisation.　The biphasic wheal-papule lesion has never been experimentally produced by an allergic reaction to foods and it is likely that it is always of parasitic origin.　The insects responsible vary with the environment.　Cat and dog fleas are common offenders: gnats, mosquitoes, harvest mites and occasionally bed bugs may be incriminated.

Diagnosis.—Papular urticaria must be differentiated from true urticaria which is not common in children and from cholinogenic urticaria which is sometimes seen in older children.　In both these conditions evanescent wheals and not persistent papules occur mainly on the trunk.

Treatment depends on tracing and eliminating the source of infestation. DDT dusting powder may be freely used and insect repellents are helpful.

§ 657. IV. Loiasis (Syn. Calabar Swellings) is due to the filarial worm loa-loa (§ 542).　It is present only in the tropical rain forests of Africa which extend from the Gulf of Guinea to the Great Lakes—but in this region it is common.

Symptoms are due to a local anaphylactic reaction caused by the adult worms which inhabit the subcutaneous tissues.　The results are seldom dangerous.　There are (i.) brawny itchy urticarial reactions, sometimes with pain: these usually last one or ' two days but sometimes persist for weeks: (ii.) other swellings are white and painless. Both types of swellings are the size of a hen's egg, and although they may occur in any area of the body they are most often found near joints or in the orbit. (iii.) When a worm migrates across the conjunctiva it causes local inflammation and the patient may see the worm crossing his field of vision.

The *diagnosis* is established by the history. There is a marked eosinophilia, and filarial antigen gives positive skin and complement fixation tests. After some months, typical sheathed micro-filariæ can be found in the blood by day (Fig. 160).

Treatment.—Diethylcarbamazine (Banocide, Hetrazan) by mouth in doses of 2·0 mg./Kg. body weight three times a day for three weeks will effect a cure.

(d) Eruptions in which SCALES are often a conspicuous feature

Common.
- I.   Psoriasis (§ 658).
- II. Seborrhœic dermatitis (§ 659).
- III. Pityriasis rosea (§ 660).
- IV. Pityriasis alba (§ 661).
- V.   Tinea circinata (§ 662) and erythrasma (§ 663).
- VI. Ichthyosis (§ 664).
- VII. Exfoliative dermatitis (§ 665).

Rare.
- VIII. Parapsoriasis (§ 666).
- IX.   Squamous syphilide (§ 667).
- X.   Pityriasis rubra pilaris (§ 668).
- XI.   Skin conditions sometimes scaly at one stage (§ 669).

§ **658.** I. **Psoriasis** is one of the commonest diseases of the skin. The first attack usually occurs between the ages of 10 and 30, but attacks can occur at any age.

Symptoms.—The lesions consist of sharply defined, slightly elevated bright red papules or plaques covered with fine dry silvery scales. When these are removed the tips of the hyperæmic papillæ are exposed. Central clearing and peripheral extension give rise to figured and annular lesions: confluence of neighbouring plaques can produce extensive sheets (Plate XIX). The site of the lesion, the age of the patient, the type of skin and other features modify the gross appearance of the lesions but the essential morphological features are usually preserved. In most cases the only disability is cosmetic and æsthetic as irritation is usually absent, but in the nervous individual irritation may be severe. Psoriasis favours traumatised areas and tends to spare those exposed to light. It is usually more severe in the least sunny months of the year. The disease may remain restricted for long periods to the sites of predilection, viz., the extensor surfaces of the knees and elbows, the scalp and the trunk, but any part of the body may be affected. A single plaque may persist unchanged for many years. Extension, generalisation and recurrences may follow a period of emotional stress and physical fatigue, an acute infection, or may occur for no discoverable reason.

Varieties: In *guttate psoriasis* a profuse eruption of small papular lesions is present on the trunk and limbs. It occurs particularly in children and young adults and is often provoked by a streptococcal infection. *Pustular psoriasis* is uncommon, involving particularly the palms and soles. Crops of sterile pustules are succeeded by brownish crusts. *Intertriginous psoriasis* involves the natal cleft, the external genitalia and the groins and is often irritable. The patients are usually past middle life. *Psoriatic arthritis* (§ 597): there is statistical and immunological evidence that the association of rheumatoid arthritis and psoriasis is not fortuitous. In some cases the arthritis is exceptionally destructive and the psoriasis unusually severe and resistant to treatment. *Psoriasis of the nails* may accompany skin lesions or may occur alone. The affected nail may show only fine pitting or may be discoloured and thickened (§ 783). *Exfoliative psoriasis* may develop as the result of overtreatment but more often there is no obvious cause for the universal generalisation of the disease.

Diagnosis is usually simple. The intertriginous form must be differentiated from other forms of intertrigo, but the sharp margination and the presence of typical lesions elsewhere are helpful. Psoriasis of the scalp may so closely resemble seborrhœic dermatitis that diagnosis is difficult but the lesions of psoriasis are circumscribed and are usually palpable whereas those of seborrhœic dermatitis are not.

Etiology.—The cause is unknown. There is frequently a family history of the disease and it is probable that psoriasis is a manifestation of an inborn defect of the epidermis. It is rare in the negro and is most common in the white races in temperate climates. Many attempts have been made to relate psoriasis to various metabolic factors but no constant association has been established. It often clears during pregnancy.

The *prognosis* is always difficult: after a single attack the patient may remain free for many years. In others an early relapse follows treatment.

Treatment.—It is unjustifiable to dismiss the patient with the statement that the disease is incurable. The tendency to this pattern of cutaneous reaction cannot be eradicated but with well-planned treatment there are very few attacks that cannot be cleared for a longer or shorter period. *Systemic treatment.* In the severe and extensive case the patient should be put to bed with sedation. Oral triamcinolone will often clear psoriasis but the benefit is temporary and the frequency of severe relapses contraindicates its use except in the generalised erythrodermic form under hospital supervision. Arsenic should not be used on account of the risk of polyneuritis and skin cancer after repeated courses. In recurrent guttate psoriasis, when each attack follows tonsillitis, tonsillectomy should be considered but operation should not be undertaken solely on account of the psoriasis. *Local treatment* is still the main line of therapy. The nature and site of the lesions, the type of skin and the feasibility of hospital treatment will influence the choice of treatment. The *mildest cases* respond to ung. acid. salicylic. (2 per cent.). The common form of *moderate severity* can be treated with an ointment containing liq. picis carb. ℔. 30, salicylic acid gr. 15 in paraffin molle 1 oz., supplemented by a course of ultraviolet light. In *extensive* or *long-standing psoriasis* more vigorous measures and hospital admission are required. The following procedure is effective but requires daily treatment at hospital with a skilled staff. After soaking in a bath containing liq. picis carb. 4 fl. oz. in 20 gallons of water the patient is exposed to an erythema dose of ultraviolet light. Lassar's paste with dithranol 0·1 to 2·0 per cent. is applied carefully and thickly to each patch of psoriasis under bandages. This routine is repeated daily. For the greatly thickened plaque of long duration the higher concentrations of dithranol will be necessary. Many other treatment procedures are useful in certain types of psoriasis and rigid standardisation is impossible. In the *acute* forms only bland local applications are required. In the *intertriginous* form greasy ointment bases are poorly tolerated and Vioform in a cream base is helpful. Triamcinolone or fluocinolone ointment is often effective in anogenital psoriasis and for the rare facial lesions, but it is useless in other sites unless applied under occlusive polythene sheeting when it is often valuable (see § 785). For the *scalp* oil of cade ℳ. 30, precipitated sulphur gr. 15, salicylic acid gr. 10 in ung. emulsificans 1 oz. is useful.

§ **659. II. Seborrhœic dermatitis** is the name given to a group of skin eruptions commonly arising in subjects of a particular constitutional make-up. The sites of predilection are the scalp, the face, the mid-line of the chest and back and the flexures. The eruption assumes several clinical forms. On the trunk dull red follicular papules covered by a greasy scale may extend to form circinate lesions with yellowish-brown centres and greasy scales around their advancing margins. This is commonly seen in men. A more acute form closely resembles pityriasis rosea but the lesions are more widely distributed and, without treatment, may run a longer course. Behind the ears and in the body folds seborrhœic dermatitis causes a form of intertrigo with sharply marginated diffuse erythema and variable scaling; in the depth of the fold there is often fissuring and crusting. A single site or many areas may be involved simultaneously. With inappropriate treatment this type of seborrhœic dermatitis may become œdematous and crusted and extend widely beyond the original site. On the genitalia of both sexes a resistant psoriasiform variety occurs.

Etiology.—In the seborrhœic state both epidermis and dermis are slightly œdematous and keratinisation is imperfect. These abnormalities together with sebaceous dysfunction diminish the normal powers of self-disinfection of the skin's surface and modify its response to trauma. Many attacks of seborrhœic dermatitis are preceded by emotional stress, fatigue, infections, dietary irregularities or digestive disturbances and these factors temporarily accentuate the abnormalities of the inborn seborrhœic state.

Treatment.—In the more *acute case* bed rest is desirable, and adequate sedation must be prescribed. Chlortetracycline or tetracycline 500 mg. 3 or 4 times daily may be given. Bland local applications—normal saline compresses and lotio. calaminæ oleosa N.F. are indicated. In *localised forms* including *acute seborrhœic dermatitis of the scalp* and *seborrhœic intertrigo* neomycin or chlortetracycline ointment should be combined with an equal part of hydrocortisone acetate ointment, 1 per cent. For *chronic scaly seborrhœic dermatitis* sulphur and salicylic acid (3 per cent. of each) in soft paraffin is usually effective. In all except the most chronic forms overtreatment is a frequent error. The scalp should always be treated (see § 777).

§ 660. III. Pityriasis Rosea is most frequent in adolescence and early adult life, but can occur at any age. It is probably of infective origin. In the typical case there is first a *herald patch*, usually larger and more conspicuous than the subsequent lesions and often situated over the lower ribs, on the upper abdomen or on the shoulders. This patch is sharply defined, round or oval in shape and covered by fine scales. About 7 to 10 days later the general eruption follows. Lesions develop in crops over a period of a few days; they are confined to the trunk and the upper third of the thighs and arms. They may be papular, especially in children, but are much more often in the form of oval medallions, with the long axis in the lines of cleavage of the skin, deep red or dull tawny pink in colour with dry furfuraceous silvery-grey scales. Spontaneous cure takes from 4 to 8 weeks, but some cases last much longer. In differential *diagnosis* seborrhœic dermatitis and secondary syphilis must be considered. *Treatment* is seldom necessary as irritation is slight or absent.

§ 661. IV. Pityriasis alba is common in young children and can occur in adults.

Symptoms.—As a result of a chronic streptococcal infection it is often associated with fissures beneath the ears or may follow an attack of impetigo or an upper respiratory infection with nasal discharge. The face is usually involved but lesions may also occur on the neck and trunk and, more rarely, on the limbs. These are round, oval or irregular patches, pink or skin-coloured with a wrinkled surface and scanty fine scales. They can persist for months and may be more conspicuous in the early summer when they do not pigment as does the surrounding normal skin on exposure to sunlight. A variant of this condition, of very similar appearance, shows no bacteriological or clinical association with streptococcal infection and is attributed to the irritant effect of cold weather, soap, etc., on sensitive skin.

Treatment.—Ichthammol and ammoniated mercury (2 per cent. of each) in zinc cream (B.P.) is usually effective: recurrences are common.

§ 662. V. Tinea circinata.—Ringworm infections of the non-hairy skin produce a wide variety of lesions. In general those fungi whose natural hosts are animals provoke a more vigorous inflammatory response than the human species. Small red discoid patches with slight scaling and with vesiculation of the advancing border are produced by *Microsporon canis*, a parasite of kittens and some other animals. Tinea capitis may be associated with this. The lesions are common in children and small outbreaks centre round the family kitten. Inflammatory lesions of greater intensity are caused by *Trichophyton verrucosum*, the common cause of ringworm in cattle, and *Trichophyton mentagrophytes*, also an animal parasite (see § 779). Well-defined dull red slightly scaly patches, sometimes showing central clearing, are caused by *Trichophyton rubrum*, a human parasite of steadily increasing incidence. The circinate form has a well-defined dull red margin and may or may not show central clearing. Another characteristic form presents as a dusky erythema with fine scaling on the palms and soles but lesions may occur elsewhere. Hyperkeratotic lesions are sometimes produced.

Tinea cruris is commonly caused by *Epidermophyton floccosum, Trichophyton rubrum* or *T. interdigitale* and is seen on the upper and inner thigh mainly in male adolescents or young adults. The vesiculation of the advancing margin is characteristic and differentiates it from lichen simplex and intertrigo.

Tinea pedis and **Tinea manuum.**—Tinea of the feet, common in young adults, is usually due to *Trichophyton interdigitale, T. rubrum* or *Epidermophyton floccosum*. There may be scaling and maceration of the interdigital skin (especially between the third and fourth toes), a vesicular eruption of the soles, or scaling and persistent dull erythema of the soles or the sides of the feet, which may be unilateral. Severe cases may be complicated by recurrent cellulitis and occasionally by phlebitis. A symmetrical vesicular eruption of the palms (cheiropompholyx) may occur as an ide (allergic) reaction to an actively inflammatory tinea pedis but this is not the common cause of cheiropompholyx. See § 672. True fungus infection of the hands was formerly uncommon: the dull red scaling of *T. rubrum* infection is met with increasing frequency on the palms or on the backs of the hands or fingers, often accompanied by nail involvement.

Diagnosis should be confirmed by microscopical examination of scrapings from *active* lesions. Many patients carry pathogenic fungi without subjective symptoms; interdigital maceration predisposes to infection but is caused by occlusive footwear. The demonstration of fungus mycelium does not exclude the diagnosis of dyshidrotic pompholyx or overtreatment dermatitis.

Treatment.—The more inflammatory the lesion the less active the treatment required. In vesicular tinea pedis the feet should be soaked in potassium permanganate 1/5,000 until the acute state subsides. During the subacute stage and in the common forms of tinea circinata and tinea cruris zinc undecenoate ointment (N.F.) may be prescribed. In chronic scaly forms Whitfield's ointment or 0·1 per cent. dithranol in Lassar's paste may be necessary. Resistant cases may be given tab. griseofulvin-forte 0·125 G. q.i.d. for 3 to 4 weeks. Relapse is of greater importance than re-infection and meticulous attention to foot hygiene, treatment of hyperhidrosis and the use of a fungistatic dusting powder may prevent further attacks.

§ 663. **Erythrasma** is a superficial infection with *Nocardia minutissimum*. Finely scaling plaques, at first reddish-brown in colour and later yellow-brown, occur in the groins, in the axillæ and beneath the breasts. *Treatment* is with erythromycin.

§ 664. VI. **Ichthyosis** is a congenital abnormality of the skin usually first evident between the ages of 2 and 4, and not present at birth. It often becomes more marked during childhood, may improve after puberty, but persists in some degree throughout life. It often accompanies the eczema/asthma complex.

Symptoms.—In its mildest form the skin is merely excessively dry and harsh (Xeroderma). In the ordinary type the whole skin surface with the exception of the flexures, palms and soles is dry, rough and scaly. The extensor surfaces are most severely affected; keratosis pilaris is often associated and the scalp is dry and scurfy. The dry skin is readily damaged by detergents and other grease-solvents. Patients are most comfortable during the warmer months of the year. Icthyosiform scaling may occur in vitamin A deficiency and chronic cachectic states. Rarely ichthyosis may occur in Hodgkin's disease.

Treatment.—Vitamin A can be prescribed but with uncertain benefit; there is a risk of overdosage in young children. The application of an emollient ointment such as acid salicylic (2 per cent.) in equal parts of glycerine and soft paraffin ointment is helpful.

ICHTHYOSIFORM CONDITIONS OF THE NEWBORN.—In **Ichthyosis congenita** the infant is covered by thick horny masses (" harlequin fœtus ") and seldom survives more than a few days. **Lamellar ichthyosis,** which may give rise to the appearance of " collodion skin," is an exaggeration of physiological desquamation and the infant's skin soon becomes normal. **Ichthyosiform erythroderma of Brocq** is exceedingly rare. Generalised erythroderma in infancy may gradually regress, leaving an ichthyosis which favours the flexures. Bullæ can occur as a complication in infancy and childhood.

§ **665. VII. Exfoliative Dermatitis** is characterised by persistent almost universal erythema (erythroderma) accompanied by *profuse and repeated exfoliation*; the nails and hair may be shed. A sensation of tightness and discomfort is more frequent than pruritus. The lymph nodes may be enlarged. The sustained erythema disturbs the mechanism of heat-regulation and patients complain constantly of cold. Loss of protein in the scales contributes to the gradual deterioration in the general condition which is common but not invariable. Untreated exfoliative dermatitis may continue for months or years.

Etiology.—This condition may be (i.) a stage of a skin disorder such as psoriasis, eczema or seborrhœic dermatitis (often as the result of over-treatment), pemphigus foliaceus or pityriasis rubra pilaris; (ii.) a drug reaction (arsenic, gold, mercury, barbiturates, etc.); (iii.) a manifestation of a reticulosis, of leukæmia or of cancer; (iv.) a disease of unknown origin, especially in elderly men.

Diagnosis.—The cause must be established by full physical examination, biopsy of skin, lymph nodes and sternal marrow and examination of the peripheral blood.

Treatment depends on the cause. Good nursing is essential. Local applications should be bland. In cases not associated with malignant disease the treatment of choice is with a corticosteroid: a small maintenance dose may be necessary for a prolonged period and careful regular supervision is obligatory.

IN INFANTS exfoliative dermatitis presents a different problem. **Ritter's disease** is the exfoliative stage of bullous impetigo (§ 674). **Leiner's disease** is generalised seborrhœic dermatitis. Exogenous dermatitis from overtreatment can generalise in infants as in adults and an exfoliative reaction to boric acid absorbed percutaneously from dusting powder, has occurred. **Ichthyosiform erythroderma** is a rare congenital abnormality in which a universal erythroderma may be present in infancy.

§ **666.** VIII. **Parapsoriasis.**—There is no uniformity in the use of this term: it is best restricted to Parapsoriasis en plaques, a rare disease of adults in which sharply marginated, very superficial yellowish-red plaques with fine scaling appear on the trunk and limbs. They are irritable and are often polycyclic or angulated. Some cases develop, often after many years, the malignant reticulosis, mycosis fungoides. To be differentiated is the more common parapsoriasis-like eruption, which usually runs a protracted but benign course and is a chronic superficial dermatitis. The patches are more scaly, are not irritable and are round or oval.

Treatment.—Thorium-X (2,000 e.s.u./ml.) may be painted on the lesions 6 or 8 times at intervals of 2 or 3 weeks.

§ **667.** IX. The **Squamous Syphilide** occurs characteristically on the palms and soles, where the thickness of the horny layer modifies the appearance of the papules. In the secondary stage the dull copper-coloured papules which are often symmetrically disposed may be covered by scanty scales. At a later stage an asymmetrical distribution of lesions grouped in segments of a circle is typical: irregular scaling and horny thickening may be present.

§ **668.** X. **Pityriasis Rubra Pilaris** is rare. Two groups of cases are met, the *familial* form which usually begins in childhood and the *acquired* form later in life.

Symptoms.—The earliest change may be the insidious onset of erythema, with scaling of the scalp and the face, resembling seborrhœic dermatitis. Scaling and later diffuse hyperkeratosis develop on the palms and soles. The characteristic lesion is a hard horny follicular papule which usually appears before the scaling is of wide extent. In the *more acute form* large numbers of papules develop very rapidly. These are most striking on the dorsal surfaces of the first phalanges and aggregate into plaques on the knees and elbows. Extensive areas of sharply marginated erythema and scaling may become confluent, forming a universal exfoliative dermatitis. The tense red scaly skin of the face may evert the lower lids to produce ectropion. The course is variable, some cases persisting unchanged for months or years, others undergoing partial or complete regression.

Diagnosis.—Partial forms of the eruption easily escape recognition, but the fully developed eruption is distinctive.

Etiology.—Many cases show a low plasma vitamin A level despite an adequate dietary intake. There appears to be some disorder of vitamin A metabolism, but its nature is still uncertain.

Treatment.—Vitamin A, 50,000–100,000 units daily for several months, is sometimes effective, particularly in acquired cases.

§ **669.** XI. Skin diseases which may be scaly at one stage.—Scaling is frequently a feature of the reparative stage of many inflammatory skin disorders. It is common in chronic and subacute eczema (§ 671) and in lichen simplex (§ 776).

GROUP II. LESIONS USUALLY MOIST
Vesicular and Bullous Eruptions

In many of these the vesicles rupture almost as soon as they are formed and the lesions are commonly observed in the exudative or crusted stage. A practical distinction can be made between conditions which are vesicular and those which are bullous, but there is no fundamental difference between the two.

§ 670. I. **Eczema** in its various forms is by far the commonest skin disorder. The terms eczema, dermatitis and eczematous dermatitis have been employed with such widely differing significance that definition of these terms is essential to a clear understanding of the subject.

ECZEMA is a mode of reaction of the skin characterised histologically by (i.) intercellular and intracellular œdema of the epidermis (spongiosis), leading to (ii.) vesicle-formation within the epidermis, and (iii.) capillary dilatation, œdema and a perivascular infiltration of lymphocytes and histiocytes in the dermis. These are represented clinically by erythema, œdema, grouped papulovesicles. In typical cases the eczema reaction evolves through well-defined stages and regression may take place at any stage. In very acute cases the earlier stages may be passed through so rapidly that they are not clinically apparent. DERMATITIS is a general term for inflammation of the skin, and unless qualified, *e.g.*, infective dermatitis, occupational dermatitis, has so wide a scope that it has no practical value. ECZEMATOUS DERMATITIS is now frequently used to designate eczema of external origin.

Symptoms.—The initial stage of eczema is erythema, which may be accompanied by marked œdema when sites such as the eyelid or scrotum are involved. Grouped papules develop on the area of erythema and becoming vesicular, rupture to cause weeping and crusting. If the reaction is very intense bullæ may form. As recovery takes place the affected area passes through a stage of erythema and scaling which finally subsides to leave normal skin. *Itching* is the predominant symptom of eczema and may be severe. Rubbing and scratching may produce *lichenification*—thickening of the skin with exaggeration of the normal skin markings and often some pigmentation. It is probable that not all skins are capable of lichenifying in response to scratching. Secondary infection, unwise treatment or recurrent attacks can modify the basic changes of the eczema reaction.

The *Etiology* of eczema is complex. Even where the role of an exogenous irritant can be clearly demonstrated this often acts merely as the trigger in a predisposed individual. Some suffer from recurrent attacks, each of which may be initiated by the same or a different factor, whilst others, apparently exposed to the same hazards, remain unaffected. *Causes.*—(*a*) Fatigue and emotional stress may predispose to an attack which is partly determined by external factors. In others emotional factors are apparently solely responsible; they can certainly play a large part in the perpetuation of an eruption which was initially exogenous. (*b*) Whereas allergic sensitisation is of fundamental importance in many cases of eczematous dermatitis (*q.v.*), the role of allergy in other patterns of eczematous reaction is doubtful. Although cases have been reported in which allergy to an ingested or inhaled antigen has been claimed to provoke a primarily eczematous eruption, many experienced dermatologists have never encountered such cases. (*c*) A process of autosensitisation can occur, the patient having become allergically sensitised to his own altered skin proteins. A typical instance is that of an eczematous eruption on the lower leg, which may explosively disseminate to other areas of the skin often as the result of over-vigorous treatment. (*d*) A phenomenon often observed is an isomorphic reaction, new lesions developing at sites of friction or trauma in a patient with an eczematous reaction originally of limited extent. (*e*) Sweat-retention is often an important factor. Sweating of thermal or emotional origin provokes crises of intense irritation in areas where partial or complete sweat duct occlusion has been produced by pre-existing inflammatory epidermal lesions. (*f*) Endocrine and nutritional factors probably play a poorly understood role in some cases.

§ 671. 1. **Eczematous Dermatitis** (including Contact dermatitis, Occupational dermatitis).

Symptoms.—The clinical features depend on the mode of response to the external agent, its nature and the intensity of the reaction. Any or all of the stages of eczema (*vide supra*) are present in varying degree: Pruritus is almost always present and is often severe. Irritability, dryness, cracking, redness, slowly increasing until eczematous breakdown occurs, suggest progressive skin damage by a chemical or physical agent. The sites most exposed to the irritant are usually the most severely affected. Irregular acute relapses suggest an allergic reaction. The dermatitis may initially involve sites such as the eyelids, penis or scrotum, remote from the sites most heavily exposed to the allergen.

It is convenient to distinguish two types of eczematous dermatitis. (i.) Primary irritants injure the skin by physicochemical action (*e.g.*, caustic, hygroscopic, etc.) and will damage any skin if in adequate concentration for a long period. (ii.) Allergic sensitisation of the skin occurs in a minority of those exposed to certain substances in concentrations in which they inflict no clinically perceptible physical or chemical damage. Some substances (*e.g.*, penicillin, procaine) induce this very readily whereas others seldom do so. After a variable period of exposure during which no reaction is provoked (refractory period) the development of sensitisation takes 7–10 days (incubation period). Thereafter exposure to the same or sometimes a chemically related substance, even in high dilution, will produce an eczematous response in 12 to 48 hours (reaction time). Although the clinical reaction to a sensitiser may be localised the entire epidermis is allergically sensitised—advantage is taken of this in the diagnostic patch test.

The PATCH TEST is employed to confirm a suspected allergic sensitisation of the epidermis. It aims at reproducing in miniature the original exposure to the allergen. Testing is postponed until the dermatitis is quiescent so as to minimise the risk of

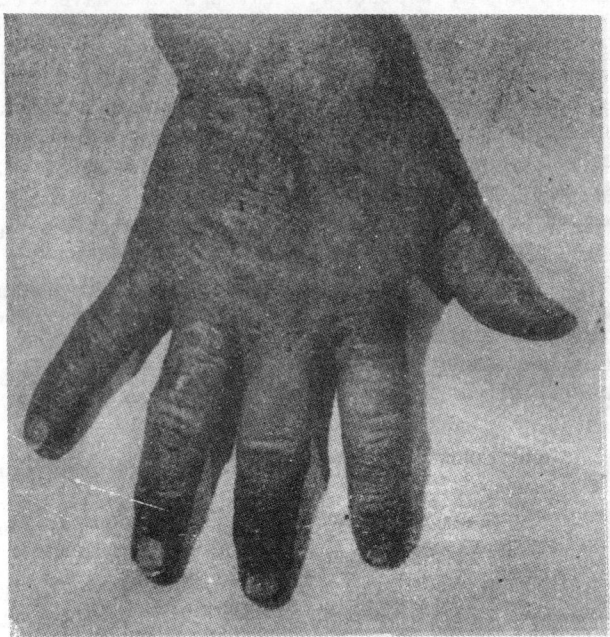

FIG. 184.—ECZEMATOUS DERMATITIS produced by the primary irritant effect of a strong disinfectant.

provoking an exacerbation or obtaining a non-specific false positive reaction. An unaffected area of skin is selected, usually the flexor surface of the forearm or the interscapular region. If the suspected substance is liquid or is soluble the concentration employed must have no primary irritant effect: [1] in case of doubt a high dilution is used initially. Solid substances, such as the leaves of plants, can be applied in their natural state provided that they are not primary irritants. A square of filter paper, ½ inch across, is saturated in the selected solution and covered with a 2-inch square of cellophane: these are held in place by a strip of adhesive plaster or by a special " patch test window " dressing. After 48 hours the patch is removed and the test is interpreted. The test site must be examined again after a further 48 hours as delayed positive reactions can occur. The result is commonly recorded as, 0 for no reaction; + erythema; + + erythema and œdema; + + + papules;

---

[1] A list of suitable concentrations of many substances employed in industry is given in " The Eczemas " by L. J. A. Loewenthal, 1954, pp. 237–251.

++++ vesicles. An even more intense reaction may be provoked and if there is much irritation the patch should be removed sooner. Considerable experience is necessary for the correct interpretation of the patch test. A true positive reaction indicates that the patient is allergic to the test substance and, provided that the clinical evidence points in the same direction, incriminates it as the cause of the dermatitis. A negative patch test does not necessarily exonerate the suspected substance as the conditions of exposure may not have been simulated.

Diagnosis.—The cause of dermatitis can often be determined only by the most detailed investigation. The exact nature of the occupational

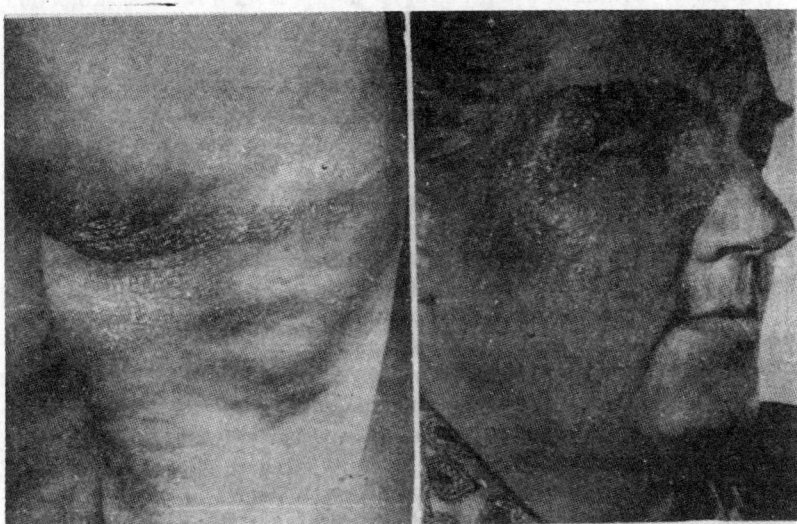

FIG. 185.—CONTACT DERMATITIS caused by allergic sensitivity to nickel suspender fastening. Nickel sensitivity is common. The eruption may later disseminate to the cubital fossæ and the neck. The diagnosis is established by applying a patch test of 0·5 per cent. nickel sulphate *after* the acute eruption has subsided.

FIG. 186.—CONTACT DERMATITIS caused by allergic sensitivity to penicillin eye drops. There may be conjunctivitis and chemosis and the condition may be wrongly considered to be infective.

hazards to which the patient is exposed must be established. This may require a visit to the work place, or a letter to the works manager. Substances handled at home, and especially cleaning agents, disinfectants, plants, clothing and cosmetics must be considered (Fig. 184). Inquiry must be made of the patient's hobbies as photography, gardening. The patient's own efforts at self-treatment may be responsible for provoking or prolonging the dermatitis. The course of the skin eruption and its site must be correlated with the time and mode of exposure to any suggested cause.

Occupational dermatitis can prove an economic disaster for a trained man and it is unjust to make this diagnosis unless it is established beyond any reasonable doubt. Many mistakes can be avoided if the following principles are observed:—(i.) The site of onset is the site of maximum contact with the alleged cause. (ii.) The pattern of skin reaction is that which this substance is known to provoke. (iii.) Removal from exposure results in improvement and re-exposure is followed by relapse. (iv.) If a sensitiser is involved, a patch test should be positive (Fig. 185). There are exceptions to these general principles; *e.g.*, some types of sensitisation dermatitis (*e.g.*, to plants and antibiotics) tend to spare the hands at first and to involve the eyelids and face (Fig. 186); or a patch test may be negative because the exact conditions of occupational exposure are not reproduced.

Etiology.—An intact and healthy horny layer provides protection. Ichthyosis, age changes, and damage by detergents, soaps, grease solvents or repeated physical trauma can all increase susceptibility of the skin to further injury.

Prognosis depends on (i.) Early and adequate treatment. (ii.) Identification and elimination of any sensitising agent. (iii.) Convalescence and rehabilitation to allow full functional recovery of the skin before return to work. (iv.) Age: the condition tends to recover slowly in the elderly. (v.) Emotional factors: it is extremely common for an eczematous dermatitis originally provoked by external agents to persist or to relapse repeatedly without re-exposure to the initiating factor, the clinical picture slowly changing to that of neurodermatitis.

Treatment.—If the dermatitis is extensive a short period of bed rest is desirable. Sedation with phenobarbitone gr. $\frac{1}{2}$ b.d. or a tranquillising drug can seldom be omitted and should be continued until cure is complete. The patient will be helped by repeated reassurance and the opportunity to discuss the problems that arise from his disability. A hypnotic such as sodium amylobarbitone gr. 3 or 6 must be given to ensure sound sleep. In very acute sensitisation dermatitis a short course of a corticosteroid is valuable. *Local treatment.*—In the acute exudative stage apply normal saline compresses with applications of lotio calaminæ oleosa N.F. or of equal parts of limewater and olive oil. In localised acute reactions particularly on the face, hydrocortisone acetate $\frac{1}{2}$-1 per cent. ointment or lotion is helpful. In the subacute stage cremor zinci (B.P.) to which ichthammol (2 per cent.) can be added is often acceptable. In the chronic forms liquor picis carbonis (4–8 per cent.) in zinc paste is indicated: for persistent lichenification small doses of X-ray may be used.

2. **Infantile Eczema** (Atopic eczema—Besnier's prurigo).

Symptoms.—In 75 per cent. of cases infantile eczema begins in the first three months of life on the cheeks, sparing the nose and central face. The scalp is usually not affected but the scaly crusted scalp of so-called seborrhœic dermatitis of infancy occasionally precedes the typical facial eczema. The lesions on the face consist of erythema, exudation and crusting which next involve the extensor surface of the limbs. Usually between 6–18 months the popliteal and cubital fossæ and the sides of the neck are involved and the face tends to clear. The course of the eruption in infancy is variable. It is often worse in the colder months of the year. Exacerbations may be provoked by teething and by gastro-intestinal disturbances which cause flushing.   The eczema tends to be more severe and persistent when the home environment is unsatisfactory.

From the third year onwards the skin lesions may assume the form of Besnier's prurigo.   The skin of the flexures, especially the popliteal and cubital fossæ, is lichenified.   Other sites may be involved including the sides of the neck, the face and the hands, but the exudative lesions of infancy no longer occur and scratching during the crises of intense irritation is responsible for the lichenification.   Some, but not all cases are worse in the winter but sweating may increase the irritation.   Fatigue and

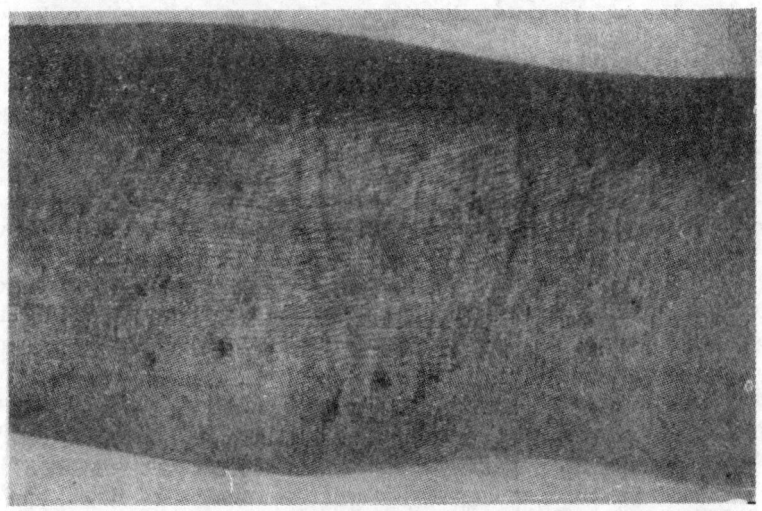

Fig. 187.—Atopic Eczema (Besnier's prurigo).   The skin of this adolescent girl's antecubital fossæ is grossly lichenified.   The thickening pigmentation exaggeration of skin markings are clearly shown.

emotional stress are very frequently incriminated by the patients as the cause of recurrences, but other factors may be concerned.

About 50 per cent. of children with infantile eczema have Besnier's prurigo at the age of 13.   It often reaches its greatest severity in girls between 13 and 15 and boys between 18 and 20, after which milder and less frequent attacks recur. in some patients.   About 50 per cent. of children with infantile eczema develop asthma, but not always the same children in whom the eczema persists.   Hay fever occurs in some 10 per cent.

Etiology.—An inborn constitutional state which afflicts a proportion of the population, estimated at 5–7 per cent., predisposes to the development of skin reactions of a special type.   This state has been labelled atopy by Coca; the term is sufficiently noncommittal to be useful in the present state of our knowledge.   The atopic state is inherited.   The atopic individual readily forms antibodies of a special type (reagins) to antigens to which he is exposed by ingestion or inhalation.   Their presence can be demonstrated by an immediate wheal reaction to intradermal or scratch tests. Atopic infants show positive wheal reactions to many foods, but over the age of 3 show fewer reactions to foods and more to inhalants. The presence of reagins is often of no clinical significance and even where ingestion of a food, especially egg-white, provokes œdema of the lips, urticaria or gastro-intestinal symptoms, it does not directly provoke eczema. Skin tests are usually therefore of little practical value in the management of infantile eczema.

In addition to this immunological anomaly the atopic state is characterised by other unusual patterns of reaction. The vascular responses of the skin are abnormal; the skin readily becomes lichenified in response to scratching and rubbing; xeroderma or ichthyosis is often present. The atopic individual is often emotionally labile and electro-encephalographic studies have revealed an unsuspectedly high proportion of tracings of epileptic type. The response to certain infections is unusual, e.g., herpes simplex and vaccinia (see §§ 675, 677). There is an association between atopy and juvenile cataract. The atopic subject shows no special liability to develop allergic contact dermatitis, but is particularly susceptible to the dangerous anaphylactoid type of drug reaction.

Infantile eczema is initiated by physical trauma which evokes this response only in the atopic infant. Too vigorous efforts to cleanse the newborn skin, soap and unsuitable local applications, rapid changes of temperature and sweating or contact with wool produce the initial changes which are perpetuated by rubbing and scratching. Despite many contrary opinions in the recent past it seems that the role of allergy in infantile eczema has been greatly over-estimated. Physical and psychological factors are of principal importance in maintaining the established skin lesions in childhood and adolescence and in provoking relapses.

Treatment.—The child's parents should be given some understanding of the nature of the atopic state, as far as it is known, and of the long-term policy to be adopted. Frequent changes of doctor and of treatment are undesirable and the parents must learn that there can be no rapid cure. The child requires a calm and restful emotional and physical environment. Feeds seldom need modification if the child is fit but if he is overweight sugar should be restricted. No important food should be omitted from the diet unless its role in perpetuating the eczema has been evaluated by trial exposure in hospital. The infant will often require sedation—chloral or phenobarbitone can be prescribed. Soap should be used as little as possible; arachis oil can be employed to clean the skin. Contact with wool must be avoided. Secondary infection can be controlled with chlortetra-cycline ointment; then Lassar's paste should be applied until the acute stage has settled. Triamcinolone ointment (0·01 per cent.) has proved a valuable temporary suppressive measure in acute and refractory cases. Later 8 per cent. liquor picis carbonis or 5 per cent. crude tar in zinc paste are still valuable preparations. If persistent scratching is preventing healing it may be necessary to secure the arms and legs with cardboard or light plastic splints and to cover the face with a mask. It is unwise to vaccinate the atopic infant unless the risk of exposure to small-pox is high. Inoculation against diphtheria, etc., need not be forbidden. In the older child Besnier's prurigo presents a very similar problem. Sedatives and the tranquillising drugs are valuable. Tar is often the most effective application. The response to treatment depends largely on the intelligent co-operation of understanding parents.

3. **Nummular Eczema** is a common variety of constitutional eczema. *Symptoms.*—The characteristic lesion is a discoid or coin-shaped plaque

of eczema. Single or multiple plaques are frequently seen on the backs of the hands and forearms of adolescent girls and young women, and less often in young men. Only one hand may be affected; relapses occur readily. In the elderly numerous plaques may develop on the extensor surfaces of the arms and legs, and sometimes on the trunk, especially the back and shoulders. Irritation is often severe. Attacks are most frequent in the winter.

Diagnosis.—The single plaque of eczema must be differentiated from ringworm.

Etiology.—Nummular and other constitutional eczemas show periods of peak incidence from puberty to 25 and in the fifth and sixth decades. Exogenous factors, for example household cleaning agents in the younger group and cold dry air and woollen clothing in older patients, are probably no more than contributory or " trigger " factors, and in a majority of cases no external agent can be incriminated. Emotional tension is usually of obvious importance but the full explanation is still unknown.

Treatment is that of eczematous dermatitis (above). Liq. picis carbonis (8 per cent.), or 4 per cent. with Vioform 1·5 per cent. in zinc paste, should be applied under protective dressings.

4. Infective Eczema (Infective eczematoid dermatitis) develops around infected abrasions, ulcers, fissures or chronic draining sinuses as a red moist dermatitis, often with a sharp margin. The oozing surface may be crusted or pustular, or in chronic forms, covered by sticky parakeratotic scales. An acute variety in the genital region occurs particularly in diabetics. A chronic form is commonly seen around hypostatic leg ulcers or extending into the scalp from fissures behind the ears. Involvement of the perianal skin in children suggests threadworms.

Diagnosis.—Differentiate from moniliasis, seborrhœic dermatitis and overtreatment dermatitis.

Treatment.—After treatment of the underlying factors apply potassium permanganate compresses 1 /5,000 if very acute. Later, and as the initial treatment in subacute cases, apply chlortetracycline or neomycin ointment alone or in combination with hydrocortisone acetate ointment (I per cent.). Vioform ointment is effective in chronic cases and is particularly suitable for children. It may prove irritating on the lower leg.

§ 672. II. **Pompholyx** is a vesicular eruption of the palms and sides of the fingers (cheiropompholyx) or less commonly the soles.

Symptoms.—Pompholyx occurs particularly in adolescents and young adults, but is not uncommon in children. Attacks are more frequent in warm weather and are preceded and accompanied by irritation, which may be intense. In the mildest cases transitory vesicles are restricted to the sides of the fingers; in more severe forms they cover the palms and soles and, by confluence, form large blisters, which readily become infected. Healing follows exfoliation, but recurrences are common.

Three groups of cases must be distinguished. (i.) The commonest form, almost always symmetrical, occurs in nervous individuals, as a reaction to fatigue or emotional stress, or without discoverable cause. It may be associated with atopic or seborrhœic dermatitis in other parts of the skin. (ii.) At the height of an actively inflammatory ringworm infection of the feet (not merely a latent infection) a symmetrical cheiropompholyx may develop as an allergic reaction (ide). The skin of the hands is not infected by the fungus and the pompholyx will subside if the feet are adequately treated. (iii.) Eczematous dermatitis of external origin may produce a pompholyx if it involves the skin of palms or soles. This is uncommon unless the contiguous skin of the dorsal surfaces is simultaneously affected.

Diagnosis.—Ringworm infection of the palms is a rare cause of a localised vesicular eruption of the palms. It is usually limited to one hand, and diagnosis must be established by discovery of the fungus mycelium in scrapings from the advancing edge. If there are crops of small pustules on the palms, particularly the thenar eminence, see § 677.

Treatment.—In the acute vesicular stage the hands should be soaked twice daily in normal saline, the blisters opened with sterile scissors and dressings of oily calamine lotion applied. In the subacute stage bland creams or soft pastes are well tolerated. In the dry scaling stage liquor picis carbonis (4–8 per cent.) in zinc paste may be applied at night and unguentum aquosum freely used by day. If there is secondary infection a sulphonamide or an antibiotic should be administered systemically. Phenobarbitone (gr. ½ b.d.) or Belladenal (tab. i t.d.s.) is helpful in relieving irritation and lessening the risk of recurrence. A tranquillising drug is valuable where there is an important nervous factor.

§ **673. III. Sudamina** and **Miliaria.**—Sweat retention is of considerable clinical importance in temperate and tropical climates. The various clinical manifestations depend largely on the level at which the sweat duct is obstructed. In SUDAMINA (miliaria crystallina) clear superficial vesicles last a few hours or at the most a day or two. This is commonly seen in acute febrile illnesses, especially in children. The sweat is retained immediately below the horny layer. In MILIARIA RUBRA (prickly heat) recurrent crops of discrete papulovesicles occur, especially in areas where the skin is subjected to friction by clothing. Here the obstruction is deeper and sweat is retained within the epidermis. In MILIARIA PROFUNDA in which absence of sweating disturbs temperature regulation the state of tropical anhidrotic asthenia occurs (§ 510 ii.). Sweat is retained in the dermis, often after repeated attacks of prickly heat.

The only effective *Treatment* of all forms of miliaria is removal to a cooler environment in which sweating is reduced. Bland local applications may be helpful and excessive soap and spirit are to be avoided.

§ **674. IV. Impetigo** is a superficial pyogenic infection.

For many years staphylococcal and streptococcal types have been recognised and this distinction may be valid, but recent investigations have been contradictory, perhaps because, whichever organism is the primary invader secondary infection occurs so rapidly. Staphylococci certainly appear to play the predominant role in both clinical forms of impetigo, and newer bacteriological techniques incriminate certain specific strains.

Impetigo contagiosa occurs mainly on the face, neck and scalp of children. Very thin-walled vesicles form on an erythematous base. They extend peripherally but rupture in the centre. Exuding serum forms " stuck-on " yellow-brown crusts. Local lymphadenitis may occur but fever is exceptional. The infection may appear in previously normal skin or as a complication of pediculosis, scabies or other skin disease. Outbreaks occur mainly in the autumn and winter months.

Bullous impetigo occurs in older children and adults as clear tense blisters, the contents of which may become purulent. Grouping of the blisters gives rise to the clinical picture of *circinate impetigo*. Fever is rare. The condition is of staphylococcal origin and attacks are commoner in the summer.

Bullous impetigo of the newborn (Syn. Pemphigus neonatorum) is also of staphylococcal origin. The first lesions may appear at the sides of the neck or in other flexures. The eruption of bullæ may become widespread, but shows no special predilection for the palms and soles in contrast with the bullous syphilide of the newborn.

Etiology.—Small epidemics occur in nurseries and the source of the infection can sometimes be traced to a nurse or a midwife. Outbreaks are more common in the warmer months of the year.

Ritter's disease is a universal exfoliative state resulting from generalisation of bullous impetigo. Such cases were often fatal before antibiotics became available.

Treatment.—Search should first be made for evidence of scabies or pediculosis, in impetigo other than on the face. Impetigo contagiosa responds rapidly to chlortetracycline or neomycin ointment. Penicillin and sulphonamide ointments are not recommended, as there is a risk of provoking a sensitisation dermatitis. If there is severe adenitis a systemic antibiotic is advisable. Bullous impetigo also responds well to topical antibiotics or may be treated with an aqueous solution of gentian violet (1 per cent.), painted on after opening the blisters. In severe bullous impetigo of the newborn an antibiotic must be administered systemically.

§ 675. V. Herpes simplex is caused by a virus. The *primary* infection usually takes place in infancy; sometimes it occurs in adults. In the majority of cases it is clinically inapparent and can be recognised only by the presence of circulating antibodies. A small proportion of primary infections are severe, producing an acute kerato-conjunctivitis, or more rarely gingivo-stomatitis or vulvo-vaginitis with constitutional symptoms. Rarely an encephalitis occurs. In an infant with atopic dermatitis the primary infection may take the form of **Kaposi's varicelliform eruption.** Once the primary infection has occurred, the virus is carried in the tissues for many years and recurrent attacks, mild and localised, may be provoked by a number of factors. Lobar pneumonia, meningococcal infections, malaria and coryza frequently provoke attacks. Recurrences are also provoked by sunlight, by certain foods, or drugs or may occur at regular or irregular intervals for no discoverable reason.

Symptoms.—Children with herpetic stomatitis are ill with fever ranging from 100° to 103° for about a week. The mouth is sore and the submental glands enlarged and tender. Whitish plaques or many small discrete superficial ulcers are present on the buccal mucous membrane, the tongue, the gums and the floor of the mouth. There is usually no leucocytosis.

Kaposi's varicelliform eruption can be caused by the virus of vaccinia as well as of herpes simplex, and consists of an eruption of umbilicated vesicles covering the areas of skin affected by infantile eczema. Constitutional symptoms may be severe and before antibiotic treatment many cases were fatal.

The common *recurrent form of herpes simplex* develops after premonitory burning or irritation as a group or groups of small vesicles on an inflamed base. The face, particularly around the mouth and nose, is the commonest site, and recurrent attacks over a period of years are common. Lesions can develop on any part of the body and when they occur on unexpected sites (*e.g.*, the hand or fingers) the diagnosis is often overlooked. Healing takes place in 7 to 10 days and leaves no scar. When lesions occur on the genitalia of either sex (*herpes genitalis*) the grouped vesicles rapidly erode to produce discrete superficial ulcers.

Treatment of recurrent herpes simplex is often disappointing and attacks continue despite all efforts to control them. Application of small doses of superficial X-ray to the site of repeated attacks, or several paintings with thorium-X sometimes appears to diminish recurrences.

§ 676. VI. **Herpes Zoster** (and see § 1021).

Symptoms.—After more or less premonitory pain or burning, groups of vesicles on an erythematous base develop in unilateral segmental distribution. The lesions heal in 7–14 days but may leave scars. In rare cases a generalised varicelliform eruption appears a few days after the zoster. Dorsal and lumbar segments are more commonly affected but trigeminal zoster is not unusual in the elderly, in whom the lesions in any site may be hæmorrhagic or gangrenous. Post-herpetic neuralgia is the only common complication. Herpes zoster is rare in childhood and becomes progressively more frequent with increasing age: the sex incidence is equal.

Etiology.—The cause is a virus, possibly identical with that of varicella.

Treatment.—Analgesics must be given to reduce the pain, adequate control of which may reduce the probability of subsequent neuralgia. In severe cases cortisone or prednisone by mouth for 4 or 5 days relieves symptoms and induces rapid healing. In milder cases local application of a dusting powder or of collodion is acceptable. For severely ulcerated lesions antibiotic ointments can be applied.

VII. **Varicella** and **Variola** must always be thought of in every case of a generalised vesicular eruption (see §§ 476, 479).

§ 677. VIII. **Orf** is a rare infection in man, contracted from sheep suffering from contagious pustular dermatitis, a virus disease.

Symptoms.—After an incubation period of about 6 days, a small red papule develops, often at the site of an abrasion. The papule is soon surmounted by a flat vesicle with indurated edges. Lesions are single or few and constitutional symptoms mild. Recovery is complete in 3–4 weeks.

Cowpox is occasionally seen in farm workers. A single vesicle develops about 2 weeks after contact. Regional adenitis and fever are usual.

Vaccinia.—Accidental vaccination is rare, but occurs in doctors and nurses from self-inoculation with vaccine lymph or in children in close contact with recently vaccinated individuals. Eczema vaccinatum, one form of Kaposi's varicelliform eruption, is a generalised vaccinial eruption which is sometimes fatal (see §§ 480, 675).

§ 678. IX. **Hydroa Aestivale** is a symmetrical eruption of vesicles and papules, in crops on areas exposed to sunlight, especially on the nose, the cheeks and the backs of the hands. It usually begins in early childhood and tends to improve after puberty. Attacks occur at intervals during the summer. *H. vacciniforme* is a more severe variety in which a necrotic reaction leads to scar formation. Porphyrinuria is sometimes present, but its relationship to the hydroa is uncertain.

Treatment.—Protection from sunlight is essential. Chemical light screens (see § 628) may be tried.

§ 679. X. **Phytophotodermatitis** is a bullous eruption observed in those who have exposed the skin to light after contact with certain plants, as in bathing on a river bank. The bullae are linear and follow the imprint on the skin of the plant stems and leaves. They are followed by pigmentation.

§ 680. XI. **Dermatitis Herpetiformis** is relatively uncommon. It is a relapsing disorder continuing for many years with periods of comparative freedom. Males are rather more often affected than females, and the peak age of onset is between 30 and 50, but cases can occur at any age.

Symptoms.—The eruption is characteristically polymorphic and of symmetrical distribution; clusters of wheals, vesicles and papules preceded and accompanied by intense pruritus develop in the scapular region, over the sacrum, on the extensor aspects of the arms, the abdominal wall and the outer thighs. In some, the eruption may consist exclusively of papules, of vesicles or of plaques of erythema, and any combination of these lesions may occur; vesicles or bullae are usually present at some stage. In infants and children the lesions may be predominantly bullous and the distribution atypical, groups of bullae developing on the hands and feet, the genitalia and the lower abdominal wall. The lesions heal to leave pigmentation. In some the severity of the attacks diminishes gradually and they may cease after a year or two, but in many they continue for years. Severe attacks may rarely be accompanied by mild constitutional symptoms. Eosinophilia is frequent.

Etiology.—The cause is unknown. There is no evidence that a virus is responsible and dermatitis herpetiformis may be a non-specific pattern of reaction with multiple causes. Histological examination of a bulla demonstrates its formation beneath an intact epidermis: the underlying dermis contains a pleomorphic infiltrate in which eosinophils are often conspicuous.

Treatment.—No treatment is curative, but it is usually possible to control the distressing symptoms for as long as treatment is continued. Liq. arsenicalis (Fowler's solution) is effective, but because of the risk of skin cancer after repeated courses the treatment of choice is now dapsone 50 mg. twice daily. Sometimes a smaller dose controls the eruption; side effects may be encountered, particularly during the early weeks of treatment, and red blood counts are advisable. As an alternative, which is slightly less effective, but which relieves some cases not responding to this drug, sulphapyridine is almost specific in doses of 0·5 G. once or twice daily; the white blood count must be watched for granulocytopenia. With either drug the minimum effective dose must be established and continued.

Herpes gestationis resembles bullous dermatitis herpetiformis but occurs in pregnancy, commonly beginning during the fifth or sixth month. It may recur in successive pregnancies. The eruption usually terminates spontaneously soon after parturition. Infant mortality is high. In severe cases therapeutic abortion may be indicated, but the eruption can usually be suppressed with prednisone or cortisone.

Pemphigoid is the term applied to a bullous eruption which had previously been confused with pemphigus: histologically it resembles dermatitis herpetiformis. The patients are usually elderly.

Symptoms.—The eruption may consist of wheals, plaques of erythema and bullæ or exclusively of large tense bullæ. It may remain localised to one region for many weeks, but ultimately generalises. The mucous membranes are rarely involved. Although it may prove fatal in a frail elderly patient it is not lethal in itself, and if the patient's condition can be maintained recovery is usual. Pemphigoid may occur as a reaction to a carcinoma and this possibility must be excluded before symptomatic treatment is given. In contrast to dermatitis herpetiformis there is no response to sulphapyridine or to sulphones, but corticosteroids will control most cases.

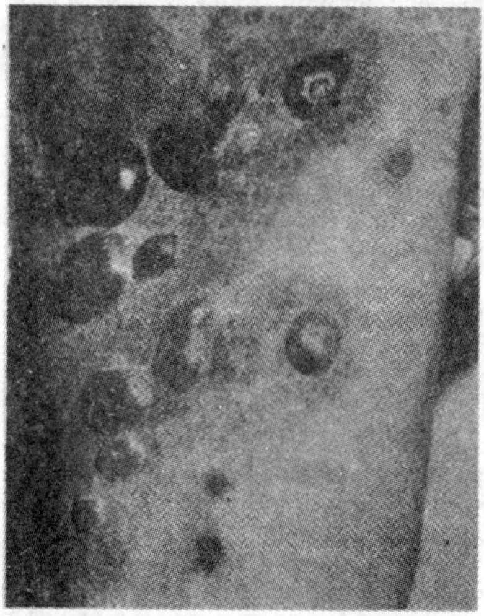

Ocular pemphigus is rare, and apparently related to pemphigoid, affecting mainly elderly women. Cutaneous lesions are few and usually restricted to the face and neck. Involvement of the conjunctiva produces essential shrinkage and the erosions in the mouth can cause severe dysphagia.

FIG. 188.—PEMPHIGOID IN AN ELDERLY MAN. Large clear tense bullæ and plaques of erythema.

§ 681. XII. Pemphigus is a rare disease affecting both sexes after 50 years of age. It occasionally occurs in younger patients and runs a rapid course. Several clinical forms are recognised, but all are manifestations of the same disease and transition from one to another is frequent.

Symptoms.—In *P. vulgaris* the onset is often insidious; a persistent stomatitis or flaccid bullæ forming recurrent soft crusts on the scalp may occur many months before a generalised bullous eruption appears. The mucous membranes are involved initially or at some stage in most cases. The eruption of large thin-walled bullæ may be almost universal, these rupturing to leave raw moist areas. The skin of apparently unaffected sites separates readily with slight friction (Nikolski's sign). The general condition deteriorates and although temporary remissions may occur without treatment death usually follows in a few months. In *P. vegetans*, moist foul-smelling vegetating masses in the mouth and lips, anogenital area, groins and axillæ mirabilis and occasionally other sites increase the patient's distress. It has a similar grave prognosis. In *P. foliaceus* the bullæ are very superficial and flaccid, rupturing as soon as they are formed and producing by their universal extension one form of exfoliative dermatitis. Untreated, most cases are fatal in a year or two. *P. erythematosus* (Senear-Usher syndrome) is a relatively benign phase of pemphigus. It may change into *P. foliaceus* or *P. vulgaris* or the latter may, rarely, regress to this partial form only to revert later to the graver phase. This benign stage may persist for many years with no deterioration of the patient's health. Bullæ appear mainly near the mid-line of the trunk or on the face and dry to form red crusted lesions which superficially resemble seborrhœic dermatitis.

In *diagnosis* of *P. vulgaris* exclude bullous drug eruptions, Stevens-Johnson syndrome, pemphigoid. Despite occasional anomalous findings histological examination is a valuable aid. A fresh bulla must be selected. The various forms of pemphigus all show a primary epidermal change in which acantholysis leads to loss of cohesion between the cells and the development of irregular clefts.

Treatment.—Admission to hospital is advisable as nursing presents great difficulties. The majority of cases show very marked improvement, or even complete regression of all lesions, when treated with ACTH or cortisone. Very large initial doses may be required, up to 1,500 mg. of oral cortisone daily, or 150 mg. of ACTH given intramusc., after which a maintenance dose of oral cortisone or prednisone must be continued. Some patients, who would otherwise have succumbed, are now leading normal lives, but any reduction of dosage below a critical level is followed by the development of new bullæ.

§ 682. XIII. **Erythema multiforme exudativum** (Stevens-Johnson syndrome, Ectodermosis erosiva pluriorificialis).—Bullæ are a feature of the iris type of erythema

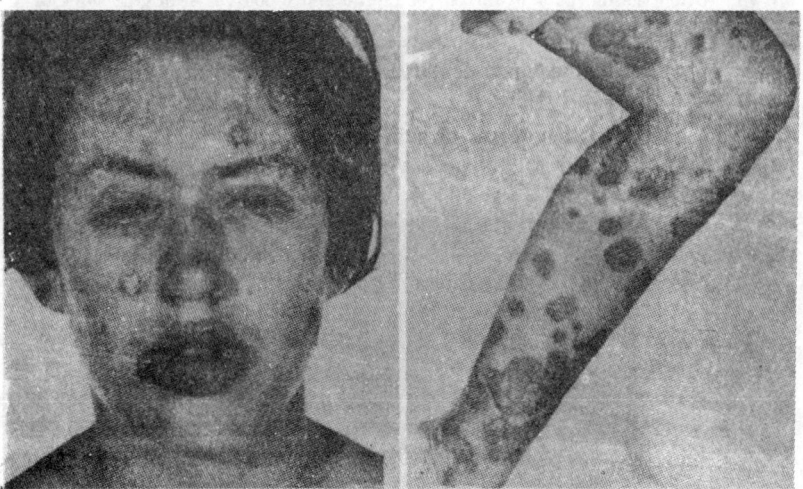

FIGS. 189 AND 190.—ERYTHEMA MULTIFORME EXUDATIVUM in a girl aged 17. The buccal mucous membrane and the vulva were severely involved.

multiforme (§ 643) but there are good grounds for differentiating as a distinct entity this syndrome which runs a characteristic course. Children and young adults are commonly affected.

Symptoms.—After variable prodomal symptoms, usually those of a respiratory infection, bullæ develop on the lips and in the mouth, on the conjunctivæ and in the anogenital region. They rupture to form superficial erosions beneath a pseudomembrane. The eye lesions, often accompanied by gross œdema of the lids, may be followed by serious ocular complications. Erythematous plaques and bullæ may occur on the trunk and limbs, but are not invariable. A pneumonitis is often associated. Fever above 103° F for several days is frequent. The cause is unknown but a virus is suspected.

Diagnosis.—A phenobarbitone eruption, which may be very similar, must be excluded. Pemphigoid and pemphigus should not cause confusion.

Prognosis.—Recovery is the rule, but occasional fatalities occur.

Treatment.—Antibiotics are useful in preventing secondary infection. The corticosteroids are usually without effect.

§ **683**. XIV. **Epidermolysis bullosa** is a rare genetically determined defect in which blisters develop at sites of trauma.

Symptoms.—There are many clinical forms; the commonest, inherited as a simple dominant character, is relatively mild. Bullæ develop mainly on points of friction, particularly in the warmer weather. The expectation of life is not reduced. In certain types, of recessive inheritance, blisters, which may be present at birth, form with trivial traumata or even spontaneously and may involve the buccal mucous membrane, interfering with feeding. Other congenital defects may be present. The prognosis is more grave.

§ **684**. XV. **Hydrocystoma** occurs in middle-aged women working in a hot moist atmosphere. Tense firm vesicles due to sweat retention appear symmetrically on the forehead, below the eyes and on the upper cheeks. They may disappear rapidly or persist for some weeks.

§ **685**. XVI. **Lymphangioma circumscriptum** is a lymphatic tissue nævus. The groups of vesicles present at birth or in early childhood, somewhat resemble frog-spawn. Often the nævus is of mixed lymphatic and blood-vessel origin: some or all of the vesicles may be hæmorrhagic.

XVII. **Other bullous** or **vesicular drug eruptions.** Some drug eruptions are bullous (§§ 624, 701).

§ **686**. XVIII. **Other forms of skin diseases** which are not commonly bullous may give rise to bullæ or vesicles in certain cases. Congenital

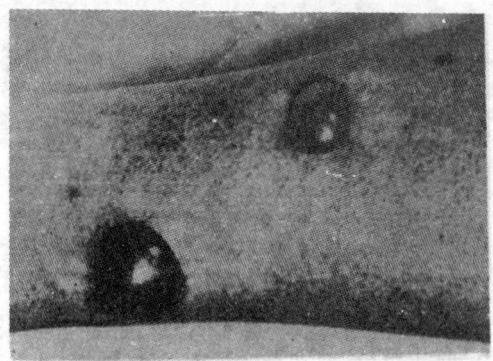

FIG. 191.—INSECT BITES. Large tense bullæ on a child's leg. Not an uncommon reaction to insect bites.

syphilis can cause a bullous eruption in the newborn, showing a predilection for the palms and soles. Scabies, especially in infants, may produce vesicles, particularly on the palms or soles. The bites of fleas and other insects may provoke a bullous reaction especially on the legs (§ 655, Fig. 191). Tinea pedis is commonly vesicular or bullous (§ 662). Bullæ may occasionally develop in lichen planus (§ 637) and in lichen sclerosus but are not likely to confuse the diagnosis. Recurrent bullæ, sometimes hæmorrhagic, may develop on a mast-cell nævus (see urticaria pigmentosa, § 764).

GROUP III.　PUSTULAR ERUPTIONS

*Eruptions which are essentially pustular or in which pustule
formation may be a conspicuous feature*

Common.

I. Furunculosis (§ 687).
II. Carbuncles (§ 688).
III. Folliculitis barbæ (§ 689).
IV. Sycosis—pyogenic (§ 690).
V. Pustular miliaria (§ 691).
VI. Impetigo of Bockhart (§ 692).
VII. Pustular acne (§ 693).
VIII. Folliculitis cheloidalis nuchæ
　　　(§ 694).
IX. Hidradenitis suppurativa
　　　(§ 695).
X. Pustular ringworm, tinea
　　sycosis and kerion (§ 696).

Rare.

XI. Pustular bacteride (§ 697).
XII. Acrodermatitis perstans (§ 698).
XIII. Kaposi's varicelliform eruption
　　　(§ 675).
XIV. Anthrax (§ 490).
XV. Impetigo herpetiformis (§ 699).
XVI. Blastomycosis (§ 700).
XVII. Drug eruptions (§§ 624, 701).
XVIII. Pustular tuberculide (§ 702).
XIX. Pustular syphilide (§ 703).
XX. Subcorneal pustular dermatitis
　　　(§ 704).

Many vesicular eruptions mentioned in Group II, including the various forms of
eczema and impetigo, may become pustular as the result of secondary infection by
pyogenic cocci. Pompholyx of the hands or feet readily becomes infected and
secondary infection of tinea pedis is common.

§ **687. I. Furunculosis** (Boils).—A furuncle is a red follicular papule
which becomes increasingly tender and painful as it enlarges. It may
subside spontaneously (blind boil) but commonly becomes pustular and
central necrosis is followed by discharge of the core. The cavity fills
with granulation tissue and heals with a scar. The individual lesion runs
a course of 1 to 3 weeks but boils are often multiple and fresh crops may
continue for months. Common sites are the face, neck, ear and anogenital
region, buttocks and thighs.

Etiology.—Boils are due to staphylococcal infection of a hair follicle
and differ from folliculitis in the extent of the perifollicular cellulitis and
the necrosis. Diabetes, anæmia, leukæmia, malnutrition, alcoholism,
nervous and physical exhaustion may be predisposing factors but in most
cases no cause for the breakdown in the normal mechanism of skin disinfection is apparent. Friction of clothing and auto-inoculation determine
the distribution.

Treatment.—The single painful boil will respond rapidly to intramuscular penicillin or to chlortetracycline (aureomycin) by mouth. The
antibiotics are seldom of permanent value in chronic furunculosis as new
lesions appear as soon as they are discontinued. The best results are
obtained from rest and sedation or recreational activity, a low carbohydrate diet with vitamin B complex and careful attention to hygiene
both of the person and of the clothes. General ultraviolet light is helpful.
Neomycin ointment applied to the nasal vestibules twice daily reduces

the nasal carriage of staphylococci which disseminate to the skin from this site. Injection of staphylococcal ambotoxoid (mixed vaccine and toxoid) or autogenous vaccines gives inconsistent results. Diabetes and other systemic disorders must receive treatment.

§ 688. II. A **Carbuncle** is formed by the confluence of deep follicular infections with extensive cellulitis of the surrounding tissues leading to necrosis and the formation of a slough. It may be regarded as a cluster of boils. The same predisposing factors are of importance as in furunculosis. Carbuncles occur mainly after the age of 40 and are usually on the neck or back. A tender dull red area of induration extends slowly for 5 to 7 days; pus first discharges from follicular points of necrosis, then the whole central area necroses and separates to leave a painful ulcer which slowly heals. *Treatment* has been revolutionised by the antibiotics: a suitable preparation to which the infecting staphylococcus is sensitive should be administered until healing is established. Attention must be paid to general measures as with furunculosis: in extensive lesions in the elderly and debilitated treatment may need to be prolonged.

§ 689. III. **Folliculitis barbæ** (Barber's rash) is extremely common. The infection of the follicle is very superficial.

Symptoms.—Redness and slight swelling of the orifice of the hair follicles are sometimes accompanied by crusting. The shaved area is involved. Indoor workers with seborrhœic skins are particularly susceptible and recurrences after apparent cure are frequent.

Diagnosis.—Pseudofolliculitis, caused by ingrowing hairs, is very common in negroes and occasionally in other races, especially on the sides of the neck.

Treatment.—The patient must keep his hands away from his face. Substitution of an electric shaver for an ordinary razor may help. Overtreatment must be avoided. Antibiotic ointments are usually effective but relapses are common when they are discontinued and their prolonged use is not advisable. The best result is given by chlortetracycline or neomycin ointment combined with hydrocortisone acetate ointment ($\frac{1}{2}$–1 per cent.). Lotio cupro-zincica (N.F.) diluted with 8 parts of water may be applied after shaving and lotio calaminæ oleosa at night. Other cases respond well to the application of quinolor ointment 1 part with zinc paste 2 parts, at night. Where seborrhœa is conspicuous sulphur precip. (2 per cent.) in lotio calaminæ can be used after shaving.

§ 690. IV. **Sycosis**—the pyogenic form differs from superficial folliculitis in the extension of the infection to the whole depth of the follicle. The beard area is most commonly affected but the pubes and other sites may be involved.

Symptoms.—Groups of œdematous indurated papules or pustules develop on the upper lip, the cheeks and the chin. They are usually limited to a small area, but may be more widely distributed. Sycosis of the upper lip can occur with a chronic sinus infection but often no obvious contributory factor is found. In one form, known as *lupoid sycosis*, the inflammatory process destroys the follicles leaving a central scar with an actively pustular advancing margin. This condition is chronic and refractory to treatment.

Treatment.—In the acute and painful cases hot compresses of mercury perchloride (1 in 2,000) should be applied twice daily; loose hairs should be epilated with forceps and a soothing application such as lotio calaminæ oleosa prescribed. In less acute cases chlortetracycline or neomycin ointment are often effective alone or in combination with hydrocortisone. Quinolor ointment may give good results. In localised chronic sycosis an epilating dose of X-ray followed by an antibiotic ointment is often curative. Associated upper respiratory infections must be treated. In severe and resistant cases a period of bed rest, a holiday or a course of general ultraviolet light may be beneficial.

§ 691. V. **Pustular miliaria.**—Crops of small non-follicular pustules may develop where sweat is retained in the epidermis (§ 673). They are usually sterile. They occur at any age, often as a complication of an inflammatory skin disorder. In infants they are seen especially in the deep folds at the sides of the neck.

§ 692. VI. **Impetigo of Bockhart** is a suppurative staphylococcal infection of the upper third of the hair follicles. Children are affected more often than adults: poor general hygiene and pruritic skin diseases such as scabies predispose. It is common in troops under active service conditions. Fomentations, plasters and over-vigorous local applications may initiate the eruption; ointments containing tar are particularly liable to do so. Any hairy region may be affected.

Symptoms.—The eruption consists of discrete superficial pustules with a red areola and a central hair. The lesions may heal rapidly or some or all may develop into furuncles, from downward extension of the infection.

Treatment demands improvement in general hygiene, regular baths and clean clothing. The skin may be painted daily with gentian violet (1 per cent.) or with mercury perchloride (1 in 2,000) in calamine lotion. Vioform ointment is also suitable.

§ 693. VII. **Pustular acne.**—An acneiform eruption, which may be pustular, can be provoked by local contact with mineral oil; the arms and the upper thighs are often affected (§ 635).

§ 694. VIII. **Folliculitis cheloidalis nuchæ** (Acne cheloid) occurs on the nape of the neck in young and middle-aged adult males. Friction of the collar is usually held responsible, often with little justification.

Symptoms.—Follicular pustules are gradually replaced by firm pink papules which coalesce to form irregular cheloid-like scars.

Treatment.—Neomycin ointment with hydrocortisone prevents the development of new pustules. The cheloid papules may respond to radiotherapy but if the scarring is disfiguring it may be necessary to combine this with plastic excision.

§ **695.** IX. **Hidradenitis suppurativa** is commonly misdiagnosed as furunculosis. Women are affected more often than men. It is an infection of the apocrine sweat glands: the axillæ are most commonly involved but lesions can occur in other apocrine areas especially the anogenital region. Shaving the axillæ may be a causative factor.

Symptoms.—Small firm nodules, deeply situated in the subcutaneous tissue of one or both axillæ, break down and discharge pus. New lesions may continue to develop for many months.

Treatment is the same as for furunculosis. X-ray therapy is helpful if given before the nodules break down.

§ **696.** X. **Pustular ringworm, tinea sycosis and kerion.** Certain species of ringworm fungus, particularly those of animal origin, may provoke a brisk inflammatory response in man, and produce pustular lesions.

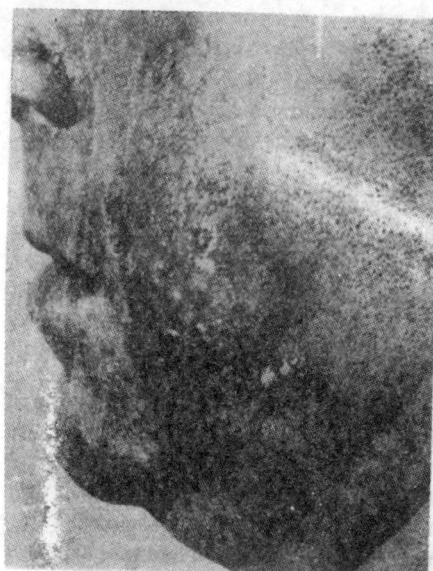

FIG. 192.—RINGWORM INFECTION OF THE BEARD. The patient was a farmer. The intense inflammatory reaction has produced the boggy mass of follicular pustules known as a kerion.

Symptoms.—Infections with *Trichophyton verrucosum* (usually contracted from calves) and *T. mentagrophytes* often give rise either to dull red plaques studded with pustules (agminate folliculitis) or on hairy regions to a kerion—a boggy œdematous mass with follicular pustules. The exposed skin of farm workers is most commonly affected and on the beard area the closely grouped œdematous pustules constitute tinea sycosis. In contrast to pyogenic sycosis there is no predilection for the upper lip. A kerion may also be produced by Microsporon infection, especially when the lesions have been too vigorously treated. The inflammatory forms of ringworm infection are self-limiting.

Treatment in the acute stage consists of hot compresses of mercury perchloride (1 in 2,000) and a fungicidal ointment such as ung. zinci undecenoate (N.F.) subsequently. Griseofulvin is required in severe cases (§ 662).

§ **697.** XI. **Pustular bacteride** is an uncommon condition in which crops of small discrete pustules develop on the palms or soles. They heal with the separation of a brown scale, but successive crops may appear for long periods. The relationship to pustular psoriasis (§ 658) is uncertain. An obvious association between the crops of pustules and an infective focus, dental or upper respiratory, is unusual but such a focus should be sought and eliminated. Local applications are of little value. Sulphapyridine or diaminodiphenyl sulphone is sometimes effective.

§ **698.** XII. **Acrodermatitis perstans** (Dermatitis repens) is rare; as the name implies it is resistant to treatment. It is probably a form of pustular psoriasis.

Symptoms.—Most cases begin as paronychial infections; a moist infective dermatitis with pustulation in the advancing margin, slowly extends up the finger. Oil fingers and toes may be similarly affected. The nails become dystrophic and are sometimes destroyed. Rarely similar patches may develop in other areas. Many cases resist all forms of treatment. Sulphapyridine and diaminodiphenyl sulphone should be tried.

XIII. KAPOSI'S VARICELLIFORM ERUPTION should be suspected if a widespread eruption of vesicles, which rapidly become pustular, develops in an individual affected by atopic dermatitis (§ 675).

XIV. **Anthrax.** *Symptoms.*— The lesion begins as a firm red papule which rapidly develops into a hæmorrhagic pustule, on an indurated œdematous base, surrounded by a zone of erythema on which are vesicles or pustules. The central pustule ruptures and a dark crust is formed. There may be severe constitutional symptoms (§ 490).

§ **699.** XV. **Impetigo herpetiformis** is extremely rare. It usually affects pregnant women, but cases have been reported in non-pregnant women and in men.

Symptoms. — Accompanied by fever and severe constitutional symptoms, groups of miliary pustules develop first in the flexures,

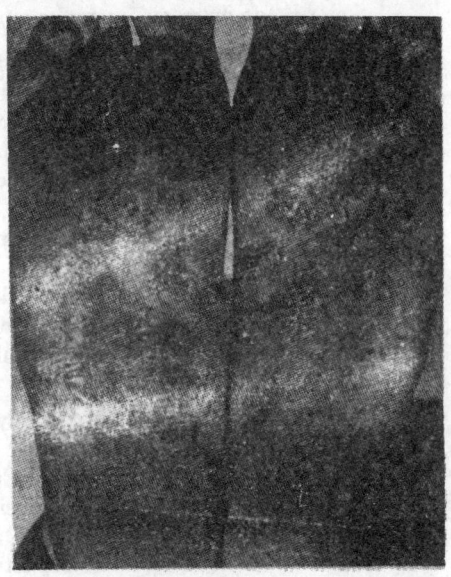

FIG. 193.—PUSTULAR PSORIASIS. The flat yellow patches dry to form brown crusts. The condition is often confused with tinea pedis.

whence they extend widely. The mortality is high. Hypocalcæmia is usual.

§ **700.** XVI. **Blastomycosis** (North American blastomycosis) is caused by the yeast-like organism *Blastomyces dermatitidis* and is almost confined to the North American continent. The skin lesions, which are soft plaques with a fungating surface and a smooth advancing border studded with micro-abscesses, are usually a manifestation of systemic infection. Iodides by mouth and X-ray therapy may be effective in local infection. Stilbamidine is given in systemic infection (§ 147).

§ **701.** XVII. **Drug eruptions.**—Bromides commonly produce a pustular eruption of acneiform type; iodides, pustules on an indurated base or moist fungating masses.

§ **702.** XVIII. **Pustular tuberculides.**—The various forms of papulonecrotic tuberculide may be pustular at times. The indolence of the lesions, their induration and the symmetrical distribution will suggest the diagnosis (see § 646).

§ **703.** XIX. **Pustular syphilides** are uncommon and occur during the first year after infection mainly by ill-nourished individuals whose standard of hygiene is low. Several clinical forms have been described, small papulo-pustular, rupioid, varioliform, etc. The pustules are indolent and heavy crust formation and ulceration are conspicuous. The characters common to all syphilitic eruptions (§ 705) assist the differentiation from other disorders.

§ **704.** XX. **Subcorneal pustular dermatitis** used to be confused with dermatitis

herpetiformis. It affects middle-aged women who develop on the trunk and in the
flexures small flat pustules clustered in groups, extending centrifugally to form gyrate
or annular patterns which eventually heal to leave pigmentation. Phases of activity
and quiescence may alternate for months or years but the general health remains
unimpaired. The cause is unknown. *Treatment.*—Many cases are controlled by the
measures used for dermatitis herpetiformis (§ 680).

GROUP IV. MULTIFORM ERUPTIONS

When an eruption consists of lesions of several different types it is often
possible on careful examination to establish that they represent merely
different stages in the evolution of the elementary lesions—papules may
evolve into vesicles and thence into pustules. Recurrent crops of new
lesions account for the polymorphism sometimes seen in varicella. In other
conditions the apparent polymorphism may be the result of changes
brought about by scratching or by secondary infection, as in scabies, or
by the reaction to treatment.

Polymorphic eruptions are particularly frequent in dermatitis herpetiformis (erythema, papules, wheals, vesicles) § 680, erythema multiforme
(erythema, papules, circinate plaques, bullæ) § 643, syphilis and pityriasis
lichenoides (§ 705).

§ 705. General Characteristics of Syphilitic eruptions: Syphilis is
notorious for the polymorphism of many of its eruptions and its ability to
simulate a great variety of disorders. Certain general characteristics are
therefore of vital importance in diagnosis: (i.) Early syphilitic eruptions
tend to be symmetrical, widespread and superficial. (ii.) Later eruptions
are less extensive, more infiltrated and often grouped in segments of circles.
Some of these ulcerate. (iii.) The papular forms have a predilection for
the face, palms and soles. (iv.) Syphilitic eruptions very rarely itch and
apart from the bullous congenital syphilide are never vesicular or bullous.
(v.) The brighter pink and red of some skin conditions are seldom encountered and syphilitic lesions are usually dull brown or yellowish-red.

Pityriasis lichenoides (Guttate Parapsoriasis) is a rare condition sometimes misdiagnosed as varicella or syphilis, which occurs mainly in young adults. *Symptoms.*—
In the *acute* form known as **pityriasis lichenoides et varioliformis acuta** the eruption,
which is commonly on the trunk, may first resemble varicella but is soon strikingly
polymorphic, consisting of vesicles, pustules, crusted hæmorrhagic ulcers and small
scars. New lesions may develop in crops for months, or the eruption of **pityriasis
lichenoides chronica** may take its place and persist unchanged for years. The chronic
form may develop *ab initio.* The papules are small, flat and reddish-brown: each is
covered by a single scale, which may be detached quite readily and is of diagnostic
value. Ultra-violet light is of temporary benefit.

GROUP V. NODULAR ERUPTIONS AND TUMOURS

A nodule may be defined as a circumscribed solid lesion in or beneath
the skin, larger than a papule. Clearly many lesions which are initially
papules may become nodules and are then classified according to their
more characteristic form.

Certain skin tumours which are not nodular are for convenience considered in this section.

Infective granulomata and other diseases

Common.

I. Erythema nodosum (§ 706).
II. Erythema induratum (§ 707).
III. Nodular vasculitis (§ 708).
IV. Lupus vulgaris (§ 709).
V. Sarcoidosis (§ 710).
VI. Rheumatoid nodules (§ 711).
VII. Xanthoma (§ 712).
VIII. Leukæmia (§ 713).

Rare. [1]

IX. Nodular syphilides (§ 714).
X. Leprosy (§ 715).
XI. Yaws (§ 716).
XII. Cutaneous Leishmaniasis (§ 717).
XIII. Madura Foot (§ 718).
XIV. Actinomycosis (§ 719).
XV. Sporotrichosis (§ 720).
XVI. Polyarteritis nodosa (§§ 98, 721).
XVII. Weber-Christian Disease (§ 722).
XVIII. Mycosis fungoides (§ 723).
XIX. Onchocerciasis (§ 724).

Tumours, nævi and cysts

XX. Squamous epithelioma (§ 725).
XXI. Basal cell epithelioma (§ 726).
XXII. Keratoacanthoma (§ 727).
XXIII. Other skin tumours of epithelial origin (§ 728).
XXIV. Sebaceous and epithelial cysts (§ 729).

XXV. Hæmangioma and lymphangioma (§ 730).
XXVI. Lipoma (§ 731).
XXVII. Histiocytoma (§ 732).
XXVIII. Granuloma pyogenicum (§ 733).
XXIX. Neurofibroma (§ 734).
XXX. Melanoma (see § 756).

Infective Granulomata and other Diseases

§ **706.** I. **Erythema nodosum** is a clinico-pathological syndrome. Most cases occur in young women between the ages of 20 and 30.

Symptoms.—Accompanied by mild fever, malaise and joint and muscle pain, one, two or three crops of dull red tender nodules develop each few days, symmetrically on the shins: they are rarely seen on other areas. The nodules fade in the course of 2 or 3 weeks to leave bruise-like staining.

Etiology.—E. nodosum is a reaction to an infection or a drug and may depend on an allergic mechanism. The provocative factors commonly encountered in Britain are: tuberculosis, the eruption developing in a primary infection at the stage of Mantoux conversion; streptococcal infection; drugs, especially sulphathiazole, iodides and bromides; and sarcoidosis. Rare causes are meningococcal infections, lymphogranuloma venereum, coccidioidomycosis and leprosy. Sometimes no cause can be established.

[1] Although rare in Great Britain many of these diseases are very common in tropical and semi-tropical climates.

Treatment.—As spontaneous resolution occurs only bed rest and analgesics are required unless the provocati.e infection demands treatment.

§ **707.** II. **Erythema induratum** (Bazin's disease) is a tuberculide. It is commonly seen in adolescent girls and young women, especially stout girls with fat legs and a sluggish peripheral circulation.

Symptoms.—Dull purplish-red subcutaneous nodules develop on the lower half of the back of the leg and persist for months. They may absorb or may break down to form indolent punched-out ulcers, which heal to leave depressed pigmented scars.

Diagnosis.—Clinical differentiation from the nodular form of perniosis, which is very much commoner, may be impossible since both conditions occur in the same type of individual but marked ulceration suggests a tuberculous origin. It is possible that circulating bacilli from a tuberculous focus are trapped in areas of stasis and actually cause the specific transformation of a perniotic nodule. The diagnosis of Bazin's disease must therefore be based on clinical or radiological evidence of tuberculosis elsewhere in the body, a positive Mantoux reaction and tuberculous changes on histological examination.

Treatment.—The response to specific chemotherapy is usually satisfactory but recurrence in subsequent winters may take place.

§ **708.** III. **Nodular vasculitis** occurs mainly in middle-aged or elderly women.

Symptoms.—Crops of tender nodules develop on the lower legs. They disappear with rest in bed but tend to recur. The *etiology* of this fairly common condition is uncertain and the terminology of this and of other nodular eruptions of the legs is confused.

Diagnosis.—Other clinical entities which must be distinguished are (i.) the crops of small bright red nodules occurring on the legs and feet in thrombo-angiitis obliterans which may precede other manifestations by many years. They may also occur in senile obliterative arteritis: (ii.) the variable symptom complexes comprising combinations of nodules, papules, bullæ and purpura which occur with chronic infections. Many names have been applied—allergic arteriolitis, polysymptome of Gougerot, etc. There is an overlap between these syndromes and cutaneous polyarteritis.

§ **709.** IV. **Lupus vulgaris** is the commonest form of skin tuberculosis.

Symptoms.—Most cases begin in childhood. The skin of the face is affected in the majority of cases, particularly the nose and cheeks, but the disease may occur anywhere. The mucous membranes of the nose, mouth and larynx may be involved. The initial lesion is a soft reddish-brown gelatinous nodule, which, on diascopy, has the appearance of " apple-jelly." Irregular plaques are formed by the coalescence of such nodules; the centre may become cicatricial but a few nodules often persist in the scar. If untreated the disease may persist throughout life, usually extending very slowly, with periods of apparent quiescence. Ulceration may result in rapid extension and destruction of underlying tissues with grossly mutilating effects. In the many clinical variants which may occur changes such as scaling or epidermal hyperplasia may modify the appearance but the characteristic nodules suggest the diagnosis. Carcinoma or sarcoma may follow; the liability to these is probably increased by X-ray therapy which was formerly employed in treatment. Associated pulmonary tuberculosis is exceptional, but bone and joint tuberculosis or tuberculous adenitis are sometimes present. In children a disseminated form may

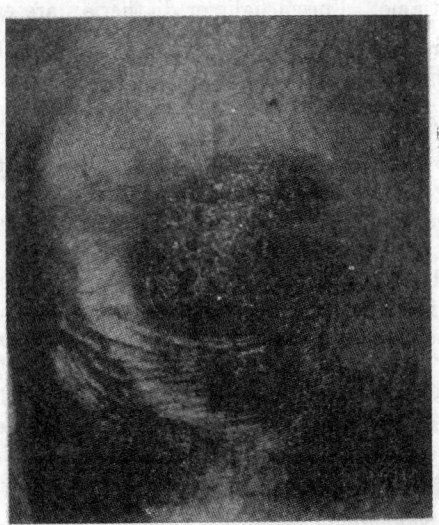

FIG. 194.—LUPUS VULGARIS. This lesion on the knee of a young man had been present since infancy. Note the scarring. Complete healing has been obtained with isoniazid.

occur very rarely; widely scattered groups of typical nodules develop especially after measles.

In *diagnosis* tertiary syphilis, sarcoidosis and lupus erythematosus must be considered. All these commonly begin in adult life. In lupus erythematosus (§ 631) no nodules are present in the plaques of erythema, but there are follicular plugs, atrophy and telangiectasia.

The *Treatment* of choice is now isoniazid 0·2 to 0·5 G. daily for at least six months. The white blood count should be examined at regular intervals, as leucopenia may be produced. When lupus nodules can no longer be detected on diascopy the dose can be reduced, but a small maintenance dose must be given for many months to reduce the otherwise high recurrence rate. Recent lesions usually respond very well, but long-standing cicatrised lesions respond less consistently. Then the treatment may be combined with streptomycin 1 G. daily for a few weeks after which the isoniazid is continued alone. The introduction of calciferol marked a great advance and it is still worth a trial when response is unsatisfactory to other measures, with which it may usefully be combined. The initial dose is 150,000 units daily: this may require reduction if toxic symptoms such as anorexia or lassitude develop. The serum calcium level must be estimated regularly. Calciferol is contra-indicated in the presence of renal or cardio-vascular disease. Clinical experience and histological and bacteriological studies all emphasise the need to keep the patient under regular supervision for several years after clinical cure.

Local measures are still occasionally required to deal with resistant nodules in scar tissue. Finsen light or diathermy are employed.

§ 710. V. Sarcoidosis.—The clinical aspects of the skin lesions must be carefully studied in conjunction with associated lesions in other systems and the results of laboratory investigations (see § 141).

Symptoms.—Skin lesions are present in 30–50 per cent. of cases of sarcoidosis; they may precede or follow other manifestations and certain forms are rarely if ever associated with systemic involvement. Several clinical forms occur—(i.) papules, nodules or plaques, mainly on the face and upper limbs: an annular configuration is sometimes seen. The lesions are brownish-red in colour, less soft and translucent than lupus vulgaris; (ii.) **Lupus pernio**—infiltrated bluish plaques on the nose, cheeks and fingers; (iii.) subcutaneous brownish-red nodules; (iv.) **Angiolupoid**—firm, rounded, rather vascular nodules, usually in the centre of the face.

The *diagnosis* of sarcoidosis must never be made solely on histological grounds, as the sarcoid type of tissue response is not specific and can be provoked by foreign bodies (silica granuloma) and has been observed in leprosy and in syphilis.

§ 711. VI. Rheumatoid nodules.—Subcutaneous nodules occur in 10 per cent. of patients with rheumatoid arthritis (§ 597). They usually develop on the extensor surface of the forearms, but also over the patellæ and other bony prominences and along tendon sheaths. *Diagnosis.*—They must be differentiated from the nodules of rheumatic fever and the very rare juxta-articular nodes of syphilis and yaws.

§ 712. VII. Xanthoma.—Cutaneous xanthomata are conveniently classified into the following groups: (i.) *Xanthoma tuberosum:* this produces yellowish nodules which are sometimes lobulated; they affect the extensor surfaces of the limbs, the buttocks, the tendon sheaths and the creases of the palms, and may appear at any age. Minor and inconstant differences may be noted between the skin lesions in the various hypercholesterolæmic disorders. *Etiology.*—It occurs in familial essential hypercholesterolæmia, idiopathic primary hyperlipæmia (in both of these there is a high incidence of early coronary disease), primary biliary cirrhosis, diabetes mellitus and occasionally in other disorders with a high serum cholesterol level. (ii.) *Xanthoma disseminatum* shows small nodules: they are often arranged in lines and involve predominantly the flexures. The serum cholesterol and total lipids are normal. (iii.) *Nævoxanthoendothelioma* is seen as irregularly distributed reddish-yellow nodules, single or few in number, which are present at birth or appear in early infancy. They disappear spontaneously in a few years. The serum cholesterol and lipids are normal. (iv.) The *cellular cholesterol disorders*, all very rare and beginning at an early age, include the Hand-Schüller-Christian disease (§ 559) and Eosinophilic granuloma.

§ **713. VIII. Leukæmia.**—Purpura, furunculosis, prurigo and other non-specific eruptions are fairly common in both acute and chronic forms. Skin involvement manifest as livid red nodules, predominantly involving the face and producing a leonine facies, may precede any evidence of systemic changes in chronic lymphatic leukæmia. In monocytic leukæmia bluish-red nodules or plaques may occur. In chronic myeloid leukæmia skin lesions are exceptional. If nodules develop they are more often on the trunk and may undergo hæmorrhagic necrosis.

§ **714. IX. Nodular syphilides** seldom develop until several years after infection.

Symptoms.—The eruption may occur anywhere, is asymmetrical and usually restricted to a single region of the body. Dull red nodules are grouped in arcs of a

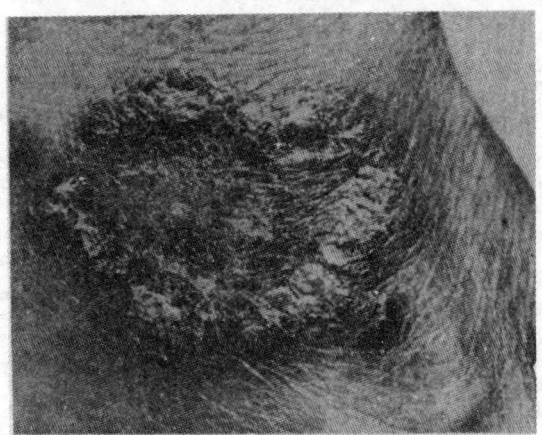

Fig. 195.—Tertiary Syphilis. The patient was an elderly woman. Note the general configuration of the lesion which was red-brown in colour.

circle and may ulcerate. They extend further in a month than does lupus in a year, leaving a soft atrophic scar. The *gumma* is a deeply situated painless nodule which extends upwards to the skin and breaks down to form a sharply marginated ulcer.

§ **715. X. Leprosy.**

Symptoms.—The older classifications of the clinical types have been largely superseded since the Fifth International Leprosy Conference of 1948. Varied prodromal symptoms such as attacks of fever, malaise and pains in the limbs may precede the development of the full clinical picture by months or years. (i.) *Lepromatous leprosy.*—Dull red infiltrated nodules develop on the face, giving the leonine facies, on the limbs and less often on the trunk. They may fuse to form large plaques. There may be early involvement of the naso-pharynx. The disease is progressive with periods of quiescence. Many bacilli are present in the lesions and patients are frequently infectious: the lepromin reaction is negative. (ii.) *Tuberculoid leprosy.*—The macular skin lesions are more superficial and pigmented and are anæsthetic

C.M.—K K

(maculo-anæsthetic form): trophic changes are conspicuous. Palpable enlargement of the peripheral nerve trunks is usually present and the muscular wasting and paralysis produce a claw-hand deformity. Trophic ulceration of the extremities may be destructive. There are few bacilli in the lesions; resistance is high and the disease tends to regress; the patients are usually not infectious. The lepromin reaction is positive. (iii.) Intermediate and indeterminate forms occur.

The *Diagnosis* is established in lepromatous leprosy by the presence of bacilli in skin biopsies and in the nasal secretions. In the tuberculoid form the positive lepromin reaction is helpful. Where the neural involvement is marked progressive muscular atrophy, amyotrophic lateral sclerosis, the thoracic inlet syndromes, scleroderma and Raynaud's disease must be differentiated.

Etiology.—Leprosy is a chronic infection due to *Mycobacterium lepræ*. It is endemic in many tropical countries, and most of the cases encountered in Great Britain are introduced from abroad. Because of the increasing influx of natives of countries in which the disease is still endemic, it is no longer of merely academic interest to the practitioner. Several cases have been reported in men who served in the tropics during World War II. Prolonged and close contact appears to be necessary for its transmission and children are particularly susceptible. The incubation period is prolonged and usually exceeds three to five years.

Treatment requires good food, good living conditions, the elimination of intercurrent disease and the prolonged administration of one of the bacteriostatic sulphone drugs. Tab. dapsone (B.P.C.) is given in very small initial doses to avoid severe toxic reactions; only two doses a week are given, these being, in the first week 25 mg., second week 50 mg., third week 75 mg., fourth week 100 mg., second month 200 mg., third month 300 mg. and if the patient can tolerate it 400 mg. twice a week in the fourth and subsequent months. Reactions necessitate temporary reduction or cessation of doses and for severe lepra reactions the use of corticosteroid. Solapsone (B.P.C.) is given intramusc. (50 per cent. solution) to replace dapsone when side effects are marked, in doses of 2–5 ml. twice a week, as it is less toxic. Inject. streptomycin is useful in patients who do not tolerate the sulphones. In any case treatment must be continued for at least 12 months and for 6 months after apparent cure.

§ 716. XI. **Yaws** (Frambœsia) is a widespread disease endemic in many tropical countries. *Symptoms.*—The primary lesion, which is extragenital and is usually on exposed surfaces, develops at the site of inoculation after an incubation period of 2 to 4 weeks as a crusted papule which enlarges and ulcerates. It may be preceded by mild constitutional symptoms. The secondary eruption appears 1–3 months later and is also accompanied by headache, bone pains and arthralgia. It consists of irregular crops of crusted papules, some of which develop into the characteristic raspberry-like nodules; others become warty, especially on palms and soles. The secondary lesions resolve in from 3 to 12 months in most cases. The tertiary stage follows after months or years; its manifestations include gummatous nodules, osteitis, periostitis and juxta-articular nodules; the cardio-vascular and central nervous system are never involved. The Wassermann reaction is positive. Goundou is a later manifestation of yaws.

Etiology.—The causative agent, *Treponema pertenue*, is indistinguishable from the spirochæte of syphilis, *T. pallidum*. Transmission is not venereal but by direct inoculation on abraded skin and perhaps by insect vectors. It affects both sexes and all ages. Spread is encouraged by unhygienic crowded conditions. There is no congenital form.

Treatment.—Give penicillin as in syphilis (§ 500). Tetracycline is equally effective.

§ 717. XII. **Cutaneous Leishmaniasis** (Oriental sore) is endemic in the Mediterranean region and the Middle East, and is caused by *Leishmania tropica* transmitted by the bite of the sandfly. The incubation period varies from 2 weeks (average 5 weeks) to over a year.

Symptoms.—The exposed sites are commonly affected. A hard bluish-red papule develops, enlarges slowly, becomes crusted and breaks down to form an ulcer around which satellite lesions may appear. Healing with scar formation takes place in a few months. A large variety of clinical forms have been described and there are apparently regional differences. In one form lupoid nodules develop from the initial papule or around the margin of a healed lesion. The duration is very variable.

Diagnosis is established by the isolation of the Leishmania from the lesions.

Treatment will depend on the stage and type of the lesion. For early lesions Castellani's paint is used. For lesions on the face mepacrine 0·05–0·10 G. dissolved in 1–2 ml. of distilled water may be injected into the lesion two or three times at intervals of 10 days. For small lesions electrocoagulation is suitable and for older chronic lesions X-ray therapy. Where numerous sores are present some give intravenous injections of pentavalent antimony compounds.

American Leishmaniasis, endemic in Central America, is caused by the morphologically identical organism *L. braziliense.* The nose and lips are often severely affected.

§ 718. XIII. Madura Foot (Maduromycosis) is a disease of tropical and subtropical regions and is characterised by indurated nodules, abscesses and sinuses of the feet. More than one species of fungus can cause the infection, which resembles actinomycosis in its pathological features. *Treatment* is surgical; sulphonamides may help.

§ 719. XIV. Actinomycosis of the skin is uncommon; more often the skin is secondarily involved as in cervico-facial actinomycosis. In the primary cutaneous form a group of firm dull red nodules eventually develops the characteristic sinuses; from the pus actinomycotic granules can be identified (and see § 337).

§ 720. XV. Sporotrichosis is an infection with the fungus, *Sporotrichium schenckii*, which is widely distributed throughout the world as a saprophyte in the soil and on vegetable matter, wood or straw. A nodule or ulcer develops at the site of inoculation and gummatous nodules later appear along the lines of lymphatic drainage. A rare systemic form, with generalised subcutaneous nodules, is recognised (§ 147). The response of the cutaneous form to potassium iodide is rapid.

§ 721. XVI. POLYARTERITIS NODOSA is uncommon (see § 98). The cutaneous manifestations of the systemic form are extremely variable: whereas urticaria, bullæ, purpura and scarlatiniform erythema are non-specific, others such as subcutaneous nodules, a racemose livedo and cutaneous gangrene afford valuable assistance in establishing the diagnosis. Recently a benign cutaneous form of polyarteritis has been described; the eruption consists of crops of nodules, often on the legs or arms, but sometimes in other sites. The recognition of this form is important, les' an unjustifiably poor prognosis be given on the strength of a histological report.

§ 722. XVII. Weber-Christian Disease (Relapsing Febrile Non-suppurative Panniculitis) is very rare and affects women more often than men.

Symptoms.—Recurrent bouts of fever are accompanied by crops of subcutaneous nodules, varying from one to several centimetres in diameter, on the thighs, arms or trunk. The skin is red at first, but later, as the inflammatory changes in the fatty panniculus subside, it regains its normal colour and dips into an underlying hollow produced by localised fat-atrophy. *Treatment.*—Cortisone is reported to be effective.

§ 723. XVIII. Mycosis fungoides.—Plum-coloured or red-brown nodules, sometimes lobulated or pedunculated and eventually ulcerating, are the characteristic lesions of the final or tumour stage of mycosis fungoides. The disease is rare, occurs mainly in men over 40, and usually runs a prolonged course. The initial lesions (premycotic stage) are commonly irritable plaques of erythema with superficial scaling (see parapsoriasis en plaques, § 666); less often they may be eczematous or erythrodermic. After an interval of many years the second or infiltrative stage appears with dull-red indurated gyrate plaques, and on these the nodular tumours develop after a few months. The disease is ultimately fatal. but the tumours are radiosensitive and carefully planned treatment with X-ray and nitrogen mustards can prolong life.

Lymphosarcoma and *Reticulum-cell sarcoma* may present as single or multiple skin nodules.

§ **724.** XIX. **Onchocerciasis** (Syn. River Blindness) is caused by the filarial worm *Onchocerca volvulus* (§ 542) which infests human beings in West and Central Africa and in Central America (especially Guatemala and Mexico). *Symptoms.*—The first to occur is pruritus of the limbs, buttocks and shoulders; this may be severe. Later micro-filariæ invade the eye and cause blindness due to choroiditis, iritis and keratitis. Also subcutaneous nodules appear, usually around the pelvic girdle or on the head, due to adult filariæ being encapsulated in fibrous tissue; later these may form cystic tumours under the skin.

Diagnosis.—This is established by demonstrating microfilariæ (larvæ) in skin shavings teased in normal saline and viewed microscopically. They can sometimes be seen in the eyes with a corneal microscope. The blood often shows a high eosinophilia and skin tests with filarial antigen are positive.

Treatment is with diethylcarbamazine (Banocide, Hetrazan) by mouth t.i.d. in very small doses at first (0·5 mg./Kg. body weight a day) increased slowly to full dosage (6–12 mg./Kg. a day) which is continued for three weeks: in addition give five intravenous injections of suramin B.P. 1·0 G. at weekly intervals. Severe exacerbations of the skin condition often occur early in treatment, which can partly be controlled by antihistamines. Severe ocular reactions are rare and require hydrocortisone eye-drops. All palpable nodules should be excised under a local anæsthetic but a further course of drug treatment is often necessary after a few months.

TUMOURS, NÆVI AND CYSTS

§ **725.** XX. **Squamous epithelioma** usually develops after the age of 50, more commonly in men than women. It can occur in younger patients, particularly as a complication of congenital cutaneous abnormalities such

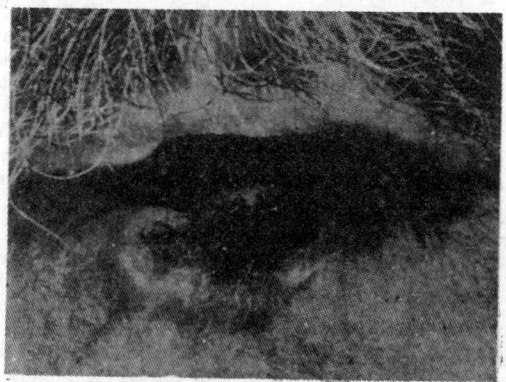

FIG. 196.—SQUAMOUS EPITHELIOMA OF THE LIP in an agricultural labourer.

as xeroderma pigmentosum. It may arise on previously normal skin, but more often it develops in precancerous lesions such as keratoses, scars and leucoplakia. Chronic irritation and occupational exposure to tar, pitch, certain mineral oils and sunlight and prolonged treatment with inorganic arsenic compounds are important provocative factors.

Symptoms.—The earliest lesion is a small firm papule or an area of induration in a pre-existing keratosis or scar, especially on the face, the lower lip, the hands and the forearms (Fig. 196). Some lesions grow rapidly, ulcerate early and metastasise to regional lymphatic glands: there may be gross local tissue destruction. In other cases enlargement is gradual with the formation of a large nodule which may become cauliflower-like, ulceration being delayed for months or years.

Diagnosis.—The main problems are to differentiate kerato-acanthoma (§ 727), and pseudo-epitheliomatous hyperplasia developing in a chronic ulcer. Whenever epithelioma is suspected a biopsy should be undertaken.

Treatment is by adequate surgical excision, by radiotherapy or by a combination of both. Regular follow-up examination is essential so that any recurrence can receive immediate attention.

§ 726. XXI. **Basal-cell epithelioma** (Rodent ulcer) occurs mainly in later life but is occasionally seen in younger patients. Prolonged exposure to sunlight is an important provocative factor.

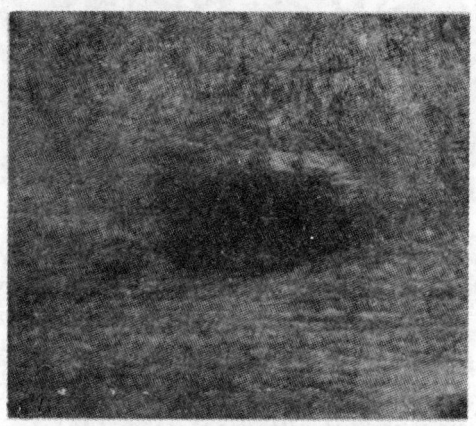

FIG. 197.—BASAL-CELL EPITHELIOMA.

Symptoms.—The initial lesion is a small nodule with a characteristic translucent pearly appearance: it occurs most commonly on the face, but sometimes in other sites including the trunk and scalp. Growth is usually slow but eventually a crusted ulcer with a cordlike pearly border forms (Fig. 197). In neglected cases there may be extensive local tissue destruction. Metastasis is very rare. The lesions are sometimes heavily pigmented and lead to a mistaken diagnosis of melanoma. In another clinical form cicatrisation produces an indurated plaque resembling morphœa. Metatypical forms may show some clinical and histological features of squamous epithelioma. The choice of *treatment* depends on the site of the lesion, its size and on other factors. Surgical excision and radiotherapy in experienced hands both give excellent results with a low recurrence rate

§ 727. XXII. **Kerato-acanthoma** (Molluscum Sebaceum) has been recognised as a clinicopathological entity only in recent years, but is not uncommon. Many cases have been regarded as squamous epithelioma.

Symptoms.—The condition usually occurs between the ages of 50 and 70 in both sexes but is also met in younger patients. Exposure to sunlight and tar are provocative factors. Some patients give a history of recent trauma but the lesion otherwise develops on previously normal skin. The exposed sites are usually but not invariably affected. A firm hemispherical papule enlarges very rapidly to reach a diameter of 1–2 cm. or more in

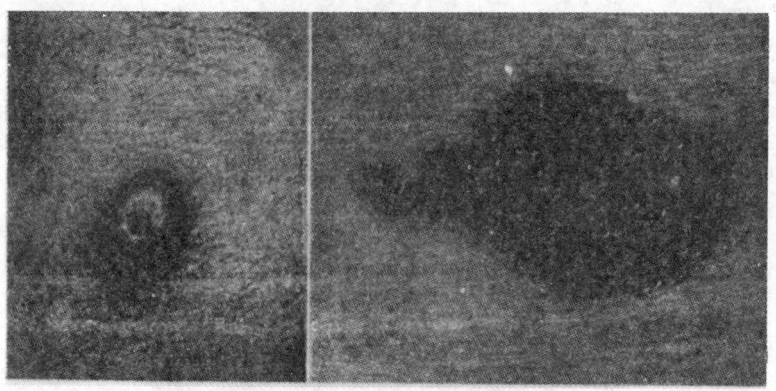

FIG. 198.—KERATO-ACANTHOMA.   FIG. 199.—BASAL-CELL EPITHELIOMA.   Superficial type.

6 to 8 weeks. No further enlargement takes place. At this stage the kerato-acanthoma is a smooth rounded nodule covered by tense shining epidermis: the summit is umbilicated and may be covered by a crust beneath which is a crater filled with horn (Fig. 198). Spontaneous regression then occurs, the lesion becomes softer and flatter and ultimately leaves a small puckered scar. This typical course is subject to some variation. The *diagnosis* from squamous epithelioma can usually be made but in every case a biopsy should be performed and when the diagnosis is confirmed the lesion can be removed with a curette under local anæsthesia, with an excellent cosmetic result.

§ 728. XXIII. **Other Epithelial Tumours of the Skin.**—(i.) **Paget's disease** in the great majority of cases affects the female nipple, but has occasionally occurred in the anogenital region. On the nipple an oozing sharply marginated area of erythema after a variable interval becomes thickened and indurated. In a large proportion of cases a duct-carcinoma of the underlying breast is present and determines both prognosis and treatment. (ii.) **Bowen's disease** consists of a plaque of red crusted papules in which after many years squamous epithelioma may develop. (iii.) **Superficial epitheliomatosis** occurs in a number of clinical and histological variants. *Symptoms.*—Single or multiple sharply demarcated erythematous plaques

develop usually on the trunk, and may show a thread-like pearly margin
if of basal-cell type (Fig. 199). They may closely resemble psoriasis. The
course is usually prolonged and benign but typical basal-cell or squamous
epithelioma may develop in one or more plaques. *Treatment* with carbon
dioxide snow is effective unless these changes have developed. (iv.) **Metastatic carcinoma** ⁻rom a growth in the breast, prostate, kidney, ovary or
other organs may occur before the presence of the primary lesion has been
suspected. Single or multiple hard red or purplish nodules appear suddenly
and enlarge rapidly, often on the trunk or scalp. A *diagnosis* is established
by biopsy which should indicate the probable site of the primary growth.

§ **729. XXIV. Sebaceous and epithelial cysts** are common lesions which
are often confused. *Sebaceous cysts* may develop at any age after puberty,
are single or multiple, are common on the face, trunk and genitalia, and
contain cheesy sebaceous material. They are sometimes the si*e of
recurrent episodes of inflammation. Rarely malignant change of basal-
cell type occurs. Larger cysts must be carefully excised. Small cysts
can be treated with the diathermy which destroys the lining epithelium.
Epithelial cysts are firm subcutaneous cysts, single or multiple, appearing
usually in middle life, often on the scalp but also anywhere on the body.
Small traumatic epithelial cysts sometimes develop on the hands and feet.
These enlarge very slowly and contain horny material. Squamous
carcinoma is a rare complication. *Treatment* is by simple excision.

§ **730. XXV. Hæmangioma and Lymphangioma.**—The commonest
type of vascular nævus is the *superficial* cavernous hæmangioma or strawberry mark, which may be present at birth, but usually appears a few days

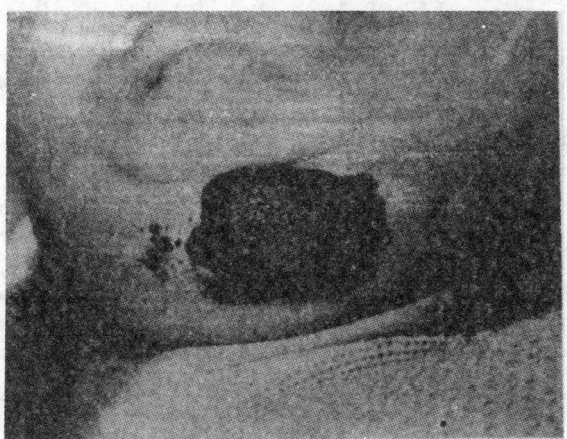

FIG. 200.—HÆMANGIOMA. This is the common superficial cavernous type of vascular nævus. It
appears soon after birth, enlarges for four or five months and then regresses spontaneously.

later. It commonly enlarges for 4 or 5 months. The elevated bright
red lesions which fade on pressure seldom cause diagnostic difficulty.

Ulceration may take place, especially in the napkin area, but healing readily occurs. After 6 months further enlargement is unusual except in proportion to the general growth of the child. Slate-coloured flecks appear on the surface, the nævus gradually becomes paler, softer and flatter and in most cases spontaneous resolution with a perfect or nearly perfect cosmetic result is complete before the age of 5 or 6 years. The *subcutaneous* cavernous hæmangioma may be associated with the superficial form or may occur independently as a soft compressible subcutaneous swelling. Spontaneous resolution is less frequent and less complete.

Before *treatment* is planned every case must be individually assessed. The small strawberry mark, not involving muco-cutaneous junctions, can safely be left alone. The larger lesions around the mouth and eyes and those with a large subcutaneous component should be inspected at frequent intervals, and also left alone if involution is proceeding satisfactorily, as the cosmetic results are generally superior to those obtained with active treatment. When intervention is considered desirable the choice lies between radiotherapy (with the risk of inflicting permanent damage to epiphyses), sclerosing injections and applications of carbon-dioxide snow.

Lymphangioma is rare. Involvement of the tongue produces a macroglossia studded with small vesicles. Lymphangioma circumscriptum presents as groups of small vesicles likened to frog-spawn; these may be hæmorrhagic. *Treatment* is by excision.

§ **731. XXVI. Lipoma.**—This soft lobulated tumour covered by normal skin presents little diagnostic difficulty. The single lipoma usually occurs in women. Diffuse lipomatosis of the neck and shoulders is seen mainly in men. Multiple symmetrical circumscribed lipomata of the arms and thighs are an inherited abnormality. Liposarcoma is very rare.

§ **732. XXVII. Histiocytoma** (Fibroma durum) is a benign lesion usually single, occurring in adults on the legs or less commonly elsewhere. The small firm nodule is adherent to the overlying epidermis which is reddened or pigmented. It is occasionally misdiagnosed clinically as melanoma. *Treatment* is by simple excision.

§ **733. XXVIII. Pyogenic granuloma** is a moist very vascular lesion, bleeding readily on minor trauma, bright red in colour, growing rapidly and often pedunculated. It may develop at the site of trauma. Common sites are the hands and face. The lesion is of pyogenic origin and consists of granulation tissue: it has been confused clinically with a rapidly growing melanoma. *Treatment* is removal by a curette and cauterisation.

§ **734. XXIX. Neurofibroma.**—Neurofibromatosis (Von Recklinghausen's disease) is a genetically determined syndrome which is seen in its complete form only in some members of a family, others presenting one or more innocuous manifestations.

Symptoms.—Skin lesions may be present in infancy or childhood, but commonly appear or become more extensive at puberty, during pregnancy or after a severe illness. Several types are encountered: (i.) molluscum fibrosum: soft pinkish swellings, sessile or pedunculated, later becoming firm and sometimes present in very large numbers; (ii.) plexiform neuroma: elongated and diffuse fibromata confined to the

skin along the course of one or more nerves; (iii.) fibroma pendulum: diffuse neurofibromatosis of nerve trunks with overgrowth of skin and subcutaneous tissues forming large pendulous folds; (iv.) *café au lait* spots: patches of pigmentation, light brown
in colour, small or of wide extent and usually on the trunk (Fig. 201). The accom-.
panying lesions of the central nervous system are considered in §§ 970, 1048, 1083.

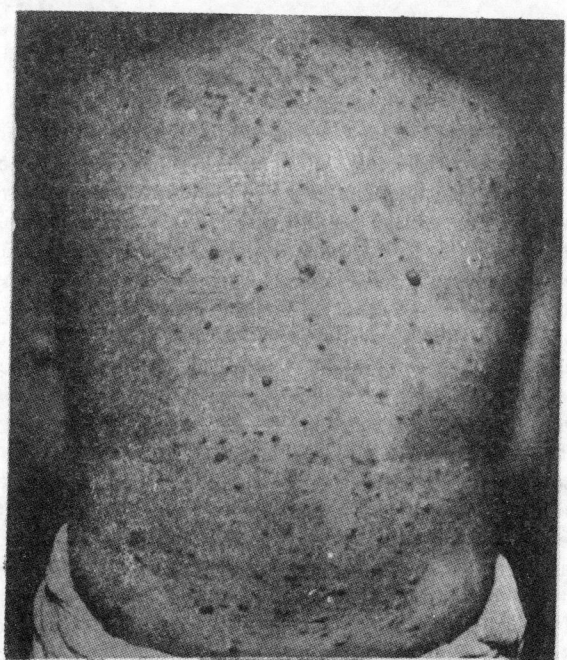

FIG. 201.—NEUROFIBROMATOSIS. The mollusca and the patches of *café au lait* pigmentation are
well shown.

Treatment, which must be surgical, may be necessary for cosmetic reasons or
because of hæmorrhage into or sarcomatous transformation of a neurofibroma.

GROUP VI. ULCERS

An **Ulcer** is a loss of substance of the whole skin and results from
destruction of the dermis by vascular, inflammatory or neoplastic processes.
It may remain superficial or may involve the deeper tissues extensively.
More than one causal factor can often be incriminated in such cases but
for practical purposes ulcers may be classified under seven headings:

I. Ulcers of vascular origin (§ 735).	IV. Infective ulcers (§ 738) (*cont.*).
(*a*) Venous and varicose.	(*b*) Syphilitic.
(*b*) Hypertensive.	(*c*) Pyogenic.
(*c*) Arteriosclerotic.	(*d*) Tropical.
II. Trophic ulcers (§ 736).	(*e*) Desert sore.
III. Neoplastic ulcers (§ 737).	(*f*) Diphtheritic.
IV. Infective ulcers (§ 738).	(*g*) Chancroid.
(*a*) Tuberculous.	(*h*) Granuloma inguinale.

IV. Infective ulcers (§ 738) (*cont.*).
    (*i*) Leishmaniasis.
    (*j*) With actinomycosis, blasto-
        mycosis, sporotrichosis.
    (*k*) Pyoderma-gangrenosum.

V. Ulcers with blood diseases (§ 739).
VI. Ulcers of chemical and traumatic
      origin (§ 740).
VII. Ulcers of unknown origin (§ 740*a*).

§ 735. I. Ulcers of Vascular Origin

(*a*) **Venous ulcers** (Syn. Hypostatic ulcers) and Varicose ulcers constitute a major social and therapeutic problem.

Symptoms.—Hypostatic congestion of the lower third of the leg is first manifest by œdema of the ankle and staining of the skin by blood pigments and by melanin. Continued œdema, aided perhaps by secondary infection, leads to an indurative cellulitis and ultimately to dense fibrosis. Ulceration is often precipitated by trauma. Ulcers of long duration may cover the entire circumference of the leg and may be surrounded by a zone of fibrosis which greatly restricts ankle movements. Malignant change is uncommon but should be suspected if heaping up of epithelium is noted at one edge of the ulcer. Hypostatic ulceration may be associated with a troublesome dermatitis or the latter may occur in the absence of an ulcer. Dermatitis of the lower leg is particularly liable to give rise to an autosensitisation eruption of the face, neck and arms.

Diagnosis.—Leg ulcers due to arteriosclerosis, hypertension, syphilis, tuberculosis and blood diseases must be excluded. There is a tendency to label eczematous eruptions of the lower leg " varicose eczema " rather indiscriminately. Contact dermatitis, especially that provoked by over-treatment, infective dermatitis, neurodermatitis and nummular eczema are all of common occurrence in this site and must be excluded.

Etiology.—An inadequate venous return results from insufficiency of the valves in the deep veins of the leg (§ 579). A functional insufficiency results from fixation of the knee or ankle.

Treatment.—Hypostatic ulcers can be controlled effectively only by measures which improve venous return. In all cases the patient should be taught exercises which increase the mobility of the ankle joint and improve the tone of the calf-muscle pump, which plays a major role in the return of the blood. In severe cases a period of bed rest may be required. When œdema has been controlled apply an elastic-web (not crêpe) bandage while the patient remains ambulant. The patient must learn the correct technique of applying the bandage and of using sorbo-rubber or felt-pads to help to keep the leg free from œdema. Local applications are of less importance; penicillin, the sulphonamides and other potent sensitisers must be avoided. If gross infection is present, chlortetracycline ointment may be used for a few days: subsequently bland applications are desirable. To treat hypostatic dermatitis the same attention must be given to relieving hypostatic congestion. Lotio calaminæ oleosa N.F. with silver proteinate ¼ per cent. is a useful application or, if the leg is very moist, gentian violet 1 per cent. in lotio calaminæ. When secondary infection has been controlled a medicated bandage such as " viscopaste " or " coltapaste " may be applied and changed at intervals of a week or more.

(b) **Hypertensive ulcers** due to arterial thrombosis occur in patients with diastolic hypertension even in the absence of venous insufficiency. They are commonly situated on the anterolateral aspect of the leg at the junction of the lower and middle thirds and may be bilaterally symmetrical. They are usually small and superficial, may be very painful and the pain is not relieved by rest.

(c) **Arteriosclerotic ulcers** commonly affect the toes or heels, especially in diabetic patients, but trauma may precipitate ulceration over the malleoli or on the anterior aspects of the lower third of the leg. The ulceration is often extremely painful and extensive, and recurrent break-down is common in cold weather. Other signs of arterial insufficiency are present but signs of venous insufficiency may be absent.

§ **736.** II. **Trophic ulcers** occur on the soles in tabes dorsalis, lumbo-sacral syringomyelia and diabetes mellitus; also on the alæ nasi after section of the sensory root of the trigeminal nerve for neuralgia; and on the hands and feet in leprosy. Decubitus ulcers are a troublesome complication of spinal cord lesions.

§ **737.** III. **Neoplastic ulcers** arise from squamous and basal-cell epitheliomata, the tendency to ulcerate being greatest when growth is rapid and outpaces the blood supply. A raised indurated border suggests a neoplastic change, which should be confirmed by biopsy (§§ 725, 727).

§ **738.** IV. **Infective ulcers.**

(a) *Tuberculous ulceration* is a feature of several forms of cutaneous tuberculosis. *Primary tuberculosis* of the skin develops at the site of inoculation as a small indolent ulcer with a raised edge, or as a bluish-red nodule after an incubation period of about 2 weeks. Regional lympha-denitis occurs after 3 to 6 weeks and the glands may persist for some time after spontaneous healing of the ulcer. *Diagnosis.—Cat-scratch disease* closely simulates primary tuberculosis of the skin (§ 508). In *scrofuloderma* the skin overlying caseating lymph nodes or infected joints becomes indurated, blue-red in colour and breaks down to form undermined irregular ulcers and sinuses. The nodule of *Bazin's disease* may ulcerate (§ 707). *Tuberculosis cutis orificialis:* painful indolent shallow ulcers of the tongue, the mucous membranes of the mouth and the anal region develop in patients with advanced tuberculosis of the lungs or intestine. *Lupus vulgaris* may ulcerate, especially around the nose and mouth in malnourished individuals (§ 709).

(b) **Syphilitic ulceration.**—The *primary chancre* presents as a small indurated ulcer and the diagnosis is readily overlooked in extragenital lesions (§ 500). *Tertiary* lesions are seen as grouped punched-out ulcers with polycyclic configuration. A *gumma* of the subcutaneous tissues pro-duces a larger ulcer with a sharp margin and purulent floor. The

" punched-out " appearance and festooned or figured outline will often suggest the diagnosis. The Wassermann reaction is positive but a clinically unsupported positive Wassermann reaction must not be allowed to impose a diagnosis of syphilis (§ 1207), as it may be a biological false positive or a coincidental finding in a patient with, for example, a carcinoma.

(c) **Pyogenic ulcers.**—*Chronic streptococcal ulcers* have red undermined irregular borders. They are uncommon. The *chancriform pyoderma* usually occurs on the face. Over the course of a few weeks an indurated ulcer develops. It may simulate an epithelioma, but only inflammatory changes are present and healing eventually takes place.

(d) **Tropical ulcer** causes serious disability and economic loss in hot humid climates. It is commonest in native men in the third decade, but can occur in both sexes at any age, except in early childhood.

Symptoms.—The early lesion is a painful bulla at the site of mild abrasions or insect bites on the legs, accompanied by fever. Within a few hours the bulla ruptures exposing a grey slough, and the ulcer rapidly extends through the skin and subcutaneous tissues, with a yellow base and an evil smell. Sometimes the ulcer extends deeply to destroy muscles, tendons and periosteum, and blood vessels, nerves and joints may become involved. In the absence of treatment death can ensue; or when the ulcer eventually heals contraction of scar tissue can cause great disability. The skin over the scar is liable to break down rapidly or may develop an epitheliomatous change.

Diagnosis is from ulcers due to yaws, syphilis, cutaneous leishmaniasis, varicose veins and desert sore.

Etiology.—The immediate cause is trauma or insect bites; poor nutrition and inadequate cleanliness undoubtedly predispose. Chronic malaria probably plays a part as the geographical line between ulcer-stricken and ulcer-free islands in the Pacific coincides with that between malarial and non-malarial islands. A mixed bacterial infection is found and Vincent's spirochætes and fusiform bacilli are almost invariably present.

Treatment is by strict bed rest and penicillin which rapidly cure early lesions. The chronic ulcer requires weeks of treatment in hospital; surgical measures such as excision, skin grafting and immobilisation in plaster are often necessary. *Prophylaxis* is by improvement in the diet and personal hygiene; when at the end of the day's work all small abrasions are cleaned and covered with collodion, the economic loss in any labour force is greatly reduced.

(e) **Desert sore** (Syn. Veld sore) occurs on exposed parts of the body in hot dry desert regions of the tropics and subtropics. The ulcers are usually multiple and differ from tropical ulcers in being shallower with a dry membrane. In most cases the Klebs-Lœffler bacillis can be isolated from early ulcers and in a proportion of cases diphtheritic paralyses occur.

Treatment is with systemic and local applications of an antibiotic (Table XXXV). In every case at least 20,000 units of anti-diphtheritic serum should be injected locally in the vicinity of the sore.

(f) **Cutaneous diphtheria** forming an ulcer is sometimes seen in Great Britain; the leg is the principal site of infection.

(g) CHANCROID (soft sore) is caused by the sexual transmission of *H. Ducreyi*; painful ragged ulcers on the genitalia may be multiple but are not usually indurated (§ 583).

(h) **Granuloma inguinale** (Granuloma venereum), caused by *Donovania granulomatis*, is usually transmitted by sexual contact. The lesions, which are usually in the anogenital region, are red papules evolving into indurated ulcers. Gross destruction and elephantiasic lymphœdema may occur. *Diagnosis* is by finding *Donovania* in mucus from the lesions. Streptomycin, chloramphenicol and chlortetracycline are curative.

(*i*) *Leishmaniasis*—see § 717.

(*j*) **Other infective granulomata** may ulcerate—Actinomycosis (§ 719), Blastomycosis (§ 700), Sporotrichosis (§ 720).

(*k*) **Pyoderma gangrenosum.**—A pustule rapidly undergoes hæmorrhagic necrosis and forms a large burrowing ulcer with a ragged undermined edge and a foul-smelling base. Multiple ulcers may develop. It occurs particularly in patients with active ulcerative colitis but may complicate other debilitating diseases. None of the many organisms which can be grown from the ulcers can be incriminated as their cause.

§ 739. V. Chronic Ulcers associated with certain Blood Diseases occur on the legs in 75 per cent. of adults with sickle-cell anæmia; also rarely in hereditary spherocytosis (acholuric jaundice) even in children and heal after splenectomy. They have been recorded in Felty's syndrome, Cooley's anæmia and polycythæmia.

§ 740. VI. Ulcers of chemical and traumatic origin.—Any caustic in contact with the skin for sufficient time and in adequate concentration will produce necrosis and ulceration. The majority of such ulcers are of accidental origin but they may be self-inflicted. Their clinical features will vary with the method employed but bizarre and irregular configuration and distribution are often present (§ 623). A distinctive type of small round indurated ulcer on the hands and in the cartilaginous nasal septum occurs in workers handling chromic acid or chromates.

§ 740a. VII. Ulcers of Unknown Origin.—(*a*) *Aphthosis.* Aphthæ are common in the mouth of older children and adults (§ 210). (*b*) *Behcet's Syndrome* is rare. Deep and persistent painful ulcers of the mouth and the vulva or scrotum are associated with conjunctivitis, keratitis and iridocyclitis. The course is prolonged and there is no effective treatment.

GROUP VII. HYPERKERATOTIC LESIONS

Lesions which are horny or warty

Common.

I. Warts (§ 741).
II. Corns and Callosities (§ 742).
III. Senile and Seborrhœic keratosis (§ 743).

Rare.

IV. Tuberculosis verrucosa cutis (§ 744).
V. Syphilitic condylomata (§ 745).
VI. Leucoplakia (§ 746).
VII. Palmoplantar keratodermias (§ 747).
VIII. Keratoderma blenorrhagica (§ 748).
IX. Acanthosis nigricans (§ 749).

§ 741. I. Warts (Verrucæ) are due to a virus infection. After experimental inoculation the average incubation period is 4 months but varies from 1 to 21 months.

Varieties.—The various clinical forms result from differences in the nature of the sites in which they occur, and perhaps from differing degrees of immunity. *V. vulgaris*, the common wart, occurs mainly on the hands and knees, but occasionally on the face and lips. *Juvenile* or *plane warts* are most frequent in childhood and may be present in large numbers on the face and backs of the hands. *V. plantaris* is seen mainly in schoolchildren, and afflicts girls twice as often as boys. It commonly develops beneath the pressure points of the heel and metatarsal arch and may be painful. *Acuminate warts* occur in the anogenital region. The individual wart is pink soft filiform and often pedunculated but when large numbers are present cauliflower-like masses may form. All types of warts may disappear spontaneously and some individuals are cured by suggestion. These facts must be remembered when the results of treatment are evaluated.

Treatment.—When only a small number of common or plantar warts is present the treatment of choice is curettage under local or general anæsthesia. A pencil of solid carbon dioxide snow or a slush of snow and acetone is useful for smaller warts and is suitable for school clinics. Plane warts may be painted with 1 in 100 salicylic acid and 1 in 1,000 mercury perchloride in spirit. Acuminate warts respond well to weekly or twice weekly application of podophyllum resin 20 per cent. in spirit. The paint should be applied by a doctor or nurse and the surrounding skin protected with soft paraffin.

§ **742. II. Corns and Callosities.**—Corns are modified callosities; downward extension of the thickened horny layer renders them tender to pressure. They develop particularly on the toes or between them when one toe is constantly pressed against another. Callosities are circumscribed thickened horny patches which develop at the sites of long-continued pressure or friction: those of the sole must be distinguished from plantar warts. If they become painful they may be pared after softening with salicylic plaster.

§ **743. III. Senile and Seborrhœic keratoses.**—Senile keratoses occur on the exposed skin—the face, hands and arms, and are particularly frequent in those who have spent their lives in outdoor occupations. The rough horny patches, firmly adherent, may undergo malignant change clinically evident as induration or ulceration. *Treatment* with phenol or pure trichloracetic acid is effective, but if neoplastic change is suspected a biopsy should be performed and the lesion excised. *Seborrhœic keratoses* (seborrhœic warts) are circumscribed rounded or oval flattened elevations covered by brown greasy scale. They may occur in large numbers around the waist, on the neck and shoulders and less commonly on the face. Although more usual in those over 50 they can occur below the age of 30. *Treatment* is purely a cosmetic problem as they are not pre-malignant lesions. Excision, curettage or destruction by diathermy may be used.

§ **744. IV. Tuberculosis verrucosa cutis** is a form of secondary inoculation tuberculosis and usually occurs in patients with chronic pulmonary tuberculosis by selfinoculation from their own sputum. An indurated pustule becomes hyperkeratotic and may extend considerably to form a large warty plaque retaining a dull red inflammatory areola which distinguishes it from virus warts. Verruca necrogenica occurs on the hands of those handling infected bodies, human or animal.

§ 745. V. **Syphilitic condylomata** develop in the secondary stage of syphilis in those parts of the body where two skin surfaces are in apposition. They are most commonly seen in the anogenital region, but can occur beneath the breasts, in the axillæ and between the fingers and toes. Initially soft flat papules, they may become hypertrophied and verrucose as the result of sweating and friction. They are covered by an offensive mucoid secretion which is highly infective.

§ 746. VI. **Leucoplakia.**—The white patches of leucoplakia may occur on the lips, the tongue or anywhere in the mouth (§ 215) and on the vulva. They may feel slightly rough to the touch, but induration is an indication of probable malignant change. They are analogous to senile or solar keratosis of the skin, and are a response of the mucous membrane to chronic irritation. Certain vulval atrophies predispose (§ 752).

Diagnosis.—In the mouth lichen planus must be differentiated; on the vulva lichen planus and lichen simplex. Biopsy is essential if the diagnosis is in doubt or if radical treatment is contemplated. *Treatment.*—The mildest forms may regress if smoking or other sources of irritation can be suppressed. Symptomatic measures are justifiable only if the patient is under close and regular supervision. Surgical excision is obligatory if there is induration or ulceration or if there is no response to local applications, as squamous carcinoma develops in a high proportion of cases.

§ 747. VII. **Palmoplantar keratodermas.**—(i.) *Congenital keratoderma palmaris et plantaris (tylosis)* is inherited as a dominant character. Diffuse thickening of palms and soles usually begins symmetrically before 2 years of age. The sharp margins are surrounded by a narrow red areola. *Treatment.*—Recently excision and split-skin grafting has been employed successfully in cases where the thickening was disabling. Another congenital variety of keratoderma occurs as discrete horny papules, somewhat resembling corns. (ii.) *Keratoderma climactericum* occurs in women of menopausal age or older. Obesity, hypertension and osteo-arthritis of the knees are often associated. Discrete sharply defined round or oval patches of hyperkeratosis tend to become confluent to form horny plaques or bands on the soles and palms. *Treatment.*—The response to œstrogens is unsatisfactory. Weight reduction and keratolytic applications give some relief. Thyroid may be given if the serum cholesterol is elevated. (iii.) *Arsenical keratoses* are a late result of arsenical medication. Fowler's solution was formerly administered for prolonged periods as treatment of many chronic skin disorders, and in bromide mixtures for nervous disorders. The lesions develop on the palms and soles as small rough horny papules. Arsenical pigmentation of other skin areas is present in about half the cases. The keratoses persist and may undergo malignant change to squamous epitheliomata. (iv.) *Keratoderma of the palms or soles* may follow a variety of skin conditions which assume hyperkeratotic forms in these sites—eczema, lichen simplex, lichen planus and psoriasis. Diffuse hyperkeratosis is present in pityriasis rubra pilaris.

§ 748. VIII. **Keratoderma blenorrhagica** is rare and affects men more often than women. As the name implies it was formerly attributed to gonococcal infection, with which it may be associated, but it also occurs in Reiter's disease. The lesions are symmetrical and develop on the palms and soles, around the nail matrix, on ankles, legs, knees, thighs, genitalia and occasionally on the mucous membranes. The primary lesion is a small vesicopustule, but small brown waxy papules, conical in shape and resembling barnacles, form rapidly and may become confluent in extensive sheets. Arthritis and iritis may be associated. Differentiation from rupioid psoriasis may be difficult or impossible.

Treatment.—The response to the antibiotics is disappointing. ACTH and cortisone are sometimes successful.

§ 749. IX. **Acanthosis nigricans** is characterised by a symmetrical eruption of pigmented warty excrescences in the flexures or the mucocutaneous junctions.

It is usually a manifestation of carcinoma of the ovaries, uterus or gastro-intestinal tract. It may precede other evidence of the neoplasm by months or years. A benign form occurs in children and adolescents in association with obesity of pituitary type.

GROUP VII. SCARRING, SCLEROSIS, ATROPHY

I. Scars and Cheloids (§ 750).
II. Sclerosis—the skin feels hardened, thickened and cannot be pinched up between the fingers (§ 751).

Common.	*Rare.*
i. Hypostatic sclerosis.	ii. Scleroderma.
	iii. Necrobiosis lipoidica.
	iv. Scleroedema.
	v. Sclerema neonatorum.

III. Atrophies—the skin is soft, smooth and finely wrinkled (§ 752).

Common.	*Rare.*
i. Senile atrophy.	v. Atrophy of subcutaneous fat.
ii. Striæ atrophicæ.	vi. Idiopathic macular atrophy.
iii. Kraurosis vulvæ.	vii. Acrodermatitis atrophicans.
iv. Lichen sclerosus.	viii. Poikiloderma.
	ix. Congenital atrophies.

§ **750.** I. **Scars** follow many skin disorders in which there is destruction of dermal connective tissue; tuberculosis cutis, tertiary syphilis, lupus erythematosus, etc. If the scars are disfiguring and the disease process is completely inactive plastic surgery may be considered. *Traumatic scars*, particularly those following burns, may be the site of squamous epitheliomata. *Atrophic* scarring, the late result of overdosage with radium or X-ray (chronic radio-dermatitis) is liable to intractable painful ulceration and to malignant change. *Cheloids* are hypertrophic scars which extend beyond the limits of the original lesion. The sites of predilection are the back and sides of the neck, the ears and the mid-chest, but cheloids can develop anywhere. They occur especially in negroes but there may be a constitutional susceptibility in those of other races. Many follow infection of operation wounds and burns but they may arise spontaneously, particularly on the trunk in women. *Treatment* is by excision combined with radiotherapy to prevent recurrence.

§ **751.** II. Sclerosis of the Skin

i. **Hypostatic sclerosis** presents as diffuse thickening and hardening of the skin of the lower leg and ankle in a gaiter distribution. Pigmentation is usual and dermatitis and eczema are frequently associated. The condition follows chronic œdema from prolonged venous insufficiency and should be treated by massage, exercises and bandaging (see §§ 579, 735).

ii. **Scleroderma** is characterised by hardening of the skin as the result of sclerosis of dermal connective tissue. It occurs in two clinical forms:—

(a) Morphœa.—Smooth, ivory-white plaques are surrounded in their active stage by a narrow lilac-tinted zone of erythema. The lesions may be small and numerous (guttate morphœa), round or oval and a few inches in diameter, elongated in the long axis of a limb or on the forehead (" coup de sabre ") or forming extensive sheets.

They may remain unchanged for months or years or, after a period of gradual extension, may regress leaving atrophy. The general health is not impaired. The sexes are equally affected at all ages, but it is rare in the elderly.

(b) SYSTEMIC SCLERODERMA (Systemic Sclerosis) commonly begins with Raynaud's syndrome with stiffening and œdema of the fingers, the skin of which becomes white and indurated (Sclerodactyly). Increasing sclerosis produces severe disability. Involvement of the face produces a mask-like appearance with a small mouth sharp nose and expressionless features. Œsophageal, colonic, pulmonary and cardiac lesions are frequently associated. Young adult women are usually affected. In the Thibierge–Weissenbach syndrome there is also a deposit of calcium salts around the phalangeal joints and even around the elbows and knees. The *prognosis* is generally unfavourable. *Treatment.*—The corticosteroids do not help. Sympathectomy may give symptomatic relief, but this is often temporary.

iii. **Necrobiosis lipoidica** occurs as well-defined smooth, shining plaques, yellowish-red in colour, with conspicuous telangiectasia: they may ulcerate. Their site on the lower leg is determined by trauma. The patients are usually diabetics. *Treatment.*—There may be some regression when the diabetes is controlled. An elastic supporting bandage is helpful; local infiltration with a suspension of hydrocortisone acetate is giving promising results.

iv. **Sclerœdema** is a rare disease of children and of adults under 50. Diffuse non-pitting œdematous thickening of the skin involves the face, neck, upper trunk and arms, and more rarely the rest of the body. Spontaneous resolution usually occurs in a few months.

v. **Sclerema neonatorum** affects premature or feeble infants in the first days of life. The skin of the calves or thighs first becomes white, smooth, firm and cold to the touch, and this change extends rapidly to most of the body. The mortality is high. The differential *diagnosis* includes fat necrosis of the newborn, sclerœdema and the general œdema of erythroblastosis. *Treatment* is not satisfactory, but the steroids may be helpful. The child should be nursed in an incubator.

§ 752. III. ATROPHIES OF THE SKIN.

i. **Senile Atrophy** is most marked on the uncovered parts of the body and occurs at an earlier age in those much exposed to sunlight. The dry inelastic skin, irregularly pigmented, may be irritable in cold weather. Keratosis and carcinoma are complications.

ii. **Striæ atrophicæ** are red, lilac or white irregular linear bands of atrophy where the skin has been subjected to tension, as on the abdominal wall in pregnancy. They are a characteristic feature of Cushing's syndrome but are occasionally seen, especially on the buttocks, thighs and upper arms in healthy adolescents of both sexes.

iii. **Kraurosis vulvæ** is a sclerosing atrophy leading to stenosis of the vaginal orifice and disappearance of the labia minora. The smooth, shining mucous membrane is usually red or yellow but may be white. Pruritus may be severe. The term kraurosis is widely used but is confusing as many cases so described are lichen sclerosus, and other pathological processes can produce similar clinical changes. *Diagnosis.*—Biopsy is useful, and is essential if radical treatment is under consideration. In lichen sclerosus (see below) the perianal skin is often involved. *Senile atrophy*, which may be accompanied by senile vaginitis, is usually symptomatic and is not complicated by leucoplakia. Leucoplakia presenting as single thickened white patches may develop *ab initio* or in kraurosis or lichen sclerosus. *Lichen simplex*, the result of prolonged and repeated scratching, is common; the white thickened areas often extend on to the upper thighs, but if localised to the vulva may be difficult to distinguish from leucoplakia. Leucoplakia, a precursor of carcinoma, is a frequent

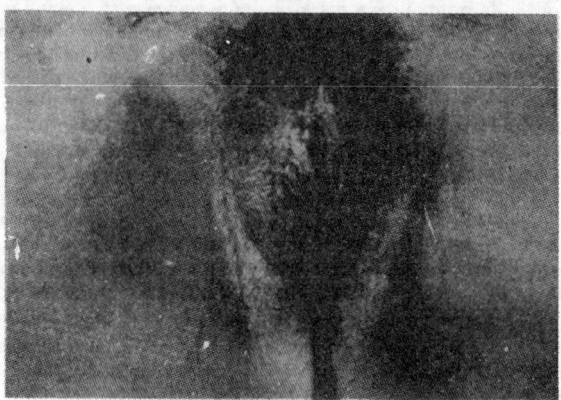

FIG. 202.—LICHEN SIMPLEX of the thighs and labia majora. Note the thickening and pigmentation and regression of normal skin markings. This condition is the consequence of rubbing and scratching, and may be misdiagnosed as leucoplakia when it is confined to the labia majora.

complication. *Treatment* is unsatisfactory; sedation and hydrocortisone ointments or bland applications will give symptomatic relief. Over-treatment is a common error. If leucoplakia develops (confirmed by a histopathologist familiar with the differentiation from lichen simplex) vulvectomy may be advisable.

iv. **Lichen sclerosus.**—Flat white papules, the surface of which shows small depressions or horny plugs, may coalesce to form plaques. The

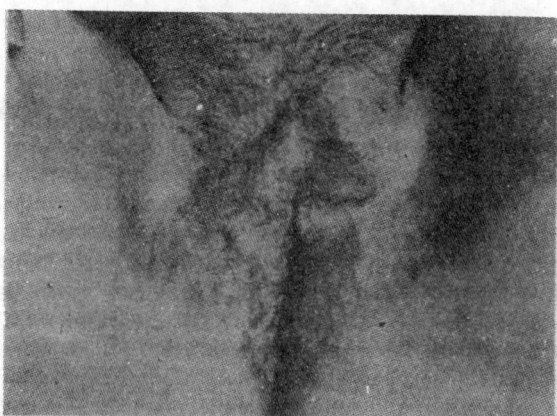

FIG. 203.—LICHEN SCLEROSUS. Note the atrophy and the involvement of the perianal skin. This patient had undergone vulvectomy for leucoplakia two years previously.

centre of the plaque flattens to leave finely wrinkled bluish-white atrophy. The usual sites are the sides of the neck, the upper trunk and the anogenital region, to which the disease may be limited. The vulva is commonly involved, with gross shrinkage of the clitoris and labia minora; the wrinkled white atrophy may extend backwards round the anus (Fig. 203). The white papules can be detected along the sharp margin. Although there may be no symptoms pruritus, soreness and dyspareunia are usual. Telangiectasia, purpura and bullæ are frequent complications and leucoplakia may develop. Middle-aged women are usually affected but the disease occurs in girls before puberty. *Diagnosis* from other atrophic states of the vulva may require biops. in the absence of lesions elsewhere. *Treatment* consists of symptomatic measures for the relief of pruritus. Regular inspection is necessary to detect the early development of leucoplakia. Prophylactic vulvectomy fails as the atrophy involves the reconstructed vulva.

Lichen sclerosus of the penis (Kraurosis penis, Balanitis xerotica obliterans) is rare, and presents as stenosis of the meatus or a sclerosing balanitis with phimosis. *Treatment* is by circumcision.

v. **Atrophy of the subcutaneous fat** presenting as circumscribed depressions in the skin, develops at the site of repeated injections of *insulin*, particularly in women and children. The incidence can be reduced by regularly changing the injection site.

Depressed areas of atrophy follow the inflammatory nodules of *Weber-Christian Disease* (§ 722). *Progressive lipodystrophy* is a very rare disease of unknown origin in which the subcutaneous fat disappears from the upper half of the body but increases in the lower half. Extensive fat loss in other distributions may also occur.

vi. **Idiopathic Macular Atrophy** (Anetoderma) is a rare disease in which localised areas of soft white atrophy, 1 or 2 cm. in diameter, develop on the trunk. They may be preceded by erythema or urticaria. It must be differentiated from secondary macular atrophy following a syphilide.

vii. **Acrodermatitis Atrophicans** mainly affects women of middle age. Œdematous red plaques on the limbs are followed by atrophy which leaves the skin soft, thin and translucent. Fibrous nodules and pseudo-sclerodermatous bands occur in some cases. The disease may be of infective origin; large doses of penicillin are effective.

viii. **Poikiloderma** is a descriptive term applied to the combination of atrophy with mottled pigmentation, depigmentation and telangiectasia. In **Poikiloderma atrophicans** of Jacobi this change develops especially around the large flexures. It may remain localised and unchanged for years or may become generalised. In some it is a manifestation of mycosis fungoides or reticulosarcoma. Extensive poikiloderma may develop in the chronic forms of dermatomyositis. **Poikiloderma congenitale** is a partial form of Rothmund's syndrome. The skin changes appear in early life on the face, buttocks and limbs. Cataracts may develop later. **Poikiloderma of Civatte**, in which the skin changes are limited to the sides of the neck and face in middle-aged women, is described with the pigmentary dermatoses below.

ix. **Congenital Atrophies.**—Atrophy is a feature of many congenital syndromes, including poikiloderma congenitale (above), xeroderma pigmentosum (§ 763) and congenital ectodermal dysplasia (§ 773). In *Acrogeria* the skin of the distal extremities is thin and soft, resembling that of the aged.

GROUP IX. *PIGMENTARY AND VASCULAR CHANGES*

The factors which determine skin colour are summarised on page 938.

§ **753.** DEFICIENT PIGMENTATION; partial or complete absence of melanin pigmentation occurs in:

I. **Albinism,** a congenital condition. It may be *partial* with single or multiple areas devoid of pigment, or *universal,* with no melanin in the skin or its appendages or in the iris. The hair is white or very pale yellow and the iris pink.

II. **Vitiligo.**—Patches of depigmentation with sharply defined convex borders develop on any part of the body, but favour the neck, hands and trunk: it is often symmetrical in distribution. The contrasting hyper-pigmentation of the surrounding skin may first attract attention. The affected areas may become sore on exposure to sunlight but the disability is mainly cosmetic. The course is variable, with partial temporary remissions and occasional spontaneous cure, but is usually prolonged. Young adults of both sexes are most commonly affected. The cause is unknown; there may be a familial factor. *Diagnosis.*—In addition to the other conditions described in this section morphœa and lichen sclerosus may need exclusion. In both the texture of the white patches is abnormal, scar-like in the former and soft and wrinkled in the latter. *Treatment* is unsatisfactory and cosmetic covering creams should be recommended. Ammoidin (8-methoxypsoralen) by mouth and by local applications may be employed under careful supervision as promising results are occasionally obtained, but the response is uncertain.

III. **Secondary** and **symptomatic leucoderma.**—Some inflammatory dis-orders such as psoriasis and lichen simplex may be followed by temporary depigmentation. It very rarely develops on the neck in secondary syphilis and in the anæsthetic lesions of leprosy. Scars may be depigmented, especially those of lupus erythematosus and syphilis.

IV. **Occupational leucoderma** of the hands and forearms has been observed in negro workers wearing gloves made of rubber containing mono-benzoyl ether of hydroquinone as an antioxidant.

V. **Pseudo-leucoderma** develops when diseased patches of skin fail to pigment on exposure to sunlight, as conspicuously as surrounding normal skin, and so appear white. The dry scaly patches on children's faces (pityriasis alba, § 661) and pityriasis versicolor (§ 761) commonly behave in this manner.

§ 754. INCREASE IN PIGMENTATION.

(a) This is *extensive* or *generalised* in:

Common.

I. Racial pigmentation.
II. Pregnancy (§ 451).
III. Cachexia, especially of neoplastic origin (§ 571).
IV. Hyperthyroidism (§ 186).
V. Addison's Disease (§ 576).

Rare in Great Britain.

VI. Malignant phæochromocytoma (§ 97).
VII. Cirrhosis of the liver (§ 342).
VIII. Sprue (§ 318).
IX. Pellagra (§ 633).
X. Kala azar (§ 506).
XI. Malaria (§ 511).
XII. Chronic arsenical poisoning (§ 318).
XIII. Silver, gold or bismuth poisoning.
XIV. Hæmochromatosis (§ 343).
XV. Scleroderma (§ 751).
XVI. Acanthosis nigricans (§ 749).
XVII. Malignant melanoma (§ 756).
XVIII. Gaucher's Disease (§ 559).

Generalised pigmentation develops in some individuals in response to prolonged and repeated scratching in chronic pediculosis (vagabond's disease); and may accompany or follow chronic inflammatory changes as in certain erythrodermas (§ 665).

(b) A *localised* alteration in skin colour from increase in pigmentation or other cause occurs with:

i. *Black, brown or slate-grey pigmentation—*

Common.

I. Ephelis and Lentigo (§ 755).
II. Nævus pigmentosus and Melanoma (§ 756).
III. Blue nævus and Mongolian spot (§ 757).
IV. Occupational and Cosmetic melanosis (§ 758).
V. Chloasma (§ 759).
VI. Post-inflammatory pigmentation (§ 760).
VII. Pityriasis versicolor (§ 761).

Rare.

VIII. Leprosy and Syphilis (§ 762).
IX. Pellagra (§ 633).
X. Von Recklinghausen's Disease (§ 734).
XI. Xeroderma pigmentosum (§ 763).
XII. Urticaria pigmentosa (§ 764).
XIII. Incontinentia pigmenti (§ 765).
XIV. Ochronosis (§ 766).

ii. *Pink, red or red-brown pigmentation—*

XV. Purpura (§ 767).
XVI. Hæmosiderosis (including Schamberg's Disease) (§ 768).

XVII. Telangiectasia (§ 769).
XVIII. Capillary nævus (§ 770).
XIX. Angioma serpiginosum (§ 771).

iii. *Yellow or orange-yellow pigmentation*—
XX. Carotenæmia (§ 772).

(i) BLACK, BROWN OR SLATE-GREY PIGMENTATION:

§ 755. I. **Ephelis** and **Lentigo.** The *ephelis* is the common freckle.
Large numbers commonly make their appearance in fair-skinned individuals in early childhood on sites exposed to sunlight. They may fade
during the winter. To be differentiated from this is the *lentigo*—a small
brown macule occurring anywhere on the body and on all types of skin,
showing no seasonal variation and almost universally present. The
number increases from early childhood to the middle thirties and then
declines. Multiple lentigines of the mucosa and peribuccal skin occur with
intestinal polyposis in the rare Peutz's syndrome. *Senile lentigines*
(" liver spots "), light brown macules of various sizes, occur on the backs
of the hands and on the face in old age. *Lentigo maligna* occurs mainly
in the elderly and most frequently on the face. A mottled patch of brown
or black pigmentation extends slowly and irregularly for many years but
may develop localised thickening or ulceration, an indication of melanomatous transformation. The *prognosis* is very much more favourable than
in other forms of melanoma and wide local excision is adequate.

§ 756. II. **Nævus pigmentosus** (Pigmented nævus, mole). At least
one or two are present in most individuals. They occur anywhere on the
body and may be present at birth or may appear later. They may be
smooth and flat, soft, raised and dome-shaped, warty or hairy and show
wide variation in size and shape. The warty, hairy and raised nævi very
rarely undergo malignant change: those which are dangerous are the small
flat heavily pigmented nævi, especially on the hands or feet or in sites
subjected to trauma; malignant change is extremely rare before puberty.

Histologically they are characterised by the presence of the distinctive nævus
cells, which are probably of neural origin, either at the dermio-epidermal junction or
deeper in the dermis.

Treatment is often requested for cosmetic reasons. Thorough destruction with the diathermy is permissible when the nævus is of the soft raised
variety or is warty or hairy. A flat nævus and any nævus on the hands
or feet should be excised: some authorities advocate this as a prophylactic
measure if the nævus is liable to be subjected to trauma.

Melanoma (Malignant melanoma).—This may arise on previously
normal skin or may develop in a pre-existing nævus, usually of the flat
smooth type. Enlargement, hæmorrhage, ulceration or increased pigmentation in any nævus calls for immediate excision and histological
examination. *Diagnosis.*—The clinical differentiation of a melanoma from
a benign nævus, histiocytoma, pyogenic granuloma, pigmented basal-cell
epithelioma and other less common lesions may be difficult. *Treatment.*—
A wide local excision and grafting and, in many cases, dissection of the

regional lymphatic glands should be undertaken. Metastasis may occur early and the prognosis is always uncertain but with early and adequate treatment long survival is possible. Diffuse pigmentation most marked on the exposed areas is a rare terminal event.

§ **757. III. Blue nævus and Mongolian spot.**—A blue nævus is a circumscribed papule usually an intense blue-black in colour. It occurs mainly on the backs of the hands or feet but may occur anywhere and is not uncommon. Melanomatous change is exceptional and if treatment is demanded on cosmetic grounds simple excision is satisfactory. Histologically rather similar is the *Mongolian spot*, an ill-defined patch of pigmentation present at birth in the sacral area of a majority of infants of Asiatic race and very rarely in others. It disappears during the early years of life.

§ **758. IV. Occupational and Cosmetic melanosis.**—(i.) Diffuse pigmentation of the exposed skin of the face, hands and arms, often associated with hyperkeratosis and follicular plugging, may develop in workers exposed to *tar* and certain hydrocarbons and sunlight. (ii.) *Berloque* pigmentation, in irregular streaks along the hair line or at the sides of the neck, is due to the photosensitising action of oil of bergamot in eau de Cologne and other perfumes.

Riehl's melanosis (Poikiloderma of Civatte) is a finely reticulate pigmentation developing slowly in women of 30–50 years. It is often preceded by erythema, extending from the temples and the sides of the neck to the forehead and cheeks, usually sparing the chin and the mid-face. Atrophy and telangiectasia are associated in variable degree. Photosensitising substances in cosmetics are probably responsible.

§ **759. V. Chloasma** consists of symmetrical patches of diffuse brown pigmentation of the mid-forehead and of the cheeks, but sparing the central area of the face. It often develops during pregnancy, disappears after parturition, but can persist for months or years. It also occurs at the menopause or with ovarian tumours, or without discernible cause.

§ **760. VI. Post-inflammatory pigmentation.**—Many inflammatory changes in the skin are followed by pigmentation for which advice may be sought by the patient, who may not have noticed the original lesion. The pattern of pigmentation may be distinctive. It is a characteristic feature of lichen planus and dermatitis herpetiformis. Irregular clusters of pigmented macules on the buttocks and thighs in children may follow insect bites. Linear streaks of pigmentation follow the bullæ of phytophotodermatitis (§ 679). Reticulate pigmentation is often seen on the lower legs of those who spend long hours near a fire, or in other sites from repeated contact with a hot-water bottle.

§ **761. VII. Pityriasis versicolor** (Tinea versicolor) is a persistent superficial skin infection with the fungus *Malassezia furfur*. It presents as irregular but sharply defined patches of dull brown pigmentation, usually on the upper trunk and commonly in adults. Fine scaling is usual but may not be conspicuous. *Diagnosis* is established by finding the fungus in direct examination of scales. *Treatment* is by the application of 20 per cent. solution of sodium thiosulphate each morning and 5 per cent. salicylic acid ointment at night.

§ **762.** VIII. **Leprosy** and **Syphilis.**—The macular lesions of leprosy may be pigmented. Anæsthesia of the lesions is diagnostic. The pigmentary syphilide is very uncommon and is almost confined to women, in whom it occurs around the back and sides of the neck.

§ **763.** XI. **Xeroderma pigmentosum** develops in infancy as dryness, roughness and redness of the exposed skin. In the third or fourth year numerous brown pigmented macules develop in these sites, and the picture is gradually completed by the appearance of white atrophic scars, telangiectasia and warty keratoses. Carcinomatous or rarely melanomatous changes may result in early death. The disease is a manifestation of an inherited susceptibility to ultraviolet light. *Treatment* consists of protection against light and early radical excision of malignant lesions.

§ **764.** XII. **Urticaria pigmentosa** may be present at birth or appear in early infancy or childhood. It is occasionally seen in adults. The lesions are commonly all of one type in any individual but macular, papular and nodular forms occur. A single lesion, or few or large numbers may be present. They are dull brown in colour and characteristically, but not invariably, urticate on friction. Bullæ may develop on the lesions. Urticaria pigmentosa was considered to be localised to the skin and entirely benign, but recently generalised mast-cell infiltration of lymph nodes, spleen, liver and bone marrow has been reported. Every case should be fully investigated for evidence of a systemic mast-cell reticulosis—X-ray of the skeleton for bony lesions, examination of the bone marrow and search for abnormalities in the clotting mechanism. In the absence of systemic lesions the prognosis is good and spontaneous cure often occurs.

§ **765.** XIII. **Incontinentia pigmenti** is rare. It is present at birth or develops within the first weeks of life. Bizarre and irregular patterns of brownish pigmentation on the trunk and limbs may be preceded by bullæ and warty papules. The pigmentation eventually fades. Congenital defects in other organs may be found.

§ **766.** XIV. **Ochronosis** is characterised by the development in middle life of grey or black pigmentation of cartilages, ligaments and tendons. The urine turns black on exposure to air (alkaptonuria, § 385). In this rare hereditary metabolic defect, the degradation of tyrosine cannot proceed beyond the stage of homogentisic acid.

(ii) PINK, RED OR RED-BROWN PIGMENTATION:

§ **767.** XV. **Purpura** is hæmorrhage into the skin or mucous membranes. It does not fade on pressure. There may simultaneously be hæmorrhages into other organs such as the joints or the retina. At first bright red in colour, as the blood pigments are broken down and later carried away by phagocytic cells this changes through purple to red-brown and then to yellow-brown. Purpuric macules are known as *petechiæ*; large irregular hæmorrhages are *ecchymoses*.

Red cells can only escape when the integrity of the capillary wall is impaired. Purpura may be the result of a capillary lesion without a defect in the coagulation mechanism, or if coagulation is defective may develop with trivial capillary damage, the nature of which may not be demonstrable. Gross coagulation defects are not of necessity always accompanied by purpura.

With rare exceptions the clinical features of the purpuric lesions themselves are not sufficiently distinctive to permit an etiological diagnosis.

Purpura is therefore an indication for a full clinical examination followed by red and white cell and platelet counts, estimation of bleeding time, coagulation time, clot retraction and the *capillary resistance test*.

This is performed by placing a sphygmomanometer cuff round the upper arm and inflating it to a pressure midway between the diastolic and systolic levels. The cuff is removed after five minutes. The test is positive if multiple petechiæ have developed on the arm below the level of the cuff.

On the basis of these tests a simple classification is:—

A. **Purpura due mainly to capillary damage** (platelets usually normal).

1. *Senile purpura* occurs on the backs of the hands and forearms and on the lower legs after the age of 60. The petechiæ are often large and are commonly associated with the atrophic appearance and irregular pigmentation of old age. They are due to weakening of the capillary wall by degenerative changes in the supporting connective tissues.

2. *Mechanical purpura* develops as the result of increased intracapillary pressure, as in chronic venous stasis, after convulsive attacks or from mechanical constriction of a limb.

3. *Scurvy.* In the skin follicular hyperkeratosis of the buttocks or calves precedes the development of perifollicular petechiæ especially on the legs. Purpura is due to weakening of the capillary walls as the intercellular ground substance is defective. (See § 560.)

4. *Anaphylactoid purpura* (Schönlein-Henoch Syndrome) usually occurs in children and young adults. The petechiæ are symmetrically distributed on the buttocks, thighs and lower legs and on the extensor aspects of the arms. They are often preceded by small wheals. Mild fever is usual. The skin lesion may occur alone or in conjunction with intestinal colic, joint pains and other internal symptoms (§ 595).

Purpura fulminans is rare, but usually fatal. It is a severe form of anaphylactoid purpura in which extensive necrosis follows an acute streptococcal infection.

5. *Symptomatic purpura* occurs during acute infections due to toxic injury to the capillary endothelium, to sensitisation or to thrombocytopenia. Purpura may complicate the *acute specific fevers*, and occurs in severe septicæmia: it is characteristic of meningococcal bacteræmia. The purpura of *subacute bacterial endocarditis* is the result of bacterial embolism. Purpura of uncertain cause is common in *nephritis* and may occur in gout. *Drug* purpura is usually the result of an allergic mechanism damaging either the capillary endothelium or the platelets. A few drugs can produce both types of purpura. Purpura caused by carbromalum, cinchophen, gold salts, quinidine, quinine and sulphonamides is usually not thrombocytopenic. *Lupus erythematosus* in its acute form may be hæmorrhagic. This is the result of vascular damage but thrombocytopenia is often also present. Purpura may also occur in *polyarteritis nodosa*.

B. **Purpura associated with quantitative or qualitative platelet deficiencies** (no gross capillary defect). See also § 541.

1. *Essential thrombocytopenia* (Primary thrombocytopenia). The

chronic form of this rare disease is characterised by a gradual onset and by continuing symptoms or complete remissions during months or years. Purpura, especially on the legs, develops only during exacerbations and at other times easy bruising, intestinal bleeding and metrorrhagia are present. Chronic leg ulcers may occur. The spleen is palpable in 10 per cent. The platelet count is low during attacks. In remissions only the capillary resistance may be abnormal. The *acute* form is rarer still. The onset is sudden with fever, extensive purpura and hæmorrhage from mucous membranes. Patients may be exsanguinated in a few hours. Capillary fragility is greatly increased and the platelet count is very low (even 10,000 per c.mm.). Both forms affect children and young adults (80 per cent. occur before the age of 25). The etiology is not proved but an immunological mechanism is probably concerned. The prognosis is good if blood loss can be effectively controlled or replaced. *Treatment.*— Transfusion may be required. Splenectomy gives reasonable results (except in the familial variety): Cortisone and ACTH may control acute episodes.

2. *Symptomatic thrombocytopenia* occurs with (*a*) bone-marrow defect, as in aplastic anæmia, leukæmia, sometimes in pernicious anæmia and after X-ray therapy; (*b*) hypersplenism: the enlarged spleen in Hodgkin's disease or in other conditions may produce excessive destruction of platelets; (*c*) hypersensitivity: drugs causing this include arsenicals, phenylbutazone, procaine, quinidine, quinine, Sedormid, sulphonamides and thiouracil. (*d*) The purpura in some infections may be thrombocytopenic.

C. **Purpura associated with defective coagulation** other than platelet abnormalities. Hæmophilia, hypoprothrombinæmia, fibrinogenopenia and other deficiencies or abnormalities of plasma coagulation factors are rarely associated with purpura, but subcutaneous hæmorrhage and ecchymosis may occur. Such cases occur particularly with liver disease.

§ **768.** XVI. **Hæmosiderosis** (Pigmented purpuric eruptions). These fairly common disorders are characterised by localised or extensive hæmosiderin pigmentation formed by discrete red-brown puncta which have been likened to grains of cayenne pepper. The underlying lesion is capillary damage insufficient to give the grosser forms of purpura. *Gravitational hæmosiderin pigmentation* of the lower third of the leg is common in venous insufficiency. Melanin pigmentation is often associated. *Schamberg's disease* may also begin on the legs, but is not of venous origin. More commonly seen in men, irregular patches of red-brown pigmentation may cover large areas of the body and may persist for many years. The capillary fragility is usually increased but no hæmatological abnormalities are present. The cause is unknown. *Purpura annularis telangiectoides* occurs as localised patches of punctate purpura slowly extending centrifugally and leaving central atrophy. The lesions, which are usually on the lower leg, foot or arm, clear after a few months. *Pigmented purpuric lichenoid dermatitis* also occurs usually on the legs but may develop on the arms or trunk. The lesions consist of grouped flat pink papules which become purpuric and telangiectatic. *Diagnosis.*—The purpura produced by certain drugs, notably the ureides (carbromalum) may be punctate. Clothing, especially khaki, may produce a purpuric dermatitis; the punctate and linear purpura is associated with small papules and erythema and is confined to sites in contact with the garment.

§ 769. XVII. **Telangiectasia** is a permanent dilatation of small bloodvessels in the skin or mucous membranes. It is often conspicuous on the cheeks in those who have lived much in the sun. It is often a feature of rosacea, lupus erythematosus, dermatomyositis, radiodermatitis. Telangiectasia of the face may occur in the later stages of systemic scleroderma. It is the most prominent feature in poikiloderma congenitale (§ 752).

Telangiectases sometimes found between the shoulder-blades in young persons are of no known significance. They may encircle the trunk at the level of the diaphragm, especially in asthmatic and chronic bronchitic subjects. Branching linear telangiectasia of the thighs in young women and symmetrical arborescent telangiectasia of the lower legs in older women are not necessarily associated with venous insufficiency.

Nævus araneus (Spider nævus) is common on the face and upper trunk in children and in women with fair skins. Small dilated vessels radiate from a central punctum, like the legs of a spider. The lesions may follow minor trauma. They may also develop in pregnancy and in cirrhosis of the liver. *Treatment.*—The central vessel can be thrombosed with a cautery point.

Hereditary hæmorrhagic telangiectasia (Osler–Rendu Syndrome) is a rare disorder with numerous telangiectases in the skin and mucous membranes; their presence on the lip and tongue is characteristic and diagnostic. The condition mainly develops after puberty, but may begin in infancy or in middle life. Epistaxis is the commonest presenting symptom and later repeated gastro-intestinal hæmorrhages may occur. The syndrome affects the sexes equally, and is inherited as a simple dominant character.

§ 770. XVIII. **Capillary nævus** (Nævus flammeus).—This common vascular nævus is usually present at birth. The colour ranges from pale pink to purple and the area from a few centimetres square to half or more of the skin surface. The nævus is flat or very slightly raised. The pale telangiectatic type present at birth over the glabella and upper eyelids fades in the first week of life; the remainder show no tendency to spontaneous cure. The darker type (port-wine marks) are very disfiguring. *Treatment.*—Tattooing or plastic procedures may be practicable. Painting with thorium-X (2,000 e.s.u. per ml.) may make the colour somewhat paler, but abrasion is the best method of treatment.

Sturge–Weber Syndrome.—A port-wine nævus of unilateral trigeminal distribution may be associated with hæmangiomatous involvement of the meninges (epilepsy, hemiparesis and mental deficiency) and of the ciliary body (glaucoma).

Klippel–Trenaunay–Weber Syndrome.—Extensive hæmangiomatous involvement of a limb is accompanied by hypertrophy of bone and soft tissues.

§ 771. XIX. **Angioma serpiginosum** is a rare nævoid disorder. Punctate telangiectasia, usually on a limb, gradually extends over the course of years, by the development and coalescence of new puncta beyond the advancing margin.

(iii.) Yellow or Orange-yellow Pigmentation:

§ 772. XX. **Carotenæmia** commonly results from the excessive consumption of foods containing carotene, especially carrots and certain other vegetables. It may also occur in myxœdema, diabetes mellitus and in liver disease. Carotene stains the horny layer of the skin and the yellowish discoloration is therefore most marked on the palms and soles. The sclera is not involved and the serum van den Bergh reaction is negative (distinguishing it from jaundice).

GROUP X. DISORDERS OF THE SWEAT MECHANISM

§ 773. **Anhidrosis,** or absence of sweating, may be generalised or localised and may be due to failure of sweat production or to obstruction of the sweat ducts. The sweat glands are absent in congenital ectodermal dysplasia: they are atrophic or destroyed in radiodermatitis, acrodermatitis atrophicans, scleroderma and other atrophic or sclerotic disorders. Generalized reduction or absence of sweating may occur in myxœdema, Addison's disease and by the use of anticholingeric drugs such as atropine.

Congenital ectodermal dysplasia is a rare inherited abnormality. The skin generally is dry, thin and smooth. Hair is sparse or absent, nails are rudimentary and teeth are defective. The depressed bridge of the nose produces a facies recalling congenital syphilis in that form of the syndrome in which sweat glands are absent, and the consequent heat intolerance may lead to heatstroke or present as pyrexia of uncertain origin in warm weather.

Localised anhidrosis can be produced by lesions in the brain stem or cord or involvement of the sympathetic fibres peripherally. It most commonly results from sweat duct obstruction, often as a consequence of previous inflammatory changes. (For the miliarial syndromes see § 673.)

§ 774. **Hyperhidrosis** is excessive sweating. When *generalised* it is a physiological response in hot climates and on physical exertion. It occurs during defervescence of many acute fevers and is often a feature of active tuberculosis and acute rheumatism. It is usual in hyperthyroidism and may occur in pregnancy and at the menopause. It is common in certain toxic states such as acute alcoholic poisoning. *Local* hyperhidrosis most commonly involves the palms, soles, axillæ and groins. Sweating in these sites is a normal emotional response and can be considered pathological only when it becomes socially or occupationally disabling. Excessive sweating may be present from very early childhood, when it is sometimes hereditary, but most commonly begins soon after adolescence. The affected sites are constantly moist and sweat profusely with excitement or anxiety; a raised environmental temperature further lowers the threshold. Hyperhidrosis of the face may be provoked by highly seasoned foods (gustatory sweating); in some normal persons it may be a symptom of a neurological lesion, which may also give rise to other bizarre patterns.

In **bromidrosis** the odour of the sweat is offensive as the result of bacterial decomposition of sebum and keratin.

In **chromidrosis** the sweat is discoloured; it is usually black, brown or grey due to pigments produced by the apocrine glands. Bacterial or mycotic infection may discolour the sweat after secretion: in *trichomycosis axillaris* there are small hard granules on the axillary hairs and the sweat may stain the clothing red or yellow.

Treatment of local hyperhidrosis is difficult. The emotional component is of paramount importance and sedation with phenobarbitone gr. ½ b.d. or with tranquillising drugs is often desirable. When there is a severe anxiety state psychiatric advice may be required. The anticholinergic drugs are useful if effective doses do not produce unpleasant side effects. Tinct. belladonna ℳ 5, Belladenal 1 tablet or probanthine bromide 15 mg., three times daily may be tried. A high standard of personal hygiene with suitable clothing and shoes are obviously essential. Local applications of temporary benefit for hyperhidrosis of the feet are a paint to the soles daily with aluminium chloride (25 per cent.) and a dusting powder containing salicylic acid (3 per cent.) in talc. Painting with formalin (20 per cent.) two or three times a week is more effective but can be irritating. In axillary hyperhidrosis a useful local application is aluminium chloride (15 per cent.), glycerine (5 per cent.) in equal parts of water and spirit.

GROUP XI. DISEASES OF THE SCALP AND HAIR

I. Alopecia (baldness) (§ 775).

II. Irritable conditions of the scalp (§ 776).

III. Scaly conditions of the scalp (§ 777).

IV. Grey or white hair (§ 778).

V. Ringworm infections (§ 779).

VI. Congenital abnormalities (§ 780).

VII. Hair dyes and waving (§ 781).

VIII. Hypertrichosis (§ 782).

§ 775. I. **Alopecia.**—When the patient complains of baldness it is important to determine whether the loss of hair is occurring more or less diffusely or in well-defined circumscribed patches, and whether the scalp in the affected areas appears normal or is cicatricial. The scarred or cicatricial scalp is smooth and white and no follicular orifices are visible.

NON-CICATRICIAL ALOPECIA

With diffuse hair loss

i. Common baldness.

ii. Alopecia in Endocrine disease.

iii. Postfebrile and postpartum alopecia.

iv. Congenital alopecia.

With patchy hair loss

v. Alopecia areata.

vi. Traumatic alopecia.

vii. Ringworm (§ 779).

viii. Secondary syphilis.

WITH DIFFUSE HAIR LOSS

i. **Common Baldness.**—The familiar male pattern of hair loss begins as bilateral recession of the temporofrontal hair margin; later hair is lost from the vertex. The age of onset, at any time after adolescence, the rate of progression and the pattern of baldness ultimately produced are largely dependent on hereditary factors. Androgenic stimulation is invariable and male pattern alopecia does not occur before puberty or in castrates. Some diffuse thinning of the hair is common in women after the menopause, and sometimes earlier in life. Less often the male pattern may develop. As in men hereditary factors are of chief importance, but relative androgenic excess may contribute. Seborrhœa is often associated with common baldness but is not its cause.

Treatment is unsatisfactory. It is a kindness to the patient to persuade him to accept his baldness philosophically. None of the hundreds of remedies recommended is of proven value.

ii. **Alopecia in Endocrine Diseases.**—Male pattern alopecia occurs in women with Cushing's disease and in suprarenal and ovarian virilism. In acromegaly the hair is coarse and there may be patchy alopecia. In hypoparathyroidism the hair is dull and brittle and may be thin and patchy. In hyperthyroidism alopecia areata may occur, but the hair is often particularly luxuriant, although it may become prematurely grey. In hypothyroidism the hair is scanty, dry and grey. In hypopituitarism the hair is dry, dull and sparse.

iii. **Postfebrile and Postpartum Alopecia.**—Extensive diffuse loss of hair may occur 8 to 10 weeks after a febrile illness and after childbirth. Complete regrowth takes place without treatment.

iv. **Congenital Alopecia** may occur alone or in association with abnormalities of the nails and teeth, or with still more extensive changes in congenital anhidrotic ectodermal defect or other rare syndromes.

With Patchy Hair Loss

v. **Alopecia Areata** is the commonest cause of patchy hair loss. It affects patients of both sexes and any age but is less common in the elderly. A single round or oval patch of complete baldness develops rapidly, usually over the vertex or in the occipital region. There are no subjective symptoms and the denuded area of scalp is of normal colour and texture. This original patch may extend slowly, when exclamation mark hairs (!) may be seen in the advancing margin. There may be only a single patch or further patches may appear at intervals of a few weeks. In some cases all the scalp hair is lost (*alopecia totalis*) or all hair on the body (*alopecia universalis*). Patches on the beard may occur alone or in association with involvement of the scalp. Ridging or pitting of the nails accompanies some severe cases. In one form (*ophiasis*) the alopecia extends as a band along the hair margin.

Diagnosis.—*Ringworm* is excluded by the presence of scaling and of broken hairs. In case of doubt direct microscopy of hairs should be undertaken. *Traumatic alopecia* is the commonest source of confusion except in ringworm epidemics. In *secondary syphilis* the scalp has a moth-eaten appearance and other signs of the disease are present. The cicatricial alopecias are excluded by careful examination.

Etiology.—The cause is still disputed. A history of acute emotional stress or anxiety preceding the onset is common and is widely accepted as a provocative factor. Errors of refraction, focal sepsis and unidentified infective agents have been suggested. The role of endocrine factors is obscure and indirect.

The *prognosis* is always uncertain. In many cases regrowth is complete in 6 or 7 months but in others may require over a year. About one-third never recover completely from the initial attack and recurrences are frequent. Alopecia totalis always has a poor prognosis, particularly if the onset is before puberty. Ophiasis is also liable to persist.

Treatment is unsatisfactory and it is doubtful whether any of the methods employed materially influence the natural course of the disease. Reassurance and, if necessary, sedation should be given. Local and general ultraviolet light may be of value. As a mild counter-irritant acid lactic ℥ 120, ol. ricini ℥ 120, spir, vin. rect. to fl. oz. 4, is clean to use. Steroids systemically cause regrowth, but the hair is lost again when treatment is discontinued, and they should not be prescribed.

vi. **Traumatic Alopecia.**—Three clinical forms of non-cicatricial traumatic alopecia are of common occurrence. In *trichotillomania* the hairs are

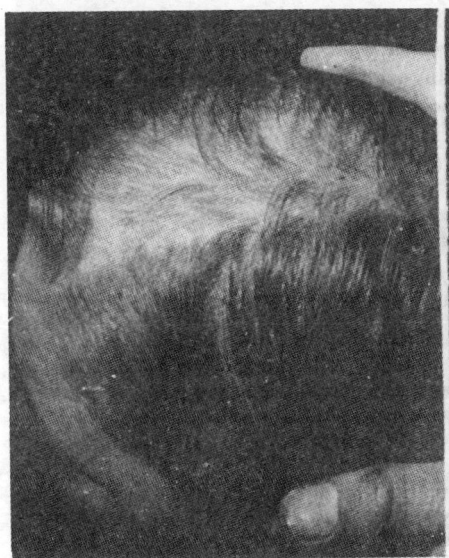 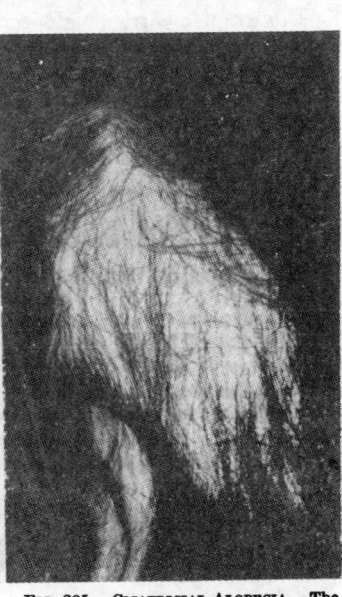

FIG. 204.—TRAUMATIC ALOPECIA in a typical site in a child. The alopecia is the result of a hair-pulling tic. The remaining hairs in the patch are broken and twisted but otherwise normal.

FIG. 205.—CICATRICIAL ALOPECIA. The scalp is smooth and white and the hair follicles are destroyed. This is an example of pseudopelade.

broken and twisted, due to a hair-pulling tic (Fig. 204). In children a habit of twisting the hair round the fingers has often been observed by the parents. The partially bald patch is frequently in the left frontoparietal region in a right-handed child and on the right in the left-handed, but may occur anywhere. The same condition occurs in adults, particularly in psychotics, in whom a large area of the scalp may be affected. In infants and small children a partially bald patch over the occiput is produced by the movements of the head on the pillow and may alarm the inexperienced mother. A third form is seen in adults as friction alopecia; large or small patches of partial alopecia with twisted and broken, but otherwise normal, hairs occur mainly on the vertex. The patient, usually a woman, but sometimes a nervous young man, admits to regular and vigorous friction with a proprietary lotion, self-prescribed. In all these forms of traumatic alopecia the hair regrows when allowed to do so.

viii. In **Secondary Syphilis** patchy alopecia may occur or there may be diffuse thinning of the hair. The patches are numerous, small and not completely bald so that the scalp assumes a characteristic " moth-eaten " appearance. Other signs are present and serological tests are positive.

CICATRICIAL ALOPECIA is relatively uncommon. The affected areas are smooth, flat and devoid of hair follicles. They may be sclerotic or atrophic and may show telangiectasia, horny plugging or irregular pigmentation according to their mode of origin. Unless the cause is evident the entire skin surface and the buccal mucous membranes should be carefully examined.

Causes of cicatricial alopecia:—

   i. Burns; overdosage with X-ray (§ 750).

   ii. Destructive infective processes; syphilides; leprosy; lupus vulgaris; herpes zoster; certain ringworm infections (favus, kerion).

   iii. Neoplastic processes; especially basal-cell epithelioma.

   iv. Nævi.

   v. Lupus erythematosus (§ 631), lichen planus (§ 637), scleroderma (§ 751).

   vi. Pseudopelade.

   vii. Folliculitis decalvans.

vi. **Pseudopelade** occurs in adults of both sexes as small circumscribed areas of cicatricial alopecia. The patches are smooth, white and atrophic with no obvious inflammatory changes (Fig. 205). By extension and coalescence of the original patches large irregular areas of scalp may be affected. The prognosis is poor as the process usually extends slowly despite treatment. Pseudopelade is not a pathological entity. It is a distinctive clinical state which may be produced by lichen planus, lichen spinulosus or the burnt-out inactive stage of lupus erythematosus. In other cases there is no evidence of the cause.

vii. **Folliculitis Decalvans** is an uncommon progressive cicatricial alopecia in which small follicular pustules are present in the advancing margins of the scarred areas. The pustules are sterile. *Treatment* is usually ineffective.

§ 776. II. Irritable conditions of the Scalp.

Pruritus may be present in many inflammatory disorders of the scalp, eczema, contact dermatitis from hair dyes or lotions, pityriasis capitis and seborrhœic dermatitis and some cases of psoriasis. It is the predominant symptom in:—

   i. Pediculosis capitis.

   ii. Neurodermatitis of the scalp.

   iii. Acne necrotica miliaris.

i. **Pediculosis Capitis** occurs mainly in girls whose standard of hygiene is low, but the diagnosis must always be excluded in cases of pruritus or impetigo of the scalp or of enlargement or tenderness of the occipital and cervical glands even in individuals whose cleanliness is otherwise above reproach. The head louse, *Pediculus capitis*, causes severe irritation, particularly in the occipital region, and secondary bacterial infection may follow scratching. The hair in this region should be searched for eggs (nits), greyish-white oval capsules cemented to the hair shafts.

Treatment.—Applicatio dicophani B.P.C. (DDT) 2 per cent. or applicatio lethani should be thoroughly rubbed into the scalp, which should be shampooed the next day and combed with a fine tooth-comb to remove the dead nits. It is not necessary to cut the hair. When there is gross secondary infection it may be necessary first to apply an antibiotic ointment for two days. Hats, caps, brushes and combs must be disinfected.

ii. **Neurodermatitis of the Scalp** (Lichen simplex chronicus) is seen mainly in middle-aged and elderly women. Patches occur most commonly on the nape of the neck, but can occur behind and above the ears, when

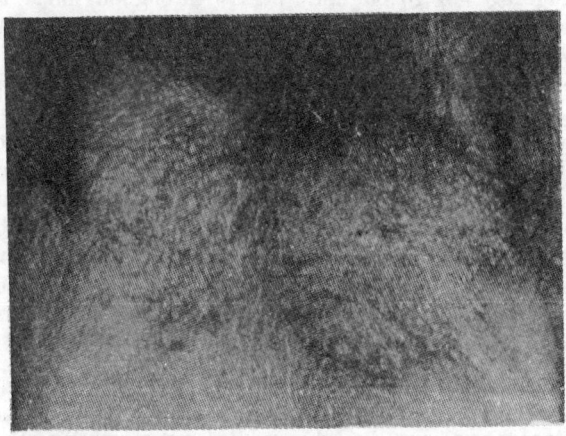

FIG. 206.—LICHEN SIMPLEX of the nape of the neck. This thickened patch of lichenification is intensely irritable. The condition is quite common in women.

they may be symmetrical. Pruritus is often intense. The skin changes which result from repeated rubbing and scratching consist of circumscribed and thickened plaques, with exaggeration of the normal skin markings visible when the patch extends beyond the scalp margin. There may be profuse psoriasiform scaling and obvious signs of secondary infection. The hair may be sparse and broken (Fig. 206). The condition is due to nervous tension and unless this can be reduced topical applications are of only temporary benefit.

Treatment.—The patient must understand that the objective changes have been produced by scratching and an attempt must be made to relieve the nervous tension. Rest and hypnotics are often necessary: chlorpromazine 10 to 25 mg. t.i.d. is helpful. Ung. hydrocortisone acetate (½–1 per cent.) often gives great symptomatic relief. In refractory cases infiltration with triamcinolone is useful.

iii. **Acne necrotica miliaris** occurs in adults, in men more often than in women. The patient complains of bouts of intense pruritus and examination reveals small follicular vesicles, or more commonly, the crusts resulting from their excoriation. *Treatment* with 2 per cent. ammoniated mercury in emulsifying ointment is often effective, as is lotio hydrocortisone (½ per cent.). Recurrences are frequent unless the underlying nervous tension can be reduced.

§ 777. III. Scaly Conditions of the Scalp.

i. Pityriasis capitis.   iv. Neurodermatitis (§ 776).
ii. Tinea amiantacea.   v. Ringworm (§ 779).
iii. Psoriasis (§ 658).

i. **Pityriasis Capitis** (Dandruff).—*Pityriasis simplex* consists of dry branny scaling of the scalp. The scales are readily detached and are not accompanied by signs of inflammation. The condition rarely develops before the age of 9 or 10 but may persist throughout life. It must be regarded as physiological. It may be transformed after puberty into *pityriasis steatoides* in which the scales become larger, greasy and more adherent and the underlying scalp red and moist. This is a form of seborrhœic dermatitis and is often associated with male-pattern alopecia, but is not responsible for the loss of hair. The *diagnosis* should never be made in childhood until ringworm has been excluded. *Treatment.*—In mild cases a weekly shampoo may be adequate. More often this must be preceded by the weekly or twice weekly application of ol. cadini ℥ 30, sulphur precip. gr. 15, acid salicyl. gr. 10, ung. emulsificans to oz. 1 which can be washed out after 5–10 hours. If this does not completely control it a few drops of a lotion containing hydrarg. perchlor. gr. 1, acid. salicylic. gr. 40, ol. ric. ℥ 20, acetone ℥ 240, spir. vini meth. to fl. oz. 4 should be massaged into the scalp each morning.

ii. **Tinea Amiantacea** (Pityriasis Amiantacea) presents as layers of adherent sticky scales, sometimes forming quite large masses. It is not a pathological entity, but a clinical syndrome which may complicate a neurodermatitis, psoriasis or infective dermatitis, and merely represents a distinctive reaction of the scalp common to various underlying disorders.

§ 778. IV. Grey or White Hair (Canities).—Greying of the hair

normally begins at the temples at about the age of 35 and may be complete by 60. *Premature canities* in which the first grey hairs appear in childhood or early adult life is inherited. It also occurs in progeria and in certain rare congenital syndromes. *Pathological greying* or *whitening* of the hair, sometimes of rapid onset, may occur in severe illnesses or after profound emotional stress. A *localised patch of white hair, poliosis*, can occur as an inherited feature (" white forelock ") which may be associated with partial albinism. If *vitiligo* involves the scalp the hairs in the affected

areas lose their pigment.   The regrown hair in alopecia areata is sometimes
white at first, but may regain its normal colour.   *Localised greying* of the
hair may occur after herpes zoster and in trigeminal neuralgia.   *Treatment.*
—No systemic treatment is effective and the patient must resort to hair
dyes if the condition causes distress or embarrassment.

§ **779. V. Ringworm infection of the Scalp** (Tinea Capitis) occurs
predominantly in the child before puberty but infections with certain
species may persist into adult life.   The species commonly concerned are
listed in Table XLIX.

Symptoms.—Circumscribed patches of alopecia, showing fine scaling of
the scalp and dull lustreless hairs broken off two or three millimetres above
the surface, are due to *Microsporon audouini*.   There may be a single
small patch or as much as one-third of the scalp may be involved.   Inflammatory changes are usually slight or absent unless they have been induced
by treatment.   Tinea circinata of the face or neck is unusual.   An indistinguishable picture results from *Microsporon canis* infections, but
inflammatory changes are more often present and associated lesions of
the glabrous skin are frequent.   Under Wood's light infected hairs in both
infections show a distinctive greenish fluorescence, not to be confused with
the white or yellow fluorescence produced by some ointments.   Diffuse
dry scaling and broken hairs interspersed with normal hairs are produced
by *Trichophyton sulphureum* infections.   The hair stumps may be so short
that they appear as black dots.   The patches of alopecia are often of
irregular rather angular outline.   There may be no obvious inflammatory
changes but some cases show folliculitis or even kerion formation.   The
infection may resolve spontaneously or persist for many years, particularly
in adults.   Scarring, which simulates lupus erythematosus, is sometimes
produced.   A " black dot " ringworm in which inflammatory reactions are
rare, can be caused by *T. violaceum*.   The animal species *T. discoides* and
T. mentagrophytes on the contrary usually provoke a briskly inflammatory
lesion which is self-limiting in a few weeks.   Occasionally more persistent
granulomatous forms are seen.

Favus is uncommon in Britain, but small outbreaks occur.   Children are usually
affected ; without treatment the infection can persist throughout life.   Within
a few weeks of infection small, firm, saucer-like crusts (favic scutula) form around
single hairs or groups of hairs.   They are not easily detached.   The scutula may
coalesce to form large friable masses, ultimately separating to leave an irregular
cicatricial alopecia.   The causative fungus *Achorion* (Trichophyton) *schöenleini* is a
human parasite.   It can be seen microscopically in the hairs, penetrating the scutula,
and is confirmed by culture.

Diagnosis.—Broken hairs are the characteristic clinical feature of scalp
ringworm infections.   They should always be sought in the presence of
scaling of the scalp in the child under 10 in whom dandruff is uncommon.
Irregular alopecia, with or without scar formation, should raise the
suspicion of ringworm at any age.   In all cases broken hairs should be
extracted, placed in 20 per cent. potassium hydroxide and examined under

the microscope for mycelium and spores. If fungus is present further hairs should be cultured as identification of the species is of value in planning treatment, tracing the source of the infection and determining the measures required to prevent its further transmission. Microsporon infections can be identified by examination under Wood's light, but this must supplement and not replace the direct examination of suspected hairs as most trichophyton infections give no fluorescence.

Etiology.—*Microsporon audouini*, a human parasite, is the most important cause of a scalp ringworm in Britain and is responsible for large epidemics in schoolchildren, among whom the disease is transmitted directly or by means of hats and caps, hair brushes, cinema seats, etc. *M. canis*, a parasite of kittens and sometimes of puppies, causes sporadic cases or small outbreaks centred round the family pet. Child to child transmission without renewal of infection from the animal source is limited. *Trichophyton discoides*, the parasite of cattle ringworm, and *T. mentagrophytes*, also an animal parasite, occasionally cause scalp infection in humans. The species of trichophyton, whose natural host is man, are less commonly encountered in Britain, but their incidence appears to be increasing in many parts of the country. *T. sulphureum* (*T. tonsurans, T. crateriforme*) is exclusively a human parasite but the infectivity is less than that of *M. audouini* and sporadic cases or small outbreaks have been commoner than large epidemics; however, the diagnosis is easily overlooked and many cases are probably undetected. *T. violaceum* infections are extremely common in many parts of the Middle East and Far East and are occasionally introduced to Britain. *T. sabouraudi* (*T. accuminatum*) occurs in France and other parts of Europe but is rare in Great Britain.

Pathogenesis and Pathology.—Slight trauma favours the initial inoculation of the scalp. From the site of infection the fungus grows radially in the horny layer infecting the majority of hair follicles in its path. Within a week after infection with *Microsporon audouini* a zone of greenish fluorescence can be detected just above the hair-bulb if hairs are pulled out. After a further five days the fluorescent zone extends above the surface of the scalp, and by the third week infected hairs break off a millimetre or two above the surface. While the infection is extending hairs with a basal fluorescent zone are present just beyond the margins of the area clinically affected. When the infection ceases to extend the hairs beyond the margin no longer show basal fluorescence; the scalp surface then presents only slight scaling. A state of host-parasite equilibrium may be maintained for some months, the fungus mycelium growing down into the hairshaft as it is formed. After a variable period spontaneous cure takes place. In infections of human origin such as *M. audouini* and *T. sulphureum* this may require many months. Infections of animal origin provoke an inflammatory response in the hair follicles which results in more rapid cure.

The relative immunity of the adult scalp to ringworm infections cannot yet be fully explained. Alterations occurring at puberty in the quantity and composition of the sebum and physiochemical changes in the hair itself may be responsible.

Treatment of Ringworm and Favus.—(i.) Parasites confined to *human beings* provoke little or no visible inflammatory reaction for months or years unless actively treated. Such include most infections with *M. audouini* and *T. sulphureum* and almost all infections with *T. violaceum* and *T. sabouraudi* and *favus*. The treatment of choice is with tab. griseofulvin, an antibiotic which is deposited in keratin and renders it resistant to invasion by ringworm. The adult dose is 1 G. daily and for children 10 mg./lb. body weight. Most cases are cured in 3 to 6 weeks, but a few require treatment for 15 weeks, until three weekly examinations under Wood's light (Microsporon infections) or by microscopy and culture have proved negative. Minor digestive disturbances with griseofulvin are avoided if it is given after meals, headaches usually subside if treatment is continued, and drug rashes and leucopenia are rare. As antibiotics do not reach infected debris in the mouths of follicles, the hair in affected regions needs shaving and application of a fungicidal ointment after a daily shampoo.

X-ray epilation has become obsolete but may be required again if griseofulvin-resistant fungi appear. It must be carried out by an experienced person and with reliable well-calibrated apparatus. It is usually advisable to epilate the whole scalp; epilation of a single area may succeed if the infection is circumscribed and has ceased to extend. If there are no good facilities for X-ray epilation, and griseofulvin is not available or has failed, local applications must be employed, combined with manual epilation of infected hairs. The hair over the entire scalp should be clipped short or shaved, the application selected thoroughly rubbed into the affected areas, or vigorously applied with a toothbrush and the scalp washed daily. Infected hairs should be carefully pulled out with forceps of Whitfield's pattern, a procedure greatly facilitated in microsporon infections by the use of Wood's light. Treatment must be continued until three weekly examinations reveal no further infected hairs, and microscopical examination of suspected hairs has given negative results. No local application is entirely satisfactory; Whitfield's ointment, ammoniated mercury ointment (5 per cent.), salicylanilide and various proprietary preparations containing undecenoic, propionic or other fatty acids have their advocates.

(ii.) Most infections of *animal origin* produce inflammatory changes which enhance the prospect of an early cure. X-ray epilation is not required. Griseofulvin is administered as described above. With mild inflammatory changes such as are common in *M. canis* infections, the hair immediately around the patches should be clipped, infected hairs epilated manually 2 or 3 times weekly and a non-irritating fungicide of the fatty acid type applied. The severe inflammatory infection with kerion formation may require compresses of potassium permanganate (1 in 5,000) or of mercury perchloride (1 in 2,000). Manual epilation accelerates cure. Powerful fungicides are not indicated.

PREVENTIVE MEASURES.—Accurate identification of the species of fungus is essential. With *M. audouini* and with other species of *human* origin the school authorities should be notified. *M. audouini* infections in close contacts from school and home will be recognised by inspection under Wood's light. Infected children should wear cotton or linen caps, which can be washed daily, and must be excluded from school until cured. A large outbreak may necessitate inspection of all pre-pubertal children in the school and the adoption of special measures to reduce spread of infection in barber's shops, children's cinema performances, etc. Infection with fungi of *animal* origin present a different problem. Many authorities allow the child to attend school provided he is under treatment and is wearing a linen cap. The animal source of infection should be looked for and treated.

§ **780. VI. Congenital Abnormalities.**—Congenital alopecia is mentioned in § 775 IV. A *localised* congenital defect may result in a single atrophic patch in an otherwise normal scalp. There are many hereditary abnormalities of the hair, most of them uncommon and some very rare. The most distinctive are:—*Monilethrix*, in which the hair shafts are beaded and break off when they have attained a length of only a few millimetres. The whole scalp or only the occipital region may be affected. Horny papules at the follicular orifices give the scalp the feel of a nutmeg grater. The condition persists throughout life, and is seldom influenced by treatment. *Pili torti*, in which the hairs are twisted repeatedly on their own axis through an angle of 180°. The occipital region is most commonly involved, the affected hairs breaking readily and showing a distinctive sheen in reflected light. *Pili annulati:* in which the hairs show alternate dark and light bands.

§ **781. VII. Conditions due to Hair Dyes and Waving.**—*Vegetable dyes,* including henna and camomile, are safe, but are relatively seldom used as their action is uncertain; *metallic dyes* are no longer popular as the shades they produce often appear unnatural. *Hydrogen peroxide* is extensively used for bleaching: short applications probably do little harm, but repeated or prolonged applications make the hair brittle. *Paraphenylenediamine,* sold under many trade names, is widely used as it can produce a variety of shades and when skilfully applied is difficult to detect. Unfortunately it can cause a severe dermatitis in women who have become sensitised by previous contact with it or with chemically related compounds. Irritation of the scalp develops within a few hours and eczematous plaques rapidly appear, sometimes associated with marked œdema and exudation, which may involve forehead and eyelids. The reaction can be distressingly severe. As soon as possible the hair should be rinsed with 15 per cent. saline solution to which hydrogen peroxide is added at the moment of application.

The conventional methods of *waving* the hair involve the use of heat and various alkaline solutions and very rarely harm the scalp or hair unless the latter has been damaged by other chemicals or the operator is very unskilled. In recent years a process of " cold-waving " has become popular. A keratolytic agent, a salt of thioglycollic acid in alkaline solution, renders the hair plastic. A " neutraliser," often a bromate, or other weak oxidising agent is applied when the waving is completed. Although adverse effects on the hair and scalp have been reported such cases are rare. Cold-waving is generally safe provided the scalp is healthy and the manufacturer's directions are carefully followed. However, dermatitis is occasionally produced and each case requires careful investigation including patch tests with solutions of the brand actually employed, on account of potential medicolegal implications. Dermatitis of the hands of the hairdresser is less uncommon as contact may be very frequently repeated, but careful investigation is equally necessary in these cases as hairdressers employ many other possible causes of dermatitis. Strong thioglycollate solutions may act either as primary irritants or as sensitisers.

§ **782. VIII. Hypertrichosis,** or excessive growth of hair, occurs in certain rare congenital syndromes. Excessive hair in women in the normal male distribution (hirsuties) is a feature of Cushing's syndrome, of suprarenal virilism and of certain virilising tumours. Such causes must always be looked for. The vast majority of cases are not associated with any gross disturbance of endocrine function and the hirsuties is largely determined by racial and familial factors. Coarse hairs may add further disfigurement to a pigmented nævus and a purely hairy nævus is occasionally seen over the lower sacrum. *Treatment* is often requested on cosmetic grounds. Coarse hairs on the chin or neck can be removed by electrolysis or with the diathermy. With the common profuse growth of fine hairs on the upper lip these procedures produce small follicular scars which may be more disfiguring than the hair. Bleaching solutions and, if necessary, an electric shaver may be recommended as it is a fallacy that shaving stimulates coarser hair growth. X-ray therapy to produce permanent epilation is dangerous and is never justifiable.

GROUP XII. DISEASES OF THE NAILS

§ **783.** Minor disorders of the nails are common but very few are pathognomonic. The nail plate may appear abnormal as the result of (i.) a congenital defect, (ii.) disease of the skin with involvement of the nail bed, (iii.) systemic disease, (iv.) reduction in blood supply, (v.) local trauma, physical or chemical, (vi.) tumours or nævi of the nail fold or nail bed, (vii.) infection of the nail fold, (viii.) infection of the nail plate. In a great many cases no cause can be discovered. Nail changes must not be falsely attributed to coincidental systemic disease without convincing supporting evidence. The diseased conditions which may be met are:—

I. THE NAIL IS DISCOLOURED.

Leuconychia occurs in 60 per cent. of normal persons. White spots or lines appear on one or more nails and grow out spontaneously. Minor trauma may be a factor. There is no evidence incriminating nutritional deficiencies, endocrine disorders or systemic disease.

The nails may be stained by many chemicals including potassium permanganate (brown), chrysarobin (yellow-brown). Black or slate pigmentation may be produced by the heavy metals given therapeutically and mepacrine may produce a bluish-violet discoloration. Subungual hæmorrhage from trauma gives rise to reddish-brown discoloration beneath the nail and splinter hæmorrhages are seen in subacute bacterial endocarditis and in trichiniasis. The appearance of unsightly discoloured patches in the nail is a frequent sign of ringworm infection.

Onychomycosis may first become clinically evident as yellow or yellow-brown patches near the lateral border of the nail. Beneath the nail masses of soft horny débris accumulate and the nail plate gradually becomes thickened, broken and irregularly distorted. Men are more often affected than women, and the toe-nails more than the finger-nails. One or many nails may be affected and there may be associated infection of the skin of the feet or elsewhere. Most infections are caused by *Trichophyton rubrum* or *T. interdigitale*. Other fungi may be found as contaminants, particularly in nails already diseased.

Diagnosis.—Psoriasis and the nail changes secondary to pompholyx most commonly cause confusion. Nail clippings and the horny material beneath the nail should be examined microscopically for fungus mycelium and cultures made.

Treatment.—Griseofulvin is the treatment of choice, but as it must be administered for from 9 to 18 months may be financially impracticable. For dosage see § 779.

As much as possible of the damaged nail should be regularly filed away and Whitfield's ointment applied. Most finger-nail infections will respond, but many toe-nails may remain infected after treatment for a year. Surgical avulsion of infected toe-nails is therefore advisable, griseofulvin being administered during regrowth. Other treatments rarely succeed and apparent successes are probably the result of spontaneous cures. If griseofulvin is not available toe-nail infections are best left untreated. An attempt may be made to treat finger-nails with topical fungicides as described in § 779.

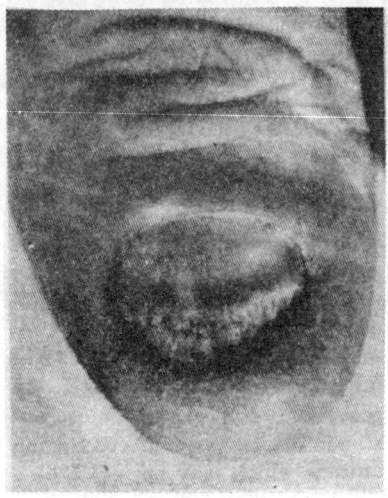

FIG. 207.—RINGWORM OF THE NAIL.

II. THE NAIL IS ABSENT OR RUDIMENTARY.

Anonychia or absence of the nails occurs as an isolated congenital defect or as part of ectodermal dystrophic syndromes such as epidermolysis bullosa. The nails may be completely lacking or may be reduced to small horny plugs. Local injury to the nail bed, excessive exposure to X-rays or radium, and reduction of the blood supply as in acrosclerosis and Raynaud's disease may also result in small deformed nails. *Onychomadesis* or shedding of the nails may occur in scarlet fever, exfoliative dermatitis and occasionally in alopecia areata. A single nail may be shed after local trauma. Recurrent shedding of one or more toe-nails is sometimes seen in adolescents and young adults, without discoverable cause.

III. THE NAIL IS THICKENED (Onychauxis) as a congenital abnormality (pachyonychia) alone or in combination with other ectodermal abnormalities, and in particular with tylosis (§ 747). The nails may be thickened as a result of repeated trauma from tight shoes or occupational injuries, in trophic disorders, in chronic eczema, psoriasis, exfoliative dermatitis, pityriasis rubra pilaris and in onychomycosis.

IV. THE NAIL IS TRANSVERSELY RIDGED.

Beau's lines—transverse ridges at the base of the nail which move distally at a rate of about 0·1 mm. daily with the growth of the nail— may be produced by a severe systemic illness, high fever, coronary thrombosis or an emotional shock. Transverse ridging can also be the result of involvement of the nail bed in local diseases such as eczema or paronychial infection, and may occur without discoverable cause.

V. THE NAIL IS LONGITUDINALLY RIDGED.—This is common in old age. It is also seen in radiodermatitis, after chemical trauma and in trophic disorders. Splitting of the free edge may be troublesome. A localised lesion of the nail bed, a subungual exostosis, or a wart of the nail fold or trauma may produce a deep ridge or an actual fissure. In *median canaliform dystrophy* there is a longitudinal ridge or groove often without apparent cause.

VI. THE NAIL IS PITTED.—This is common. Irregular pitting, often associated with transverse ridging, may follow any inflammatory skin disease in the region of the nail bed. It may be a sequel to an attack of pompholyx which, if mild, the patient may have forgotten; and is also seen in lichen planus and alopecia areata. It is a characteristic feature of **psoriasis** of the nail. The pits are usually small, numerous and of uniform size. There may also be areas of yellow discoloration, thickening and crumbling of the nail and hyperkeratosis beneath it. Psoriasis of the skin is usually present, but the nails alone may be affected. Nail involvement is particularly common and severe in psoriatic arthritis (§ 597).

VII. The Nail is abnormally Curved or Flattened.

In **onychogryphosis** the nails of one or both great toes are grossly thickened and are curved downwards and backwards to resemble an animal's claw. It is seen most often in the elderly and results from a combination of trophic changes and neglect.

Clubbing of the fingers, with thickening and increased curvature of the nails (*Hippocratic nails*) and *Koilonychia,* with flattened, thin spoon-shaped nails, are described in § 578*a.*

VIII. The Nail is Soft and Brittle.

This is common in women. The free edge of the nail may readily develop longitudinal splits or may occasionally separate in horizontal lamellæ. More rarely the nails are soft and thin. In some excessive use of nail cosmetics and of solvents and in others a recent eczema of the fingers may appear to be responsible. In most cases no cause is discoverable. Such nail changes are not a manifestation of deficiency of calcium or any other nutritional factor. *Treatment* consists in avoiding exposure to potentially injurious substances.

IX. The Nail is Separated from the Nail Bed.

Many lesions beneath the nail plate cause this. In **onycholysis,** however, the nail is separated from its bed in its distal third in the absence of any evident local abnormality. It may be produced by occupational trauma, *e.g.,* removing labels from bottles or peeling oranges, or by excessive zeal in manicuring; more often it is the result of a nervous tic in which the nails are picked. Frequently no cause is found. When the affected fingers are protected from trauma many cases recover spontaneously.

X. Diseases of the Nail Fold.

Paronychia or inflammation of the nail fold is common. In the *acute* form a painful tender swelling of part of the nail fold soon results in pus formation and is essentially a surgical problem. The *chronic* form, increasingly common in women, is characterised by indolent bolster-like swelling of one or more nail folds. The swelling is tender and periodically discharges pus. There is some secondary deformity of the nail plate. Occupational trauma, chemical or physical, or wet work of any kind may be a predisposing factor. A poor peripheral circulation is a common finding and recurrences in the colder weather are frequent. Staphylococci or monilia are the usual infecting organisms. The form occasionally seen

C.M.—L L*

in infants is usually of monilial origin. *Treatment.*—The hands should be kept as dry and warm as possible. If the peripheral circulation is poor give nicotinic acid 50 mg. t.i.d. Rest and sedation are of even greater value in the tired housewife. Surgery is neither necessary nor desirable; but apply a paint such as pigmentum resorcin—resorcin 1·5, acetone 1·0, boric acid, 1·0, water to 60 to the nail fold with a brush nightly.

Many conditions may involve the nail folds. Warts (§ 741), pyogenic

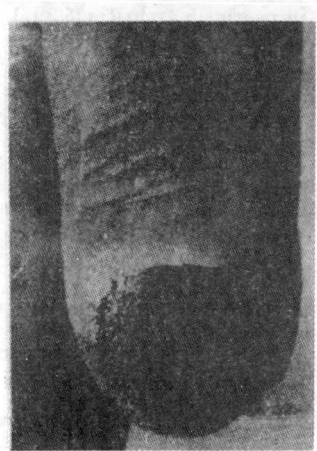

granuloma (§ 733), commonly do so. The syphilitic chancre (§ 738) may occur in this site. Telangiectasia and atrophy of the nail fold are a characteristic lesion of lupus erythematosus (§ 631). Smooth wart-like periungual fibromata are a manifestation of epiloia (§ 649). Osler's nodes in bacterial endocarditis may involve the nail folds together with the tips and side of the fingers (§ 50a).

XI. TUMOURS UNDER THE NAIL.

Subungual exostosis appears as a fibrous nodule the size of a pea beneath the inner margin of either great toe-nail. The usual age of onset is between 12 and 30, in women more often than men. *Treatment* is surgical.

FIG. 208.—CHRONIC PARONYCHIA with secondary nail changes.

Melanoma under or around the nail is rare but of great importance. It may simulate a pyogenic granuloma. Pigmentation may not be conspicuous. Early amputation is essential.

Glomus tumours may develop under the nail. The small red nodule is very painful with paroxysms after minor trauma. Treatment is by simple excision.

The **common wart** often develops beneath the free edge of the nail.

§ 784. General Principles of Treatment.—Patients with skin disorders frequently suffer from a surfeit of local applications, many of them illogical and even potentially irritating and sensitising. The skin has remarkable powers of recovery and treatment should be planned on physiological lines, to assist the normal reparative processes; too often it merely places a further burden on an already irritated organ.

In all cases of skin disease the patient must be reassured about the infectivity of his lesions; his doubts and fears concerning their origin and prognosis must be relieved; he must be given such sedation as may be required and an hypnotic to ensure sleep. Most therapeutic failures are the result of overtreatment of the skin and undertreatment of the patient.

The treatment of many of the individual skin disorders has been summarised in earlier sections. The general principles determining the choice of a local application are reviewed here to emphasise that the vehicle or base plays a most important role and must be selected with as much thought as the active ingredients.

1. *Lotions* are either simple aqueous solutions or unstable suspensions of powder in an aqueous solution or in water. Lotions, which can be applied as wet dressings, are valuable in acute exudative and crusted conditions in which they have a cleansing action and by free evaporation of water produce cooling and consequent reduction

of exudation with relief of itching—normal saline, potassium permanganate (1 in 5,000) or Burow's solution (1 in 40), are in common use. In shake lotions, such as calamine lotion, the powder delays the evaporation of water and prolongs the cooling action. They should not be applied to oozing or crusted surfaces, as the powder forms hard lumps with the serum and the patient's discomfort is increased.

2. *Powders* can be used to absorb excess moisture and prevent maceration of the skin. Talc does not adhere well to the skin, and has to be combined with zinc oxide which, used alone, is too heavy to spread evenly. It is better to avoid powder containing starch, which ferments, for prolonged application to intertriginous areas.

3. *Liniments* are unstable emulsions of oil and water with or without incorporated powders. Lotio calaminæ oleosa (B.P.C.) is useful, alternating with wet dressings, in acute inflammatory conditions or alone in subacute states.

4. *Hydrocarbon ointment bases*, such as soft paraffin, are stable and chemically inert but greasy and unpleasant to use. They form an occlusive layer on the skin impermeable to sweat and to exudates; they should never be prescribed in acute inflammatory disorders. However, in psoriasis and certain other chronic scaly dermatoses the macerating effect of an impermeable film is an advantage and dithranol ointment (B.P.C.) and tar, salicylic acid and ammoniated mercury ointments (B.P.C.) are in soft paraffin bases.

5. *Creams* are emulsions of oil and water. Medicaments incorporated in emulsion bases come into closer contact with the epidermis than in other vehicles. There are two types of emulsion base, oil-in-water, and water-in-oil; in an oil-in-water emulsion droplets of the oil are dispersed in water which form the continuous or external phase: in a water-in-oil emulsion the oil forms the external phase. Maximum penetration of added medicaments is obtained when they are soluble in the external phase. Both types of emulsion are cosmetically pleasant and evaporation of the aqueous phase produces cooling, and both readily wash off the skin. Water-in-oil creams are useful in subacute inflammatory conditions: examples are zinc cream (B.P.) and lanoline, but this latter is sticky and malodorous. Unguentum alcohol lanæ (B.P.) contains wool alcohols with soft and liquid paraffin and is a valuable base: its paraffin content causes it to leave a thin greasy film on the skin which prevents drying. Unguentum aquosum (B.P.) contains additional water. Emulsifying ointment (B.P.) is an oil-in-water emulsion and is a useful base for scalp preparations, as it is readily washed out. It is a " vanishing cream " and has a drying effect on the skin, which is helpful in seborrhœic conditions. Many proprietary creams contain polyethylene glycols (carbowax) which also form oil-in-water emulsions.

6. *Pastes* contain a large proportion of solid matter in the form of powder. Lassar's paste contains 50 per cent. of powder, but many pastes are softer with a powder content of 20–30 per cent. Pastes are not as occlusive as ointments and can absorb sweat and secretions. They exert a protective and " splinting " action which is particularly helpful in conditions such as nummular eczema.

§ **785. Antibiotics and Steroids.**—The topical application of antibiotics is valuable in many superficial infections, but their prolonged use involves the risk of sensitising the patient and of increasing the percentage of strains of the organism in question resistant to an antibiotic. Penicillin and chloramphenicol readily sensitise the skin and are seldom recommended for topical use. The tetracyclines very rarely sensitise and neomycin does so infrequently: they have a wide antibacterial range and are usually the first choice. It is seldom necessary to apply them for more than a week.

In many chronic infections Vioform, Quinolor, sulphur, the aniline dyes and mercurial preparations are of value and are often to be preferred to antibiotics.

The Steroids.—Systemic treatment with ACTH, cortisone, prednisone or prednisolone may be life-saving in pemphigus, pemphigoid and systemic lupus erythematosus. It is of doubtful and inconsistent value in dermatomyositis, scleroderma and polyarteritis. In exfoliative dermatitis it controls the symptoms, but a maintenance dose may be required for a long period. Small doses of prednisone shorten the course of drug reactions and of acute contact dermatitis and if, after careful examination of the patient, no contra-indications are established, may be given in severe cases. Very acute lichen planus may be treated with cortisone, prednisone or triamcinolone. The steroids should not be given in most cases of chronic eczema or in psoriasis.

Topical hydrocortisone is sometimes grossly over-prescribed. It is a most valuable preparation in the treatment of infantile eczema, other forms of eczema of the face and anogenital region, lichen simplex, anogenital pruritus and otitis externa. When infection is present it may be combined with neomycin or chlortetracycline. It is ineffective or no better than conventional applications in eczema in other parts of the body or in most other conditions. If a concentration of 1 per cent. proves effective, it is usually possible to continue treatment with 0·5 per cent.

Triamcinolone 0·01 per cent. is the most economical application for routine use in chronic eczema. Fluocinolone (Synalar) ointment 0·025 per cent. is effective in chronic lupus erythematosus and psoriasis because it is absorbed well, but for this reason should not be prescribed for widespread conditions, especially in infants. The efficacy of topical triamcinolone or fluocinolone is greatly enhanced by application under occlusive dressings of polythene sheeting, indicated in psoriasis and chronic eczema.

Intralesional injection of hydrocortisone or triamcinolone suspension is the treatment of choice in lichen simplex, verrucous lichen planus and very chronic circumscribed psoriasis. It is of some value in granuloma annulare, necrobiosis lipoidica, discoid lupus erythematosus and some other conditions.

§ 786. *Treatment of pruritus.*—The empirical relief of this symptom should where possible be combined with logical treatment of its cause. Local antipruritic applications include coal tar, phenol (to be avoided in infants) and menthol. Local anæsthetics of the procaine series are effective, but are potent sensitisers and should not be employed for more than a few days; antihistamine creams are of questionable value and may also cause dermatitis. Hydrocortisone (0·5–1 per cent.) as a lotion or ointment is valuable in relieving pruritus in inflammatory conditions, especially on the face and in the anogenital region. Antihistamine drugs by mouth may relieve the irritation of urticaria, but are not otherwise strikingly effective. Aspirin alone, or in combination with bromides or a barbiturate, is usually preferable.

TABLE XLIX.—THE COMMON DERMATOPHYTES. LESIONS IN MAN

Genus	Species	Natural Host or Source	T. capitis	T. barbæ	T. corporis	T. cruris	T. pedis	T. unguium	Comments
Microsporon	audouini	Man	+++		+				Infected hairs give green fluorescence under Wood's light.
,,	canis	cat, dog	+++		+				
,,	gypseum	soil	+		+				
Trichophyton	rubrum	Man	+	+	++	++	++	+++	Very chronic infections. Resistant to treatment.
,,	mentagrophytes	animals rodents	+	++	+				Acutely inflammatory lesion — lesion of beard or scalp.
,,	interdigitale	Man	+		+	++	+++	+	The commonest cause of T. pedis.
,,	verrucosum	cattle	+	+++	++				Acutely inflammatory "cattle ringworm," in man. Kerions in hairy regions.
,,	violaceum	Man	+		+			+	"Black dot" ringworm of scalp.
,,	sulphureum	Man	++		+++	++	+		
,,	schœnleini	Man							Favus.
Epidermophyton	floccosum	Man			+	++		++	

CHAPTER XIX

THE NERVOUS SYSTEM

THE student will find the arrangement of this chapter conforming to the method pursued throughout the book. An account of the applied anatomy and physiology of the nervous system is followed by:

At the outset certain principles applied to disease processes in the nervous system may be stated:

(1) The nervous system may be visualised as consisting of a number of physiological levels, the functions of the lowest or spinal level (most automatic) being comparatively well organised at birth, the highest or cortical (most voluntary) continually organising throughout life. The higher levels inhibit or control the lower levels. For example, a destructive lesion of the pyramidal tract will cause loss or impairment of voluntary movements below the level of the lesion—the *negative* symptom. We also observe new phenomena not present before the onset, viz.—muscular hypertonus and an extensor type of plantar response. These are *positive* symptoms due to release of intact extra-pyramidal mechanisms which have escaped from pyramidal inhibition.

(2) In disease the functions first acquired in development are the last to be destroyed. Thus when speech function is destroyed by a cortical lesion, the ability to gesture, which is acquired chronologically before speech, invariably remains. In acquired dementia the memory for recent events has gone, while the patient may still remember events of earlier life.

(3) The more rapid the destruction the greater the dissolution. *Acute* lesions (*e.g.*, a blow on the head) produce at first widespread loss of function, complete loss of consciousness, flaccid paralysis and incontinence. These " shock phenomena " are usually transient.

(4) *Chronic* lesions of the nervous system at first irritate and later paralyse function. Thus a slowly growing meningeal tumour compressing the motor cortex usually at first causes a focal (Jacksonian) convulsion (irritative sign), later a monoplegia (paralytic sign).

(5) Nerve-cells once destroyed do not regenerate. Their function however may be carried on or taken over by residual undamaged nerve-cells. This *compensation* is particularly observed in man after destruction of parts of the cerebral cortex or of the cerebellum where compensation for destruction may take place to a remarkable extent.

APPLIED PHYSIOLOGICAL ANATOMY OF THE NERVOUS SYSTEM

The central nervous system consists of vast numbers of *Neurones*, both *Afferent* and *Efferent*. A neurone is a nerve-cell with its dendrites and axon. The *nerve-cells* are found in the grey matter of the cortex, basal ganglia and nuclei, the central grey matter of the spinal cord and in posterior root ganglia. The *axons* are collected into bundles or tracts and run mostly in the white matter and peripheral nerves. The *nervous impulse* travels at different rates in different nerves. A *synapse* or junction between two neurones will allow an impulse to pass in one direction only. At the synapse a chemical change occurs. Acetyl-choline may be released in central synapses by the passage of the impulse and is split by an enzyme, cholinesterase. This effect is also observed at the end-organs of many peripheral neurones: *e.g.*, the neuro-muscular junction. Not all central synapses however are cholinergic: the mediator in non-cholinergic synapses is not known.

The brain is provided with a number of *enzymes* which serve its metabolism. Some of these regulate the supply of glucose to brain cells by oxidising carbohydrate. Carbohydrate is broken down to pyruvic acid, before being oxidised to carbon dioxide and water. By a second path pyruvic acid is not an intermediary product of carbohydrate breakdown. An absence of aneurine (which acts as a catalyst) from the diet will lead to accumulation of pyruvates in the blood and cerebro-spinal fluid. In brain-cell metabolism protein and amino-acids seem to be of less importance, although recent work suggests that glutamic acid (an amino-acid) plays an important role. Concerning the metabolism of lipoids and myelin we know very little.

Neurones are extremely sensitive to oxygen-want (anoxia) and alterations in the blood supply produce many disturbances of function in neurones. Cerebral and spinal tumours produce signs not so much by distortion or disruption of nerve-tracts as by causing *local anoxia*. Again, certain inorganic poisons or organic toxins are *selective* in action and exert their effects by picking out particular groups of neurones or muscles, *e.g.*, lead commonly affects the neurones proceeding from the seventh cervical segment, producing wrist-drop, whilst the toxin of diphtheria picks out the ciliary and the bulbar muscles. This selective action is also observed in infection with viruses, the virus of acute poliomyelitis affecting the anterior horn cells or their bulbar homologues, and that of herpes zoster the cells in the posterior root ganglia. An acute toxic lesion (*e.g.*, polyneuritis) may produce widespread recoverable paralysis without demonstrable structural changes in the neurones.

The activity of the cortical nerve-cells can be studied with the Electro-encephalograph; with this, cortical action currents are led off by electrodes placed on the intact scalp, amplified by wireless valves and recorded by a cathode-ray oscillograph (§847).

§ 790. The Cerebral Cortex.—The laminated human cortex is much more highly developed than in anthropoid apes. Its area is much increased by convolutional infoldings.

Considerable areas of the human cortex are excitable, *e.g.*, the pre- and post-central gyri and the calcarine cortex. Stimulation of these areas causes positive symptoms, *e.g.* discrete movements of parts of the body or limbs, paræsthesiæ, or crude visual auræ. In the pre-central cortex there exists one of several " suppressor bands " stimulation of which causes diminution of muscular tone and cessation of movements on the opposite side of the body. Large areas of the cortex called " association areas " are irresponsive to stimulation. Study of epilepsy and focal cortical lesions indicate their possible function in integration. During development and the acquisition of learning, cortical areas for speech, hand-skills and the recognition and discrimination of sensory impulses are established, but these are less clearly defined than the motor, sensory and visual areas.

Dominance.—"Handedness" is probably genetically determined. In right-handed individuals the speech centres are formed in the left or " dominant " hemisphere. The contra-lateral hemisphere is termed " minor." This tendency for certain functions to be concentrated in the left cerebral hemisphere is one conspicuous phenomenon distinguishing the brain of man from that of lower animals.

Cortical areas receive afferent impulses and project efferent impulses. Certain areas can be limited and defined as subserving specific functions. (1) Post- and precentral somatic sensory areas. (2) Calcarine visual areas. (3) Superior temporal auditory areas. (4) Uncinate (and anterior to this) olfactory areas. (5) The Motor areas, too, can be mapped with precision.

THE MOTOR AREAS (Fig. 209) lie in the pre-central gyrus and the posterior part of the frontal convolutions immediately in front of this (" area 6 "). *Here are represented not muscles but movements.* Topographically, the movements of the foot are

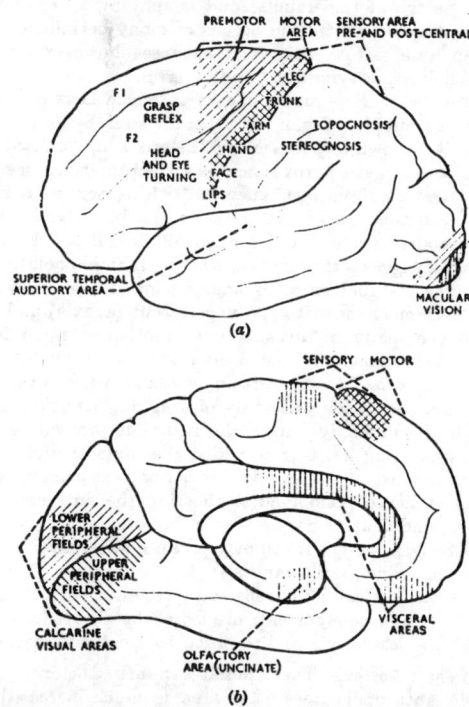

FIG. 209.—CORTICAL LOCALISATION OF FUNCTION. (*a*) Lateral and (*b*) Medial aspect of the left hemisphere. The sensory cortex spreads into the pre-central gyrus. On the medial aspect of the hemisphere the sensory and motor areas for toes and foot are hatched. The SPEECH AREAS are shown in Fig. 239.

represented at the upper end of the motor cortex; those of the leg, trunk, arm, hand, neck, face, lips and tongue, in that order from above downwards. It will be noticed that the complicated movements of the face and hand have a relatively large cortical representation, a good example of adaptation of structure to function. Irritative lesions of these areas cause focal *Jacksonian fits.* Jacksonian fits commonly commence in one of three foci—(*a*) the thumb and index finger, (*b*) the angle of the mouth, or (*c*) the big toe, and are followed by the " paralytic sign," a transient monoplegia. Such a fit begins with clonic convulsions of one of these parts and (*a*) may remain local, or, (*b*) more commonly, spreads in an orderly march in accordance with the cortical representation of the parts affected, so that face, arm and leg on one side of the body are involved and eventually all the muscles of the body. So long as the convulsion is localised consciousness may be preserved, but when it is generalised consciousness is lost. It is possible to distinguish between (a) the motor area and (b) the premotor area, on the basis of stimulation experiments. Local slight stimuli to the motor area evoke discrete movements. Much stronger stimuli are required for activating the premotor area and the movements evoked are more generalised. Destruction of the premotor cortex causes a spasticity which is more marked and permanent than that produced by destruction of the motor area. At the posterior end of the second frontal gyrus is an area for the *conjugate movement of the head and eyes* to the contra-lateral side (oculogyric area). An area at the posterior end of the first and second frontal gyri is connected with the *grasp reflex, i.e.,* stroking the palm of the contra-lateral hand or stretching the flexors of the fingers produces a tonic closure of the fist. Lesions extending deeply into the substance of the motor areas produce a *monoplegia* or *hemiplegia*.

The SENSORY AREAS (Fig. 209) occupy the post-central gyrus and the parietal cortex, extending forwards to overlap the motor areas in the precentral gyrus. The parietal cortex receives afferent fibres from the lateral nucleus of the thalamus. It is believed that the pattern of pyramidal activity is continuously moulded by auxiliary afferents, sensory (thalamo-cortical) and non-sensory (cerebello-frontal), as well as by visual afferents in the performance of learned movements of skill and precision. Sensory areas for the contra-lateral foot, toes and perineum are represented on the medial aspect of the hemisphere in the paracentral lobule (Fig. 209b). Sensory areas for the contra-lateral leg, trunk, arm, hand, neck, face, lips, tongue are represented in that order from above downwards on the lateral aspect of the hemisphere in the post-central gyrus. Sensory impulses from the lips and tongue are believed to have a bilateral cortical representation. *Irritative lesions* of the post-central gyrus cause sensory Jacksonian fits, a numbness or tingling which spreads rapidly from the thumb or angle of the mouth in an orderly march (according to the arrangement of cortical areas) to the shoulder, trunk and leg. *Destructive lesions* of the posterior parietal cortex destroy the discriminative aspects of sensation; thus the patient fails to recognise or localise certain forms of sensation (especially sense of position) in the contra-lateral limbs. These cortical sensory anomalies may be discrete and confined to part of a limb if the lesion is discrete. The parietal cortex is not only concerned with awareness of the body surface and its parts, but also with the relationship of the body to its environmental surroundings. There may be (1) Loss of ability to estimate the size, shape and consistency of objects held in the opposite hand (Astereognosis), and (2) Impaired ability to localise tactile stimuli (Atopognosis) and to discriminate two simultaneous touches with compass points. Defective sense of position and sense of spatial recognition leads to inco-ordination of the affected contra-lateral limbs (sensory ataxia). Sensations of pain and temperature are often intact, but there is difficulty in appreciating the intensity of stimuli. (3) In destructive posterior parietal cortical lesions, in the dominant hemisphere moreover, we encounter inability to recognise visual symbols (letters, words, digits, printed music and other symbols), disturbances of the body image (inability to name the fingers correctly, and to identify right and left) and a tendency to ignore the contra-lateral side of the body and any stimuli arising there.

In lesions of the supramarginal gyrus there may be defective comprehension of words and phrases causing a state of considerable mental confusion.

Further back is the VISUAL AREA (Fig. 209b) represented in the upper and lower lips of the calcarine fissure on the medial aspect of the occipital lobe, and extending on the lateral aspect of the occipital lobe as far as the lunate sulcus. The corresponding halves of the visual fields are represented in the contra-lateral occipital cortex. The upper quadrants of the fields are represented on the lower lips of the calcarine fissure and the lower quadrants of the fields on the upper lips of the fissure. Macular (central) vision is represented at the tip of the occipital pole and peripheral vision more anteriorly along the calcarine fissure (Fig. 219). *Irritative lesions* of the visual cortex cause visual Jacksonian attacks in the form of visual hallucinations of hemianopic distribution. In lesions far back in the occipital cortex these hallucinations take the form of moving lights, " sheets of flame." With lesions involving the occipital and temporal cortex the visions may be more complex, taking the form of scenes, " play acting." *Paralytic lesions* of the visual cortex cause a homonymous hemianopia of the contra-lateral visual fields (" a hemiplegia of the visual fields "). Lesions of the upper lip of the calcarine fissure will produce homonymous lower quadrantic defects. Lesions of the angular gyrus (visual association area) cause loss of stereoscopic vision and failure to recognise objects seen (visual agnosia).

AUDITORY AREAS (Fig. 209a) exist in the superior temporal cortex in both hemi-spheres. Cortical deafness is excessively rare; irritative lesions of these areas may cause tinnitus or auditory hallucinations.

OLFACTORY AREAS (Fig. 209b) are situated in the uncinate cortex and the grey matter anterior to this. *Irritative lesions* cause " uncinate fits " characterised by spitting and champing movements of the jaws, gustatory hallucinations and a transient disturbance of consciousness called a " dreamy state."

SPEECH AREAS (Fig. 239) are located in the dominant hemisphere in the posterior parts of the second and third frontal (verbal speech and writing), the superior temporal (auditory) and angular gyri (visual). Lesions of these cause various types of *aphasia.*

BILATERAL CORTICAL LESIONS are more likely to be accompanied by personality changes, intellectual impairment, apraxia and agnosia. This is seen in cortical atrophy due to organic dementia, arteriosclerosis, or atrophy consequent on severe brain trauma.

VISCERAL AREAS (Fig. 209b). Autonomic afferents and efferents proceed from the hypothalamic nuclei to the orbito-frontal and cingulate gyri. In some cases the cortical representation of visceral function overlaps the motor. Thus salivation is observed when the area for the lips and tongue is excited.

§ 791. The Pathway for Voluntary Movements.—All impulses for voluntary move-ment are transmitted by the Pyramidal Tracts or Upper Motor Neurones. Damage to the pyramidal tract produces (1) *Impairment or loss of voluntary movement* from interruption of the conduction of motor impulses. The resulting paralysis is termed a Monoplegia (paralysis of one limb), Hemiplegia (paralysis of face, arm and leg on one side of the body), Paraplegia (paralysis of both lower limbs), or Diplegia (paralysis of all four limbs). (2) *Release of extra-pyramidal motor phenomena,* viz., increase of tone and exaggeration of the tendon reflexes, with the appearance of the extensor type of plantar response.

The Pyramidal Tract or Upper Motor Neurone (Fig. 210) extends from pyramidal cells of the motor and premotor cortex to the contra-lateral anterior horn cells of the spinal cord. The cells of origin are motor cells in the fifth layer of grey matter of the ascending frontal convolutions and part of the cortex (area 6 of Brodmann) anterior to this. From the cortical cells the fibres converge through a fan-shaped radiation, the corona radiata, to the internal capsule, which lies between the lentiform nucleus externally and the caudate nucleus and thalamus internally. The motor fibres occupy the genu and portion just anterior to this, and the anterior two-thirds of the posterior limb of the internal capsule. Here the fibres have undergone some rearrange-ment since leaving the cortex, for the order from before backwards is now face, shoulder, elbow, fingers, trunk, hip, knee and toes. Behind the motor fibres in the posterior limb of the internal capsule are the sensory and auditory fibres, and behind these the visual fibres of the optic radiations (Fig. 211).

From the internal capsule, the pyramidal tract descends through the ventral part of the crus cerebri (near the oculomotor nerve), spreading out a little in the ventrally situated nuclear masses of the pons (the motor nucleus of the trigeminal is in the middle of the pons, and the abducent and facial nuclei in the lower part of the pons). On reaching the upper part of the medulla, the pyramidal tracts converge as the two ventrally and medially placed pyramids. Below this, nearly all the cortico-spinal fibres decussate to form the Crossed pyramidal tract which descends in the opposite lateral column of the cord. Some pyramidal fibres end directly in the cells of the anterior horn, others terminate in the region of the posterior horn, whence short intermediary neurones connect to the anterior horn cells.   A small proportion of pyramidal fibres

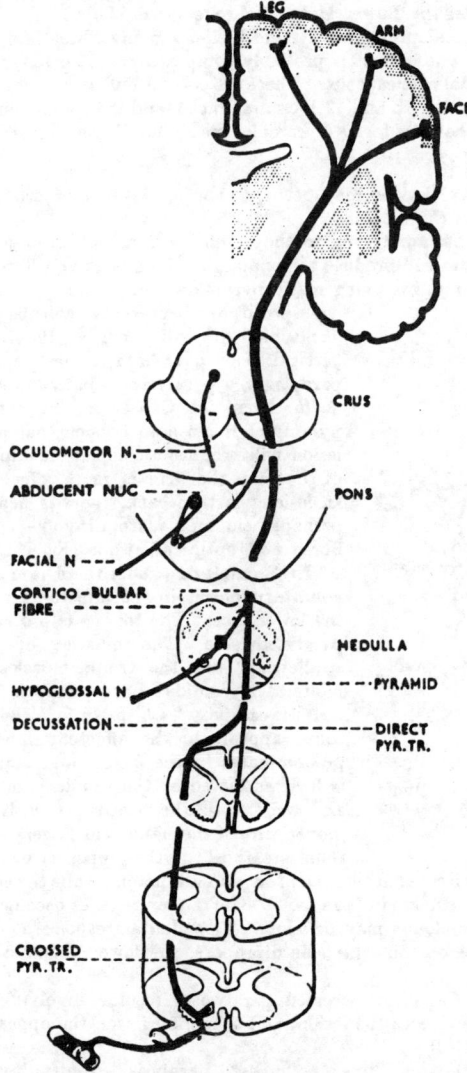

Fig. 210.—Diagram of the Right Pyramidad Tract showing its course through the brain, brain-stem and spinal cord.

are continued down the ipsilateral side of the cord as far as the mid-thoracic region lying near the anterior median fissure (the Direct pyramidal tract), but these fibres too eventually decussate to the opposite anterior horn cells.

All the motor nuclei of the cranial nerves receive fibres bilaterally from both pyramidal tracts, except the hypoglossal and that part of the facial nucleus connected with movements of the lower face. These receive fibres from the pyramidal tract of the contra-lateral side only. From the cells of the anterior horns and the cranial nerve motor nuclei the Lower Motor Neurones arise (Fig. 210).

The cortico-spinal projection system includes many fibres beside those just described. The pyramidal tract is probably complex, including fibres other than those arising in pyramidal cortical cells. There are cortico-bulbar bundles with " aberrant " fibres which reach the 7th and 12th cranial nuclei, and the spinal neurones. It is only for convenience that the terms Pyramidal tract and Upper Motor Neurone are used synonymously.

§ 792. Pyramidal lesions may occur at various levels and produce the following clinical symptoms (Fig. 210):

(a) CORTICAL LEVEL: Owing to the extensive distribution of motor cells on the cortex a focal lesion will produce a monoplegia which is at first flaccid. If the lesion extends more deeply, involving many pyramidal fibres, the symptoms will be more widespread and spasticity will be present. Motor Jacksonian fits will occur as the irritative sign. A vertical lesion over both cortical leg areas will cause paraplegia, a paralysis of both lower limbs.

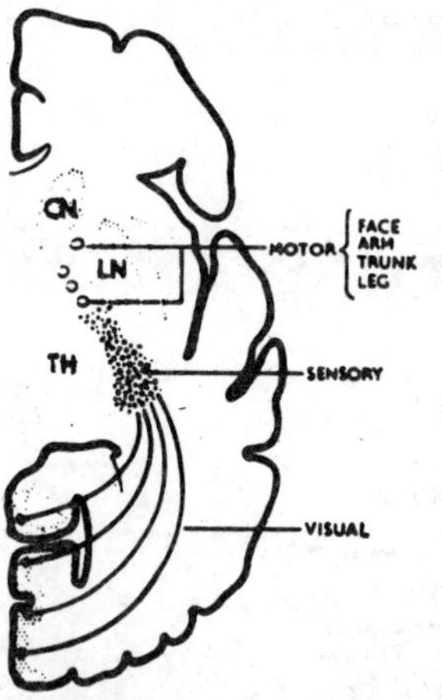

(b) INTERNAL CAPSULE: The convergence of the pyramidal fibres here is such that a relatively small lesion will produce a complete hemiplegia. In lesions of the genu the arm is more affected than the leg. In lesions farther back, there is hemianæsthesia and perhaps hemianopia, from involvement of the sensory fibres and optic radiations (Fig. 211).

In Hemiplegia (§ 901) there is a unilateral loss of voluntary power in the affected arm and leg and in the lower face. The tongue is protruded towards the paralysed side. The muscles of mastication and swallowing and the trunk muscles, which have a bilateral pyramidal nerve supply from the cortex usually escape. " Clasp-Knife " rigidity with hypertonus appears in the affected limbs; in the arm it predominates in the flexors and adductors so that it is held adducted at the shoulder, flexed at the elbow and wrist with the forearm slightly pronated. The movements of the hand and fingers are more affected than are those of the upper arm. In the legs the

FIG. 211.—DIAGRAM OF RIGHT INTERNAL CAPSULE showing the arrangement of the motor and sensory fibres.

hypertonus predominates in the extensors and adductors, while the chief loss of movement is that of dorsiflexion of the foot. The tendon reflexes become exaggerated and ankle and patellar clonus may develop. The plantar response is extensor and the abdominal reflexes on the same side disappear, the lower abdominal reflexes before the upper.

(c) LEVEL OF CRUS: A " crossed paralysis " results, involving the oculomotor nerve on the same side as the lesion, and a hemiplegia on the opposite side (Weber's Syndrome) (Fig. 210).

(d) LEVEL OF LOWER PONS: A "crossed paralysis " results, involving the facial and abducent nerves on the same side as the lesion, and a hemiplegia on the opposite side (Millard-Gubler Syndrome).

(e) LEVEL OF SPINAL CORD: A spastic paralysis of the leg on the same side results. Lesions above the fifth cervical segment involve the arm as well as the leg.

To summarise: upper motor neurone lesions produce, on the side affected: (1) Loss of voluntary power. (2) Spasticity of the " clasp-knife " type. (3) Increased tendon reflexes with ankle and patellar clonus. (4) Extensor plantar responses with absent abdominal reflexes.   (5) Normal electrical reactions in the affected muscles.   (6) No muscular wasting.

§ 793. **Striatal Mechanisms.**—The corpus striatum (basal ganglia) consists of the CAUDATE and LENTIFORM NUCLEI (the latter composed of the putamen and globus

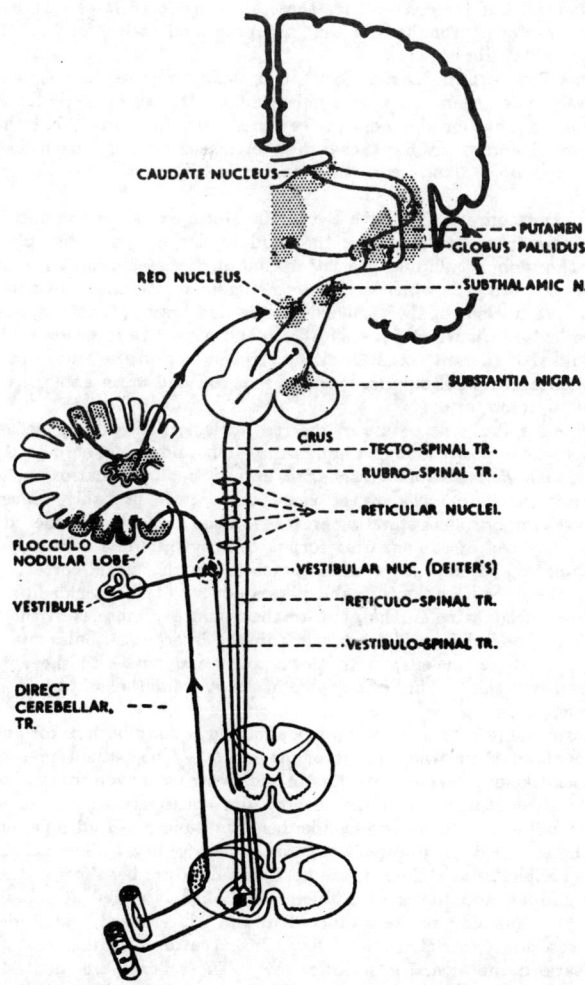

CAUDATE NUCLEUS

PUTAMEN
GLOBUS PALLIDUS

RED NUCLEUS

SUBTHALAMIC N.

SUBSTANTIA NIGRA

CRUS
TECTO-SPINAL TR.
RUBRO-SPINAL TR.
RETICULAR NUCLEI.

FLOCCULO NODULAR LOBE

VESTIBULAR NUC. (DEITER'S)

VESTIBULE

RETICULO-SPINAL TR.

VESTIBULO-SPINAL TR.

DIRECT CEREBELLAR. TR.

FIG. 212.—DIAGRAM OF THE EXTRA-PYRAMIDAL MOTOR TRACTS showing their origin in subcortical masses of grey matter and ultimate endings in the anterior horn cells.   The cerebellar afferent fibres are shown in green.

pallidus).   These important nuclei and other masses of grey matter, notably the Red Nucleus, Substantia Nigra and the Subthalamic body (Corpus Luysii) of the midbrain, and the Vestibular (Deiter's) nucleus in the pons, send efferents (Extra-pyramidal tracts) extending by one or more links to the anterior horn cells (Fig. 212).

The corpus striatum represents, in part, a motor mechanism concerned with the involuntary control of subsidiary motor centres, and through them with the striated muscles. It seems to act in conjunction with cortical and other systems in man, and clinical evidence suggests that it plays an important part in involuntary postural adjustments and fixations, and with muscular reactions to emotion.

The Cerebellum and its connections may be considered as part of the Extra-pyramidal systems, but for convenience these are considered later. It will be seen that the Lower motor neurone is thus the " final common path " for both pyramidal and extra-pyramidal fibres.

The EXTRA-PYRAMIDAL MOTOR SYSTEM probably represents a motor system phylogenetically older than the pyramidal system. It was formerly believed that the extra-pyramidal system did not receive fibres from the cortex, but the work of Dusser de Barenne and others has shown that cortico-striate fibres from the premotor and other " suppressor " bands exercise some degree of cortical control over the basal ganglia.

The internal anatomy of the Extra-Pyramidal Motor System is complex (Fig. 212). Short axons pass from the putamen, the caudate nucleus and probably from the thalamus to the globus pallidus; the latter contains large pyramidal or multipolar cells like anterior horn cells which give rise to efferent fibres (ansa lenticularis) which end in (1) the red nucleus of the same side of the mid-brain, (2) the substantia nigra and (3) the reticular formation of the mid-brain and pons. In these areas of the brain stem they link with efferent tracts from the cerebellum and the labyrinth which are particularly concerned with equilibration. From the mid-brain and pons four chief extra-pyramidal tracts arise:

(1) the *Rubro-spinal tract* arises in the red nucleus, immediately decussates and passes through the opposite side of the pons, medulla and spinal cord to the anterior horn cells. (2) The *Reticulo-spinal* tract arises in the reticular formation and terminates around the anterior horn cells of the same side. It is probably concerned with postural reflexes important in standing erect. (3) The *Tecto-spinal* tract arises in the mid-brain at the level of the superior corpus quadrigeminum where it has received impulses originating in the retinæ which reach it via the visual cortex. The tract decussates in the dorsal tegmentum and passes down to the anterior horn cells conveying impulses originating in the eyes, to the voluntary muscles of the trunk and limbs. (4) The *Vestibulo-spinal* tract arises in the lateral vestibular nucleus of the VIIIth nerve (Deiter's nucleus) in the lower pons and passes to the antero-lateral region of the same side. This is an efferent tract from the mid-brain subserving muscular tone.

In **Parkinsonism** (§ 914) there is rigidity affecting equally both flexor and extensor muscles throughout their whole range of movement. The patient presents a characteristic mask-like expression, with loss of the swinging movements of the arms on walking. On attempting to move the affected limbs passively, *e.g.*, at the wrist-joint, the examiner will encounter resistance like bending a piece of lead-pipe, or turning a cog-wheel, the so-called " lead-pipe " or " cog-wheel rigidity." The patient assumes an attitude of slight general flexion, the head and neck are bent forwards, the gait is shuffling or gliding, and the arms adducted and slightly flexed at the sides of the trunk (Fig. 5). The fingers are adducted in the " interosseal " attitude. All the movements are slow, restricted and delayed in execution. Rather coarse rhythmic tremor appears in the arm, leg or lower jaw. The reflexes are unalter. 1.

Involuntary Movements—Tremor, Chorea, Athetosis. Three main types of involuntary movements occur in voluntary musculature. They are never present when the muscles are completely paralysed, *i.e.*, there must be relative integrity of the pyramidal tracts. They are: (1) *Tremor*—Involuntary, rhythmical oscillations of one or more parts of the body, resulting from the alternate contraction of muscle groups and their antagonists. (2) *Chorea*—Irregular and spasmodic involuntary movements of groups of muscles, occurring during rest, and also super-imposed upon voluntary movements, which they render inco-ordinate. (3) *Athetosis*—Involuntary movements of a writhing, or (in the face) grimacing type, slower and more stereotyped than the movements of chorea. Between the periods of increased spasm the limbs are frequently hypotonic (§§ 913, 925).

The pathogenesis of these involuntary movements is obscure. In congenital athetosis and chorea, the lesions are found chiefly in the caudate nucleus and putamen. Acute focal lesions of the *sub-thalamic body or corpus Luysii* (Fig. 212) are known to produce hemichorea of the contra-lateral half of the body, and choreiform movements are known to follow lesions of the superior cerebellar peduncle and the thalamus. In this connection, it should be remembered that the cerebellum is part of the extra-pyramidal motor system. The consensus of opinion is that these involuntary movements are due (in part) to uncontrolled activity of lower *motor mechanisms important in postural fixation.*

§ 794. The Lower Motor Neurone consists of an anterior horn cell or its homologue in the brain stem. With its dendrites, axon and end-plate it terminates upon the group of striated muscle-fibres which it innervates. The lower motor neurone is the basic motor element of the reflex arc subserving muscular tone. It is the final common pathway for all motor impulses, pyramidal and extra-pyramidal. *Destructive lesions of the lower motor neurone.* When the motor nerve supply to a muscle is destroyed, the muscle shows (1) flaccid paralysis, and later (2) atrophy. During the stage of active destruction of the anterior horn cell small groups of muscle fibres show irregular twitchings known as (3) fasciculation. At the onset the muscle is usually tender, and the patient may complain of such sensory phenomena as subjective pain and cramp, although the lesion is purely motor and there is no sensory loss. (4) The tendon reflex of the affected muscle diminishes and finally disappears. In the last stages the atrophic muscle shortens and is said to undergo (5) contracture. (6) *Reaction of degeneration* is the term applied to the altered state of electrical excitability in a skeletal muscle completely cut off from its nerve supply. It is present some three weeks after the onset of the lesion and foreshadows contracture. *Irritative* lesions of the facial nerve may produce clonic twitchings of one side of the face. The same phenomenon (facial hemispasm), may be seen in conditions of partial destruction of the facial nerve. Other motor nerves do not show such clonic spasm.

§ 795. Muscular Tone.—" Tone " refers to the slight constant tension which is characteristic of living muscle. The normal constantly varying tension of striped muscle is due to a number of reflexes, spinal and cerebral, physiologically described as " stretch reflexes," " standing and postural reflexes," " righting reflexes." Stretch and postural reflexes are subserved by proprioceptive receptors in tendons and muscles, and afferents from these pass up the spinal cord in the antero-lateral and posterior columns to the mid-brain, where the reflex centres are probably the red nucleus and the reticular formation. The receptors for righting reflexes (concerned with balance) are in the labyrinths. The efferents of all these mid-brain reflexes are the *extra-pyramidal tracts* (rubro-spinal, reticulo-spinal, vestibulo-spinal tracts, Fig. 212) terminating in the anterior horn cells.

Lower motor neurone efferent fibres to striped muscle are of two kinds: (1) large-sized alpha-fibrils (70 per cent.), stimulation of which causes striped muscle contraction; and (2) smaller gamma-fibrils (30 per cent.), stimulation of which at their special rate causes no muscular twitch. The latter are motor fibres for the intra-fusal fibrils of the *muscle spindles.* By stimulation they cause local contraction of

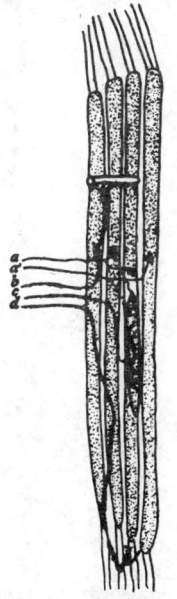

FIG. 213.—END ORGANS IN SKELETAL MUSCLE. *a, a'* are *motor* nerve fibres, innervating muscle fibres and a muscle spindle. *b, c, d* are afferent fibres from arteriole, muscle spindle and tendon respectively.

the intrafusal muscle fibres, which then excite the sensory endings of the spindle without causing any contraction of the muscle as a whole. The afferent discharge of the spindle is thus increased. The gamma-efferents and spindle afferents maintain a considerable tonic discharge in striped muscle. Gamma-fibrils may be stimulated to activity from the motor cortex (Fig. 213).

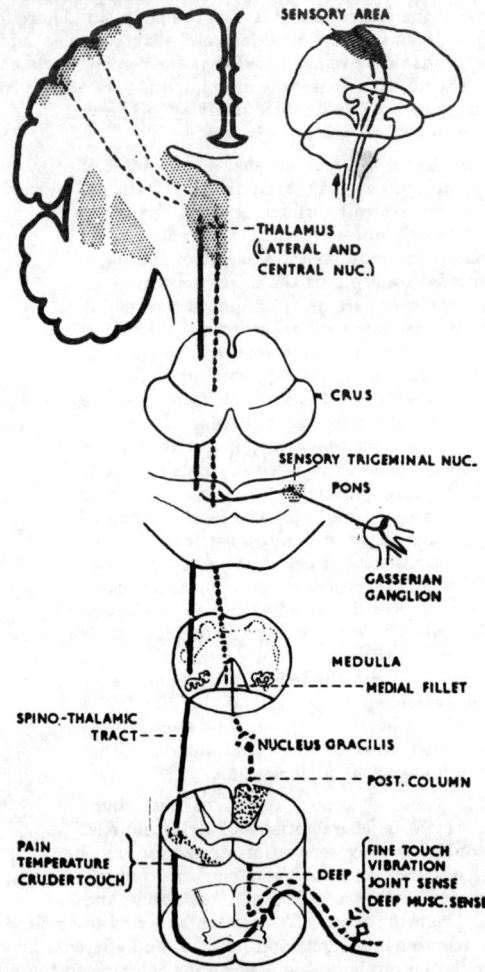

FIG. 214.—DIAGRAM OF THE SENSORY PATHWAYS TO THE BRAIN. (The inset shows the sensory cortex.)

Normal skeletal muscle tone is increased by startle (sudden sights or sounds) and by heightened attention. or emotional tension (especially misery or weeping). It is diminished in states of apathy, laughter and somnolence. When movement is about to be made, the prime movers increase in tone and later contract whilst their antagonists relax (reciprocal innervation). A cortical " suppressor band " has been demonstrated in the premotor area, stimulation of which causes relaxation of postural contraction.

Increase of muscle tone in disease. (1) Spasticity is the term employed for the " clasp-knife " rigidity characteristic of pyramidal disease. On attempting to move the affected limbs passively, resistance is encountered which suddenly yields to continuing pressure. (2) To describe the uniform resistance observed on passively flexing and extending the limbs in Parkinsonism, the term Rigidity is employed. (3) " Irritative " or " discharging " motor lesions, *e.g.*, meningeal irritation or epilepsy, cause increased muscle tone. (4) Cramp and myotonia are examples of local changes in muscle causing increased tone. (5) Certain drugs, *e.g.*, strychnine, cause skeletal muscle hypertonus. (6) In hysterical spasm the resistance met with an attempted passive movement is proportional to the force used to overcome it (§ 1034).

Decreased muscle tone in abnormal states is observed (1) As a shock effect, cerebral or spinal, in upper motor neurone lesions, (2) In lesions of the lower pons including the reticular formation (loss of consciousness and loss of muscle tone). (3) In acute cerebellar and vestibular lesions tone is lost in the ipsilateral muscles. (4) In disease of the posterior columns of the spinal cord and of the parietal cortex, *e.g.*, tabes dorsalis, subacute combined degeneration, parietal tumours. (5) In lesions of the lower motor neurone, or muscle. (6) After injection of drugs, *e.g.*, procaine, curare.

§ 796. Sensory Pathways.—A mixed peripheral nerve contains fibres subserving every aspect of sensibility, cutaneous and deep. The *Cutaneous* sensory impulses are those of (1) Touch, (2) Pain, (3) Temperature. The *Deep* (Proprioceptive) sensory impulses are (1) Vibration of a tuning-fork on bone, (2) Sense of passive movement of joints, (3) Sense of position, (4) Deep muscular sensibility, and (5) Tendon sensibility to deep pressure. All these sensory impulses, cutaneous and deep, enter the spinal cord through the posterior roots (Fig. 214).

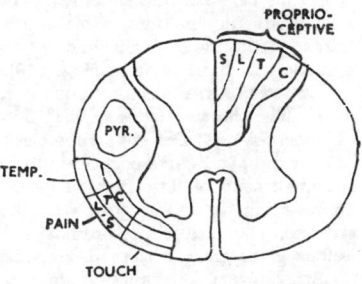

The fibres for *Pain, Temperature* and cruder forms of Tactile Sensation are freshly relayed in the posterior horn and, crossing over immediately on entering the cord in the *anterior commissure*, ascend directly in the SPINOTHALAMIC TRACT of the opposite

FIG. 215.—DIAGRAM OF THE POSITION OF LAMINATING FIBRES in the chief sensory pathways of the Spinal Cord (*after Gordon Holmes*).
C. = Cervical; T. = Thoracic; L. = Lumbar; S. = Sacral; Pyr. = Pyramidal tract.

side to the lateral nucleus of the thalamus. In the spinal cord the spino-thalamic tract lies in the lateral column, just ventrál to the pyramidal tract (Fig. 215). The fibres for *Deep Sensibility* (viz., Vibration, Sense of passive movement and position, Deep muscular sensibility, and Tendon sensibility) together with some fibres subserving Tactile Discrimination, ascend without relay in the POSTERIOR COLUMNS of Goll (fasciculus gracilis) and Burdach (fasciculus cuneatus) of the same side, to the ipsilateral nucleus gracilis and nucleus cuneatus in the medulla. Here they are freshly relayed and ascend in the decussating *medial fillet* (medial lemniscus) to reach the thalamus of the opposite side. So that, eventually, all the afferent impulses, whether cutaneous or deep, undergo a decussation either immediately on entering the cord or later, in the fillet, and terminate in the contra-lateral thalamus. It will be noted that there are two pathways for touch. Tactile fibres, on entering the cord, ascend both in the contra-lateral spino-thalamic tract and in the ipsilateral posterior columns.

In the cord we have both crossed and uncrossed sensory pathways. In the spino-thalamic tracts (crossed) and in the posterior columns (uncrossed), the longest posterior root fibres, which ascend from the coccygeal and sacral segments, lie nearer the mid-line. As fibres enter at higher segmental levels they are conveyed in a lamellar fashion so that the fibres derived from lower segments are displaced inwards by those entering at higher levels (see Fig. 215). Furthermore, the fibres for touch, pain and temperature, entering the cord to cross to the spino-thalamic tract, decussate in the anterior commissure in a diagonal fashion; the fibres for pain and temperature crossing in the mid-dorsal region in the space of one segment, those for touch crossing more slowly, the decussation occupying two or more segments. At higher segmental levels the crossing is more and more oblique. In the spino-thalamic tracts the " pain " fibres are situated separately from the " temperature " fibres in the lateral part of the tract.

The *spino-thalamic tract*, containing pain, temperature and touch fibres, ascends through the formatio reticularis of the medulla to join the crossed medial fillet, in the pons, ultimately reaching the thalamus. The fibres for temperature and pain diverge in the medulla from the tactile fibres and pass to the outer side of the olive, subsequently converging to the mid-line and joining the fillet (see Fig. 214).

The fibres of the *posterior columns* are relayed in the nucleus cuneatus and nucleus gracilis, the latter more medial nucleus receiving fibres from the lower limbs; from these nuclei arise the fibres of the *medial fillet* which terminate in the lateral nucleus of the thalamus (vide supra). The *fillet*, in the pons, passes along the inner side of the sensory nucleus of the trigeminal nerve of the same side. The *thalamus*, situated in the lateral wall of the third ventricle, receives all the sensory impulses of the body, with the exception of the olfactory impulses, which have a direct connection with the cortex of the uncus. The thalamus registers the crude affective sensations of pain, heat, cold, producing emotions of pleasure or pain, and visceral sensations of hunger and thirst. From the thalamus afferent impulses are relayed to the *sensory cortex*, where sensation is discriminative (Fig. 216).

LESIONS OF THE SENSORY CORTEX do not affect crude sensations of temperature or pain. The characteristics are: (1) Loss of ability to localise tactile cutaneous stimuli (Atopognosis), (2) Defective appreciation of the size, shape and consistency of objects held in the hand (Astereognosis), (3) Light touches may be imperfectly felt, (4) there is impairment of Two-Point Discrimination (Compass-test), and (5) difficulty in appreciating the intensity of stimuli. The loss of these discriminative features of sensation may lead to inco-ordination of the affected limb. Sensory testing in cortical lesions gives great variety of response and threshold.

SUB-CORTICAL LESIONS produce a hemianæsthesia, affecting the contra-lateral face, arm, leg and trunk. At the level of the sensory nucleus of the trigeminal nerve a lesion will produce a crossed hemianæsthesia, affecting the face on the same side as the lesion (from the proximity of the fillet to the ipsilateral sensory fifth nucleus) and the upper and lower limbs and trunk on the opposite side (Fig. 223).

LESIONS OF THE THALAMUS, see § 797.

CENTRAL CORD LESIONS (such as syringomyelia or intramedullary tumour) involve the fibres for pain and temperature, which cross in the anterior commissure, together with the fibres subserving cruder forms of tactile sensation, which cross in this region. Touch, as we have seen, has a double pathway ; some of the fibres ascend in the posterior columns and consequently escape. The resulting cutaneous anæsthesia was termed by Charcot " Dissociated anæsthesia," *i.e.*, there is loss of sensation to pin-prick, hot and cold (pain and temperature), while touches with cotton-wool can still be felt. In *Central Bulbar lesions* similar dissociated sensory changes involve the face as well as the trunk and limbs.

LESIONS OF THE POSTERIOR COLUMNS produce sensory ataxia from loss of sense of position (Joint sense). There is loss of vibration sense and the finer types of tactile sensibility on the ipsilateral side. Hypotonia may be present. If the root entry zone is affected the tendon reflexes will be abolished from interference with spinal reflex-arcs.

HEMISECTION OF THE CORD, see § 799.

LESIONS OF THE SENSORY ROOTS AND PERIPHERAL NERVES. All the forms of sensibility within the distribution of the root or nerve are affected, but lesions are usually *partial*, so that the extent of the cutaneous sensory impairment is much lessened. There is commonly a focus of complete cutaneous anæsthesia surrounded by a zone of partial loss; in the latter zone pin-pricks have a diffuse burning quality.

§ 797. The **Thalamus**, unlike the Corpus Striatum, is largely sensory, not motor. It is a great relay station receiving streams of afferent impulses, sensory and non-sensory, from the contra-lateral half of the body, relaying them to the parietal and sensory cortex. It also receives visual (lateral geniculate body) and auditory impulses (medial geniculate body) which are relayed to the striate area and superior temporal convolutions of the cortex respectively. It may be said indeed that various thalamic nuclei project to all parts of the cortex. The thalami, two ovoid masses of grey matter, lie on either side of the third ventricle and approach one another anteriorly over the roof of the mid-brain. Each is divided by a Y-shaped *internal medullary lamina* of white matter into several nuclei. (1) The *ventral nucleus* (" lemniscus nucleus ") receives afferents from the medial fillet (lemniscus), the spino-thalamic tracts and the trigeminal fillet. Cerebellar (dento-rubro-frontal) fibres are here relayed to the motor cortex. (2) The *lateral geniculate body* is the main site of termination of the optic tract. (3) The *medial geniculate body* receives auditory impulses. As

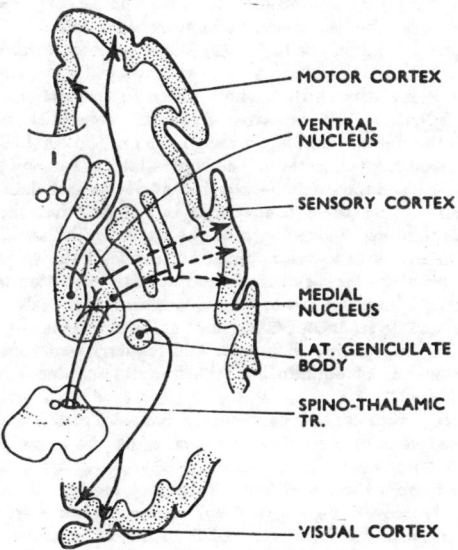

FIG. 216.—THE THALAMIC NUCLEI AND THEIR PROJECTIONS (*after Prof. W. J. Hamilton*).

well as these, there are the (4) medial, (5) anterior and (6) central nuclear masses whose functions are not clearly defined. The anterior nucleus connects with the cingulate gyrus (visceral cortex, Figs. 209b and 216). (7) Connections between the thalamus and the corpus striatum are probably of great clinical importance.

LESIONS OF THE VENTRAL PART OF THE THALAMUS cause (1) Transient slight impairment of cutaneous sensibility on the contra-lateral side of the body, with often permanent loss of deep sensations (joint sense and vibration) and resultant *sensory ataxia*. Characteristically these symptoms are accompanied by persistent severe pain in the affected parts (" thalamic pain "). (2) Spontaneous pain over one half of the body may be associated with over-reaction to painful and thermal stimuli and to tickling. (3) Ataxia and choreo-athetotic movements, not wholly accounted for by the loss of joint sense, may be observed on rare occasions. The pain and over-reaction to sensory stimuli are now believed to be due to a " discharging " or irritative lesion of the thalamus. Loss of sense of position may be so profound that the patient loses awareness of the affected half of his body—" auto-topagnosia."

Somatic (Proprioceptive) Afferents. Impulses arising in muscles, tendons and joints do not all ascend in the dorsal columns and so reach consciousness. Some are directed to the *Cerebellum*. Proprioceptive neurones entering the posterior horn pass to the nuclei of Clarke's column at the base of the posterior horn. From thence secondary neurones arise to ascend in the *dorsal* or *ventral spino-cerebellar tracts* to enter the cerebellum by the inferior and superior peduncles respectively (Fig. 212). Other non-sensory afferents have to do with mid-brain reflexes concerned with the *maintenance of tone* (reticular substance, red nucleus and extra-pyramidal tracts). Non-sensory afferents from the cerebellum are projected via the superior peduncle to the mid-brain and thence to the thalamus and cortex. They are believed to be concerned with the co-ordination of willed movements.

In a disease of the afferent system of projection fibres (such as tabes), besides loss of proprioceptive sensations there are present also symptoms referable to destruction of these reflex-arcs—*e.g.* hypotonia, loss of tendon reflexes and inco-ordination.

§ 798. The Cerebellum is " the head ganglion of the proprioceptive system " (Fig. 212). *Afferents:* (1) The cerebellum receives non-sensory *spinal* afferents from the trunk and limbs on the same side (spino-cerebellar tracts). These pass chiefly to the anterior lobe of the cerebellum. (2) Other afferent *cerebral* connections are from the contra-lateral frontal and temporal cortex relayed by pontine nuclei. (3) The flocculo-nodular lobe receives and transmits fibres to the *vestibular* nuclei and their efferent tracts. *Efferents:* All messages from the cerebellar cortex are relayed indirectly through the dentate and other deep nuclei of the cerebellum. The cerebellum is linked to the prefrontal cortex of the contra-lateral hemisphere by fibres which pass via the superior peduncle to the pontine nuclei and thalamus and are thence relayed to the cortex. By these connections it appears that the cerebellum helps to mould willed and skilled movements of the limbs by influencing their rate and regularity. (2) The efferents to the anterior horn cells in the spinal cord are all also indirect and pass from the cerebellum to the reticular formation and red nuclei and thence by the extra-pyramidal tracts to the anterior horn cells.

The cerebellum and its tracts appear to have three functions:—(1) the maintenance of muscular tone, (2) the control of the rate and regularity of voluntary movements, and (3) the maintenance of equilibrium (the flocculo-nodular lobe acting with the vestibular mechanisms).

LESIONS OF THE CEREBELLUM, particularly if *acute*, cause ipsilateral hypotonia. Some of the clinical signs of cerebellar dysfunction can be explained on the basis of hypotonia. Owing to defective tone, unsupported parts of the body such as the outstretched limbs drift from their position. Voluntary movements are often jerky and irregular in rate. Moreover the range of willed movements is frequently inaccurate and the hand overshoots its objective. Disturbance of innervation in the synergic muscles and antagonists cause oscillation of the finger if it is directed purposively to a point. The coarse rhythmical tremors of the head and limbs which are seen in chronic cerebellar diseases are not all easily explained by existing knowledge.

In lesions of the *flocculo-nodular lobe* (the deep posterior lobe of the cerebellum in the mid-line) vestibular connections are interrupted, and we find unsteady gait without much else (" Trunk ataxia "). *Irritative* lesions of the lateral lobes of the cerebellum produce a vestibulo-ocular group of phenomena with notable hypotonia in the ipsilateral voluntary muscles, nystagmus, reeling or forced movements, the trunk rarely tending to rotate on its long axis. In less acute cases there is a " cerebellar " attitude of the head and inco-ordination of voluntary movement. There is deviation from the straight line when the patient attempts to walk, the sound side, as it were, pushing him over to the side of the lesion. The patient past-points to the side of the lesion (see § 934). Skew deviation of the eyes, a rare symptom, seems to depend on irritative lesions of the deep (dentate) nuclei of the cerebellum.

In *destructive* lesions of the cerebellum in man (*e.g.*, cerebellar atrophy) there is often absence of ocular phenomena and the only symptom may be a loss of the power of regulating willed movements (cerebellar ataxia). In patients who lost the whole of the cerebellum through war wounds, after months of recovery the only residual findings were a general clumsiness of movement, intention tremor and slight slurring of speech. The inference is that if the cerebellum is destroyed, the cerebral cortex can make itself independent of normal cerebellar adjustments.

Ataxia (Inco-ordination of Movement). Any lesion of the spinal cord, brain-stem, thalamus or cerebral hemisphere which interrupts afferent impulses subserving sense of position and the appreciation of passive movement (joint sense), will produce *Sensory ataxia*. It will be remembered that these impulses are conveyed in the posterior columns to the contra-lateral thalamus and are thence relayed to the cortex. Clinically such ataxia is well exemplified in diseases in which the posterior columns are affected, *e.g.*, tabes dorsalis, sub-acute combined degeneration and certain cases of diabetic neuropathy. It may also result from peripheral neuropathies or disease of the sensory cortex. This form of ataxia is increased when the patient's eyes are closed, from loss of information given by the eyes as to the position of the limbs.

Cerebellar ataxia is commonly encountered in lesions of the cerebellum or its con-nections. A characteristic phenomenon is "intention tremor," to demonstrate which the patient is asked to touch his nose with his forefinger. The finger oscillates about its objective just before it is reached but the nose is touched correctly even

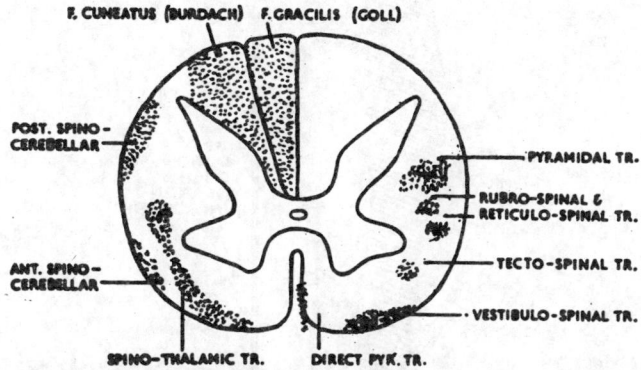

FIG. 217.—ASCENDING AND DESCENDING TRACTS IN THE SPINAL CORD. The afferent tracts are represented in blue on the left, and the efferent tracts in red on the right.

if the eyes are shut. Disease of the flocculo-nodular lobe of the cerebellum affects balance and equilibrium, and the unsteadiness is apparent when the patient rises to his feet (trunk ataxia). Cerebellar ataxia in uninfluenced by closure of the eyes.

Ascending and Descending Tracts in the Spinal Cord (Fig. 217).—The *Posterior Columns* are composed of the ascending *Tracts of Goll and Burdach* carrying uncrossed fibres subserving Deep Sensibility (viz., Postural Sense, Sense of Passive Movement of Joints, Vibration Sense, Deep Muscular Sensibility and the uncrossed fibres for finer Touch). These all pass to the nucleus gracilis and cuneatus, whence they are relayed in the medial fillet to the contra-lateral thalamus.

The *Lateral Columns* contain the descending *Crossed Pyramidal Tract* and, just ventral to this, the *Rubro-Spinal Tract* and *Reticulo-spinal Tract*, the chief extra-pyramidal motor tracts. These motor fibres are all relayed to the anterior horn cells. The periphery of the lateral columns is occupied by two ascending cerebellar tracts, the *Posterior (Direct)* and *Anterior Spino-Cerebellar Tracts*, containing cerebellar afferents relayed from the cells of Clarke's Column.

The *Ventral Columns* contain the descending *Direct (Uncrossed) Pyramidal Tracts* and two extra-pyramidal motor tracts, the *Vestibulo-Spinal* and *Tecto-Spinal Tracts*. These descending motor tracts all pass direct to the anterior horn cells. The ascending *Spino-thalamic Tracts* lie in the antero-lateral region of the cord, carrying crossed fibres subserving Cutaneous Sensibility (viz., Pain, Temperature and most of those for Touch) to the fillet and ipsilateral thalamus.

§ 799. **Hemisection of the Cord** (Brown-Séquard Syndrome)—(1) On the side of the lesion dorsal column sensibility (joint sense and vibration with some touch) will be lost below the level of the lesion. There will be spastic paralysis of the ipsilateral leg with increased tendon reflexes, clonus and an extensor plantar response from destruction of the pyramidal tract on the same side. (2) On the side opposite to the

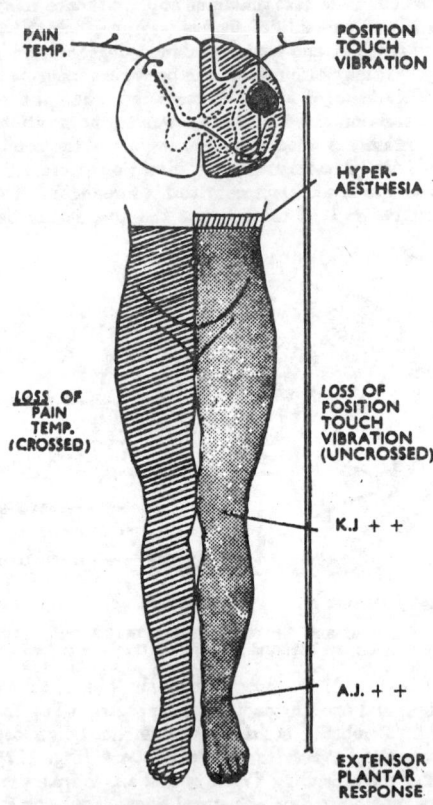

PAIN
TEMP.

POSITION
TOUCH
VIBRATION

HYPER-
AESTHESIA

LOSS OF
PAIN
TEMP.
(CROSSED)

LOSS OF
POSITION
TOUCH
VIBRATION
(UNCROSSED)

K.J + +

A.J. + +

EXTENSOR
PLANTAR
RESPONSE

FIG. 218.—THE BROWN-SÉQUARD SYNDROME. Diagram showing the effects of the left-sided hemisection of the dorsal part of the spinal cord.

lesion pain and temperature are lost and touch is blunted for two to three segments below the level of the lesion. (3) At the upper level of the lesion there may be a zone of root hyperæsthesia.

Segmentation in the Spinal Cord.—Each spinal segment or metamere has its anterior (motor) and posterior (sensory) roots. The spinal nerves are formed by fusion of one anterior and posterior spinal root. The spinal nerve then divides into a ventral and a dorsal *primary division*. Each of these divisions contains motor and sensory fibres, and ultimately supplies the cutaneous segment (Fig. 244) and the muscles (Table LVIII) developed in connection with its corresponding metamere. So far as the limbs are concerned the cells to the proximal muscles lie nearest to the central median fissure. The extensors and the flexors are represented separately in the anterior horns.

The **Pathways for the Special Senses.** The peripheral organs for vision, hearing, taste and smell are paired, and in man the sensory fibres proceeding from them to the cortex all exhibit a hemi-decussation, so that the cortex of one hemisphere sub-serves both organs in the case of each of these senses.

§ 800. I. The Visual Mechanisms.—Together with the great Sensory and Motor projection systems the Visual projections are of great importance in regional diagnosis. We may consider here (a) Visual pathways, (b) The Pupil, (c) Eye movements.

(a) **The Visual Pathways and Visual Field Syndromes** (Fig. 219). The pathways extend from the optic nerve heads to the striate cortex, the radiations within the tem-poral and occipital lobes making wide sweeps. Each *Optic Nerve* passes backwards from the eye globe into the cranial cavity through the optic foramen. The constituent fibres divide into medial and lateral groups. The medial portion decussates at the *Optic Chiasma* which lies just in front of the pituitary fossa. Each medial division, as it crosses, fans out a little in the opposite optic nerve before it joins with the uncrossed lateral division of the opposite side to form the *Optic Tract*. Throughout their course from the retina to the striate cortex the visual fibres are grouped according to the retinal quadrants in which they arise. Thus those fibres from the upper quadrants of the two retinæ lie dorsal to those from the lower quadrants. This arrangement main-tains throughout the whole length of the visual pathway. Behind the chiasma each tract and radiation contains all the fibres from the corresponding halves of both retinæ. Fibres of macular origin maintain a central position in the tract and radiation.

The Optic Tract bends round the lateral aspect of the mid-brain to terminate in the *primary visual centres*—the *lateral geniculate body* of the thalamus and the *superior corpus quadrigeminum*. Each optic tract contains the fibres from the uncrossed temporal and the crossed nasal half-fields. The fibres terminating in the lateral geniculate body carry visual impulses which will pass by the optic radiations to con-sciousness. The fibres ending under the superior corpus quadrigeminus (pre-tectal nucleus) have to do with the pupillary light reflex.

The Optic Radiations are relayed from the lateral geniculate bodies (as secondary afferent neurones), passing through the internal capsule behind the somatic afferents to end in the Striate Cortex (Fig. 219). Each optic radiation contains fibres relayed from the corresponding lateral halves of both retinæ. The *dorsal bundle* of fibres contains fibres relayed from the corresponding superior quadrants of both retinæ and passes directly backwards to the cuneus or upper lip of the post-calcarine fissure. The *ventral bundle* of the optic radiation, containing fibres from the corresponding inferior quadrants of both retinæ runs first downwards towards the uncus then, turning round the tip of the descending horn of the lateral ventricle ("temporal knee"), runs back-wards to reach the lingual gyrus. The fibres of the temporal knee thus represent the lower homonymous retinal quadrants.

The *macular fibres* undergo a decussation in the chiasma and are relayed from the lateral geniculate body to the tip of the occipital pole. The cortex of the tip of each occipital pole contains fibres relayed from the corresponding halves of both maculæ. The projection of the retina on the *Visual Cortex* (area striata) is of a point-to-point order. The superiorly placed cuneus subserves the corresponding superior quadrants of both retinæ and the inferiorly placed lingual gyrus the correspond-ing inferior quadrants of both retinæ.

A LESION OF THE OPTIC NERVE will cause blindness of that eye, pallor of the optic disc (optic atrophy), loss of direct pupillary light reflex, with preservation of the consensual light reflex from the opposite eye.

A LESION OF THE OPTIC CHIASMA will abolish the function of the nasal halves of both retinæ and produce blindness of both temporal fields (bitemporal hemianopia). Damage from behind the chiasma (e.g., pituitary or basal lesions) will cause upper quadrantic temporal field defects which gradually become hemianopic. The lesion may extend along one optic nerve producing blindness in one eye.

LESIONS OF THE OPTIC TRACT will abolish the functions of the corresponding halves of both retinæ, producing blindness of the contra-lateral halves of the visual fields (homonymous hemianopia).

LESIONS OF THE OPTIC RADIATION affect the "temporal knee," thus producing

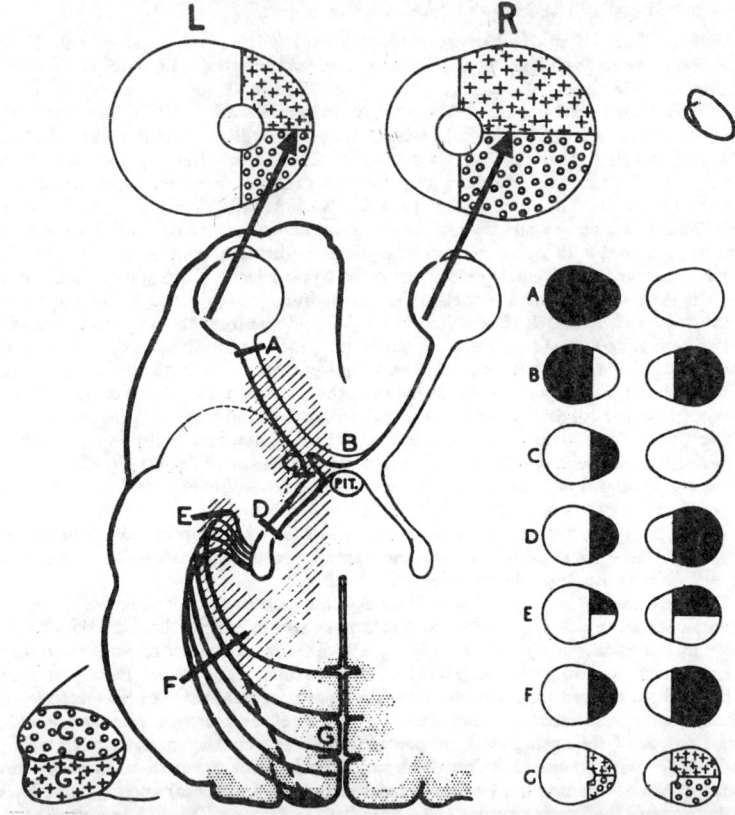

FIG. 219.—THE VISUAL PATHWAYS. L and R represent the left and right visual fields. Letters on the diagram of the visual pathways indicate the position of lesions; all, except B, left-sided. Corresponding letters to the right of the diagram indicate the effect of the various lesions on the visual fields. The hatched area on the brain diagram represents the lateral ventricle. The interrupted line in the optic radiation indicates the course of the fibres concerned with central vision. Inset G represents the left visual cortex (area striata) with macular vision represented most posteriorly. (*After Homans, Fulton.*)

     A = Optic nerve (Blindness in left eye).
     B = Chiasma (Bitemporal hemianopia).
     C = Para-chiasmal lesion (Left nasal hemianopia).
     D = Lateral geniculate body or optic tract (Right homonymous hemianopia).
     E = Genu (lower fibres) of optic radiation (Right upper quadrantic hemianopia).
     F = Optic radiations (Right homonymous hemianopia).
     G = Visual cortex (Right homonymous hemianopia, sparing the macula).

a crossed homonymous defect of upper quadrants of the visual fields. Such defects tend to be congruous, *i.e.*, they can be superimposed one on the other exactly. The farther back they are situated in the hemisphere the more congruous the defects. Lesions involving the whole of the radiation lead to a crossed homonymous hemianopia —" a hemiplegia of the fields of vision."

LESIONS OF THE STRIATE CORTEX cause crossed homonymous defects just like lesions in the radiations. Homonymous central hemiscotoma, quadrant defects, and complete hemianopia all occur. They are often accompanied, when progressive, by cortical discharges manifested as hemianopic hallucinations of flashing or coloured lights. Visual inattention arises from lesions in the lateral surface of the hemispheres with disturbance of spatial orientation in the visual fields. Lesions of the lateral surface of the occipital cortex in the dominant hemisphere may cause visual agnosia and the memory of topography may be lost.

(b) The Pupil.—The *tonic constrictor* of the pupil is the Oculomotor nerve which innervates the circular fibres. The *tonic dilator* of the pupil is the Cervical Sympathetic, innervating the radial fibres. (Fig. 227.)

The optic nerves not only carry visual fibres; certain fibres are non-visual, constituting the afferent paths of mid-brain reflexes concerned in pupillary reactions to light.

The LIGHT REFLEX (Fig. 220). Impulses pass from the retina by the medial portion of the optic nerve to the superior corpus quadrigeminum and *pretectal nucleus* of the same side. Here secondary neurones arise which decussate round the aqueduct. The third neurone lies within the oculomotor nerve and, passing through its branch to the inferior oblique muscle, terminates in the ciliary muscle of the pupil (short ciliary nerves via the ciliary ganglion). Each oculomotor nucleus receives light impulses from both retinæ. When a beam of light is thrown into one eye, not only does the pupil of that eye contract, the contra-lateral pupil contracts also (consensual reflex).

LESIONS OF THE OPTIC NERVE do not usually affect the size of the pupil, but abolish the direct light reflex in the affected eye as the afferent path from the retina is destroyed. The consensual reflex from the opposite eye is preserved. In retro-bulbar neuritis, where there is a partial lesion of the optic nerve, the pupil contracts to light, but the contraction is not maintained, although the eye is exposed to light. This is called the "neuritic" reaction.

LESIONS OF THE THIRD NERVE NUCLEUS, the efferent fibres to the ciliary ganglion or the short ciliary nerves, disturb the reaction of the pupil to light. The pupil will dilate owing to the unopposed action of the cervical sympathetic unless the dilator fibres are also involved.

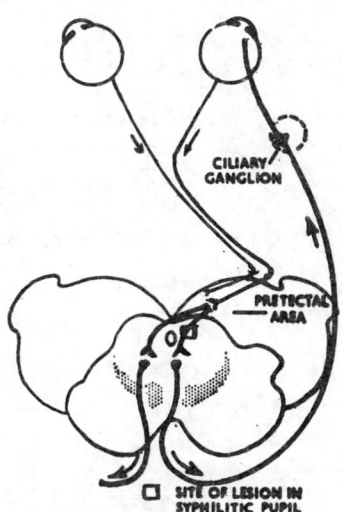

FIG. 220.—PATHWAYS INVOLVED IN PUPILLARY LIGHT REFLEX (*after Gordon Holmes*).

CONVERGENCE ACCOMMODATION is an associated or synkinetic phenomenon helping to increase the depth of focus. It is probably produced by proprioceptive impulses arising in the adductor muscles of the eyes and acting through the medial nucleus of Perlia.

(c) External Eye Movements are normally conjugate movements, i.e., the eyes are moved laterally, or are elevated or depressed with the visual axes in parallel. The eyes normally converge on accommodation. Such movements are all willed movements, but, in fact, are usually carried out reflexly; they involve reciprocal innervation—fixing by prime-movers and synergists and relaxation of antagonist muscle pairs.

The cortical areas for ocular movements lie in the second frontal convolution anterior to the motor areas for the trunk and limbs (Fig. 209a). Subsidiary reflex

C.M.—M M

centres for reflex conjugate movements exist in the mid-brain. From these areas, motor neurones are projected upon the various oculomotor nuclei and these *supra-nuclear fibres* are homologous with upper motor neurones.

The origin of the oculomotor nerve is from various nuclear masses in the floor of the aqueduct. The fibres to the pupil arise in the most anterior part (Edinger-Westphal's Nucleus). Behind this arise the fibres to the superior recti, next those to the internal recti, and behind these, the fibres to the depressors (inferior recti). The trochlear nucleus supplies the superior oblique which is a depressor. From these nuclei and the paired sixth nuclei in the pons the *lower motor neurones* pass to individual ocular muscles. The medial longitudinal bundle connects these various nuclei with reflex centres in the pons for lateral gaze and head-turning movements.

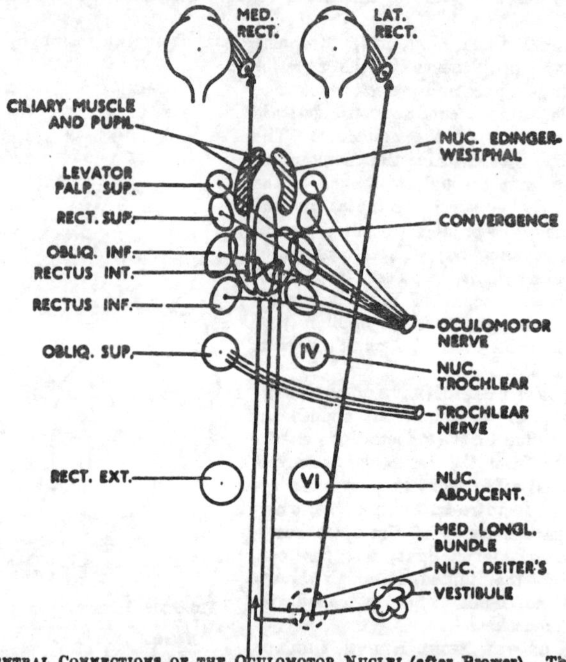

FIG. 221.—CENTRAL CONNECTIONS OF THE OCULOMOTOR NUCLEI (after Brower). The distribution of the nuclei and of the fibres to separate ocular muscles is shown diagrammatically. The pathway involved in lateral gaze to the right is indicated in red. Note the connections with the vestibular (Deiter's) nucleus.

CORTICAL LESIONS. In an epileptic fit we may see the head and eyes turn to the side opposite to the lesion with tonic and clonic contraction of the contra-lateral limbs.

SUPRANUCLEAR LESIONS produce paralysis in terms of conjugate movements, not of muscles. Paralysis of elevation of the eyes is sometimes associated with bilateral loss of the pupillary reflex to light and occurs in lesions of the quadrigeminal area and tectum of the mid-brain (Parinaud's syndrome). In *acute hemiplegia* we may see conjugate deviation of the head and eyes towards the side of the lesion with loss of lateral gaze to the opposite side as a transient phenomenon.

SUPRANUCLEAR AND NUCLEAR LESIONS not infrequently exist together in lesions of the mid-brain. A lesion of the medial longitudinal bundle produces isolated palsy of the internal recti in lateral deviation only, not on convergence (seen in small embolic lesions and in multiple sclerosis). *Nuclear lesions* affect (from before backwards) (1) pupillary light reactions, (2) elevation of the eyes, (3) lateral movements and

(4) depression of the eyes. An isolated lesion of the sixth nerve nucleus produces an external rectus palsy, usually associated with facial palsy on the same side from the proximity of the VII to the VI nucleus.

INFRANUCLEAR LESIONS produce paralysis of individual muscles, commonly but not of course always unilateral. Oculomotor palsy results in ptosis, a dilated fixed pupil with the eye in abduction. There is paralysis of the superior, inferior and internal recti, the striped portion of levator palpebral superioris with ptosis, and the pupillary constrictor fibres with inactivity of the pupil to light.

§ 801. II. AUDITORY SENSE.—The Eighth Cranial Nerve consists of a sensory or Cochlear division concerned with hearing, and a non-sensory or Vestibular portion concerned with equilibrium.

(a) *Cochlear nerve fibres* arise from cells in the SPIRAL GANGLION situated in the central pillar of the cochlea, their peripheral terminations ending in the hair-cells of the organ of Corti. Centrally, the cochlear nerve passes to the brain through the internal auditory meatus and enters the lower border of the pons to terminate in the dorsally-placed *Cochlear nucleus* (tuberculum acousticum) which lies in the lower pons just external to the restiform body. From here, the fibres decussate as the *striae acousticae* and run in the *lateral fillet (lemniscus)* to the Medial Geniculate Body and Inferior Corpus Quadrigeminum (*Primary Auditory Centres*). The former is concerned with impulses of hearing ascending to conscious level, the latter with unconscious auditory reflexes. From the Medial Geniculate Body a fresh relay of fibres arises, which passes to the higher auditory areas in the superior temporal gyrus of the cortex.

Destruction of the Cochlea or the cochlear nerve produces *nerve-deafness*, irritative lesions produce *tinnitus*. Lesions of the cochlear nucleus in the pons, or the lateral fillets (lemnisci), will have a similar effect, but brain-stem deafness is rare. Lesions of the superior temporal gyrus do not destroy hearing because each ear has a bilateral cortical representation. In right-handed people, a lesion of the left superior temporal gyrus abolishes the comprehension of words and sounds heard (word-deafness).

(b) *Vestibular fibres*, see § 802.

III. GUSTATORY SENSE.—Smell and Taste are described in §§ 1104, 1105. Loss of taste on the anterior two-thirds of the tongue occurs in lesions of the facial nerve in the aqueductus Fallopii involving the geniculate ganglion.

§ 802. The Mechanism of Equilibrium.—*Equilibrium* is dependent on perfect co-ordination of certain afferent impulses. These impulses are set up by: (1) movement of the limbs acting through the muscle-spindles, joints and tendons, (2) vision and (3) gravity, the latter acting through the vestibular apparatus.

The Vestibular Apparatus consists of: (a) The UTRICLE and SACCULE, containing sensitive hair-cells in contact with small crystals, the otoliths. The position of the otoliths with regard to the hair-cells varies with gravity, and impulses are set up in the saccules when the head is moved *vertically* or *horizontally*. (b) SEMICIRCULAR CANALS, containing sensitive hair-cells which respond to movement of the endolymph. Impulses are set up in the semicircular canals by *angular* displacement of the head.

Impulses are constantly being received from the vestibular apparatus telling the position of the head in space. The cells of origin of the *vestibular nerve* are in Scarpa's ganglion in the internal auditory meatus. Fibres pass centrally to the lateral *vestibular (Deiter's) nucleus*, which lies ventrally in the pons in the outer part of the floor of the fourth ventricle (Figs. 212, 222). Efferent fibres connect this nucleus with (1) the flocculo-nodular lobe of the cerebellum, (2) the anterior horn cells (vestibulo-spinal tract) and (3) the ocular nuclei (medial longitudinal bundle). Deiter's nucleus receives afferents also from the cerebellum. *Disturbances of the vestibular mechanism* produce: (1) subjective vertigo, (2) hypotonia on the side of the lesion, (3) forced movements and falling, and (4) nystagmus.

In a normal subject certain manœuvres (*e.g.*, sudden cessation of rotation, rocking) will cause maladjustment of postural reflexes and a sense of mild confusion. If a normal individual is rotated in a rotating chair which is suddenly checked and tilted backwards, the whole vestibular mechanism is so disturbed that the person may collapse or be flung out of the chair. For a time he will have no conception of how to orient himself in space. Ewald found that ablation of the vestibule causes hypotonia of the ipsilateral half of the body. A similar result follows section of the vestibular nerve but passes off in three or four weeks or less.

§ 803. Anatomy of the Brain-Stem.—The Brain-Stem comprises the Mid-Brain, Pons and Medulla. Here are grouped (1) the Sensory and Motor Pathways, (2) the Cranial Nerve Nuclei, (3) Important Reflex and Association Nuclei, *e.g.*, red nucleus, reticular nuclei, superior corpus quadrigeminum, vestibular nuclei.

(1) MOTOR AND SENSORY PATHWAYS.—These have already been considered.

(2) CRANIAL NERVE NUCLEI.—The student is advised to study the diagram (Fig. 222) which indicates the position of the various cranial nerve nuclei in the pons

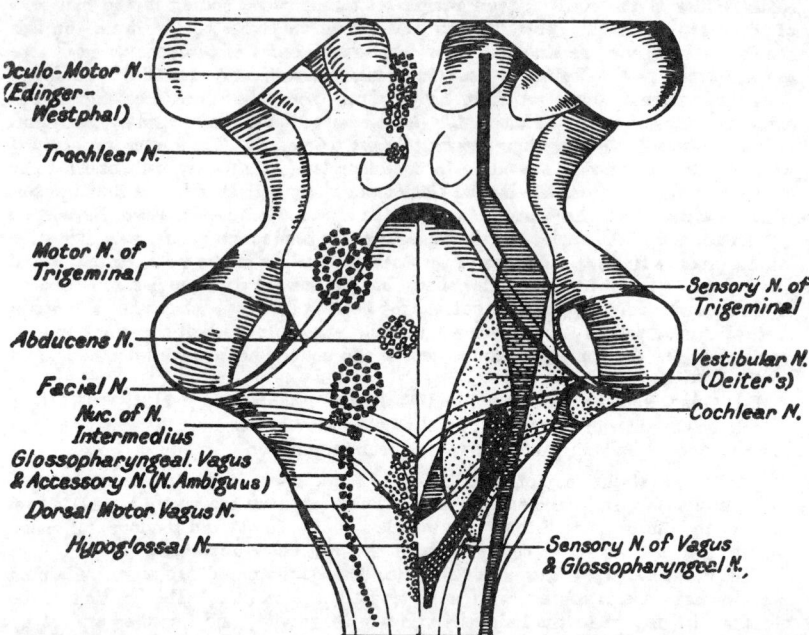

FIG. 222.—DIAGRAM OF THE CRANIAL NERVE NUCLEI (Motor Nuclei on Left, Sensory on Right).

and medulla. The *trigeminal nuclei* are two, a motor and a sensory, and they are of great clinical importance, both from their extent and position. The ventral *motor nucleus* lies in the floor of the fourth ventricle and is concerned with the innervation of the muscles of mastication. The main *sensory nucleus* is of wide extent, and in the pons lies lateral to the medial fillet. As the fibres enter the pons they arrange themselves in a short ascending and a long descending portion. The ascending part ends in the upper sensory nucleus of the trigeminal nerve in the pons and subserves touch and proprioception from the entire trigeminal area. The descending part forms the *nucleus of the spinal tract* and extends caudally into the cervical cord as low as C3 where it becomes continuous with the substantia gelatinosa; this subserves pain and temperature sensation of the whole trigeminal area but is arranged in a peculiar fashion in that its lower extremity is connected with pain and temperature sensation in the upper face and cornea, while its upper extremity is concerned with these sensations over the distribution of the ·mandibular (third) division of the fifth nerve. The sensory nucleus as a whole is concerned with sensation in the face, scalp, cornea, conjunctiva, tongue and nasal mucosa. The motor and sensory roots emerge from the ventrolateral aspect of the pons, and on the sensory root is the Gasserian ganglion.

The movements of the face and tongue may be mentioned here. The *facial nucleus* lies in the lateral aspect of the pons, its nerve-fibres turning round the abducent nucleus under the floor of the fourth ventricle before emerging to supply the facial muscles. The *hypoglossal nucleus* is purely motor and concerned with the movements of the tongue. It lies lowest of all the cranial nuclei in the floor of the fourth ventricle near the mid-line (Fig. 223). All the cranial nerve nuclei receive supranuclear pyramidal (cortico-bulbar) fibres from the motor cortex of both hemispheres *except* the part of the facial nucleus supplying the lower facial muscles, and the hypoglossal nucleus, which receive fibres from one hemisphere only, the contra-lateral. In hemiplegia, due to a focal lesion in the internal capsule, all the cranial nerve nuclei escape paralysis owing to their bilateral innervation, except these two nuclei. We thus observe, in hemiplegia, a weakness of the lower face (the upper face is spared) and deviation of the tongue to the hemiplegic side when it is protruded.

The sensory *cochlear nucleus* is situated on the dorsal and outer aspects of the pons. The motor *glossopharyngeal-vagus-accessorius* nucleus (n. ambiguus) lies in the

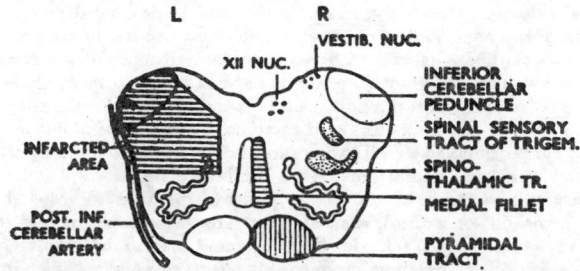

L　　　　　　　　　R
VESTIB. NUC.
XII NUC.
INFERIOR CEREBELLAR PEDUNCLE
SPINAL SENSORY TRACT OF TRIGEM.
INFARCTED AREA
SPINO-THALAMIC TR.
MEDIAL FILLET
POST. INF. CEREBELLAR ARTERY
PYRAMIDAL TRACT

FIG. 223.—CROSS-SECTION THROUGH THE LOWER MEDULLA. The area of infarction in thrombosis of the Left Posterior Inferior Cerebellar Artery is hatched in red. This produces a crossed dissociated hemianæsthesia affecting the left face and the right half of the body.

medulla and is concerned with the innervation of the muscles of the pharynx, larynx, palate, sternomastoid and trapezius. The motor nucleus of the spinal accessory nerve reaches as low as the fifth cervical segment. The *dorsal motor nucleus of the vagus* supplies the unstriped muscle of the alimentary tract and air passages. There is also a *sensory glossopharyngeal-vagus* nucleus in the medulla, concerned with common sensation from the ear, mouth, pharynx and afferents from the abdominal and thoracic viscera.

Syndromes of the Brain-Stem. LESIONS OF THE MID-BRAIN. There may be an oculomotor palsy on the side of the lesion with contra-lateral hemiplegia from pyramidal involvement. Signs of paralysis or irritation of the ocular sympathetic may be present (viz., constricted pupil with enophthalmos, or the reverse). If the superior cerebellar peduncles are involved, ataxia may be present. Lesions of the tectum produce *defective conjugate elevation of the eyes* with *ptosis* and loss of pupillary light reflex.

LESIONS OF THE PONS produce sixth and seventh nerve nuclear palsies associated with pyramidal, sensory, cerebellar or vestibular signs.

LESIONS OF THE MEDULLA produce ninth, tenth, eleventh or twelfth nerve palsies in association with pyramidal and sensory long tract signs usually bilateral (for the " unilateral bulbar syndrome " see §§ 809, 936, Fig. 223). The following bulbar functions depend on the integrity of *cortico-ponto-bulbar mechanisms*. Some like the *enunciation of speech* or *emotional expression* are controlled and normally inhibited by the cortex. Others like swallowing or respiration are less voluntary and more automatic. (1) *Enunciation of speech*—singing, whistling, humming. (2) *Emotional expression*—giggling, laughing, sobbing, weeping. (3) *Swallowing of solids and liquids*—choking, vomiting. (4) *Respiration*—sighing, yawning, coughing, sniffing, hiccough.

BILATERAL SUPRANUCLEAR LESIONS affect these mechanisms and the bulbar nuclei; these escape in ordinary hemiplegia owing to their innervation from both hemispheres. The jaw-jerk in these cases is increased.

LOWER MOTOR NEURONE LESIONS OF THE BULB cause wasting of the associated muscles, which may show fasciculation. There is diminution or loss of bulbar functions and of the jaw-jerk.

(3) REFLEX AND ASSOCIATION NUCLEI OF THE BRAIN-STEM.

Superior Corpus Quadrigeminum (Tectal Area). This reflex centre in the mid-brain receives afferents from the optic tracts and from the visual cortex and, through its efferents the oculomotor nerves and the tecto-spinal tracts, effects pupillary alterations, ocular movements, protective blinking and turning away from sudden visual stimuli. Lesions produce loss of upward movement of the eyes, with disorder of the pupillary reactions.

The Reticular Formation consists of an elongated band of scattered collections of grey matter intersected by nerve-fibres running in several directions. The formation extends from the thalamus (intralaminar nuclei) along the floor of the aqueduct in the mid-brain (separate from the red nucleus), and is prolonged downwards in the dorsal region of the pons, and in the medulla oblongata to its junction with the cord. It receives cortical fibres as well as fibres from the red nucleus and cerebellum and sends an extra-pyramidal tract (the reticulo-spinal tract) downwards in the lateral columns of the cord to the anterior horn cells. It influences muscular tone. Extravagant claims have been made for its functions. Besides its influence on muscle tone, the lateral portion has a facilitating function on the anterior horn cells and their reflex systems, and the medial portion an inhibitory function.

Consciousness and the Brain-Stem. A patient who fails to respond to sensory stimuli (from without or within), such as might arouse a sleeper, is said to be unconscious. A variety of lesions (anoxic, traumatic and neoplastic) involving the brain-stem and posterior hypothalamus produce this effect, especially lesions involving the hypothalamic region. The mechanisms causing this are not understood. A " waking centre " which may alert the cortex has been postulated in the most cephalic part of the reticular formation but adequate proof of this is lacking.

Red Nucleus. This nucleus and the substantia nigra, both in the mid-brain, subserve reflex tone in the voluntary muscles. It is a head ganglion in a series of proprioceptive reflexes whose afferents come from (1) the cerebellum, controlling through the rubro-spinal tract the co-ordination of the limbs, and (2) from the globus pallidus, governing the performance of automatic association movements, *e.g.*, swinging the arms when walking. Lesions of the red nucleus may produce involuntary movements and ataxia. In animals, section of the mid-brain through the red nucleus produces the phenomena of " decerebrate rigidity," due to the destruction of pyramidal control and the release of the extra-pyramidal mid-brain centres for reflex tone in the voluntary muscles.

The Lateral Vestibular (Deiter's) Nucleus in the pons receives fibres from Scarpa's ganglion (vestibular nerve), proprioceptive afferents from antero-lateral columns of the cord and from the cerebellum, and transmits, through the vestibulo-spinal tract to the anterior horn cells, impulses regulating contractile tone and equilibrium. Lesions of this nucleus produce hypotonia and loss of balance.

(4) AUTONOMIC CELLS AND FIBRES.—Disturbance of the sympathetic innervation of the eye, with irritative signs (midriasis, exophthalmos or lid-reaction) or paralytic signs (miosis, enophthalmos and pseudoptosis) follow upon lesions of the posterior longitudinal bundle in the mid-brain, pons or medulla (Fig. 227).

THE HYPOTHALAMUS, THE AUTONOMIC NERVOUS SYSTEM AND THE PITUITARY GLAND

§ 804. The **Hypothalamus** has been called "the head ganglion of the Autonomic Nervous System." It is formed by the floor and the lateral walls of the third ventricle. It lies in the mid-line in the diencephalon or "'tween brain" between the hemispheres. It consists of lateral masses of grey matter, the *mammillary bodies, tuber cinereum, paraventricular* and *supra-optic* nuclei. It is largely concerned with the control of the visual and metabolic activities of the body, and is morphologically and physiologically associated with the hypophysis (pituitary gland). A large fibre tract runs from the supra-optic nucleus to the posterior lobe of the hypophysis (supraoptico-hypophyseal tract). This probably conducts antidiuretic hormone and oxytocin elaborated in the cell bodies of the paraventricular and supra-optic nuclei to the posterior pituitary gland where they are stored. When the tract is destroyed, diabetes insipidus follows. This contrasts with the purely chemical mechanism by which the anterior pituitary body receives its stimuli from the hypothalamus by purely vascular channels.

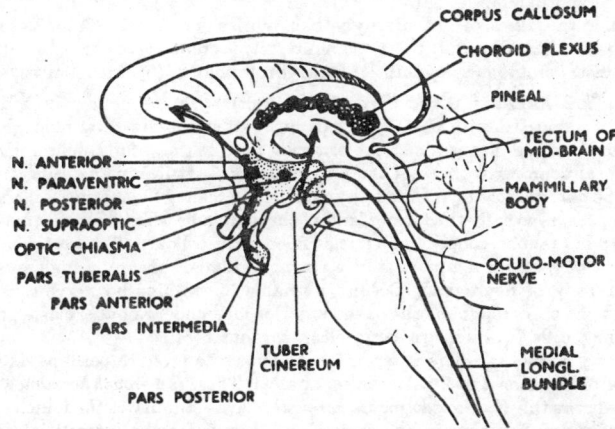

FIG. 224.—HYPOTHALAMIC AND PITUITARY CONNECTIONS. A medial sagittal section of the hypothalamus and pituitary gland. The shaded area in the wall and floor of the third ventricle represents the hypothalamic nuclei. From the *paraventricular* nucleus a tract descends to the *supraoptic* nucleus, thence by the *supraoptico-hypophyseal tract* to the posterior lobe of the gland.

The hypothalamus has cortical projections especially to the orbitofrontal cortex and to the cingulate gyri on the medial aspect of the brain via the mammillo-thalamic tract. From the mammillary body also arises the median longitudinal bundle which descends to the bulb supplying parasympathetic fibres to certain nuclei of the brainstem, especially the oculomotor nuclei, the facial nuclei and to the dorsal nucleus of the vagus.

The hypothalamus has had many functions ascribed to it. (1) It is important in connection with *homeostasis, i.e.,* regulation of body temperature, metabolism, rhythms of sleeping and waking, and of sexual activity. (2) It integrates autonomic and cerebro-spinal reactions involved in *emotional expression.* Stimulation of the posterior and lateral parts of the hypothalamus evokes motor excitement with sympathetic effects—dilatation of the pupils, flushing, sweating, alterations in salivary secretions, etc. During operations on the hypothalamic region in man it has been repeatedly observed that stimulation of the posterior part is followed by excited talk and behaviour. Stimulation of the anterior and tuberal parts of the hypothalamus produces effects which are predominantly parasympathetic, viz., bradycardia, somnolence, lowering of body temperature.

Lesions of the Hypothalamus and Fronto-thalamic Fibres cause apathy, loss of initiative, social indifference, lack of emotion, and often drowsiness. These symptoms may be observed in frontal or suprapituitary tumours, or after the operation of leucotomy. It is recognised that nuclei in the anterior part of the hypothalamus may play a part in the maintenance of wakefulness and consciousness.

Acute Lesions of the Hypothalamus may be associated with *Diabetes insipidus.* Hæmatemesis due to acute œsophageal or gastric ulcers is observed. Hyperthermia occurs after head injuries or operations involving the hypothalamus.

Chronic Lesions of the Hypothalamus cause interference with the following functions: (1) *Renal excretion:* Diabetes insipidus results from lesions of the supraoptico-hypophyseal tract. (2) *Sexual functions:* Genital hypoplasia with lack of secondary sexual characteristics (or regression of these) occurs with impotence or amenorrhœa. Lesions of the posterior hypothalamus in children cause precocious puberty (pineal tumours). (3) *Growth:* Infantilism and Dystrophia adiposo-genitalis are rarely associated with hypothalamic lesions. (4) *Sleep:* Somnolence may be prominent, especially if there is obesity or depression of metabolism. *The Laurence Moon-Biedl Syndrome* is probably hypothalamic (§ 18).

The known *causes* of chronic hypothalamic lesions are (1) Trauma to the base of the brain; (2) Suprapituitary tumours, *e.g.,* cranio-pharyngioma; (3) Chronic meningitis, tuberculous or syphilitic; (4) Hydrocephalus; (5) Encephalitis.

§ 805. The **Pituitary Gland** (Syn. **Hypophysis**) with its hollow infundibulum is intimately connected with the Hypothalamus. It is the most vascular gland in the body and a venous plexus along the anterior part of the infundibulum connects the hypophyseal veins with those of the hypothalamus. It lies in the sella turcica (Fig. 224). The *anterior lobe* (syn. Adeno-hypophysis) is made up of eosinophil and basophil secretory cells, especially the former, and of chromophobe cells which are non-secretory. The *intermediate* lobe consists of vesicles filled with colloid. The *posterior lobe* (Syn. Neuro-hypophysis), developmentally an evagination of the hypothalamus, consists almost entirely of neuroglia. Despite its name it contains no nerve-cells. During pregnancy the chromophobe cells of the anterior lobe undergo hyperplasia and become "pregnancy cells" which are large clear agranular cells.

Pituitary hormones. The anterior lobe is known to produce perhaps six hormones, the posterior lobe stores two. ANTERIOR LOBE (1) There is a *growth hormone* stimulating epiphyseal growth. (2) *Gonadotrophic hormones.* One stimulates the follicles, the other has a luteinising function in the female and stimulates the interstitial cells in the male. (3) A *thyrotrophic hormone.* (4) *Adrenocorticotrophic hormone* (ACTH) when used clinically must be injected intramuscularly. It is useless as replacement therapy in Addison's disease, unlike cortisone. Not itself a steroid substance ACTH stimulates the adrenal cortex to secrete various steroids; these are metabolised in the liver and excreted in the urine as corticosteroids and 17-ketosteroids. (5) A *lactogenic* hormone stimulates milk secretion. (6) A *diabetogenic* hormone is described but may be the same as the growth hormone.

POSTERIOR LOBE. This contains two hormones which are probably produced in the hypothalamic nuclei (*vide supra*). (1) *Oxytocin* has a specific constrictor effect on uterine muscle. (2) *Antidiuretic hormone* controls the secretion of the renal tubules and the osmotic pressure of the blood plasma. It is no longer believed that *vasopressin* is produced as a separate hormone; oxytocin in large doses has a vasopressor effect.

The PARS INTERMEDIA probably produces a *melanophore stimulating hormone* which perhaps contributes to the pigmentation of pregnancy.

HYPERPITUITARISM results from multiplication of eosinophil cells in the anterior lobe with hypersecretion of the growth hormones causing *Gigantism* and *Acromegaly. Cushing's Syndrome* may occur with a basophil adenoma of the anterior pituitary but it is usually due to adrenal cortex hyperplasia.

HYPOPITUITARISM from disease or destruction of the anterior lobe in childhood causes *Infantilism. Simmond's disease* is due to destruction or to sudden post-partum necrosis of the anterior lobe (see § 570).

§ 306. The Autonomic Nervous System consists of (1) Sympathetic and (2) Parasympathetic Divisions, which are anatomically and physiologically separate.

The confusion of nomenclature of different writers is troublesome to the student and the following scheme may be found helpful.

Vegetative = AUTONOMIC = Involuntary

Sympathetic
or Thoracolumbar
(from Th1–L2)

Parasympathetic
or Cranio-sacral
(from oculomotor,
facial, glosso-
pharyngeal, vagus,
accessory and S2–4)

The Autonomic Nervous System (Fig. 228) innervates structures which are not under direct voluntary control. These include *smooth muscle* organs, the iris, and *tubular viscera* such as the bronchi, gastro-intestinal and genito-urinary tracts, the lachrymal, sweat and digestive *glands*, the *heart* and *blood-vessels*. Many of these structures have a dual innervation from the sympathetic and parasympathetic divisions, which are physiologically in a state of balanced opposition. When one division is excited, the other is inhibited. Sympathetic stimulation causes a diffuse reaction in several organs, but the result of parasympathetic stimulation is more specific and local.

The *Sympathetic fibres* innervate sweat-glands, constrict the blood-vessels of the skin and viscera, dilate the blood-vessels of muscle and cause erection of the hairs (" goose-flesh "). They also relax the walls and constrict the sphincters of the various hollow viscera, accelerate the heart-rate, deepen respiration and dilate the pupils.

Parasympathetic stimulation causes effects antagonistic to those produced by sympathetic stimulation. Therefore we find contraction of hollow viscera with relaxation of the sphincters (e.g., emptying of the urinary bladder), slowing of the heart-rate, and constriction of the pupil. Blood vessels are little influenced.

I. The **Sympathetic Division** consists of (a) Ganglion cells situated in the lateral horn of the grey matter of the spinal cord extending from the Th1 to L2 level (lateral column); (b) The paravertebral *Sympathetic Chains* lying close to the vertebral column on the two sides and (c) Peripheral *Sympathetic Nerves* (greater, middle and lesser splanchnic nerves) and *Collateral Plexuses* (cardiac, coeliac and hypogastric plexuses). The sympathetic chains and the peripheral plexuses are all that may be seen by the naked eye of the casual dissector. In the thoracic region each ganglion of the chain is connected to its anterior spinal nerve root by two little *rami communicantes*.

Histologically, the sympathetic division is made up of a number of reflex arcs with afferent, intercalary and efferent neurones, as in a spinal reflex arc (Fig. 225). The *afferent neurone* has its cell in the posterior root ganglion and enters the spinal cord to terminate in cells of the lateral column of grey matter. From this column the *intercalary neurone* arises, and passes out of the cord, within the anterior nerve root, which it leaves to enter the corresponding ganglion of the sympathetic chain. The *efferent neurone* arises in the ganglion and joins the anterior nerve root to be distributed with it peripherally. The sympathetic intercalary neurone is called the *white* (myelinated) ramus; the efferent neurone is called the *grey* (unmyelinated) ramus. The student will find it easy to remember that the grey ramus passes *away* from the ganglion. To the naked eye the grey and white rami are indistinguishable, the difference is histological.

The SYMPATHETIC CHAINS consist of 24 ganglia: superior, middle and inferior cervical (stellate) ganglia, 12 ganglia in the thoracic, 4 in the lumbar and 5 in the sacral region. The chains fuse below in front of the coccyx (ganglion impar) and above they break up over the internal carotid arteries. The outflow of intercalary neurones (white rami) from the spinal cord is between Th1 and L2 segments only. These intercalary neurones, when they enter the sympathetic chain ganglia, behave in one of three ways (Fig. 226):—(1) They may terminate here and anastomose with an efferent neurone (e.g., fibres to sweat-glands or blood-vessels). (2) They may pass upwards or downwards in the sympathetic chain to terminate in a ganglion above or below (e.g., fibres from Th1 and 2 passing to the cervical ganglia, and from L1 and 2 passing to the lumbar and sacral ganglia). (3) They may branch in the ganglion of the chain and pass through it to form peripheral sympathetic nerves (e.g., splanchnic) and plexuses (e.g., cœliac).

It is characteristic of the sympathetic division—that there is always a ganglion

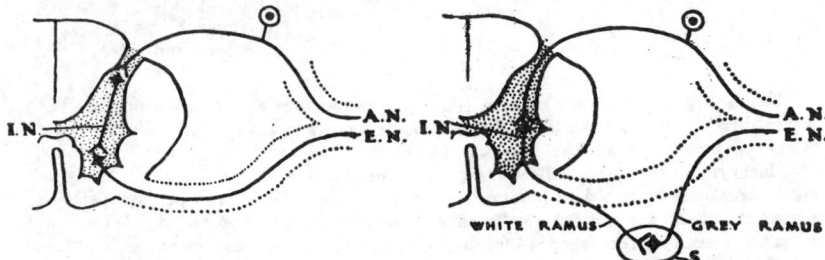

FIG. 225.—Diagram showing AFFERENT (A.N.), INTERCALARY (I.N.) and EFFERENT (E.N.) Neurones in (i.) a spinal and (ii.) in a sympathetic reflex arc. S. indicates the sympathetic ganglion of the paravertebral chain.

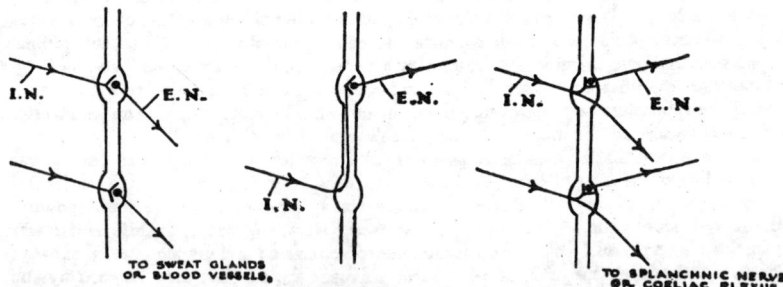

FIG. 226.—Diagram to show the three possible arrangements of intercalary neurones on entering the paravertebral sympathetic chain.

between the cord and the viscus, blood-vessel, or gland supplied by the efferent neurone. The intercalary neurone entering the ganglion is sometimes called the *pre-ganglionic* fibre, the efferent neurone the *post-ganglionic* fibre.

The cells of the lateral column are brought into relationship with the *hypothalamus* through the medial longitudinal bundle and the vestibulo-spinal tract.

CERVICAL SYMPATHETIC fibres (Fig. 227) leave the cord at the Th1 and 2 level to ascend in the cervical sympathetic chain in the dorsal wall of the carotid sheath to the superior cervical ganglion. Here efferent neurones arise and ascend in the carotid plexus into the skull. Thence they pass into the ophthalmic division of the fifth nerve and run via the long ciliary nerves to the eyeball. The cervical sympathetic is the tonic dilator of the pupil. The pupil-dilating fibres have a special course. Arising from a paraventricular nucleus in the hypothalamus they traverse the brain-stem, descending in the lateral column of the spinal cord to emerge as preganglionic fibres through the ventral roots of Th1 and 2. Thence they enter the inferior cervical ganglion of the sympathetic chain as white rami communicantes ascending as post-ganglionic fibres in the cervical chain to enter the skull. The pupillary fibres (pupillo-dilator) pass along the ophthalmic division of the trigeminal to the cavernous plexus, and via the long ciliary nerves to the radial fibres of the pupil. They traverse but are not relayed in the ciliary ganglion. The middle cervical ganglion gives fibres to the thyroid gland, and the stellate and upper thoracic ganglia furnish accelerator fibres to the heart and vaso-constrictor fibres to the arms. The Stellate ganglion is formed by the fusion of the Inferior Cervical and 1st Thoracic ganglia.

Destruction of the cervical sympathetic occurs from damage to the medulla, cervical cord, Th1 and 2 spinal roots and to the carotid sheath in the neck. The resultant HORNER'S SYNDROME consists of a small pupil, narrowing of the ocular fissure

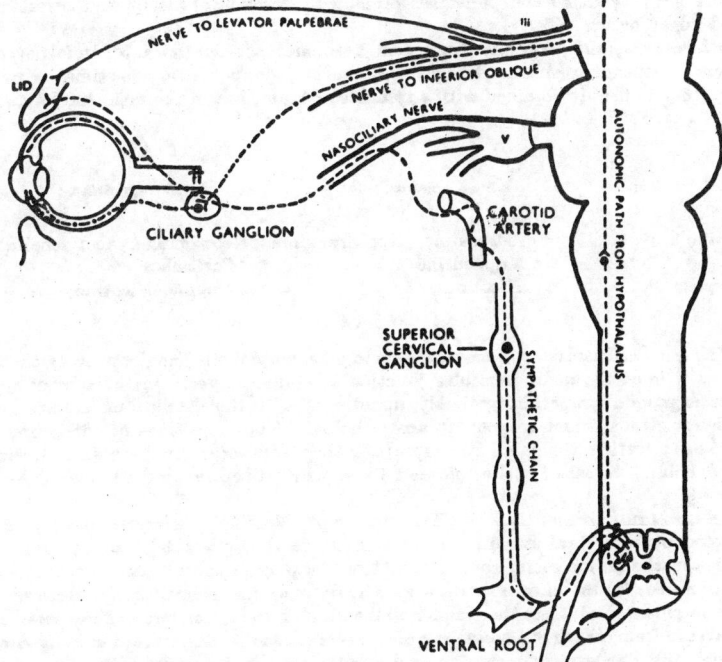

FIG. 227.—Diagram of the course of the oculo-sympathetic fibres. (From Gordon Holmes, *Introduction to Clinical Neurology.* E. & S. Livingstone, Edinburgh.)

from paralysis of the unstriped muscle of the levator palpebræ superioris, apparent but not real enophthalmos and vasodilatation with absence of sweating on the face and neck. Irritative lesions of the cervical sympathetic cause opposite effects. Excision of the *stellate ganglion* will cause in addition similar changes in the blood vessels and sweat glands in the upper limbs, with insignificant slowing of the heart.

II. The **Parasympathetic Division** has two main outflows from the central system:
(a) The Cranial Outflow and (b) The Sacral Outflow. (Fig. 228.)

(a) The CRANIAL OUTFLOW occurs through the oculomotor, facial, glossopharyngeal, vagus and accessory nerves, the ganglion cells being situated in the mid-brain in the oculomotor (Edinger-Westphal) nucleus, and in the medulla in the superior and inferior salivary nuclei and the dorsal nucleus of the vagus. Most bodily structures innervated by the sympathetic have also a parasympathetic innervation, but the blood-vessels have usually only a sympathetic supply. It is through the vast ramifications of the vagus nerve that the parasympathetic is brought into communication with most of the viscera.

(b) The SACRAL OUTFLOW leaves the spinal cord with S2 and 3 nerves in the cauda equina. They leave the spinal nerves, do not pass through the sacral sympathetic chains, but, forming the nervi erigentes, run directly into the hypogastric ganglia and thence to the walls of the pelvic viscera. As with the sympathetic, there is always a ganglion between the cord and viscus supplied. In the case of the parasympathetic, however, the ganglia lie in the walls of the viscera, so that the preganglionic fibres are long and the post-ganglionic fibres very short.

Stimulation of the parasympathetic causes effects antagonistic to those caused by sympathetic stimulation. The pupil is constricted, the heart rate retarded, the bronchioles constricted and peristalsis promoted; secretion of insulin and lowering of blood sugar occurs.

Pharmacologically, various drugs and hormones act on the autonomic nervous system. Depending on the dosage, sometimes a sympathetic, sometimes a parasympathetic effect is obtained with any one substance, but in the main the following table is true:—

	Sympathetic	Parasympathetic
Stimulating	Adrenaline, Noradrenaline, Ephedrine	Neostigmine, Acetylcholine, Carbachol
Depressing	Nicotine	Atropine, Nicotine

The chemical mediator of transmission in parasympathetic ganglia is acetylcholine just as it is at the neuro-muscular junction in spinal nerves. In the case of sympathetic ganglia sympathin (probably, noradrenaline) is the chemical mediator except for sweat-glands, which respond to acetylcholine. Thus injections of adrenaline do not cause sweating though all other sympathetic effects occur. Nerves which liberate acetylcholine are called *cholinergic* and those which liberate sympathin are termed *adrenergic*.

INNERVATION OF THE URINARY BLADDER (Figs. 228, 229). Micturition is normally initiated by a cerebral stimulus which travels via the pyramidal tracts to activate centres in the lumbo-sacral cord. The MOTOR supply of the bladder involves three sets of fibres: (1) the most important are the detrusor (parasympathetic) fibres which carry impulses to contract the bladder wall and relax the sphincters. These leave the sacral cord from cells in S2-3 segments and travel via the pelvic nerves (nervi erigentes), through the hypogastric plexus to end around cells in intramural plexuses in the bladder wall; from these, short post-ganglionic fibres arise to supply the bladder muscles. (2) The inhibitor (sympathetic) fibres come from cells in the grey matter of the lower dorsal and upper lumbar cord (chiefly D12, L1 and L2), and pursue a very long course through the sympathetic chain and then by devious routes (some via the coeliac and superior mesenteric plexuses, others direct from L3 and L4 ganglia) to collect as the presacral nerves in front of the upper sacrum. These continue as the two hypogastric nerves to end in the hypogastric ganglia on the lateral aspects of the rectum. Here the final cell stations arise to supply the bladder. The activity of the sympathetic helps to retain urine in the bladder. (3) The pudic (internal pudendal) nerves (S3-4) are somatic and supply the prostatic urethra and the external sphincter. The SENSORY nerve supply from the bladder is believed to pass chiefly by parasympathetic fibres upwards with sacral nerve roots (S2-3-4); a less important path is by sympathetic fibres to the paravertebral chain and so to the lumbar cord. Damage to the sacral segments of the spinal cord causes loss of all kinds of bladder sensation. *Bladder pain* can be (a) bursting due to muscle spasm and ischaemia vaguely located suprapubically and in the perineum: and (b) stabbing pain due to mechanical irritation of the trigone or the bladder mucosa and accurately referred to the tip of the penis and the perineum. *Lesions of the Frontal Cortex:* Patients empty their bladder in epileptic fits, in petit mal attacks, as well as in major fits. Patients with frontal lobe tumours who have lost their social sense and have become apathetic pass urine in their clothes. In senile, demented patients the bladder may fill up (retention with overflow) and leak,

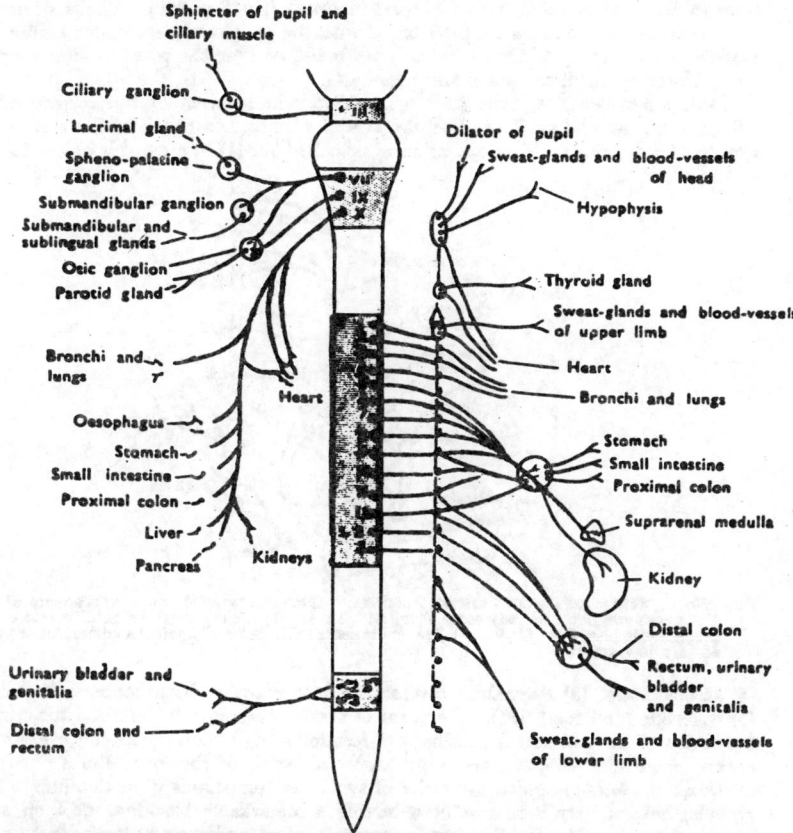

FIG. 228.—SCHEME OF GENERAL ARRANGEMENT OF AUTONOMIC NERVOUS SYSTEM. Pre-ganglionic fibres of the parasympathetic system are in *blue* and of the sympathetic system in *red*. Post-ganglionic fibres of both systems in *black*. Afferent fibres are not included. (From *Cunningham's Textbook of Anatomy.*)

a dangerous state of affairs for which we must always be on the watch in frontal lobe lesions. *Lesions of the Spinal Cord:* In the stage of spinal shock after *acute lesions* there is retention of urine with overflow incontinence. Later on reflex incontinence occurs, *i.e.*, partial relaxation of the sphincter with incomplete evacuation of the bladder. With reflex incontinence there is always *residual urine* which invariably becomes infected. In *chronic lesions* of slow onset (*e.g.*, cord compression) retention with overflow occurs except in " system diseases " of the cord in which the bladder escapes, *e.g.*, motor neurone disease, spino-cerebellar ataxia.

Lesions of L1 and 2 roots (as in cauda equina lesions) cause overflow dribbling. In sacral tabes sensory parasympathetic fibres are damaged and there is incomplete emptying of the bladder from loss of bladder sensation.

INNERVATION OF THE BLOOD-VESSELS OF THE LIMBS is controlled by both nervous and humoral factors. Vaso-constriction is effected through sympathetic pathways (cortico-hypothalamic-spinal) and thence through pre- and post-ganglionic fibres. (a) *Those for the Upper Limbs* leave the spinal cord via the ventral roots from Th2–8. The upper level of the outflow may include Th1. (b) *Those for the Lower Limbs* issue in the ventral roots from Th11–L2 inclusive (see Fig. 228). The majority of these post-ganglionic fibres are distributed with the peripheral nerves, but a minority reach the main artery of the limbs as direct branches from the paravertebral ganglia. Vaso-dilator mechanisms are mainly humoral.

Stellate ganglionectomy produces sympathetic denervation of the corresponding half of the head and neck and ipsilateral upper limbs except the axilla. Horner's syndrome also results. This operation is practised for (1) hyperidrosis of the hands,

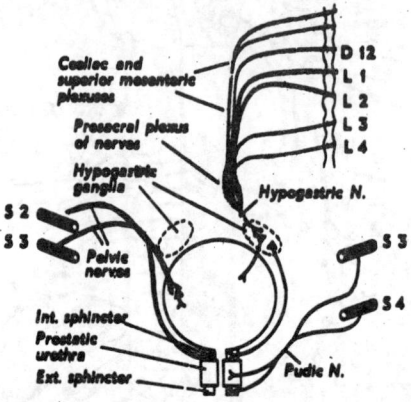

Cœliac and superior mesenteric plexuses

Presacral plexus of nerves

Hypogastric ganglia

Hypogastric N.

D 12
L 1
L 2
L 3
L 4

S 2
S 3

Pelvic nerves

S 3

S 4

Int. sphincter
Prostatic urethra
Ext. sphincter

Pudic N.

FIG. 229.—INNERVATION OF THE URINARY BLADDER. Afferents are not shown. (a) The sympathetic fibres (pre-ganglionic in red) come from D12, L1–4. (b) The parasympathetic detrusor (pre-ganglionic in blue) from S2, 3. (c) The pudic nerve to the external sphincter comes from somatic S3, 4 spinal nerves.

(2) acrocyanosis, (3) Raynaud's disease, (4) late vascular disturbances of frostbite, (5) causalgia (and see § 821). Removal of the *lumbar chain* is practised for trophic ulceration of the feet and legs, blue cold feet following poliomyelitis and other vaso-spastic conditions affecting the superficial circulation of the lower limbs.

Ganglion blocking agents. A series of synthetic compounds (" methonium " compounds) has recently been produced having a remarkable blocking effect on autonomic synapses. Hexamethonium, pentamethonium and mecamylamine act in this way and produce lowering of the blood pressure by reducing vaso-motor tone. In surgery where profuse hæmorrhage might be a hazard, *e.g.*, vascular surgery, these drugs lower blood pressure and paralyse the functions which conserve heat. The body temperature may thus be lowered to about 30° C by extreme cooling, reducing cell metabolism and the need for oxygen (hibernation technique).

§ 807. The Cerebral Ventricles.—In each cerebral hemisphere lies a *lateral ventricle* having three horns meeting in the parietal region. The anterior horn is deeply indented on its lateral surface by the head of the caudate nucleus. The temporal or descending horn is smaller and extends into the temporal lobe. The occipital or posterior horn is very inconstant in size and length. The anterior horns in their posterior two-thirds are separated only by the thin septum lucidum. The occipital horns are somewhat widely separated, while the temporal horns diverge more markedly *from one another.* The lateral ventricles communicate through small apertures called interventricular foramina (of Monro) with a single median cavity, the *third ventricle*, which lies between the thalami. The third ventricle communicates with the infundibulum or pituitary stalk, and posteriorly by the long narrow aqueduct through the mid-brain with the *fourth ventricle* which lies between the bulb and cerebellum. The fourth ventricle opens into the subarachnoid space by three foramina, one in the median dorsal line (foramen of Magendie) and two laterally near the flocculi of the cerebellum (foramina of Luschka).

The Cerebrospinal Fluid.—The central nervous system is enclosed in the bony case of the skull and vertebral column, and is suspended in a water-cushion of cerebrospinal fluid (C.S.F.). This fluid is formed by the ependymal-covered choroid plexuses of the lateral, third and fourth ventricles, by a process of dialysis. The total amount of fluid normally present within the cranio-spinal dura mater is 120–150 cu. ml. From the lateral ventricles the fluid passes through the foramina of Monro into the third ventricle and thence by the aqueduct of Sylvius to the fourth. It leaves the ventricular system by the medial foramen of Magendie in the roof of the fourth ventricle and the bilateral foramina of Luschka, one in each lateral recess of the fourth ventricle.

Within the subarachnoid space, the cerebrospinal fluid bathes the whole surface of the brain and spinal cord. The fluid circulates forward through the basal cisterns, passes through the opening between the tentorium and the brain-stem and upwards over the surface of the hemispheres, to be absorbed directly into the cranial venous sinuses by way of the arachnoid villi. These villi are invaginations of the subarachnoid space through the fibrous dural wall of the sinuses and project into their lumen. It is possible that some absorption may take place through perivascular spaces, into the cerebral capillaries, but this is of subordinate importance.

The *subarachnoid space*, in which the cerebrospinal fluid circulates, is traversed by numerous delicate trabeculæ stretching from the arachnoid on the outer side to the pia on the inner. Within this space lie the cerebral and spinal blood-vessels, and it is crossed by the cranial and spinal nerves. All these structures, like the walls of the subarachnoid space, are covered by flattened mesothelial cells.

The subarachnoid space dips into the sulci and is continued as sleeve-like channels surrounding the pial vessels into the brain substance. These perivascular spaces were first described by Virchow and Robin, and they are called *Virchow-Robin Spaces*. They subdivide with the blood-vessels, and eventually communicate within the cerebral substance with pericellular spaces about the nerve cells. The Virchow-Robin spaces normally empty into the subarachnoid space, and, in inflammatory conditions affecting the central nervous system, they are packed with cells. Seen on a cross-section, they present the so-called " perivascular cuffing " appearance.

It is possible that the C.S.F., when secreted, contains neither cells nor protein, these being added to it in the course of its circulation, from the perivascular spaces. It is possible also that the lymph from the peripheral nerves may pass into the subarachnoid space by way of the nerve-roots.

Normal cerebrospinal fluid is clear and colourless. Whereas the ventricular fluid is almost non-albuminous and cell-free, the fluid obtained normally from the dependent spinal theca by lumbar puncture contains not more than 4 lymphocytes per cubic millimetre, 0·025 to 0·03 per cent. protein, 0·05 to 0·08 per cent. glucose and 0·725 per cent. chlorides (Table LXVI). Spinal fluid, obtained by lumbar puncture, is normally under a pressure of 60 to 150 mm. of water (§ 1201) when the patient is horizontal.

Certain deep expansions of the subarachnoid space, called *Cisterns*, exist at the base of the brain. Of these the most important are (1) the *cisterna magna*, situated between the inferior vermis and the medulla, and extending outwards on each side beneath the cerebellar hemispheres; and (2) the *cisterna basalis*, in the neighbourhood of the interpeduncular space, in which lie the Circle of Willis and the third nerves. The subarachnoid space sends important funnel-shaped prolongations along the spinal nerves as far as their foramina of exit from the dura mater, and within the cranium there are important prolongations (*a*) along the trigeminal nerve; so that the Gasserian ganglion is enclosed in a tiny pool of cerebrospinal fluid, the cave of Meckel. The perilymph of the internal ear communicates through a special cochlear aqueduct with the cerebrospinal fluid in the subarachnoid space.

Surface Markings.—The *Central* (*Rolandic*) *Fissure* is identified by taking a point midway between the nasion (root of the nose) and the external occipital protuberance, and drawing a line from a point 1 cm. behind this, downwards and forwards, at an angle of 67½ degrees, *i.e.*, three-quarters of a right angle (easily obtained by folding the square edge of a card appropriately) with the mid-line.

The *Spinal Cord* terminates in the conus medullaris, which is opposite the first lumbar spinous process, while the *spinal theca* and subarachnoid space reach as low as the level of the second sacral spinous process.

§ 808. The Cranial Venous Sinuses.—The walls of the venous sinuses consist of dura mater. They drain blood from the brain and meninges, and cerebro-spinal fluid passes into these sinuses through the Pacchionian bodies. They empty into the internal jugular vein and communicate with the veins of the head and neck through the orbital vein and various emissary veins, the most important of which is the large mastoid emissary vein. The chief sinuses are the Superior Longitudinal, the Lateral, the Straight and the Cavernous. The basal sinuses, *e.g.*, Lateral and Cavernous, communicate freely, but the *Superior Longitudinal Sinus*, which drains the cortical veins, opens only into the Torcular Herophili, and obstruction of this sinus leads to widespread bilateral cortical necrosis, characterised, clinically, by a paraplegia from destruction of the cortical motor leg areas.

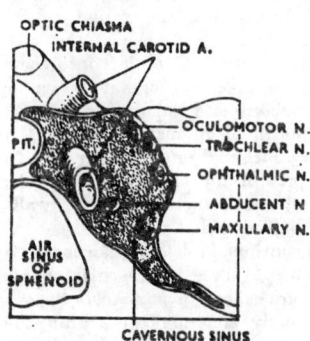

OPTIC CHIASMA
INTERNAL CAROTID A.
PIT.
OCULOMOTOR N.
TROCHLEAR N.
OPHTHALMIC N.
ABDUCENT N
MAXILLARY N.
AIR SINUS OF SPHENOID
CAVERNOUS SINUS

Fig. 230. Oblique Section through the Right Cavernous Sinus.

The Straight Sinus runs medially between the two halves of the tentorium cerebelli, draining the choroidal veins and the great vein of Galen.

The Lateral Sinus drains the veins of the posterior fossa and runs from the external occipital protuberance, in an arched fashion forwards and downwards, to open into the internal jugular vein through the jugular foramen. It occupies a groove in the mastoid part of the temporal bone (sigmoid sinus) and communicates with the mastoid emissary vein.

Obstruction causes œdema over the mastoid process.

The reticulated *Cavernous Sinuses* lie on either side of the sphenoidal air cells, draining the veins at the base of the brain and the orbital veins. They communicate with one another by means of the circular sinus, anteriorly with the ophthalmic and facial veins and posteriorly through the superior and inferior petrosal sinuses with the lateral and sigmoid sinuses. Thrombosis of the lateral sinuses may thus spread into first one cavernous sinus and then the other. On the medial wall of the cavernous sinus lies the internal carotid artery, with the abducent nerve. The oculomotor, trochlear and ophthalmic divisions of the trigeminal nerve pass forwards, on the lateral wall of the sinus, to enter the orbit through the sphenoidal fissure. These structures are separated from the blood in the sinus only by its lining membrane (Fig. 230). *Occlusion or compression of the cavernous sinus* causes proptosis (protrusion of the eyeball) with orbital œdema, ocular palsies, and pain and sensory loss over the first and second divisions of the trigeminal nerve.

The Jugular Foramen: This important aperture in the anterior and medial part of the floor of the posterior fossa of the skull transmits not only the internal jugular vein, but also the glossopharyngeal, vagus and spinal accessory nerves.

§ 809. Spinal and Cerebral Arteries and their Syndromes.—The Vertebral

ARTERIES, before entering the foramen magnum, give off the *anterior spinal* and two *posterior spinal arteries*. These run downwards the entire length of the cord, forming, with their anastomoses, a vascular chain reinforced by branches of the intercostal and lumbar arteries, entering the vertebral column through the intervertebral foramina, and running along the anterior and posterior nerve roots. The ANTERIOR SPINAL ARTERY supplies all the structures within the cord except the dorsal portions of the posterior columns and the tip of the posterior horns of grey matter (posterior spinal arteries). Occlusion of the anterior spinal artery leads to a partial transverse softening of the spinal cord extending over several segments. On entering the foramen magnum, the Vertebral arteries give off the *Posterior inferior cerebellar arteries* and unite at the lower border of the pons to form the BASILAR ARTERY (Fig. 231).

The *Posterior Inferior Cerebellar Artery* supplies the lateral aspect of the medulla, including the superior cerebellar peduncle, part of the " nucleus of the spinal tract " of the trigeminal (§ 803), the lemniscus, the decussating arcuate fibres of the lemniscus, and the glossopharyngeal-vagus nucleus. Lesions of this artery produce " Cerebellar Apoplexy " with acute vertigo and hemiataxy, paralysis of the pharynx, soft palate and vocal cord, with sympathetic oculo-pupillary signs all on the side of the lesion, with a dissociated anæsthesia so that pain and temperature sensation is lost on the opposite side of the body but on the same side of the face; touch sensation is unaffected in both areas (*unilateral bulbar syndrome*) (Fig. 223).

The *Basilar Artery* supplies branches to the pons, and two large branches, the *superior cerebellar arteries*, to the upper cerebellum, and divides at the level of the crura of the mid-brain to form the two POSTERIOR CEREBRAL ARTERIES (Fig. 231). A sigmoid tortuous basilar artery may compress the vagus nerve, causing a recurrent laryngeal palsy. *Stenosis of the basilar artery* may cause attacks of vertigo and impaired consciousness lasting some minutes in which the patient staggers or falls and is temporarily bereft of speech, basilar insufficiency. Occlusion of the basilar artery may result in a contra-lateral hemiplegia with paralysis of the ipsilateral external rectus and facial muscles from involvement of the sixth and seventh nerve nuclei. Other cases show conjugate ocular palsies.

The Internal Carotid Artery (Fig. 232) enters the skull just laterally to the posterior clinoid processes of the pituitary fossa and gives off the *ophthalmic artery* supplying the globe and orbit. *Complete occlusion of the internal carotid artery* (" carotid hemiplegia ") should (in theory) result in ipsilateral blindness from its ophthalmic branch, with contra-lateral sensory and motor hemiplegia (with aphasia if the lesion is in the dominant hemisphere). Owing to the development of compensatory circulation, and to other causes, partial lesions are seen more frequently than complete occlusions. Anastomoses occur between the ophthalmic artery and branches of the external carotid, the middle and posterior cerebral arteries, and between one internal carotid and the other through the Circle of Willis. The internal carotid arteries divide into MIDDLE and ANTERIOR CEREBRAL ARTERIES, supplying roughly the anterior two-thirds of the cerebral hemispheres (Fig. 233 *a, b, c*).

The anterior, middle and posterior cerebral arteries are connected to form the CIRCLE OF WILLIS in the subarachnoid space at the base of the brain. This circle is occasionally incompletely developed (Fig. 231). It surrounds the optic chiasma and pituitary stalk. One anterior communicating artery unites the two anterior cerebral arteries, branches of the internal carotids. The internal carotids communicate posteriorly by the two posterior communicating arteries with the posterior cerebral arteries (branches of the basilar). Upon the integrity of this hexagon or circle depends the circulation of a cerebral hemisphere when its ipsilateral carotid artery is occluded by thrombosis or by ligature.

The ANTERIOR CEREBRAL ARTERY (Fig. 231) passes anteriorly into the great median fissure, and, curving round the genu of the corpus callosum, runs backwards upon the superior aspect of this structure, supplying its anterior seven-eighths and giving off branches to supply the medial surfaces of the hemispheres as far back as the parieto-occipital fissure, and supplying, in this territory, the cortical areas for the foot

and leg at the top of the pre-central gyrus. The anterior cerebral artery sends perforating branches inwards towards the caudate nucleus. *Obstruction of an anterior
cerebral artery* gives rise to a crural monoplegia or hemiplegia, with sensory impair-

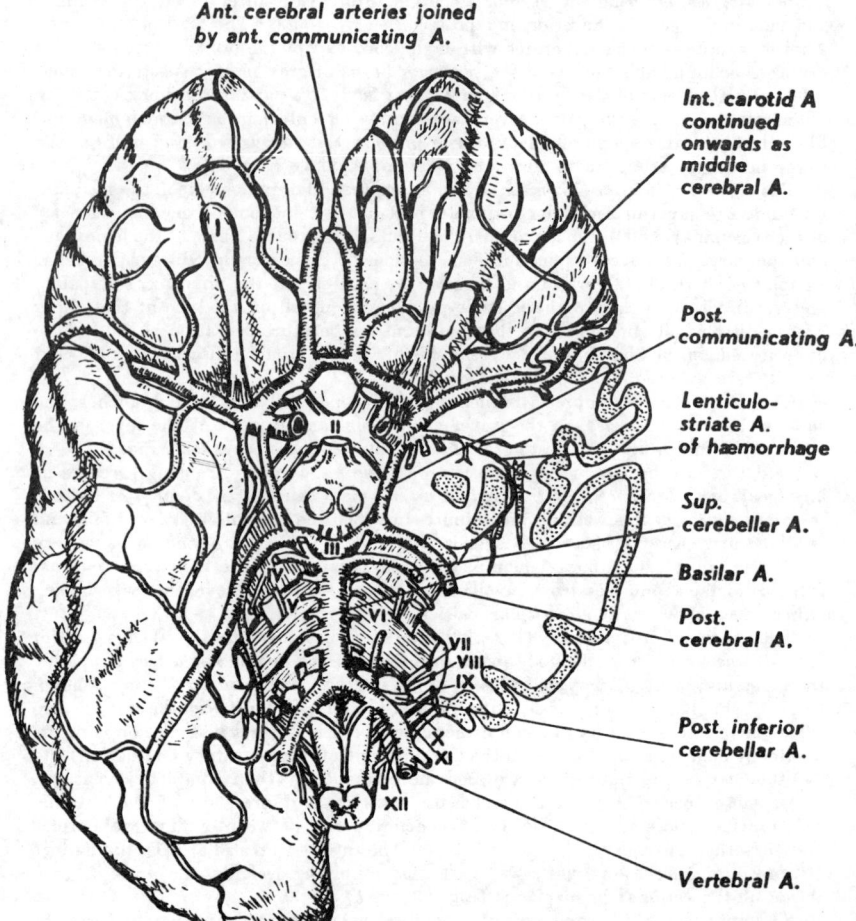

**Ant. cerebral arteries joined
by ant. communicating A.**

**Int. carotid A
continued
onwards as
middle
cerebral A.**

**Post.
communicating A.**

**Lenticulo-
striate A.
of hæmorrhage**

**Sup.
cerebellar A.**

Basilar A.

**Post.
cerebral A.**

**Post. inferior
cerebellar A.**

Vertebral A.

FIG. 231.—THE BASE OF THE BRAIN, showing the arterial distribution and the cranial nerves.—In the
oblique section of the left hemisphere are seen from without inwards—grey matter of the insula and of
the claustrum (grey); external capsule (white); lentiform nucleus (grey); internal capsule (white)
with artery of hæmorrhage; and caudate nucleus (grey). I. Olfactory lobe; II. optic chiasma;
III. bifurcation of basilar artery between the third nerves; IV. (on right crus cerebri), beside
fourth nerve; V. (on pons Varolii), beside fifth nerve; VI. sixth nerve (abducent); VII. facial
nerve; VIII. auditory nerve; IX. glossopharyngeal nerve; X. vagus; XI. spinal accessory; XII.
hypoglossal nerve.

ment, most marked in the leg with apraxia of the left arm from involvement of the
corpus callosum.

The Middle Cerebral (Sylvian) Artery supplies most of the convexity of the cerebral
hemisphere, including the motor, sensory and speech areas of the cortex. Leaving
the Circle of Willis, it gives off several small but important perforating arteries, which

pierce the anterior perforated substance to supply the corpus striatum, thalamus and region of the internal capsule.   These are terminal arteries, without anastomoses, and they are termed the *lenticulo-striate* and *lenticulo-optic* arteries (Fig. 233a, b, c). The middle cerebral artery then runs along the Sylvian fissure to supply the whole of the convexity of the cortex, with the exception of the area supplied by the anterior cerebral artery.   At the occipital pole of the hemisphere it anastomoses over the cortical area for central vision with the posterior cerebral artery.   The middle cerebral artery also supplies, by penetrating branches, the major part of the centrum ovale, including the " temporal knee " of the optic radiations and external capsule. *Occlusion of the middle cerebral artery* may cause severe contra-lateral hemiplegia, hemianæsthesia and hemianopia, with aphasia, sensory agnosia and apraxia if the lesion is in the dominant hemisphere.   It is commoner to meet with partial lesions. When the branch to Broca's area (see p. 1153) is alone affected an isolated motor aphasia results.   The cortical divisions of the middle cerebral artery are called (1) posterior temporal, (2) posterior parietal, and (3) the artery to the angular gyrus (" the Sylvian Group ").

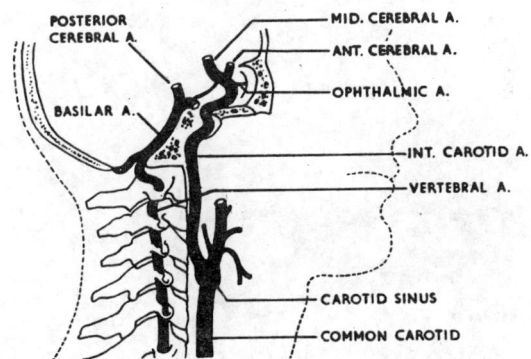

FIG. 232.—THE VERTEBRAL AND CAROTID ARTERIES IN THE NECK.

The Posterior cerebral artery (Fig. 231) winds round the crus, supplying the mid-brain nuclei (corpora quadrigemina, red nucleus, etc.), and the inferior medial surfaces of the temporal and occipital lobes, the uncus, and posterior seventh of the corpus callosum.   It anastomoses, with the middle cerebral artery, over the convexity of the occipital pole (area for central vision).   It gives off an important branch, the *calcarine artery,* to supply the cuneus and lingual gyri, above ana below the calcarine and post-calcarine fissures.   In *obstructive lesions of the posterior cerebral* artery, whilst peripheral vision is destroyed from destruction of the calcarine cortex, the anastomosis with the middle cerebral artery over the occipital pole ensures a blood supply to the area of central vision which, therefore, escapes.   When the deep branches are occluded in addition to contra-lateral hemianopia the *thalamic syndrome* may develop; viz., contra-lateral hemianæsthesia with intolerable spontaneous pain over the affected half of the body.   The thalamus is also supplied by the middle cerebral artery.

The *choroid plexuses* of the lateral ventricles, which have to do with the formation of spinal fluid, are supplied by the choroid branches of the internal carotid and middle cerebral arteries.   The choroid veins drain backwards to join the great vein of Galen, draining into the anterior extremity of the straight sinus in the tentorium cerebelli.

Inhalations of 5–7 per cent. carbon dioxide increase the cerebral circulation by 75 per cent.; whereas high concentrations of oxygen markedly reduce the circulation.

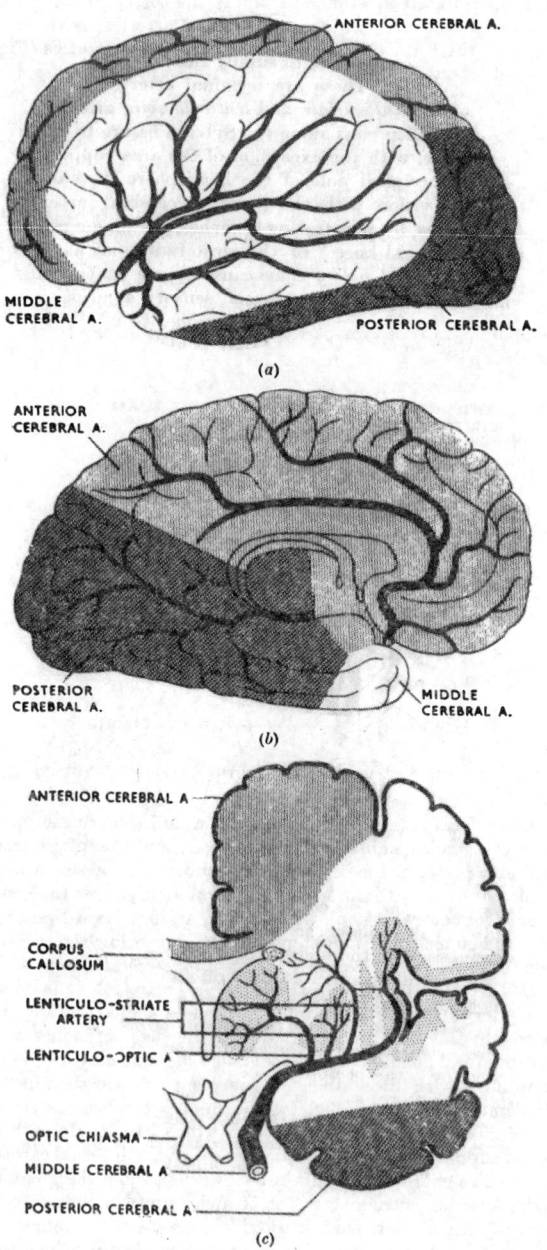

FIG. 233. DISTRIBUTION OF THE CEREBRAL ARTERIES. (*a*) Lateral aspect of left hemisphere, (*b*) Medial aspect of left hemisphere, (*c*) Coronal section of the right hemisphere.

PART A. SYMPTOMATOLOGY

The *subjective* symptoms complained of by patients with neurological disease are for the most part sensory—viz., pain, paræsthesiæ, disordered vision. In many cases, however, the patient will complain of the external indication of his neurological lesion, *e.g.*, loss of power, falling about, unsteadiness in walking. These complaints, whether mainly subjective or mainly objective, are generally of considerable localising value, with the exception of a complaint of headache. The *distribution* of this symptom and its *character*, give information anatomically suggestive which can be fully evaluated in the light of the subsequent detailed physical examination which is essential in all cases. In infants, children and in confused, stuporose, amnesic or dysphasic patients, the antecedent symptoms must be obtained from relatives or friends. When there has been a fit or faint a witness's account, if available, is essential.

Many patients with organic disease have coexistent functional symptoms. This may sometimes be seen in patients with disseminated sclerosis, or in cases of organic dementia in elderly patients.

The chief subjective symptoms of neurological disease are:—

    I. Headache and Neuralgia (§ 810).
   II. Nervousness and Exhaustion, Tremulousness (§ 819).
  III. Pain, Numbness, Tingling in a limb (§ 820).
   IV. Unsteadiness in walking, Falling about, Giddiness (§ 825).
    V. Fainting spells, " Blackouts," Swoons (§ 832).
   VI. Disordered vision—loss of vision, double vision (§ 834).
  VII. Weakness, Stiffness or Difficulty in controlling one or more limbs (§ 835).
 VIII. Disordered sleep (§ 836).

§ **810. I. Headache** is the name given to any feeling of discomfort in the head, not necessarily pain. The stimuli causing headache are believed to arise in the walls of the blood-vessels. *Vaso-dilation* of dural arteries, *displacement* or *traction* on sensitive basal blood-vessels or dural sinuses can evoke pain, although the brain itself, the pia arachnoid and the bones of the skull are all insensitive.

The cause of most headaches can best be elucidated by a full and accurate history and by routine general examination of the whole patient.

Investigation of Headaches: Inquire if there have been previous headaches. Then ask the character of the discomfort (whether it is more pain or more a feeling of pressure); follow these by asking the distribution, the time of onset, whether continuous or periodic. What precipitates and what relieves the symptom. Are there accompaniments, such as vomiting, visual or sensory disturbances. What is the total duration of an attack, and what symptoms occur between the headaches, if any. Is there a family history of headache; or a personal history of head injury, sinusitis, operations, loss of weight. Look for local causes, stiff neck, ocular hypertension or inflammation, sinus tenderness. Listen for an intracranial bruit. In all cases examine the fundi, take the blood pressure and examine the urine.

In chronic or recurrent headaches, X-rays of the nasal sinuses, skull or cervical spine may be revealing. A blood count or blood Wasserman reaction may help.

A *Classification* of headache is difficult. An etiological classification might recognise *psychogenic, vascular, traumatic, toxic, intracranial hypertensive, meningeal, sinus* and *ocular* headaches.

Clinically we recognise (1) Chronic and progressive headaches, (2) Recurrent paroxysmal headaches, and (3) Acute episodic headaches. These categories include headaches due to neurological and general causes. (4) A fourth group clinically contains headaches due to purely *local causes.*

CAUSES OF HEADACHE

(1) *Chronic, progressive headache* (often increasing intracranial pressure or toxæmia).
  (a) PSYCHOGENIC STATES.
  (b) INTRACRANIAL NEOPLASM, ABSCESS OR SUBDURAL HÆMATOMA (including pituitary tumour).
  (c) Uræmia, diabetes and other toxic states.
  (d) Syphilitic meningitis.
  (e) Industrial toxæmia (lead and other poisonings).

(2) *Recurrent paroxysmal headaches* (often vascular).
  (a) MIGRAINE.
  (b) UNRESOLVED CEREBRAL CONTUSION.
  (c) CEREBRAL ARTERIOPATHY (including Temporal Arteritis § 98).
  (d) Arterial hypertension.
  (e) CERVICAL SPONDYLOSIS (Occipital headache).

(3) *Acute episodic headaches* (nearly always organic).
  (a) ONSET OF FEVER, influenza, malaria.
  (b) ALCOHOLIC EXCESS. " Hangover."
  (c) HEAD INJURY.
  (d) SUBARACHNOID HÆMORRHAGE.
  (e) INTRACRANIAL HYPOTENSION (lumbar puncture).
  (f) Heat exhaustion (§ 510).

(4) *Local causes of headaches.*
  (a) Ocular causes—uncorrected refractive error, iritis, glaucoma.
  (b) SINUS DISEASE or abnormality—sinusitis.
  (c) Disease of the skull bones—osteitis deformans, syphilitic osteitis, secondary neoplasm.

(1) CHRONIC PROGRESSIVE HEADACHES. See also Group XV.

A patient constitutionally predisposed to breakdown presents with DISCOMFORT IN THE HEAD PERSISTING FOR DAYS, WEEKS OR MONTHS. *There are no organic signs.—The condition is likely to be a* PSYCHOGENIC STATE.

§ 811. I (a) PSYCHOGENIC HEADACHES: In these the discomfort is continuous and lasts weeks, months, or years. It is described with the use of florid adjectives (" agonising," " appalling "), and metaphor (" like a tight band round my head "). It is often said to be more a sense of pressure than a pain, although pain may occur. It is unrelieved by the usual analgesics such as aspirin or codeine. Such headaches may be the presenting symptom in affective disorders (depression, anxiety), or in hysterical states; but it must never be forgotten that they are met with also in persons who are the subject of organic neurological disease, *e.g.,* arteriopathy or intracranial tumour. Moreover headaches following upon *head injury* may closely resemble psychogenic headache, although due to unresolved bruising of the brain tissue and œdema.

When the HEADACHE *comes on in the early morning, it is so* SEVERE *that the patient holds his head in his hands and vomits, and it passes off during the day only to recur again, suspect increasing* INTRACRANIAL PRESSURE *or* CHRONIC TOXÆMIA.

(*b*) INTRACRANIAL NEOPLASM, ABSCESS OR SUBDURAL HÆMATOMA: Seen during such a headache, the patient says little, as talking makes it worse. Such headaches are accompanied by papilloedema and slowly increasing focal signs. As the headache increases in severity, the patient becomes more and more apathetic, and eventually stuporose. The possibility of a primary neoplasm in the bronchi, stomach or rectum should be kept in mind. *Pituitary tumour* is characteristically associated with bitemporal headache and a feeling of bursting pressure behind the eyes.

(*c*) *Uræmic* headaches may be diagnosed after a comprehensive examination of the patient has shown albuminuria, arterial hypertension, œdema, retinopathy. Diabetic headaches also are revealed by examination of the urine and the retinæ.

(*d*) *Syphilitic meningo-encephalitis* may be revealed by finding an Argyll-Robertson pupil, by a history of exposure to infection or family history of lues and by finding appropriate serological reactions in the blood and spinal fluid.

(*e*) *Industrial toxæmias*, *e.g.*, lead, methylbromide, etc., cause symptoms similar to those of uræmia.

(2) RECURRENT PAROXYSMAL HEADACHES.

An adolescent or young adult with a FAMILY HISTORY *of similar attacks, complains of recurrent paroxysm of* UNILATERAL *spreading head pains,* PHOTOPHOBIA *and " BILIOUSNESS," preceded perhaps by transitory visual aura. The condition is probably* MIGRAINE.

§ 812. (*a*) **Migraine** (Syn. Sick headaches, bilious attacks).—The headaches are paroxysmal, recurrent and date from adolescence. Each attack lasts 4 to 48 hours or longer. In typical migraine two phases can often be distinguished—(i.) the aura, (ii.) the headache. (i.) The *aura* lasts 15–20 minutes. The commonest aura is *visual* and consists of glittering zig-zag lines, curved or straight castellated or " fortification " figures, often in movement in one half of the field of vision (teichopsia, visual spectrum). There may be a scotoma or hemianopia blotting out part of the vision. Scotoma or scintillations may occur singly or together affecting sometimes one half of the visual field, sometimes the other. *Paræsthesiæ* constitute a less frequent aura. If they occur in the right hand and round the lips and tongue in right-handed people, there may be transient difficulty in finding words (dysphasia) or in writing (dysgraphia). Much less commonly transient *vertigo* or *double vision* lasting 2–3 minutes are met as a migrainous aura.

(ii.) The *headache* succeeds, or is contemporary with the aura; it never precedes it. Typically the headache starts in one frontal region, spreading to the opposite side of the head: sometimes, however, it remains a " hemicrania," confined to one half of the head. It is accompanied by photophobia, flushing, pallor, or by *vomiting* or faint feelings. The pain lasts

4 to 48 hours and may leave the patient exhausted if the attack has been unduly prolonged. During an attack unequal pupils may be observed. Attacks may be heralded by bouts of euphoria, anxiety or depression. They may be precipitated by menstruation, eyestrain, or dietetic indiscretions. Paroxysms occur at varying intervals and may consist of (1) recurrent headaches, (2) recurrent headaches with vomiting, (3) the aura with a subsequent headache, or (4) the aura alone.

SPECIAL TYPES OF MIGRAINE. (1) *Abdominal migraine*—Attacks of colic due to tonic spasm of the colon occur singly or alternate with classical migraine headaches. (2) *Trigeminal migraine*—The pain radiates to the face or supra-orbital region, *sometimes on one side, sometimes on the other.* It may be retro-orbital and accompanied by suffusion of the eye or ptosis. Such cases, if the pain is always on one side, raise the suspicion of retro-orbital aneurysm or tumour. First attacks may simulate the pain of glaucoma, iritis or trigeminal neuralgia. (For Migrainous Neuralgia see § 818.) (3) *Transient hemiparesis* is very rare. Unless the patient is a child, suspect a focal intracranial cause, *e.g.*, vascular anomaly or tumour. There may be a family history of this condition. The hemiplegia is often thought to be due to head injury sustained playing some game, but it is transient, lasting a few hours only, and recurs on one or other side of the body. (4) *Permanent visual field changes* (*e.g.* hemianopia) are rare and are usually due to prolonged spasm of the retinal or cerebral arteries. Listen for an intracranial bruit and suspect a focal cause if the vessels of the fundi are normal. (5) *Status migrainosus.* The headache in such cases may last for days and there may be evidences of emotional upset. In order not to confuse these cases with *leaking cerebral aneurysm* or *meningitis* it may be necessary to perform spinal puncture. (6) *Ophthalmoplegic migraine* (§ 1067).

SYMPTOMATIC MIGRAINE. A migraine syndrome may betoken focal or general disease. It may be due to intracerebral neoplasm, leaking saccular aneurysm of the brain or an angiomatous malformation. (1) When a *migraine syndrome* is encountered for the first time in middle age, or (2) if the pain or aura is constantly referred to one side, suspect a focal intracranial cause. This is confirmed if there is fever, neck stiffness, a permanent residual weakness of limbs or alteration in the reflexes, or if an intracranial bruit on auscultating the skull can be heard. In *epilepsy* and *polycythæmia* attacks like migraine occur. In emotional patients, subject to eyestrain and tension, migraine-like attacks may occur as an occupational disorder, and they improve or disappear when the environment is changed.

Diagnosis.—Headaches resembling migraine occur in tumours of the occipital lobe and in chronic nephritis with uræmia. The diagnosis of migraine is made on the recurring paroxysms of headache, the unilateral character of the headache, the accompanying phenomena, and the absence of objective signs of disease. The slowness of the aura in migraine is of great value in the diagnosis from Jacksonian, visual or other epilepsy, as the duration of an epileptic aura is but a few seconds.

Etiology.—Markedly hereditary and familial in most cases, the disease may be associated also with allergy or epilepsy in siblings. The pain of migraine which is temporarily abolished by pressure on the ipsilateral carotid is believed to be due to dilatation of the vessel walls of the external

carotid artery.   The pain is increased by intravenous injection of histamine..
The neurological symptoms of migraine in contrast with the headache are
thought to be due to initial vascular spasm.

Exciting causes of attacks are (1) psychological stress, (2) anoxia, (3)
fatigue, (4) uncorrected refractive errors, (5) cervical spondylosis, (6)
chronic infection or anæmia.   Precipitating factors are extremely variable,
dietetic indiscretions, driving at night, exposure to glare or prolonged
eyestrain are mentioned as "triggers" by those who suffer from the
malady.   Anxiety is the commonest cause of a sudden increase in the
severity or duration of the attacks.   There is often an exacerbation at
the menopause.

Prognosis.—No radical treatment is possible and attacks tend to last
throughout life.   Many sufferers have years of freedom from attacks.

Treatment.—1. *Unless attention is paid to psychological and environmental factors, treatment may be of little avail.*   The cause of increased
severity of attacks rarely lies in the teeth, sinuses, or in uncorrected errors
of refraction, although these should be reviewed.   In older patients co-
existent cervical spondylosis or supervening cerebral arteriopathy may
intensify the headaches.

2. *Prevention of Attacks.*   The object of treatment is to break the
sequence of the attacks.   If they are not disabling all that may be
necessary is reassurance that these symptoms, though alarming, are not
dangerous.   In cases where the attacks are disabling give phenobarbitone gr. ½–1 at bedtime throughout periods of stress, or until the patient
has been free of severe headaches for several months.   For patients who
cannot take phenobarbitone, give nightly soluble aspirin, gr. 10, with a
morning alkaline drink, *e.g.*, sodium bicarbonate gr. 30 in a wineglassful
of water.   Thrice daily glucose, ½ oz. with meals, helps some.   A vaso-
dilator and sedative such as Gower's mixture is worth trial:—sod. bromidi
gr. 10, liq. trinitrini ℳ 1, liq. strychninæ ℳ 3, acid hydrochlor. dil. ℳ 10,
tinct. gelsemii ℳ 5, aq. chloroformi ad fl. oz. ½ t.i.d., p.c.   Tab. methysergide (Deseril) 1 mg. is often helpful for severe recurrent attacks.

3. *In the Attacks.*   When an attack begins, oral ergotamine tartrate
1–2 mg. with hot coffee or tea helps many.   Drugs given by mouth are
frequently vomited or are ineffective; then use 1–2 suppositories of Cafergot.
In all severe cases ergotamine tartrate 0·25–0·50 mg. (½–1 ml.) oily solution
should be injected from a warmed ampoule under the fascia lata of the
thigh.   Patients may be taught to give themselves the injection, which
often diminishes the severity and duration of the attacks.   In *status
migrainosus* give soluble phenobarbitone gr. 3 (180 mg.) intramuscularly,
in addition to repeated injections of ergotamine tartrate 8-hourly.

Ergotamine tartrate should not be given to hypertensive patients or
during pregnancy or menstruation as it is liable to cause uterine colic.
In sensitive individuals ergotamine may produce vomiting, diarrhœa,
paræsthesiæ in the limbs or cramps in the abdomen.   In these cases
give dihydroergotamine tartrate 1 mg. orally or by injection, with caffeine

by mouth. Powders or tablets containing antipyrin are dangerous when used repeatedly, producing agranulocytosis.

§ **813.** (*b*) **Unresolved Cerebral Contusion** (Syn. Post-contusional syndrome).—*After minor closed head injuries* the symptoms are (1) localised headaches intensified by exertion, noise or alteration in posture, (2) giddiness, (3) inability to concentrate. There may be accompanying local tenderness of the scalp. Slight facial weakness, pupillary abnormalities and alteration in the reflexes may be present. Tolerance for alcohol is diminished. If there is a dilated fixed pupil, suspect a subdural clot. The symptoms are due to cerebral œdema persisting round the bruised area of the brain. Owing to the lack of elasticity of the dura the reactionary swelling does not resolve as in a superficial contusion, say of the skin, but may persist for many months. *Treatment.*—Contusion headaches may be prevented by adequate bed rest after head injury. Rest the patient in bed propped into the position which affords greatest relief. Sedation is usually necessary, phenobarb. gr. ½, twice or thrice daily, with a morning saline aperient. Convalescence should be graduated with progressive increase of physical and mental activity. When patients develop such headaches during convalescence from head injury, it is an indication for one to three weeks' further bed rest. If the pretraumatic personality is good, the prognosis is usually favourable. Occupational therapy helps during convalescence.

If there is litigation pending, patients who have suffered head injuries may develop *Compensation* or *traumatic hysteria* (§ 1174). The doctor may not be told at first about the litigation. These cases have other symptoms, *e.g.*, sleeplessness, loss of weight, irritability. Here the prognosis is unfavourably influenced by the overlying neurosis.

After severe generalised *Contusion of the brain*, personality change, memory defect, emotional lability, occur with evidence of focal damage, dysphasia, agnosia, hemiparesis, hemianopia. The mental changes may be transient or develop into a chronic *Traumatic psychosis*.

§ **814.** (*c*) **Cerebral Arteriopathy.**—Cerebral arteriosclerosis is common and headaches in hypertensive subjects may well be due to some other cause, *e.g.*, intracranial neoplasm or aneurysm. In Malignant hypertension (§ 79) the headache is accompanied by giddiness, effort dyspnœa, hypertensive retinopathy, albuminuria and nitrogen retention. The course is progressive and interrupted by convulsive attacks or focal symptoms, from which the patient may make an apparently good recovery until terminal uræmia or cerebral hæmorrhage occur.

(*d*) ARTERIAL HYPERTENSION (Hypertensive encephalopathy). A further rise in an already high blood pressure precipitates a hypertensive crisis. The headache when accompanied by papillœdema raises the suspicion of an intracranial space-occupying lesion. Sudden and transient paralyses occur—Jacksonian attacks, dysphasias, hemianopias which clear rapidly, leaving little or no trace (see § 851).

(e) CERVICAL SPONDYLOSIS. Degeneration of the disc tissue and vertebral bodies of the cervical spine causes painful stiffness of the neck and recurrent attacks of pain which may be referred to the occipito-cervical region (§ 596, 5). Numbness and tingling in the occipital area may be present. Some cases have radicular and long tract signs (§ 1018).

(3) ACUTE EPISODIC HEADACHES.

(a) *Fevers* particularly associated with headache are influenza, typhoid, smallpox, malaria, dengue, and those producing meningitis.

(b) The headache of a " hangover " following *Alcoholic excess* is of the vascular type and is associated with depression, nausea and remorse. Chronic alcoholics may suffer from morning headaches and vomiting.

(c) *A minor head injury* may cause an acute episodic headache.

(d) *Subarachnoid hæmorrhage* may commence with acute episodic or recurrent acute headaches if due to a " leaking " aneurysm.

§ 815. (e) **Lumbar Puncture Headache** (Syn. *Intracranial Hypotension*). The headache is orthostatic, *i.e.*, relieved by the patient adopting the horizontal position. Slight neck stiffness, vomiting and photophobia may be present for 7 to 10 days after the puncture. Meningeal infection or irritation should be suspected if the symptoms continue when the patient is in the horizontal position, or if the temperature is elevated. Lumbar puncture headaches are common in disseminated sclerosis, rare in neurosyphilis; they are believed to be due to leakage of spinal fluid through the puncture hole in the dura.

Prevention.—Use a fine lumbar puncture needle recently sharpened and bevelled. After the puncture keep the patient strictly horizontal for 24 hours, see that meals are taken lying down, from a tray at the bedside, and raise the foot of the bed.

Treatment.—Give 50–100 mg. pethidine intramusc. with 0·5 ml. Pitressin, and fluids by mouth. Sometimes sterile normal saline 10–30 ml. given intrathecally may help. If there is infection, treat systemically for meningitis; culture the organism and determine its sensitivity to antibiotics.

(4) THE LOCAL CAUSES OF HEADACHES are mostly connected with diseases of the eyes or sinuses or the bones of the skull.

(a) *Ocular headaches* may be due to (i) uncorrected refraction errors such as hypermetropia and astigmatism, and defective convergence; (ii) prolonged use of the eyes under conditions of emotional strain or where there is close work; (iii) some develop symptoms in picture galleries, cinemas or looking at television; (iv) iridocyclitis and glaucoma are painful eye diseases causing headache (§§ 1109, 1110, 1120).

(b) SINUS HEADACHE. Disease of the nasal accessory sinuses is an important cause of pain referred to the supra-orbital region or to the teeth. These headaches are intermittent, and are characteristically accompanied by œdema of the orbital tissues (in frontal sinusitis) or of the face (in antral suppuration) and are relieved by a gush of pus from the nose. Local tenderness is often present on palpating or percussing the wall of the sinus, or in the case of the frontal sinus, on upward pressure from the orbit on the floor of the sinus. Fœtor may be present. The sinus affected does not transilluminate clearly. Suppuration in the ethmoidal sinuses is characterised by pain over the nasal bridge, behind the eyes or over the temples (and see § 179).

(c) *Diseases of the skull bones.* *Osteitis deformans* (Paget's disease of bone) may cause retro-orbital headaches long before there is any enlargement of the skull. Inflammatory or neoplastic infiltration of the skull bones may cause local swelling, tenderness and headache.

HEADACHES IN CHILDREN are due to similar causes. Migraine with its variant Cyclical vomiting, Head injury, Increasing intracranial pressure are important. Brain tumours are not infrequent in childhood. Look for infection of the nasal sinuses, and for Urinary infection. After a nocturnal fit a child may waken with a headache. Psychogenic headaches occur as in adults, but should not be lightly diagnosed.

§ 816. **Neuralgia** is a term popularly applied to pains in the face and neck. These pains tend to follow a peripheral nerve distribution; one or other division of the trigeminal, the sensory branches of the glossopharyngeal or vagus nerves, or the sensory divisions of C1–3 roots.

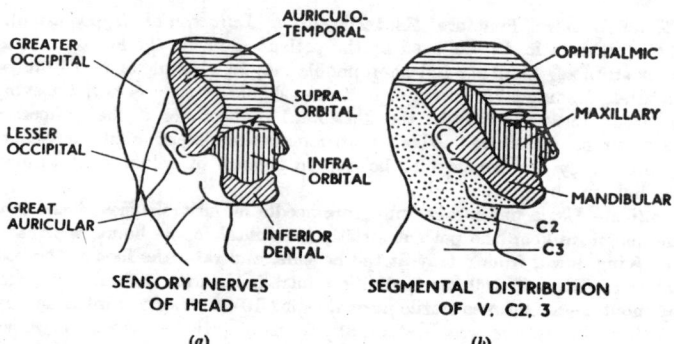

FIG. 234.—SENSORY AREAS OF THE HEAD AND FACE. (a) Distribution of the peripheral sensory nerves; (b) the sensory segmental distribution of the three divisions of the trigeminal nerve, and of C2 and C3.

(a) POST-HERPETIC TRIGEMINAL PAIN. Following an attack of herpes zoster in an elderly or aged person, pain persists after the vesicles disappear. The pain is confined to the distribution of the trigeminus, usually the first division. It is constant and accompanied by paræsthesiæ, a feeling of burning, rawness or prickling with the pain. Debility and continued pain cause intense depression.

Treatment.—Codeine phosphate gr. ¼ 6-hourly or chlorpromazine help the pain. These may be supplemented by daily injections of 1,000 μg. of cyanocobalamin B.P. (vitamin B$_{12}$) or vasopressin (B.P.), 10 units, intramusc. If, after three to four months the pain continues and is making life unbearable, deep X-ray treatment to the Gasserian ganglion should be tried. Alcohol injection of the ganglion is ineffective. In the worst cases frontal leucotomy may be considered as a last resort.

§ 817. (b) **Trigeminal Neuralgia** (Syn. Tic Douloureux) is a complex neuralgia characterised by (1) paroxysms of repetitive and intense pain in the distribution of one or more divisions of the fifth cranial nerve; (2) clonic twitchings of the facial muscles on the side affected, and (3) unilateral lachrymation, rhinorrhœa or sialorrhœa with flushing of the face during the paroxysms of pain. The condition runs a cyclical course with re-

missions over a great number of years. It is a disease of the aged, though
rarely it may occur in middle life. Females are more often affected than
males. Major and minor types of the neuralgia occur. *Symptoms.*—
The pain commonly commences in the second division, less often in the
third (see Fig. 234*b*) and rarely in the first division. It is described as
stabbing " like red-hot needles or wires," " like an explosion of fireworks
on my face ! " This pain of truly awful severity is brought on by cold air,
blowing on the cheek, talking, eating, washing the face, or a sudden jar
when walking. Pressure on certain " trigger-zones," the red margin of
the lip, the angle of the ala nasi and cheek may start off a bout of pain.
Such sufferers leave off wearing dentures, they walk rigidly and gingerly,
speak without moving their jaws and indicate the site of the pain with the
forefinger held over the cheek, but rarely touching it. They cannot shave
or wash the face; and the cheek or eyebrow on the affected side may show
an accumulation of desquamated epithelium and dirt. In third-division
neuralgias unilateral furring of the tongue may be present owing to its
relative immobility in the mouth. In severe bouts, which may last two
to three weeks, the patient wastes rapidly from lack of food and sleep.
After many years the pain may affect the other side of the face.

Diagnosis.—The diagnostic criteria are (1) the pain is confined to the
anatomical boundaries of the fifth nerve, and (2) is strictly unilateral,
(3) no objective impairment of sensibility is present, (4) cranial nerve
palsies are absent. The explosive character of the pain is characteristic.
BILATERAL facial pains and paræsthesiæ are due to vascular disease or
angioneuroses. UNILATERAL pain with sensory impairment over the first
and second divisions of the trigeminal nerve with unilateral ophthalmoplegia occurs in *saccular aneurysms* in the cavernous sinus. Recurrent
trigeminal pain in the young without signs suggest *trigeminal migraine.*
Trigeminal pains and paræsthesiæ occur in *disseminated sclerosis,* a diagnosis which is suggested by finding other neurological signs (§ 952). Trigeminal pain and ocular palsies (often abducent) may occur in *carcinoma
of the nasopharynx* or other tumours of the base of the skull. *Maxillary
sinusitis* may cause pain closely resembling trigeminal neuralgia. After
thrombosis of the posterior inferior cerebellar artery trigeminal pain with
dissociated sensory loss on the face occurs. *Disease of the pons, medulla
or lateral recess* cause neuralgic pains with bulbar cranial nerve palsies
or long tract signs. In *tabes dorsalis* facial pains occur.

Etiology.—The pathology is obscure apart from cases associated with
disseminated sclerosis which are related to a plaque of demyelination in
the pons at the entry zone of the sensory root.

Treatment.—(*a*) In the *minor* types of neuralgia, the patient should
remain indoors in a uniform temperature, taking warmed liquid food
through a glass tube. Give tinct gelsemii ♏ 15, sod. bromidi gr. 10, liq.
arsenicalis ♏ 2, in peppermint water thrice daily. Phenytoin gr. 1½
(mg. 100) thrice daily may tide a patient over an attack. Large doses of
cyanocobalamin (vitamin B_{12}) should be given intramuscularly. In severe

cases give pethidine hydrochlor. (50–100 mg.) intramusc., pending consideration of surgical treatment. (b) In all *major* cases some destructive operation on the nerve roots or ganglion must sooner or later be undertaken when paroxysms frequently recur and render life a burden. Younger patients and those who have to go abroad far from help are best treated *surgically* by retro-Gasserian section of the sensory root as it leaves the pons. For aged patients *alcohol injection* of the ganglion is probably best. A well-placed injection made by an expert will give freedom for five to seven years. With either procedure 20–25 per cent. of patients develop a subsequent keratitis. Then the lids of the eye on the affected side have to be sutured for months to prevent corneal ulceration.

(c) DENTAL NEURALGIA (see § 205).

Dental Causalgia. Following dental operations a burning, continuous pain may arise within the territory of the third or second division of the trigeminal nerve. Psychological factors may be present. These cases should never be injected or operated upon. Sedation and sedative galvanism are sometimes helpful.

Costen's Syndrome. Persistent overclosure of the jaws damaging the temporo-maxillary joint, may cause a third-division neuralgia, affecting the temple, cheek, lower jaw and also felt deep in the ear. A burning pain may occur on the affected side of the tongue. Relief may follow the provision of dentures which widen the bite.

§ 818. (d) **Migrainous neuralgia** is a term applied to facial pain of trigeminal distribution in migrainous subjects. In RECURRENT SUPRAORBITAL NEURALGIA and in the severe FRONTAL NEURALGIA of Harris the pain is paroxysmal, often retro-orbital or over the first division of the fifth nerve. It lasts days, weeks or even months at a time with intervals of freedom between bouts. It occurs in persons of highly strung personality. Pupillary anomalies, *e.g.*, inequality, may occur. It may be allied to migraine and respond to injection of ergotamine tartrate 0·25–0·5 mg. or to tab. methysergide (Deseril) given night and morning for five consecutive days a week. If Gasserian block with procaine relieves the pain, alcohol injection of the first division may be undertaken in severe and intractable cases.

(e) **Glossopharyngeal Neuralgia.** The pain occurs in the region of the tonsillar fossa, deep in the ear and in front or behind the auricle, which may be hyperæsthetic. The possibility of malignant disease of the pharyngeal region must be excluded. Minor cases respond to sedation with phenobarbitone and analgesics, but severe cases may require intracranial section of the glossopharyngeal nerve (see § 1084).

(f) OCCIPITAL NEURALGIA. In *younger individuals* occipital neuralgia may be due to tension and faulty posture at work, migraine, head injury, exposure to cold, sinusitis, or follows lumbar puncture (§ 815). In patients *after middle life* spondylosis may cause occipital pain. The pain is associated with neck stiffness and creaking. The headaches and pains of cervical spondylosis are often worse after a night's rest (§ 596, 5). In *later life* " temporal " arteritis may affect the occipital arteries (§ 98). Rarely a persistent severe occipital pain is a symptom of posterior fossa neoplasm (*e.g.*, acoustic fibroma). *Treatment.*—Rest and fixation of the neck, with heat or deep injections of procaine into the tender muscles will help. If there is doubt as to the diagnosis avoid neck traction. Antihistamines reduce muscle spasm.

Benign myalgic encephalomyelitis occurs in epidemics or sporadically. The symptoms are malaise, vertigo, nausea, occipital headache and pain in the neck and shoulders. The posterior cervical muscles are in spasm and small firm glands can be felt in the posterior triangles. Relapses occur over months.

Atypical facial neuralgias are often psychogenic (§ 1076, V).

§ 819. II. Nervousness and Exhaustion. Tremulousness.—Patients presenting these symptoms should on no account be diagnosed as " neurotic " until after careful and painstaking physical examination. The finding of a persistent tachycardia, an enlarged thyroid and lid-retraction with raised basal metabolic rate may reveal *Hyperthyroidism.* Such symptoms may also be complained of in individuals addicted to *Alcohol* or *Drugs*, while *B. coli* infection or early *Pulmonary tuberculosis* may manifest themselves first by these symptoms. For *Industrial poisoning* see § 919.

Tremulousness may be *familial.* Physiologically it occurs in the head *in old age.* In disease it is a common finding in *Striatal Disease*, notably Parkinsonism (see § 914). The general picture of rigidity and slowness of movement may escape the doctor's notice. General tremulousness is a common finding in the early stages of *General Paralysis of the Insane* (an Argyll-Robertson pupil, or tremor of the face and tongue and tremulous articulation, in such cases, are easily missed (§ 1190)). The early symptoms of *Cerebral arteriosclerosis* may resemble those of functional disease, but the retinal arteries show atherosclerotic changes, and other signs of arterial degeneration are present.

§ 820. III. Pain, Numbness, Tingling in a limb.

Pain.—A careful observer will always investigate four important features of a pain. (1) The exact *distribution and sites of radiation.* (2) Its *character and degree*—whether throbbing, burning, stabbing, aching, etc. (3) The *factors which increase the pain, e.g.*, coughing, sneezing, deep breathing, or movement in a particular direction. (4) Its *constancy, i.e.*, whether persistent or paroxysmal. Local examination of the painful part should never be omitted. A patient's own diagnosis of " rheumatism " should not be accepted without question. The lightning pains of tabes dorsalis, which commonly precede all the other symptoms of that disease by years, may be wrongly diagnosed as rheumatic on insufficient examination. Painful affections of the spinal roots and nerves are dealt with in Group XIII (p. 1270).

For pain in the limbs and trunk due to *non-neurological causes* see Table LXI. When a *neurological cause* is suspected, physical signs in the early stages may be lacking. We are then dependent for diagnosis on the patient's account of the character and distribution of the pain and discomfort. Pain is more characteristic of root lesions than of peripheral nerve affections. Root-pains are made worse by coughing, sneezing, straining to defæcate, by straight leg raising from the horizontal position when the neck is flexed. Do not be deterred from diagnosing a root pain if it does not occupy the whole cutaneous distribution of its segment. A C7 root lesion due, say, to prolapse of the C6 disc may cause pain and numbness in the middle finger only and not be felt in the arm. Pain and tenderness in the muscles supplied by the corresponding cord segment are fairly usual in root-lesions.

UNILATERAL PAIN referred to *one root only* suggests disc prolapse, post-herpetic neuralgia or neurofibroma. If pain and numbness in the arm in the distribution of one or more roots is accompanied by coldness, deadness, heaviness in the feet or legs, or dragging of a leg, suspect cord compression.

BILATERAL *pains and paræsthesiæ* affecting more than one root occur in cervical spondylosis. Pains due to secondary malignant disease of the vertebræ are often bilateral, exceedingly severe, resisting ordinary analgesics. In the lower limbs bilateral sciatic pain should always arouse the suspicion of a cauda equina lesion.

Peripheral nerve pains and paræsthesiæ occur in the carpal tunnel syndrome (due to median nerve compression at the wrist) and are felt in the three middle fingers of the hand, never the little finger and rarely the thumb. Accidental jarring of a finger in this condition will cause a shock-like pain which runs up the arm as high as the elbow.

Burning pain occurs in thalamic and central cord lesions (§§ 797, 970 (12)) and after partial injury to a peripheral nerve (causalgia). In such cases the pain is burning, deep or superficial and intolerable. Diffuse burning sensations vaguely localised to one or other half of the body occur in central cord disease or in disease of the thalamus. In the latter case the patient characteristically " overreacts " to peripheral stimuli. For " Burning feet syndrome " see §§ 590, 983 and Alcoholism § 1184.

The patient who has evidence of a PARTIAL NERVE INJURY (*median, sciatic*) *complains of* CONSTANT AND SEVERE BURNING PAIN. *The affected extremity is cold, sweating and blue and trophic changes are present. Psychological changes often exist.* The condition is CAUSALGIA.

§ 821. **Causalgia** follows partial lesions of the peripheral nerves, especially median and sciatic. It is rare except after wartime or industrial injury. *Symptoms.*— (1) The pain is characteristically burning and continuous. (2) It sometimes exceeds the anatomical distribution of the affected nerve. (3) Some patients are of psychopathic constitution and may become addicted to narcotics. (4) Examination of the affected limbs is made with great difficulty owing to extreme hyperæsthesia. (5) Trophic changes and contractures occur in old-standing cases. Spontaneous remission may occur. Causalgic pain may be felt in an amputation stump, or in a " phantom limb " after amputation for injury. *Treatment.*—The limbs should be wrapped with damp dressings. No drug of addiction should be prescribed owing to the risk of addiction. Sympathectomy may be undertaken if sympathetic ganglion-block gives any relief.

For **Herpes Zoster** see § 1021.

SECONDARY CARCINOMA OF THE VERTEBRÆ gives rise to severe and persistent root pains, without marked objective neurological signs or local abnormality in the spine. Two years or more after an operation for cancer (commonly mammary carcinoma), the patient, while making some physical effort, suffers sudden intense pain in the back. These " alarm pains " become increasingly frequent and persistent, and, with increasing cachexia and sleeplessness, may be the only symptoms present. Radiograms of the vertebræ often appear normal. Such deposits occur mostly in the lumbar vertebræ, but signs of compression of the cauda equina (§ 969) are late, and the patient may die of secondary deposits in other organs before they appear.

MYELOMATOSIS may present with sciatic pain. The initial X-ray changes are easily overlooked (§ 613).

§ 822. **Acroparæsthesia** is a common condition characterised by numbness and pain, tingling and " pins and needles " and often disagreeable burning sensations in the palmar surfaces of the ends of the fingers, and less commonly in the toes.   The fingers may be clumsy but they do not alter profoundly in colour.   The intrinsic muscles of the hands are often tender and there may be slight blunting of superficial sensation to cotton wool and pin-pricks over the pads of the fingers.

The commoner known causes are partly skeletal, partly neurological. (a) " The carpal tunnel syndrome," (b) Cervical spondylosis, (c) Irritative lesions of the brachial plexus including cervical rib.

Raynaud's disease (§ 589) is a spasmodic vascular condition with marked colour changes in the fingers.   Some cases occur in persons using vibrating tools or those affected by myxœdema or scleroderma.

A woman of 40-60 years, or more rarely a man, complains bitterly of NOCTURNAL PARÆSTHESIÆ, *usually in the pads of the index and middle fingers, although all the distribution of the median nerve may be affected.   The arm jerks are present and equal and there are no long tract signs.   During the day symptoms are minimal.   The condition is the* " CARPAL TUNNEL SYNDROME."

§ 823. (a) **Carpal Tunnel Syndrome** (Syn. Compression of the Median Nerve in the Carpal Tunnel).—*Symptoms.*   The sufferer complains of waking in the night with painful paræsthesiæ referred to the palmar surfaces of several fingers, often the index and middle.   Some patients have difficulty in defining the distribution of the paræsthesiæ but the little finger escapes and the area of palmar skin supplied by the median nerve tingles in whole or in part.   Attacks of painful numbness last 15–30 minutes or longer and to relieve the suffering the patient hangs the arm out of bed or walks up and down the bedroom.   Aching may extend up the forearm. One or both hands may be affected.

In the morning the fingers are stiff, clumsy and sometimes swollen but this soon passes off.   There may be difficulty in fastening buttons and if objects are suddenly touched a shocklike feeling like electricity may run from the finger pads up the arm.   An aching pain at the elbow is often felt.

In the stage of more permanent damage the fingers feel constantly numb and patients cannot easily identify objects in their pockets or handbags.   The fingers may be slightly swollen.   There is difficulty in turning doorknobs, winding clocks and watches and all processes of laundering (wringing clothes, ironing) and sewing are impaired.

On examination there may be tenderness of the small muscles of the hand and objective impairment of sensibility to cotton wool, pin-pricks, compass tests over the pads of the fingers supplied by the median nerve. The sensory impairment is usually slight except in late cases.   In these it may be severe with " partial thenar atrophy," *i.e.*, wasting of the abductor and flexor pollicis brevis.   Percussion of the median nerve at the wrist with the hand extended may induce the disagreeable feelings in the fingers of which the patient complains.   The arm jerks are brisk and equal and there are no long tract signs. Soft tissue swelling may be seen over the flexor aspect of the wrists, worse on the more affected side.

Etiology.—The soft tissue swelling seems to involve not only the median nerve within and proximal to the carpal ligament but also the surrounding connective tissue. (*a*) Some cases are occupational in strenuous or un-accustomed manual work. (*b*) Pregnancy is a precipitatory factor and in such cases watch should be kept for toxæmia with œdema. (*c*) Old Colles fracture or arthritis of the wrist may be contributory. Many have associated cervical spondylosis; and hypochromic anæmia, myxœdema or acromegaly may coexist.

Treatment.—Most are cured by the use at night only of a light dorsal plastic splint for the forearm, wrist and back of the hand which fixes the wrist joint in the slightly flexed position. Such a splint should be worn for six weeks. Injection of hydrocortisone into the tendon sheath, and repeated if necessary, is well worth a trial. At first until lost sleep is made up and the symptoms controlled, hypnotics and sedatives may be necessary. If the symptoms are bilateral the worse hand is splinted at night; the other may remit spontaneously. Oral diuretics such as the chlorothiazides may help pregnancy cases. Should hypochromic anæmia be present give ferric ammon. citrate (30 gr. diluted) t.i.d. by mouth. Thyroid will help myxœdematous patients. If the symptoms are not relieved by a splint a surgical opinion should be sought. Relief by division of the flexor retinaculum (transverse carpal ligament) is often prompt and lasting.

(*b*) CERVICAL SPONDYLOSIS (§§ 596, 1004) is a common cause of uni-lateral or bilateral paræsthesiæ in the hands, usually at a later age than in the carpal tunnel syndrome.

There are PAINS AND PARÆSTHESIÆ *of root distribution over the ulnar border of the hand and forearm* (*Th8, C1*). CERVICAL SYMPATHETIC OCULAR PALSY *is often present and* WASTING OF THE INTRINSIC HAND MUSCLES, *especially flexor brevis, and adductor pollicis. The irritative lesion of the lower cord of the brachial plexus is due to the* THORACIC INLET *or the* RIB PRESSURE SYNDROME.

§ 824. (*c*) In the **Thoracic inlet** and **Rib Pressure Syndromes** the symptoms are similar. Blueness and swelling of the hand and fingers occur. No cervical rib is found on X-ray. Middle-aged women about the menopause suffer mostly, and fatigue and states of debility are causal factors. The shoulder girdle muscles sag owing to loss of muscular tone, and the neuro-vascular bundle of brachial plexus, subclavian artery and vein, becomes compressed by the normal first rib. The lowest cord of the brachial plexus (C8, Th1) suffers most. *Treatment* is by rest in bed from one to three weeks with the forearm and elbows supported on pillows. Later, shoulder raising exercises to improve the tone of the shoulder-girdle muscles may be prescribed. Sedatives and an œstrogen help meno-pausal cases (and see § 596).

Be reluctant to attribute neurological signs to a *cervical rib* even if the X-rays show such a rib. Incomplete ribs are more likely to cause symptoms. In all cases the presence of malignant and Hodgkin's nodes in the brachial plexus or infiltration of the cervical spine or apex of the lung with new growth must be excluded.

CERVICAL RIBS may require operation by a skilled neurosurgeon if causing progressive disability.

TABLE L

	Carpal Tunnel Syndrome.	Cervical Spondylosis.	Brachial plexus Conditions, e.g., cervical rib or thoracic inlet syndrome.
Age.	40-60 years.	Over 60 years.	Often at menopause.
Distribution of paræsthesiæ.	Median nerve, i.e., all except little finger.	Bilateral in hands and fingers.	C8, Th1 chiefly.
Pain.	"Electric shocks" on touching objects. As high or higher than elbow.	Stiff neck and cervical root pains.	Ulnar muscles of hands and forearms.
Wasting.	"Partial thenar atrophy," i.e., abductor and flexor pollicis brevis.	Intrinsic muscles of the hands.	Small muscles of hands especially interossei.
Cervical sympathetic palsy.	Absent.	Absent.	Present.
Arm reflexes.	Present.	Inversion of supinator jerks, or absent arm jerks.	Present.
Long tract signs.	Absent.	May be extensor response.	Absent.

(d) **Meralgia Paræsthetica.** In this condition there is numbness and tingling with cutaneous hyperæsthesia on the outer aspect of the thigh in the distribution of the lateral cutaneous nerve. The cause is probably mechanical, some derangement of the nerve where it pierces the fascia lata of the thigh, and is often associated with gain in weight. *Treatment* is that of obesity, and in severe cases necessitates incision of the fascia lata from the neural opening in the fascia to the inguinal ligament.

PARÆSTHESIÆ are more characteristic of peripheral nerve or spinal cord disease. They do not occur in visceral or somatic disease and are therefore characteristic of neurological lesions.

When the distribution is bilateral in the upper limbs, think of Cervical spondylosis (see § 1004). Disseminated sclerosis (§ 952) may cause paræsthesiæ in the limbs or below the level of a spinal cord plaque. In the cervical region when there is disease, either of the posterior roots or posterior columns, flexion of the neck on to the chest produces tingling in the trunk and lower limbs (L'Hermitte's Sign). In polyneuritis (§ 974), subacute combined degeneration (§ 950) and myxœdema (§ 575), paræsthesiæ in the fingers of both hands are characteristic.

Patchy numbness, chiefly peripheral, occurs in polyneuritis, e.g., in nodular leprosy. The " girdle-sensation " of tabes is a feeling as if a cord were tied round the waist; it occurs too in cord compression. When nerve trunks or roots are compressed, *e.g.*, in the rib pressure syndrome, paræsthesiæ may precede the onset of pain. Numbness along the ulnar borders of the hand is a usual complaint in ulnar neuritis.

Attacks of "pins and needles" which spread in an orderly march, often from the thumb and index towards the lips and tongue, occur in Jacksonian Epilepsy, in migraine and in hypertensive encephalopathy.

§ 825. IV. Unsteadiness in walking. Falling about.

Patients with sensory *ataxia* and *cerebellar ataxia* complain of unsteadiness in walking, and falling about. When *vertigo or giddiness* accompanies the loss of balance there is probably disease of the labyrinths or vestibular pathways.

SENSORY ATAXIA is due to loss of sensory impulses from the joints, tendons and muscles, and it is increased when the eyes are shut. The range and direction of movements are impaired and there is hypotonia. It occurs in disease of the posterior columns of the cord, *e.g.*, disseminated sclerosis, tabes, subacute combined degeneration, but it is seen also in mixed or sensory polyneuritis (§§ 948, 974).

CEREBELLAR ATAXIA is due to loss of non-sensory proprioceptive impulses. It is uninfluenced by closure of the eyes. The ataxia may be unilateral or bilateral, and nystagmus, dysarthria, intention tremor and hypotonia are often present. It occurs in gross lesions of the cerebellum (abscess, neoplasm) and in degeneration of the cerebellar or spino-cerebellar tracts. It is acute and unilateral with crossed and dissociated sensory changes in thrombosis of the posterior inferior cerebellar artery. It is acute and bilateral in barbiturate or hydantoin poisoning (§§ 934, 935).

§ 826. In **Vertigo** (1) the senses are deceived into feeling or seeing movement either of self or surrounding objects, (2) balance is upset, the gait unsteady and the patient clutches for support. Do not mistake for true vertigo feelings of insecurity or lack of confidence, often described as " giddiness " or " dizziness," occurring in psychoneurotic states.

Clinical Investigation of Vertigo. Inquire for a history of ear discharge, deafness, tinnitus, or upper respiratory infection, for head injury or taking of barbiturate. Test the hearing, corneal reflexes, look for nystagmus. Look at the eardrums and fundi. Test the tone of the limbs and examine them for ataxia and past-pointing. Test the reflexes; examine the heart, take the blood pressure and look for albumen in the urine. Take blood for a W.R. where there is nerve deafness. In severe or recurrent cases special investigations will be required: (*a*) measurement of hearing by audiometry, (*b*) differential caloric tests of the labyrinths.

CASES OF VERTIGO

(*a*) Motion sickness (sea-sickness).

(*b*) Acute Labyrinthine failure— Vestibular neuronitis.

(*c*) Postural vertigo and benign positional nystagmus.

(*d*) After head injury.

(*e*) Acute labyrinthitis.

(*f*) Ménière's syndrome.

(*g*) Posterior inferior cerebellar artery thrombosis.

(*h*) Acoustic neurofibroma.

Vertigo occurs as an *aura* of migraine and may last for several minutes before the onset of incapacitating headache. It may be the aura of an epileptic fit; in this case when the patient recovers consciousness the vertigo has gone. In the absence of disease it occurs while syringing the ear with hot or cold liquids (§ 1143).

VERTIGO, *with* VOMITING, *sweating, pallor and depression occur only at sea, in cars, trains, lifts, roundabouts, swings or flying. The condition is* MOTION SICKNESS.

§ 827. (a) **Motion Sickness.** *Symptoms.*—In addition to vomiting and nausea the patient may complain of vertigo, faint feelings, apathy or depression and may show sweating, pallor or flushing of the face, salivation, tachycardia or diarrhœa. In sea-sickness prolongation of bad weather may cause prostration; ketosis and fluid depletion from prolonged vomiting may result. As air journeys are shorter these secondary effects are not seen in air sickness which occurs only on bumpy flying.

Diagnosis depends on the specificity of the symptoms to the circumstances of motion. Gastro-intestinal, renal and cerebral disease will have to be excluded in cases where the symptoms are prolonged.

Etiology.—The cause is the effect of accelerations, linear, angular, vertical, etc. on the labyrinths. Deaf-mutes are immune. A personal idiosyncrasy exists and whilst it is rare in infants it is common in migrainous subjects.

Prognosis.—Symptoms may persist for hours after landing. Many adolescents adapt, especially to air travel; this is less likely to occur in sea-sickness.

Treatment, see § 271.

The patient is seized with INTENSE GIDDINESS *causing* STAGGERING GAIT, *reeling or even falling, with nausea,* OFTEN VOMITING *or faintness. The cause is usually* ACUTE LABYRINTHINE FAILURE *due to epidemic vertigo, circulatory or toxic causes affecting the peripheral labyrinth.*

§ 828. (b) **Acute Labyrinthine Failure.** In severe attacks consciousness may be momentarily lost, but *on recovering consciousness the vertigo is persistent.* In the horizontal position in bed the patient lies, pallid and sweating, with closed eyes. He is usually more comfortable lying on one particular side. When he opens his eyes the room seems to be in motion. If he changes his position or sits up, he may vomit. There may be occipital pain, or diarrhœa may accompany the vertigo. Vertigo not infrequently comes on while asleep at night. The condition lasts for minutes, hours or days. Examined during this period the patient may show horizontal nystagmus, coarser on looking to the side of the lesion with ipsilateral hypotonia, ataxia and past-pointing. In most cases the vertigo passes completely away, but the patient may be left with unsteadiness on bending or on rapid changes of posture or in traffic. In other cases the vertigo is recurrent. Nearly all such cases are *Peripheral* and due to some disorder of the labyrinth or vestibular nerve.

Vestibular Neuronitis (Syn. Epidemic Vertigo) may occur from upper respiratory infections, tonsillitis, sinusitis. It is a benign condition and the symptoms, which are those of labyrinthine vertigo, last for some days only. The hearing is not affected (§ 1151). During the illness treat any respiratory infection, give phenobarbitone gr. ½ t.i.d., with nicotinic acid

50 mg., twice or thrice daily. During convalescence the patient may take Dramamine, 50-100 mg., for attacks of vertigo, or 100 mg. (suppositories) may be given per rectum during the acute phase of the illness.

Vertigo lasting a minute or two occurs on change of posture.

§ 829. (c) POSTURAL VERTIGO occurs in *hypertension* and cerebral *arteriosclerosis* from defective blood supply to the labyrinths. Similar vertigo may occur in *severe anæmia* or during *convalescence* and other states of vaso-motor instability, *e.g.*, menopause. It may be due to a *toxic* cause, *e.g.*, alcoholic poisoning. A firm abdominal support helps some cases. The patient should be warned against sudden change of position and should walk with a stick and ferrule.

Benign Positional Nystagmus may be peripheral or central in origin. When the patient is laid flat on a couch and the head tilted over the edge a coarse nystagmus on lateral gaze appears with feelings of vertigo. The condition lasts some months and usually disappears. Such patients should be kept under observation as the phenomenon has occurred as an early symptom with a cerebral tumour.

(d) After *Head Injury* paroxymal positional vertigo is common (§ 813). It usually passes off with rest and mild sedation. More severe cases may be due to labyrinthine or to severe cortical damage.

§ 830. (e) *Severe episodic vertigo occurs with sudden perceptive deafness and tinnitus.* (1) ACUTE LABYRINTHITIS may be *suppurative or non-suppurative* in otitis media or in meningitis. The inflammatory process extends into the cochlea and causes deafness (§ 1150). (2) TRAUMA: Deafness or vertigo may be due to concussion of the labyrinth and cochlea. (3) TOXIC: *Streptomycin* and dihydrostreptomycin, especially in the elderly, may cause deafness and vertigo. Dihydrostreptomycin being more toxic is now rarely used. (4) GENICULATE HERPES: When herpes attacks the geniculate ganglion, vertigo, deafness, tinnitus and facial palsy may result. In mild cases the facial palsy may recover, but in severe infections the facial palsy and deafness are severe and permanent.

The VERTIGO *is recurrent and associated with* DEAFNESS *of the perceptive type and* TINNITUS. *The cause is either* MÉNIÈRE'S SYNDROME, *or* OTOSCLEROSIS.

§ 831. (f) **Ménière's Syndrome** occurs between the ages of 30-60 years. Attacks of acute labyrinthine failure are paroxysmal with recurrent vertigo and vomiting, and each attack leaves the patient with increasing deafness. Between the attacks there is tinnitus in the affected ear. The disease is essentially bilateral, although one ear is affected before the other. Between the attacks, physical examination reveals no neurological abnormality apart from the nerve deafness and defective labyrinthine responses. As deafness increases the attacks become less severe. The disease runs its course over a period of months or years. It is probably due to recurrent hydrops of the labyrinth; gross dilatation of the endolymph system in such cases was first observed by Cairns and Hallpike.

Diagnosis.—The residual deafness and tinnitus distinguish the condition from *epilepsy* and from *migraine*. The caloric test will show a semicircular canal paresis and occasionally directional preponderance to the opposite side (§ 1143). The audiogram shows in early cases a nerve deafness with a hearing for *low* tones.

Treatment.—*The acute attack:* Inflation of the Eustachian tubes helps some patients. Give phenobarbitone gr. ½, twice or thrice daily, or soluble aspirin gr. 10 at bedtime. Restriction of fluids to 2½ pints daily and diuretics may help. Intramuscular injection of histamine acid phosphate may be given twice weekly during active phases of the disease. In the belief that acute attacks are due to vasospasm some advocate tab. nicotinic acid 100 mg., t.i.d. before meals, and even cervical sympathectomy. Balancing exercises seem to expedite recovery as soon as the patient can sit up in bed. The patient should not be allowed to swim, and should probably not drive a car or ride a bicycle until free of attacks for six months. If syphilis, either congenital or acquired, is present it should be treated.

Recurrent attacks: When the attacks render the patient's life a misery, destruction of the labyrinth may be contemplated. If there is no useful hearing in the ear the labyrinth may be destroyed by alcohol injection into the external semicircular canal or by labyrinthotomy by an expert—both these measures completely destroy labyrinthine and cochlear functions. If the hearing is useful it may be preserved by surgical division of the vestibular nerve only or by the local effect of ultrasonic sound waves applied to the external semicircular canal.

OTOSCLEROSIS gives rise to similar paroxysmal vertigo. The deafness however is obstructive, or mixed in type (§ 1149).

The vertigo is persistent and accompanied by vertical nystagmus, persistent diplopia, cranial nerve palsies, e.g., absent corneal reflexes, facial palsy, long tract signs such as cerebellar ataxia, and crossed sensory changes in the limbs. The cause is CENTRAL.

(*g*) An unusual cause is infarction of the *posterior inferior cerebellar artery* (see § 936). Other causes are inflammatory (bulbar encephalitis), neoplastic (auditory neurofibroma, medullo-blastoma, secondary growths in the brain-stem or cerebellum), demyelinating lesions (disseminated sclerosis). In central lesions there are sensory changes in the limbs, often crossed or dissociated, with cerebellar and pyramidal signs. The cranial nerves most often affected after the oculomotor nerves, are sensory V, motor V, VI, VII. These neurological findings distinguish such cases from the labyrinthine groups.

(*h*) ACOUSTIC NEUROFIBROMA (see § 1083).

§ 832. V. Fainting Spells, " Blackouts," Swoons.

In the investigation of obscure attacks of swooning a careful history and an eye-witness's account are usually more valuable than an E.E.G. Remember *faints may be of emotional origin* but suspect epilepsy if there is a bitten tongue, a bruised lip, or injury or burns are sustained in the attack.

In *hysterical hyperventilation, carotid sinus sensitivity* and *hypoglycæmia* it may be possible to reproduce an attack.

Ancillary investigations used in the elucidation of obscure swoons include X-ray of the skull, estimation of blood sugar (after a dose of insulin), electrocardiography in patients suspected of *intermittent heart block*, and E.E.G. with hyperventilation techniques (and see § 847).

When EPILEPSY is suspected turn to § 859.

§ 833. Syncope (Fainting).—In predisposed individuals faints due to *postural hypotension* occur after prolonged standing especially under conditions of emotional tension, *e.g.*, concerts, ceremonial parades. The blood pressures taken with the patient standing and then reclining may point to the nature of the attack. Exercises to improve muscular tone in the limbs and abdominal muscles may help in prevention. In states of VASO-MOTOR INSTABILITY, *e.g.*, during convalescence, in anæmia, syncope may occur or it may be a symptom of *aortic stenosis* or *insufficiency*, or of hypertension if the cerebral blood pressure falls. CAROTID SINUS SYNCOPE occurs typically in elderly arteriopaths. Pressure on the carotid sinus by tight collars may cause a sudden faintness or loss of consciousness. SENILE SYNCOPE occurs on too rapid change of posture in elderly patients with carotid and basilar artery insufficiency. DROP ATTACKS are unexpected, short-lived sudden falls without loss of consciousness. They occur especially in menopausal and elderly women and they are a cause of great embarrassment and of danger from fracture of bones. The E.E.G. is normal and the attacks are not helped by anticonvulsant drugs. The suggested cause is ischæmia of the reticular formation due to basilar artery atherosclerosis. Some faint after PHYSICAL OVEREXERTION.

Many faints are EMOTIONAL and occur on feeling sudden pain, after hearing bad news, listening to medical lectures, at the sight of blood etc. (§ 35). These " situations " are possible triggers for epileptic fits as well as for faints.

COUGH SYNCOPE occurs in chronic bronchitis. The extreme rise of intrathoracic pressure after a bout of coughing diminishes the venous return to the heart and precipitates unconsciousness or convulsions. Similar attacks may occur after a bout of uproarious laughter or after choking. When loss of consciousness follows a single cough the cause is probably epileptic. A patient who falls in a syncopal attack may sustain a head injury, causing loss of consciousness of prolonged nature.

VERTIGO bears a superficial resemblance to fainting. If vertigo is the aura of an epileptic fit, it will have disappeared when the patient regains consciousness. This is not so in the disturbance of consciousness which sometimes accompanies severe vertigo—the illusion of rotation of objects goes on after the patient has recovered his senses.

" **Blackouts.**" The word is sometimes used by migrainous subjects to describe their *visual auras*; these are prolonged and last 10–20 minutes (§ 812). Spreading half-headache usually but not invariably follows. Patients can draw their visual spectra. Usually, however, the word

" Blackout " implies (1) *an episodic disturbance of function in the nervous system* either due to a psychogenic cause or to epilepsy, (2) *a disturbance of blood supply to the brain,* either in the amount of blood or its composition.

Causes of Blackouts

(*a*) Psychological illness.

(*b*) Head injury.

(*c*) Epilepsy.

(*d*) Hypertensive encephalopathy.

(*e*) Basilar and carotid insufficiency.

(*f*) Hypoglycæmia.

(*g*) Paroxysmal tachycardia.

(*h*) Hyperventilation syndrome.

(*a*) *Psychogenic " Blackout."* Patients with affective disorder (anxiety, depression) may refer to attacks of depersonalisation or feelings of unreality as " blackouts." Between the attacks other symptoms of their illness will be present, *e.g.*, melancholy, anxiety, retardation of thought, inability to concentrate, sleeplessness, lack of appetite. Alcoholics who have confusional episodes may refer to these as " blackouts " and in such cases an episodic fit may occur.

(*b*) *Following head injury* attacks of vertigo and faintness occur, often precipitated by sudden change of posture. These may go on for weeks or months and have to be distinguished from post-traumatic epilepsy.

(*c*) *Psychic fits.* In Epilepsy, psycho-motor fits (Temporal lobe attacks) occur. These are brief " absences," followed by transient automatism, often bizarre behaviour, with subsequent amnesia for the attack (§ 864).

(*d*) *Hypertensive cerebral disease* may cause disturbance of consciousness in various ways—from falls in blood pressure with ischæmia, from brain swelling in encephalopathy, from transient vascular occlusions.

(*e*) In conditions of *arterial narrowing, e.g.*, aortic or carotid stenosis, syncopal attacks are sometimes produced. With basilar artery stenosis (" basilar insufficiency ") the patient may be for several minutes ataxic and bereft of speech. The stenosis may be demonstrated by angiography.

(*f*) *Hypoglycæmic attacks* occur in diabetic patients after an overdose of insulin. They are usually slow in onset and are relieved by a carbohydrate meal or injection of dextrose. *Spontaneous hypoglycæmia* due to hyperinsulinism is sometimes seen (§ 425).

(*g*) Attacks of *paroxysmal tachycardia* cause rather prolonged agitation and mental perturbation but rarely loss of consciousness.

(*h*) The *hyperventilation syndrome* occurs as the result of emotional stress and in psychoneurotics overbreathing may become a habit. The patient overbreathes for some minutes " trying to get air," and this induces paræsthesiæ round the lips and tongue, in the fingers, and even attacks of tetany (§ 1030) from the induced alkalosis. The fingers and toes pass into carpo-pedal spasm and there may be disturbances of consciousness.

§ 834. VI. Disordered Vision.—Blurring of vision or double vision are common neurological complaints.

The patient complains of PAINLESS DOUBLE VISION. If there is a *paralytic squint* the diplopia will be greater when the patient turns his gaze in the direction of traction of the paralysed muscle, *e.g.*, to the right in cases of right abducent palsy (§ 1065). Most squints require elucidation by an ophthalmologist, who will use diplopia tests and Sim's charts to identify the paralysed muscle or muscles. Sudden painless diplopia occurring in younger adults (often without frank squint) may be due to *disseminated sclerosis*. *Neurosyphilis* is a rarer cause and there is usually a frank squint. In the elderly, ocular palsies involving one or more nerves appear suddenly due to *cerebral ischæmia* or hæmorrhage into the nerve sheath peripherally from an adherent *atheromatous artery*. Many of these recover after a few weeks or months. Any unexplained unilateral or bilateral external ophthalmoplegia may be due to a purely muscle disease such as *myasthenia gravis*; the neostigmine test will help in the diagnosis. Sudden diplopia may be due to proptosis in exophthalmic ophthalmoplegia. In childhood a latent squint may suddenly become manifest. Persons with *errors of muscle balance* (heterophoria) may have transient diplopia when fatigued or under stress. True diplopia disappears if one eye is covered.

The patient complains of DIPLOPIA, WITH PAIN *often of trigeminal distribution and corresponding sensory changes.* If there is complete ptosis and on lifting the lid there is a dilated inactive pupil and an abducted eye, there is oculomotor nerve paralysis. The most likely cause is *Saccular aneurysm* on the internal carotid artery. Pain and numbness may be present over the first and second divisions of the trigeminal nerve. Thrombophlebitis of the cavernous and petrosal sinuses can cause diplopia with pain in association with sinus infections and infections of the apex of the petrous temporal bone.

In childhood, squint of the paralytic type appearing suddenly, whether painful or not, may be due to meningeal infection (tuberculous meningitis, sinusitis with intracranial extension) or to a tumour or other space-occupying lesion.

The patient complains of SUDDEN LOSS OF VISION (*a*) *in one eye,* (*b*) *in both eyes.* In (*a*) the cause is probably intraocular (§ 1118), or due to Retrobulbar neuritis. In (*b*) the cause is probably some non-neurological condition (§ 1120). In all cases the fundi must be carefully examined, the blood pressure estimated and the urine tested for albumen and sugar.

The patient complains of TRANSIENT FLASHING LIGHTS OR SCINTILLATING FIGURES OR BLOTTING OUT OF PART OF THE VISUAL FIELD. The cause is probably Migraine. The aura in migraine is slow, lasting 10–30 minutes. A visual Jacksonian attack is usually much shorter, but can persist for hours.

§ 835. VII. **Weakness, Stiffness, or Difficulty in controlling one or more limbs.**

In painful conditions, *e.g.*, injured limbs after road accidents, the patient will not want to move the painful part. Do not confuse this with paralysis. Loss of power in the limbs is due to disease in one of four situations: (1) the pyramidal tract, (2) the anterior horn cells and their axons, (3) the myoneural junction, (4) the muscles themselves.

Pyramidal weakness (flaccidity, later spasticity) is characterised by increased tendon reflexes, absent abdominal reflexes and extensor plantar responses. *Lower motor neurone weakness* causes a flaccid paralysis of individual muscles, loss of tendon reflexes and muscle atrophy. In a mixed peripheral nerve lesion the distribution of the paralysis and sensory loss will conform to the anatomical distribution of the nerve. *Disease of the myoneural junction* (myasthenis gravis) is characterised by fatigue paralysis, recovering after rest or after injection of edrophonium (Tensilon) or neostigmine (§ 988). *Muscle disease* is a cause of weakness sometimes forgotten. In the myopathies the distribution of the wasting and weakness in the muscles of the face, shoulders and pelvic girdles is highly characteristic; muscle hypertrophy or myotonia may be present (§§ 1008, 1027).

Parkinsonism, with its rigidity of facial expression, loss of blinking, loss of swing of the arms in walking and the gliding gait, is sometimes more easily diagnosed by seeing the patient walk than by examining him on a couch or in bed, as these signs may not be evident until the patient performs active movements (and see § 914).

Loss of tone in an arm or leg on the same side without loss of power is seen in cerebellar lesions and in flaccid chorea in children.

Difficulty in controlling one or more limbs can occur from loss of joint sense due to disease of the posterior columns, *e.g.,* disseminated sclerosis, or peripheral nerves, *e.g.,* polyneuritis. It can be due to cerebellar ataxia or to involuntary movements (chorea, athetosis).

§ 836. VIII. Disorders of Sleep.—The *amount* of sleep required in healthy individuals varies with the age of the person and the individual peculiarity. In general, it may be said that infants require about sixteen hours, adolescents ten hours, the middle-aged eight, and the aged five hours. Some families and individuals are notoriously poor sleepers and do not seem to suffer in health or comfort on this account. Man can exist without sleep for about the same time that he can do without food, viz., three to four weeks, but he cannot live without it.

In *normal sleep* the power to make voluntary movements is first lost, then the use of the special senses disappears, hearing being the last to go and the easiest to evoke on arousing the patient. General muscular relaxation with ptosis develops, the eyeballs turning upward and becoming slightly divergent. Respiration becomes slower and noisier, and tends to periodicity in the very young and the very aged. The pulse frequency lessens, the blood pressure falls with cerebral anæmia, and the general body temperature falls. Temporarily, the knee-jerks are abolished and the plantar responses become extensor. Two important features of normal sleep are: (1) Its fixed periodicity in the rhythm of sleeping and wakefulness. (2) The sleeper can be roused from sleep to normal activity, unlike the comatose or stuporose patient.

We have no precise knowledge of the *physiology of sleep.* Pavlov believed it to be a state of *active inhibition* of the cortical mechanism. Its function is to protect the nerve-cells so that they can recuperate from fatigue and recover their normal functions. In the region of the *hypothalamus* and *the grey matter of the floor of the third ventricle* there is a nervous mechanism intimately connected with sleep. Damage to this area, by tumours or other structural disease, usually results in excessive drowsiness. There is some evidence for the existence of an " alerting " or " waking " mechanism in the *reticular formation* of the pons.

Sleep may be (A) *Diminished in Quantity* (insomnia), (B) *Defective in*

TABLE LI.—HYPNOTICS

Sleeplessness due to	Hypnotic.	Single dose.	Max. dose.
Mental stress	Acetylsalicylic acid (Aspirin) tab.	5 gr.	15 gr.
	Diphenhydramine hydrochl. (Benadryl) caps.	25 mg.	100 mg.
	Haust. Chloral et Pot. Brom. (B.P.C.) (freshly prepared mixture)	30 ml. (1 oz.)	45 ml.
	Dichloralphenazone (Welldorm) tab.	10 gr.	30 gr.
	Glutethimide (Doriden) tab.	250 mg.	500 mg.
	Quinalbarbitone sod. (Seconal) tab.	50 mg.	200 mg.
	Amylobarbitone sod. (Sod. amytal) tab.	50 mg.	300 mg.
	Butobarbitone (Soneryl) tab.	100 mg.	200 mg.
	Phenobarbitone tab.	30 mg.	120 mg.
	Barbitone sod. (Medinal) tab.	320 mg.	500 mg.
	Inj. Amylobarbitone sod. (B.P.C.) intravenous ampoule	0-3 G.	1 G.
Pain	Tab. Codeine Co. (B.P.)	1 tab.	2 tab.
	Tab. Codeine Phosph. (B.N.F.) (may be given with Barbiturate or Chlorpromazine)	15 mg.	60 mg.
	Tab. Paracetamol (Panadol)	0-5 G.	1-0 G.
	Alioral tab.(Aprobarbital 50 mg., Propylphenazone 110 mg.)	1-2 tab.	up to 6 tabs. daily
	Pethidine hydrochloride tab.	50 mg.	100 mg.
	Inj. Pethidine hydrochloride (100 mg. in 2 ml.) ampoule intramusc.	2 ml.	2 ml.
	Inj. Methadone hydrochloride (Physeptone) (10 mg. in 1 ml.) ampoule	5 mg.	10 mg.
	" A.P.H. Powder " [1]	For occasional use only	
	" Brompton Cocktail " mixture [2]	½ oz.	
Restlessness	Inj. Chlorpromazine hydrochlor } may be combined intraven. or intramusc.	25 mg.	50 mg.
	Inj. Phenobarbitone sod. (B.P.) } (ampoules)	60 mg.	200 mg.
	Inj. Paraldehyde (B.N.F.) intramusc. ampoule	5 ml.	10 ml.
Cardiac Dyspnœa	Inj. Papaveretum (B.P.C.) (Omnopon) intramusc. ampoule	0-5 ml.	1 ml.
	Inj. Morphine sulphate (B.P.) intramusc. ampoule	8 mg.	20 mg.
Senile and arteriosclerotic conditions	Alcohol (whisky, brandy, rum in milk)	1 oz.	
	Amylobarbitone sod. (Sod. amytal) tab.	50 mg.	300 mg.
	Pentobarbitone sod. (Nembutal) tab. or caps.	50 mg.	200 mg.
	Haust. chloral B.P.C.	15 ml.	22 ml.
	Promazine hydrochlor. (Sparine) tab.	25 mg.	200 mg.

[1] " A.P.H. Powder " = Aspirin gr. 10, Amidopyrine (Pyramidon) gr. 5, Diamorph. hydrochlor. (Heroin) ¹⁄₁₂–¼ gr. for root pains.

[2] " Haustus Euphoriens " = Morphine hydrochloride gr. ⅓, Cocaine hydrochloride gr. ⅙, gin 60♏, honey 60 ♏, Chloroform water to ½ fl. oz. For pains of secondary carcinoma in terminal stages.

Quality (disturbed sleep), (C) *Increased in Quantity* (protracted sleep). (D) *Sleep Rhythm* may be Inverted or Disturbed.

A. **Sleeplessness (Insomnia).**—The chief cause of sleeplessness is (1) *Psychical*, but there are many other causes. Sleeplessness may arise (2) as the result of *pain* anywhere in the body, or *discomfort*, such as is caused by flatulence in the stomach or intestine, or by dyspnœa in cardiac disease or dropsy. (3) In *febrile conditions*. (4) In *organic brain disease*. In *Encephalitis Lethargica* absolute sleeplessness, lasting several days, may be met, especially in children. Sleeplessness is an early symptom of

General Paralysis of the Insane, when the patient is restless or excited (later, drowsiness and apathy are common). In *cerebral arteriosclerosis*, especially when the blood pressure is high, the patient may fall off to sleep, but wakens in the early morning unable to sleep again. (5) In many forms of *chronic toxæmia*, *e.g.*, *uræmia* and *alcoholism*, sleeplessness may be present in the early stages.

The *Psychical Causes*, owing to their relatively great importance, must be considered in detail. They may be divided into three groups: (1) The patient is unable to sleep because of *anxiety* (by far the largest group). (2) The patient is unable to sleep because of some *bad habit of thought*, anxious preoccupation with affairs of the past, present or future, visualising of scenes, rehearsing of conversations, etc. (3) The patient, usually a bad sleeper, is *obsessed* with the idea of sleeplessness, or "insomnia" as he calls it. Persistent insomnia may be the prelude to the development of a psychosis.

Treatment of Insomnia.—(1) The *factors underlying the neurosis* should be elucidated. Bad sleepers are nearly always apprehensive that the lack of sleep will cause insanity, or that if they take hypnotics they will become drug-addicts. Such patients should be reassured. (2) In slight cases *physical treatment* is prescribed—comfort, quiet, warmth, change of surroundings, hot baths followed by massage, hot packs, hot drinks, last thing at night, may suffice to restore the lost sleep habit. Heavy meals and over-fatigue, emotional or intellectual strain should be avoided late in the evening. Some sleep better at the seaside, some at a higher altitude. A period of rest in bed, away from home and its distractions and worries, helps the poorly nourished and tired-out patient. A dry biscuit and a Thermos-jug of hot milk by the bedside will sometimes help those who waken in the night to fall asleep again. (3) *Hypnotics* (Table LI). In more severe cases, where the continued loss of sleep is rendering the patient panicky and less and less capable of dealing with his anxieties, the insomnia should be immediately relieved by hypnotics. The *rules for prescribing a hypnotic* are: (1) It should first be explained to the patient that he is not being drugged, and that it is better for him to obtain sleep with a sedative than to go on having sleepless and wearying nights without it. (2) It should be prescribed *for a stated initial period*, *e.g.*, alternate nights for a week, or a fortnight. (3) The *hour at which it is to be taken* must be definitely stated. The additional anxiety of having to decide when to take the hypnotic is bad for the patient. (4) If possible, the patient should not know what hypnotic he is having. (5) It must be given in adequate dosage to produce sleep. (6) If the patient says that it is losing its effect, the same dose should be given in divided quantities, every quarter of an hour, before it is decided to increase the dose or change the hypnotic.

When the patient has difficulty in falling asleep give a short-acting hypnotic, *e.g.*, sod. quinalbarbitone or sod. amylobarbitone. If the patient tends to wake in the night give a longer-acting hypnotic, *e.g.*, butobarbitone or phenobarbitone. For patients who wake in the early morning with agitation and anxious ruminations give a hot drink at bedtime, and on wakening sod. pentobarbitone which is a quick but relatively short-acting barbiturate. An antihistamine such as diphenhydramine (Benadryl) 25–50 mg. is useful for those who cannot take barbiturate; or try chloral hydrate, dichloralphenazone or glutethimide (see Table LI).

Paraldehyde is a safe hypnotic, but has an unpleasant taste and a persistent and offensive smell. It can be given by mouth (2–8 ml.) or by intramuscular injection (5 ml.) to restless wakeful patients (*e.g.*, alcoholic patients with pneumonia, cases of head injury) where other hypnotics might cause medullary depression. For extreme restlessness in acute psychosis some give hyoscine hydrobromide 0·6 mg. with morphine 8–20 mg.: lesser degrees will be helped by chlorpromazine (50 mg.) with sod. phenobarbitone (200 mg.) given intravenously and repeated in 6 to 8 hours intramuscularly.

Potassium bromide and chloral hydrate (G. 0·9 of each) combined in a draught (Haust. Chloral et Pot. Brom.) is time-honoured and useful especially to wakeful worrying patients, but the danger of bromide intoxication should be borne in mind, as it is cumulative in elderly and arteriosclerotic patients. Morphine or its derivatives may cause death from respiratory depression and anoxia in *status asthmaticus*. Preparations containing amidopyrin or apronal (Sedormid) are liable to cause anæmia and purpura. Chloral hydrate is a hypnotic which can be given with safety to children (0·3–0·5 G.) by mouth.

Persons who sleep badly notoriously exaggerate this symptom. In severe cases the physician may have to ask the nurse to chart the number of hours of sleep. Sleeplessness due to severe affective disorder (anxiety, depression) may yield quickly to electro-convulsive therapy.

B. **Defective Sleep.**—(1) *Nightmares or Night-Terrors* may be due to physical or psychical causes. In *children* the cause is commonly some unhappiness in the child's domestic or school environment, an over-anxious, bullying or quarrelsome parent, or memory of some emotional trauma. Physical causes also operate, *e.g.*, thread-worms, gastro-intestinal fermentation, adenoids severe enough to impede respiration. In *adults* night-terrors are commonly the result of a psychoneurosis; disturbed sleep and frequent waking up may also occur in advanced cardiac disease, chronic uræmia and other toxæmias. (2) *Somnambulism* or sleep-walking is a condition in which the sleeper rises apparently asleep and behaves automatically. It is commoner in children than in adults. Contrary to popular belief, patients may do themselves serious damage by climbing out of windows, or falling over stairs whilst sleep-walking.

C. **Protracted Sleep.**—Pathological drowsiness (stupor) is met in (1) Lesions affecting the hypothalamic area and the grey matter of the floor of the third ventricle, and the reticular formation, *e.g.*, anoxia, after asphyxiation, tumours of the *pituitary stalk*, *encephalitis lethargica* and *trypanosomiasis* (African sleeping sickness). (2) Increasing intracranial pressure, from any progressive intracranial lesion, *e.g.*, cerebral tumour.

After a *head injury* the patient may sleep for several hours. (3) Chronic toxæmias, such as uræmia and diabetic ketosis, lead to drowsiness and later, coma. (4) Obesity, such as the obesity of *myxœdema* and *pituitary disease*, is often accompanied by sleepiness. (5) After an *epileptic* fit the patient may sleep for many hours. (6) In the *Kleine-Levin Syndrome*, affecting young males, episodes of sleep lasting one to three weeks are associated with excessive appetite for food. The cause is unknown and no organic lesion has been demonstrated.

(7) *In* TRANCE STATES *of psychopathic origin* the patient appears to sleep but resists if one attempts to open the eyelids. Trances may be acute or subacute in onset and may last for weeks or months. They are met in schizophrenia, in confusional states and other psychoses, and in hysteria. Recurrences are frequent.

§ 837. **Encephalitis lethargica** (Syn. Epidemic Encephalitis, " Sleepy Sickness ") is now an exceedingly rare disease. Between 1918–1930, however, it was common in Europe and the United Kingdom, appearing as a febrile illness with continued drowsiness and ophthalmoplegia. In neurological practice at present (1962) it is seen as post-encephalitic Parkinsonism with or without oculogyric crises, a late sequel of an attack often unrecognised, or misdiagnosed as "influenza" or meningitis in the 1918–1930 epidemic.

Symptoms.—After a period of general malaise lasting several days the patient becomes aware of persistent double vision and increasing *drowsiness* when he should be awake. Some hours later persistent somnolence sets in which continues by day for three to six weeks with delirium at night. During this acute phase various internal and external *ophthalmoplegias* are observed—variations in the size of the pupils and in their reaction to light. Bilateral ptosis and squints occur with nystagmus. Loss of pupillary reaction on accommodation-convergence may be observed during conscious periods. Pyramidal signs and coarse rhythmic tremors are not infrequent. In rare cases myoclonic movements, root pains and persistent hiccough may be observed. The *cerebro-spinal fluid* is normal in one-third of the cases; the others show increased pressure, 10–100 lymphocytes per c.mm. with a normal chloride and glucose content. The colloidal gold curve is usually normal.

Diagnosis.—Persistent lethargy with squints occurs in barbiturate intoxication, chronic bromism and in cerebral anoxia. Wernicke's hæmorrhagic encephalopathy found in patients with nutritional neuropathy and alcoholism causes drowsiness, ptosis and ocular palsies. Hypothalamic tumours, posterior fossa tumours and basal leptomeningitis are differentiated by their spinal fluid findings or by the use of contrast radiography. Epidemic encephalitis is more easily diagnosed during an epidemic.

Etiology.—The disease is due to a virus which probably remains active for years in the central nervous system. Economo claims to have transferred the disease from human brains to monkeys.

Prognosis.—One-third of the cases die. A considerable proportion of those who survive develop sequelæ. In children mental symptoms of bizarre pattern, personality changes, delinquency and dementia may follow. In adults sequelæ may ensue as long as twenty years after an attack. The commonest sequel in adult life is *Post-Encephalitic Parkinsonism* (§ 915). Oculogyric crises in which the eyes turn upwards or to one side in prolonged paroxysms accompany this disorder as well as evidences of hypothalamic disorder and brain stem symptoms, especially sialorrhœa and various respiratory tics such as violent yawning, sighing, hyperventilation with tetany. Diplopia and squint usually clear up, but the pupillary abnormalities and slight ptosis are often permanent and together with tremors tend to afford valuable diagnostic marks of the disease.

Treatment.—The acute illness is notifiable. Cases need not be isolated, as the incidence of case-to-case infectivity is not high. Behaviour disorders in children following encephalitis are usually serious and may call for special schooling or institutional care. In post-encephalitic Parkinsonism tincture of stramonium ℳ 12–20 t.i.d. or Artane 2–5 mg. t.i.d. helps the rigidity. In oculogyric crises give *d*-amphetamine sulphate 5–10 mg. soon after waking.

D. **Disturbances of Sleep Rhythm.**—In *Encephalitis Lethargica*, especially in children, the patient falls into a heavy sleep during the day but at night-time becomes wakeful and restless, often destructive, *e.g.*, tearing the bedclothes into shreds.

§ 838. In **Narcolepsy** the patient is periodically overcome by an irresistible desire to sleep. He can be roused, but, if left undisturbed, may slumber for half an hour or longer, waking to normal consciousness. Dreams may occur. The attacks may occur several times a day and the depth of sleep varies, as in normal sleep. There is often abnormal slowness in waking up after normal sleep. Associated with this is a phenomenon known as *Cataplexy.* Whenever the patient feels a strong emotion, after hearty laughter, after anger, or when intensely interested in something, a sudden weakness overcomes him and he sinks helpless to the ground, retaining full consciousness but unable to utter a sound. The element of *surprise* in the emotional situation seems to be important in precipitating an attack. The whole attack lasts only a second or two and during this, the knee-jerks are abolished and the plantars are extensor in type. Narcolepsy occurs as an idiopathic disease; it may occur as a sequel of encephalitis lethargica, in cases of idiopathic epilepsy, with obesity and genital atrophy, after head injuries and in cerebral tumours, especially in the hypothalamic region. The E.E.G. is usually normal, awake or asleep.

Treatment.—The patient should be advised not to drive any vehicle, swim or ride, or work at a height from the ground. Caffeine citrate 5 grains may be prescribed twice daily. Dexamphetamine sulphate, 5–10 mg., given on waking and at midday, will in many cases avert the sleep attacks. A larger dose may be required for a time. Continuous daily administration of this substance over long periods is not advised. If taken in the evening it is likely to interfere with the patient's normal sleep.

PART B.　CLINICAL INVESTIGATION

§ 839. The acquisition of a proficient technique in examining patients, and routine in applying it, is essential for solving neurological problems. The examiner must secure the patient's co-operation by explaining the objects of the tests used. The examination must be thorough and accurate, otherwise the deductions will be erroneous. Experience in neurological disease never absolves one from the necessity of careful examination, for the case history, without the physical signs, may be entirely misleading.

GENERAL CONSIDERATIONS.—Ambulatory patients should be examined while lying on a couch in a good light. In eliciting reflexes one tries to secure good muscular relaxation. Later the patient should be asked to walk, whenever possible, for inspection of the gait.

In writing case-notes on neurological cases remember the following points: (1) *Put down your observations categorically* and systematically under the various headings. (2) *Never omit to record regative as well as positive findings:* if the pupils are equal, central, circular, and react to light directly and consensually, say so. It may be as important in the final diagnosis as the finding of a fixed pupil. (3) Only certain abbreviations are permitted. These are SJ, BJ, TJ, KJ, AJ, for supinator, biceps, triceps, knee-jerk and ankle-jerk, respectively. AC and PC may be used for ankle-and patellar-clonus. + signifies a reflex elicited, + + an exaggeration of a reflex, O an absent reflex. The signs > greater than, < less than, are also permissible (*e.g.*, KJ's R̲ > L). In sensory testing C.W., P.P., V.S., J.S., and T° are used for cotton-wool, pin-prick, vibration sense, joint-sense, and temperature respectively. R and L underlined are used to indicate Right and Left; thus V.R. = 6/6 indicates that the visual acuity of the Right eye is six-sixths.

No neurological examination is complete without a full examination of other systems, including the urine. Progress notes should always be made. In certain cases a spinal puncture with examination of the cerebro-spinal fluid will be necessary. The ordinary methods of clinical examination—palpation, percussion, are not available in examining the nervous system. Special methods are used, requiring special tools, and the observer should provide himself with one of the heavier types of reflex-hammer, a tuning-fork (C 128) for testing vibration sense, and a good electrical ophthalmoscope. A skin pencil for marking out areas of diminished sensation is useful.

THE HISTORY.—The *mode of onset* of the symptoms is of the greatest importance in diagnosing the cause of the lesion. Thus, a hemiplegia coming on in a few seconds is commonly due to cerebral hæmorrhage or embolism, one coming on in a few minutes or hours to a cerebral thrombosis, whilst a hemiplegia developing gradually over weeks or months is commonly caused by a slowly-forming tumour or abscess. In a chronic disease like disseminated sclerosis, the first symptom may have occurred in early adult life, and neurological histories often cover the major part of the patient's lifetime. Events should be set down chronologically, using a fresh paragraph for recording the occurrence of each fresh symptom in the story. Experience is necessary to avoid inclusion of irrelevant matter. Important points may be missed if leading questions are not asked. The examiner should never omit to ask for a history of double vision, precipitancy of micturition, frequency or incontinence, since through shyness a patient may suppress important facts. A history of double vision, elicited in response to a leading question, should not be accepted too readily: most patients can recall what was the first object seen as a double image. It is often necessary to obtain additional history from *relatives* or *friends*, to supplement, corroborate, or amend the patient's story. In cases of epilepsy we should, whenever possible, obtain a description of the attack from an eye-witness.

Previous History.—A history of recurrent headache in adolescence and cyclical vomiting in childhood may be important in cases of migraine. In cases of fits we should inquire for teething convulsions in infancy, bed-wetting, or night-terrors. A history of head injury may be forgotten. Rheumatism, diphtheria, severe influenza, aural discharges, operations for malignant disease, may all have a bearing on the patient's illness. Ask for disturbances of vision in earlier life where disseminated sclerosis is a possibility. A history of stillbirths or absence of pregnancies over a long period of married life may suggest syphilitic infection when no history of this is volunteered. In cases of cerebral diplegia or infantile hemiplegia ask for a history of anoxia following birth, icterus gravis neonatorum (where the mother is Rh negative) which may cause athetosis in later life, or birth injury.

Family History is particularly important in neurological disease, as some neurological diseases, e.g., Friedreich's ataxia, dystrophia myotonica, Huntington's chorea, are heredo-familial, whilst others, e.g., Hepato-lenticular degeneration, are familial. The patient should be asked regarding the occurrence of headaches, fits or nervous illness in his brothers or sisters, parents, uncles, aunts, cousins, etc. The health of his wife and of his family should be ascertained.

Habits and Occupation.—Inquiry should be made as to past residence abroad. Soldiers infected in India with cysticercosis develop fits in later life. If alcoholism is suspected, the patient's own statement must be accepted with " philosophic doubt."

Tobacco addiction may cause a retrobulbar neuritis.   The patient's occupation often has a close bearing on his illness.

THE EXAMINATION

SCHEME FOR ROUTINE NEUROLOGICAL EXAMINATION. Build and general appearance. Temperature. Pulse rate. Body weight.

PSYCHICAL FUNCTIONS: (*and see Chapter XXI*).

Intelligence, Attentiveness, Memory, Orientation, Emotional State—Phobias, Hallucinations, Delusions—Sleep, Delirium, Coma.

SPEECH AND ARTICULATION.

Is the patient right- or left-handed ?   Aphasia, Apraxia, Articulation.

CRANIAL NERVES.

Smell—Visual acuity; Fields of Vision; Optic Discs and Fundi—Pupils; External ocular movements; Nystagmus; Oculo-pupillary sympathetic phenomena—Corneal reflexes; Sensation over face; Masseters, Temporals—Facial movements and symmetry of face—Hearing—Palate; Tongue; Sterno-mastoids and Trapezii.

MOTOR FUNCTIONS.

(1) Power; (2) Co-ordination; (3) Tone; (4) Wasting and Fasciculation, Hypertrophy of muscles; (5) Involuntary movements and Fits.

EXAMINATION OF GAIT.

SENSORY FUNCTIONS.

Cutaneous Sensibility—(1) Touch (cotton-wool); (2) Pain (pin-prick); (3) Temperature.

Deep Sensibility—(4) Joint Sense; (5) Vibration; (6) Sensibility of Muscles and Tendons to Deep Pressure.

Stereognosis, Tactile Localisation, Compass Tests.

REFLEX FUNCTIONS.

Tendon Reflexes—Biceps, Triceps and Radial (Supinator) Reflexes. Knee-Jerks and Ankle-Jerks.   Presence of Clonus.

Cutaneous Reflexes—Epigastric Reflexes, Upper and Lower Abdominal Reflexes.   Plantar Reflexes.

Visceral Reflexes—Micturition and Defæcation.

Tonic Reflexes—Kernig's Sign, Neck stiffness.

SPINE AND CRANIUM.

Deformities or Tenderness.   Presence of bruit on auscultation of skull.

TROPHIC CHANGES.

Skin—Bed-sores, perforating ulcers.   Nævi, pigmented patches.

Bones and Joints—Arthropathies, pes cavus.

SPECIAL EXAMINATIONS.

(1) Cerebro-spinal Fluid—Dynamics, Cells, Total Protein, Globulin, Sugar, Chlorides, Wassermann Reaction, Lange Curve, Culture.

(2) Blood—Wassermann Reaction, Blood Counts and Sedimentation Rate (E.S.R.) may be required.

(3) *X-ray examination*, including contrast radiography.

(4) *Electroencephalography*—E.E.G.

(5) *Electrical and other exploratory examinations of nerve and muscle, electromyography.*

(6) *Muscle or cerebral biopsy.*

For Examination of COMATOSE PATIENTS turn to § 850.

EXAMINATION OF OTHER SYSTEMS.

Psychical Functions.—Note the patient's intelligence, comprehension, attentiveness, his memory for recent and remote events, and whether he is oriented in space and time. Note his behaviour throughout the examination and record delusions, hallucinations, phobias or obsessions (see § 1162 *et seq.*).

Psychometry.—Where progressive mental deterioration or mental defect is suspected (*e.g.*, after a head injury, or in dementia) mental testing carried out by an experienced psychologist is often invaluable.

For less precise examination the *intelligence* and *attentiveness* of the patient can be gauged by hearing him tell the history of his illness. *Memory* for recent and remote events may be tested by obtaining confirmation of the history from a reliable relative. *Memory span* is tested by asking the patient to repeat seven digits forward or five backwards. Ask him to repeat a sentence of 28 syllables, *e.g.*, " Walter likes very much to go on visits to his grandmother, because she always tells him many funny stories." Ask the patient to memorise the name of a flower, the name of a piece of furniture and a simple street address, and note if he remembers these three minutes later. Ask the patient to recall the names of Monarchs or Prime Ministers. Tests for *reasoning* or *calculation* may be helpful—ask the patient to subtract aloud serial sevens from a hundred and note his speed and accuracy. *Orientation* in space is tested by asking the patient " What place is this ? " " How did you come here ? " etc., and in time, " What month (or year) is this ? " " How long have you been here ? " *Drawing tests* with pencil and paper are instructive.

Do not mistake aphasia or apraxia due to organic focal brain disease for mental illness.

§ 840. Speech and Articulation.—(*a*) **Aphasia and Apraxia.**—The tests for these are described in §§ 869, 872. In certain cortical lesions the patient has difficulty in translating his thoughts into words, either spoken or written, or difficulty in comprehending spoken or written speech. This is aphasia. An apraxic patient recognises objects, *e.g.*, a key or a pipe, but cannot demonstrate how to use them, although he is aware of their proper use and is not paralysed or ataxic.

(*b*) *Articulation.*—This has to do with the peripheral speech mechanism. Dysarthric patients have difficulty " in getting their tongues round words." This is tested by getting the patient to repeat certain catch-phrases, *e.g.*, " Biblical criticism," " Methodist Episcopal," " West Register Street," " Baby Hippopotamus."

(*c*) The occurrence of speech areas in the left cerebral cortex in right-handed people, and in the right hemisphere in left-handed people, renders it necessary that you should know whether the patient is right- or left-handed.

§ 841. Cranial Nerves.—I. OLFACTORY.—You ask the patient to close his eyes. *Each nostril* is tested separately, by applying a smelling-bottle of peppermint or lavender oil to the nostril tested while closing the other with your finger. It is sufficient if the patient can recognise differences in odour. Odours need not be named specifically. Ammonia, or substances containing it, such as smelling-salts or sal volatile, should not be used, because they stimulate the fibres of the trigeminal in the nasal mucosa, *i.e.* common sensation. Ask the patient " Do you smell anything ? " " Of what does this smell ? " " Is it different from this ? "

II. OPTIC.—You must make three examinations:

(a) Visual acuity.

(b) Fields of vision—peripheral and central.

(c) Ophthalmoscopic examination.

(a) *Visual Acuity* is normally tested by "Snellen's types" at a distance of 6 metres (to exclude accommodation so far as possible), or by Jaeger's test card for near vision (§ 1116).

Poorer vision is expressed by the distance at which he can count fingers (" C.F. = 1 metre "), or perceive hand movements (" H.M."). Poorer vision near blindness means usually only perception of light (" P.L.").

(b) *Fields of Vision* are tested (i.) by confrontation, (ii.) by mechanical perimetry, (iii) by Bjerrum's screen.

(i.) *Confrontation* is the method used in a routine neurological examination. The patient, who has his back to the light, sits opposite the examiner, their eyes separated by a distance of one metre. In examining the right field the patient's left eye is covered. You then say, " I want you to look directly at my left eye," pointing to your left eye and closing your right eye. Tell the patient you wish to test his visual field and demonstrate this to him. Now, fixing the patient's pupil with a steady gaze so that you can note any deviation of the eye you are examining, hold your hands almost at arms' length at a place midway between yourself and the patient. Then tell the patient, " I want you to point to anything you see moving." Move the thumb of one hand rapidly once and, if the movement is seen, the patient will point to the moving object. The moving thumbs are in this way brought from the periphery of the visual field towards the centre, testing all four quadrants of the visual field. You can thus compare the patient's field with your own. If any defect is suspected a careful perimetric chart should be made with a reliable perimeter. Visual inattention may be present when no gross field defect exists: a patient will then fail to notice your moving finger in the affected fields, there being no formal field defect. Central vision is tested with a 5-mm. white or red object, on a black rod held in the centre of the visual field, midway between one's own and the patient's eye. For convenience, a fragment of blotting-paper stuck in the nib of a pen is often used. If a central blind spot or scotoma is present the patient will not see the object until it is moved radially outwards. If a field defect exists it should be charted accurately by Mechanical Perimetry or Bjerrum's Screen.

(ii.) *Mechanical Perimetry* is used to make a permanent record of the fields of vision; and (iii.) Bjerrum's Screen maps out central and paracentral defects (scotomata). These are described in § 1117.

(c) *Ophthalmoscopic Examination.*—The optic discs and retinæ must be examined in every case of nervous disease. Every physician must know how to use an ophthalmoscope, and to recognise papillœdema, optic atrophy, and the commoner pathological appearances in the retina and its vessels (§ 1126 *et seq.*).

III, IV, VI. OCULOMOTOR, TROCHLEAR, ABDUCENT.

These nerves supplying the internal and external ocular muscles are conveniently examined together. The *Oculomotor* supplies the superior, inferior and medial recti and inferior oblique, the striped muscle of the levator palpebræ superioris, and contains efferent autonomic fibres supplying the tonic constrictor fibres of the sphincter pupillæ and ciliary muscle. The *Trochlear* supplies the superior oblique muscle and the *Abducent* the lateral rectus alone. The *Cervical Sympathetic* supplies the tonic dilator fibres of the pupil, the unstriped part of the levator palpebræ superioris and unstriped muscle at the back of the orbit.

(a) *Pupils.*—You must note if the pupils are equal, central, circular, oval, or irregular in outline. Observe their reactions to light, tested directly, consensually and on accommodation. Examine the external ocular movements for paresis and diplopia, look for nystagmus and note any inequality in the size of the ocular fissures, proptosis or enophthalmos (sinking of the eye into the socket). *The normal pupil dilates to shade, and contracts briskly when light falls on the same eye (direct reflex)* or on the opposite eye (consensual reflex). The *light reflex* is best tested by covering and unshading first one eye of the patient and then the other as he looks at the light. Each eye must be observed separately. Watch the effect on the pupil of shading and uncovering the opposite eye. Another way of testing the pupillary reflex to light is: turn the patient's face away from the light and (observing one pupil at a time) throw a beam of light from an electric torch first into the one eye and then into the other. Loss of direct reflex to light with preservation of pupillary contraction to accommodation constitutes the *Argyll-Robertson phenomenon.* Test the *accommodation-convergence reaction* (near reflex) of the pupils by asking the patient to look first at a distant object in the room, and then suddenly to look at your forefinger held about a foot from his eyes. The normal pupil contracts briskly as the eyes converge.

Tonic pupils (Adie) contract very slowly on accommodation. The contraction is long sustained and may last for half a minute or more. *Fixed pupils* react neither on accommodation nor to light stimuli.

(*b*) *External Ocular Movements.*—Steady the patient's chin with your left hand, in order to fix the head. Then raise the forefinger of your right hand at a distance of more than 20 inches from the patient's eyes and say, "I want you to follow my finger closely with your eyes." Move the finger to the extreme right, and pause in order to see if there is lack of movement in one or other eye, or the presence of nystagmus. Test both eyes together on lateral gaze to the right, on lateral gaze to the left, on elevation and on depression. Ask in each case if the vision is clear or blurred.

Nystagmus is an involuntary rhythmic oscillation of the eyes, usually appearing when the gaze is directed to a fixed point, *e.g.*, the examiner's finger held some distance away from the patient beyond the rest point of the eyes. Nystagmus may be *pendular,* or *rotatory* or *jerking.* In the case of jerking nystagmus the quick phase is taken to indicate the direction of the nystagmus. Thus if the quick phase is to the subject's right, and the slow phase his left, the convention is to label this *nystagmus to the right.* Note the amplitude whether coarse (large) or fine (small) and the *rate*— slow or rapid. Three degrees of *jerking nystagmus* are recognised. Thus in a patient with nystagmus to the right, if it appears only on gaze to the right, it is of first degree. If it appears on gaze to the right and on gazing ahead it is *of second degree,* and if it appears on gaze to the right, gaze ahead and gaze to the left it is *of third degree.*

	Gaze to the Right	*Gaze ahead*	*Gaze to the Left*
1st Degree	+	−	−
2nd Degree	++	+	−
3rd Degree	+++	++	+

— no nystagmus; + small amplitude; ++ large amplitude; +++ very large amplitude. For the *Causes* of nystagmus see § 1073.

V. TRIGEMINAL.—This nerve supplies sensory fibres to the anterior part of the scalp, eyes, face, nose, mouth, and parts of the ear and tongue, as well as the dura mater (see § 1076). The motor root supplies the muscles of mastication, masseter, temporals, pterygoids, mylohyoid, anterior belly of digastric, tensor palati and tensor tympani muscles.

You must make three examinations: (*a*) corneal reflex, (*b*) sensation over face, (*c*) the muscles of mastication.

(*a*) The *corneal reflex* is tested by asking the patient to look upwards and touching the cornea from outwards and below with a long pointed strand of cotton-wool. The reflexes should be compared on the two sides. Care should be taken to touch the cornea, not the conjunctiva. (*b*) *Sensation over the face* is tested with cotton-wool, pin-pricks and tubes of hot and cold water. Where there is diminution or loss of sensation, this is mapped out with a skin pencil, working from the dull to the sensitive area. (*c*) *The muscles of mastication* are tested by asking the patient to clench his jaws, when the masseters and temporals can be palpated as they contract on the two sides. In unilateral lesions, when the patient opens his mouth, the jaw deviates to the side of the lesion, being pushed over by the healthy external pterygoid muscle of the opposite side. Wasting of the masseters or temporals should be looked for.

VII. FACIAL.—Test the *voluntary movements* of both the upper and the lower face and the reflex *emotional movements*, e.g., facial movements on smiling. Taste on the anterior two-thirds of the tongue is conveniently tested with this nerve, as taste fibres for this part of the tongue are distributed with the chorda tympani (Fig. 262).

Voluntary movements of the *upper face* are tested by asking the patient to wrinkle up his eyebrows and screw up his eyes. Slight degrees of weakness can be observed by the difference in burying of the eyelashes on the two sides, or by comparing the effort needed to open with your thumb the screwed-up eyelids. Voluntary movements of the *lower face* are tested by asking the patient to show his teeth, blow out his cheeks, or whistle. Slight degrees of facial weakness are shown by widening of the ocular fissure on the affected side, and flattening of the naso-labial fold. In upper motor neurone lesions only the lower face is affected.

Emotional movements are tested by asking the patient to smile and noting the difference in the angles of the mouth, or they may be observed during the general examination. *Taste* is best tested with a weak galvanic current; the wire electrode on the taste-sensitive areas produces a metallic taste. Or the patient is asked to protrude his tongue and to keep it out, and to nod if he tastes anything. Powdered sugar, salt, citric acid or quinine are then rubbed on the tongue with a clean glass rod. If the patient tastes the substance he nods and is allowed to withdraw the tongue and describe the taste.

VIII. AUDITORY.—The sensory or cochlear component subserves *hearing*, the vestibular non-sensory component subserves reflexes concerned with *equilibrium*. The clinical examination and methods of testing are described in § 1143.

IX, X, XI. GLOSSOPHARYNGEAL, VAGUS AND SPINAL ACCESSORY.—
These nerves are intimately related in their central connections; they leave the skull by the jugular foramen and are conveniently tested together. (*a*) *Sensory tests:* Tickling the soft palate or posterior pharyngeal wall with cotton-wool on the end of a probe will normally produce reflex movements (Glossopharyngeal). Fibres of the glossopharyngeal nerve supply taste to the posterior third of the tongue. (*b*) *Motor Tests:* (1) *Palate:* The patient is asked to open his mouth and say, " A-Ah." When the patient phonates the soft palate will rise in the mid-line; if one side is paralysed the palate will be deviated to the sound side. Bilateral palatal palsy produces a characteristic nasal intonation, with regurgitation of fluids through the nose on swallowing. (2) *Pharynx:* In unilateral paralysis, the posterior pharyngeal wall moves like a curtain pulled over to the sound side (" curtain movement ") when the patient phonates. (3) *Larynx* (see § 164). (4) *Sterno-mastoids and Trapezii:* Examine the sterno-mastoids by asking the patient to turn his head forcibly to the right and then to the left, or by asking him to push his forehead downwards against the resistance of the palm of your right hand. The trapezii are tested by asking the patient to shrug his shoulders against the resistance of your hands placed on his shoulders. In all cases the muscles should be inspected and palpated for wasting.

The visceral functions of this group of nerves are described in the examination of the other systems.

XII. HYPOGLOSSAL.—Ask the patient to protrude the tongue and to push it first into the right cheek and then the left. The protruded tongue is examined for spasticity, fasciculation, atrophy or wrinkling (§§ 216, 217). If one side of the tongue is paralysed and the patient attempts to protrude the organ, the tip is pushed round to the paralysed side, in a sickle-shaped curve, by the healthy side (§ 1088).

§ 842. Motor Functions.—It is advisable to have the patient in pyjamas, or stripped and in a dressing-gown. First, examine the upper limbs, then the trunk, and then the lower limbs, and the results are recorded in that order. You should note especially if the limbs are strong and steady, also examine their tone, and look for wasting and fasciculation, or hypertrophy of muscles.   Then proceed as follows:—

(1) POWER.—The hand-grips are conveniently tested by crossing one's forearms and giving one finger or your three middle fingers, shaped in the form of a cone, to the patient to squeeze as hard as he can.   The flexors of the fingers can be tested by asking the patient to hook the flexed fingers of his right hand round the flexed fingers of your right hand and then you attempt to extend his fingers against resistance.   The dorsiflexion of the feet is similarly tested against resistance by asking the patient, when recumbent, to cock his feet upwards.   You then attempt to plantar-flex them whilst he resists.   In these tests the power is compared on the two sides.   Each joint and each movement should be tested separately, fixing the proximal part of the limb and instructing the patient to perform various movements—flexion, extension, rotation outwards, inwards, etc., separately.   If the weakness is marked, support the limb in the optimum position for action of the particular muscle or group of muscles you are investigating.   In *lower motor neurone* lesions list in columns the muscles affected, and indicate by a numerical index whether the loss of power is slight, moderate or severe.   Full power may be indicated by 5 and lesser degrees by a descending scale down to complete loss of power = 0.   Inability to relax the hand-grip for some seconds is characteristic of *tonic innervation* or *myotonia*.

(2) CO-ORDINATION.—In the " finger–nose " test the patient, keeping his eyes open, moves his forefinger alternately to his nose and then to the examiner's finger, which is held about one metre in front of him.   He is asked to repeat this movement several times.   When " intention tremor " is present the movement is jerkily performed and a coarse oscillation of the forearm and hand appears just before the objective is reached.   When ataxia is present the finger misses the nose by a greater or smaller interval.   You should notice if the unsteadiness is increased when the patient shuts his eyes.   Co-ordination of the fine finger movements is tested with the " thumb–finger " test, the patient being asked to touch the tip of each finger in rapid succession (beginning with the fourth) to the tip of the thumb of his same hand.   Other useful tests are picking up a pin, fastening the buttons of a coat, etc.   In the " heel–knee " test the patient is placed in the recumbent position and is asked to place the heel of one foot on the opposite knee and to slide the heel slowly down the front of his shin.   Here, too, you should notice if ataxia is increased on shutting the eyes.   Other tests in the lower limbs are made with examination of the *gait*.   Special cerebellar tests are described in § 934.

(3) TONE.—*Hypotonia* is tested by shaking the relaxed limbs like a flail and comparing the resistance of the two sides, or attempting to fling the patient's hand on his chest.   In another test the hands are passively dorsiflexed and the angle made with the forearm on the two sides compared; the knee-joints are passively hyperextended, etc.   *Hypertonus* or rigidity is of three main types: (*a*) " Clasp-knife " rigidity; (*b*) " Cog-wheel " or " Lead-pipe " rigidity; (*c*) Hysterical Spasm.

(*a*) " Clasp-knife " rigidity is seen typically in a residual hemiplegia.   The arm is flexed at the elbow and pronated.   When you attempt to undo the flexion, resistance is encountered until the elbow is almost extended, when the resistance suddenly " gives " as in the opening of a clasp-knife.   This is characteristic of pyramidal disease.   (*b*) " Lead-pipe " or " Cog-wheel " rigidity is characteristic of extrapyramidal disease and is seen typically in Parkinsonism (§ 914).   When you attempt to extend the elbow-joint, resistance is felt like the bending of a piece of lead-piping.   Or on attempting to flex and extend the patient's wrist-joint, a feeling like turning a cogged wheel is met.   (*c*) In Hysterical Spasm the prime-movers and antagonists are simultaneously innervated by the patient so that little or no movement results—*e.g.*, when he attempts to use his hamstrings, the quadriceps, instead of relaxing reciprocally, tighten up.   The spasm increases with the amount of force used to overcome it .

(4) WASTING AND FASCICULATION.   HYPERTROPHY.—By inspection and palpation

you observe if the muscles are increased in bulk (hypertrophy) or wasted (atrophy). Sometimes hypertrophied muscles are feeble in their performance (pseudo-hypertrophy). *The names of the affected muscles are recorded.* You should carefully inspect all aspects of the limb and the back as well as the front of the patient. Whenever wasting is present you should look for *fasciculation* in the atrophied muscles. This is a flickering or quivering of muscle-fibres or bundles, best seen when the muscles are relaxed. It is seen too in states of fatigue and toxæmia. Direct percussion of a muscle with a reflex hammer may show in certain pathological conditions the appearance of a dimple, which is persistent for some seconds—*myotonia on percussion.*

(5) INVOLUNTARY MOVEMENTS.—*Tremor* is best seen when the arms and fingers are extended. It may be coarse or fine. Tremor never exists in flaccid limbs; it usually ceases during sleep, and can often be controlled by an effort of will. *Choreic movements* are irregular, non-rhythmic, spontaneous but purposeless movements of groups of muscles. In organic disease they are more marked on one side than the other, and in the facial muscles they occur bilaterally. *Athetoid Movements* (athetosis) are slow, irregular, writhing movements, seen in hemiplegic limbs, more often in children than in adults (Fig. 241). The limbs are never completely paralysed: the movements are more marked peripherally and usually greater on one side than the other, and are bilaterally distributed in the face. The movements are intensified by emotion and by voluntary movements, and, between the accesses of mobile spasm, the limb is generally hypotonic. *Myoclonus* is a sudden shock-like contraction occurring regularly or irregularly in various muscles. *Tics* are sudden clonic jerks of a stereotyped character in people of neuropathic constitution, increased by emotion.

§ 843. Examination of the Gait.

Except in patients confined strictly to bed the gait should always be examined. This is frequently forgotten by students. The patient is asked to walk away from you to a given point, to turn round and then come back. It is advisable to pull or pin up the clothing or pyjama-trousers so that as much as possible of the legs can be seen. The patient walks on a strip of carpet with bare feet. Look for dragging of the legs, reeling or tottering, especially in turning, whether the patient deviates from the straight line and if so to which side he deviates, and whether he swings both arms as he walks. Where cerebellar or posterior column disease is suspected ask the patient to heel-and-toe a straight line, to stand or hop, first on one leg and then on the other. Where myopathy is suspected the patient (usually a child) is laid flat on the floor and asked to stand upright. The various motions performed in accomplishing this are characteristic. The following are:

TYPES OF ABNORMAL GAIT

(1) In *Spastic Gait* the toes are dragged on the ground. This occurs in pyramidal disease, *e.g.*, disseminated sclerosis, residual hemiplegia. Where extensor rigidity is combined with adductor rigidity, a " crosslegged " or " scissor-gait " is met, the patient walking on the toes, *e.g.*, in cerebral diplegia in children.

(2) *Spastic Ataxic Gait* is met in combined disease of the pyramidal tracts and posterior columns, *e.g.*, disseminated sclerosis, subacute combined degeneration, spinal tumour.

(3) *Ataxic or Reeling Gait* occurs in cerebellar, vestibular or posterior

column disease, *e.g.*, cerebellar tumour, Friedreich's hereditary ataxia, labyrinthine disease or tabes dorsalis.

(4) *A Festinant or Shuffling Gait*, in which the patient glides forward with little running or shuffling paces, occurs in striatal disease, *e.g.*, Parkinsonism. In this condition the normal swing of the arms is lost and the patient turns *en bloc*. It is seen in the general muscular rigidity of cerebral arteriosclerosis.

(5) *Waddling Gait* is met when there is weakness of the pelvic muscles, *e.g.*, myopathy; or from deformities, *e.g.*, congenital dislocation of the hip.

(6) *High-stepping Gait* occurs in conditions of foot-drop, *e.g.* polyneuritis; or from loss of joint sense, as in tabes, in which the feet are lifted high and the heels banged on the ground.

(7) *Jaunty Gait* is seen in chorea.

(8) *Limping Gait* may result from poliomyelitis or any injury or joint affection confined to one side.

(9) *Bizarre Gaits*, in which the patient walks with bent knees or trunk, or in zig-zag fashion, are seen in hysteria. A gingerly insecure gait, where the patient seeks support from the walls, furniture or the observers, is common in that disease.

§ **844. Sensory Functions.**—In order to make sensory testing accurate it is desirable to gain the intelligent co-operation of the patient, and each test should be briefly explained before it is carried out. The room should be as quiet as possible and the patient's eyes closed in order to shut out extraneous stimuli.

The following rules should be observed: (1) Test each variety of sensation separately over the whole body before proceeding to the next; (2) *Always compare the sensibility over corresponding areas on the two halves of the body*; (3) Whenever possible chart the findings on an outline diagram; (4) Avoid suggesting the presence of a sensory change to the patient by the manner in which commands or questions are put, *i.e.*, first find out if the patient can feel the stimulus and then explore any difference in quality of the sensation. The following are useful approaches which suggest little to the patient: " Shut your eyes and say ' Yes ' every time I touch you " (C.W.). " What does this feel like ? " (P.P.). " Is there any difference in the feeling here, and here ? " (P.P.).

CUTANEOUS SENSIBILITY.—(1) *Touch* is tested with a wisp of long-fibred cottonwool. In mapping out anæsthetic areas, proceed from the area of impaired sensibility towards normal skin and from below upwards on the trunk. The point at which sensation becomes normal is recorded on the skin by a single dot made with a skin pencil. A number of these dots are made, and they can subsequently be connected, as in a graph, to outline the area. An anæsthetic area so mapped out should be recorded on the chart and shaded. Vertical hatching is used conventionally in diagrams for recording impairment of touch.

(2) *Pain* is tested with the prick of a sharp steel pin. To obtain a uniform stimulus the pin should be held with the point just projecting between the pads of the thumb and middle finger. *Dragged pin* is used to map out areas of hyperæsthesia, the pin being lightly dragged across the skin from the less to the more sensitive area.

Loss of pain sensation is termed *analgesia* and is represented in outline diagrams conventionally by horizontal hatching; *hyperæsthesia* or exalted sensibility to pain is represented by a series of small crosses. The distinction should be made between " impaired sensibility " and " total analgesia." In mapping out sensory levels on the trunk remember that the segmental distribution of the spinal nerve roots runs downwards anteriorly, and upwards posteriorly, towards the mid-line. Horizontal upper levels of sensory loss are found only in hysteria and are produced by suggestion. The hysterical nature of a totally anæsthetic area may sometimes be demonstrated by Janet's " Yes-No " test. The patient is instructed to close his eyes and say " Yes " every time he feels a pin-prick and " No " every time he does not feel it. In hysteria the patient will say " No " every time he is touched over the apparently totally anæsthetic area, thus demonstrating that he is really able to feel but does not comprehend that he feels.

(3) *Temperature* is tested with tightly stoppered metal tubes or corked test-tubes of cold and warm water (60° C). The results are recorded on outline diagrams using conventional oblique hatching (Rt. to Lt. = Loss to Hot; Lt. to Rt. = Loss to Cold), Loss of sensation to temperature is called Therm-anæsthesia. In centrally situated diseases of the brain-stem and cord, such as Syringomyelia, the patient may feel the lightest touches with cotton-wool but cannot appreciate painful or thermal stimuli —this was called by Charcot " *dissociated anæsthesia*."

DEEP SENSIBILITY.—(4) *Joint sense* comprises the sense of passive movement of the joint surfaces on one another, and the sense of position. In testing, the patient closes his eyes, or they are covered. In order to avoid sensations of pressure, you grasp the digit you are testing, *laterally*, with your thumb and forefinger. *When testing sense of passive movement* wait a few moments, then move the joint gently, having previously asked the patient to say " Yes " when he feels any movement. In testing *sense of position* ask the patient to say " Up " or " Down " every time you move the joint, showing him first what is meant by " Up " and by " Down." You then passively move the joint in either direction, waiting for the patient's reply after each movement. Corresponding fingers and toes are tested on the two sides.

(5) *Vibration* is tested by placing a low-pitched tuning-fork (C.128) on the radial styloids and tibial malleoli. Other bony prominences may be used. Vibration sensibility may be diminished or lost very early in disease of the posterior columns or posterior roots.

(6) *Sensibility of Muscles and Tendons to Deep Pressure.*—An increased sensitiveness of the calf muscles to deep pressure of your thumb is common in polyneuritis —i e , the *deep muscular sensibility* is increased. In tabes dorsalis, as an early sign, the normal sensibility of the tendo Achillis to pressure may be diminished or lost (A adie's sign).

Stereognosis is tested by placing various objects—e.g., key, coin, rubber, in the hand or against the sole of the patient, whose eyes are closed, asking him to describe the shape, size and consistency of the object used. For true stereognosis to be present, cutaneous sensibility in the hand or foot tested should not be impaired. *Tactile localisation* (topognosis) is tested by asking the patient, who has his eyes closed, to point to where he has been touched with a pin. Normally the localisation is exact to a fraction of an inch. *Compass Tests* are performed with small blunt-pointed calipers (Head's compasses). The patient, who has his eyes closed, states whether he has been touched with one or two points, while the distance between the limbs of the calipers is gradually narrowed.

Sensory inattention is a phenomenon sometimes found in patients with parietal lobe lesions. Ask the patient to close his eyes, then test simultaneously (and separately) corresponding skin points on the patient's right and left sides. The patient is asked to say if he feels the touch on the right or left, or on both sides together. In sensory inattention the patient ignores touches on the affected side when identical mirror points are tested simultaneously. The condition may be present in the absence of any formal sensory loss.

§ 845. Reflex Functions.

In routine examinations you must test the TENDON REFLEXES, certain CUTANEOUS REFLEXES, including the PLANTAR REFLEXES, and you must note the condition of certain VISCERAL REFLEXES, *e.g.*, micturition, defæcation. TONIC or POSTURAL REFLEXES, *e.g.*, Kernig's Sign, are also used in clinical diagnosis.

1. **Tendon Reflexes.**—These are elicited by percussing the tendons of insertion of certain muscles.

	Method of Eliciting.	Response.	Segmental Distribution.
Biceps-Jerk.	Tapping biceps tendon.	Biceps contracts.	C5–6.
Triceps-Jerk.	Tapping triceps tendon.	Triceps contracts.	C6 7.
Supinator-Jerk (Radial reflex).	Tapping above radial styloid.	Brachioradialis contracts.	C6 7.
Knee-Jerk.	Tapping patellar tendon.	Vastus medialis, etc., contract.	L2–4.
Ankle-Jerk.	Tapping tendo Achillis.	Calf muscles contract.	S1 2.

In UPPER MOTOR NEURONE disease these reflexes are exaggerated and may be accompanied by sustained *clonus*, a rhythmic series of involuntary muscular contractions, produced by the sudden stretching of the tendon. In LOWER MOTOR NEURONE disease and in the MYOPATHIES, the deep reflexes are diminished or abolished in the affected muscles.

The *Biceps-Jerk* (C5–6) is elicited by supporting the patient's forearm with his elbow loosely flexed. Your thumb is placed over the biceps tendon and the thumb percussed with a hammer. The resultant jerk of the biceps is both felt and seen. The *Triceps-Jerk* (C6–7) is then investigated by abducting the patient's arm loosely and percussing the triceps tendon. The *Supinator-Jerk* or *Radial reflex* (C6–7) is elicited by tapping just above the radial styloid, the patient's forearm supported in a semi-supinated position, the elbow loosely bent to a right-angle. The resultant contraction of the supinator and flexors of the elbow is looked for. *Inversion of the radial reflex*, often associated with cord lesions at the C5/6 segmental level, occurs when the usual contraction of the brachioradialis is lost or reduced. A brisk contraction of the finger flexors on tapping the radial styloid is obtained instead. In testing the knee-jerks and ankle-jerks it is best to have the patient in the recumbent position to ensure muscular relaxation. To elicit the *Knee-Jerks* (L2–4) the recumbent patient's knees are slightly flexed, resting loosely on your arm, while you percuss the patellar tendons on the two sides and look for the resulting contraction of the vastus medialis. To elicit the *Ankle-Jerk* (S1–2) the lower limb is then rotated outwards at the hip and the knee-joint slightly flexed, the sole is grasped and slightly dorsiflexed to stretch the tendo Achillis and the tendon percussed. If difficulty is encountered in eliciting the ankle-jerks in this way the patient should be asked to kneel on a *padded* chair with the calf muscles relaxed and the feet dangling over the edge. When the tendo Achillis is percussed a brisk contraction of the calf muscles results, which can be felt as well as seen if you are slightly dorsiflexing the foot with your left hand to stretch the tendon. In eliciting deep reflexes the responses on the two sides should be compared with the greatest care and noted. Always use the *minimal stimulus*, especially when testing knee-jerks. Never use much force, otherwise no accurate comparison of the two sides can be obtained.   In testing sluggish knee- and ankle-jerks it may be necessary to use *reinforcement*; ask the patient to look to the roof and clench his hands tightly, or ask him to attempt to pull apart the interlocked fingers of the two hands.   The presence of sluggish deep reflexes may thus be made evident.

Patellar-clonus is elicited in spastic limbs by sudden downward traction on the patella, with the knee extended. *Ankle-clonus* is elicited with the knee passively flexed; the ankle is then suddenly dorsiflexed by light upward pressure on the sole. True clonus is always sustained and accompanied by an extensor type of plantar response.

2. Cutaneous Reflexes.—These are elicited by stimulating certain areas

of skin or mucous membrane.   The cutaneous reflexes of greatest practical importance are the Plantar Reflexes and the Abdominal Reflexes.   These must be tested in every case.   In upper motor neurone lesions these cutaneous reflexes alter profoundly.   This is most strikingly seen in the disappearance of the abdominal reflexes, first the lower and then the upper, in pyramidal disease.

The EPIGASTRIC (Th6–8), and UPPER (Th8–10) and LOWER (Th11–12) ABDOMINAL REFLEXES are elicited by stroking the lower anterior chest wall and the upper and lower quadrants of the abdominal wall respectively on the two sides.   These reflexes are elicited with difficulty when the abdominal wall is obese or flaccid.   In a healthy young adult they are constantly present.   In pyramidal disease these reflexes are diminished, tire easily or are lost on the affected side.   The lower reflexes go before the upper.   An absent abdominal reflex is an important early sign of disseminated sclerosis.   In suspected disease of the cauda equina or lowest segments of the cord you have to test three other cutaneous reflexes: the Cremasteric (L1–2), Bulbo-cavernosus (S3–4) and Superficial Anal (S4–5).

The CREMASTERIC REFLEX (L1–2) is the reflex drawing up of the testis, on down-ward stroking or firm pressure, applied on the inner side of the thigh.   The BULBO-CAVERNOSUS REFLEX (S3–4) gives valuable information about lesions of the third sacral segment.   It is elicited by placing one finger on the perineum and pricking the dorsum of the glans penis.   Normally, the bulbous urethra can be felt to contract briskly.   The SUPERFICIAL ANAL REFLEX (S4–5) is obtained by watching for the contraction of the external sphincter when the skin of the perineum is pricked.

A GRASP-REFLEX is elicited in the fully conscious patient in the contra-lateral palm, in lesions of the posterior ends of the first and second frontal gyri.   To obtain this you draw your fingers across the patient's palm near the thenar eminence.   The patient's fingers contract reflexly and, when you attempt to withdraw your hand, the involuntary tonic contraction of the fingers increases and may take seconds to relax.

The PLANTAR REFLEXES are of the utmost importance in clinical neurology, and the student should be thoroughly conversant with the correct technique of eliciting them.   The patient should be in the recumbent position with the lower limb slightly rotated outwards at the hip and the knee slightly flexed, and the feet comfortably warm.   Normally, firm stroking along the *outer* border of the sole of the foot with one's thumb nail or the end of a penholder produces flexion of the great toe—*flexor plantar response*.   In pyramidal disease, however, when we stroke the outer margin of the sole there results a dorsiflexion of the great toe, associated with dorsiflexion and fanning of the other toes—*extensor plantar response* (Babinski).   This extensor movement is part of a general withdrawal reflex of the whole lower limb from a painful stimulus and is often accompanied by an associated contraction of the hamstring muscles.   Plantar responses may be *flexor, extensor, equivocal* or *absent* at the toes. When, therefore, the plantar responses are equivocal, the hamstrings should be palpated for contraction, while the sole of the foot is being stimulated.

The *flexor* plantar response is associated with plantigrade functions associated

	Method of Eliciting.	Response.	Segmental Distribution.
Epigastric.	Stroking lower anterior chest wall.	Epigastrium dimples.	Th6–8.
Upper Abdominal.	Stroking below costal margin.	Rectus abdominis contracts.	Th8–10.
Lower Abdominal.	Stroking above Poupart's ligament	Obliquus abdominis contracts.	Th11–12.
Cremasteric.	Stroking inner side of thigh.	Testis is drawn up.	L1–2.
Bulbo-cavernosus.	Pricking dorsum of glans penis.	Bulbo-cavernosus contracts.	S3–4.
Superficial Anal.	Pricking skin of perineum.	External anal sphincter contracts.	S4–5.
Plantar.	Stroking outer border of sole of foot.	Plantar flexion of the hallux.	L5–S2.

with standing and walking. It is a cortical reflex. In infants who have not learned to walk the normal plantar response is of the extensor type. This *extensor* reflex is of spinal origin, and in later life when the infant learns to walk, is normally inhibited by cortical control. When the cortical control is removed by pyramidal disease the more primitive spinal extensor response is re-established. In spastic paraplegia the receptive field for this reflex spreads over the skin of the whole limb and an extensor response can be obtained by scratching or pinching the skin (especially above the outer malleolus of the ankle). An *extensor* response may be observed during sleep or deep coma from any cause, and after epileptic fits.

3. The **Visceral Reflexes** of clinical importance are those concerned with micturition and defæcation.

MICTURITION.—(*a*) Precipitancy of micturition is a frequent early symptom of cord lesions, *e.g.*, disseminated sclerosis, slow cord compression, etc. (*b*) Difficulty in commencing micturition and dribbling incontinence of urine, especially at nights, occurs in tabes dorsalis when the bladder is anæsthetic and distended. (*c*) Retention, with overflow dribbling, occurs in coma, or during the initial three weeks of spinal shock following an acute transverse cord lesion, *e.g.*, myelitis, fracture-dislocation; and in the later stages of total transverse cord lesions. (*d*) Involuntary periodic micturition may occur, in which the bladder empties reflexly but never completely. (*e*) In patients with frontal lobe lesions there is loss or impairment of social sense and such patients frequently wet or soil their clothing and are unembarrassed by this.

DEFÆCATION.—Incontinence of fæces is commonly due to anæsthesia of the rectum from paralysis of the afferent nerves from the rectum, *e.g.*, in tabes or lesions of the cauda equina. In such cases, the internal anal sphincter, if felt by rectal examination, is flaccid. In spinal cord lesions, above the spinal centre in the conus, the internal sphincter retains its tone, and there is intermittent rectal incontinence, the patient being aware of the passage of fæces. Mentally confused patients are commonly incontinent.

4. Certain **Tonic** or **Postural Reflexes** are used clinically. In cases of

suspected meningitis or meningeal irritation, you test for reflex tonic contraction of the hamstrings (Kernig's sign) and posterior cervical muscles (Brudzinski's sign). *Kernig's Sign* is a reflex tonic contraction of the hamstring muscles, made evident by passively flexing the hip to a right-angle and at the same time extending the knee. *Brudzinski's Sign* is a tonic neck reflex. When the head is passively flexed on the chest the lower limbs become flexed at the hips and knees. In hemiplegia, rotation or lateral flexion of the head towards the paralysed side may cause extension of the paralysed limbs. Movement of the head to the normal side has the reverse effect. This is *Magnus and de Kleijn's tonic neck reflex.*

Straight leg raising. The patient raises each leg separately until stopped by pain. This test is of value in *assessing the severity* of pain in a disc lesion. Repeated tests will show improvement or deterioration and help in *prognosis.* Normally straight leg raising can be carried out to 90°. We note the angle each limb makes with the horizontal and record this in degrees.

Spine and Cranium.—Examine the patient's spine and cranium for *tenderness or deformity.* Neglect of this procedure may lead to your missing the fact that a patient's paraplegia is due to early Pott's disease. In suspected fracture of the skull look for bruising over the mastoids and elsewhere. When a vascular malformation is suspected *auscultate* the skull with a stethoscope or by direct application of your ear. Bruits are best heard over the mastoids, the occipital or frontal bones or orbits.

Trophic Changes.—The *skin* should be examined for perforating ulcers and bed-sores. The *bones and joints* may show arthropathy, *e.g.,* Charcot joints; or deformity, *e.g.,* pes cavus. Look too for pigmented areas, nævi, herpetic scarring.

EXAMINATIONS OF OTHER SYSTEMS.

The Cardio-vascular, Respiratory, Alimentary and Genito-urinary Systems should be examined and the urine tested in all cases.

§ 846. RADIOLOGICAL EXAMINATIONS AND CONTRAST RADIOGRAPHY.

PLAIN X-RAYS OF THE SKULL necessitate (1) postero-anterior, (2) lateral, and (3) basal (submento-vertical) views. (4) Towne's antero-posterior projection is also most valuable and will demonstrate the petrous crests, internal auditory meati, dorsum sellæ, foramen magnum and occiput.

Normal Findings.—(1) "Convolutional markings" in the vault are of little diagnostic importance. (2) Rarefaction of the posterior clinoid processes is common in normal skulls after middle life. (3) The pineal and choroid plexuses are often calcified in adults. (4) Hyperostosis frontalis interna, an irregular proliferation of the inner table of the frontal bone, is common in women at the menopause and does not indicate intracranial disease.

Abnormal Findings.—(1) If the pineal is calcified its displacement more than 3 mm. from the mid-line (in a well-centred film of Towne's projection) is pathological, and is valuable evidence of an expanding lesion in one hemisphere. (2) If there is rarefaction and erosion of the pituitary fossa this is abnormal and may be due to increased intracranial pressure; or if the sella is "ballooned," to a chromophobe pituitary adenoma. (3) Abnormal calcification may be seen in slow-growing neoplasms, cortical degeneration, vascular anomalies and parasitic invasions. (4) Increased vascular markings, if gross, generalised and symmetrical, may indicate the presence of a meningioma. (5) Bony defects either in the vault or base occur in invasive and metastatic growths, reticuloses, lipoidoses and inflammatory lesions.

Stereoscopic views of an abnormal pituitary fossa are often helpful. To visualise the optic foramina special oblique projections are necessary.

X-RAYS OF THE VERTEBRAL SPINE (antero-posterior, lateral and oblique views) will be required where spinal cord compression, disc lesions, cervical ribs, spondylosis, myelomatosis or congenital deformities are suspected. Unexpected evidences of tuberculous disease, osteitis deformans, primary or secondary neoplasms, or fracture may be revealed if routine radiography is performed in cases with neurological symptoms, especially where there is a possibility of root or cord compression.

Widening or erosion of the pedicles visible on an antero-posterior film may give the clue to the presence of an intraspinal tumour. When a spinal tumour is suspected good plain X-rays of the vertical spine should be taken before any attempt is made to do a spinal puncture.

Tomograms of the spine may help with injuries, congenital deformities.

CHEST X-RAYS must be taken as a routine in all cases where a brain tumour is suspected as a bronchial carcinoma is so often found. In myasthenia gravis the thymus may be enlarged. X-RAYS OF THE SKELETAL MUSCLES, *e.g.*, thigh muscles, may be required in suspected cysticercosis.

CEREBRAL ANGIOGRAPHY.—(a) *Carotid.* A percutaneous injection of 35 per cent. diodone (5–8 ml.) is made into the internal carotid artery and antero-posterior and lateral pictures are taken soon after the end of the injection and a few seconds later. Arterial and venous phases of filling are observed. This injection will fill the carotid syphon, the branches of the middle cerebral, and usually the anterior cerebral. In only a quarter of the cases will it fill the posterior cerebral, which normally fills from the vertebral artery. This gives useful information in (1) tumours of the cerebral hemispheres, (2) cerebral aneurysms and angiomatous malformations, (3) meningiomata, which show a "blush," (4) thrombosis or stenosis of the internal carotid artery.

(b) *Vertebral.* Vertebral angiograms are helpful in diagnosing (1) tumours in the posterior fossa, (2) angiomatous malformations and saccular aneurysms, (3) thrombosis or stenosis of the basilar artery.

Dangers and Reactions. Hæmatoma in the carotid sheath causes stiff neck and bruising, and occasionally cervical sympathetic palsy. Rare cases of hemiplegia (sometimes persistent) and rarer cases of coma (sometimes fatal) are described in association with gross cerebral disease. Allergic reactions and iodism are observed, *e.g.*, swelling of the face, lips and tongue, more uncomfortable than dangerous. The examination is, however, relatively safe in expert hands.

LUMBAR ENCEPHALOGRAPHY.—With the patient in the sitting position lumbar puncture is performed. The cerebro-spinal fluid is allowed to escape slowly and is replaced by air, 5 ml. at a time until 20–30 ml. have been injected. In cases of cerebral atrophy amounts as much as 100–200 ml. have been injected. All parts of the ventricular system can normally be visualised, including the descending horns of the lateral ventricles which are filled by manipulating the head, the aqueduct of Sylvius and the fourth ventricle. This procedure is of value in the investigation of epilepsy of late onset, in the diagnosis of cortical and cerebral atrophy and in tumours of the mid-line and posterior fossa. Space-occupying lesions and unilateral atrophic lesions cause displacement of the ventricular system to one or other side. In non-obstructive hydrocephalus due to brain atrophy the ventricles are symmetrically dilated and filled. Encephalography is sometimes followed by severe headache and a meningeal reaction lasting some hours or days.

VENTRICULOGRAPHY may be carried out by a surgeon prior to operation on a tumour or where subdural hæmatoma is suspected. Air is introduced into the ventricles by needles inserted through posterior parietal burr holes. It is not uncommon for ventriculography to precipitate the development of tentorial or medullary pressure cones in cases of raised intracranial pressure, and it is therefore extremely dangerous when performed where expert surgical help is not immediately available.

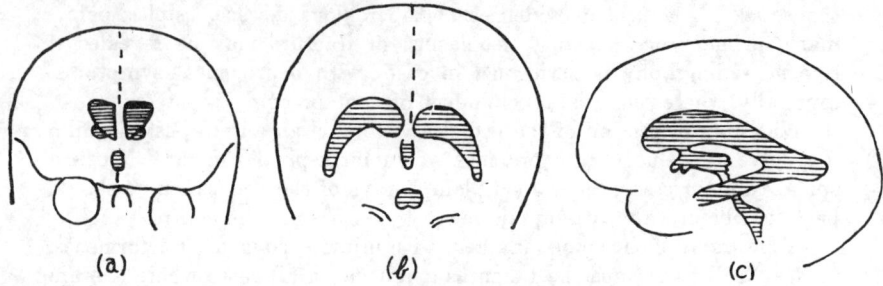

FIG. 235.—DIAGRAMS OF NORMAL AIR ENCEPHALOGRAMS: (*a*) Antero-posterior, (*b*) postero-anterior, (*c*) lateral views.

MYELOGRAPHY.—3 ml. of C.S.F. are withdrawn by lumbar puncture and then 3 ml. of Myodil or other iodised oil is introduced into the spinal theca. The heavy contrast medium sinks or rises in the subarachnoid space and by examining the patient on a tilting table it is possible to demonstrate the existence of spinal block, by screening and radiography (Fig. 245). The upper level of such a block may be demonstrated after cisternal injection, or (when the block is incomplete) by allowing the opaque medium to flow upwards from below. If the patient has recently had spinal puncture, it is advisable to let three weeks elapse after the last spinal puncture before myelography is undertaken, otherwise the injection may be made subdurally instead of into the subarachnoid space and the examination is then worthless.

OTHER SPECIAL EXAMINATIONS

(1) *Cerebro-spinal Fluid.* It is necessary to examine the spinal fluid in many cases of neurological disease by performing *Lumbar puncture* (1201).

Manometric observations on the spinal fluid-pressure must be made during the puncture, and the effect of compression of both jugular veins duly noted. The naked-eye appearance of the fluid should be observed in all cases. In sending fluids to the laboratory the following tests are made as routine: (1) Cell-count, (2) Total Protein, (3) Globulin content, (4) Wassermann Reaction, (5) Lange's Gold Reaction (Gold Curve). Where infection of the nervous system is suspected the C.S.F. must be examined bacteriologically as well as serologically and the chlorides and glucose content estimated. *Cisternal* (or *Ventricular*) *puncture* (1201) should not be practised by those unfamiliar with the technique: they are not without serious danger.

(2) *The Blood Wassermann Reaction* is usually necessary in diagnosis.

§ 847. (3) **Electro-encephalography.**—The activity of cortical nerve-cells can be studied with the electro-encephalograph by means of which cortical action currents are led off by electrodes placed on the intact scalp, amplified by wireless valves and recorded by a cathode-ray oscillograph.

The electro-encephalogram (E.E.G.) of a normal adult usually shows various waves which are regular in amplitude and frequency (Fig. 236a). Rhythmical waves of approximately 10 cycles per second and 0·5 to 1·0 millivolt amplitude are observed in the occipital region, when the subject is at rest with the eyes closed (alpha waves). Alpha waves are inhibited by visual attention, *i.e.*, opening the eyes to gaze, by concentration on a problem, by hyperventilation, hypoglycæmia, certain

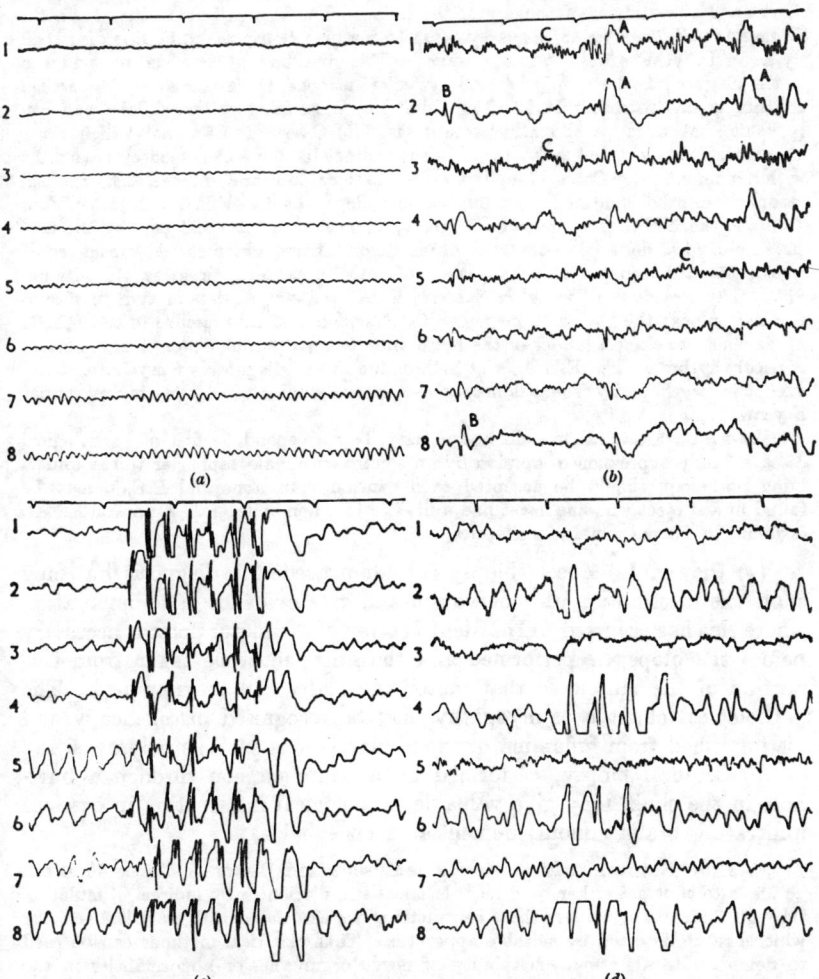

Leads. 1. R. anterior frontal; 2. L. anterior frontal; 3. R. posterior frontal; 4. L. posterior frontal; 5. R. parietal; 6. L. parietal; 7. R. occipital; 8. L. occipital.

FIG. 236.—(a) A normal E.E.G. showing alpha rhythm 9 c/sec. most marked in leads 7 and 8; (b) E.E.G. from an epileptic child showing generalised dysrhythmia with bouts of high-voltage slow waves (A), sharp waves (B), and bursts of fast activity (C); (c) E.E.G. from a child of 11 with petit mal. All leads show bursts of high-voltage spike and wave lasting 2·5 secs.; (d) High-voltage slow waves and spikes most marked over the left temporal lobe in a case of temporal lobe epilepsy. (Dr. B. G. Parsons-Smith.)

drugs and sleep. Beta waves of a frequency of 14 to 15 cycles per second are also obtained from the fronto-central areas of the adult cortex.

The E.E.G. of a child is quite different, and shows a variety of rhythmical high-voltage slow waves called delta (1 to 4 per second) or theta (4 to 8 per second) waves. This pattern is gradually replaced by the adult one and the transition is usually complete by the age of 15 years.

VALUE IN CLINICAL NEUROLOGY.—Records must be interpreted in the light of the clinical findings. The interpretation is a matter for an expert, and any conclusions drawn must necessarily be of a limited kind, for the record throws little direct light on the underlying pathology of the lesion. The E.E.G. is of value: 1. *In the Diagnosis and Treatment of Epilepsy.* (a) In major epilepsy the E.E.G. is disturbed by a rapid rhythm of fast and large waves. This gives helpful confirmatory evidence in the diagnosis between epilepsy and hysterical attacks, for in the latter the cortical rhythm is undisturbed. It is often helpful in diagnosing temporal lobe epilepsy (psychic fits) from psychopathic conditions. (b) Cases of petit mal which show alternating slow and fast spike-like episodes and are likely to be helped by treatment with troxidone. (c) Cases of epilepsy due to focal cerebral disease, e.g., cortical atrophy, may be identified from idiopathic epilepsy by the E.E.G. 2. *After Head Injuries,* the E.E.G. may indicate a liability to post-traumatic epilepsy, by the persistence of focal delta (slow wave) or other abnormalities, which should subside some weeks after the injury. The changes are of value in assessing progress and outlook. 3. *Rapidly Progressive Cortical or Subcortical Disease,* e.g., abscess or tumour if subcortical or near the thalamus may give focal evidence of its presence in the E.E.G. 4. Various *pathological lesions* of the brain and *abnormal mental states* yield abnormal cortical rhythms. The E.E.G. is of little value in the diagnosis of psychotic states except in psychopathy where it may give a record similar to that of children under 5 years of age.

Fallacies.—Electrical foci do not necessarily correspond to foci of pathological disease. Any expression of opinion by an electro-encephalographer as to the underlying pathology should be accepted with caution. An abnormal E.E.G. may be found in a subject who has never had a fit, *i.e.,* in a non-epileptic. A normal E.E.G. is found in 20 per cent. of epileptics.

(4) **Biopsy.** (a) Muscle biopsy is seldom needed in diagnosis but may show the distribution of denervation and give evidence of re-innervation where this has occurred. The identification of the motor point is necessary before the biopsy is performed and the fibres must be taken from this portion of the muscle so that motor end-plates can be examined. The pathological changes of myopathy may be recognised histologically and distinguished from inflammatory muscular lesions such as polymyositis.

(b) Cerebral biopsy, performed by a neuro-surgeon through a burr-hole in the skull, may give valuable pathological information in cases of infiltrating brain tumour, dementia or encephalitis.

§ 848. (5). ELECTRICAL EXAMINATION OF MUSCLES AND NERVES. Muscle fibres can be made to contract either by direct electrical stimulation or by indirect stimulation through their motor nerves; these contractions are associated with electrical activity which can be detected by suitable apparatus. Thus electrical methods can be used to demonstrate abnormal excitability of nerve or muscle, or abnormalities in the electrical activity associated with contraction. Diagnosis of the condition which is the cause of the abnormalities observed must often depend on other evidence—e.g., the history, clinical examination, laboratory and radiological examination—the electrical tests being merely confirmatory. On occasion, however, the abnormalities themselves may be sufficiently characteristic to be diagnostic. The tests may help in assessing the prognosis. If reliable results are to be obtained scrupulous attention to technique is essential and experience is required for the interpretation of the results. Almost all the abnormalities observed are quantitative rather than qualitative, and a sound knowledge of the normal, which may differ from muscle to muscle in different parts of the body, is required. For detailed information, specialised literature on electrodiagnosis should be consulted : here a general account of the methods in use is given.

Electrical Stimulation of Muscle.   Apparatus and Methods.—The electronic stimulator is now in general use for direct or indirect stimulation of muscle: this is capable of delivering electrical pulses of abrupt onset and termination (" square waves "), the duration, strength (voltage or current) and frequency of which can be selected by the operator. It is common to use pulse durations varying from 300 to 0·01 milliseconds (ms.), starting at zero volts and increasing to 150 volts, repeating these either once every two seconds or five times a second. After removing surface grease to reduce electrical resistance, and ensuring that the part to be examined is warm, stimulation is usually effected by means of a small electrode making contact with the skin through a pad soaked in saline and placed directly over the muscle to be tested, the other lead from the stimulator being connected to a large " indifferent " or " dispersive " electrode with a similarly moistened pad placed on the skin at a distance from the muscle. Contractions may be detected by watching for the movement of the stimulated muscle belly, but palpation of the tendon is sometimes a more sensitive method, and where identification of the contracting muscle is otherwise difficult, this may be effected with certainty by electromyography (see below). In routine testing, a short-duration weak stimulus is first applied over the approximate position of the " motor point " of the muscle to be tested and its strength is increased until a contraction of the muscle is detected. The electrode is then moved a short distance, first in one and then in another direction, until the exact motor point at which the muscle is most effectively stimulated is found. (When stimuli are applied at the motor point, not only is discomfort for the patient minimised, but spread of current to surrounding muscles is reduced.) If no contraction is obtained with any stimulus which the patient can tolerate, a longer duration pulse is tried.

The motor point owes its high excitability to the fact that it overlies the most excitable part of the motor nerve fibres at their terminations in the motor end-plates. Thus when a muscle is completely denervated, and its motor nerve has degenerated, no motor point can be found. Only direct stimulation of the muscle fibres is then possible, and, for this, longer duration stimuli are required (1 ms. or longer). This is known as the " *Reaction of Degeneration* ": when it is present stimulation through two small electrodes placed near the ends of the muscle tested is often preferable to the electrode arrangement described above.

Diagnostic Use.—Electrical stimulation is most commonly of value in detecting denervation and estimating its degree. Serial tests can be made in order to follow progression of a nerve lesion or its recovery. Most information is obtained by plotting a " *Strength/Duration Curve* ". Stimuli are applied to the motor point (if this can be located). Starting with stimuli of the longest duration and repeating with those of progressively shorter duration, the strengths (measured in volts or milliamps) of stimuli required to produce just detectable contractions are measured and the results plotted to form a curve (Fig. 237). It will be seen that from both normally innervated and completely denervated muscle, smooth curves are obtained but in the latter the curve is displaced to the right: short stimuli are less effective in exciting denervated muscle. When denervation is partial, normally-innervation fibres respond to the short duration pulses and denervated fibres respond to the longer duration pulses : a discontinuous curve is obtained. During re-innervation the discontinuity (or discontinuities) shift to the left (Fig. 237) and finally disappear, so that serial tests can be used to follow recovery. The older method of testing electrical reactions using as stimuli the output from the faradic battery (induction coil) and galvanic battery (source of intermittent direct current) employs stimuli of brief (about 1 ms.) and long duration and so provides some of the information obtainable from a Strength/Duration curve, but neither the faradic/galvanic test nor any of the measurements suggested as estimates of excitability (chronaxie, tetanus/twitch ratio, etc.) provide as much information about the state of innervation as the full curve.

Denervation is not detectable by the direct electrical testing of muscle until degeneration of the terminal fibres of the motor nerve is complete; this may take up to three weeks. If, in the presence of complete paralysis from damage to a peripheral nerve (as, for example, in facial palsy) the Strength/Duration curve remains normal for more than this length of time, a temporary failure of nerve conduction without destruction of the nerve axons (neurapraxia) is indicated and full recovery can be

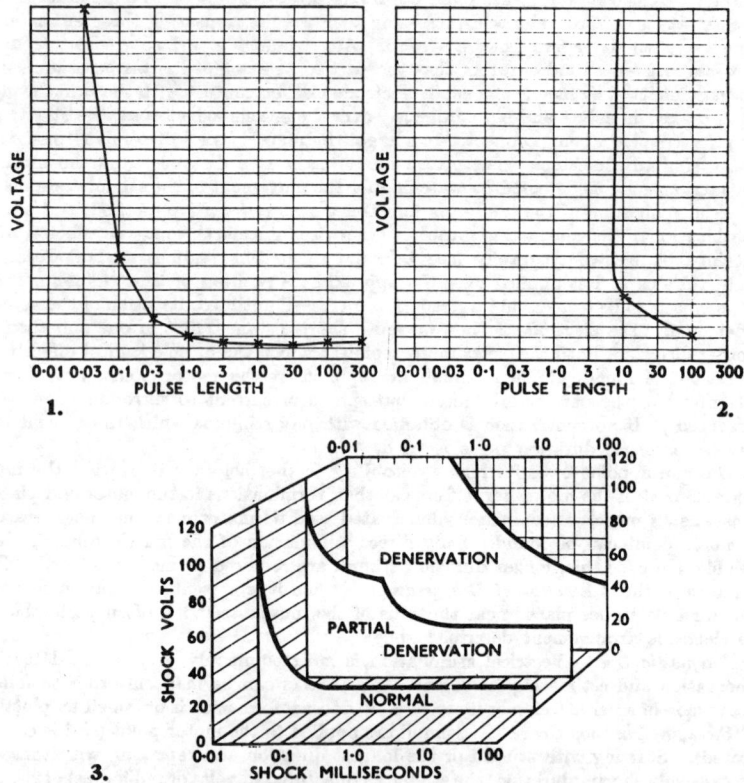

FIG. 237.—Strength/duration curves from orbicularis oculi muscle. (1) Normal—(2) Denervation — (3) Course of recovery in denervated muscle.

expected. The appearance of discontinuities on a Strength/Duration curve from a muscle which has previously shown complete denervation (*e.g.*, following nerve injury or poliomyelitis) may precede by several weeks the first signs of voluntary contraction and indicates early re-innervation. If, however, the return of voluntary contraction is then unduly delayed, the prognosis for recovery of useful function is poor.

Electrical testing may also be used in the investigation of other conditions. In *myasthenia gravis* prolonged repetitive stimulation of suitable muscles (*e.g.*, orbicularis oculi) with short duration pulses will demonstrate the gradual failure of neuro-muscular transmission; when the stimulation is stopped, excitability rapidly returns. In *motor neurone* disease and similar slowly progressive conditions in which nerve degeneration occurs, denervated muscle fibres become re-innervated by the sprouting of surviving motor nerves, and change in Strength/Duration curves is prevented. In the *myopathies,* such muscle fibres as retain their excitability respond normally: their innervation is intact. In *central nervous diseases not affecting the lower motor neurone* and in *hysteria* the Strength/Duration curves are normal.

Electromyography.—The electrical changes which occur during muscle activity may be picked up either by electrodes placed on the skin or by needle electrodes inserted directly into the muscle. They are of small potential and must be greatly amplified before they can be displayed on the cathode-ray tube of the electromyograph. Meticulous attention to detail of technique is necessary, for the small potentials resulting from movement of the electrodes on the skin, or picked up from neighbouring electrical apparatus by the patient or the leads connecting him to the electromyograph which are subsequently amplified, may produce interference sufficient to make interpretation difficult or impossible. When skin electrodes are used mild abrasion of the skin surface and the application of electrode jelly is essential to ensure good contact and a connection of the patient to earth is usually necessary. It is sometimes necessary to operate inside an earthed screening cage. When needle electrodes are used, these and the skin surface must be sterilised. Every electromyographic examination should include observations made with the patient relaxing, contracting lightly, and contracting maximally, the muscle under examination.

Skin electrodes overlie many muscle fibres and the potentials they pick up represent the pooled output from a considerable bulk of muscle. They may therefore detect activity when only a small proportion of the fibres of a muscle are contracting but are only of use when the muscle to be examined is superficially placed. Further, with skin electrodes, accurate localisation of the active muscle fibres is impossible. Activity may be detected over inactive muscles by reason of spread from active muscles in the neighbourhood or even as far away as the opposite side of a limb. *Needle electrodes* are essential for the accurate localisation of activity and when a detailed analysis of action potentials is required. Potentials of short duration (1–2 ms.), " fibrillation potentials," are dissipated in the tissues between the active fibres and skin electrodes and as these potentials are a most important electromyographic finding, needle electrodes must, in most cases, be used.

The unit from which all muscle potentials are made up is the action potential of the single muscle fibre, but normally muscle fibres rarely contract singly. In response to nerve impulses, the smallest group of fibres to contract together is that supplied by a single motor nerve fibre—the group in a single motor unit. When a needle electrode is initially inserted into a normal muscle, a burst of small (10–300 mV) potentials of short duration (1–2 ms.) is observed, producing a rapid succession of ticks in the loud-speaker. These are due to mechanical stimulation of single muscle fibres and are identical in appearance (and sound) with the single muscle fibre potentials seen in pathological conditions. Unlike these, however, they rapidly subside. They are known as " insertion potentials ". Once they have disappeared, the normal resting muscle shows " electrical silence ". On minimal contraction, motor unit activity makes its appearance. Though a motor unit contains many muscle fibres, the potential produced is only some 2–5 times larger than the muscle fibre potential. This is because active fibres relatively remote from the tip of the electrode are able to make little contribution to the potential and the potentials do not all reach the electrode quite synchronously. For the latter reason, the duration of the motor unit potential is prolonged and may last up to 7 ms. The sound made in the loud-speaker is a pop. On maximal contraction, a complex pattern of potentials, never returning to the baseline, and represented on the loud-speaker by a sound reminiscent of a drum-roll, is produced—the normal " interference pattern."

In the *myopathies,* the contractile mechanism of the muscle fibre degenerates more rapidly than its surface membrane (upon which electrical potential generation depends). Weakness may therefore be marked at a stage when little or no abnormality can be detected in the electromyogram. Later on, the motor units become depleted of

excitable muscle fibres, and the motor unit potentials become " disintegrated."
These, seen in isolation during gentle voluntary contraction, are usually reduced in
voltage, and consist of a group of more or less discrete potentials. As the disease
progresses, the number of potentials in each group decreases. In contrast to this
picture, in complete *denervation*, no response of any kind is obtained even to maximal
voluntary effort. Following acute denervation, complete electrical silence is found
(*e.g.* acute *poliomyelitis, nerve section*). Then within about two weeks spontaneous
short-duration low-voltage potentials make their appearance, indicating that the
integrity of the motor unit has been destroyed by the degeneration of the motor nerve.
These spontaneously occurring muscle fibre potentials are known as " Fibrillation
potentials." Where, in a peripheral nerve lesion, electrical silence persists, even
though voluntary power does not at once return, the prognosis is good. In the
absence of regeneration following denervation, fibrillation persists until the muscle
fibres atrophy, when it gradually disappears. Also when re-innervation occurs,
fibrillation ceases. Gradually, small groups of brief, low-voltage potentials on maximum voluntary effort make their appearance. These are " nascent motor units " and
represent re-innervation of small groups of fibres. As re-innervation progresses, motor
unit activity of normal appearance supervenes, but, combined with this, " polyphasic
potentials " are seen. These represent the formation of giant motor units by the
innervation of many muscle fibres by recovering nerve fibres. Early electromyographic evidence of nerve regeneration may be obtained up to eight weeks before
there is any clinical evidence of recovery of function. The changes described as
occurring during denervation and re-innervation occur together in many slowly
degenerative diseases affecting the motor nerves—*e.g.*, *motor neurone disease, peripheral
neuritis* and *syringomyelia*, re-innervation from collaterals sprouted by surviving nerve-
fibres occurring simultaneously with the degenerative process, so that polyphasic
potentials and fibrillation are both seen. The same may be true of the nerve-root
lesions seen following *intervertebral disc protrusion* or resulting from *spondylosis*. The
distribution of fibrillation as between different muscles has been used as a guide to
the level of root involvement. Perhaps the most clearly diagnostic findings by
electromyography are obtained in *myotonia*, for the insertion of a needle electrode into
muscle precipitates a rapid stream of potentials of fibrillation size. The frequency of
these potentials is regular and slowly declines, producing a sound in the loud-speaker
suggesting a dive bomber. Following voluntary contraction of the muscle, an after
discharge occurs; this may even be of greater intensity than that of the voluntary
contraction which preceded it.

In many conditions, diagnostic electrical stimulation and electromyography are
complementary and on occasion they may be combined. By the use of the electromyograph, the time of onset of contraction in a muscle can be accurately gauged, and
the " latency " between electrical stimulation of a nerve trunk and the resultant
contraction can be measured. The latency may be increased when a nerve is constricted, as in the carpal tunnel syndrome.

*PART C.   DISEASES OF THE NERVOUS SYSTEM.   THEIR DIAGNOSIS,
PROGNOSIS AND TREATMENT*

§ 849. Routine Procedure and Classification.

DIAGNOSIS.—(1) Having examined the patient it should be possible,
in the light of what we know of physiological anatomy, to come to some
conclusion concerning the ANATOMICAL DIAGNOSIS, *i.e.*, the diagnosis of
the seat of the disease. We should always try to make an anatomical
diagnosis from the clinical findings, for they may be less misleading than
special ancillary techniques, especially in the early stages of disease.

(2) The PATHOLOGICAL DIAGNOSIS, *i.e.*, the nature of the disease, is a far more difficult problem. We must know the likeliest possibilities for each site and the rate at which the symptoms developed. We may be helped by signs of disease in other organs; by the character and mode of onset of the symptoms, the age of the patient, or hereditary features. The following clinical classification is based on presenting *signs*.

GROUP I. COMA OR STUPOR

§ 850. *The patient is attacked with deep, persistent and* PROLONGED UNCONSCIOUSNESS *from which he* CANNOT BE ROUSED *by shaking or calling.* The case is one of COMA. Lesser degrees are called STUPOR. The stuporose patient can be aroused by a vigorous stimulus to such an extent that he responds by behaviour which appears to indicate awareness of his surroundings.

Four levels of consciousness may be distinguished. (1) *Patient unrousable.* (2) Patient rousable by application of painful stimuli, *e.g.*, squeezing the tendo Achillis and pricking the soles of the feet. (3) Patient conscious but confused and disoriented, often irritable. (4) Patient fully conscious. During states of partial consciousness patients may exhibit automatic behaviour.

Symptoms.—The Coma is of *sudden onset* when due to head injury, or to hæmorrhagic or embolic lesions within the brain substance. A *subacute onset* over minutes or hours occurs in a hypertensive attack, an occlusion of a cerebral vessel by thrombosis, when a meningeal vessel bleeds, or in hypoglycæmia. *Unconsciousness persisting in the morning after sleep* suggests cerebral infarction, or intoxication from hypnotics.

In Coma the limbs are flaccid, the corneal reflexes are absent. In deep coma the pupils are inactive to light; food and fluids placed in the mouth remain unswallowed, there is retention of urine, or incontinence of urine and fæces. The tendon reflexes vary greatly, but in deep coma they are usually absent. As a transient phenomenon extensor plantar responses may be present. The persistence of this sign for an hour or so after the patient has regained consciousness does not necessarily mean a gross focal cerebral or spinal lesion.

The causes of Coma are here considered in two clinical groups: A, those with signs which are mainly *unilateral*; B, those with signs which are mainly *bilateral* and symmetrical.

TABLE LII.—CAUSES OF COMA

(all these may also cause symptomatic epilepsy)

A With signs which are mainly UNILATERAL.

I. CEREBRO-VASCULAR ACCIDENTS
(a) Cerebral hæmorrhage, (b) Thrombosis, (c) Embolism, (d) Subarachnoid hæmorrhage, (e) Hypertensive encephalopathy, (f) Thrombosis of venous sinuses.

II. EFFECTS OF HEAD INJURY
(a) Cerebral contusion (§§ 813, 852) and laceration, (b) Extradural (middle meningeal hæmorrhage) (§ 852), (c) Subdural hæmamatoma (§ 1052).

III. EXPANDING LESIONS
(a) Primary and secondary intracranial neoplasms, (b) Abscess.

B With signs which are mainly BILATERAL and SYMMETRICAL.

IV. SUBARACHNOID HÆMORRHAGE

V. EPILEPSY—post-epileptic coma.

VI. Cerebral concussion, basal trauma; and other physical causes, *e.g.*, electric shock, heat exhaustion.

VII. DIABETES, Diabetic coma, Insulin hypoglycæmia.

VIII. ENDOCRINE STATES OTHER THAN DIABETES
Acute suprarenal failure, Hypopituitarism, Myxœdema.

IX. BIOCHEMICAL STATES
Uræmia, Eclampsia, Hepatic coma, Avitaminosis.

X. INFECTIONS
Meningitis, *e.g.*, Tuberculous, Meningococcal, Encephalitis, Cerebral malaria, Syphilis, Typhoid, Typhus, Cholera.

XI. ANOXIC STATES—Chronic bronchitis and Emphysema, Asthma, Obstructed airway, Respiratory failure.

XII. PSYCHOGENIC CAUSES—Anergic stupor, Hysterical trance.

XIII. POISONING—Alcohol (delirium tremens), Barbiturates, Aspirin, Tranquillisers, Carbon monoxide, Morphine.

CLINICAL INVESTIGATION OF UNCONSCIOUS PATIENTS (see Table LIII)

Obtain any history of preceding ill-health (Hypertension, Diabetes) or fits (Epilepsy) from relatives, neighbours or police. Was the patient depressed or suicidal (Poisoning) or subject to headaches (Cerebral neoplasm) ? Did the unconsciousness come on suddenly (Cerebral hæmorrhage) or gradually (Hypoglycæmia) ? Observe the age of the patient. Coma in *childhood* is due to Meningitis, Epilepsy, Intracranial neoplasm or Abscess; after middle age suspect Cerebral hæmorrhage. If possible keep the patient warm throughout the examination and examine in a good light.

1. *General Examination.*—Look at the scalp for local trauma, the mastoids for bruising and note any escape of blood or fluid from the nose or ears (fractured base of the skull). Listen to the breathing (stertor in Apoplexy, sighing in Diabetic coma). Smell the breath for acetone (Diabetes) and note the colour of the skin (yellow in Hepatic coma, pink in Carbon Monoxide poisoning). Observe any scars on the face, tongue or limbs (Epilepsy) and marks of hypodermic punctures (Hypoglycæmia, Morphinism).

2. *Neurological Examination.*—Note the size of the pupils (pinpoint in Opium poisoning and Pontine hæmorrhage) or the presence of neck rigidity (Meningitis or Subarachnoid Hæmorrhage). Next look at the optic discs (papillœdema in brain tumour or Hypertensive encephalopathy, albuminuric retinopathy in Renal uræmia) and

TABLE LIII.—DIAGNOSIS OF UNCONSCIOUS STATES

General Examination

	Routine Examination.	*Probable Diagnosis.*
History.	High blood pressure.	Apoplexy.
	Headache, vomiting.	Intracranial neoplasm.
	Falling about or recent injury.	Subdural hæmatoma.
	Fits.	Epilepsy.
Surroundings.	Domestic Gas.	Carbon monoxide.
	Tablets or their containers.	{ Barbiturates. / Aspirin.
Injury.	Lacerations, bruises on scalp or mastoids.	Concussion.
	Bitten tongue, blood in mouth.	Epilepsy.
	Escape of C.S.F. or blood from ears.	Fractured Base of Skull.
Hypodermic Punctures.	Thighs, arms (insulin, morphine)	{ Diabetes. / Hypoglycæmia. / Addiction (morphia).
Colour of face.	Grey.	Hæmorrhage.
	Pink.	Carbon monoxide.
	Jaundice.	Acute yellow atrophy of liver.
	Suntanned.	Malaria, heat-stroke.
	Cyanosed, congested.	Apoplexy (cerebral hæmorrhage).
Pulse and heart.	Slow.	Rising intracranial pressure.
	Auricular fibrillation.	Embolism.
Blood pressure.	Raised.	Cerebral hæmorrhage.
	Much raised.	Hypertensive encephalopathy.
Respiration.	Stertor.	Cerebral hæmorrhage.
	Sighing " Air Hunger."	Diabetic coma.
Temperature.	Rectal T° rising.	Heat-stroke.
	Hyperpyrexia.	{ Cerebral malaria. / Meningitis. / Pontine lesions.

Neurological Examination

Neck stiffness.	Kernig's sign present.	{ Meningitis. / Subarachnoid hæmorrhage.
Hemiplegia.	Conjugate deviation of the head and eyes. }	Intracerebral hæmorrhage.
	Facial asymmetry.	
Monoplegia.	Unilateral flaccidity of limb.	Meningeal hæmorrhage.
Pupils.	Dilated pupils.	Alcohol, Aspirin, Belladonna.
	Pin-point pupils.	Pontine lesion, Morphine.
	A fixed dilated pupil.	Subdural hæmatoma.
	Unequal pupils.	Cerebral vascular accident.
Fundi.	Papillœdema.	Cerebral tumour or Malignant hypertension.
Ears.	Otorrhœa with drum perforation.	Cerebral abscess.

Special Tests

Stomach lavage.	For barbiturate, or Alcohol.	Barbiturates. / Alcohol.
Catheterise and test urine.	Albumen.	Uræmia.
	Sugar.	Diabetes.
	Barbiturate.	
	Aspirin.	
Blood (1) films, (2) spectroscope.	Parasites.	Cerebral malaria.
	Carboxyhæmoglobin.	Carbon monoxide.
Spinal puncture.	Cells.	{ Meningitis, Encephalitis.
	Organisms. }	Poliomyelitis.
	Chloride.	Subarachnoid Hæmorrhage.
	Sugar.	

examine the ears for suppurative disease (Sinus thrombosis, intracranial abscess). Lift the limbs and let them fall one by one, noting increased flaccidity on one or other side. Prick the soles of the patient's feet and observe the absence of reflex withdrawal on the paralysed side.

3. *Special Examinations.*—Estimate the blood pressure. Obtain a specimen of urine (by catheter if necessary) and test it for albumen or sugar: in all cases this examination is essential. Finally remember that a diagnostic spinal puncture may reveal the cause—blood (in Meningeal or Ventricular Hæmorrhage) or turbidity (in Meningitis).

When *Poisoning* is suspected treat the patient at once for this (§ 856) or if hospital is easily reached send the patient there with all tablets, or vomitus found nearby.

The comatose patient smelling of alcohol.—All such cases should be admitted to hospital or detained until the diagnosis is perfectly clear. Small amounts of ingested alcohol readily induce fits or coma in patients with organic brain disease (*e.g.*, tumour, recent head injury). Alcohol may precipitate coma in a diabetic patient; or an attack of hypertensive encephalopathy, or subarachnoid hæmorrhage in a person with arterial disease. Patients who are intoxicated and fall are very liable to serious head injury, such as concussion, fracture of the skull base, or middle meningeal hæmorrhage. The risk of sending from hospital a patient with undiagnosed cerebral disease or unsuspected skull fracture in these circumstances is considerable; the patient's subsequent rapid deterioration and death may lead to legal inquiries.

The commonest causes are—Epilepsy, Cerebro-vascular accidents including Subarachnoid hæmorrhage, Hypertensive encephalopathy, Brain trauma, Diabetes, Accidental or attempted suicidal poisoning.

A. THE SIGNS ARE MAINLY UNILATERAL.—Such unilateral signs are unequal pupils, conjugate deviation of the head and eyes to one side, asymmetry of the mouth or face or a recent cranial nerve palsy, absolute flaccidity of the limbs on one side compared with the other, or unilateral fits. When such signs exist the cause is usually some focal intracranial lesion. Occasionally transient unilateral signs occur from focal brain swelling in coma due to a generalised cause.

I (a). *A middle-aged or elderly subject, often hypertensive, suffers* BRIEF *premonitory* HEADACHE *or unilateral paræsthesiæ and within a few moments develops* RAPIDLY DEEPENING COMA *with* STERTOROUS BREATHING *and* HEMIPLEGIA. The cause is likely to be INTRACEREBRAL HÆMORRHAGE.

§ 851. **Cerebral Hæmorrhage.**—The term apoplexy, or "stroke," is used to indicate a sudden loss of consciousness due to a vascular lesion—hæmorrhage, embolism or thrombosis—within the skull. The *extent* and the *suddenness* of the vascular lesion, rather than its nature, determine the occurrence of coma. Cerebral hæmorrhage is most frequent between fifty and seventy, but it may occur even in children.

Symptoms.—Initial Stage. The attack may be ushered in by a stage of headache or giddiness, lasting a few days, connected doubtless with associated high blood pressure; or it may come on suddenly without warning. Vomiting or a convulsion with turning of the head and eyes to the contra-lateral side sometimes occurs. Sometimes the paralysis comes on with faintness and vertigo only; or it may develop more gradually, followed later by unconsciousness (ingravescent apoplexy). Sometimes it comes on during sleep.

Stage of shock. In severe cases the patient is deeply comatose, cyanosed, and the breathing is stertorous, the skin is cold and covered with sweat. The muscles are completely flaccid, the flaccidity being greater on the paralysed side. The paralysed angle of the mouth drops, and the cheek flaps in and out with respiration. The patient is incontinent and when in coma blisters may develop on the heels, buttocks and sacrum. The pupils may at first react to light, later the pupil and tendon reflexes are commonly absent. A larger pupil may be present on the side of the cerebral lesion. The pulse is slow and the temperature subnormal.

TABLE LIV.—CEREBRAL HÆMORRHAGE, THROMBOSIS AND EMBOLISM

	Cerebral Hæmorrhage.	*Cerebral Thrombosis.*	*Cerebral Embolism.*
Age.	Middle and advanced life.	Middle and advanced life or any age.	Any age, but frequent in early life.
Causes.	1. Arteriosclerosis with high blood pressure. 2. Blood diseases. 3. Acute infections and septicæmia.	1. Cerebral arteriosclerosis. 2. Syphilitic endarteritis. 3. Acute infections. 4. Exhausting conditions, phthisis, anæmia. 5. Cardiac enfeeblement.	1. Cardiac lesions, especially mitral stenosis, auricular fibrillation and bacterial endocarditis. 2. " Fat embolism " in fracture of long bones.
Onset.	Coma usually sudden, with convulsions.	Onset usually gradual with premonitory vertigo. Sometimes convulsions, rarely coma.	Instantaneous loss of consciousness.
Time of onset.	During emotional excitement or physical exertion.	Often during sleep.	During exertion.

Diagnosis of Cerebral Hæmorrhage.—The *sudden* onset of profound coma in a person of middle age, with the presence of unilateral signs, are points of great diagnostic significance. It should be remembered that cerebral hæmorrhage frequently supervenes in the course of chronic interstitial nephritis, and therefore uræmia and apoplexy may be concurrent. The diagnostic features of the greatest value are the state of the pupils, particularly their inequality and the loss of the conjunctival reflex. The diagnosis of the various *causes of vascular lesion* is given in Table LIV. It is usually impossible to diagnose hæmorrhage from thrombosis by measuring the blood pressure of the comatose patient. Unless he is collapsed and moribund it will probably be found to be above normal in most cases. If instead of getting worse the patient unexpectedly recovers, the condition is probably a crisis of hypertensive encephalopathy (§§ 97, 851).

As regards the *locality* of the hæmorrhage, the usual position (about 70 per cent.) is the *external* or *internal capsule.* The hæmorrhage comes from the lenticulo-striate artery (Figs. 231, 233c), especially the left side, producing hemiplegia on the side opposite to the lesion. In most of the cases of hæmorrhage into the *ventricles* there is deep coma and head retraction with paralysis or rigidity of all four limbs, and blood in the spinal fluid: the condition is fatal.   Marked contraction of both pupils, convulsions and vomiting, with paralysis of all four limbs, and rapid rise of temperature to the level of hyperpyrexia, suggest hæmorrhage into the *pons*.   Hurried or Cheyne-Stokes' respiration often accompanies hæmorrhage in this site, and death ensues.   *Conjugate deviation of the head and eyes* towards the paralysed side is frequent when the hæmorrhage involves the motor tract.

Etiology.—Cerebral hæmorrhage is more frequent in males than females. Alcoholism or a hereditary tendency to vascular disease may be underlying factors.   In middle life or later the causes are: (1) Hypertensive vascular disease; (2) Arteriosclerosis with hypertension; (3) Occasionally an angiomatous malformation bleeds into the brain; (4) Hæmorrhage into an unsuspected vascular brain tumour occurs at any age.   In younger subjects (5) a saccular aneurysm buried in the Sylvian fissure or between the frontal lobes, or one adherent to the base of the brain, may bleed intracerebrally.   Brain hæmorrhage occurs also in : (6) Severe head injury, (7) in acute specific fevers and septicæmia, (8) as a terminal event in blood diseases (*e.g.*, acute leukæmia, purpura) in young adults.   (9) In infants, birth injury may be a cause.

Prognosis.—Most cases are fatal in two to ten days.   Slow intracerebral bleeding occurs in hypertension and the patient may survive longer.   The depth and duration of the coma are fair measures of the extent of the mischief, and therefore of the prognosis.   As regards *locality*, ventricular hæmorrhage and hæmorrhage into the pons are the most serious.

Treatment.—The nursing and management of a comatose patient is described in § 858.   In rare cases of cerebral hæmorrhage, where the patient's condition stabilises within the first few days, ventriculography may be carried out.   If ventriculograms show the presence of a space-occupying lesion a clot may be surgically evacuated.   This is most often possible in younger patients who have bled from a congenital aneurysm or angiomatous malformation.

I (*b*). CEREBRAL THROMBOSIS may or may not cause disturbance of consciousness.   If there is coma it is more gradual in onset than in cerebral hæmorrhage (§ 902).

I (*c*). CEREBRAL EMBOLISM.—The coma in such cases is transient, and where the embolism has not occluded a major vessel the paresis tends to lessen in its severity and distribution within a few hours or days after the onset (§ 905).   For *Fat Embolism* see § 905.

I (*d*). SUBARACHNOID HÆMORRHAGE.—Unilateral symptoms, *e.g.*, oculomotor palsy, may be present when the onset is gradual.   When there is associated intracerebral bleeding, signs of hemiplegia will occur.   In most cases, however, the signs are bilateral and symmetrical (§ 853).

I (*e*). HYPERTENSIVE ATTACKS (hypertensive encephalopathy) occur in patients with very high blood pressures (§ 97).   The symptoms (due to acute brain swelling) are severe headache, vomiting, drowsiness, fits, hemiplegia and coma.   Bilateral papilloedema helps to differentiate cases of sudden onset from cerebral hæmorrhage.   The paralytic symptoms are usually transient, and this may be the first indication that the case is not one of cerebral hæmorrhage. The symptoms develop more rapidly than in intracranial tumour. Treatment of the hypertension is urgently required (§ 97) and for fits give sod. phenobarb. 3 gr. intravenously or paraldehyde 3–6 ml. intramuscularly.

I (*f*). THROMBOSIS OF THE CEREBRAL SINUSES may give rise to coma and all the symptoms of apoplexy. It may arise from caries of the skull (syphilitic or tuberculous), extension from an intracranial abscess, *e.g.*, in suppurative ear disease, and occasionally from the pressure of an aneurysm, gumma or other tumour; or in association with meningitis. It occurs in the puerperium and with the feeble cerebral circulation of cachetic conditions (chronic diarrhœa, typhoid fever, and marasmus in children). *Septic thrombosis* and the differential diagnosis of thrombosis of the lateral, cavernous and longitudinal sinuses are described in § 892.

§ 852. II. EFFECTS OF HEAD INJURY. With unilateral signs there may be:

(*a*) CEREBRAL CONTUSION AND LACERATION.—In severe head injuries the brain may be lacerated and intracerebral hæmorrhage may occur. In such cases paralytic signs will be present, and the spinal fluid will contain blood. The prognosis is grave and a worsening state may call for surgical treatment.

(*b*) EXTRADURAL (MIDDLE MENINGEAL) HÆMORRHAGE (delayed traumatic apoplexy).—The patient partially recovers from the initial concussion and collapse. With the rise of blood pressure within a few hours, stupor or coma supervene with focal convulsions and rapidly progressive monoplegia or hemiplegia. The cause is usually *rupture of the middle meningeal artery* with extradural hæmatoma.

(*c*) SUBDURAL HÆMATOMA from rupture of cortical veins occurs after a long latent interval (§ 1052). *Treatment* of both conditions is surgical.

III (*a*). PRIMARY or SECONDARY INTRACRANIAL NEOPLASMS may cause coma. There is sometimes pleocytosis in the spinal fluid, and then the condition simulates encephalitis.

(*b*) INTRACRANIAL ABSCESS (see § 891).

B. THE SIGNS ARE MAINLY BILATERAL AND SYMMETRICAL.—Coma may be caused by damage to the upper brain-stem, and hypothalamus (reticular formation), or to the brain generally. The lesions may be hæmorrhagic or demyelinating or they may be due to a great variety of general states, ischæmic, anoxic, endocrine, infective and biochemical; or to poisoning and psychogenic illnesses (see Table LIII, § 851).

There is a SUDDEN SEVERE HEADACHE *or pain at the back of the neck, with* NECK STIFFNESS *and a positive Kernig's sign followed by deepening coma or convulsions.* The cause is likely to be SUBARACHNOID HÆMORRHAGE.

§ 853. IV. Subarachnoid Hæmorrhage from rupture of a basal saccular aneurysm is common. It occurs usually between the ages of 40–60 years, but also occurs in children and young adults. There may be a previous history of migraine or recurrent unilateral headaches.

Symptoms.—The headache may start in the supra-orbital region, but is

characteristically occipito-cervical.   It is *sudden* in onset and accompanied
by rigidity of the posterior cervical muscles and spine and vomiting.   The
temperature soon becomes elevated.   Headache with photophobia may
pass into restlessness and irritability, confusion, status epilepticus or
stupor; coma follows.   Pains in the back, trunk and lower limbs occur from
irritation of blood in the theca.   The plantar responses are usually extensor
and Kernig's sign is positive.   Retinal hæmorrhages or massive subhyaloid hæmorrhage may be observed on ophthalmoscopy.   During the
first 48 hours there may be transient albuminuria or glycosuria.   Retention of urine with overflow may occur.

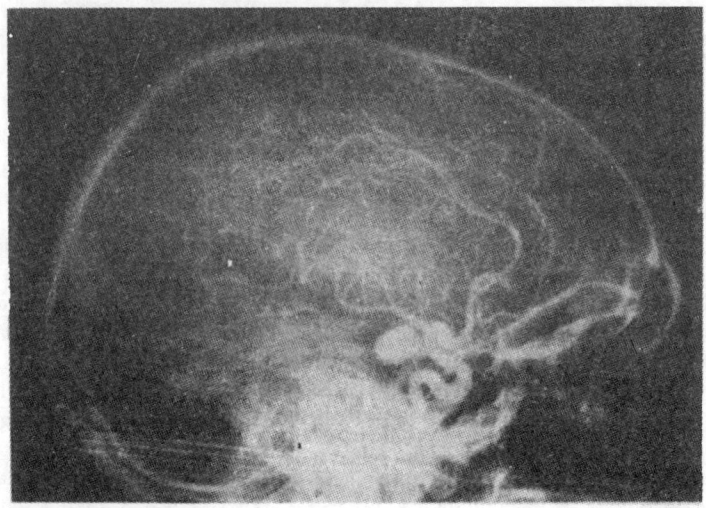

FIG. 238.—RIGHT CAROTID ANGIOGRAM.   A large bilocular saccular aneurysm projects backwards
   from the internal carotid; it probably arises from the posterior communicating artery.
   (Dr. Charles MacLean.)

Diagnosis.—The occurrence of such sudden headache with neck stiffness, coma and raised temperature, is sufficient indication to perform
spinal puncture.   Two successive samples, each of 1 ml. spinal fluid, are
withdrawn and put into separate tubes.   Each will show an equal amount
of blood deposit with the supernatant fluid stained red by " laked "
blood; soon the C.S.F. becomes yellow (§ 1204).   When the blood is
due to trauma at the time of the puncture successive tubes will show
progressively less and less blood.   If traumatic subarachnoid bleeding
is suspected examine the mastoids for bruising and X-ray the skull.

Etiology.—Most saccular aneurysms are on the internal carotid (Fig.
238), or middle or anterior cerebral arteries near where they form the Circle
of Willis.   Those on the middle cerebral in the Sylvian fissure may bleed
initially into the brain substance.   In the younger age-group these saccular aneurysms are often multiple and occur from herniations at the

division of an artery, a site of muscular weakness—("congenital" aneurysms). In older patients they may be due to dilatation and herniation of arteriosclerotic vessels.

Prognosis.—About a third of the patients die in the first attack. After a few weeks the symptoms tend to disappear, although a second hæmorrhage may occur within the first two weeks. Once basal aneurysms have bled they tend to become adherent to the pia covering the brain or to the dura, and subsequent hæmorrhage may then be intracerebral or extradural. Further hæmorrhages, either from the same aneurysm or another, commonly occur weeks or years after the first bleeding. Confusional states similar to Korsakow's psychosis may occur during convalescence from stupor.

Treatment.—Give an injection of morphine gr. ⅓ repeated once or twice at intervals of six hours, record the pulse, temperature and respiration on an hourly chart. Keep the patient on absolute bed rest and watch for retention of urine and pneumonic complications. Bilateral carotid angiograms and a vertebral angiogram may be necessary to demonstrate the source of the bleeding; these are undertaken at the end of the first week or sooner if active surgery is contemplated, but in 20–30 per cent. no aneurysm can be demonstrated. Ligature of the internal carotid in the neck or a more direct intracranial attack on the aneurysm may be possible. After bed rest for six weeks return to work should be gradual and heavy lifting or violent exercise avoided.

Other Varieties of Hæmorrhage into the Subarachnoid Space.—(1) *Perforation of the arterial wall* under an atheromatous plaque. (2) *Intracerebral hæmorrhage* may leak through the cortex or into the lateral ventricle. (3) *Fracture of the base of the skull* sustained accidentally or in a fit or faint. (4) *Vascular tumours* bleed into the subarachnoid space. (5) *Hæmorrhagic diseases*, *e.g.*, leukæmia and *septicæmia*, are rare.

V. Post-epileptic Coma.—If there is no history we may have to rely on the finding of old scars for evidence of previous attacks. The coma is usually of short duration but may be followed by deep sleep. Transient hemiplegia is occasionally seen after an attack (§ 863).

There is COMA *with* BILATERAL FLACCID PARALYSIS *and the patient has been subjected to a head injury, an electric current or to excessive heat.* The condition is likely to be CEREBRAL CONCUSSION, or due to an ELECTRIC SHOCK or HEAT EXHAUSTION.

§ 854. VI. Cerebral Concussion. *Symptoms.*—The unconsciousness follows immediately after the head injury without any latent interval. The patient is pale and collapsed, with weak pulse, shallow respiration, pale face, dilated pupils, sweating, flaccidity of the limbs and low blood pressure. In other cases he is merely dazed. In severe concussion there may also be a focal or more general contusion or bruising of the brain; the coma or stupor lasts hours or days and is followed by a reactive stage ushered in by vomiting or convulsions. The temperature rises to 100° F or higher, the pulse becomes full and bounding and the respirations deeper. There is intense headache and photophobia with hypersensitiveness to noise, and the patient lies curled up in bed with his limbs flexed, resentful of interference. This is termed " cerebral irritation " and these symptoms may last for days or weeks, perhaps accompanied by disturbed automatic behaviour or hallucinations. Steadily rising temperature to 104° or 105° is a sign of grave omen, indicating extensive contusion. The occurrence of *cerebral compression* from intracranial hæmorrhage may be indicated by (1) progressive deepening of unconsciousness, (2) progressive loss of tone or power in the limbs on one side, (3) progressive slowing of the pulse, (4) progressive discrepancy in the size of the pupils—the hæmorrhage being usually on the side of the slowly dilating pupil, which does not react to light (see §§ 851, 1052).

Post-traumatic Amnesia is that interval of forgetfulness which may elapse between the moment of impact and the time of subsequent recovery of continuous awareness of surroundings. " Islands " of memory may exist within the span of post-traumatic amnesia. As the patient recovers, the duration of post-traumatic amnesia tends to shrink. During this period apparently rational actions may be carried out and then forgotten.

Retrograde Amnesia may also be present for the events immediately preceding the injury. Long retrograde amnesias of months or years, or total amnesia of all events prior to the injury, occur usually in hysterical personalities. (For Unresolved Cerebral Contusion see § 813.)

Prognosis.—The duration of post-traumatic amnesia is usually a fairly reliable guide to the severity of the brain injury and may be used to estimate prognosis except in cases which are complicated by compensation hysteria. If the post-traumatic amnesia lasts minutes, the brain injury is minor. When it lasts 1 to 3 hours, the brain injury is moderate and complete recovery may be expected in from six to eight weeks. When the post-traumatic amnesia (P.T.A.) lasts a week or more, the brain injury is severe and intellectual insufficiency or personality change may result as a temporary or permanent finding. Complete recovery in such cases may take three to six months or longer. Other factors to be taken into account in estimating the prognosis are—(1) the pre-traumatic personality of the patient, (2) associated damage to cranial nerves and other structures, and (3) the type and circumstances of the injury. Most patients with *cerebral contusion*, even when aphasic, recover without operation. Convalescence should be graduated with slow, progressive increase of the field of mental and physical effort. Many will be able to leave their bed at the end of three weeks and return to work in four to six weeks' time. Others continue to suffer from liability to physical and mental fatigue, difficulty in concentration, headaches, giddiness, sleeplessness and other symptoms of unresolved cerebral contusion (§§ 813, 852).

Complications.—A fit occurring within the first ten days of a severe head injury probably does not have the same significance as regards recurrence as fits occurring months or years afterwards (see Traumatic epilepsy). Other complications are post-contusional headaches, and various psychological *post-traumatic syndromes*, viz. amnestic, affective, confusional or psychotic.

Treatment.—As soon as possible the patient should be laid in bed in the semi-prone position with the head to one side, and warmth applied to the body to counteract shock and heat loss (see § 858). If there is a bleeding scalp-wound, hæmorrhage should be arrested by a pad and tight bandage, or by deeply suturing the scalp. If there is a depressed fracture of the skull, operation will probably be necessary (*e.g.*, if there is an overlying scalp wound, which might admit infection to the underlying structures). Search must be made for gross injuries of the limbs and spine, and as soon as the patient has recovered from initial shock, X-ray photographs of the skull are essential. Noise and light should be excluded from the sick room. Watch the bladder for retention. Morphine and alcohol must on no account be given. Thirty-six hours after a severe head injury lumbar puncture should be performed and the fluid pressure estimated by a mano-meter. If the pressure is *above* 150 mm., fluid should be withdrawn until that pressure is reached; this may have to be repeated. Saline purgatives and 2 to 4 fl. oz. of a 50 per cent. solution of magnesium sulphate run into the rectum with a tube and funnel will help to dehydrate the œdematous brain. When the C.S.F. pressure is *below* 100 mm., no fluid should be withdrawn, but the foot of the bed needs to be raised on 6-inch blocks. When return to consciousness is delayed for days or weeks (traumatic stupor), the question of decompression has to be considered.

§ 855. **Electric Shock.**—In many cases sudden death occurs from ventricular fibrillation. The attendant circumstances and the presence of burns will point to the diagnosis. Give artificial respiration in all cases. Distinguish between the effects of the shock and any neurological injury the patient has sustained from falling from a ladder or scaffold.

Heat Exhaustion occurs in tropical climates (§ 510) and in those who work in very hot atmospheres, *e.g.*, near furnaces. Hyperpyrexia, dry skin and albuminuria are present with stupor or coma. Except for diminished chlorides the spinal fluid analysis is normal.

VII. Diabetic Coma (§ 423).—The cause is usually intercurrent ill-ness or infection. The patient is often known to be diabetic. In mid-brain damage from subarachnoid hæmorrhage or injury remember that transient glycosuria may occur.

Hypoglycæmia may be (1) idiopathic or (2) it follows an overdose of insulin in a diabetic (§ 425).

VIII. Endocrine States other than Diabetes.—In Addison's disease, with acute infections (*e.g.*, meningococcal septicæmia (§ 504)) and in patients during with-drawal of cortisone therapy, *acute adrenal failure* may occur with coma. An injection of cortisone can be life-saving. In patients with acute anterior pituitary deficiency a similar condition may develop (§ 570). Coma in *myxœdema* or *thyrotoxicosis* is rare and occurs only in advanced cases.

IX. Biochemical States.—Uræmia (see § 372). There may be albuminuric retinitis, or œdema about the face and legs. A catheter specimen will show albumen, casts, and the blood urea is high. Uræmia produces stupor rather than coma, the deep reflexes can be obtained, there is usually no incontinence and the plantars are flexor. Uræmic twitchings or convulsions may be observed. The muscles are hyper-excitable to gentle tapping with a reflex hammer. Deep coma with unilateral signs is usually due to cerebral hæmorrhage, to which these patients are especially liable.

ECLAMPSIA in pregnancy or the puerperium. The examination of the blood pressure and urine will establish the cause of the coma (§ 410).

HEPATIC COMA.—*Acute liver failure* occurs in (1) infective hepatitis, (2) Eclampsia and (3) Weil's disease. Jaundice supervenes with various cranial nerve palsies, delirium and episodic convulsions. *Portal systemic encephalopathy* is found in patients with cirrhosis, who have developed portal-systemic venous anastomoses (§ 342).

Avitaminosis.—In comatose elderly persons who have been subsisting on an inadequate diet for long periods suspect avitaminosis. High-concentrate vitamin injections are always worth a trial if no focal symptoms are present and if the cause is obscure.

X. INFECTIONS.—The cause of the coma will often be found after diagnostic spinal puncture. Acute encephalitis (§§ 893–897) and dementia paralytica are possible diagnoses. Polio-encephalitis in childhood may cause coma with convulsions and rapidly developing hemiplegia. In fulminating cases of meningococcal meningitis skin petechiæ or joint swellings may be present with meningeal signs (§ 504). When CEREBRAL MALARIA is suspected look for *P. falciparum* (malignant tertian) in the blood (§ 542), and perform spinal puncture to exclude hæmorrhage. Coma may occur in severe cases of typhus, typhoid and cholera.

XI. ANOXIC STATES with coma may occur in patients with chronic bronchitis and emphysema (especially during prolonged oxygen administration (§ 143)). Asthmatic patients given morphine may rapidly die in coma (§ 127). Patients allowed to develop obstruction of the air-passages during anæsthesia are liable to remain unconscious subsequently and to die of respiratory failure.

XII. PSYCHOGENIC CAUSES such as *Trance states* (§ 836C) should never be mistaken for true coma. The breathing is never stertorous, the pupils react to light and the patient forcibly resists attempts to open the eyes. In the katatonia of *Schizophrenia* there is mutism, refusal of food and general diminution of activities. Such patients allow their limbs and bodies to be placed in awkward positions which are maintained indefinitely (§ 1182). There is apathy but no unconsciousness. *Traumatic* and *Anoxic Stupors may be very prolonged.* Cases of hypothalamic neoplasm may have behaviour disorder as well as *anergic stupor*.

§ 856. XIII. Poisoning by Alcohol, Barbiturates, Aspirin, Tranquillisers, Carbon Monoxide or Morphine.

In all forms of severe narcotic poisoning the deep reflexes are lost and the plantar responses may become extensor.

(a) ALCOHOL is perhaps the best-known cause of coma. The flushed face, dilated pupils, stertor and ethylic odour of the breath are readily noted. The danger is not that alcoholism will be missed, but that coma due to some other cause may be attributed to drunkenness.

(b) BARBITURATE.—An overdose of several different barbiturates may be taken by a confused patient or with suicidal intent. An initial stage of excitement may precede coma followed by signs of depression of the mid-brain and bulbar functions. The pulse is rapid. Complete absence of deep reflexes and small inactive pupils are signs that the poisoning is severe. Cyanosis is usually a late sign. There is a great tendency to hypostatic pulmonary œdema.

(c) ASPIRIN is rarely fatal. There is profuse sweating, coma and the deep sighing respiration of acidosis. The pupils are dilated. Urine tests may lead to a false diagnosis of diabetic coma; large quantities of salicylates reduce Fehling's and Benedict's solutions and with the ferric chloride test there is a purple colour to be distinguished from that due to diacetic acid. Rothera's test for acetone is often negative.

(d) TRANQUILLISERS are not infrequently swallowed by infants who are attracted by the bright colours of the capsules.

(e) CARBON MONOXIDE.—The patient suffering from coal gas poisoning has a feeble pulse, the breathing is heavy, there is gross cyanosis and fixed contracted pupils. The body is usually icy cold. A cherry-red complexion is usually seen. Spectroscopy with the finding of the bands characteristic of carboxyhæmoglobin will confirm the diagnosis. Accidental poisoning may occur from leaking gas pipes or faulty water heaters of the geyser type. *Sequelæ* develop in some cases after hours, days or weeks of stupor—(i.) intellectual and emotional insufficiency due to diffuse brain damage or (ii.) Parkinsonism due to focal vascular damage to the basal ganglia.

(f) The coma of MORPHINE causes pin-point pupils. Scars of hypodermic punctures (often septic) are found on the arms and thighs, and burns from cigarettes which have fallen on the chest or limbs.

The *Prognosis* in cases of poisoning with prolonged coma is always grave and depends on the amount of the drug taken and upon the promptitude and efficiency of the treatment. The immediate dangers are respiratory and circulatory failure, and later the development of pulmonary complications. In poisoning by alcohol, belladonna or aspirin, the outlook is much better than with barbiturates. In carbon monoxide poisoning death may occur when coma is prolonged more than 2–3 days.

Treatment.—If transfer to hospital means long delay the patient must be treated at once. (1) Empty the stomach by gastric lavage with 8–12 pints of warm water, with the patient semi-prone and the head held over the edge of the couch. Before withdrawing the tube leave in the stomach a pint of warm water in which magnesium sulphate 1 oz. has been dissolved. (2) When coma is deep a cuffed endotracheal tube connected with an anæsthetic machine should be inserted before the stomach is washed out. (3) Keep the patient well wrapped up to combat heat loss. (4) Raise the foot of the bed and give normal dextrose-saline or plasma intravenously for shock in all but the mildest cases. (5) Cyanosis and mucus accumulating in the bronchi require oxygen and bronchoscopic drainage. Sometimes a respirator is necessary. (6) Prophylactic penicillin injections help to prevent lung infection. *Specific antidotes* are: *Barbiturate poisoning* —administer through the intravenous tubing bemegride (Megimide) 50 mg. *every five minutes* until signs of consciousness appear. *Aspirin poisoning* requires 1–2 litres of either compound injection of sodium lactate, B.P. (Hartmann's solution) or isotonic sod. bicarbonate (1·4 per cent.) intravenously. For *Morphine poisoning* give nalorphine 10 mg. intravenously: the dose may be repeated three times in the course of four hours. In *Carbon monoxide* poisoning move the patient, well wrapped, into the fresh air and commence artificial respiration; also give oxygen, or a mixture of oxygen and 5 per cent. carbon dioxide to inhale.

§ 857. **Coma in Children,** apart from injury, may be due (in order of frequency) to poisoning, tuberculous meningitis, meningococcal and purulent meningitis, encephalitis and encephalopathy, diabetes, post-epileptic stupor and cerebral neoplasm, especially hypothalamic tumour. Syphilitic pachymeningitis, sinus thrombosis and hæmorrhage, abscess and intracranial cysts are rare causes. The history, mode of onset and associated symptoms aid the diagnosis. Tuberculous meningitis is a frequent cause (§ 886). Cerebral hæmorrhage or embolism occurs chiefly in association with the specific fevers, such as small-pox and whooping cough, also with severe rickets and scurvy. In marasmic conditions, thrombosis of the longitudinal sinus (§ 892) may ensue, together with meningeal hæmorrhage, giving rise to convulsions followed by coma. Thrombosis of the vein of Galen and lateral sinus thrombosis (§ 892) in association with ear infections may cause coma.

§ 858. Care of the Unconscious Patient.

—For days or weeks the patient may remain comatose, or restless and unco-operative. In the first few days the chief dangers are respiratory obstruction and shock. Bladder infection, pulmonary œdema or general dehydration may develop; later we must watch for thrombo-phlebitis, pneumonia or bedsores.

Hourly Records.—The doctor who first sees the patient should assess the *basic state* as regards the patient's conscious level, the presence of any focal paralysis, the pupils, pulse rate and blood pressure. Any change from the basic state will be more quickly seen if the nurse keeps hourly records, charting (i.) *pulse rate* (slowing indicates cerebral compression), (ii.) *blood pressure* (falling diastolic level in shock), (iii.) *level of consciousness*, (iv.) *pupils* (inequality suggests a focal intracranial lesion), (v.) the presence of *fits* or other phenomena, (vi.) the temperature and the respiratory rate.

Nursing.—At first the patient should be laid semi-prone with the head turned to one side and lowered to prevent aspiration of secretions. The patient should preferably be nursed on a " ripple-bed," rolled from side to side two-hourly to prevent hypostasis and bedsores, and no hot bottles are allowed. If the patient is restless use cot-sides, and restraining cuffs made of thick white felt threaded with bandage for the wrists. Nurses should be taught to recognise signs of respiratory obstruction and of shock. A syringe and catheter, or a suction apparatus, help to keep the air-passages clear of mucus. If the tongue falls back and obstructs breathing it may be necessary to pull it forward by a stitch inserted 1 cm. behind the tip. Eight-hourly catheterisation is usually essential, using an aseptic technique, or in a male patient insert a Gibbon's catheter draining into a sealed bottle (Fig. 246). Give no aperients; an enema every third day will keep the rectum empty and avoid the risks of fæcal incontinence. The eyes and mouth must be kept clean and free from accumulations. If there is deep coma do not attempt tube feeding but give dextrose-saline intravenously and see that the patient is not dehydrated.

Prolongation of coma after 7–10 days may mean nasal feeding and nursing the patient in a propped-up position. If the airway is obstructed or if there is respiratory paralysis, tracheostomy and a mechanical respirator may have to be used. *Bladder:* In male patients insert a Gibbon's or a 16–18 French Foley catheter with 5 ml. balloon and connect this to a bottle with sealed (continuous) drainage. In female patients use a self-retaining Malecot catheter. Spigots should not be used except temporarily during bedmaking. *Feeding:* If nasal feeding is required, the doctor (not the nurse) passes a No. 6 Portex plastic nasal tube. This is done with the patient sitting up after spraying the nose and pharynx with local anæsthetic.

Drugs.—(i.) Give prophylactic benzylpenicillin 500,000 units intramusc. twice daily until the cough reflex is active and respiration normal. (ii.) If high concentrations of penicillin are being given urinary antiseptics are unnecessary. (iii.) Restless patients may be given chlorpromazine 50 mg. and sod. phenobarbitone 200 mg. intravenously; repeated in 6 hours intramusc. as necessary. Paraldehyde 6 ml. intramusc. is a useful hypnotic. Never give morphine.

If the temperature rises.—(i.) Examine the chest clinically and by X-ray; (ii.) culture the urine; (iii.) look at the legs for thrombo-phlebitis; (iv.) obtain C.S.F. by lumbar puncture and have it cultured and examined for cells, chlorides, sugar; and (v.) determine the sensitivity of any bacteria cultured to antibiotics and chemotherapeutic substances.

GROUP II. FITS, CONVULSIONS OR RECURRENT DISTURBANCES OF CONSCIOUSNESS

In fainting due to SYNCOPE consciousness may be so deeply lost that there are clonic movements of the limbs and incontinence of urine. In such cases we must suspect epilepsy and a recurrence of attacks may confirm this suspicion. No clear line of distinction exists between " faints " and " fits "; both may be due to a transient disturbance of cerebral function or to an alteration in the blood, or the blood-supply to the cerebrum.

EPILEPSY may be defined as an abrupt and transient disturbance of cerebral function. Loss of consciousness does not necessarily occur, but it is usual whenever the cerebral disturbance is widespread. In general, epileptic fits are more related to internal rhythms such as sleeping, waking or menstruation, whilst emotional faints are more " situational " and more reactive to factors outside of the subject. This distinction is, however, by no means absolute. NON-EPILEPTIC CAUSES of fainting, swooning and of "blackouts " are described in §§ 35, 832.

§ 859. Convulsions (Syn. Fits, Epilepsy) may be (A) Idiopathic, (B) Symptomatic or (C) Hysterical. Such a classification is not entirely satisfactory, for organic factors are present in most cases. Attention to the manifestations of attacks gives the best evidence as to the area of cerebrum involved.

(A) Idiopathic Convulsions are almost invariably due to Epilepsy. The attacks may be generalised or focal, and nearly always make their appearance before adult life is reached. They commonly start in infancy, at puberty or during adolescence. The attacks tend to occur at certain times of day and are often related to rhythms of sleep or menstruation. They occur singly or in groups, after rising in the morning, in the night during sleep, or at other times, especially when the patient's attention is unoccupied. They can be related sometimes to emotional upset, or to over-indulgence in food or alcohol.

Epileptic attacks usually recur at intervals throughout life, but in some cases they disappear spontaneously either for years or permanently. Occasionally isolated fits may not be repeated.

FORMS OF EPILEPTIC ATTACKS

I. Major Epilepsy (Grand mal).
II. Status Epilepticus.
III. Minor Epilepsy (Petit mal).

IV. Jacksonian (Focal) Fits.
V. Psychic (" Temporal Lobe ").
VI. Myoclonic Epilepsy.

§ 860. INVESTIGATION OF CASES OF FITS.—When the doctor arrives the fit is usually over and the patient is either confused and restless with headache, or else is in post-epileptic stupor. The fit may have been due to idiopathic epilepsy, subarachnoid hæmorrhage, apoplexy or hysteria. If the case is one of idiopathic epilepsy the patient may have had previous fits, known to relatives or friends. Look for evidences of head injury, posterior cervical rigidity (subarachnoid hæmorrhage) and make a brief examination of the nervous system, looking for *unilateral signs—e.g.*, weakness of face or limbs on one side, a difference in the deep reflexes or an extensor response on one side. Take the blood pressure. It is probably wise to *regard all doubtful cases as possibly epileptic until subsequent progress makes the diagnosis clear.*

It is important to calm the relatives. Arrange for the patient to be watched for several hours in case other fits occur. A knotted handkerchief placed between the premolar teeth will prevent cheek or tongue biting. The nurse or watcher should provide a written description of any further fits which may occur.

To obtain the necessary diagnostic information, if you have not observed the attack yourself, *it is essential to interrogate an eye-witness of the attack in addition to the patient.* In talking to the patient you should be careful not to speak of " fits " but of " attacks " or " seizures."

1. *Interrogation of the Eye-witness.*—The eye-witness should be asked to describe the attack in his own words. Questions are then put—Is there any sound before he falls ? What is his breathing like in the attacks; is it snoring ? What is the colour of his face in the attacks ? Does the patient reply to questions in his attacks ? How long do they last ? These questions can be answered only by an eye-witness.

2. *Interrogation of the Patient.*—This should include direct questions as—Do you fall in the attacks ? Do you get any warning ? Has there ever been any blood in your mouth after the attack ? Have you ever wet yourself in an attack by passing water ? Have you ever hurt yourself in an attack ? (An examination of the face, scalp, tongue or limbs may reveal cicatrices, evidences of injury in the fits.) At what time of day or night do your attacks mostly occur ?

When observing a fit, push the edge of a handkerchief into the patient's mouth, stand back and watch the distribution and spread of the convulsion. If the patient is in bed, throw back the bedclothes. After the convulsion is over, examine the limbs for flaccidity, examine the pupils and test the tendon reflexes and plantar responses.

Later the *urine* will have to be tested and the ocular fundi examined. An electro-encephalogram, X-ray of chest and skull, and blood Wassermann reaction may be helpful. When cases of epilepsy of late onset show any lateralising neurological sign, lumbar encephalography or angiography may have to be undertaken.

There are REPEATED ATTACKS *of* SUDDEN DISTURBANCE OF CONSCIOUS-NESS *with* CONVULSIONS *and falling.* The condition is likely to be MAJOR EPILEPSY.

§ 861. I. **Major Epilepsy** (Syn. Grand Mal) may occur alone or alternate with petit mal attacks. Few epileptic fits correspond in all respects to the classical form; great variations are possible.

Symptoms.—" Stages " may be recognised in a grand mal convulsion. (1) *Prodromata*—sudden jerkings, persistent giddiness, irritability, ravenous appetite may warn the relations that an attack is impending in some hours or days. (2) *Aura*—in many cases a warning or aura precedes the attack, and lasts a few seconds. Auræ are classified as: (*a*) Visceral—a sensation rising from the epigastrium, or nausea; (*b*) Sensory—" a wave passing over the body," sounds and sights becoming faint, ringing in the ears, momentary vertigo or faintness occur; (*c*) Motor—twitching of a limb, " the jerks," as patients call this; or (*d*) Psychic—feelings of familiarity, fear, dreamy states, hallucinations are common in temporal lobe epilepsy and may influence the patient's behaviour, *e.g.*, he may begin to run, or call for help. (3) *Loss of consciousness and falling* may succeed the aura so quickly that the patient may not have time to place himself out of harm's way. The fit proper follows. (4) *Tonic Stage.*—As the patient falls the muscles usually go into tonic spasm, and he may give a weird unearthly hollow cry produced by inspiratory spasm drawing in air over the nearly closed vocal cords. In the tonic stage the breath is held, the hands clenched, the back rigid and the legs extended. One arm may be raised slowly and flexed and the head and eyes directed to one side; this should not be interpreted as a focal discharge. After about half a minute (5) the *clonic stage* ensues. Clonic movements involve the whole body and are sometimes of great violence, consisting of rapid extension and flexion of the limbs, opening and shutting of the eyes and jaws. The interference with respiration during both the tonic and clonic stages causes apnœa or stertor and an ever-increasing blueness and congestion of the face. The tongue or lower lip is often bitten, and conjunctival hæmorrhages may occur. The pulse is rapid and strong. As the convulsion passes off the period of apnœa ceases and the respiration returns, urine and fæces may be voided and saliva may issue from the mouth as a fr hy foam, sometimes churned up with blood from injury to the tongue. Swallowed blood from an injured mouth may subsequently be vomited. (6) *The stage of flaccid coma (post-epileptic stupor)* succeeds the convulsions and the patient passes from it into deep sleep or recovers consciousness at once. Examination is possible in the stage of flaccid coma and will show that the pupils are dilated and inactive to light, the corneal reflexes diminished or absent, the tendon reflexes diminished or abolished and the plantar responses temporarily extensor. The reflexes rapidly become normal again. On waking from sleep the patient, who has no recollection of the attack, may recognise that he has had a seizure by the following signs: (*a*) bitten tongue, (*b*) blood on the pillow, (*c*) wet bed or disarranged bedclothes, (*d*) severe headache or aching muscles.

Mental changes in epilepsy.—Since treatment with bromides was stopped intellectual and emotional dullness, forgetfulness and irritability are rarely seen. Drug idiosyncrasy with newer anticonvulsants shows itself soon after treatment is initiated, usually as confusion or drowsiness.

There is no foundation for the popular belief that chronic epileptics inevitably deteriorate mentally. If major fits are uncontrolled and frequently repeated, anoxic cerebral lesions sustained in the attack may eventually cause dementia. Most epileptic outpatients are able to earn their living in sheltered employment. Rather more than a quarter of such cases will show a greater or lesser degree of mental or emotional insufficiency, usually due to an organic cause, *i.e.*, the epilepsy is symptomatic of underlying brain damage. Such mental deterioration may be *non-progressive* after birth-injury, anoxia, a cerebro-vascular accident, or *progressive*, as in cases where a congenital, inflammatory, neoplastic, traumatic or degenerative cerebral lesion, itself progressive, is associated with fits.

A few patients, perhaps because of their hallucinatory experiences in fits, become fanatically religious. Paroxysms of odd behaviour of brief duration are believed by some to be atypical seizures (" equivalents "). During states of automatism or in despair after an attack, epileptic patients occasionally consume lethal doses of anti-convulsant drugs. Epilepsy may be associated with psychopathic personality and delinquency, with obsessive-compulsive personality or with hysteria or affective disorder. *Psychoses* in epileptic patients are varied. (1) Transient states of *post-epileptic confusion* have been alluded to above. (2) Post-epileptic "furor" with destructive and homicidal behaviour is happily very rare. (3) Post-epileptic depressive states are common. (4) A more prolonged psychosis of schizophrenic type, often paranoid, occurs with slow dementia (for Personality changes and automatism in temporal lobe attacks see § 864).

Rarer Varieties of Major Epilepsy.—(1) *Tonic Fits* occur in mid-brain lesions and in lesions of the vermis of the cerebellum, *e.g.*, medullo-blastoma. Other kinds of brain damage, *e.g.*, encephalitis, may cause these attacks, which are often associated with coma. The head is retracted, the upper limbs flexed and the lower limbs extended as in decerebration. (2) In *Flaccid* (Inhibitory) Epilepsy there is loss of consciousness with falling. Clonic and tonic movements are absent, the muscles being flaccid and limp. These attacks, which are epileptic and may last minutes, have to be distinguished from *momentary "Drop seizures"* (§ 833) and *Cataplexy* (§ 838) in which no loss of consciousness occurs. The two latter conditions are probably not epileptic. (3) *Reflex Epilepsy.* Local or general convulsions with loss of consciousness start as the result of a specific peripheral stimulus. Focal attacks may be precipitated in this way; thus pinching or pricking the sole of the foot may start a Jacksonian attack. The phenomenon may occur with focal cortical lesions. An attack may be prevented by tying a tight band round the limb or gripping it firmly above the area stimulated. Stranger still are the cases in which a sudden loud noise or a bright flash of light will cause a patient to fall to the ground in a fit.

Cerebrospinal Fluid. In about 10 per cent. of cases the protein of the spinal fluid is slightly raised (45–90 mg.) especially after an attack.

EPILEPSY OF LATE ONSET. If attacks begin after the age of twenty the possibility that they are *symptomatic* is very considerable, especially if there are neurological signs between the attacks (see Symptomatic Convulsions, p. 1149).

A SOLITARY FIT. Isolated fits occur in predisposed individuals as the result of (*a*) hydration and alcoholic excess, (*b*) severe emotional stress, (*c*) the onset of infection, *e.g.*, pneumonia. It is probably better not to put these cases on anticonvulsants at once but to wait for a further attack to occur before diagnosing epilepsy.

II. **Status Epilepticus,** a rather rare, but occasionally fatal complication of epilepsy, occurs when a patient has more than two fits without recovering consciousness. Often a series of fits occurs over a period of hours or days without consciousness being regained. The rectal temperature may rise to 108° F and death may occur from myocardial failure. Status epilepticus may be the first symptom of *subarachnoid hæmorrhage or encephalitis.* After the convulsions have been controlled or cease, post-epileptic coma may continue, or stupor may pass into a confusional state lasting some days or weeks. (For Treatment see § 864.)

When there is a MOMENTARY DISTURBANCE OF CONSCIOUSNESS *or " absence" without falling,* the condition is probably MINOR EPILEPSY.

§ **862.** III. **Minor Epilepsy** (Syn. Petit Mal).—The attack in about half the cases is preceded by some sensory aura or warning such as precedes

major epileptic fits. Petit mal may be characterised only by loss of consciousness lasting a second or two. The patient resumes his occupation
or conversation where he left off, as if nothing had happened. An observer
may note, however, that his expression is vacant or his gaze fixed, he
may not reply to questions, he may pause in his conversation or babble
in speech for a second or two, his head may drop, incontinence of urine
may occur, or things held in his hands (e.g., knife and fork) may be dropped.
There may be slight visible spasm such as stiffening and shaking of the
whole body for a second or two, or quasi-purposive fumblings or other
gestures may occur. Sometimes there is pallor of the face at the moment
of an attack: commonly the face later becomes flushed. After an attack
is over the patient may be well at once or he may be stupid and dull
for a short time. Rarely some familiar action may be performed in a
dreamlike automatic manner. When he recovers he has no recollection
of the attack or of the period of automatism, if such has occurred. He
may only realise he has had an attack from the expressions and utterances
of those around him.

Varieties of Petit Mal.—In *Juvenile petit mal* there may be as many as twenty to
forty or more attacks during the day, each lasting a second or two. The child looks
vacant for a second, may fumble with the hands, or recovers at once. This type of
petit mal is further distinguished by the " spike and wave " in the E.E.G. Consideration should be given to a trial of anticonvulsants of the dione group if the
attacks do not react to less toxic substances. *Pyknolepsy:* In children between the
ages of 4 and 12 years attacks of minor epilepsy occur up to the number of fifty daily.
No mental deterioration occurs and the attacks cease at puberty. The condition
cannot be diagnosed with any confidence until spontaneous cessation of all fits has
occurred. Most believe that this is the same condition as Juvenile Petit Mal. *Apparent mental deterioration* in epileptic children lasting days, weeks or months may be
due to " minor epileptic states "—epileptic discharges, often subclinical, follow so
quickly one on the other that the child has no time to recover. Ataxia, dysarthria,
slobbering and loss of sphincter control may occur. This is a reversible condition.
In other cases intoxication by anticonvulsants may be the cause of a reversible
pseudo-dementia in a child.

§ 863. IV. The **Jacksonian (Focal) Fit** is characteristic of an isolated cortical
lesion, but may occur in idiopathic epilepsy. (a) Motor, (b) Sensory, (c) Visual,
(d) Auditory and (e) Uncinate attacks are described. The cortical area most excitable
is that for the index and thumb and the adjacent area for the angle of the mouth.

(a) *Motor Jacksonian Fits* commence unilaterally in the thumb or index finger,
the corner of the mouth or the big toe. The attack *spreads in an orderly march,*
according to the arrangement of centres for movements in the motor cortical area
(Fig. 209a). The onset is with tonic spasm. Later, broken or tonic twitchings occur,
the whole attack occupying, perhaps, twenty minutes. The movements are confined,
for a long period, to one limb or one side of the body and consciousness is retained.
Jacksonian attacks may terminate in a generalised convulsion, with loss of consciousness. The Jacksonian fit may be followed by a transient local paralysis (usually a
monoplegia) or, if the convulsion is right-sided, accompanied by temporary aphasia:
this is known as *Todd's paralysis*, and may last hours or days after the fit. (b) *Sensory
Jacksonian fits* occur in parietal cortical lesions with numbness and tingling, starting
locally and spreading in an orderly march. These may be followed by transient
astereognosis. (c) *Visual attacks*, blinding flashes of light of hemianopic distribution,
followed by transient hemianopia, occur in occipital and temporal cortical lesions,

and (d) *Auditory attacks*, sudden hallucinations of sound, followed by transient deafness, in temporal lobe lesions.　(e) *Uncinate fits* occur in lesions of the uncinate gyrus or lesions in its neighbourhood (*e.g.*, in pituitary neoplasms) and consist of (i.) an intensely unpleasant flavour or odour, (ii.) champing or spitting movements, (iii.) a characteristic " dreamy " state.　*Etiology*, see Symptomatic Convulsions.

§ 864.　V. **The Psychic** (Temporal-lobe) **Attack** is a variety of focal seizure.　In many cases an organic cause exists.　There is (1) transient loss of consciousness like that occurring in petit mal, (2) preceded in some cases by a visual, auditory or *psychic aura* (" dreamy state ").　One common form of aura is a feeling of familiarity (*déja vu* phenomena) as if the sufferer were passing through or were about to experience some familiar experience.　Other psychic auræ are feelings of fear, ecstasy, or depression of mood.　(3) The patient may resume normal activity at once.　(4) Temporal lobe epilepsy is sometimes associated with *personality* disorders, *e.g.*, *psychopathy*.　If there is *recent change* of personality suspect a focal lesion.　Irritability and episodes of aggressive behaviour, forgetfulness and loss of social sense may occur.　(5) Automatism can follow a temporal or petit mal attack; this seems to be related to mental stress.　In this " twilight " state of altered consciousness the patient's behaviour may be automatic and irrational (post-epileptic automatism).　Undressing in public, walking into furniture or against windows, doors or walls, or walking unheedingly into the traffic may occur.　During this phase, which may last minutes (or more rarely days or weeks), the patient may commit aggressive or violent acts for which there is subsequent *amnesia*.　Such an attack may have medico-legal significance when an epileptic accused of a criminal act pleads this condition as his defence.　(6) *E.E.G. changes* are characteristically present in one temporal lobe but not everyone agrees that they are specific.　Temporal " spike and wave " discharges in sleep records may occur.　Slow, high-voltage, square-topped waves 2–4 per second with superimposed fast waves may be obtained in the waking state (Fig. 236).　Taken with (1) the typical clinical history, (2) abnormal calcification in plain X-rays or ventricular distortion in air studies, these findings may indicate a focal organic lesion.　For the *Causes of Convulsions* see Symptomatic Epilepsy.

VI. Epileptic Myoclonus.—Many epileptic patients suffer at times from sudden shock-like clonic contractions of groups of voluntary muscles (" the jerks ") without gross disturbance of consciousness.　Some authorities attribute certain " drop attacks " to such myoclonus.　Myoclonus occurs temporarily in adults during withdrawal of hypnotic or sedative drugs (see § 931).

The *Diagnosis of Epilepsy* is best made from a witness's description of a fit.　Tongue-biting, incontinence of urine, stertor and blueness, history of injury, are signs indicating a severe and sudden degree of loss of consciousness.　For the diagnosis of epilepsy to be established it may be necessary to wait for recurrence of a fit.　Look for scars of burns or for bruising or scars on the buccal surface of the lower lip.　If neurological and general clinical examination reveals a possible focal or general cause the condition is *symptomatic* epilepsy (see p. 1149).　All cases where the onset of the first fit occurs after the age of 25 years must be suspected of a focal cause.　If reflex changes exist on one side or lateralising neurological signs, air studies or contrast radiography may be required.　For the diagnosis of syncopal attacks, swoons and " blackouts " see §§ 35, 832, 833.

Hysterical fits are uncommon nowadays.　Patients of hysterical personality may have bizarre attacks which if stereotyped may be epileptic.　Patients with " psychic " epileptic fits may wrongly be thought to be hysterical. Where there is any doubt it is best to have the patient under observation in hospital for a short time and to try the effect of various anticonvulsants. An electro-encephalogram showing specific epileptic abnormalities (§ 847) is against the diagnosis of hysteria.

ELECTRO-ENCEPHALOGRAPHY in Epilepsy.—The description of an attack by a reliable witness is much more valuable than an E.E.G. The records are not specific as are those obtained from electrocardiography. In epilepsy—(1) the resting record is *normal* in about 33 per cent. of epileptics. A normal record renders unlikely any gross *focal* cause for the attacks. (2) The record may show a diagnostic abnormality; subclinical attacks may be observed, or the " spike and wave " record seen in juvenile petit mal attacks (Fig. 236). (3) The record may show a non-specific abnormality. In the latter case examination (i.) after overbreathing for several minutes, or (ii.) after administration of a rapidly acting analeptic or barbiturate drug, may bring out latent epileptic features not previously noted.

Etiology of Idiopathic Epilepsy.—The cause is unknown. Males and females are equally affected. Popularly it is thought to be hereditary, although it follows no genetic law. Direct inheritance is exceptional. A history of nervous instability and migraine may be found in the family; of epilepsy less commonly. Metabolic and endocrine factors may exist. In some individuals there appears to be a predisposition, perhaps inherited. In these perhaps " normal " individuals, epileptic fits or faints can be induced by hyperpnœa, alkalosis or excessive hydration.

Prognosis of Idiopathic Epilepsy.—Convulsions in infancy are not necessarily followed by epilepsy in adult life. " *Pyknolepsy* " is said to disappear completely at puberty. In some cases one or two fits occur in adolescence and then a long remission follows. In exceptional cases isolated major fits may occur in adult life and not recur. Most confirmed epileptics are able to live a normal working life under selected conditions away from potential dangers (machinery, furnaces, heights), and to marry and have healthy children. In a few established cases the fits can be completely controlled by anticonvulsant drugs. When the fits are all nocturnal the employment of the patient presents fewer problems.

Treatment.—During the attack put a knotted handkerchief between the teeth, loosen clothing round the neck, remove spectacles and false teeth and prevent the patient damaging himself in the clonic stage. For *Status Epilepticus:* Give intramusc. paraldehyde 5–10 ml. (2–3 ml. for a child), repeated in an hour if the fit continues, or give intramusc. sodium phenobarbitone 3–6 gr. Chloroform inhalations may be used. Feed parenterally or by nasal tube, taking care not to overhydrate the patient. A rising temperature and falling blood pressure are ominous signs and require treatment. Positive-pressure anæsthesia in hospital will save many cases who otherwise may die.

Between the Attacks. (1) The patient should not ride a bicycle, drive a car, or swim. All open fires in the house should be screened. Certain exciting factors should if possible be avoided, viz.: (*a*) constipation, (*b*) overeating, (*c*) large amounts of alcoholic or other fluids, (*d*) emotional strain. No special diet is advised. (2) *Choice of occupation:* Sedentary occupation on the ground level carries least risk. If possible, epileptic children should be guided into suitable occupations. Nursing, service life, engineering, building, motor- or engine-driving, cooking are highly unsuitable. It is surprising how occupation in sheltered surroundings helps epileptic patients. Mental lethargy induces fits. (3) *Marriage and family:* Marriage has no effect on epilepsy. The other contracting partner must (in English Law) have full information about the patient's epilepsy before the marriage. If the partner's family history and E.E.G. is normal the risk of children being affected is said to be less, but direct transmission of the disease to children is exceptional. Some doctors advise " protected " marriage. Sterilisation for epilepsy is illegal. During pregnancy the attacks may disappear or become more frequent. (4) *Drugs:* If two or three attacks have occurred, continued anticonvulsant treatment will be required. Having discovered the most suitable remedy and the adequate dose, the treatment must be continued without reduction until the patient has been free of attacks for at least three years. If fitness to drive a vehicle is in question a further period of 2–3 years off all medicines with freedom from an attack will be required. Patients sometimes foolishly break the continuity of treatment after a bout of attacks, attributing the seizures not to the malady, but to the " drugs " they are taking. In prescribing for epilepsy try to time the dose of the medicine to precede the occurrence of the attacks. If the fits are nocturnal, the larger dose should be given before bedtime; if they occur on waking, the medicine should be taken before rising; if the fits occur at the menstrual periods, the dose may have to be increased at these times. Table LV shows the drugs most suited to different types of seizure. Major fits usually respond best to *phenobarbitone*. Children tolerate it well in doses of $\frac{1}{4}$ to $\frac{1}{2}$ gr. twice daily. A few patients with idiosyncrasy develop a scarlatiniform or moribilliform rash, or drowsiness. If phenobarbitone alone does not control the attacks the *hydantoins* (tab. phenytoin sodium) should next be used, preferably with phenobarbitone. A useful tablet contains soluble phenytoin gr. $1\frac{1}{2}$, phenobarbitone gr. $\frac{3}{4}$. This two to one proportion tends to be more effective than when either substance is used alone. Toxic effects are—hypertrophy of the gums, unsteady gait, diplopia and rashes. Should albumin or urobilin appear in the urine the dose should be diminished. If toxic effects arise with hydantoins, give a combination of two other preparations in smaller doses. If toxic symptoms persist or the fits are not controlled, try *Primidone* B.P. up to four or five tablets a day, beginning with 125 mg. once daily. *Bromides* have gone out of favour but are still useful in some cases in doses of 10–15 gr. twice or thrice daily. *Diones:* Although petit mal attacks are usually very resistant to anticonvulsants, begin treatment as for major epilepsy. Troxidone B.P. in 5-gr. capsules may be effective in cases of petit mal showing a " spike and wave " formation during the attacks. Give 1–4 capsules daily for an adult and 1–2 capsules daily for a child of ten years.

Troxidone is toxic and as it may cause agranulocyotosis it should only be given under expert supervision, and with weekly blood counts for the first weeks of treatment. It may precipitate major attacks. Ethosuximide (Zarontin) 250 mg. capsules four times daily is under trial for petit mal. In epilepsy, if the administration of drugs is suddenly stopped, status epilepticus may ensue.

TABLE LV.—ANTICONVULSANT DRUGS

	Dose, twice or three times a day	Maximum daily dose: Child. Adult.		Toxic Side-effects.
(A) *Major and minor epilepsy*				
(1) Phenobarbitone (Luminal, Gardenal).	¼–½ gr. 16–30 mg.	1½ gr. 100 mg.	3 gr. 200 mg.	Drowsiness, rashes.
(2) Phenytoin sodium (Epanutin).	¾–1½ gr. 50–100 mg.	3 gr. 200 mg.	6 gr. 400 mg.	Dizziness, rashes, ataxia. Hypertrophy of gums. Megaloblastic anæmia (rare).
(3) Combination of these.	{ Phenobarbitone ¾ gr. Phenytoin Sod. 1½ gr. each	2;	4 tablets	
(B) *Psychic and temporal lobe attacks*				
(1) Phenytoin sodium.	see above	see above		
(2) Phenytoin sodium and phenobarbitone.	see above	see above		
(3) Primidone (Mysoline).	2–4 gr. 125–250 mg.	8 gr. 0·5 G.	30 gr. 2 G.	Drowsiness, ataxia, vomiting. Megaloblastic anæmia (rare).
(C) *Juvenile petit mal* Troxidone (tridione).	5 gr. 300 mg.	8 gr. 0·5 G.	30 gr. 2 G.	Photophobia, rashes, vertigo, drowsiness. Agranulocytosis.
Tridione Solution (Oral).	150 mg. in 60 ℳ (4 ml.)	180 ℳ for a child (12 ml.)		

(B) In Symptomatic Convulsions the fits may be (1) Focal or (2) Generalised. Symptomatic epilepsy should be suspected (1) in all cases with neurological signs; (2) where general examination of the other systems reveals a possible cause for fits; (3) in cases with focal (Jacksonian) fits, especially if the fits are followed by increasing weakness of a limb; (4) in cases of epilepsy of late onset; (5) in cases showing cutaneous nævi or pigmented moles or the skin lesions of epiloia. The commonest findings are cortical atrophy due to trauma or cerebral arteriosclerosis, congenital malformations of the brain and its blood-vessels (including angiomatous malformations), intracranial cysticercosis, or cerebral syphilis. Febrile (infantile) convulsions may be symptomatic.

The causes of symptomatic epilepsy are numerous: they may be classified as (i.) Atrophic lesions and (ii.) Expanding (space-occupying) lesions. Of 2,000 cases of epilepsy at all ages Lennox found no cause for the seizures in 77·6 per cent. Of the remaining 22·4 per cent., cerebral injuries, congenital defects, cerebral infections, cerebral neoplasms and cerebral circulatory defects were the most common.

CAUSES OF SYMPTOMATIC CONVULSIONS

(All causes of COMA are possible causes of symptomatic convulsions (§ 850).)

I. Traumatic epilepsy (§ 865).
II. Focal cortical atrophy (§ 866).
III. Subdural hæmatoma (§ 1052).
IV. Cerebral diplegia.
V. Infantile hemiplegia.
VI. Congenital angiomatous malformations (§ 1047).
VII. Presenile dementia (§ 1188) and Dementia paralytica (§ 1190).
VIII. Acute encephalitis and Meningitis.
IX. Cerebral vascular syphilis.

X. Cerebral abscess (§ 891).
XI. Cerebral cysticercosis.
XII. Cerebral malaria (§ 512).
XIII. Intracranial neoplasm.
XIV. Cerebral circulatory defects, Stokes Adams' syndrome.
XV. Alcoholism and Drugs.
XVI. Asphyxia.
XVII. Biochemical disorders.
XVIII. Industrial poisoning.

Also Hypoglycæmia (§ 425), Porphyria (§ 415), Hyperpnœa (§ 832).

§ 865. I. Traumatic Epilepsy.—Following upon open head injuries (often with sepsis) or more rarely closed head injuries, fits may occur. Fits in the first six weeks after head injury are usually due to the acute lesion and may disappear. Serial E.E.G. examinations may help in assessing their significance. A head injury may occur in the first of a series of idiopathic epileptic fits or of fits due to cortical atrophy. *Etiology.*—The usual cause of epilepsy is either scar-formation or brain atrophy coming on years after the injury, but in some patients constitutional factors are evident. *Treatment* is as for idiopathic epilepsy. In rare cases surgery may help.

§ 866. II. Focal Cortical Atrophy.—The cause of this condition is not known with certainty. It occurs after head injury or as an early symptom in dementia: cerebral arteriosclerosis may be a factor. The age incidence is 30–60 years. Memory defect of a progressive kind accompanies the fits. The signs resemble those of a slowly expanding lesion in that they may be focal and progressive, but air-studies show the atrophic area with ventricular shift towards the side of the lesion. *Treatment* is as for idiopathic epilepsy.

III. *Subdural hæmatoma* (see § 1052).

IV. In *Cerebral Diplegia* (§ 972) and (V) *Infantile Hemiplegia* the fits can often be controlled by anticonvulsants. In *Tuberose Sclerosis* (Epiloia) (§ 1194c) dementia and fits are found with the cutaneous lesions characteristic of adenoma sebaceum. For *Cerebro-macular degeneration* see § 1194c.

VI. CONGENITAL ANGIOMATOUS MALFORMATIONS.—For *Sturge-Weber Syndrome* (i.e., extensive nævus of scalp or face with fits), see § 1047f.

VII. PRESENILE DEMENTIA (§ 1188) and Dementia paralytica (§ 1190) may commence with epilepsy of late onset.

VIII. *Acute Encephalitis* and *Meningitis* may begin with general or focal fits, or fits may be a sequel of such an illness (see §§ 882, 893).

IX. CEREBRAL VASCULAR SYPHILIS, active or healed, is a cause of symptomatic epilepsy (§ 907).

X. *Cerebral Abscess* (see § 891).

§ 867. XI. **Cerebral Cysticercosis** (*T. Solium*) is a cause of symptomatic general-ised convulsions to be suspected in patients who have served in India and the Far East. The condition is due to eating " measly " pork infested with the tapeworm eggs. If man ingests these the resulting cysticerci invade the brain and skeletal muscles, and calcify, giving rise to recurrent generalised fits. X-rays of the muscles will show calcified cysts flattened by muscular contraction; or skull X-rays· may reveal the circular shadows of calcified cysts.

XII. *Cerebral Malaria* (see § 512).

XIII. INTRACRANIAL NEOPLASM, either a primary growth (glioma, meningioma) or a secondary (often from bronchial carcinoma), causes symptomatic convulsions. So often does bronchial carcinoma first show its presence by cerebral symptoms that it is now usual to X-ray the chest as routine in adult males with unexplained cerebral symptoms. For months generalised or focal fits may be the only symptom of a brain tumour. Headache and papillœdema often come later (and see § 1041).

XIV. *Cerebral Circulatory defects*, *e.g.*, hæmorrhage, thrombosis, em-bolism, hypertensive attacks, internal carotid occlusion, basilar insuffi-ciency, Stokes-Adams' syndrome.

CEREBRAL ARTERIOSCLEROSIS AND HYPERTENSIVE ENCEPHALOPATHY (§ 97) cause focal or generalised epilepsy of late onset. Examination of the fundi may reveal arteriosclerotic retinopathy. In hypertensive cases the blood-pressure will show readings of the order of 230–240 mm. systolic and 140–120 mm. diastolic. Brain tumours occur in arteriopaths and the differential diagnosis of these causes may be clinically very difficult. Progressive rapid deterioration is more suggestive of neoplasm. Epilepsy may occur after a CEREBRAL THROMBOSIS with hemiplegia.

STOKES-ADAMS' SYNDROME.—In *heart-block* in elderly arteriosclerotic patients extreme slowing of the pulse causes cerebral anoxia with transient falling, loss of consciousness and convulsions (§ 71).

XV. ALCOHOLISM AND DRUGS.—A fit may herald delirium tremens or other psychosis in an alcoholic patient. Withdrawal of narcotic drugs in addicts causes symptomatic episodic fits or myoclonus.

XVI. ASPHYXIA from a foreign body in the trachea may give rise to unconscious-ness with fits, especially in children.

XVII. *Biochemical disorders* such as uræmia (due to renal disease, persistent vomiting or diarrhœa or dehydration), hepatic disease, alkalosis, hypoglycæmia, eclampsia (in pregnant or puerperal women) are all causes of fits.

XVIII. *Industrial poisoning.*—Chronic encephalopathy due to lead, methyl bromide and other industrial poisons may cause fits.

Diagnosis of Symptomatic Convulsions may depend on (1) a history of brain trauma, birth injury, progressive headaches, " strokes," excessive consumption of alcohol, loss of weight, a previous operation for a growth. When the fits come on *after* childhood or adolescence be suspicious of a slowly developing intracranial focal lesion. Diagnosis will also depend on (2) *careful neurological examination* for focal signs or signs of increased intracranial pressure and a *thorough general examination* for evidence of cerebro-vascular disease, bronchial carcinoma, carcinoma elsewhere, or hepatic disease.   The urine must be examined in every case.   (3) *Blood*. Where a tropical illness is in question blood films for malaria, blood counts and E.S.R. may be required.   The W.R. in the blood and perhaps in the spinal fluid will often be necessary.   (4) Most valuable are the plain X-rays of the chest for bronchial carcinoma, and of the skull for displacement of the calcified pineal (over 3 mm. is significant) in basal projections. X-rays of the muscles may show calcified cysticerci.   (5) E.E.G. records are often helpful if taken with the clinical findings.   (6) Air-studies and angiograms are required in cases with focal signs.

Treatment.—If the cause cannot be found and removed by (*a*) medical or (*b*) surgical means, the treatment is that of idiopathic epilepsy.   These cases require periodic examination over the years as focal symptoms may suddenly appear.   Psychotic epileptics, those with suicidal or homicidal tendencies, and deteriorated and destructive patients, may require treatment in mental hospitals.

(C) **Hysterical fits** are uncommon nowadays.   Patients of hysterical personality may have bizarre attacks which if stereotyped may be epileptic. Patients with " psychic " epileptic fits may wrongly. be thought to be hysterical.   Where there is any doubt it is best to have the patient under observation in hospital for a short time and to try the effect of various anticonvulsants.   An electro-encephalogram showing specific epileptic abnormalities is against the diagnosis of hysteria (and see § 1173*e*).

§ **868. Infantile Convulsions.**—A convulsion in infancy has probably a less serious significance than in adult life.   The convulsive threshold appears to be lower in infancy and is said to increase with maturation of the nervous system.   In infancy febrile states such as teething, exanthemata, gastro-intestinal infections are frequent causes of convulsions. If a single fit occurs there is little cause for alarm, but if fits recur in recurrent illnesses or if they are repeated without adequate cause epilepsy becomes a much more likely diagnosis.   The rectal temperature is often much raised in the attacks.

CAUSES OF INFANTILE CONVULSIONS

A. *In the first 6 months of life.*
  1. Birth injury, *e.g.*, subdural hæmatoma.
  2. Acute infections.
  3. Cerebral malformations, *e.g.*, hydrocephalus, infantile hemiplegia, cerebral diplegia.
  4. Congenital syphilis.
  5. Cerebro-macular degeneration (see § 1194*c*).

B. *From 6–18 months of life.*
  6. Acute fevers (pertussis, pneumonia, measles).
  7. Other infections (bacilluria, tonsillitis, otitis media).
  8. Reflex causes (gastro-enteritis, constipation).
  9. Breath-holding fits.
  10. Tetany and rickets.
  11. Meningitis and Encephalitis.

C. *After the age of 2-3 years.*
   As B., but the likelihood of epilepsy as a cause of repeated unexplained fits
   is greater.

Treatment.—(1) *Control the convulsions* and reduce fever.   Immerse the
infant in a warm bath for 10–15 minutes, then place in a warm bed.   Give
an enema or glycerine suppository.   Bromethol B.P. per rectum, the rectal
instillation of chloral hydrate gr. 4 and sodium bromide gr. 5 in 1 oz.
warm water or after the age of 1 year sod. phenobarbitone ½ gr. intramusc.
may control the fits.   It may be repeated in one hour.   Inhalations of
chloroform are effective but one or two drops only on a mask are necessary.
(2) *Investigate the cause*—(*a*) Question the mother or nurse about the
diet with special attention to the question of overfeeding, unsuitable
food or constipation.   (*b*) Search for a history or signs of rickets and tetany.
(*c*) Make a general physical examination of the child for a rash, any source
of sepsis (throat and ears), examine the chest.   Look for head retraction,
squint or Kernig's sign, and lastly (*d*) Examine the stools and urine.

GROUP III. DEFECTS OF SPEECH AND ARTICULATION

The elements of speech are words, phrases or sentences either spoken or
written.   These are arranged or analysed in the cerebral cortex.   Defects
of speech of CORTICAL origin are called *Aphasia* or *Dysphasia*, and receptive and expressive forms are described.   The lips, tongue and palate which
are under the control of lower bulbar centres mould the sounds made by the
larynx on phonation into articulate speech.   Defects of these BULBAR or
peripheral mechanisms cause *Dysarthria* or *Dysphonia*.   Absence of speech
due to psychical causes is called *Mutism.*

Applied Physiology of Speech Mechanisms.

The acquisition of speech in childhood: About the thirteenth month, *gesture* appears,
in the form of shaking the head from side to side as a sign of negation.   (In conditions
which damage the speech functions in later life gesture is the last to be destroyed.)
The child understands much of what is heard or seen before words are uttered.   Sounds
are recognised by their association with objects handled (*word-hearing*); thus an area
for the memory of spoken words begins to be developed in the superior temporal
gyrus of the left side in right-handed children.   The speech areas are probably
developed bilaterally, but are chiefly left-sided in right-handed children.   By eighteen
months the child has a small vocabulary of thirty to forty words.   Between the
second and third years he can understand what is said and make himself understood
by others.   The acquisition of *reading* and *writing* comes later.   The visual symbols
(letters, words in written or printed combinations) are recognised by education of
the angular gyrus (" word-seeing ") and afterwards they can be reproduced in writing
or drawing by education of the posterior part of the second frontal convolution.
Like all speech processes, writing is sense-guided and governed.   The angular gyrus
has a guiding influence on writing and drawing.   Later, as further communicating
pathways between cortical areas are opened up, the child begins to read aloud, recite,
sing, write from dictation, copy print, etc.   These speech areas are shown in Fig. 239.
Vascular supply: The speech areas are supplied by the (left) *middle cerebral artery,*
the anterior branch of which supplies the second and third frontal gyri and the insula.
Occlusion of this branch causes an almost pure motor dysphasia (Fig. 233a).   The

posterior branch running in the Sylvian fissure supplies the remainder of the speech area, those parts concerned with the production of word-blindness and word-deafness. Lesions of the calcarine branches of the *posterior cerebral artery* cause homonymous hemianopia with sparing of macular vision. The branches to the lateral cortex of the occipital lobe anastomose with branches of the middle cerebral artery. In spite of this, lesions of the left posterior cerebral artery may cause word-blindness as well as hemianopia.

Cerebral dominance: Handedness, which is probably genetically determined, plays a large part in the laying down of speech function in the left hemisphere in right-handed persons. Slight damage to speech areas in the left hemisphere in young children may be recovered from in 1–2 weeks; in adults speech seems to be more totally represented in the left hemisphere (if the individual is right-handed). The left hemisphere in this case is called the *dominant* hemisphere. It has to do not only with speech, but with all more voluntary and less automatic activities. The *minor* hemisphere in the adult may have some function in speech, for in severely aphasic patients certain emotional interjections are preserved when all other speech is lost. If a left-handed child is taught to write with the right hand, stutter may develop. A classical symptom of left-handedness is the ability to write backwards with the left hand, the resultant script being legible in a mirror, so-called " mirror writing."

Uttered speech is of two kinds: (a) *Propositional or referential speech* (voluntary)

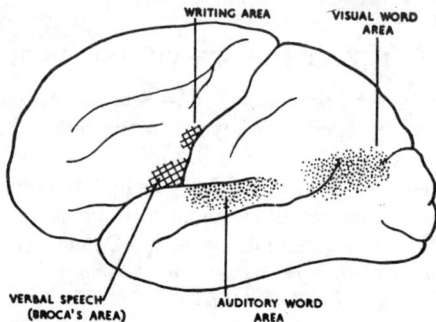

FIG. 239.—SPEECH AREAS IN THE LEFT HEMISPHERE.

which we use when we express our ideas or intellectual processes as statements, (b) *Emotional speech* which is used to express our feelings. This we do chiefly by exclamations, swear-words, or interjections, which have a variable emotional content, *e.g.*, " Not on your life !," " God help us !," " By Heavens ! " Emotional speech is more automatic. For propositional speech volition is required to will our thoughts into appropriate language; in emotional speech the will is needed not to effect expression, but to restrain it.

Internal speech: Between an idea and its utterance, or an uttered sentence and its comprehension, there may be an internal revival of words or of thought. This is most marked in reading, where the lips of some persons can be seen to frame the words although nothing is articulated. Deliberate thought is, however, possible without internal speech.

The speech areas of the brain comprise a U-shaped area of cortex in the left hemisphere (see Fig. 239). The anterior limb is related to " motor " speech, the remainder is connected with " sensory " speech. Certain aspects of speech function are related to *association areas* of cortex. Thus the area for *verbal speech* (Broca's area) is in the posterior end of the third frontal convolution and insula, near the areas for the lips and tongue. The area for *writing* is the posterior end of the second frontal convolution near the hand area. The area for *word hearing* is the superior temporal gyrus, near the auditory cortex, and the area for *word seeing* is the angular and supramarginal gyri adjacent to the visual cortex, but in the lateral aspect of the hemisphere.

Verbal speech, facial expression and *gesture*, all have different pathways. *Efferents* from (1) the posterior part of the third frontal gyrus (verbal speech) and (2) from the posterior part of the second frontal gyrus (written speech) proceed with the motor tracts to the bulbar nuclei and spinal cord. *Afferents* from (3) the striate visual cortex pass to the angular and supramarginal gyri (word-seeing) and from (4) the temporal projection of the auditory fibres to the superior temporal convolution (word-hearing). (5) Thalamo-cortical pathways exist carrying proprioceptive impulses from the lips and tongue essential for articulation and the storage of patterns of speech movements. *Lesions of the cortical areas for speech* or the *white matter immediately subjacent* cause *Aphasia*.

I. *The patient has* DIFFICULTY IN EXPRESSING HIS IDEAS *in* SPEECH *or* WRITING; *or you are unable to communicate with him because he cannot recognise words spoken to or written for him. The condition is* APHASIA. DYSPHASIA *is a milder degree of aphasia.*

§ 869. Aphasia.—In *Motor (Expressive) Aphasia* there is loss of power to exteriorise thought in spoken or written words—the patient knows what he wishes to say, but cannot say it, although the peripheral neuro-muscular mechanism of articulation is intact. In *Sensory (Receptive) Aphasia* there is defect of comprehension of spoken speech (word-deafness) or written speech (word-blindness) in the absence of deafness or blindness. The words are heard or seen by the patient, but they convey imperfect ideas or nothing at all to him.

Nearly all aphasias are mixed, Sensory and Motor, a combined defect; so that no classification is absolute. Destruction of the speech areas always produces (1) some loss of speech, (2) derangement of whatever speech is preserved. The elements of speech retained may be altered in form or arrangement. Emotional or interjectional speech may be retained when propositional speech is destroyed. All power of expression is never lost. Aphasia may be combined with *confusion of general thought, or intellectual deficit.*

CLINICAL INVESTIGATION OF APHASIA.—If possible the patient suspected of aphasia should be given a separate interview. For the investigation of aphasia and apraxia a printed card like that shown below is useful, as are pencil, writing pad and various easily handled objects, *e.g.*, key, scissors, india-rubber, coin, wrist-watch. The

1. WHAT IS YOUR NAME ?	1. LIFT UP YOUR HAND.
2. HOW OLD ARE YOU ?	2. CLOSE BOTH YOUR EYES.
3. WHERE WERE YOU BORN ?	3. PUT OUT YOUR TONGUE.
4. WHERE DO YOU LIVE ?	4. CLENCH YOUR FIST.
5. WHICH DAY FOLLOWS MONDAY ?	5. PRETEND TO KNOCK AT A DOOR.
6. TELL ME THE MONTHS OF THE YEAR.	6. PLAY THE PIANO.
	7. PLAY THE VIOLIN.

patient should be comfortable and relaxed. In applying the tests explanation and encouragement should always be used, and we should remember that by no movement or glance should we or anyone else present indicate to the patient what is required of him. Gestures and facial movements are rapidly and easily interpreted by such patients. *We must know accurately the condition of the patient's vision and hearing. We should know whether he is right- or left-handed. We must ascertain if general mental confusion is present and, if so, in what degree.*

A. *Tests for Motor (Expressive) Aphasia.*

1. **Encourage the patient to** *talk spontaneously* by asking him " How are you to-day ? " " I hear you are interested in . . ."
2. Show and ask him to name common objects, *e.g.*, penny, button, handkerchief, pencil, wrist-watch, fountain pen, cuff links, etc.
3. Ask him to write spontaneously—*e.g.*, an account of the weather. Ask him to write to dictation, *e.g.*, " Three cheers for St. Christopher's Hospital."

B. *Tests for Sensory (Receptive) Aphasia.*

4. *Give a series of verbal commands.* These should be of increasing complexity, *e.g.*, " Close your eyes," " Take hold of my hand." " When I put my hands in my pockets, but not before, hold up your left hand " (Word-deafness).
5. *Show a written request* on the card or in legible printing or handwriting, *e.g.*, " Open your mouth," " Put out your tongue." These tests should be of increasing complexity. " When I lift my right hand above my head, but not before, pick up the pencil " (Word-blindness).
6. *Ask him to read aloud* from the card, or a paragraph from a book or newspaper.

A. Motor (Expressive) Aphasia. *Symptoms.*—Verbal speech may be almost lost together with the ability for writing, even when there is no paralysis of the hand. The remaining speech in less severe cases may be deranged not only in respect of its quantity, but in respect of its use. " Yes " and " No " may be used wrongly. Unintended words may be used. There may be difficulty in constructing words or sentences, or speech may be telegraphic " Tell—John—come." Emotional or interjectional speech may remain " Oh my ! ", " I'm all right ! " Recurring utterances may be noted, often interjections, " Hold back there ! " Meaningless repetitions of words or parts of words (perseveration) is usual.

AGRAPHIA, loss of the ability to write, is never found as an isolated defect. The loss may be absolute without paralysis of the hand. Letters may be formed, but combined at random, " cg ng Kgig " or words, syllables, or letters may be repeated in a meaningless way—"Maiddddd" (perseveration). A patient can sometimes write his own name and nothing else. Errors in writing are usually greater than in verbal speech. Agraphia can also result from a lesion of the angular gyrus which destroys the visual patterns of written words. In NOMINAL APHASIA the patient can recognise an object held before him and describe or demonstrate its use, but he cannot remember what it is called. Shown a penny he will use a circumlocution—" That is what you pay with, put it in the slot," but he cannot name it. If a list of words is told him, including the word " penny," he will nod and smile when that word is reached in the list, *i.e.*, he recognises the sound of the word he lacks.

B. Sensory (Receptive) Aphasia.—In WORD-DEAFNESS the patient is not deaf in the ordinary sense; he hears sounds and noises, but spoken words are not understood and appear to him like an unknown language. There is not much total speech deficit, but words are wrongly formed and arranged. The defect is usually severe. The patient is thrown back on his motor memory which misleads him as it is no longer under sensory control. Speech may sound like unintelligible jargon—" Jargon Aphasia, " and it is important not to mistake this for the more general mental confusion of insanity. In lesser degrees the patient understands familiar words or phrases, but not the less familiar. He understands signs when he does not understand speech and he may anticipate your command by observing your expression or gestures. Asked to shut his eyes, he may continue to shut his eyes in response to subsequent different requests (perseveration). A patient may have aphasia for a recently acquired language and not so much for the language of his childhood or one to which he is strongly bound by an emotional tie.

In WORD-BLINDNESS (Alexia) the patient can see, but the printed characters convey nothing to him. Some words may be comprehended, others are missed, or words are wrongly interpreted. The patient may be able to read imperfectly, but cannot say afterwards the meaning of what he has read. Patients may have inability to comprehend other visual symbols, *e.g.*, mathematical symbols (acalculia), musical notation, etc. One form of agraphia is due to loss of the visual memories for written words. Pure word-blindness is rare; usually the lesion extends deeper than the angular gyrus into the white matter of the occipital pole and there is an associated right homonymous hemianopia.

In the normal individual ideas are evoked by activation of auditory or visual mechanisms in the cortex, if we listen or read. Blind and dumb persons can absorb ideas from symbols (*e.g.*, Braille) and finger movements, using tactile mechanisms only. This has been called Tactile Speech (§ 878).

INTELLECTUAL IMPAIRMENT.—Not only do we find aphasia in patients who are generally mentally confused or demented, but *severe* aphasia itself produces some degree of intellectual deficit. In transient dysphasias this is not so, especially if there is no associated hemiplegia. Apparent intellectual deficit is most marked in cases of word-deafness, where there is confusion of speech intelligence (semantic aphasia). PERSEVERATION is the meaningless repetition of words in speech, letters in writing, or the reiterating of the initial response to subsequent requests, *e.g.*, the patient goes on shutting his eyes when you are now asking him to show his teeth. It is characteristic of all forms of aphasia.

Etiology of Aphasia.—The lesions are usually *cortical* or *subcortical*—the causes are *Acute* or *Gradual* in onset or *Transient*.

CAUSES OF APHASIA

A. Aphasia of SUDDEN Onset:
    (1) Cortical softening (thrombosis or embolism).
    (2) Cerebral hæmorrhage.
    (3) Head injury.
    (4) Syphilitic meningo-encephalitis.
Signs of involvement of the motor, visual or sensory tracts in the affected hemisphere are usually found in varying degree in all such cases.

B. Aphasia of GRADUAL Onset:
    (1) Subdural hæmatoma.
    (2) Cerebral tumour.

(3) Temporal lobe abscess.

(4) Meningo-encephalitis (tuberculous, syphilitic).

Hemiplegia, hemianæsthesia or hemianopia will occur in varying degrees, but in the following causes such findings are rare and the speech loss is associated with memory defect and increasing childishness.

(5) Dementia (presenile or G.P.I.).

(6) Alzheimer's or Pick's Disease.

§ 870. Alzheimer's Disease is a form of presenile dementia in which there is widespread cortical shrinkage. It comes on between the ages of 40 and 60, and epileptic attacks may occur. Intelligence in many cases fails, there is aphasia and apraxia and loss of social sense and initiative. Emotional expression may be defective.

§ 871. Pick's Disease, also a form of presenile dementia, is characterised by bilateral symmetrical and circumscribed areas of cortical atrophy, chiefly frontal and temporal. These two diseases are pathologically dissimilar but clinically indistinguishable.

C. TRANSIENT Aphasia may be due to

(1) Migraine.

(2) Epilepsy.

(3) Hypertensive encephalopathy.

(4) Head injuries (especially in young children).

(5) Hypoglycæmia.

(6) Uræmia.

(7) " Congestive attacks " of G.P.I.

(8) Recurrent ischæmic episodes due to falls in blood pressure.

(9) Carotid stenosis.

POST-EPILEPTIC DYSPHASIA occurring after a fit is always highly suggestive of an organic lesion involving the speech cortex in the left hemisphere. It calls for detailed investigation, clinical, serological and radiological. It occurs in tumours, arterial disease and cerebral syphilis.

The *Prognosis in Aphasia* depends upon (1) whether the cause is removable or not, (2) the extent of the damage and its duration. Cases due to subdural hæmatoma or meningioma do well. In head injury and vascular disease no assessment of the degree of aphasia can be made for two or three weeks, until the shock effects have passed off. Young children below the age of six years make good recovery from severe aphasia, usually within a few weeks. In adults little recovery is seen after the first few weeks.

Treatment.—When the aphasia is due to pressure on the cortical area by a blood clot (subdural hæmatoma), superficial abscess, meningioma or a depressed fragment of skull it may be possible by surgical operation to afford relief. In other cases treatment should be directed to treating syphilis if it is a cause or to re-education of the patient, using the physiological and anatomical pathways which are still open. The best results are obtained with children under the age of seven years.

APRAXIA AND AGNOSIA

II. *The patient,* KNOWING THE NATURE OF SOME FAMILIAR OBJECT *and having neither paralysis, ataxia, nor sensory loss,* CANNOT PERFORM THE MOVEMENTS APPROPRIATE *to the use of that object.* The condition is APRAXIA.

§ 872. Apraxia.—A patient cannot carry out purposive movements when requested to do so, although he may perform the movements required unwittingly. He knows what he wants to do but cannot do it. Asked

to put out his tongue, *he may be unable to do it to order*, though a second
or two later he puts out his tongue to moisten his lips.   Apraxia may be
specific for certain learned movements, *e.g.*, dressing, shaving, feeding
with a knife, fork and spoon and his muddled attempts at carrying out
these actions may lead you to suspect apraxia.   In other cases the apraxia
is only revealed by the use of special tests.

Tests for Apraxia: Much may be learned from the *history*: how the patient can
dress himself or use a knife and fork, etc.

1. Ask the patient to show how he would use scissors, toothbrush (naming the
   object in each case as it is handed to him).
2. Ask him to fold paper and put it in an envelope.
3. Ask him to make a fist, clap his hands, snap his fingers. Ask him to do two
   things at the same time, *e.g.*, close his eyes and make a fist.
4. Ask him to wink, salute, wave goodbye.
5. Ask him to pretend to knock at a door, play a piano.
6. Give him matches and ask him with these to construct a square, triangle, and a
   triangle on top of a square.

Constructional apraxia is shown by drawing anomalies in simple tests, when the
patient attempts to draw a square, a house, an engine.   He cannot reproduce simple
geometric patterns with matches or bricks.   This condition may be independent of
any defect in general intelligence and the patient usually realises his mistake.   In
" dressing apraxia " the patient is unable to dress himself and becomes entangled
in his clothes or is unable to start to dress or to continue after being helped.   In
ideational apraxia the patient recognises an object shown him, *e.g.*, scissors, names it
yet cannot imagine its use.   In *ideo-motor apraxia* the patient knows the object and
can say what its purpose is, yet cannot translate the idea of use into action.   Patients
with apraxia show perseveration. Apraxia is commonly bilateral, but may be unilateral.

Etiology.—It occurs in disease of the parietal lobes, especially bilateral
disease, *e.g.*, in bilaterally situated chronic *subdural hæmatoma, tumour* and
in *focal cortical atrophy*.   It is also observed in different degenerative
diseases affecting the cortex as in *dementia paralytica* and *cerebral arteriosclerosis*.   In lesions of the anterior cerebral artery a left-sided apraxia
occurs in right-handed persons.   The left hemisphere in such cases controls the right cortex through the corpus collosum.

*The patient appears unable to recognise the nature of familiar afferent
impressions.*   The condition is AGNOSIA.

Agnosia.—Word-deafness and word-blindness are examples of agnosia.
Sensory agnosia or *astereognosis* is inability to tell the size, shape, or consistency of an object placed in the hand when sensibility is intact.   Such
a patient, shown a key and asked to use it, may put it in his mouth
and try to smoke it like a cigarette.   Agnosia is common in parietal lobe
lesions especially when these are bilateral: they may be due to bilateral
vascular or expanding (space-occupying) lesions or to cortical atrophy.
Patients with agnosia may neglect sensory stimuli from one half of their
bodies.   Neglect of one half of visual space, or disowning of hemiplegic
limbs (" anosognosia for hemiplegia ") occur.   In " finger agnosia " the
patient cannot tell individual fingers. Such patients may confuse the
right and left sides of their bodies.

III. (*a*) *There is defective movement due to paralysis or ataxia of the lips, tongue and palate, so that the patient cannot articulate or else articulates indistinctly.* The condition is DYSARTHRIA. *When voice sounds made by the larynx are defective,* the condition is DYSPHONIA.

§ 873. Dysarthria is a defect of the peripheral neuromuscular mechanisms of the larynx, lips, tongue, palate or pharynx. The patient " cannot get his tongue round words." It is tested by observing the patient's spontaneous speech or by asking him to repeat test sentences appropriate to his educational standard, *e.g.,* " Biblical criticism," " Methodist Episcopal." In the most severe cases the patient can make only moaning noises and has to communicate by writing on a pad. The lesion may be in the upper or lower bulbar motor neurones, cerebellum or striatal pathways, or in the muscles themselves. According to the type of disorder the dysarthria may be called spastic, flaccid, ataxic, etc.

In DYSPHONIA the voice is hoarse or reduced to a whisper.

Etiology.—Causes of DYSARTHRIA are: Dementia paralytica, pseudobulbar palsy, progressive bulbar palsy, and a variety of lesions affecting the bulb (syringobulbia), lower motor neurones (acute bulbar poliomyelitis, hypoglossal nerve paralysis, § 1088), or muscles (myopathy, myasthenia gravis). Dysarthria is commonly seen in states of *Intoxication* from alcohol or a barbiturate, and in *painful conditions of the mouth.*

There is SLURRED INDISTINCT SPEECH, DIFFICULTY IN SWALLOWING *and* EMOTIONALISM, *with signs of generalised cerebral arteriosclerosis.* The condition is PSEUDOBULBAR PALSY.

§ 874. Pseudo-bulbar Palsy. *Symptoms.*—There is usually a history of repeated slight " strokes," none of which has been followed by persistent severe hemiplegia. At rest the patient presents an expressionless face; the saliva which the paretic feeble lips cannot hold drops from the mouth. Speech is a low indistinct moaning, often unintelligible. When the patient attempts to talk or after being presented with stimuli which are inappropriate or inadequate he becomes emotional; the expression is contorted into something between sorrow and mirth and he bursts into a curious spastic wail which is imperfectly controlled or into uncontrolled laughter. Mental childishness and some degree of intellectual deterioration are often present. Bilaterally innervated muscles are most affected, *e.g.,* those of the tongue, palate, pharynx, larynx. The tongue is small and spastic and usually cannot be protruded beyond the line of the teeth. Tongue wasting and fasciculation may be seen. Swallowing produces choking and spluttering and coughing is laboured. There may be nasal regurgitation of fluid and solid food stays in the mouth. Signs of slight bilateral hemiplegia may be present in the limbs, *i.e.,* loss of power and exaggerated deep reflexes. The jaw-jerk is increased. The plantar responses may, however, be flexor.

Diagnosis.—In motor neurone disease the tongue is grossly atrophic and fasciculation is marked; but with no history of " strokes " and no dementia or memory defect.

Etiology.—Most cases are due to small bilateral softenings in both hemispheres or in the bulb. Any bilateral hemisphere lesion, if deep, may cause this picture. It occurs in auricular fibrillation after emboli in both hemispheres, and after acute specific fevers, *e.g.,* pneumonia, due to bilateral demyelinating lesions.

Prognosis.—If the causal condition is progressive, further " strokes " are likely to occur or the patient will die of intercurrent disease. In embolism and in post-infective cases the prognosis is better. In all there is a tendency to improvement after the first few days of the illness.

Treatment.—So long as feeding is possible with a spoon do not resort to a nasal tube. Benzhexol hydrochlor. 2 mg. (Artane) crushed and given in liquid tends to diminish salivation and rigidity. A food mincer or pulveriser is an asset in feeding.

There is SLURRED, INDISTINCT SPEECH *of insidious onset associated with a* WASTED FASCICULATING TONGUE *and an exaggerated jaw-jerk.* FASCICULATION AND MUSCULAR ATROPHY *may be seen in the skeletal muscles.* The condition is PROGRESSIVE BULBAR PALSY.

§ 875. **Progressive Bulbar Palsy** is a variety of Motor Neurone Disease (§ 1001). *Symptoms.*—There is slowly increasing difficulty in speaking and swallowing. Atrophic and spastic types occur. In the *Spastic Atrophic type* the tongue lies in the floor of the mouth in a pool of saliva, shrunken, wrinkled and fasciculating. The patient may have to write to make himself understood. Later the laryngeal muscles, the muscles of the floor of the mouth, the palate and lips are affected. Saliva drips from the mouth and fluids regurgitate from the nose and with involvement of the pharyngeal muscles swallowing becomes difficult. The atrophy and fasciculation of the muscles of the limbs may be combined with exaggerated tendon reflexes and extensor plantar responses. In the later stages the abductor and adductor muscles of the larynx are affected. In the *Spastic type* wasting is not marked, the jaw-jerk is much increased and there may be emotionalism with spastic laughing and wailing as is seen in pseudo-bulbar palsy. Sensory changes are entirely absent.

Diagnosis.—The spastic type may be confused with pseudo-bulbar palsy, but a history of " strokes " is lacking and there is no dementia. In *Syringobulbia* there may be wasting of the tongue, but it is accompanied by dissociated analgesia to pin-pricks and temperature over the face and trunk, and the corneal reflex is often absent. There are long tract signs and signs of a focal bulbar lesion. Primary and secondary *Neoplasms* in adults cause severe pain and sensory changes. Mistakes are more likely to be made with *Chronic Bromism* or *Barbiturate Poisoning* or with a *Toxic Polyneuritis, e.g.,* Diphtheria causing a transient paralysis of the bulbar muscles. *Vascular bulbar lesions* are sudden in onset and cause long tract signs. In all cases a blood Wassermann reaction should be carried out as *Syphilis* is a possible cause of similar progressive bulbar motor symptoms. *Myopathy* occasionally attacks the lips and tongue. *Myasthenia gravis* causes bulbar palsies relieved by neostigmine injection.

Etiology.—The cause of this progressive degeneration of the bulbar motor nuclei and their communications with the cortex is unknown. The disease is common in males over forty. Hereditary and familial factors are absent.

Prognosis.—Cessation of progress may occur for a week or two, but inevitably the disease progresses to death from respiratory failure within 2–3 years. Suspect the diagnosis to be wrong in cases who have survived longer.

Treatment.—Foods should be minced or pulverised. Give tinct. belladonna ♏ 10–15 or benzhexol hydrochlor. (Artane) 2 mg. an hour before meals to control salivation. Spoon feeding is often possible until the last few days or weeks. No specific remedy has yet been discovered.

III. (*b*) *On attempting to speak the sound of the voice is reduced to a whisper.* The condition is DYSPHONIA.

§ 876. In **Dysphonia,** the hoarseness or whispered articulation isproduced by laryngeal or respiratory failure. The laryngeal muscles by altering the tension and length of the vocal cords alter the pitch of the voice. Respiratory muscles help phonation by creating a forceful blast of air. A laryngeal palsy produces little defect in speech—a hoarseness or huskiness of the voice; the patient has difficulty in humming and coughing. The condition of the vocal cords must be examined with a laryngoscope. For *Etiology* and *Treatment* see §§ 166–176.

HYSTERICAL DYSPHONIA causes the patient to speak in a scarcely audible whisper. On coughing the patient phonates in a startlingly paradoxical fashion. Laryngeal examination is essential and shows the cords are not sufficiently approximated to produce a sound on attempted phonation (§ 176e). *Treatment* is difficult and relapse is common; the help of a psychiatrist and speech therapist will usually be required.

IV. *Speech and phonation are absent.* The condition is MUTISM.

§ 877. **Mutism** occurs when the patient is wordless, *e.g., Schizophrenia,* in *Hysteria,* and other psychiatric conditions. The dysphasic patient is never completely word-less. The acquired mutism in schizophrenia is helped by insulin coma treatment.

§ 878. *Deaf-mutism* is usually due to congenital peripheral stone-deafness which prevents the child learning to talk. A few patients have associated retinitis pig-mentosa, and become blind as well. Mental retardation can be present, but typically the congenital deaf-mute is bright and clever. Many use a " sign-language " in which they become highly expert, as do their associates.

Etiology.—Congenital cases are usually due to malformation of the cochleæ. A normal infant after severe head injury or an attack of meningitis or encephalitis may be left with stone-deafness. Such speech as existed may disappear and the patient is left deaf and mute.

Treatment.—Children can nowadays be taught to speak at special schools by patient " lip-reading " and other methods requiring a highly skilled individual teacher. Speech thus acquired rarely sounds normal.

The following speech defects in children may raise suspicion of mental retardation.

§ 879. **Congenital Aphasia.**—CONGENITAL WORD-BLINDNESS (Dyslexia) may be familial. It is often associated with left-handedness. It should be distinguished from other causes of difficulty in learning to read in children which are much commoner, *e.g.,* non-reading due to general dullness of intellect, or to emotional causes. With suitable education and management (usually at home) children with congenital dyslexia grow up able to fend for themselves. In CONGENITAL WORD-DEAFNESS, the child may, owing to the difficulty in understanding spoken words, be regarded as imbecile. Talk, if attempted, is babbling. Signs of hearing must be shown to exist before the condition is diagnosed. The child learns the use of common objects by visual perception, has normal habits and may be able to draw objects accurately, but cannot name them. With suitable education word-deaf children may grow up to be mentally normal.

Retarded speech in children may be due to emotional causes or to mental dullness. Some apparently normal children may make no attempt to talk until the third year of life. When the child uses baby talk until the age of five years or later the cause may be sought in the parents, who wish the child to preserve attractive baby-like ways. A severe illness in childhood may retard speaking.

LALLING, or infantile speech, is that in which the letters difficult to pronounce —*e.g.,* R, L, C, Sh—are avoided; " British " is pronounced " Bitty." It persists only when the child is mentally retarded.

In IDIOGLOSSIA the child has a speech of its own, which is unintelligible except to those accustomed to the child. It is due to an inability to reproduce the sounds of words said to him. It may be a variety of congenital Aphasia. Speech training may improve the condition where the intelligence of the child is normal.

ECHOLALIA is the senseless echoing of phrases: sometimes the last words put to the patient are repeated. In other cases parts of words are reiterated as in Palilalia seen in Parkinsonism. These symptoms may occur in children learning to talk and in schizophrenia, in presenile and arteriosclerotic dementia in adults.

Some Disorders of Articulation

§ 880. 1. Stammering and Tics of Articulation.—There are various spasmodic defects of articulation leading to a sudden check in the utterance; of these stammering is the commonest. The affection is not congenital. Between the ages of 3 and 4 years it may be physiological. It appears as a pathological symptom towards puberty, and much more commonly in boys. Often a family history of the complaint is ascertained. The patient sticks over the *consonants*, particularly explosives and labials, B, D, P, T, K or G. The consonant is repeated " P-P-P-Please ! " In a rarer minority of cases the patient sticks over the *vowels*, the mouth remaining open and the face contorted. After the difficulty is overcome the words may appear with a rush. The trouble is accentuated in conditions of excitement. Stammerers can sing and whisper normally, and the defect disappears when the patient is talking to himself. There is want of co-ordination between the respiratory, laryngeal and labio-lingual components of articulation. It is common in left-handed children and may apparently be provoked by teaching left-handed children to write with the right hand.

Treatment by (a) psychotherapy and (b) daily speaking exercises should be undertaken early. It is most important to endeavour to correct errors in the environment. The child's relationship to the parents, brothers and sisters and school-teachers should be ascertained, and the co-operation of all these individuals enlisted. Speech training classes are now run in connection with most neurological clinics. The patient is directed to fill his chest with air, speak slowly with a resonant voice, and when he comes to a word on which he sticks, he is to sing it, accentuating the second part of the word with a raised voice. These daily exercises should first be performed alone and, later, with an audience. Breathing and singing exercises and gymnastics or dancing may be used in treatment.

In Lisping there is defective enunciation of certain consonants, *e.g.*, S becomes Th, Th becomes V. It is due to faulty articulation and occurs normally in infants learning to speak. In adult life it is due to bad habit of articulation or defective conformation of the mouth. Speech training, with an expert, can remove it in most cases.

2. In *Tremulous Articulation* coarse tremors of the lips, lower facial muscles and tongue are seen and the articulation is slurred. When syllables are jumbled as in advanced Parkinsonism it may be due to toxic causes or arterial disease and is met with in *Alcoholic Intoxication* or poisoning from narcotic drugs, *e.g.*, after large doses of bromide or barbiturate. Its presence is often the clue to the diagnosis of *General Paralysis of the Insane*; when a patient presents himself with a shaking voice and tremor of the lips and tongue always carefully examine the pupils and question the relatives for a history of character changes (§ 1190). In this type of dysarthria, from the disease of the cortex which causes it, syllables are often misplaced, or wrong words are used. The paretic makes the same mistake in spelling as he does in articulation. A similar picture may be

seen in other organic dementias, *e.g.*, arteriosclerotic. In psychoneurotic anxiety states and hyperthyroidism, the articulation is occasionally tremulous, but syllables are normally placed and the patient's writing shows no mistakes or omissions although it may be shaky.

3. A *thin, monotonous voice*, which tails away at the end of sentences, is produced by the rigidity of *Parkinsonism*.

4. "*Scanning Speech*" (Ataxic dysarthria), in which syllables are separated staccato-fashion or eleided (slurred), occurs in lesions of the cerebellum or its medullary connections. It is found in *Disseminated Sclerosis* (§ 952) and is a very characteristic finding in *Friedreich's Ataxia* (§ 945). It is found in *tumours and abscesses, vascular lesions* and *degenerations of the cerebellum*, especially when these involve the vermis.

5. *Indistinct Articulation* may result from flaccid paralysis of the lips, palate or tongue (progressive bulbar palsy or pseudo-bulbar palsy) or cleft palate. In severe *Bell's palsy* (§ 1079) articulation may be impeded. In *Diphtheria* the palate may be paralysed so that " B " sounds are produced like " M " sounds, and there may be nasal regurgitation of fluids. *Myasthenia gravis* may affect the lips, tongue or palate, producing a flaccid palsy varying in degree from time to time and accentuated by fatigue. In certain types of *Myopathy* the face and even the tongue may be affected (myotonic dysphasia). If the hypoglossal nerve is damaged during operation on the tongue or throat a clumsy, slowed articulation ensues which the patient learns to overcome. *Intoxicants* and *abuse of barbiturates* also cause slurred speech.

6. *Jerking or gasping* articulation occurs in severe *Chorea* from involuntary movements of the respiratory, tongue and facial muscles. In bilateral congenital chorea or Athetosis, the grimaces of the face and the rolling movements of the tongue cause the patients to " chew their words " so that articulation may be almost unintelligible.

GROUP IV. PYREXIA WITH NEUROLOGICAL SIGNS

In diseases of the nervous system transient fever may occur from INFECTION OF THE BLADDER, INFECTED BED-SORES, PULMONARY INFECTIONS or THROMBO-PHLEBITIS of the lower limbs. Pyrexia occurs with a variety of *non-infective* conditions. Patients with the remitting type of Disseminated Sclerosis will often give a history of " influenzal attacks " which are pyrexial attacks doubtless associated with the laying down of fresh plaques. Fever may occur after EPILEPTIC FITS, especially in children, or after fits in dementia paralytica. In **acute** cerebral lesions of any kind, notably intra- or extra-cerebral (*e.g.*, especially subarachnoid) HÆMORRHAGE, cerebral contusion or laceration, the temperature is subnormal during the initial stages of collapse, but subsequently rises above normal. In hæmorrhage into the pons hyperpyrexia is frequent, and may be as high as 108° F; convulsions occur, affecting chiefly the legs, with coma, bilateral extensor responses and strongly contracted pupils, and death occurs rapidly. Acute non-infective lesions of the hypothalamic region and the tuber cinereum may cause hyperpyrexia.

The nervous system may be invaded by a variety of bacteria, viruses, yeasts, spirochætes, protozoa and metazoa. Of these, the commoner infections are those due to the *meningococcus* and other pyogenic bacteria,

M. tuberculosis, Tr. pallidum (meningovascular and parenchymatous syphilis), and the *viruses* causing anterior poliomyelitis. All the others are rare. An unusual complication of the exanthemata is acute encephalomyelopathy (sometimes termed " acute encephalomyelitis "); this is probably not an infective but an allergic reaction of the central nervous system to a systemic virus invasion.

Clinically acute and subacute infections of the central nervous system may be chiefly (A) Meningeal, (B) Cerebral or (C) Spinal in their manifestations, but there is much overlap in symptomatology.

Infections of the Nervous System

A MENINGEAL

    I. Acute Purulent Meningitis   ..   .. § 882
    II. Tuberculous Meningitis .. .. § 886
    III. Syphilitic Meningitis .. .. § 887
    IV. Benign Lymphocytic Meningitis .. .. § 888
    V. Subacute Meningitis (Sarcoidosis, Blastomycosis, Behcet's Syndrome) .. .. §§ 889, 890

B CEREBRAL

    VI. Intracranial abscess .. .. § 891
    VII. Intracranial Thrombo-phlebitis .. .. § 892
    VIII. Virus Encephalitis .. .. § 893
    IX. Post-infective Encephalomyelopathy .. .. .. § 895
    X. Cerebral forms of Malaria, Syphilis, Toxoplasmosis, Trypanosomiasis, Schistosomiasis, Trichinosis, Cysticercosis .. .. § 896

C SPINAL

    XI. Acute Poliomyelitis .. .. § 898
    XII. Spinal Epidural Abscess ... . § 899
    XIII. Post-infective Myelopathy .. .. § 895
    XIV. Acute Infective Polyneuritis .. .. § 976
    XV. Acute Myelitis .. .. § 955
    XVI. Paralytic Brachial Neuritis .. .. § 998

CLINICAL INVESTIGATION.—(1) Obtain a complete *Personal and Family history*, especially with regard to tuberculosis, previous suppurative ear disease, bronchiectasis, pneumonia, empyema, etc. In tuberculous meningitis there is often a history of preceding weeks of malaise. A history of a rigor or fit may indicate the formation of a cerebral abscess. (2) The *age* of the patient is of some importance. Postbasic meningitis is almost confined to infants under one year. (3) Look for *signs of meningeal irritation*, e.g., stiffness of the posterior cervical muscles, positive Kernig's Sign, etc. (4) Make as detailed a *neurological examination* as possible with special reference to the cranial nerves, tendon reflexes and plantar responses, signs of paresis in the limbs. Examine the fundi for optic neuritis (intracranial abscess), hæmorrhages (subarachnoid hæmorrhage) or tuberculous deposits (tuberculous meningitis). (5) Examine the *scalp, cranial bones, mastoid and other air sinuses, the skin* for exanthematous rashes, herpetic vesicles, etc., *the ears, throat and lungs* for evidence of infection. Œdema of the face, scalp or neck should be noted. Suppurative sinus disease is accompanied by facial œdema, extradural abscess by Pott's puffy tumour of the scalp, and sinus thrombosis by orbital œdema or œdema of the neck. (6) In all cases it is necessary to obtain by *lumbar puncture* fresh specimens of spinal fluid which should be collected in sterile containers and sent immediately to the laboratory. The meningococcus dies very rapidly. The pressure of the fluid should be estimated manometrically. Note the naked-eye appearance of the specimen before dispatch to the laboratory (turbidity, xanthochromia, clot). The fluid must be examined for Cells, Glucose, Chlorides, Total Protein, Organisms, W.R. The laboratory findings should be tabulated on the patient's notes so that comparison of successive samples obtained on different occasions may be made at a glance. (7) Four-hourly *tempera-ture records* will be required. If simulation of fever in malingering is suspected it may be helpful to take mouth, axillary and rectal temperatures simultaneously, and note untoward discrepancies between the various readings.

A. *The patient has* PYREXIA, HEADACHE, PHOTOPHOBIA, NECK STIFFNESS *and positive* KERNIG'S SIGN. *The cause is either* MENINGEAL IRRITATION *(Meningism) or* MENINGITIS.

§ 881. In **Meningism** these symptoms are coincident with the onset of many acute infections *in infancy or childhood*. The pyrexia, posterior cervical rigidity and vomiting simulate meningitis and may cause much anxiety and perplexity. But ocular palsies, unequal pupils and weakness of the limbs such as are relatively common in meningitis are not seen, and the spinal fluid is entirely normal. Meningism occurs in apical pneumonia, in the exanthemata, in otitis media and acute pyelitis. In a sick child, especially when the meningeal symptoms persist, after the temperature has lessened, a spinal puncture will be necessary in order to exclude acute meningitis or pre-paralytic poliomyelitis. *Hysteria* may cause an analogous picture but there is no fever and there is often a history of previous attacks. In adults *meningeal carcinomatosis* due to invasion by secondary carcino-matous deposits causes fever and clinical serological signs like those of chronic meningitis. *Subarachnoid hæmorrhage* produces sudden headache, usually followed by loss of consciousness with meningeal signs: the diagnosis is made by the C.S.F. findings (§§ 853, 1204).

§ 882. I. **Acute Purulent Meningitis** may be caused by the meningo-coccus, pneumococcus, *H. influenzæ*, streptococcus or staphylococcus.

Symptoms.—(1) There is intense occipito-cervical headache of subacute or acute onset and of such severity that the patient cries out with pain. There is pain in the back, photophobia and intolerance of noise. (2) The patient is irritable, later drowsy and finally comatose. He lies on his side, curled up, and may be resistive if disturbed. In the early stages retention of urine is a common feature. In severe cases with stupor there may be a monotonous wailing cry. (3) On examination the posterior cervical muscles are contracted and rigid. This may be demonstrated as follows: (i.) Ask the patient if conscious to put his chin on his chest, or to " kiss his knees." (ii.) Rest your elbows gently on the patient's chest with your hands cupped under the occiput. Now gently try the tension of the posterior cervical muscles. Infants may show severe head retraction with opisthotonos. (4) *Kernig's Sign* is commonly present, *i.e.*, inability to. extend the knee when the thigh is flexed to a right-angle on the abdomen. *Brudzinski's Sign* is the appearance of similar flexion of the lower limbs, and sometimes also of the upper limbs, when the head is acutely flexed on the chest. (5) There may be ocular palsies, inequality of pupils, squints, paralysis of the limbs, loss of knee- and ankle-jerks or unequal tendon reflexes, and extensor plantar responses. (6) Some degree of inflammation of the brain, cord and nerve roots always accompanies meningitis: these reflex changes and palsies are due to associated encephalitis or radiculitis. (7) Added to these neurological signs there are signs of general infection and toxæmia. Always look for a rash, characteristically petechial in meningococcal meningitis.

Types of Purulent Meningitis (Leptomeningitis).

For MENINGOCOCCAL MENINGITIS, see Cerebro-spinal fever (§ 504).

§ 883. **Pneumococcal Meningitis** (due to pneumococcus type I, II or III) may be secondary to otitis media, nasal accessory sinus infection, fractured skull, empyema, pneumonia, lung abscess or pneumococcal peritonitis. The spinal fluid is sometimes too thick to flow through a lumbar puncture needle: it is greenish-yellow and contains abundant polymorphonuclear leucocytes amongst which the pneumococcus is found. The condition develops rapidly, coma supervenes early and before the introduction of sulphonamides the disease was nearly always fatal. In many cases there is an associated blood infection. The mortality is still high; the cases following fracture of the skull and those with no ascertained source of infection do best.

§ 884. **Influenzal Meningitis** (due to *Hæmophilus influenzæ*) is a rare cause of purulent meningitis in infants and childrɔn, in whom it is primary. In adults it is usually secondary to fracture of the skull, sinusitis or otitis media, but 90 per cent. of the cases occur before the age of five years.

§ 885. **Streptococcal Meningitis** may be secondary to middle-ear or mastoid disease, erysipelas, or other infections of the scalp, face or cranial air sinuses. It is rare.

Meningitis due to organisms of low pathogenicity—*B. proteus*, *E. coli* or *B. pyocyaneus*—occurs in head injuries or in accidental contamination during spinal puncture or brain operations.

Diagnosis of Purulent Meningitis.—When symptoms of meningeal irritation are present spinal puncture must be carried out. The pressure of the fluid will be found elevated. Two or three specimens of fluid, each at least 1 ml., are withdrawn into sterile test-tubes and sent at once for culture and smears. If one of the specimens is retained for examination it may be turbid or purulent and may clot on standing. The total protein and globulin and the cells are much increased, the majority being polymorphs. Glucose is rapidly destroyed by pyogenic organisms. The chloride level is usually between 600–700 mg. per cent. (normal 720–750 mg. per cent.).

Etiology.—The organisms may reach the meninges by the blood-stream (meningococcus, pneumococcus, *H. influenzæ* and in staphylococcal osteomyelitis). A direct spread from a neighbouring focus of infection, either through veins or through the dura, occurs in infections of the ears and accessory nasal sinuses (pneumococcus, streptococcus and staphylococcus). In head injuries the organism may be introduced directly through a dural tear or by spinal puncture (*B. proteus*, *E. coli* or *Ps. pyocyaneus*). A non-infective or chemical meningeal reaction may follow the intrathecal injection of air, opaque media (as in myelography), antibiotics and antisera.

Prognosis.—The discovery of sulphonamides, penicillin and streptomycin has revolutionised the prognosis in pyogenic meningitis. If the meningitis is secondary it may be treated at once and the focus of infection dealt with later on. Nowadays it is common for cases of pneumococcal, *H. influenzæ* and streptococcal meningitis to recover. Rarely, fits may develop after recovery from meningitis. Collections of sterile serous fluid between the cortex and the meninges may be present, producing irritative cortical symptoms (subdural empyema).

TABLE LVI. TREATMENT OF MENINGITIS

(Combinations of Sulpha Drugs with one or other Antibiotics)

Organism.	Therapeutic Substance.	Daily Dose.	Route.	Duration.
Pneumococcus and Hæmolytic Streptococcus.	Sulphadimidine with Benzyl penicillin.	Adult 2–4 G. then 2 G. 4-hourly. 1–5 million units (divided). 20,000 units in N-saline 2 ml.	Intravenous. Oral. Intramusc. or Intravenously. Intrathecally.	4 days. 14 days. 10 days.
	or Chloramphenicol.	Adult 1·5–3·0 G. Child 50–100 mg./Kg.	Oral in 4-hourly doses.	6 days.
H. Influenzæ.	Chloramphenicol with Sulphadimidine.	As above. As above.		6 days. 4–6 days.
Staphylococcus.	Benzylpenicillin or Chloramphenicol or Erythromycin.	1–5 million units (in divided doses). As above. Adult 3·0 G.	Intramusc. Oral in 4-hourly doses. ,,	5 days. 6 days. 10 days.
Tuberculosis.	Streptomycin with Isoniazid and Sodium Amino-salicylate (P.A.S.).	Adult up to 2 G. Child 50 mg./Kg. Also 50–100 mg. in 5–10 ml. N-saline. Adult 200–300 mg. Child 10 mg./Kg. Adult 10–20 G. Child 0·4 G./Kg.	Intramusc. in 12-hourly doses. Intrathecal each 1–2 days. Oral in 8-hourly doses. Oral in 4-hourly doses.	Until C.S.F. is normal. 12 months. 12 months.
E. coli.	Streptomycin or Chloramphenicol with Sulphadimidine	Adult 3 G. As above. 4 G.	Intramusc. in 4-hourly doses. Oral. Oral in 4-hourly doses.	2–4 days. 2–4 days. 2–4 days.
Ps. pyocyaneus Proteus vulgaris	Streptomycin or Polymyxin B.	Adult 3 G. Also 100 mg. in 5 ml. N-saline. Adult 1·5 million units. Child 15,000 units/Kg. Also 20,000–100,000 units in 5–10 ml. N-saline (for Adult or Child over 4 years).	Intramusc. in 8-hourly doses. Intrathecal daily. Intramusc. in 4-hourly doses. Intrathecal daily.	Until C.F.S. is normal. Until C.F.S. is normal.

Treatment.—Effective treatment depends upon the isolation of the infecting organism from the spinal fluid and testing its sensitivity to sulphonamides and to antibiotics. Treatment should not wait for laboratory results once the disease has been diagnosed. If the patient is unconscious, drugs will have to be given by nasal tube passed by the doctor into the stomach, or intramuscularly (Table LVI). By a nasal tube adequate amounts of fluid can be given to prevent dehydration. For an adult give sulphadimidine by mouth or via the tube. Over-concentration of sulpha drugs in the renal tract with renal blockage requires ample fluid (5 pints daily for an adult) with an alkaline mixture, *e.g.*, sodium citrate and sodium bicarbonate āā gr. 20 well diluted with each dose. Sulphonamides pass into the C.S.F.—never give them intrathecally. Benzylpenicillin (B.P.) may be given intramusc., and since it does not pass freely into the C.S.F. it needs also to be given by the lumbar, cisternal or ventricular route. For the " penicillin-resistant " staphylococcus give methicillin (intramusc.) instead. ACTH or prednisolone may be required for severe collapse. If the patient is delirious and restless, give to adults intramusc. phenobarbitone gr. 3, or paraldehyde fl. oz. ¼–½ by mouth. Lumbar puncture relieves severe headache.

These cases have to be nursed with cot-sides to the bed. The nurse must chart the fluid intake and output, and should palpate the abdomen periodically for retention of urine, which is frequent in comatose patients.

When mild fever persists with stupor, convulsions, signs of increased intracranial pressure, or if the patient has persistent focal signs, suspect the presence of a cerebral abscess, or a subdural empyema or hygroma (a subdural collection of pus or yellow or blood-stained fluid). In these cases air-studies or arteriography will be required, with subsequent aspiration by a neuro-surgeon and surgical care.

Pneumococcal and *Hæmolytic Streptococcal Meningitis* require treatment by sulphadimidine and penicillin and perhaps chloramphenicol (see Table LVI). A focus in the middle ear or elsewhere may later require treatment. *Influenzal Meningitis* is relatively insensitive to penicillin. Give sulphadimidine and chloramphenicol.

After a week or so of malaise a CHILD *or* YOUNG ADULT *develops* FEVER, SIGNS OF MENINGEAL IRRITATION *with drowsiness, squints and diminution or exaggeration of the tendon reflexes. There may be a history of tuberculosis or exposure to infection. The disease may be* TUBERCULOUS MENINGITIS.

§ 886. II. Tuberculous Meningitis.—The *early Symptoms* are most insidious. The child loses appetite, becomes thinner, peevish and apathetic. A slight irregular fever and constipation are common and occasional vomiting occurs. Complaints of pain or discomfort in the neck should never be ignored. Such symptoms persist over a period of several weeks and then become rapidly worse. It is in this early stage that treatment may help the patient. The *irritative stage* follows—Headache, neck rigidity, vomiting and photophobia occur. Kernig's sign is present.

The pulse rate slows, and squints, alteration in size of the pupils, or transient weakness of limbs occur. Focal signs may be transient due to inflammatory change, or permanent due to occlusive tuberculous arteritis. *Obstructive hydrocephalus* may supervene from thickening of the meninges round the basal cisterns. When this happens vomiting becomes persistent and papillœdema, stupor, coma and incontinence occur. Choroidal tubercles should be looked for in the fundi, the pupils having been previously dilated. In 20–25 per cent. of cases, when the spread is miliary, these pale yellow areas can be seen: they are rather flat, about a quarter of the size of the disc or larger. Later, they are surrounded by black pigment. X-rays of the chest may show miliary tuberculosis or a pulmonary focus. The Mantoux test is usually positive.

Diagnosis, whether presumptive or absolute, is made by examination of the spinal fluid (Table LXVI). The C.S.F. is clear or opalescent and under pressure: yellow fluid suggests an arachnoid block. When a tube of fluid is allowed to stand and cool a " spider web " clot (fibrinogen) may form, in the meshes of which tubercle bacilli may be entangled. The tubercle bacilli may also be found in the centrifugalised deposit. The cell count varies from 50–500 per c. mm.; the cells are nearly all lymphocytes, but polymorphs may be present up to 30 per cent. The total protein is raised to 100–200 mg. per cent. Higher protein values suggest hydrocephalus. The chloride level frequently falls to 650 or 600 mg. per cent., and may be as low as 500 mg. per cent. These low chloride readings are very characteristic (normal is 720–750 mg. per cent.). A fall in/ the glucose content is a constant early sign and sugar tends to fall progressively as the disease advances. The absolute diagnostic test is the finding of the tubercle bacilli in the spinal fluid, and for this several successive specimens may have to be examined. In all suspected cases cultures should be made from the spinal fluid and a guinea-pig inoculated.

Etiology.—Tuberculous meningitis is part of a generalised blood-borne miliary tuberculosis (§ 515), the meningeal signs overshadowing the others. It also may occur from the dissemination of a microscopic or caseous focus in the brain into the ventricles or subarachnoid space. It is commonest in children (rare under six months), but it occurs also in young adults, in whom it tends to be more benign. Over 85 per cent. of all cases occur before the age of 40.

Prognosis.—Once regarded as fatal in three weeks, it now tends to recovery since Waksman discovered streptomycin (1944). In young adults 20–30 per cent., perhaps more, recover clinically and serologically, but there is danger of relapse later. In cases treated with streptomycin, isoniazid and P.A.S. the progress of the disease is greatly slowed, the general condition of the patient improves and in many cases, especially in young children, cure may occur. At least 50 per cent. of all cases treated still die. The incidence of relapse is not at present known. The disease may run a course of three to six months, or much longer. *Sequelæ* are blindness due to optic atrophy, squint, mental confusion or deficit, or dysphasia, hemiplegia, paraplegia, deafness (perhaps due to streptomycin). These are due to obstructive hydrocephalus or ischæmic softening from arteritis.

Treatment.—After diagnosis the patient is preferably transferred to a special hospital centre for the treatment of tuberculous meningitis. Treatment is given continuously for at least three months, or until the C.S.F. is normal. Streptomycin is used intramuscularly, and also intrathecally each 1–2 days, six hours after an intramusc. injection (Table LVI). Isoniazid has been used alone successfully in treating this disease; it should be given for at least a year. Sodium aminosalicylate (P.A.S.) also is given. Usually all three drugs are given simultaneously. Toxic effects of streptomycin, viz., tinnitus, deafness, nystagmus and ataxia, are not indications to stop using it. If signs of intrathecal block or hydrocephalus develop, air-studies will be required, and the streptomycin will have to be given into the ventricles through burr holes in the skull. Comatose patients may be helped by prednisolone or cortisone. Prolonged sanatorium treatment is advisable after the mcningitis is controlled; relapses may occur.

§ 887. III. **Syphilitic Meningitis** (Meningovascular syphilis) due to *Tr. pallidum* may cause pyrexia and (*a*) diffuse leptomeningitis and hydrocephalus, increased intracranial pressure or cranial nerve palsies or (*b*) focal cerebral symptoms due to a localised gummatous meningitis. The latter form is rare (see § 907).

§ 888. IV. **Benign Lymphocytic Meningitis** (Lymphocytic choriomeningitis) occurs in children and young adults. Invasion of the bloodstream by the virus causes what is at first presumed to be an upper respiratory or gastro-intestinal infection. Within a week fever (99°–104°) with meningeal symptoms appear—severe headache, vomiting, drowsiness with stiff neck, Kernig's sign and depressed or hyperactive reflexes simulating bacterial meningitis or pre-paralytic poliomyelitis. There is a leucocytosis in the blood. The cerebro-spinal fluid, which may be under pressure and may form a clot, contains an excess of lymphocytes numbering 30 to several thousands per c. mm. The protein is raised but the chloride and glucose content are normal. The *Diagnosis* can be established with certainty by finding antibodies in the serum. *Etiology.*—Most cases are sporadic but epidemics may occur. The virus which causes experimental lymphocytic choriomeningitis in mice has been blamed for the human infection, so has infection with Coxsackie and other viruses. *Prognosis.*—Complete recovery is usually established after one to four weeks although an excess of lymphocytes may persist for weeks after all clinical signs have disappeared. *Treatment* is symptomatic.

Other causes of a relatively benign lymphocytic meningitis are (1) Mumps, with its parotitis or orchitis, (2) Infective mononucleosis, with enlarged lymphatic glands, (3) Herpes zoster, with its characteristic eruption and (4) Infective hepatitis, with jaundice.

Lymphocytic meningitis of grave import may occur in (1) tuberculous meningitis, (2) spirochætal infections, *e.g.*, *S. pallida*, *L. ictero-hæmorrhagica*, *L. canicola*, (3) trypanosomiasis, (4) acute poliomyelitis, (5) cerebral abscess, (6) infection with yeasts (torulosis), (7) carcinomatous invasion of the meninges.

§ **889. V. Subacute Meningitis** may occur due to rarer causes:

(a) SARCOIDOSIS (§ 141). The small nodules which characterise the disease and are usually found in the skin, lungs, lymph nodes and spleen, may invade the nervous system. The disease affects the cranial nerves, causing facial palsies with inflammation of the uveal tract of the eye and parotid swellings, or retro-bulbar neuritis with secondary atrophy may occur. Sensory and motor peripheral nerve palsies and focal signs of invasion of the brain and spinal cord are found. There is a mild meningeal reaction with 10-200 lymphocytes per c. mm. and the blood shows a leucocytosis with eosinophilia. Tuberculin tests are negative. The diagnosis can only be made by biopsy of a skin nodule or lymph node. Some cases die of tuberculosis. *Treatment* is by ACTH or corticosteroids.

(b) BLASTOMYCOSIS rarely invades the meninges. The primary focus may be the nasal accessory sinuses or respiratory tract. Meningeal signs with ocular palsies and evidences of long tract involvement appear. The course of the disease is subacute or chronic. Examination of the spinal fluid shows a pleocytosis, which may be considerable, increase of protein, and a diminished chloride and glucose content. " Peculiar cells " may be seen in centrifugalised specimens of fluid and when cultured on Sabouraud's medium these prove to be yeast organisms. The disease simulates tuberculous meningitis, brain tumour and Hodgkin's disease (and see § 147).

§ **890.** (c) **Behçet's Syndrome** is rare. It is characterised by (1) recurrent genital ulcers (prepuce or vulva) or anal ulcers; (2) relapsing uveal tract inflammation (iritis, choroiditis); and (3) signs in the nervous system *resembling those of disseminated sclerosis*, viz., retro-bulbar neuritis, dysphasia, cerebellar ataxia, pyramidal signs. Remissions and relapses occur over a number of years. Marked visual failure may be caused by keratitis or vitreous hæmorrhage. There is a low-grade fever and the spinal fluid shows a pleocytosis, often marked in degree (up to 5,000 lymphocytes per c. mm.) and a moderate increase in the protein content. The cause is not definitely established, but Evans, Pallis and Spillane claim to have isolated a virus from the brain and spinal fluid in one case. No effective treatment is yet known.

B. CEREBRAL INFECTIONS.

There is DELIRIUM *and mental confusion with* PYREXIA, HEADACHE, NECK STIFFNESS, *and later* CRANIAL NERVE PALSIES and LONG TRACT SIGNS. INVOLUNTARY MOVEMENTS *such as myoclonus or epileptiform convulsions may be present; and the* C.S.F. CONTAINS *an* EXCESS OF LYMPHOCYTES. *The disease may be* ENCEPHALITIS.

§ **891. VI. Intracranial Abscess** (Purulent encephalitis).—Encapsulated or free pus forms in the cerebral or cerebellar parenchyma or in the brain-stem. Brain abscesses vary greatly in size and are often multiple and loculated. The infecting organism may be *Staph. aureus, Strep. viridans,* or *Strep. hæmolyticus. Entamœba histolytica* is a possible but infrequent cause. Subdural collections of pus (subdural empyema) also occur and like intracerebral abscesses these may be sterile.

Symptoms.—Very rarely the formation of a pyæmic brain abscess causes a rigor with meningeal or focal neurological signs. In almost all cases of otitic and pyæmic abscess the signs are latent for several weeks. The earliest changes are an alteration in the patient's mental and general condition. Apathy, defective attention, difficulty in expressing ideas and defect of memory are found. The patient begins to look ill, to lose flesh and the tongue becomes coated. There may or may not be elevation of temperature. In intracerebral abscess the pulse is slow; in extra-dural abscess the pulse rate is raised. Papilloedema is a late sign and headache is rarely marked. *Local Symptoms* are never marked in *Temporal Lobe Abscess*. Slight paresis of the lower face, diminished or absent abdominal reflexes and extensor plantar responses on the contra-lateral side may be found. Abscesses extending backwards in the temporal lobe involve the optic radiations with production of upper quadrantic hemianopic field defects. If the abscess is in the left temporal lobe and the patient is right-handed there will be dysphasia, sometimes " jargon aphasia." Jacksonian fits may occur from cortical irritation. Occasionally signs of mid-brain compression are present—squint with diplopia or paralytic dilation of the ipsilateral pupil. In *Cerebellar Abscess* coarse horizontal nystagmus may be present on looking to the side of the lesion. Flaccidity of the ipsilateral upper limb with undue extensibility of the muscles may be present. There is no alteration in the tendon reflexes and the upper and lower abdominal reflexes remain brisk; a point which may be valuable in distinction from temporal abscess. The progressive apathy and drowsiness of the patient soon render the patient's co-operation in clinical examination almost impossible. The blood may show no polymorphonuclear leucocytosis but the E.S.R. is often raised. *Spinal fluid.*—Cells are perhaps 5–30 per c. mm. and are mostly lymphocytes with a few polymorphs. This is the characteristic finding, but if the abscess is thick-walled the cytology of the fluid may be normal. Protein may be increased. Glucose and chlorides are normal unless the abscess leaks, when signs of recurrent meningitis become apparent clinically, with fall in the cerebrospinal fluid chlorides and rise in cell count. Rupture into the ventricle will cause signs of acute meningitis.

Diagnosis.—The *electro-encephalographic changes* are similar to those which are found in other space-occupying (expanding) lesions (§ 847). In infants straight X-rays of the skull may show separation of the sutures, in adults a calcified pineal shadow may be displaced. Remember that examination of blood and urine are normal unless there is activity in the septic focus or unless complications are present. *Air-encephalography* (§ 846) will show displacement of the lateral ventricles and septum lucidum in temporal lobe or frontal lobe abscess. Meningeal Hydrops (Otitic Hydrocephalus) is a benign condition causing papilloedema. Ventriculography in such cases is normal. *Thrombosis of the lateral sinus* following middle-ear or mastoid infection causes convulsions and increased intracranial pressure, but in abscess focal neurological signs are present.

Etiology.—Usually brain abscess is due to direct extension of a suppurative focus in the middle ear or nasal accessory sinuses. There may be complicating extradural or subdural suppuration or infective thrombosis of the venous sinuses. Rarely mastoid suppuration is blood-borne into the contralateral cerebral hemisphere. Thus temporal and cerebellar abscesses are often due to suppurative otitis media, and frontal lobe abscesses to frontal sinusitis, especially in children and young adults. Infected missiles or other objects which penetrate the skull may bring pyogenic organisms with them, and abscess may occur after an infected compound fracture of the skull. The residuum of a pyogenic meningitis treated by antibiotics may be a cerebral or subdural abscess, perhaps sterile. *Metastatic abscesses* are sometimes multiple and usually secondary to bronchiectasis, lung abscess or infective endocarditis. Two per cent. of infants with congenital heart lesions develop cerebral abscess. It may follow tonsillitis or osteomyelitis. In other cases the cause is not apparent.

Prognosis.—If untreated the condition is likely to prove fatal. The mortality is highest when the primary infection is in the lungs. The mortality has greatly lessened in recent years, especially in cerebellar abscess.

Treatment.—Medical treatment prior to surgical removal is that of purulent meningitis. The antibiotics and sulphonamides favour the formation of a capsule and their use should be continuous before, during and after operation. Surgical treatment consists of repeated aspiration, or aspiration followed by excision of the capsule of the abscess. The denser the capsule the better the chance of extirpation. Convulsive seizures are not infrequent after such operations on a cerebral hemisphere, and in all cases prophylactic anticonvulsant drugs should be given for a year or more.

§ 892. VII. Intracranial Thrombo-phlebitis occurs as (*a*) Sinus thrombosis, (*b*) Cortical thrombo-phlebitis or (*c*) Meningeal hydrops.

(*a*) *Pyogenic Sinus Thrombosis* causes (1) severe headache, vomiting and high fever of a pyogenic type, accompanied by rigors and sweats (see Fig. 154), (2) optic neuritis supervening in a day or two, and often photophobia, (3) drowsiness, deepening into coma and, if operative measures are not prompt, ending in death. The use of sulphonamides and antibiotics to combat ear infections has greatly reduced the incidence of sinus thrombosis.

In *lateral sinus thrombosis* there are pain and tenderness in the mastoid region, together with other signs of suppurative otitis media; the inflammation spreads down the jugular vein on the same side, and backwards behind the mastoid; consequently there is generally some hard brawny swelling in these positions. If there has previously been a discharge from the ear it usually ceases. When the *sagittal sinus* is thrombosed the localising signs consist of œdema of the scalp, distension of the veins over the forehead and sometimes strabismus, associated with convulsions at the onset. There may be a spastic paraplegia or bilateral hemiplegia. With pyogenic thrombosis, the cause is usually some septic lesion of the face or scalp. When the *cavernous sinus* is affected the localising signs are œdema of the eyelids and root of the nose, sometimes also of the pharynx, exophthalmos and paralysis of the third, fourth, ophthalmic division of the fifth and sixth nerves. There may be blindness from infarction of the retina, with retinal hæmorrhages and thromboses. Pyogenic thrombosis of this sinus may arise from some septic lesion of the orbit, nose, pharynx or face. The *Diagnosis* of pyogenic sinus thrombosis is difficult unless the local signs are pronounced. In uncomplicated lateral sinus thrombosis there may be papillœdema, and this is not necessarily a sign of co-existing cerebral abscess. It may clear up when the sinus has been opened and drained and the jugular vein ligatured. The *Treatment* of lateral sinus thrombosis is a matter for an aural surgeon. In cavernous sinus thrombosis the mortality is lowest when conservative treatment is employed. In septic cases, penicillin and sulphonamides are of great value.

(b) *Cortical Thrombo-phlebitis* is a cause of fever and hemiplegia in puerperal women, or in association with septic lesions in veins or tissues elsewhere (§ 908).

(c) *Meningeal Hydrops* (Syn. Otitic Hydrocephalus) causes fever, headache and papilloedema without focal signs (§ 1036).

VIRUS DISEASES of the nervous system have long been suspected, as with rabies, poliomyelitis, herpes zoster and encephalitis lethargica. However, precise knowledge of the etiology of this group of diseases is of recent origin (1930). Apart from herpes zoster and acute poliomyelitis neurological virus diseases are uncommon in man. Viruses which specifically invade nervous tissue are termed " neurotropic."

§ 893. VIII. **Virus Encephalitis** occurs in (a) epidemic and (b) non-epidemic forms.

(a) EPIDEMICS are usually localised—such as have occurred in Japan (mortality 60 per cent.), St. Louis (mortality 20 per cent.) and elsewhere. Infants and young children and the elderly are specially vulnerable. *Symptoms.*—There is sudden onset of headache, drowsiness, stupor or convulsive seizures. Vomiting, stiffness of the neck and cranial nerve palsies may suggest meningitis. Myoclonus, dystonia and other involuntary movements are seen. Focal signs of mid-brain involvement are common but long tract signs are not marked. The severity of symptoms varies from case to case and in different epidemics. The C.S.F. pressure is raised and the fluid contains a slight or moderate lymphocytosis. There may be a paretic type of gold curve. *Diagnosis.*—The epidemic character of the disease may suggest the diagnosis, especially if the cases show myoclonus or dystonia; but diagnosis cannot be established with certainty during the acute phase of the illness with the clinical methods now available. In non-fatal cases the virus may be identified by (1) the injection of blood, cerebrospinal fluid, saliva, nasal washings or excreta into susceptible animals; and (2) the application of complement fixation or neutralisation tests. It is necessary to show that antibodies are absent or are only present in a high titre at a proper interval following the onset of symptoms. In fatal cases the injection of suspensions of material from the brain or spinal cord into susceptible animals is used. The diagnosis is a highly specialised matter requiring the assistance of a trained virologist.

Etiology.—The causal viruses in epidemics have been those of equine encephalomyelitis (Western, Eastern and Venezuelan types), St. Louis, Japanese B. and Russia Far East encephalitis. In the U.S.A. epidemics have been caused by the Coxsackie and enteric cytopathogenic orphan (ECHO) viruses—these two are benign. *Treatment.*—There is at present no specific therapy for any of these infections.

Virus Meningo-encephalitis. In a recent epidemic amongst London hospital nursing staff symptoms of meningo-encephalitis accompanied by enlargement of lymph nodes and muscular pains were observed. Convalescence was prolonged. *Infectious mononucleosis* (glandular fever, § 498) may present with transient early meningeal or encephalitic symptoms: Cranial nerve palsies and polyneuritis occur as in acute infective polyneuritis (§ 976). Encephalitis Lethargica (§ 837), first described by Von Economo in 1915, spread over the entire world for over a decade but has now disappeared.

(b) NON-EPIDEMIC VIRUS ENCEPHALITIS is seen in Rabies (§ 1032) and very rarely in Herpes Zoster (§ 1021).

§ 894. **Inclusion Body Encephalitis,** described by Dawson in 1934, is a slowly progressive and subacute sclerosing encephalitis occurring sporadically in children and adolescents, probably due to a virus. *Symptoms.*—Three stages are described. At first the child is febrile, listless and forgetful, with behaviour disorder and major and minor epileptiform convulsions. In the second stage inco-ordination of the limbs with myoclonic jerkings appear. Dysphasia, dyspraxia and dementia herald the terminal third stage with rigid tetraplegia. Blindness and chorioretinitis are described. The E.E.G. shows diffuse changes with spike and wave complexes 2–4 per second, sometimes synchronous with the myoclonic jerkings. The C.S.F. is normal except for a mildly paretic type of colloidal gold curve. Patients rarely survive longer than six months. At post-mortem the affected nerve-cells show acidophil inclusion bodies. There is demyelination with secondary gliosis. Inclusion bodies are also seen in encephalitis due to herpes simplex. No effective *treatment* is known.

ENCEPHALOPATHY indicates a pathological cerebral reaction to a systemic infection or toxæmia. It is in contrast to ENCEPHALITIS, which denotes invasion of the brain by an infective agent.

§ 895. IX. **Post-infective Encephalo-myelopathy** (Syn. " Encephalomyelitis ") is a demyelinating affection of the nervous system due to various causes similar in its pathological manifestations, whatever the nature of the original acute infection. *Symptoms* are very variable and occur during the first or second week of the acute infection. The fever recurs, the child may become restless, drowsy and stuporose with headache and vomiting. Any of the following manifestations may occur— (1) Meningeal symptoms may be seen. (2) In the Encephalitic form fits, myoclonus, delirium, retention of urine and mental changes are seen with dyspraxia, dysphasia and pyramidal signs. (3) A Hemiplegic form causes infantile hemiplegia. (4) Cerebellar syndromes are characterised by slurred speech, nystagmus and hypotonia with intention tremor and ataxic gait. (5) Spinal syndromes, sensory and motor, with retention of urine, occur; and paralysis may be of the ascending type. (6) Papillœdema is present in some cases. The spinal fluid shows a lymphocytic meningeal reaction (15–250 cells per c. mm.) with slightly raised protein and normal sugar and chloride content. Diffuse abnormalities in the E.E.G. may persist after clinical recovery.

Varieties.—*Measles encephalitis* is fairly common. *Post-vaccinal encephalo-myelitis* occurs in less than 1 in 100,000 vaccinations with glycerinated calf-lymph (§ 480). If recovery ensues it may be complete. The mortality is between 30–50 per cent. After *acute poliomyelitis inoculation* cases of transient localised paralysis (*e.g.*, of trapezius or deltoid) rarely are seen. The cause probably is an allergic radiculopathy. Peripheral nerve or root palsies or a generalised polyneuritis may occur.

In *Acute Disseminated Encephalo-myelitis* the cause is not apparent but the symptoms suggest a scattered demyelination of the brain and spinal cord. Some of these cases are diagnosed as acute disseminated sclerosis. There is a strong tendency to recovery and relapses are rare. The spinal fluid shows an excess of lymphocytes and perhaps a paretic gold curve.

Diagnosis.—When neurological signs occur 10–12 days after the onset of an exanthematous fever or after vaccination the diagnosis is likely, especially if there are spinal fluid abnormalities.

Etiology.—The disease occurs following (1) Exanthematous fevers, *e.g.*, measles, German measles, chicken-pox, small-pox, mumps and influenza, (2) Vaccination against small-pox or rabies, (3) Inoculation against typhoid or with anti-tetanic serum. An allergic factor has been postulated, for the onset of the neurological symptoms corresponds with the appearance in the blood of antibodies against infection.

Prognosis.—Recovery can be hoped for in many cases and is usual if the patient survives the first two weeks of the illness. Death occurs in 10–15 per cent. of cases. In others residual fits or intellectual, emotional or neurological deficits occur.

Treatment with prednisone 10 mg. three or four times a day probably reduces the severity of the neurological signs.

§ **896.** X. CEREBRAL FORMS of the following diseases are described due to invasions of the brain by the parasite—malaria (§ 512), toxoplasmosis (§ 509a), trypanosomiasis (§ 521), schistosomiasis (§ 315), trichiniasis (§ 606), cysticercosis (§ 867).

Cerebral malaria due to the malignant tertian parasite (*Plasmodium falciparum*), occurs in less than 2 per cent. of patients with malaria. Cerebral manifestations usually appear in the second or third week of the illness and have no relationship to the height of the fever. The *Symptoms* are those of encephalitis; psychic manifestations such as delirium, disorientation, amnesia, resistive behaviour are present in a large percentage of the cases; paralysis, hemianopia or ataxia may occur. Psychotic manifestations also occur in the course of mepacrine treatment of malaria but disappear if quinine is substituted and the mepacrine withdrawn. Cerebral malaria may simulate heat exhaustion or sunstroke. *Diagnosis.*—The *Plasmodium falciparum* is found in the blood. The spinal fluid is under pressure and may be xanthochromic and contain an excess of lymphocytes and protein. The blood W.R. may be positive but this test is negative in the spinal fluid. *Treatment.*—Sedation with intramuscular par-aldehyde 5 ml. may be necessary in disturbed or delirious patients. Give transfusions of whole blood or plasma. Quinine dihydrochloride 0·65 G. (gr. 10) in 20 ml. of normal saline should be injected very slowly into a vein. If given too quickly it may cause circulatory collapse. Otherwise give intravenous chloroquine sulphate 200 mg. intravenously (§ 512).

CEREBRAL SYPHILIS.—In secondary syphilis, pyrexia with severe and persistent headache usually is due to *meningeal* involvement. Fever may also accompany cerebral *vascular* syphilis. In the early stage of dementia paralytica (syphilitic encephalitis) transient fits, or dysphasias, occur with rise of temperature. Patients with dementia paralytica who also have been treated with malaria may show inter-mittent fever due to persistence of malarial infection.

§ 897. TOXOPLASMOSIS affects children and adults and causes encephalitic lesions; most human infections are mild and may be unnoticed. Infection occurs usually *in utero* or in early infancy and childhood; in adults active infection often is missed and occasionally proves fatal; there is encephalitis, prolonged fever, pneumonitis and an erythematous skin rash (§ 509a).

Trypanosomiasis (see § 521). *Schistosoma japonicum* (§ 315) is a rare cause of cerebral granulomata producing symptoms of a space-occupying (expanding) lesion. *Trichinosis* may invade the nervous system producing confusion, delirium, focal neurological signs with œdema of the eyelids and a marked eosinophilia (§ 606).

CYSTICERCOSIS.—*Tænia solium* or *Tænia saginata* cause cysts in the brain. Calcified cysticercus cellulosæ, the cysticercus stage of *Tænia solium*, is a cause of epilepsy (§ 867). Within the cerebral ventricles, especially the fourth ventricle, cysts may form like bunches of grapes, giving symptoms like those of a posterior fossa tumour. Single large cysts have been removed from the cerebral hemisphere surgically, but removal of cyst-clusters in the posterior fossa is not usually possible.

C. SPINAL INFECTIONS.

A patient shows PYREXIA *followed by* FLACCID PARALYSIS *of one or more limbs. There are no sensory changes and the spinal fluid shows a lymphocytic pleocytosis. The condition may be* ACUTE POLIOMYELITIS.

§ 898. XI. **Acute Poliomyelitis** (Syn. Infantile Paralysis) is a con-tagious infection due to a virus. No age is exempt; there is a relative immunity during the first year of life and the disease is uncommon after middle age. The major incidence is in children between two and ten years. Lately in epidemics a bulbar type affecting young adults has been seen. The incubation period varies between three days and five weeks. A systemic infection (viræmia) is followed in most cases by invasion of the nervous system (perhaps via the nerve-fibres). The virus has a selective affinity for the ventral horn cells of the spinal cord, their motor homologues in the bulb and the reticular substance in the pons. This results in loss of power and flaccid paralysis, more or less widespread; recovery may occur in partially damaged cells.

Symptoms.—In about 40 per cent. of cases there is (1) a minor illness, with fever, sore throat, headache or nasal catarrh.   The disease may abort at this stage.   In others, this is followed by the major illness, which comprises *Pre-paralytic* and *Paralytic Stages.*   (2) The *Pre-paralytic Stage* closely resembles influenza; with severe headache, backache, pains in the chest, abdomen and thighs, sore throat, vomiting or diarrhœa.   There may be joint pains.   Neurological symptoms are often present with cutaneous hyperæsthesia, muscle tenderness, neck rigidity, retention of urine, vertigo and disturbed vision due to jerking movements of the eyes. Muscle fasciculation may be seen.   Restlessness, irregular respiration, delirium, may occur.   These symptoms last two to seven days, then in many cases paralysis becomes evident.   If muscular exercise is taken during the pre-paralytic stage, it may determine the degree and distribution of the subsequent paralysis.

(3) *Paralytic Stage.*   The patient is irritable and apprehensive of being moved.   (i.) The muscles affected show flaccid paralysis to a variable degree.   To ascertain severe paralysis the patient is asked to tighten the muscle by a voluntary effort whilst the observer palpates the contraction. It is then unnecessary for the subject to move the limbs.   (ii.) Gentle kneading of the muscles will reveal tenderness.   (iii.) The corresponding tendon reflexes are lost.   (iv.) There is no sensory loss.   The paralysis may ascend or descend or spread in a patchy way for three to four days after it has appeared, but no further spread occurs after the temperature has been normal for one week.   Retention of urine may be seen and in severe cases lasts up to three weeks.   The initial paralysis is always much more widespread and severe than the final residual paralysis.

Respiratory paralysis may be due to (1) involvement of bulbar respiratory centres, (2) diaphragmatic paralysis (C3) or (3) paralysis of the intercostal muscles (Th1–12).

Varieties of Paralysis.—(1) The *Bulbar type* occurs alone or associated with spinal paralysis.   A feeble voice or cough, spluttering or choking over drinks, or mucus collecting in the throat and producing a rattle in a conscious patient, are ominous signs which require prompt and energetic action.   Laboured breathing portends respiratory failure and if anoxia occurs it will increase the paralysis.   A jerky type of nystagmus may be seen.   Paralysis of the muscles of the face, jaw, palate and pharynx and complete paralysis of the ocular muscles is rare.   The signs may be unilateral.   (2) In the *Spinal type* the paralysis is asymmetrical and is a true flaccid lower motor neurone paralysis.   It may ascend or descend or spread by " jumps," especially in adults.   This type tends to be severe from its tendency to produce respiratory paralysis, from involvement of the intercostal muscles and diaphragm.   Constipation and retention of urine occur.   (3) *Polio-encephalitis:* Mental confusion and restless delirium persist for some days after the fever has subsided.   (4) *Abortive* and (5) *meningeal* types exist, in which no paralysis occurs, but changes are present in the spinal fluid.   These can be diagnosed accurately in epidemics.

Diagnosis.—The remarkable preservation of full consciousness whilst

the neurological symptoms are developing is most striking. In the early
stages the *blood* shows a polymorphonuclear leucocytosis which may reach
30,000. The *C.S.F.* shows most marked changes in the pre-paralytic
stage. The pressure is not usually raised but cell counts of 50–300 (mostly
lymphocytes) per c. mm. with only slightly raised protein, normal sugar
and chlorides are characteristic, particularly when there is a leucocytosis
in the blood. In the paralytic stage the *C.S.F.* may show raised pressure
and protein, especially if there is respiratory failure. The cell count
gradually falls to normal. *Epidemic myalgia* and *acute dermatomyositis*
may simulate poliomyelitis, but in these the spinal fluid is normal.
Especially in infants, painful conditions of a limb, *e.g.*, *acute arthritis* and
infantile scurvy, where the affected limbs are tender and swollen, cause
difficulty. In *acute infective polyneuritis* high C.S.F. protein readings sometimes may be a characteristic and persistent finding, as in poliomyelitis,
but sensory changes may occur. In *acute myelitis* sensory loss also occurs
but with a sensory level, and bedsores tend to develop rapidly. The
differential diagnosis from *tuberculous meningitis* is made by finding in
poliomyelitis normal amounts of chloride and glucose in the spinal fluid,
and a polymorphonuclear leucocytosis in the blood. Clear fluid and a
spider-web clot are common to the two conditions. In a*cute purulent
meningitis* the meningeal symptoms increase and the C.S.F. is purulent and
contains the infecting organism.

Etiology.—The disease is due to one of the smallest filterable viruses
known (Noguchi and Flexner, 1913). The virus can be found in the naso-
pharyngeal mucosa, in the wall of the gut and in the fæces of patients
and of healthy carriers. Three types are described and are designated as
the Brunhilde, the Lansing and the Leon types. The only method of
demonstrating the virus is by injection of emulsions of suspected material
into certain monkeys, thus producing disease in the inoculated animals.
The virus is believed to spread from the oro-gastro-intestinal tract to the
nervous system via the V, VII, IX, X cranial nerves and visceral afferents,
but in the early stages of the disease there is always a viræmia. The virus
is found in the brain and spinal cord of fatal cases, and also in the alimentary canal; fæcal excretion can continue for three weeks after the paralysis
has appeared. The disease is spread by *carriers*. *Epidemics* occur in the
warmer months and in the autumn. No race or country is exempt, but
it is more common in the white races. It appears in countries with a
high standard of hygiene and sanitation, *e.g.*, Northern America, Scandi-
navia, Switzerland. The disease is infectious in that several cases may
appear in a community at about the same time. Case-to-case infection
is rare. Males are affected rather more frequently than females, but
pregnant women are specially liable to infection. The fæces and handkerchiefs which may contain the virus should be treated as infective. They
must be destroyed, for common disinfectants do not kill the virus.

Prognosis.—The mortality rate in epidemics ranges from 7 to 25 per
cent. and is greatest in the bulbar and spreading forms of the disease

affecting young adults.   Death is due to respiratory paralysis or pulmonary complications and is partly due to cardio-vascular failure and hypotension. The severity of the paralysis bears a clear relationship to physical activity after the onset of the major illness.   Patients who have developed paralysis must be kept at complete rest.   Muscles incompletely paralysed will certainly recover.   Many cases of bulbar poliomyelitis make excellent functional recoveries after periods spent in a respirator.   The final prognosis as to ability to use the affected limbs or limb depends on whether the muscles affected perform essential functions in walking or prehension and on certain orthopædic considerations.   Only 2 per cent. are completely disabled.   No case should be considered hopeless until months or years have elapsed, as recovery is often long delayed.   If the paralysis occurs during the growth period, shortening of the affected limb may occur.   For electro-prognosis, see § 848.   Second attacks, though rare, may certainly occur after 3–4 years, perhaps due to a different strain of virus.

Treatment.—The virus is not affected by any known antibiotic and no specific remedy is known. *Suspected cases* raise difficult decisions; but all seriously ill suspects, and all unconscious or confused patients should be sent to hospital.   Contacts in the home should be advised to avoid hard physical exercise.   If the disease is diagnosed *in the Pre-paralytic Stage* (this is often possible in epidemics) complete rest in bed must be enforced at once.   If the diagnosis is uncertain spinal puncture is essential.

In the early *Acute Paralytic Stage*, if the disease is severe and the paralysis spreading, the case should be transferred to a special poliomyelitis unit.   The first few weeks may be most anxious and expert care by a team is often required.   Under epidemic conditions mobile teams from Infectious Diseases Hospitals, supplied with respirators and equipment for transport, are sometimes available.   Where the paralysis seems localised and static there is something to be said for keeping a very frightened patient at home but most are best in hospital.   *Rest and Posture.*   Absolute physiological rest is essential, emotional as well as physical.   The patient should be fed and washed in bed, and must use a urinal and bedpan.   During the first two weeks of paralysis, stretching out for drinks on the side table, the holding of a book, and unnecessary visiting must be prohibited.   A padded foot-board serves to protect the legs from the pressure of bedclothes and keeps the feet at 90 degrees.   In *Bulbar Poliomyelitis* (especially in children) the patient should be nursed in the semi-prone ("tonsillectomy") position.   The foot of the cot or bed should be raised on blocks to an angle of 15 degrees with the horizontal, to keep the airway clear of mucus.   The patient should be turned from one side to the other every few hours.   Postural drainage and a sucker to remove mucus in the throat may be life-saving. Give prophylactic penicillin to prevent respiratory infection.   Train the patient to count from one upwards at a fixed rate whilst slowly breathing out, after taking the deepest breath possible.   A fall in the count indicates a decrease in vital capacity and pulmonary ventilation, indicating possible anoxia.

Respiratory Failure. The use of a respirator is strongly advised for anoxia even when the weakness of the respiratory muscles is only moderate. This will limit paralysis, save lives and probably lessen the severity of after-effects. Terror of the respirator may affect an inexperienced physician as well as the patient but this must not cause delay, which may be fatal. An experienced nursing team, medical and engineering staffs used to respirator work will add greatly to the patient's chances. It is often best to perform early tracheostomy inserting a cuffed hooded tube to prevent suction of secretions into the lungs. Intermittent positive pressure respirators are now available operating with a face mask, as in closed-circuit anæsthesia. In most cases, however, after a period in a tank-type intermittent pressure respirator, the patient may be graduated to a cuirass-type respirator, which leaves the limbs and neck free. Thence progress can be made to unassisted breathing. Should bilateral abductor paralysis of the vocal cords develop tracheostomy is essential. Where there is dysphagia, nasal feeding must be undertaken. *Retention of urine* will require eight-hourly catheterisation, using a " no-touch " technique. Avoid all strong aperients. Watch for signs of dehydration and treat this by parenteral dextrose or saline.

For *Pain* give soluble aspirin, tab. codein co., or apply hot fomentations well wrung out to painful muscles in spasm. Restlessness may indicate anoxia: *Sleeplessness* may require a sedative (*e.g.*, sod. amylobarbitone).

After the first two to three weeks the danger of aggravating the spinal cord condition has passed and *Re-education* becomes of paramount importance. Any voluntary movement performed by the patient is of much greater value than the same movement performed passively by a masseuse. Massage is never an adequate substitute for active exercises. Faradism cannot hasten recovery; it should never be used in the painful stage, nor can it replace re-educative exercises. Immersing the limbs in a brine bath or exercises in a swimming bath assist re-education by affording additional support to the moving limbs. A walking machine on skids or wheels helps to recover power in the legs. Occupational therapy is valuable. When contractures have appeared, they should be dealt with by passive manipulation and stretching, and later by tenotomy and other orthopædic measures. In old paralysed limbs cyanosis, œdema and chilblains may be relieved by lumbar sympathectomy. In young children the regime of passive movements, massage and exercises advocated by Sister Kenny seems to produce good results, and physiological reflex systems underlying posture and tonus are kept active by this. Resisted movements with the affected limbs suspended in a canvas sling attached to a stout spring and Balkan frame are useful in promoting recovery in affected limb muscles. If possible sheltered *schools* for the physically handicapped should be avoided. If the child can attend an ordinary school and mingle with normal children the results are usually excellent; but this is not possible in severely handicapped cases.

Prophylaxis.—During epidemics children should avoid swimming pools and crowded places, over-exertion and the operation of tonsillectomy. If an epidemic breaks out in a boarding school the prevailing custom is to quarantine the school for three weeks. Parents are given the option of leaving their child at school or removal home. Many will choose the latter, and then the child should be kept away from younger members of the family for three weeks. Cases which develop the disease should be rigidly isolated, treated as contagious and nursed with precautions as for typhoid fever. Nurses should wear gauze masks; the patient's stools and handkerchiefs, eating utensils and bedding are treated as infective. *Vaccination.*—Inactivated virus vaccine from each of the three types is used. Those at risk between six months and forty years of age should receive the recommended three doses by deep subcutaneous injection or otherwise by mouth (§ 525). For children starting school between the ages of five and eleven years a fourth " booster " dose may be given. A previous attack of poliomyelitis does not imply immunity to all three types. At present it is suggested that about 70 per cent. at risk will be protected. It is possible that in a vaccinated population the clinical manifestations of the disease will be modified by the acquired immunity. In very rare cases vaccination may cause an allergic radiculopathy affecting the motor roots corresponding to the site of the injection. Symptoms of this are mild and transient.

§ 899. XII. Spinal Epidural Abscess is rare. It occurs at any age. The infection reaches the epidural space by direct extension from a suppurating focus in the skin, a perinephric abscess or from a penetrating wound of the back. More rarely the infection comes from infective thrombophlebitis or a septicæmia. The *Symptoms* are headache, pain in the back, high fever, weakness of the lower limbs and finally complete paraplegia. The blood shows a leucocytosis. The spinal fluid findings are characteristic—there is manometric evidence of spinal block, the fluid is xanthochromic or cloudy, there is a moderate pleocytosis and high protein content (100–1,500 mg. per 100 ml.). Pus may be withdrawn during spinal puncture which, if the condition is suspected should always be done, applying steady suction with a syringe during the puncture. Prompt treatment with sulphonamides and antibiotics have lessened the mortality but surgical treatment is usually necessary. Residual paraplegic symptoms are common.

XIII. Post-infective Myelopathy may be of the ascending type (§ 895).

A patient shows Pyrexia *followed by* rapidly ascending paralysis. *There may be sensory changes, and the spinal fluid is either normal or shows excess of protein with slight pleocytosis. The condition may be* (a) Acute Infective Polyneuritis *or* (b) Acute Myelitis.

XIV. Acute Infective Polyneuritis (§ 976). Following a febrile illness a motor paralysis appears and may affect the cranial nerves. Unlike poliomyelitis there is only slight increase of cells in the spinal fluid but a high protein reading in the fluid without manometric evidence of spinal block are characteristic (§ 969).

XV. Acute Myelitis (§ 955). XVI. Paralytic brachial Neuritis (§ 998).

GROUP V. STROKE AND HEMIPLEGIA

There is more or less SUDDEN PARALYSIS *affecting* ONE SIDE *of the body;* MOTOR, SENSORY, VISUAL *or* SPEECH *functions are affected.* *The condition is a* STROKE.

§ 900. A Stroke (Syn. Cerebro-vascular attack, Ictus) is usually due to disease of the *Intracranial vessels*, but the cause is often primarily *Extracranial, e.g.*, Embolism, Carotid or Vertebral occlusion, Hypertension, essential or renal, Hæmorrhagic disease or Pyæmia. The underlying cerebral pathological changes are (A) Ischæmia, (B) Hæmorrhage, (C) Acute Brain Swelling.

(A) ISCHÆMIC LESIONS result from arterial occlusions by thrombosis from atheroma or arteritis, or embolism. Thrombosis most usually affects the cerebral and cerebellar arteries, but it is frequent in the internal carotid or vertebral arteries. In these latter vessels stenosis may occur due to atheromatous or traumatic narrowing or to an organised mural thrombus. Cerebral emboli come from the heart, or the pulmonary veins in lung diseases. Sudden falls in blood pressure (*e.g.*, in coronary occlusion) can cause focal cerebral ischæmia of rapid onset, causing a transient or more permanent hemiparesis. There is evidence that cerebral ischæmia can also occur with prolonged vascular spasm, and in severe anæmia.

(B) HÆMORRHAGIC LESIONS within the skull may be *intra-* or *extracerebral*. Bleeding occurs from atheroma with hypertension, or from rupture of atheromatous or congenital aneurysms. Traumatic rupture of healthy arteries complicates severe head injury. Infections with hæmolytic bacteria and blood diseases, *e.g.*, leukæmia, are rarer causes.

(C) ACUTE BRAIN SWELLING occurs in hypertensive encephalopathy and in cerebral tumours with focal cerebral symptoms resembling stroke.

The occurrence of loss of consciousness will depend not only upon the extent and suddenness of the lesion but also on its site. Unconsciousness is common in basal lesions. " Shock effects " at the onset of such an illness are commonly seen (*e.g.*, flaccid paresis of the limbs affected) and much recovery may take place in a few hours or days. A final prognosis should not be given in a cerebral vascular accident until at least two to three weeks have elapsed for shock effects to pass off.

§ 901. Hemiplegia is the commonest manifestation of a " stroke," with paralysis affecting the face, limbs and trunk on one side of the body. *Symptoms.*—(a) *Stage of Onset.* If the responsible cerebral lesion is acute the paralysis is at first flaccid (shock effect). In complete hemiplegia the arm is affected more than the leg and the distal movements suffer more than proximal ones. The lower face is more affected than the upper. A transient conjugate deviation of the head and eyes towards the unparalysed side may be observed for a few days. The trunk muscles are weakened on the affected side but the ocular muscles and those of mastication escape, as they have a dual innervation from both hemispheres. *If the patient is unconscious* we recognise the paralysis by lifting the limbs and letting them drop in turn. We may notice blowing out of the angle of the mouth on the affected side, or a narrowing of the ocular fissure. The abdominal reflexes are abolished on the affected side: the plantar response is usually extensor from the first. *If the patient is conscious* we observe on the affected side weakness of closure of the eye and the orbicularis muscle, weakness of the lower face when the patient is asked to show his teeth with flattening of the naso-labial fold (emotional movements of the face sometimes escape) and the base of the tongue may be higher. In slighter cases we find weakness of dorsiflexion of the wrist and clumsiness of the fine finger movements with the thumb–finger test, weakness of the extensors of the fingers and elbow-joint; and in the leg there is inability to dorsiflex the affected foot as powerfully as that on the unaffected side, with weakness of the flexors of the knee and hip. The tendon reflexes may be abolished for some hours but they become exaggerated within the first ten days as *spasticity* develops.

(b) *Stage of Recovery* (Residual hemiplegia).—In chronic progressive lesions and in the stage of recovery of acute lesions there is: (1) Spasticity of the affected limbs, of the " clasp-knife " variety. (2) The upper limb is held with the arm adducted at the shoulder, and flexed at the elbow, wrist and fingers, with the forearm slightly pronated. (3) The lower limb is extended at the hip- and knee-joints, and (4) the gait is characteristic, the paralysed leg being dragged round in a semi-circle, the toes scraping the floor. (5) There is weakness of the affected side of the face in smiling, and food collects round the teeth on the paralysed side, but the patient can screw up both eyes normally. (6) The tongue is protruded to the affected side, owing to the unbalanced action of the genio-hyoglossus. (7) There may be also certain involuntary " associated movements " in the affected limbs. Thus, if the patient yawns, he may extend his paralysed wrist and fingers and raise his hand in front of his face, performing involuntarily movements which he cannot voluntarily achieve.

Power returns first, with hypertonus, to the flexor muscles of the arm, in accordance with the physiological principle that primitive function (in this case prehension) is the last to be destroyed and the first to recover. Thus the patient may soon be able to elevate and abduct the affected upper limb at the shoulder, and to flex the elbow, fingers and wrist. In the leg, power returns first to the extensors of the hip and knee, and to the adductors (maintenance of erect posture). Power may return almost completely, with the exception of ability to dorsiflex the foot and perform fine finger movements. The upper abdominal reflex returns before the lower, the plantar reflex may become flexor. The recovery of aphasia, if present, usually precedes recovery of paralysis.

Other symptoms may be present: (1) *Aphasia*, in right-handed people, if the lesion is in the left hemisphere; (2) *hemianæsthesia* if the posterior part of the internal capsule is affected (see Fig. 211); (3) *hemianopia* if the lesion is still farther back in the internal capsule; (4) some *mental impairment*, apart from aphasia, often results from a " stroke." (5) *Involuntary movements* are apt to appear when hemiplegia occurs in childhood; they take the form of athetosis or chorea.

For the syndromes produced by obstruction of the various intracranial arteries see § 809.

The *Varieties* of hemiplegia depend on the site of the lesion. (1) Crossed hemiplegia (see § 792) occurs in lesions of the crus, pons or medulla. (2) " Hemiplegia dolorosa " occurs in thalamic lesions and is characterised by intractable pain, and by overreaction to exteroceptive stimuli over the affected half of the body. (3) Flaccid hemiplegia is rare and may indicate a lesion involving the pre-motor cortex. (4) Residual hemiplegia. In some cases the recovery is only partial; the affected limbs remain spastic and weak, and the deep reflexes increased. The paralysed limbs are blue and cold, and fibrosis occurs in the muscles, especially of the upper limb, with contractures at the shoulder and elbow and arthritic changes. The muscles show no wasting, apart from that due to disuse.

For Diagnosis, Prognosis and Treatment of hemiplegia see §§ 910–911.

The *Causes* of hemiplegia can be divided into three groups according to their mode of onset or course: (A) Hemiplegia of Sudden Onset, (B) Transient and Recurrent Hemiplegia, (C) Hemiplegia of Gradual Onset.

(A) CAUSES OF HEMIPLEGIA OF SUDDEN ONSET

I. Cerebral thrombosis (" cerebro-vascular accident ") (§ 902).
II. Internal carotid thrombosis or stenosis (§ 903).
III. Basilar and carotid insufficiency (§ 904).
IV. Cerebral embolism (§ 905).
V. Cerebral hæmorrhage (§ 851).
VI. Hypertensive encephalopathy (§ 906).
VII. Cerebral tumour (§ 1041).
VIII. Cerebral vascular syphilis (§ 907).
IX. Cortical thrombo-phlebitis (§ 908).
X. Acute encephalitis (§§ 893–897).

HYSTERIA, the great stimulator of organic disease, may produce signs superficially resembling those of a stroke (see § 912).

A middle-aged or elderly subject, who may have suffered in the past from headaches or dizzy spells, develops within the space of a few hours a UNILATERAL PARALYSIS, HEMIANÆSTHESIA OR HEMIANOPIA. *In some, but not in all cases, there may be* GRADUALLY DEEPENING UNCONSCIOUSNESS. *The condition may be* CEREBRAL *or* CAROTID THOMBOSIS.

§ 902. I. **Cerebral Thrombosis.**—(i.) *Premonitory Symptoms* are common and exist for hours, days or months before the onset of paralysis. They are headache, giddiness, slurred speech, memory failure or irritability. Transient attacks of numbness or weakness on one side, sometimes limited to one limb, often correspond to the site of the subsequent paralysis. (ii.) *Focal Symptoms of Occlusion.* Loss of consciousness at the onset is not invariable but may be profound in basilar lesions and if the vessel affected is large. Coma or delirium may last for hours or days: initial convulsions are rare. When there is no loss of consciousness there is usually sudden headache, giddiness and incoherence, followed by paralysis.

Focal symptoms commence in two ways: weakness or numbness lasts for a few hours or days before sudden hemiplegia; or a person, apparently in good health, may waken conscious but with a hemiplegia. At the onset the limb or limbs affected are flaccid, with absent or depressed tendon-reflexes, there is weakness of the affected lower face; and perhaps conjugate deviation of the head and eyes. In other cases the picture is that of hemianopia, aphasia, ataxia, appearing in the course of one or two hours. In some cases no focal symptoms occur. Rarely the focal symptoms, especially hemiplegia, come on before the coma.

The obstruction usually involves the middle, anterior or posterior cerebral arteries, the internal carotid, the posterior inferior cerebellar or the basilar arteries. The middle cerebral artery and its branches are much the most frequently affected. For the symptoms following upon obstruction of each of these arteries see § 809. *Bilateral obstruction* of large vessels is rare; it occurs in quick succession and causes bilateral signs with increasing coma and death. Lesser degrees cause pseudo-bulbar palsy (§ 874).

Other Symptoms.—The fundi may show the changes of hypertensive retinopathy (§ 1134). The blood pressure is usually elevated but thrombosis may occur in patients with normal or subnormal pressures. The cerebro-spinal fluid shows a normal or slightly raised pressure (200–250 mm.) and the cells and protein are normal unless syphilis is the cause. After an extensive thrombosis near the ventricular wall the C.S.F. may be faintly xanthochromic for a few days.

Diagnosis.—The cause of the arterial disease should be determined as well as the site of the lesion. Isolated aphasia or partial hemiplegia are more common in thrombosis than hæmorrhage. Occlusion of the posterior cerebral artery due to *temporal arteritis* may cause sudden hemianopia. Remember the lesion may be *extracranial* in the carotid or vertebral artery. Suspect *Subdural hæmatoma* if the patient is elderly, the loss of consciousness is gradual with variable mental confusion, and paralytic signs are present but less marked than the severity of the mental state would indicate. A history of trauma may be absent. When in *Cerebral tumour* softening occurs the symptoms and signs are slowly progressive over days and weeks, with signs of increasing intracranial pressure. *Syphilitic thrombosis* is recognised by finding Argyll-Robertson pupils or positive serological tests in the blood or C.S.F. In *Hypertensive attacks* the paresis with multiple softenings clears up very rapidly: hypertensive retinopathy may be present and the diastolic blood pressure is raised. In CHILDREN AND YOUNG ADULTS a softening from tumour or angioma occurs, or it may be a manifestation of a systemic disease, *e.g.*, pneumonia, streptococcal septicæmia.

Etiology.—The commonest cause is atheroma. Latent or active syphilis is less frequent nowadays but may cause endarteritis and thrombosis. Temporal arteritis (" giant-celled " arteritis), polyarteritis nodosa and severe general infections are rare causes.

Prognosis.—It is rare for the condition to be immediately fatal. Previous coronary attacks or " strokes," advanced age, deep and prolonged coma are bad signs. Lesions in the cerebellum may show almost complete recovery between episodes. In more severe cases of hemiplegia partial recovery is the rule. The large joint movements recover better than fine hand skills, which are usually permanently affected. Syphilitic cases have a better prognosis especially as regards life and future attacks. *Basilar thrombosis*, occlusion of *both* internal carotids or *both* middle cerebrals means imminent danger to life. *Post-hemiplegic* convulsions or tremors rarely occur. Visual Jacksonian fits sometimes persist after middle cerebral thrombosis.

Treatment.—Milder cases require complete bed-rest for a week or so, with graduated convalescence. Anticoagulants, such as heparin, are not advised as they may precipitate hæmorrhage. For treatment of syphilitic cases see § 500. When consciousness is severely depressed (see § 858) nikethamide B.P. (Coramine) may be used as a respiratory stimulant. For Treatment of Hemiplegia see § 911.

§ 903. II. **Internal Carotid Artery Thrombosis.** The artery may be *stenosed* from atheroma near its origin from the aorta. In other cases a thrombosis occurs above the bifurcation of the common carotid or inside the carotid syphon within the skull. The condition occurs in the fifth and sixth decades and five out of every six cases are male patients.

Symptoms may rarely be quite absent. Usually there are premonitory symptoms similar to those of cerebral thrombosis. Previous syncopal attacks are common (§ 833). The fully developed syndrome is exceptional (§ 809). Substantial recovery may occur from restoration of circulation through collaterals and through the Circle of Willis: this will be evident within a week of onset of the symptoms of occlusion. In other cases the thrombosis propagates or portions of clot are detached and form emboli. Bilateral carotid thromboses may occur. The *diagnosis* is difficult on clinical grounds. Absence of pulsation on the affected side is not a reliable sign; a localised systolic murmur over the artery is often audible when partial stenosis is present. Angiography will show stenosis or occlusion (Fig. 240). Early unilateral cases diagnosed by carotid angiography when the lesion is due to focal stenosis have been dealt with successfully by surgical removal of the clot. Resection of portions of the vessel has been carried out with success. Anticoagulants are of problematic value and may precipitate cerebral hæmorrhage. Some believe in stellate ganglion block, but there is no proof that it improves the prognosis.

§ 904. III. **Basilar or Carotid Artery Insufficiency** due to repeated falls of blood pressure in patients with atheromatous narrowing of the cerebral arteries causes transient hemiplegia or transient ataxia so that he may fall. The attacks may last some minutes and the patient may for a time be bereft of speech. Attacks are precipitated by fatigue, starvation, or tilting the head backwards. In many cases the attacks will pass off after a local or general improvement in the circulation.   Vasoconstrictor drugs, *e.g.*, methylamphetamine, should be avoided.

A patient known to have mitral disease, auricular fibrillation or subacute bacterial endocarditis suddenly develops a HEMIPLEGIA *which tends to recovery after a few hours.   The condition may be* CEREBRAL EMBOLISM.

§ 905.   IV. Cerebral Embolism.—The embolus is usually a clot or a vegetation (perhaps infected) from the left side of the heart or pulmonary circulation.   *Symptoms.*—Embolism of a larger artery is characterised by *instantaneous* loss of consciousness.   When a small cortical vessel is blocked, giddiness or a Jacksonian attack followed by monoplegia may

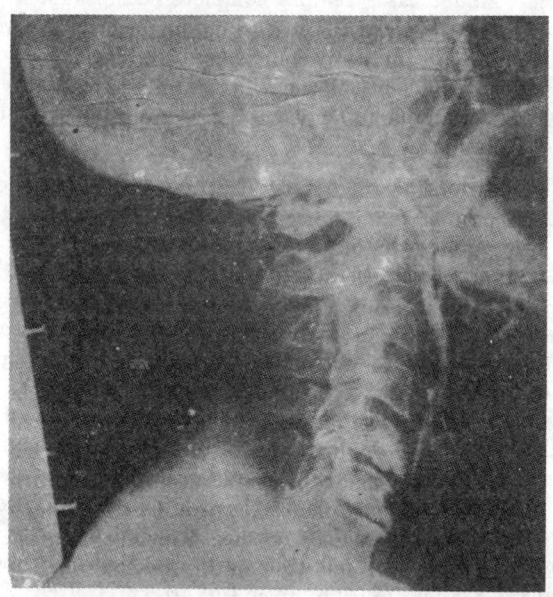

FIG. 240.—RIGHT CAROTID ANGIOGRAM SHOWING INTERNAL CAROTID STENOSIS.   The needle which carried the injection is seen in the neck, but only the branches of the External Carotid have filled with the contrast medium.   (Dr. Charles MacLean.)

replace loss of consciousness.   Usually the middle cerebral artery is affected, with hemiplegia, dysphasia or sensory changes.   When the posterior cerebral artery is affected hemianopia results.   Partial thrombosis of a large vessel, *e.g.*, the internal carotid or vertebral, may soften and discharge emboli which lodge in its more distal branches; these cause slight and transient paralytic attacks in the course of convalescence from the initial attack and endanger life.

Etiology.—Embolism may occur in young persons with cardiac disease. Usually the cause is evident: signs of auricular fibrillation, mitral or aortic disease (often infective endocarditis) or suppurative lung disease may be present.   Infected emboli (*e.g.*, in bronchiectasis, infective endocarditis) give rise to cerebral abscess, single or multiple.   Air from punctured veins (perhaps during pleural or lung puncture) may act as an embolus.

Prognosis.—In young patients the effects of lodging of a single small embolus in the cerebral circulation, at first alarming, may soon improve. In auricular fibrillation when emboli are likely to be repeated, or in patients when the embolus is infected, the prognosis is much more serious.

Treatment.—When the embolus is infected the focus of origin must be treated.   When the embolus is aseptic, measures to promote vaso-dilatation have been tried with alcohol or nicotinic acid by mouth, tolazoline (Priscol) into the carotid artery or surgical stellate ganglion block.   These measures have been attended with little success.   Anticoagulants can be used in aseptic cases and may prevent retrograde propagation of the clot from the embolus (§ 52).   Mitral stenosis with embolism often calls for valvotomy.

Fat Embolism follows a few hours after fracture of a long bone. The fat globules lodge first in the lungs, producing cyanosis and pulmonary œdema. Some of the globules may make their way through the pulmonary capillaries to the cerebral vessels, with delirium, coma and localised cerebral palsies.

V. CEREBRAL HÆMORRHAGE often causes hemiplegic symptoms and signs but its most striking feature is Coma (§ 851).

§ **906.** VI. HYPERTENSIVE ENCEPHALOPATHY (Syn. Hypertensive attack).—Patients with benign or malignant hypertension, besides suffering from cerebral softenings, may develop a hypertensive crisis (§§ 97, 851).

VII. CEREBRAL NEOPLASM.—The presence of a hitherto unsuspected growth may become apparent when hæmorrhage suddenly occurs within its substance.   Such vascular tumours are primary or secondary vascular malignant growths or angiomatous malformations (§ 1039 *et seq.*).

§ **907.** VIII. **Cerebral Vascular Syphilis** due to endarteritis of the cerebral vessels with thrombosis and softening, causes hemiplegia and dysphasia.

Symptoms are similar to those of cerebral thrombosis but *premonitory* symptoms are more frequent. Headache, giddiness, slurred or hesitant speech, loss of memory, irritability, sleeplessness, may be present for some weeks or months before the onset of focal signs. *Focal signs* occur usually without loss of consciousness but fits are common before the onset of paralysis. Hemiplegia and dysphasia are frequent manifestations. Syphilitic pupils may be present and there may be a history of the disease or of exposure to infection. *Diagnosis* is simpler in a younger patient but many cases are middle-aged or elderly. The blood W.R. is usually positive. The condition is diagnosed from dementia paralytica by the suddenness of onset and by the persistently paralytic or dysphasic signs. The C.S.F. shows a moderate lymphocytosis, increased protein, and sometimes a positive W.R. The colloidal gold curve is different to that found in dementia paralytica (Table LXVI).

Etiology.—Males are mostly affected and the incubation period may be several years. The syphilitic endarteritis is accompanied by a meningo-encephalitis.

Prognosis.—The danger to life is less than in atheroma unless a large vessel, *e.g.*, the basilar, is occluded, or when complicating aortic or renal disease is present.

Treatment is by intramuscular penicillin giving 1 mega unit daily for 14–20 days. The treatment of residual lesions is symptomatic.

§ **908.** IX. **Cortical Thrombophlebitis.**—Some cases of hemiplegia and other cerebral symptoms in women during the puerperium or after abortion (confusional states) are attributed to venous occlusions in the sagittal sinus and cortical veins. Associated pelvic and femoral thromboses are often present. Hemiplegia or bilateral hemiplegia comes on with convulsions or coma. The C.S.F. is under increased pressure but is normal in composition. A similar condition may occur in closed head injuries. In association with suppurative otitis media and mastoid infection a spreading non-suppurative thrombosis of the sinuses and cortical veins can occur, causing foci of superficial encephalitis and softenings. The physical signs and spinal fluid findings are indistinguishable from those of intracerebral abscess formation. In most cases, however, the condition resolves and the patient recovers.

X. ACUTE ENCEPHALITIS.—In children after vaccination or an acute specific fever or other demyelinating encephalopathy a hemiplegia may occur (§ 893 *et seq.*).

(3) CAUSES OF TRANSIENT OR RECURRENT HEMIPLEGIA

I. Post-epileptic hemiplegia.
II. Migraine.
III. Cerebral vascular accidents (embolism, thrombosis).
IV. Internal carotid artery stenosis.
V. Hypertensive attacks.
VI. Cerebral contusion.
VII. Dementia paralytica.
VIII. Encephalitis, abscess and cerebral thrombo-phlebitis.
IX. Cerebral neoplasm.
X. Disseminated sclerosis.
XI. Diabetic coma.

§ 909. I. POST-EPILEPTIC HEMIPLEGIA (Todd's paralysis) usually follows a Jacksonian fit (§ 863). After lasting some hours it may pass off completely. Patients showing this sign are likely to have a focal expanding or atrophic cerebral lesion, and may require ancillary investigations.

II. In MIGRAINE transient hemiplegia is rare: but it may occur as a familial form of the disease. In elderly migrainous subjects it often indicates cerebral arterial disease.

III. CEREBRAL VASCULAR ACCIDENTS cause transient hemiplegia from focal ischæmia, embolism, infarction, sudden fall of blood pressure, or spasm of a cerebral artery.

IV. INTERNAL CAROTID THROMBOSIS OR STENOSIS may cause transient attacks of hemiplegia. If they are accompanied by visual impairment on the side opposite to the hemiplegia (the ophthalmic artery is given off before the vessel supplies the hemisphere) the condition may be diagnosed clinically. Carotid angiography may be required to elucidate this cause. Similar attacks occur in *vertebral* or *basilar insufficiency* in atheromatous patients.

V. HYPERTENSIVE ATTACKS, see §§ 97, 851.

VI. In CEREBRAL INJURIES hemiplegia is nearly always due to intracranial hæmorrhage, only rarely to contusion of the brain.

VII. In DEMENTIA PARALYTICA transient hemiplegia constitutes one form of " congestive attack " (§ 1190).

VIII. ENCEPHALITIS, non-suppurative and suppurative, or intracranial thrombo-phlebitis are rare causes of transient hemiparesis.

IX. In CEREBRAL NEOPLASM transient hemiplegia is usually a post-epileptic phenomenon.

X. In DISSEMINATED SCLEROSIS the paresis takes some days or weeks to pass off.

XI. DIABETIC COMA. Transient recoverable hemiplegia is a rare complication.

(C) CAUSES OF HEMIPLEGIA OF GRADUAL ONSET

I. Intracranial neoplasm.
II. Chronic subdural hæmatoma.
III. Cerebral abscess.
} Onset over a period of days, weeks or months.

IV. Meningitis acute and chronic. Onset over a period of days.

§ 910. I. INTRACRANIAL NEOPLASM.—(1) The *progressive* character of the hemiplegia, coming on insidiously over a period of days, weeks or

months, suggests tumour.   When a hæmorrhage into the growth or sudden
œdema occurs, sudden hemiplegia may occur, but symptoms have usually
been present in the affected limbs previously.   (2) The occurrence of
Jacksonian attacks during the slow progress of the hemiplegia is strong
evidence of an expanding lesion, especially in the presence of (3) headaches,
vomiting and papillœdema.   Any or all of these latter symptoms may
be absent.   Existing arterial disease does not rule out tumour.   A primary
bronchial carcinoma should be sought in these cases.   Intense papillœdema with hæmorrhages and exudates occurs in conditions other than
intracranial tumour, viz., hypertensive encephalopathy, uræmia.   These
conditions, however, seldom cause *progressive* hemiplegia (§ 1035).

II. Chronic Subdural Hæmatomata occur more commonly in the
elderly.   The history of previous head injury may be missed; the bleeding
may be bilateral.   In young adults a subdural hæmatoma may follow
trauma or rupture of a saccular aneurysm.   The hemiplegia progresses
slowly and signs may be bilateral.   There is often mental confusion,
dyspraxia, agnosia, and remissions in the mental state are characteristic.
A *fixed, dilated pupil* on the side of the hæmorrhage is highly characteristic.
The spinal fluid is usually clear, rarely bloodstained.   The investigation
and treatment of these cases requires surgical help (§ 1052).

III. Cerebral Abscess may produce hemiplegia.   There is a history
of meningitis, infected head wound, infected nasal sinus or middle ear,
or chronic sepsis in the lung or abdomen (§ 891).

IV. Meningitis.—Hemiplegia in the course of meningitis is usually due
to cerebral softening from arteritis.   *Syphilitic meningomyelitis* is an
important cause of hemiplegia in persons under the age of 40.

Diagnosis of Hemiplegia.—Most cases of acute hemiplegia are due to
cerebro-vascular accidents.   In many cases it is not possible to differentiate
at the onset between cerebral hæmorrhage, thrombosis of a cerebral artery,
or thrombosis of the internal carotid or vertebral artery.   Embolism is
easier to recognise from the abrupt onset and the associated heart lesion.
Neck stiffness and a positive Kernig's sign may indicate subarachnoid
hæmorrhage.   If necessary the pupils should be dilated to inspect the
ocular fundi; papillœdema may mean increased intracranial pressure, renal
disease or a hypertensive attack.   If papillœdema is absent C.S.F. may
be withdrawn for analysis after manometry.   Carotid or vertebral angiography may help diagnosis, especially in cases of progressive or recurrent
hemiplegia with progressive signs.

Prognosis of Hemiplegia.—Intracerebral hæmorrhage is usually fatal
within hours or days but cases which survive undoubtedly occur.   Patients
may recover from subarachnoid hæmorrhage but there is danger of recurrence of the bleeding, especially in the first six weeks.   In cases of embolism
the neurological lesion is often slight and recovery rapid.   In internal
carotid artery thrombosis the thrombus may propagate as high as the Circle
of Willis, but in spite of this the establishment of a collateral circulation

in the affected hemisphere may enable reasonable recovery to occur in some cases. In intracerebral thrombosis, whether due to atheroma or syphilitic arteritis, the prognosis is always anxious during the first three to four weeks. In hemiplegia of slow onset the prognosis is ominous. *Complications.*—(1) Bedsores over the sacrum and heels. (2) Contractures of the shoulder, wrist and fingers, knees and ankles. (3) Broncho-pneumonia.

§ 911. **Treatment of Hemiplegia.**—(*a*) Acute Hemiplegia. Treatment in the early stages is similar to the Care of the Unconscious Patient (§ 858). Venesection is not advised, except in cases due to hypertensive encephalo-pathy. Anticoagulant drugs are not often used as they may precipitate bleeding from cerebral vessels, except in cases of embolism. As soon as is feasible the patient should be lifted out of bed into a chair for an increas-ing period each day. (*b*) Residual Hemiplegia. Energetic rehabilitation is contra-indicated where there has been coronary thrombosis, or other severe heart disease. Improvement may be expected to continue for six months in cases with non-progressive lesions. From the first, movement of all the joints of the affected limbs should be carried out daily, special attention being devoted to the shoulder. A slightly cocked night-splint for the fingers and wrist and a foot-board will prevent contractures. If the patient can lift the lower limbs from the bed, it is probable that he will be able to walk. Later on walking exercises with a nurse and between parallel bars are helpful. A cardboard cylinder under the flexed hand enables the hand to be slid across the bar and used as a support. The patient should be taught to swing the right arm forwards with the left leg, and *vice versa*. Walking with a stick is the next step. All exercises should be graduated, more being attempted each day. The arm must not be neglected; exercises with the arm in a sling attached to an overhead pulley can be carried out by the patient using his sound arm to hoist the spastic limb. Or he can grasp his spastic arm by the wrist with his good arm and push it above his head, routinely three or four times a day.

A " frozen shoulder " is best treated by gentle daily manipulation, with heat and massage (§ 604). Some few cases are benefited by a toe-raising spring or a brace which counteracts inversion of the foot. Extensive flexion contracture in hemiplegic limbs may be helped by section of anterior roots or tenotomy.

§ 912. **Hysterical Hemiplegia** is rare and is distinguished by: (1) in hysteria the reflexes show no qualitative change, the abdominal reflexes remain normal and the plantar responses are either absent at the toes or of the normal flexor type. (2) The paralysis or spasm in the affected limbs shows paradoxes and inconsistencies, and " stocking " or " glove " anæsthesia may be present. Early slight hemiplegic weakness in *Disseminated Sclerosis* is sometimes diagnosed as hysteria. Look for differences in the tendon reflexes on the two sides, absent abdominal reflexes, diminished vibration sense over the tibial malleoli or an extensor plantar response (§ 952).

§ 913. Infantile Hemiplegia may be present at birth or is acquired in the early years of childhood.

Symptoms.—Two-thirds of the cases give a history suggestive that the hemiplegia was present at birth. In the remainder the child is normal at birth; (1) the onset follows a febrile illness which is succeeded by convulsions, and on recovering consciousness hemiplegia of varying degree is found. (2) If speech had been acquired, aphasia may result but this usually returns to normal in weeks or months. (3) The residual hemiplegia affects the arm more than the leg and athetosis is fairly common. (4) There may be proprioceptive sensory changes on the affected side. (5) In later life the affected limbs may be shortened. (6) Epilepsy or mental defect may remain. Whereas the leg recovers quickly the hand improves little, and this and the fits interfere with normal education.

Etiology.—The causes of the prenatal cases are unknown. The post-natal cases are due to: (1) vascular occlusions and cerebral softening, (2) meningitis, (3) head injury, (4) subarachnoid and intracerebral hæmorrhage. " Polio-encephalitis " is blamed.

Treatment.—Education should, if possible, be given at a school for physically handicapped children or at a small private school. Epilepsy is treated with anti-convulsant drugs. The children grow up tending to use the normal hand only. In adult life most have to be supported and cared for by relatives, but a few show remarkable ability in spite of handicaps. In selected cases with *fits, and behaviour disorders* of severe degree, hemispherectomy has been performed; it is claimed that removal of the diseased hemisphere diminishes or abolishes epilepsy and behaviour disorders, and affects power and sensation in minimal degree. It leaves the patient with a permanent homonymous hemianopia and is suitable only for carefully selected cases.

GROUP VI.   PARKINSONIAN RIGIDITY

A patient at or past middle age shows a COARSE RHYTHMIC TREMOR *of the arm and/or leg on one side of the body ; the affected limb or limbs also show* MUSCULAR RIGIDITY AND WEAKNESS *and the face has a* FIXED EXPRESSION. *The condition is* PARKINSONISM.

TYPES OF PARKINSONISM

I. Paralysis Agitans (Idiopathic Parkinsonism).
II. Symptomatic Parkinsonism.
    (*a*) Post-encephalitis lethargica.
    (*b*) Arteriosclerotic muscular rigidity.
    (*c*) Hepato-lenticular degeneration.
    (*d*) Poisoning by carbon monoxide, mercury, manganese, or over-dosage with rauwolfia, chlorpromazine and other tranquillising drugs.

§ 914. I. Paralysis Agitans (Syn. Idiopathic Parkinsonism) is a common degenerative disease, first described by a London doctor, James Parkinson (1817), who aptly called it " Shaking Palsy." The onset is usually between 40 and 60 years, rather more often in men than women.

Symptoms.—The onset is most insidious and the patient's family may notice little wrong until the condition is established. Patients complain that their walking has become a conscious effort, that dressing in the morning takes much longer, or that they can no longer swing a golf club with freedom, or deal a hand at cards. Their subjective complaints of " rheumatism," " cramp," " fibrositis " must not be taken at their face value.

If the patient is examined in bed it is easy to miss the diagnosis for there are no changes in the tendon reflexes or plantar responses, no gross paralysis and no sensory changes. But a physician, who sees the patient walking towards him, is at once struck by the inexpressive, staring face, the unblinking eyes, the low monotonous voice, the slow tremulousness of the movements and the gliding gait. (1) *Tremor* is the earliest symptom in most cases. At first it is unilateral, with coarse rhythmic movements (3–5 per sec.) due to alternating contractions in prime mover and antagonist muscles. It usually commences in the forefinger and thumb, or may affect all the fingers, the hand, even the forearm or whole arm. A " pill-rolling " type of tremor is sometimes seen. The tremor may start in the foot or leg, and as the patient sits in his chair a rhythmic tapping of his heel on the floor may be noticed. It may affect the lower jaw or more rarely the head. The eyelids flicker tremulously when the lids are lightly closed. The great characteristic of the tremor, as Parkinson pointed out, is that it continues during rest. The hands go on moving as they rest on the patient's knees and the legs continue to move when he is sitting. The tremor may appear only when the limb is in action, but it is rarely increased by the " finger–nose " test. It can often be controlled for a short time by an effort of will or by voluntary supination of the forearm. It disappears during sleep and fatigue or emotion increase it. The tremor can be demonstrated thus: (*a*) Ask the patient to put his hands lightly on his thighs and lightly to close his eyes. Look for the tremor in the hands and eyelids. (*b*) As the patient writes the letters may be fully formed but every line is a zig-zag. In slight cases a magnifying lens is required to see the irregularity. Later, rigidity causes micrographia and a tendency for the lines to slope from right to left. The irregularity of the writing may be brought out by asking the patient to draw one or more spirals. (*c*) The " glabellar sign ": With the patient's eyes open tap with a reflex hammer lightly on the glabella and watch for the blink which accompanies each tap. This is not a normal finding. (2) *Muscular Rigidity* is also at first usually unilateral in distribution, later it becomes bilateral. It produces the " mask-like " facies, the slowness of movements, *e.g.*, dressing, fastening buttons, tying shoelaces, shaving, the lack of swing of the arm in walking and the gliding gait. The rigidity does not affect ocular movements, but the muscles of articulation may suffer, hence the low monotonous voice devoid of normal inflections. It causes a characteristic *attitude* (Fig. 5)—one of slight general flexion, the arm being adducted and slightly flexed at the elbow, the forearm held between supination and pronation, the fingers usually slightly flexed in the position of interosseal extension (" interosseal attitude "). The rigidity may be demonstrated thus: (*a*) Passively flex and extend the hand on the forearm at the wrist-joint on the affected side. Diffuse rigidity different from the unaffected arm will be evident along with " cog-wheel " rigidity if there is coarse tremor as well as stiffness. (*b*) Ask the patient to walk without holding his clothes and look for the lack of swinging of one arm. *Muscular weakness* accompanies the rigidity but it is never severe or complete.   (3) The *Disorder of gait* is highly characteristic and is one of the chief disabilities.   The patient walks with a shuffling, gliding gait.   In turning, his head turns with his body *en bloc* and rapid turning is difficult.   Later the steps are short with a tendency to become quicker and quicker, and then to run (festination), with a tendency to fall, from the forward inclination of the body (propulsion).   Trousseau said that " the patient has to run after his centre of gravity," but a similar tendency to totter backwards (retropulsion) is seen, and even laterally.   (4) All movements become *slow and deliberate*: only one thing can be done at a time and in an unhurried fashion.   Turning over in bed becomes difficult without help, dressing-time becomes prolonged, and, in later stages, if the patient has been sitting long in a low chair, he may have to be pulled out with expenditure of considerable effort, and his knees, trunk and shoulders have to be straightened before he can stand.   (5) *Nutrition* suffers in the later stages, quite apart from the possible decreased food intake due to slowness of eating.   Marked loss of weight follows.   (6) *Respiratory and Autonomic symptoms* are common, quite apart from the use of drugs with an atropine-like effect.   Sighing, feelings of heat and flushes, increased perspiration, salivation (not only due to decreased swallowing), tachycardia, constipation and abdominal distension occur.   In the later stages incontinence of urine may occur in bed.   (7) *Mental changes.*   A feeling of *restlessness* is common, the patient demanding an arm or leg to be moved passively even a centimetre to ease his tension.   Severe *depression* is usually reactive; suicide may be attempted.   Periods of *mental vagueness* and delusions with ideas of persecution occur.   *Mental confusion* is often due to the cumulative effect of some remedy which the patient is taking regularly, *e.g.*, benzhexol in doses of 15 mg. or more daily.   Anarthria and stupor are terminal symptoms in uncomplicated cases.

Diagnosis.—*Senile tremor* begins in the head; head tremor is rare in Paralysis agitans.   *Hyperthyroidism* and *alcoholism* cause a finer and more irregular tremor, and other signs are present.   *Myxœdema* and *cervical spondylitis* may cause poverty of movement or rigidity and altered gait.   The hand wasting, paræsthesiæ and changes in the arm reflex in cervical spondylosis should be remembered.   A few, because of the tremor, or because of infrequent speech and bent attitude, are deemed to have primary anxiety or depressive states.   Occasionally the unilateral stiffness and weakness leads to needless investigations in neurosurgical centres because of a suspicion of brain tumour.

Etiology.—The cause is probably degenerative.   Widespread atrophic changes occur, especially in cells of the vegetative nuclei of the hypothalamus, brain-stem and medulla, but are most marked in the substantia nigra and globus pallidus.   The pigmented cells in the brain-stem show hyaline inclusions.   Gowers traced heredity in 15 per cent. of his cases. No convincing evidence exists that trauma is a causative factor.

The *Prognosis* regarding recovery or cessation is bad.   Rigid patients are liable to fall and may be unable to rise unaided.   After 10–15 years many are chairbound and helpless.   Even after surgical treatment the progressive nature of the disease will reassert itself, but often advance is so slow that the patient dies of intercurrent disease.   If *vascular hemiplegia* supervenes the tremor will cease on the paralysed side, only to return as the hemiplegia recovers.   Cramps in the feet and legs are very common.   *Œdema* of the feet and legs complicates sedentary cases.   *Contracture* may occur in the hands or arm muscles or elsewhere.   Parkinsonism coexisting with tabes or other chronic neurological diseases is a fortuitous event.

   Treatment.—All treatment is palliative and may be considered under three headings.   (1) *General management.*   The patient should continue at work as long as he can.   Daily walks short of fatigue, or daily car or bus rides, help physically and mentally and improve the morale.   Tremulous patients can often drive their cars, but when slowness of movement is present this should be discouraged.   Patients with tremor tend to become sensitive and anti-social, and visits to understanding friends are to be encouraged.   Alcohol and a warm climate lessen stiffness.   Daily massage and exercises in which all joints are moved actively or passively should be given to prevent contractures and œdema.   A course of intensive physiotherapy in hospital for two weeks may temporarily abolish discomforts.   Many get help from " zipp " fasteners, " collar-attached " shirts and buckled or " casual "-type shoes.   A stout rope suspended from a Balkan frame over the bed helps the patient to turn in the night.   High chairs and a hard mattress are preferable.   (2) *Medicinal treatment.*   Not all cases can take muscle-relaxant drugs.   Formerly hyoscine hydrobromide gr. $\frac{1}{100}$ t.i.d., or tinct. stramonii ♏ 10–15 t.i.d. after meals, were used but these cause a dry mouth, blurred vision and even spells of confusion.   They have been supplanted by newer muscle-relaxants and antihistamine preparations which tend to make patients drowsy.   The ideal substance has yet to be found.   Begin with benzhexol hydrochlor. (Artane) 2 mg. daily for a week, then increase the daily dose by 2 mg. each week until 2 mg. three or four times a day is being taken.   Such a dose will have to be continued.   If dry mouth or blurred vision occurs, reduce the dose for a time; never attempt to increase it too rapidly.   On no account should the drug be stopped suddenly, as intensification of tremor and rigidity then occurs, so disabling and alarming to the patient that he usually thinks he has become paralysed.   Other substances used have been ethopropazine hydrochlor. (Lysivane) 50 mg. t.i.d.; benztropine methanesulphonate (Cogentin) 1–2 mg. as a single morning dose—this is slowly excreted and may cause rashes and nausea; orphenadrine hydrochlor. (Disipal) 50 mg. three or four times daily.   In the writer's hands these have had no advantages over benzhexol.   Inevitably, increased manifestations of the disease will appear, more slowness or tremor.   The tendency is to increase the dose of benzhexol to 15 mg. daily (the limit of tolerance for most).   But before doing this try the effect of benzhexol 2 mg. 3–6 doses a day with phenindamine (Thephorin) 25 mg. at bedtime.   The combination of benzhexol with morning *d*-amphetamine (Dexedrine) 5–10 mg. may be tried. *Tremor* is little influenced by medicine but its effects may be mitigated by amylobarbitone 16 mg. thrice daily, or chlorpromazine 25 mg. three or four times daily. For *sleeplessness* give aspirin and barbitone, or diphenhydramine hydrochlor. (Benadryl) 50 mg. at bedtime. *Depression* demands guarding the patient against suicidal risk. Attention to sleep, altered regime, occupation and psychological attention help. Chlorpromazine or an analogous substance may be tried. Imipramine hydroch. (Tofranil) or iproniazid (Marsilid) are for use in skilled hands, as they are toxic. Convulsive therapy may have to be considered and where there are no cardio-vascular changes or hypertension, muscle relaxants may render this treatment possible by experts.

(3) *Surgical treatment.* Destructive lesions in the globus pallidus or the postero-medial nucleus of the thalamus may temporarily alleviate rigidity or tremor on the opposite side. These operations (" pallidectomy," " thalamectomy ") are done under local anæsthesia through a burr-hole in the skull: the lesions are produced by injecting alcohol or by electro-coagulation assisted by a stereotaxic metal frame clamped to the skull. The operation has been most successful in mitigating progressive symptoms in those under 60 years, some post-encephalitic cases, or where the tremor is very violent and confined to one side. The criteria for operation are not yet clearly defined and a final assessment of the value of such operations cannot be made. The mortality is less than 3 per cent. in expert hands. Dysarthria, dysphagia, pulmonary complications and hemiplegia are transitory post-operative complications. Bilateral operations are not advised on elderly patients; six months should elapse between operations on the two sides.

II. Symptomatic Parkinsonism.

§ 915. (*a*) **Post-encephalitis Lethargica.**—As a result of infection with the virus of Encephalitis Lethargica, Parkinsonism appears in more than a third of all cases. There may be no history of an " acute attack " (§ 837), the onset of the Parkinsonism being the only sign of the progressive activity of the virus in the mid-brain extra-pyramidal nuclei (substantia nigra and sub-thalamic region). The rigidity may be the residuum of an acute attack, or may follow complete recovery from such an attack 10–20 years previously. The condition may remit but rarely improves. *The course is much more benign and prolonged* than in Paralysis Agitans, but sudden exacerbations may occur. Post-encephalitic Parkinsonism is distinguished by the following features: (1) The patient may be of any age from childhood upwards. (2) Owing to the disease in the mid-brain, involvement of the ocular mechanisms occurs early. The ocular signs persist, and are valuable evidence of the encephalitic origin of the Parkinsonism. Any known abnormality of pupillary reaction may be met, including the Argyll-Robertson phenomenon and its converse. Protracted attacks of upward or lateral conjugate deviation of the eyes, lasting minutes or hours (oculogyric crises), are highly characteristic. (3) Bizarre and complicated involuntary movements of the voluntary muscles may be present, and, when these involve the respiratory mechanisms, " respiratory tics " occur, paroxysms of tachypnœa, faint breathing, yawning, etc. (4) An extensor plantar response may be present. (5) The skin of the face may be excessively greasy, and sialorrhœa is common. *Treatment* is that of Paralysis Agitans. Behaviour disorders in children occur mostly without Parkinsonism: many tend to improve with special care and schooling (§ 1194).

§ 916. (*b*) **Arteriosclerotic Muscular Rigidity.**—In subjects of Cerebral Arterio-sclerosis, with high blood pressure and evidences of arterial disease in the retinal or systemic arteries, Parkinsonian-like rigidity may appear. The plantar responses in such cases may be extensor and fits may occur, both of which are rare in idiopathic Parkinsonism. Other senile mental changes are present (§§ 574, 1187). This condition does not usually react to the drugs useful in Paralysis Agitans, although they may be tried. It may be part of the picture of Pseudo-bulbar Paralysis (§ 874).

§ 917. (c) **Hepato-lenticular degeneration** (Syn. Wilson's disease) is a rare and fatal familial affection of adolescents where cirrhosis of the liver accompanies signs of basal ganglia damage. *Symptoms.*—(1) There is widespread and slowly developing striatal rigidity of the voluntary muscles resembling that of Parkinsonism. (2) In other cases a " flapping " coarse tremor of the upper limbs only is seen. Dystonic movements and variable rigidity like athetosis are common. (3) Spasmodic " pathological " weeping or laughter may occur with dysphagia and dysarthria, and there may be mild dementia as in pseudo-bulbar states. The reflexes are qualitatively unaltered and there is no true paralysis of muscles. (4) When the cornea is examined by a slit-lamp the characteristic greenish-brown zone of pigment in granular form is shown at the corneo-scleral junction (Kayser-Fleischer ring) in 50 per cent. of cases. (5) Abnormalities of liver function revealed by biochemical tests are present only in exacerbations of the disease. Biochemical tests may show an increase in copper excretion in the urine, reduced ceruloplasmin content of the serum and complex abnormalities in the pattern of amino-acid excretion in the urine.

Etiology.—The disease is due to an inborn error in metabolism of copper. Copper in blood serum is normally bound to a specific protein called ceruloplasmin. In hepato-lenticular degeneration copper is absorbed in normal or in excessive amounts from the gut, but because of a low ceruloplasmin level it cannot be retained in the serum and is deposited in the basal ganglia, the liver and kidneys. Copper is a powerful enzyme inhibitor and this accounts for the basal-ganglia lesions, the nodular cirrhosis of the liver, the complex abnormalities in amino-acid excretion in the urine, and renal failure. The condition is familial but not hereditary. It occurs between the ages of 11 and 25 years in both sexes.

Prognosis.—Partial remissions occur but the disease is usually fatal in 4-10 years.

Treatment is by drugs which increase the excretion of copper and by a low copper-containing diet.

§ 918. (d) **Toxic Parkinsonism** is in most cases reversible. A few cases after recovery from coma due to severe carbon monoxide poisoning gradually develop signs of permanent Parkinsonism. Mercury (in barometer cleaners and testers) and manganese can be inhaled or ingested. Parkinsonian tremors occur but in most cases recovery will result after removal from exposure. Patients receiving large doses of rauwolfia, chlorpromazine or other tranquillising drugs may develop toxic Parkinsonism which clears up when they are withdrawn.

GROUP VII. INVOLUNTARY MOVEMENTS

The three main types of involuntary movements met with clinically are: 1. TREMOR, 2. CHOREA and 3. ATHETOSIS. Other types of involuntary movements are 4. TIC (§ 927), 5. SPASMODIC TORTICOLLIS (§ 929), 6. FACIAL HEMISPASM (§ 1080), 7. EPILEPSIA PARTIALIS CONTINUANS (§ 930), 8. MYOCLONUS (§ 931) and 9. FASCICULATION (§ 932).

(1) *The patient comes to you with rhythmical* SHAKING *of some part of the body. The condition is* TREMOR.

§ 919. **Tremor** is an involuntary rhythmical oscillation of one or more parts of the body, resulting from alternate contraction of muscle groups and of their antagonists (Purves-Stewart).

CAUSES OF TREMOR

Toxic.	*Functional.*

Toxic.

I. Hyperthyroidism.
II. Chronic Alcoholism.
III. Nicotine Poisoning.
IV. Mercurial Poisoning.

Functional.

XII. Anxiety Neurosis.
XIII. Hysteria.

Organic Affections of the Brain.

V. Parkinsonism.
VI. Hepato-lenticular Degeneration.
VII. General Paralysis of the Insane.
VIII. Disseminated Sclerosis.
IX. Cerebellar Ataxia.
X. Cerebral Tumour.
XI. Senile Tremor and Progressive Cerebellar Degeneration.

Familial.

XIV. Familial Tremor.

In Infants.

XV. Spasmus Nutans.

CLINICAL INVESTIGATION OF TREMOR.—The (1) Amplitude, (2) Rate, (3) Distribution of the movements should be noted with (4) Factors increasing the tremor or diminishing it (voluntary movement, effort of will, sleep, etc.) and (5) whether the tremor is accompanied by " cog-wheel " rigidity, as in Parkinsonism. (6) The age of the patient is important. Tremor in children is familial, or due to cerebellar disease, or follows Encephalitis, sometimes syphilitic. In early adult life it is due to Hyperthyroidism, Encephalitis, Disseminated Sclerosis or Psycho-neurosis. After middle life it may be due to Paralysis Agitans, General Paralysis of the Insane, Hyperthyroidism, or it may be Senile.

(a) Tremor may be **Toxic** in origin. Toxic tremors are best demonstrated by asking the patient to hold his hands out horizontally, with his fingers widespread, when the tremor can be seen or felt by light palpation of the dorsum of his hands. Toxic tremor is characteristic of: I *Hyperthyroidism*, in association with tachycardia, thyroid enlargement, lid-retraction, exophthalmos and wasting: II *Chronic Alcoholism*: III *Nicotine Poisoning* from excessive cigarette smoking: IV Poisoning by heavy metals, especially *Mercurial Poisoning*.

(b) Tremor may be due to **Organic affections** of the cerebrum, brain-stem or cerebellum. It is seen in association with Striatal Rigidity in V *Parkinsonism* (see § 914) due either to *Paralysis Agitans, Encephalitis Lethargica, Arteriosclerosis* or a Toxic Cause, and in VI *Hepato-Lenticular Degeneration*. In VII *General Paralysis of the Insane* spontaneous tremors of an irregular type occur in the lips and tongue, or can be demonstrated by asking the patient to write. They are often mistaken for simple nervousness, but the diagnosis can usually be made from the jumbling of syllables and slurred dysarthria, the irregular or unequal pupils, often of the Argyll-Robertson type, and the history of apathy, unreasonable irritability, or mistakes made at work. In doubtful cases, C.S.F. examination will clear up the diagnosis (Table LXVI). General *tremulousness* is seen in VIII *Disseminated Sclerosis*, as well as the " intention tremor " and titubation met in this disease (§ 952). Tremor, intention tremor and titubation are also met with in IX *Cerebellar Ataxia*, accompanied by absence of the tendon reflexes, extensor plantar responses, scanning speech, and pes cavus or scoliosis. In X *Cerebral Neoplasms* of the frontal lobes, mid-brain or corpus callosum, tremor, often unilateral, may occur. XI *Senile* tremor, or rhythmical head-nodding, occurs in the aged and in Progressive Cerebellar Degeneration (see § 941).

(c) XII **Functional** Tremors occur in *Anxiety Neurosis*. XIII *Hysterical* tremors are sometimes very difficult to differentiate from organic disease. They are, however, usually (1) sudden in onset, following emotional trauma, (2) variable and diminished or abolished by suggestion, (3) if rigidity is present, it is of the hysterical type, *i.e.*, on passive movement, the greater the force used to overcome it the greater is the resistance.

(d) XIV **Familial** Tremor is sometimes encountered. It may be of the "intention" type and is not disabling.

(e) XV In debilitated infants **Spasmus Nutans,** a rhythmic head-nodding, with nystagmus, is seen. It resembles titubation and may be due to defective ocular fixation or to cerebellar agenesia. The prognosis is good with improvement in general health. Vitamins and sunshine, with suitable feeding, may be given with advantage.

(2) *Irregular and spasmodic involuntary movements of groups of muscles occur during rest and are increased by exertion. They are bilaterally distributed in the face, producing grimaces, and tend to be of unilateral distribution in the limbs. Voluntary movements are inco-ordinate. The condition is* CHOREA.

§ 920. Chorea.—Choreic movements are irregular, jerking, wriggling and grimacing involuntary movements. Chorea occurs in association with a number of neurological conditions.

TYPES OF CHOREA

I. Rheumatic Chorea.   IV. Senile Chorea.
II. Huntington's Chorea.   V. Apoplectiform Chorea.
III. Encephalitis.   VI. Hysterical Chorea.

§ 921. I. Rheumatic Chorea (Syn. Sydenham's Chorea).—This is a rheumatic encephalitis, with a tendency to recur and to cause cardiac damage, seen usually in children or young adults between the ages of 5 years and 20 years, and in girls three times more often than in boys.

Symptoms.—A history of rheumatic " growing pains," recurrent sore throat, rheumatic nodules or erythema, is elicited in most cases. The earliest symptom is (1) emotional instability, and the child becomes fretful, wakeful and easily tired. (2) General motor restlessness ensues, the child drops things or bumps clumsily against the furniture. (3) Spontaneous involuntary movements of groups of muscles appear, hemiplegic in distribution in the limbs, but bilaterally distributed in the face and motor cranial nerves. These jerky involuntary movements appear at rest, or they are superimposed upon voluntary movements, rendering them inco-ordinated. Thus, in picking up a pin, the choreic child will stretch out the hand, but just before the thumb and forefinger can close on the pin, the supinators of the wrist contract suddenly, jerking the hand away from the pin. After several attempts, success may be obtained. (4) In most cases, there is definite general muscular weakness. (5) Excitement and emotional instability persist through the illness, in varying degree. All types of spasmodic movement are seen in the facial, lingual and bulbar muscles, leading to grimacing, grotesque squinting, dysarthria and dysphagia. The pupils are normal, or are rarely unequal and show hippus. The hand-grip is poorly sustained, and when the arms are outstretched, the wrists become flexed and the fingers hyper-extended (the " choreic hand "). The knee-jerks may become pendular, viz., during the eliciting of the knee-jerk the quadriceps tendon suddenly contracts and holds the leg suspended in the air for a second before it flops back. Any known abnormality of the knee-jerks may be met; they may be diminished, increased or absent. The cutaneous and plantar reflexes are always normal. Tachycardia and slight cardiac dilatation are common; endocarditis may develop during or between recurrent attacks in at least a third of cases. Uncomplicated chorea is an apyrexial disease.

Flaccid Chorea (Syn. Chorea mollis). Here the movements are absent and the child is brought because " She has suddenly lost the use of her arm or leg," *i.e.*, muscular weakness predominates. Do not fall into the trap of diagnosing hemiplegia, even although the symptoms are unilateral in distribution. The plantars are flexor, the abdominals brisk, and careful physical examination will rarely fail to show slight choreic movements in the face or fingers. The paralysis, moreover, is never more than slight, although the flaccidity and lack of spontaneous movement are great.

Chorea Gravidarum is the same disease as rheumatic chorea, met in young pregnant women during the first three months of pregnancy. The disease may be serious, with great motor restlessness and delirium, and is rarely fatal.

Etiology.—The disease is a manifestation of acute rheumatism; most believe it to be a form of encephalitis.

Prognosis.—Most cases recover in from six weeks to six months; severe cases may last longer. Recurrences, with cardiac complications, are always to be feared. The incidence of rheumatic endocarditis is 20 per cent. Embolic phenomena may occur.

Treatment.—This comprises the following essentials: (1) Absolute rest in bed, with interesting adult companionship and isolation from other children. (2) Protection from injury through the violence of the movements, attained by padding the limbs or arranging pillows around the patient. (3) Systematic over-feeding with milk and farinaceous foods, in addition to the ordinary diet. In the early stages, a rubber tube should be fitted round the tube of a china feeding-cup which may otherwise be bitten off; an enamelled feeding-cup is safer. (4) Of drugs the best is aspirin. A child of ten can take 0·6 G. (10 gr.), *i.e.*, 2 tablets of soluble aspirin thrice daily after food. Older children can take 1 G. (gr. 15) thrice daily. No other drug is a substitute for aspirin unless the patient has an idiosyncrasy. With it phenobarbitone (16–30 mg.), or syrup of chloral (2 ml.) may be given for sleeplessness. In cases with great excitement give inj. phenobarbitone sod. (200 mg.) by intravenous or intramuscular injection with chlorpromazine 25 mg. thrice daily by mouth for an adult or adolescent. Morphine should not be given. If possible, the child should rest in bed until all movements have ceased for several weeks. Thereafter, a restricted life is necessary for at least six months with a convalescent holiday. Tonsillectomy should only be undertaken after complete recovery, never while movements are present. Routine tonsillectomy greatly increases the likelihood of relapse of chorea. In chorea gravidarum termination of pregnancy is seldom necessary.

§ 922. II. **Huntington's Chorea.**—This is a heredo-familial disease, characterised by (1) Bilateral Chorea and (2) Progressive Dementia. It is more common than was once supposed and it is calculated that there are 2,000 cases in England and Wales alone. It comes on gradually between the fourth and sixth decades, the commonest age of onset being 35 years. *Symptoms.*—Early dysarthria is invariably followed by coarse choreiform and jerky movements, with clumsiness of the fingers, altered handwriting and ataxia of gait. Irregular respiration and grimacing are seen. Mental deterioration is usual later but may be an early symptom. JUVENILE HUNTINGTON'S CHOREA, which is excessively rare, may produce a picture like Parkinsonism in children. There is a marked family history of the disorder (it is genetically dominant, affecting both males and females). *Diagnosis* from psychoses with multiple tics may be difficult if a family history cannot be elicited or is suppressed. *Prognosis.*—Most cases finish their lives in mental hospitals and death is usual 10–15 years from the onset. There is no certain means of telling which children in such families will develop the disease. *Treatment* is symptomatic. Chlorpromazine 25–50 mg. thrice daily may diminish the movements and calm irascibility.

III. ENCEPHALITIS (§ 893).—Cases of lethargic and other forms of encephalitis may manifest themselves first with symptoms of chorea and pains in the limbs. A careful watch should be kept for the advent of ptosis, ophthalmoplegia, or lethargy, which differentiate these cases from rheumatic chorea.

§ 923. IV. **Senile Chorea** is probably a variant of Huntington's chorea with a later age of onset. Mental symptoms are mild or absent.

§ 924. V. **Apoplectiform Chorea.**—This is due to a thrombosis in the neighbourhood of the corpus Luysii (subthalamic body) or substantia nigra. When the patient recovers from the stroke, violent choreiform movements remain, which are strictly unilateral in distribution (Hemiballismus).

VI. HYSTERICAL " CHOREA " can usually be easily diagnosed by the absence of choreic movements in the face. These are constant in all other varieties.

(3) *Slow involuntary writhing and stereotyped movements occur in one or more limbs and sometimes produce bilateral grimacing of the face, and dysarthria. The condition is* ATHETOSIS *and the onset is usually in childhood.*

§ 925. The slow, writhing movements of **Athetosis** are most commonly observed in (1) *Infantile hemiplegia* (§ 913), due to trauma at birth, encephalitis following an acute specific fever, or polio-encephalitis. The movements occur in the hemiplegic limbs, which retain some degree of power. They are spasmodic and initiated by emotion or attempts at voluntary movement. Athetosis is seen also in (2) *Cerebral diplegia* (§ 972), where it may be unilateral or bilateral in distribution. Erythroblastosis foetalis (congenital hæmolytic jaundice) is responsible for some of these cases. Commonly, the movements affect one side of the body more than the other.   Cases of (3) *Congenital Bilateral Athetosis* occur without signs of pyramidal disease, and show to the naked eye degenerative changes and a marbled appearance of the caudate nucleus and putamen of the lenticular nucleus (" status marmoratus ").   (4) Athetosis coming on in adult life is rare and is usually the result of vascular disease (especially embolism), encephalitis, syphilis, or neoplasm affecting the basal ganglia.

§ 926. In **Dystonia musculorum** the muscular movements are like those of athetosis but the spasms differ in three respects: (1) they are more prolonged, (2) they involve the muscles of the trunk, neck, chest and face, causing gross and varying distortions of the head, trunk and limbs and rendering the child helpless, (3) they occur proximally in the muscles of the pelvic and shoulder girdles.   (*a*) *Symptomatic* dystonia occurs after encephalitis or birth injury (anoxia).   (*b*) *Idiopathic* dystonia musculorum is a heredo-familial disease allied to hepato-lenticular degeneration coming on in childhood. There are no signs of mental deficiency nor of pyramidal disease, and power and

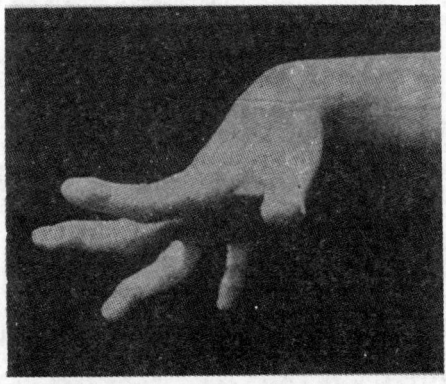

FIG. 241.—ATHETOSIS in the hand of a child with infantile hemiplegia.   The figure shows " mobile spasm " of the fingers and wrist of the right hand.

sensation are unaffected.   The disease slowly progresses and the patient is usually bedridden before adolescence.   *Treatment.*—Surgical operations in the basal ganglia or cortex may be considered, but few cases are helped by such procedures.

(4) *There are recurrent, involuntary, localised and stereotyped tricks of movement.   The condition is* TIC.

§ 927. A **Tic** is a spasmodic involuntary movement.   The pattern of the movement may be one associated with irritation, but in others the movements are often of a defensive character, *e.g.*, sudden blinking of the eyes, with or without retraction of the head, wriggling of the shoulder, shaking or tossing of the head.   The movements are violent and irregular; they do not interfere with, but are rather improved by voluntary effort.   A minor form of Tic is *Habit Spasm*, occurring usually in children between 5 and 10 years of age.   Although it may appear that the movements have originated as a habit from some peripheral source of irritation, *e.g.*, refractive errors, coryza, ill-fitting clothes, etc., it cannot be sufficiently emphasised that tics are central in origin and are not cured by removal of teeth or tonsils, nor by circumcision. The condition is sometimes associated with an Obsessive-Compulsive Neurosis (§ 1175).

The following *Types of tic* are encountered:

1. *Simple Tic.*—Sudden blinking (blepharospasm), tossing of the chin, grimacing, wriggling, jerky stereotyped movements of the arms or, less commonly, of the legs. Respiratory grunts, barks, sudden explosive laryngeal sounds also occur. (2) *Con-vulsive Tic.*—The movements are highly complex and purposeful, *e.g.*, " salaaming " or explosive and defensive movements of the whole body. 3. *Psychical Tic.*—There is no spasmodic movement, but the patient is compelled to make an explosive utterance of words or sentences, often obscene. The patient may be a child. 4. *Co-ordinated Tic.*—The patient feels impelled to execute some apparently meaningless, highly co-ordinated act, *e.g.*, twiddling a piece of string, in conditions of mental stress or boredom. 5. *Post-Encephalitic Tics.*—Following an attack of Encephalitis Lethargica (§ 837), various respiratory tics are met, *e.g.*, polypnœa, yawning, even to the extent of jaw dislocation, grunting or barking largyneal noises. Any form of tic may appear in a patient after this disease. The Post-Encephalitic tics appear to have an organic origin; some of them, in the young, are possibly associated with the psychical disturbances which follow the disease.

6. *Post-Choreic Tics.*—After an attack of rheumatic chorea, the patient may be left with a transient simple tic. The prognosis is good.

§ 928. **Blepharospasm** is an intractable state of tonic and chronic spasm in the orbicularis oculi muscles. It may follow a painful eye disease. It is seen in the elderly, as a form of facial tic in obsessional-compulsive psychoneurosis, in Miner's nystagmus (§ 1074) and in compensatory hysteria.

Diagnosis.—Tics should not be confused with *Chorea*. In tic (1) the movement is localised and stereotyped, not generalised like the irregular varied movements of chorea, (2) objects are not dropped, and (3) the hand-grip is not irregularly sustained as in chorea. Facial tics are often bilateral and must be clearly separated from Facial Hemispasm (see § 1080).

Treatment.—(1) Attend to environmental factors. Often simple removal of the child from a faulty home or school environment is necessary. (2) Psychotherapy may help, even if it is of a very simple kind. (3) Criticism of the habit is to be avoided. (4) Re-educative exercises in front of a mirror, breathing and gymnastic exercises, will help: (5) In an adult dexamphetamine 10 mg. before breakfast is worth a trial. (6) In severe exacerbations, rest in bed, with complete freedom from emotional strain, should be enjoined. In tics occurring after the age of 40, a cure is almost impossible. Psychoses may develop later.

§ 929. (5) **Spasmodic Torticollis.**—In this disease tonic and clonic contractions of the deep and superficial muscles of the neck occur, causing spasmodic turning of the head to one side and upwards, or there may be tonic extension. It occurs, like other tics, in neuropathic subjects or after encephalitis lethargica. It may result from emotional strain.

Spasm appears first in the sternomastoid and may be tonic or clonic, or both. The contra-lateral splenius capitis and trapezius are next involved, and, later, the other deep cervical muscles. Bilateral affection of the splenii causes tonic or clonic retraction of the head (retrocollic spasm). True hypertrophy of the affected muscles is frequently seen. The patient may make a " corrective gesture," touching the cheek with a finger or pushing his chin forwards when the spasm occurs. Spasms are initiated by voluntary effort (*e.g.*, lifting a chair) or emotional causes. Writer's cramp may co-exist. The disease, like other tics, is chronic, with spontaneous remissions. It should be distinguished from *congenital wry-neck*, due to birth injury of the sterno-mastoid muscle, which is contractured, with co-existing slight facial asymmetry. In *rheumatic torticollis*, there are no clonic spasms, nor do these occur in *stiff-neck* due to *cervical Pott's disease*, retro-pharyngeal abscess, or *cervical glands*.

Treatment is unsatisfactory. The disease runs a remitting course and removal from environments of tension will occasionally help. A light plastic collar may be tried, but many will not wear it. In a number of cases the tic eventually disappears. Surgical operations (section of the spinal accessory, greater and lesser occipital nerves) meet with temporary, rarely permanent success. After these operations the spasm tends to spread to other muscles. Massage, relaxation exercises and a graduated suspension of the neck have been tried. In psychological cases, psychotherapy may help.

WRITER'S CRAMP. See § 1033.

(6) FACIAL HEMISPASM (§ 1080) may follow severe Bell's palsy, or it may occur during gradual compression of the facial nerve, *e.g.*, by auditory neurofibroma. Persistent fasciculation may be seen in the muscles of the chin after severe facial palsy.

§ 930. (7) **Epilepsia partialis continuans** is a continuous form of motor cortical discharge producing coarse irregular jerkings of the limbs without disturbance of consciousness. It is associated with epileptic discharges in the E.E.G. and is found in focal cortical disease, often as an atrophic process.

(8) *There are sudden shock-like contractions of individual muscles. The condition is* MYOCLONUS.

§ 931. **Myoclonus** is the name given to shock-like contractions occurring in various muscles throughout the body. As many as ten to fifty such shocks per minute may be observed. It is seen (1) In normal individuals falling off to sleep; (2) In epileptic patients as a variety of motor petit mal, or when anticonvulsants are being withdrawn or changed. The movements may throw the patient to the floor. *Myoclonic Epilepsy* is a rare special familial form of epilepsy associated with dementia and myoclonus. (3) It is a characteristic finding in encephalitis and encephalopathy. Thus it occurs in inclusion body encephalitis, post-vaccinial encephalopathy, Schilder's disease and cerebro-macular degeneration. (4) During withdrawal of barbiturate drugs from habituated patients myoclonus as a transient symptom may cause much distress. Myoclonic jerkings may be accompanied by characteristic E.E.G. " spike and wave " discharges, some synchronous with the movements, others independent.

CLONUS. Knee or ankle clonus may be very persistent in states of spasticity. It is usually initiated by peripheral stimuli and general apprehension. Sedation and a bed-cradle help in some cases.

(9) *Flicking or quivering movements of individual muscle bundles are present. The condition is* FASCICULATION.

§ 932. **Fasciculation** or twitching of muscle bundles may be felt as " flutterings under the skin " or pass unnoticed by patients until their attention is directed to the condition. It arises in a variety of conditions affecting ventral horn cells, peripheral roots, or muscles. (1) It occurs as a transient phenomenon in *normal* muscles after fatigue or exposure to cold and in states of debility. (2) When associated with *atrophy* of muscles of segmental or spinal distribution, or extensor plantar responses, the implication is much more serious and suggests a progressive phase of motor neurone disease, peroneal muscular atrophy or syringomyelia. In progressive bulbar palsy it is seen at the crenated edges of the wasted tongue. (3) It occurs in a variety of radiculo-pathies, *e.g.*, cervical spondylosis, thoracic inlet syndrome, and disc lesions. In *myopathy* and *myasthenia gravis* it is usually absent.

GROUP VIII. INCO-ORDINATION OR ATAXIA

The patient shows NO PARALYSIS, *but reveals a* CLUMSINESS *or* UNSTEADI-NESS ON MOVING THE LIMBS, *especially with movements of precision. The* BALANCE *is Upset and the* GAIT IS UNSTEADY *or* REELING. *The condition is* ATAXIA.

In conditions of flaccid paralysis of muscles weakness may be so great that the patient may move the affected limbs in an awkward fashion simulating ataxia. In the absence of defective sense of position or cerebellar signs the clumsiness can be attributed to muscular paresis. *Choreic movements* render patients ataxic but should be easily recognised for they occur with the limbs at rest or supported. For *Disorders of Gait* see § 843.

Ataxia, clinically considered, may be of three types:—(A) VESTIBULAR, (B) CEREBELLAR or (C) SENSORY.

§ 933. (A) **Vestibular Ataxia** is typically *acute* in onset and accompanied by vertigo, vomiting and disordered balance. It is usually *paroxysmal* but it may be continuous for weeks. Commonly the patient cannot stand up or even sit up and there is gross ataxia of movement, with loss of tonus in the ipsilateral limbs. Jerking lateral nystagmus and subjective vertigo are present. See Vertigo (§ 826). The commonest causes are *peripheral*: (1) VESTIBULAR NEURONITIS (§ 828); (2) ACUTE LABY-RINTHITIS (§ 828); (3) MÉNIÈRE'S SYNDROME (§ 831). In AUDITORY NEUROFIBROMA (§ 1083) the ataxia and vertigo may be paroxysmal or continuous. When the cause is *central, e.g.*, tumour of the medulla or cerebellum, there are added signs of involvement of the brain-stem (vertical nystagmus and diplopia), or of the cerebellar peduncles (forced rotation of the trunk).

§ 934. (B) **Cerebellar Ataxia** causes an unsteadiness and lack of balance which is unaffected by closure of the eyes. Cerebellar signs are present which depend on specific tests.

The CLINICAL SIGNS OF CEREBELLAR LESIONS and irritative signs are:—

ACUTE lesions of the cerebellum produce ipsilateral hypotonia with ataxia of movement. In CHRONIC destructive lesions of the cerebellum, rhythmical jerking and inco-ordination of purposive movements of the limbs (intention tremor) is seen. This also produces disturbances of the rate and rhythm of alternating movements of the limbs, *e.g.*, pronation and supination of the wrists.

HYPOTONIA of the ipsilateral voluntary muscles is such that the extended arm cannot maintain its posture on the affected side; it sags and becomes pronated. The affected limb, if grasped firmly at the forearm, can be shaken like a flail. Excessive passive hyperextension at the wrists or elbow joints compared with the normal side can be demonstrated.

JERKING NYSTAGMUS is present with a slow, coarse movement, on looking to the side of the lesion, and a rapid, finer nystagmus on looking from the side of the lesion. This lateral horizontal nystagmus is often accompanied by defective conjugate movement of the eyes, *e.g.*, there may be coarse horizontal nystagmus of the right eye on looking to the right, with defective inward movement of the left eye, or a general unwillingness to look to the side of the lesion. Vertical nystagmus on upward or downward movement of the eye occurs in lesions of the brain-stem. The fixation jerking nystagmus of cerebellar disease is probably dependent on lack of tone in the ocular muscles. A rare phenomenon in acute lesions is " skew-deviation " of the eyes.

CEREBELLAR ATTITUDE. The occiput on the affected side is turned downwards and the chin tilted to the opposite side. Occasionally this position of the head is reversed. In lesions of the posterior vermis, the head may be tilted backwards, with a tendency for the patient to fall backwards.

TITUBATION is a rhythmical tremor of the unsupported head. It is seen in chronic degenerative cerebellar diseases and in disseminated sclerosis.

CEREBELLAR SPEECH. The articulation assumes a syllabic-staccato quality, or articulation is slurred.

INTENTION TREMOR is shown by the " finger–nose " or " heel–knee " test. As the moving finger or heel approaches its objective a coarse oscillation develops, preventing precise execution of the test.

DYSDIADOCHOKINESIS. There is difficulty in performing rapidly alternating voluntary movements, *e.g.*, clenching and unclenching the fingers, shaking the forearms, tapping the knees with the palms of the hands. On the affected side the movements are slower, irregular in rhythm and the patient moves many other muscles in the affected limb in the attempt to overcome this.

DYSMETRIA. The inco-ordination of voluntary movement may show itself by a tendency to overshoot the mark with the " finger–nose " or " heel–knee " test.

PAST-POINTING (Bárány). The patient is asked to stretch out one arm and point the forefinger. He is then made to move the arm in the vertical plane and with closed eyes bring his finger back to its original position. After a unilateral cerebellar lesion the arm deviates outwards on the side of the lesion.

GAIT.—This is staggering or reeling. It may be noticed especially when the patient turns in walking. On attempting to walk in a straight line he deviates to the affected side. There is greater difficulty in balancing on the leg of the side affected.

When the upper limbs are outstretched, the one on the affected side tends to fall away or, if it is briskly tapped, it bounces or oscillates abnormally compared with the sound side.

In lesions of the *vermis* or *flocculo-nodular lobe* (a) the symptoms tend to be bilateral in distribution and most marked in the lower limbs, (b) there is ataxic dysarthria, and (c) retraction of the head may be present if the lesion is far back.

CEREBELLAR ATAXIA may be *Acute, Subacute* or *Chronic* in onset.

CAUSES OF CEREBELLAR ATAXIA

Acute.

I. Basilar artery insufficiency.
II. Toxic poisoning.
III. Disseminated sclerosis.
IV. Acute encephalomyelopathy.
V. Cerebellar vascular Accidents.
VI. Meningo-vascular syphilis.
VII. Cerebellar abscess.

Subacute or Chronic.

VIII. Posterior fossa tumours.
IX. Progressive cerebellar degeneration (Olivo-ponto-cerebellar atrophy).
X. Syringobulbia.
XI. Platybasia.
XII. Spino-cerebellar ataxias, especially Friedreich's ataxia.

In Infants.

XIII. Cerebellar developmental defects.

Acute Cerebellar Ataxia

§ 935. I. BASILAR ARTERY INSUFFICIENCY.—Patients with atheromatous narrowing of the vertebral, basilar and internal carotid arteries may have attacks of ataxia with dysarthria and dysphagia; if the disturbance of balance is severe the patient may fall (§ 904).

II. Toxic poisoning with alcohol, barbiturates or hydantoin drugs causes ataxia and disturbed balance. It is abolished by withdrawing the toxic substance. The signs may closely simulate those of an acute or chronic cerebellar lesion.

III. Disseminated Sclerosis. In a few cases vertigo and unsteady gait may be the first symptoms. The diagnosis then may be confusing unless there is evidence of changes in parts of the nervous system other than the cerebellum (§ 952). The plaques causing these symptoms are often symmetrically placed in the pons or medulla and involve the cerebellar tracts. The outlook in these cerebellar cases is poor. In late cases cerebellar ataxia, nystagmus and slurred speech are often present.

IV. Acute Encephalomyelopathy. Following an exanthematous fever, inoculation or vaccination acute cerebellar signs may appear (§ 895).

V. Cerebellar Vascular Accidents. *Thrombosis* may occur in a cerebellar artery from atheroma. *Hæmorrhage* results from atheroma, saccular aneurysm or an angiomatous malformation. Blood usually escapes into the meninges with signs of Subarachnoid Hæmorrhage (§ 853).

The patient is suddenly seized with intense Vertigo, Vomiting *and* Diplopia *and often reels or falls to the ground without losing consciousness. Crossed dissociated sensory changes are found with ipsilateral cranial nerve palsies. The condition is* Thrombosis of the Posterior Inferior Cerebellar Artery.

§ 936. Thrombosis of the Posterior inferior cerebellar artery (Syn. Cerebellar apoplexy). The symptoms are quite unlike those of other vascular lesions. The artery supplies a wedge-shaped area in the superior quadrant of one side of the medulla. Within the area of softening lie: (1) the fibres of the direct cerebellar tract and inferior cerebellar peduncle, (2) the lower part of the sensory nucleus of the trigeminal, (3) the spino-thalamic tract, (4) nuclei of lower cranial nerves, (5) autonomic fibres descending to the cervical sympathetic (Fig. 223 and § 809).

Symptoms.—The onset is sudden, with vertigo, reeling or falling and double vision. Sudden facial pain of trigeminal distribution may herald the attack. Consciousness is rarely lost. The patient cannot sit up because of vertigo and is usually dysarthric and dysphagic from paralysis of the palate, pharynx and vocal cord on the side of the lesion. The corneal reflex on the side of the lesion is abolished; and sensitivity to pain and temperature is impaired on that side of the face, and the opposite half of the body. Touch sensation is unaffected. Horner's syndrome (enophthalmos, ptosis of the upper lid and small pupil) is seen on the side of the lesion. There is jerking nystagmus to the affected side, and hypotonia and ataxia of the ipsilateral limbs. The plantar responses are flexor as the pyramids are supplied by the anterior spinal artery.

Diagnosis.—The patient is much more ill than with an attack of vestibular neuronitis. The ipsilateral cranial nerve palsies and crossed dissociated hemianæsthesia to pain and temperature are pathognomonic in a lesion of sudden onset.

Etiology.—Signs of systemic atheroma or hypertension may be absent. Women are more affected than men. The age incidence is 40-60 years.

Prognosis.—Most cases recover in a remarkable way after some weeks or months, but a partial residual crossed and dissociated anæsthesia may remain, with a small pupil and drooping eyelid on the side of the lesion. Cerebellar signs disappear soon after the patient begins to walk and may vanish completely. Death is rare and due to propagation of clot into the basilar artery.

Treatment.—Persistent vomiting at the onset may require injections of chlorpromazine 50 mg. intramusc. or prochlorperazine (Stemetil). Pain in the face or headache if severe is alleviated by pethidine 25–50 mg. intramusc. Nasal feeding may be required at the onset and care should be taken to see that the patient does not become dehydrated. It is advisable to get the patient out of bed as soon as his equilibrium and strength permit.

§ 937. In **Thrombosis of the Anterior Inferior Cerebellar Artery** the symptoms are similar but *deafness* and *facial palsy* also occur, simulating a lesion in the lateral recess.

VI. MENINGO-VASCULAR SYPHILIS (§§ 887, 907) rarely affects the cerebellum. The diagnosis is made by the coexistence of syphilitic pupils or by examining the blood and C.S.F.

§ 938. VII. CEREBELLAR ABSCESS is a complication of acute suppurative mastoiditis now rarely seen. The onset of an otitic abscess is often extremely insidious. Nystagmus, ophthalmoplegia, ipsilateral cerebellar signs, occipital headache and papilloedema may be late in appearing (§ 891).

Subacute and Chronic Cerebellar Ataxia

VIII. POSTERIOR FOSSA TUMOURS may be (*a*) intra-cerebellar, or (*b*) extra-cerebellar.

§ 939. (*a*) **Intra-cerebellar Tumours, Angiomata and Tuberculomata.**—In CHILDREN cerebellar tumours are relatively common; they are mostly of two types: (1) The malignant *Medulloblastoma*, growing in the mid-line from the roof of the fourth ventricle and killing the patient within a year. (2) The more benign cystic *Astrocytoma* or the vascular and cystic *Hæmangioma*, usually in a lateral lobe. This latter is sometimes associated with angioma of the retina and cysts and cavernomas of the liver (Lindau).

Symptoms.—Papilloedema is intense, headache and vomiting occur early due to hydrocephalus. The signs are those of mid-line, or sensory fifth cranial nerve or bulbar palsies; and bilateral pyramidal signs may be present. In children the knee-jerks and ankle-jerks disappear and there may be great hypotonia. In ADULTS *Astrocytoma* and *Hæmangioma* also occur, and *Metastatic Carcinoma* is a common intra-cerebellar growth. *Angiomatous malformations* are rare at all ages. *Treatment* is surgical. Preliminary tapping of the ventricles may relieve symptoms until decompression can be undertaken. *Tuberculoma* and *Cerebellar abscess* (§ 891) can be successfully treated surgically, without supervening meningitis, if appropriate antibiotics are used.

§ 940. (*b*) **Extra-cerebellar Tumours,** usually in adults, are either benign *á coustic* neurofibromata or Meningiomas. Signs of involvement of the eighth, seventh or fifth cranial nerves often precede the appearance of cerebellar signs for years. A ACOUSTIC NEUROFIBROMA (see § 1083) may cause cerebellar or vestibular ataxia in those of 30–50 years of age. Progressive nerve deafness, tinnitus and early diminution or loss of the labyrinth response to hot and cold water (§ 1143) are characteristic of this tumour.

§ 941. IX. **Progressive Cerebellar Degeneration.**—Two chief forms occur sporadically between the ages of 50 and 70 years. (*a*) **Olivo-ponto-cerebellar atrophy** (Dejerine and Thomas) causes progressive cerebellar ataxia of the trunk and extremities in late middle life. Balance is defective and the patient begins to fall about. Titubation of the head may be seen, with slurred speech and occasionally nystagmoid jerks. Sustained nystagmus is rare. Extensor plantar responses may occur and the knee- and ankle-jerks are occasionally absent. *Diagnosis.*—The condition may be confused with tabes dorsalis or with subacute combined degeneration of the cord (Table LVII). *Etiology.*—There is degeneration of the olives, pontine nuclei and cerebellum of unknown origin. The *Prognosis* is poor and the patient deteriorates to a chairbound state in five to ten years. Mental vagueness may occur. *Treatment* fails to prevent progress. Care should be taken to protect the patient from the effects of falls.

(*b*) **Parenchymatous Cerebellar Degeneration** (Gordon Holmes) in which the cerebellar cortex and Purkinje cells chiefly suffer, occurs in middle life. It may be associated with chronic alcoholism or carcinoma. Dysarthria, ataxia, intention tremor, titubation of the head and grossly unsteady gait are present and are slowly progressive. In cases where alcohol is a factor, its withdrawal is said to stop the disease progressing. There is no specific therapy.

§ 942. X. SYRINGOBULBIA and MEDULLARY NEOPLASMS.—By interference with the cerebellar tracts, the pyramidal and sensory projection fibres, bulbar nuclei and oculopupillary fibres, these diseases produce characteristic anatomical lesions, bilateral in distribution. They are slow in onset. Characteristic of *syringobulbia* is the dissociated anæsthesia, and there may be evidence of syringomyelia, wasted hands, painless whitlows and scoliosis (§ 1005). Signs of increasing intracranial pressure, headache and vomiting, may be late in *pontine or medullary tumours*. These tumours are usually infiltrating gliomas.

§ 943. XI. **Platybasia** is a rare condition of hypoplasia and softening of the skull base so that the basi-occipital bone becomes " mushroomed " into the posterior fossa by the atlas. Ataxia, nystagmus, bilateral extensor plantar responses and somatic signs like those of Syringomyelia in the upper limbs develop as the result of traction and distortion of the medulla, cerebellum and lowest cranial nerves. The *Diagnosis* is made radiologically. Spinal puncture may show subarachnoid block. *Treatment* by sub-occipital decompression has met with a measure of success.

§ 944. XII. **Spino-cerebellar Ataxias.**—(*a*) *Heredo-familial* and (*b*) *Acquired* forms are described. (*a*) There are a number of different syndromes in which heredo-familial factors are evident. These affect in varying degrees the cerebellum and cerebellar tracts, pyramidal tracts, posterior columns and optic nerves. All except Friedreich's Ataxia are very rare.

An adolescent with CLUB-FOOT *and* SCOLIOSIS *gradually develops a progressively disabling* ATAXIA *of the limbs and trunk,* DYSARTHRIA, *and absence of tendon reflexes. The disease is* FRIEDREICH'S ATAXIA.

§ 945. **Friedreich's Ataxia.**—*Symptoms* develop insidiously in childhood or early adult life, or become apparent after an acute illness. (1) Pes cavus and kypho-scoliosis have usually been present since early childhood; claw-toes are often seen. (2) An unsteady, reeling gait gradually develops and the patient is soon confined to a wheel-chair. The speech becomes " scanning " or syllabic, a fine nystagmus may be evident and often rhythmical shaking of the head (titubation). Intention tremor is present in the arms and there is ataxia of the legs. (3) Claw-hand with wasting of the intrinsic muscles may occur, and the legs may be wasted below the knees. (4) The tendon reflexes disappear early, from disease of the posterior columns, but there is seldom any loss of proprioceptive sensation until late in the disease. (5) The pyramidal responses are extensor, and absent or diminished abdominal reflexes are found: the legs, however, are usually not spastic. (6) Rarely optic atrophy is found. Heart-block due to myocardial disease may occur. The *Diagnosis* from juvenile tabes dorsalis is made by finding kypho-scoliosis, pes cavus and cerebellar signs. In disseminated sclerosis these orthopædic deformities are not found, and the tendon reflexes are rarely absent. The condition is closely allied to peroneal muscular atrophy. *Etiology.*—There is degeneration of the dorsal spino-cerebellar tracts, the posterior columns, the pyramidal tracts and the cells of Clarke's column. *Prognosis.*—Death often occurs in middle life from intercurrent disease connected with the patient's bedridden state. *Treatment* is symptomatic.

§ 946. **Hereditary Ataxia** (Marie) is much rarer and resembles Friedreich's Ataxia in the occurrence of cerebellar ataxia, ataxic dysarthria, deformities and pyramidal signs. The differences are three: (*a*) the onset is always in *adult* life, (*b*) the tendon reflexes are always exaggerated, and (*c*) optic atrophy is common. Occasionally Argyll-Robertson pupils are found in this disease.

§ **947.** (*b*) **Acquired (Carcinomatous) Degeneration of Cerebellar and Spinal tracts** may occur in association with carcinoma of the lung, stomach or ovary. The neuropathy affects the Purkinje cells of the cerebellar cortex; the brain-stem, spinal cord and peripheral nerves may also be involved. This carcinogenic spino-cerebellar degeneration is not due to invasion by secondary malignant deposits, but is a toxic or nutritional change. Dermatomyositis may be found in the skeletal muscles, and this too has a high correlation incidence with carcinoma, especially of the bronchus.

XIII. In **Infants** cerebellar signs may appear after *Acute Encephalo-myelopathy* or may be due to *Developmental defects* (*e.g.*, Arnold-Chiari Syndrome, Agenesis of the Cerebellum) or *Birth Injury* (Cerebro-cerebellar Diplegia). *Anti-convulsants* cause toxic ataxia in epileptic children. In *Cerebellar Tumour* the signs are steadily progressive.

§ **948.** (C) **Sensory Ataxia** occurs in lesions of the proprioceptive sensory afferent fibres, whether in the peripheral nerves, posterior columns of the spinal cord, thalamus or cerebral cortex. It is usually possible to demonstrate loss of joint-sense (sense of position and passive movement). Voluntary movements are executed in an irregular fashion and it is characteristic of this form of ataxia that it is increased when the patient's eyes are closed.

CAUSES OF SENSORY ATAXIA

I. Tabes Dorsalis.
II. Subacute Combined Degeneration of the Cord.
III. Sensory Polyneuritis (Metabolic, Toxic, Nutritional or Carcinomatous).
IV. Disseminated Sclerosis.
V. Spinal Cord Compression.
VI. Toxic Encephalopathy.
VII. Parietal Lobe Lesions.
VIII. Thalamic Lesions.

§ **949.** I. TABES DORSALIS (Syn. Locomotor Ataxy) should be diagnosed in the *Pre-ataxic Stage* if treatment is to be effective. The presenting symptom in the *early stages* is usually the characteristic " lightning-pains " (§ 1022). In the *later* stages the tabetic is ataxic because of the loss of afferent sensory impressions from his muscles and joints. At first there is remarkable compensation for the loss of joint-sense and the patient, by concentrating his attention on his movements, is able to make great use of his remaining powers. In these cases the ataxia is latent but may be revealed by the heel–knee or finger–nose tests when the patient's eyes are shut, or by asking him to walk backwards or sideways, stand on one foot or turn round quickly. In the last stages the ataxia is manifest. The gait is wide-based and staggering, support is needed in walking, and the patient holds on to the furniture in turning. In walking, the eyes are fixed on the ground for additional visual control of movement and the legs are lifted high in the air and stamped on the heels, owing to loss of joint-sense. The diagnosis of tabes in this stage rarely presents any difficulty.

A middle-aged, sallow-complexioned patient complains of PINS AND NEEDLES IN THE FINGERS AND FEET *and a* SORENESS OF THE TONGUE.

The GAIT IS UNSTEADY. *There is* ACHYLIA *and the blood count shows* MEGALOCYTIC ANÆMIA. *The disease is* SUBACUTE COMBINED DEGENERATION OF THE SPINAL CORD.

§ 950. II. Subacute Combined Degeneration of the Spinal Cord is a disease of gradual onset in middle-aged or elderly persons, usually associated with the blood picture of a megalocytic (pernicious anæmia) (§ 548). *Symptoms.—(a) Polyneuritic stage.* The patient comes for his nervous symptoms and not his anæmia. Only rarely does the disease develop in patients who are being treated for pernicious anæmia. (1) Pins and needles and numbness in the hands and feet are early symptoms. The patient may sit rubbing his fingers and thumbs together as he tells of these sensations. (2) Tenderness of the calf muscles is an extremely common early symptom. When it is present, and the plan ar responses are flexor, it probably indicates that the disease is in the polyneuritic stage and treatment may be curative. (3) Objective sensory impairment to all forms of sensibility occurs, of " stocking and glove " distribution in the periphery of the limbs. Girdle pains round the waist and under the costal margins are not uncommon. Deep forms of sensibility are particularly affected, producing (4) Sensory Ataxia from loss of joint-sense. (5) Flaccidity of the lower limb muscles is common. (*b*) *Spinal stage*—the appearance of extensor plantar responses indicates that the disease now involves the spinal cord. The tendon reflexes may be increased or diminished, depending on the relative degree of pyramidal and peripheral nerve or posterior column involvement. In the late stages hesitancy and dribbling after micturition appear, also overflow incontinence of urine and incontinence of fæces. The gait exhibits a combination of spasticity and ataxia—the spastic-ataxic gait. The toes are dragged, the feet are lifted jerkily from the ground and the patient staggers when he turns or walks, holding on to furniture. The patient at the end of his illness may show a spastic or flaccid paraplegia which renders him bedridden. Transient local œdema of the extremities occurs. Optic atrophy has been described. In the later stages (now very rarely seen) hæmorrhages occur in the retina, due to the severe anæmia. The *spinal fluid* is usually normal. *Mental and other Symptoms.*—In association with marked polyneuritic symptoms, and in the late stages of the disease, mild mental confusion may occur. Korsakoff's psychosis may be met (§ 1184).

Clinical Types.—(1) *Flaccid type*—the muscles of the legs are tender and flaccid, the tendon jerks abolished, with absence of sense of position and vibration in the feet and toes. The symptoms resemble those of polyneuritis, but eventually an extensor plantar response appears. (2) *Spastic type*—the legs show clasp-knife rigidity, increased tendon jerks with clonus, and extensor plantar responses. Cutaneous sensitivity is impaired in minor degree over the distal parts of the limbs or hyperæsthesia is present. In the final stages the spastic legs become flexed, and there is incontinence of urine. When the process is most marked in the pyramidal tracts, the spastic picture predominates, when more in the posterior and lateral columns and peripheral nerves, the limbs become flaccid.

Diagnosis.—The combination of tenderness of the small muscles of the feet, with sensory ataxia and extensor plantar responses is characteristic. Look for atrophic glossitis with soreness of the edges of the tongue. Achylia gastrica is almost invariable. The blood and bone marrow show the findings of pernicious anæmia (§ 548); the serum B_{12} is below 100 $\mu\mu$g./ml. In other types of severe anæmia and in *Sprue* neurological signs resembling subacute combined degeneration may be found, but these are probably caused by peripheral neuropathy. In gastric, bronchial and other *Carcinoma* and in some Nutritional Disorders a myelopathy may occur, as well as changes in the peripheral nerves and muscles. It is wise to limit the name subacute combined degeneration to cord changes found with pernicious anæmia. *Spinocerebellar ataxia* and *Progressive cerebellar degeneration* may both produce ataxia, with absent tendon reflexes and extensor responses.

Etiology.—The disease commences in most cases as a polyneuritis (" demyelination neuritis"), but the characteristic lesions are found in the spinal cord, particularly in the posterior columns, the pyramidal tracts and, to lesser extent, in the spinothalamic tracts (Fig. 242). The cord lesions are focal, with ascending and descending degeneration proceeding from the diseased foci (" funicular myelopathy ").

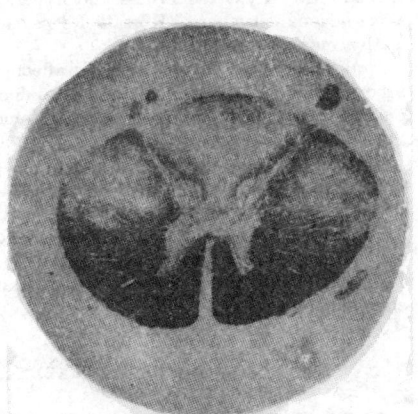

Fig. 242.—SUBACUTE COMBINED DEGENERATIO: OF THE SPINAL CORD showing degeneration in the posterior and lateral columns (Weigert-Pal stain for myelin).

Prognosis.—Improvement in the neurological signs usually begins within two months of starting treatment. In almost all cases, in those diagnosed in the early stage complete recovery is the rule.

Treatment.—(a) *Specific.* Give cyanocobalamin B.P. (vitamin B_{12}) 100 micrograms intramuscularly daily for 10 days and twice weekly for 6–8 weeks. Often larger doses will be found necessary before the paræsthesiæ disappear. A maintenance dose will be needed for the rest of the patient's life and it should be impressed on all that omission of treatment will result in relapse of the anæmia and of the neurological symptoms. If iron deficiency exists this should be treated by an oral iron preparation. Folic acid has no place in the treatment of subacute combined degeneration of the cord, for the neurological symptoms are not influenced and may be accelerated by it. (b) *General.* Rest in bed will be necessary at first. In bed the patient's feet may have to be lightly splinted to avoid dropping.   A bed cradle is advised.   Frenkl's bed and walking exercises will help ataxic patients during convalescence.

III. SENSORY POLYNEURITIS.   Purely sensory forms of polyneuritis are rare: but in polyneuritis due to diabetes, alcohol, porphyria, nutritional defects and carcinoma sensory ataxia may occur, as well as in other types (see § 974).

(a) *Diabetic neuropathy* in the early stages causes little except absent ankle-jerks, cramps and tingling in the limbs, skin abrasions and ulcers which heal slowly.   In more advanced cases there are posterior column and peripheral nerve changes, "diabetic pseudo-tabes" with arthropathies, perforating ulcers and sensory ataxia (see § 980).

(b) *Alcoholic neuropathy* may cause sensory ataxia.   A history of alcoholism can be confirmed if the patient has morning nausea or vomiting, or chronic looseness of the bowels.   Great tenderness and hyperæsthesia of the limbs may be present and a confusional psychosis (Korsakoff's psychosis) is common.   Wernicke's encephalopathy may be present (§ 979).

(c) *Intermittent Acute Porphyria* affects women more than men and is due to an inborn error of metabolism.   Sudden abdominal pain simulates intestinal obstruction or peritonitis, and neurological symptoms include confusional states and absent knee- and ankle-jerks (§ 415).

(d) *Nutritional neuropathy* occurs in (1) persons living on an ill-balanced diet (not necessarily small amounts of food), in aged persons living alone and also in war-time prison camps, (2) in Pellagra, (3) in Beri-beri (§ 981).

(e) *Carcinomatous neuropathy* is a rare form of sensory polyneuritis (rarely motor) due to a metabolic or toxic cause and not to infiltration of nerves with carcinoma cells. Remissions may occur.   There is a primary growth in the lung, breast, ovary or elsewhere (§ 984).

TABLE LVII

	Subacute Combined Degeneration of the Cord.	Polyneuritis.	Tabes Dorsalis.	Friedreich's Ataxia.
Age.	Usually middle-aged and elderly.	Any age.	Any age (Juvenile Tabes).	Patient a child or young adult.
Speech.	Speech normal.	Speech normal.	Speech normal.	Ataxic dysarthria.
Sensory symptoms.	Pins and needles in the fingers and feet.	Cramp in legs.	"Lightning Pains."	Painless.
Muscular tenderness.	Muscular tenderness.	Marked muscular tenderness in most cases.	Muscles and tendons insensitive to deep pressure.	No muscular tenderness.
Reflexes.	Plantars usually extensor.	Plantars absent.	Plantars flexor.	Plantars extensor.
Special characteristics.	Achylia and often picture of pernicious anæmia.	Glycosuria in diabetic neuritis.	Characteristic spinal fluid findings in 65 per cent.	Pes cavus and scoliosis.

IV. In DISSEMINATED SCLEROSIS, a patch of disease in the posterior columns or fillet will cause sensory ataxia, acute or gradual in onset.   The diagnosis is made by other symptoms and signs: viz., (1) transient attacks of uselessness in the limbs, of paræsthesiæ, of diplopia or of blindness, or (2) evidence of disseminated lesions in the nervous system, *e.g.*, pallor of the temporal halves of the optic discs, nystagmus (§ 952).

V. SPINAL CORD COMPRESSION. Tumours and cervical spondylosis compressing the posterior columns of the spinal cord or the cerebellar tracts cause an ataxic gait. Persistent root pains on one or other side often precede the objective sensory changes. A sensory level should be sought clinically, spinal puncture with manometry, withdrawal of C.S.F. for analysis and myodil radiography may be undertaken prior to surgical exploration.

VI. TOXIC ENCEPHALOPATHY due to chronic alcoholism, abuse of barbiturates or sensitivity to anticonvulsant drugs in epileptics, the cumulative effects of antispasmodic drugs in Parkinsonism and inhalation of industrial poisons, may cause ataxia of the limbs with mental confusion.

VII. PARIETAL LOBE ATAXIA in an unco-operative patient may closely simulate cerebellar ataxia. Sense of position is defective in the affected limbs with astereognosis and impairment of other discriminative aspects of sensation. Infiltrating gliomata or cerebro-vascular accidents may be causal.

VIII. THALAMIC LESIONS produce a sensory hemiplegia affecting chiefly pain and temperature. Burning causalgic pain may occur in the analgesic limbs, especially if they are lightly touched or stroked. Sensory ataxia is present from defect of the sense of position.

Treatment of Sensory Ataxia.—After removal or treatment of the cause, if this is possible, much can be done by re-education of existing healthy mechanisms to improve the residual ataxia. The exercises designed by Frenkl are of great use. These need the co-operation of a skilled teacher, but much can be done by the patient at home. (1) *Bed exercises*—Lying on his bed or on a couch, the patient should be taught to bring his great toe accurately on to various squares drawn on a smooth inclined board, placed under his feet. Sitting up, with the board flat, he does the same movements with each heel. (2) *Walking exercises*—Now, getting up, he practises walking on footmarks chalked on the floor, or painted on a strip of linoleum. Later, walking sideways, walking on tiptoe, heeling and toeing a line are practised. Weighting the boots may give increased security. The hands are trained by means of chessmen or draughts and a draught-board, or with marbles on a solitaire board.

GROUP IX. MONOPLEGIA

There is gross paralysis of one arm or leg.   The condition is MONOPLEGIA.

§ **951.** MONOPLEGIA results from a cerebral, spinal or peripheral (plexus or nerve) lesion. The lower face is sometimes affected along with the arm —FACIOBRACHIAL MONOPLEGIA. When the leg is affected, we speak of CRURAL MONOPLEGIA.

The onset may be (A) Sudden, or (B) Gradual. Cerebral causes are commoner than spinal or peripheral.

CAUSES OF MONOPLEGIA

(A) Sudden in Onset.

I. CEREBRAL VASCULAR ACCIDENT, e.g., embolism, or middle or anterior cerebral artery thrombosis.
II. POLIOMYELITIS.
III. DISSEMINATED SCLEROSIS.
IV. Ischæmic paralysis of arm or leg.
V. Encephalitis and Rheumatic chorea.
VI. Brachial or Sacral plexus injury (e.g., Obstetrical).

(B) Gradual in Onset.

VII. PRIMARY OR SECONDARY CEREBRAL NEOPLASMS.
VIII. SUBDURAL HÆMATOMA.
IX. SPINAL TUMOUR.
X. MOTOR NEURONE DISEASE.
XI. Paralytic brachial neuritis.
XII. Infiltrating lesions of the brachial plexus, e.g., carcinoma or Hodgkin's disease.

XIII. HYSTERICAL MONOPLEGIA is sudden or gradual in onset (§§ 952, 1173).

Clinical Examination.—Many cases are seen after sleep or unconsciousness following head injury or surgical anæsthesia. Cerebral lesions in the stage of flaccidity may cause perplexity. If the lesion is thought to be cerebral look for (1) lower facial asymmetry, (2) dysphasia, (3) weakness of dorsiflexion of the ipsilateral foot, (4) hemianopia, (5) diminished abdominal reflexes or (6) an extensor response on the side of the monoplegia. Lesions of the brachial plexus produce segmental paralysis of muscles. Always palpate the axilla, supraclavicular region and pelvis.

(A) SUDDEN *Monoplegia.*

I. CEREBRAL VASCULAR ACCIDENT. Make certain, by looking for lower facial weakness, increased tendon reflexes or absent abdominal responses, that the weakness is cerebral and not due to a cerebellar lesion with hypotonia. Embolism or thrombosis affecting the cortical or subcortical branches of the middle cerebral or anterior cerebral artery may cause monoplegia—crural in anterior cerebral occlusion (§ 809). Embolism may occur in auricular fibrillation, infective endocarditis, or from suppurative lung disease (§ 905). Following head injury, suspect acute extradural hæmatoma from damage to the middle meningeal artery.

II. ACUTE POLIOMYELITIS (§ 898).

A young adult complains that: " My leg has suddenly begun to drag," or " My arm has suddenly become useless " ; there may have been double vision or precipitancy of micturition. The disease is probably DISSEMINATED SCLEROSIS.

§ 952. III. **Disseminated Sclerosis** (Syn. Multiple Sclerosis) is due to scattered areas of demyelination in the spinal cord, brain stem, optic nerves and cerebellum appearing at intervals over many years, commencing between the ages of 20–45.

Symptoms.—Sudden loss of power in an arm or leg may be the presenting symptom but other initial complaints are common: (1) sudden onset of double vision, " I can see two of everything, doctor "; (2) sudden temporary unilateral blindness (retro-bulbar neuritis) (see § 1129); (3) numbness, tingling, or pins and needles in a limb, and (4) weakness of the urinary bladder with precipitate micturition. The essential characteristics of the lesions in this disease are (i.) their *acute development at irregular intervals* and (ii.) their *scattered distribution*. It will be realised that any conceivable type of neurological symptoms or sign can occur in this disease, *e.g.*, (5) intention tremor, (6) sensory ataxia, (7) cerebellar ataxia, (8) nuclear or supranuclear cranial nerve palsies, (9) scanning speech, (10) fits and even hemianopia.   The speech is often characterised by slow separation of the syllables, like the scanning of prosody, with slurring of the articulation.   The *intention tremor* merits special description; it appears on voluntary movement, not during the active phase of the movement, but when the object is about to be attained.   Thus in the finger–nose test the finger is brought accurately to the neighbourhood of the nose, then violent oscillations appear before the nose is eventually touched.   A random involuntary movement made by the affected limb may however show no oscillation or tremor.   This ataxia is not increased by closing of the eyes.   When the complaint is of " uselessness " in the limbs, sensory ataxia with dysmetria increased by closing the eyes may be found to be present, with impairment of sense of position.   Slight monoplegic weakness is often entirely missed through insufficient examination; " neuritis," writer's cramp, " rheumatism " or hysteria is diagnosed erroneously.

When such cases are examined for one or other of the following signs not many cases of disseminated sclerosis will be missed: (1) One or other plantar response may be extensor.   (2) Rapid tiring or diminution of abdominal reflexes, especially the lower, should always be looked for. (3) Examine the optic discs for pallor of the temporal halves.   (4) Test vibration sensibility over the tibial malleoli; it is frequently diminished or absent.   (5) Look for nystagmus.   Nystagmus, as an isolated sign, is of little use in diagnosis, but combined with any of the above signs it affords valuable evidence of organic disease.   The difficulties of diagnosis are often increased by the patient's suggestibility, or by her making light of the symptoms.

In early *remitting* cases the initial symptom is often acute in onset and severe in degree.   It lasts, however, only a few weeks, then slowly clears up, perhaps with no residual physical signs.   The recovery may be complete in early days, but subsequent lesions leave behind them residual weakness and physical signs, often an intensification of the original symptoms with signs of spread.   In the *chronic progressive* type the symptoms slowly develop from the onset.

In the *later stage of the disease* the gait becomes spastic and ataxic, and the patient holds on to the furniture in walking, or walks with one or two sticks, or is bedridden.   Flexor spasms are added to ankle and patellar clonus in the lower limbs and interfere with sleep.   Precipitancy, even incontinence of urine occur.   Ataxia, either sensory or cerebellar, is manifest, with intention tremor, nystagmus, titubation (oscillation of the head) and scanning speech.   Remissions cease to occur; finally, contracture of the flexor muscles sets in with great loss of power, incontinence of urine and fæces, and bedsores.   Advanced cases often show characteristic cheerfulness, lack of insight, and emotional unrestraint such as may sometimes be seen in the early stages of the disease. Lack of insight into the seriousness of the symptoms, combined with a certain jocularity or hilariousness, is referred to as *Euphoria*. The patient laughs in unrestrained fashion when asked to touch the nose with the forefinger. But other affective states are common; depression or irritability, occasionally psychoses or dementia may occur.

Cerebro-spinal Fluid.—The spinal fluid is often normal, but some cases show abnormal results and especially a positive Lange colloidal gold curve. The Wassermann reaction is negative. A typical C.S.F. analysis might read—cells = 2 per ml., protein = 30 mg. per cent., Nonne-Apelt test positive, Lange = 0112100000. A slight lymphocytosis of 10–30 cells per ml. is most often seen with acute lesions either in the optic nerve, near the ventricles, or on the surface of nervous structures in contact with the subarachnoid space. Marked increase of protein is rare and should always arouse the suspicion of spinal cord compression. In some cases gamma globulin is increased. In 50 per cent. of cases or more the spinal fluid shows a " paretic " type of Lange curve, or some other modification (Table LXVI). Examination of the C.S.F. may be unnecessary when the diagnosis is clear from the history and signs. It may be required, however, to exclude cord compression, syphilis or other conditions simulating disseminated sclerosis.

Diagnosis.—At the onset of the disease or in a remission *hysteria* is often erroneously diagnosed. Patients with disseminated sclerosis are highly suggestible and hysterical signs may exist with those of organic origin. Diagnosis of the disease is based on: (1) The acute development of symptoms at irregular intervals. (2) The presence of symptoms and signs of multiple lesions in the central nervous system. Multiple lesions also occur in *cerebro-spinal syphilis, multiple emboli, polyarteritis, metastatic tumours* (Behçet's syndrome, § 890). Difficulty is likely to occur in early mono-symptomatic cases.

(a) *The patient, a young adult, complains of sudden unilateral, transient loss of vision, and the signs of retro-bulbar neuritis* (§ 1129) *may be found.* Retro-bulbar neuritis rarely occurs from sphenoidal or other nasal accessory sinus infection, but is extremely frequent in early disseminated sclerosis.

(b) *The signs are those of a pure pyramidal lesion, either monoplegic or paraplegic in distribution.* The disease may be *motor neurone disease* or *syphilitic spinal paralysis of Erb.* Examination of the C.S.F. may show the slight increase of globulin with paretic type of Lange curve and a negative Wassermann reaction, which is characteristic of disseminated sclerosis. The finding of muscular wasting or fibrillation, or bulbar paralysis, favours *motor neurone disease*, while the serological reactions of the blood or C.S.F. may indicate syphilis.

(c) *Cervical spondylosis* when it involves the cord may closely simulate disseminated sclerosis. Many cases previously termed chronic progressive disseminated sclerosis are due to cervical spondylosis. The age of onset in this condition is over 50. Root pains and paraesthesiae, wasting of the small hand muscles, inversion of the radial reflex, stiff neck, absence of remissions, are all characteristics of spondylosis. Plain or myodil X-rays may demonstrate the lesion. In cervical spondylosis the symptoms may respond to extension or immobilisation of the neck.

(d) *There is a spastic paraplegia, with sensory loss, up to a segmental level.* Increased protein and evidence of block on spinal manometry indicate *Spinal cord compression,* perhaps from tumour.　Acute paraplegia develops rapidly in association with extensive bilateral central scotomata in *neurolomyelitis optica* (§ 1121), which closely resembles disseminated sclerosis.

(e) Diplopia, cerebellar symptoms and pyramidal signs indicate a *focal lesion in the pons.* In pontine neoplasm, papilloedema is late and in disseminated sclerosis papilloedema is excessively rare and slight.　The diagnosis in such cases can often be settled only by the ultimate progress of the case.

However protean the manifestations of the disease, certain symptoms are so rare that their presence in a case of supposed disseminated sclerosis warrants revision of the diagnosis.　These are (1) *Pain,* rare in disseminated sclerosis apart from the muscular cramps and backache of the early stiffness and the paroxysmal pain associated with flexor spasms in the later stages of the disease.　Trigeminal pain may occur (§ 1076) but root pains in the limbs or trunk suggests spinal compression.　(2) *Muscular wasting* is rare in disseminated sclerosis, but occurs in syringomyelia, motor neurone disease and some spinal forms of syphilis.　(3) *Absence of tendon reflexes* is rare in disseminated sclerosis, whereas the knee- and ankle-jerks are lost early in Friedreich's ataxia.

The *Etiology* is unknown.　There is little evidence to support the view that the disease is due to a virus.　The current opinion inclines to the view that the condition is a non-specific allergic manifestation, although a history of allergy is not obtained with greater frequency in such cases.　The disease may have to do with enzyme systems in the brain and cord. Females are more liable than males.　The disease is more common in colder climates, excessively rare in the East.　Familial cases, according to McAlpine, vary from 3 to 7 per cent.

Pathology.—Scattered areas of demyelination for which there is no evident cause appear in the white matter, sometimes overlapping into the grey matter.　They vary in size from a lentil to a pea and are rarely symmetrically distributed.　The axis cylinders persist long after the myelin is destroyed.　There is a secondary gliosis or " sclerosis," hence the name (Fig. 243).

Prognosis.—(1) The outlook is better in patients with retrobulbar neuritis, posterior column signs or facial paræsthesiæ.　(2) Remitting cases do well at first until remissions cease to occur.　A remission may last as long as 20 years, but is usually much less.　(3) Purely motor symptoms, or motor and cerebellar symptoms combined, tend to be progressive.　(4) Exacerbation and progression of symptoms may occur during pregnancy or lactation, but this may be fortuitous.　Many women with the disease avoid pregnancy.　Most patients who have the disease can have a successful pregnancy and are prepared to take the risk.　Death occurs usually in 20 years or more after the onset, but respiratory or urinary infections terminate life sooner in some patients.

Treatment.—In acute exacerbations bed-rest is advisable for short periods.　Prolonged bed-rest does harm.　Prednisolone 5 mg. twice daily may be given *for short periods of 5–7 days* in selected cases; or antihistamine preparations, promethazine hydrochloride (Phenergan) 25 mg. night and morning. In the remitting and chronic stages of the disease short intramuscular courses of cyanocobalamin (50 micrograms weekly for 6 weeks) every 3 or 4 months may be given, or liq. arsenicalis ℥ 1 with tinct. belladonnæ ℥ 7 in a mixture thrice daily for short periods. A negative policy with regard to treatment does much harm and encourages the patient to drift from one doctor to another. For *precipitancy of micturition* give a pill containing extract of belladonna ¼ gr. twice or thrice daily. *Stiffness.*— Strychnine increases spasticity. Meprobamate or oral procaineamide (Pronestyl) occasionally lessen stiffness. *Sensory ataxia* is helped by Frenkl's exercises, but in cerebellar ataxia, physiotherapy is of little help.

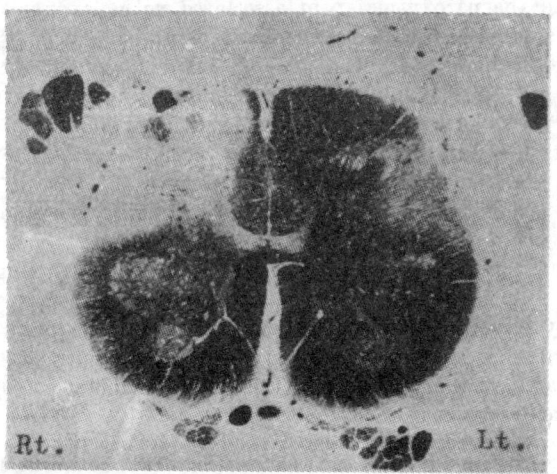

Fig. 243.—DISSEMINATED SCLEROSIS. Section through the lumbar spinal cord showing areas of demyelination in the right posterior and in both lateral columns. On the right side the plaque involves the grey matter of the posterior horn. Note the demyelination in the posterior commissure.

Intensive short courses of physiotherapy are well worth while and the patient can go on practising exercises to improve co-ordination and help balance and relaxation at home. *Intercurrent infections* of the chest or bladder must be treated promptly and vigorously as they may endanger life. A daily dose of a long-acting sulphonamide by mouth may prevent re-infection. During *pregnancy* the patient should have extra rest and vitamin supplements. Nursing the baby for longer than a few weeks is not advised. Many improve in a warm climate.

The *social implications* of the disease—loss of employment, break-up of marriage, financial worry—have a most adverse effect on the course of the illness and often seem responsible for intensification of symptoms.

IV. *Ischæmic paralysis* follows the deep sleep of alcoholic intoxication or overlong application of a tourniquet.

V. *Rheumatic chorea* (" chorea mollis ") rarely presents with flaccidity

Classification of the Demyelinating Diseases

	Incidence.
I. Disseminated sclerosis (§ 952).	Sporadic chiefly in northern hemisphere. Rarely familial. First half of adult life.
II. Neuromyelitis optica (§ 1121).	Sporadic, acute or subacute, rarely self-limited.
III. Acute disseminated encephalo-myelopathy (§ 895).	Acute or subacute, perhaps relapsing later.
IV. Acute encephalo-myelopathy following exanthemata, vaccinations and inoculations (§ 895).	Acute and self-limited.
V. Encephalitis periaxialis diffuse (Schilder's disease) (§ 1194c).	Produces progressive cerebral illness with cortical blindness in children and young adults.
VI. Toxic encephalopathy—carbon monoxide, cyanide, spinal anæsthetics, arsphenamine.	Self-limited and acute, often fatal.

of an arm or leg. Other forms of *encephalitis* following acute specific fevers produce cerebral monoplegia (see § 895).

VI. *Brachial or Sacral Plexus Injuries* are usually associated with fractured clavicle or pelvis. The brachial plexus may be damaged by stretching injuries when the patient is unconscious. For OBSTETRICAL PARALYSIS in newly born infants see § 994.

BEHÇETS SYNDROME (§ 890) and SARCOIDOSIS (see § 889) may cause scattered neurological lesions.

(B) GRADUAL *Monoplegia* may be due to:

VII. PRIMARY OR SECONDARY CEREBRAL NEOPLASMS cause slowly progressive monoplegia. Jacksonian fits may be associated when the lesion involves the cortex —e.g., focal fits, commencing in the foot in parasagittal meningioma (§ 1044).

VIII. SUBDURAL HÆMATOMA should be suspected in elderly persons or alcoholics with a history of falling about. A large *inactive* pupil on the side of the lesion is often found (§ 1052).

IX. SPINAL TUMOUR often produces root pains (see § 968).

X. MOTOR NEURONE DISEASE is sometimes confined to one limb for weeks or months before its inevitable spread (§ 1001).

XI. PARALYTIC BRACHIAL NEURITIS. Following neuritic pain in the neck, shoulder or arm, segmental paralysis and wasting appear. The condition occurs after surgical operations, after injection of sera or vaccines, or in small epidemics (§ 998).

XII. Infiltrating lesions of the brachial plexus or sacral plexus should always be searched for. They may co-exist with cerebral secondaries in carcinomatosis, rendering the signs puzzling. Enlarged nodes in Hodgkin's disease cause monoplegia.

XIII. HYSTERICAL MONOPLEGIA may be sudden or gradual in onset. It is seen in war injuries and in " compensation " cases. The weakness is variable, and " stocking and glove " areas of anæsthesia of varying and variable extent exist with normal tendon reflexes (§ 1173). A co-existent organic lesion, e.g., disseminated sclerosis, is common.

GROUP X. PARAPLEGIA

There is WEAKNESS OF BOTH LOWER LIMBS *and a* DRAGGING GAIT. *Bladder disturbances are frequent. The condition is* SPINAL PARAPLEGIA. *When all* FOUR LIMBS *are affected* (a) *from a spinal cord lesion the condition is termed* QUADRIPLEGIA, (b) *from a cerebral cause* DIPLEGIA (§ 972).

§ 953. In **Paraplegia** the onset may be (A) Acute, or (B) Gradual. When weakness affects both legs it is probable that the lesion is in the *spinal cord* or sometimes in the *brain* stem, especially if there is bladder disturbance. When bilateral pains in the lower limbs exist with weakness, the lesion is probably in the *Cauda Equina*.

Symptoms.—(a) *Stage of Spinal Shock and Flaccidity.* In acute cases there is usually flaccidity and loss of power in the affected limbs with sensory impairment below the level of the lesion, with retention of urine. In cases of cervical injury the legs may be spastic and the arms flaccid, or all four limbs may be flaccid. The tendon reflexes are at first absent, so usually are the plantar and abdominal reflexes. A sensory level should be sought, but at first it may not extend as high as the upper level of the lesion. Dissociated sensory loss or a picture of the Brown-Séquard type (§ 799) is usual. If the lesion is very acute, a low blood pressure, sweating, pallor and coldness of the extremities are present because of associated systemic shock (§ 239). Respiratory failure may occur. The patient who has defective temperature sensation may be burnt with hot-water bottles. (b) *Stage of Paraplegia in Extension and Spasticity.* After a variable period of time (often three to six weeks) tonus reappears in the paralysed limbs and the tendon reflexes return. Spasticity with an extensor plantar response appears and the legs become rigidly extended and adducted. In other cases we may see extensor or flexor spasms in the legs with spontaneous clonus: their appearance does not of course imply recovery. (c) *Stage of Paraplegia in Flexion.* The thighs become drawn up towards the abdomen and the knees flexed so that the heels press against the buttocks. Voluntary extension is minimal and much force is required to extend the legs. Reflex spasm becomes continuous. The knee- and ankle-jerks tend to disappear. Bedsores and incontinence of urine and fæces are present in this final irreversible condition.

Diagnosis.—The *Segmental diagnosis* of the level of the lesion is made by a study of the segmental innervation of the muscles paralysed, the sensory level and the reflexes abolished (Table LVIII). *Differential diagnosis.* Cases of acute high cervical paraplegia are frequently thought to be hysterical but in organic lesions the tendon reflexes are abolished and bladder disturbances occur.   In *Hysteria* the tendon reflexes are present, the patient is not shocked and the sensory changes are variable and paradoxical.   *Acute Poliomyelitis* causes a purely motor flaccid paraplegia, usually asymmetrical and transient.   Bladder disturbance is frequent. The history of tenderness of affected muscles, the age of the patient and the C.S.F. changes are characteristic.   *Polyneuritis* may cause paraplegia with absent tendon reflexes and increased protein in the C.S.F., but the muscles are tender, and manometry shows a free rise and fall on jugular compression.

In all cases where a block is thought to exist, plain X-rays of the spine should be taken in the first instance: look especially for erosion of the pedicles.   *Spinal puncture* is essential when poliomyelitis or spinal cord compression is suspected.   In both polyneuritis and spinal cord compression, the fluid may be yellow with excess of protein (Froin's Syndrome). *Myelography* may be necessary to exclude a spinal block and to localise the level of the lesion (§ 846).   When manometry is normal myelography is unlikely to show a block.   In cases of extradural spinal cord compression, myelograms are sometimes normal.

Prognosis.—If the lesion is traumatic or inflammatory, and recovery is to occur, it will show before the third week.   In cases other than those due to removable tumour only the passage of time will show what recovery is likely.   The prognosis for recovery is bad with high cervical cord lesions and in cases where compression of the cord has existed for months or years. *Complications.*   Burns, bedsores, hypostatic pneumonia, pyelonephritis and amyloidosis are all theoretically preventable.

Treatment.—If the cause is neoplastic a surgical opinion must be sought. For the *Management of Paraplegia* see § 971.

(*A*) **Paraplegia of Acute Onset** may be due to:

I. Spinal cord injuries.	V. Spinal vascular syphilis.
II. Demyelinating diseases especially	VI. Post-infective myelopathy.
Disseminated sclerosis.	VII. Vascular lesions of the spinal cord.
III. Acute myelitis.	VIII. Neoplasm.
IV. Cervical spondylosis.	IX. Caisson disease.

§ 954. I. **Spinal Cord Injuries** produce CONCUSSION, CONTUSION or LACERATION.— The *symptoms* are those of acute spinal paraplegia.   In *Spinal concussion* the lesion is often in the midcervical or cervicodorsal region.   During the stage of concussion the patient complains of paræsthesiæ up to a segmental level, there is a variable degree of limb paresis and there may be transient retention of urine.   After some hours or days these symptoms pass off, usually completely.   In *Spinal contusion or laceration* the cord may be pulped at the site of the lesion.   The symptoms are those of profound and permanent transverse section of the cord.

Diagnosis is made from the history of the injury and the presence of organic signs of spinal cord damage.

Etiology.—Direct injury by missiles or stab wounds are rare in civil practice. The vertebræ most commonly fractured or dislocated are C4, 5 (cord segments C5, 6), and L1 under which vertebral body lies the conus and roots of the cauda equina. Severe cord damage in the *cervical* region is often found without any X-ray evidence of fracture or dislocation. In patients with cervical spondylosis or cervical disc lesions, relatively slight injuries, *e.g.*, falling down stairs or a blow on the chin, may cause paraplegia; so may injudicious attempts to mobilise a stiff neck in patients with vertebral disease. Cervical injuries result from acute forward flexion of the neck with application of force to the vertex (*e.g.*, somersault) whilst *Lumbar* injuries are usually caused from falls on the buttocks.

Prognosis.—In contusion most patients show recovery after some days or weeks; a few are left with wasted or clumsy hands, inversion of the radial reflex and spastic weakness of the legs. In some the symptoms may progress due to vascular softening after the injury. In cases of *cervical spondylosis* with paraplegia some recovery can be anticipated. In *spinal cord laceration* the prognosis for recovery of lost function is poor.

Treatment.—The patient must be lifted *en masse* by three or four assistants, or rolled on to a firm stretcher, taking special care not to let the head fall forwards or backwards. Open surgery is rarely called for. Traction will be necessary where there is cervical dislocation.

II. DEMYELINATING DISEASES.—In *Disseminated sclerosis* an acute paraplegia may occur, but signs will usually exist elsewhere (*e.g.*, nystagmus, intention tremor) or there is a history of retro-bulbar neuritis (§ 1129). In *Neuromyelitis optica* (§ 1121) sudden bilateral dimness or loss of vision due to retro-bulbar neuritis precedes or accompanies the signs of paraplegia.

§ 955. III. Acute Myelitis is more common before the age of 45. It may be (*a*) non-suppurative or (*b*) suppurative.

(*a*) In *non-suppurative myelitis*:

Symptoms.—(1) Marked paraplegia develops in association with fever, (2) pains in the back and (3) numbness, tingling or a sense of *girdle constriction* round the body at the level of the lesion. (4) At the onset there is flaccid paraplegia with absence of tendon reflexes and retention of urine. (5) Sensory loss is present up to the level of the lesion. (6) Later, the paralysis becomes spastic, with reflex incontinence, the tendon reflexes are exaggerated, with clonus, and the plantars are extensor. Bedsores develop. The paralysis and anæsthesia may ascend.

The *spinal fluid* may show the syndrome of Froin (*i.e.*, yellow coloration with hyperalbuminosis, formation of clot and relatively little pleocytosis), due to the formation of a zone of arachnoidal thickening and adhesion around the inflamed portion of the cord. If the spinal block persists, the syndrome may continue indefinitely in the spinal fluid.

Diagnosis.—The Wasserman reaction should be carried out in the blood and C.S.F. If on manometry partial block is observed, this may be due to transient cord swelling or to compression. It should be repeated with myelography in 3–4 weeks' time unless the patient is improving. Sudden collapse of a vertebral body infiltrated by *metastatic carcinoma* or vertebral *lymphosarcoma* causes similar symptoms but pain is much more severe. Acute myelitis must be differentiated from other causes of acute paraplegia. (1) In *disseminated sclerosis*: evidence of disseminated lesions may be present clinically or ascertained by a careful history of previous illness (see § 952). (2) In *spinal vascular syphilis* the Wassermann reaction is usually positive in blood and C.S.F. (3) In the aged, sudden thrombosis of diseased arteries and veins, *myelomalacia*, occurs (§ 957). (4) In *spinal cord compression*, particularly that associated with extension of tuberculous or pyogenic osteomyelitis of the vertebræ, the diagnosis may be difficult, but is usually made by the slower onset of the symptoms.

Etiology.—In most cases the cause is unknown. An association with infection has been postulated. Thrombo-phlebitis of the veins of the cord may cause similar symptoms. The known causes are rabies, syphilis and chemical substances introduced by injection, *e.g.*, spinal anæsthetics, sacral epidural injections (which affect the roots of the cauda equina) or aortic arteriography, where cord symptoms are produced by chemotoxicity.

(b) *Suppurative myelitis* (spinal abscess) is due to metastatic blood infection with purulent organisms (see § 899).

Prognosis of Acute myelitis.—Recovery of function is poor in all cases.

Treatment is symptomatic and general (see § 971). With a suppurative lesion antibiotics are required, then exploration to exclude the presence of subdural abscess.

IV. IN CERVICAL SPONDYLOSIS quadriplegia may follow a sudden fall. Many of these cases of acute paraplegia with spondylosis recover to a remarkable degree (§ 1004).

§ 956. V. **Spinal Vascular Syphilis** causes signs of acute paraplegia, sensory and motor. Syphilitic pupils, or a history of infection months or years before, may lead to the diagnosis, or the condition may complicate treatment of neuro-syphilis (tabes or meningo-myelitis) with penicillin or pentavalent arsenicals. It is commonest in young or middle-aged males. *Diagnosis.*—The blood Wasserman reaction is almost always positive. The spinal fluid shows a moderate lymphocytic increase; there is moderate increase of protein and globulin with a luetic type of colloidal gold curve. The *Prognosis* is poor if symptoms of paraplegia are severe. *Treatment* (see § 500).

VI. POST-INFECTIVE MYELOPATHY (§ 895) is due to virus disease or follows on the exanthemata.

§ 957. VII. VASCULAR LESIONS OF THE SPINAL CORD are all very rare as primary diseases. They result in softening of an ischæmic area of cord, termed *myelomalacia*.

(a) **Myelomalacia** occurs in many conditions. In cervical spondylosis the anterior and posterior spinal arteries may be strangled by meningeal fibrosis with resultant medullary ischæmia. Thrombophlebitis of the spinal veins may result from acute infections or from injection of irritant substance into the theca (*e.g.*, spinal anæsthetics or contrast media). Anterior spinal artery thrombosis occurs rarely in atheromatous or hypertensive patients and may cause an acute transverse cord lesion: the posterior columns (supplied by the two posterior spinal arteries) escape. Myelomalacia occurs from spinal vascular syphilis, tuberculosis and after aortography.

(b) **Hæmatomyelia** implies hæmorrhage into the substance of the spinal cord. This almost always is due to trauma, *e.g.*, injury to the cervical cord by high diving with acute flexion or extension of the head; this can occur in healthy individuals, or those with cervical spondylosis. The *Symptoms* produced are those of acute paraplegia, both sensory and motor. Dissociation of sensation below the level of the lesion may be marked and a Brown-Séquard syndrome may be present. The *Diagnosis* is clinically difficult but the condition may be suspected if a patient recovers from a cervical cord contusion with signs resembling those of syringomyelia (§ 1005). *Treatment* consists in attempting to limit the hæmorrhage with morphine or chlorpromazine, and the nursing of the associated paraplegia. Hæmatomyelia has been found at operation for decompression of the cervical spine after injury, and at post mortem. Some postulate a pre-existing angioma in cases which appear to be spontaneous.

§ 958. VIII. ACUTE PARAPLEGIA FROM NEOPLASM.—In metastastic tumours, *e.g.*, carcinoma, vascular tumours (*e.g.*, angiomata) and in invasive malignant tumours of bone sudden paraplegia may occur from cord compression, from spinal vascular occlusion or from medullary hæmorrhage. Plain X-rays of the spine often are most helpful in diagnosis and should always precede spinal puncture or myelography.

§ 959. IX. **Caisson Disease** (Syn. " Diver's Paralysis," Compressed-Air Illness) is a form of acute paraplegia occurring in divers, workers in diving bells and in underground tunnellers, working at high atmospheric pressure. Too rapid decompression causes the excess of nitrogen in solution in the tissues and body fluids to be released as bubbles of gas in the tissues, especially in the central nervous system. If decompression is gradual, the nitrogen is liberated into the blood and excreted by the lungs, and symptoms do not occur.

Symptoms depend on the localisation of the bubbles of nitrogen and their size. They occur thirty minutes to several hours after decompression is complete. Severe root-pains, " the bends," are common at the onset, then a paraplegia, transient or permanent, results. The paraplegia is never complete and the arms are rarely affected as much as the legs. Anæsthesia and sphincter paralysis only occur in the graver cases. Auditory vertigo, tinnitus, hæmorrhage from the nose, lungs and other parts sometimes occur, with abdominal distension, pain and vomiting.

The *Prognosis* is favourable; pain and paresis pass off in a few days to six weeks. A few cases have died.

Treatment.—The patient should immediately be put in a compressed-air chamber and exposed to the same pressure as that under which he was working. This results in reabsorption of the nitrogen, with relief of symptoms, and decompression can then take place very gradually. *Prophylaxis* consists in adopting precautions for gradual decompression. Snell recommends ten minutes' decompression for each atmosphere of pressure. The obese and alcoholic are more liable to the disease.

The signs of ACUTE PARAPLEGIA *may pass into those of* CHRONIC SPASTIC PARAPLEGIA *when the " shock " effect of the lesion wears off. In most chronic myelopathies, however, the lower limbs are spastic from the outset, e.g.,* motor neurone disease, slow spinal cord compression. In cases where there is pure posterior column disease, *e.g.,* subacute combined degeneration of the cord or some cases of disseminated sclerosis, the lower limbs may show a combination of flaccidity with increased tendon reflexes and extensor plantar responses. This also is seen in motor neurone disease when the upper and lower motor neurones to the lower limb muscles are affected.

(*B*) Paraplegia of Gradual Onset may be due to:

I. DISSEMINATED SCLEROSIS.
II. AMYOTROPHIC LATERAL SCLEROSIS.
III. CEREBRAL ARTERIOSCLEROSIS.
IV. CERVICAL SPONDYLOSIS.
V. Syphilitic Meningomyelitis.
VI. Subacute Combined Degeneration of the Cord.
VII. Nutritional Neuropathy.
VIII. Syringomyelia.
IX. Congenital Paraplegia.
X. Heredo-familial Paraplegia.
XI. SPINAL CORD COMPRESSION.
XII. Lesions of the Cauda Equina and Conus.

Symptoms.—(1) Weakness appears first in the dorsiflexors of the feet, usually more marked on one side than the other. The patient drags the foot, " Clasp-knife " rigidity develops with increased tendon reflexes and extensor plantar responses. The lower abdominal reflexes disappear before the upper ones. The legs are adducted and are extended rigidly in spasm. When such limbs are being examined they may show spontaneous clonus. This condition is called *paraplegia in extension.* The weakness is the result of pyramidal damage, the hypertonus to release of reflex systems which subserve extensor tone. If the lesion is confined to the upper motor neurones, *e.g.,* motor neurone disease, this picture will persist and increase. (2) When sensory as well as motor tracts are seriously damaged and when infection of the skin and bladder are present *paraplegia in flexion* occurs.

HYSTERICAL PARAPLEGIA may be of sudden or gradual onset (§ 1173). The tendon reflexes are unaltered. In this condition various paradoxes are found, *e.g.,* gross weakness of the limbs when the patient is in the horizontal position in bed, but not on standing. The feet may appear to be " glued to the ground," or one leg may be trailed behind the patient, who progresses by bizarre hops. The tendon reflexes and the abdominal responses are unaltered, while the plantar reflexes are usually absent.

§ 960. I. DISSEMINATED SCLEROSIS.—The earliest symptom may be a weakness of one limb with an extensor plantar response (§ 952). The diagnosis must be based on clinical evidence of recurrent isolated lesions in various parts of the nervous system over a period of time.

§ 961. II. AMYOTROPHIC LATERAL SCLEROSIS (Syn. Motor Neurone Disease) should be suspected if the signs are purely motor. This disease cannot be diagnosed with certainty until there is evidence of anterior horn cell involvement—muscular atrophy and fasciculation. If there are spastic lower limbs in an adult with bilateral extensor responses and no other signs, the diagnosis from other cord conditions may be difficult (§ 1001). Sensory changes are entirely absent in motor neurone disease, and the abdominal reflexes tend to be retained although the plantar responses are extensor. Spinal puncture and myelography may be necessary to differentiate such cases from spinal cord compression or cervical spondylosis.

§ 962. III. CEREBRAL ARTERIOSCLEROSIS.—Weakness and stiffness of the lower limbs so that the subject walks with short shuffling steps (*marche à petits pas*) occurs in those with arteriosclerotic muscular rigidity. Extensor plantar responses sometimes occur. The signs of pseudo-bulbar palsy may be present with memory failure for recent events and progressive narrowing of interests (§§ 574, 916).

§ 963. IV. CERVICAL SPONDYLOSIS in patients over 50 years of age may cause stiff neck with spastic weakness of the lower limbs and extensor responses, or symptomless pyramidal signs.

Symptoms.—(1) Pain and paræsthesia of root distribution in the arms, with hyperæsthesia and hyperalgesia, or diminution of touch and pain sensation; (2) Muscular wasting, often in the hands; and (3) Inversion of the radial reflexes are frequent concomitant findings (and see § 1004).

Diagnosis.—X-ray changes can be very deceptive as they may be found co-existing in patients with spinal cord disease such as disseminated sclerosis, amyotrophic lateral sclerosis, spinal cord tumours, syringomyelia, subacute combined degeneration. The C.S.F. is usually normal, but exceptionally partial block and slightly raised protein are found.

Prognosis.—In many cases the paraplegia becomes stationary; 50 per cent. of those treated conservatively by rest, neck traction or with immobilisation of the neck by a plastic collar show improvement.

§ 964. V. SYPHILITIC MENINGOMYELITIS should be suspected if a slowly increasing paraplegia occurs with a history of syphilis, or with a syphilitic or Argyll-Robertson pupil. Root-pains or girdle sensations round the trunk or limbs with numbness in the feet and signs of spastic paraplegia occur early (§ 1025).

Two rare forms of spinal syphilis require special mention.

§ 965. (1) Syphilitic amyotrophy is due to chronic meningeal and vascular syphilis affecting the cervical cord and nerve roots. Amyotrophy of the small hand muscles or muscles of the upper limbs is found with diminution or loss of arm-jerks as in motor neurone disease. Argyll-Robertson pupils are commonly present, together with pyramidal signs. The condition is sometimes seen associated with tabes dorsalis. Cervical spondylosis may cause similar symptoms in patients with latent syphilis. Syphilitic amyotrophy is a chronic process which may be arrested by treatment.

§ 966. (2) Erb's paraplegia is an extremely chronic and slowly progressive condition. A mild paraplegia exists with minimal sensory changes. The arms are rarely affected. The condition is uncommon and is not much helped by treatment. A primary pyramidal affection in a man past middle life with a history of syphilis is likely to be due to this form of vascular and meningeal syphilis.

VI. Subacute Combined Degeneration of the Cord.—The paraplegia is accompanied by signs of polyneuritis. Paræsthesiæ of the fingers and hands occur with absent knee- and ankle-jerks, tenderness of the small muscles of the feet and hands (§ 950) and signs of pernicious anæmia (§ 548).

VII. Nutritional Neuropathy.—During periods of famine, especially in India, spastic paralysis of the legs occurs due to poisoning by flour made from *lathyrus sativa*, a chick-pea. Changes in the pyramidal tracts and to a lesser degree in the posterior columns are described. The symptoms are permanent and do not respond to any known treatment.

VIII. Syringomyelia.—Recognised by the dissociation and suspended areas of sensory impairment on the trunk and limbs, is often diagnosed in adolescence. Trophic ulcers and neuropathic joints occur. The paraplegia is slight or moderate and the disease is in many cases compatible with gainful occupation (see § 1005).

IX. Congenital Spastic Paraplegia occurs in infancy, producing extensor and adductor spasm of the lower limbs. It is a form of *Cerebral Diplegia* (see § 972).

§ 967. X. Familial and Heredo-familial Paraplegia.—Familial Spastic Paraplegia is a rare condition with a purely motor spastic paraplegia and extensor responses. A relationship with Addison's disease has been described. Friedreich's Ataxia is recognised by the ataxic dysarthria, nystagmus and titubation, absent tendon reflexes, pes cavus and scoliosis (§ 945).

Cerebro-macular degeneration (§ 1194c) and *Niemann-Pick's* disease (§ 559) are rare familial conditions due to an inborn error of lipoid metabolism. *Symptoms* occur in early life and include paraplegia and mental deficiency.

There are Pains or Paræsthesiæ of Root Distribution *followed by* Sensory Changes *below the level of the lesion and* Dragging of the Legs. Manometry *of the spinal fluid shows a* Partial *or* Complete Block *and its protein content is raised. The cause is* Spinal Cord Compression.

§ 968. XI. Spinal Cord Compression.—The *Symptoms* are usually gradually progressive. There is pain due to distortion of sensory roots or to involvement of sensitive dura or periosteum. There are also signs of motor and sensory disturbance indicating an involvement of the spinal cord tracts below a given level, usually that at which the pain occurs.

(1) *Local Effects.*—Where sensory roots are involved, pain of root dis-

TABLE LVIII.—SYMPTOMS OF SPINAL CORD COMPRESSION AT VARIOUS
SEGMENTAL LEVELS

(For corresponding Cutaneous Root Areas, see Fig. 244.)

Cord Segment.	Clinical Picture.	Muscles chiefly Paralysed.	Reflexes Abolished.	Other Features.	Level of Spinous Process.
C.3–4.	Brachial Paraplegia.	Lower part of Trapezius. Supraspinatus. Infraspinatus. Diaphragm.		Relative analgesia and thermanæsthesia of face.	C.III
C.5.	Brachial Paraplegia.	Rhomboids. Biceps, Deltoid, Brachioradialis. Supinator.	Biceps jerk (C.5–6). Radial jerk inverted.	Triceps jerk+ +	C.IV
C.7.	Paraplegia.	Triceps and Extensors of Wrist and Fingers. Costal pectoralis major. Latissimus dorsi.	T.J. and S.J. (C.6–7).		C.VI
C.8–Th.1.	Paraplegia.	Flexors of Wrist and Fingers. Small muscles of Hand.		Paralysis of ocular sympathetic. Arm jerks +	C.VII
Th.6.	Paraplegia.	Intercostals. Upper Rectus abdominis.	Epigastric (Th.6–8).	Spastic paralysis of trunk muscles and lower limbs.	Th.IV
Th.9–10.	Paraplegia.	Lower Rectus abdominis. Obliquus abdominis.	Upper Abdominal (Th.8–10).	Umbilicus deviates upwards.	Th.VIII
Th.12–L.2.	Paraplegia.	Adductors of thigh. Sartorius.	Lower abdominal (Th.11–12). Cremasteric (L.1–2).		Th.X
L.3–4.	Paraplegia.	Iliopsoas. Quadriceps femoris.	Knee-jerk (L.2–4).	Flexion of wasted hip preserved.	Th.XI
L.5.	Paraplegia.	Hamstrings. Ext. long. hallucis.			
S.1.	Paraplegia.	Glutei. Calf muscles.	Ankle-jerk (S.1–2).	Anal and Bulbocavernosus reflexes preserved.	Th.XII
S.2.	Paraplegia.	Anterior Tibial muscles. Peronei. Small muscles of foot.	Ankle-jerk (S.1–2).		
S.3–4.	No motor symptoms in legs.	Perineal muscles. Levator ani.	Bulbocavernosus (S.3–4). Superficial anal. (S.4–5).	Retention of urine and fæces. Motility of lower limbs and deep reflexes normal.	L.1

tribution will occur. It will be made worse by coughing, sneezing or
straining. The pain may be accompanied by cutaneous hyperæsthesia to
dragged pin of segmental distribution. As the lesion increases in size
and compresses the root, the pain tends to disappear and a segmental

root area of hypoalgesia or hypoæsthesia will take its place. Root-pains and paræsthesiæ are the most valuable evidences of the level of the lesion. Fig. 244 indicates the segmental zones in which root-pains occur.

Involvement of the motor roots causes muscular wasting, flaccidity or, more rarely, spasm. Interruption of the reflex arcs from the spinal reflexes will cause diminution or absence of the tendon reflexes.

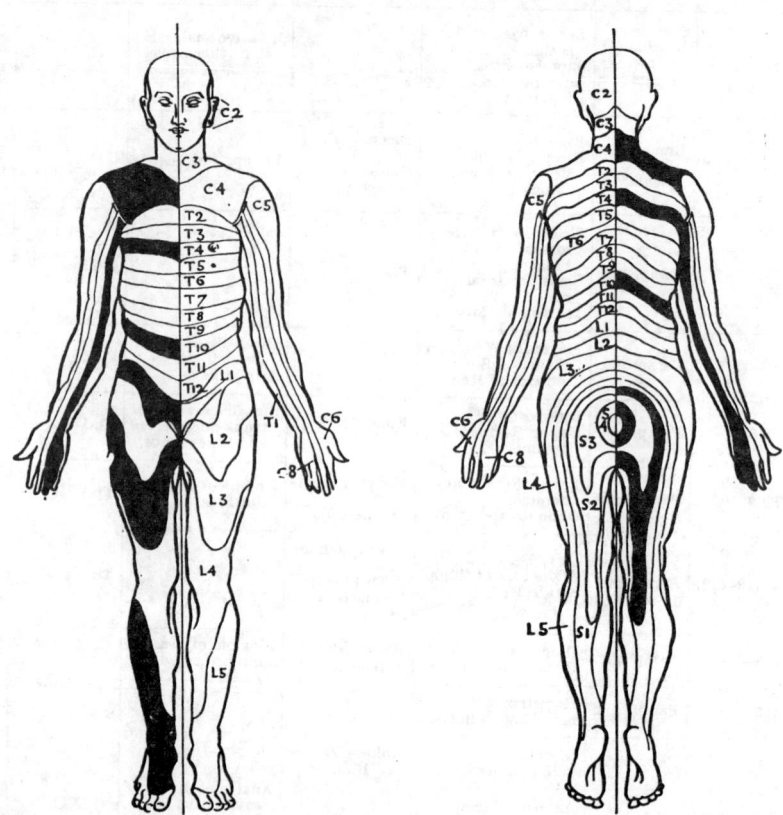

Fig. 244.—Distribution of the Sensory Spinal Roots on the Body Surface. The student should memorise the shaded segmental areas.

(2) *Remote Effects.*—Cord symptoms next occur due to involvement of the long sensory and motor tracts, with accompanying motor, sensory and reflex changes below the level of the lesion. Spastic paralysis may be noticed first in the lower limbs on the side of the lesion, from pressure on the homolateral pyramidal tract. It spreads, and a spastic paraplegia develops with increased tendon reflexes, patellar- and ankle-clonus and extensor plantar responses. At first the lower limbs show *paraplegia in extension* from interruption of local spinal reflex arcs. Later, when the long mid-brain reflex arcs subserving tonus in the extensor muscles are

involved, *paraplegia in flexion* occurs, with involuntary flexor spasms. Sensory changes develop in one of two ways. (1) Sensory loss may begin in the lowest sacral segments with anæsthesia over the " saddle-area," or (2) Sensory loss commences in the periphery of the limbs. Whatever the mode of onset, it gradually spreads up to the segmental level of the lesion, involving all forms of sensibility In testing cutaneous sensibility at the level of the lesion we find the level highest for touch, lowest for pain (pin-prick) with temperature intermediate, owing to the oblique crossing of the fibres going to the spino-thalamic tracts. Not uncommonly, an incomplete *Brown-Séquard Phenomenon* is observed. The pyramidal weakness and loss of deep sensibility (joint sense and vibration) is greater on the side of the lesion, with loss of sensation to pain, heat and cold in the contra-lateral lower limb. At first, there is hesitancy of micturition; later, reflex incontinence or overflow with dribbling occurs and incontinence of fæces. The abdominal reflexes disappear if the lesion is above the thoracic region. The tendon reflexes, which lie in the compressed segment or segments, are abolished. Below the level of the lesion they are increased with clonus. Cord lesions involving C8 and Th1 segments, or above this, may be associated with oculo-pupillary sympathetic paralysis (miosis, enophthalmos and narrowed ocular fissure) on the side of the lesion. Lesions of the cauda equina are described in § 969. Unless the paraplegia is relieved, irreparable ascending and descending degenerations occur in the spinal cord tracts. Such degenerations occur after a year of compression and, when the stage of paraplegia in flexion is reached, they are well established. Death, in such cases, takes place from infection, bedsores or ascending pyelonephritis.

Diagnosis of the Level of the Lesion.

The guide is the upper limit of the signs. The *root symptoms* are of paramount importance in this respect (Fig. 244). The root area of anæsthesia at the level of compression must be carefully mapped out and its upper limit defined with a skin pencil, testing each form of cutaneous sensibility in turn, working from the anæstheti: to the normal skin and carefully charting the observations in each case. In this connection, root areas of hyperæsthesia at the upper limit of sensory loss are as important as anæsthesia, and may indicate the necessity for a localisation above the upper limit of sensory loss. Any local loss of power, due to pressure on anterior roots, is of the greatest use in localisation of the level of the lesion. Wasting of an intercostal muscle may be observed. Lesions of the 9th Thoracic segment produce paralysis of the lower rectus with deviation of the umbilicus upwards and to the contra-lateral side when the patient attempts to sit up. Lesions of the 11th Thoracic segment spare the rectus but paralyse the obliquus abdominis, with bulging in the affected flank when the patient attempts to sit up. Abolition of the tendon reflexes occurs in those reflexes seated in the affected cord segments. The upper limits of the *tract anæsthesia* often merges with the root anæsthesia but should always be carefully charted. The characteristic findings at different segmental levels are given in Table LVIII.

§ **969.** XII. **Lesions of the Cauda Equina and Conus** require a special description. The cauda equina consists of L2–S5 nerve roots, motor and sensory.

The sciatic pain which is often the initial symptom differs in two respects from the pain of disc lesions—(1) it is often referred to both lower limbs, (2) it is distributed over more than one sacral segment. Numbness over the saddle area and loss of feeling on defæcation and micturition occur. In *lesions of the lower cauda equina* (1) sensory changes will be present over the saddle area, *i.e.*, buttocks, perinæum and genitalia and a strip down the posterior aspect of the thigh (S2–4) on one or both sides.   (2) Flaccid paralysis below the knee with foot-drop, wasting and fasciculation may be present.   (3) The ankle-jerk disappears.   (4) Bladder disturbance and impotence in the male are late symptoms.   (5) Over the analgesic areas minor abrasions may lead to chronic ulcers.   (6) The superficial anal and bulbocavernosus reflexes disappear.   In *lesions of the upper cauda equina* the picture is not so characteristic.   (1) There is an area of sensory loss over the foot and the posterior and outer aspect of the leg (L5, S1) and (2) Weakness of the long extensor of the big toe may be present.   *Lesions of the conus* cause bladder disturbance, rectal and urethral anæsthesia, much pain and dissociated analgesia to pin-prick and temperature.

Diagnosis of Spinal Cord Compression.—Cases of spinal tumour are likely to be treated as disc lesions or as brachial neuritis unless the possibility of a tumour is kept in mind.   Many spinal tumours grow very slowly and are relatively benign.   Cases of cord compression with flaccid lower limbs and high protein in the spinal fluid simulate polyneuritis, but in that condition manometry of the spinal fluid shows a free rise and fall. Multiple spinal neurofibromata producing an asymmetrical " polyradiculitis multiplex " with a high spinal fluid protein may be misdiagnosed as polyneuritis.   If a case thought to be disseminated sclerosis gives a history of root-pain be suspicious of the diagnosis unless it is well founded on a history such as of retro-bulbar neuritis.   Cases of multiple myeloma and metastatic tumours often masquerade as sciatica in their earlier stages, and the X-ray changes may not at first be easily observed.

Radiological Diagnosis.—If a spinal tumour is suspected, in all cases the chest as well as the spine should be X-rayed.   In bronchial carcinoma the spinal cord signs may precede the pulmonary signs.   Multiple myeloma and secondary growths cause local destruction or rarefaction in the vertebral bodies or their processes.   Lateral and antero-posterior films should be taken; and oblique views as well in the case of the cervical spine.   These X-rays should precede lumbar puncture.   Look for (1) erosion of the pedicles, (2) separation of the pedicles in antero-posterior films, (3) enlargement of an intervertebral foramen, especially in cervical neurofibroma (" dumb-bell tumour ").   (4) Paraspinal masses are seen in chest films when there are dumb-bell neurofibromas.   Look for congenital malformation, *e.g.*, a hemivertebra.   In some cases *tomograms* help.   *Myelography* (§ 846) cannot be undertaken for two weeks after a spinal puncture otherwise the injection of contrast medium may be made subdurally and the test will be useless.   It is often best to have plain X-rays of the vertebræ and if the clinical and X-ray findings still require further elucidation perform spinal puncture and myelography together.   The latter will show intra- and extra-medullary tumours and angiomatous malformations.   Calcification occurs in disc lesions but is rare in spinal tumours, except in occasional meningioma (" psammoma ").

The Spinal Fluid.—A block in the subarachnoid space is produced by a tumour. The spinal fluid below the level of the block ceases to circulate and the congested spinal veins leak protein and hæmoglobin into it. (*a*) *Manometry.* If the block is complete manometry with the patient in the lateral position will show absence of the normal respiratory oscillations of the fluid in the manometer. Moreover, jugular vein compression (Queckenstedt's test) produces no elevation in pressure, and after withdrawal of 5 ml. of fluid the pressure falls and will not rise again. Partial block is however more common. In this condition there is a slow and limited excursion and slow fall away after jugular vein compression, holding the breath, coughing or abdominal compression. A normal Queckenstedt test may be found in cases of cauda equina tumours, cervical tumours and with extradural growths compressing the cord. (*b*) *Froin's "loculation" syndrome* (also present in polyneuritis) is (1) A primrose yellow coloration of the fluid (xanthochromia) seen on holding the specimen against a sheet of white paper in a good light; (2) Increase of the normal protein content (25–50 mg. per cent.) to a value of at least 100 mg. per cent. (in some cases the fluid coagulates spontaneously); (3) Normal cell count (*i.e.*, up to 7 per c. mm.). (*c*) *Unusual C.S.F. findings.* Normal protein readings may be found in cervical cord compression and in extradural lesions. In some tumours within the cord the rise in protein is slight. A rise in cell count to 25–100 per c. mm. may occur but is exceptional unless the lesion is inflammatory.

Causes of Spinal Cord Compression

I. *Vertebral*

(1) Metastatic carcinoma.
(2) Fracture.
(3) Herniation of Nucleus Pulposus.
(4) Tuberculous and other forms of Osteomyelitis.
(5) Myelomatosis.
(6) Erosion by Thoracic Aneurysm.
(7) Sarcoma.
(8) Osteitis Deformans.

Meningeal

(9) Meningioma.
(10) Circumscribed Arachnoiditis.

Nerve Roots

(11) Neurofibroma.

Intramedullary

(12) Glioma.
     Ependymoma.

Extra-vertebral

(13) Hodgkin's disease.

Other causes

(14) Dermoid cyst.
(15) Angioma.

(1) Metastatic Carcinoma usually comes from a peripheral bronchial, mammary, prostatic, thyroid or ovarian carcinoma. The onset of *Symptoms* of cord compression may be sudden. *Treatment* by radiotherapy, œstrogens, steroids, etc., relieves many cases for a time. Surgery is not usually indicated unless it seems likely that the lesion is an isolated one. Previous deep X-ray therapy to the spine contra-indicates the making of a surgical incision, which will then be unlikely to heal.

(2) Fractures and fracture dislocations occur usually in the body of L.1 or C.5, 6.

(3) Herniation of the nucleus pulposus and cervical spondylosis are rare causes of paraplegia.

(4) Tuberculous and other forms of osteomyelitis are associated with fever and cachexia.

(5) MYELOMATOSIS begins with sciatic pain. The urine may show the presence of Bence-Jones' protein (§ 613). The condition is usually fatal in one to two years.

(6) Erosion by Thoracic aneurysm is rare.

(7) Periosteal sarcoma is a disease of young adults. *Treatment* is by radiotherapy.

(8) Osteitis deformans at the other extreme of life may cause much collapse of the spinal column but rarely cord compression.

Meningeal Causes

(9) MENINGIOMA is a fairly common benign lesion growing slowly from the dura whence it obtains its blood supply. In the region of the cauda equina these tumours may become very large and adherent to the nerve roots. In the thoracic region they cause erosions of the pedicles and

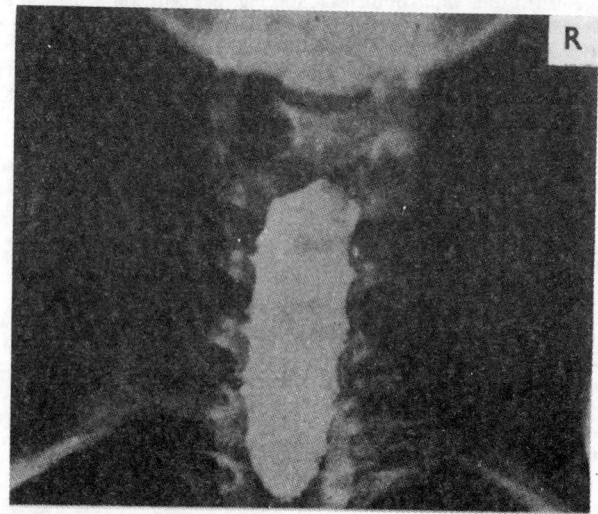

FIG. 245.—MYELOGRAM. Patient tilted 45° forward on an X-ray tilting table. There is erosion of the body of C3 and its articular process on the right side. The column of contrast medium is held up at the C4 level due to complete obstruction at the lower border of a neurofibroma.

widening of the space between them. The removal of the tumour with its dural attachment in most cases relieves the paraplegia.

(10) CIRCUMSCRIBED ARACHNOIDITIS is an encystment of fluid in thickened pia-arachnoid. It may follow upon injury, meningitis (infective or chemical) or hæmorrhage. Signs of cord compression extend over several segments. Surgical treatment, often undertaken for supposed neurofibroma, is not followed by much improvement, as the underlying cord is atrophic.

Nerve Root Causes

(11) NEUROFIBROMATA are benign rather common lesions growing very slowly from the sheath of Schwann of the nerve root, to which they become firmly attached. Unlike meningiomas they do not calcify but they erode and cause separation of the pedicles (Fig. 245). They may be (*a*) solitary or (*b*) multiple (" deep " neurofibromatosis) (see § 970). In an intervertebral foramen they form a " dumb-bell " tumour, widen the foramen and produce on X-ray films a paravertebral circular or ovoid shadow. Within the spinal cord they become elongated and can extend upwards and

downwards to compress the cord over several segments. Removal may mean cutting the parent root. Results are excellent in solitary cases, but less good in multiple cases where signs keep recurring as new fibromas grow.

There are signs of SPINAL CORD COMPRESSION; *there may also be* NEUROFIBROMATA ON THE PERIPHERAL NERVES—*and/or* EIGHTH NERVE DEAFNESS, *associated with multiple pedunculated or* SESSILE TUMOURS OF THE SKIN *which shows a* " CAFÉ AU LAIT " PIGMENTATION. *The condition is* NEUROFIBROMATOSIS.

§ 970. Neurofibromatosis (Syn. von Recklinghausen's disease) may be familial. *Symptoms.*—There are tumours in the spinal cord, on the nerve roots, in the brain or on peripheral nerves; those in the mesentery (ganglion-neuromata) can cause severe disability. In the superficial form of the disease soft subcutaneous tumours can be felt to be freely movable under the skin and hypertrophy of nerves produces plexiform neuroma. The disease may cause auditory neurofibromata and deafness (§ 1083). The tumours of the skin and the skin pigmentation are described in § 734. Other changes occasionally seen are in the pituitary, kyphosis and scoliosis, cysts in the ends of the long bones and elephantiasis. *Prognosis.*—There is no shortening of life unless sarcomatous metaplasia occurs. *Treatment* is by removal of the neurofibromata from the spinal roots or when they occur intraspinally or intracranially.

Intramedullary Causes

(12) GLIOMATA of various types occur extending upwards and downwards within the cord over several segments. Nothing is to be gained by attempting to remove these. EPENDYMOMA is a gliomatous tumour growing from the conus or filum terminale. Such growths are only relatively benign and are difficult to remove without damage to the cauda equina.

Extra-vertebral Causes

(13) HODGKIN'S DISEASE spreading from the mediastinum through the intervertebral foramina may cause sudden or gradual spinal cord compression. The operation of scraping the extradural lymphadenomatous tissue gives good results for several years if there has been no previous radiotherapy; subsequent radiotherapy will be needed.

Other Causes

(14) Dermoid cysts and (15) Angiomata are rare causes of compression which may be diagnosed radiographically. Angiomata produce a characteristic myelogram.

§ 971. Treatment of Paraplegia.—(1) The *cause* should be treated. Where an innocent spinal tumour exists, laminectomy must be undertaken, otherwise the condition will lead to complete paralysis and death. (2) *Nursing care.* The patient should be nursed on a sponge-rubber bed on fracture boards or on a " ripple bed " and the posture changed every three hours by gentle rolling on the side. The greatest care should be taken to avoid wrinkles in the sheets under the patient, and he should always be lifted not dragged along the bed. A bed-cradle sufficiently high to clear the legs even when in flexor spasm will be necessary, with rubber rings for the heels and pads, bandages and pillows to protect pressure points. The feet should be kept from rotating outwards and they should be dorsiflexed and supported with light splints and sandbags. Adductor spasm will require a firm pillow between the knees. Hot-water bottles should have thick covers free from holes. They should never be placed in direct contact with the skin as they may burn an insensitive or unconscious patient through two layers of blankets. Breathing exercises and frequent change of posture tend to prevent hypostatic pneumonia. Give procaine penicillin 500,000 units intramusc. each day to prevent chest and bladder infection. The *skin* should be washed twice daily with soap and water, carefully dried and rubbed with spirit, then powdered with zinc oxide and starch. Back blisters should be aspirated and deep sloughs curetted. Separation of sloughs in bedsores may be helped by compresses of hydrogen peroxide applied for half-an-hour twice a day. Saline or sterile paraffin dressings well covered with Elastoplast needs to be changed daily. Systemic antibiotics may help to sterilise a sore. Zinc oxide and castor oil ointment (B.P.) is useful in treating clean bedsores, as is silicone ointment. Excessive sweating sometimes responds to tab. benzhexol hydrochlor. 2–5 mg. (3) *Nutrition.*—In patients with bedsores, sweating and bladder sepsis, general measures to replace protein loss and dehydration are indicated. Anorexia, muscle wasting and low metabolism lead to anæmia. A high protein diet, drinks of fruit juice and glucose should be given. Blood transfusion by drip may help dehydrated and anæmic patients. (4) *Bowels.* Avoid aperients by mouth. Give twice weekly a soap and water enema or a bowel lavage with plain water. Manual removal of fæces with a gloved finger is sometimes necessary. (5) The *care of the bladder* is of paramount importance. A few may be able to empty the bladder by suprapubic pressure. Catheterisation eight-hourly with a " no-touch " technique should always be used (and see § 858). If retention is prolonged this will often mean in a male patient the insertion of a Gibbon's plastic catheter

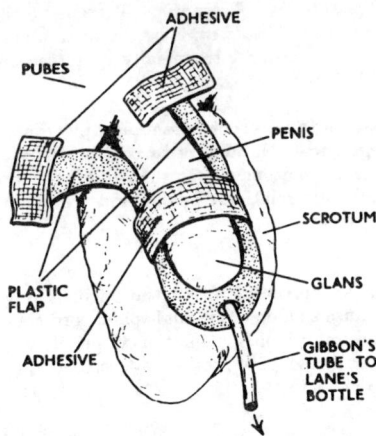

FIG. 246.—GIBBON'S TUBE IN POSITION. The plastic flaps are attached 30–35 cm. from the vesical end of the tube and are fixed to the penis and pubis by strapping. The tube drains into a closed drainage system. These tubes must be changed weekly with strict aseptic precautions.

to drain into a closed bottle hung at the side of the bed below the bladder level (Fig. 246). The urine should be kept acid with acid sodium phosphate gr. 30–60, ammonium chloride gr. 5–60, or ammonium mandelate gr. 50. Sulpha-drugs are not necessary if the patient is on penicillin. In other cases a morning dose of a long-acting sulphonamide, sulphamethoxypyridazine (Midicel), with 5 pints of fluid daily will be required. When the patient begins to get up the Gibbon's catheter is drained into a rubber container attached to a belt. Large intraurethral plastic or rubber catheters cause balanitis and urethritis and are not advised. High suprapubic cystotomy may be required later in those who do not recover bladder function. (6) *Pain* in the early stages is due to damage to nerve roots or to the conus, or it arises in the sensitive dura. Give pethidine 50 mg. with chlorpromazine 25 mg. or codein phosphate gr. ½–½. Tab. codein co. four-hourly is useful. In the later stages painful flexor spasms will have to be treated and this is not easy. A high bed-cradle helps. Tinct. gelsemii ℳ. 20 in a mixture and phenobarbitone gr. 3 intramuscularly may be tried. Hyoscine hydrobromide gr. 1/100 under the tongue at bedtime helps some. Muscle relaxants are not very effective. Intrathecal injections of alcohol or phenol in myodil, section of ventral roots or chordotomy is kept for cases of malignancy and " hopeless " paraplegics and may bring great relief of pain. They tend however to disturb bladder function and where control is good should not be lightly undertaken. (7) *Physiotherapy*. The joints of the paralysed limbs should be moved passively at least twice a day. Tilting the patient on a board at an angle with the feet supported and head up will encourage weight-bearing. While in bed, the bones quickly decalcify. Voluntary movements should be encouraged with the limbs suspended in slings. Many can be taught to walk at first between parallel bars and later with elbow crutches and toe-raising springs. (8) *Rehabilitation*. By developing the physiological residue of muscle power in the upper limbs and trunk, and by mechanical aids the health and morale of many cases can be enormously improved. All are taught independence and many become fit for sedentary occupations and recreation in spite of disability. Mechanically propelled chairs should not be ordered for patients who have defective vision, poor arm control or a tendency to fits.

The paraplegia is due to CEREBRAL *disease or bilateral hemiplegia. The condition is* DIPLEGIA (Syn. Cerebral Palsy).

Lesions of the medulla and pons produce brachial paraplegia in which the arms are affected. Bilateral hemiplegia occurs in cerebral arterio-sclerosis (§§ 574, 916).

A CHILD *has been* STIFF FROM BIRTH, *is unable to suck properly, has a feeble cry and may have fits; or after a few months of nearly normal development it* FAILS TO HOLD ITS HEAD UP, TO SIT UP OR TO STAND *at the normal age,* AND HOLDS ITS LEGS IN RIGID EXTENSION AND ADDUCTION; *the condition is* CEREBRAL DIPLEGIA.

§ 972. **Cerebral Diplegia** (Syn. Little's disease, Cerebral palsy) is relatively common. There is spastic paralysis of both legs and in many cases a milder affection of the arms. A lesser or greater degree of mental deficiency is present in most cases.

Symptoms are noticed at birth (pre-natal) or within the first three years of life (post-natal). The infant never learns to walk correctly. The extensor plantar response of infancy may be perpetuated, and the legs are spastic and adducted, the arms flexed across the chest and adducted at the shoulders. When an attempt is made to put the child to the ground, stepping may be attempted, but the legs tend to cross in front of one another (scissor-gait). Bilateral equino-varus is present. The degree of intelligence varies but is commonly subnormal and speaking is often delayed. The post-natal cases tend to progress, the pre-natal ones to improve. Microcephaly, internal squint and contractures are frequently present. The head is symmetrical, the distribution of the spasticity is rarely perfectly symmetrical.

CLINICAL INVESTIGATION.—Inquire for the pre-natal history, history of prolonged labour or precipitate delivery (prematurity, cyanosis, pallor, collapse), the use of oxygen, Rh incompatibility and jaundice at birth, and the birth weight. Also whether the infant was spastic or flaccid, the developmental progress and were there any fits ? On examination notice the posture and response to objects. Measure the head circumference and note the condition of the fontanelles. Examine the eyes for squint or pupillary anomalies (fundus examination usually requires a general anæsthetic). Note spasticity or flaccidity of the limbs and the tendon and cutaneous reflexes.

Varieties.—Spastic, athetoid and ataxic types occur.

(1) SPASTIC DIPLEGIA is the commonest type. The arms and the legs are all affected. The condition may be asymmetrical. Fits and athetoid movements may be present. Squints are common and severe. The psychological handicap is greater in this group. In *Infantile hemiplegia* (§ 913) cortical sensory loss and hemianopia may be present. Intelligence is normal or mediocre.

(2) SPASTIC PARAPLEGIA.—The legs only are affected, they are spastic and so adducted that perhaps they cross one another. The spinal and neck muscles are weak. Supporting the child by the armpits will reveal flexion of the head and a " scissor " attitude of the legs. Ankle and patellar clonus with clasp-knife rigidity of the legs is ·

found. The abdominals are often present: extensor responses are difficult to elicit. The mentality is often within normal range.

(3) ATHETOID DIPLEGIA.—Some of these cases are due to partial destruction of the basal ganglia by icterus gravis neonatorum. The cortex is usually unaffected and intelligence is normal. Choreo-athetotic movements interfere with speech, the acquisition of hand skills and with walking. Deafness may be present in cases due to jaundice.

(4) ATAXIC DIPLEGIA with hypotonia and nystagmus is described. The tendon reflexes can be elicited, unlike cases of polyneuritis and amyotonia congenita.

Etiology.—This is a syndrome, the end result of many factors damaging the embryonic and developing brain. Known factors are mostly post-natal and include, (1) Birth injury, (2) Anoxia, (3) Sagittal sinus thrombosis, (4) Meningeal hæmorrhage, (5) Congenital hæmolytic jaundice (which causes disease of the basal ganglia), (6) Toxoplasmosis. We know little of pre-natal causes but it seems likely that they are due to infections, metabolic disorders, toxæmia or exposure of the mother to radiation during pregnancy.

Prognosis.—In severe cases early death from intercurrent infection is common. In the absence of gross mental defect and severe sphincter disturbance, education should be undertaken. Most cases improve—even patients with episodic fits, severe squints and mild degrees of mental retardation. Cases of spastic paraplegia do best. Those with congenital athetosis, if symptoms are mild, may be educated to earn their living.

Treatment.—Epilepsy must be treated. Special care and schooling helps selected patients, especially those who show signs of initiative and eagerness to reach an objective. Patient physiotherapy and speech therapy will be necessary in most. Stereotaxic surgery for involuntary movements and spasticity is on trial but not all patients are helped.

GROUP XI.   FLACCID PARALYSIS AND PERIPHERAL NERVE LESIONS

§ 973. **Flaccid Paralysis** is usually due to a lesion of the lower motor neurone. The dendrites of a single axon branch and ramify widely amongst individual fibres in a muscle bundle (Fig. 213). Lesions affecting the *Lower Motor Neurones* cause flaccid muscle paralysis, with loss of muscle tone and tendon reflex due to the abolition of the stretch reflex. Atrophy of muscle fibres and the reaction of degeneration follow. Such findings are seen in traumatic lesions of a motor nerve, *e.g.*, serratus anterior palsy (long thoracic nerve) or in purely motor forms of neuropathy (*e.g.*, lead palsy), or in acute lesions of the anterior horn cells as in acute poliomyelitis. When the *anterior horn cell* undergoes chronic progressive degeneration (*e.g.*, motor neurone disease) fasciculation may be seen in the affected muscles before they become wasted and paralysed. Lesions at the *myoneural junction* (as in myasthenia gravis) are characterised by a fatigue paralysis which disappears after rest, perhaps due to a disturbance of choline metabolism. Paralysis due to primary *Disease of the Muscles* is seen in myopathy, polymyositis, dermatomyositis. *Biochemical disorders, e.g.*, (1) potassium depletion, (2) disorders of choline and cholinesterases are rare causes of diffuse reversible flaccid paralysis (see Family Periodic Paralysis (§ 990), Primary Aldosteronism (§ 991)).

In acute *Upper Motor Neurone* lesions transient flaccid paralysis of the affected limbs may be seen as a temporary shock effect. The distribution is characteristic.

There is BILATERALLY SYMMETRICAL FLACCID PARALYSIS of the limbs, usually with TINGLING, NUMBNESS AND PERIPHERAL SENSORY LOSS. The muscles are extremely tender to gentle kneading and the TENDON REFLEXES DISAPPEAR. Cranial nerves may be affected. The condition may be POLYNEURITIS.

§ 974. Polyneuritis (Syn. Multiple Symmetrical Peripheral Neuritis, Peripheral Neuropathy) is a relatively common disease. The lesions in the peripheral nerves are partly biochemical, partly degenerative. In some cases the posterior columns of the cord are also affected. The commonest known causes are alcoholism, diphtheria, diabetes mellitus, pernicious anæmia and beri-beri. In the majority of cases the cause is unknown. A large and ever-increasing list of toxic substances used in medicine and industry may cause the disease. With polyneuritis due to alcoholism, lead poisoning, diabetes mellitus and carcinoma the lesions are widespread in the central and peripheral nervous systems and the posterior columns, cerebrum, cerebellum and (in the case of carcinomatous and diabetic neuropathy) the skeletal muscles may be affected.

CAUSES OF POLYNEURITIS

I. *Infections*—Diphtheria, Acute Infective Polyneuritis, Bacterial toxins and bacteria.

II. *Metallic Substances*—Lead, Arsenic, Mercury and " Pink " Disease.

III. *Drugs and Industrial Poisons*—Alcohol, Isoniazid, Carbon bisulphide, Triorthocresyl phosphate (" Jake "), Trinitrobenzene, Aniline, Methyl bromide, etc.

IV. *Metabolic*—Diabetes mellitus, Porphyria.

V. *Deficiency diseases*—Beri-beri, Subacute combined degeneration, Pellagra, Steatorrhœa, Hyperemesis Gravidarum, Nutritional neuropathy of prisoners.

VI. *Growths*—Cancer of the lung and elsewhere.

VII. *Other disease states*—Allergic conditions (serum sickness), Sarcoidosis, Myxœdema, Immersion in the sea.

MONONEURITIS MULTIPLEX is the term used to describe *asymmetrical* pathological affection of multiple peripheral nerves. This occurs in leprosy, amyloidosis, neurofibromatosis, progressive hypertrophic neuritis and periarteritis nodosa.

Symptoms of Polyneuritis.—The onset is usually subacute over a period of weeks, but in acute infective polyneuritis the onset is sudden within a day or two. (1) *Sensory symptoms* usually come first. They are aching or burning pains and paræsthesiæ, numbness and tingling in the periphery of the limbs. In alcoholic neuritis, the soles of the feet, although numb, are hyperæsthetic. (2) There is diminution of cutaneous sensitivity to light touches, pin-prick and temperature over the periphery of the limbs of " glove " and " stocking " distribution, with hyperæsthesia to stroking or handling. (3) Sensory ataxia may occur from impairment of deep sensitivity (joint sense). (4) *Motor paralysis* affects the extensors of the wrists and fingers, producing wrist-drop; or the anterior tibial and peroneal muscles, producing foot-drop. Symmetrical paralysis of the diaphragm, respiratory and trunk muscles, facial or bulbar palsies occur in severe cases. If the condition becomes chronic, atrophy may occur in the paralysed muscles with contracture and fibrosis. Cranial nerves are rarely affected except in acute infective polyneuritis. Paralysis of accommodation is characteristic of diphtheritic polyneuritis. (5) The affected muscles (and the Achilles tendons) are often extremely tender to palpation or gentle kneading. (6) The tendon and superficial reflexes are diminished or absent. (7) *Autonomic paralysis* may cause the affected limbs to be œdematous, blue and clammy. (8) *Myocardial signs* are common—tachycardia, extrasystoles or dilatation of the heart from myocardial changes; death may occur from ventricular fibrillation. (9) *Mental symptoms.* Confusion and disorientation with amnesia and confabulation (Korsakoff's psychosis) is common in alcoholic polyneuritis, and it occasionally occurs in other forms, *e.g.*, polyneuritis of pregnancy. Pathological stupor or lethargy with ocular palsies occurs in Wernicke's syndrome due to aneurine deficiency. (10) The *spinal fluid* in many cases is unaltered, but in others may show the most profound changes. Xanthochromia, massive coagulation of the fluid, great increase of protein (100–1,000 mg. per cent.) without increase of cells (Froin's syndrome) may be found. A slight pleocytosis is rare.

Blood pyruvate estimations can provide useful information regarding advanced cases of aneurine deficiency, *e.g.*, beri-beri, alcoholic neuropathy, and the neuropathy of chronic gastroenteritis. The fasting blood pyruvate is 0·6–1·4 mg. per 100 ml. of whole blood. After withdrawing a fasting specimen of blood 50 G. of glucose is given by mouth followed 30 minutes later by a second dose of 50 G. Blood specimens for pyruvate estimation are taken 30, 60 and 90 minutes after the first dose and if the values are above 2·0 mg. 100 ml. of whole blood there is aneurine deficiency.

Diagnosis.—The ataxic cases have a superficial resemblance to tabes dorsalis, but the (1) tenderness of muscles, (2) absence of Argyll-Robertson pupils, (3) absence of sphincter disturbance, and (4) C.S.F. findings usually make the diagnosis from tabes easy (Table LVII). In diagnosing the cause, the history of infection or of exposure to poisoning is important.

Etiology.—The biochemical causes underlying peripheral neuritis are not fully understood. Half of the cases show incomplete breakdown in the carbohydrate metabolic cycle on which nerve-cells depend so much for respiration. In these cases pyruvic acid accumulates in the blood but restoration of the biochemical fault by aneurine injection does not cure the peripheral neuropathy. In *mononeuritis multiplex* the cause is either microscopically visible on nerve biopsy, or characteristic organic lesions of the nerve are present, *e.g.*, leprosy (lepra bacillus), amyloidosis, neurofibromatosis, progressive hypertrophic neuritis, polyarteritis nodosa.

Prognosis.—The illness lasts many months. Unexpected death from sudden cardiac failure may occur in diphtheritic neuritis. Acute infective polyneuritis may run a rapidly fatal course in spite of artificial respiration. Acute porphyria is sometimes fatal and patients with carcinomatous neuropathy do not survive long. In other forms recovery is usual unless there is complicating broncho-pneumonia, or Korsakoff's psychosis.

Patients with diphtheritic neuritis usually make a complete recovery. In older patients with chronic neuropathies recovery is incomplete with persistent wasting, weakness and absent tendon reflexes.

I. *Polyneuritis due to Infections.*

In **Botulism** (§ 1068), **Diphtheria** (§ 975) and **Tetanus** (§ 1031) the cause is a qacterial exotoxin. In **Leprous neuritis** (§ 985) bacilli are found in the nerves.

§ **975. Diphtheritic Neuritis** due to the exotoxin of the *C. diphtheriæ* is now rare in the United Kingdom due to immunisation campaigns and the early use of antitoxin. *Local* paralysis occurs in muscles and parts anatomically related to the site of infection, *e.g.*, palatal paralysis in faucial diphtheria, in the leg muscles in case of infected sores on the leg. The *specific* paralysis is of accommodation. The *generalised* neuritis affecting the periphery of the limbs comes on in the third to the sixth week (§ 497). Sensory changes are inconspicuous but sensory ataxia is almost always present.

Prognosis.—Recovery is the rule although progress is slow. It may be six months before strength is fully recovered in the affected limbs.

§ **976. Acute Infective Polyneuritis** (Syn. Landry's paralysis, Guillain-Barré Syndrome). *Symptoms.*—Following a short febrile attack lasting some hours with respiratory or gastro-intestinal symptoms, spreading flaccid paralysis of muscles rapidly appears; pain, muscle tenderness, numbness, tingling and pins and needles in the trunk and limbs occur early. Occasionally fever is absent. The paralysis is said to affect the proximal more than the distal muscles: facial diplegia is common: retention of urine may complicate the first ten days of the illness. Papillœdema is occasionally seen. If the disease ascends a flaccid quadriplegia with bulbar symptoms will appear in a few days and the use of a respirator and a team of skilled nurses will be required. *Spinal fluid pressure on manometry* is normal. A characteristic finding in many cases is a very high protein reading (1,000 mg. per cent.) with xanthochromic fluid and spontaneous coagulation after withdrawal. Usually the cells are not increased but a slight excess of lymphocytes (10 to 100 per c. mm.) is rarely found.

Diagnosis from acute ascending poliomyelitis is made by (1) the presence of paræsthesiæ and sensory changes, (2) the usual absence of lymphocytosis in the spinal fluid in polyneuritis. Diphtheritic neuritis and neuropathy of acute porphyria may simulate acute infective polyneuritis.

Etiology.—The cause is unknown. Any age may be affected and the sexes are attacked equally.

Prognosis.—The mortality rate is high, especially in older patients; death may occur in the first few days from respiratory failure or toxic myocarditis. In children the disease may run a slowly remitting course and a bulbar extension of the paralysis can occur as late as the sixth week.

II. *Polyneuritis due to Metallic Substances.*

§ **977. Lead poisoning** (Syn. " Plumbism ") produces motor neuropathy, anterior horn cell degeneration, myopathy and encephalopathy. *Symptoms.*—(1) Bilateral wrist-drop appears with paralysis of the extensors of the fingers and thumbs characteristically sparing the extensor ossis metacarpi pollicis and the brachioradialis muscles. There is occasionally foot-drop from paralysis of the anterior tibial and peroneal muscles. (2) Cramps, tremors and pains may be present in the limbs but no sensory changes occur. (3) Lead encephalopathy may co-exist with headache and papillœdema. (4) Rare cases of anterior horn cell and cord damage are described resembling amyotrophic lateral sclerosis. (5) There are other signs of plumbism (§ 568).

Etiology.—The poisoning may be industrial or accidental. *Prognosis.*—Gradual recovery in adults is the rule following removal from the source of poisoning.

§ **978. Arsenical** Neuritis is rare but may still be seen from accidental poisoning from weed-killer. Arsenic still remains a favourite with poisoners—often females. The neuritis produces foot-drop, associated with pigmentation on the skin of the abdomen, hyperkeratosis of the palms and soles in chronic cases, and diarrhœa and vomiting in acute cases. In suspected poisoning arsenic may be found in the hair, nails or urine.

ERYTHRŒDEMA POLYNEURITIS (Syn. " Pink disease ") in infants under four years of age is probably due to mercurial salts in teething powders. Polyneuritis, intense erythema with photophobia characterise the complaint (§ 591).

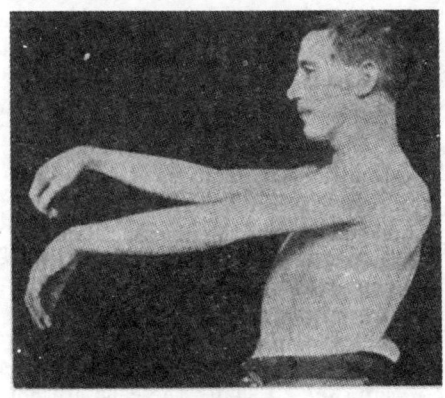

FIG. 247.—BILATERAL WRIST-DROP in a patient with polyneuritis due to lead poisoning.

III. *Polyneuritis due to Drugs and Industrial Poisons.*

§ **979. Alcoholic Neuropathy** is the commonest type of peripheral neuritis. It is much more frequent in men than women, usually in those of 40 to 70 years. It is not known with certainty whether the damage is due to nutritional disorder (aneurine deficiency) secondary to alcoholic gastro-enteritis and hepatic disease, or to the toxic action of ingested alcohol.

Symptoms.—The onset is usually subacute but may be acute after an infection or a drinking bout with abstention from food. The patient is often a solitary drinker. The polyneuritis is associated with *great tenderness of muscles and hyperæsthesia of the soles of the feet*. The lower limbs are affected more than the upper and " stocking " and " glove " anæsthesia of the skin may be present. Ankle- and knee-jerks are often absent. Mental changes are common—(1) confusional states (delirium tremens), (2) dementia (due to cortical atrophy, Korsakoff's psychosis or necrosis of the corpus callosum), or (3) lethargy, ptosis and external ocular palsies (Wernicke's syndrome).   Nystagmus and cerebellar ataxia may be observed as temporary or more permanent signs.

Prognosis.—The course is prolonged and contractures are prone to occur in paralysed muscles.

Isoniazid Neuritis is seen during the treatment of pulmonary tuberculosis with isoniazid.   It is believed to be due to interference with the metabolism of pyridoxine and can be prevented by giving tab. pyridoxine hydrochlor. 20 to 200 mg. (gr. ⅓ to 3) daily.

OCCUPATIONAL POISONING may cause neuropathy from *mercury* (in barometer makers tremors, sponginess of the gums), *carbon bisulphide, trinitrobenzol, aniline, methyl bromide* (fire extinguishers, etc.).   Acute and chronic widespread lesions are found in fatal cases.

" *Jake* " *paralysis* due to ingestion of triorthocresol phosphate occurs in small outbreaks; Jamaica ginger extract or aircraft oils may be the vehicles of poisoning.

IV. *Polyneuritis due to Metabolic Diseases.*

§ 980. Diabetic Neuropathy, chiefly seen in those whose diabetes is not properly controlled, may be mild or severe. *Symptoms.*—In mild cases there are paræsthesiæ in the extremities and absence of the ankle-jerks. The muscles of the calves are often tender to pressure.   Orthostatic hypotension and fainting may occur from autonomic paralyses.   In the severe type (diabetic pseudo-tabes), the patient is ataxic from loss of sense of position, and perforating ulcers and arthropathies may be present in the feet and toes.   Pupillary abnormalities are frequent.   In arteriosclerotic diabetics, mononeuritis multiplex affecting particularly the sciatic or femoral nerves, or unilateral or bilateral external ocular palsies may occur. A myopathy affecting the proximal shoulder and pelvic girdle muscles is rarely seen.

Prognosis.—The disease bears no clear relationship to the diabetic state and may progress after control is established.   The paralysis of elderly arteriosclerotic diabetic patients may be permanent.

In **Porphyria,** recurrent abdominal colic with absence of ankle- and knee-jerks raises the suspicion of tabes or of intestinal obstruction.   Some have mental symptoms. Attacks may be precipitated by barbiturates or sulpha-drugs and examination of the urine will demonstrate porphyrins (§§ 415, 950).

V. *Polyneuritis due to Deficiency Diseases* (Nutritional Neuropathies).

In deficiency states polyneuritis, mental changes, Wernicke's encephalopathy (§ 1070), cranial nerve palsies, burning feet, spinal ataxia and spastic paraplegia may occur.

§ 981. Beri-beri is a vitamin B_1 (aneurine) deficiency disease especially affecting rice eaters in the tropics.   It shows œdema in the legs and polyneuritis, producing paraplegia.

The *Symptoms* are of two kinds: (*a*) those referable to the neuro-muscular system associated with polyneuritis; (*b*) those referable to the cardio-vascular system associated with neuritis of the vagus and sympathetic nerves and interstitial œdema of the heart muscle.   Either form may occur alone, but generally there is gastro-intestinal trouble and polyneuritis as well as œdema and other evidence of cardiac failure; many cases do not fall into either of these categories. The onset is gradual and the incubation period two to three months.

In (a), known as " dry beri-beri," there is no œdema, the dominant features being wasting and weakness of the muscles. The knee-jerks are at first exaggerated, then lost, the ankle-jerks are lost and there is cutaneous sensory loss below the knees and wrists. The calf-muscles are tender and areas of hyperæsthesia develop on the soles. High-steppage gait and wrist-drop occur and the patient cannot rise from a squatting position.

In (b), known as " wet beri-beri," various grades of œdema involve the feet, legs and later the serous cavities. Dyspnœa, dilatation of the right heart associated with systolic murmurs and perhaps tachycardia, and a rapid, low-tension pulse develop. The urine is free from albumen and casts as a rule. Signs of polyneuritis are generally also present.

(c) Acute fulminating cardiac beri-beri (Shöshin) has been studied by Hawes in Malaya. The patient is extremely breathless, with vomiting, epigastric pain and great restlessness, and, unless appropriately treated by intravenous injections of pure vitamin B_1, dies in a few hours. The heart is greatly enlarged, the cervical veins engorged, but the pulse does not often exceed 120–130 per minute. The systolic pressure is well sustained until just before death; the diastolic always drops with the onset of severe symptoms.

(d) Infantile beri-beri is found in breast-fed infants of mothers with latent or clinical beri-beri. It occurs in acute and chronic forms in Japan and the Philippine Islands. Cardiac œdema and gastro-intestinal symptoms such as nausea, vomiting, diarrhœa or constipation are characteristic.

Diagnosis.—Wet beri-beri has to be diagnosed from severe ankylostomiasis, cardiac failure and nephritis, and the dry form from alcoholic and arsenical neuritis, tabes, etc. The dietetic history and the occurrence amongst Orientals of widespread poly-neuritis should arouse suspicion.

Prognosis.—The fulminating cases of cardiac beri-beri were invariably fatal until dramatic cure was found to follow pure vitamin B_1 given intravenously. Ordinary cases recover with extra supplies of vitamin B_1 by mouth.

Etiology.—Beri-beri occurs in the rice-eating population of Oriental countries, and is also endemic in Newfoundland and Labrador where white wheaten flour is used. It is due to deficiency in the antineuritic vitamin B_1 which is removed from the rice grain by the polishing process and from flour when refined. The use of under-milled rice and whole wheat prevents its development. Vitamin B_1 influences carbohydrate metabolism and controls the conversion of pyruvate into oxidation products like CO_2 and H_2O: in fulminating beri-beri pyruvic acid increases in the blood, cerebro-spinal fluid and urine, especially in the presence of fever, muscular work and carbohydrate intake, all of which intensify metabolism; normal levels follow the administration of pure vitamin B_1. In some instances, however, disturbances appear to have reached the stage at which recovery cannot be effected merely by supplying adequate amounts of vitamin B_1, and in " dry atrophic " types of beri-beri pyruvic acid may not be demonstrably increased.

Treatment.—Cardiac cases should immediately receive pure vitamin B_1 intra-venously in a dosage of 5–10 mg. As much as 50 mg. of the crystalline substance may be necessary in profoundly ill patients: vene-section may be advisable and the bowels should be kept open with salines. Absolute rest in bed is essential. Later on, and in less severely ill patients, pure vitamin B_1 can be injected or given in doses of 3–5 mg. t.d.s. *per os.* At first small feeds, including marmite, eggs and milk, are given two-hourly, and later a dry diet rich in vitamin and low in carbohydrate. Foods rich in vitamin B_1 include yeast, liver, sheep brains, heart muscle, haricot beans, lettuce, wholemeal or brown bread, undermilled rice and rice polishings.

§ 982. STEATORRHŒA (including sprue, and chronic infective colitis), and HYPER-EMESIS GRAVIDARUM (rarely), may all be associated with peripheral neuritis.

The deficiency in most cases is complex, and attempts to link these conditions with specific vitamin defects not entirely successful. Thus aneurine deficiency causes beri-beri and alcoholic polyneuritis in man; *pantothenic acid* deficiency " Burning Feet "; *nicotinic acid* deficiency Pellagra; and *cyanocobalamin* (B₁₂) deficiency subacute combined degeneration (§ 950). Parenteral or oral vitamin therapy may improve the patient's general health without influencing the neuritis, which responds much more slowly.

§ **983. Nutritional Neuropathy.**—In prisoners of war on an ill-balanced diet, symptoms of neuropathy may appear. Central scotomata, optic atrophy, nerve deafness and laryngeal palsies may accompany absent tendon reflexes, loss of joint sense and ataxia. The " Burning Feet Syndrome " (§ 590) is one type of clinical picture (related to pantothenic acid deficiency); spastic paraplegia is rarer. Recovery is slow; permanent visual or auditory defects and absent jerks remain. Similar symptoms occur in conditions of chronic malnutrition due to ill-balanced diets, *e.g.*, elderly persons living alone, mental patients refusing food, chronic alcoholics.

VI. *Polyneuritis due to Malignant Growths.*

§ **984. Carcinomatous Neuropathy** is chiefly seen in patients with bronchial carcinoma but also in cases of carcinoma of the stomach or ovary. The neurological symptoms may precede discovery of the growth and have nothing to do with metastases; one theory is that they are nutritional in origin. Peripheral neuropathy, postero-lateral cord changes, posterior column or cerebellar degeneration and myopathy may sometimes occur. All are rare.

VII. *Polyneuritis due to other Causes.*

Allergic Neuropathy is occasionally seen with serum sickness and urticaria (§ 652).

Sarcoidosis (§§ 141, 889) is a rare cause of peripheral neuropathy. Enlargement of the parotid glands associated with iritis and facial palsy was formerly termed " uveoparotid paralysis " (§ 9). Other cranial nerves may be affected. Meningeal and central lesions have been described. *Diagnosis* is by biopsy of nodules and by the Kveim test (§ 141). *Prognosis.*—The condition is usually benign and recovery of the cranial nerves and peripheral palsies may be aided by steroid therapy.

MYXŒDEMA may cause (1) " carpal tunnel syndrome," (2) peripheral neuropathy and (3) " drop-attacks." The facies is characteristic (§§ 9, 575).

Immersion in the sea for days on inadequate food supplies may be followed by a chronic severe peripheral neuropathy.

MONONEURITIS MULTIPLEX.

§ **985. Leprous Neuritis** causes diffuse or nodular thickening of peripheral nerves. The ulnar, great auricular, anterior tibial and external popliteal nerves are often picked out. Patchy anæsthesia to pin-prick and cotton-wool is found over the cutaneous distribution of the affected nerves, or motor paralysis (ulnar palsy or foot-drop) appears. Trophic ulcers may be present on fingers or toes. Patchy anæsthesia of the face occurs when the trigeminal nerve is affected. Cutaneous lesions or ulceration of the nasal septum may be present (§ 715). Children and young adults are especially liable.

Diagnosis from syringomyelia or other hypertrophic forms of neuropathy (amyloidosis, progressive hypertrophic neuropathy) can be made easily if the possibility of leprosy be considered in those patients from Burma, Nigeria, China and other areas where the disease is prevalent.

The bacillus should be sought in nasal mucus, in scrapings from skin lesions or nerve biopsy.

Etiology.—This is a true neuritis due to the presence of *mycobacterium lepræ* in the substance of the nerve affected.

In **Amyloidosis** there may be thickening of peripheral nerves due to intraneural deposits of amyloid material. There is albuminuria (§ 409) with chronic diarrhœa (see § 318).

Neurofibromatosis (see § 1083).

§ 986. Progressive Hypertrophic Neuritis is a rare heredo-familial disease, producing thickening of the peripheral palpable nerve-trunks, *e.g.*, superficial cervical nerves, with distal atrophy of muscles and sensory loss of posterior column type. It is probably allied to Neurofibromatosis.

§ 987. Polyarteritis nodosa produces an asymmetrical mononeuritis multiplex in a third of the cases, possibly due to ischæmic changes in the nerve-trunks (§ 98). This *diagnosis* should be considered in a patient with a low-grade continued pyrexia who has symptoms of an asymmetrical neuropathy.

Treatment of Polyneuritis.—(1) Remove the patient from the cause if this is possible. When alcoholism is in question this will mean preliminary detoxication treatment in a home for a week or two; limiting alcoholic consumption is of no use. (2) Chelating agents are used in metallic poisonings. Thus in lead poisoning give sodium calciumedetate (§ 568). (3) Aneurine parenterally is of value in beri-beri, in alcoholic neuropathy (including Wernicke's syndrome) and in the neuropathy of chronic gastrointestinal disease, *e.g.*, steatorrhœa. Give aneurine hydrochlor. 10–50 mg. intramusc. daily for Wernicke's encephalopathy and later vitamin B complex by mouth. Cyanocobalamin 1,000 micrograms has been given with benefit in gastro-intestinal neuropathy; others use concentrated injections of vitamin B complex (" Parentrovite ") in dextrose-saline for intravenous injection, or with an added local anæsthetic for intramuscular injection. (4) Rest in bed with careful nursing is required in all cases until the pulse rate is normal and until the limbs have regained enough strength to bear the patient's weight. (5) Bed cradles, sandbags, light splints, passive movements, warm packs and aspirin will help to relieve pain and to prevent contractures. (6) After the painful stage, light massage and re-educative exercises will help the patient to regain strength. Electrical treatment is rarely required. A full, palatable and nourishing diet should be given. Cortisone in acute or subacute cases may be helpful, *e.g.*, in fulminating acute infective polyneuritis. In acute ascending or bulbar cases respiratory failure should be forestalled by early tracheostomy, and the use of an intermittent positive pressure respirator.

Recurrent Temporary Flaccid Paralysis occurs in

I. Myasthenia gravis.
II. Potassium deficiency.
III. Family Periodic Paralysis.
IV. Primary Aldosteronism.
V. Disseminated Sclerosis.
VI. Sarcoidosis.

The patient complains of EXHAUSTION *and shows* EXTERNAL OPHTHALMOPLEGIA *with* BILATERAL PTOSIS, FACIAL WEAKNESS, NASAL OR FEEBLE VOICE.

The symptoms are abolished wholly or in part by an injection of neostigmin or Tensilon. The condition is MYASTHENIA GRAVIS.

§ 988. I. **Myasthenia Gravis,** characterised by fatigue paralysis of the striped ocular, bulbar and skeletal muscles, is believed to be due to a lesion at the myoneural junction. The disease may occur at any age, in infants and even in late life, but most often in the third decade; men and women are equally affected.

Symptoms.—The onset is insidious: rarely it follows thyroidectomy or an acute infection. The patient complains of abnormal fatigue, especially when extra effort is made, *e.g.,* after hard manual work. Towards the end of the day, the waitress begins to drop trays, the commercial traveller may be aware of dragging his legs as he climbs stairs, the lecturer's voice may become nasal or may fall to a whisper at the end of his discourse; after a short period of rest recovery ensues, but the paralysis recurs on slight exertion. The ocular and bulbar muscles are selectively affected, usually bilaterally. *Ocular Symptoms.*—Variable ptosis (with compensating backward tilting of the head and wrinkling of the forehead) and extreme ophthalmoplegia occur in 40 per cent. of cases. Variable squints and diplopia occur. The pupils are unaffected. Weakness of the orbicularis oculi is common and it is easy to force the lids apart when the patient tries to screw them together. Weakness of the *lower face* causes difficulty in whistling and a peculiar feeble " transverse smile." *Bulbar Symptoms.*—Increasing feebleness of mastication may end in dropping of the jaw. The head falls forwards or backwards after long sessions at the television or cinema. Paralysis of the palate results in nasal voice, and if the pharyngeal muscles are affected there will be dysphagia. *The skeletal muscles* are involved in a third of the cases and in these focal muscular atrophy may be seen. The characteristic " fatigue paralysis " can be demonstrated by appropriate tests, *e.g.,* squeezing a dynamometer, or against resistance. *Sensory changes* are absent and the tendon reflexes are not affected.

Specific tests.—(1) Give inj. neostigmine methylsulphate (B.P.) subcutaneously 2 ml. (0·5 mg. in 1 ml.) together with atropine sulphate 0·16 mg. (to counteract intestinal colic caused by neostigmine). If the paralysis is myasthenic considerable increase of power in the affected muscles with disappearance of ptosis will result within 20 to 30 minutes and last for some hours. (2) Alternatively give 2 mg. edrophonium chloride (Tensilon) intravenously, and if no reaction occurs after 30 seconds give a further injection of 8 mg. This substance produces a similar but more transient effect on the striped muscle palsies of myasthenic patients within 5 minutes of injection; the effects on autonomic ganglia (*e.g.,* colic) are less marked than with neostigmine. (3) Electrical faradic stimulation of nerve produces at first brisk contractions but on rapid repeated stimulation the excitability becomes less and less and finally disappears (" Myasthenic reaction of Jolly ").

Diagnosis depends on the finding of variable paralysis increasing on exertion, diminishing with rest or after injection of neostigmine or Tensilon. The presence of normal tendon reflexes and normal sensation differentiate this from other causes of motor flaccid paralysis. *Any bilateral bulbar paralysis without wasting, or any obscure bilateral external ophthalmoplegia may be myasthenic.* X-rays of the chest in less than half the cases will show evidences of hyperplasia of the thymus or of a thymic neoplasm.

Etiology.—Recently anatomical changes in the nerve endings of the end-plates have been demonstrated. It is believed that there is either a defect in the production of acetylcholine, or an excess of cholinesterase at the myoneural junction. The occasional association of the disease with thymic enlargement, thymic tumours and its occasional occurrence after thyroidectomy suggest an endocrine factor. The muscles contain an excess of glycogen. Small foci of mononuclear cells (lymphorrhages) are found post mortem in the striped muscles, myocardium and liver.

Prognosis.—Remissions may occur lasting for years. In nearly all cases, however, the course is slowly progressive. Death may result from respiratory infection or sudden respiratory failure after great muscular effort. The prognosis for life is best in patients where the limbs are chiefly involved, poorest in those with bulbar paralysis.

Treatment.—Ephedrine hydrochlor. 30 mg. twice or thrice daily, or amphetamine sulphate 10 mg. at similar intervals, helps mild cases but may cause sleeplessness. Many patients can live a reasonably active life whilst on a maintenance dose of tab. neostigmine bromide 15 mg. The dose and method of administration is a matter for trial in individual cases and should be worked out whilst the patient is in bed and later when leading an active life. Usually the tablets are given sublingually; 10 to 20 may be required daily, the first dose being taken before rising. An overdose causes epigastric ache, sweating and blurred vision, but atropine sulphate (0·3 mg.) by mouth or tincture of belladonna may abolish these effects. Mestinon tablets (pyridostigmine bromide) each 60 mg. is an analogue of neostigmine which may render the use of atropine unnecessary. Potassium chloride 1–2 G. thrice daily may be given with neostigmine or Mestinon. *Thymectomy.* The operation is certainly not curative in most cases; generally patients who have been operated upon feel stronger and may be able to live with less medication than before. A few surgically treated patients have been able to dispense with neostigmine completely.

§ 989. II. **Potassium deficiency.**—Excessive loss of potassium by vomiting, diarrhœa or diuresis may result in flaccid paralysis of the limbs. Excessive excretion of potassium with sodium retention results from high doses of cortisone and ACTH. Potassium is concentrated in the intracellular fluids, and estimation of plasma potassium is not necessarily a reliable measure of deficiency. Potassium salts must be given intravenously with caution, as a sudden rise in extracellular potassium may stop the heart. Give potassium chloride 1–2 G. by mouth or per rectum, using 5 per cent. dextrose solution containing 30 mEq. of potassium (and see § 547).

Recurrent weakness due to potassium deficiency occurs also in Family Periodic Paralysis and Primary Aldosteronism.

§ 990. III. **Family Periodic Paralysis** is a very rare heredo-familial disease affecting males more than females and developing during infancy or adolescence.

Symptoms.—Fleeting attacks of paralysis come on after a night's rest, especially if a high carbohydrate meal has been taken before retiring. There may be only slight weakness of the legs which the patient can " walk off " or severe paralysis of the limbs and respiratory muscles lasting hours or days. In the affected muscles the tendon reflexes wane and the electrical excitability disappears. Bradycardia with partial or complete heart block may accompany the attacks. In between attacks these patients are well.

The *Etiology* is unknown. The muscular paralysis is associated with a severe fall in the serum potassium and a rise in sodium: there is no actual loss of potassium from the body, the fall in serum potassium being due to its transfer from the extracellular to the intracellular tissues. Increase of urinary aldosterone with retention of sodium may precede the attacks (Conn).

Treatment.—Attacks may be prevented by giving potassium chloride 2–4 G. in 25 per cent. solution by mouth three or four times daily. Restriction of carbohydrates is advisable. In the attacks potassium salts may be given by mouth or per rectum.

§ 991. IV. In **Primary Aldosteronism** (Conn's Syndrome), due to hyperactivity or tumour of the adrenal cortex, an excessive amount of aldosterone is excreted in the urine and low blood potassium levels are found.

Symptoms.—Recurrent attacks of muscular weakness like those seen in family periodic paralysis occur with hypertension, tetany and polyuria (and see § 263).

The *Treatment* is removal of the cause.

HYSTERICAL FLACCID PARALYSIS may occur with normal tendon reflexes, " stocking and glove " anæsthesia of the hysterical type, and paradoxical posture of the affected limbs.

Peripheral Nerve Lesions

There is a UNILATERAL FLACCID PARALYSIS *with* SENSORY LOSS, *involving completely or in part the distribution of a* NERVE ROOT, PLEXUS OR PERIPHERAL NERVE. *The condition is a localised* PERIPHERAL NERVE LESION.

§ 992. Isolated lesions of individual nerves.—For the most part peripheral nerve paralyses are not painful. There is *flaccid paralysis* of the muscles supplied by the nerve distal to the injury with muscular tenderness. The affected muscles waste and altered electrical reactions occur after three weeks. The tendon reflexes subserved by the paralysed muscles are diminished or disappear. The area of *sensory loss* does not always correspond to textbook pictures, there is commonly a focus of analgesia within a wider area of impaired sensibility over which pin-pricks have a diffuse and painful quality. The *skin* becomes atrophic and the nails may break; in severe cases ulcers may appear on the anæsthetic areas.

Functional disturbance does not necessarily run parallel with anatomical damage, *e.g.*, there may be complete loss of conduction in a nerve with extensively damaged axons which are not necessarily anatomically divided.

CAUSES.—(1) Trauma—perforating wounds, traction or crushing injuries; (2) Prolonged ischæmia from pressure in sleep, anæsthesia or by a tourniquet; Involvement by (3) Fractures or callus formation, (4) Arthritis producing periarticular changes; (5) Growths primary or metastatic, enlarged lymph nodes, (6) Misplaced deep injections; (7) Allergic (serum) reactions; (8) Toxic and metabolic disease.

INVESTIGATION OF PERIPHERAL NERVE LESIONS.[1]—Inquire for a *history of compression* of the nerve. The patient's *occupation* may give a clue to compression or traumatic lesions. Always *palpate* the nerves in their course for thickening and neuromata. Examine the axilla, supraclavicular region, femoral canal and triangle and pelvis for masses of growth or glands. The *urine* should always be tested for sugar and albumen.

Muscle charts of progress should be kept and each muscle separately tested every 4–6 weeks. The state of power of each muscle may be charted as follows: 0 = no contraction, 1 = Flicker or trace of contraction, 2 = Active movement with gravity eliminated, 3 = Active movement against gravity, 4 = Active movement against gravity and resistance, 5 = normal power.

In testing *sensation* on the skin proceed from the anæsthetic towards the normal area. Hairy parts may have to be shaved. Electrical tests of muscles or nerves performed at intervals of time may give valuable information regarding recovery. In treating such cases orthopædic surgical help is usually required.

Upper Limb Paralyses.   (See Fig. 248a and Table LIX.)

§ 993. Brachial Plexus Lesions (C5–Th1).—Two types occur: (a) UPPER PLEXUS TYPE (Erb-Duchenne) and (b) LOWER PLEXUS TYPE (Klumpke). In (a) the muscles affected are those supplied by C5, 6 roots, viz., deltoid, biceps, brachialis anticus, supinator longus, supra- and infra-spinatus, serratus magnus, subscapularis, latissimus dorsi and the clavicular part of pectoralis major. The scapula is winged, the

---

[1] The reader is advised to consult "Aids to the Investigation of Peripheral Nerve Injuries," (M.R.C. War Memorandum No. 7, H.M. Stationery Office, London).

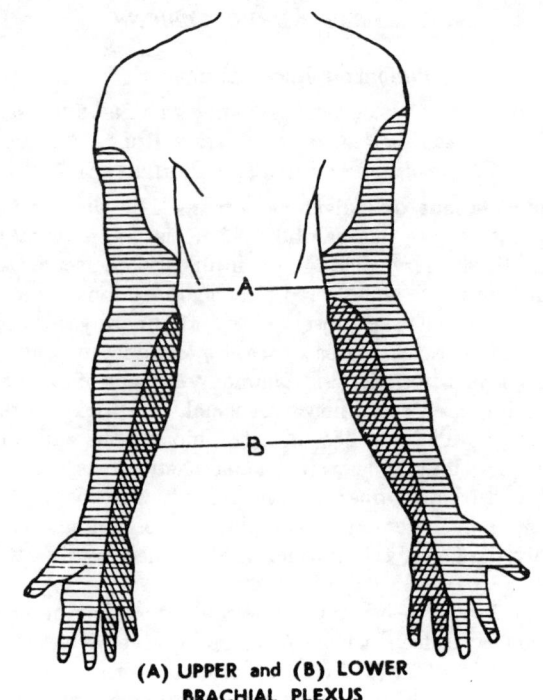

**(A) UPPER and (B) LOWER
BRACHIAL PLEXUS**

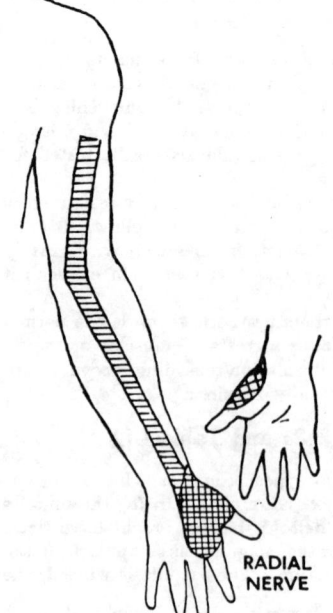

**RADIAL
NERVE**

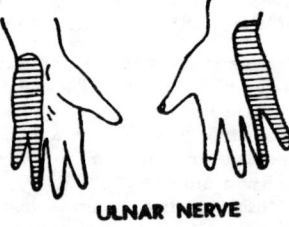

ULNAR NERVE

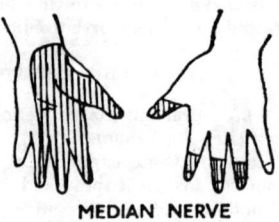

MEDIAN NERVE

(a)

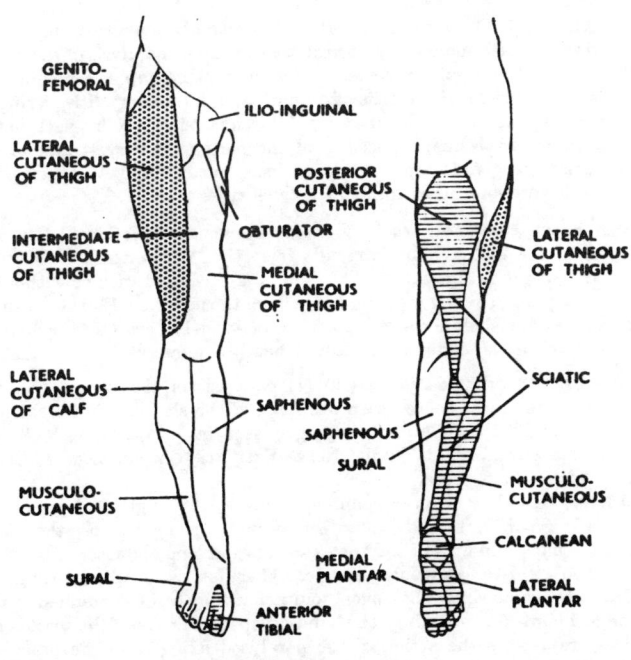

FIG. 248.—Approximate areas of CUTANEOUS SENSATION supplied by peripheral nerves. (a) Upper limb, (b) Lower limb.

arm cannot be flexed at the elbow (flexors of elbow) nor raised and abducted (deltoid). The movements of the wrist, and the hand-grasp and finger movements are unimpaired. Sensory loss involves the outer aspect of the shoulder and runs along the outer border of the whole limb. In (b) the hand and fingers are paralysed, and the ulnar border of the forearm and hand is anæsthetic from involvement of the C8, Th1 root supply, viz., the intrinsic muscles of the hand and flexors of the wrist and fingers. From involvement of the first thoracic root, oculo-pupillary phenomena may occur (pupillary miosis, enophthalmos and narrowing of the ocular fissure) from damage to the cervical sympathetic fibres.

If the lesion is near the intervertebral foramina. the long (posterior) thoracic nerve (to the serratus magnus) will be involved, with winging of the scapula. This nerve leaves C5-7 roots immediately after their exit from the intervertebral foramina.

The Causes of Brachial Plexus Lesions are usually (1) Traumatic crushes or wrenches of the upper limbs, including obstetric injuries in which the roots may be avulsed from the cord; (2) Enlarged supraclavicular glands in malignant disease, tuberculosis, Hodgkin's disease; (3) Paralytic brachial neuritis (§ 998); (4) Cervical rib; (5) Vertebral disease, tuberculous caries, spondylitis or neoplasms; (6) Syphilitic pachymeningitis.

§ 994. **Obstetric Paralysis,** usually of the upper plexus type, occurs during delivery in head presentations where lateral traction is made on the head, separating it from the shoulder, or in breech presentations when similar lateral traction is made on the trunk, the head being fixed in the pelvis.   The attitude of the limb in the later stages is typical, the arm being rotated inwards at the shoulder (from paralysis of the supra- and infra-spinati), the forearm is extended and the hand pronated (from paralysis of the supinator longus and brevis).   It is the attitude of a waiter " receiving a tip." Less commonly the lower type of brachial plexus injury occurs.

Phrenic Nerve (C3–5) paralysis causes: (1) Dyspnœa on exertion. (2) During deep inspiration the abdomen does not protrude, owing to paralysis of the diaphragm. (3) Paradoxical diaphragmatic movement is found on radiographic screening. Causes of paralysis are: (1) lesions of the cells of origin, C3, 4, 5 (poliomyelitis, syringomyelia, spinal compression, motor neurone disease); (2) lesions of the roots—pachymeningitis, vertebral caries or neoplasms; (3) lesions of the peripheral nerve-trunk in the neck or thorax (enlarged glands, thoracic aneurysm, mediastinal tumour, pericardial effusion), diphtheritic and other forms of polyneuritis.

DELTOID PALSY commonly results from Circumflex nerve lesions. Great wasting and weakness of the deltoid muscle results from the " Frozen shoulder syndrome."
Circumflex Nerve (C5, 6) lesions.—The deltoid is paralysed with or without sensory loss over an oval patch of skin covering the belly of the muscle. Elevation and abduction of the arm at the shoulder are limited. *Causes.*—(1) Paralytic brachial neuritis, (2) Dislocation of the shoulder or fractured head of humerus.

WINGING OF THE SCAPULA is seen in (1) paralysis of the Long Thoracic nerve C5–7, (2) and in much less degree with dropping of the shoulder in Spinal Accessory Nerve paralysis (§ 1086). Bilateral winging is seen in Myopathy (§ 1008).
WRIST-DROP occurs from (1) Radial Nerve Palsy, (2) Chronic Lead Poisoning and after lesions of C6, 7, 8 roots.
Radial Nerve (C5–8) lesions are common owing to its length and exposed course.
(a) If the nerve is damaged below the branch to the triceps, the supinators, extensors of the hand and fingers and the extensors and long abductor of the thumb are paralysed. The triceps and anconeus escape. There is wrist-drop. The fingers cannot be extended at the metacarpo-phalangeal joints, but they can be extended at the distal interphalangeal joints (interossei). The hand-grasp is weak, but if the wrist is passively dorsiflexed to reproduce the action of the paralysed fixing (synergic) muscles, there is very little disability. Supination of the forearm is lost (brachio-radialis). Sensory changes are inconstant, but they occur on the dorsum of the hand between the thumb and index fingers. (b) In lesions high in the axilla (e.g., " crutch paralysis ") the triceps and anconeus also are involved, with diminution or loss of the triceps jerk.
Causes.—(1) " Crutch palsy," (2) from pressure against a hard object in sleep (usually alcoholic sleep " Saturday night palsy," or during anæsthesia), (3) after prolonged application of a tourniquet, (4) Paralytic brachial neuritis (§ 998), (5) Fracture of the shaft of the humerus or involvement by callus, (6) Chronic lead poisoning. In lead poisoning the paralysis is usually bilateral and the extensor of the metacarpal of the thumb and the supinator longus escape. *Prognosis.*—Unless the nerve is severed or the damage is prolonged and severe, recovery is the rule. *Treatment.*—The hand and fingers should be placed in a cock-up splint with active daily exercise. In alcoholic patients abstention from alcohol will hasten recovery.
Ulnar Nerve (C7, 8, Th1), paralysis is not infrequent and recovery is unusual except in slight or partial lesions. The hand assumes a characteristic attitude. The two ulnar fingers are hyperextended at the metacarpo-phalangeal joint and flexed at the interphalangeal joints. The hypothenar muscles and the interossei are paralysed with the flexor carpi ulnaris, medial half of flexor profundus digitorum and the abductors of the thumb. Note that the first dorsal interosseus as well as the six other interossei is supplied by the ulnar nerve. If the patient is asked to grasp a piece of card with both hands between the fingers and thumb, the thumb of the affected hand will become flexed at the thenal-interphalangeal joint. This is because the patient compensates for the loss of the abductor pollicis by using the flexor muscle of the thumb. With the hand and fingers flat on the table, the patient has difficulty in abducting the outspread fingers. Sensory loss may exist over the ulnar border of the hand, the little and ulnar half of the ring finger on the palmar and dorsal aspect; sensory loss does not extend higher than the wrist.
Causes.—(1) In repeated trauma to the nerve behind the medial epicondyle of the humerus in draymen, etc., the nerve may be palpably thickened, (2) Hypertrophic

TABLE LIX.—INNERVATION OF MUSCLES BY NERVES

Only muscles commonly tested are given.

Nerve.	Muscles Supplied.	Defective Movement.	Deformity Produced.
Accessory Nerve. C3–4	Trapezius.	Shoulder cannot be shrugged or braced back. Arm cannot be elevated above the head.	Dropped shoulder with "winging" of the vertebral border of the scapula.
Brachial Plexus. C5–Th1	Rhomboids. Serratus anterior. Pectoralis major. Supraspinatus. Infraspinatus. Latissimus dorsi.	Loss of adduction and of lateral rotation of arm at shoulder. Arm cannot be raised above horizontal position.	Atrophic shoulder girdle with winging of the vertebral border of the scapula.
Circumflex Nerve. C5–6	Deltoid.	Arm cannot be abducted nor elevated backwards or forwards.	Contours of shoulder become flattened; later, shoulder-joint relaxes.
Musculo-cutaneous Nerve. C5, 6, 7	Biceps.	Forearm flexed with difficulty in the supinated position.	Depression on outer surface of arm between insertion of deltoid and origin of supinator.
Radial and Posterior Interosseous Nerve of forearm. C5–8	Triceps. Brachio-radialis. Extensor carpi radialis longus. Supinator. Extensor digitorum. Extensor carpi ulnaris. Abductor pollicis longus. Extensor pollicis longus. Extensor pollicis brevis. Extensor indicis.	Elbow, wrist and basal phalanges of fingers cannot be extended; grip weakened; impaired flexion of forearm if supinator is involved.	"Wrist-drop," fingers flexed at metacarpophalangeal joints; thumb opposed to fingers and depressed somewhat.
Median Nerve. C6–Th1	Pronator teres. Flexor carpi radialis. Flexor digitorum sublimis. Flexor pollicis longus. Flexor digitorum profundus I and II. Flexor pollicis brevis. Abductor pollicis brevis. Opponens pollicis. Lumbricals I and II.	Power of flexion of hand defective. Ulnar deviation on flexion of hand. Fingers cannot be properly flexed at first inter-phalangeal joint, while flexion of terminal phalanges only practicable in 3 ulnar fingers. Thumb cannot be opposed and its terminal phalanx cannot be flexed.	Wasting of the thenar muscles and of the muscles of the palm of the hand.
Ulnar Nerve. C7, 8, Th1	Flexor carpi ulnaris. Flexor digitorum profundus III and IV. Abductor digiti minimi. Opponens digiti minimi. Adductor pollicis. Flexor pollicis brevis. Palmar interosseous I. Dorsal interosseous I.	Radial deviation on flexion of hand. Terminal phalanges of the ulnar fingers cannot be flexed nor thumb adducted. Basal phalanges of two ulnar fingers cannot be satisfactorily flexed nor their middle and distal phalanges be extended. Abduction and adduction of fingers impossible.	"Claw-hand" most pronounced in fourth and fifth fingers. First phalanges of fourth and fifth fingers in extreme extension and second and third phalanges flexed; atrophy of hypothenar eminence and interossei.

TABLE LIX (continued)

Nerve.	Muscles Supplied.	Defective Movement.	Deformity Produced.
Femoral Nerve. L2–4	Ilio-psoas. Sartorius. Rectus femoris. Vastus lateralis. Vastus intermedius. Vastus medialis.	Inability to flex the hip or extend the knee. Absence of knee-jerk.	Gait disturbed. Patient drags leg.
Obturator Nerve. L2–4	Gracilis. Adductor magnus. Adductor longus.	Adduction, and to slight extent rotation, at hip impaired.	—
Inferior Gluteal Nerve. L5–S2	Gluteus maximus.	Extension at hip-joint impaired; also abduction.	Pelvis is tilted in walking to swing leg.
Superior Gluteal Nerve. L4–S1	Gluteus medius and minimus. Tensor fasciæ latæ.	Loss of abduction and circumduction of thigh.	
Sciatic, Medial Popliteal and Posterior Tibial Nerves. L4–S3	Semitendinosus. Biceps (long head), and ½ Adductor magnus. Semimembranosus. Gastrocnemius. Soleus. Tibialis posterior. Flexor digitorum longus. Flexor hallucis longus. Abductor hallucis. Abductor digiti minimi. All interossei.	Loss of flexion of knee and plantar flexion of the foot and toes. Patient unable to walk on his toes.	Claw position of toes (pied en griffe). pes calcaneus or valgus.
Sciatic, Lateral Popliteal and Anterior Tibial Nerves. L4–S2	Biceps (short head). Tibialis anterior. Extensor digitorum longus. Extensor hallucis longus. Extensor digitorum brevis.	Foot falls from its own weight, and cannot be raised nor can first phalanx of great toe be extended. Patient cannot walk on heels.	Foot-drop. Toes scrape the floor in walking.
Sciatic. Lateral Popliteal and Musculo-cutaneous Nerves. L5–S2	Peroneus longus. Peroneus brevis.	Foot cannot be everted.	Foot in varus position.

arthritis of the elbow-joint, (3) Fractures of the medial epicondyle of the humerus, (4) " Toxic " interstitial neuritis, (5) Leprosy, (6) Periarteritis nodosa.

Prognosis.—There is little disability except that the little finger tends to get in the way and may suffer trophic change. Recovery is slow and minimal in severe lesions.

Treatment.—Elbow pads may help to prevent repeated trauma. In cases of compression at the epicondyle, transplantation of the nerve to the anterior aspect of the elbow should be considered.

Median Nerve (C6, 7, 8, Th1). Lesions cause paralysis of the flexors of the fingers and the radial flexor of the wrist. Partial thenar atrophy occurs from wasting of the flexor pollicis brevis, abductor pollicis and opponens pollicis. Opposition of the thumb is lost and the palm of the hand becomes flattened. Flexion of the thumb, index and middle fingers is lost, but the ring and little fingers can still be flexed.

Pronation is lost and flexion of the wrist is feeble with ulnar deviation. Sensory changes occur on the palmar aspect of the hand and fingers, within an area bounded by a line drawn through the middle of the ring finger and obliquely from the wrist to the metacarpal of the thumb. On the dorsum of the hand only the distal portions of the fingers are anæsthetic.

Causes.—(1) Trauma, (2) Occupational palsy in hand workers from pressure of a file, screwdriver, iron, etc., on the palmar branch, (3) Compression may occur in the carpal tunnel ("Carpal Tunnel Syndrome," (§ 823)), (4) *Median causalgia* follows incomplete division of the nerve by injury. Burning pain of median distribution with trophic changes occurs in the hand.

Prognosis.—Severe lesions cause great disability from loss of opposition of the thumbs. Recovery is slow and rarely complete. *Treatment.*—In old traumatic lesions surgical exploration with resection of the scarred area and re-suture may help.

Lower Limb Paralyses.   (See Fig. 248 (*b*) and Table LIX.)

LESIONS OF THE CAUDA EQUINA. See § 969.

§ 995. **Sacral Plexus** (L4–S5).—Lesions of the plexus are relatively rare, owing to its protected situation. The sciatic nerve L4–S3, owing to its size, is the trunk most affected in traumatic and pressure lesions, and its peroneal branch suffers most. The common symptoms are foot-drop, with paralysis of the peronei and dorsiflexors of the foot, and sensory loss over the outer aspect of the leg and dorsum of the foot. The hamstrings are rarely affected.

Causes of Sacral Plexus Lesions: (1) Traumatic, from fracture of the pelvis, with subperitoneal effusion of urine or blood. (2) Pressure Lesions. (*a*) Pressure of the fœtal head in transverse presentations. (*b*) Pressure of pelvic neoplasms or infiltration by malignant or Hodgkin's glands, or rectal neoplasms. (3) Acute Radiculitis. (4) Sacro-iliac tuberculous caries, spondylitis or vertebral neoplasms.

Femoral nerve (L2–4) **lesions** cause paralysis of extension of the leg and weakness of flexion of the thigh. Standing erect with the knees braced the patient shows only wasting of the thigh, but if he makes the slightest flexion movement the knee gives way. It is difficult to climb stairs in the normal way. The muscles paralysed are the iliacus, psoas magnus, pectineus, sartorius and the quadriceps femoris. The adductor longus is also affected. The knee-jerk disappears. There is sensory impairment over the front of the thigh.

The *cause* is often obscure. Some cases are due to fracture of the pelvis, pelvic neoplasm or enlarged lymph nodes, constriction of the nerve in the femoral sheath, syphilis.

FOOT-DROP most commonly results from a pressure lesion of the lateral popliteal nerve. It may occur in radiculopathies due to disc lesions and other causes, as well as sciatic nerve palsy.

Sciatic Nerve (L4–S3) *lesions.*—The medial popliteal fibres lie more medially than the lateral popliteal fibres which are more vulnerable, and division of the nerve takes place at any point in the thigh between the sciatic foramen and lower third of the thigh. A lesion of the sciatic trunk high up often produces paralysis limited to the lateral popliteal, the ankle-jerk being absent.

In *total paralysis* "flail foot" and total paralysis of the muscles below the knee result. If the branches to the hamstring muscles and ischial part of the adductor magnus given off in the thigh are affected, these muscles also may be paralysed. The ankle-jerk is lost, but the knee-jerk is unaffected. Sensory loss may be present over the lateral and posterior aspect of the lower two-thirds of the leg, over the external malleolus and the tendo Achillis. Usually there is a *partial lesion* of the nerve and the lateral popliteal fibres are those affected.

The **Lateral Popliteal (Peroneal) Nerve** (L4–S1) winds round the head of the fibula and divides into the anterior tibial nerve and the musculo-cutaneous nerve to the perone:. Lesions cause paralysis of the anterior tibial and peroneal muscles, with foot-drop and loss of ability to evert the foot. The knee- and ankle-jerks are present. The patient can walk on the toes, but not on the heel of the affected foot. Sensory loss will be present over the outer aspect of the leg and the dorsum of the foot.

Causes of Sciatic and Lateral Popliteal Lesions.—(1) Lumbar spondylitis. (2) Pelvic neoplasms. (3) Compression during pregnancy and after parturition. (4) Misplaced intramuscular injections of sulphonamides and certain other drugs may cause complete and permanent palsy. (5) Interstitial neuritis. (6) Gunshot wounds and fractures of the pelvis or femur. (7) After anæsthetics and labour, when the knees have been held up in slings. (8) Compression of the peroneal nerve from prolonged crossing of the knees. (9) Ischæmic paralysis in arteriosclerosis and diabetes. (10) Prolonged kneeling may affect the *Anterior Tibial Nerve* where it pierces the fascia to enter the anterior tibial compartment. All the muscles in that compartment waste profoundly and there is severe foot-drop.

Prognosis.—The common foot-drop from prolonged crossing of the knees or after anæsthetics usually recovers quickly. Other more serious lesions of the nerve take up to eighteen months to recover.

Treatment.—Care must be taken that the tendo Achillis does not develop a contracture. If the degree of foot-drop is severe enough to cause difficulty in walking a toe-raising spring and a night-shoe of plastic felt will be required.

Posterior Tibial (Medial Popliteal) Nerve (L4–S2) **lesions.**—The calf muscles and plantar muscles are paralysed and wasted and the ankle-jerk disappears. There is sensory loss over the sole of the foot and the posterior aspect of the leg in its lower third. The *cause* is usually a penetrating injury and nerve suture should be considered. (For Causalgia and other painful lesions see § 821.)

GROUP XII. MUSCULAR WASTING AND MUSCULAR ATROPHY

The bulk of a normal muscle is related to the age, activities and state of nutrition of the subject. For its maintenance it requires adequate exercise of its contractile power, a sufficient blood supply, integrity of its nerve supply and of the myofibrils of which it is composed. When one or other of these factors is disturbed muscular wasting and even atrophy results. Deprived of its motor neurone, muscle becomes flaccid and loses its contractile power, its tendon reflex tends to disappear and fasciculation of muscle bundles may be seen, especially if the atrophy is due to disease of the anterior horn cell or anterior root.

§ 996. DISEASES OUTSIDE THE NERVOUS SYSTEM. The causes of *generalised* wasting are described in §§ 569–573. *Local* muscular wasting occurs in arthritis, *e.g.*, in the hand muscles in rheumatoid arthritis. It is seen when the blood supply to muscle groups is obstructed, viz. ischæmic paralysis (seen in the hand and forearm muscles after too tight splinting, and, rarely, in the muscles of the anterior tibial compartment in those who kneel a great deal). *Disuse* atrophy may occur in functional and organic disease.

NEUROLOGICAL CAUSES OF MUSCULAR ATROPHY

Group A. *Localised Muscular Atrophy* due to

 I. Spinal cord lesions (with no sensory changes)
　　Acute Poliomyelitis (§ 898).
　　Motor Neurone Disease (early stages) (§ 1001).
 II. Root lesions, with root pain and later segmental wasting
　　Paralytic Brachial Neuritis (§ 998).
　　Rib pressure syndromes (§ 999).
　　Herpes Zoster (§ 1021).
　　Disc lesions (§§ 1018–1020).
 III. Peripheral nerve lesions with characteristic wasting and sensory changes
　　(§§ 992–994).

Group B. *Localised Muscular Atrophy with Long Tract signs.*

    IV. Motor Neurone Disease (§ 1001).
    V. Infantile Progressive Spinal Muscular Atrophy (§ 1002).
    VI. Syphilitic Amyotrophy (§ 965).
    VII. Spinal Cord Compression from Tumour (§§ 968, 1003) or Spondylosis (§ 1004).
    VIII. Syringomyelia (§ 1005) and Syringobulbia (§ 1006).
    IX. Peroneal Muscular Atrophy (§ 1007).

Group C. *Symmetrical and bilateral wasting and weakness of shoulder and pelvic girdle muscles which may be slowly progressive over years.*

    X. Muscular Dystrophy and Myopathy (§ 1008).
    XI. Infantile Myopathy—Amyotonia Congenita (§ 1012), Benign Congenital Myopathy (§ 1013).
    XII. Symptomatic Myopathy due to Carcinoma, Thyrotoxicosis, Myasthenia gravis, Diabetes mellitus; menopausal and exophthalmoplegic (§ 1014).

§ 997. CLINICAL INVESTIGATION OF MUSCULAR ATROPHY

In the diagnosis of *neurological and myopathic causes of wasting,* the following points should be considered:

(*a*) *The Age and Family History* are important in myopathies and in peroneal muscular atrophy.

(*b*) *Mode of Onset.* A *rapid onset* after a febrile attack occurs in *post-paralytic atrophy, e.g.,* after acute poliomyelitis or paralytic brachial neuritis. A *more gradual onset* after a febrile attack or sore throat occurs in diphtheritic and other forms of polyneuritis. In motor neurone disease atrophy generally precedes wasting and the onset is insidious.

(*c*) *Distribution of the Paralysis.* In muscular atrophy of *Spinal Cord origin* (myelopathy) the paralysis and wasting are predominantly distal, affecting chiefly the peripheral limb muscles and the bulbar muscles. *Myopathic wasting* is characteristically proximal and bilaterally symmetrical, sparing the distal muscles and affecting those of the shoulder and pelvic girdles and sometimes those of the face. In myopathy, pseudo-hypertrophy or myotonia may be present. In *Root lesions, e.g.,* due to prolapsed intervertebral disc, spondylosis or spinal cord compression, the weakness and wasting are of root distribution. In *Peripheral Nerve lesions,* motor and sensory changes will be present in the territory of the affected nerve. Long-standing atrophy in one limb is generally due to a peripheral cause, *e.g.,* a disc lesion or a cervical rib. When long-standing or severe muscular atrophy is more generalised it may be due to *myasthenia gravis*: the weakness is reduced or abolished by inject. prostigmine.

(*d*) *Presence of Visible or Palpable Phenomena in the Affected Muscles or Nerves.* Fasciculation in association with progressive atrophy is highly characteristic of motor neurone disease. In healthy subjects it occurs in fatigue and toxic states. It is seen in disc lesions, syringomyelia and peroneal muscular atrophy. *Tenderness of muscles to pressure or gentle kneading* is characteristic of acute lesions of the lower motor neurone, *e.g.,* polyneuritis (especially alcoholic), acute poliomyelitis. *Myotonia* occurs only in the myopathies in association with myopathic wasting. *Thickening of peripheral nerves* occurs in the ulnar nerve at the elbow as a result of trauma. It occurs in leprosy, amyloid disease and hypertrophic neuritis. *Peripheral neuroma* should be sought for in all cases of peripheral nerve lesions; it may be solitary, or multiple in neuro-fibromatosis.

(*e*) *Extensor Plantar Responses* indicate spinal cord disease. They will be found in cases of muscle atrophy due to motor neurone disease, cervical spondylosis or other form of cord compression, syringomyelia, peroneal muscular atrophy.

(*f*) *Sensory Changes and their distribution.* The finding of objective sensory changes excludes motor neurone disease. In *Spinal Cord disease* there will be a sensory level, or evidences of a Brown-Séquard type of lesion or of posterior column sensory loss.

Root and Peripheral Nerve lesions have their appropriately restricted sensory patterns. In polyneuritis the loss of sensibility is global and of the " glove and stocking " variety.

Progressive muscular wasting with pain and sensory changes, whether unilateral or bilateral, should lead to a search for evidences of a vertebral or spinal lesion by radiography. When spinal cord compression is suspected, lumbar puncture and myelography are often required prior to operation.

Group *A*. THE MUSCULAR ATROPHY IS LOCALISED

I. *Spinal cord* lesions causing this are Acute Poliomyelitis and Motor Neurone Disease in its early stages.

Root lesions include Herpes zoster, Disc lesions and Paralytic Brachial Neuritis.

Following severe and persistent ROOT PAINS IN THE NECK AND ARM *the patient develops* MUSCULAR WASTING *of one or more muscles* ROUND THE SHOULDER GIRDLE. *C.S.F. changes are absent. The condition may be* PARALYTIC BRACHIAL NEURITIS.

§ 998. II. Paralytic Brachial Neuritis (Syn. Neuralgic Amyotrophy).

Symptoms.—Pain starts acutely and appears round the shoulder-blade and down the back of the arm as far as the elbow. The pain is severe and lasts from two days to two weeks. Fever and constitutional signs are absent and the C.S.F. is normal. As the pain disappears muscle wasting and paralysis become evident. Serratus anterior (long thoracic nerve), spinati (suprascapular nerve), deltoid, or the muscles supplied by C5, 6 roots are affected. Sensory changes are slight and inconspicuous and soon pass off. In one-third of the cases the changes are bilateral.

Diagnosis.—The presence of sensory changes, the absence of fever and a normal C.S.F. are against the diagnosis of acute poliomyelitis. These cases resemble closely " serum neuritis " following inoculation with anti-tetanic or other sera (see § 524).

Etiology.—Epidemics of this disease appear in young male adults under conditions of military service, often in hospital whilst convalescing from pneumonia, malaria or some minor operation (Aldren Turner).

Prognosis.—Bilateral pains at the onset do not always mean bilateral paralysis. Electrical testing of the affected muscles should be carried out by an expert after the first 3 weeks. Most cases recover in 6–12 weeks but in a few with reaction of degeneration little or no recovery occurs.

Treatment.—Rest in bed, tab. codeine co. for the pain and later splinting of the weakened muscles to prevent overstretching should be prescribed.

§ 999. Rib Pressure Syndromes are usually produced by compression of the inner cord of the brachial plexus (which contains fibres originating in C8, D1 roots); occasionally the plexus is prefixed and then fibres arising from C7, C8 are involved. Although the abnormalities producing the compression are bilateral and congenital, symptoms are *unilateral* and do not show themselves until adult life. Women are much more often affected than men. Neuritic, vascular and cervical sympathetic symptoms are encountered.

Symptoms.—(1) Localised pains and tingling occur along the inner side of the forearm and hand, in the distribution of the first thoracic root. This pain is relieved by raising the arm above the head, thereby relaxing the compressed nerve cord. (2) Localised wasting of the abductor and opponens pollicis occurs, so that the normal convexity of the thenar eminence is replaced by hollowing of the soft parts and exposure of the metacarpal of the thumb. Whenever localised pain or atrophy of this distribution has existed for over a year in one hand, this syndrome should be suspected. Symptoms occur when the muscular tonus is diminished by fatigue so that the shoulder girdle drops. (3) Coldness of the hand is frequently observed and (4) the radial pulse may be diminished. (5) There may be oculo-pupillary sympathetic phenomena on the affected side.　(6) An abnormal rib may be visible or palpable as a bony swelling in the neck.　(7) X-rays sometimes reveal the presence of an abnormal rib or transverse process.

Diagnosis.—Many cases of acroparæsthesiæ with partial thenar atrophy formerly supposed to be due to cervical rib are now believed to be due to the *carpal tunnel syndrome* (§ 823).　Indeed the finding of a cervical rib in the X-ray of such a case does not necessarily mean that it is the cause of the symptoms.　In all doubtful cases treat the case as a carpal tunnel syndrome in the first instance.　Cervical ribs occur in syringomyelia, but in these cases sensory impairment is dissociated and transgresses the C8, Th1 segmental limits.　If a single muscle is affected the cause may be in the peripheral nerve or root.　In such cases think of trauma or virus infection (herpes zoster) as a possible cause.　See also Table LIX.

Etiology.—Compression of the inner cord of the brachial plexus may be due to (1) an enlarged transverse process of the seventh cervical vertebra, (2) a fibrous band uniting such a transverse process or an abnormal cervical rib to the first rib, (3) a cervical rib articulating posteriorly with the transverse process of the seventh cervical vertebra and anteriorly with the first rib, or (4) hypertrophy of the scalenus anticus muscle.

Treatment.—Bed-rest for 2-3 weeks with the arm on a pillow will cure some cases. Shoulder-raising exercises, support of the elbow and forearm on a level with the shoulder and the wearing of a sling help ambulant patients.　Operations of various kinds (removal of the cervical rib or band, section of the first rib or of the scalenus anticus, etc.) are rarely performed nowadays.　Operation is only indicated where there is severe pain and progressive wasting and must be performed by a neurosurgeon.

SEGMENTAL WASTING of the *arm muscles* may be due to malignant metastasis in axillary and supraclavicular glands, or disease of the cervical vertebræ, *e.g.*, cervical spondylosis, tuberculosis, osteitis deformans.　Wasting of the *muscles of the lower limbs* is seen after acute poliomyelitis, and in cases where there is disease of the lumbar or sacral spine, or a cauda equina lesion (disc lesions or tumour).　Wasting may follow herpes zoster of the lumbar or sacral roots, after injuries to the spine and pelvis, and after pressure of the fœtal head on the sciatic nerve in obstructed labour.

BRACHIAL PLEXUS LESIONS affecting the lowest cord C8, Th1 (*e.g.*, dislocation of the shoulder with rupture or contusion of the nerve root) cause paralysis of the thumb and intrinsic hand muscles with possibly cervical sympathetic paralysis.

§ 1000. Wasting of a Hand.—ARTHRITIC ATROPHY of the interossei and thenar muscles is seen in rheumatoid patients with swollen joints.　The accompanying ulnar deviation of the wrist and fingers is characteristic.

PARTIAL THENAR ATROPHY due to wasting of the abductor and opponens pollicis may be unilateral or bilateral and occurs in a variety of conditions.　The radial aspect of the thenar eminence becomes flattened or scooped out and the first meta-carpal, denuded of its muscular coverings, is visible and can be palpated beneath the skin throughout its extent.　(a) *Without symptoms* partial thenar atrophy may be due to a radiculopathy of C8, Th1 roots in cervical spondylosis (§ 1004).　(b) *With pain referred to the index, middle and possibly the ring finger,* which radiates up the arm. " like electric shocks " when the patient touches objects, the cause is possibly compression of the median nerve in the carpal tunnel (§ 823).　In severe median nerve lesions there is loss of power of opposing the thumb so that it falls backwards to the plane of the other digits, rather like an ape's hand.　(c) With *vaso-motor changes,* such as swelling of the fingers, coldness, cyanosis, differences in the radial pulses on the two sides, the cause may be a rib pressure syndrome (§ 999) from compression of the neurovascular bundle upon a normal first rib as it enters the thoracic inlet or upon a cervical rib.　*Selective wasting with tenderness of the wasted muscles* is char-acteristic of the carpal tunnel or the rib pressure syndrome.

CLAW-HAND due to paralysis of the interossei and lumbricals is most often due to lesions of the ulnar nerve below the level where it gives off its branch to the flexor profundus.　The proximal phalanges are hyperextended whilst the distal ones are flexed and clawed. The clawing is most marked in the two ulnar fingers, for the radial lumbricals have an additional nerve supply from the median nerve. In peripheral ulnar and median lesions sensory loss does not extend above the wrist. In brachial plexus and root lesions it may extend up the forearm. An *ulnar type of wasting* may be caused by repeated trauma to the ulnar nerve behind the medial epicondyle, rib-pressure syndromes or cervical disc lesions.

Acute Poliomyelitis and *Paralytic Brachial Neuritis* may affect the hand muscles. In *Amyotrophic lateral sclerosis* the wasting for months may be confined to one hand. But the wasting in these cases is not selective, it is global, the muscles are not tender and there is no history of pain down the limbs. Objective sensory changes are entirely absent. Fasciculation may be seen in the atrophic hand muscles.

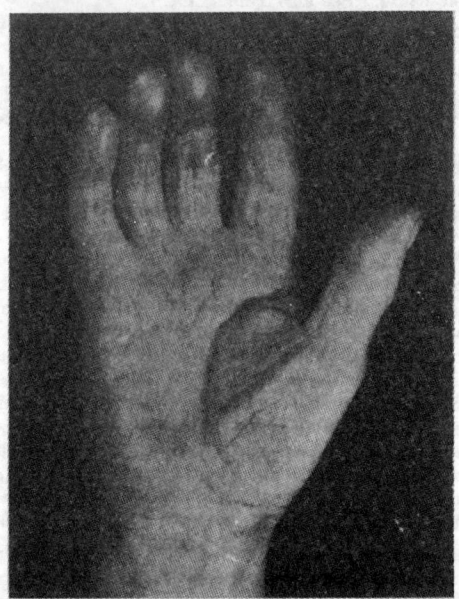

Fig. 249.—PARTIAL THENAR ATROPHY from a case of Cervical Spondylosis. There is flattening of the radial side of the thenar eminence due to wasting of the abductor and flexor brevis pollicis. The metacarpal bone of the thumb is easily palpable under the skin.

Syringomyelia may be unilateral at onset, but the finding of dissociated sensory changes (temperature and pain loss with preservation of light touch) and painless burns or whitlows will suggest the diagnosis (§ 1005).

If there is progressive wasting with pain referred to one root and sensory changes, suspect *spinal neurofibroma or cervical disc prolapse.* X-rays and C.S.F. examination may be necessary in such cases to confirm the clinical diagnosis.

III. *Peripheral Nerve lesions* have wasting and sensory nerve changes which are characteristic (§ 992 *et seq.*).

Group *B.* THE MUSCULAR ATROPHY IS ASSOCIATED WITH LONG-TRACT SIGNS

There is PROGRESSIVE MUSCULAR WASTING *which is not segmental, but affects the upper or lower limbs of one or both sides; there is no sensory loss, and ultimately* PYRAMIDAL SIGNS APPEAR. *The condition may be* MOTOR NEURONE DISEASE.

§ **1001. IV. Motor Neurone Disease** (Syn. Amyotrophic Lateral Sclerosis, Progressive Bulbar Palsy) is a relatively common systemic degeneration of upper and lower motor neurones. It may affect: (1) the pyramidal cells of the precentral gyrus and their axons (cortico-spinal and cortico-bulbar tracts), (2) the bulbar motor nuclei and their axons, *i.e.*, facial, hypoglossal, motor cells of the vagus-glossopharyngeal-accessorius, (3) the anterior horn cells of the spinal cord and their axons.

The disease usually commences in the anterior horn cells of the cervical cord and later on produces pyramidal signs in the lower limbs (AMYOTROPHIC LATERAL SCLEROSIS). When it commences in the upper or lower motor neurones of the bulb it is called PROGRESSIVE BULBAR PARALYSIS.

Symptoms.—(1) The patient is usually a man over 40 years of age who has probably noticed wasting of the muscles of one hand. There is little weakness at this stage, for wasting precedes weakness. He may not have noticed that the small muscles of his other hand are beginning to be similarly affected. The wasting is global, affecting all the muscles equally, the interossei and the muscles of the thenar and hypothenar eminences. Depressions appear on the dorsum of the hands between the metacarpals ("guttering"), and a hollow appears between the thumb and index due to wasting of the first dorsal interosseous muscle. On flattening the palms of the hands the flexor tendons become prominent. The fingers cannot be abducted and the power to oppose the thumb is gradually lost. Occasionally the wasting first appears in the muscles of the shoulder girdle. The triceps, latissimus dorsi and the lower part of pectoralis major tend to show the wasting later than other muscles of the hands and arms: the last to waste is often the upper portion of the trapezius (the "ultimum moriens"). In some cases weakness and wasting appear first in the periphery of the legs with foot-drop. Usually, however, in the stage of hand-wasting only a slight degree of spastic weakness and wasting is found in the legs. (2) When the patient is undressed coarse *fasciculation* of the wasted muscles is seen especially when the limbs are cold; it is present also in muscles which are not yet wasted or paralysed. The fasciculation is most evident when the disease is active; it signifies degeneration of the lower motor neurone. The combination of progressive weakness and wasting of the small muscles of the hand and other peripheral muscles, with fasciculation and brisk tendon jerks, is highly characteristic (tonic atrophy). Direct percussion of wasted muscles results in a brisk twitch or a ridge of contraction of muscle fibres which lasts a second or two. (3) The combination of upper and lower motor neurone lesions gives rise to muscular atrophy accompanied either by spasticity or flaccidity, spasticity tending to preponderate where the lesion is largely pyramidal. (4) *Objective sensory changes are entirely absent* and there is no tenderness of muscles. The finding of objective sensory changes immediately calls for revision of the diagnosis. *Subjective sensory complaints* are, however,

common—aching pains and painful cramps, stiffness, coldness, numbness
or, rarely, tingling.   These feelings are referred to affected muscles and
have no objective concomitant on sensory testing.   (5) The *tendon reflexes*
are usually lively and the jaw-jerk is commonly increased.   If the lesion
is predominantly in the lower motor neurones, however, the tendon jerks
in the arms may be depressed or absent.   The plantar responses are
extensor.   The abdominal reflexes may be retained until a late stage of
the illness.   Paraplegia in flexion does not occur.   (6) The sphincters are
unaffected.

TYPES OF MOTOR NEURONE DISEASE.—(*a*) *Amyotrophic Lateral Sclerosis* (*vide
supra*).

(*b*) *Progressive Muscular Atrophy.*—The wasting and weakness usually starts in
one or both hands.   More rarely it may start in the lower limbs as a dropped foot
with progressing wasting, fasciculation and brisk tendon jerks.   Occasionally it starts
in the proximal muscles of the limb girdles.   The muscles of the neck, splenius capitis
and complexus may be the first affected.   The head drops forwards in a characteristic
posture and the spinous processes of the lower cervical and upper dorsal vertebræ
are unduly prominent because of the wasting and flexion of the neck.   These cases
simulate cervical spondylosis.

(*c*) *Progressive Bulbar Paralysis.*   Atrophic and spastic types of bulbar paralysis
occur according as to whether the cortico-bulbar or bulbar neurones are most affected.
The muscles of the tongue, the mylohyoid and the digastric in the floor of the mouth,
and the elevators and depressors of the hyoid bone are involved.   Slurring dysarthria,
nasal and later monotonous moaning speech develop, phonation is never entirely lost.
Salivation and difficulty in swallowing may be intense.   Spastic and uncontrolled
weeping or laughter may occur in these cases when bilateral pyramidal signs are
present.   The tongue lies in the floor of the mouth and it cannot be protruded or
thrust into either cheek.   Its surface is thrown into wrinkles by the atrophy and
its substance is found to be thinned on palpation.   The jaw-jerk is increased and the
pharyngeal reflex is commonly active.

(*d*) *Primary Lateral Sclerosis.*   In rare cases bilateral extensor plantar responses
and dragging of the legs is the first symptom.   These cases may be wrongly diagnosed
as Disseminated Sclerosis.

Diagnosis.—One should be reluctant to diagnose this disease in its early
stages unless clear evidences of progressive disease are present: mistakes
are sometimes made which the passage of time renders evident, and
recoverable lesions, *e.g.*, motor neuritis, may simulate this hopeless malady.
Spinal cord compression is diagnosed by the characteristic finding of a
spinal block and the raised protein in the C.S.F.   In motor neurone disease
the fluid is normal.   *Syphilitic amyotrophy* often presents with Argyll-
Robertson pupils; and pleocytosis, a positive Wassermann reaction and
a luetic Lange curve may be found in the C.S.F.   The signs of *cervical
spondylosis* may closely simulate those of amyotrophic lateral sclerosis,
but sensory changes are present and the condition runs a more benign
course.   *Pseudo-bulbar paralysis* in cerebral arteriosclerosis has a more
gradual onset with a history of "faints" or strokes, the patients are
emotionally unstable with spastic weeping or laughing: fasciculation of the
tongue is absent as a rule.   *Motor polyneuritis* occurs rarely in malignant

disease (*e.g.*, bronchial carcinoma).   *Lead amyotrophy* with wasted hands, dropped wrists and extensor plantar responses is rarely seen nowadays.

Etiology.—The cause is not known.   It is rarely a late sequel in those who have suffered earlier in life from acute poliomyelitis.

Prognosis.—Chronic progressive and intermittently progressive types of the disease occur.   The latter runs an irregular course, but both types succumb to respiratory failure in two to four years or less.   Generalised atrophy with fasciculation is of evil omen.

Treatment.—Treatment is symptomatic.   Rest, warmth and careful feeding are indicated.   Care should be taken to prevent falls, respiratory infections and aspiration of food particles.   Injections of calcium gluconate and parathyroid by mouth may help cases with cramps.   Salivation is helped by a belladonna mixture.   Strychnine tonics are commonly prescribed, but have no known direct effect on the progress of the disease.   Faradism exhausts already weakened muscles.   Steroids do not influence the disease.   Careful splinting of the hands and feet at night with passive movements of the joints night and morning may prevent contractures.   In the later stages, dressing and feeding the patient and getting him into a chair every day is a very considerable burden for the relatives.

§ 1002. V. Infantile Progressive Spinal Muscular Atrophy (Syn. Werdnig-Hoffman disease) is very rare and sometimes familial.   It starts in the first year of life and progresses rapidly over months.   The proximal and trunk muscles are first affected, with hypotonia and loss of tendon reflexes.   Later bulbar palsy appears with fasciculation and atrophy of the tongue.   Rarely the condition is arrested spontaneously; most children die in infancy of respiratory failure.   As in adult Motor neurone disease sensory changes are absent.   The lesion is an atrophy of the anterior horn cells not amenable to treatment.   The disease may be confused with Benign congenital myopathy (§ 1013).

VI. Syphilitic Amyotrophy (see § 965).

VII. Spinal cord compression from Spinal tumour (see § 968) or other causes (*e.g.*, Cervical Spondylosis).

§ 1003. Cervical cord compression in the region of C8 and Th1 segments produces atrophic paralysis of the wrist and fingers and of the small muscles of the hands.   The arm-jerks are unaffected.   Evidences of spinal block will be present with a high C.S.F. protein.   The *upper cervical cord* may be affected by cervical spondylosis or tumours; they cause pain and dissociated anæsthesia in the face from involvement of the sensory nucleus of the trigeminal, which lies in the substantia gelatinosa of Rolando as low as C3 segment.   Paralysis of the diaphragm, or hiccough, may be noted.

There are bilateral or unilateral root pains *and* paræsthesiæ *extending from the neck, down the arms to the fingers involving more than one cervical root; sometimes* wasting *of the intrinsic muscles of the hands and* reduced tendon reflexes.   *There is often* chronic neck stiffness *with characteristic degenerative changes in X-rays of the cervical spine.   The condition is probably* Cervical Spondylosis.

§ 1004. **Cervical Spondylosis** (Syn. Cervical Osteoarthritis).—Apart from the arthritic symptoms already described (§ 596), this is the cause of a number of neurological symptoms, especially those previously termed brachial neuritis. It is common after the age of 50 and is due to a degenerative condition affecting the middle and lower cervical vertebræ and the intervening disc tissue with compression and ischæmia of the nerve roots in

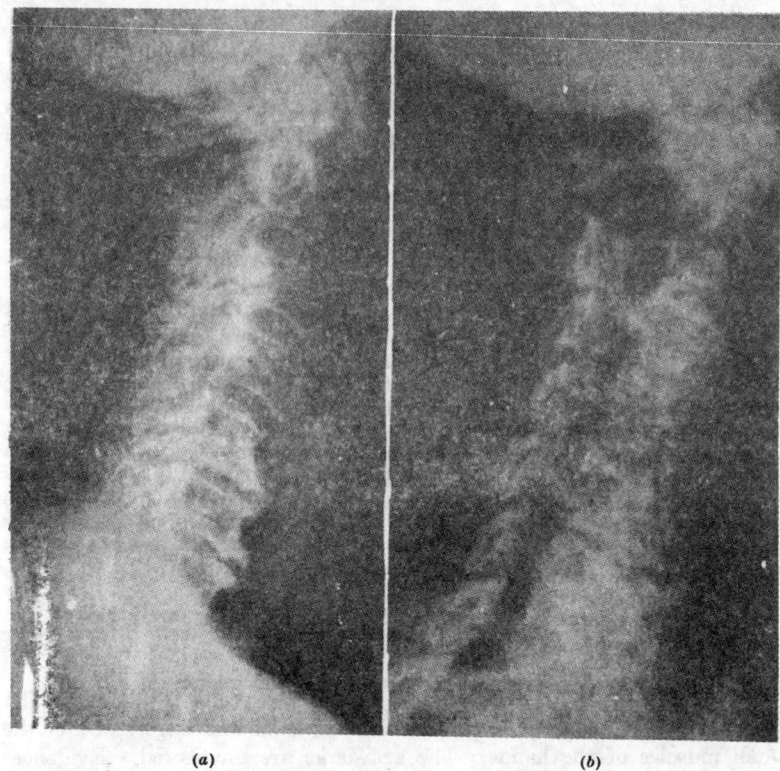

(a)   (b)

FIG. 250.—X-RAYS OF SEVERE CERVICAL SPONDYLOSIS. (a) Lateral view, with gross narrowing of C5, 6 and 7 disc spaces and anterior osteophytes causing " bridging " of the vertebral bodies. (b) Oblique view of same spine shows posterior osteophytes projecting into the intervertebral foramen between C3, 4. (Dr. David Sutton.)

the intervertebral spaces. Although other areas can be affected the 5th and 6th discs involving the 6th and 7th cervical roots are the most usual.

Symptoms are usually gradual in onset over weeks or months. *Early symptoms* comprise (1) painful stiffness of the neck with creaking and grating on movement but these may pass unnoticed in elderly patients. (2) Root pains and burnings or tinglings extend especially along the radial border of the forearms and hands; the distribution corresponds to the nerve roots involved (Fig. 250) and in 75 per cent. all the fingers are affected (acroparæsthesiæ). The symptoms are worse on waking, and are intensified by lateral flexion of the head to the painful side, by rotation of the head and by coughing and sneezing. (3) Tenderness may be present over the lower cervical spine. *Late symptoms* are not common. These may be evidence of severe compression of the cervical nerve-roots (§ 1018) with (4) sensory impairment and blunting of pin-prick over the painful fingers, or hyperæsthesiæ; (5) decrease in the tendon reflexes; (6) wasting of the thenar muscles or " guttering " of the dorsal interossei and (7) rarely fasciculation of the wasted muscles. Muscular weakness is slight and paralysis should throw doubt on the diagnosis.

Diagnosis.—X-ray examination of the cervical spine with antero-posterior, lateral and oblique views shows narrowing of the intervertebral disc spaces, anterior or posterior osteophyte formation, loss of the normal alignment and curve of the vertebræ in lateral views, or subluxation of degenerated vertebræ. Such changes may occur in the absence of symptoms and can coexist with other conditions, *e.g.*, motor neurone disease, syringomyelia. *Motor neurone disease* shows marked muscle wasting, fasciculation and presents no sensory impairment. The age incidence of spondylosis, 50–80 years, is later than that of the *carpal tunnel syndrome* (§ 823); cases with paræsthesiæ in the fingers and hands may simulate *subacute combined degeneration* of the spinal cord; remitting cases resemble *disseminated sclerosis. Angina pectoris* may be wrongly diagnosed when pain is referred to the pectoral area and down the outer side of the upper arm.

Etiology.—In osteoarthritis of the spine there are multiple projections around the margins of the annulus fibrosus of the cervical discs which stimulate osteophytic outgrowths from the edges of the adjacent vertebral bodies. Symptoms arise when these cause pressure on the nerve roots in the intervertebral spaces; ischæmia aggravates this by producing meningeal thickening and " root-sleeve fibrosis."

Prognosis.—Remission of symptoms may last 6 months or more but recurrences are common, especially after minor injuries. *Complications* arise when there is simultaneous prolapse of an intervertebral disc (§ 1018).

Treatment is difficult. A period of rest in bed in the horizontal position may give relief. In addition, manual, or gentle continuous or intermittent traction of the head by a halter and pulley with a 5–10 lb. weight may help. Not all patients tolerate traction. Short-wave diathermy aids some if combined with rest and analgesics. A collar may have to be prescribed for patients who are not helped by bed-rest.

The patient has wasted hands, and INJURES OR BURNS *his* FINGERS *and palms* WITHOUT FEELING PAIN; *the fingers may be livid and swollen. There is* LOSS OF PAINFUL AND THERMAL SENSITIVITY *over the face, upper limbs and trunk with preservation of sensitivity to light touch. The condition is probably* SYRINGOMYELIA.

§ 1005. VIII. **Syringomyelia** is a slowly progressive disease due to a congenital cavitation and gliosis of the cervico-dorsal cord. The brain-stem may also be affected (syringobulbia). It often presents with a wasted hand in a young adult together with "dissociated" and "suspended" thermanæsthesia and analgesia and pes cavus and kyphoscoliosis.

Symptoms.—The constant anatomical distribution of the lesions produces a characteristic clinical picture. Six chief groups of symptoms commonly occur: (1) *Sensory symptoms* are so highly characteristic that they will be first described. Subjectively deep boring *pains* are felt in the neck, shoulders and upper limbs, when the spino-thalamic tracts are invaded. "Dissociated anæsthesia" arises from interruption of the fibres subserving pain, temperature and tactile cutaneous sensibility, as they cross in the anterior commissure of the cord to attain the spino-thalamic tract (Fig. 214). Touch has two pathways: thus the fibres for the cruder forms of touch and those subserving proprioception and deep forms of sensation (vibration, joint-sense) are often intact. Consequently over the affected areas the patient is unable to feel pinpricks and hot objects; and often sustains blisters and burns from touching lighted cigarettes, matches or lighters, or hot stoves. Yet *light touches* with cotton-wool are felt over the analgesic areas and joint and vibration sense may be normal. Cavitation or gliosis of one posterior horn will cause loss of pain and temperature sensation on the same side, whereas a centrally placed lesion will cause bilateral therm-anæsthesia and analgesia. In the later stages all forms of sensation may be affected. The distribution of the cutaneous sensory impairment is commonly that of a "sleeved jacket," as the disease notably affects the cervical enlargement. There is always (*a*) an upper and usually (*b*) a lower level to the sensory loss whether it is unilateral or bilateral, and Cl or 2, to Th6 or 7 segments are often affected. If the cavity extends above C3 level in the posterior horn the spinal nucleus of the trigeminal will be destroyed, with "dissociated" sensory changes over the periphery of the face. At first when the upper and lower borders of sensory loss are clearly defined the area may be said to be "suspended." As gliosis spreads into the antero-lateral columns, sensory tracts from the lower limbs become affected and the lower level is difficult to define. (2) *Motor symptoms.* The intrinsic hand muscles waste early, perhaps on one hand but later bilaterally but rarely before the selective sensory loss has appeared. The atrophy is global and may also affect the muscles of the forearm or of the shoulder girdles. Fasciculation is sometimes seen in affected muscles. The atrophy of the hand muscles may produce a "claw hand," or it may be hidden by a curious blue œdema of the hands and fingers with diffuse thickening of the subcutaneous tissues. Grasping such a hand gives a feeling of "a bag of bones." The distribution of the muscular atrophy depends upon the destruction of ventral horn cells. (3) *Spastic paraplegia* is due to compression of the pyramidal tracts in the lateral columns of the cord. Spasticity of a lower limb on one side with impaired temperature and pain sensibility on the opposite lower limb (Brown-Séquard phenomenon) is due to a laterally placed cavity. Sphincter changes and incontinence are rare and only occur when cavitation extends to the lumbar enlargement. (4) *Skeletal deformities* often date from birth, viz., scoliosis, pes cavus, cranial asymmetry, cervical rib and spina bifida. (5) The *hands and fingers* are blue, swollen and fleshy, with diffuse thickening of the subcutaneous tissues (*main succulente*). In manual workers they become scarred, necrosed, blistered or ulcerated, as the result of painless whitlows, infected abrasions and burns; clerical workers are less likely to show such lesions. (6) *Painless fractures and arthropathies*, either atrophic or hypertrophic (Charcot joints), are due to trauma of the affected limbs. (7) *Cervical sympathetic lesions* with ptosis and small pupil result from lesions at C8, Th1 level. Owing to vaso-dilatation on the affected side of the face, the beard, moustache and eyebrow may grow more profusely on that side. (8) Any known neurological abnormality may occur in syringomyelic patients. Fits are rather infrequent. Slight raising of the C.S.F. protein is common, but any greater amount, *e.g.*, 100–400 mg. per cent., should arouse suspicion of an associated spinal tumour.

Diagnosis.—*Cervical rib* (§ 999), either unilateral or bilateral, is a common finding in syringomyelia. When in a case of atrophy of hand muscles thought to be due to cervical rib any physical sign is found outside the territory of the upper limb and neck, syringomyelia should be suspected. Cavitation of the cord with syringomyelic symptoms occurs in connection with certain spinal cord tumours, and a high C.S.F. protein reading should suggest the presence of neoplasm.

Etiology.—The disease is probably congenital, but the symptoms are rarely noticed before the age of 15 years or over the age of 30. Two-thirds of the cases occur in males. Familial cases are rare. To the naked eye, the cord on section shows a central gelatinous mass of glial tissue, containing an irregular cavity, usually most marked in the cervico-dorsal and lumbar enlargements; it may extend into the floor of the fourth ventricle or mid-brain (§ 1006). Surrounding normal structures are compressed by the enlarging cavity and proliferating cells.

Prognosis.—The disease runs a very slow but progressive course; the patient may live to an old age or may die of some intercurrent disease. If the disease extends rapidly upwards, death may occur from respiratory paralysis; or a sudden hæmorrhage into a cavity may cause rapid increase in the severity of the symptoms (*Hæmatomyelia*, § 957*b*). With spastic paralysis of the legs and sphincter disturbance there may be great incapacity, but in most cases the incapacity is only moderate.

Treatment.—Protect the affected hands from changes of temperature and from trauma. Splinting at night prevents deformities from contracture. The postural scoliosis is improved by appropriate exercises. Deep X-ray to the cervical spine may relieve the aching pain and other symptoms of the disease, but is not curative.

§ **1006. Syringobulbia** occurs when the lesion presents or extends to the brain-stem. There may be (1) nystagmus from involvement of the posterior longitudinal bundle, (2) hemiatrophy of the tongue with palatal, pharyngeal or laryngeal paralysis from disease of the bulbar nuclei, and (3) selective " dissociated " sensory changes affecting pain and temperature over the periphery of the face with loss of the corneal reflex due to involvement of the descending root of the trigeminal nerve. (4) A drooping eyelid and small pupil occur when sympathetic tracts in the bulb are invaded.

The atrophy is bilaterally symmetrical in the feet and legs with claw-feet, absent ankle-jerks and long-tract signs; the condition is painless and very slowly progressive with little disability. The disease is probably PERONEAL MUSCULAR ATROPHY.

§ **1007. IX. Peroneal Muscular Atrophy** is a rare, heredo-familial (or sometimes sporadic) disease affecting the ventral horn cells and the dorsal columns of the spinal cord. The motor fibres of the peroneal nerves atrophy with interstitial reactive changes. The disease produces deformity rather than disability. The patients are usually male.

Symptoms.—In the *earlier stage* a symmetrical wasting of the peroneal muscles and intrinsic muscles of the feet is seen in childhood or adolescence. Many patients first seek orthopædic advice for dropping or clawing of the feet; the ankle-jerks are absent and extensor plantar responses may be found with slight posterior column loss (diminished vibration). This " forme fruste " of the disease may not progress further. *Later stage.*—In most cases the wasting of muscles progresses slowly in an extremely characteristic fashion, inch by inch up the limbs until the junction of the middle and lower thirds of the thigh is reached, producing thighs like inverted champagne bottles. Similar atrophy is seen later in the intrinsic muscles of the hands, producing claw hands and spreading upwards to the upper forearms. Fasciculation in affected muscles is slight. The gait is high-stepping from dropped foot but a great degree of muscular power remains in the wasted muscles owing to the deposition of yellow elastic tissue which follows upon the atrophy. These patients are able to follow useful occupations, and may even play games. All forms of sensation, especially deep sensation, may be impaired in slight degree in the wasted limbs. The ankle-jerks are lost early, later the knee-jerks may diminish or disappear. The plantar responses are not obtained, owing to the atrophy of the toe muscles.

Treatment is symptomatic. Specially made shoes or boots may prevent trophic sores on the feet; toe-raising springs help some with severe foot-drop. Surgical operations on such feet must be avoided.

Group C. X. *There is* SYMMETRICAL AND BILATERAL WASTING AND WEAKNESS *of the* SHOULDER AND PELVIC GIRDLE MUSCLES *and perhaps the face—slowly progressive over the years.* PSEUDO-HYPERTROPHY *or myotonia exist in heredo-familial cases. These findings suggest* MUSCULAR DYSTROPHY.

The term MYOPATHY is often applied to *acquired* types of this syndrome.

§ 1008. **Muscular Dystrophy** has a gradual onset in infancy, childhood, or early adult life, and produces symmetrical bilateral wasting and weakness of the *proximal* muscles of the limbs, the muscles of the shoulder and pelvic girdles and the face. Fasciculation is rarely seen. The tendon reflexes are qualitatively diminished in the affected muscles, according to the degree of disease present. The condition is primarily in the muscles themselves, and no signs of central nervous disease can be demonstrated, clinically or pathologically. The disease is usually heredo-familial, and any of the following characters may be inherited: (1) simple atrophy, (2) pseudo-hypertrophy, (3) true hypertrophy, (4) myotonia, (5) slight mental impairment, (6) dystrophic phenomena, cataract, premature baldness, testicular atrophy. Varying combinations of these characters produce bizarre clinical types. A *distal* type is excessively rare. "**Symptomatic**" **myopathies** are described where similar muscular syndromes occur in association with systemic disease.

The various clinical types of myopathy have received special names; much confusion arises in terminology.

TYPES OF MYOPATHIC DISEASE

HEREDO-FAMILIAL TYPES (Muscular Dystrophy).

   a. Pseudo-hypertrophic (Duchenne).
   b. Facio-scapulo-humeral (Landouzy-Déjérine).
   c. Limb-girdle type (Erb).
   d. Dystrophia myotonica (myotonic muscular dystrophy), see §§ 1028, 1029.

INFANTILE MYOPATHIES (" India-rubber " or " Floppy " Baby).

   e. Amyotonia congenita, § 1012.
   f. Benign congenital myopathy, § 1013.
   g. Infantile progressive spinal muscular atrophy (Werdnig-Hoffman), § 1002.

SYMPTOMATIC MYOPATHIES.

   Carcinomatous, Thyrotoxic, Myasthenia gravis, Diabetes Mellitus, Menopausal, Ophthalmoplegic.

HEREDO-FAMILIAL TYPES.

§ 1009. (*a*) **Pseudo-hypertrophic Muscular Dystrophy** is a disease of early childhood (onset usually 4–5 years of age) affecting little boys. Small girls are rarely affected. The disease is transmitted by the mother, who does not suffer from the malady (as in hæmophilia and congenital night-blindness). The patient usually dies before he can transmit the disease; several brothers in a family, affected in varying degree, are usually seen.

Symptoms.—A waddling gait and enlargement of the calves draw attention to the disease. In a few years the child is bed-ridden. The gait is wide-based and the body lurches from side to side, with a rolling motion to clear the toes from the ground.

There is great lordosis. When the patient is laid on his back on the floor, he rolls over on to his face, gets on to hands and knees and proceeds to climb up his legs by moving his hands alternately upwards on his thighs, to extend his hip-joints. These symptoms are due to weakness of the pelvic girdle muscles, the glutei, hamstrings and other hip extensors. In the shoulder girdle, the muscles chiefly affected are the lower part of the trapezius and pectoralis major, serratus magnus, biceps and triceps, producing winging of the scapula and " loose shoulders," the child tending to slip through one's hands when lifted by the axillæ. Pseudo-hypertrophy is most often seen in the calf muscles and infraspinati but may occur elsewhere (Fig. 6). Contractures develop with the progress of weakness, especially when the child becomes confined to a chair. Death occurs in adolescence from involvement of the respiratory muscles. Only in this type of myopathy are the serum aldonase and serum transaminase readings considerably raised. Creatine and creatinine are in excess in the urine. These findings are probably due to destruction of muscle and throw no light on the cause of the disease.

§ 1010. (b) **Facio-scapulo-humeral Muscular Dystrophy** (Landouzy-Déjérine) usually commences in late childhood or adolescence. *Symptoms.*—The facial muscles become wasted: it is easy to force open the patient's eyes when he screws them up and the weakness of the lower face renders the mask expressionless; whistling and blowing out the cheeks are difficult. The limb girdle muscles waste symmetrically and involvement of the paraspinal muscles render it difficult for the patient to rise from the horizontal position without help. There is lordosis and a rolling gait. Stair-climbing is impeded by the proximal muscular weakness. In a few cases electrocardiographic changes indicate alteration in the state of the cardiac muscle.

The *prognosis* improves the later the age of onset. The mentality is usually normal and life may be prolonged for many years. In pregnancy labour may have to be assisted. Contractures increase the disability.

§ 1011. (c) **Limb-girdle Muscular Dystrophy** (Erb) may be late in onset and is very slowly progressive. Winging of the scapulæ and lordosis occur from wasting and weakness of the shoulder and pelvic girdle muscles. When long muscles, such as the biceps femoris, are attacked " cricket-ball " hardenings may be observed when the muscle contracts, as the ends of the muscle have undergone dystrophic changes. The deep reflexes tend to disappear in proportion to the degree of muscular atrophy. Sensory and sphincter changes are absent; myocardial changes may occur.

(d) MYOTONIC MUSCULAR DYSTROPHIES are described in §§ 1028, 1029.

XI. INFANTILE MYOPATHIES.

§ 1012. (e) **Amyotonia Congenita** is a familial and possibly hereditary condition of extreme flaccidity of the muscles, which are small and soft to touch. The onset is probably pre-natal, the mothers of children with this disease usually giving a history of absence of " quickening " at mid-term. The disease is, however, usually not noticed until an attempt is made to teach the child to walk; then some abnormal mode of progression is often adopted, e.g., sitting on the buttocks and " rowing " with the heels. The joints are flail-like and the limbs can be hyperextended into bizarre attitudes. The disease differs from all other myopathies in its tendency to gradual but incomplete recovery. In adult life the muscular power is never normal.

The *diagnosis* from the hypotonia of *rickets* and *diphtheritic paralysis* is made by the history and associated findings. The diagnosis from *cerebellar diplegia* may be very difficult, but the hypotonia of this type of diplegia is not as marked, nystagmus may be present, there is no family history, and diplegia is progressive.

§ 1013. (f) **Benign Congenital Myopathy** produces similar symptoms in infants. " Rag-doll " or " india-rubber " baby are popular terms to indicate the grotesque attitudes which these children may be made to assume owing to the loss of tone in the muscles. There is a strong tendency to recovery. These conditions are probably *syndromes* due either to (1) atrophic myopathy, (2) infantile polyneuritis or polymyositis, (3) congenital myasthenia gravis, or (4) congenital atonic diplegia. Some. of these cases tend to improve as adult life is reached. The *diagnosis* is exceedingly difficult in early childhood; *muscle biopsy* may be helpful.

§ 1014. XII. Symptomatic myopathy should be suspected when a myopathic type of wasting appears late in life. It has been observed (1) in association with malignant disease, *e.g.*, bronchial carcinoma, (2) thyrotoxicosis, (3) myasthenia gravis, and (4) diabetes mellitus. (5) Menopausal myopathy and (6) a myopathy causing progressive external ophthalmoplegia (Nevin) are described.

Diagnosis of Myopathic Disease.—Diagnostic difficulties arise chiefly in cases of muscular dystrophy of *late onset*. Fasciculation is rare in dystrophy. In *motor neurone disease* extensor responses, a brisk jaw-jerk and active tendon reflexes are found. *Dermatomyositis* is a recoverable form of muscular disease which produces tenderness as well as atrophy of the affected muscles. Biopsy may show cellular infiltration of the muscle fibres.

Etiology.—The cause of muscular dystrophy is unknown; it has been ascribed to an inborn developmental defect (abiotrophy). It is not, however, usually apparent at birth. The age of onset varies from two to sixty years.

Treatment.—The congenital and heredo-familial forms have been treated with glycine or vitamin E, but there is no evidence that these are effective. Menopausal myopathy occasionally improves with prednisolone 5–10 mg. twice or thrice daily. Thyrotoxic cases improve after thyroidectomy and diabetic myopathy reacts slowly to stabilisation of the diabetes. Cases of carcinomatous myopathy run a fluctuating course and the patient usually dies of the associated neoplasm.

GROUP XIII. NEURITIC PAIN IN THE LIMBS AND TRUNK

In this section are considered diseases presenting symptoms of pain or sensory disorder. The investigation of pain has been briefly considered in § 820. Apart from neuralgia, the following types of pain in neurological disease can be recognised:

Table LX

Type of Pain.	Distribution.	Accompaniments.
(1) Peripheral Nerve Pain.	Follows cutaneous distribution of particular nerve involved. Fig. 248.	Paræsthesiæ, often sensory impairment and tenderness of nerve and muscles on pressure.
(2) Root Pain.	Follows cutaneous distribution of corresponding spinal nerve root. Fig. 244	Intensified by coughing and sneezing.
(3) Central Pain.	When due to disease of Thalamus is of hemiplegic distribution.	Persistent aching or burning.
(4) Referred Pain.	Referred to cutaneous Root Area corresponding to segmental supply of affected viscus.	Visceral disease, *e.g.*, coronary disease.
(5) Psychalgia.	Of no fixed anatomical distribution.	Psychoneurosis, *e.g.*, Anxiety State or Hysteria.

In the investigation of any pain, make it an invariable rule never to omit a careful local examination of all that part of the body to which the pain is referred.

(1) **Pain due to Peripheral Nerve Disease.** These pains follow the distribution of the particular nerve involved. In simple *Neuralgia* sensory loss and paralysis are absent. In *Neuritis*, or inflammatory disease of single peripheral nerves, the following characteristics are present: (*a*) pain over the cutaneous distribution of the nerve and slight impairment of cutaneous sensibility; (*b*) tenderness of the affected nerve on pressure, and pain when it is passively stretched; (*c*) cutaneous hyperæsthesiæ or paræsthesiæ (sensations of crawling under the skin, numbness or pins and needles) in the distribution of the affected nerve; (*d*) deep tenderness of the muscles supplied by the nerve, slight wasting and perhaps fasciculation. There is never great wasting and there is no true weakness; (*e*) diminution of the corresponding tendon reflexes in the later stages. For Polyneuritis, see § 974. In *Pressure Lesions* of peripheral nerves there is muscular paralysis and the wasting is much more profound.

(2) **Root Pains.** These follow the cutaneous distribution of the corresponding spinal segments (see Fig. 244). They are intensified by coughing or sneezing and may be accompanied by tingling or feelings of constriction accurately localised to root areas and hyperæsthesia of the skin to dragged pin over the affected areas. The aggravation of the pain on coughing or sneezing is due to the distension of the pial sheath of the posterior nerve root, occasioned by the raised cerebro-spinal fluid pressure. Such root pains are met with in *tabes dorsalis*, in *meningeal inflammations, e.g.*, syphilitic meningomyelitis, *extra-medullary spinal tumours*, in *spondylitis* (associated with creaking and stiffness in the spine and lipping of the edges of the vertebral bodies seen in radiograms of the vertebræ), in secondary *deposits of carcinoma* in the vertebræ, *Pott's disease*, and in *herpes zoster* before the vesicular eruption.

(3) **Central Pain.** (*a*) *Spinal Cord.* In certain central lesions of the spinal cord (*e.g.*, syringomyelia, intramedullary growths) spontaneous inveterate pain (in the limbs and trunk but rarely the face) may be met, possibly due to irritation of the adjacent spino-thalamic tracts. (*b*) *Thalamus.* In thalamic thrombosis and in neoplasms involving this structure, pain of similar character may be met. It is of hemiplegic distribution, including the face, associated with perverted perception of cutaneous sensibility (hemiplegia dolorosa) and, perhaps, involuntary movements—the " thalamic syndrome " of Déjérine and Roussy. Central pain is difficult to alleviate.

(4) **Referred Pains.** Familiar examples of this are the pain occurring in the throat and down the inner side of the left arm in angina pectoris, and in the pain referred to the tip of the corresponding shoulder in diaphragmatic pleurisy, subphrenic abscess, liver abscess, and cholecystitis. In these cases, the pain is referred to the cutaneous root-areas corresponding to the segmental supply of the affected viscus.

(5) **Psychalgias.** These are pains of mental origin; they do not follow anatomical boundaries, are constant and are accompanied by a disordered mental make-up. They are produced by suggestion, are perpetuated by anxiety and can be influenced by suggestion. Such are the bilateral facial pains following dental extractions, or pains in the body associated with phobia of cancer or tuberculosis.

It should be borne in mind that pain in a limb may be due to disease of the muscles, bursæ, blood-vessels, bones, joints, peripheral nerves or central nervous system, or may be referred, as in coronary disease. Each of these structures should be examined systematically, palpating the bones, vessels and peripheral nerves, testing the mobility of the joints, testing sensibility and the tendon reflexes. A general examination of all the systems is necessary, together with testing the urine and often an X-ray examination for evidence of arthritis, cervical rib, or spondylitis. Spinal puncture may be necessary to exclude spinal cord compression.

TABLE LXI.—SOME COMMON CAUSES OF PAIN IN THE LIMBS

Cause in.	*Upper Limbs.*	*Lower Limbs.*
Muscles.	Fibrositis. Trauma.	Fibrositis. Cramp and heat-cramp.
Blood-vessels.	Raynaud's disease.	Intermittent claudication. Thrombo-angiitis obliterans. Syphilitic endarteritis.
Bones.	Periostitis or Osteomyelitis. Neoplasm.	Periostitis or Osteomyelitis. Neoplasm. Osteitis deformans.
Joints.	Periarticular adhesions. Arthritis (especially shoulder-joint). Cervical spondylosis. Pott's disease.	Disease of sacro-iliac or hip joints (Osteo-arthritis, tuberculous disease, acute rheumatism, etc.). Lumbar spondylosis. Prolapsed intervertebral disc.
Peripheral nerves.	Rib pressure syndromes. Pressure lesions (enlarged supraclavicular glands, fibrositis, etc.). Brachial neuritis. Median and ulnar neuritis. Causalgia. Radiculitis. Referred pains in coronary disease.	Sciatic neuritis. Pressure lesions, *e.g.*, pelvic tumours. Meralgia paræsthetica. Diabetic and other types of polyneuritis.
Spinal cord.	Acute cervical disc herniation. Spinal tumour (primary and secondary). Meningomyelitis. Tabes dorsalis.	Primary and secondary growths in the cauda equina. Meningomyelitis. Tabes dorsalis.

Causes of pain are considered (A) in the UPPER LIMBS, (B) in the LOWER LIMBS, (C) in the TRUNK AND LIMBS.

§ 1015. (*A*) **Pain in the Upper Limbs.**—Periarticular adhesions round the shoulder-joint, or *subacromial bursitis and fibrositis* (§ 604) are common causes of neuralgic pains. Such pains are increased by movement of the neck, shoulder-joint or arm in certain directions, and there are limitation of movement and tender points in these structures.

NEUROLOGICAL CAUSES OF UPPER LIMB PAIN

I. Brachial neuritis.
II. Paralytic brachial neuritis.
III. Acute cervical disc herniation.
IV. Cervical spondylosis.
V. Rib pressure syndrome.
VI. Carpal tunnel syndrome.
VII. Herpes zoster.
VIII. Malignant metastases in the vertebræ.
IX. Tabes dorsalis; hypertrophic cervical pachymeningitis.
X. Syringomyelia.
XI. Tumour of cervical cord.

§ 1016. I. BRACHIAL NEURITIS causes stabbing or burning pains with paræsthesiæ from the shoulder or neck to the fingers. Most cases are due to acute cervical spondylosis or disc protrusions.   But the condition may be traumatic or due to an infection.

§ 1017. II. PARALYTIC BRACHIAL NEURITIS affecting several roots is followed by segmental paralysis and atrophy (see § 998).

SUDDEN PAIN IN THE DISTRIBUTION OF ONE NERVE ROOT *in the upper limb follows trauma or coughing.   The corresponding tendon reflex may be diminished.   The condition may be* ACUTE HERNIATION OF A CERVICAL DISC.

§ 1018. III. **Acute Cervical Disc Herniation** is one of the common causes of " acute brachial neuritis."   The fifth and sixth discs are chiefly affected, producing monoradicular signs referred to the C6 and C7 roots respectively.

Symptoms.—The onset is usually sudden and about half the cases give a history of trauma—sudden lifting strain, a fall, twisting the neck, coughing violently.   Paræsthesiæ are prominent and *root pain* is felt not only in the cutaneous segment supplied by the sensory root, but also in muscles supplied by the corresponding motor root.   The neck may be held stiffly and the head tilted.   Movement is very limited and increases the pain.

When C6 root (C5 disc) is involved pain radiates from the neck across the shoulder down the outer side of the arm and forearm into the thumb and index finger, with numbness and decreased sensation to cotton wool and to pin-prick over this same nerve root distribution (Fig. 244).   The scapular muscles may be tender.   There is weakness, wasting, tenderness, perhaps fasciculation in the deltoid, biceps, extensor carpi radialis and in the thumb muscles.   The biceps and supinator jerks are diminished or lost; eliciting the supinator jerk may cause an exaggerated flexion of the fingers (" inversion of the radial reflex ") so characteristic of damage at this level.

When C7 root (C6 disc) is involved the pain radiates from the neck down the back of the shoulder and arm into the middle finger (and sometimes the ring finger) of the hand (Fig. 244).   Numbness, paræsthesiæ and impairment to light touch and to pin-prick may be demonstrated in the painful area or in the pad of the middle finger. There is weakness, tenderness, wasting and fasciculation, perhaps in the triceps and extensor carpi radialis, with weakness of the grasp and of the extensors of the fingers; the triceps and supinator jerks are diminished or abolished.

A *large herniation extending towards the mid-line* can cause spinal cord compression with extensor plantar responses or a Brown-Séquard syndrome. On rare occasions these can occur without symptoms in the neck or arms.

X-ray examination, undertaken as in cervical spondylosis (§ 1004), shows narrowing of the disc spaces between C5–6 or C6–7, often in association with osteoarthritic changes in neighbouring areas; views taken with the head flexed are often valuable.   The *C.S.F.* is usually normal on manometry and analysis; 15–20 per cent. of cases show evidence of partial spinal block.   *Myelography* is sometimes called for and shows indentation of the column of Myodil opposite the protruding disc (Fig. 251).

Diagnosis depends on the *sudden* onset of symptoms with pain, paræsthesiæ, motor, sensory and reflex evidence of involvement of either the sixth or the seventh cervical root.   A *neurofibroma* of the nerve root produces similar symptoms, but X-rays will show the intervertebral foramen of the affected root to be enlarged and in antero-posterior views the pedicles may be eroded. *Spinal cord compression* may be caused not only by a large disc herniation but also by a neoplasm. In the *thoracic inlet syndrome* vascular symptoms are prominent and more than one nerve root is involved.

Etiology.—Trauma, age and infections are factors influencing herniation. The nucleus of the disc is suddenly protruded in a dorso-medial, dorso-lateral or intraforaminal direction (Fig. 252).

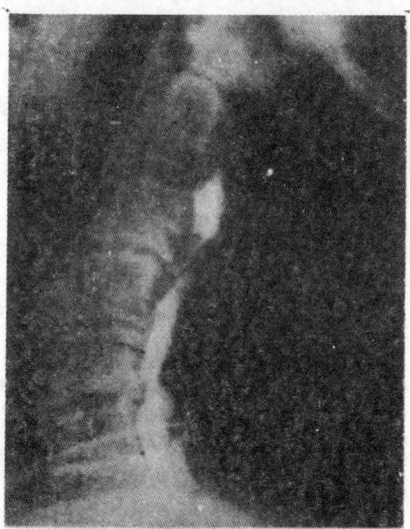

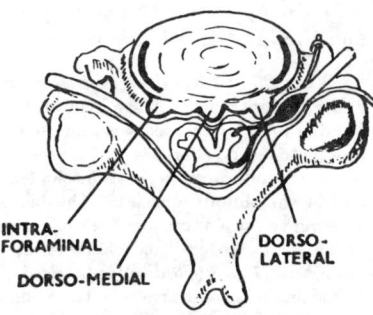

FIG. 251.—MYELOGRAM FROM A PATIENT WITH A PROLAPSED CERVICAL DISC causing quadriplegia. The column of Myodil is broken opposite C3, 4 and indented opposite C5, 6 from disc protrusions and posterior osteophytes. Note the cervical spondylosis and posterior subluxation of C3. (Dr. David Sutton.)

FIG. 252.—A CERVICAL VERTEBRA WITH ITS DISC showing three types of disc herniation: (*a*) Intraforaminal, (*b*) Dorso-medial (central), (*c*) Dorso-lateral.

Prognosis.—Most cases recover after 2–6 weeks. Recurrences are fairly frequent and may be incapacitating.

Treatment.—Rest in bed for several days or a week or more is essential; enough pillows to support the head and elbow will curtail pain and incapacity. Later the arm should be carried in a sling which supports the elbow but this must not drag across the lower neck; on sitting down the elbow can rest on the arm of an armchair. Tab. codeine co. (B.P.) 4 to 6 in 24 hours, inject. pethidine or inject. papaveretum (Omnopon) may be necessary at first. Moist heat with towels thoroughly wrung out of boiling water and applied to the neck and shoulder, and infiltration of tender areas in painful muscles with lignocaine 1 per cent. relieve spasm. Radiant heat is less helpful. In acute disc lesions gentle traction may be tried, but massage increases the pain. After this has abated, gentle movements of the neck and shoulder may be tried, and traction manually or with a collar and weight (§ 1004) often give relief. Mobilisation under anæsthesia is not advisable. Intractable cases are usually those who have refused initial bed-rest; they often have to wear a plastic collar. Myelography followed by operation may be necessary if there are signs of advancing cord compression or if recurrent attacks of disabling pain occur; a simple laminectomy can prove helpful.

IV. CERVICAL SPONDYLOSIS is closely allied to disc herniation. It is more chronic and causes unilateral or bilateral pains and paræsthesiæ involving more than one root, often several roots (§ 1004).

V. RIB PRESSURE SYNDROME (§ 999).

VI. THE CARPAL TUNNEL SYNDROME is a common cause of recurrent pain and paræsthesiæ in the hands and fingers, sometimes extending as high as the elbow. The symptoms are worst at night or on waking and pass off during the day in most cases (§ 823).

VII. HERPES ZOSTER (see § 1021).

VIII. MALIGNANT METASTASES are usually extra-dural. The onset of symptoms and signs is sudden; root pain is common. This is sometimes followed by a sudden and total paraplegia; and a tendency for the patient to lose strength and weight in which case general cachexia follows. Often there is no radiological evidence of collapsed vertebræ and the symptoms must be attributed to the deposits infiltrating blood-vessels of the cord. Mammary and prostatic carcinomata commonly metastatise in the spine. *Treatment*, see § 571.

IX. TABES DORSALIS; hypertrophic cervical pachymeningitis (§ 1025).

X. SYRINGOMYELIA may cause deep boring and aching pain in the cervical and occipital regions and shoulders (§ 1005).

XI. A NEOPLASM OF THE CERVICAL CORD is usually a Neurofibroma or Meningioma. In the arm, weakness, wasting and fasciculation are seen in muscles innervated from the cervical root or area of the cord involved. A spastic weakness of the leg may appear first on the same side as the tumour, then in the opposite leg and finally in the opposite arm. X-rays of the cervical spine (including lateral and oblique views), C.S.F. examination, often followed by injection of radio-opaque Myodil, help to confirm and localise the tumour.

(*B*) **Pain in the Lower Limbs** may be due to lesions of skeletal, vascular or visceral structures. Do not forget to test the urine or to make a rectal examination. Pain, in association with *chronic arthritis of the hip-joint*, may be referred to the knee (§ 596).

NEUROLOGICAL CAUSES OF LOWER LIMB PAIN

I. Sciatic neuritis.
II. Acute lumbar disc herniation.
III. Lumbar spondylosis.
IV. Cauda equina tumours.
V. Malignant Metastases (§ 969).
VI. Myelomatosis.
VII. Tabes dorsalis (§1022).
VIII. Occlusive vascular disease "Claudication" (see § 586).

§ 1019. I. Sciatic Neuritis (Syn. Sciatica) may follow an attack of lumbago causing pain of sciatic distribution in one limb, associated with paræsthesiæ. The pain is made worse by coughing or sneezing. It is a disease of early and middle life and occupational causes may be evident (exposure to damp, continued pressure in long-distance lorry drivers, etc.). Slight attacks last a week or two. Severe sciatica is usually due to (1) Acute lumbar disc lesions, (2) Malignant disease (secondary deposits or myelomatosis), (3) Diabetes mellitus.

The patient who is young and muscular is suddenly seized with IMMOBILISING PAIN, SHOOTING DOWN THE LEG *in the distribution of a lower lumbar or upper sacral root. The condition is probably* ACUTE LUMBAR OR LUMBO-SACRAL DISC HERNIATION.

§ 1020. II. **Acute Lumbar or Lumbo-sacral Disc Herniation** may cause a unilateral or bilateral sciatic syndrome, following extrusion of the nucleus pulposus of an intervertebral disc through its annulus.

Symptoms.—There is often sudden immobilising pain in the lower back. Other cases are more chronic and give a history of remitting attacks. The condition occurs in active, athletic individuals often of muscular build. The patient walks with a limp and has difficulty in sitting on the affected buttock. *When Lumbar 4 root is affected* (Lumbar 3 disc), there is pain over the anterior surface of the thigh and medial aspect of the lower leg. It tends to extend to the medial side of the foot (Fig. 244). There is tenderness and weakness of the quadriceps and the knee-jerk is diminished or lost. This disc is less commonly prolapsed than the others. *When Lumbar 5 root is affected* (Lumbar 4 disc), pain radiates down the lateral and posterior aspect of the thigh, the lateral side of the leg, and across the dorsum of the foot to the great toe (Fig. 244). Sensory impairment to cotton-wool and pin-prick exists on the lateral aspect of the lower leg. There is weakness of extension of the great toe, less commonly dorsiflexion and eversion of the foot; and foot-drop may occur. The reflexes are normal. *When Sacral 1 root is affected* (Lumbar 5 disc), pain will radiate down the posterior aspect of the thigh and lower leg to the outer side of the foot. Sensory impairment is almost always over the outer toes and border of the foot (Fig. 244). The gastrocnemius muscle wastes and the ankle-jerk is absent or diminished. Rarely more than one root is affected.

Other Signs.—(1) When the patient is in the horizontal position, on a couch or on the floor, ask him to do *straight leg raising.* This test, which may show limitation of straight leg raising owing to pain caused by stretching the affected roots, is most useful (i.) *diagnostically* to assess the severity of the pain, (ii.) *prognostically* to assess the results of treatment. (2) In many cases the lumbar spine will have lost its normal lordosis and will be flattened. The patient will tilt his pelvis sometimes to one side, sometimes to the other, producing a compensating scoliosis. (3) *C.S.F.*—There may be slight increase in the protein content. This examination is usually not necessary unless spinal cord compression is suspected; then myelography should be undertaken when the puncture is made. (4) X-ray of the lumbar spine may show narrowing of a disc space or the findings may be normal.

Diagnosis.—In all cases a rectal examination should be made, the urine tested for sugar and the spine X-rayed. Radicular pain in the lumbar or sciatic region may be the first symptom of malignant disease, tuberculous disease of the spine or myelomatosis.

Etiology.—Trauma, infection and degenerative changes are causal factors. In the later weeks of pregnancy or after parturition increased vascularity of the lumbar and sacral discs may cause herniation quite apart from pressure of the foetal head on the sciatic nerve.

Prognosis.—Favourable cases rested absolutely in bed recover in 4-6 weeks, but recurrences are frequent. Foot-drop seldom recovers completely.

Treatment of Sciatic Neuritis and Lumbar Disc Lesions.—The patient should be rested in bed absolutely and not allowed to get up for bath or toilet. For the pain give tab. codeine co. (B.P.) 4 to 6 in 24 hours or aspirin. Tablets containing propylphenazone, phenacetin and caffeine (Saridone) are suitable for short-term use in doses of 1 to 2 tablets twice daily. Stronger analgesics such as allyl-isopropyl-barbitone (Allonal) or the opium alkaloids may be needed for severe pain. Chlorpromazine (Largactil) 25 mg. by mouth thrice or four times daily potentiates analgesics. A long Liston splint may be applied from the axilla to the ankle, or the patient put in a plaster jacket or shell. If he wishes to be treated at home, a plaster spica to fix to the lumbar spine, hip and knee, may be applied for four to six weeks. When the patient will not tolerate fixation, try sacral epidural injection of 50–100 ml. of 0·5 per cent. procaine in normal saline. Relief may be obtained by infiltrating tender areas in the muscles with 1 per cent. procaine hydrochlor. No manipulation should be carried out during the active phase of the disease but pelvic traction helps some cases with disc lesions. Massage and heat are comforting and useful.

In cases who do not improve after weeks of bed-rest, or who have recurrent disabling attacks, surgical removal of the disc by an expert may be considered; the results are not always immediately curative and this must be made clear to the patient before operation is undertaken. Residual mobility of the vertebræ may require fixation by a bone graft.

III. LUMBAR SPONDYLOSIS as a cause of pain with neurological signs in the limbs is briefly mentioned here. It is a common cause of lumbago, sciatic pains and anterior femoral neuritis. More than one root is involved and the symptoms are often, but not invariably, bilateral.

IV. In CAUDA EQUINA LESIONS pain is early, often severe and bilateral, down the back of both thighs, and accompanied by numbness and paræsthesiæ in the saddle-area or the soles of the feet (§ 969). Lesions of the lumbo-sacral cord show a similar picture with the addition of (1) pyramidal signs, (2) dissociated sensory loss.

Etiology.—(1) The commonest lesion is a fracture dislocation of L1 vertebra with backward displacement into the vertebral canal. (2) Prolapsed disc (especially central protrusions), (3) Benign tumours, (4) Malignant secondary deposits, (5) Myelomatosis also occur.

Treatment depends on accurate diagnosis of the cause.

V. MALIGNANT METASTASES (§ 969).

VI. MYELOMATOSIS (§ 613) may involve a single vertebra. The earliest X-ray changes seen when the disease presents as sciatica are easily missed.

(*C*) **Pain in the Trunk and Limbs** due to muscular or aponeurotic fibrositis, spondylosis, tuberculous caries or neoplasms of the vertebræ, intrathoracic growths or aneurysms and pleurisy are discussed elsewhere. The *referred* pains of renal and biliary colic and of coronary disease are discussed in their appropriate sections. Chronic *pain under the left breast* complained of by many women is usually part of an anxiety neurosis.

NEUROLOGICAL CAUSES

I. Herpes zoster.
II. Tabes dorsalis.

III. Syphilitic meningo-myelitis.
IV. Spinal cord compression (see § 968).

The patient develops a UNILATERAL INTENSE BORING PAIN OF ROOT DISTRIBUTION. *There is* MALAISE *and* PYREXIA *and about the fourth day the skin reddens and small vesicles begin to appear over the painful dermatome. The disease is* HERPES ZOSTER.

§ 1021. I. Herpes Zoster (Syn. "Shingles").—*Symptoms.*—*Pre-eruptive phase.* The patient feels an intense boring pain with hyperæsthesia of the skin, which is unilateral and segmental in distribution. There is malaise and a temperature of 100–102°. *Eruptive phase.* The first crop of vesicles, which are related to nerve endings in the skin of the affected dermatome, appear about the fourth day. This is followed by others all on the same side so that many coalesce. The skin around the vesicles becomes hyperæmic: the vesicles rupture, then gradually dry up with scabbing of the surface. The lymph nodes draining the affected area enlarge and the C.S.F. shows a lymphocytic reaction. *Stage of Healing.* Secondary infection may occur. If the loss of tissue is deep, white or pigmented scars may be left. Over the affected dermatome hyperæsthesia may coexist with analgesia to light touch and pin-prick.

Varieties.—(1) *Zoster of the trunk and limbs* is commonest over Th3–5 segments. Zoster of C4–5 may be accompanied by paresis of the deltoid and spinati, D11 by paralysis of the oblique abdominal muscles and L3 by quadriceps paralysis, but these are rare. (2) *Visceral herpes* may cause cystitis, pleurisy, arthritis. (3) *Trigeminal herpes* affects the supra-orbital division and vesicles appear on one side of the forehead, on the cornea and down the nose (naso-ciliary branch) (Herpes ophthalmicus, § 1076). Keratitis, ophthalmoplegia or optic atrophy may result in rare cases. (4) *Geniculate herpes.* Facial palsy may occur when herpes zoster affects the geniculate ganglion (Ramsay-Hunt syndrome). The initial patch of vesicles may be on the auricle simulating erysipelas, inside the mouth or on the skin of the neck (§ 1080). (5) *Meningo-encephalitis*, with confusion and focal cerebral or spinal cord signs, *e.g.*, paraplegia is very rare. (6) SYMPTOMATIC ZOSTER occurs in relationship to trauma, vertebral carcinomatosis, leukæmia, tabes, after irradiation and intrathecal contrast radiography. In such cases the virus is probably carried by the host in the nerve tissues affected.

Diagnosis.—Skin lesions on the face may simulate erysipelas, those on the trunk or groin may simulate eczema, and the pain of abdominal zoster may simulate that of an abdominal emergency.

Etiology.—The disease is much more common after the age of 50 years and both sexes suffer. It is due to a filtrable virus similar to that causing varicella. It is now believed to affect the central nervous system as a whole and no longer regarded as a localised radicular lesion. Although the posterior nerve root ganglion and the grey matter of the particular horns over one or more dermatomes are principally affected, it is fairly common to find motor paralysis and even involvement of the long tracts. One attack usually confers immunity against subsequent attacks.

Prognosis.—Most patients are able to resume normal life after three weeks but recovery may be delayed by infection of the vesicles. For post-herpetic neuralgia see § 816.

Treatment.—There is no specific remedy. See § 676.

The patient complains of attacks of ACUTE STABBING PAINS IN THE LIMBS, *usually the legs, which are paroxysmal and are not related to effort; the* PUPILS MAY BE UNEQUAL *with* LOSS OF THE LIGHT REFLEX. *The condition is likely to be* TABES DORSALIS.

§ 1022. II. **Tabes Dorsalis** (Syn. Locomotor Ataxia) is much less common since the introduction of effective treatment for syphilis. It is characterised by (*a*) disturbances of sensation in the form of lightning pains, paræsthesiæ and anæsthesiæ; (*b*) loss of the tendon reflexes and muscular hypotonia; (*c*) sensory ataxia; (*d*) loss of the pupillary light reflex; and (*e*) disorders of micturition. Muscular power usually remains intact until near the end. Ten years is the average date of onset after the primary syphilitic sore; it rarely begins within five years of infection.

The *Symptoms* run a prolonged course over many years and usually last all the patient's lifetime. The development of the disease is most insidious and it may not be apparent until it is well established. There is no disease of the nervous system which is so frequently missed; yet it is relatively common. The patient will only rarely come for his ataxia. He comes before this because of his " *rheumatism* " (lightning pains), *bladder troubles,* hesitancy or dribbling after micturition, *acute abdominal pain and vomiting* (" crises "), *failure of vision* and *diplopia,* or a *fracture, dislocation or swollen joint* (Charcot joint). Attention is focused on the local condition and the diagnosis may be missed. Remember that it is possible to make the diagnosis from *the characteristic lightning pains alone* and to confirm it by further clinical and serological examinations. The symptoms can be discussed categorically in order of frequency of their early appearance.

(*A*) *Those referable to Disease of the Posterior Roots or Columns.* (1) *Lightning Pains* (" rheumatism ") are the commonest early symptoms. They may precede all the other symptoms by years, and occur in no other disease. They may be unilateral or bilateral, and are described as stabbing, burning, tearing or bursting pains. They are commonly in the legs (since tabes usually starts in the lumbo-sacral region) and like " stabs with a knife " seem to *pierce the transverse axis* of the limbs. They are *paroxysmal* and vary with the weather, a point which must not lead to a mistaken diagnosis of rheumatism. They are diagnosed, not by the severity of the pain, but by their (i.) paroxysmal character, (ii.) distribution in the legs, especially in the calves and heels, (iii.) " transverse " direction. Pins and needles, and " girdle-sensations " of constriction round the trunk, occur. (2) *Sensory Impairment.*—All forms of sensibility are affected, cutaneous and deep. Cutaneous impairment occurs as (*a*) a " cuirass " over the thorax and down the inner aspect of both upper limbs, including the ring and little fingers. (*b*) A " butterfly-area " over the nose and cheeks (*masque tabétique* of Duchenne), (*c*) on the soles of the feet and perinæum, in sacral tabes. Deep sensibility is affected early; especially common are loss of pain sensibility of the tendo Achillis to pressure (Abadie's sign), and loss of vibration sense over the tibial malleoli or sacrum. Pressure over the ulnar nerves at the elbow may fail to produce the normal " funny-bone " sensation in the ring and little fingers (Biernacki's sign) and the lateral popliteal nerve as it winds below the head of the fibula may be similarly insensitive (Sarbo's sign). (3) *Diminution or Loss of Tendon Reflexes and Hypotonia.*—The disappearance of the ankle-jerks (S1, 2) precedes the disappearance of the knee-jerks by years, because tabes commences in the sacral roots. The arm-jerks are retained late, except in cervical tabes. The cutaneous and plantar reflexes are normal, unless tabes is complicated by another form of neuro-syphilis. In uncomplicated tabes the plantars are always flexor. The disease in the posterior roots interrupts spinal reflex-arcs subserving muscular tone as well as those connected with the tendon reflexes, and hypotonia with ability to hyperextend the knee-joints or hip-joints into grotesque attitudes, may be present. (4) *Sensory Ataxia* is due to disease of sensory and non-sensory afferents concerned with joint sense and posture. It is usually, in the early stages of the disease, compensated for by the patient, and the ataxia may only be made manifest by the heel–knee or finger–nose test, the patient's eyes being closed. Romberg's sign is fallacious; it may occur in nervous individuals who are organically sound. In the later stages the ataxia is manifest, the gait wide-based, the heels being brought down jerkily with a stamp and the feet lifted high in stepping, owing to errors in projection of the limbs. The eyes are fixed on the ground for additional visual guidance (§ 949).

(*B*) *Those referable to other parts of the Nervous System. Pupillary and Ocular Phenomena.*—(*a*) *The pupils* gradually become smaller and irregular in outline, often oval. They become eccentrically placed, usually to the nasal side of the iris. They are commonly unequal. Miosis is not constant, one pupil may be widely dilated. Later, the pupils, whether dilated or contracted, fail to react to light but preserve the accommodation-converg-

ence reaction—the *Argyll-Robertson phenomenon*; this may occur in large
or small pupils, in one eye or both.   The consensual reflex may be lost.
" Fixed pupils " are also met, which do not react to light, nor accommodation (§ 1059, Fig. 220).   (b) *Diplopia*, in the early stages, is caused by
transient weakness of the external ocular muscles and lasts a few days.
Later, permanent frank external ophthalmoplegias occur.   (c) *Pseudo-
ptosis* is due to paralysis of the cervical sympathetic, and is bilateral, with
compensatory wrinkling of the forehead, producing the " tabetic facies."
(d) *Optic Atrophy* usually progresses to complete blindness.   For years it
may be confined to one eye.   The earliest sign is pallor of the disc, with

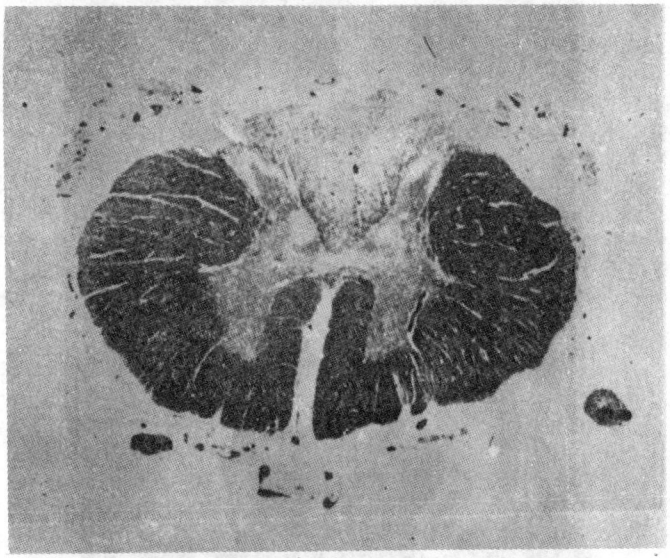

FIG. 253.—TABES DORSALIS.   Cross-section of spinal cord showing degeneration of the posterior
columns and of the posterior roots (Weigert-Pal stain for myelin).

peripheral constriction of the visual fields, when perimetrically charted.
Later, the disc shows a typically clear-cut yellow appearance, the colour
of candle wax (Plate XXII).   Tabetics with optic atrophy rarely show
advanced tabetic signs elsewhere (Benedict's Law).

  Vesical and Sexual Disabilities.—Hesitancy and dribbling of urine after
micturition appear early.   Nocturnal incontinence may occur.   Residual
urine easily becomes infected, leading to cystitis with ascending pyelonephritis.   Impotence is an early symptom in sacral tabes.   Incontinence
of fæces may occur, especially after aperients.

  Visceral Crises.—Acute abdominal pain may occur, with vomiting of
pints of acid gastric juice, lasting days; this can be mistaken for an acute
abdominal catastrophe (§ 271).   The pains of gastric crises are in no way
related to food.   Crises occur in other organs, *e.g.*, spasm in the larynx,

the colon or rectum, producing tenesmus; or in the bladder, with painful micturition or retention.

Trophic Changes.—(a) *Charcot joints.* This arthropathy is probably always occasioned by local trauma. The joint becomes swollen, but pain, heat and redness are absent. Several joints may be affected. Recurrent effusions cause great disorganisation and may produce a flail-limb or genu recurvatum, if the knee-joint is involved. The spine (Fig. 254) or the thumb or finger-joints may be affected. Usually it is large joints in the lower limbs (*cf.* syringomyelia, in which the large joints of the upper limbs

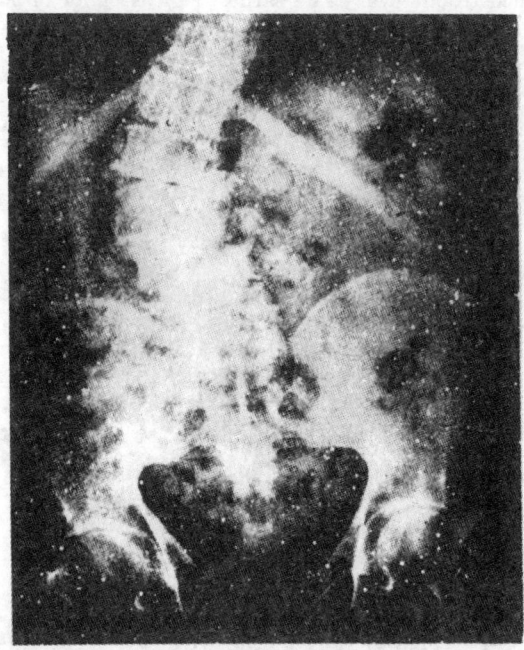

FIG 254.—CHARCOT ARTHROPATHY OF THE LOWER LUMBAR VERTEBRÆ from a case of tabes dorsalis.

are similarly affected). Hypertrophic and atrophic changes occur. X-ray shows great rarefaction, irregular large osteophytes, erosion, linear fractures or a dislocation. (b) *Perforating ulcers* occur in the ball of the great toe; they become keratinised and covered over temporarily; then the callosity sloughs out leaving the cylindrical cavity unhealed as before. They may extend into the joint. *Painless ulceration* may occur in the nail-bed.

TABES ASSOCIATED WITH OTHER FORMS OF NEUROSYPHILIS.—Dementia paralytica (§ 1190) may co-exist, with tremor of the lips and tongue, dysarthria and character change—*Tubo-Paresis*. *Syphilitic Amyotrophy* may be present (§ 965) with local wasting of the peripheral upper limb muscles.

VISCERAL SYPHILIS.—Aortitis, thoracic aneurysm, or syphilitic aortic regurgitation, occur in about a third of the cases (§ 80). Recurrent laryngeal paralysis may be present, however, apart from aneurysm (§ 176).

Diagnosis.—The presence of lightning pains alone is sufficient to make the diagnosis, combined with evidence of past syphilis as, *e.g.*, when the patient admits infection (usually imperfectly treated). Patches of leuko-plakia on the palate, tongue or cheeks are suggestive, also repeated still-births or absence of pregnancy after many years of marriage. The diagnosis rests on clinical grounds and is confirmed by examination of the blood and C.S.F. The Wassermann reaction is positive in the blood in 65 per cent. of cases, and in the C.S.F. in about the same percentage. The C.S.F., when positive, shows lymphocytic pleocytosis, 10–80 cells per c.mm. (corresponding to the degree of meningeal inflammation present), increased globulin, protein 0·03 to 0·08 per cent., and a " luetic " type of Lange curve—viz., 1233210000. The *tonic pupil* (§ 1060) with absent tendon reflexes is a benign condition without pains in the limbs, sometimes confused with tabes dorsalis. In *polyneuritis* (alcoholic or diabetic) absent knee- and ankle-jerks are found: occasionally these reflexes are absent as an isolated and unexplained finding in an otherwise normal individual. For *Differential Diagnosis*, see Table LVII.

Etiology.—(1) As with dementia paralytica, tabes usually begins between 25 and 40 years of age. It is a rare result of congenital syphilis. (2) The majority of cases are males. Husband and wife may both be affected (conjugal tabes). (3) The disease is at first meningo-vascular, and is due to the *Treponema pallidum* affecting the posterior root between the ganglion and the spinal cord. The sensory fibres are involved earliest in the sacral region. (4) Spinal cord degenerations follow in the posterior column as high as the nucleus gracilis and nucleus cuneatus; the spino-thalamic fibres, being relayed afresh on entering the posterior horn, are unaffected (Fig. 253). (5) Degenerative changes may occur in the optic nerves. (6) The Argyll-Robertson pupil is thought to be due to degenera-tion of the colliculo-ocular fibres in the mid-brain (Fig. 220).

Prognosis.—Effective treatment of primary syphilis probably prevents the later onset of tabes. Cases treated late may develop tabes or dementia paralytica in spite of treatment. The longer the period elapsing between infection and the first tabetic symptom the milder will the tabes be. The disease probably never completely dies out, but periods of quiescence may last for years, when the patient is untroubled by lightning pains or visceral crises and the signs in the nervous system are at a standstill. The disease appears in these cases to have burnt itself out. Activity is possible as long as the C.S.F. shows pleocytosis; but in serologically negative cases symptoms may progress when intercurrent illness or injury necessitates prolonged rest in bed. It is relatively easy in most cases by anti-syphilitic treatment to produce a normal or almost normal C.S.F., but this does not mean the disease is arrested, or that lightning pains and crises, if ameli-orated, have ceased. The blood and C.S.F. Wassermann reactions sometimes remains persistently positive after full courses of treatment; further treatment in such cases is not usually indicated.

Ocular palsies may be transient, but optic atrophy almost invariably progresses to total blindness. Bladder and other intercurrent infections and the aortic complications of the disease are liable to cause death.

Treatment.—(a) Anti-syphilitic Treatment.—In patients with progressive symptoms, those with pleocytosis in the spinal fluid, increased globulin or changes in the Lange curve, treatment by penicillin usually causes marked improvement in the patient's general and neurological condition. It is doubtful, in other cases, if anti-syphilitic treatment radically influences the course of the disease. Many benign and quiescent cases have had little or no treatment. For details of the treatment of Neurosyphilis see § 500.

(b) Symptomatic Treatment.—(i.) For *lightning pains* or *visceral crises* never give drugs liable to cause addiction (morphine, methadone, pethidine). Aspirin gr. 10–20, or codeine gr. $\frac{1}{4}$ repeated if necessary, should first be tried. Chloretone gr. 10 in a cachet may be given and repeated. For visceral crises give atropine sulphate gr. $\frac{1}{100}$ repeated as necessary with phenobarbitone gr. 3 intramusc. Short courses of penicillin intramusc. or neoarsphenamine intravenously in small doses given over three or four weeks may cut short bouts of pain. Chordotomy is only to be advised in the most severe and intractable cases. (ii.) For *optic atrophy* malarial therapy may be tried to check the progress of blindness but its value is doubtful. (iii.) *The bladder.* The patient should be taught to empty the bladder every three hours, whether he feels the need or not, by suprapubic manual expression of the contents. Cystitis is usually due to residual urine and needs appropriate treatment (§ 418): vesical calculi are sometimes present. For retention avoid catheterisation. Inj. carbachol B.P. (0·25 mg. in 1 ml.) may be given in 2 ml. doses subcut. If the prostate is hypertrophied, a wedge resection or prostatectomy may help. Continuous bladder drainage by a urethral or a suprapubic tube may be required, or in males the use of a portable rubber urinal for dribbling. (iv.) *Charcot's Joints.*—The acute stages are best treated by rest in bed. Even large effusions will become absorbed without aspiration. Heavy calipers are of doubtful value and some patients cannot wear them. Using the joint invariably causes erosion of bone fractures, usually painless and with much bony hypertrophy. An orthopædic opinion should be obtained at an early stage in each individual case. (v.) *Perforating ulcers* on the feet will seldom heal until the patient is put to bed for 4–6 weeks. They should be curetted and covered with strapping, having been dressed with gauze soaked in one of the following—zinc and castor oil, red lotion, acriflavine, sulphonamide cream, sterile paraffin or cod-liver oil. (vi.) *Ataxia* is markedly improved by a course of Frenkl's exercises.

§ 1023. **Juvenile Tabes** is rare and may be combined with signs of paresis. The symptoms are congenital, but may not show themselves until after the first decade. The younger the patient at the onset of symptoms, the more severe the disease.

Choroido-retinitis, bilateral deafness, Hutchinsonian teeth, sabre-shaped tibiæ and rhagades may be present; otherwise the disease is identical with the adult form.

TYPES OF NEUROSYPHILIS

I. ASYMPTOMATIC.

II. MENINGOVASCULAR:
  (a) Meningomyelitis (§ 964).
  (b) Cerebral vascular (§ 907).
  (c) Spinal vascular (§ 956).
  (d) Amyotrophy, (§ 965).
  (e) Hypertrophic cervical pachy-
      meningitis (§ 1025).

III. PARENCHYMATOUS:
  (a) Tabes dorsalis (§ 1022).
  (b) Dementia paralytica (§ 1190).
  (c) Erb's paraplegia (§ 966).

§ 1024. I. In **Asymptomatic Neurosyphilis** there are no clinical symptoms except for abnormality of the C.S.F.; when there is pleocytosis, raised globulin, a positive Lange curve, the case should be treated as indicated in § 500.

§ 1025. **Hypertrophic Cervical Pachymeningitis** produces severe root pains, radiating down the upper limbs and across the neck, with wasting and weakness of the hand and weakness of the hand and forearm muscles, sensory changes and alteration in the tendon reflexes. In the later stages the legs become spastic. Protein is greatly increased in the C.S.F., but cellular increase is slight or absent. The Lange curve is of the luetic type and the Wassermann reaction is often strongly positive.

GROUP XIV.　CRAMPS

Cramps are intermittent spasms affecting groups of voluntary muscles, usually but not always painful. Stiffness and loss of power of the affected part may be experienced while the cramp lasts. They are tonic contractions involving one or more muscles and they may occur " spontaneously " or reflexly. Sometimes they appear only on attempted movement. Skilled movements, such as writing or playing the violin, may be the only ones affected. We know little of the causes of cramp. It may be a symptom of muscular, metabolic, infective, vascular or psychical disorder.

CAUSES OF CRAMP

Vascular Disease.
  I. Intermittent Claudication (§ 586).
Muscle Disorders.
  II. Myotonia including
      Dystrophia Myotonica (§ 1028).
      Myotonia Congenita (§ 1029).
Metabolic Disorders.
  III. Heat cramp (§ 510, IV).
  IV. Diabetes Mellitus (§ 423).
  V. Tetany (§ 1030).

Following Infections.
  VI. Tetanus (§ 1031).
  VII. Hydrophobia (§ 1032).
Psychical Disorders.
  VIII. Writer's cramp (§ 1033).
  IX. Hysterical spasm (§ 1034).
Other Causes.
  Flexor spasms (see § 953).
  Facial hemispasm (see § 1080).
  Spasmodic Torticollis (§ 929).

Cramp due to ischæmia of the muscle is painful and to a swimmer dangerous. Healthy individuals may be seized during violent exercise, *e.g.*, tennis, squash, swimming. Some persons are affected by cramp throughout life on light provocation such as lying in bed at night. *Symptomatic treatment.* Quinine sulphate orally gr. 5 or sod. bicarbonate gr. 60

at bedtime may produce freedom from nocturnal cramps. Tablets of quinine and ascorbic acid (Kina-Redoxon) or quinine sulphate gr. 3 with tinct. gelsemii ℳ 15 in a mixture at bedtime may be tried.

Cramp is associated with signs of Vascular Disease.

§ 1026. I. Intermittent Claudication due to muscular ischæmia causes painful cramps in the legs on walking or in bed. It occurs mainly at or after middle age and accompanies occlusive arterial disease (§ 586).

Cramp is associated with Muscular Wasting or Weakness.

§ 1027. II. **Myotonia.**—There is inability to relax the muscle after a voluntary effort or reflex muscular contraction with a peculiar prolonged tonic spasm of the muscle. It is painless and is probably due to a biochemical neuro-muscular disorder with disturbance at the myoneural junction and elsewhere. Direct percussion of the muscles affected, *e.g.*, the thenar muscles or the tongue, produces prolonged dimpling at the site of percussion (myotonia on percussion). Myotonia in the respiratory muscles may appear when the patient sneezes, or in the facial muscles if he yawns or screws up his eyes (reflex myotonia). Myotonia is characteristically precipitated by exposure to cold and helped by warmth and alcohol: it is increased by neostigmin and decreased by quinine salts. The symptom is heredo-familial and may be associated with a muscular and endocrine dystrophy (dystrophia myotonica), or with generalised muscle hypertrophy, or psychotic disturbances (myotonia congenita).

§ 1028. **Dystrophia Myotonica** (Syn. Myotonia Atrophica) is a rare heredo-familial disorder developing especially in males between 20–25 years of age.

Symptoms.—(1) Myotonia is usually seen in the muscles of the hands when the patient makes a forceful hand-grip. The patient tries to straighten his fingers (which are flexed in spasm) on his chest or knees. Many patients are so used to the phenomenon that they do not mention it or attempt to conceal it. If in such circumstances the sufferer is accepted for military service, the discipline of drill soon renders his disability evident. (2) Muscular atrophy and weakness is seen in the sternomastoids, the facial muscles and the muscles supplied from the bulb. There is bilateral ptosis and lack of emotional movement in the face (myopathic facies) with falling forward of the head. The muscles of the limbs are small and feeble. Weakness is present in the atrophied muscles, but when the wasting is confined to the sternomastoids the patient may not notice it. (3) Cataract is present in a third of the cases, or patients give a history of cataract in relations. It may be seen only by examination with a slit-lamp. (4) Endocrine changes are marked; testicular atrophy, impotence, premature baldness, functional hypopituitarism are commonly seen. (5) A few are mentally retarded. Other abnormalities may co-exist. The affected muscles give the characteristic prolonged tonic contraction on galvanic stimulation, relaxing slowly after the stimulus ceases. *Diagnosis* depends on the recognition of myotonia accompanied by characteristic wasting of the sternomastoid and facial muscles, and endocrine signs. The grasp reflex is a different phenomenon (§ 845(2)). *Etiology.*—Often several in a family are affected. The descent is equally through males and females. Earlier generations may betray the disease by a history of cataract, frequent celibacy, childless marriages, dying out of certain branches of the family, a steady decline, generation after generation, in the family fortunes, from affluence to poverty.

Prognosis.—The progress is very slow and many live to old age without serious incapacity. Some become confined to a chair.

Treatment.—Quinine bisulphate tablets 300 mg. (5 gr.) may be given twice or thrice daily to relieve the myotonia. Procainamide (Pronestyl) tablets may relieve the myotonia, but also slow the ventricular rate. Injections of ACTH have lessened myotonia in occasional cases. Testosterone injections may help the endocrine deficiency in male patients. Cataracts must be treated surgically.

§ 1029. **Myotonia Congenita** (Thomsen's Disease) is probably a variant of Dystrophia myotonica but is much more rare. *Symptoms* are: (1) Hypertrophy of muscles, (2) muscular weakness (which may be profound), (3) myotonia, and (4) slight mental impairment are the inherited factors. Psychosis may occur. True or pseudo-hypertrophy of muscles, focal or generalised, may be met, the large muscles contrasting with the patient's poor muscular strength. Myotonia is demonstrated on voluntary effort, not in slight but in more powerful movements. The patient has difficulty in relaxing the grip on shaking hands, cannot open his eyes after he has screwed them up, etc. Violent reflex actions, such as coughing or sneezing, produce transient tonic spasm in the muscles concerned. Myotonic dimpling is present on direct percussion of the tongue or affected skeletal muscles, and myotonic spasm is produced with mild faradic currents. Repetition of the movement tends to abolish the myotonia. The disease is slowly progressive and death may occur from sudden asphyxia during coughing.

Cramp is associated with a disturbance in metabolism.

III. HEAT CRAMP affects the muscles of the limbs and abdomen (§ 510, IV).

IV. DIABETES MELLITUS also causes cramps in the legs due to salt depletion.

§ **1030.** V. **Tetany** (Syn. Spasmophilia) is an increased irritability of the neuro-muscular apparatus causing paroxysmal stiffness of the hands, feet and facial muscles, caused by disease usually outside the nervous system.

Symptoms.—Paroxysmal stiffness affects the forearms, hands and feet (carpo-pedal spasms). The attitude of the fingers, compressed into a cone (the accoucheur's hand), has been emphasised, but other attitudes occur. The paroxysms last from a few seconds to an hour or so. In severe cases there is no intervening relaxation; moreover, all the muscles of the body are affected and there may even be opisthotonos. The spasms are painful if prolonged. In children it may be associated with laryngismus stridulus (§ 177) and in infants convulsive seizures with loss of consciousness. Many grades of severity are seen; the disease may only last two days, or two or more months, recovery being the rule. Three signs are described (1) *Chvostek's sign* is a brisk contraction of the facial muscles on one side on tapping in front of the ear with a reflex hammer. (2) *Trousseau* described: spasm in the hands and fingers after the application of an inflated blood-pressure cuff which presses on the nerves and vessels. (3) *Erb's sign* is a lowered threshold of excitability of the peripheral nerves to electrical and other stimuli. These may be elicited when infantile convulsions are the only sign of tetany. *Diagnosis* is made by the characteristic carpo-pedal spasms and laryngo-spasm. Where these are absent and the infant has convulsions only, look for Chvostek's and Trousseau's signs between the fits. Laryngeal stridor occurs with laryngitis stridulosa in some highly strung children.

Etiology.—Tetany may result from (A) any condition in which there is decrease in the serum calcium, *e.g.*, some cases of rickets, hypoparathyroidism, (B) alkalosis, (C) hyperpnœa.

(A) *Decrease in serum calcium:*
    (1) In infants with low calcium rickets; the serum phosphate is often low.
    (2) In steatorrhœa, cœliac disease and sprue.
    (3) In hypoparathyroidism when the parathyroids are damaged during thyroidectomy; the serum phosphate is elevated.
Idiopathic chronic hypoparathyroidism is rare; neural defect, recurrent epileptic fits and calcification of the basal ganglia occur.
    (4) During lactation.
    (5) In chronic renal disease.
(B) *Alkalosis:*
    (6) In pyloric stenosis with vomiting.
    (7) Overdosage with alkali.
(C) *Hyperpnœa:*
    (8) Habitual overbreathing will cause alkalosis and tetany.

Prognosis.—A fatal issue is rare. Infantile convulsions due to this cause may not recur.

Treatment.—If convulsions are present these must be controlled (§ 868). Calcium gluconate (10 per cent. solution) may be given intravenously in doses of 5–10 ml. Give to adults vitamin D_2 as tab. calciferol (B.P.) or to infants calcium with vitamin D tablets (calciferol compound tablets B.P.C.) orally, controlling the doses by serum calcium tests or by Sulkowitch's test for urinary calcium. Some prefer dihydrotachysterol.

Cramp follows upon an infected wound or injury.

§ 1031. VI. **Tetanus** (Syn. Lockjaw) is a severe disease characterised by paroxysms of tonic and sometimes clonic spasms, due to the inoculation into a scratch or wound of the tetanus bacillus (*Cl. tetani*), the chief habitat of which is highly manured earth and the excreta of herbivora.

Symptoms.—(1) Within 2–14 days after the injury the patient complains of stiffness of the jaw and back of the neck. In some the incubation period may, however, measure weeks, even months in cases who have had a prophylactic anti-tetanic serum injection. (2) Very soon the jaw and neck muscles become rigid. The spasm of the jaw-muscles is known as trismus or lockjaw. A similar tonic spasm spreads to all the muscles of the trunk, and in a less degree of the extremities. The back is rigid, sometimes arched in the position of *opisthotonos*, in which only the head and buttocks rest on the bed. Or there may be flexion to one side—*pleurosthotonos*, or bending forward of the body—*emprosthotonos*. The angles of the mouth are drawn down and the eyebrows are elevated—"*risus sardonicus.*" (3) Reflex spasms supervene from time to time, in which the already rigid muscles become still more contracted, causing agonising pain. The slightest touch may excite these. In severe cases these spasms become more frequent, leading to death from involvement of the laryngeal or respiratory muscles. (4) The temperature may be normal or slightly raised throughout, and may rise to 108° F just before death. There is often retention of urine. The mind is clear to the last. A *local form* due to head wounds is described, with paralysis of the facial muscles and difficulty in swallowing. A single case may show (i.) tonic spasms, (ii.) reflex spasms, (iii.) peripheral palsies.

After an injection of antitetanic serum to prevent the disease, temporary localised spasm or paralysis may result, *e.g.*, in one arm if the wound is in the hand.

Diagnosis.—In *strychnine poisoning* the muscles relax in the intervals between the spasms and the spasms involve the extremities to a greater degree. In *meningitis* there is a temperature and there is no trismus. *Tetany* is not likely to be mistaken for tetanus. In *hysterical opisthotonos* there are other evidences of hysteria. Trismus is rarely seen in medullary neoplasms and bulbar poliomyelitis, with periostitis of the jaw, disease of the temporo-maxillary joint, or other *local irritation*, such as quinsy or the cutting of a tooth; but the course serves to differentiate these from tetanus.

Etiology.—The disease is due to the *Cl. tetani*, a spore-forming anærobic bacillus. It may contaminate catgut. Introduced into the body through an abrasion or wound, it produces, locally, an exotoxin, which travels up the axis cylinders of a contiguous nerve and affects the motor cells, spinal or cranial, at first causing local spasm, then general spasm, or paralysis.

Prognosis.—The earlier serum is given the better the outlook. The fatality rate when the case is in experienced hands is now 20 to 30 per cent. (Garland). Death, however, may occur from the effect of the toxin on the respiratory centre, even when convulsions are well controlled. An incubation period of five days or less is grave and if the time between the first symptom and the first convulsion (" onset period ") is less than 48 hours death is likely.

Treatment.—Whenever possible the patient should be transferred to hospital or to a special centre. In the meantime (1) *Local Treatment.*—Excise and clean the wound; (2) *Antitoxin.*—Give tetanus antitoxin B.P. 50,000 units intramuscularly and 100,000 units intravenously (never intrathecally). Anaphylaxis may occur in those who have had previous A.T.S. Further doses of 25,000 units should be given weekly. (3) *Spasms.*—Where facilities are available produce complete paralysis of all voluntary muscles (Garland uses laudexium methylsulphate as a curarising agent, given intramuscularly 20–30 mg. approximately 2-hourly, which does not affect cardiac muscle), using an intermittent positive pressure apparatus and a cuffed endotracheal tube to control respiration. Tracheal secretions have to be aspirated by a sucker. When curarisation is no longer needed, it is replaced by fairly large doses of chlorpromazine, which must be withdrawn gradually. Others use 1–2 per cent. mephenesin by intravenous drip, or acetylpromazine (3–5 mg/Kg. intramusc. or intravenously) not more often than 2-hourly. Continuous sedation by 5–10 ml. paraldehyde orally or intramusc. every 2 to 3 hours will produce amnesia. (4) Prophylactic penicillin (2 megaunits daily) is needed to prevent pulmonary infection. (5) Feeding through a nasal tube using a balanced diet of at least 2,500 calories is advised. (6) Daily electrolyte assessment will be needed during any regime of muscular paralysis. (7) Anæmia can arise rapidly and 50 per cent. of patients will require transfusion. Active immunisation is needed before the patient leaves hospital.

In *neonatal* cases Adams gives chlorpromazine injections 25 mg. 4–6-hourly with sod. phenobarbitone injected in doses of 60 mg. 6–8 hourly.

The help of a consultant anæsthetist and a surgeon as well as a skilled nursing team is necessary to carry out such regimes efficiently.

Prophylaxis.—Give tetanus antitoxin B.P. (A.T.S.) 1,500 units after thorough cleansing of the wound. This dose may be repeated weekly for three weeks. When giving A.T.S. *a solution of 1 : 1,000 adrenalin should be available in case of anaphylaxis.* After the injection is given the patient must be kept under observation for half an hour. For the precautions when there is *a history of previous injection of A.T.S.* see § 524.

§ 1032. VII. **Hydrophobia** (Syn. Rabies) is a fatal disease, transferred to man by inoculation by the infected saliva of an animal (dog, vampire bat, wolf, fox, jackal, skunk, or other warm-blooded animal) suffering from the disease. It is characterised by spasms and paralysis of the muscles, notably those of deglutition and respiration. The causative filterable virus travels along the axons centripetally to the central nervous system from the area of the bite.   The disease is non-existent in Great Britain but common in S.E. Europe, Asia and the U.S.A.

Symptoms.—(1) After an incubation stage, which is generally about 6 weeks, never less than 12 days, and sometimes as long as 12–18 months or more, there is an insidious onset of malaise and lethargy with perhaps slight fever and, sometimes, tingling in the wound.   (2) With or without premonitory symptoms, paroxysms of painful spasms of the pharynx supervene, at first brought on by any attempt to swallow, or even the sight of fluid; hence the name hydrophobia.   (3) These clonic spasms later become tonic, lasting 15–30 minutes at a time, and spread to the muscles of respiration and of the neck.   The attacks produce excruciating pain and agony of mind.   The mind is quite clear, but in the intervals there is prostration and general hyperæsthesia.   (4) Paralysis ensues in 3–4 days, first of the muscles of the lower jaw and of respiration; death follows within a week from the onset.

Prognosis.—Cauterisation of the wound, if performed immediately after the bite, helps to prevent the disease.   Once the disease is established it is invariably fatal: serum does not cure.   Not all biting animals in the East have rabies; if the suspected carrier animal can be shot and its brain examined by a skilled pathologist the presence or absence of rabies can be determined: 5–10 per cent. of cases of rabid dog-bites develop rabies: with rabid wolves the incidence is higher.   If the bite is inflicted through clothing which soaks some of the infected saliva from the jaws of the animal the incidence is less.

Treatment is entirely prophylactic (see § 525).

ENCEPHALO-MYELITIS following immunisation treatment for rabies occurs in 1 in 600 cases.   Myoclonic jerkings and meningeal, cerebral, brain-stem or spinal cord symptoms occur.   Prednisone 10 mg. thrice daily for a week may reduce the severity of symptoms.

Cramp in Psychical Disorders.

§ 1033. VIII. **Writer's Cramp** is probably a disorder of cerebral origin, unlike ordinary cramp, and consists essentially of (1) spasm and (2) cramp-like pain in the affected muscles when writing is attempted.   For all other movements of similar complexity, *e.g.*, shaving, the hand and fingers move normally.   It is this specificity that stamps the disease.   It affects adults, usually those who write with the intrinsic hand muscles only, not from the wrist, elbow or shoulder.   The pen is at first grasped with undue firmness. The onset of spasm and cramp-like pain produces great ataxia in the writing; the pen suddenly flies from or is driven through the sheet.   The writing becomes smaller and more indecipherable, and the lines slope upwards or downwards, not running horizontally across the sheet.   In diagnosing the condition the physician should be careful not to fall into the pitfall of mistaking early Parkinsonism, a cervical disc or peripheral nerve lesion, or tenosynovitis, for this disease.   In these the symptoms are not solely determined by the act of writing and occur when the hand is used for other purposes.

Treatment.—Absolute rest from writing is essential for not less than six months.   During this time the patient should learn to use a type-writer.   If the left hand is educated to write, the cramp usually appears in it also.   Re-education is attempted with a large pen, or the pen is thrust through a solid rubber ball, which is grasped in the patient's hand.   He then learns to write from the wrist, elbow or shoulder, using fresh groups of muscles. In the majority of cases the disease tends to recur, but not invariably. Change of occupation has often to be advised.

Occupational Cramps are met among factory workers, drapers, dressmakers (in using scissors), musicians, violinists and others—in short, amongst those following any occupation necessitating the constant repetition of one particular movement.

§ **1034.** IX. In *Hysterical Spasm* the prime movers and antagonist muscles contract simultaneously. The spasm is variable and proportional to the force used to overcome it. The distribution of the spasm does not correspond to any anatomical or physiological grouping and the reflexes are all normal. The plantar responses may be absent and an ill-sustained ankle clonus elicited. Hysterical " stocking " or " glove " analgesia may co-exist. Evidence of hysterical personality can usually be obtained except in " compensation " cases or war neurosis.

GROUP XV. HEADACHES WITH PROGRESSIVE MENTAL CHANGES

A patient without previous neurological disease develops one or more of a group of symptoms—fits, increasing headache, vertigo, lethargy, papillœdema and vomiting. The condition may be RAISED INTRACRANIAL PRESSURE.

§ **1035. Raised Intracranial Pressure** arises from brain-swelling, aqueduct obstruction, brain herniation or from compression of intracranial venous channels. It also accompanies intracranial bleeding or inflammation.

Symptoms.—(1) *Mental changes.* Increasing apathy or torpor and dulling of mental alertness are common. It is often difficult to hold the patient's attention during the examination as he keeps losing interest and dropping off to sleep. He may be observed to rub his nose with undue frequency. In posterior fossa neoplasms, however, the patient's mentality is often clear even when the intracranial pressure is high. (2) An unexpected *epileptic* fit is often the presenting symptom. The fit may be generalised or focal. A Jacksonian fit followed by transient paresis of the limbs which have been convulsed does not always mean a focal lesion. Transient giddy spells or slight attacks of disturbed consciousness are late symptoms of increased pressure. True vertigo, however, may be early and have an important localising significance. (3) *Increasing headache,* an insistent dull pain with paroxysms of great intensity, is early and severe, especially in posterior fossa and pituitary neoplasms. In the former pain may be occipital, in the latter bitemporal and retro-ocular. The headache may wake the patient early in the morning, and he may hold his head in his hands and rock himself in distress. Headache occurs early in only 20–25 per cent. of cases of neoplasm but is ultimately present in most patients. Distortion of and traction on blood-vessels is a factor in causation, and the pain is worsened by coughing, sneezing, on bending down or defæcation. It is abolished by rest and by dehydration. Analgesics give only partial and temporary relief. Constant " pressing " feelings in the head are characteristic of psychogenic states, but a neurotic patient suffering from increased intracranial pressure may describe his headache in such terms. (4) *Vomiting* occurs late and is often due to obstructive hydrocephalus; it is not necessarily projectile and may be preceded by nausea. (5) *Papillœdema* (§ 1127) (Plate XXI) should be looked for in every case of headache or when raised intracranial pressure is suspected. The pupils should be dilated with homatropine if the discs cannot be seen clearly in a darkened room. Papillœdema tends to be early in cerebellar neoplasm, but is often absent in abscess, subdural hæmatoma or neoplasms of the brain-stem. It may rapidly appear when there is sudden ventricular obstruction, sudden intracranial hæmorrhage or thrombophlebitis. *C.S.F.* In suspected raised intracranial pressure examination of the fluid should be made with extreme caution and never at all in the presence of papillœdema. Growths may exist without elevation of manometric pressure. High-protein readings occur in lateral recess tumours (auditory neurofibromas). Tumour cells are rarely found in centrifugalised C.S.F. *Focal signs* (§ 1038) may or may not be present.

CAUSES OF INTRACRANIAL HYPERTENSION

I. Cerebral injuries.
II. Cerebral vascular accidents.
III. Intracranial neoplasms.
IV. Hypertensive encephalopathy.

V. Intracranial inflammation.
VI. Progressive toxæmia.
VII. Meningeal hydrops.
VIII. Congenital Hydrocephalus.

I. CEREBRAL INJURIES.—Central contusion (§ 813) is often accompanied by a degree of brain-swelling, with headache, vomiting and mild papillœdema. Severe degrees of papillœdema following head-injury may be due to traumatic subarachnoid, subdural or extradural hæmorrhage or to intracranial venous thrombosis (see § 892).

II. INTRACRANIAL VASCULAR ACCIDENTS.—Slow intracranial bleeding, usually productive of convulsions and coma, is considered in § 852. Common causes are spontaneous subarachnoid hæmorrhage from a ruptured saccular aneurysm or intracerebral oozing from an atheromatous arteriole. Papillœdema is common in subarachnoid hæmorrhage, rare in cerebral and carotid thrombosis.

III. HYPERTENSIVE ENCEPHALOPATHY (see § 97).

IV. INTRACRANIAL NEOPLASMS (§ 1041 et seq.).

V. INTRACRANIAL INFLAMMATION.—Encephalitis does not cause a marked rise of intracranial pressure unless *obstructive hydrocephalus* or some other complication occurs. FOR SUBDURAL HYGROMA see § 1054 and INTRACRANIAL ABSCESS § 1055.

VI. PROGRESSIVE TOXÆMIA.—*Chronic renal disease* with uræmia may cause headache, vomiting and papillœdema. Advanced papillœdema with hæmorrhages and exudates closely simulates albuminuric retinitis. In such cases focal ischæmic softenings of the cerebrum may occur gradually, simulating the march of symptoms of a neoplasm. Very high blood-pressure readings and marked albuminuria are more characteristic of renal disease than neoplasm. *Eclampsia* either before or after delivery is usually easy to diagnose. *Industrial Toxæmia, e.g.,* chronic poisoning with lead (§ 568) or methyl bromide used in fire-extinguishers causes evidence of raised intracranial pressure.

§ 1036. VII. **Meningeal Hydrops** (Syn. Otitic, or Toxic " hydrocephalus ") causes headache, vomiting and papillœdema without localising signs in children and young adults. There is no ventricular dilatation so the name " hydrocephalus " is a misnomer. The C.S.F., although under pressure, is sterile and free from excess of cells or protein. This syndrome occurs in association with chronic suppurative ear conditions and suppurative lesions elsewhere in the body. It is believed to be due to a partial thrombosis of the sagittal sinus. The course is benign, and the hydrops will subside spontaneously without specific treatment, § 892.

§ 1037. VIII. **Congenital Hydrocephalus** causes rapid enlargement of the head, leading in some cases to primary optic atrophy and blindness. The sutures separate, the fontanelles bulge and the eyes are depressed from pressure on the orbital plates. The skull gives a cracked-pot sound on percussion, and the brain and skull may be so thinned that transillumination is possible. Most cases develop mental defect and paralysis, but the patient may survive into adult life. The severe progressive cases are associated with spina bifida and a sacral meningocele containing nerve roots. *Etiology.*—In infancy the cause is often the Arnold-Chiari malformation, *i.e.*, a deformity of the cerebellum in which tongues of the lateral cerebellar lobes project downwards through the foramen magnum into the cervical canal. *Treatment* is unsatisfactory. In a few cases valvular drainage of the lateral ventricles into the internal jugular veins is possible, prolonging life and sparing the mental faculties.

In *adolescence* hydrocephalus may develop from stenosis of a congenitally malformed aqueduct of Sylvius. The signs produced are those of a posterior fossa tumour.

ACQUIRED HYDROCEPHALUS usually results from meningitis or neoplasm obstructing the iter or the basal cisterns. X-rays show absorption of the clinoid processes and a scaphoid enlargement of the pituitary fossa. There is persistent headache, vomiting, mental impairment, fits and either papillœdema or optic atrophy. Relief has been achieved in a few cases by drainage of the lateral ventricles through a catheter into the cisterna magna.

Megencephaly, a condition of simple " large-headedness," may occur without neurological hydrocephalus. There are no signs. The condition is benign. When due to *osteitis deformans* signs of basilar compression and cranial nerve palsies (optic atrophy, deafness) may occur.

§ **1038.** FOCAL SYMPTOMS OF INTRACRANIAL DISEASE *may accompany signs of raised intracranial pressure.* These, like the general symptoms, may be progressive. They are commonly due either to circulatory changes in the neighbourhood of a growth, anoxia, or distortion of nerve tracts or blood-vessels. Thus after successful removal of an encapsuled tumour the symptoms may rapidly disappear as the circulation is restored to surrounding tissues. *The earliest symptoms and signs have the greatest localising value.* They vary with the site and extent of area of brain involved.

Frontal Lobe.—(1) The patient's personality may change. A previously normal person may show memory failure, childishness, lack of judgment and carelessness (*e.g.*, in dress), loss of social sense, incontinence of urine, euphoria. A tendency to " wisecrack " is seen in such patients, with shallowness of emotional feeling, " Witzelsucht." (2) Unilateral anosmia occurs in meningiomata, pituitary tumours, or large aneurysms involving the cribriform plate. (3) Unilateral proptosis occurs from circulatory changes or invasion of the orbit. (4) Contra-lateral pyramidal signs are usually monoplegic. (5) In lesions of the posterior parts of the first and second frontal convolutions the " grasp reflex " occurs. It has localising value when observed in fully conscious patients. (6) The motor or sensory cortex may be involved with irritative or paralytic signs—Jacksonian fits or monoplegia. The tumours usually found are gliomata, secondary growths, forward extensions of pituitary tumour, meningiomata and large saccular aneurysms.

Temporal Lobe.—(1) Quadrantic hemianopia or a homonymous hemianopia of the contra-lateral fields is often found. Complex visual hallucinations may occur in the affected fields. (2) Facio-brachial monoplegia may be present. (3) Lesions on the left side involving the speech areas produce " word deafness " or " jargon aphasia " in right-handed persons (§ 869). (4) Personality changes, irritability and aggressive behaviour may occur. (5) "Temporal lobe" epileptic fits occur with an aura of unpleasant smell or taste; masticatory fits with champing, spitting and salivation or a transient "dreamy state" with subsequent automatism are frequent. Uncinate (masticating) fits tend to occur with para-sellar lesions. The tumours usually found are gliomata, secondary carcinoma, extensions of pituitary growths, meningiomata and angiomatous malformations.

Parietal Lobe.—(1) Some degree of hemiplegia with sensory changes of the discriminative kind is present, i.e., loss of joint sense, defective two-point discrimination tested with compasses, or astereognosis. (2) Sensory Jacksonian fits may occur. (3) In left-sided cortical lesions the patient has usually receptive dysphasia and dyslexia. (4) Unawareness of the contra-lateral half of the body or of space shows itself by various tests, e.g., of objects in contra-lateral visual fields, "dressing apraxia," confusion of left and right, inability to draw or construct in two or three dimensions, and inability to name fingers in the affected hand (finger agnosia). Such symptoms are probably dependent on interruption of sensory pathways and failure of sensory cortical integration. When simultaneous pin-pricks are applied to two halves of the body the patient pays attention only to those on the unaffected side, the others are ignored. Such patients may lose sense of direction and lose themselves in familiar surroundings. Similar symptoms occur in demented patients.

Occipital Lobe.—(1) Irritative lesions involving the calcarine cortex produce visual Jacksonian attacks ("sheets of flame," "moving lights") of hemianopic distribution and lasting only a few seconds. (2) Paralytic cortical and deep lesions cause homonymous hemianopia or quadrantic hemianopia of which the patient may or may not be aware. Altitudinal hemianopia may occur with migraine or interhemispherical lesions involving the occipital lobes. (3) Dyslexia will occur in left-sided lesions when the angular and supramarginal gyri are involved. (4) Contra-lateral sensory or pyramidal signs may exist. The tumours most often found invading the occipital lobes are gliomata, secondary growths, angiomatous malformations and meningiomata.

Corpus Callosum.—Early apathy or fits occur with bilateral pyramidal signs, rarely symmetrical, and yellow cerebro-spinal fluid. Apraxia may occur in lesions of the genu or of the splenium in a few cases. Later there is dementia. Malignant gliomata infiltrate the corpus callosum, spreading into the contra-lateral hemisphere.

Third Ventricle and Superior Colliculi.—Tumours in this region produce internal hydrocephalus from obstruction of the foramen of Monro. Paroxysmal headache or even progressive dementia may ensue from recurrent hydrocephalic attacks. Pineal tumours with precocious puberty (chiefly in boys) are associated with loss of conjugate elevation of the eyes, pupils which do not react to light, and external ocular palsies. Lesions involving the floor of the third ventricle cause obesity, amenorrhœa, diabetes insipidus, lethargy and prolonged sleep, cataplectic attacks, i.e., sudden loss of muscular tone with falling. Tumours here may be congenital, such as hypophyseal duct tumours (cranio-pharyngioma), gliomata, meningiomata, angiomatous malformations, pinealomata or pituitary growths.

Brain-stem.—(1) "Crossed" paralysis involving a cranial nerve on one side and pyramidal tracts on the other, or a crossed and sometimes dissociated sensory paralysis involving the face and contra-lateral limbs may be seen. (2) Vertical nystagmus on upward gaze is pathognomonic of a brain-stem lesion. (a) In lesions of the *Crus Cerebri* oculomotor palsy on one side with contra-lateral hemiplegia (Weber's Syndrome) occurs. There may be hemiataxy from involvement of the cerebellar peduncle or mesial fillet. (b) *Pontine* lesions cause very varied symptoms. Trigeminal, abducent and facial nerves may be paralysed on one side with crossed hemiparesis (Foville's Syndrome). If the lateral fillet is involved there will be crossed hemianæsthesia and thermanæsthesia. Bilateral pyramidal signs are present with ataxia. (c) *Medulla.* Unilateral or bilateral paralysis of the lowest cranial nerves and nuclei from the ninth to the twelfth may occur—producing dysarthria and dysphagia. The lateral bulbar syndrome is observed from vascular lesions rather than tumours. Medullary symptoms with long-tract signs, sensory and motor, may be secondary to tumours of the fourth ventricle, vermis or pons: these growths are often gliomata.

Cerebellum (see § 934 *et seq.*).

§ 1039. Space-occupying Lesions in the Cranial Fossæ produce symptoms which can be grouped according to their origin in the anterior, middle or posterior fossæ.

Anterior Cranial Fossa.—(1) Anosmia, (2) Unilateral exophthalmos and diplopia, (3) Primary optic atrophy with papillœdema of the opposite eye (Foster Kennedy syndrome), (4) Mental deterioration and fits, (5) Contra-lateral pyramidal signs may occur. The tumour is commonly a meningioma of the falx or an extension of a frontal glioma.

Middle Cranial Fossa.—(*a*) *Region of Optic Chiasma:* (1) Endocrine Pituitary disturbances—Acromegaly, Gigantism or Infantilism from anterior pituitary tumours and Fröhlich's syndrome from hypophyseal stalk tumours. (2) Chiasmal defects— central scotomata, quadrantic temporal defects in the visual fields, the upper quadrants being first affected when the lesion is below the chiasma. (3) Unilateral optic atrophy with contra-lateral papillœdema. (4) Unilateral proptosis and (5) Uncinate fits occur from meningiomata and pituitary growths. (*b*) *Cavernous Sinuses:* (1) Complete ophthalmoplegia from paralysis of third, fourth and sixth cranial nerves, (2) Anæsthesia in the distribution of the ophthalmic and maxillary divisions of the trigeminal nerve with loss of corneal reflex and (3) proptosis of the affected eye occur. The cause is either a large saccular aneurysm or a meningioma. (*c*) *Base of Skull:* Various cranial nerves may be paralysed in succession, often more on one side. Curiously some escape and long-tract signs are often absent. There is usually no increase of intra-cranial pressure. This is seen with chordomas and meningioma *en plaque*.

Posterior Cranial Fossa.—Lesions in the lateral recess (cerebello-pontine angle) cause (1) increasing nerve-deafness with tinnitus, (2) loss of corneal reflex and anæsthesia in the face, (3) facial hemispasm, (4) ipsilateral ataxia. Headache and papillœdema are often absent. The usual cause is an auditory neurofibroma.

§ 1040. False Localising Signs.—(i.) Unilateral or bilateral *abducent palsy* in suspected brain tumour is often a false localising sign. The long intracranial course of the sixth nerves renders them particularly liable to be damaged by stretching when the intracranial pressure rises. (ii.) *Herniation of the brain* within the cranium also causes false localising signs, and the resultant ophthalmoplegia may distract attention from the actual site of the lesion. (*a*) Tentorial herniation occurs when the medial hippocampal portion of the temporal lobe prolapses downwards over the free edge of the tentorium cerebelli, thus compressing and displacing the crura cerebri. Symptoms of transient oculomotor palsy may thus be produced, or a fixed dilated pupil on the side of the lesion from compression of the third nerve or its nucleus in the crus. Displacements of the crus and its compression against the tentorial edge on the other side may cause ipsilateral pyramidal signs. (*b*) In foraminal herniation the cerebellar tonsils prolapse through the foramen magnum, producing occipital pain, headache, vomiting and stiff neck. (iii.) *Brain swelling* may produce a transient hemianopia or hemiplegia. Sometimes frontal lobe lesions may present with contralateral cerebellar signs. The use of rectal hypertonic solutions may abolish these false localising signs. The advent of contrast radiography has made the localisation, as well as the pre-operative pathological diagnosis of intracranial tumours, much more precise.

SPACE-OCCUPYING (Expanding) LESIONS WITH FOCAL SIGNS

I. Intracranial Neoplasms (§ 1041).
II. Subdural Hæmatoma (§ 1052).
III. Subdural Hygroma (§ 1054).

IV. Intracranial Abscess (§ 1055).
V. Unruptured Aneurysm (§ 1047).

§ 1041. I. Intracranial Neoplasms are as common as mammary growths. They occur in infancy, childhood and in adult life but become rarer in old age. Such tumours may be present within the skull for weeks, months, or even years before producing focal signs. The condition should be suspected: (1) When *epileptic fits of " late " onset* (over 20 years) occur, especially if such fits are Jacksonian or focal (*e.g.,* " temporal lobe " attacks), with transient residual palsies or permanent changes in the reflexes. (2) In cases of *increasing headache and vomiting in a person who has never had severe headache before.* The vomiting need not be projectile, nor is it necessary that *papillœdema* should be present. (3) In any *progressive* focal lesion of the nervous system, *e.g.,* progressive hemiplegia, progressive nerve deafness or advancing visual failure not due to ocular causes. (4) When there is *pituitary* or *pineal* endocrine disturbance.

INVESTIGATION OF SUSPECTED SPACE-OCCUPYING (EXPANDING) LESIONS

A careful history from a relative or friend should be followed by a detailed neurological examination including the fields of vision. Look for nævi, swellings on the scalp or skull, and listen for an intracranial bruit. Examine the patient generally for loss of weight or presence of tumour elsewhere, take the blood pressure and examine the urine. Difficulty in getting the co-operation of a lethargic apathetic patient in a full neurological examination demands patience. 60 ml. of 50 per cent. solution of magnesium sulphate in warm water and retained per rectum, may help to improve the conscious level. *X-ray* examination of the chest should be carried out as well as of the skull (pineal shift, abnormal calcification). *E.E.G.* examination is often helpful. In many cases *contrast angiography* will give valuable information as to the site, size and nature of the growth. *Air encephalography should never be carried out in suspected tumour cases unless a neurosurgeon is at hand to proceed with craniotomy.* In all cases with papillœdema and signs of increased intracranial pressure, lumbar puncture is potentially dangerous and may cause respiratory failure from tentorial herniation.

TYPES OF INTRACRANIAL TUMOURS

(*a*) Glioma.
(*b*) Secondary Carcinoma.
(*c*) Meningioma.
(*d*) Auditory Neurofibron a.

(*e*) Pituitaryand Hypothalamic Growths.
(*f*) Blood-vessel Tumours.
(*g*) Neurofibromatosis.
(*h*) Granulomata.

§ 1042 (*a*). A **Glioma** occurs in varying degrees of malignancy and forms 40 per cent. of all intracranial tumours. It is a tumour of the glial " supporting " tissues. The *Astrocytoma* is found in the temporal and frontal lobes and also in the lateral lobes of the cerebellum. This growth may undergo degeneration, forming a cyst containing yellow fluid and on its wall there is a mural nodule of tumour tissue. Characteristically these are tumours of childhood or early adult life and many cerebellar growths at this age are of this type. They occur also in middle life and for years the only symptom of a cerebral astrocytoma may be temporal lobe epilepsy or generalised fits until some alteration in size due to growth, vascular change or cystic degeneration produces focal neurological signs, often rather abruptly. Occasionally a localised growth in the minor (non-dominant) hemisphere or in the cerebellum may be removed with some success, but anaplastic change in tumour tissue left behind after operation tends to cause recurrence and so deep X-ray treatment is usually advised after operation. The survival period after operation varies from weeks to some years. The highly malignant *Glioblastoma* occurs in the cerebral hemisphere of patients in late adult life, as a reddish purple infiltrating mass surrounded by brain swelling and softening. These growths are vascular and the rapid development of focal signs and increased intracranial pressure, due to hæmorrhage or softening within the growth, may suggest the diagnosis of secondary carcinoma, or (if signs of increased pressure are absent) cerebral or internal carotid thrombosis. There may be several hemiplegic episodes before the diagnosis is apparent. The clinical history in cases of glioblastoma is usually short, perhaps a few weeks, and epilepsy occurs in 80 per cent. of cases when the growth is fronto-parietal. Progressive " strokes " in elderly persons may be due to this cause. Progressive dementia is an important symptom and may be due to invasion of the frontal lobes or to slowly progressive hydrocephalus. Air encephalography in such cases carries a high risk, and angiography is preferable. The angiogram is often characteristic; biopsy may be used to confirm the diagnosis if it is not evident. Surgical removal is not possible and the results of radiotherapy poor. Life is rarely prolonged beyond 12–15 months. *Oligodendroglioma* is a tumour of adult life found chiefly in the cerebral hemispheres, often fronto-parietal; it is relatively benign and tends to calcify. It is a rare tumour, but is important for there is a good chance of survival after surgical removal. The *Medulloblastoma* is a rapidly growing tumour of the vermis in children (§ 1050). *Gliomata* also occur in the optic nerve or chiasma, usually in children and young adults; these are highly malignant.

§ 1043 (*b*). **Secondary Carcinoma** forms about 20 per cent. of all intracranial tumours. Symptoms are usually those of a single tumour, although deposits are most often multiple. The primary tumour is so often an unsuspected carcinoma in a peripheral bronchus that X-ray of the chest should be performed as a routine in all cases where an intracranial growth is diagnosed. Mammary carcinoma and hypernephroma are also common primary sites. The *Symptoms* may be those of increased intracranial pressure, of focal cerebral or cerebellar disease; or when the meninges are infiltrated, of meningeal irritation. Pleocytosis in the spinal fluid may lead to an erroneous diagnosis of encephalitis. An exploratory biopsy may be justified as there is sometimes a possibility that the cerebral growth is benign. Where the secondary growth is solitary and slow-growing (over three months), surgery may be contemplated, but death usually occurs in a few weeks or months. The results of radiotherapy are poor.

§ 1044 (*c*). A **Meningioma** (15 per cent. of all intracranial growths) is a benign tumour, rarely multiple, arising in the arachnoid villi on the walls of the dural sinuses, the venous tributaries of which become adherent to the tumour mass. It is often highly vascular, supplied by dural arteries (external carotid). A meningioma does not invade but indents the brain; it tends, on the other hand, to invade the overlying skull bones, and to cause reactive changes therein, and these bony changes together with enlarged diplœic venous channels near the growth may be visible on a straight X-ray. Meningiomata are found over the vertex (para-sagittal) and elsewhere, or in all the cranial fossæ at the base of the brain. The latter type of growth may be flattened *en plaque* and not rounded like the para-sagittal meningiomata.

Symptoms may have been present as focal or generalised fits for as long as 8–10 years. The sudden appearance of focal symptoms or those of increased intracranial pressure does not rule out the diagnosis of a meningioma, as the growth in such cases may be of some size and probably " silent " for years. Mental defect and psychoses occur in association with meningioma of the cerebrum. Meningiomas of the anterior fossa can cause depression of the orbit and anosmia. Those in the middle fossa cause proptosis, ophthalmoplegia and optic atrophy and may simulate pituitary growths. Those at the base of the brain may cause paralysis of many cranial nerves one after the other, only on one side. Posterior fossa meningiomata may attain a large size, invading several dural compartments of the skull before they are diagnosed. The growth absorbs contrast medium and its outline may be seen on angiography (Fig. 255). *Prognosis.*—Growths unremoved will eventually cause death. Partially removed

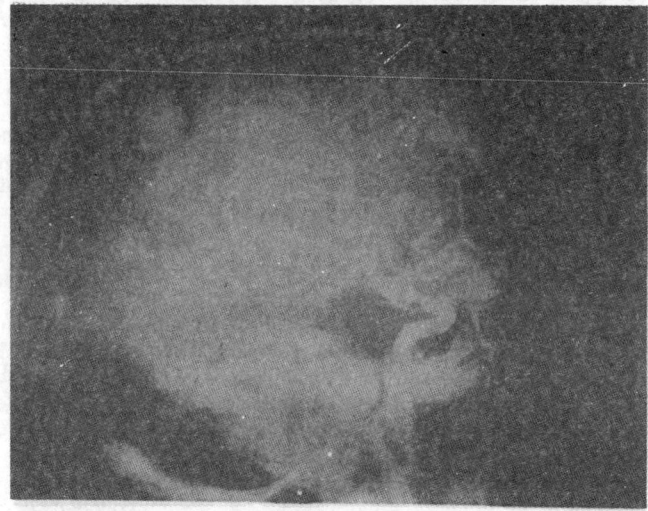

(*a*)

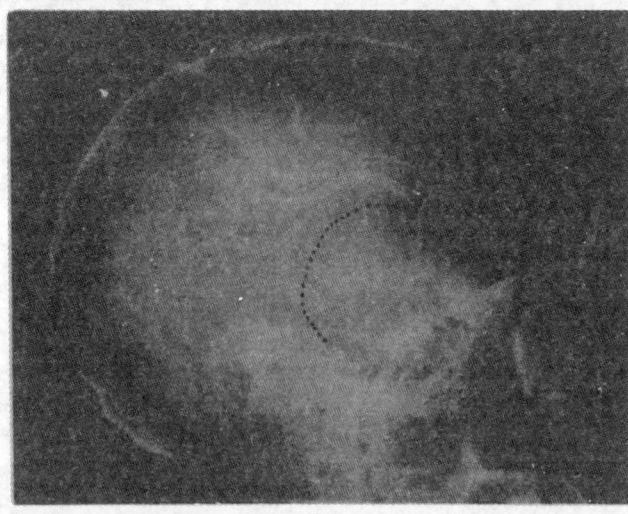

(*b*)

FIG. 255.—CAROTID ANGIOGRAMS. (*a*) A normal angiogram showing the int. carotid artery and its anterior and middle cerebral branches. (*b*) A meningioma in the middle fossa is considerably elevating the middle cerebral artery and its branches so that they are projected over the ant. cerebral group. (Dr. Charles MacLean.)

growths may recur locally.   Usually the results of surgery are good but thrombosis of cortical veins following tying of vessels during removal may cause extensive cortical necrosis (sagittal sinus syndrome, see § 892).   Not only the growth but the surrounding dura and overlying bone may have to be removed at operation.   Post-operative epilepsy should be guarded against by prescribing anticonvulsants for one or two years.

§ 1045 (d). Acoustic Neurofibroma (Syn.   Auditory Neurofibroma) is a benign tumour growing from the Schwann sheath of the eighth cranial nerve just within the porus acousticus, which it enlarges.   For symptoms see § 1083.

§ 1046 (e). Pituitary and Hypothalamic Tumours.—*Chromophobe* and *chromophil adenomata* occur in the anterior pituitary and compress the chiasma from below. A *basophil adenoma* is rare.   The pituitary gland may be the seat of *secondary malignant deposits.   Hypophyseal.duct tumours* (craniopharyngiomas) growing on the pituitary stalk from embryonic buccal " rests " contain calcareous matter and portions of the enamel organ of teeth.   They grow into the hypothalamus, compressing the chiasma and sella from above or behind.   *A meningioma* may arise from the diaphragma sellæ.

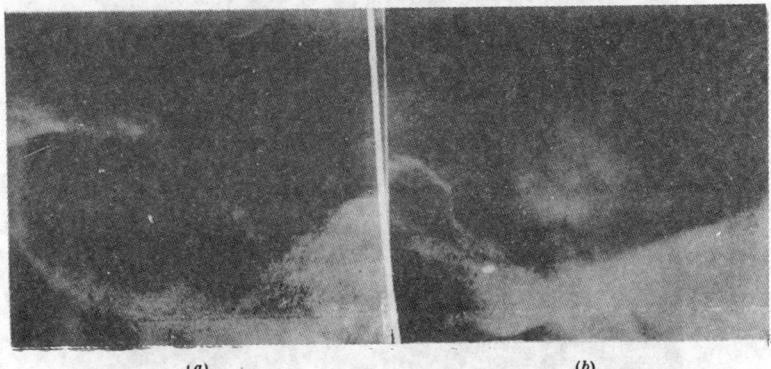

(a)   (b)

FIG. 256.—RADIOGRAPHS OF THE SELLA TURCICA. (*a*) Normal sella. (*b*) Abnormal sella—the posterior clinoid processes are eroded, the sella is scaphoid and above it is an extensive area of abnormal calcification. From a case of hypophyseal duct tumour (craniopharyngioma). (Dr. David Sutton.)

" Cystic arachnoiditis " in the region of the chiasma may produce symptoms like those of a pituitary growth as may aneurysms of the internal carotid.

Symptoms produced by pituitary growths are those of (1) Neighbourhood symptoms from infiltration or compression of surrounding structures—the chiasma, temporal lobe, frontal lobe or hypothalamus.   Upper temporal or bitemporal field defects are seen.   There may be gross impairment of visual acuity due to optic atrophy.   Polyuria, infantilism and stupor may occur from infiltration of the hypothalamus, and hemiplegia from extension into the lateral hemisphere.   (2) Increased intracranial pressure. Obstructive hydrocephalus causes papilloedema and optic atrophy.   (3) Endocrine disturbances.   Acromegaly when due to a growth is always caused by an *eosinophil adenoma* of the anterior lobe of the pituitary.   A *chromophobe adenoma* of the anterior lobe may or may not be associated with signs of hypopituitarism.   Amenorrhœa is common in women.   Both these growths produce an asymmetrical or bitemporal hemianopia beginning with quadrantic defects in the upper temporal quadrants of the fields, or central scotomata.   Optic atrophy will occur with blindness as the growth increases.   A chromophobe adenoma causes obesity and infantilism in childhood and in later life regression of sexual functions, amenorrhœa and obesity.   A basophil adenoma is usually microscopic; it may occur with adrenal growths and hypertension (Cushing's Syndrome).   A craniopharyngioma is found characteristically in children and young adults.   *X-ray* films of the skull (if possible stereoscopic) provide valuable information of supracellar calcification in many cases. There is deepening of the pituitary fossa, excavation under the anterior clinoid process in glandular growths and erosion of the posterior clinoid processes (Fig. 256). Chronic hydrocephalus from any cause may produce a closely similar picture. Ventriculography or air encephalography will give evidence of the upward extension of these growths into the third ventricle. Angiography, will demonstrate anterior or lateral extension, or an unsuspected saccular aneurysm. It will sometimes delineate a meningioma.

§ 1047 (*f*). **Blood-vessel Tumours.**—(*a*) A *Hæmangioblastoma* is a cystic tumour (with a mural nodule) in the lateral lobe of the cerebellum, occurring mostly in children but at all ages. These cavernous tumours may also occur in the cerebral hemispheres. When it is associated with angiomata in the retina, cysts of the kidneys and pancreas, the family history of such an illness can often be obtained (Von Hippel-Lindau syndrome). Surgical removal of an isolated tumour in the cerebellum gives an excellent result. (*b*) A *Large Saccular Aneurysm* may produce the symptoms of an isolated basal

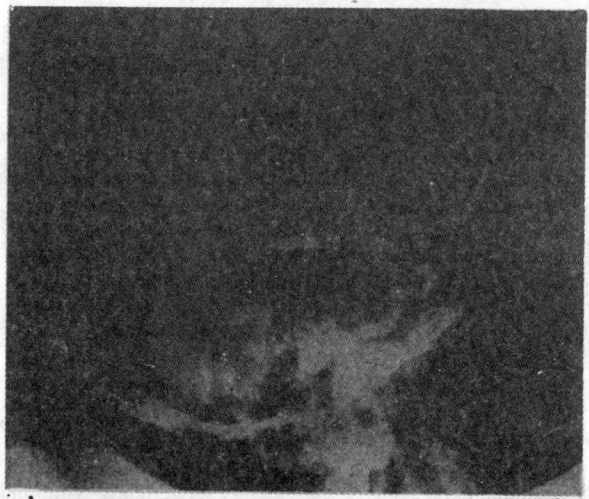

FIG. 257.—ANGIOMATOUS MALFORMATION. Right carotid angiogram showing a cirsoid aneurysm on the middle cerebral artery.

meningioma. (*c*) *Angiomatous Malformations* are often cirsoid aneurysms, mostly venous but partly arterial, occurring on the surface of the brain or deeply in its parenchyma (Fig. 257). They may communicate through openings in the skull with angiomatous varicosities on the scalp. Although such lesions are congenital, symptoms may not arise until the third or fourth decades. *Symptoms.*—(1) Subarachnoid hæmorrhage, (2) paralysis—viz. hemiplegia, monoplegia, hemianopia, (3) epilepsy, are the usual manifestations. In some cases compression of the jugular veins in the neck may cause proptosis or filling of extracranial dilated vascular channels. A bruit may be heard by the patient, or on auscultation by the physician. A bruit without signs rarely means an angioma or vascular tumour. *Treatment.*—Surgical removal of superficial cortical angiomata is possible and the results are good; but the deep parenchymatous forms are irremovable and do not react to radiation. Fits may require anticonvulsants, but the condition is compatible with long life. (*d*) In the *Sturge-Weber Syndrome* a trigeminal nævus on the scalp, face or neck is associated with intracranial calcifications on the surface of certain underlying atrophic cerebral convolutions. Focal epilepsy, mental retardation, contra-lateral hemiplegia or hemianopia are present in a high proportion of cases. Skull X-rays show sinuous shadows

with a double contour corresponding to the convolutional calcifications and atrophy
Treatment is symptomatic, as for epilepsy.

Soft mobile SUBCUTANEOUS TUMOURS *and sessile or pedunculated* MOLLUSCUM
FIBROSUM *are found in and under the skin with areas of " café-au-lait " pigmentation
associated with* CRANIAL NERVE OR SPINAL ROOT PARALYSES.   *The conditions is* NEURO
FIBROMATOSIS (Von Recklinghausen's disease).

§ 1048 (*g*). The soft tumours which stud the peripheral nerves may cause multiple
cranial and spinal nerve palsies, and may compress the spinal cord.   Within the skull
they are a cause of bilateral auditory neurofibromata.   Some cases show endocrine
changes, *e.g.*, pituitary enlargement, and cysts at the ends of the long bones.   It
may be a familial or hereditary disease but many cases are sporadic (§§ 734, 970).

MENTAL DEFECT *and epilepsy exist with the* ADENOMA SEBACEUM *on the skin of the
face.   The condition is* EPILOIA.

§ 1049. Epiloia (Syn. Tuberose Sclerosis).—This rare condition is a cause of mental
defect and fits in children and adolescents, and is probably allied to neurofibromatosis.
Tumours exist in the brain, deforming the ventricles.   Retinal examination may
show gliomatous tumours (phakamata) allied to those seen in the Von Hippel-Lindau
syndrome.

(*h*). A GRANULOMA is usually not suspected until operation reveals it.   A *Tuberculoma*, once common, is now much rarer in regions where tuberculosis is disappearing.
The *gumma* is now almost unknown.   A brain tumour with positive serological
reactions in blood and C.S.F. is more likely to be a glioma in a patient with latent
syphilis than a gumma.   *Torula histolytica* may cause granulomatous tumours; so
may *schistosoma* in those living in Egypt or Japan.

§ 1050. INTRACRANIAL TUMOURS IN CHILDREN differ in some ways from those in
adults.   They are much more common sub-tentorially (cerebellum, fourth ventricle
and brain-stem) than in the cerebrum.   Pituitary adenomata, meningiomata and
auditory nerve growths are almost exclusively tumours of adult life and not of childhood.   As in adults *gliomata* predominate.   The *Medulloblastoma* is a highly malignant
type of glioma found in the roof of the fourth ventricle or in the pons.   Early signs
are diplopia with squint and unsteady gait; glossopharyngeal pain, palatal palsy; stiff
neck and papilloedema may be present.   Local metastases occur and although the
lesion is radiosensitive at first few cases survive longer than a year.   In the cerebellum
of children and young adults *Cystic Astrocytoma* occurs, a more benign lesion which
may in a few cases be cured surgically (§ 1042).   A *Hæmangioblastoma* is usually
cerebellar (§ 1047).   *Hypophyseal duct tumours* occur in children and adolescents
(§ 1046).   *Pinealomas* in boys cause precocious puberty with iridoplegia, defective
elevation of the eyes and other ophthalmoplegias.

§ 1051. The DIAGNOSIS of INTRACRANIAL TUMOUR has to be made from:
(1) *Conditions causing progressive cerebral lesions.*   Cases of slowly propagating *thrombosis* of a diseased cerebral artery or internal carotid artery,
or of slowly progressive *cerebral hæmorrhage* may be very perplexing.
Arteriography may demonstrate stenosis of the carotid, a lack of filling
of a cerebral artery or a saccular aneurysm.   When angiography shows
lateral displacement of the anterior cerebral arteries, this may be due to
brain swelling around softened or hæmorrhagic brain tissue or to a growth
in the hemisphere, and surgical exploration may be required to exclude
a tumour.   Brain tumours occur in persons who already have cerebral
vascular disease.   A *subdural hæmatoma* can often be demonstrated by
arteriography which usually shows a filling defect in the para-sagittal area

on one or both sides. *Focal atrophic lesions* due to atheroma, early presenile or Pick's dementia, or following upon injury may cause progressive
symptoms like those of tumour, but signs of increased intracranial pressure
are absent; then air studies will show dilated ventricles and air over the
convolutions of the diseased hemisphere, with the septum lucidum displaced *towards* the side of the lesion. In suspected *meningovascular
cerebral syphilis* Argyll-Robertson pupils are not always found and a
cautious lumbar puncture may be necessary. A positive blood W.R. due
to syphilis is occasionally found in patients with brain tumours and seldom
indicates the presence of a cerebral gumma. (2) *Conditions causing
increased intracranial pressure and papilloedema* other than tumour or
abscess may have to be considered. In *Meningeal hydrops in young
adults, papilloedema is the only sign and focal signs are absent*. Papilloedema
without focal signs is a rare finding in cases of *pulmonary emphysema*
with venous hypertension and anoxia. *Hypertensive encephalography* is
diagnosed by the associated retinopathy and extreme hypertension; and
uraemia by the albuminuria and raised blood urea. *Toxic encephalopathy*
due to industrial poisoning by lead or methyl bromide may cause papilloedema. (3) The cause of *epilepsy of late onset*, especially " temporal
lobe fits," may for many years not be apparent until signs of a tumour
suddenly appear. In this condition if any focal signs co-exist air encephalography and sometimes arteriography should be carried out.

SPECIAL INVESTIGATIONS IN THE DIAGNOSIS OF INTRACRANIAL TUMOURS

X-rays.—In all cases radiograms of the chest and skull should be obtained. Chest
X-rays may show an unsuspected bronchial carcinoma and skull X-rays a lateral
displacement of a calcified pineal shadow in basal projections. Displacements of over
3 mm. in accurately centred films are significant. Enlargement of the pituitary fossa
may occur in pituitary neoplasm or hydrocephalus. Abnormal calcification (not to
be mistaken for calcified plaques in the dura) may be seen in hypophyseal duct tumours
and oligodendrogliomata; indeed, any slowly growing brain tumour may calcify.
In suspected acoustic neurofibroma special projections of the skull to show the internal
auditory meatus may be required. Erosion of the inner table of the skull or hyperostosis with enlarged diploeic channels is seen with some meningiomata. The optic
foramen may be enlarged by a local tumour, causing optic atrophy, and this will
require a specially projected film as the optic foramina are not visible in ordinary
antero-posterior films of the skull.

Angiography is of most value where vascular tumours (meningiomata, saccular
aneurysms, angiomatous malformations) are suspected, and it may outline a meningioma. The feeding and draining vessels of such masses can be demonstrated.
Angiography in glioma may show displacement of vessels by the growth, or abnormal
vascular patterns of vessels within a vascular tumour. Often bilateral carotid angiograms and perhaps a vertebral angiogram will be necessary. Angiography has the
advantage that it gives information not only about the site and size of the lesion,
but also about the type of tumour (Figs. 255, 257).

Lumbar encephalography is the method of choice in cases of epilepsy of late onset
where no tumour is suspected, viz. in suspected cortical atrophy, post-traumatic
states and congenital brain lesions. It may also reveal a space-occupying (expanding)
lesion (Fig. 258). In other cases a *Ventriculogram* performed by the neurosurgeon
through burr-holes is safer. *Myodil ventriculography* is sometimes used to demonstrate suprapituitary growths invading the third ventricle or distortion of the aqueduct

of Sylvius in auditory nerve fibromata; in the latter cautious lumbar puncture may be undertaken if there is no papilloedema, as a protein reading over 100 mg. per cent. is characteristic.

Radioactive tracer substances have recently been used in an attempt to visualise intracranial growths; this method is still in the experimental stage.

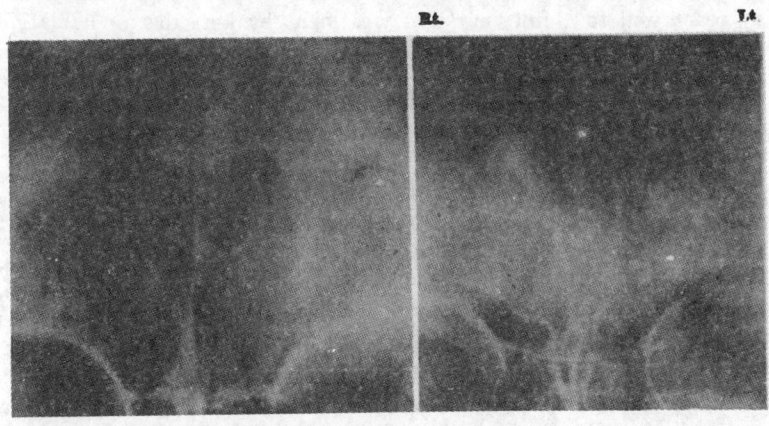

(a)   (b)

FIG. 258.—AIR ENCEPHALOGRAMS (antero-posterior views after lumbar encephalography). (a) Normal. (b) Tumour of the Right Basal Ganglia displacing the septum lucidum and elevating the floor of the right lateral ventricle. (Dr. David Sutton.)

Etiology.—The brain is a commoner site for neoplasms than is generally supposed. Intracranial tumours form about 1·5-2 per cent. of all tumours admitted to general hospitals. They are common in children and in males more than females. Brain tumours not infrequently develop from embryonic tissue " rests."

DISTRIBUTION OF INTRACRANIAL TUMOURS (Adson)

Supratentorial 70 per cent.

Frontal 16·8	22·3	Temporal	13·6
Anterior fossa 5·5		Parietal	11·8
Corpus callosum	11·8	Occipital	2·7
Pituitary	2·7	Mid-brain	0·9
Third ventricle	1·3	Multiple	2·3

Infratentorial 30 per cent.

Cerebellum	12·7	Fourth ventricle	6·8
Cerebello-pontine angle	10·4		

Prognosis.—Coma and death ensue if the tumour is inoperable, and blindness may occur very rapidly with papilloedema. Cases of tuberculoma may heal with streptomycin and isoniazid. Ventriculography carries a much greater risk than angiography. Sudden coma occurring before operation is of the gravest omen. Cases of inoperable glioma may survive as long as two years.

Treatment.—(a) A neurosurgeon should be consulted in every case as removal is sometimes possible. Operative results are good in auditory neurofibromata, parasagittal meningiomata, hæmangiomata and pituitary growths. (b) X-ray treatment is palliative and needs accurate localisation of the tumour beforehand; a cerebral biopsy helps to indicate the nature of the tumour and whether it will respond to X-ray therapy. Certain meningiomata, vascular and pineal tumours, and oligodendriomata may react well to a full course of treatment by an expert. Palliative treatment is by rectal retention of a 50 per cent. solution of magnesium sulphate twice daily—this will relieve headache and lessen symptoms due to brain swelling prior to operation. Intravenous hypertonic solutions are not advised as they may cause. reactionary cerebral œdema.

§ 1052. II. Subdural Hæmatoma results from traumatic tearing of the small cortical veins which drain into the superior longitudinal sinus, or occasionally of those veins draining into the lateral sinus. A slow venous oozing between the dura and the arachnoid membranes then occurs, increased by anything which raises the intracranial venous pressure—e.g., coughing, sneezing, straining at stool. The effused blood clots and becomes encysted. The "blood cyst" increases in size, indenting the cortex, usually over the para-sagittal area. In approximately 15 per cent. of cases such hæmatomata are bilateral. Acute or Chronic Subdural Hæmatomata are described. The former occur after recent trauma.

Symptoms.—The history of head injury preceding most cases is often missed. Either the injury was considered trivial at the time, or the patient's subsequent illness may have made him forgetful. After days, weeks (or more rarely months), headache, vomiting, papillœdema, and progressive apathy appear, the lethargy characteristically varying from day to day. Focal Jacksonian fits or hemiparesis with dysphasia occur, and bilateral pyramidal signs with dyspraxia when there are bilateral hæmatomata. The pulse is often slow even in the early stages. A fixed dilated pupil appears on the side of the lesion. This pupillary sign is due to herniation of the uncus through the tentorial opening, compressing the oculomotor nerve or its nucleus in the crus cerebri. A large pupil which reacts to light has not this diagnostic significance.

The Diagnosis should be seriously considered in all stuporose patients who may have suffered a head injury if there are (1) fluctuations in the level of consciousness, (2) slight persistent pyrexia, or (3) if recovery from stupor is unduly delayed or (4) if a fixed dilated pupil appears. The C.S.F. is usually colourless but may be tinged yellow from altered blood. Normal manometric readings are common. X-ray of the skull may show displacement of a calcified pineal. E.E.G. tracings may show depression of cortical electrical activity on the side of the lesion. Carotid angiograms show filling defects and depression of the middle cerebral vessels.

Etiology.—Hæmatomata may occur as the result of trauma in those with a normal brain, but they are often associated in older patients with conditions of brain atrophy due to arteriosclerosis, alcoholism, senile or syphilitic dementia when after a trivial injury the shrunken brain is thrown rapidly backwards and forwards inside the cranium, thus rupturing the cortical venous tributaries of the sagittal sinus. In young adults a saccular aneurysm in the Sylvian fissure, if adherent to the meninges, may in rupturing cause a subdural clot.

§ 1053. Subdural Hæmatomas in Infancy are commonly bilateral and they produce bulging of the head, often asymmetrical, with its fits or stupor. Pyrexia, bulging fontanelles and papillœdema may be present. The cause is injury to the head before, during or after birth.

Prognosis.—If untreated, death may occur or else the hæmatoma may calcify. The results of surgical drainage are usually excellent but in a few cases with atrophic brain tissue permanent ischæmic cerebral changes occur with hemiplegia, confusion or dementia.

Treatment is surgical. In adults bilateral burr-holes are made and the clot is washed out. In infants repeated aspirations through the intact skull may have to be followed by craniotomy to remove clot and fibrotic membrane, thus allowing the underlying brain to expand.

§ 1054. III. Subdural Hygroma.—A patient who has suffered from pyogenic meningitis treated with antibiotics develops Jacksonian fits with focal cortical disturbances, *e.g.*, hemiparesis, dysphasia. The cause of such residual symptoms may be an encysted subdural collection of turbid or xanthochromic fluid, usually sterile. It can be diagnosed by air encephalography and should be treated surgically by drainage and extirpation under antibiotic cover.

§ 1055. IV. INTRACRANIAL ABSCESS.—Since the use of antibiotics in the treatment of middle-ear, mastoid and pulmonary infections the signs of formation of an intracranial abscess may be most insidious (§ 891). There may be no pyrexia, no leucocytosis in the blood and papillœdema may be late. The presence of an abscess should be suspected in all cases of pyogenic mastoid or pulmonary disease where cerebral symptoms have occurred. A quadrantic defect in the visual fields caused by a temporal lobe abscess is easily missed. A full neurological examination with analysis of the C.S.F. should be carried out before attributing cerebral symptoms of subacute onset in pyrexial patients to a vascular lesion.

GROUP XVI. THE CRANIAL NERVES

§ 1056. The **Olfactory Nerve** consists of 15–20 filaments which arise in the upper nasal mucosa, penetrate the cribriform plate of the ethmoid bone and terminate in the olfactory bulbs. The sense of smell is described in § 1104.

§ 1057. The **Optic Nerve** leaves the orbit through a special aperture, the optic foramen, which lies in front of and medial to the anterior clinoid process. This foramen also transmits the ophthalmic artery. In X-rays of the skull the optic foramina are visible only on special oblique projections. The anatomy of the visual pathway and the symptoms referable to lesions at different sites have been considered already (§ 800).

For Clinical Investigation see § 841. The Optic Nerve is examined by testing (*A*) the Visual acuity, (*B*) the Fields of vision and (*C*) by Examining with an ophthalmoscope.

(*A*) The VISUAL ACUITY is measured with Snellen's Test Types at 6 metres in good light, with a Jæger's test card, or by the counting of fingers held up at 1 metre. These are fully described in § 1116.

TABLE LXII.—CRANIAL NERVES AND THEIR FUNCTIONS

No.	Name.	Components.	Functions.
I	Olfactory.	Afferent.	Smell.
II	Optic.	Afferent.	i. Sight (via lat. geniculate body to visual cortex). ii. Light reflex (via pretectal nucleus).
III	Oculomotor.	Efferent. *i. Somatic.* *ii. Parasymp.* Afferent.	To all extrinsic eye muscles (except sup. obliq. and ext. rectus) and lev. palpebræ superioris. Ciliary and sphincter pupillæ. Pupillary constriction and accommodation. Proprioceptive (via mesencephalic V) from external ocular muscles.
IV	Trochlear.	Efferent. Afferent.	Sup. oblique muscle of eye. Proprioceptive.
V	Trigeminal.	Efferent. Afferent. *i. Ophthal-mic* *ii. Maxillary* *iii. Mandibu-lar*	Muscles of mastication, anterior belly of digastric, mylohyoid, tensor palati and tensor tympani. Proprioceptive from muscles of mastication and expression; and tongue. Forehead and anterior scalp, bridge of nose, upper lid, eyeball. Cheek, lower eyelid, side of nose and upper lip, teeth and gum of upper jaw, mucous membrane of roof of mouth and nose, maxillary sinus. Lower lip, anterior two-thirds tongue, lower teeth and gum.
VI	Abducent.	Efferent. Afferent.	Ext. rectus of eye. Proprioceptive.
VII	Facial.	Efferent. *i. Branchial.* *ii. Parasymp.*	Muscles of face and scalp and elevations of hyoid bone. Facial expression. Secreto-motor and vaso-dilator to salivary, lacrimal glands.
VIII	Auditory.	Afferent.	i. From duct of cochlea. Hearing. ii. From utricle and ampullæ. Equilibration.
IX	Glossopharyngeal.	Efferent. *i. Branchial.* *ii. Parasymp.* Afferent.	Middle constrictor stylo-pharyngeus movements. Secreto-motor and vaso-dilator to parotid gland. Taste (post. one-third tongue). General sensibility of pharynx, tonsil and tympanic cavity. To carotid body and carotid sinus.
X	Vagus and cranial part of accessory.	Efferent. *i. Branchial.* *ii. Parasymp.* Afferent	Palatal muscles. Pharyngeal muscles. Muscles of larynx for phonation and respiration. Plain muscle of small gut, heart (depressor), broncho-constrictor. Larynx and respiratory passages, lungs. Wall of alimentary canal. General and visceral sensibility.
XI	Accessory (Spinal Root).	Efferent.	Trapezius and sternomastoid muscles.
XII	Hypoglossal.	Efferent.	Muscles of tongue.

(*B*) The VISUAL FIELDS may show defects (voids or gaps) which are revealed by confrontation (§ 841), by mechanical perimetry, or by the use of Bjerrum's Screen (§ 1117). The physiological anatomy and clinical investigation of the visual fields have been considered in § 800. Central

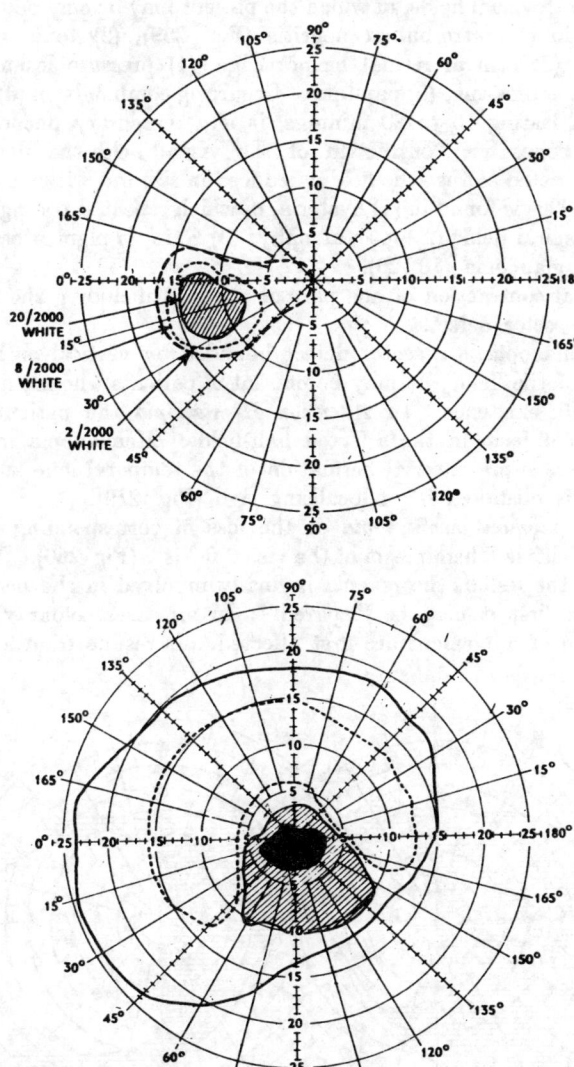

FIG. 259.—Fields of vision of left eye charted on Bjerrum's screen. Top shows a central scotoma in acute retrobulbar neuritis from a case of disseminated sclerosis; and bottom a caecocentral scotoma in tobacco amblyopia.

Examination was done with test objects of different sizes: the central black area shows complete loss of vision, the shaded areas considerable loss of vision and those within the broken lines slightly depressed vision.

opacities in the lens or cornea must be excluded before perimetry is undertaken.

(1) **Central Scotoma,** or more usually a centro-cæcal scotoma (*i.e.*, extending from the normal blind spot into the macula), is a blind patch in one or both visual fields, of which the patient may or may not be aware. It occurs in (1) retro-bulbar neuritis (Fig. 259), (2) toxic amblyopia (Fig. 259), (3) central retinal hæmorrhage, (4) pressure lesions on the optic nerve or chiasma, (5) papillitis. Occurring commonly in (6) migraine as an aura lasting 15 to 20 minutes, it is a temporary phenomenon.

(2) In **Concentric Contraction** of the visual field the periphery is equally restricted so that the field is reduced in size but without alteration in shape. This is found in (1) hysteria, in which repeated testing may also produce a spiral field; (2) optic atrophy; (3) retinitis pigmentosa (§ 1139) and in (4) glaucoma (§ 1120).

(3) Local contraction of one part of the field including the periphery is called a **sector defect.**

(4) **Hemianopia** is a sector defect bounded by vertical or horizontal diameters of the field. It may be present in patients who are not always aware of its existence. In *Attention Hemianopia* the patient appears unaware of objects in the affected half-fields. Hemianopia may occur when there is supratentorial herniation of the temporal lobe and lead to error if it is mistaken for a localising sign (Fig. 219).

(*a*) *Homonymous hemianopia* or the loss of corresponding halves of the visual fields is " hemiplegia of the visual fields " (Fig. 260). Whatever the site of the lesion, the macula is finally involved in the hemianopia, although at first it may be " spared." In all cases colour vision and appreciation of movement are first affected. It results from a lesion in

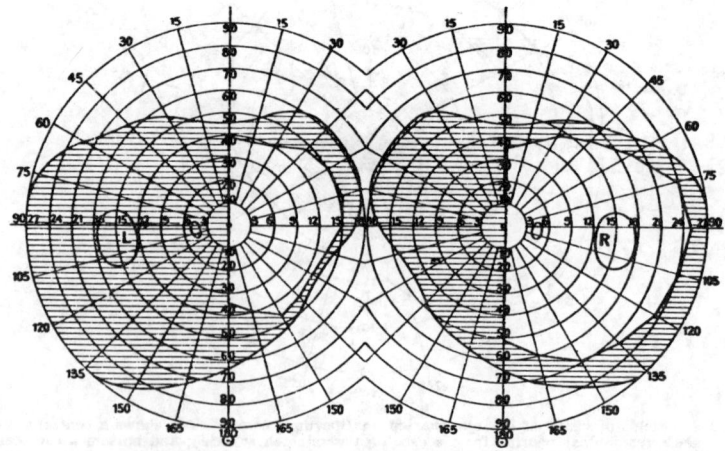

FIG. 260.—VISUAL FIELDS SHOWING LEFT HOMONYMOUS HEMIANOPIA from a case of right-sided temporo-occipital glioblastoma involving the optic radiations. The blind areas are shaded.

the contra-lateral (i.) Optic tract or (ii.) Optic radiation. Tract hemianopia begins peripherally. Radiation hemianopia due to a lesion in the temporal lobe gradually enlarges to become a complete crossed homonymous defect. (b) In *Quadrantic hemianopia* only one quadrant, upper or lower (instead of one half), of corresponding half-fields is blind. This is generally due to a lesion of the optic radiation in the temporal lobe involving the temporal " knee." Less commonly it is due to a lesion of the striate cortex. A lesion above the post-calcarine fissure causes an inferior quadrantic hemianopia, a lesion below the calcarine and post-calcarine fissures an upper quadrantic lesion in the crossed half-fields. (c) *Bitemporal hemianopia* or loss of the temporal halves of both visual fields results from a lesion of the optic chiasma (Fig. 261). (d) *Altitudinal hemianopia* is loss of the upper or lower halves of both visual fields. It may occur in migraine or from bilateral lesions of the visual cortex. (e) *Nasal hemianopia* in one eye may occur from a lesion affecting the lateral fibres of the chiasma on the same side.

PATHOLOGICAL CAUSES OF FIELD DEFECTS.—Field defects may be due to (i.) trauma, (ii.) cerebro-vascular accidents (hæmorrhage, thrombosis, embolism), (iii.) space-occupying (expanding) lesions (tumour, aneurysm, angiomatous malformation), (iv.) inflammatory lesions (abscess, syphilis, meningitis), (v.) demyelinating and toxic lesions. When due to tumour, abscess or a progressive demyelination the defect gets worse or is static. When due to a benign vascular lesion or trauma the defect tends to improve. Variable defects suggest a functional illness. When the field changes are due to supratentorial herniation of the temporal lobe or brain swelling, hemianopia may be a " false localising sign."

(a) Homonymous hemianopia is usually due to a cerebral vascular accident or to the presence of an infiltrating neoplasm (primary or secondary). Angiomatous malformation and abscess are less frequent; it is uncommon in demyelinating disease except in the encephalo-myelopathies. If combined with a nasal defect in one field a chiasmal lesion is likely, e.g., tumour, saccular aneurysm.

(b) Quadrantic hemianopia—If homonymous, a vascular accident or infiltrating tumour of the temporal lobe is likely. If bitemporal, a pituitary adenoma, meningioma, a hypophyseal duct tumour or a saccular aneurysm are possible causes.

(c) Bitemporal hemianopia indicates a chiasmal lesion due to a pituitary adenoma, hypophyseal duct tumour, meningioma, large saccular aneurysm or arachnoiditis (Fig. 261).

(d) Altitudinal hemianopia is rarely seen except as a temporary phenomenon in migraine. It can occur in basal chiasmal lesions.

(e) Nasal hemianopia may be due to dilatation of the internal carotid artery external to the chiasma, but is usually part of a homonymous hemianopia perhaps obscured by blindness of one eye.

(C) OPHTHALMOSCOPIC EXAMINATION reveals changes in the optic discs and fundi. The student must make himself familiar with the normal appearances and the changes found in disease (§§ 1126–1140).

§ 1058. Optic atrophy (Syn. Primary Optic Atrophy).—Vision fails progressively and blindness follows. Ophthalmoscopy shows a pale white porcelain-like disc smaller than normal whose outline is sharply defined. The greyish-white lamina cribrosa is visible. The retinal arteries and veins are narrow. Visual acuity is affected in marked cases. The changes in the visual fields depend on the cause of the atrophy.

In the mild atrophy which follows retro-bulbar neuritis the pallor is most marked on the temporal side of the disc due to vascular ischæmia.

CAUSES.—Optic atrophy may occur *with retinal disease*, such as retinitis pigmentosa, amaurotic family idiocy in lipoidoses (§ 1127) or other forms of extensive choroido-retinal disease ("Consecutive" atrophy), due to damage to the parent ganglion cells of the retina. NEUROLOGICAL CAUSES of Primary optic atrophy are: (1) tabes dorsalis and dementia paralytica, (2) Expanding lesions pressing on the optic nerve within and behind the orbit (tumours and aneurysm), (3) fracture of the anterior fossa, (4) methyl alcohol and industrial poisonings, (5) following the administration of pentavalent arsenicals, *e.g.*, tryparsamide, (6) in the hereditary ataxias (§ 945), and in (7) Leber's disease (§ 1058a), (8) hydrocephalus, (9) oxycephaly and (10) in severe anæmia. Antisyphilitic treatment has no effect on the progress of syphilitic atrophy. The importance of obtaining good plain X-rays of the optic foramina can thus be realised, for tumours and aneurysms are the only removable causes of optic atrophy.

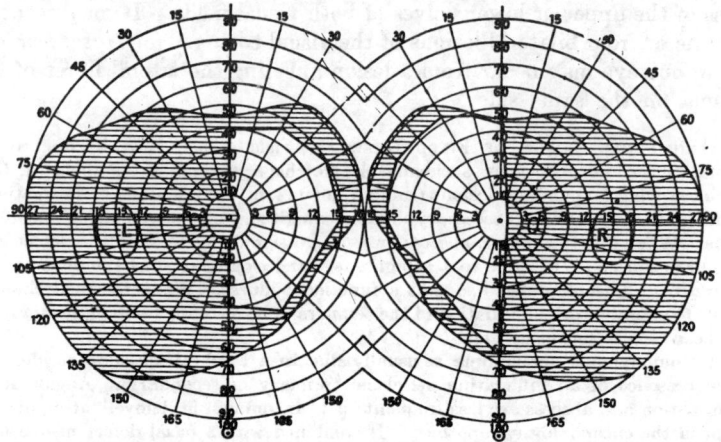

FIG. 261.—VISUAL FIELDS SHOWING BITEMPORAL HEMIANOPIA. Case of Acromegaly due to an eosinophil adenoma of the pituitary in a woman aged 30 years; two years duration. The blind areas are shaded.

§ 1058a. Leber's Hereditary Optic Atrophy usually begins as a retro-bulbar neuritis with central scotoma and slight swelling of the disc or discs. The resultant optic atrophy and visual failure are rarely complete and useful vision is retained. The condition is not always confined to the optic nerves. Nystagmus or ataxia may rarely co-exist. It is an inherited condition affecting men six times more than women, but transmitted only by women. Clinically the symptoms resemble those of tobacco amblyopia. The age of onset is in the third decade, whereas tobacco amblyopia comes later.

§ 1059. Condition of the Pupils.—The tonic dilator of the pupil is the cervical sympathetic (supplying the dilator pupillæ); the tonic constrictor of the pupil is the oculomotor nerve (supplying the ciliary muscle and sphincter pupillæ). Each of the three muscles may be paralysed separately: paralysis of the last two is known as *ophthalmoplegia interna*. The pupils must be tested with regard to their size, shape, equality, reaction to light, direct and consensual, and to accommodation (§ 841).

ABNORMAL DILATATION OF THE PUPIL (mydriasis), when *bilateral*, may be noted in fear states, hyperthyroidism, after the use of mydriatic drugs, *e.g.*, homatropine or cocaine, and in deep coma.

A *unilateral* dilated pupil which does not react to light is seen in partial oculomotor nerve palsy. Coming on soon after a severe head injury it may mean the presence of a subarachnoid or subdural clot on the side of the large inactive pupil. The clot causes herniation of the temporal lobe through the tentorium with pressure on the third nerve nucleus in the mid-brain. A large pupil which reacts to light has not this significance and may result from sympathetic irritation. Unilateral dilatation of the pupil occurs in optic atrophy, glaucoma and after local trauma to the eye (traumatic mydriasis). It is a rare occurrence in migraine during the attack, when the presence of a saccular aneurysm may be suspected.

ABNORMAL CONTRACTION OF THE PUPIL (miosis) occurs in old age, in bright light, after the use of miotic drugs such as eserine, pilocarpine or opium, in iritis, in pontine hæmorrhage and in tabes dorsalis and dementia paralytica.

INEQUALITY OF THE PUPILS may be due to (1) congenital or acquired cervical sympathetic palsy (with a narrowed palpebral fissure), (2) old iritic adhesions, (3) neurosyphilis (if the pupil does not react to light but reacts on accommodation-convergence), (4) glaucoma, (5) tonic pupils (§ 1060). Slight inequalities of the pupils may be observed in health, especially as the result of unequal illumination of the two eyes or a refractive error. In hippus the iris may be observed to contract and dilate rhythmically. It is seen in normal eyes or in some cases of chorea.

IRREGULARITY OF OUTLINE OF THE PUPIL may be due to (1) old iritic adhesions, (2) or may result from previous iridectomy or trauma. (3) Deviations from the circular shape occur in syphilitic pupils, (4) Glaucoma and (5) Coloboma iridis cause irregularities of outline. In coloboma there is a congenital defect in the development of the iris, usually in its lower part, which may be continued backwards to involve the choroid below and even the optic nerve. Vision is impaired.

ECCENTRIC PUPILS (Ectopia pupillæ) may be congenital. It is seen after iritis. It may occur in mid-brain lesions, *e.g.*, syphilis, encephalitis, neoplasm.

The **Pupillary Light Reflexes** (direct and consensual) depend on the integrity of the retina, the optic nerve, the chiasma, the optic tract, the intermediate cells starting in the mid-brain and posterior commissure, the colliculo-ocular (Meynert's) fibres, the nuclei of the third nerves situated around the aqueduct. The fibres of the third nerve pass to the ciliary ganglia and thence to the sphincter pupillæ in the short ciliary nerves (Fig. 220).

The pupil reactions, besides involving pupillary contraction to light, comprise also dilatation to shade and darkness. The latter reaction is brought about through a sympathetic pathway (Fig. 227).

As the pupil is also governed by accommodation-convergence pathways it is important in testing the light reflex to be sure that the patient's gaze is fixed on some point in the middle distance so that a sudden convergence contraction is not mistaken for a light reaction.

LOSS OF THE PUPILLARY REACTION TO LIGHT (light iridoplegia) may be produced by a lesion situated anywhere in these afferent or efferent tracts. The phenomenon described by Argyll-Robertson was (1) loss of direct reflex to light with (2) preservation of pupillary contraction on convergence accommodation, and he noted its association with (3) small pupils. Such pupils may be called truly " Argyll-Robertson pupils." Syphilitic pupils may have characteristics other than those noted by Argyll-Robertson. Thus they may be (4) large, (5) unequal in size, (6) irregular in outline, (7) eccentrically placed in the iris. (8) They may be surrounded by an atrophic zone of paler pigmentation in blue irides. Fixed pupils are those which react neither to light nor to accommodation-convergence.

Causes of Argyll-Robertson Pupil: Clinically: the Argyll-Robertson pupil is found in syphilis affecting the vicinity of the aqueductus of the mid-brain (Fig. 220) and the superior colliculi. Apart from the syphilitic lesion, non-reacting pupils have been observed and reported as a clinical rarity in the following conditions: non-specific encephalitis (*e.g.*, encephalitis lethargica), mid-brain tumours, syringobulbia, in traumatic lesions of the mid-brain, in alcoholic polyneuritis and diabetes mellitus.

The *anatomical* basis of the Argyll-Robertson phenomenon is obscure. The condition may be met with in: (1) lesions of both optic nerves, (2) lesions of both optic tracts, and (3) central lesions of the colliculo-ocular fibres which pass to the anterior end of the third nucleus in the mid-brain. (If one is to insist on small pupils as described by Argyll-Robertson the third situation is the only one possible.)

§ 1060. Tonic pupils (Syn. Myotonic pupils of Adie) are pupils which react only to very strong light, and on convergence-accommodation may contract slowly, remaining contracted for some seconds, before very slowly dilating again: in 80 per cent. of cases only one eye is affected. The condition is usually found in women between 20 and 30 in association with absence of tendon reflexes (Adie's syndrome), and may simulate tabes dorsalis, if the true condition of the pupils is not recognised.

CONVERGENCE-ACCOMMODATION REACTION (Near Reflex).—When looking at a near object the eyes are converged, the ciliary muscles contract (causing increased convexity of the lens) and the pupils narrow. These ciliary and pupillary reactions constitute accommodation (§ 800). Loss of pupillary contraction on accommodation occurs in: (1) Traumatic lesions of the mid-brain, (2) Diphtheria (with palatal paralysis or loss of tendon reflexes), (3) Poisoning with atropine or belladonna, (4) lesions of the oculomotor nerve, (5) following encephalitis or encephalopathy.

The **Cervical Sympathetic** is the tonic dilator of the pupil. Lesions may be due to (a) Paralytic, or (b) Irritative causes.

(a) *Paralytic* lesions produce (i.) small pupil, (ii.) loss of cilio-spinal reflex, (iii.) enophthalmos, (iv.) narrowing of the palpebral fissure with pseudo-ptosis, and (v.) increased sweating on the corresponding side of the face and forequarter (stellate ganglion and Th2).

(b) *Irritative* lesions produce (i.) dilated pupil, (ii.) brisk cilio-spinal reflex, (iii.) lid retraction and (iv.) increased sweating on the corresponding side of the face and forequarter.

The *Causes* of such lesions are (1) Congenital cervical sympathetic lesions, (2) Brain-stem vascular lesions (*e.g.*, basilar or posterior inferior cerebellar occlusion), (3) Mid-brain lesion (syringobulbia). (4) In the neck development of a cervico-sympathetic palsy may accompany thrombosis of the internal carotid artery, and as a complication of carotid angiography. (5) At the base of the skull near the jugular foramen metastic tumours or enlarged lymph nodes are rare causes. (6) At the lung apex and thoracic inlet bronchial carcinoma, apical fibrosis in tuberculosis, and sub-clavian aneurysm, cervical rib, the thoracic inlet syndrome and other lesions of the lowest trunk of the brachial plexus may all cause sympathetic palsy. (7) Of the spinal causes, remember spinal tumours at the Th1–2 level and syringomyelia.

§ 1061. Disorders of External Ocular Movements and Muscles.—The external muscles of the eyeball (as distinct from the internal or involuntary muscles of the eye) are six in number and are supplied by three cranial nerves: the medial, superior and inferior recti and the inferior oblique by the third (oculomotor) nerve (which also supplies the levator palpebræ, the sphincter fibres of the iris and the ciliary muscle); the superior oblique by the fourth (trochlear) nerve; and the external rectus by the sixth (abducent) nerve. It therefore follows that:

Complete paralysis of the third nerve (oculomotor) is attended by { Ptosis; external strabismus; pupil dilatation and immobility; loss of accommodation; inability to move the eyeball inwards or upwards, and only imperfectly downwards; slight protrusion of the eyeball: crossed diplopia.

Paralysis of the fourth nerve (trochlear) is attended by { Slight deviation of cornea upwards; homonymous diplopia on looking downwards.

Paralysis of the sixth nerve (abducent) is attended by { Internal strabismus; inability to move the eye outwards; homonymous diplopia.

Defects in the ocular muscles prevent the eyeballs moving synchronously so that objects cannot be focused on the retinæ in a normal manner. A squint is produced when the muscular defect is pronounced. Two conditions ensue: (1) A squint without diplopia. This is considered under Diseases of the Eye (§ 1125). (2) Diplopia (double vision) occurs when the lesion is recent; if the muscle weakness is slight, a squint is not obvious. There may also be (3) Vertigo; and (4) sometimes an abnormal carriage of the head.

§ 1062. **Diplopia** is sometimes due to *local causes* which alter the visual axes, *e.g.*, unequal proptosis or fracture of the orbit. Usually it is due to *neurological disease* involving the third, fourth or sixth cranial nerve nuclei, the nerves which arise from these (Oculomotor, Trochlear or Abducent) or their myoneural junctions (in myasthenia gravis). When diplopia is slight the recognition of which muscles are weakened is often a matter for the oculist, who uses special tests (§ 1124); but when diplopia is marked and there is a considerable muscle paralysis these are not necessary, and a squint develops.

There is marked PTOSIS OF AN EYELID *and on lifting this* THE EYE *is seen to be* ABDUCTED. *The* PUPIL IS DILATED AND INACTIVE TO LIGHT. *The condition is* OCULOMOTOR (THIRD NERVE) PARALYSIS.

§ 1063. **Oculomotor Nerve Paralysis.**—*Symptoms.*—The upper lid droops and may completely cover the eye, due to paralysis of the levator palpebræ superioris. When the upper lid is lifted, the eyeball is seen in the abducted position, pulled outwards by the lateral rectus muscle (supplied by the abducent nerve). Usually no elevation, depression or adduction are possible. The pupil will be dilated and inactive to light if tested by the direct and consensual reflexes. Accommodation is not possible. Occasionally a slight downward and outward movement is made by the superior oblique muscle (supplied by the trochlear nerve). Partial oculomotor paralysis is more common than complete paralysis.

There is DOUBLE VISION, *greatest when the patient looks* DOWNWARDS AND OUTWARDS. *Special tests are usually required to ascertain paralysis of the Superior Oblique muscle. The condition is* TROCHLEAR (FOURTH NERVE) PARALYSIS.

§ 1064. **Trochlear Nerve Paralysis.**—Most cases of superior oblique palsy in middle-aged or elderly persons are due to cerebro-vascular causes. Many clear up after a few weeks or months.

There is DOUBLE VISION *when the patient* DIRECTS HIS GAZE TO THE SIDE. *The condition is* ABDUCENT (SIXTH NERVE) PARALYSIS.

§ 1065. **Abducent Nerve Paralysis.**—There is internal strabismus and inability to abduct the affected eye.

NEUROLOGICAL CAUSES OF OCULAR NERVE PARALYSES AND DIPLOPIA

may be due to (*A*) lesions in the Peripheral Nerves, (*B*) Nuclear or Supranuclear causes, or (*C*) they may be muscular.

(A) PERIPHERAL NERVE LESIONS outside the brain-stem are caused by

1. Trauma.
2. Arteriosclerosis.
3. Intracranial Neoplasm.
4. Neuritis.
5. Polyneuritis.
6. Subarachnoid Hæmorrhage.
7. Intracranial Aneurysm.
8. Syndrome of the Orbital (Sphenoidal) Fissure.
9. Cavernous Sinus Thrombosis.
10. Meningitis.
11. Herpes Ophthalmicus.
12. Gradinegro's Syndrome.
13. Ophthalmoplegic Migraine.
14. Botulism.

1. TRAUMA.—Blows without a fracture, or fractures involving the anterior or middle cranial fossæ may cause damage to the third, fourth or sixth nerves. Diplopia may follow spinal anæsthesia and frontal sinus operations.

2. ARTERIOSCLEROSIS.—Isolated nerve palsies may be caused by pressure of a distorted arteriosclerotic artery, particularly on the sixth nerve in its long intracranial course (lateral rectus palsy).

3. INTRACRANIAL NEOPLASM.—Tumours of the base of the skull, primary or secondary growths, or suprasellar extensions of pituitary tumours growing laterally, may cause ocular palsies. With increasing intracranial pressure, sixth nerve paralysis on one or both sides may be the first sign, *e.g.*, in intracranial neoplasm or hydrocephalus.

4. NEURITIS occurs in children or young adults causing a sudden paralysis similar to Bell's palsy. It normally involves the sixth nerve, but there may be paralysis of more than one ocular muscle, with severe pain in the face and in the eye itself. Complete recovery is frequent.

5. POLYNEURITIS of alcoholism, diphtheria, lead, etc. (§ 974) may be accompanied by external ocular palsies.

6. SUBARACHNOID HÆMORRHAGE may be massive with unconsciousness, and the patient may develop a paralytic squint with diplopia.

7. INTRACRANIAL ANEURYSMS.—A small aneurysm on the internal carotid or other arteries may cause unilateral headache and paralysis of one of the ocular nerves; after some weeks or months recovery may follow.

8. SYNDROME OF THE ORBITAL (SPHENOIDAL) FISSURE.—There is acute pain in the forehead and in the eye, followed by signs of paralysis of the third, fourth or sixth cranial nerves. Some proptosis may be present and there may be sensory impairment over the ophthalmic (and sometimes the maxillary) division of the trigeminal nerve. Ultimately there may be complete ophthalmoplegia, proptosis and anæsthesia of the eye and forehead with severe pain, but this complete syndrome is rare. The cause is usually an aneurysm of the internal carotid artery in the cavernous sinus, but trauma, syphilitic periostitis or a tumour behind or in front of the orbital fissure (*e.g.*, a nasopharyngeal growth from below, or a meningioma on the lesser wing of the sphenoid) may produce similar signs.

9. CAVERNOUS SINUS THROMBOSIS (see § 892).—In pyæmic conditions, with rigors and high fever, sudden unilateral proptosis develops with œdema, external ocular paralysis of the nerves running in the cavernous sinus (Fig. 230), blindness and retinal hæmorrhage. The symptoms usually become bilateral within a few hours or days.

10. MENINGITIS, whether purulent, syphilitic, tuberculous or due to chronic infection by yeasts, may produce ophthalmoplegia, usually bilateral, when the basal meninges are diseased. Sometimes a meningeal deposit from carcinoma of the bronchus produces an early ocular palsy.

11. HERPES OPHTHALMICUS in rare cases may be followed by external ocular palsies, pupillary abnormalities or even by optic atrophy.

§ **1066. 12. Gradinego's Syndrome.**—In association with acute suppurative mastoiditis in children, an external ocular palsy develops (usually the lateral rectus muscle) with pain referred to the distribution of the trigeminal nerve on the face. Other cranial nerves, *e.g.*, facial, hypoglossal, may be affected on the same side. The syndrome is believed to be due to localised meningitis or granulations at the tip of the petrous temporal bone spreading into the posterior fosse. The symptoms clear up completely some days or weeks after surgical treatment of the mastoid infection. These cases have to be distinguished from toxic neuropathies occurring with suppurative sinusitis, which are also transient and reversible.

§ **1067. 13. Ophthalmoplegic Migraine** is a very rare condition characterised by periodic attacks of headache beginning in early life associated with paralysis of the third nerve, which lasts a few days. Permanent paralysis of the third nerve may eventually develop. A familial incidence is reported. These cases may be due to compression of the third nerve by a dilated artery or aneurysm, and angiography should be performed in all suspect cases to exclude this. Not all cases have this etiology.

Following upon CONSUMPTION OF ARTIFICIALLY PRESERVED FOOD *one or more persons develop* HEADACHE, SQUINT *and* DOUBLE VISION *and* DYSPHAGIA. The condition is likely to be BOTULISM.

§ **1068. 14. Botulism** is a very rare severe disease which follows the consumption of artificially preserved food infected with *Cl. botulinum*. Under anærobic conditions the organism or its spores multiply and produce a very powerful exotoxin which is absorbed from the alimentary tract and produces paralysis of striated muscle fibres. The toxin is readily destroyed by reheating the food. It occurs in small localised epidemics.

Symptoms occur 24–48 hours after ingestion. Gastro-intestinal symptoms are rare and usually those first noticed are diplopia, complete ptosis, internal and external ophthalmoplegia with failure of accommodation. General muscular weakness ensues. There is usually no headache and the temperature is subnormal. Later the tongue cannot be protruded, dysphagia and dysarthria follow and there is general severe muscular asthenia; there are no sensory changes and the mind is clear. Death is due to cardiac or to respiratory failure and occurs in 50 to 100 per cent. of cases.

Diagnosis.—The disease bears a superficial resemblance to acute myasthenia gravis and acute encephalitis lethargica. The history of the disease in other consumers of the same tinned food, the subnormal temperature and the rapid development of the ocular signs and general muscle weakness make the diagnosis clear. Neostigmine does not help.

Treatment.—Wash out the stomach and colon repeatedly and keep the bowels open with saline aperients. Alcohol should be given early. An antitoxic serum is available and should be given as soon as possible, but its value is not yet proved. The patient may have to be placed in a respirator and fed artificially.

§ **1069.** (B) NUCLEAR LESIONS in the brain-stem with paralysis of the nerve and muscles on the side of the lesion and a contralateral hemiplegia (Weber's Syndrome, Fig. 210, and the Millard-Gubler Syndrome) are described in § 792. A lesion involving the third nerve, as well as the red nucleus in the mid-brain, may give rise to Benedikt's syndrome—oculomotor palsy and tremor of the opposite arm. These occur with cerebral thrombosis or tumours involving the crus. Infranuclear lesions, often involving the long tracts, are common due to disseminated sclerosis; and in the case of the third nerve a saccular aneurysm of the posterior cerebral artery will cause diplopia (Fig. 231).

SUPRANUCLEAR LESIONS give rise to a Squint and *defective Conjugate Movement of Both Eyes.* The diplopia is not marked but there may be associated pupillary abnormalities. The functions of the oculomotor nuclei in the mid-brain from before backwards are: (1) Pupillary reflex to light, (2) Convergence-accommodation mechanism,

(3) **Upward**, (4) **Downward**, and (5) **Lateral** movement of both eyes. In mid-brain and pontine tumours these functions are often paralysed (Fig. 221).

Paralysis of Conjugate Movement may occur in (1) Vascular Lesions, (2) Tumours, (3) Injuries, (4) Encephalitis or encephalopathy involving the supranuclear fibres to the oculomotor nuclei in the mid-brain.

PARINAUD'S SYNDROME is paralysis of conjugate elevation of the eyes with ptosis, and loss of the pupillary light reflex. It is usually seen in cerebral arteriosclerosis. Signs of pseudo-bulbar palsy (§ 874) may be present and there will often be a history of repeated strokes. Tumours of the posterior hypothalamus (*e.g.*, pinealomas, § 1050) may show this syndrome.

§ 1070. Wernicke's Encephalopathy ("Polioencephalitis Superior").—*Symptoms.*— Ptosis, drowsiness, internal ophthalmoplegia, defective conjugate elevation of the eyes and ataxia may be present with a complicating neuropathy in the limbs or a confusional state. The condition simulates the signs caused by a hypothalamic tumour. It occurs in states of alcoholic poisoning or with nutritional or carcinomatous neuropathy, and is now considered to be a toxic or metabolic condition, not inflammatory. Under the floor of the third ventricle in the mammillar. region and elsewhere are areas of capillary hæmorrhage and demyelination. *Treatment* with parenteral vitamin B_1 effects a rapid improvement in the ocular condition in many cases. Give aneurine hydrochlor. 100 mg. intravenously daily, with vitamin B complex by mouth.

OCULOGYRIC CRISES ("tonic eye fits") occur in patients with post-encephalitic Parkinsonism. The patient's eyes suddenly become fixed in a position of conjugate deviation, usually upwards. The eyes can be brought to the resting position by an effort of will, but only for a few seconds, and may remain tonically deviated for minutes or hours until the spasm relaxes.

In INTER-NUCLEAR OPHTHALMOPLEGIA one or other medial rectus fails to act when the eyes are abducted, but acts normally on convergence-accommodation. The condition is seen in disseminated sclerosis and in small vascular lesions of the pons.

(C) *The patient complains of* PAINLESS DOUBLE VISION AFTER FATIGUE, *with partial paralysis of movement. One or both eyes may be affected unequally. The cause may be* MUSCULAR.

§ 1071. MYASTHENIA GRAVIS causes chronic unilateral or bilateral ophthalmoplegia not conforming to the distribution of any of the oculomotor nerves. Ptosis is an accompaniment and may increase after fatigue or towards the end of the day. The diagnosis is made by noting the degree of ocular movement in all directions and then injecting "Tensilon" intravenously or neostigmine subcutaneously (§ 988).

FATIGUE STATES in patients with disorders of muscle balance (phorias) may render a latent diplopia manifest, with variable squint.

Myopathic Ophthalmoplegia is a rare condition of primary muscle disease involving the external ocular muscles and orbicularis oculi. The condition spreads gradually, and eventually wasting and weakness of the muscles of the face, neck and upper limbs appears. The onset occurs at any age, but mostly in early adult life.

For *Exophthalmic ophthalmoplegia* see § 1114.

§ 1072. Conjugate deviation of the head and eyes occurs after vascular and other sudden lesions of the brain, and in epilepsy. The patient may lose the power of turning his eyes to the contra-lateral side and the eyes and head are deviated to the side of the lesion. Irritative lesions of the second frontal gyrus cause conjugate deviation of the head and eyes to the contra-lateral side.

SKEW-DEVIATION of the eyes is a transient state of loss of parallelism of the visual axes, so that they cross, the homolateral eye looking down and in and the other up and out. It occurs in acute lesions of the middle cerebellar peduncle.

Diagnosis of Diplopia.—This necessitates a careful history of the onset and a full neurological examination. It is often necessary to undertake plain X-rays of the skull, the blood W.R., and a spinal puncture.   Only angiography will make possible the absolute diagnosis of saccular aneurysm, the commonest cause of oculomotor palsy.   Sinusitis and toxic polyneuritis are rare causes.   Doubt is now cast on the existence of a periostitis of the sphenoidal fissure.   Painless oculomotor nerve palsy should always raise the suspicion of myasthenia gravis, even if the symptoms are confined to one eye: the lesion is usually incomplete.

§ 1073. **Nystagmus** is a rapid involuntary jerking of the eyeballs, usually from side to side (lateral nystagmus), occasionally in a vertical direction (vertical nystagmus) or in a circular direction (rotatory nystagmus).   Both eyes are usually involved, though each eye should be separately examined (§ 841).   The movements may be constantly present, but slighter degrees can only be brought out by causing the patient to follow your finger or a small bright object.   Very slight nystagmus can be discovered by direct ophthalmoscopic examination, when the image of the fundus, becoming magnified about fifteen diameters, shows the slightest movements of the eyeball.   It may occur from lesions in the cerebrum, cerebellum, brain-stem and upper cervical cord. It may also arise from toxic causes.   Nystagmus may be divided into pendular nystagmus which is almost always ocular in origin and jerking nystagmus which is almost always labyrinthine, neurological or physiological (optico-kinetic).   In very ill patients, physiological end-nystagmus is sometimes observed.

CONGENITAL NYSTAGMUS is pendular, the two phases being equally fast.   It occurs in association with other congenital abnormalities, and also when some condition (*e.g.*, local ocular disease) has prevented the child using his eyes during the first few weeks of infancy when co-ordination of the extrinsic muscles is usually acquired.   It is seen in albinos where, from want of pigmentation, the retina has never received definite images and cannot therefore acquire the power of fixation and muscular co-ordination.

VESTIBULAR NYSTAGMUS is a jerking nystagmus although it may have a rotatory component as well.   This sign together with violent vertigo may be induced in normal persons by irrigating the ears with hot or with cold water (caloric tests), by rotation or by galvanic stimulation applied to the mastoid.   Absence of such induced nystagmus is pathological (§ 1143).   In irritative diseased conditions of the labyrinths (*e.g.*, labyrinthitis, hydrops), horizontal jerking nystagmus may be present.   Together with absence of the corneal reflex, deafness and facial hemispasm, jerking nystagmus may occur in lesions in the lateral recess (§ 1083).

BENIGN POSITIONAL NYSTAGMUS will appear when the patient is tilted suddenly backwards into the horizontal from the sitting position on a couch, and the head tilted over the side of the couch at an angle of 30° (the " critical " position).   Patients with benign positional nystagmus suffer spontaneous vertigo after certain changes of position, and when the head is at a certain angle.   These movements they learn to avoid. The condition may last for months.   It is occasionally found to be associated with central lesions.

CEREBELLAR NYSTAGMUS is seen most characteristically in acute lesions.   Fixation is poorly sustained on looking to the side of the lesion; the gaze keeps falling away from the fixation point (slow component).   A rapid movement (quick component) restores the gaze to the fixation point.   The nystagmus is a rhythmic jerking movement most marked on looking to the diseased side.   There may be a rotatory element as in vestibular nystagmus.   But nystagmus may be absent in extensive degenerative cerebellar disease and occasionally in expanding lesions.   Lateral jerking nystagmus is sometimes observed in high cervical cord lesions.

VERTICAL NYSTAGMUS on upward gaze is characteristic of brain-stem lesions. Long-tract signs are usually present.

TOXIC NYSTAGMUS is seen in chronic barbiturate intoxication, chronic alcoholism, chloroform and coal-gas poisoning, and in morphine addiction; it occurs in epileptics treated with hydantoinates and is then a sign of intolerance. The symptom disappears a few days after discontinuing the causal drug if it is due to a toxic and not to a degenerative condition.

§ **1074. Miner's Nystagmus** is a variety of occupational nystagmus. Four stages are described: Latent, subacute, acute and neurasthenic. The latent form is found after leaving work and is elicited on rotation. The subacute is found at work; there are headache, complaints of dazzling and giddiness. Nystagmus and a defect in visual acuity by day and poor vision at night are present. In the acute stage all the above symptoms are aggravated and complicated by photophobia and spasm of the lids; the fourth stage is similar to the acute but general nervous symptoms develop. Bad illumination and poor ventilation have been blamed, but the causes are probably largely psychological, *i.e.*, hysterical symptoms superimposed on congenital or acquired instabilities of the ocular mechanisms.

Two varieties of nystagmus which can be induced in healthy eyes may be mentioned. RAILWAY NYSTAGMUS appears when a healthy person is gazing out of a carriage window at the telegraph poles " going by." The eyes fix on one pole and as it passes from the visual field the eyes jerk rapidly back to fix the succeeding pole.

OPTICO-KINETIC NYSTAGMUS occurs in normal subjects when they gaze at a slowly revolving drum on which are painted alternating thick white and black bands.

§ **1075. The Trigeminal Nerve.**—The *motor* and *sensory* nuclei of this, the largest of the cranial nerves, have been described in § 803. The motor and sensory roots leave the ventro-lateral surface of the pons in a sheath of dura mater called the cavum Meckelii. The sensory root before it joins the ganglion lies close to the seventh and eighth cranial nerves in the cerebello-pontine angle. In Meckel's cave, on the tip of the petrous portion of the temporal bone, lies the trilobed trigeminal (Gasserian) ganglion. The ganglion divides into three nerves—(1) The Ophthalmic division, which enters the orbit; (2) The Maxillary division, which leaves the skull by the foramen rotundum; and (3) The Mandibular division, which is joined by the motor root and leaves the skull by the foramen ovale. The first two divisions are purely sensory and lie for part of their intracranial course in the wall of the cavernous sinus; the third is a mixed nerve.

(1) *The Ophthalmic division* supplies the eyeball and conjunctiva (corneal reflex), the skin of the forehead and scalp up to the centre of the vertex, a median cutaneous strip on the nose, the meninges and the mucous membrane of the upper nasal cavity and lachrymal glands (Fig. 234).

(2) *The Maxillary division* supplies the skin of the face on the lateral aspect of the nose, on the cheek, from the upper lip to the lower eyelid inclusive and, laterally, as far as the pinna, the upper jaw and its teeth, pharynx and tonsil, and the lower part of the nasal cavity.

(3) *The Mandibular division* supplies the skin of the posterior aspect of the temple (auriculo-temporal branch), the upper part of the pinna and side of the face (not the angle of the jaw, C1), the tongue, lower cheek and gums and the Eustachian tube. The motor fibres supply the masseter, temporal, pterygoids, mylohyoid, anterior belly of digastric, tensor palati and tensor tympani muscles.

The methods of examination are described in § 841.

TYPES OF TRIGEMINAL NERVE LESION.—These may be Acute or Chronic.

§ **1076.** (*A*) ACUTE TRIGEMINAL NEURALGIA (Syn. Tic Douloureux) in middle-aged and elderly subjects causes paroxysms of explosive unilateral stabbing pain of trigeminal distribution. There is *no sensory loss or motor paresis* and long-tract signs are usually absent (see § 817).

Trigeminal Migraine (§ 812) and Sensory Jacksonian Fits (§ 863) cause transient numbness of the face, sometimes on one side, sometimes on the other.

(B) CHRONIC. I. OBJECTIVE SENSORY LOSS OVER THE FACE *and wasting and* WEAKNESS *of the* MASSETERS AND TEMPORAL MUSCLES *are present. There is probably a* LESION OF THE TRIGEMINAL NERVE *in the pons, lateral recess, Gasserian ganglion, cavernous sinus or orbit.*

Symptoms.—Lesions of the fifth nerve produce sensory loss, diminution or loss of corneal and conjunctival reflexes on the side of the lesion, and paræsthesiæ over the anatomical distribution of the nerve and, if the motor root is involved, paralysis of the muscles of mastication. Slowly progressive lesions are painless and produce, as their earliest sign, diminution of the corneal reflex. Wasting of the masseter and hollowing of the temporal fossa often precede loss of power in the muscles affected. When the jaw is opened it is pushed over to the paralysed side by the healthy lateral pterygoid muscle of the other side.

The CAUSES are: i. *Trigeminal paræsthesiæ,* pain, sensory impairment over the face *with long-tract signs,* either motor or sensory or both, occur from lesions in the PONS. Thus in disseminated sclerosis trigeminal pain and paræsthesiæ may be found with extensor plantar responses. This form (" Medullary sclerosis ") contradicts the aphorism that severe pain does not occur in disseminated sclerosis. In posterior inferior cerebellar artery occlusion the infarcted wedge of medulla contains not only the sensory trigeminal nucleus but the spinothalamic tract carrying pain and temperature from the contra-lateral half of the body. Thus we find crossed dissociated sensory changes on the opposite side of the body with ipsilateral cerebellar signs, cranial nerve palsies and sometimes Horner's syndrome (§ 809). Tumours of the pons (*e.g.,* glioma) and syringobulbia commonly cause squint and diplopia and the trigeminal signs tend to become bilateral. High cervical lesions may cause pain and paræsthesiæ on the face. In syringomyelia and in tabes dorsalis the sensory trigeminal involvement is bilateral and affects mostly the central " butterfly area," *i.e.,* over the nose and eyes.

ii. *Motor paralysis* of the masseters, temporal muscles and mylohyoids occurs in bilateral SUPRANUCLEAR lesions, *e.g.,* pseudo-bulbar palsy. When the masseters and temporals are wasted and the jaw-jerk is markedly increased the cause is probably motor neurone disease (progressive bulbar palsy). Poliomyelitis and polyneuritis rarely involve these muscles. In myasthenia gravis severe weakness of the jaw muscles is common. There is often associated weakness of the facial or ocular muscles and paralysis disappears after injection of " Tensilon " or neostigmine (§ 988).

iii. *Severe trigeminal pain and paralysis (sensory and motor)* of all three divisions is characteristic of destruction of the ROOTS and GASSERIAN GANGLION. This occurs when secondary growths of the base of the skull or naso-pharyngeal carcinomata involve the ganglion. Benign neurofibromas or meningiomas of the ganglion or its coverings are rare causes of pain.

iv. *Loss of the corneal reflex* and *numbness* of the cheek with ipsilateral *facial paresis* or hemispasm, *perceptive deafness* and *tinnitus* characterise lesions IN THE CEREBELLO-PONTINE ANGLE, especially *acoustic neurofibromas* (§ 1083).

v. *Trigeminal pain and paræsthesiæ above and below an eye* together with severe *ophthalmoplegia* occur with lesions in the CAVERNOUS SINUS and orbit, viz. saccular intra-cavernous aneurysms or orbital tumours. Supra-orbital or infra-orbital numbness follows fracture of the maxilla.

vi. *Bilateral facial numbness* occurs in polyneuritis, pontine neoplasms and following injections or inhalations of toxic substances, *e.g.,* trichlorethylene.

II. *There are* NO SENSORY OR MOTOR SIGNS *but there is* PAIN OF ACHING THROBBING OR BURNING CHARACTER *in the trigeminal distribution or part of it.*

This may be due to : i. COSTEN'S SYNDROME. Third division pain occurs in osteo-arthritis of the temporo-mandibular joint and in mal-occlusion of the teeth (§ 817). It causes great distress which is sometimes helped by a dental splint or special denture.

ii. DENTAL NEURALGIA is a deep ache on one side of the upper or lower jaw; it may be increased by hot or cold, or by sweet or salt food (§ 205).

iii. Suppurative sinusitis or carcinoma of the antrum produce pain which may closely resemble that of trigeminal neuralgia.

iv. HERPES OPHTHALMICUS is an inflammation of the Gasserian ganglion, due to the virus of herpes zoster (§ 1021). It is a disease of maturity, but may occur in young adults. Vesiculation and pain occur over the distribution of the ophthalmic division only. Keratitis and corneal ulceration may be present, and vesicles occur also in the upper nasal cavity. The vesiculation in the forehead may be followed by permanent scarring and often by intractable supra-orbital neuralgia and sensory impairment. The trophic corneal lesions may cause blindness. External ocular palsies, pupillary abnormalities, iritis, even optic atrophy may occur.

v. ATYPICAL FACIAL NEURALGIAS. These give rise to aches, pulsations, flushings, burnings and paræsthesiæ vaguely described and not localised within the trigeminal area and accompany certain psychoneuroses. These discomforts are constant, sometimes bilateral and their association with flushing suggests a vascular origin. Sometimes the simulation of trigeminal neuralgia is so close that a diagnostic ganglion block with lignocaine is required : this will temporarily abolish the pain of true tri-geminal neuralgia. " PSYCHALGIA " is pain which transgresses the limits of the trigeminal nerve and is helped by sedatives and sometimes convulsive therapy rather than analgesics.

III. *A* DEVELOPMENTAL ANOMALY *of trigeminal distribution is suggested in two conditions.*

i. STURGE-WEBER SYNDROME. A " port-wine stain " nævus over one or other divisions of the fifth nerve is associated with intracranial calcification of underlying cerebral convolutions, mental defect, contra-lateral hemianopia and fits (§ 770).

§ 1077. ii. **Progressive Facial Hemiatrophy** (Syn. Parry-Romberg Syndrome) is rare and is characterised by atrophy of the skin, its hairs and follicles, subcutaneous tissues, muscles, bone and cartilage within the territory of the trigeminal nerve. There is no sensory loss or paralysis. A vertical furrow on the forehead makes the transition from the atrophic to the normal side. The eye may be involved. The earlier the age of onset in the growing period the greater the deformity.

Treatment by plastic surgery may be undertaken when growth of the facial bones is complete (*e.g.*, late adolescence) if the condition is severely disfiguring.

§ 1078. **The Facial Nerve.**—Of all the nerves of the body the facial is the most frequently affected by paralysis. It is peculiar in having a long tortuous course through a bony canal, the aqueductus Fallopii. During the onset of slow paralysis, or during slow recovery, clonic or fibrillary twitches may be observed in the paralysed muscles: these are seen in the case of no other nerve in the body.

Motor and *sensory* roots are described. The *motor root* arises from a nucleus in the lower part of the pons and the fibres bend round the sixth nucleus before emerging from the brain-stem at the junction of pons and medulla. The nerve passes forwards and outwards with the auditory nerve to enter the internal auditory meatus, where it is joined by the sensory root (n. intermedius). In the aqueduct of Fallopius, the nerve pursues a curved course. To it is attached the geniculate ganglion of the n. intermedius. The nerve within the petrous temporal bone gives off a nerve to the stapedius muscle and runs down behind the tympanum. A quarter of an inch above its emergence from the stylo-mastoid foramen, it gives off the chorda tympani which joins the lingual nerve. On emerging from the stylo-mastoid foramen the nerve passes forwards in the substance of the parotid gland to supply all the facial muscles of

expression and the platysma. The *sensory root* (n. intermedius of Wrisberg) is really
a separate nerve with its own ganglion (geniculate ganglion) functionally related to the
glossopharyngeal nerve. From the geniculate ganglion, fibres run centrally to the
nucleus of the tractus solitarius in the medulla and peripherally with the facial, then
into the chorda tympani with which they are distributed to the anterior two-thirds
of the tongue, supplying this with taste fibres (Fig. 262).

CLINICAL INVESTIGATION: Note how much the eyelids can be closed, the eyebrows
elevated and the teeth shown on maximum effort. The degree to which the lids can
be approximated should be assessed, and the number of upper incisor teeth shown on
maximum effort noted. Improvement can thus be recorded, as with increasing power
the range of these movements improves. Make a general neurological examination.
Test the sense of taste on the anterior two-thirds of the tongue with sugar, salt and
quinine solution. Test the external ocular movements. Look at the ear-drums and
test for deafness. Look inside the pinna and the mouth for herpetic vesicles. No
electrical testing should be undertaken until the third week after the onset of paralysis.

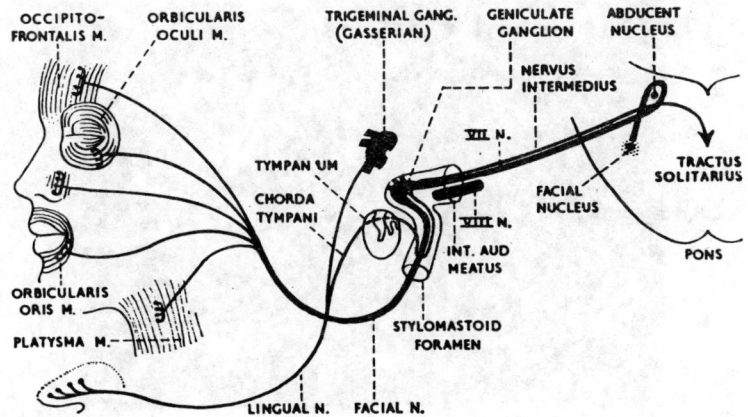

FIG. 262.—DIAGRAM OF FACIAL NERVE, showing the motor and sensory fibres.

Facial weakness may be due to lesions in (*A*) the Upper Motor Neurone,
(*B*) the Lower Motor Neurone, (*C*) or is Bilateral.

(A) Upper Motor Neurone Facial Weakness

A **Supranuclear lesion** of the facial nerve produces asymmetry of the
lower face; the eyelid movements are scarcely weakened, but the angle
of the lip droops and cannot be elevated. The naso-labial fold on the
weakened side is less distinct. When the patient opens the mouth the
asymmetry may be more evident. The commonest *cause* is a cerebral
vascular accident with simultaneous involvement of the hand, or upper
and lower limbs. Usually the facial paralysis is for voluntary movements
only and emotional movements are relatively unaffected, but in some
cases, *e.g.*, deep temporal lesions, " mimic " paralysis of the lower face
occurs, and emotional movements on one side of the lower face are lost.
The value of this latter sign is problematical, as some normal persons
smile only on one side of the face.

In *Pontine* lesions supranuclear fibres or the facial nucleus or nerve may be damaged. The lateral rectus muscle of the eye on the same side is also affected, and there are contra-lateral long-tract signs. This may occur in children and adults in glioma of the pons, or in vascular and inflammatory lesions.

(*B*) *Lower Motor Neurone Lesions* cause weakness of the upper and lower face in varying degree. The commonest cause is Bell's palsy.

After exposure to cold the patient complains of PAIN BEHIND THE EAR *and within a few hours notices* INABILITY TO CLOSE THE EYE *on the same side. The condition is* BELL'S PALSY.

§ **1079. Bell's Palsy.**—*Symptoms.*—For some hours before the onset of paralysis, the patient may complain of pain behind the ear and in front of the mastoid; some swelling may exist in the region of the parotid for

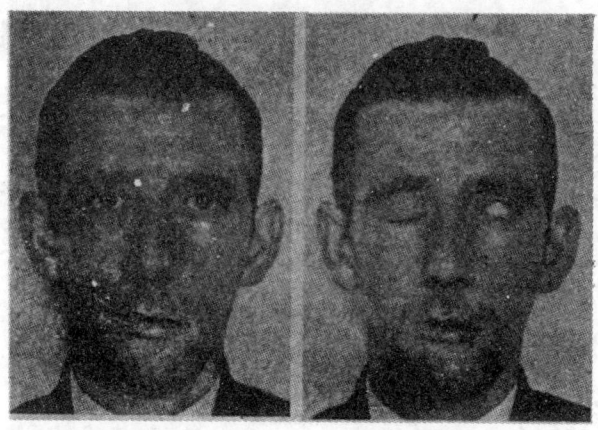

(*a*)   (*b*)

FIG. 263.—LEFT-SIDED FACIAL PALSY. (*a*) At rest. Observe the facial asymmetry with widened ocular fissure and drooping of the angle of the mouth on the left side. (*b*) On attempting to shut the eyes the patient merely rolls the eyeball upwards and outwards on the affected side so that the cornea passes under cover of the upper lid.

one or two days. Occasionally a lymphatic gland is palpable behind the angle of the jaw. The onset of the paralysis is rapid; the patient notices stiffness of the affected side of the face; he cannot close the eye properly and tears trickle from the flaccid lower lid (Fig. 263). Articulation is at first indistinct, fluids are spilled in drinking and food collects between the cheek and the gum. In less severe cases the patient cannot on the paralysed side quite close the eyelids, show the teeth, whistle or puff out the cheeks. In severe cases there is complete immobility of the upper and lower face on the affected side and no voluntary or emotional movement is possible. The paralysis becomes most evident when the patient tries to laugh; the normal side of the face moves into laughter, the paralysed side is stiff and mask-like. In old people the effect of the paralysis is to smooth out the wrinkles on the affected side and the palsy reproduces " the unseared features of earlier age " (Gowers). Epiphora occurs from paralysis of the tensor tarsi (part of the orbicularis). The zygomatici draw the mouth far over to the sound side when the patient tries to laugh. When an attempt is made to close the eyes, the globe on the affected side turns upwards and outwards more than on the normal side, and this is apparent as the lids cannot be approximated on the paralysed side (Negro's sign). The platysma is commonly paralysed. Taste is usually lost on the anterior two-thirds of the tongue. This occurs if the nerve is affected between the geniculate ganglion and the distal point at which the chorda tympani leaves the facial nerve (Fig. 262). Paralysis of the stapedius may cause hyperacusis or clicking in the ear.

Diagnosis.—Peripheral facial palsy may occur in herpes, parotid tumours, poliomyelitis, diphtheria, tetanus, leprosy and sarcoidosis (uveoparotitic paralysis). When the paralysis is due to petrous temporal disease, deafness, otorrhœa and perforation of the tympanum will co-exist. Intracranial lesions should always be considered when other nerves are paralysed, or when long-tract signs are found.

Etiology.—The condition follows exposure to cold and it is thought to be due to an inflammation of the nerve in its fibrous sheath within the stylomastoid foramen. Small epidemics have been attributed to infection with herpes virus. Very occasionally the paralysis spreads to the other side of the face to become bilateral, when a general toxic cause should be suspected.

Prognosis.—The paralysis may increase in severity during the first two weeks. The prognosis on seeing the patient in the first week should therefore be very guarded. The degree of recovery can be measured by the amount of approximation of the eyelids on the affected side, the elevation of the eyebrow, or the number of teeth shown. When observing these, make sure the patient is making the maximum voluntary effort. The upper face is usually the first to recover. Slighter cases without loss of tone in the facial muscles and where the lids can be moved, begin to recover in 3–4 weeks. Complete recovery may take weeks or months. Those who have to make public appearances, speakers and concert artists, may be unable to work for weeks or months. If after three months there is no visible sign of recovery, restoration of movement may take over a year and may be incomplete. In cases which recover imperfectly a curious contracture occurs and voluntary movements, whilst less in degree, spread too widely over the face, so that the eye closes unduly in smiling and the corner of the mouth is drawn up when the eye is closed. This contracture deepens the naso-labial fold; the normal side of the face may be the smoother of the two and until the voluntary movements are observed there may be doubt as to which is the paralysed side. The wide extent of these facial movements has been explained by misdirection of regenerating bundles of regenerating fibres. With such contracture, fasciculation (especially around the angle of the mouth and in the platysma) and occasional clonic hemifacial spasms may be seen on the paralysed side. Epiphora may cause the eye to water in old cases; or else the eye waters when savoury food is eaten ("crocodile tears"). *Recurrence.*—Bell's palsy may recur on the same side or on the opposite side, but this is rare.

Electrical testing should be deferred until all the damaged nerve fibres have degenerated, *i.e.*, the third week. If possible a qualitative method of testing should be used, and the reaction should be repeated at intervals. Such testing is quite useless unless performed by an expert. If in the third or fourth week after the onset some faradic response is present, early recovery of function is to be expected (*i.e.*, within 3 months). Where the reaction of degeneration is present at the end of the fourth week, only partial recovery may be expected.

Treatment.—Explanation of the condition will tend to allay the patient's anxieties. As recovery often takes weeks or months encouragement will be needed. The mouth should be washed out after meals to prevent accumulation of food in the cheek. Instruct the patient to wipe the watering eye upwards and inwards so as to lessen the danger of epiphora. In severe cases, where the cornea is exposed, a nightly eyebath will prevent conjunctivitis and a light woven straw "basket" type of eye-shield may be worn in dusty, windy weather. After the patient has been out in the cold, he should hold a flannel, or sponge wrung out of hot water, to the affected side of the face. Voluntary re-educative exercises should be practised for ten minutes by the clock, night and morning, in front of a mirror; the patient should attempt to elevate and depress the eyebrows, close and open the eyelids, wrinkle the nose, show the teeth, blow out the cheeks, whistle, etc. Facial massage is of use and radiant heat in skilled hands is of value. Faradism is said by some to increase the risk of contracture. At the onset of a severe case some give vitamin preparations or short five-day courses of prednisone 10 mg. twice daily. In severely flaccid cases a piece of transparent plaster or "Sellotape" from the temple to the angle of the mouth, which includes a fold of skin of the cheek, will make the deformity less noticeable. A piece of copper wire covered with rubber tubing can be bent over one ear with a chain and plastic hook to lift up the angle of the mouth on the flaccid, drooping side. This may be worn during the day only if it does not cause soreness of the angle of the mouth. These splints are not used ordinarily in young persons. In cases where the nerve has been destroyed, or when there is no recovery after a year, a plastic operation is probably best. An attempt is made to lessen the deformity by supporting the paralysed muscles with strips of fascia turned down from the temporal muscle and inserted subcutaneously. Anastomosis of the facial nerve to the twelfth or to the eleventh cranial nerve may otherwise be performed.

§ 1080. **Facial Hemispasm.**—There is intermittent unilateral spasm of the face with slight weakness of the affected muscles. Tonic contraction is interrupted by clonic spasms. In the intervals the facial muscles relax partly or completely. This condition usually affects elderly persons and may cause great embarrassment. In the common idiopathic form no cause is apparent. Rarely the hemispasm may be symptomatic of increasing pressure on the peripheral facial nerve by an aneurysm, a parotid or auditory tumour, or an inflammatory lesion and a thorough search should always be made for these, *e.g.*, an acoustic neurofibroma. Hemispasm occurs in chronic Bell's palsy with partial recovery. The facial nerve is the only motor nerve to show this phenomenon. *Treatment* is unsatisfactory unless the cause can be found. Exposure of the nerve at the angle of the jaw and partial destruction of the fibres so as to produce partial facial palsy will stop the movements for a time, but most prefer to endure the movements. Sedative (anodal) galvanism and sedative drugs help some patients when given intermittently.

Facial tic and *Blepharospasm* (§§ 927, 928).

In *Cerebello-pontine* angle (" Lateral Recess ") lesions peripheral facial weakness is accompanied by facial hemispasm with ipsilateral nerve deafness, tinnitus, diminished or absent corneal reflex and numbness of the face. The usual causes are Acoustic neurofibroma or much more rarely meningioma or arachnoiditis.

Lesions in the *Petrous Temporal Bone* (Facial Canal) cause peripheral facial palsy with deafness, tinnitus, and impairment of taste on the anterior two-thirds of the tongue.

The causes are (1) *Fractures* of the petrous temporal bone causing contusion or compression by blood clot. Laceration of the facial nerve is rare and recovery is usual. (2) *Pyogenic* infections of the middle ear or injury during operation on the mastoid. The onset of paralysis may be delayed by some days after the head injury. (3) *Tumours* involving the petrous temporal bone, *e.g.*, Cholesteatoma (epidermoid tumour), carcinoma of the middle ear, Glomus jugulare tumour (§ 1081), or metastatic growths. (4) In surgical operations for the removal of malignant parotid growths or intracranial acoustic fibromas the facial nerve may have to be sacrificed by the surgeon.

There are VESICLES ON THE FACE, NECK, EXTERNAL AUDITORY MEATUS, *or* ON THE HARD PALATE *or* PHARYNX, *with* SEVERE PAIN IN THE EAR, FACIAL PALSY, DEAFNESS AND VERTIGO. *The condition is* GENICULATE HERPES (Syn. Ramsay Hunt Syndrome) (§ 1021). In the milder form a transient facial palsy occurs, but in many cases the condition is severe, causing absolute nerve deafness and severe facial paralysis.

§ 1081. A Glomus Jugulare Tumour arises in the jugular bulb from cells akin to those forming the carotid body. The growth invades the middle-ear, producing deafness with bloodstained aural discharge and vascular polypi in the ear. The facial and vestibular nerves may be affected and a bruit can sometimes be heard over the mastoid. *Diagnosis* is made by aural biopsy. *Treatment* is by radiotherapy. In some cases partial surgical excision is possible.

(*C*) *Bilateral Facial Weakness* if recent in onset should arouse the suspicion of *Myasthenia Gravis* (§ 988). It occurs also in *Myopathy*, *Muscular dystrophy* (§ 1008) and in Uveo-parotitic paralysis (§ 9). In Acute Infective Polyneuritis, and rarely in Bell's palsy, the facial nerve lesion may be bilateral.

§ 1082. Auditory and Vestibular (Eighth) Nerves.—There are two distinct portions with separate functions—(A) the *cochlear* portion concerned with hearing, and (B) the *vestibular* portion concerned with equilibration.

CLINICAL INVESTIGATION (see § 1143).

(A) **Causes of Deafness.**—Two kinds of Deafness are recognisable: **Obstructive deafness,** due to some disease in the middle ear or external auditory passages; and **Nerve (Perceptive) deafness,** due to lesions of the cochlear apparatus or auditory nerve pathways. Mixed types occur. These are described under Diseases of the Ear (§§ 1149, 1150).

Two NEUROLOGICAL CAUSES of Deafness with Neurological Signs are I. Acoustica Neurofibroma, and II. Central Lesions.

§ 1083. I. Acoustic Neurofibroma causes progressive nerve-deafness, tinnitus and vertigo, with loss of the corneal reflex on the ipsilateral side in individuals of 30 to 50 years of age. The tumour mass lies mainly in the lateral recess of the posterior fossa between the cerebellum and the medulla and near the trigeminal nerve. The facial nerve is often stretched over the growth. The fibrous tumour contains very few axons.

Symptoms.—(1) There is a long-standing history of deafness extending over many years, of the type of nerve deafness. (2) Tinnitus has been present intermittently, before the patient is seen by the doctor. (3) There is diminution or absence of the corneal reflex on the side of the nerve deafness. This symptom merits the closest attention; it is due to pressure upon the sensory root of the trigeminal nerve. (4) In some cases there is facial hemispasm or peripheral facial weakness, due to involvement of the facial nerve. (5) Cerebellar signs, including a cerebellar attitude of the head, are present in the ipsilateral limbs. (6) Signs of increasing intracranial pressure—vomiting and papilloedema—are late in appearing. The headache is sometimes early and characteristically localised to the occipital region, with agonising pain and retraction of the head.

Diagnosis.—*Audiometry* shows a nerve deafness. (These tumours are sometimes bilateral.) *Caloric tests* evoke no induced nystagmus, for the labyrinthine fibres are destroyed at an early stage. *X-rays* of the skull taken with a suitable projection may show enlargement of the internal auditory canal. The *C.S.F.* shows evidence of block on manometry with high protein readings—often over 150 mg. per cent. To clinch the diagnosis before operation an opaque contrast medium (Myodil) may be injected into the lateral ventricles of the brain to visualise the aqueduct which is pushed to the contra-lateral side.

Treatment is surgical, but complete removal is not always possible, and the facial nerve, often adherent to the capsule, has to be cut. The resultant complete facial palsy is treated by plastic surgery. In skilled hands the result of both neurosurgical and plastic operations are good, leaving only permanent unilateral deafness.

II. CENTRAL LESIONS, *e.g.*, pontine gliomata, do not usually produce deafness owing to the hemi-decussation of auditory fibres there. Encephalitis and Syringobulbia occasionally produce bilateral central deafness. Long-tract signs and often vertical nystagmus will be present.

Cortical lesions cause inability to comprehend spoken speech (word-deafness), sometimes jargon speech (§ 869B). There may be difficulty in recognising tones and musical configurations of sounds, or in localising sounds in space.

Diplacusis occurs when distorted hearing arises from inequality of acuity on the two sides. For *Deaf Mutism* see § 878.

(B) **Vestibular** lesions cause Vertigo, T nnitus and Nystagmus. The lesions may be (1) in the vestibule itself, the vestibular nerve fibres, in the brain-stem or cerebral cortex, (2) the peripheral organs which initiate the reception of impulses concerned with balance—the vestibule and semi-circular canals. These are described in §§ 826, 1073, and in Tinnitus (§ 1152).

§ 1084. The **Glossopharyngeal, Vagus and Accessory Nerves.**—The afferent and efferent nuclei, visceral and somatic, form a continuous series in the bulb (medulla) and the three nerves leave the skull through the jugular foramen. They are usually affected together. Supra-nuclear lesions of these nerves (pseudo-bulbar palsy) are associated with an exaggerated jaw-jerk.

The **Glossopharyngeal (Ninth) Nerve** contains afferent fibres from the tonsillar fossa and pharynx, and taste fibres from the posterior third of the tongue. Its motor nucleus with that of the vagus supplies the pharyngeal muscles. There are secreto-motor fibres in it from the parotid gland.

CLINICAL INVESTIGATION. Look for reflex " gagging " on tickling the posterior pharyngeal wall with cotton-wool on a probe.

GLOSSOPHARYNGEAL NEURALGIA (see § 818).

Symptomatic Glossopharyngeal pain is felt in the tonsil, pharynx, back of the tongue and deep in the ear. It occurs in invasive and expanding lesions of the brainstem (*e.g.*, medulloblastoma), posterior fossa (metastases) or tongue (carcinoma). Application of 5 per cent. cocaine hydrochloride solution to the tonsillar fossa will temporarily abolish the pain. This test can be used diagnostically prior to the intracranial section of the nerve, sometimes practised for intractable pain.

§ 1085. The **Vagus (Tenth) Nerve** supplies the (1) soft palate, (2) laryngeal muscles, (3) pharyngeal muscles.

CLINICAL INVESTIGATION. Ask for a history of nasal regurgitation of fluids and observe any nasal pronunciation of " B " and " G " sounds in suspected palatal palsy (and see § 841).

Symptoms.—Acute bulbar nuclear lesions, *e.g.*, poliomyelitis, may cause paralysis of the vocal cords in adduction, with such stridor and obstruction of respiration that tracheostomy is necessary. Slighter cases produce hoarseness and dysphagia. In chronic lesions of the nuclei or the corticobulbar tracts (progressive bulbar palsy, pseudo-bulbar palsy) there will be dysphonia and dysphagia. In lesions of the nerve trunks, the nearer the lesion to the bulb the more likely are both abductors and adductors of the larynx to be paralysed, with the cords fixed in the cadaveric position (Fig. 74).

COMBINED BILATERAL PALATAL AND PHARYNGEAL PALSIES are seen in (*a*) myasthenia gravis (§ 988), (*b*) bulbar poliomyelitis, (*c*) progressive bulbar paralysis (§ 875), (*d*) pseudo-bulbar paralysis (§ 874), (*e*) syringo-bulbia (§ 1006). A UNILATERAL lesion suggests a periphereal focal cause.

LARYNGEAL PARALYSIS produces (1) hoarseness, (2) obstruction to breathing and swallowing, (3) lack of movement on inspection with a laryngoscope. Abductor paralysis is usually the result of a lesion in the chest involving the recurrent laryngeal nerve (§ 176). Laryngeal paralysis also occurs in dystrophia myotonica, tabes dorsalis and in sigmoid deformity and fusiform dilatation of the basilar artery.

§ 1086. **Accessory (Eleventh) Nerve** has two distinct portions, spinal and bulbar (accessory to vagus). The spinal portion (Cl–5) innervates the Trapezius and Sternomastoid muscles.

CLINICAL INVESTIGATION (see § 841).

Symptoms.—Paralysis of the spinal portion causes dropping of the shoulder from trapezius palsy. The inferior angle of the scapula rotates away from the mid-line and all movements of the arm lack force. The affected sternomastoid muscle wastes. Trapezius palsy may be seen in penetrating wounds of the retro-mastoid region, in invasion of the base of the skull by metastatic deposits, in poliomyelitis, bulbar encephalitis and progressive bulbar palsy. *Bilateral* sternomastoid wasting is seen in myotonia dystrophica, due not to a nerve lesion but to myopathy.

§ 1087. **Combined lesions of Glossopharyngeal, Vagus and Accessory Nerves** may occur in the (1) Posterior fossa, (2) Jugular foramen, (3) Neck.

(1) Lesions in the *posterior fossa* cause occipital pain, pain in the throat and ear, with paralysis of the palate, laryngeal muscles, sternomastoid and trapezius. The cause may be (*a*) traumatic (a fracture of the posterior fossa), (*b*) an invasive tumour, or (*c*) pressure from an aneurysmal dilatation.

(2) LESIONS AT THE JUGULAR FORAMEN (Syn. Jugular Foramen Syndrome). The glossopharyngeal, vagus and accessory nerves pass through the jugular foramen. Lesions here may cause unilateral palatal and pharyngeal paralysis with anæsthesia, laryngeal paralysis, sternomastoid palsy and partial trapezius paralysis. The jugular vein may be injured or compressed. The " jugular foramen syndrome " is found in neck injuries and in growths at the base of the skull. Lesions due to trauma to the neck tend to be nerve contusions and improve rapidly.

(3) In the *neck*, especially in the retro-parotid region, the three nerves, together with the hypoglossal and cervical sympathetic, may be involved. Not only is the shoulder dropped and the sternomastoid and one half of the palate and larynx affected, but there is a hemiatrophy of the tongue and Horner's syndrome on the affected side. This may be caused by (*a*) enlarged lymph nodes, Hodgkin's glands or malignant growths or (*b*) invasive tumours of the parotid.

§ 1088. **The Hypoglossal Nerve** leaves the skull through the anterior condylar foramen and runs forwards above the hyoid bone resting upon the hyoglossus muscle, to the under surface of the tongue. It is a purely motor nerve and supplies all the muscles of the tongue, intrinsic and extrinsic. CLINICAL EXAMINATION (see §§ 216, 841).

Symptoms of a *unilateral* hypoglossal palsy are atrophy and fasciculation of half of the tongue. The affected side of the organ shrinks and the tongue cannot be pushed into the contra-lateral cheek. At first there is a slight articulatory defect which the patient may overcome. Atrophy and fasciculation occur in nuclear and infranuclear lesions. *Bilateral* lesions are more common. Spasticity of the tongue causes slurred speech and arises from supranuclear lesions of the cortico-bulbar tracts. Saliva is not swallowed and accumulates and overflows.

Etiology.—*Unilateral* palsies are seen in (1) bulbar poliomyelitis, (2) progressive bulbar palsy, (3) syringobulbia, (4) trauma during surgical operations on the neck or throat, or damage to the nerve in the tongue by anæsthetic equipment, (5) medullary tumours, (6) syphilitic basal meningitis, (7) metastases in the anterior triangle, under the mandible or at the base of the skull. *Bilateral* palsies are seen in pseudo-bulbar palsy, double hemiplegia, and as a transient condition in myasthenia gravis.

CHAPTER XX

THE SPECIAL SENSES

THESE comprise the senses of smell and of taste, the vision and the hearing. Investigation of these is of considerable importance from the standpoint of general medical disorders. Apart from the disabilities which result from partial or complete loss of function of these senses, their investigation often reveals the presence and even the nature of disease elsewhere. The peripheral organs for each of these senses are paired and in man the sensory fibres proceeding from them to the cerebral cortex all exhibit a hemidecussation so that the cortex of one hemisphere subserves both organs for each of these senses.

Senses of Smell and Taste (Gustatory Sense)

Smell and Taste are difficult to separate in man, in whom the older rhinencephalon or " smell-brain " has lost much of its function. Many people who for some reason or other have lost their sense of smell are apt to think (wrongly) that their sense of taste is affected. This is well illustrated by the great impairment of taste during a common cold.

THE SENSE OF SMELL is concerned with the appreciation of odours and flavours.

The *olfactory organs* lie at the roof of the nose; impulses received from the delicate olfactory hairs on the surface of the mucous membrane pass directly to bipolar nerve cells in the mucous membrane, the deep or central processes of which penetrate the cribriform plate of the ethmoids to terminate in the olfactory bulbs. Here fibres are relayed in the olfactory tracts, each of which divides into a medial and a lateral portion. The medial portions decussate and join with the uncrossed lateral portions to terminate in the *uncus* and *hippocampal gyri* on the medial aspect of the temporal lobe (Fig. 209).

The METHODS OF EXAMINATION are described in § 841.

§ **1104.** *Disorders of the Sense of Smell.*—Many otherwise normal persons have little or no sense of smell. *Anosmia* is loss of smell. *Bilateral Anosmia* may arise (i.) from smoking tobacco or from other local conditions in the nose (§ 179 *et seq.*). (ii.) During a severe head injury the delicate olfactory nerve fibres may be torn as they traverse the cribriform plate, usually with permanent loss of smell. The patient runs risks from being unable to smell escaping gas or petrol fumes. (iii.) Temporary loss may occur with migraine. (iv.) Inflammation in the anterior and middle fossæ of the skull is a rare cause. (v.) A pituitary, suprasellar or frontal lobe tumour may compress the olfactory bulbs or stalks. *Unilateral anosmia* is rare and is not complained of by the patient; when revealed by testing it is usually due to a local nasal cause; when there is also primary optic atrophy, first on one side but later bilateral, this suggests meningioma of the olfactory groove, or sometimes an early frontal lobe tumour. *Hysterical anosmia* is usually associated with diminution of all the special senses, perhaps on one side (and see § 1173). Anosmia does not occur from cortical lesions. *Parosmia* or perversion of the sense of smell, with normal olfactory acuity, occurs especially after head injuries. A subjective unpleasant sense of smell and taste associated with champing of the jaws, smacking of the lips and a transient diminution of consciousness occurs with an uncinate epileptiform fit (§ 863).

§ **1105.** THE SENSE OF TASTE is concerned with sensations that are more crude than those of smell; there are four primary tastes, sweet, sour, bitter and salt. Some add to these a metallic taste.

The *taste-buds* are most plentiful on the dorsum of the tongue, but also exist on the inner surface of the cheek, the palate, fauces and the pharynx. The sensations they receive are quite separate from the " common sensations " which arise from the mucous membrane of the mouth, viz., pain, touch, heat and cold; but substances taken into the mouth *in solution* usually stimulate the senses of taste and of common sensation—thus a fluid may be described as sweet and as hot at the same time. From the taste-buds the special sensations are transmitted to the cortex by two distinct routes. (i.) Taste from the anterior two-thirds of the tongue is carried centrally first by the chorda tympani which runs with the lingual nerve until it separates to enter the geniculate ganglion in the aqueductus Fallopii (Fig. 262). Thence the taste-fibres travel in the nervus intermedius to the dorsal nuclei of the seventh and ninth cranial nerves (nucleus of the tractus solitarius) in the hinder part of the pons and in the medulla. (ii.) From the posterior third of the tongue, taste fibres travel along the glossopharyngeal nerve to their cell station in the petrous ganglion, and thence they reach the same nucleus of the tractus solitarius in the medulla. From here both sets of taste fibres run together in a second relay which crosses to join the opposite medial lemniscus, to end in the thalamus. Then a third relay carries the sensations to the lower part of the post-central cortex close to the cortical area receiving sensation from the face. Therefore all the sensory fibres from the tongue, palate and pharynx (of taste and of common sensation) follow a closely similar course to the thalamus and to the cortex—it is no longer believed that the cortical representation of taste resides in the uncus and hippocampal gyri.

The *Methods of Examination* are described in § 841, VII.

Disorders of the Sense of Taste.—By utilising this sense a useful and pleasant article of food is accepted for mastication and swallowing and a harmful food is rejected. Richter believes that this sensation may be altered to suit the requirements of the body; thus an adrenalectomised animal will seek sodium chloride and a parathyroidectomised subject will seek calcium salts. *Altered* sensations of taste are due to local conditions in the mouth. Loss of taste on the anterior two-thirds of the tongue occurs in lesions of the facial nerve in the aqueductus Fallopii involving the geniculate ganglion. Cortical lesions seldom cause loss of taste because of its bilateral representation but irritative lesions of this area may cause hallucinations of taste (Uncinate fits, § 863).

Vision and the Eyes

The Visual Mechanism consists of the eyeballs and the complicated structures therein, the extrinsic ocular muscles, the optic nerves and the nerve pathways in the brain to the cerebral cortex. Here we are concerned only with the eyes themselves—the many different neurological conditions have already been dealt with in Chapter XIX.

SYMPTOMATOLOGY.—The chief symptoms which reveal disease of the eye are:

    I. Pain (§ 1106);

    II. Superficial Alterations, especially (a) Redness; (b) Exophthalmos; (c) Changes in the Eyelids (§§ 1107–1115).

    III. Defects or Loss of Vision (§§ 1116–1140).

§ 1106. I. **Pain in the Eyes** is not infrequently absent in ocular affections. Eyestrain may give rise to headache, eye-ache or neuralgia. Glaucoma is a serious cause of pain in the eye and its neighbourhood. Retrobulbar neuritis causes pain which is aggravated by movement of the eyeball, and tenderness to light touch. Dental disorders may not only give rise to reflex pain, but also to both functional and organic affections of the eyes. Among subjective sensations other than pain may be noted muscæ volitantes (black specks) and scintillating scotoma or zigzag lines. The former may be normal, but evident to the patient because of eye-strain or poor health, or they may be pathological and due to vitreous opacities. The latter occurs in association with migraine.

ASTHENOPIA, with painful itching of the eyes and lachrymation, is associated with some degree of photophobia and blepharospasm. Often an expression of allergy, there may be a contributory refractive error. When constant, dust and feathers, or otherwise dogs, cats and horses are causal; when seasonal, pollens. (§ 179, IV.)

THE CLINICAL EXAMINATION of the Eye consists of: Noting any Superficial Alterations (§ 1107); Testing Defects of Vision including the Visual Acuity and Refraction (§ 1116) and the Fields of Vision (§§ 841, 1117); Examining the Pupils (§§ 841, 1059), the Ocular Movements (§§ 841, 1124) and the Fundi (§ 1126).

§ 1107. II. **Superficial Alterations** require careful examination preferably with a strong pencil of light directed into the eye. A *Binocular Loupe* and a *Hand Lens* permit magnification of the structures in the front of the eye—the cornea, sclerotic, iris, lens and the aqueous humour.

The *Slit Lamp* enables us to make an even more detailed examination. It consists of a binocular microscope carried on an arc and working in concert with a source of light shedding an intense beam on the part examined. By its means the minutest alterations in the anterior parts of the eye (including the anterior vitreous) can be examined, and the detailed progress of pathological phenomena noted.

IIa. REDNESS may affect one or both eyes. *Generalised* redness is usually due to conjunctivitis, iritis, acute glaucoma or to polycythæmia; whereas *localised* redness suggests corneal ulceration, episcleritis or a subconjunctival hæmorrhage.

§ 1108. **Conjunctivitis** may develop fairly rapidly.
Symptoms.—(i.) The eye is uncomfortable but not painful. (ii.)

Photophobia is present. (iii.) There is a discharge which may be purulent, muco-purulent or rarely watery. (iv.) The palpebral and bulbar parts of the conjunctiva are equally affected, but owing to gravity the lower part of the eye is at first redder than the upper part. (v.) The hyperæmia is superficial and there is no circumcorneal congestion as can be shown by applying pressure to this area through the lower lid—when the lid is quickly drawn downwards the vessels can be shown to be momentarily emptied. (vi.) The intra-ocular tension, the size and reactions of the pupil and the vision are unaffected.

Etiology.—Conjunctivitis showing a purulent or muco-purulent discharge is usually due to infections by streptococci, staphylococci, pneumococci, *C. xerosis* and sometimes by gram-negative bacilli; the gonococcus is sometimes causal. Acute catarrhal conjunctivitis can be caused by the Koch-Weeks or the Morax-Axenfeld bacillus. Non-purulent cases with a very acute onset may be due to a virus such as that which causes acute kerato-conjunctivitis, in which case the pre-auricular lymph glands are swollen; or otherwise to a foreign body, excessive exposure to heat or to light, or to allergy.

Ophthalmia Neonatorum is due to infection of the conjunctiva of the newly-born during the passage through an infected cervix and vagina. Formerly it was due to the gonococcus, but now many other organisms (and especially staphylococci) are causal. A few cases are due to a virus, causing the condition known as inclusion blennorrhœa; epithelial scrapings show inclusion bodies under the microscope.

Treatment is by washing away a purulent exudate and then instilling penicillin, neomycin, chloramphenicol or sulphacetamide eye-drops (B.P.C.) each two hours by day. In severe cases oral sulphonamides may also be given. Muco-purulent cases usually respond to penicillin eye ointment (B.P.) applied two-hourly. In allergic cases hydrocortisone or adrenalin eye-drops are helpful. For inclusion blennorrhœa give systemic sulphadiazine.

§ 1109.—**Iritis** is frequently associated with inflammation of the ciliary body (irido-cyclitis). In the acute variety usually only one eye is affected, but in chronic cases both eyes are likely to be involved. The term uveitis signifies inflammation of the iris, ciliary body and the choroid.

Symptoms.—(i.) Pain is a prominent feature and is often severe enough to prevent sleep. (ii.) The eye is congested, especially in the circumcorneal area where tenderness can be elicited through the closed upper eyelid. (iii.) Photophobia and lachrymation are present. (iv.) The affected pupil is smaller than normal, reacts sluggishly to light and the affected iris changes colour. (v.) Visual acuity is not necessarily diminished. (vi.) As inflammation advances a sticky exudate forms adhesions between the iris and the lens (posterior synechiæ) and with the aid of the +12 lens of an ophthalmoscope the normally circular red reflex shows irregular projections at the circumference. When *cyclitis* is present deposits of inflammatory material can be made out on the back of the cornea (keratitis punctata): these are best seen with a binocular loupe and a condensing lens. The chief *complication* in severe cases is the development of posterior synechiæ; secondary glaucoma is rare. In chronic cases the pupil may be occluded by the density of the exudate.

Etiology.--The known causes fall into three main groups. (1) There may be local trauma or extension from conjunctivitis or keratitis. (2) Systemic conditions include focal infection from teeth, tonsils, urethra, etc., tuberculosis, syphilis, leprosy, the infectious fevers and rheumatoid disease, including ankylosing spondylitis in young adults and Still's disease in children. (3) Metabolic disease such as gout or diabetes mellitus. In many cases the cause cannot be found. After traumatic cyclitis sympathetic irido-cyclitis (sympathetic ophthalmia) sometimes occurs in the sound eye at the height of the disturbance in the affected eye.

Treatment. The eyes need protection by dark glasses, and severe pain is usually relieved by aspirin 10-15 gr. In order to rest the inflamed eye and prevent the formation of synechiæ, persistent dilatation of the pupil must be ensured with drops of atropine sulphate (1·0 per cent.) into the conjunctival sac—in severe cases a careful watch must be kept for the occurrence of secondary glaucoma. Hydrocortisone eye-drops (1 per cent.) applied four-hourly limit the local inflammatory reaction while the primary cause is being sought and appropriate treatment given, but in protracted cases systemic steroids may be required. In recurring iritis, not associated with cyclitis (keratitis punctata), iridectomy in the quiescent stage may be required. If complete annular synechiæ form, iridectomy should be undertaken to prevent secondary glaucoma. Some still use injections of tuberculin.

SARCOIDOSIS may affect any part of the eye, but irido-cyclitis is the most important lesion, with keratitis punctata and nodules on the iris. (See also §§ 141, 710, 889.) Blindness may result.

§ 1110. **Acute Glaucoma** signifies an increase in the intraocular tension and is much more common after the age of 50. For diagnosis and to watch the progress of the disease, inspection by an ophthalmic loupe and a good source of light are essential.

Symptoms. (i.) Pain and tenderness of the eye vary with the severity of the attack, but in severe cases the pain and tenderness are violent; pain is frequently referred via the ophthalmic division of the trigeminal nerve to produce a severe hemicrania. (ii.) Within a few hours the patient complains of misty vision and of seeing " rainbows " or haloes around bright lights. Loss of vision may be rapidly progressive. (iii.) The chemosis of the affected eye is more extensive than in iritis and is of a dark, even purple, colour. (iv.) The eye waters freely and is œdematous. The lids are frequently swollen. (v.) The cornea is cloudy, has lost its sheen because of œdema and is relatively insensitive to cotton wool. (vi.) The pupil is seen through a haze to be irregularly dilated and it is frequently oval vertically. These give the eye a look of blindness with a curious grey-green colour. (vii.) The pupil fails to react to light or to accommodation. (viii.) The optic disc and the retina are often rendered invisible by the clouded media. (ix.) The patient is in considerable distress as a result of the pain, loss of sleep and loss of vision, and vomiting is frequent. (x.) The intraocular tension, taken with the two index fingers or by a tonometer, is very high.

Etiology.—The raised intraocular tension is due to interference with filtration of the aqueous humour through the canal of Schlemm from which it enters the ophthalmic veins. The cause of primary glaucoma is undecided. Secondary glaucoma is usually due to previous irido-cyclitis which results in adhesions; it may follow some weeks after thrombosis of the central retinal vein, and on occasions is due to intraocular growths or to a venous congestion resulting from a retro-orbital tumour.

Treatment.—An ophthalmic surgeon should see the patient as soon as the diagnosis is suspected, for irreparable blindness may occur. Medical treatment consists of keeping the pupil persistently contracted, by the regular and constant instillation into the conjunctival sac night and morning of guttæ pilocarpinæ (B.P.C.) or physostigminæ (B.P.C.), but the latter may cause local irritation. Tab. dichlorphenamide (Daranide) 25–50 mg. given once, twice or thrice daily in conjunction with such miotics, is sometimes preferable to acetazolamide (Diamox); it has a relatively quick action and usually reduces intraocular tension in all types of glaucoma. Surgical treatment embraces a number of different measures and especially trephining.

§ **1111. Corneal Ulcers** cause a local lesion with localised redness.

Symptoms.—(i.) The eye is painful; (ii.) photophobia and blepharospasm are marked. (iii.) The eye waters freely. (iv.) The floor of the ulcer readily stains with fluorescein eye-drops (B.P.C.) and there may be an area of infiltration around the margins of the ulcer with corresponding cloudiness of the cornea. (v.) In severe cases there is a tendency to perforation of the cornea.

Etiology.—Primary ulcers are due to local trauma such as an abrasion, burn, foreign body or ingrowing eyelash. Secondary ulcers are the result of the same causes as produce conjunctivitis, and are much more common in debilitated persons. In either case infection may be present.

Treatment is by removing the cause when possible and by attending to the general health. Two-hourly drops containing neomycin sulphate and hydrocortisone are often effective. Sometimes local cauterisation is needed.

§ **1112. Episcleritis** signifies inflammation of the episcleral tissue which lies between the sclera and its conjunctival covering; nodules are usually seen with this.

Symptoms consist of inflammation and redness of a sector of the sclerotic, usually quite near the cornea. When the cornea is invaded the condition is called sclerosing keratitis. Discomfort, tenderness and watering are also present. The pupil and the vision are unaffected.

Etiology.—Systemic factors are believed to be causal, such as focal infection, articular rheumatism and sometimes tuberculosis or syphilis.

Treatment is by the regular use of hydrocortisone drops.

§ 1113. Subconjunctival Hæmorrhage may be localised, or massive and diffuse so that a part or the whole of the sclerotic is covered by dark red blood. The cornea and the iris are unaffected so that the sight and pupillary reactions are normal. The condition is painless.

Etiology.—Hæmorrhage is usually the result of trauma, but it may be due to spontaneous rupture of vessels in elderly persons who are healthy.

Treatment.—Reassurance is all that is needed.

§ 1114. II*b*. EXOPHTHALMOS (proptosis) is an undue prominence of one or both eyeballs and may be detected by standing behind the patient and looking down over the forehead. Apparent exophthalmos may be seen in high myopia.

. *Symptoms.*—The patient or the relatives notice the protrusion of the eyes, which may be more marked on one side than on the other. A white band of sclerotic is seen above and below the margins of the iris (Fig. 3). In severe cases double vision is also present, due to paresis of the extrinsic ocular muscles (ophthalmoplegia); the intrinsic muscles are not affected. Œdema of the eyelids may be seen; and when the eyelids cannot meet corneal ulceration is likely to occur.

Etiology.—Patients with *bilateral proptosis* fall into two groups. (1) EXOPHTHALMIC GOITRE (hyperthyroidism) is the commonest cause and the appearance of protrusion is usually aggravated by upper lid retraction. The exophthalmos is at least in part due to excess of fat which is deposited in the retro-orbital tissues and the extrinsic muscles. (2) In MALIGNANT EXOPHTHALMOS, a rare condition which may at first affect only one eye, this fatty change becomes extreme and is associated with lymphocytic infiltration and œdema so that the muscles become 5 to 10 times their normal size. Great weakness of the muscles (exophthalmic ophthalmoplegia) results. It often follows thyroidectomy or the drug treatment of hyperthyroidism, but in many cases the thyroid is not enlarged, and it usually occurs in patients who are euthyroid. Previously it was thought to be due to excess of circulating thyroid-stimulating hormone of the pituitary (TSH) but excess of TSH in the blood in myxœdema and in acromegaly is not accompanied by exophthalmos; also patients with malignant exophthalmos who are not hyperthyroid show no excess of circulating TSH. The condition may be due to some hormone from the anterior lobe of the pituitary other than TSH. *Unilateral proptosis* may be due (1) to the same causes as produce bilateral changes. Other causes are (2) Aneurysm or tumour in or behind the orbit, (3) Irritation of the Cervical Sympathetic in the neck or thorax, (4) Orbital cellulitis or periostitis, (5) Cavernous sinus thrombosis, (6) Facial asymmetry, and (7) Nasopharyngeal tumour.

Treatment is often disappointing. Small doses of thyroid with liq. iodi aquosus have been used to depress the formation of TSH and cortisone has been tried for its local and central action. The best results have been claimed by deep X-ray therapy to the orbits while shielding the eyeballs. Tarsorraphy is necessary if corneal ulceration is threatened and removal of the superior cervical ganglion of the sympathetic will allow ptosis of the upper lid. In severe cases decompression of the roof of the orbit may be necessary (Naffziger's operation).

ENOPHTHALMOS (Recession of the eyeballs) occurs in paralysis of the cervical sympathetic (Horner's syndrome), the other symptoms of which are pseudo-ptosis, narrowing of the ocular fissure, contraction of the pupil, loss of the cilio-spinal reflex

(reflex dilatation of the pupil when the skin of the neck is pinched) and absence of sweating over the face and the forequarter of the corresponding side.

§ 1115. IIc. THE EYELIDS are puffy in renal disease, cardiac dropsy, angioneurotic œdema, after violent coughing or vomiting, in eye-strain, arsenical poisoning, insect bites, trichinosis, frontal sinus suppuration, Graves' disease and mongolism. *Ptosis*, or drooping of the upper eyelid, may be partial or complete, and unilateral or bilateral. It is most commonly *congenital* and often familial in origin. When *acquired* it may be due to (i.) Paralysis of the unstriped muscle of Müller in the upper lid (cervical sympathetic palsy), (ii.) Paralysis of the striped levator palpebræ superioris muscle when it is part of an Oculomotor nerve palsy due to tabes, aneurysm in the cavernous sinus, encephalitis lethargica, herpes ophthalmicus and mid-brain tumour, (iii.) Ophthalmoplegic migraine, (iv.) Myopathy affecting the face, (v.) Myasthenia Gravis or (vi.) Hysteria. Ptosis is usually accompanied by a compensatory over-action of the frontalis muscle, except in myasthenia gravis (where the frontalis is also paralysed) and hysteria. *Blepharospasm* is an involuntary clonic twitching of the eyelid (§ 928). *Inability to close the eyelids*—Lagophthalmos— is due to weakness of the orbicularis oculi and is met with in Bell's (facial) palsy, myopathy and myasthenia gravis.

LAGGING BEHIND OF THE UPPER EYELIDS when the patient looks down constitutes Von Graefe's sign in exophthalmic goitre (see § 186). In *Lid Retraction* a band of white sclerotic is seen between the upper lid margin and the iris. In *Proptosis* a white band of sclerotic is also visible between the iris and the margin of the lower lid.

III. **Defects of Vision** may consist of (1) defective visual acuity, (2) alteration in the field of vision, (3) defective sense of colour.

§ 1116. (1) VISUAL ACUITY indicates (i.) an ability to appreciate light, and (ii.) an ability to recognise the form of objects. (i.) When vision is very defective it may not be possible to perceive light (" P.L.") from darkness, in which case the person tested is blind. The eyes must be examined separately, as a defect may have existed in one eye for a long time without the person knowing it. Such gross defects are tested by asking the patient to count the number of fingers (" C.F.") held up before him. If these are not recognised a hand is moved (" H.M.") in front of the eye being tested; if even this is not recognised a bright light is shone in front of the eye—failure to recognise this means total blindness in that eye. (ii.) The ability to recognise the form of objects depends on a normal transparency of the media, a normal retina and optic nerve, and on the ability to focus letters on the retina. The most sensitive part of the latter is the macula or " point of distinct-vision"; when only macular vision is lost the remainder of the retina can still appreciate light and movement, especially with weak illumination. By far the most common loss of a sense of form is due to an error of refraction. The *symptoms* which result are those of eye-strain. The protracted over-action of the intrinsic muscles of the eye is manifested by headache, Vth nerve neuralgia, eye-ache, blepharitis and styes, blinking (in children) and conjunctival hyperæmia.

TESTING ERRORS OF REFRACTION is undertaken by asking the patient to read letters on a chart at a given distance, testing each eye separately. *Snellen's test-types* are usually used at a distance of 6 metres, the card has one large letter at the top, with rows of letters of a progressively smaller size below; the healthy emmetropic eye should be able to read the letters in each row at a distance which is recorded under each line of letters. The visual acuity of the patient is recorded as a fraction, the numerator being the distance from the test card (6 metres) and the denominator the smallest line of letters which he can read. Thus if he can only read the top letters the fraction is $\frac{6}{60}$, but if he can read the bottom line of small print the vision is $\frac{6}{5}$. To ascertain the error of refraction, the ciliary muscle and iris are paralysed beforehand with homatropine, and then various lenses are placed in the trial spectacle frame until it is found which of them corrects the error. Convex lenses are indicated by the sign $+$, concave by the sign $-$ The defect is measured by the focal length of the lens required to correct the error, and is expressed in dioptres, indicated by the sign D. A lens of one dioptre has a focal length of 1 metre. Thus, a $+3$ D. lens indicates a convex lens with a focal length of $\frac{1}{3}$ metre, being three times as strong as a lens of $+1$ D. *Jaeger's Test Card* with print of different sizes, each on a separate line, is of great practical use in testing the visual acuity of each eye for near vision, but cannot be used in eye-testing to correct refractive errors.

Retinoscopy is a more accurate method of testing refractive errors. A plane mirror is used. No details of the fundus are visible in this way, but an evenly red field is seen—the red reflex. On tilting the mirror up and down or from side to side the red reflex will be found to move in the direction of the tilting in Hypermetropia and against the tilting in Myopia. In Hypermetropia this movement will be neutralised by a plus sphere of a power one dioptre more than the degree of Hypermetropia present, this difference being due to the fact that one works at a distance of one metre. Therefore, a movement in a patient with a Hypermetropia of 2 dioptres will be neutralised by a $+3$ D. lens and an Emmetrope will require a $+1$ D. lens to neutralise the movement. The use of a lens of a higher power will produce an artificial Myopia and therefore reverse the movement. No movement and no lens represents a Myopia of 1 dioptre, and neutralisation of movement against will be brought about by a lens 1 dioptre less powerful than the measure of the Myopia present. Similarly, the use of a minus lens of a higher power would produce an artificial Hypermetropia with reversed movement.

In astigmatism the reflex tends to be rectangular in shape and is neutralised by different lenses at opposite axes; the difference in power of the lenses is the measure of the patient's astigmatism.

The movement of the red reflex is accompanied by the movement of a shadow, and the movement of this shadow may be observed instead of following the reflex, but most observers find the latter to be the more satisfactory method.

Opacities in the media may be seen as dark shadows upon the red field. Thus the radiating streaks of commencing cataract or moving opacities in the vitreous are detected; the former stop moving when the movement of the eyeball ceases.

VARIETIES OF ERRORS OF REFRACTION. In *myopia* (or near sight) the image is formed in front of the retina, and the patient cannot see distant objects clearly. In *hypermetropia* (or far sight) the image is formed on a plane behind the retina, and the patient has to accommodate power-fully for near objects. Both may be due to defective shape of the globe. Concave lenses are used to correct myopia, and convex to correct hyper-metropia. In *presbyopia* the rigidity of the lens renders it either difficult or impossible to accommodate for near objects; it generally shows itself after the age of 45. The far vision of presbyopes may be good, though they cannot read or see near objects distinctly without convex glasses. *Astig-matism* is a non-correspondence of the curve in the principal meridians of the cornea, the curvature being similar to that of the bowl of a spoon. In *simple* astigmatism one meridian is myopic or hypermetropic; in *compound* astigmatism the error of the two meridians, though of the same kind, differs in degree; in *mixed* astigmatism there is a myopic error in one meridian, and a hypermetropic error in the other meridian; in *irregular astigmatism,* usually the result of scarring, the curves of the cornea vary even in the same meridian. Astigmatism is detected accurately by a skilled examination with retinoscopy, with the ophthalmometer or better still with a crossed cylinder.

Treatment.—When the lenses necessary to correct errors of refraction have been determined, the patient is fitted with lenses in a spectacle frame or with contact lenses. The latter are usually made of glass and are particularly useful in high myopes or when necessary for cosmetic reasons.

§ 1117. (2) THE FIELD OF VISION is the extent to which indistinct or peripheral vision can be seen by each eye while looking straight ahead. Within that field there is normally no vision in an area corresponding to the nerve head, producing a " blind spot "; in disease, other areas of local loss of vision are known as scotomata, *e.g.,* a central blind area in the middle of the field is known as a central scotoma.

Methods of Testing.—(1) The *confrontation method* is a rough method in common clinical use: it is described in § 841.

(2) The Perimeters in common use are those of Lister and Traquair; they give a much more accurate outline of the visual fields and enable a permanent chart to be constructed. Test objects of varying sizes and colours (1–60 mm. in diameter) and separate charts for the right and for the left eye will be required. One eye is covered with a shade and the patient places his chin on the chin-rest. He must keep his eye steadily fixed on the spot opposite, while the operator, by turning a handle, moves the test object along the arc of the perimeter from periphery to centre. The position at which the patient can first see the test object (while looking fixedly all the time at the central spot) is then marked on the chart by an automatic pricker (Figs. 260, 261). The perception of colours in the

peripheral field varies normally in extent with the different colours.   Thus, from without inwards they are seen in the following order : white, blue, yellow, red, green.   The perimeter is not sufficiently accurate for detecting minute central and paracentral scotomata, such as are met in retrobulbar neuritis and pituitary enlargements.

(3) The *Bjerrum's screen* is used only to map out such scotomata, and is of particular value in determining the arcuate scotomata of chronic glaucoma or in demonstrating any increase in the size of the blind spot. The screen consists of a large square of black cloth 2 metres wide with a central fixation spot.   With the chin support on a rest 2 metres away, a white test object 4 cm. wide is moved from the periphery to the centre along eight to twelve different meridians.   This is repeated using a 1-mm. or a 2-mm. object, again working from the periphery to the centre.   A permanent record can be made on a special chart (Fig. 259).

DEFECTS OF THE VISUAL FIELDS, producing peripheral field defects (Hemianopia) or central or paracentral scotomata, have been dealt with in § 1057.

(4) COLOUR VISION may be tested by matching coloured wools, by the Edridge Green lamp or by Ishihara test cards.   The lamp is used in Great Britain for testing the colour vision of engine drivers.

Colour blindness (achromatopsia) is a symptom in some diseases of the retina and also occurs in optic atrophy.   Red-green blindness as a congenital or familial deficiency is common: yellow-blue blindness is rare.   In tobacco blindness and in some other forms of retrobulbar neuritis, anything from minute scotomata for red and green to complete colour blindness may occur (§ 1129, Fig. 259).

§ 1118. Defective vision which is not due to errors of refraction (and therefore cannot be corrected by lenses) may be considered under 1. UNILATERAL BLINDNESS, 2. BILATERAL BLINDNESS, 3. NIGHT BLINDNESS and 4. DEFECTS OF THE VISUAL FIELDS.

AMBLYOPIA indicates diminished vision, usually without discoverable changes in the fundi; it usually refers to *amblyopia ex anopsia* which is found so frequently in an eye with an old squint.   It may also be functional, hysterical or due to some lesion of the visual paths.

1. UNILATERAL BLINDNESS may be rapid or gradual.

(a) *Rapid unilateral blindness* occurs in
   (i.) Retrobulbar Neuritis (§ 1129).
   (ii.) Thrombosis of the Central Retinal Vein (§ 1135).
   (iii.) Embolism or Spasm of the Central Retinal Artery (§ 1135).
   (iv.) Acute Glaucoma (§ 1110).
   (v.) Temporal Arteritis (§ 98).
   (vi.) Occlusion of the Internal Carotid Artery (§ 903).
   (vii.) Sudden Intraocular Hæmorrhage.
   (viii.) Detachment of the Retina (§ 1131).
   (ix.) Hysteria.

(b) *Gradual unilateral blindness* may result from
   (i.) Cataract (§ 1119).
   (ii.) Chronic Glaucoma (§ 1120).
   (iii.) Retrobulbar Neuritis (§ 1129).

(iv.) Tumour of or Pressure on the Optic Nerve (§ 1120).

(v.) Optic Atrophy (§ 1058).

(vi.) Local disease of the Choroid or Retina (Choroido-retinopathy) (§§ 1131–1140).

(vii.) Amblyopia ex anopsia (see above).

(viii.) Orbital Neoplasm.

(ix.) Unruptured Intracranial Aneurysm (§ 1047).

§ 1119. **A Cataract** is an opacity in the crystalline lens of one or both eyes.

Symptoms.—There is usually diminution or loss of vision. During the development of the opacity diplopia may occur. Usually the lens of one eye is first affected, but sooner or later both are likely to be involved. Especially in the young, the change may be non-progressive, but in the common senile form the lens of one or both sides ultimately develops a complete opacity and becomes grey or greyish-white in colour.

Diagnosis.—In the early stages the changes in the lens may be seen with the + 12 lens of the ophthalmoscope, but much more detail is obtained with the slit-lamp. The early opacities will be seen to occupy varying positions—subcapsular, cortical or central (nuclear). Subcapsular opacities which remain stationary often cause little damage to the sight, in marked contrast with the effect of nuclear changes.

Etiology.—A cataract is sometimes *congenital* or *juvenile*, in which case changes are seen in the development of the teeth and of other organs; in these patients there is often an inherited tendency. It also occurs in babies with congenital galactosæmia, those whose mothers have had rubella in the early months of pregnancy and premature babies who have been exposed to excess of oxygen in the incubator. *Acquired* disease may result from excessive exposure to brilliant sunlight, ultraviolet rays, radium or X rays, to chemical agents such as naphthalene, thallium and other occupational hazards and in hypoparathyroidism. A traumatic cataract follows a contusion or a penetrating wound of the eyeball; and irido-cyclitis is sometimes causal. The origin of the common " senile " type occurring after the age of 50 is unknown; it is more common in those with diabetes mellitus, especially if the patient is not properly stabilised.

Treatment.—No effective medical treatment is known. When the patient has been seen at an earlier stage and the retina found to be healthy, the best treatment is operative removal when the cataract is " ripe." If the patient is not seen until the opacity is well developed, a healthy retina is presumed when the position of a bright source of light projected from different positions is accurately localised by the affected eye. Before operation all carious teeth should be removed, the nasal sinuses examined and any infection of the lacrymal sac treated.

§ 1120. **Chronic Glaucoma** is rare before 40 years of age, but becomes increasingly common with advancing years. The severity of the condition may vary from time to time in the same patient.

Symptoms.—There may be attacks of unilateral frontal headache associated with blurring of vision; rainbow-coloured haloes may appear around lights with the blue colour next to the light. Ophthalmoscopic examination shows " cupping " or excavation of the optic disc so that the vessels are seen to bend abruptly over the margins of the disc. At this stage enlargement of the blind spot or a central scotomata are found when the visual fields are plotted on a Bjerrum's screen. Later there is marked pallor and atrophy of the nerve head, and the retina and its vessels also show atrophic changes.

Treatment is less urgent than for acute glaucoma but is on similar lines.

Infantile glaucoma or *buphthalmos*, fortunately rare, is due to faulty development of the angle of the anterior chamber with poor excretion and increased tension: the globe enlarges as the pressure increases. Trephining offers the only hope, but the prognosis is bad.

Optic Nerve Compression from tumours or aneurysms rarely causes sudden visual failure, but may do so by invading or compressing the ophthalmic artery.

2. BILATERAL DETERIORATION OF SIGHT OR BLINDNESS may also be *rapid* or *gradual*.

(a) *Rapid bilateral blindness* may occur in
- (i.) Faints or " blackouts " including those of aerobatics (§ 832).⎫
- (ii.) Migraine (§ 812) ⎬temporary.
- (iii.) Exposure to glare ⎭
- (iv.) Insulin hypoglycæmia (§ 425).
- (v.) Uræmia (§§ 370–372).
- (vi.) Toxic Amblyopia (§ 1122).
- (vii.) Local cerebral trauma to the calcarine cortex and occipital lobes (§ 790).
- (viii.) Sudden copious hæmorrhage as from the stomach, duodenum or uterus.
- (ix.) Acute Methyl Alcohol poisoning, by ingestion (§ 1184) or by inhalation.
- (x.) Optic Nerve Compression.
- (xi.) Neuromyelitis optica (§ 1121).
- (xii.) Leber's Hereditary Optic Atrophy (§ 1058a).
- (xiii.) Hysteria (§ 1173).

(b) *Gradual bilateral blindness* may be due to
- (i.) Cataract (§ 1119).
- (ii.) Chronic Glaucoma (§ 1120).
- (iii.) Tobacco Amblyopia (§ 1122).
- (iv.) Toxic Amblyopia (§ 1122).
- (v.) Senile Macular Degeneration (§ 1138).
- (vi.) Local disease of the Retina (§ 1131 *et seq.*) or of the Optic Nerve (Optic Atrophy) (§ 1058).
- (vii.) Pituitary Tumour or Suprasellar Cyst (§ 1046).
- (viii.) Amaurotic Family Idiocy (§ 1194).
- (ix.) Schilder's disease (§ 1194).
- (x.) Leber's Hereditary Optic Atrophy (§ 1058a).
- (xi.) Optic Nerve Compression.
- (xii.) Hysteria (§ 1173).
- (xiii.) In prematuie infants the commonest cause is Retrolental Fibroplasia in one or both eyes due to prolonged use of oxygen for resuscitation.

Faints or " blackouts " are usually vaso-vagal in origin (§§ 35, 833) and cause temporary cerebral ischæmia. Air pilots performing aerobatic steep turns at high speeds, or pulling out abruptly after a steep dive, may get transient visual failure due to similar retinal or cerebral ischæmia.

Exposure to glare of snow or direct sunlight may cause temporary blindness unless dark glasses are worn.

§ 1121. Neuromyelitis Optica (Devic's Disease) begins acutely with bilateral blindness or dimness of vision (due to bilateral retrobulbar neuritis) and acute paraplegia. The paraplegia may precede the visual loss. In the most severe cases the paralysis spreads rapidly. The spinal fluid may show pleocytosis (200 lymphocytes per c.mm.) and the protein increase may be marked (160 mg. per cent.). The E.S.R. is raised. In other cases the vision returns and the patient improves, usually with a permanent paraplegia, perhaps with residual fits and defective vision. *Etiology.* —In fatal cases a necrotising myelitis is found, with scattered demyelination, especially marked in the cervical cord. The lesions resemble those of disseminated sclerosis. *Prognosis.*—Rapid progression of the symptoms is a bad sign. In the majority of cases partial recovery occurs. *Treatment.*—Prednisone, blood transfusions, etc., have no certain effect on the illness, but are worth a trial.

§ 1122. Tobacco Amblyopia is often accompanied by Chronic Alcoholic Poisoning. The former occurs sometimes in hard smokers of over three or four ounces per week, or in debilitated persons and in women from a smaller quantity. In both tobacco and alcoholic cases the patient first complains of defective vision in bright light; he sees better at dusk than at noon and mistakes silver for copper coins. The defect is slowly progressive, becoming most marked in the *central* field, and there is a central colour scotoma, especially for red and green (Fig. 259). At first there may be no changes in the fundi, then the discs become slightly congested in the earlier stages, and pale and atrophied, especially on the temporal side, in the later stages. Defective vision is the earliest symptom to attract the patient's notice. It arises from a chronic retrobulbar neuritis. The pupil reaction, both in chronic and acute retrobulbar neuritis, is characteristic. The pupil contracts normally to light, but does not remain contracted under the same light stimulus and rapidly dilates.

Treatment consists of total abstention from tobacco and from alcohol. Vitamin B complex and vaso-dilator drugs have been used.

Toxic Amblyopia is exemplified in uræmia and diabetes (§§ 370, 423). It may also be produced by large doses of quinine, carbon bisulphide, trichlorethylene, chloroquine and tryparsamide. *Treatment.*—Unless seen early, when removal of the cause and functional rest to the eye may lead to recovery, little can be done to help.

HYSTERICAL BLINDNESS was seen in " shell-shock " of the First World War. In civil practice it is very rare. Reference has been made to its concentrically constricted or " spiral " fields of vision. The diagnosis of hysterical blindness should never be made unless with the help of a highly skilled ophthalmologist. Normal fundi and reactive pupils occur with organic cortical blindness, *e.g.*, in disease of the posterior cerebral arteries, Schilder's disease and after occipital lobe trauma.

§ 1123. 3. NIGHT BLINDNESS (hemeralopia) is defective vision in dim lights. Dark adaptation is mainly due to visual purple (rhodopsin) in the rods of the retina. Although the macula is responsible for vision in bright lights it is less sensitive than the rest of the retina in a dim light. Night blindness is a feature of (i.) retinitis pigmentosa in particular. Rare causes are (ii.) congenital deficiency of rods, (iii.) xerophthalmia in which there is severe deficiency of vitamin A, (iv.) syphilitic retinitis and (v.) hysteria. Night vision is particularly important for night-flying and is aided by wearing red goggles before " taking off." It may be estimated by a special instrument known as an adaptometer. Improvement of function may be influenced by the generous administration of vitamins A, B and C.

§ 1124. Ocular Movements.—When there is *recent* weakness or paralysis of one or more of the external muscles of the eyeball the patient becomes very conscious of double vision (diplopia, § 1061). This also produces an erroneous projection, *i.e.*, an error in judging the position of objects, and vertigo. It is important to be able to detect which muscles are involved.

Deficient movement of the eyeball				*Indicates paralysis of*
outwards	..	..	..	.. lateral rectus—sixth nerve.
inwards	..	..	..	.. medial rectus—third nerve.
upwards	..	..	..	$\begin{cases} superior \text{ rectus} \\ inferior \text{ oblique} \end{cases}$ third nerve.
downwards	..	..	..	$\begin{cases} inferior \text{ rectus—third nerve.} \\ superior \text{ oblique—fourth nerve.} \end{cases}$

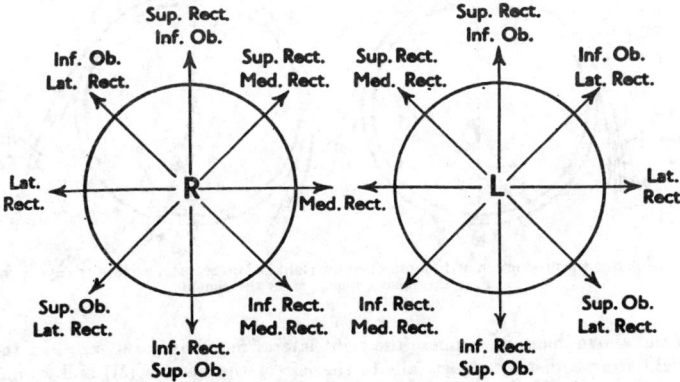

FIG. 264.—Diagram showing muscles concerned in ocular movements. Lateral movements—one muscle. Vertical and oblique movements—two muscles.

Method of Detecting the Affected Eye and Paralysed Muscle.—Place a red glass before the patient's right eye, and hold a small source of light before him in a dark room, on a level with his eyes at 2 yards distance. Suppose that it is found that the red image overlaps, or is a little to the right of the white image, and both images are on the same level, to determine which muscle is affected the light must be moved to the left and to the right, and we must notice *in which direction the distance between the images becomes increased*. On moving the light to the left the images approach till only one light is seen and, on moving to the right, the distance between the true and false images increases. Bearing in mind the rule that the weakened muscle is on the same side as the direction in which diplopia increases, it is evident that either the right external rectus or the left internal rectus is affected. Ask then on which side the red image appears. If on the right of the white image, homonymous diplopia is present; therefore the right *external* rectus is the paralysed muscle. If, however, the red image is to the left of the white image, crossed diplopia is present; therefore the left *internal* rectus is the paralysed muscle. The reason is that the movement of the eye with the paralysed muscle is arrested whereas the other continues to follow the light and sees it where it actually is; this is the true image. The affected eye, however, places the light where it appears to be in relation to the visual axis of that eye; this is the false image (Fig. 265). Paralysis of the superior or inferior rectus, and of the superior or inferior oblique, gives rise to vertical diplopia. The former causes crossed diplopia, the latter homonymous diplopia. Loss of motion upwards is due to paralysis of the third nerve; loss of motion downwards may be due to paralysis of the inferior rectus (third nerve) or the superior oblique (fourth nerve). Diplopia occurs when, due to a paralysed muscle, an eye fails to move fully in the direction intended. The subject is not aware of the lack of movement and thus makes a faulty estimate of the disposition in space of the object of regard.   The separation of the two images in diplopia is maximal when the eyes are looking in the direction of action of the paralysed muscle and the false image is shifted in the direction of action of the paralysed muscle.   This means that it is always the furthest *out* in a horizontal diplopia, the furthest *up* in a diplopia occurring in upward gaze and the furthest *down* in a diplopia occurring in downward gaze.

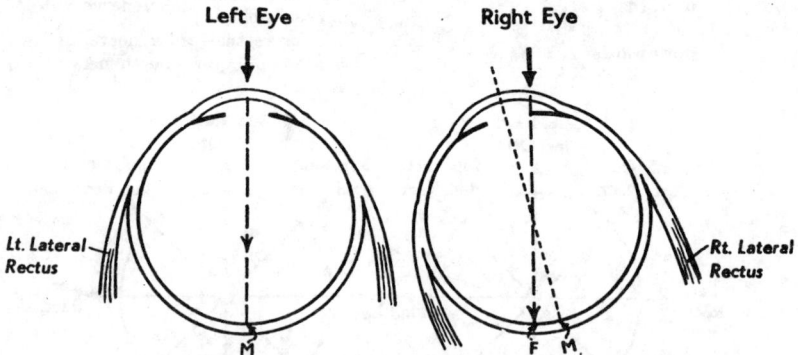

Fig. 265.—Shows the production of diplopia when the right lateral rectus muscle of the eye is paralysed. F is the false image. M is the macula.

In the above diagram, suppose the right lateral rectus is paralysed.   In the right eye, light from a distant object falls to the left of the macula (M) and stimulates a point on its retina (F).   The subject is unaware that the eye is deviated and thinks the object is in the position indicated (F).   Therefore the false image is projected to the right half of the visual field, *i.e.*, in the direction of action of the paralysed muscle.

§ 1125. **Squint** or strabismus is a want of parallelism between the visual axes when looking at a distant object.   It is called *convergent* when one eyeball looks inwards and *divergent* when one eyeball looks outwards. In *children* it is chiefly associated with some error of refraction—hypermetropia (internal strabismus, the commonest in children), or myopia (external strabismus).   In many cases the patient or a parent is left-handed : the refractive error may be small and a psychological factor may be of great importance.   In adults or children, squint of recent acute origin is due to definite paralysis of an ocular nerve (§§ 1061–1071).

Clinical Investigation of Squint.—There are three steps.   (1) Diagnosis of the Type of Squint, (2) Diagnosis of the Affected Muscle, (3) Diagnosis of the Position of the Lesion and its cause.

(1) Diagnosis of the Type of Squint.—Squints are of three kinds: (A) Concomitant, (B) Alternating and (C) Paralytic.

(A) *Concomitant Squint* is met with most frequently in children.   (i.) It comes on slowly.   (ii.) Each eye, when the other is covered, moves perfectly in all directions, there being no paralysis but, when examined together, the squint is present in all positions of the eyeball.   (iii.) Spontaneous diplopia is absent.   (iv.) The affected eye follows the sound eye with equal defect in all directions (hence the name " concomitant "), so that the defect of parallelism is the same in all directions. It is due, in about 90 per cent. of cases, to hypermetropia or other error of refraction, or to a defect in the fusion faculty.

(B) *Alternating Squints* are nearly always associated with left-handedness in the patient or family, and sometimes with stammering.

(C) *Paralytic Squint* is met in children or adults. (i.) It usually appears suddenly. (ii.) It is always accompanied by double vision. (iii.) There is limitation of movement of the globe corresponding to the direction of traction of the paralysed muscle. Paralytic squints are due to ocular paralyses resulting from intracranial or other serious mischief and are described in § 1061 *et seq.*

(2) DIAGNOSIS OF THE AFFECTED MUSCLE.—In *Paralytic Squint* the affected muscles *can usually be recognised by simply testing the external ocular movements as described* in § 841.

In cases of slighter weakness, and in *Concomitant Squint*, tell the patient to look at an object straight in front of him, that being the normal position of the eyes at rest, and fix some object. The eye with which he fixes is the normal eye. The deviation of the affected eye from the middle line is known as the " primary deviation." Now partially cover the sound eye and let him fix with the affected eye. The sound eye will now be found to deviate (" secondary deviation "). In concomitant squint the primary and secondary deviations are equal, but in paralytic squint, the secondary exceeds the primary. The patient unconsciously turns his face *towards the side of the weak or paralysed muscle.*

Treatment of Squint.—In concomitant squint the visual refractive error is corrected, and afterwards attempts are made to develop binocular vision by orthoptic training—with special exercises to promote fusion and increased amplitude of movement. In paralytic squint, to relieve diplopia, the false image should be excluded by covering the affected eye; but the cause must always be looked for and treated.

MONOCULAR DIPLOPIA is recognised by the persistence of diplopia when one eye is closed. It is met in (i.) Hysteria and in (ii.) Malingering. (iii.) It may arise from defects of the media, *e.g.*, a developing cataract, or with vitreous opacities.

§ 1126. The Ocular Fundi are best examined by an electric ophthalmoscope.

Taking each eye in turn, commence with a + 12 lens in the aperture and examine with its aid the cornea, aqueous and lens; by rotating the battery of lenses to a lower number of dioptres any opacities in the vitreous can be noted and when the fundus comes into focus the number of the lens in the aperture should be observed. This gives a rough measure of the refraction of the eye. Estimation of visual acuity without a knowledge of the patient's refraction is bound to mislead.

When the fundus is in focus, first the purple red retina and then the optic disc are seen. The disc represents the entrance of the optic nerve in the centre of which is the physiological cup-like depression. The disc is circular or slightly oval with a clearly defined border, especially at the outer edge; it appears oval and may appear partly out of focus in astigmatic eyes. The colour of the disc is a paler red than the rest of the fundus. The central artery and vein enter and leave the eye in the middle of the disc; the artery divides almost immediately into upper and lower nasal and upper and lower temporal branches, the veins running along with the arteries; normally the arteries are narrower (two-thirds) than the veins, are a trifle paler, and have a broader and more continuous light stripe (" central light reflex ") running along the middle. Whereas the optic disc is incapable of receiving light impulses and forms

C.M.—X X

the blind-spot, the macula lutea and its most central part, the fovea centralis, are the areas of most distinct vision. The macula lies exactly at the posterior pole of the eye, at a distance about twice the width of the optic disc to the outer side of the disc; it has a pale yellow colour and the fovea is devoid of all blood vessels.

ABNORMALITIES IN THE FUNDI.—(a) *Physiological Variations.* Opaque white fibres are seen to spread out from the margins of the disc in a fan-shaped manner when the medullated sheaths covering the nerve fibres continue for a distance into the substance of the retina. In others the margin of the disc is partially surrounded by a black ring of choroidal pigment. Neither of these conditions interfere with vision.

(b) *In Disease* the ophthalmoscopic examination of each eye should be directed in succession to (i.) changes in the optic disc, (ii.) the colour of the retina and the presence of hæmorrhages, exudates and abnormal pigmentation, (iii.) the condition of the retinal arteries and veins and (iv.) abnormalities in and around the macula.

(i.) *Optic disc.* The *level* of the disc is important, but a little difficult to gauge. If when using the ophthalmoscope, the surrounding *retina* can be seen clearly without the aid of any lens placed in the mirror hole, but the *disc* cannot be seen clearly without the aid of the lens, it must be at a different level. If a weak — lens is necessary to see the disc under these circumstances, then the disc must evidently be behind the retinal level (cupping). If, on the other hand, a weak + lens is necessary, then the disc is on a level anterior to the retina (swelling). One can gauge the amount of swelling or cupping in this way, for roughly each 3 D. = 1 mm. of swelling or cupping. Thus, supposing it is necessary to use + 1 D. to focus the retinal vessels precisely, and + 4 D. to focus the disc, then there must be 3 D. or 1 mm. swelling. This is an accurate method of measuring, provided the observer is able to *relax his own accommodation thoroughly.* The *edge* of the disc is normally clearly defined, but is obscured when there is œdema of the papilla (papillœdema). The *colour* of the disc becomes greyish-white or a china-white colour in optic atrophy.

(ii.) *Retina.* The colour becomes uniformly pale in anæmia. *Hæmorrhages* vary greatly in size and shape; they may appear as small red spots when more superficial or as larger flame-shaped hæmorrhages when they spread out in the direction of the nerve fibres. Massive hæmorrhages in the region of the macula, in the subhyaloid space anterior to the retina (subhyaloid hæmorrhage), are characteristic of a subarachnoid hæmorrhage. Retinal hæmorrhages occur in a great variety of conditions including (a) blood diseases and especially acute leukæmia, aplastic anæmia, pernicious anæmia and thrombocytopenia, (b) toxic conditions such as chronic nephritis, uræmia and diabetes mellitus, (c) severe and especially malignant hypertension. *Exudates* also vary greatly in size and may be as large as the disc. They are either greyish-white or almost pure white in colour and may have clearly defined edges or give a " cotton-wool " appearance. They are found in chronic nephritis, when they often assume a radiating or star shape around the macula, in diabetes mellitus, arteriosclerosis, papillœdema, syphilitic and non-syphilitic chorio-retinitis. Widespread scarring is seen in long-standing retinal detachment. *Pigmentary changes* are seen when black pigment granules are carried through a degenerate retina by phagocytes. This occurs with choroidal degeneration, uveitis, macular degeneration, retinal detachment and in retinitis pigmentosa.

(iii.) The *Retinal Arteries and Veins* give a clue to many diseases which also affect other areas of the body. The *arteries* sometimes pulsate in raised intraocular pressure and in aortic regurgitation. They are uniformly narrowed in optic atrophy and in retinitis pigmentosa. Irregular narrowing and tortuosity of the arteries with kinking and nipping of the veins at the arterio-venous crossings are characteristic of arteriosclerosis. In more advanced cases the arteries become "copper-wired" or "silver-wired" due to an increased reflection of light from the middle of the vessel wall, and still later small hæmorrhages and hard exudates appear, especially around the macula. A general narrowing of the arteries with areas which appear to be in spasm is characteristic of the early stages of hypertension (and see § 1134). Occlusion of a main artery or vein of the retina produces characteristic changes (§ 1135). The veins are engorged in the early stages of increased intracranial pressure, and become plum-coloured and wider in polycythæmia.

(iv.) The *macular area* is particularly prone to damage. Exudates and hæmorrhages are especially liable to occur with diseases of the blood vessels (*vide supra*), and temporary local œdema may follow a direct injury to the eye. Degeneration of the macula can also follow such an injury, but is more common with arteriosclerosis. A cherry-red spot is seen at the macula in sudden arterial occlusion, and in children with amaurotic family idiocy (Tay-Sachs disease) and in Niemann Pick disease.

(v.) *Other changes in the retina and choroid* which are distinctive include (i.) the various types of Retinopathy (§ 1132 *et seq.*); (ii.) Retinal detachment (§ 1131); (iii.) Acute and chronic tuberculosis (§ 1137); (iv.) Atrophic patches in the choroid.

Examination of the Ocular Fundi will reveal the following conditions:—
  I. Papillœdema (§ 1127).
  II. Optic Neuritis (§ 1128) (*i.e.*, Retrobulbar Neuritis and Optic Papillitis).
  III. Optic Atrophy (§ 1058): and Leber's Hereditary Optic Atrophy (§ 1058a).
  IV. Detachment of the Retina (§ 1131).
  V. Retinopathy, especially (*a*) Albuminuric Retinopathy (§ 1132).
                            (*b*) Diabetic Retinopathy (§ 1133).
                            (*c*) Hypertensive Retinopathy (§ 1134).
                            (*d*) Occlusion of a main Artery or Vein (§ 1135).
                            (*e*) Various Septic and Toxic states (§ 1136).
                            (*f*) Acute and Chronic Tuberculosis (§ 1137).
  VI. Senile Macular Degeneration (§ 1138).
  VII. Retinitis Pigmentosa (§ 1139).
  VIII. Choroiditis Disseminata; Atrophic patches in the choroid (§ 1140).

§ 1127. I. **Papillœdema** is œdema of the optic nerve head (or "papilla") as it enters the globe. At first the main retinal veins become engorged and the disc reddened by increased vascularity; in this early stage the upper nasal edge of the disc soon becomes blurred and develops a fluffy look. Then the physiological cup is filled up, the entire edge of the disc becomes œdematous, the arteries become narrower and the veins still further engorged and tortuous; continuity of the vessels disappears as they curve over the œdematous edge. Later the retina surrounding the edges of the disc becomes spattered with small hæmorrhages (Plate XXi. 4). These œdematous changes may gradually subside or may advance to consecutive atrophy (Plate XXII. 6).

Even when papillœdema is marked *the acuity of vision may be undisturbed*, except for occasional dimming (" Obscurations "), though the visual field may show enlargement of the blind spot. Disturbance of vision generally becomes more marked as the acute stage subsides. In severe papillœdema visual failure may occur with catastrophic rapidity; the vision may be saved in such cases by subtemporal decompression; this should not be delayed, even if the cause is not evident. In papillœdema with preservation of vision, the pupils react to light. BILATERAL PAPILLŒDEMA is especially common in : (i.) *Intracranial neoplasm* in which it is present at some stage in 85 per cent. of cases. It is especially common in cerebellar tumour but is rare in cerebral hæmorrhage and embolism. (ii.) *Increase of pressure from other causes—e.g.*, malignant hypertension, subarachnoid hæmorrhage, toxic encephalopathy or after a head injury. It is uncommon in acute meningitis; venous hypertension in pulmonary emphysema, temporal arteritis and acute syphilitic hydrocephalus are rare causes. UNILATERAL PAPILLŒDEMA may indicate disease (i.) in the orbit, from malignant exophthalmos, thrombosis of the central retinal vein, periarteritis nodosa, orbital tumour; or (ii.) behind the orbital fissure from paranasal sinus infections, cavernous sinus thrombosis, aneurysm of the internal carotid artery.

§ 1128. II. **Optic Neuritis** may develop in any part of the optic nerve and is usually associated with loss of visual acuity and a central scotoma. The condition is clinically recognisable in two forms: (i.) The disease most commonly affects the nerve behind the optic disc and is then known as *Retrobulbar Neuritis*. (ii.) More rarely the nerve-head is involved by inflammation—*Papillitis*; this is more chronic and leads to visual failure.

§ 1129. (i.) **Retrobulbar Neuritis** (Syn. Acute Optic Neuritis) is much more commonly due to a patch of demyelination than to inflammation.

Symptoms are : (1) Sudden visual failure particularly affecting macular (central) vision. (2) Retro-orbital or temporal pain and tenderness of the eyeball. (3) A central or paracentral area of complete or relative blindness (often complete for colours). (4) The pupil may be slightly dilated. While a beam of light is held focused upon it the pupil contracts, stays contracted for a second, and then dilates again in a jerky fashion (the " neuritic reaction "). The consensual light reflex and the pupillary reaction to accommodation are normal. (5) If the lesion is near the

PLATE XX

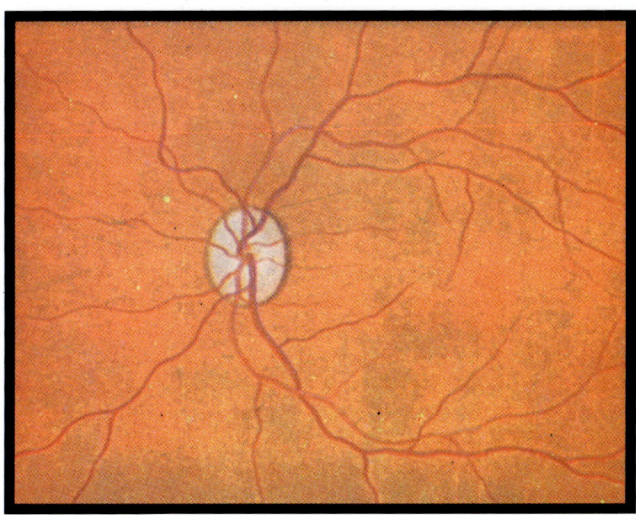

1. NORMAL.

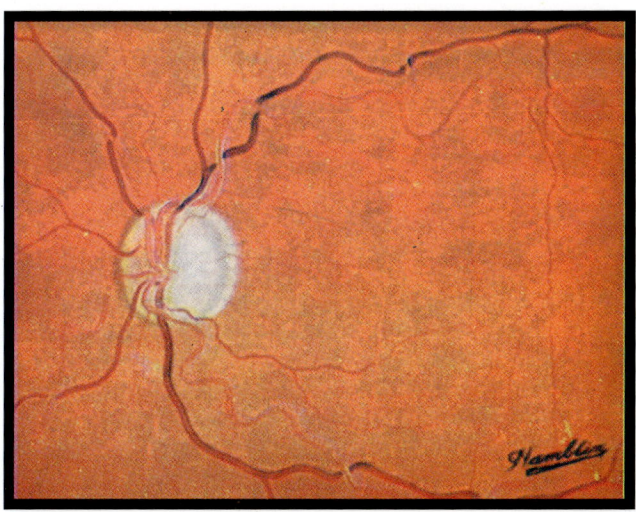

2. ARTERIOSCLEROSIS.

Arteries tortuous and irregularly narrowed, with light reflex marked, and loss of transparency. Veins kinked and their course deviated where crossed by arteries.

PLATE XXI

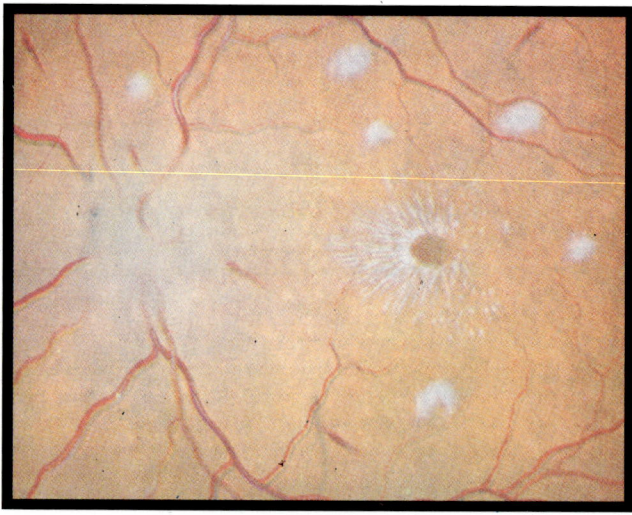

3. CHRONIC NEPHRITIS.
Later stage.
Disc—Swollen and margin blurred. Macula—Radiating lines of white dots resembling the Star of India. Fundus—Flame-shaped haemorrhages disposed radially to the disc; White woolly patches.

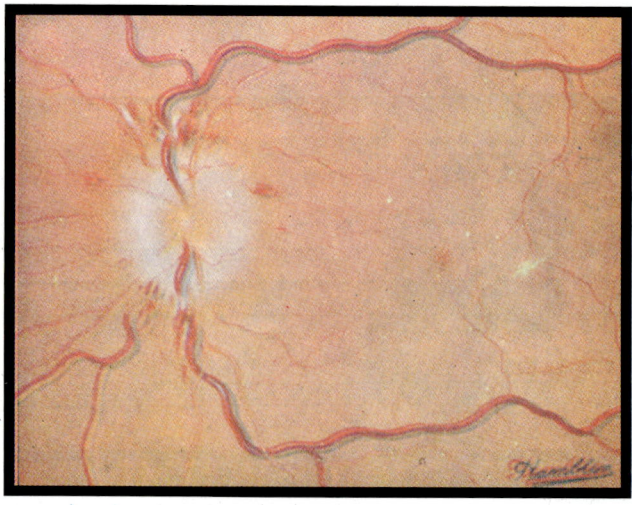

4. PAPILLOEDEMA.
Mushroom-like swellings of disc with blurring of margins due to lymphatic stasis; engorgement of veins. Vessels bent by swelling and partly covered up. Haemorrhages variable. No loss of visual acuity in early stages.

PLATE XXII

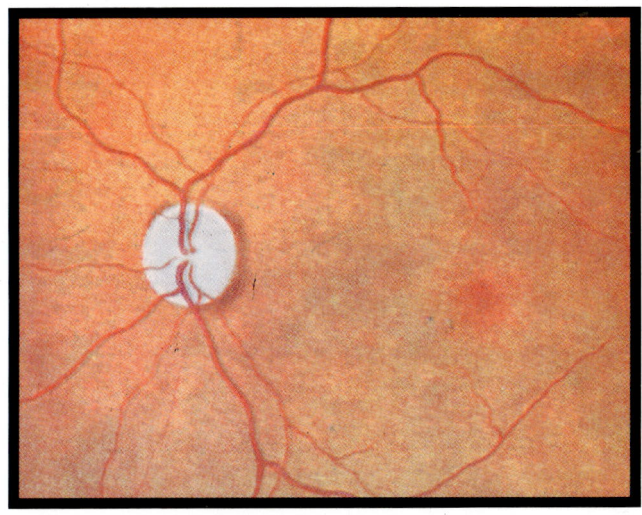

5. PRIMARY OPTIC ATROPHY.
Clear cut blue white disc with fine vessels.

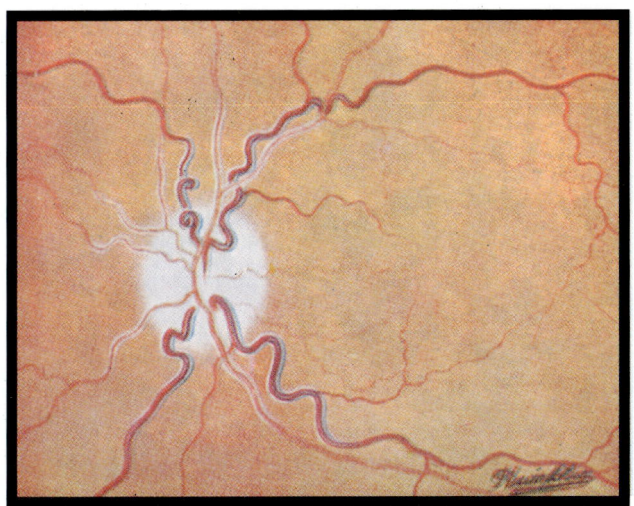

6. SECONDARY OPTIC ATROPHY.
White disc blurred by deposition of fibrous tissue which may extend along the vessels, giving them a fibrous sheath. Tortuosity of vessels near disc.

nerve-head the optic disc may be swollen (papillitis). Later, when the effects subside, the temporal half of the disc is paler than the rest (" temporal pallor "), and there may be a central or cæco-central scotoma, especially for colours. The C.S.F. during the active stage shows a mild lymphocytic reaction in many cases. *Causes :* UNILATERAL RETROBULBAR NEURITIS : (1) In a young adult the commonest cause is disseminated sclerosis. In about a third of the cases it is the first symptom of the disease and, whilst usually unilateral, one eye may be affected after the other. Do not, however, diagnose this disease until evidence of multiple lesions is present. (2) Less common causes are suppurative disease of the para-nasal sinuses, and pressure on the macular fibres from a pituitary tumour   v : 1 behind the sphenoidal fissure. X-rays of the pituitary fossa, nasal accessory sinuses and a blood Wasserman reaction will be necessary. BILATERAL RETROBULBAR NEURITIS may occur in neuro-myelitis optica (§ 1121) and other demyelinating diseases (§ 952); nutritional neuropathies in prisoner-of-war camps (§ 981); pernicious and other severe anæmias; diabetes; and as a result of poisoning from quinine or tobacco, combined with alcoholic excess. Syphilis is a rare cause. In Leber's hereditary optic atrophy (§ 1058a) there is a family history of visual failure in middle life. For Toxic Amblyopia see § 1122.

Thus, the cause may be (1) demyelinating, (2) inflammatory or (3) due to selective axon degeneration in toxæmia.

Prognosis.—When confined to one eye the vision gradually clears in a few weeks and the scotoma disappears, leaving the disc pale but with normal visual acuity. In a few cases vision is permanently affected and a scotoma persists. In poisoning by methyl alcohol and in Leber's hereditary optic atrophy the vision is seriously and permanently affected.

Treatment is by resting the eye with a shade for some weeks. Prednisolone 10 mg. may be given twice daily for a week at the onset.

§ 1130. (ii.) **Papillitis** is a condition similar to retrobulbar neuritis but the optic papilla is much swollen, reddened, with blurred edges and there is a central scotoma. It occurs in lead poisoning and methyl bromide intoxication and, if this diagnosis is proved, the neuritis if severe should be treated by subtemporal decompression. It occurs also in renal disease and in intracranial inflammation, *e.g.*, meningitis, sinusitis, abscess, syphilis.

POST-NEURITIC (SECONDARY) ATROPHY.—The disc edges are blurred and there are pigmentary disturbances around the margin. The physiological pit is filled up with exudate and this tends to hide the lamina cribrosa. The vessels are sheathed in fibrous tissue and narrowed. The amount of visual failure depends on the severity of the primary lesion. Blindness may be complete. It is seen after optic neuritis in expanding intracranial lesions, and after attacks of hypertensive encephalopathy.

§ 1131. (IV) **Detachment of the Retina** is in most cases accompanied by a hole in the retina.

Symptoms consist of a rapid diminution or loss of vision in the affected eye. These are sometimes preceded by flashes of light, transient attacks of decreased vision or by floating specks in front of the eye. Detailed examination of the retina can only be undertaken after full dilatation of the pupil; a crescentic tear is the most frequent, and the hole in the retina is accompanied by a devascularised area which gives a greyish-red colour to the surrounding retina. Numerous floating vitreous opacities are usually present.

Etiology.—The cause may not be found. Those recognisable are (i.) previous trauma, particularly in those with high myopia; (ii.) extensive areas of inflammation, especially with œdema of the choroid; (iii.) intra-ocular growths. A solid detachment due to a new growth may be accompanied by a fluid detachment; (iv.) conditions which cause contraction of the vitreous.

Treatment involves the production of an adhesive choroiditis around the hole by means of coagulation or perforating diathermy, electrolysis or a combination of these coupled with evacuation of the subretinal fluid. Detachment complicating inflammation is not suitable for such treatment.

§ 1132. (V*a*) **Albuminuric Retinopathy** may occur in any form of renal disease, but is most frequently associated with chronic nephritis. The changes are fourfold : (i.) Œdema which commences at the margins of the disc and later may involve the whole disc (papillœdema); (ii.) hæmorrhages into the retina, usually flame-shaped and most plentiful around the disc or near the vessels; (iii.) small or large cotton-wool patches with fluffy margins; and (iv.) usually at a later stage, white shiny spots with a sharp outline which are usually most marked around the macula, often in a star-shaped formation. One or other of these features is sometimes missing, but in its typical form this kind of retinopathy is sufficiently characteristic to diagnose renal disease before examining the urine. In the elderly the changes of arteriosclerosis are also often present. Albuminuric retinopathy is of grave significance, the patient seldom surviving more than twelve months after its appearance; albuminuric retinopathy of pregnancy is an exception to this, recovery often following parturition.

§ 1133. (V*b*) **Diabetic Retinopathy.**—Apart from the arteriosclerotic changes found in the retina of elderly diabetics distinctive changes are liable to occur in adults of all ages. The disc usually appears normal but optic atrophy can occur. Hæmorrhages may be numerous, deep in the retina and round or irregular. A characteristic feature of diabetic retinopathy is the presence of small red dots scattered over the posterior pole of the retina due to micro-aneurysms of the capillaries. Sausage-like dilatation of the veins may be seen. Diabetic exudates are white and sharply defined, like pieces of china, or are sometimes yellowish. In uncontrolled diabetics the larger hæmorrhages in the retina may become adherent to the vitreous, and as they become organised they develop bands of fibrous tissue and new blood vessels which pull on and detach the retina (*Retinitis proliferans*).

§ **1134.** (V*c*) **Hypertensive Retinopathy** indicates the changes found in both eyes in the varying grades of hypertension. Keith and Wagener's four stages form a useful method of classification. (i.) Grade I changes are seen in the early stages of benign hypertension. The arteries are narrowed, rather tortuous and show areas of constant " spasm " producing a thread-like appearance. (ii.) In Grade II these changes are more marked and at the arterio-venous crossings the arteries distort and nip the veins as they cross in front of them. (iii.) In Grade III there are superficial flame-shaped hæmorrhages and deeper small hæmorrhages associated with fluffy " cotton wool " and harder pale grey exudates. All these are more marked at the posterior poles of the eyes and around the maculæ. (iv.) In Grade IV where papillœdema is present the picture is that of malignant hypertension.

§ **1135.** (V*d*) **Occlusion of a Main Artery or Vein.**—*Arterial occlusion* occurs with an embolus in auricular fibrillation or infective endocarditis, and a thrombosis in vascular sclerosis due to atheroma, temporal arteritis, syphilitic endarteritis and internal carotid thrombosis. Occlusion of the central artery causes sudden blindness with a pale œdematous retina; the arteries are emptied of blood and become very narrow, but the veins are little affected. On the other hand the macula shows up as a cherry-red spot surrounded by a large pale area. After several weeks the retinal appearances may become more normal although the vessels remain small and the disc pale. Occlusion of a branch of the central artery produces similar changes confined to the distribution of the affected vessel. *Venous occlusion* of the central vein causes great distension and tortuosity of the veins distal to the block. The engorged capillaries rupture, producing masses of small and medium-sized hæmorrhages; exudates appear and the margins of the optic disc become swollen, indistinct or lost. Thrombosis of a branch of the main vein produces similar changes in the area of its tributaries. Gradually the thrombus canalises, permitting absorption of the hæmorrhages and exudates, but when one of the temporal veins has been occluded central vision is likely to be permanently decreased. The other eye may be involved later. The majority of cases occur in those with arteriosclerosis.

§ 1136. (V*e*). In **Various Septic and Toxic States,** arising from focal infection in the teeth, tonsils, nasal sinuses and other areas, papillœdema and retinal degeneration are found. The changes are due to the toxins produced or may be the result of bacteræmia or septicæmia. The picture depends on the stage at which the examination takes place, the age of the patient and on the condition of the blood vessels at the time of onset of the retinal disease.

§ 1137. (V*f*). **Miliary tuberculosis** can be identified by pale yellow slightly raised areas in the choroid comparable to those found in the lungs and elsewhere. The CHRONIC FORM of tuberculosis bears some resemblance to the disseminated choroiditis of syphilis.

§ 1138. (VI). **Senile Macular Degeneration** occurs in elderly persons with arterio-sclerosis. Fairly sudden loss of central vision occurs first in one eye and often in the other. The ophthalmoscope reveals pigmentary changes at the macula; there may also be exudates through diseased capillaries.

§ 1139. (VII) **Retinitis Pigmentosa** is frequently inherited and consanguinity is often present. It affects both eyes in childhood and may involve several members of the same family. The chief *Symptom* is night blindness; later, vision in daylight is affected, the peripheral field of vision is contracted but central vision is affected relatively late. Examination reveals narrowing of the lumen of the retinal and choroidal vessels, secondary atrophy of the optic nerve with a waxy looking disc, and the characteristic deposition in the periphery of pigment in aggregations which resemble bone-corpuscles. The *Prognosis* is poor, but total blindness may not occur.

§ 1140. (VIII). **Choroiditis Disseminata,** like other manifestations of advanced congenital or acquired syphilis, is now comparatively rare in Great Britain. When present, discrete white atrophic patches with irregular black edges are found scattered over the fundus, *most marked at the periphery.* **Atrophic patches in the Choroid** with retinal involvement occur in the secondary changes of progressive myopia; the macular region is especially apt to suffer.

TOXOPLASMOSIS produces in the newborn signs of encephalomyelitis, hydrocephalus and often small eyes (microphthalmia). After a few weeks choroido-retinopathy and vitreous opacities may develop, leading to severe visual loss. The disease is due to a protozoa, *Toxoplasma gondii*, derived from an unsuspected infection in the mother (§ 509a).

The Ears and Hearing

Sound waves, after passing along the external auditory meatus, reach the tympanic membrane, causing it to vibrate. These vibrations are transmitted across the middle ear by the three ossicles (malleus, incus and stapes) to the inner ear (cochlea). The frequency of the sound waves is analysed by the cochlea which then sends nervous impulses along the auditory nerve to the brain. A diagram of the essential structures in the ear is seen in Fig. 266. The neurological pathways have already been dealt with in § 801.

Healthy young adults are capable of hearing sound within the frequency range 16 to 25,000 cycles per second (c.p.s.). In later life the ability to hear high-frequency sounds diminishes. Deafness, especially if it is of gradual onset, may not be apparent until there is moderate hearing loss for sounds within the normal speech range (250 to 4,000 c.p.s.). An intelligent person may learn to lip read and thus overcome a severe hearing loss.

PART A. SYMPTOMATOLOGY

The *Principal Symptoms* complained of are pain, discharge from the ear, deafness, vertigo and tinnitus.

§ 1141. **Pain in the Ear** may be Acute or Chronic. It is important to try and localise the site of the pain for it may originate in the ear itself or be referred to the ear from other structures in the vicinity. Acute diseases are likely to be accompanied by pyrexia, and when pain originates in the ear deafness is almost certain to be present simultaneously.

Acute Pain in the Ear may be due to (1) disease in the external meatus, such as a furuncle (boil) or eczema. When the former is present movement of the pinna causes pain. (2) Disease in the middle ear, with deafness, some pyrexia, congestion and perhaps bulging of the membrane, indicates acute otitis media (§ 1147).

Chronic Pain in the Ear may be reflex in origin. Thus a carious, unerupted or impacted molar tooth, tonsillitis, temporo-mandibular arthritis (Costen's syndrome), tuberculous laryngitis and advanced carcinoma of the tongue or of the pyriform fossa, may all produce this.

Pain in the Mastoid Region may be due to (1) Mastoiditis which is accompanied by redness, swelling and tenderness, deep throbbing and constitutional disturbance. It may follow acute or chronic suppuration. (2) A furuncle on the posterior wall of the meatus may give rise to a swelling behind the auricle. (3) A tender post-auricular gland may be found with local sepsis or pediculi capitis.

Pain more or less Generalised over the Head, accompanied by *Pyrexia*, may be associated with the following diseases of the ear: (1) Acute middle-ear suppuration, which is relieved by the release of pus, (2) Acute meningitis. (3) If the temperature is continuously high it may be due to retention of pus, extradural abscess, or meningitis. (4) If the temperature oscillates, there may be sinus thrombosis and pyæmia (§§ 516, 892). (5) If the temperature after an initial rise is normal or subnormal, and there are headache, slow pulse, and delayed cerebration, suspect abscess of the temporo-sphenoidal lobe or cerebellum (§ 891). (6) Labyrinthitis (with nystagmus, giddiness, vomiting and pyrexia) is rare (§ 830).

PART B. PHYSICAL EXAMINATION

EXAMINATION OF THE EAR is part of the routine investigation of the patient as a whole. The student should lose no opportunity to examine the ear in health as well as in disease, in children and in adults. The anatomical structures concerned in hearing are represented in Fig. 266.

Inspection.—The best method is to have a mirror on the forehead of the examiner (as in laryngoscopy, § 152) and to use this to reflect light from a lamp at the side of the patient's head into the meatus; otherwise an electric auroscope may be used. First examine the meatus without a speculum; to see this passage more clearly, pull the auricle gently upwards and backwards, at the same time as the tragus is pulled forward by making traction with the thumb on the skin in front of it. Note the presence of cerumen, which is dark brown in colour and often of soft consistency. Then see if there is a discharge present, and if so record its character. If wax needs removal soften it with warm oil a few hours beforehand and then gently syringe the ear with warm saline or with sodium bicarbonate (2 teaspoonsful to the pint) at 100° F. To examine the deeper parts of the ear a speculum should be used. The auricle should be held between the middle and ring fingers of the left hand (for the patient's right ear) as the speculum is gently inserted inwards, and slightly downwards and forwards with the right hand. The speculum can then be held between the thumb and forefinger of the left hand. Pay particular attention to the tympanic membrane in the depth of the ear; note whether it is indrawn (due to block of the Eustachian tube), bulging, congested, thickened, and whether it has lost its lustre or shows perforations or areas of atrophy.

§ 1142. **Discharge from the Ear** may be serous, hæmorrhagic, muco-purulent or purulent. In a child with a high temperature, wax may melt and cause an apparent discharge from a healthy ear.

A *Serous Discharge* occurs in acute eczematous otitis externa. There is often swelling of the meatus which prevents inspection of the tympanic membrane. This type of infection is more commonly seen in hot climates, and often follows swimming in polluted water. Following head injury cerebro-spinal fluid may flow from the ear.

A *Hæmorrhagic Discharge* will follow rupture of the tympanic membrane whether due to trauma or to acute otitis media. In the latter case pus will be mixed with the blood. Bleeding from the meatus may follow head injury and fracture of the middle fossa. If a hæmorrhagic discharge is present with a history of purulent discharge of long standing, then it is due to granulation tissue formed in chronic middle-ear disease. An offensive sanious discharge, with fungating granulations, acute radiating neuralgia and enlargement of the neighbouring lymph nodes is character-istic of malignant disease of the ear.

A *Muco-purulent Discharge* is usually copious and associated with an upper respiratory tract infection; it may be caused by infection in the middle ear originating from the Eustachian tube. (There are no mucus-secreting glands in the tympanum.)

A *Purulent Discharge* (a) *which is* or has been *copious*, and associated with deafness from the beginning of the symptoms, is due to acute or chronic suppuration of the middle ear. When associated with chronic suppuration, its chronicity may be due to the presence of polypus, granu-lations, or cholesteatoma, caries of the malleus, incus or temporal bone, disease of the mastoid, antrum or naso-pharynx, or to constitutional causes, such as diabetes mellitus, tubercle or syphilis. (b) *A Purulent Discharge which is never copious*, together with deafness, may be due to acute or chronic disease of the external ear. A patient may deny that the ear does discharge, while admitting a rapid accumulation of " wax "; it is therefore important to be sure that any wax removed is free from smell; if an offensive odour is detected in soft wax, underlying suppurative disease must be suspected.

The Nose, Throat and Naso-Pharynx should then be examined especially for (1) the activity of the palatal muscles; (2) the condition of the tonsils; (3) the Eustachian tubes and back of the nose by posterior rhinoscopy; (4) the patency of each nostril and (5) the presence of pus or other abnormality in the nose.

Patency of the Eustachian Tube may be tested by *Valsalva's method* of auto-inflation. The patient pinches his nostrils firmly and makes an expiration as if to blow his nose but without letting any air escape. At the same time the examiner observes the tympanic membrane. The postero-superior part of the membrane may be seen to bulge if the tube is patent. Failing this *Politzer's method* is used. The nozzle of the rubber bag is inserted into one nostril and both nostrils are closed between the thumb and finger of the operator. The patient is then directed to swallow or to say " hic " and at the same time the air from the rubber bag is forced into the nose. Deglutition raises the palate and opens the Eustachian tube, and the air, having no other outlet, is forced into it. A tube connecting the ear of the patient with that of the operator will enable the latter to hear an audible " pick " if the middle ear is inflated, and this will reveal the patency of the Eustachian tube. A second point to

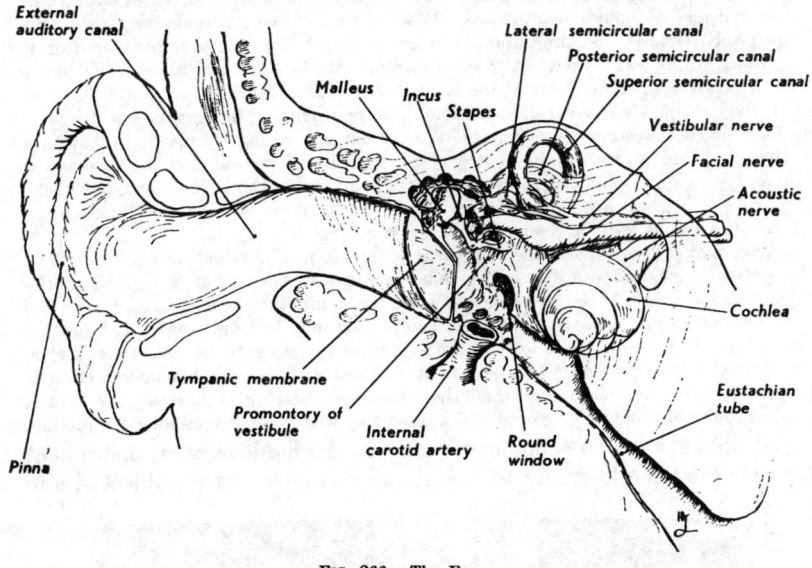

External
auditory canal

Lateral semicircular canal

Posterior semicircular canal

Superior semicircular canal

Malleus   Incus

Stapes

Vestibular nerve

Facial nerve

Acoustic
nerve

Cochlea

Tympanic membrane

Eustachian
tube

Promontory of
vestibule

Internal
carotid artery

Round
window

Pinna

FIG. 266.—The Ear.

note is the effect which inflation has upon the symptoms—deafness and tinnitus. The hearing is temporarily improved in middle-ear or Eustachian disease and it is unaltered in otosclerosis and nerve deafness. The *Eustachian catheter* is also used to inflate the ear for diagnosis or treatment. It is not a difficult operation, but requires a little practice. Pass it tip downward very gently along the floor of the nose to the edge of the hard palate, the patient being directed to breathe through the nose so that the soft palate may droop. Immediately the tip of the catheter has reached the edge of the hard palate turn it upwards and outwards, and it will enter the Eustachian orifice. It may be aided by the patient swallowing at the same time. The nozzle of Politzer's bag may now be carefully introduced into the catheter and inflation performed as before.

§ **1143.** The **Hearing** may be tested by the voice, the tuning-fork and the audiometer. Wax in the external meatus must be first removed, and if necessary the ear should be syringed with warm saline (38° C) after the wax has been softened with warm olive oil. The patient's ability to hear a forced whisper and the conversational voice enables the examiner to test the hearing by air conduction. The patient sits with the ear to be tested towards the examiner. The opposite ear is occluded by the patient or by an assistant. Commencing 20 feet from the ear the examiner advances slowly until the patient is able to repeat accurately each word or number whispered or spoken. In a quiet room the conversational voice should be heard at 20 feet and a forced whisper at 10 feet. Numbers are usually heard more easily than words.

Rinne's Test.—In a normal person a tuning-fork (256 double vibrations per second) placed on the mastoid bone until no longer heard in that situation, can still be heard by him if removed and held opposite the meatus (Rinne's test positive), hearing by air-conduction being more prolonged than by bone-conduction: it indicates an absence of any considerable middle-ear disease. When the middle ear or conducting apparatus is definitely diseased the tuning-fork cannot be heard opposite the meatus after it has ceased to be heard when held on the mastoid (Rinne's test negative). If Rinne's test is positive in a deaf ear there is probably nerve deafness present.

Weber's Test.—To ascertain whether an impairment of hearing is due to *nerve deafness* or to *obstructive deafness*, test the per-osseus hearing by placing a watch or a vibrating tuning-fork on the centre of the patient's forehead. If the deafness is due to disease of the auditory nerve it will be heard not in the affected ear, but in the good ear. This indicates nerve deafness. If the deafness is due to obstructive ear disease the sound will be heard *on the defective side.*

Schwabach's Test is performed by placing the stem of a vibrating tuning-fork on the patient's mastoid process and, when he ceases to hear it, it is applied to the observer's mastoid. If the observer still hears the sound, there is said to be diminution of bone-conduction. On the other hand conduction may be lengthened. A vibrating tuning-fork is held on the observer's mastoid till it ceases to be heard; it is then transferred to the patient. If the patient still hears the sound, bone-conduction is longer than normal (assuming that the observer's hearing is normal). A watch applied to the mastoid may be used in the same way to give an idea of bone-conduction.

AUDIOMETRY.—The audiometer is a standardised electrical instrument by which hearing loss may be accurately measured. The subject sits in

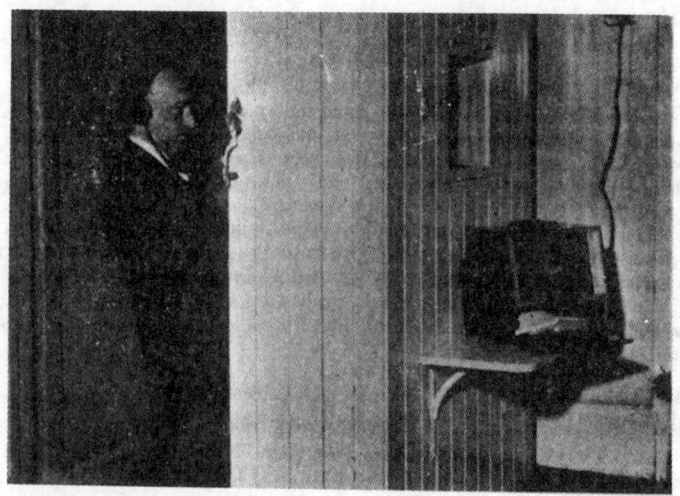

FIG. 267.—Audiometry test.

a sound-proof room to exclude interference from extraneous noise. Sound is transmitted from the audiometer via headphones for air-conduction, and a receiver placed on the mastoid process for bone-conduction. Either the ability to hear pure tones or speech may be determined. *Pure-tone audiometry:* The hearing is tested by both air and bone conduction over a range of tones from 125 to 8,000 cycles per second. The lowest intensity of each tone just audible (the threshold) is recorded. The pure-tone audiogram provides not only a record of hearing function, but assists in diagnosis. There is a characteristic pattern of hearing loss for many ear diseases. The results are recorded as shown in Fig. 268.

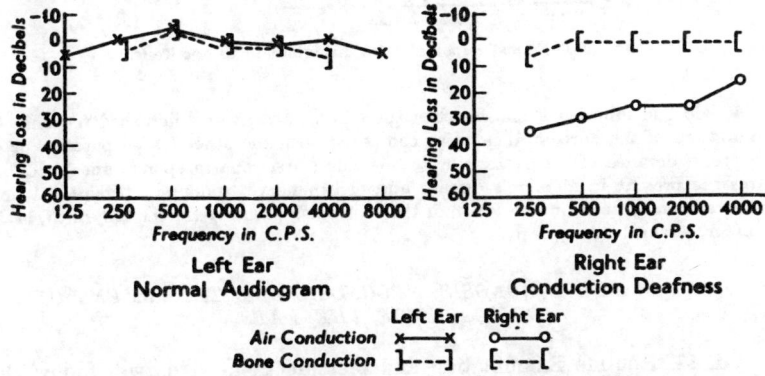

FIG. 268.—Audiograms for normal hearing and conduction deafness.

Deafness is of two types, which may be differentiated by the above tests : Obstructive (conduction) deafness is due to disease in the middle ear or external auditory passages; and Nerve (perceptive) deafness is due to lesions of the cochlear apparatus or auditory nerve pathways. Mixed types also occur.

TABLE LXIII.—DIAGNOSIS OF TYPE OF DEAFNESS

Obstructive (Conduction) Deafness	*Nerve (Perceptive) Deafness*
Loss of air-conduction only with negative Rinne and Weber's test to deaf ear.	Diminution of air- and bone-conduction, with positive Rinne and Weber to good ear.
Better hearing in noise (paracusis).	Decreased hearing in noise.
Audiogram shows by air conduction either low tone loss or uniform hearing loss; bone conduction normal.	Audiogram shows by both air and bone conduction a high tone loss.

The **Labyrinth** is tested by *Labyrinthine Function Tests*. The labyrinth may be stimulated by rotation or by hot or cold water syringed into the external auditory meatus. Nystagmus results if the labyrinth is active.

The *Caloric Test* is in common use but is unsuitable for patients who have a perforation of the tympanic membrane. The patient lies on a couch with the head raised

30° so that the horizontal semicircular canals are vertical. Using a douche can and a small catheter, water is run into the ear for 40 seconds and the duration of the nystagmus is recorded. Each labyrinth is stimulated by hot water (44° C) and then cold water (30° C), five minutes being allowed between tests to allow the ear to return to body temperature. The results are plotted thus (Normal Calorigram):

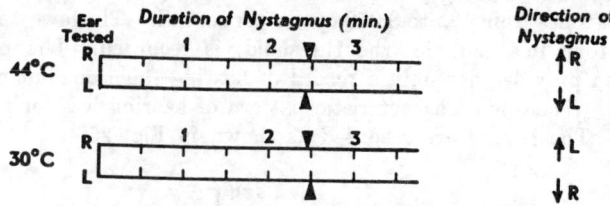

FIG. 269.—Normal response of the Labyrinth to Caloric Tests.

A defect in function is shown when there is an absent or diminished response to stimulation of one horizontal canal as compared with the other (canal paresis), or in the preponderance of the nystagmus to one side (directional preponderance). Canal paresis is present in Ménière's disease and eighth nerve tumours. Directional preponderance may occur in any lesion of the vestibular pathway (in the labyrinth, brain stem or cerebral hemispheres).

PART C. THE DIAGNOSIS, PROGNOSIS AND TREATMENT OF DISEASES OF THE EARS

§ 1144. Routine Examination and Classification.—This will follow the pattern of investigations performed elsewhere:—

First ask the patient for the LEADING SYMPTOM or SYMPTOMS.

Second, take a careful HISTORY of the development of the symptoms in chronological order.

Third, examine the EXTERNAL EAR, THE NOSE AND THROAT, THE HEARING AND THE NERVE PATHWAYS associated with the Cochlea and Labyrinth.

Diseases of the Ear may be conveniently divided into (A) those of the External Ear; (B) the Middle Ear and (C) the Inner Ear; this corresponds to the methods adopted in the routine examination of the Ear.

(A) DISEASES OF THE EXTERNAL EAR (Syn. Otitis Externa) may be *localised* or *diffuse*.

§ 1145. Furunculosis is localised to one part of the external ear.

Symptoms.—First there is discomfort or irritation. Soon acute pain develops and trismus may occur. Deafness is the result of the meatus becoming occluded by swelling. A purulent otorrhœa follows spontaneous rupture of the boil.

Diagnosis.—In furunculosis deafness occurs late after the onset of pain and not early as in otitis media and acute mastoiditis. Also there is pain on moving the pinna but not on pressure over the mastoid process, unless the post-auricular glands are inflamed.

Etiology.—There is a staphylococcal infection of a hair follicle in the cartilaginous meatus. Recurrent boils may indicate diabetes mellitus.

Treatment is by a wick soaked in 10 per cent. ichthammol in glycerin inserted gently into the meatus to reduce œdema and relieve pain. Local heat is comforting and analgesics will be required. Systemic treatment with antibiotics is disappointing.

§ 1146. **Diffuse Otitis Externa** is often bilateral and the eczema may spread to the pinna and to the post-auricular sulcus.

Symptoms.—The patient complains of irritation in the ears and in acute cases the discharge is of a serous nature. In chronic cases there is a scanty desquamative accumulation. Deafness occurs when the meatus is blocked by œdema and the discharge.

Diagnosis is by examining the lining membrane of the meatus. Middle-ear disease must be excluded by syringing the ear with saline so as to obtain a good view of the tympanic membrane. The two conditions may co-exist.

Etiology.—Different varieties of gram-negative organisms may be isolated from the discharge. The presence of *E. coli* indicates unhygienic habits. A seborrhœic diathesis may be present.

Prognosis.—Recurrence is likely if the etiological factors are not eradicated.

Treatment is directed to the local removal of all discharges, by syringing if necessary, and to the topical application of antiseptics or antibiotics. Ichthammol (10 per cent. in glycerin) is effective in most cases. Neomycin-hydrocortisone drops may be needed in resistant cases. The patient's hands must be kept clean, the finger-nails short and seborrhœa of the scalp will need treatment (§ 777 (i.)).

(B) Diseases of the Middle Ear.   The chief of these are:

§ 1147. I. **Acute Otitis Media** is due to a spread of infection from the naso-pharynx along the Eustachian tube to the middle ear. It may be catarrhal, muco-purulent or purulent.

Symptoms.—Deafness, tinnitus and a pulsating discomfort occur first. Then pain is likely to follow; should perforation of the drum and otorrhœa take place there is rapid relief from pain. Pyrexia is often present in adults and is invariable in children. Infants normally present only constitutional symptoms—a high temperature, irritability, vomiting, neck stiffness and sometimes convulsions. The symptoms may be masked by the administration of an antibiotic.

Diagnosis is by examination of the ear-drums. In more severe cases the drumhead is markedly hyperæmic and bulges outwards. Care must be taken to exclude a co-existent acute exanthem in children.

Etiology.—The infection may be with catarrhal organisms, but in severe cases coagulase-positive staphylococci, streptococcus pyogenes or pneumococci are present. Infection may follow traumatic rupture of the tympanic membrane.

Prognosis.—Most cases of acute otitis media resolve completely without complications or sequelæ if prompt and adequate treatment is given.

Complications.—*Acute mastoiditis* is due to a spread of infection into the mastoid air cells. It must be suspected if pain, pyrexia and discharge continue after perforation of the membrane. Tenderness and/or swelling over the mastoid process with opacity of the air cells on X-ray examination confirm the diagnosis. Untreated mastoiditis may lead to a subdural or temporo-sphenoidal abscess, or to meningitis. Thrombosis of the lateral sinus followed by pyæmia is now rare.

Treatment.—The patient must go to bed and the nasal passages should be decongested with ephedrine nasal drops (B.P.C.) every two or three hours during the day. Pain is relieved by local heat and analgesics. Systemic benzylpenicillin should be given for a full five-day course. If after twenty-four hours the pain, raised pulse rate and temperature persist, the advice of an otologist should be sought, for myringotomy will probably be necessary. Other surgical measures may be required if complications threaten. In *Acute Catarrhal (Secretory) Otitis Media* when the middle ear is full of clear straw-coloured fluid, if ephedrine drops to the nose or Eustachian catheterisation do not give relief it may be necessary to incise the tympanic membrane.

§ 1148. II. **Chronic Otitis Media** may follow acute otitis media or commence insidiously after a sub-clinical inflammation of the middle ear. It is much less common in Great Britain than it was a few decades ago and commonly starts in childhood or early adult life.

Symptoms.—There is a chronic perforation of the ear-drum; loss of hearing may be severe or so slight as to be hardly appreciated; discharge from the ear may be persistent, purulent and fœtid, or may be recurrent and mainly mucoid. Pain is always a serious symptom and tinnitus and vertigo are occasionally present. Two types can be distinguished—(a) the benign and (b) the serious forms.

(a) *Benign chronic otitis media* is due to persistent upper naso-pharyngeal infection involving the middle ear via the Eustachian tube. This causes a recurrent muco-purulent discharge from the ear, often without pain. The principal diagnostic feature is the presence of a *central or anterior perforation* of the ear-drum without destruction of the bony rim (annulus). The perforation may be small or large (Fig. 270); the discharge is not likely to be of thick or fœtid pus but the ossicles may atrophy, in which case considerable obstructive deafness will be present. *Treatment* is by eradicating nasal sepsis. Spirit ear-drops (B.P.C.), or chloramphenicol or neomycin ear-drops will sterilise the middle ear. In some cases

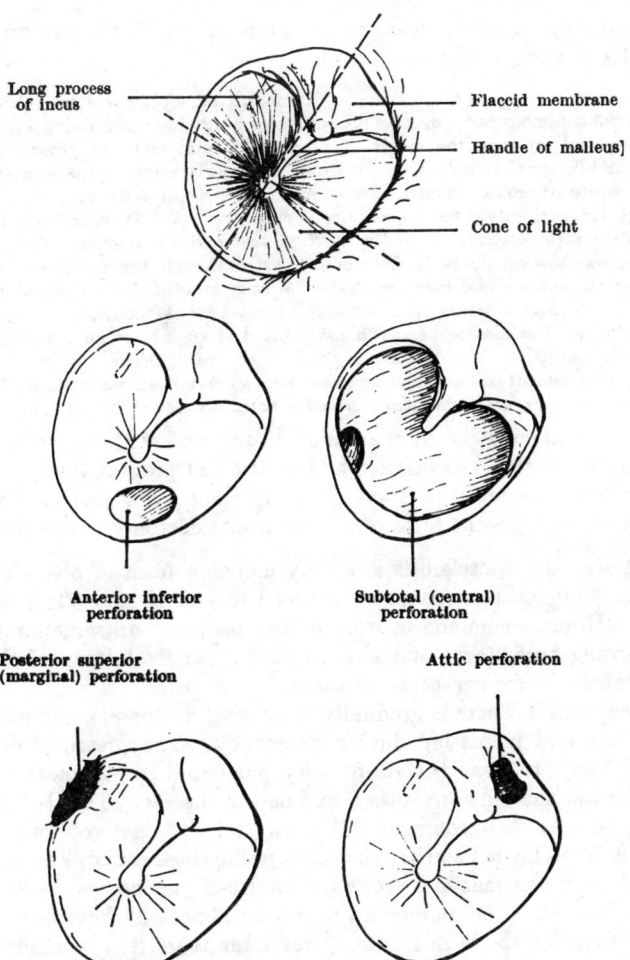

Long process of incus

Flaccid membrane

Handle of malleus]

Cone of light

Anterior inferior perforation

Subtotal (central) perforation

Posterior superior (marginal) perforation

Attic perforation

FIG. 270.—Diagram of Right Ear showing the normal appearance and the types of perforation which can occur in the tympanic membrane.

it is possible to improve the hearing by applying a skin graft to the defect in the tympanic membrane (Myringoplasty).

(b) *Serious or potentially dangerous otitis media* is present when there is either a *marginal* perforation in the posterior superior quadrant of the ear-drum, or a perforation of the attic (Shrapnell's) membrane (Fig. 270). This indicates disease in the attic or mastoid antrum. Such perforations may be obscured by dried pus which may appear to be debris arising from otitis externa. There is often a history of slight deafness and scanty otorrhœa for many years. Pain, vertigo or facial palsy may make the patient seek medical advice for the first time. A blood-stained discharge indicates that granulations are present and these may be seen pouting through a perforation; occasionally a granulation fills the external meatus, forming a variety of aural polyp.

A common *Complication* of this is formation of a *cholesteatoma* (cholesteatosis). This is not a tumour but a mass of desquamated epithelium containing a small amount of cholesterol crystals, the result of a low-grade inflammatory process in the attic of the middle ear. It only occurs with an attic perforation and is seen as a mass of pearly white or cream-coloured cheesy material in the middle ear; when it projects through the perforation the appearance is characteristic. It causes chronic suppuration in the attic, often associated with *B. proteus* and a foul smell. A cholesteatoma which grows to a considerable size erodes the structures in the middle ear, may invade the mastoid antrum and may penetrate the bony wall of the horizontal semicircular canal, producing a fistula with attacks of severe but momentary vertigo. It is probable that the disease begins in early life and smoulders for many years before becoming manifest. The deafness is progressive and of the mixed type—obstructive due to involvement of the ossicular chain and a nerve deafness when the inner ear is affected. Intracranial complications and a brain abscess still have a high mortality.

Treatment must be in the hands of an aural surgeon whose object is to prevent further hearing loss and to try and prevent further discharge. Untreated cases are a constant threat to the hearing and even to the life the patient. Some form of radical mastoidectomy is usually required.

§ 1149. III. **Otosclerosis** is a very common form of obstructive deafness in young adults (usually starting between 18 and 30 years of age), and much more common in women than in men. In some families there is a strong hereditary tendency, so that a family history of the disease is obtained in 50 per cent. of cases.

Symptoms.—There is gradually increasing deafness, commencing at an early age and increasing during pregnancy. The presence of paracusis —an ability to hear better in noisy surroundings—is more marked in otosclerosis than in any other middle-ear disease. Tinnitus is marked but giddiness is uncommon. Rinne's test is negative; and bone-conduction is prolonged so that the C256 tuning-fork can still be heard when placed over the mastoid process even when the normal person can no longer hear it. The audiogram shows an almost uniform loss of hearing to all tones in the earlier stages, but later there is a marked high tone loss due to additional nerve-deafness. Examination of the ear-drum sometimes shows it to be rather more transparent than normal, and occasionally a flamingo-pink flush is seen through the membrane, due to hyperæmia of the inner wall of the middle ear.

Etiology.—There is an overgrowth of spongy vascular bone which prevents the footplate of the stapes articulating in the oval window of the cochlea; the cause of this is unknown.

Prognosis.—The disease is progressive, tending to get less active in later life. The earlier the onset of the disease the greater the ultimate hearing loss is likely to be. The deafness may be not purely obstructive. The spongy bone may involve the cochlea, producing a nerve deafness in addition.

Treatment.—The disease process cannot be arrested. Of the variety of surgical procedures designed to overcome the obstructive deafness, the fenestration operation was the first; it by-passed the ankylosed stapes and allowed sound to enter the cochlea via the horizontal semicircular canal. More recent surgical techniques aim at enabling the ossicular chain to function physiologically, especially by mobilisation of the stapes (Rosen's operation); in other cases the stapes is removed and replaced by a plastic or other prosthesis.

Obstructive (Conduction) Deafness may be (a) Sudden or (b) Gradual in onset. The causes are:

<table>
<tr><td>(a) Sudden onset</td><td>(b) Gradual onset</td></tr>
<tr><td>I. Impaction of Wax.
II. Impaction of a foreign body in the meatus.
III. Acute Eustachian catarrh and catarrhal otitis media.
IV. Acute suppurative otitis media.
V. Secretory otitis media.</td><td>VI. Chronic Eustachian catarrh with adhesions in the middle ear.
VII. Otosclerosis.
VIII. Perforation or cicatrices of the drum from previous middle-ear suppuration.</td></tr>
</table>

(C) DISEASES OF THE INNER EAR cause Nerve (Perceptive) Deafness, Vertigo and Tinnitus.

§ **1150. Nerve Deafness** may be of (a) Sudden or (b) Gradual in onset.

(a) Nerve Deafness of *sudden onset* may be due to:

I. Ménière's Disease.
II. Acute Labyrinthitis—Mumps, Influenza.
III. Concussion of the Cochlea.
IV. Small Hæmorrhagic or Vascular Lesions.
V. Syphilis.
VI. Septic Meningitis.
VII. Hysteria.

I. MÉNIÈRE'S DISEASE (see § 831).

II. **Acute Labyrinthitis** may result from acute or chronic otitis media and is more often suppurative than non-suppurative. The inflammatory process, by spreading to the cochlea, produces permanent nerve deafness. The involvement of the labyrinth produces severe constitutional disturbances, symptoms and signs of labyrinthine vertigo, fever and pleocytosis in the spinal fluid. A cholesteatoma may be present in the middle ear (§ 1148). Non-suppurative inflammation of the cochlea and labyrinth may also result from influenza in adults and from mumps in children; the loss of hearing may not be discovered until the child goes to school.

Treatment is by controlling any suppuration with a suitable antibiotic, and after recovery from the acute phase a radical mastoid operation may be necessary to prevent recurrence.

III. **Concussion of the Cochlea** results from open or closed head injuries, explosions and loud noises or too forceful syringing of the ear. When the petrous temporal bone is fractured there may be associated facial palsy. Improvement in hearing may occur when the damage is partial.

IV. **Small Hæmorrhagic or Vascular Lesions.**—Hæmorrhage into the cochlea is a rare complication of leukæmia and other hæmorrhagic diseases. In thrombosis of the Anterior Inferior Cerebellar Artery deafness may occur (§ 937).

V. Syphilis, Acquired or Congenital.—A syphilitic neuritis of the cochlear nerve or syphilitic neuro-labyrinthitis may occur a few weeks after infection. This may be bilateral (Table XXXII) and is more sudden than syphilitic meningitis, which may be unilateral or bilateral. During treatment a Herxheimer reaction may cause sudden deafness, tinnitus and vertigo.

VI. Septic Meningitis, once an important cause of nerve-deafness, is now rare since the use of sulpha drugs and antibiotics.

VII. Hysterical Deafness can be sudden in origin following an emotional shock. (i.) Blinking of the eyes occurs if sudden loud noises are made near the patient and (ii.) even if he appears stone-deaf it may be possible to waken him from sleep by calling his name.

(b) Nerve Deafness of *gradual onset* may be due to :

I. Senile Deafness.
II. Occupational Deafness.
III. Drugs and Antibiotics.
IV. Acoustic Neurofibroma.

V. Central lesions (*e.g.*, Pontine glioma).
VI. Meningitis.
VII. Syphilis—congenital or acquired.
VIII. Deaf-mutism.

I. **Senile Deafness.**—A certain amount of nerve deafness is very common in one or both ears in old age. The loss is for high tones. It may be combined with a time lag in the interpretation of sounds so that the listener has to listen more intently; this causes fatigue. A characteristic of senile deafness is the phenomenon of *recruitment* whereby the cochlea does not respond to sounds of low intensity, but loud noises are heard as well by the deaf ear as by a normal ear. Hence when talking to an old person who has senile deafness, one must speak very clearly but must not shout.

II. **Occupational Deafness** may occur from repeated loud noises of machinery or guns. Boilermaker's deafness was the first of this type to be described; the noise from jet air engines is a twentieth-century hazard. The audiogram is characteristic, and shows almost normal hearing except for frequencies around 4,000 c.p.s.

III. **Drugs and Antibiotics** do not usually cause serious deafness, but *quinine* and *salicylates* often cause it temporarily. Prolonged courses of *dihydrostreptomycin* can produce permanent deafness, especially after middle age, even when the course has been completed; for this reason its use has been largely given up. *Streptomycin* is more liable to produce vestibular damage (ataxia), but can also cause deafness.

IV. Acoustic Neurofibroma and V. Central Lesions are described in § 1083.

VI. **Meningitis** due to suppurative middle-ear disease (circumscribed serous meningitis) or following cerebro-spinal fever (§ 504) produces local changes in the lateral recess and may cause gradual nerve-deafness.

VII. **Syphilis** in its congenital form is a cause of chronic nerve-deafness in children (§ 500); and the acquired disease may produce a local pachymeningitis.

VIII. Deaf-mutism is described in § 878.

Combined Obstructive and Nerve-Deafness.—Such cases may be due to:

(1) Suppurative otitis media spreading to the labyrinth. There is

a history or presence of a discharge and nerve-deafness gradually follows the symptoms of obstructive deafness.

(2) An old CATARRHAL OTITIS MEDIA is followed by..disease of the cochlea.

(3) In advanced cases of OTOSCLEROSIS, the uniform loss of hearing to all tones is later followed by a loss to high tones when the nerve is affected.

Treatment.—Specific treatment to remedy nerve-deafness is 'seldom effective. Whatever the cause, a hearing aid may be of assistance when deafness becomes a social handicap. The prejudice against wearing such aids is diminishing as the design of the aids is improved and the public are educated to use them. Compact transistorised models with a high output are often valuable in the very deaf. An aid is to be recommended when the hearing loss exceeds 30 decibels as measured by an audiometer. An insert receiver (worn in the meatus) is superior to the type worn behind the ear even in a patient with marked obstructive deafness. As the hearing aid is fitted to the ear with the better hearing, less amplification is necessary and less distortion of sound occurs.

§ 1151. Vertigo is a hallucination of movement which may be rotatory or a sense of rocking or swaying. In *healthy persons* it is produced by spinning round, by syringing an ear with water which is more than a few degrees above or below body temperature and by instilling cold drops into the ear. This may cause the patient to abandon the instillation of any drops prescribed and is corrected by warming all drops before use.

The *Causes* of vertigo are described in §§ 826, 933. The common aural causes are (1) Ménière's disease (§ 831); (2) Acute Labyrinthitis (§ 1150); and (3) Vestibular neuronitis (Epidemic Vertigo (§ 828)) caused by a lesion of the vestibular nerve or nucleus, but without deafness. The caloric test usually shows a canal paresis (see § 1143).

§ 1152. Tinnitus is a ringing or a noise in the ear. It is very common, especially in middle age or in the elderly. Two varieties occur: (*a*) The usual variety is subjective and only heard by the patient. (*b*) Rarely it is objective and can be heard by the physician.

(*a*) SUBJECTIVE TINNITUS. *Symptoms.*—The patient complains of a hissing, whistling, buzzing " like a bell," or roaring sound in one ear. Occasionally the other ear is affected to a lesser extent. The intensity of the sound varies from day to day and may only be heard at night when all is quiet. Depending on the cause some deafness may be present, and if the tinnitus is loud and continuous it may make hearing difficult even without loss when tested by an audiometer. Severe tinnitus leads to insomnia and a psychoneurosis.

Etiology.—Often the cause cannot be found; but it may be caused by diseases of the ear (especially the middle ear), the nerve pathways or in the temporal lobe. (i.) In the external ear wax, a foreign body or perforation of the tympanic membrane are causal. (ii.) In the middle ear acute or less often chronic otitis media, temporary Eustachian obstruction or a cholesteatoma are found; otosclerosis is a frequent cause. (iii.) The cochlear apparatus may be affected by Ménière's disease, chronic inflammation, anæmia, trauma or a damaged skull, or by drugs such as quinine, salicylates or streptomycin. Fatigue or degeneration of the nerve endings occurs in those exposed to artillery fire or to occupational noises. (iv.) The auditory nerve may be irritated by an acoustic neurofibroma for years before other symptoms arise. (v.) The brain may be the site of origin, for the symptom can persist after destruction of the cochlea, the labyrinth and the auditory nerve. Important causes of this are cerebral arteriosclerosis and vascular changes associated with menopause. Tinnitus is always worse when the mental or physical condition is depressed.

Pulsating Tinnitus synchronous with the heart-beats, checked by compression of the carotid artery, is due to arteriolar dilatation in the middle or external ear.

(*b*) OBJECTIVE TINNITUS is rare. It is also vascular in origin.

Symptoms.—A pulsating low-pitched sound is heard by the patient and is audible as a bruit when a stethoscope is applied to an area of the head. This indicates a vascular malformation such as an intracranial aneurysm or a vascular tumour (§ 1047); the cause is verified by cerabrel angiography.

Prognosis of Tinnitus.—In idiopathic cases it may gradually cease when the general health is improved and with the passage of time. When it is accompanied by deafness it often ceases when total deafness develops.

Treatment is by removing the cause when this can be found. It is important to explain the condition to the patient and to relieve insomnia. Sodium amylobarbitone 15–30 mg. twice daily, one of the antihistamines, trifluoperazine (Stelazine) or nicotinic acid 50–100 mg. twice or thrice daily may be tried. Operative measures to relieve tinnitus *per se* are not successful.

HEAD NOISES are likely to be due to cerebral arteriosclerosis, presenile or senile dementia, or to a depressive state. *Auditory hallucinations* are usually associated with mental illness, but may be caused by local or diffuse disease of the temporal lobe of the brain.

CHAPTER XXI

PSYCHOLOGICAL DISORDERS

THE importance of this group of disorders is indicated by the fact that in general practice in England at the present time about 10 per cent. of patients attend for a conspicuous psychiatric disability. In recent years considerable progress has been made in the study, treatment and prevention of this group of illnesses. A much more enlightened attitude is apparent and is reflected in the recent legislation dealing with these problems.

The forms of illness to be considered, while related in varying degrees to the behaviour of the individual, represent a failure to make a satisfactory adaptation to life, environment and the other members of the community. All students of general medicine have been impressed by the influence of emotional factors in physical illnesses and how they influence their duration. Here we are concerned only with those illnesses in which psychological symptoms predominate. These can be studied in common with all other forms of illness, and failure to do so results, inevitably, in a lack of understanding of the factors involved. The major forms of mental illness have acquired for the student a sense of mystery, aggravated by the conflicting views and theories of the various schools of thought. The less severe forms include neurotic, emotional and personality disorders: individuals vary in their types of reaction to various forms of stress. Therefore many factors, constitutional, environmental, physical, biochemical and psycho-biological may be involved; the significance of each can be evaluated only in relation to the other factors.

§ 1160. **Psychopathology.** In order to understand the nature of psychological symptoms one must have some knowledge of *mental mechanisms*. The following account is a brief summary, involving the minimum of theory. Mental health depends upon the maintenance of a state of equilibrium between the conscious and the unconscious. Normally, these work in harmony and the individual adapts himself to his environment. The experience and stress of everyday life, with its struggles between desires and their gratification, within limits that allow a satisfactory adjustment of the personality, inevitably give rise to a state of mental *conflict*. Conflict is then a condition of normal mentation which is maintained by the formulation of a satisfactory solution. Difference of opinion has arisen regarding the nature of the conflicting forces. Freud originally considered they had a sexual basis, but it is obvious that this limitation is erroneous. Conflicts are accompanied by emotional *tension* and are the cause of much waste of mental energy. Most are solved successfully on the conscious level, are finally disposed of and give rise to no symptoms. Unfortunately, for various reasons inherent or acquired, many patients are unable to deal with their conflicts in this manner, and devise various methods to maintain the state of equilibrium above-mentioned. These methods are common, invariably uniform in pattern, and are described as *mental mechanisms*.

Suppression and *repression* are the most common methods. Suppression is a conscious effort to forget what is unpleasant and is always accompanied by a focusing of the attention on something else. Repression is an attempt to expel from consciousness the factors that offend; they are transferred to the level of the unconscious. There they continue to exist and seek expression. Each repressed thought with its emotional component constitutes what we speak of as a *complex*. Invariably the personality elaborates methods on the conscious level to prevent expression of the repressed ideas; consequently exaggerated personality traits become prominent. Prudishness, for instance, results from the repression of normal sexual impulses; prejudices are developed by the individual to prevent the expression of repressed ideas. The establishment of such mechanisms need not disturb the mental equilibrium, but certain types of interaction of these forces give rise to various nervous symptoms: persistent anxiety, fatiguability, hysterical or obsessional manifestations.

In all cases the energy remains latent and expression cannot be allowed an outlet unless in disguised form. This is achieved by *sublimation*. By this mechanism the energy is directed into some other activity combined invariably with an altruistic motive, such as religion, art and music. Another method of obtaining expression is by *rationalisation*. This is an unconscious mechanism and leads to the elaboration of various explanations in defence of beliefs or actions which are really the result of unrecognised motives. An attempt is made to justify such beliefs or actions by reasoning and great emotion may be displayed in their defence. The tendency to rationalise with regard to politics, religion, alcohol, tobacco are examples in everyday life. *Compensatory* mechanisms occur psychologically as well as physiologically: the aggressive, boisterous manner unconsciously adopted to compensate for excessive shyness is very familiar.

All mental life is influenced by *symbolisation*, often to such a degree that we fail to appreciate its significance. Music and art are symbolic representations of the feelings and ideals of the various artists. Similarly much of the play activity of children is symbolic. One method whereby repressed complexes achieve expression is when they are symbolised and submitted in disguised form. Many symptoms can be thus explained. Many dreams are symbolic, but the interpretation of such symbolisation is often exceedingly difficult.

Another form of defence mechanism is known as *projection*. Here the complex is regarded by the personality as no longer belonging to itself but as the product of some other real or fictitious person. By this method the activities of others are interpreted by the motives that determine the patient's own conduct. To explain their behaviour they project on others their own motives. This is the basis of many delusional ideas. The chronic alcoholic readily develops delusions regarding his wife and family and may attribute to them his own behaviour. Sometimes the desires are projected into imaginary persons. The aim of this, as of other mechanisms, is to make life more pleasant and avoid tension.

The method of repression may be replaced by that of *dissociation*. The mind becomes disintegrated, portions are separated off and function independently. On this basis are explained somnambulism and fugues. In the case of the psychotic, delusional ideas may be dissociated; this explains how patients with gross delusional ideas of their high status in life will perform most menial tasks.

The elaboration of excessive *phantasy* formation constitutes a common mental mechanism. Some degree of phantasy or imagination is common in normal life. Such elaborations in health remain subject to conscious criticism. It is also frequently seen in childhood with the elaboration of imaginary playmates. In certain forms of mental illness, particularly schizophrenia, it assumes an objective reality and thus repressed complexes attain an imaginary fulfilment.

The above-described mental mechanisms are substitutes for a logical adjustment, and may tend to produce deviation from reality; this is particularly evident in the pernicious mechanism of phantasy. The greater the degree to which they are developed the more profound are the symptoms, and the more serious the outcome.

§ 1161. General Factors. Effects of constitution and environment are not readily separated; their influence varies according to the balance of the other factors and may vary at different periods in the life history. Similarly there is a constant inter-reaction between physical factors and the nervous mechanism. It is important to appreciate that mental ill-health is the sum total of a number of factors, and not the result of any one alone. The occurrence of mental illness in members of the same family has drawn attention to the influence of heredity. There is evidence that, as in certain forms of physical illness, there is probably inherited a diminished resistance to the development of certain types of mental illness. Of these the manic-depressive variety shows the greatest family incidence; the schizophrenic to a lesser degree. Mendelian researches suggest that the former is due to a dominant gene and schizophrenia to a recessive.

Psychotic illnesses are rare before adolescence, when physiological changes are marked; conflicts between instinctive desires and social standards then become much more active and demand fresh adaptations. At this age the incidence is high and remains so for some years. Similarly there is an exacerbation at the involutional period, when further endocrine changes occur, with marked emotional components. The association of mental illness and pregnancy led formerly to the classification and description of puerperal psychoses. It is now generally accepted that such a physiological event acts by reducing the general resistance, and that a mental illness developing at this time is determined by the previous personality and the other factors already discussed.

Apart from toxic-infective conditions, physical factors in themselves are rarely direct causes of mental illness. Exceptions are found with disorders resulting from trauma, which produces direct injury to the brain, and those due to vascular changes, generally of an arteriosclerotic nature. Acute general infections may give rise to delirium followed, as in the case of influenza, by lassitude and depression. Such an illness may also release other symptoms, of a schizoid or cyclothymic nature, depending on the personality and make-up of the individual. Divergent views exist as to the role of focal sepsis and the frequency with which it is responsible for the development of mental symptoms. That such arises in certain cases, and must be dealt with, is agreed, but unless there is clinical evidence of toxæmia, improvement may not follow surgical treatment. The role of alcohol in the production of mental illness is limited: the acute alcoholic psychoses and Korsakoff's psychosis are the direct results of alcohol. A detailed investigation of the history and personality of the individual will generally show chronic indulgence in alcohol to be symptomatic rather than causative of a mental illness.

PART A. SYMPTOMATOLOGY

It is often alleged that symptoms of mental illness are much less clearly defined than those of bodily illness. Such symptoms represent the reactions of the individuals as an integrated whole, not of single mental processes. Consequently in their interpretation attention must be paid to all factors in order to appreciate fully the setting in which the symptoms have appeared. The fact that symptoms may have a symbolic meaning tends to confuse the student, but no matter how disguised, these symptoms are always germane to the mental state.

The more important symptoms may be considered as they involve predominantly behaviour, consciousness, emotion, thought-processes, sensation, memory and personality.

1. Behaviour   .   Overactivity, stereotypy, retardation, negativism, morbid impulses.
2. Consciousness .   Confusion, dream states, delirium, disorientation, stupor.
3. Emotion .   .   Elation, euphoria, depression, anxiety, apathy, emotional instability.
4. Thought .   .   Delusions, obsessions, ideas of reference.
5. Perception   .   Hallucinations, illusions.
6. Memory .   .   Amnesia, hyperamnesia, paramnesia.
7. Personality   .   Depersonalisation, transformation of personality, dissociation, fugues, multiple personality.

§ 1162. Disorders of Behaviour. *Overactivity* is characteristic of all forms of excitement, mania, schizophrenia and general paralysis. The activity is invariably purposeful, but not necessarily productive. In states of mania there is a concomitant talkativeness; distraction by external stimuli is profoundly exaggerated in the form of *flights of ideas*. Rhyming and punning are frequent accompaniments. In schizophrenic behaviour repetition of movement or speech may occur over a prolonged period and is known as *stereotypy*. Repetitive movements cause *mannerisms* to develop in the form of gestures and the embellishment of various ordinary movements. *Perseveration* should be distinguished from stereotypy: even against his own will there is an inability in the former to avoid repeating an action or a word which the individual has just used. Perseveration is a frequent symptom in organic brain disease. *Retardation* of psycho-motor activity is seen typically in melancholia. It may be accompanied by *negativism*—a refusal on the part of the patient to co-operate, even to the extent of doing the opposite of what he is told to do. Profound degrees of retardation may merge into a state of *stupor*: then *flexibilitas cerea* may develop. It is so called because of the wax-like position of the limbs which may be maintained in the most uncomfortable position for prolonged periods. *Morbid impulses* are the result of an irresistible urge to carry out some action. Failure to do so is accompanied by tension and restlessness; its performance is usually devoid of reflection or of any consideration for the interests of themselves or others. Among such impulsive forms of behaviour are pyromania—impulse to set on fire; kleptomania—impulse to steal; dipsomania—impulse to drink to excess; these are variations of obsessional behaviour.

§ 1163. Disorders of Consciousness. Consciousness implies ability to be aware of ourselves and our environment, involving the ability to synthesise and integrate as well as evaluate new experiences. It is dependent, in part, on attention. If the power of attention is impaired there develops *confusion*, perplexity and bewilderment. Such is found in the most acute stages of mental illness and in the toxic-infective group of psychoses. *Dream states* and *twilight states* are usually of psychogenic origin and last for varying periods of time. The disturbance of consciousness may be sufficient to cause the individual to lose knowledge of his surroundings, as in epilepsy and hysteria. In hysteria fugues or dissociated states may follow. *Delirium* may be psychogenic but is most frequently of toxic origin. All degrees of clouding of consciousness may develop, together with vivid hallucinations, visual and auditory. Invariably there is marked *disorientation*, indicating an inability of the individual to appreciate his position in respect of time, or place, or his relationship to other persons. Profound degrees of delirium are usually followed by a complete amnesia for the acute periods. In *stupor* there is an absence of all spontaneous activity or of any response to stimulation. It may develop in benign melancholia, the catatonic form of schizophrenia, certain toxic states, epilepsy and hysteria. In the psychogenic variety, rapid emergence from stupor to activity may be seen, once the precipitating factors have ceased.

§ **1164. Disorders of Emotion.** Emotional disturbances are assessed by the intensity, duration and degree of harmony between the mood and the content of thought. *Exaltation* is an exaggerated degree of elation, typical of mania when it is accompanied by psychomotor overactivity. *Euphoria* implies, in addition, an abnormal feeling of wellbeing. Feelings of *depression*, characterised by hopelessness or despair, may be of all degrees: the less severe are apparent in the neuroses, whereas in melancholia the degree may be profound. When depression develops as the result of obvious external factors it is termed reactive. *Anxiety* implies more than fear. The latter ceases when the danger passes, whereas in anxiety the danger is usually described as being within. *Apathy* indicates a lack of either pleasure or sorrow. On the other hand the response may be apparent but may show a marked deviation from that normally seen, *e.g.*, news that would cause sorrow to the average person may be the occasion for elation and laughter. This inappropriateness of affect is typically found in schizophrenia. *Emotional instability* is characterised by rapid variations in the affective state without any apparent cause; it occurs in organic conditions.

§ **1165. Disorders of Thought.** A *delusion* is a false belief, quite impervious to argument or reason, and one that would not be shared by persons of the same race, education and status in life. Various psychological mechanisms have been elaborated in an effort to explain such ideas. In certain cases the significance of the delusional idea and its method of elaboration are obvious; in many they remain a matter of speculation. Hallucinations may frequently form the basis of subsequent delusional ideas. They are classified for descriptive purposes as delusions of unworthiness, self-reproach, poverty—depressive ideas; of grandeur, mania, G.P.I.; of persecution—paranoid. When the delusions are based around a central theme from which deductions have been logically made to form a coherent organisation of ideas, the delusional system is said to be systematised. *Insight* is the degree of conscious appreciation which the patient has of his abnormal symptoms and the nature of his illness and is measured by the extent to which he is prepared to discuss these symptoms and recognises them as abnormal. An *obsession* is an idea that obtrudes into the mind, the individual being perfectly aware of its absurdity and control over his will. It differs from a delusion in that the nature of the idea is recognised as absurd, and the patient endeavours to rid himself of it. *Ideas of reference* are misinterpretations; the patient becomes convinced that various happenings or things recorded in the press relate to himself. When he believes that some force or other agency directs his activities so that he may perform certain acts even against his will, such are described are *passivity feelings*—commonly found in schizophrenia. *Nihilistic* ideas are associated with a marked disturbance of affect and take the form of beliefs that the individual has no body, that he is dead or that the world has ceased to be.

§ **1166. Disorders of Perception.** *Hallucinations* are sensory perceptions without any external cause. This contrasts with *illusions,* in which real perceptions are misinterpreted. Illusions are experienced by all at some time or other, and are common when there is clouding of consciousness. Hallucinations are frequent in the early stages of mental illness and are particularly common in toxic-infective conditions. Although physical factors may be present, the content is often influenced by previous psychological experiences. Hallucinations without any disturbance of consciousness—in other words, occurring in a clear setting—are of more serious import: in organic conditions hallucinations may show a nocturnal frequency. Hallucinations affect all senses, those of hearing are by far the most common. They may consist of indeterminate noises, but more often consist of words spoken by voices which may or may not be recognisable. In schizophrenia these voices may be said to arise from within and may be attributed to one of the internal organs. Hallucinations of sight are less frequent and usually occur with some clouding of consciousness; they often accompany toxic-infective illnesses, particularly delirium tremens, in which the hallucinatory experiences are very vivid and accompanied by intense fear. Hallucinations of smell are found in more chronic types of illness—chiefly schizophrenia; they are usually unpleasant and are associated with a sense of guilt. Hallucinations of taste are uncommon and are often associated with those of smell. Illusions of taste are more frequently experienced. Hallucinations of touch—haptic or tactile—occur in toxic-infective conditions, especially delirium tremens and cocaine addiction.

§ **1167. Disorders of Memory.** Loss of memory is known as *amnesia* (§§ 854, 1173). This may be for limited periods, not necessarily always sharply defined, and is then accompanied by some disorder of consciousness. It is a common result of head injury, a seizure or a hysterical attack. Amnesias connected with events the recollection of which is unpleasant, are frequent in hysteria. Anterograde amnesia denotes a loss of memory for recent events—retrograde that for remote events. An anterograde amnesia not accompanied by any disorder of consciousness is usually indicative of an organic syndrome. Generalised loss of memory is found in secondary dementia.

Paramnesia indicates a falsification of memory. In certain illnesses, particularly Korsakoff's psychosis, the memory deficiencies are filled in by the patient without any relation to fact; this is *confabulation*. *Hyperamnesia* denotes an abnormally acute memory. Incidents with a strong emotional colouring may be recalled with greater ease. It is seen in hypomania, in paranoid states, and in certain prodigies, and may be seen even in gross mental defect.

§ **1168. Disorders of Personality.** With *depersonalisation* the patient ceases to believe in his own existence: not only do external things appear unreal or strange—*derealisation*—but there is a subjective feeling that he has lost his own reality. He does not believe that he is someone else—*transformation of personality*—but rather he has ceased to identify his own personality. *Splitting of the personality* is seen in schizophrenia. There is a disintegration of the personality coupled with independent activities of their functions so that grotesque incongruities of thought and action become possible. *Dissociation* is a mental mechanism to avoid conflict whereby a group of mental processes may be separated from the stream of consciousness and so functions on its own. Examples of dissociation are somnambulism, automatic writing and fugues. In *fugues* the secondary personality may generate such activity as takes the individual varying distances from his usual habitat. More complete degrees of dissociation give rise to *double* or *multiple personality*, in which the patient assumes a new disposition and character which may alternate with his normal recognisable self. The personalities then produced display, as it were, a complete ignorance of each other.

PART B. CLINICAL INVESTIGATION

As in the investigation of other bodily systems it is imperative to adopt some scheme of examination. To obtain an adequate understanding of the patient's mental make-up we largely depend on our ability to get the patient to talk of his problems; this must be encouraged and directed by judicious stimulation and questioning. The personal factor enters into the examination to a greater degree than in the investigation of other systems. Whether the patient is co-operative or not, make it a constant rule to interview the relatives or friends in order to obtain an independent account of the patient's illness. Keep an open mind on the problem, and remember that statements of relatives need not necessarily be correct.

The close interrelationship between mental and bodily illnesses makes obvious the necessity for a detailed physical investigation.

Collect all data in an orderly manner and in chronological sequence even though the interpretation may be difficult.

§ 1169. The first requirement is a clear understanding of the patient's *symptoms* and the development of these from the earliest time that any abnormality was noticed. Find out how far the present condition differs from his previous character and conduct: behaviour which indicates madness in one person is only eccentricity in another. Ascertain, where indicated, any peculiarities of behaviour, over-activity, violence, depression, suicidal preoccupations, excessive phantasy formation, etc. Investigate any *etiological factors*, domestic, business or financial difficulties, etc., so that you may judge whether or not such are adequate to cause the symptoms. Details of the *family history* must be obtained, particularly as to the incidence of alcoholism, drug addiction, a family tendency to eccentric behaviour or peculiar personalities, and other evidence of mental illness. The *previous medical history* and any earlier mental breakdown must be noted: obtain details of the previous personal history, *i.e.*, early development, the presence of neurotic traits, school career, work record and habits. The *environment*, particularly during early life, should be inquired into especially with regard to (a) parental over-anxiety for the patient's health in early childhood, (b) lack of harmony in the family, quarrels, separation of parents, (c) faulty education or upbringing, spoiling, temper outbursts, (d) ethical and religious training, sexual development in adolescent and adult life.

Finally inquire into the patient's *previous personality*: Was he of (1) the syntonic type, popular, a good mixer and sociable; (2) the schizophrenic type, reserved, shy, given to day-dreaming; or (3) the paranoid, inclined to be suspicious and see hidden meanings in things? Endeavour to get an impression of the patient as a whole, so that you may form an opinion as to his endowments and make-up. All such points are of enormous importance in evaluating the prognosis of a mental illness.

The success or failure of a psychiatric examination is often dependent on the physician's mode of approach. Never be in a hurry: any careless, inept, insistent or rapid questioning will only confuse and silence the patient and defeat your object. Endeavour to gain his confidence. To overcome this reserve, let him talk about things in general, then of his thoughts and feelings and finally of any hallucinations or delusions. Allow the patient to give his own account of his symptoms and their development. In making a mental examination, the following scheme is suggested as a guide; from the results thus obtained you are able to make any necessary judgments.

(1) Record your observations on the *patient's reaction* to the interview. Does he look ill? Pay attention to his facial expression and to his dress. Is there over-activity or retardation? If retarded in his movements, does he resist passive movements; is there negativism; flexibilitas cerea; are mannerisms evident? (2) Consider next the *patient's conversation*. Is the enunciation clear; is there evidence of slurring, as in G.P.I.? Note the stream of mental activity; are questions answered promptly and relevantly? Is there excessive volubility; jumping from one topic to another (flight of ideas); are there self-invented words (neologisms) or there may be diminished volubility, with evidence of retardation of the mental processes? In stupor, the patient may refuse to speak or answer questions—mutism. (3) From the patient's appearance, one may get an impression as to the *mood or affective state*. If it is constant, is it appropriate to the emotional state? Carefully note any discrepancy or fluctuation in the mood, such as a smile in a situation which should produce a depressive response. Augment observation by direct inquiry—" How do you feel? How are your spirits? " etc. (4) Much may be obtained from the *content* of the patient's conversation. He is therefore encouraged to talk freely. General inquiries should be made to determine his reaction to those with whom he comes in contact. Are delusional ideas present? What is the patient's reaction to his environment? Is he suspicious? Does he think that he is treated badly or in any special way? Is he persecuted?—paranoid. Are there passivity feelings, that people can influence him to do things? Does he feel that his thoughts can be read? Can he read those of others?—schizophrenic. Are there grandiose ideas—of enormous power or wealth—mania, G.P.I.? Are there depressive ideas such as

those of self-reproach, that he has done great wrong, committed the unpardonable sin, that there is no hope, that life is not worth living, found in melancholia ? Is there evidence of illusions or of hallucinations ? The type, degree of vividness, time of occurrence and content must be noted as also the patient's impression of these. Ascertain if there is obsessional preoccupation either in thought or action. How far do such control activity: do they emanate from within the mind or from an outside force ? In regard to delusions, illusions or hallucinations, estimate how far such perversions of the mind influence or are likely to influence the acts or conduct of the individual.

Ascertain if the patient is correctly orientated as to time, place or person. Determine any memory defects both as regards recent and remote events. What is his attitude towards such—does he fill in the gaps by confabulation (Korsakoff's) ? What is his level of general information; is it adequate, considering his social class; is there evidence of deterioration from the former level ? Finally, does the patient regard his condition as an illness for which treatment is desired ? Has he any insight ? This is of value in assessing the prognosis and in recommending treatment. The essential facts in the illness can now be summarised and an opinion formed as to diagnosis, prognosis and treatment.

PART C.　DIAGNOSIS, PROGNOSIS AND TREATMENT OF MENTAL ILLNESSES

§ 1170. Classification.

PSYCHONEUROSES and PSYCHOSES in their characteristic forms may appear to be distinct entities, easily differentiated from one another. However, in some cases the line of demarcation is not always so clearly defined, and the one may merge into the other. The essential difference is the degree to which the personality is involved: in *psychoneurotic illnesses* the personality remains intact, there is ability to differentiate between reality and subjective experiences and the patient retains insight into the nature of his illness and is anxious to get well. The *psychotic patient*, on the other hand, shows distortion and disintegration of his personality, he loses his sense of reality, frequently lives in a world of phantasy, and his beliefs are not amenable to reasoned explanation.

The resultant forms of illness are not to be regarded as disease entities, but rather as *types of reaction* to various forms of stress. These may appear in several forms:—

GROUP I.—COMMON MINOR MENTAL ILLNESSES.

GROUP II.—MAJOR MENTAL ILLNESSES.

IN CHILDREN.

GROUP I. COMMON MINOR MENTAL ILLNESSES

Psychoneurotic illnesses comprise mental disturbances (anxiety, fugues, phobias) or physical symptoms (paralyses, anæsthesiæ)—for which no organic cause can be discovered. They are in general terms the result of mental conflict, dealt with by repression. The conflicting forces can often be traced to instincts of self-preservation, gregarious or herd instincts, to reproductive instincts, or to ethical teachings implanted in childhood. The various methods have been discussed already by which such repressed factors obtain expression and produce different types of neurotic symptoms.

The patient complains of loss of interest, inability to concentrate and various fears. The condition is ANXIETY NEUROSIS.

§ 1171. I. Anxiety Neurosis (Synonym: Psychoneurotic Anxiety State) is the commonest form of Psychoneurosis. Anxiety reactions are frequently displayed in normal adaptation to environmental stress, *i.e.*, before examinations or making a speech. The effect of such stimuli is diminished generally on repetition and when increased confidence has been achieved. Many cases, diagnosed Neurasthenia, are really examples of Anxiety Neurosis.

Symptoms.—(1) Anxiety is the chief symptom, and this, acting through the autonomic nervous system, produces all kinds of visceral symptoms. There is a great sense of insecurity and problems are magnified. Fears of bodily or mental illness, of suicide or death, are common. Acute panics, lasting minutes or hours, characterised by paroxysmal terror and emotional distress, occur. Between these panics the patient's emotional tone is one of anxiety. He fears to meet people, fears to walk in the traffic, and may sit in the house all day. Sleeplessness, arising from his anxiety, adds to the patient's distress; when sleep occurs, nightmares are often present. (2) Visceral symptoms, visceral reactions secondary to the panics and prevailing anxiety, are almost constantly present. Besides the physical concomitants of fear (viz., dry mouth, shaking, tachycardia, frequency of micturition) all kinds of gastro-intestinal symptoms may arise—vomiting, nausea, diarrhœa, water-brash, constipation, etc. Seminal emissions, blurring of vision, twitchings of muscles also occur. Digestive disturbances and loss of sleep often give rise to physical deterioration. To these morbid fears, which are of infinite variety, various names have been given—fear of open spaces (agoraphobia), fear of closed rooms and buildings (claustrophobia). These are not different diseases but are part of an anxiety state, varying according to the patient's history. Fear of dirt, of knives and scissors, of medicines, of travelling in tubes, lifts, omnibuses, etc., are also met. The patient cannot explain why he dreads these things, but realises their absurdity.

Effort Syndrome is the name given to a clinical picture that may develop in a variety of nervous conditions. The symptoms comprise breathlessness, giddiness, palpitation, tachycardia, sweating, pain and exhaustion, and these develop during or are aggravated by exercise (§ 34). They occur most frequently with anxiety or with varying degrees of depression, but they may be superadded to a hysterical or a psychopathic personality. The physical methods of treatment, graduated exercises, occupational therapy, etc., will obviously be augmented by psychological treatment of the primary disability.

Diagnosis.—Anxiety as a symptom is common in *obsessional neurosis, melancholia* and *schizophrenia*. The presence of the other characteristic features of these conditions simplifies the diagnosis. Anxiety neurosis results when the reaction produced is out of proportion to the cause, real or fictitious. It is the commonest form of psychoneurosis.

Etiology.—(i) Hereditary, constitutional and environmental factors. (ii) The patient is emotionally unstable; (iii) A sexual basis was propounded by Freudians to explain such reactions, but there is no doubt that anxiety neuroses may develop from mental conflicts arising from many sources, of which the chief are domestic, financial, sexual and business worries.

The *Prognosis* is better than in any other form of psychoneurosis. Apart from psychological treatment much will depend on how modifiable the other etiological factors may be. *Treatment* is described in § 1172.

The patient complains of tiredness, lack of concentration, irritability, feelings of pressure in the head, and other subjective symptoms for which you can find no organic cause. The disease is NEURASTHENIA.

§ 1172. II. Neurasthenia (Synonym: Chronic Nervous Exhaustion) as a clinical entity is rare, and the term is one of the most abused in medicine. Mainly characterised by fatigue, some degree of anxiety is also usually present, and the relative importance of each has to be assessed.

Symptoms.—(1) The chief symptom is tiredness, a ready mental fatigue and physical prostration without discoverable lesion. The tiredness of the neurasthenic differs from ordinary exhaustion in that it is not relieved by a night's rest, and it is not always precipitated by factors which cause exhaustion in the normal individual. (2) There is fatigue of cortical inhibition and control, manifesting itself by abnormal irritability over trifles, lack of emotional control and motor restlessness. All kinds of visceral sensations, normally inhibited by cortical control from reaching the sensorium, become manifest and the patient is conscious of the beating of his heart, peristaltic movements of his intestines, etc. (3) The patient becomes egocentric and introspective, the whole of his consciousness filled with his abnormal physical sensations. So full is he of his illness that he cannot devote his attention to outside affairs and he suffers from lack of concentration, which he wrongly attributes to mental failure. (4) There is a peculiar kind of headache, which is described as a pressure rather than a pain, or an aching tightness radiating from the frontal region into the back of the neck or the spine. At other times the feeling in the head is described as a " woolliness " or " cloudiness." The discomfort is never actual pain, but is described as something worse and less bearable than pain. (5) Sleeplessness adds to the patient's misery. (6) Symptoms referable to the autonomic nervous system and endocrine glands occur, tachycardia, tremor, vaso-motor instability and loss of weight. The blood pressure is invariably lowered in severe cases, with giddiness, coldness and clamminess of the extremities and tachycardia, pallor or syncope on suddenly assuming the erect position. (7) The menstrual periods in women may be irregular. All kinds of disturbances in the sexual sphere occur and may dominate the clinical picture. Sexual impotence, premature ejaculations, spermatorrhœa, all occur in men. The urine usually contains a heavy deposit of phosphates and is alkaline. Phosphates may be deposited in the bladder and appear in the urine at the end of micturition, the patient mistaking the phosphate deposit for seminal fluid and imagining that his virility is draining away.

Diagnosis from the other psychoneuroses is generally not difficult. Fatigue may be a hysterical conversion symptom. It is more difficult to differentiate between neurasthenia and a depressive illness. Fatigue is prominent in both, but there is more affective disturbance in depression; the previous history and familial incidence often aid diagnosis. Early schizophrenia and neurasthenia are not always easy to distinguish.

Etiology.—Psychological factors are the primary cause. Neurasthenia should not be accepted as the diagnosis until adequate mental phenomena have been elicited to account for the symptoms. Opinions vary as to whether the constitutional factors present are contributory or secondary to prolonged emotional conflict. Overwork is not causative; lack of occupation and of emotional outlet may be predisposing causes.

Treatment of Anxiety Neurosis and Neurasthenia.—It is essential to appreciate the psychological origin. (i) At the outset obtain a detailed account of the patient's illness and of the development of his symptoms; and at the same time his own ideas on his illness. (ii) So often he fears physical disease that the next step is a *complete physical examination*: this must be thorough, so that when negative you can reassure the patient with confidence that there is no physical basis for his symptoms. (iii) It is important to explain that recovery takes place in irregular fashion, good days being followed by bad days, until eventually the bad days disappear. By this time the confidence of the patient should have been obtained, an essential factor for progress. (iv) Next, try to trace the cause of the anxiety; for this a knowledge of mental mechanisms is generally necessary. Nevertheless by patient inquiry and encouragement each symptom can usually be traced to its origin. Advise as to the effect on the general health of an emotional upset and demonstrate how the symptoms have developed during such periods. Make it clear that you do not consider the symptoms are imaginary, but that they originate from genuine causes. For example, the exhaustion which often accompanies these psychoneuroses can be explained in terms of anxiety or emotional perturbation, the anxious preoccupation preventing the patient from using his available store of energy. Sexual impotence may be traced to false ideas of physical damage resulting from past habits of masturbation, rendered more distressing by associated feelings of remorse. (v) If environmental factors operate largely in the etiology, or if the symptoms are severe, it may be necessary to remove the patient for a time from the atmosphere of his conflicts. If isolation is practised, it should be complete, the patient being allowed to see no one but his doctor and nurse, to write and receive no letters. In slighter cases it is sufficient to re-educate the patient to face up to his difficulties and make whatever adjustments are possible.

Sleeplessness.—It is essential to ensure adequate sleep. Sleeplessness is to be treated on the lines laid down in § 836. It is better that the patient, by using an effective hypnotic, should secure sufficient sleep, than that he should go on having nights filled with wakeful, anxious preoccupation. *Occupational therapy.*—If the patient is unable to concentrate on reading, the periods of rest prescribed may be usefully employed in the practice of rug-making or some handicraft. Occupational therapy of this kind helps to restore confidence (§ 1192). *Diet* —If the patient is physically below par, careful feeding with extra amounts of cream and milk foods, and small doses of malt and cod-liver oil are indicated. *Massage.* —Daily massage and exercises will build up the general muscular tone. For stronger patients exercise in the fresh air, short of fatigue, will be helpful. *Drugs.*—If anxiety is acute and complete rest essential, then a course of prolonged narcosis may be beneficial (§ 1178). The majority respond to sedative or tranquillising drugs, either regularly or symptomatically as occasion requires. Alcohol is seldom advisable and tobacco should be limited. Strychnine, in even small doses, nearly always makes the patient worse by increasing general hypersensitiveness. *Change of*

Environment.—When the patient has recovered sufficiently, a holiday in a dry, warm climate may be prescribed. He should not be rendered anxious by needless restrictions and warnings.

To summarise, the methods of treatment are: (1) *Explanation* and analysis of the symptoms, (2) *Persuasion,* by all kinds of encouragement and reassurance, and, lastly, (3) *Re-education,* by general methods, until the patient's adaptations to his environment are normal.

There are physical signs of loss of function but without signs of organic disease. The disease is HYSTERIA.

§ 1173. III. Hysteria.—The results of a hysterical type of reaction to a distressing situation are extremely varied but present a clear clinical picture. The hysterical reaction is a manifestation of a childish need for dependence on others, and the hysterical individual solves her problem usually by the production of some physical symptom, with unconscious desire that it will remove her from the scene of her difficulties. She is, however, entirely unaware how her symptoms have arisen. The temporary solution of the problem brings her a characteristic composure and indifference ("la belle indifférence" of Janet) and a measure of mental relief, wrongly attributed by her friends to fortitude or resignation. Such patients are commonly extremely egocentric and selfish; there may be an outward show of great emotion, but there is probably very little real emotional content.

Clinically, the disease shows characteristic physical and mental symptoms:

(1) PHYSICAL SYMPTOMS, characteristically produced by suggestion, curable by suggestion and without objective evidence of structural nervous disease. The mimicry of organic nervous disease may be very close but is never complete, and there is usually some paradoxical phenomenon present, revealing the true cause of the symptom, *e.g.*, hoarseness may be present in speaking, yet the cough is clear.

(2) MENTAL SYMPTOMS such as amnesia, delirium, twilight-states, stupor, fugues, somnambulism, and self-mutilation.

It should never be forgotten that hysteria and organic disease may co-exist in the same patient. This is especially true of the traumatic cases.

1. PHYSICAL SYMPTOMS.

(*a*) MOTOR SYMPTOMS.—When *Rigidity* is present it is proportional to the force used to overcome it, on attempted passive movement. The associated contraction of the antagonistic muscles can be palpated when the patient attempts voluntary movement. *Flaccid hysterical palsies* are commoner than rigidity. When the leg is affected it trails behind the patient, who hops on the sound limb with the dorsum of the affected foot dragging on the floor behind him. All kinds of bizarre *hysterical gaits* are met with, which may be associated with remarkable spinal curvatures occasionally simulating hip-joint disease. In these conditions (i.) there is never any alteration, either quantitative or qualitative, in the deep or cutaneous reflexes, although the plantar response may be absent at the toes. (ii.) the muscles react normally to electrical stimulation, and (iii.) there is no wasting, apart from that occasioned by disuse.

Hysterical tremors and tics vary in degree and are increased by attention. Hysterical tremor may closely simulate the tremor of paralysis agitans or disseminated sclerosis, but other features of these diseases are absent. Paroxysms of violent tremor may pass over into hysterical fits. Slighter forms accompany paralysis and rigidity of hysterical origin. *Hysterical blepharospasm* is fairly common.

In *Hysterical Aphonia* the patient whispers but can phonate normally on coughing. On laryngoscopic examination the cords are not sufficiently approximated to produce a sound.

In *Mutism* there is complete abolition of speech, although the organs concerned are used normally for clearing the throat, coughing and mastication.

Hysterical recurrent cough is fairly common.

(b) SENSORY SYMPTOMS.—Sensory loss affects only *cutaneous sensibility* and is usually complete. Sense of position (which is outside the patient's knowledge) is unaffected, as evidenced by accurate co-ordination of movement. Sensory loss may be of the " stocking " or " glove " distribution in the limbs. The upper level of a hysterical analgesia has the following characters: (i.) It is horizontal. (ii.) It varies from time to time on successive examinations. (iii.) The transition from analgesia to normal skin is abrupt, without any area of impaired sensibility or hyperæsthesia, as in organic disease. In hysterical hemianæsthesia the corneal reflexes remain intact and the sensory loss ceases abruptly at the mid-line in front; whereas in organic disease it is continued for a short distance across the mid-line in front. In hysteria there is often affection of all the spinal senses on the side of the hemianæsthesia. For Janet's " Yes-No " test, see § 844.

Hysterical blindness is often sudden in onset and may be complete or incomplete. In the complete form the patient commonly avoids obstacles placed in his path. In the incomplete forms perimeter charts show an unequal constriction of the visual fields in the two eyes (hysterical amblyopia) or a spiral " fatigue " field. Diplopia can be produced by pressure displacement of one eye. The pupils and optic discs are always normal. *Hysterical deafness* can be recognised by the fact that the patient can be wakened from sleep if called by name, but when awakened he cannot hear. *Hysterical anosmia* is common in plumbers after gas explosions, and includes loss of sensation to ammonia vapour, which is a function of the fifth, not the first nerve.

(c) VISCERAL SYMPTOMS.—Digestive disturbances are not infrequent and to the relatives most alarming. *Hysterical globus* is the sensation of a lump in the throat interfering with swallowing. *Hysterical ærophagy* may lead to enormous abdominal distension with simulation of pregnancy or of an ovarian cyst. *Hysterical vomiting* is seldom accompanied by any profound loss of weight: there is no nausea and the expulsion of certain foods from the stomach will not prevent the retention immediately afterwards of others more palatable. In a few cases nothing is retained and progressive emaciation results. In diagnosing these conditions great care must be taken to exclude the presence of organic disease. The chronic abdominal pains of hysterical women are often the cause of repeated laparotomies, for " adhesions," " fixation," etc. The patient, unaware of the true cause of her malady, often invites operation with amazing eagerness.

Anorexia Nervosa is characterised by loss of appetite or a persistent refusal of food. It is a more serious condition, found more frequently in young women, and progressive emaciation may develop even to the point of death. The refusal of food is at first involuntary but soon all desire for food is lost. The condition should be distinguished from the anorexia seen in melancholia and from the cachexia of endocrine origin. Psychogenic factors are prominent and conditions usually develop out of some conflict. Effective treatment in early stages usually promotes recovery (and see § 569).

(*d*) CUTANEOUS SYMPTOMS.—Blueness, coldness, variable œdema are all met in hysterically paralysed limbs. Dermographism is common. Anomalous skin eruptions may be produced by the patient by rubbing, corrosives or by burning (§ 623).

(2) MENTAL SYMPTOMS.

Hysterical amnesias are frequently for limited periods of time and follow a marked emotional disturbance. Similarly *delirious states* follow an emotional upset; the degree of confusion is variable and the flow of talk is of a nonsensical type. The *twilight state* (Ganser syndrome) occurs essentially among prisoners and represents an attempt to appear irresponsible; the purposeful nature is obvious. *Stupor* may be maintained for prolonged periods but terminates rapidly once the precipitating factors have ceased to exist. *Amnesias, fugues* and *somnambulism* are evidence of dissociation. The dissociated portion of the personality functions independently and for the time being controls the patient's activities. *Self-mutilation* is met and suicidal threats and attempts may be made; the latter are invariably-dramatic.

(*e*) HYSTERICAL FITS never occur between definite hours of the day, as do epileptic fits, and never during sleep. They take place in the presence of an audience, there is never any incontinence or tongue-biting, and the patient never injures herself, although others may be injured. The eyes are usually screwed up and the hands clenched, and the movements are " purposive." Hysterical fits may follow upon true epileptic fits. They may be accompanied by outbursts of unrestrained laughing and crying.

Etiology.—(i.) Constitutional factors are important. (ii.) Hysteria often occurs in families with a history of schizophrenic, alcoholic or other psychopathic disorders. (iii.) It is more common in adolescence and at the menopause, and (iv.) in females than males. (v.) It occurs in a hysterical type of personality, characterised by egotism and an attitude of posing or make-believe. Such patients show a marked emotional susceptibility and are readily influenced by and imitate those who appeal to them. (vi.) Mental stress is the exciting factor; the symptom achieves some aim or desire (often not consciously appreciated by the patient) and thus allows a maintenance of self-respect otherwise impossible.

Prognosis.—Individual symptoms are usually easy to cure but the liability to recurrence is great. The prognosis depends on how far the personality can be modified and the etiological factors readjusted.

Treatment.—Treatment directed merely to the relief of local symptoms is inadequate, though by suggestion, persuasion and re-education it may be temporarily effective; somatic symptoms respond readily to suggestion.

It is not, however, enough to remove the symptoms; efforts must be made to elicit their mechanism; until this is discovered and treated no permanent benefit is derived. The employment of all psychotherapeutic methods (§ 1192) may be necessary at some time or another to achieve this end. The chief obstacle to effective treatment is the mental indifference of the patient; this prevents an appreciation of the causes which have led to the development of the symptoms. Environmental factors must be considered and readjusted as far as possible. The thought of return to the arena of conflict is, in some cases, insupportable, e.g., the childless woman will not return to her drunken husband. In such cases, you must do what you can to make the patient's environment more tolerable. In all cases, she should be encouraged to do some kind of useful work.

§ 1174. IV. **Traumatic Hysteria** (Synonym: Traumatic Neurasthenia).— The symptoms of this neurosis must be carefully distinguished from those of *Unresolved Cerebral Contusion* (see § 813).

Immediately following upon an accident, which may be trivial, or more usually some days or weeks after the accident, the patient develops hysterical symptoms. The condition is particularly likely to occur in injuries to the head or spine. There is always an additional element of anxiety in the symptoms, due to the uncertainty in the patient's mind as to the outcome of litigation and the possibility of his return to work. It occurs in workmen, especially those engaged in dangerous occupations and who work at a height from the ground. Such cases often come into Court in connection with the Workmen's Compensation Act.

Symptoms.—Mentally, the patient becomes extremely introspective, with a profound conviction of the seriousness of his complaint. He becomes sleepless and irritable, and his anxieties are increased by his uncertainty of his ultimate recovery and return to work, and the financial straits into which his illness throws him. Physically, all kinds of hysterical phenomena are met, tremors, paralysis, spasms, including convergent ocular spasm, hysterical gaits and attitudes, and hysterical affections of the special senses and cutaneous sensibility. There is commonly loss of weight, tachycardia and low blood pressure. Pains of all kinds are complained of, and these may indeed be due to associated organic disease, e.g., Spondylitis. The distinction from malingering is often difficult. In malingering there is conscious attempt to deceive others for gain; unlike the hysteric, the patient is not deceived as to the mechanism of his symptoms.

Treatment.—A period of rest in bed for two weeks, with a full neurological and X-ray examination, will prepare the way for cure. If no organic disease is found the patient should be informed of this and his symptoms should be tactfully explained to him. Hypnotics and sedatives may be necessary to secure the sleep essential in treating such cases. Explanation should be combined with reassurance and re-education. Graduated gymnastic exercises, physical work, ladder-climbing, weight-lifting, may all assist in the cure. The symptoms, however, do not usually entirely clear up until legal proceedings are finally settled, and the patient has proved or failed to prove his case against those he deems responsible for his illness. Even after such a settlement, symptoms occasionally persist, owing to the anxiety occasioned by his illness.

The patient is dominated by some thought or action recognised as senseless and accompanied by a feeling that it must be resisted. The condition is OBSESSIVE COMPULSIVE NEUROSIS.

§ 1175. V. **Obsessive Compulsive Neurosis** (Syn. Psychasthenia).—Almost everyone has experienced at some stage in life obsessions or compulsions of a mild degree. They are frequently present in minor degree in childhood and are rarely to be taken seriously then. The condition is an attempt to ward off unknown evil by a process akin to magic. When present in later life they are of much greater significance and may be so severe that the greater part of the patient's life is spent in attending to these symptoms. The condition is characterised by: (1) *Anxious preoccupation with some obsessive idea.* The patient may ask himself over and over again some religious or metaphysical question, *e.g.*, " What was the beginning of everything ? " Some are disturbed by the reiteration of certain words or phrases in their mind. These are frequently symbolic and may be so severe as to exclude other interests. (2) *Morbid compulsions.* It is easy to appreciate how ritualistic actions may develop as a means of combating the fears associated with the obsessive ideas, *e.g.*, a fear of dirt and contamination may necessitate constant washing and scrubbing of the skin to ensure cleanliness. Patients may feel compelled to touch objects, to do things in a certain order, to steal something intrinsically worthless, which they do not need (kleptomania), to commit homicidal acts or sexual assaults, to take alcohol (dipsomania) or drugs. There is, sometimes, only fear that these imperative acts will be committed, and the act is never actually carried out.

Prognosis.—When the onset is insidious and there is no marked affective disturbance the prognosis is poor. The course of the illness is invariably prolonged. It has been frequently stated that it is not uncommon for obsessional-compulsive states to be followed by a psychosis. This seems doubtful. If the obsessional symptoms are part of a depressive illness and accompanied by the other characteristic features of an affective disorder the prognosis is reasonably good.

Treatment.—The hereditary basis is marked. When the morbid impulse or obsessional idea is part of a depressive illness, the treatment is as for melancholia. The more severe forms of insidious onset are not readily amenable to psychotherapy, which is necessarily prolonged. When all other methods of treatment have failed, consideration should be given to a modified prefrontal leucotomy operation especially if tension and anxiety are prominent concomitants. Considerable benefit may be achieved in selected cases.

The patient exhibits ANOMALIES OF BEHAVIOUR, *characterised by* INADEQUATE SOCIAL ADAPTATION, ANTAGONISM TO OTHERS, *or by* PATHOLOGICAL SEXUAL IMPULSES WITHOUT *gross* PSYCHOTIC SYMPTOMS *or intellectual impairment. The condition is* PSYCHOPATHIC PERSONALITY.

§ 1176. VI. **Psychopathic Personality.**—In the Mental Health Act (1959) psychopathic disorder is defined as a persistent disorder or disability of mind (whether or not including subnormality of intelligence) which results in abnormally aggressive or seriously irresponsible conduct on the part of the patient and requires, or is susceptible to, medical treatment. Three groups are generally recognised, (i.) aggressive, (ii.) passive, (iii.) creative. Electroencephalographic records are of interest in the aggressive irritable group, and tend to show more frequently than the average a demonstrable theta-rhythm even in the resting state.

Symptoms often appear in early life, generally in the form of excessive emotional displays, temper tantrums, pathological lying, and antisocial behaviour of a criminal kind, stealing, wilful destruction, etc. (§ 1194). As puberty normally requires numerous fresh adaptations between instinctive desires and social standards, at this time the expression of a psychopathic personality invariably becomes more pronounced. Antisocial actions become more frequent, more acute, and are generally of an episodic nature and quite uncontrollable: they are devoid of reflection or any consideration for feelings of themselves or others, and their execution produces no sense of remorse. These abnormal acts generally occur in a setting of clear consciousness with no other abnormal psychotic manifestations, so that it is extremely difficult to exercise control. The intellectual level is invariably within normal limits.

Etiology.—The chief etiological factors seen are the effects of heredity and environment. A similar picture may be seen associated with organic diseases of the brain, *e.g.*, epilepsy, encephalitis lethargica.

Prognosis.—The prognosis is serious, particularly if treatment is not instituted before adult life.

Treatment.—This as it applies to problems in childhood is described in § 1194. At this stage prevention offers the greatest measure of success. Ascertain the factors that determine or aggravate the outbursts. If environmental factors are prominent, effect a change in this direction. Where antisocial acts of conduct are serious, admission to hospital may be necessary. The provision of colonies for the supervision and treatment of these patients has been repeatedly advocated. Once adult life is reached the results of psychotherapeutic treatment are disappointing.

GROUP II. THE MAJOR MENTAL ILLNESSES

§ 1177. I. States of excitement and exaltation. Acute mental excitement may be a **transient** phenomenon in the following conditions, where it is clearly traceable to some bodily disorder.

Delirium	§§ 469, 1186
Alcoholic and Drug Addiction	§§ 1184, 1185
Head Injuries	§ 854
Thyrotoxic Crises	§ 186
Epilepsy (" Equivalents ")	§ 861

Continuous mental excitement is found in:—mania (§ 1178) where the mental condition is the only, or at any rate, the principal symptom; Agitated melancholia (§ 1180), where the agitation is accompanied by severe depression; ACUTE TOXIC CONFUSIONAL PSYCHOSIS, where hallucinations and delusions are prominent features of the excited state, together with symptoms of profound exhaustion; SCHIZOPHRENIA (§ 1182), when it is accompanied by delusional ideas frequently grotesque in nature; and in GENERAL PARALYSIS (§ 1190), when accompanying physical signs are apparent.   When a patient is confused and delirious, investigate for drug intoxication, such as that following the cumulative effects of a sedative, especially bromides, taken for weeks or months; URÆMIA may produce similar symptoms (§§ 370, 371).

The patient is continuously excited, restless, garrulous, showing flight of ideas, or lacking in control.   The disease is MANIA.

§ 1178. **Mania** is classified as " Simple," " Acute," and " Chronic."

Simple Mania.—In this mild form of excitement one of the principal features is a loss of self-control.   This is accompanied by an exaggerated sense of well-being.   The patient is talkative, restless, and optimistic. Often he is interfering and irascible.   There is a general failure of judgment and instability of purpose.

Acute Mania may supervene suddenly—(1) during convalescence from exhausting diseases (as previously mentioned); (2) in the course of other diseases of the nervous system—*e.g.*, G.P.I.; (3) in the course of some other form of mental illness.   Its onset is usually rapid, tongue-tremor being often met in the early stage.   The stage of excitement is soon reached—loquaciousness, sleeplessness, continual restlessness, incoherence in which delusions and ideas succeed each other with great rapidity, sometimes relating to moral and religious, at other times to intellectual topics.   After lasting some weeks or months, recovery (sometimes quite suddenly) ensues; sometimes it is followed by moral or mental obliquity or dementia; it may pass into chronic mania.   The temperature is normal throughout.   In many cases there is a tendency to relapse and sometimes an alternation with melancholia.

Chronic Mania is suspected when a patient's restless excitement, incoherent conversation, and disordered conduct continue, although sleep and appetite have fully returned and are accompanied by improvement in the physical state   Delusions become more prominent and auditory hallucinations may be a feature.   The condition is rare before middle life.

Acute Delirious Mania is an acute maniacal condition which may follow upon one of the other varieties of mania or develop suddenly in a person in apparent health.   It is attended by pyrexia, usually running a rapidly fatal course, no lesions being found after death.   It is happily rare.   The symptoms come on abruptly, and quickly amount to frenzy, accompanied by outbreaks of great violence and refusal of food.   The temperature ranges irregularly from 100° to 104° F, and in the course of one to three weeks the disease terminates in great bodily prostration, and often in death.   The majority of these cases are nowadays better described as

Acute Toxic Confusional Psychosis. The toxic nature of the illness is evidenced by the rise in temperature, the vivid numerous and fleeting hallucinations, the intense confusion, and the state of muttering delirium which supervenes. The patient has all the appearance of one suffering from toxæmia, the complexion is pale and muddy with perhaps a malar flush, the mouth and tongue are dirty, and there is sordes on the lips. From acute mania it is known by the fever, the rapid wasting, and more rapid and fatal termination. It resembles some cases of typhoid fever, pneumonia and acute meningitis, but their distinguishing signs are absent.

The *Treatment of mania* consists mainly of rest in bed, preferably in the open air, and in the administration of food. Milder forms are controlled by sedatives and tranquillisers. Prolonged narcosis can be induced by barbiturates, *e.g.*, sodium amylobarbitone 6 gr. each 4-hours. It should be remembered that the threshold between the therapeutic and toxic doses is low and complications may readily ensue. To prevent such, the administration of glucose and insulin has been recommended; the degree of success achieved thereby is, however, not always complete. The treatment of choice is convulsive therapy, electrically induced, combined with a muscular relaxant. The number of treatments required varies usually between four and eight; invariably the response is dramatic. The successful management of manic patients depends on tactful and patient handling. The danger to life has been very much reduced by the physical methods of treatment now available. By such means it is usually possible to ensure adequate nourishment and rarely is tube feeding necessary. The principal indications in the treatment of *acute toxic confusional* psychosis are to control the extreme restlessness by hypnotics, to promote elimination as freely as possible and to maintain the patient's strength. The bowels should be well washed out with a high enema at least twice weekly, and the patient should be given copious fluids, by a nasal tube if necessary. The mouth should be kept clean and the general medical and nursing indications are similar to those required in the treatment of any acute toxic and febrile illness.

§ 1179. II. MENTAL DEPRESSION and RETARDATION may occur in: (1) MELANCHOLIA, where the signs and symptoms of depression are constant, and are the dominant features of the illness; (2) SCHIZOPHRENIA, where the affective change is inadequate, or bizarre delusional ideas are prominent; and (3) GENERAL PARALYSIS, in which disease the accompanying *physical signs* are the determining features.

The patient is continuously depressed, self-reproachful and hopeless. The disease is MELANCHOLIA.

§ 1180. **Melancholia** is a morbid condition of miserable self-consciousness and self-abnegation without hope. The onset is usually insidious, and commences with extreme self-consciousness, combined with sadness, as indicated by depression, without adequate cause, and the patient is irritable when remonstrated with. He loses interest, finds increasing difficulty in concentration, develops fears of impending calamity which cannot be named and becomes sleepless. Self-reproachful ideas are conspicuous and often refer to minor events that may have occurred years previously. The diagnosis is strengthened by a history of a previous attack, or an intervening period of high spirits and bounding energy. A family incidence of depression puts the diagnosis beyond doubt. Always regard such patients as potential suicides. The degree of affective response differentiates such patients from those suffering from hypochondriasis.

Melancholia may be simple, acute, or chronic. (1) **Simple Melancholia** is characterised by a lack of interest, loss of feeling for others, inability to concentrate as before and a dulling of the mental processes. It consists simply of misery, sleeplessness, self-reproach, and inability to continue at work. This form is common in the over-worked or much-worried, and in women at the climacteric. There are no hallucinations, but self-reproachful, depressive ideas are common and characteristic. Suicidal preoccupations are usual and they constitute a large proportion of the suicides that occur each year. Adequate precautions, which are sometimes neglected on account of the simplicity of the affection, should not be omitted. Otherwise the prognosis is favourable. (2) **Acute Melancholia.**—The symptoms already mentioned are present but to a more marked degree. There is marked psychomotor retardation and the picture is that of the most profound misery. Delusional ideas are marked and are of a self-accusatory nature, *i.e.*, they think they are the most wicked individuals, that they have committed the unpardonable sin, etc. Hypochondriacal ideas are also prominent and refer to alleged dysfunction of bodily organs. Auditory hallucinations may be prominent. Food is frequently refused because of ideas of unworthiness and the general condition deteriorates. Insomnia is marked. (3) **Chronic Melancholia.**—In this condition, the symptoms of depression persist, but they are obviously less acute than in the other forms. Although the patient still has the same despairing attitude towards life, sleep returns, food is taken satisfactorily and the physical state improves.

(4) In some cases **Melancholic** or **Benign Stupor** is met. The patients lie in bed speechless, motionless, and are often negativistic. Their habits are faulty; in some retention of urine and fæces has to be specially watched for. Their limbs may be flaccid or in cataleptic rigidity. Although they may appear oblivious to external stimuli they retain as a rule a surprising degree of appreciation of their environment while in this state. They resist external interference, but are not usually violent. It is equally common in both sexes, but is more frequent in the young than in the old. Sometimes it follows a severe and exhausting illness, and sometimes it follows acute mania. (5) **Agitated Melancholia.**—The characteristic picture is that of severe depression without retardation.—The age of onset is usually the involutional period though an earlier incidence is not unknown. Anxiety is marked and is accompanied by extreme motor restlessness. The patient paces up and down wringing his hands and repeating the same despairing remarks over and over again. Auditory hallucinations and delusional ideas are prominent. The absence of retardation increases the degree of suicidal risk. The general physical condition deteriorates because of the difficulty in feeding and the expenditure of much energy.

Recurrent Mania and **Recurrent Melancholia.**—In many instances there is a tendency for a patient to have repeated attacks of mania or melancholia. In such cases it is often remarkable how faithfully reproduced are the general symptoms and the individual peculiarities which have characterised former attacks. For many years it has been recognised that there is a close alliance between mania and melancholia. In the history of almost every attack of depression one finds evidence of an elated phase having been experienced, and similarly, attacks of elation may be preceded or followed by depression. For this reason both mania and melancholia now come under the one classification, namely, **Manic Depressive Psychosis.**

Course and Prognosis of Melancholia.—The melancholic process is longer than the maniacal one. The duration varies considerably but lasts an average of some three to twelve months. However, cases of melancholia may recover even after a very long time—up to fourteen years has been recorded. Relapses are frequent. Heredity is an important factor and the nutrition of the body at the time is another. The danger of exhaustion and intercurrent infection is great in the agitated variety; about 10 per cent. of such terminate fatally in spite of the most careful attention. The presence or absence of an adequate cause, the type of onset, the form of the illness and the absence of other features (arteriosclerosis, etc.) are the important factors to consider in estimating the prognosis. The slower the advent of the disease, the slower is the recovery. There is a distinct suicidal tendency in all cases of melancholia. The risk is less if the degree of retardation is marked, but is greatly increased in the convalescent stage. Never relax observation because the patient says he will not attempt to injure himself; most attempts to commit suicide are of an impulsive nature.

Etiology.—Hereditary factors are prominent and have already been discussed. There is a distinct constitutional basis in the majority of these patients as characterised by their pyknic build: their bodies are round with an abundance of fat, poor muscular development, a rather broad face on a short neck and small hands and feet. The predominant disposition may be either pessimism or optimism and unbounded confidence. These characteristics do not explain the etiology; much depends on the degree of stress to which an individual, so endowed, is subjected. An important factor is a general depression of the vital powers from bodily disease, *e.g.*, fevers, heart disease, and in particular, influenza. The illness is more frequent in women than men. The first attack of mania develops invariably before 30, whereas depression is more frequent at or after middle life.

Treatment of Melancholia.—In the simpler cases, such as those referred to under Simple Melancholia, a few weeks' rest under supervision and away from the conditions under which the disease developed will generally set the patient right. One of the anti-depressant drugs (§ 1192) should be given, either alone or in combination with convulsive therapy, electrically induced.   Prolonged narcosis (§ 1178) is frequently very beneficial, particularly in the less acute forms.   Convulsive therapy, electrically induced and combined with a muscular relaxant, is again the treatment of choice. A favourable response in the depressive phase is usually more easily achieved than in the manic.   The number of treatments required varies usually between four and eight, and the course of the illness is very materially shortened.   Suicide can only be prevented by adequate and constant supervision, either at home or in hospital.   Operative measures —prefrontal leucotomy—have been carried out in certain cases where anxiety and agitation have failed to respond to other methods of treatment. Beneficial results have been obtained.

§ 1181. **Hypochondriasis,** though it cannot accurately be isolated as a clear-cut neurotic or mental disorder, frequently gives rise to such a characteristic clinical picture that a description of the condition is warranted. It is an abnormal condition of the nervous system which has features common to both melancholia and to some of the neuroses.

The patient suffers from prolonged emotional disturbance interpreted in terms of general malaise and of particular physical symptoms.   Although most hypochondriacs may be shown to suffer originally from a depressed reaction to their environment, it is usually found that they also have some underlying physical disability.   They refer all their difficulties to this, and in time become intensely preoccupied with the numerous abnormalities which they discover in their state of health.   Thus, while we must presume that most hypochondriacs are badly adjusted to their environment, we can recognise that most of their symptoms are based in the first instance upon very real somatic disturbances arising from such conditions as chronic dyspepsia, visceroptosis and " floating kidney."   Very soon the whole lives of such patients are coloured by their ideas regarding the deficiencies of their internal organs.   Many of them go from doctor to doctor reciting their symptoms and gleaning from each a few fresh catchwords about their state.   Male hypochondriacs appear to be excessively worried most frequently about their sexual functions and fear impotence.   Female hypochondriacs are more usually concerned with peritoneal adhesions and " floating kidney."   Many such women contrive to be operated upon frequently in order to be relieved from a condition which is basically due to emotional disturbance and maladjustment.

Diagnosis.—It is impossible to enumerate all the symptoms of hypochondria, and it must be understood that a great number of neurasthenics and true melancholics are intensely hypochondriacal.   Nevertheless, it can be recognised that there exists a definite number of patients whose symptoms appear to be purely those described above.

Etiology.—Hypochondriasis is occasionally seen in women, about the menopause, but more often in men of middle age.   It is rare before puberty or before 30, and generally makes its first appearance between 30 and 40. There is often a neurotic family history, including insanity.   Digestive disorder (gastro-intestinal or hepatic) is always present, and may be looked upon as its most frequent cause—a fact of interest in connection with the marked prostration and depression which attend gastric and abdominal disorders. Flatulence and dilatation of the stomach are common.

Treatment is difficult unless one has the time to examine thoroughly the patient's mental state, his environmental circumstances, and to discover the reasons for his failure to react adequately towards these. The dyspepsia should be relieved, the bowels should be carefully regulated. Such treatment, with regular exercises, change of environment and cheerful society, may break through the vicious mental attitude if they are supplemented by reasonable discussions with the patient on his circumstances and his method of adjustment to them. Anti-depressant drugs should be tried but have not as yet been of much benefit in this condition.

The patient becomes apathetic, withdraws from outside interests, daydreams continuously or develops delusional ideas. The disease is SCHIZO-PHRENIA.

§ 1182. III. **Schizophrenia** (Synonym: Dementia Præcox).—This form of mental illness is characterised by an abnormal emotional reaction, accompanied by varying degrees of apparent deterioration in the personality. It has been reported in early life, but is more frequent between the ages of 15 and 35. See § 1194 B for symptoms in adolescence. There is frequently a family history of nervous or mental disorders, and the patient may show one or more stigmata of degeneration, *e.g.*, deformities of the ears. The onset is invariably insidious and no adequate cause can be demonstrated. The previous personality is that of a reserved, unsociable individual of few interests. Four types are found. (1) *Simple:* The characteristic feature is the gradual loss of interest in the environment. As time goes on such patients withdraw further from reality and substitute a world of phantasy, showing itself in indifference and apathy. Delusional ideas and hallucinatory experiences are infrequent and many of these patients lead a simple life outside hospital care. (2) *Hebephrenic:* Here delusions and hallucinations are prominent. The oddity of the delusional ideas—that half of their body has ceased to function, that their blood has gone—and the indifference with which they recite such, are characteristic. Hallucinations are both auditory and visual. Attacks of depression alternating with acute outbursts of excitement occur in the course of the illness. During the latter suicidal or homicidal attacks may be made. Other symptoms frequently seen are echopraxia and echolalia in which the actions or words of bystanders are imitated, although questions may not be answered. (3) *Katatonic:* The progress of the illness is more rapid in this form. Extreme affections of volition are found and vary from outbursts of excitement to depression and a stage of stupor. In the stuporose state no interest is displayed in anything. The patients sit in one position; if the limbs are placed in an awkward position they will remain there for an indefinite period (flexibilitas cerea). Such patients have to be dressed and undressed and require attention in all respects. They pay no need to the calls of nature, and may require to be tube fed for long periods. Although indifferent and apparently insensitive they are nevertheless able to appreciate what is going on in the environment. From this state they will pass into one of excitement, possibly without warning. Impulsive attacks, homicidal or suicidal in nature, are frequent and must be guarded against. (4) The *Paranoid* form is characterised by prominent delusional ideas. They are not systematised as in paranoia, are much more bizarre in nature and are accompanied by hallucinatory experiences. It is more common to meet this type after 30 years of age than before.

Etiology.—Hereditary and constitutional factors are again conspicuous. In stature these patients are thin, long-limbed and of poor physique. Their mental make-up is that of a reserved, shy individual with few interests and friends. The symptoms may not become manifest till after some debilitating illness or period of mental stress.

Prognosis.—In the main the outlook is poor. Such patients constitute 40 per cent. of the chronic cases in mental hospitals. Remissions occur of comparative or complete return to health; in others the degree of improvement is less marked. Of the clinical types the katatonic variety is the most favourable. A sudden onset, a previously good personality and an adequate cause, when found, make the prognosis less ominous.

Treatment.—When the illness has developed, then hospital treatment is advisable for the safety of the patient and the community. Excitement can be controlled by sedation, tranquillisers and convulsive therapy, electrically induced. Efforts must be made to prevent further deterioration in habits. In this respect occupational therapy, properly directed, is of the greatest value. Various special forms of therapy have been advocated at different times, by the induction of fever (malaria, pyrifer), vaccines, polyglandular extracts and continued narcosis. The variety of such testifies to their inefficacy.

In recent years, active therapeutic measures have included (a) electrically induced convulsions, (b) hypoglycæmia, (c) tranquillisers, (d) operation —prefrontal leucotomy. The first two require the closest supervision and should be given only by experts. A combination of both methods is sometimes used, the convulsion being induced after a light degree of hypoglycæmic coma has been attained. Convulsive therapy is more effective where the affective disturbance is marked and hypoglycæmia where there are gross delusional ideas. Early treatment gives a much better therapeutic result. (a) *Convulsive therapy, electrically induced,* is given by means of electrodes placed on the head, a small electrical current is passed through the brain (100–150 volts for 0·2 sec.) and a convulsion follows at once, with tonic and clonic phases, the period of unconsciousness lasting a few minutes. These are induced at three-day intervals; improvement is unlikely if it is not apparent after 10 to 12 treatments. Complications such as fractures and dislocations are prevented when the treatment is combined with a muscular relaxant. (*b*) In treatment by *Hypoglycæmia*, the aim is to produce a severe reaction by the introduction of insulin. The average dose of insulin to produce coma appears to be 60–80 units, but over 200 units have been necessary in some cases. The coma may be allowed to last for 1½ hours. It is terminated by a nasal feed of 33 per cent. glucose, or, if necessary, the giving of intravenous dextrose. This form of treatment is given on successive days with one day's rest a week, and the course of treatment consists of 60 coma doses. This method is much more dangerous than the former; in both, the presence of physical disease is a contra-indication. (*c*) *Tranquillising drugs* are discussed in § 1192. They have proved very effective in both acute and chronic forms of schizophrenia, though they are not without risk. Their action is to allay excitement and make the patient disinterested and rather apathetic. Hallucinations and paranoid delusional ideas become less prominent and cease to affect behaviour. The optimum dose has to be found for each patient. Chlorpromazine, 25 mg. t.i.d., is increased as required, sometimes as high as 200 mg. t.i.d. Reserpine is given in 0·5 mg. t.i.d. doses and may be increased to 2–3 mg. daily if necessary. In chronic patients aggressive behaviour and faulty habits are improved enormously, and a greater degree of co-operation in rehabilitative measures is achieved. Many of these patients have been able to leave hospital and resume a useful life in the community. Results show that the responses from these drugs is equal to that from hypoglycæmic coma. The drugs are easier to administer, can be more readily controlled and repeated when necessary. The use of hypoglycæmic treatment has been much curtailed, therefore, but is still employed after failure from medicinal measures. (*d*) *Prefrontal leucotomy* is a surgical procedure. The prefrontal area is exposed and association fibres are severed. Though the method is unscientific and destructive certain patients have improved. It should be considered only after all other methods of treatment have failed.

All the thinking processes of the patient are permeated by an idea of persecution. Such an idea may be logical. The disease is PARANOIA.

§ 1183. IV. **Paranoia** is the term used for a variety of mental illness in which the patient's whole mental life is dominated by a delusion— usually one of persecution. Disorder of judgment is the characteristic feature, and in consequence the patient interprets every incident which he observes or takes part in as fresh proof of a plot against him. There are two classes of paranoiacs. In the first, which is of a milder character and rarely needs care in a mental hospital, the patient's own personality does not take any part in the delusion, but he is possessed by some wild theory which he preaches in and out of season; in the second class, which is a grave form of mental illness, the patient's own personality is all-important, and delusions of persecution are common. This delusion is liable to lead the patient to assassination of some prominent person or even to attempt suicide in order to call attention to his case. Megalomania is apt to develop as the disease progresses. Hypochondriasis, in which the patient's attention is focused on his health or lack of it, is sometimes a' sub-variety of paranoia, but does not lead to any disorder of conduct likely to cause harm to the community. *Folie à deux* is a condition in which one patient, usually a paranoiac, persuades another with whom he or she is very intimate of the reality of the supposed plot against their lives or characters. The second patient, sometimes called the passive element, though mentally ill, is more likely to recover. In true paranoia there is no recovery, although occasionally a remission occurs. When the paranoiac disorder is dominated by active hallucinations it is called **Paraphrenia,** and mostly arises in patients past middle life.

The patient is addicted to alcohol or to a drug, or the brain is affected by a toxæmia. The disease is ALCOHOLISM, DRUG HABIT *or* DELIRIUM.

§ **1184.** V. **Addiction to alcohol,** opium or other drugs, may be symptomatic of an anxiety neurosis, obsessive-compulsive neurosis, psychopathic personality, manic-depressive psychosis or general paralysis. Others have a schizoid personality, or may be paranoid or homosexuals. A family history of alcoholism is common. The continual abuse of the drug leads to a gradual deterioration of the personality, although this seldom advances to the stage of certifiable mental disease. Excessive indulgence in alcohol occurs clinically in five forms—(1) Acute alcoholism, (2) Chronic alcoholism, (3) Dipsomania, (4) Delirium Tremens, (5) Korsakoff's Psychosis.

(1) **Acute Alcoholism** is due to an excessive quantity taken in a few hours. It gives rise to mental disturbance, ataxia and even a temporary flaccid paresis of the limbs. Later, narcosis with a marked lowering of body temperature may develop. From a medical point of view the effects of an acute alcoholic debauch are so transient as to be of no importance except in medico-legal cases. Acute drunkenness must not be confused with diseases causing cerebellar or sensory ataxia (see p. 1206) or Ménière's disease (§§ 829–831, vertigo). Certain neurotics are abnormally sensitive to small doses of alcohol, and, for months after severe head injuries, even small doses of alcohol may produce intoxication. The stupor of concussion, apoplexy, uræmia, opium poisoning, etc. (§ 850), and the muttering delirium (§ 469) of pneumonia and other diseases, may be mistaken for drunkenness, a serious error which is best avoided *by keeping the patient under observation in bed* and suspending your judgment.

(2) **Chronic Alcoholism** is due to the persistent imbibition of moderate doses of alcohol over a long period. It acts as a poison on the nervous, muscular (voluntary and involuntary) and epithelial elements, and hinders tissue oxidation, thus leading to fatty degeneration. The patient is able to take alcohol in quantities which, in a normal person, would produce drunkenness.

Symptoms are both mental and physical. Early *mental* effects are (i.) loss of complete self-control and so the patient becomes extroverted, with a fluent and even a garrulous vocabulary. (ii.) Irritability, even violence, and progressive deterioration of personality appear, especially when the patient is amongst his family circle. (iii.) Intellectual deterioration follows with loss of insight. Lack of concentration and of judgment become evident in the patient's work, he becomes untrustworthy and will attempt to cover up his mistakes by deliberate lying; (iv.) he may strongly resent any suggestion that these failings are due to alcoholism. (v.) Later, *other mental symptoms* appear, such as alternating depression or excitement, unfounded suspicions or delusions of persecution; the patient ceases to speak the truth and dementia gradually develops. Delirium tremens (see below) supervenes from time to time, and sometimes epileptiform convulsions. (vi.) The *physical* symptoms are (*a*) the facies is often plum-coloured with red conjunctivæ; (*b*) there is anorexia for food and morning vomiting due to gastric catarrh; (*c*) the liver becomes large and later may shrink as portal cirrhosis ensues (§ 342); (*d*) coarse tremors of the hands, tongue and lips develop with tremulous dysarthria; (*e*) myocardial and arterial degeneration occur and the patient often becomes much older than his age; (*f*) the kidneys may show chronic nephritis. (*g*) There is often obesity and œdema of the ankles, or the gastritis or the cirrhosis lead to marked loss of weight. (*h*) There is a reduced resistance to infections of all kinds and pneumonia, chronic bronchitis or chronic pulmonary tuberculosis are prone to occur. (*i*) Gouty symptoms are greatly aggravated.

Secret drinking is the term applied to chronic alcoholism occurring in persons who are thought to be " above suspicion." It occurs especially in women about the menopause, who commonly secrete empty bottles in the wardrobe, under the bed, etc.

(3) **Dipsomania** or paroxysmal drinking is frequently symptomatic of a psychopathic personality or of manic-depressive psychosis. It is also found sometimes in epileptics. The condition is often hereditary and may develop in middle life. Between the paroxysms the patient may be quite normal with no desire for alcohol, or even a distaste for it. Then come depression and an uncontrollable craving for alcohol. The attacks may show a definite periodicity.

(4) **Delirium Tremens** arises in chronic alcoholics: (1) after a debauch, (2) with pneumonia or other acute infection, or (3) after sudden withdrawal of alcohol, *e.g.*, when the patient is sent to hospital for treatment of a fracture. The *symptoms* are: (1) restlessness and complete insomnia, (2) terrifying visual hallucinations of animals, especially insects, spiders, rats, snakes (zoöpsia), producing intense fear and impulsive outbursts, (3) occupational delirium with disorientation in space and time, and (4) coarse tremors of the fingers, face and tongue. (5) The temperature is usually slightly raised, and (6) furring of the tongue, dryness of the mouth and anorexia are usual. A first attack will last three to five days,

the patient waking to consciousness with amnesia for his delirious period. Second attacks may last two or three weeks.

The *Diagnosis* of delirium tremens is referred to in § 469. The history of alcoholism and the type of hallucinosis are of value but care should be taken not to overlook an acute pneumonia, especially of the apex. The *Prognosis* of delirium tremens is generally favourable if the temperature is not much elevated, and the strength of the patient can be maintained. Second and third attacks are commonly longer in duration and may leave residual mental impairment.

(5) **Korsakoff's Psychosis** occurs most frequently in chronic alcoholics past middle life, but may follow an attack of delirium tremens. It is met in other toxic conditions also and is frequently seen after a severe head injury. It affects women more frequently than men and is invariably accompanied by neuritis.

Symptoms.—(1) Memory defects are characteristic. There is a gross impairment for recent events; the gaps are made up by confabulations, frequently of a most plausible nature; (2) disorientation in space and time; (3) auditory and visual hallucinations; (4) moods fluctuate rapidly between one of euphoria and one of anger and irritability, and (5) signs of polyneuritis. The *Prognosis* is frequently not good, some impairment of memory and of the intellectual faculties persists. The duration of the illness extends over months.

The *Prognosis* of *chronic alcoholism* is such that about one-third may be cured, one-third will refuse adequate treatment and one-third will relapse after apparent cure.

The *Treatment* of *acute alcoholism* consists in washing out the stomach or giving an emetic, *e.g.*, apomorphine, gr. $\frac{1}{10}-\frac{1}{6}$ hypodermically. The collapse is treated with injections of nikethamide or of amphetamine sulph., and by warm blankets and hot-water bottles, care being taken that the patient is not burned before he recovers consciousness.

Treatment of the *chronic types* is impossible unless the patient wishes to co-operate. (i.) The only method of ensuring abstinence is by institutional treatment, where one can be satisfied that the patient will not obtain alcohol. Complete withdrawal is essential—partial withdrawal rarely succeeds. (ii.) At first, rest in bed is necessary because withdrawal symptoms, restlessness, varying degrees of depression and insomnia may be troublesome; day and night supervision is essential. (iii.) Sedatives will be necessary—paraldehyde ♏ 120–240 or sodium amylobarbitone 3–6 gr. (iv.) A single intravenous dose of hydrocortisone 100 mg. is often of great help in preventing delirium tremens. (v.) Careful feeding with ample supplements of vitamins B and C improves the general health. (vi.) Aversion treatment with repeated injections of apomorphine should only be given under hospital conditions as severe reactions may be produced, the chief of which is circulatory collapse. The aversion to alcohol lasts varying periods, but unless combined with other supportive treatment tends to wear off. Disulfiram B.P.C. (Antabuse) is more effective. It impedes the metabolism of alcohol and if alcohol is taken subsequently the concentration of acetaldehyde in the blood rapidly rises, producing acetaldehyde poisoning. This causes very unpleasant symptoms—sweating, tachycardia, palpitation, nausea and vomiting—and in severe reactions cardio-vascular failure, with considerable distress and low blood pressure. The patient must be kept off all alcohol for three days and paraldehyde avoided. The disulfiram is given in doses of 0·5 G. on the first day, followed by 0·5–1·0 G. daily for a week; on the fifth day and while the patient is in hospital he is given 1 fl. oz. whisky, gin or brandy and the patient's reaction to this carefully watched; if there is no effect within half-an-hour the dose may be repeated once or twice at 30-minute intervals. The severe symptoms produced cause a marked impression and even fear on the patient and demonstrate what happens if alcohol is taken subsequently. A morning maintenance dose of disulfiram (0·25 G.) should be taken daily for 6–12 months. This treatment requires the co-operation of the patient; it must be given with great caution if severe hepatic or cardio-vascular disease is present. (vii.) The social aspects of alcoholism require consideration and effective treatment must provide additional interests for leisure. " Alcoholics Anonymous," an association of former addicts—with a religious background—has helped to provide the social contacts and support that has enabled many to lead useful lives again.

In *delirium tremens*, alcohol can usually be withdrawn at once completely; only rarely, in debilitated patients, need alcohol be given in the early stages and gradually tapered off. The main objectives are to improve the physical state, control the restlessness and obtain sleep. Small allowances of liquid nourishment at frequent intervals are necessary to maintain strength; glucose drinks are especially useful. Such patients frequently endeavour to get away from their hallucinatory experiences and in so doing may be a danger to themselves. The closest degree of observation and tactful management are therefore essential and must be insisted upon (two or even three nurses if necessary). Sleep is essential and great variations will be found in the response to sedatives. It may be necessary, therefore, to change these at intervals. Paraldehyde by mouth (♏ 120–240) or by injection (8–10 ml.), sodium pentobarbitone 4½ gr. or sodium amylobarbitone 3–6 gr. by mouth, or hyoscine hydrobromide $\frac{1}{100}$ gr. subcut. may be tried. Hot packs help to secure sleep. Massive doses of vitamins B or C intravenously (such as high potency Parentrovite) often produce dramatic improvement.

Methylated spirit contains methyl alcohol and is a cheap substitute for ethyl alcohol. Those who drink it often mix it with cheap red wine or follow it with cider.

Symptoms consist of abdominal pain, vomiting, restlessness, diarrhœa and coma; inebriation is not usual as it is with ethyl alcohol. Severe acidosis results from the production of formic acid. Serious sequelæ are dimness of vision or permanent blindness.

Treatment is similar to that of alcoholism, but large doses of intravenous M/6 sodium lactate or 5 per cent. sodium bicarbonate are necessary to correct acidosis.

§ 1185. Morphinism (Synonyms: Morphia Habit, Morphinomania) and

other **drug habits.**—Hypodermically, **morphia** in small doses induces a feeling of contentment and well-being; but in the course of 24 hours reaction and craving for more occur, particularly when pain is present, and by degrees the dose has to be increased until in the course of a few months twenty to one hundred times the normal dose is necessary to produce a feeling of satisfaction, and can be easily tolerated. The only *signs* by which the *morphine habitués* can be detected are contracted pupils, pallor of the face, loss of weight and the frequency with which they withdraw to satisfy their craving—a difference being observed in their depression before and their gaiety and brightness afterwards.

If such a patient is suddenly deprived of the drug, the following *withdrawal symptoms* set in. The pulse, which was previously normal, becomes rapid and of low tension, and the patient prostrate, suffering agonies from tingling in the limbs, sweating, sneezing, lachrymation, diarrhœa, vomiting, uncontrollable restlessness, faintings, "sinkings in the pit of the stomach," extreme wakefulness, and a host of horrible and indescribable somatic sensations resembling extreme neurasthenia.

Consequences of the morphia habit. Enormous doses may be taken by gradual increase. At first the patient is always gay, and has great capacity for mental and bodily endurance. But if the habit be continued, the character gradually becomes altered. The patient alienates his friends by tempers and unreliability; and, one by one, truth, reverence and honesty disappear. If there be difficulty in procuring the drug, great craftiness is exhibited. In course of time the mental powers gradually deteriorate, and suicide is not infrequent in those who desire, but are unable, to rid themselves of the thraldom. The body also suffers, and the patients become pale and emaciated. They get careless in the use of their syringe, multiple abscesses form and death may result from septicæmia.

Prognosis.—Since most morphine habitués are psychopathic the prognosis is always serious. It is worst in doctors, dentists, chemists and nurses, who have easy access to the drug. In these, as in all cases, relapse is very common, and the permanence of cure depends on continued supervision and the possibility of the patient being able to lead a sheltered life, free from all care. After a cure there is a tendency towards alcoholism. The morphine habit probably shortens life, and death may occur from over-dosage. A habit of short duration is easier to cure than one of long duration: the actual quantity of morphia taken per diem is of little account. If carcinoma or some other cause of an incurable and recurrent pain be present, it may be impossible to ease the pain in any other way.

Treatment.—(a) To break the habit the patient must be willing to place himself in a Home or institution and in bed. A night and day nurse will be necessary. The closest supervision is needed to ensure that the dose of morphia during the withdrawal period is controlled, and that no morphine is secreted by the patient. Unless this is accomplished, methods of deception will be practised that nullify all efforts. Sudden cessation of morphine causes intense suffering unless steps are taken to control this: such sudden withdrawal is particularly dangerous in elderly or debilitated patients. To alleviate the withdrawal symptoms the doses of morphia injected are rapidly lowered to a level at which withdrawal symptoms first appear (headache, weakness, vomiting, diarrhœa, sweating, restlessness). The morphia is then stopped and for every 4 mg. injected in the 24 hours 1 mg. of methadone is substituted, given orally in divided doses each 6–8 hours. This dose of methadone is continued for a week and then withdrawn over a period of 3-5 days; methadone addiction is uncommon and withdrawal symptoms are comparatively slight. (*b*) If vomiting occurs during this treatment, tab. chlorpromazine (Largactil) 50 mg. t.i.d. by mouth or by injection is very helpful. Treat sleeplessness with paraldehyde ℥ 120–240 per rectum, ℥ 60–120 by mouth or 5–8 ml. intramusc., or with sodium amylobarbitone 3–6 gr.; prolonged hot baths are very beneficial. Injections of soluble insulin will improve the appetite, and doses short of producing coma have a sedative effect. (*c*) When the convalescent stage has been reached psychotherapeutic treatment will be required, thereby to help the patient achieve a better method of solving his emotional problems and difficulties. Prolonged supervision and care is essential during which period occupational therapy is valuable. The patient should not return to an occupation or environment where it is easy to obtain the drug. For treatment of acute morphine poisoning, see § 856.

A **heroin** habit can cause as serious symptoms as a morphia habit and is still more difficult to overcome. Addiction is treated by the method outlined above, but the dose of methadone is 1 mg. for each 2 mg. of heroin each 6–8 hours by mouth.

The **cocaine** habit leads to many of the troubles of the morphia habit, but there is a greater tendency to mental symptoms and deterioration. Morphia and cocaine are often taken together; in such cases the cocaine may, with comparative ease, be first withdrawn. Then the morphia can be reduced as above described.

Amphetamine sulphate is a stimulant producing a sense of well-being and increased activity. Tolerance is readily acquired and the drug is liable to habit formation. The unpleasant depressing effects of the hangover leads to ever-increasing doses producing on the one hand restlessness and overactivity, and exhaustion, fatigue and depression on the other. Morphine and amphetamine are often taken together.

Indian hemp (Marihuana) addiction from smoking cigarettes produces a pleasant euphoric mental state. Immediate withdrawal does not give unpleasant symptoms.

The psychosis is associated with a general infection; the condition is
DELIRIUM.

§ 1186. VI. The causes of **delirium** were considered in § 469, and need only be enumerated here.

Clinical Investigation.—The first and most important point in any given case of delirium or mental excitement to which you may be called for the first time is to ascertain the temperature. Secondly, it is important to make a thorough and complete investigation of all the organs of the body, to ascertain whether there be any local inflammatory disorder, such as pneumonia, with which delirium may be connected, either directly or indirectly. The urine also should be carefully examined for albumen, sugar, or other abnormality. Thirdly, inquiry should be made into the history of the illness and of the patient, especially as regards the consumption of alcohol and sedative drugs, particularly bromides. The latter are cumulative, and patients vary greatly in their degree of susceptibility. The bromide replaces the chloride ion in the blood plasma and quantitative estimations of the blood bromide can be easily made. With reference to the etiology of delirium, three important *predisposing causes* have to be borne in mind. First, there is a marked predisposition in some nervous people to develop delirium with a slighter cause than would affect others. Secondly, there is a marked hereditary tendency towards the same vulnerability; and thirdly, excessive drinking of alcohol predisposes to the occurrence of delirium after an injury, operation and many diseases which are not usually so attended.

Febrile.	*Non-Febrile.*
Diseases of the brain—especially meningitis, cerebral malaria and dementia paralytica.	Delirium tremens.
	Chronic renal disease.
Acute visceral inflammations — *e.g.*, pneumonia, pericarditis, pyelitis.	Post-epileptic delirium.
	Cardiac failure.
Acute specific fevers, especially typhoid.	Drugs—*e.g.*, bromide, Medinal, hyoscine.
Delirium tremens (rare cases).	

The clinical form is not dependent on the type of infection, and the reaction to the same toxin may vary in different individuals. On the other hand, such physical illness may release a latent mental illness of the schizophrenic or manic-depressive varieties. Hence the variety of symptoms seen after childbirth and the variations in ultimate outcome.

Symptoms.—*During fever:* (i.) the commonest clinical picture is that of a delirium characterised by confusion, (ii.) disorientation for time and space, (iii.) illusions develop, followed by (iv.) hallucinations of sight and hearing. The hallucinatory experiences are very vivid and arouse great fear and restlessness, (v.) transient delusional ideas of a persecutory nature. *After fever:* (i.) exhaustion and great fatigue, (ii.) varying degree of depression, especially common after influenza, and risk of suicide, (iii.) an amnesia for the acute stages; the greater the degree of confusion the more complete the amnesia. A neurasthenic condition may form the basis of more ominous psychotic illness.

A similar mental picture may be seen following *severe physical stress, pregnancy, parturition* or *severe hæmorrhage.* Mental abnormalities after *parturition* occur most frequently in those who have had a febrile reaction after labour. There is no clinical entity characteristic of this type as was formerly described.

In *cerebral syphilis* the confusional picture is typical of any delirium, and there is a marked loss of memory for recent events. Paroxysmal headaches, sleeplessness and symptoms indicative of transient involvement of the cranial nerves, *e.g.*, squint, ptosis, dimness of vision, are common. Blood and C.S.F. investigations will confirm the diagnosis.

The *prognosis* is good if the patient recovers from the physical illness. Those who subsequently develop a schizophrenic illness have displayed abnormal personality changes previous to the physical upset.

Treatment is directed to the primary physical condition; otherwise it is symptomatic, and the objective is to secure adequate rest and nourishment. If the confusional state is due to bromide intoxication the drug should be omitted and the intake of sodium chloride greatly augmented. A period of some weeks may be necessary before the bromide is eliminated.

There is progressive mental deterioration associated with ORGANIC SIGNS *or with* FITS. *The disease is* DEMENTIA.

VII. **Dementia** is an organic condition of the brain with severe and often progressive deterioration of the mental faculties. In the later stages the patient becomes stuporose and finally comatose.

TABLE LXIV.—CAUSES OF DEMENTIA

Common		Rare	
1. Advanced Schizophrenia	.. § 1182	8. Cerebral Tumour .. .. § 1038	
2. Senile and Arteriosclerotic		9. Post-traumatic Dementia	
Dementia .. .. .. § 1187		(including Punch Drunken-	
3. Presenile Dementia .. .. § 1188		ness) .. .. .. § 1189	
4. Epileptic Dementia .. .. § 1188		10. General Paralysis of the	
5. Chronic Alcoholism .. .. § 1184		Insane .. .. .. § 1190	
6. Huntingdon's Chorea .. § 922		11. Schilder's disease .. .. § 1194c	
7. The late stages of Chronic Nephritis,		12. Prolonged Insulin or Carbon Mon-	
Liver failure and Right-sided		oxide poisoning.	
Heart failure.			

1. ADVANCED SCHIZOPHRENIA is by far the commonest cause of chronic dementia in the young and middle-aged. It is described fully in § 1182.

2. § 1187. **Senile and Arteriosclerotic Dementia** are difficult to separate from one another. Both occur more commonly and at an earlier age in men than in women and become increasingly frequent after 60.

Symptoms arise insidiously. There is a characteristic loss of memory for recent events, particularly for names and places; with this there is frequent repetition of events of years ago. A gradual and progressive failure of the mental faculties becomes evident, with loss of the ability to formulate new ideas or to make decisions. Soon there becomes apparent a difficulty in giving prolonged attention to a difficult problem—the patient often falls asleep as he loses interest. Mental and physical fatigue are noticed by the patient and by his relatives. Later emotional control is impaired, patience is lost and sudden outbursts occur over failure to perform what was previously a simple task. Gradually there is loss of interest in his personal appearance, he becomes tremulous, careless at meal times, and the speech becomes halting, slurred and monotonous. Longer hours are spent in bed or in a chair, there is little inclination to take exercise, and as the memory further disintegrates periods of mental confusion occur and urinary control is diminished or lost especially during sleep; constipation and impaction of fæces in the rectum often ensue. In the final stages there is little interest in the surroundings and dementia becomes complete. Particularly in those who have shown psychopathic tendencies in their younger years, other symptoms may arise. Some adopt a suspicious attitude and paranoid delusional ideas may be prominent. Others become restless and anxious, spending their nights wandering about the house. Varying depths of depression may result in involutional melancholia. In some, sexual urges are not controlled and this may lead to misdemeanours.

It is unusual for this condition to progress in a uniform manner. After a period when the mental and physical condition has remained stationary sudden deterioration occurs. The elderly are particularly susceptible to the effects of infection, whether it be inter-current or of a chronic nature as from a dental focus or chronic bacilluria. Small cerebro-vascular accidents produce irreparable damage and even after a small lesion of the brain the mental capacity is hardly ever as good as before its occurrence. The cerebral changes can, by electroencephalography, be shown to be diffused through the cerebral hemispheres.

Physical symptoms which accompany these mental states are described. in § 574.

Etiology.—The atrophy of the brain cells, especially in the frontal, temporal and parietal lobes is either primary, or secondary to vascular occlusion. The result may be a diffuse softening of the brain or this may occur in local patches with replacement by neuroglia. Heredity plays a leading role in the early occurrence of this condition and hypertension and alcoholism are aggravating factors. Symptoms often progress more rapidly in the colder weather.

Treatment.—So long as their essential needs can be met, patients should be left in their home surroundings; then institutional care in homes for the aged or in geriatric wards will be necessary. Even then they should be given simple tasks to perform. Food needs to be nourishing, easily digested and at regular intervals; an extra supply of vitamin B complex often appears to help. Sleeplessness and especially nocturnal restlessness require a hypnotic, remembering that arteriosclerotic and alcoholic patients are relatively intolerant to barbiturates. A small quantity of whisky or brandy at bedtime often aids sleep and chlorpromazine is useful in promoting mental relaxation. A watch must be kept for infections for these are badly tolerated and may produce little rise in temperature. Anæmia must be corrected. Impaction of fæces is insidious and produces local discomfort and considerable constitutional effects; manual removal is usually necessary.

3. § **1188. Presenile Dementia** occurs more commonly in women than in men, usually between 35 and 60 years of age. It runs a more rapid course and leads to death within five to ten years. Two varieties have been described, by Alzheimer and by Pick, more easily differentiated pathologically than clinically. Extensive degeneration of the grey matter occurs chiefly in the frontal lobes; plaques being found in Alzheimer's disease but not in Pick's disease. Progressive memory impairment, aphasic disturbances and epileptiform attacks are the prominent features. Electroencephalography reveals diffuse changes in the cerebral cortex.

4. **Epileptic Dementia.**—About 10 per cent. of epileptics become so far unmanageable as to be regarded as insane. The mental aberration may be (1) pre-paroxysmal, (2) post-paroxysmal, (3) associated with petit mal only or as an epileptic equivalent. Such symptoms are invariably those of excitement, confusion, delirium, stupor or a general mental deterioration.

5. CHRONIC ALCOHOLISM is described in § 1184.

6. HUNTINGDON'S CHOREA is an inherited condition with choreic

movements and slowly progressive dementia.   It usually starts soon after the age of thirty years and is described in § 922.

7. CHRONIC NEPHRITIS, LIVER FAILURE AND RIGHT-SIDED HEART FAILURE in their advanced stages produce dementia, sometimes accompanied by fits.   These are the result of intoxication and/or anoxia of the cortical cells of the brain.

8. A CEREBRAL TUMOUR, particularly in the frontal and temporal lobes, produces progressive changes in personality which may be overlooked unless it is borne in mind.   Focal symptoms and signs and ophthalmoscopic examination of the ocular fundi aid diagnosis (§§ 1035, 1038 *et seq.*).

Rare Causes

9. § 1189. **Post-traumatic dementia** is invariably accompanied by personality changes, especially if there is severe injury to the prefrontal region.   The patient becomes disinhibited, jocular and tactless.   Alternatively the personality changes may produce a querulous aggressive state, difficult to manage.   *Punch drunkenness* is the result of repeated small injuries to the brain.   Unsteadiness of the limbs, slurring of speech, impairment of memory and intellectual deterioration are the characteristic features; epileptic attacks may develop.

10. § 1190. **General Paralysis of the Insane** (Syn. G.P.I.; Paralytic Dementia) is characterised by progressive muscular weakness and tremor, accompanied by mental symptoms, often of a grandiose character, occurring most frequently in men of middle age.   The *Treponema pallidum* can be demonstrated in the cortex of the brain and in the subcortical tissues, at some distance from the blood-vessels.   The disease is due to parenchymatous infiltration and destruction caused by this organism.   The more intensive and effective treatment of the early stages of syphilis has greatly reduced the incidence of this condition so that it is now rarely seen.

Symptoms.—Paralysis of the limbs may sometimes exist for many years without mental symptoms (*vide infra*).   The characteristic symptoms and signs are changes in the personality, impairment of memory, delusional-ideas, tremors, pupillary changes, speech defects, and finally convulsions and generalised weakness.   Invariably mental deterioration is the earliest symptom; in some objective neurological signs, *e.g.*, Argyll-Robertson pupils, optic atrophy or slurring articulation, are prominent from the first.   The course of the illness has been regarded as showing three stages, but these are not always clearly defined, more particularly since the introduction of modern treatment.

(1) *The Early Stage* produces *Mental Changes.*—The earliest clinical manifestations are increased irritability with or without headaches, irrational behaviour and insidious changes of character.   The insidious onset often confuses the diagnosis.   Impairment of the power of attention develops, so that activities requiring any degree of mental concentration are evaded.   Memory begins to fail, particularly for recent events, though this defect may escape recognition unless looked for.   Impairment of judgment develops, and with this, conduct becomes more grossly involved.   Irresponsible decisions are made and wild speculations may result.   Indifference is apparent and the patient becomes careless and untidy in his personal appearance.   In the classical *euphoric variety* delusional ideas are prominent.   These are of a grandiose type and generally accompanied by much overactivity.   The patient believes himself to be all-powerful, of royal descent, or exceedingly wealthy so that he may squander his resources, and delay in recognition of the cause may leave his family in penury. It is now more usual to encounter symptoms of *simple progressive deterioration.* Sometimes *great depression*, sullenness, delusions of death, self-mutilation or even suicide with a marked loss of energy are predominant.

Various *Physical Changes* accompany, precede or follow the mental symptoms. The most common are: (i.) tremors (fine, small and rhythmical) of the face and lips, also of the hands (giving rise to characteristic writing), and coarse tremors of the tongue produce a characteristic slurring of the speech (dysarthria); (ii.) the pupils in this stage are usually small, unequal and irregular in outline. They fail to react to light, but react on accommodation (Argyll-Robertson pupil); (iii.) primary optic atrophy is common; (iv.) the tendon reflexes are invariably increased and the plantar reflexes may be extensor in type. Sometimes symptoms of tabes are present in addition (tabo-paresis).

Serological changes: The blood Wassermann reaction is positive. Examination of the cerebro-spinal fluid shows various pathological changes. The Wassermann reaction is positive in 99 per cent. of cases; the cell count is increased and may be as high as 400 per c.mm. (lymphocytes). The globulin and total protein are increased and the discoloration of the test tubes in the Colloidal Gold reaction (Table LXVI) is characteristic (paretic curve).

(2) *Later stages* of the illness are characterised by (i.) mental enfeeblement (dementia) which replaces the mental changes in the first stage; (ii.) increasing muscular weakness, difficulty in walking any distance, and especially in the act of turning, sometimes combined with giddiness; (iii.) fits (congestive attacks) are almost invariably present at some period of the illness; they vary in character, but are usually syncopal or epileptiform, with or without the loss of consciousness. Sometimes they consist of attacks of numbness of the limbs, or aphasia, or coma. They sometimes occur in the early stages and may constitute the initial symptom.

(3) The *final stage* is that of progressive dementia. The speech becomes inarticulate, the paralysis extreme and accompanied by contractures, so that the patient cannot feed himself. His mind undergoes progressive extinction, and there is loss of all its faculties. The urine and fæces are passed involuntarily.

Several varieties may be differentiated:—(1) The Expansive manic variety forms the basis of the above description. It is seen less frequently than formerly reported. G.P.I. should always be considered as the cause of a first attack of excitement in a patient over 30 years of age. (2) The Depressive variety presents a picture difficult to distinguish clinically from melancholia. The impairment of memory, the presence of physical signs and the serological findings differentiate the two conditions. (3) The Simple variety is characterised by childishness, apathy and indifference. Such patients are fatuous and express no gross delusions. The process is a simple progressive deterioration. (4) The Tabo-paretic variety includes those who show physical signs of tabes in addition to mental changes. (5) A Juvenile variety, occurring up to the early twenties, due to congenital syphilis (see § 1194*b*).

Diagnosis.—On account of the great variety of symptoms presented by G.P.I., its diagnosis may be difficult. It is distinguished from (*a*) other forms of *mental disorder*, especially *chronic alcoholic psychosis* and *presenile dementia*, chiefly by the tremor, speech, the pupillary changes and the spinal fluid findings; (*b*) disorders attended by tremors and other neuro-muscular symptoms, such as *disseminated sclerosis, pseudo-bulbar paralysis* and *paralysis agitans*. Chronic *alcoholism* and *polyneuritis* are sometimes difficult to differentiate; they are recognised by examination of the spinal fluid. *Cerebral arteriosclerosis* is associated with retinal changes and there may be a raised blood pressure. *Lumbar puncture is essential before a certain diagnosis of G.P.I. can be made.* The diagnosis from *tabes dorsalis* is not usually difficult.

Etiology.—Adult men are more commonly affected than women in a proportion of 4 : 1. The disease may occur at any age but is more frequent between 30 and 50. It develops 10–12 years after infection. The disease is a syphilitic inflammation and degeneration of the nerve cells and blood vessels, with an overgrowth of neuroglia. The cerebral convolutions are shrunken (especially in the frontal and temporal lobes) and there may be a localised cortical atrophy. The sulci are widened and an internal hydrocephalus results. The skull is thickened and the dura mater fibrous and adherent to the brain substance. Treponemata are present throughout the brain.

The vessels show syphilitic endarteritis and infiltration of the perivascular spaces with lymphocytes and plasma cells.

Prognosis.—The duration of untreated cases varies from a few months to four years. The earlier the onset of the disease after the primary infection, the more rapidly progressive will it be. Intermissions of comparative or complete return to health are characteristic of the disease. It is rare for the duration of such remissions to exceed two years. The prognosis in treated cases is dependent on (*a*) the duration of symptoms prior to treatment, (*b*) the form of the illness, (*c*) the age of the patient. It is imperative to make an early diagnosis as the chances of a successful outcome after treatment diminish in direct ratio to the duration of the symptoms prior to treatment. This probably accounts for the fact that the expansive type responds better to treatment than the others, as such symptoms early attract attention. Alcoholic, sexual and other excesses, anxiety and mental fatigue aggravate the disease.

Treatment with the arsenicals and the older antisyphilitic drugs is of no avail once the disease has fully developed. Penicillin must be given in large doses, 12 to 14 mega-units over a period of two weeks. This has replaced fever therapy for the ordinary case, the latter now being used only if there is a failure to respond to penicillin. The fever may be induced by the inductotherm or with malaria. Malarial inoculation may be effected by mosquitoes or by injecting defibrinated malarial blood subcutaneously, intramuscularly or intravenously. The incubation period varies from one to thirty days; when the patient develops rigors he is allowed to have eight bouts of fever unless evidence of cardiovascular weakness, jaundice, persistent vomiting or fits develop. The fever is terminated by administering quinine sulphate gr. 10 twice a day for ten days. The patient must remain under regular observation and progress assessed by the degree of clinical and serological improvement, repeat courses of penicillin being given if necessary.

11. SCHILDER'S DISEASE is seen in children and in adults and produces considerable dementia, especially when there is involvement of the frontal lobes. The classical picture is loss of vision of cortical origin with normal pupillary responses (§ 1194c).

12. **Coma due to Insulin or Carbon Monoxide,** when prolonged for many hours, causes changes in the nerve cells of the brain which may be irreversible (§ 425). The prolonged hypoglycæmia in patients who have taken a large dose of insulin, often with suicidal intentions, and the prolonged anoxia of carbon monoxide poisoning (§ 856) can result in permanent dementia.

§ **1191. The Prognosis of Mental Illness.**—The *Course* and *Prognosis* in several of the various forms of mental disorders have been referred to. In general terms the chief points on which the prospect of recovery depends are (1) the absence of heredity, especially direct heredity; (2) the personality and make-up of the individual; (3) the presence of an adequate cause; (4) the rate of onset of the attack, being more favourable in a rapid than a slow, insidious onset; (5) the duration of the illness prior to treatment; and (6) the clinical form of the illness.

Under the Matrimonial Causes Act, 1937, mental defect and unsoundness of mind are grounds of petition for divorce. It must be shown that the person concerned is incurably of unsound mind and has been continuously under care and treatment under certificate for a period of at least five years immediately preceding the presentation of the petition.

§ **1192. The Treatment of Mental Illness** in detail has been referred to under the different forms; the general principles resolve themselves into (1) Physical methods, (2) Drug Therapy, (3) Psychological methods, (4) Occupational therapy, and (5) Social factors.

(1) PHYSICAL METHODS include the control of excitement, insomnia, the prevention of self-injury, adequate feeding, prolonged narcosis, hydrotherapy, endocrine preparations, and the treatment of any physical defect discoverable. They also include such specific methods as malarial, convulsive and hypoglycæmic therapy.

(2) DRUG THERAPY has in the last few years become an increasingly important method of treatment. (i.) *Anti-depressants.* The mono-amine oxidase inhibitors are of value in relieving mild depression. Phenelzine (Nardil) 15 mg. t.i.d. and isocarboxazid (Marplan) 10 mg. t.i.d. have few untoward effects, hypotension being the only significant one. Iproniazid is a powerful anti-depressant which may produce toxic jaundice and should not be used outside hospital. The phenothiazine derivative imipramine (Tofranil) 25–75 mg. t.i.d. is very useful in cases of severe depression— hypotension and jaundice are possible complications. For the relief of tension and anxiety meprobamate 400 mg. t.i.d. or chlordiazepoxide (Librium) 10 mg. t.i.d. are sometimes effective and relatively safe. (ii.) *Tranquillisers* are drugs which in therapeutic doses exert a calming effect without producing drowsiness. The number that have been synthesised is legion—the results claimed for many unjustified. A knowledge of the action of those of proved value is advisable, while keeping an open mind on newer compounds as they appear. Chlorpromazine (Largactil) is anti-adrenergic, parasympatholytic and anti-emetic. Its psychiatric effect results from its action on subcortical areas—the reticular alerting system of the brain stem and the hypothalamus though precise knowledge of its site and mode of action is not yet defined. It controls tension, agitation and disturbed behaviour, particularly in schizophrenia and the senile psychoses, but it does not relieve depression. The usual maintenance dose is 25–50 mg. t.i.d. Large doses—800 mg. daily—may be given in hospital initially, thereafter reduced when the minimum effective dose is established. Intramuscular administration is painful. The chief complications are hypotension, Parkinsonism, agranulocytosis and jaundice. Hypersensitivity reactions include dermatitis with photosensitivity. Promazine (Sparine) is less potent but does not produce jaundice. It can be used in chronic alcoholism with liver damage. Perphenazine (Fentazin) and trifluoperazine (Stelazine) are more potent and less toxic than chlorpromazine, but Parkinsonism is more troublesome. Thioridazine (Melleril) and Haloperidol are new compounds which show initial promise. Reserpine, derived from *Rauwolfia serpentina*, is not chemically related to the phenothiazines; its main action is probably at the hypothalamic level and its chief value is in controlling psychotic behaviour due to hallucinations or delusions. The usual dose is 2–3 mg. a day but larger doses are used in hospitals; maintenance doses may be required subsequently for long periods. Complications are hypotension, nightmares, diarrhœa, extrapyramidal rigidity and tremors. Agitated melancholia may occur after prolonged use and the drug must then be withdrawn.

(3) PSYCHOLOGICAL METHODS are employed by the physician in every-

day practice. The results depend in large measure on the degree of rapport between patient and physician, the influence of the latter being a dominant factor. They assume a belief by the patient that the illness can be cured. *Reassurance, persuasion, suggestion, group therapy* and *analytic methods* are employed.

Reassurance: Often a free discussion with the patient of his symptoms and his problems, with an explanation as to their development and a reassurance as to their significance, will effect considerable improvement.

Persuasion: Here the aim is to convince the patient of the absence of any organic basis for his symptoms and such to be effective is accompanied by emotional force. No attempt is made to treat the cause of the symptoms; consequently a recurrence in a fresh site is not uncommon.

Suggestion is a process of implanting ideas of a corrective nature; by this means mental improvement ensues. The impressions desired to be made on the mind may be implanted when the patient is awake or in a drowsy hypnotic state. Many believe that suggestions are reinforced by *hypnosis*, which may be defined as a condition of partial consciousness resembling sleep, in which the subject's capacity to receive and to act upon suggestions is greatly improved. This increased suggestibility is made use of by the operator for the implanting of new and healthy conceptions and the removal of morbid ideas, the object being to influence the body through the mind. Only by trial can one determine whether a person is able to be hypnotised. Various methods of inducing hypnosis are available and details of these may be obtained in text-books on the subject. The method should be used only by medical men and with proper precautions. The consent of the patient and his relatives should be obtained; often a third person should be present during the treatment. In competent hands no bad effects result from its employment even over prolonged periods, but much moral and physical evil follow the abuse or misuse of this powerful agent. Its use for purposes of public exhibition should be forbidden by law. Hypnotism has been employed to restore memory in cases of hysterical amnesia, to reform alcoholics and moral perverts, to cure various neuroses, and to relieve various hysterical manifestations such as anæsthesiæ or paralyses.

Group therapy has become popular as a method of helping a relatively large number of patients, and is particularly effective when the illness results from a failure of social adaptation. Exploratory lectures and discussions are encouraged to promote a better understanding of the etiology and mechanism of symptoms. Patients are encouraged to take a more active part in therapy by composing and acting plays based on episodes from their own lives (psycho-drama). This gives the physician the opportunity to discuss factors in relation to the patient's own problems, as well as those of general significance for the group forming the audience.

Psycho-analysis is a method of investigation of the unconscious mind which has been advocated by Freud and modified subsequently by his pupils. It consists of a minute study of the patient's previous life by special methods—dream analysis, hypnosis, and free association. The patient is requested to state every thought and word that casually occur to him whilst under examination, in the hope of discovering some hidden psychic trauma of early life. Freud emphasises unduly the sexual content of the unconscious mind: he considers that dreams have definite symbolic meaning requiring special interpretation, and that complexes are discovered by their elucidation. Jung has extended the method by " word-associations," using 100 selected stimulus words and observing the character and time of the words of response. Any delay in reaction as shown by a stop-watch indicates that a repressed complex has been affected which when brought to consciousness and fully explained assists in curing the patient. The results of analytic treatment are difficult to assess, but the method is more successful in psychoneurotic than psychotic forms of illness. Psycho-analysis is not employed in patients past 50 years of age or those with organic disease. It requires a certain degree of intelligence and ability to co-operate on the part of the patient and its application is limited owing to the time and expense involved—many cases requiring an hour's sitting daily over a period of months. Although possessing therapeutic value in some cases otherwise intractable, psycho-analysis occasionally upsets patients and does harm. It is therefore best left in the hands of experts of acknowledged experience and repute.

(4) OCCUPATIONAL THERAPY has been defined as the treatment under medical care of physical or mental disorders by the application of occupation and recreation with the object of promoting recovery, of creating new habits and of preventing deterioration. The value of work in health is generally conceded, and much time and energy is now spent in directing healthy adolescents into their appropriate sphere of activity. In the treatment of the sick, occupational therapy includes more than mere occupation. It should find expression also in the social and recreational outlets of the hospital. Occupation should consist of much more than the mere doing of something " diversional "; being busy is not necessarily therapeutic. When properly applied the method arouses interest and the successful completion of some form of work naturally helps self-confidence. This is particularly seen in those suffering from depressive illnesses. In the schizophrenic much may be done to delay and prevent the development of deterioration. Since World War II its application in the treatment of physical diseases and injuries has received a great stimulus, but still more remains to be achieved with this.

(5) SOCIAL FACTORS: Because of the great frequency of environmental factors in the etiology of mental illness, it is generally necessary, at an early stage, to decide where the patient is to be treated. No hard and fast rules can be elaborated as to when the patient should enter hospital.

§ 1193. **Procedure for Treatment.**—The question of removal to a nursing home or mental hospital depends on many things, chiefly (i.) the manageability of the patient; (ii.) the means at home for control; and (iii.) the character of the mental disorder and its potentiality for homicide or suicide.

INFORMAL ADMISSION.   By far the majority of patients now entering a psychiatric hospital do so without formality, as they would enter a general hospital or nursing home.   They are free to leave at any time.   If medical opinion is that further treatment is imperative, *i.e.*, the patient is a danger to himself or to others, then an application for observation or treatment may be made.

COMPULSORY ADMISSION.   This may be for (*a*) Observation, (*b*) Treatment.

(*a*) *Admission for Observation.*   The application may be made on the grounds that (i.) the patient is suffering from mental disorder of a nature or degree which warrants detention in hospital under observation for at least a limited period.   (ii.) That he ought to be so detained in the interests of his own health or safety, or for the protection of others.   The application is made to the Managers of the hospital to which admission is sought, either by the nearest relative or by the Mental Welfare Officer who must have seen the patient within 14 days.   It must be supported by two medical recommendations; one of these must be given by a physician approved for this purpose by a local health authority and either he or the physician must, if practicable, be one who is already acquainted with the patient.   The patient may be detained for observation for 28 days.

In cases of *urgent necessity* an application for admission for observation for a period of three days may be made.   This should be made by the relative or by the Mental Welfare Officer on the appropriate form and supported by one medical recommendation, if practical by a physician who has had previous acquaintance with the patient. If a second medical recommendation is obtained before the expiration of the three-day period, the patient may be detained for a total of 28 days from the date of admission.

(*b*) *Admission for Treatment.*   The application may be made on the grounds that (i.) the patient is suffering from mental disorder, this being (*a*) in the case of a patient of any age, a mental illness or severe subnormality; (*b*) in the case of a patient under 21 years a psychopathic disorder or subnormality; and that the said disorder is of a nature or degree which warrants the detention of the patient in a hospital for medical treatment under this section; and (ii.) it is necessary, in the interests of the patient's health or safety or for the protection of other persons, that the patient should be so detained.   The forms required are similar to those necessary for admission for observation, with an application by the nearest relative or by a Mental Welfare Officer, supported by two medical recommendations.   The patient may be detained for treatment, if necessary, for a period of twelve months in the first instance.

Psychopathic Disorder and Subnormality.   A patient who suffers from either of these disabilities, who is over the age of 21 years, cannot be compulsorily detained unless there is some super-added mental disorder—then he can be admitted for treatment.   Such patients must be discharged when they have recovered from this mental condition.   Patients suffering from psychopathic disorders over 21 can be detained in hospital under an Order of the Court.

Guardianship under the Mental Health Act, 1959, replaces, with modifications, the similar provisions under the Mental Deficiency Acts.   It may also be used as a form of control over mentally ill patients for whom it is not necessary to provide hospital care.   Placing a patient under Guardianship merely provides powers of control over his residence and his normal day-to-day life, which are necessary for the welfare of such a patient or for the protection of others.

Transport.   Where it is necessary to provide special transport, it is the duty of the local authority to provide a car or ambulance.   Should the patient be unwilling to be moved, the person making the application should provide the ambulance authorities with written authority for the removal.   The Mental Welfare Officer will make all the necessary arrangements.   While it is no part of his duty to undertake private cases these officers, if approached tactfully, are usually willing to help in any way possible.   They can supply the statutory forms required.

It should be noted that the magistrate takes no part now in authorising the patient's detention in hospital.   If dissatisfied, the patient or the nearest relative may apply to a Mental Health Review Tribunal for his discharge within six months of his admission. The Review Tribunal is composed of three groups of members— legal, medical and other members who possess the appropriate experience, *i.e.*, social services, etc. They are appointed by the Lord Chancellor and each tribunal must consist of at least one from each group. The Chairman is the legal member.

COURT ORDERS FOR TREATMENT.—Under the Criminal Justice Act, 1948: (*a*) A Court may include in a Probation Order a requirement that an offender shall submit to treatment in a mental hospital for a period not exceeding 12 months from the date of the Order. (*b*) A Court of Summary Jurisdiction has the power to make an Order for the detention of an offender in a mental hospital. This Order has the same effect in law as a Summary Reception Order.

The procedure in Ireland and Scotland is somewhat different, as is also that under the Mental Health Act, *vide* § 1194c.

Testamentary Capacity.—A knowledge of what constitutes the testamentary capacity of a patient is of great importance to the practitioner, because it is often on his evidence that courts of justice decide such matters. The testamentary capacity of a person of unsound mind, in practice, depends on three questions:

1. Did he at the time understand the nature of a will and its effects, and did he understand the extent of the property of which he was disposing?

2. Did he provide for his relatives, or, if not, why did he leave them out?

3. Had he any delusion bearing on testamentary matters?

If these questions can be satisfactorily answered and proven, the will is valid, however eccentric the patient may have been, or even if he was at that time certified as of unsound mind. The fourth question—undue influence—is a non-medical question.

The patient is a child, showing signs of MENTAL DISORDER.

§ 1194. Mental Abnormalities in Children may be classified as:

A. PSYCHONEUROSES and BEHAVIOUR DISORDERS.
B. PSYCHOSES.
C. MENTAL SUBNORMALITY.

A. (1) The *nervous child* corresponds in childhood to the anxiety neurosis in the adult. Anxiety is frequently displayed by children. It may occur in the form of acute anxiety attacks with concomitant signs and symptoms to the adult; more often it appears to become absorbed into the constitution. Such children are generally the offspring of nervous parents from whom the children absorb their anxiety. In the majority of children with such symptoms, there is nothing intrinsically wrong; the condition is the result of environmental factors. Hysterical manifestations of a minor degree are common; headache, nausea and vomiting; usually they are the result of suggestion. Marked symptoms, such as paralysis, anæsthesia. etc., are much less frequent; when they do occur, the psychological mechanisms are usually superficial. Having satisfied oneself as to the absence of a physical cause, disregard of the hysterical symptom, and refusal to allow any gain from it, are often sufficient to cause the symptom to cease. Obsessive compulsive features are present in minor degree in most children, and are rarely to be taken seriously. Simple explanation and reassurance are usually adequate.

(2) *Habit disorders* of varying degree form a large proportion of children's problems of psychiatric interest. In the earliest stages habit training comes from parents, later from the school influence and school companions. Morbid as well as healthy reactions may be impressed. The most frequent habit disorders are enuresis, nail-biting, stammering and sleep-walking. Hubert has drawn attention to the pronounced hereditary tendency so frequently found in these conditions. Enuresis often occurs in several members of a family; it may be the result of anxiety, lack of education or negativism. Sleep-walking also commonly occurs in more than one member of a family; when psychological in origin the goal usually suggests the interpretation. Stammering is common in timid, over-anxious children, factors

already increased by their disability. Speech training is advocated together with the readjustment of psychological difficulties. Amongst the grosser forms of behaviour abnormalities come lying, unmanageability, temper tantrums, stealing and truancy. Isolated instances probably occur, at some time or other, in the life of all children; but their repeated occurrence makes them pathological and renders further investigation necessary. Lying may be of two varieties: (a) defensive to protect from consequences, (b) the result of phantasy, and is then a projection of wishes and desires into realisation in words. Temper tantrums are usually the result of methods of handling, and are developed as a means of achieving some end.

These problems in children indicate, as a rule, some difficulty in adaptation, and a frustration of some desire. Beyond obtaining, in a general way, the child's attitude towards the problem, in most cases it is undesirable and unprofitable to submit the child to a more detailed psychiatric investigation; very rarely is this necessary. More can be gained by a study of the environmental factors, the setting in which the child moves, and the attitude adopted towards him, by those with whom he comes in contact. Indirect investigation by allowing the child to talk of general matters—their dreams, phantasies and imaginary friends—can be of great value; similarly a study of their drawings, modelling and play will help. The latter has been developed extensively and conditions created to observe behaviour to special situations. The keen observer will learn much from the actual performance during tests, apart from the factual results. Educational difficulties are responsible for numerous problems. Some are the result of varying degrees of retardation, but on the other hand great intellectual capacity is not synonymous with good mental health. These difficulties are investigated by means of psychological tests (see § 839). The value of such an investigation is seen particularly in studying delinquency. Many of these children show difficulty in school adjustment, and the restlessness and discouragement thus created play no small part in determining their conduct.

The detailed investigation of adult psychiatric problems now employed has revealed the great frequency of neurotic symptoms in childhood. The " problem " adult is frequently the end result of the " problem " child. Consequently greater attention must be paid to these symptoms while it is possible to eradicate them. Discrimination is necessary as to how much the child should be treated, and how much the environment. Only in a few cases is psycho-therapeutic treatment called for. A readjustment of the environment is frequently necessary ; to obtain this, the temporary removal of the patient to new surroundings may be necessary. One should endeavour, then, to modify the conditions that either suggest ideas of misconduct, or that may reawaken the ideation which creates the impulse to misconduct.

B. **Psychoses.**—Psychoses in children are rare. Especially is this so prior to the development of secondary sexual characteristics. Thereafter affective disorders, manic-depressive and schizophrenia, are sometimes met. The clinical picture in the former condition is the same as that found in adults (§ 1180). Where children are affected there is usually a strong family history of depressive conditions. Schizophrenia is characterised by an abnormal emotional reaction. Such patients lose interest and become apathetic; news that previously would have caused sorrow now provides cause for laughter. The most prominent feature is the incongruity between the emotional state and the thought processes. These patients withdraw from reality; phantasy formation becomes prominent and acquires for them an objective reality. Numerous theories have been elaborated to account for the condition. There is no definite evidence of organic changes. The onset is in most cases of an insidious nature, beginning in childhood; the previous personality is that of a reserved, seclusive type with few friends and interests. During childhood peculiarities of behaviour occur which separately seem of no importance, but, viewed collectively later, they show their true significance. Meyer has suggested that the condition is the result of inadequate adaptation of the individual to his environment; that it is the result of faulty habits of reaction whereby the problems of life are inadequately dealt with, culminating later in the substitution of phantasy for activity. Insufficient attention has been paid to these oddities of behaviour, and when advice has been sought the patients have been unable to co-operate in treatment. The aid of the specialist should be sought before the stage of readaptation is past.

Congenital forms of *General Paralysis* may occur after the age of 7, in the offspring of adult general paralytics. The condition is characterised usually by deterioration in a previously alert and active child. Memory changes occur, and marked intellectual impairment develops in a short space of time. The younger the child when the symptoms appear the more chronic the course of the condition. Physical signs in the form of speech abnormalities, Argyll-Robertson pupils, tremors and active tendon reflexes are found. Serological examination gives the same findings as in the adult (§ 1190). Treatment by penicillin and/or malaria is less effective than in adults. Unless the condition is diagnosed and treatment instituted in the early stages the prognosis is very poor.

Behaviour difficulties of all degrees of severity may be sequelæ of encephalitis lethargica (§ 837). The milder forms are characterised by nocturnal wakefulness and excitability, disobedience, irritability, stealing and outbursts of temper entirely unprovoked. Young children show a greater degree of mental impairment, whereas older children show a moral change. In the Apache group the children become aggressive, untruthful, quarrelsome and often subject to outbursts of acute excitement. Many of these require institutional treatment, and the ultimate prognosis is not good.

Under the Mental Treatment Act, 1930, provision is made for the reception into Mental Hospitals as voluntary patients, of children under 16 years of age whose condition is such that they are likely to benefit from treatment there. Application must be made by the parent or guardian, and it must be accompanied by a medical recommendation by the family physician, or by a physician approved for the purpose by the Minister of Health.

C. **Mental Subnormality.** Whereas in the Mental Deficiency Act of 1913 three grades of intellectual defect were recognised, there are only two groups recognised in the Mental Health Act, 1959—SEVERE SUBNORMALITY and SUBNORMALITY. The provisions for treatment in hospital of subnormals is the same as for mental illness (§ 1193). The two groups are clearly defined. SEVERE SUBNORMALITY means a state of arrested or incomplete development of mind, which includes subnormality of intelligence, and is of such a nature or degree that the patient is incapable of living an independent life or of guarding himself against serious exploitation, or will be so incapable when of an age to do so. SUBNORMALITY means a state of arrested or incomplete development of mind (not amounting to severe subnormality) which includes subnormality of intelligence, and is of a nature or degree which requires or is susceptible to medical treatment or other special care or training of the patient.

Classification of mental defect has always been incomplete, due to our ignorance of the pathology. The genetic basis has been established (§ 1217) but environmental factors contribute. There are two broad groups: (a) those where the defect, generally severe, arises from a definite pathological condition and (b) a larger group not related as yet to any known pathology where the degree of defect is less. The two groups vary according to mental capacity and are differentiated by means of *special psychological tests*. As the result of numerous experiments carried out on normal school children, these tests have been grouped according to the period of life at which accomplishment may be reasonably expected, and they have been elaborated into a definite scale (§ 839). For each year of life a combination of tests is employed, the average of which gives a more representative value than any one test alone. If the child cannot do the tasks proper to its age, but can only accomplish those proper to a younger child, its mental age is reckoned to be that of the younger child, in other words, so much less than its real age. Normally the mental age and the chronological age should correspond; the ratio of the one to the other is termed the *intelligence quotient*. Apart from the actual results achieved by the child, valuable data are obtained from a study of its application in the performance of the various tasks. It may be taken that idiots have a mental age under 3, imbeciles under 7, and feeble-minded under 12.   If the child has attended a Primary School in England a rough indication of its ability may be formed by ascertaining the standard to which it reached.   Thus the average age in the infants' school is under 5 years and in Standard I 7 to 8 years, with an increment of one year for each succeeding standard, Standard VII being reached by normal children at 13 or 14.

CONGENITAL APHASIA (§ 879) though uncommon is of considerable importance, as the sufferer may be wrongly regarded as mentally defective.

CLINICAL VARIETIES: 1. *Idiocy*—a large group without characteristic features enabling it to be subdivided.   It includes children without any obvious abnormality of the cranium or limbs, only in the face or palate.   In some the facial expression may be fairly intelligent, but most of the lower grade present an animal expression, thick lips, pug-nose, large coarse ears, broad, thick, depressed bridge of nose, narrow or hairy forehead and underhung jaw.

2. The *Mongol* type of congenital deficiency (Syn. Down's syndrome) is so called from the resemblance of the face to that of the Chinese, the palpebral fissures sloping downwards and inwards.   With flat face, flat back to the head, and constant protrusions of the tongue, this form of idiocy presents an unmistakable physiognomy. The fingers also are stunted and the little fingers incurved.   Congenital heart disease occurs in about 30 per cent.   These children are imitative, and therefore educable to a limited extent, but they make no progress beyond a certain point.   They may be regarded as " unfinished " children, as they are often born of mothers who have suffered from continued ill-health during pregnancy; sometimes they are the youngest of a large family, or born of parents advanced in life.   A genetic factor is now established.   Recent cytological work has shown the presence of abnormalities in the autosome pairs of chromosomes (§ 1217).

3. *Microcephalic idiocy* includes children whose heads have a smaller circumference than the normal, which averages about 19 inches.   The head may measure 17, 15, or even 12 inches; the forehead is narrow, and slopes backwards, corresponding with the deficiency of the frontal development of the brain.   The small skull is the expression and not the cause of the small brain.   The features are frequently normal, eyes large, and nose aquiline.   These children rarely make much improvement, for they have but little power of attention, though some of them are imitative.   The majority are imbeciles.

4. *Sclerotic amentia* due to an overgrowth of neuroglia occurs in two forms—(*a*) nodular (tuberose), and (*b*) diffuse.   (*a*) *Tuberose sclerosis* is characterised by mental defect, epileptiform attacks, and adenoma sebaceum, a skin eruption appearing on the face as a rule between 4–6 years of age (§ 1049).   (*b*) *Diffuse sclerosis* may give rise to an increase in the size of the brain, producing what is frequently described as hypertrophic amentia.   The condition may be differentiated from hydrocephalus by the level of maximum enlargement; also in hydrocephalus the enlargement is generally more marked and is accompanied by a bulging of the fontanelles and sutures. Weakness, epileptiform seizures, and varying degrees of mental defect are the conspicuous features.

5. *Oxycephaly* is accompanied by a marked deformity of the skull (§ 13).   As the sutures are united prematurely, the cranium is expanded upwards so that the frontal region is greatly increased in height, and the head is short from before backwards.   The bones of the skull are abnormally thin and ocular changes are frequent.   There may be synostosis of the fingers and toes.   Varying degrees of mental defect are not infrequent, but the changes in the cranium may exist without any mental defect. The condition may occur in more than one member of a family.

The main clinical varieties with a known pathology are:—

6. *Hydrocephalic,* often due to the occlusion of the foramina of Magendie or Monro, causing distension of the ventricles with fluid and atrophy of the cortex.   The bones become widely separated and the head is globular in shape.   Most cases are quiet

and docile and there is frequently muscular weakness or paralysis. Epileptiform convulsions are frequent, but tend to decrease as the condition becomes stationary (§ 1037).

7. *Epileptic.*—Infantile convulsions, indistinguishable in many cases from those of ordinary epilepsy, may result from many causes. Where no cause can be ascertained it is looked upon as idiopathic. A large proportion of such occur in the offspring of epileptic, psychotic or psychopathic individuals. When the fits develop in early life, before the age of 7, intellectual development is arrested and mental defect frequently results (§ 861).

8. *Paralytic.*—The majority of cases in this group result, as a rule, from trauma at birth and only very occasionally from an injury during early life. There is some support for the view that certain cases are of intra-uterine origin, and not dependent, merely, upon the result of intra-cranial hæmorrhage. The resultant lesion is dependent on the site and degree of damage. Accordingly hemiplegia, diplegia, or epileptiform attacks may be concomitant symptoms. Sometimes these cases are associated with spasticity or choreiform movements and symptoms are produced due to a cerebral scar (§ 972).

9. *Inflammatory.*—This follows from encephalitis and meningitis, from scarlet fever or other exanthema, and the mental defect may not supervene till later.

10. *Syphilitic.*—Signs of congenital syphilis are often present; in some there is evidence of gross brain damage such as paralyses, seizures, deafness, and blindness. The degree of defect consequently varies greatly and treatment offers little hope of improvement (§ 500).

11. *Amaurotic Family Idiocy* (Syn. Cerebro-macular degeneration) occurs chiefly, though not entirely, in Jews, often in more than one member of the same family, sometimes in successive generations. The onset is at three to six months of age (Infantile type) or in the first three years of life (Juvenile type). The *Symptoms* are those of progressive diplegia, with rapid mental deterioration leading to idiocy with repeated slight epileptiform convulsions. The visual failure may pass unnoticed. The *Diagnosis* is made from other forms of ataxic diplegia or mental defect by the finding of a cherry-red spot at the macular region of both fundi in the infantile type (§ 1126), and a " pepper-and-salt " appearance of the macula in the juvenile type. Primary optic atrophy occurs in both types. Death occurs rapidly in 6–12 months. The brain cells are greatly distended by a group of lipoids called gangliosides, the accumulation of which is probably due to enzyme deficiency.

12. *Schilder's Disease* is a rare condition which may occur in various members of one family. The symptoms may appear in early life or during childhood in those previously of normal mental development. Mental enfeeblement, fits, bilateral cortical blindness, deafness and a progressive spastic paraplegia are the conspicuous symptoms. The optic nerves may be affected. The disease is the result of extensive cortical demyelinisation which usually commences in the occipital poles and rapidly extends forward in the white matter. There is no effective treatment.

13. *Gargoylism* resembles achondroplasia but mental defect, optic atrophy and sexual infantilism occur. By contrast those with achondroplasia alone are bright, intelligent and fertile (§ 616).

14. *Mental defect from deprivation of the senses.*—The mind is cut off from environmental stimuli owing to sight and hearing being affected from acute infections, trauma or hæmorrhage. The defect may be remedied by means of special training.

15. *Cretinism* may be endemic or sporadic. The head is usually large, flat at the top, spread out at the sides. The hair is coarse and dry and the voice squeaky. Under treatment by thyroid these cases make remarkable progress (Figs. 9*a*, *b* and *c*), but the treatment must be continued during the whole of life. And see § 192.

16. *Phenylketonuria and Galactosæmia* have recently been detected at an early stage by examination of the urine (§§ 381, 386). The former is due to a metabolic change and failure in the break down of phenylalanine leading to a reduced oxidation and possibly to poisoning of neurones. It is usually associated with mental defect

often of severe degree. A diet low in phenylalanine has been beneficial. Galacto-sæmia is a rare condition, affecting infants due to a defect in metabolism of galactose. Growth is impaired and there may be mental defect dependent on the degree of brain damage. A lactose-free diet offers promising results if started early.

Etiology of Mental Subnormality.—The influence of heredity is noticeable in these children; they frequently come from a neuropathic stock. Their family history invariably shows varying degrees of mental abnormality in both the immediate and more remote members. The exact influence of syphilis is difficult to assess. A positive Wassermann reaction is rare. It has been suggested that the association of tuberculosis and mental deficiency is indirect, probably dependent on the intermediation of poverty. Minor etiological factors are injury, anxiety and worry. There is support for the belief that the early application of forceps is preferable to an indefinitely prolonged labour. Of the factors operating after birth the chief are glandular deficiencies, epilepsy, brain disease, injuries, sense deprivation and infectious diseases.

The *prognosis* of mental subnormality is always grave. The degree of defect, the clinical type, and the environmental factors are the chief points to be considered. The variety of simple aments do better than the special forms. Many backward children are made more defective by the home atmosphere, and much would be achieved if relatives would treat such children from the point of their mental maturity rather than their actual age and physique.

Treatment of Mental Subnormality in all cases consists in utilising to the best advantage what abilities there are. Recovery cannot be expected. Idiots and imbeciles usually require institutional treatment or private care. The results of training are, in some cases, surprisingly good. Much can be accomplished for feebleminded children in Special Schools; the conditions there permit of a great amount of individual attention. The aim is to emphasise the physical and personal training, and to organise the behaviour of such children into helpful and useful activity. It may be necessary to try several forms of occupation before one is found in which the child takes an interest. The general approach now is in favour of community rather than institutional care, with greatly increased facilities for occupation, sheltered workshops and after-care. Much attention has been given to the question of sterilisation. The Departmental Committee recommended recently that voluntary sterilisation should be legalised in the case of (a) one who is mentally defective or has suffered from mental disorder, (b) one who is believed to be likely to transmit mental defect or disorder. In certain European countries and in some of the States in the U.S.A., compulsory sterilisation has been enforced. The proposal, so far as this Country is concerned, is to create facilities for performing the operation only on those persons who agree to it. As yet sterilisation is illegal, except as a therapeutic measure.

CHAPTER XXII

EXAMINATION OF PATHOLOGICAL MATERIAL

IN this chapter the methods of obtaining various pathological specimens are first described. Then a brief account is given of the methods used to examine the specimens, and of the significance of the results obtained. For a more detailed account special textbooks must be consulted.

Examination may be requested (1) to assist in making a diagnosis, or in some patients to make a diagnosis; (2) for guidance in assessing the progress of a patient's illness; (3) to enable the antibiotic sensitivity of an infecting micro-organism to be determined; or (4) to demonstrate the association of bacteria or pathological changes with disease.

§ 1200. **Sterilisation of Syringes.**—Because of the risk of infection, particularly with the virus of serum hepatitis, a fresh sterile syringe and needle should always be used for every injection or aspiration. Ideally syringes should be processed and sterilised by dry heat in a syringe service department. If dry heat is not available steam under pressure in an autoclave can be used, but precautions have to be taken to ensure that steam reaches all parts of the syringe, and the process of sterilisation is more inconvenient and difficult than is sterilisation by dry heat. Boiling is not recommended unless it is the only method available, when syringes should be kept in boiling water for at least five minutes. If syringes are boiled during mass inoculation, the use of two or more sterilisers saves time and avoids mixing sterile and unsterile syringes. For some purposes disposable plastic syringes, sterilised by the makers with ethylene oxide or gamma-radiation, can be convenient.

§ 1201. **Collection of Pathological Specimens.**—A proper technique is an essential precursor of laboratory examination. This cannot be stressed too strongly for the work of the most able laboratory staff may be rendered valueless if the person collecting the specimen is careless or does not understand what should be done. Each specimen must be *labelled* and accompanied by a written request which gives sufficient clinical information to guide the pathologist in his examination.

Throat swabs are taken in a good light from membrane or ulcers, or in their absence from the tonsil or tonsillar fossa.

Post-nasal swabs are taken either with a curved swab passed over the depressed tongue and upwards behind the soft palate, or more conveniently as a per-nasal swab passed through the nose to the post-nasal space.

Wound swabs should be charged generously with pus.

Pus from an abscess may be sampled with a swab but whenever possible pus should be collected in a pipette or tube. If actinomycosis is suspected this is essential as sulphur granules may be lost in the interstices of a wool swab.

Urine.—Clean mid-stream specimens are adequate in male patients for bacteriological examination: where necessary the prepuce should be retracted. Because of the risk of infecting the bladder by the passage of a catheter, clean specimens are being increasingly used for the examination of urine from female patients. In either case the external urethral orifice should first be cleaned with soap and water and a sterile container used to collect the *middle* part of the stream of urine. Owing to the rapid

1416

rate at which bacteria multiply the results of examination of these specimens may be misleading unless the urine is examined or refrigerated within an hour of collection.

Fæces.—If possible the pathologist should be given the opportunity of examining the whole stool and selecting for himself the portion for microscopical examination and culture. Failing this, the person sending the specimen should, after careful inspection, select any abnormal portion, looking with especial care for streaks of blood-stained mucus or pus. Some organisms, *e.g.*, salmonellæ, will survive in fæces for a considerable time. Dysentery bacilli on the other hand die rapidly in fæces and every endeavour should be made to send the stool for examination as soon as possible. Stools which are suspected to contain dysentery bacilli or *Entamœba histolytica* should be kept at body temperature until they are examined.

Sputum.—Specimens labelled as sputum frequently consist of material from the mouth or post-nasal space and are useless if the physician wishes to know the organism responsible for the chest infection. The patient should be instructed first to clear his mouth and throat, to discard this material and then to cough into a container. Disposable containers made of waxed paper or plastic are preferable to metal pots, unless the specimen has to be sent any distance. The laboratory can give no help if the patient cannot be persuaded or is unable to produce a satisfactory specimen; it may be possible, particularly in children, to collect sputum by holding the tongue in a cloth and passing a bent swab over the tongue down towards the vocal co.ds. Badly collected specimens are largely responsible for the widely held but erroneous view that sputum examination has little to offer in the diagnosis and treatment of acute respiratory infections.

Syphilitic chancre.—The surface of the sore should be cleaned with a dry swab until the slough is removed and serum wells up. If a dark ground microscope is available serum should be transferred with a platinum loop to a thin slide, covered with a glass slip and examined. If the material has to be sent elsewhere it should be allowed to run by capillary attraction into a capillary tube, which is then sealed at both ends. To protect himself the operator should wear rubber gloves.

Swabs for the diagnosis of Gonorrhœa.—As gonococci will not survive on ordinary swabs, if culture is required a charcoal-tipped swab should be used to collect the specimen, and it should be sent to the laboratory in a screw-cap bottle containing Stuart's medium.

Specimens for the diagnosis of virus infection.—For the detection of antibodies in the blood, serum is required. The requirements for isolation of viruses differ considerably and the laboratory undertaking the investigation should be consulted.

Fluid from the serous cavities or from joints can be removed with a syringe and needle with aseptic precautions. To prevent clotting and so facilitate the estimation of the protein content, cytological examination, demonstration of tubercle bacilli, etc., a portion can be added to a sterile tube containing a small amount of sodium citrate or to a sequestrin bottle.

Pleural and Pericardial Fluids are obtained by the methods described in § 119 and § 46.

Peritoneal Fluid.—The **peritoneal** cavity is explored for fluid by **paracentesis abdominis** midway between the umbilicus and pubes, or in the right iliac fossa midway between the anterior superior iliac spine and the umbilicus. The puncture must be made over a dull area and with an empty bladder. The patient is propped up in bed with two or three pillows; a many-tailed bandage is placed around the abdomen, and tightened to maintain the abdominal pressure as the fluid drains away: otherwise the patient may collapse from the rapid dilatation and congestion of the splanchnic area. After sterilisation of the skin, anæsthetise it and the subjacent abdominal wall with 2 per cent. procaine at the proposed site of puncture. A small incision is made in the skin with the point of a sterile scalpel. Then insert a small trocar and cannula into the abdominal cavity. The trocar is withdrawn and, if fluid escapes, sterile rubber tubing is attached to drain the fluid into a receptacle at the side of the bed. The cannula is fixed in position with gauze and strapping. If the flow of fluid stops, and ascites is still present, alter the direction of the cannula in an attempt to restart it, or turn the patient towards the right if the puncture is in the right iliac fossa. When no more fluid can be obtained, the cannula is withdrawn, the site of puncture painted with tincture of iodine and covered with a sterile collodion dressing.

Liver Biopsy may reveal conditions such as Kala-azar, Boeck's sarcoidosis, cirrhosis, hæmochromatosis, primary or metastatic growth and reticulo-endothelial disorders. Using a Gillman or Terry's instrument, insert the needle under local anæsthesia through the 7th right intercostal space in the anterior axillary line, the patient holding his breath during the puncture. A core of liver tissue 3 cm. in length is obtained and suitably fixed for histological section. With a hæmorrhagic tendency, estimate the prothrombin level of the blood beforehand and give Vitamin K when necessary. Only experienced operators should undertake the biopsy—fatalities or complications are occasionally met.

Liver Aspiration for the presence of pus or of Leishman-Donovan bodies is undertaken with a needle where indicated, or in the mid or anterior axillary line with a needle not longer than 90 mm. to avoid possible injury to the portal vein. When staining for Leishman-Donovan bodies, spread the contents of the needle on a glass slide. Liver aspiration must not be performed if a hydatid cyst is suspected, for fear of dissemination in the peritoneum.

Pleural Biopsy can only be undertaken when there is a pleural effusion. It is particularly helpful in malignant and tuberculous effusions where biopsy can be diagnostic in rather more than 50 per cent. of cases.

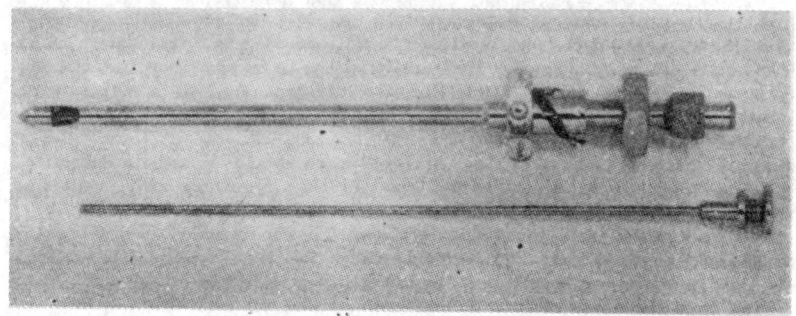

FIG. 271.—PLEURAL BIOPSY PUNCH.

(*G.-U. Company*)

Method.—After infiltration with a local anæsthetic down to the pleura, an Abram's needle (Fig. 271) is inserted through a small skin incision and advanced into the pleural cavity. A syringe is attached to the inner tube, and when this is rotated anticlockwise it opens the end of the needle so that fluid can be aspirated for analysis. Then the indicator knob (and biopsy opening) are pointed downwards or sideways (to avoid damage to the subcostal vessels), and the needle withdrawn until the biopsy opening is felt to catch against the pleura. Clockwise rotation of the inner tube will snip off the nipple of pleura caught in the opening; second and third pieces for biopsy may be taken—these biopsy specimens remain in the needle and when it is withdrawn they can be sent for histological examination.

Spleen Puncture is used in the diagnosis of Kala-azar, and Gaucher's disease: it should only be resorted to after other methods have failed. Leukæmia or a hæmorrhagic tendency is a contra-indication. *Method.*—With the patient flat on his back and hands folded beneath the head an assistant holds the spleen firmly against the diaphragm and ribs. The skin over the intended site of puncture is sterilised with

70 per cent. alcohol or liq. iodi mit. B.P. Puncture is carried out with a direct firm thrust using a No. 14 size needle and a dry syringe, the patient holding his breath. Without delay forcible aspiration is made and the needle then immediately withdrawn sharply in one motion. The patient is kept recumbent for 1½ to 2 hours and the pulse rate checked at intervals for signs of hæmorrhage.

Gland Puncture is employed to detect plague bacilli, trypanosomes and *Treponema pallidum*. The technique is similar to that of puncture in any other region.

Vene-Puncture.—Blood may be required for serological, cultural, chemical and other purposes. Vene-puncture is also necessary for transfusions, intravenous medication and simple bleeding. The most convenient site is one of the superficial veins on the front of the elbow. Apply a tourniquet to the upper arm just sufficiently firm to obstruct the venous return, and ask the patient to clench his fist. The veins stand out clearly; in fat persons the veins are often felt even when not seen. In difficult cases, warm the limb in hot water or by a hot towel. Cleanse the skin with 70 per cent. alcohol. Introduce the needle into the vein in a direction nearly parallel to the skin surface. Fill the all-glass syringe; loosen the tourniquet and withdraw the needle, cover the puncture hole with collodion on a pad of wool. The blood is transferred to a suitable sterile tube, dry if serum is required, containing an anti-coagulant if whole blood is wanted. Bayer's venules are convenient in practice. In infants the external jugular vein is used. The nurse holds the child on her lap, with the head low and turned to one side. Crying distends the vein further.

If *blood is required for culture* 10 ml. should be withdrawn and either added to a flask of 50 ml. of nutrient broth or to a tube containing sodium citrate, leaving the pathologist to make his own dilutions in the laboratory. If typhoid fever is suspected 2 ml. of blood should be added directly to a tube of ox-bile.

Blood parasites.—For malarial parasites both thick and thin films should be made. Similar stained films may also be examined for trypanosomes and micro-filariæ. For these two types of parasite wet films—4 drops of blood covered with a coverslip—will be found helpful (and see § 542).

Sternal Puncture: Bone Marrow Biopsy.—The introduction of aspiration (needle) biopsy has produced a valuable new diagnostic method, and has tended to move the focus of interest in the study of hæmopoietic disorders from the peripheral blood to

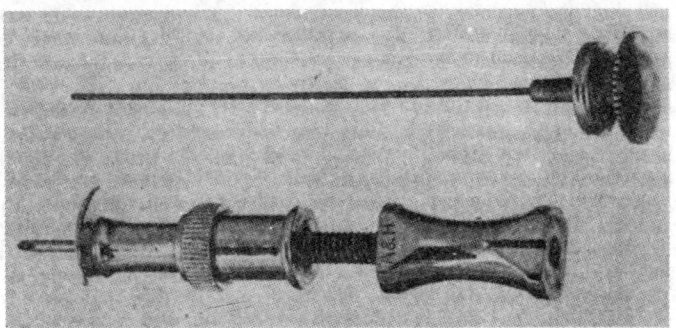

FIG. 272.—STERNAL PUNCTURE NEEDLE (Klima's Pattern).

the bone marrow. *Method.*—In young children syrup of chloral by mouth, paraldehyde per rectum or intravenous sod. hexobarbitone (Evipan) may be needed to produce a temporary drowsiness; adults do not require sedation, but men may require the removal of surplus hair from the upper sternal area. The special Salah or Klima needle (Fig. 272) and a 2 ml. syringe must be dry sterilised before use; these needles have a stout wide-bore and a short-bevelled point, a well-fitting stilette and an adjustable guard to avoid over-penetration. The usual site of entry is the upper part of the body of the sternum; after infiltration of the skin, subcutaneous tissue and periosteum with a small amount of local anæsthetic, the guard on the needle is set 1·0–1·5 cm. above the tip of the needle (depending on the amount of subcutaneous fat) and the needle is driven slightly obliquely into the upper part of the body of the sternum with a steady boring movement: penetration of the outer diplöe of the bone is appreciated when the resistance to the needle suddenly decreases. After removal of the stilette, not more than 0·25 ml. of marrow material is aspirated into the syringe, or otherwise undue dilution with blood will occur. In infancy and up to four years of age the antero-medial aspect of the tibia just below the level of the tibial tuberosity is used; and in childhood the iliac crest just behind the anterior superior iliac spine is often considered to be less disturbing to the patient. In adults, instead of the sternal bone marrow some obtain bone marrow from the iliac crest (by using a modified Klima pattern needle, the stilette of which is attached to a long stout handle) or from the ribs or the spinous processes of the third or fourth lumbar vertebræ; but the sternum contains actively hæmopoietic marrow well into old age and has a conveniently thin anterior covering of compact bone. Occasionally a *trephine biopsy* may produce more useful information as in myelosclerosis or Hodgkin's disease; a small disc of bone and underlying marrow is obtained—this is bisected, fixed, decalcified and sections are made.

Lumbar Puncture is employed to (1) collect specimens of the cerebro-spinal fluid for examination, (2) relieve intracranial and intrathecal pressure, (3) for myelography to determine the site and sometimes the nature of a spinal subarachnoid block, and (4) as a preliminary to the injection of sera, drugs and antibiotics. It is advisable that all patients should remain in bed after lumbar puncture for twelve to twenty-four hours. In certain conditions, notably cerebral tumour and disseminated sclerosis, this should be made an absolute rule, and the patient should not even be allowed to sit up for several hours afterwards. Lumbar puncture should be performed with the patient lying on his side with his back over the edge of a firm couch or bed. The head is on the same level as the sacrum and is flexed well forwards; the knees are drawn up and the back arched. The best site for the puncture is the interspace between the third and fourth lumbar vertebræ. A line joining the highest points of the iliac crests crosses the spine at this level. After sterilising the skin at the intended site of puncture, anæsthetise it with an intradermal injection of 2 per cent. procaine hydrochlor. and then infiltrate the subjacent tissue. The operator, after sterilising his hands, presses deeply into the interspace between the third and fourth lumbar spines and pushes the point of the lumbar puncture needle through the anæsthetised skin either directly in the middle line, or slightly to one side of it. The needle, with the bevel downwards, is then passed forwards and slightly upwards towards the spinal canal which it should reach at a depth of 4 to 6 cm. without encountering any resistance except at the ligamentum flavum. When it is felt that the needle has entered the spinal canal the stylet should be withdrawn, and after a few seconds the first drops of cerebro-spinal fluid should appear. If no flow results the stylet is replaced, and the needle pushed a little farther on. If the needle strikes bone, it should be withdrawn a short distance and inserted in a slightly different direction. When the puncture is made solely for diagnostic purposes as little fluid as possible should be removed, and the sample should be free from blood. The fluid normally runs out slowly (about one drop per second): but when under increased pressure, as in hydrocephalus and meningitis, it may spurt out; the intrathecal pressure can be roughly judged by the rate of flow; an accurate reading is obtained with a special manometer. In normal patients in the horizontal position the pressure varies from 60 to 150 mm. of cerebro-spinal fluid. For examination (§ 1204) 5 ml. are enough, but for treatment (below) 10 ml. up to 50 ml., according to indications, may be removed. The following precautions are essential: (1) strict asepsis; (2) the rate of withdrawal should be slow, not more than 4 or 5 drops a second; and (3) the patient should lie down for several hours afterwards. An additional safeguard is the employment of the smallest possible needle, which will inflict the minimum injury on the spinal theca, and so prevent the escape of cerebro-spinal fluid. There is one contra-indication. When there is increased intracranial pressure due to a cerebral tumour, the sudden reduction of this pressure in the cavity of the spine which results from the withdrawal of fluid may cause the descent into the foramen magnum of a part of the cerebellum. Especially is this so when the cerebellum has already been moulded to form a " cerebellar cone " in its efforts partially to slip into the foramen magnum to relieve the intracranial pressure. Tentorial pressure coning may also occur and is as dangerous as coning through the foramen magnum. When this accident occurs, there may be direct compression of the medulla, the symptoms of which range from syncopal attacks to sudden death. A further danger is that the reduction of the pressure may start hæmorrhages into a soft growth, or allow arrested bleeding to begin again.

Cisternal Puncture is useful when the spinal subarachnoid space is blocked by tumour or adhesions and occasionally to determine the presence or absence of block by the introduction of opaque substances. It is a potentially dangerous procedure which should not be attempted without previous practice under expert supervision.

§ 1202. Examination of Pathological Specimens.—Much may be learnt from the naked-eye inspection of pathological material, and this should always be done by the clinician before a specimen is sent to the laboratory. Many of the tests which are in everyday use in hospital require special apparatus or training which may be outside the experience of the doctor working by himself. No attempt will be made in this Section to describe such tests. There remain, however, certain basic laboratory procedures which need little apparatus and may be of considerable help.

Preparation of films may be for examination (*a*) in the wet state or (*b*) after drying and staining. (*a*) For the cytological and bacteriological examination of urine, pleural, peritoneal fluids, etc., the fluid is placed in a conical tube and spun in a centrifuge. The supernatant fluid is discarded or kept for chemical tests. The deposit should then be resuspended in a minimal amount of fluid and a drop or drops placed on a slide and covered with a glass slip. Examination with the low-power objective of the microscope and then the high-power follows.

(*b*) To prepare stained films of the deposit a drop should be spread on a slide and fixed, *e.g.*, by passing the slide through a flame until the heat can only just be borne on the back of the hand. Stained films are also made directly from such specimens as sputum and pus. To do this a selected portion of the material is placed on a slide and either spread with a platinum loop or crushed between two slides which are then drawn apart. Films which are to be stained for tubercle bacilli should be thicker than normal; these films also need fixing.

Staining of films.—In routine bacteriology the Gram stain and the Ziehl-Neelsen stain for tubercle bacilli are most used.

(1) *Gram staining.*—As nearly all pathogenic bacteria are either Gram-positive or Gram-negative the use of this stain is usually the first step in the identification of an organism, and used alone it may provide a clue to the nature of the infection. The technique is as follows: (i.) Cover the film with a solution of 0·5% methyl-violet B or crystal violet and allow this to act for 1 minute. (ii.) Drain off, and flood the slide with Gram's iodine solution, leaving this on for 1 minute. (iii.) Drain off and treat the film with alcohol, continuing until no more stain comes out of the preparation. (iv.) Wash in water. (v.) Pour on dilute carbol fuchsin and leave 1 minute. (vi.) Wash, blot and dry. When examined with the high-powered objective and an oil immersion lens Gram-positive bacteria are seen to be dark blue and Gram-negative bacteria red. Table LXV lists the more important Gram-positive and Gram-negative organisms.

TABLE LXV.—COMMONER GRAM-POSITIVE AND GRAM-NEGATIVE BACTERIA

Gram-Positive	Gram-Negative
Staph. aureus and albus	N. gonorrhœæ, meningitidis and catarrhalis
Strep. pyogenes, viridans, fæcalis	B. Friedlanderi
Strep. pneumoniæ	Salmonellæ (typhi, paratyphi and food poison-
C. diphtheriæ	ing members)
B. anthracis, subtilis	Shigellæ
Clostridia (tetani, welchii, etc.)	Proteus
Actinomyces isræli	Ps. pyocyanea
	H. influenzæ, pertussis
	V. choleræ
	P. pestis
	Br. melitensis, abortus, suis.

(2) *Ziehl-Neelsen Stain for Tubercle Bacilli.*—Flood the slide with filtered strong carbol fuchsin and heat gently until steam rises. Allow the preparation to stain for five minutes, heat being applied at intervals to keep the stain hot. Do not allow the stain to evaporate and dry on the slide. Wash with water, and immerse the slide in 25 per cent. sulphuric acid for a few minutes, and then in 70 per cent. spirit for a similar period. Repeat this process of decolorisation until after washing with water the film is colourless or of a faint pink tinge only. Counterstain with methylene blue or dilute malachite green for 10 to 20 seconds: then wash, blot, dry and examine with the oil immersion objective. The tubercle bacilli stain bright red, whilst cells and other organisms are stained blue or pale green.

§ 1203. **Characters of Pathological Fluids and Special Tests.**—In the pleural, pericardial and peritoneal cavities, inflammatory effusions (exudates) are to be distinguished from dropsical effusions (transudates). The presence of a large jelly-like clot formed rapidly on standing, a specific gravity above 1016, a protein content over 2 per cent., and a relatively high cellular content indicate an exudate. In a transudate, clot formation is slight or absent, the specific gravity usually below 1012, the protein content under 1 per cent., and the cytological content small. The transudate of cardiac œdema has a higher protein percentage than that of renal œdema. Blood in distinct amount in these cavities suggests neoplasm, but occurs with tuberculous disease of the pleura and with peritonitis associated with cirrhosis of the liver. A few blood cells, sufficient to give the fluid a rosy tinge, may occur with simple acute inflammation. The character of the cells in a pleural fluid may aid diagnosis of the cause of the effusion; thus, an excess of lymphocytes points to tuberculous pleurisy, the predominance of polymorph cells to pyogenic or other causes.

Guinea-pig inoculation of a sterile pleural effusion may establish its tuberculous origin when tubercle bacilli cannot otherwise be demonstrated in it. The clot ground up in normal saline in a sterile mortar, or the centrifuged deposit, form the best material for inoculation. A positive result is obtained only in about 70 per cent. of cases, whose subsequent history proves to be tuberculous; in some cases several animals should therefore be used. Cultivation of the deposit or clot on a medium specially selective for tubercle bacilli, such as that of Lowenstein-Jensen, is successful in a high percentage of cases and in a shorter time than a positive animal inoculation result.

§ 1204. **Cerebro-Spinal Fluid** in health is a clear, colourless, watery fluid, alkaline in reaction and with no clot formation. A trace of albumen (25 mg. per cent.) is normally present, and also a trace of sugar (partial reduction of Fehling's solution). In acute meningitis the fluid may exhibit varying degrees of *cloudiness*, from slight turbidity to almost pure pus, and in pyogenic infections the causal organism may be demonstrated in stained films. The presence of *blood* may result from a head injury, subarachnoid hæmorrhage, cerebral hæmorrhage or trauma of the venous plexus on the posterior surface of the vertebral canal at the time of the lumbar puncture. Recent hæmorrhage (as in the latter) can be distinguished from old hæmorrhage by centrifuging some of the fluid; if the supernatant layer be clear, with no sign of hæmolysis, the blood present is probably the result of trauma at the time of the lumbar puncture; old hæmorrhage is almost always associated with some degree of hæmolysis, and the supernatant fluid is tinged yellow. Further, if the blood-stained cerebro-spinal fluid is collected in successive small amounts in three or four test-tubes, in recent hæmorrhage caused by trauma at the time of the puncture that in the first one or two tubes will be more deeply blood-stained than in the third or fourth. In old hæmorrhage the blood admixture in all tubes will be about equal.

BACTERIOLOGICAL EXAMINATION OF THE C.S.F. is important and urgent, as in pyogenic infections the recovery of the patient depends on the use of the correct drug in treatment which in turn may depend on the identification of the organism responsible. The centrifuged deposit should be examined in a direct film under the microscope and by culture. Particularly when meningococcal meningitis is suspected the C.S.F. should reach the laboratory as quickly as possible and must be kept at body temperature until cultures are made. Other organisms which may be found include pneumococci, *H. influenzæ*, streptococci, staphylococci and various Gram-negative bacilli. Tubercle bacilli are often found most easily in the spider web clot which forms in the fluid on standing. This organism may grow on Lowenstein-Jensen medium or the fluid can be inoculated into a guinea-pig.

CYTOLOGY OF C.S.F.—The normal content is 2–4 mononuclear cells (lymphocytes or endothelial cells) per c.mm. The total cell count is best made with the Fuchs-Rosenthal counting chamber. It is well to stain the fluid before, as a differential count can then be made at the same time as the total number per c.mm. is estimated. To 0·50 ml. of the cerebro-spinal fluid in a clean dry test-tube add 0·05 ml. of a 0·2 per cent. solution of toluidin blue or methyl violet. Shake the tube and allow the mixture to stand for ten minutes. This gives a dilution of ten parts in eleven of the cerebro-spinal fluid, which can be allowed for in the subsequent calculation. The nuclei of the lymphocytes and polymorphonuclear cells take up the stain and can be distinguished by their characteristic shape; the red cells are uninfluenced.

A *differential count* can also be performed on a Leishman stained film of a centrifuged deposit of fluid. A slight *increase in lymphocytes* (5–10 per c.mm.) in the cerebro-spinal fluid occurs in any form of syphilitic nervous disease after the earlier stages and especially in the more chronic forms, such as tabes or chronic meningeal syphilis. It may also occur in disseminated sclerosis, cerebral tumour and abscess, poliomyelitis, encephalitis lethargica and some forms of polyneuritis. A greater increase in lymphocytes (10–50 per c.mm.) is common in syphilitic nervous disease of all forms during the onset or the progress of the disease. It also occurs in tuberculous meningitis and in the other conditions mentioned above. A slight increase of both lymphocytes and polymorphonuclear cells (5–10 per c.mm.) is characteristic of brain abscess or of inflammation of the cranial sinuses with involvement of the dura mater. A larger increase comprising both these types of cell occurs in tuberculous meningitis. Marked polymorphonuclear increase is the rule in all forms of cerebro-spinal meningitis, whether due to pyogenic cocci, the meningococcus, or to any of a variety of bacillary forms, *e.g.*, *H. influeuzæ*. In these conditions the causative organism can usually be demonstrated in the fluid.

CHEMICAL TESTS OF THE C.S.F.—For these, the clear fluid obtained after centrifuging should be used. *Protein*.—Mestrezat's method is preferable. In this the degree of opalescence produced by the precipitation of the protein in the fluid by trichloracetic acid is compared with that of a series of standards ranging from 10 to

100 mg. per cent.; 2 ml. of the fluid are put into a tube of similar weight and diameter to those used for the standards, 0·3 ml. of 30 per cent. trichloracetic acid is added; the tube is set aside for twenty to thirty minutes, then shaken up and compared with the standard scale. The normal protein content is 20–50 mg. per cent.

Globulin.—The Nonne-Apelt reaction consists in pouring 1 ml. of the cerebro-spinal fluid on to the surface of 1 ml. of a neutral saturated solution of ammonium sulphate. A normal fluid gives a faint opalescent ring at the junction of the two surfaces. A definite opacity indicates an increase of globulin.

Chlorides.—These are estimated against a standard silver nitrate solution, using potassium chromate as an indicator. The chlorides are precipitated as insoluble silver chloride and the indicator, potassium chromate, forms red silver chromate as soon as all the chloride is used up. The silver nitrate solution is made by dissolving 5·814 G. of pure silver nitrate in a litre of distilled water (or 2·5 G. $AgNO_3$ in 430 ml. of distilled water). This solution keeps indefinitely in a brown bottle. For the test exactly 2 ml. of cerebro-spinal fluid is measured by a delivery pipette into 15 or 20 ml. of distilled water, and 2 drops of 10 per cent. potassium chromate added. The silver nitrate solution is run in from a graduated burette with constant stirring. A permanent change of colour from lemon to orange yellow indicates the end point. Each ml. of silver solution then used indicates 100 mg. of chloride per 100 ml. of C.S.F. The normal chloride content should fall between 725 and 750 ml. per 100 ml. of fluid.

Sugar.—A routine qualitative test is sufficient. One ml. of the cerebro-spinal fluid is boiled with 0·25 ml. of Fehling's solution. Normal fluids give a heavy reddish-yellow precipitate which on standing sinks to the bottom of·the test-tube, leaving the supernatant fluid pale blue.

Lange's Colloidal Gold Reaction.—Normal cerebro-spinal fluid causes little or no alteration in a colloidal gold solution, but precipitation of the gold may occur with cerebro-spinal fluid from cases of general paralysis of the insane, tabes and some forms of meningitis (Table LXVI). Precipitation in these conditions occurs in different dilutions, though these to some extent overlap. Ten dilutions of cerebro-spinal fluid are used in the test, ranging from 1 in 10 up to 1 in 5120. Numbers denote various appearances of fluid depending on the degree of gold precipitation. 0 denotes no change (rose-red colour); 1, very slight change to deeper red, scarcely lilac; 2, lilac to purple; 3, deep blue; 4, light blue with purplish precipitate; and 5, complete decolorisation of the top fluid with a heavy bluish precipitate.

A report 0011100000 would be the reading of a normal cerebro-spinal fluid, and indicates that there is no gold precipitation in most of the dilutions, but a very slight one in the dilutions 1 in 40, 1 in 80 and 1 in 160. In the paretic response—typical of general paralysis of the insane—precipitation occurs in the eight strongest dilutions, diminishing gradually, e.g., 5555443200. In the luetic response, seen in tabes and cerebro-spinal syphilis, precipitation occurs in the higher middle dilutions, e.g., 1233210000. A positive curve of either response may be given by some cases of disseminated sclerosis; the Wassermann Reaction here is negative.

Special Tests that may be valuable if laboratory facilities are available will now be briefly described.

§ 1205. Bacteriological Examinations.

A Throat swab.—Cultures will show the presence of hæmolytic streptococci or diphtheria bacilli. In Vincent's infection a stained film will show the characteristic Gram-positive bacilli and Gram-negative spirochætes.

A Post-nasal swab is used for the isolation of meningococci, or *H. pertussis* in patients with whooping-cough.

A *Wound swab and Pus from an Abscess.*—Organisms commonly present include *Staph. aureus, Str. pyogenes* and various Gram-negative bacilli such as coliform bacilli, Proteus and *Ps. pyocyanea.* Culture will enable sensitivity tests to antibiotics to be carried out. In specific infections, e.g., anthrax and actinomycosis, the responsible organism will be isolated. In the latter sulphur granules, colonies of the streptothrix

TABLE LXVI.—CEREBRO-SPINAL FLUID

Condition.	Appearance of Fluid.	Pressure of Fluid in Recumbent Posture.	Protein mg. per cent.	Cells per c.mm.	Type of Cells.	Organisms.	Wassermann.	Colloidal Gold Curve.	Sugar per cent.	Chlorides in mg. per cent.
Normal.	Clear, colourless; no clot on standing.	60-150 mm. water.	20-50	0 5	Lymphocytes.	None.	Negative.	0000000000 or 0011100000	0·05 0·07	720-750
Tuberculous meningitis.	Clear, colourless; spidery clot on standing.	Increased.	Up to 300	10-400	75 per cent. lymphocytes.	Tubercle bacilli in clot.	Negative.	Normal.	Diminished.	Fall to below 660.
Benign lymphocytic meningitis.	Clear or hazy with spidery clot on standing.	Increased.	50-300	30 to several thousand.	Lymphocytes.	None.	Negative.	Normal or meningitic.	Normal.	Normal or a little reduced.
Cerebro-spinal meningitis.	Hazy or turbid; dense clot on standing.	Increased.	Up to 300	10-2000 or more.	Polymorphs.	Intra-cellular Gram-negative diplococci.	Negative.	Normal.	Diminished or absent.	600-700
Pneumococcal, streptococcal and staphylococcal meningitis.	Hazy, turbid or purulent; dense clot on standing.	Increased.	Up to 300	10-1000 or more.	Polymorphs.	Gram-positive cocci.	Negative.	Normal.	Diminished or absent.	600-700
General paralysis of insane.	Normal.	Increased.	50-100	20-400	Lymphocytes.		Positive in over 99 per cent.	Curve such as 5555443200.	Normal.	Normal.
Tabes dorsalis.	Normal.	Normal.	30-80	10-80	Lymphocytes.		Positive in 70 per cent.	Curve such as 1233210000.	Normal.	Normal.
Meningo-vascular syphilis.	Normal.	Normal.	30-80	10-80	Lymphocytes.		Positive in 50 per cent.	Curve such as 0014320000.	Normal.	Normal.
Encephalitis lethargica.	Normal.	Usually increased.	20-50	0-10	Lymphocytes.		Negative.	Normal or luetic.	Normal or slightly raised.	Normal.
Disseminated sclerosis.	Normal.	Normal.	Normal or slight increase.	Normal or slightly increased.	Lymphocytes.		Negative.	Normal to 5555443200.	Normal.	Normal.
Acute anterior Poliomyelitis.	Normal.	Normal or increased.	Raised to 100 from end of first to end of sixth week.	10-1000 from pre-paralytic stage to end of second week.	Polymorphs, then Lymphocytes.		Negative.	Curve such as 0123210000.	Normal.	Normal.
Spinal blockage (Loculation or Froin's syndrome); and some forms of polyneuritis.	Clear, straw to amber; dense clot.	Diminished or normal below block.	300 4000	Normal, or slight increase.	Lymphocytes.	None.	Negative unless due to syphilis.	Normal.	Normal.	Normal.

growing in the pus, should be looked for with the naked eye. In gas gangrene and in tetanus, clostridia will be present, but the finding of these organisms in a wound does not by itself mean that the patient is suffering from gas gangrene as clostridia are frequently found in wounds, causing only local infection.

In Urine common infecting organisms are coliform bacilli, *Str. fæcalis, Staph. aureus, Staph. albus,* Proteus and *Ps. pyocyanea.* Resistant strains of these bacteria are met so frequently that rational chemotherapy can only be based on sensitivity tests. When indicated, tubercle bacilli should be looked for and great care should be taken not to confuse them with the smegma bacilli which are found in many clean specimens of urine from women.

Fæces.—Pathogenic organisms which can be isolated on culture include members of the enteric family—*S. typhi* and *S. paratyphi* A, B and C, the food poisoning salmonellæ and dysentery bacilli; and from infants pathogenic strains of *E. coli.* The examination of stained films should be used for the diagnosis of staphylococcal enterocolitis and may be used to identify tubercle bacilli, although great care must be taken to exclude non-pathogenic acid-fast bacilli which have been swallowed in the food.

Microscopical examination of wet films may show the presence or absence of pus and red cells and of the cysts and ova of the various intestinal parasites. In patients with amœbic dysentery motile *E. histolytica* may be seen.

Sputum from patients with acute pneumonia is most likely to contain the pneumococcus. In rare cases hæmolytic streptococci or Friedlander's bacilli may be present. Pneumonia due to *Staph. aureus* is rarely seen except as a complication of influenza, in patients with a raised blood urea, or in late stages of chronic bronchitis. *H. influenzæ* is very commonly present in the sputum of patients with bronchitis and bronchiectasis. Every sputum examination should include the search of a Ziehl-Neelsen film for tubercle bacilli.

§ 1206. Serological Examinations.

Specimens for the diagnosis of virus infections.—Facilities for virus examination differ throughout the world and practitioners should find out what services are available in their own area. In some diseases, *e.g.*, smallpox and poliomyelitis, identification of the virus can be made rapidly. In many, diagnosis depends on determining the antibody content of the blood during the acute phase and again some three weeks later. When this is done the result may be of no value in the treatment of the individual patient who has frequently recovered before the diagnosis is made. although it may be of considerable epidemiological interest.

§ 1207. The Wassermann and other blood tests for Syphilis.—Patients with syphilis form a number of different antibodies. Many tests have been used for their detection. The three most usefully employed now are the Wassermann reaction (W.R.), the Reiter protein complement fixation test (R.P.C.F.) and the treponemal immobilisation test (T.P.I.) of Nelson, all of which detect different antibodies.

The **Wassermann reaction** depends on complement fixation and employs as its antigen an alcoholic extract of heart muscle with added cholesterol. It becomes positive in the patient's serum shortly after the appearance of the primary chancre (§ 500). If treatment is undertaken in the primary or secondary stages of syphilis the W.R. will usually become negative. If treatment is not begun until later the W.R. will probably remain positive. This is quite compatible with cure, representing residual antibody formation in the same way that patients who have had typhoid fever may have detectable antibodies to typhoid bacilli in the blood for many years. The W.R. will occasionally give *false positive* results in patients for whom the diagnosis of syphilis can be excluded. These biological false positive reactions are becoming of greater importance now that syphilis is becoming less common in Great Britain and routine blood testing is done more often. They are of two types. *Acute* false positives are of short duration, lasting at the most six months. They follow some acute infections, notably malaria and glandular fever, and may be seen after immunisation, particularly vaccination against smallpox. *Chronic* false positives may persist for years. Many of the patients in whom this finding has been made have later developed systemic lupus erythematosus.

The **Reiter Protein Complement Fixation test** is also a complement fixation reaction, the antigen used being an extract of the Reiter treponeme. This organism can be cultivated and is regarded by many as a saprophyte, although some believe it to be an adapted strain of *Treponema pallidum*. The test may also occasionally produce false positives.

The **Treponemal immobilisation test** is the most sensitive and specific test for syphilis. The antigen consists of a suspension of living *T. pallidum*, which in a positive test are immobilised by the patient's serum. The test is complex both in preparation and performance and is only done in reference centres: it is not suitable for routine use. It should normally be reserved for occasions on which it is desired to differentiate between a biologic false positive W.R. and a positive W.R. due to syphilis.

None of the serological tests distinguishes between infection caused by different species of treponema, and it is therefore not possible to separate syphilis from, for example, yaws in this way.

§ 1208. **Widal's Serum Reaction** illustrates the phenomenon of immunity (§ 523). An infecting organism acts in the human body as an antigen, a substance which stimulates the formation of antibodies. These antibodies are of various types; among them are agglutinins which cause the infecting organisms to mass together in clumps, *i.e.*, to agglutinate. The test, originally described for typhoid fever, is now applied to many other bacterial infections, notably the paratyphoid fevers, Malta fever, food poisonings and infections with *Br. abortus*. A somewhat similar technique is used for typing the pneumococcus and meningococcus. In typhoid the reaction may occur any time after the first week, rarely by the third day, and persists for several years (§ 496). Inoculated persons may give a positive result for many years.

§ 1209. **Paul-Bunnell Reaction.**—This is a diagnostic test for glandular fever dependent on the discovery that the blood in this affection contains heterophil antibodies in the form of an agglutinin for sheep's red cells. Normal serum may possess agglutinin to a titre of 1 in 16: in glandular fever the titre is usually 1 in 64 or higher by the end of the first week, and remains high during the active phase of the disease (§ 498). Sometimes it is only transient, occasionally delayed, and rarely absent. This latter suggests that glandular fever is caused by different viruses some of which do not give the typical serological reactions. The patient's serum is inactivated by heating for fifteen minutes at 55° C and is then put up in serial dilutions, to each of which is added a known volume of a 2 per cent. suspension of freshly washed sheep's cells. The test is read after incubation in a water bath or incubator for one hour at 37° C followed by refrigeration overnight at 2–4° C. A raised titre occurs in serum sickness, but apart from this the reaction is specific for glandular fever.

Other Tests which assist in Diagnosis and Treatment follow.

§ 1210. **Erythrocyte Sedimentation Rate.**—The sedimentation rate of the red cells was first studied by Fahræus, but there have been many subsequent modifications in technique. *Method.*—The Westergren method is the one most commonly used. 1·6 ml. of blood is mixed with 0·4 ml. of 3·8 per cent. sodium citrate solution, and some of the mixture drawn up into a standard Westergren tube; the latter is 2·5 mm. in diameter and closely resembles a 1 ml. pipette, but is calibrated in mm. of length. The zero mark is exactly 200 mm. from the point, and the blood is drawn up to this mark. The tube is then set upright in a special stand and the red corpuscles begin to settle down, leaving a clear supernatant plasma. At the end of one hour, the result is read as the distance sedimented in mm. by the top of the red cell column. In men the normal range is 3–5 mm. and in women and children 4–7 mm.; these values are higher in those past middle age. An increased sedimentation rate is present in pregnant women after the third or fourth month, in localised acute inflammations, in rheumatoid arthritis, in active tuberculosis and in active rheumatic disease of children (rheumatic fever, carditis, etc.). In tuberculosis, the degree of sedimentation is of some value in prognosis as it increases with the activity of the disease; in rheumatic disease of childhood, an increased rate points to a latent activity even in the absence of physical signs, and indicates continued rest to limit cardiac damage. The sedimentation rate is apparently dependent on the ratio of albumen, globulin and fibrinogen in the plasma. The test is of more value in prognosis than diagnosis, and in all cases should be interpreted in conjunction with other clinical and laboratory investigations. When the E.S.R. is over 100 mm. in 1 hour the diagnosis is likely to be myelomatosis, rheumatoid arthritis, periarteritis nodosa, disseminated lupus erythematosus, disease of the liver or kidney or a late stage of a hypernephroma.

§ 1211. The **Xenopus Pregnancy Test** (Toad ovulation test) depends on the production of ovulation in female *Xenopus lævis*—an African toad—following the injection of the anterior-pituitary-like hormone in the urine of pregnant women. Three or four toads are inoculated with 2 ml. of urine into the lymph sac under the dorsal skin, and a positive result is indicated by the shedding of eggs in 12 to 24 hours. The reliability of the test does not differ from that of the Zondek-Aschheim or the Friedman reaction, and the animals need not be killed to obtain the result. A related test is by injection of 10 ml. of a patient's untreated urine into the dorsal lymph sac of the adult male toad *Bufo arenarum* Hensel indigenous to South America. In 2–4 hours masses of spermatozoa in the toad's urine indicate a positive result.

§ 1212. **Examination for Lupus Erythematosus (L.E.) Cells.**—In disseminated lupus erythematosus, L.E. cells can be demonstrated in over 80 per cent. of cases. Although a negative result does not exclude the diagnosis, their presence should be looked for repeatedly; steroid therapy reduces the number of positive findings. The test is usually regarded as specific, as true L.E. cells have only rarely been described in other conditions, *e.g.*, chronic discoid lupus erythematosus, rheumatoid arthritis, in other collagen diseases, penicillin hypersensitivity, chronic hepatitis and after prolonged hydralazine therapy.

The L.E. cell is a neutrophil leucocyte that contains in the cytoplasm a large rounded structureless body staining purple with Romanowsky stains. These bodies consist of nuclear material liberated from lysed neutrophil leucocytes and phagocytosed by the containing cells (Plate XVII). The factor responsible for the L.E. phenomenon has been shown to be a gamma-globulin fraction of the plasma. A technique to demonstrate L.E. cells is to allow clotted blood to stand for two hours and then mash through a sieve, centrifuge, remove the buffy layer which is recentrifuged in a hæmatocrit tube and films made from the final buffy layers.

§ 1213. **Examination for Malignant Cells.**—*Direct* smears of sputum or vaginal fluid are fixed and stained by Papanicolaou's method. Centrifuged deposits of fluids, *e.g.*, pleural, peritoneal, cerebro-spinal, are stained with Leishman stain.

Malignant cells from different sites vary in appearance and considerable experience is necessary to recognise them. Features of malignant cells include variation in size, atypical nuclei including the presence of nucleoli, an increased nuclear cytoplasm ratio, clumping of cells, degeneration and the presence of mitotic figures.

§ 1214. **Basal Metabolism.**—The determination of the basal metabolic rate is of value in diagnosis, prognosis and in estimating progress at various stages of treatment. In cases of exophthalmic goitre it establishes with certainty the degree of toxicity due to the thyroid condition. In cases of hypo- or hyper-thyroidism it is of value as a guide to treatment. It may be defined as a measure of the capacity of the individual to consume oxygen under certain definite conditions which by precise adjustment permit of comparison with a standard normal.

There are several methods of determining the basal metabolic rate. For general clinical purposes, a method carried out by a physician and at the bedside is of practical value. Such a method is offered by the portable Benedict apparatus. The precautions necessary are:—(a) That the patient should be fasting and should have been resting in bed for the preceding 12 or 14 hours; (b) That he should practise for a day or two the use of the nose-piece and mouth-piece. These are at first uncomfortable; but after a little practice he will grow thoroughly accustomed both to the method of breathing and to the strangeness of the mechanical devices in the mouth and nose. This precaution is of the first importance—for mental or physical unrest at the time of the test will materially impair its accuracy.

The apparatus consists of a cylindrical spirometer with the necessary attachments to the mouth-piece and for administering the supply of oxygen. It also contains soda lime, through which both the inspired oxygen and the expired air pass—thus removing all the CO_2. The readings on the scale represent accurately the amount of oxygen consumed. These readings are interpreted by means of a table which accompanies the apparatus and which makes allowance for variations of temperature, barometric pressure, height, weight, age and sex. One is then able to ascertain the percentage of oxygen consumed per minute above or below the normal. This is expressed as the B.M.R. (basal metabolic rate), plus or minus, as the case may be.

§ 1215. **Prothrombin Time.**—Blood from a vein (1·80 ml.) is added to 0·20 ml. sodium citrate solution (3·8 per cent.) and then centrifuged to separate off the plasma. The estimation should be done within 2 hours of withdrawing the blood. Into standard sized tubes (such as 76 mm. × 6 mm.) are put 0·1 ml. plasma and 0·1 ml. reconstituted thromboplastin (thrombokinase) solution; this and 0·1 ml. calcium chloride solution (anhydrous 2·77 G. in 1 litre of distilled water) are warmed in a water bath (37° C) for 1 minute; the calcium chloride solution is added to the plasma-thromboplastin solution. At the same moment a stop-watch is started, and is stopped on the first appearance of a fibrin web. Each estimation of the time of coagulation is done at least twice and the average time taken is compared with a control estimation using normal plasma.

§ 1216. **Schilling Test for Pernicious Anæmia.**—When a normal person is given a small dose by mouth of radio-actively tagged vitamin B_{12} (e.g., 1 mc. of Co^{58} vit. B_{12}) followed by a large dose of ordinary vitamin B_{12} by intramuscular injection, during the next 24 hours 15–30 per cent. of the oral dose is excreted in the urine. In pernicious anæmia, due to malabsorption of the oral B_{12}, less than 7 per cent. is excreted in the 24-hour urine, unless intrinsic factor (such as hog's stomach) is also given. Excretion is also diminished in sprue and in renal disease.

§ 1217. **Chromosome Abnormalities in relation to Disease.**—Since it was found in 1956 that the chromosome number of man was 46, not 48, a great deal of work has clarified the cause of several anomalies of somatic, intellectual and sex development; among these are mongolism (Down's syndrome), ovarian dysgenesis and Klinefelter's syndrome. The most important advances are (a) the better techniques used to study human chromosomes, particularly during the metaphase of mitosis of cells grown *in vitro*. (b) The discovery by M. L. Barr in 1949 of the sex chromatin of nuclei of somatic cells.

The *sex-chromatin mass* is seen at the nuclear membrane of tissue cells such as those scraped from the oral mucosa of normal females (chromatin positive) and represents one of their two X chromosomes. In abnormal conditions, when more than two X chromosomes are present, the number of sex-chromatin masses in the somatic cells increases but there is always *one less mass than there are X chromosomes* (Fig. 273). In normal males, whose sex chromosomes are an X and a shorter Y, no sex-chromatin mass is visible in the somatic cells (chromatin negative), in keeping with the above rule.

The normal human chromosome complement is of 23 pairs (one chromosome of each pair is of paternal, the other of maternal origin): 22 pairs of autosomes plus one pair of sex chromosomes. In the female the two sex chromosomes are identical and quite large (XX) but in the male they are dissimilar (XY). The chromosomes, the carriers of the genes which control inherited characteristics, are studied under the light microscope after staining, or in unstained preparations by phase contrast microscopy; they can be counted in the cells and an attempt made to recognise them

(A)   (C)

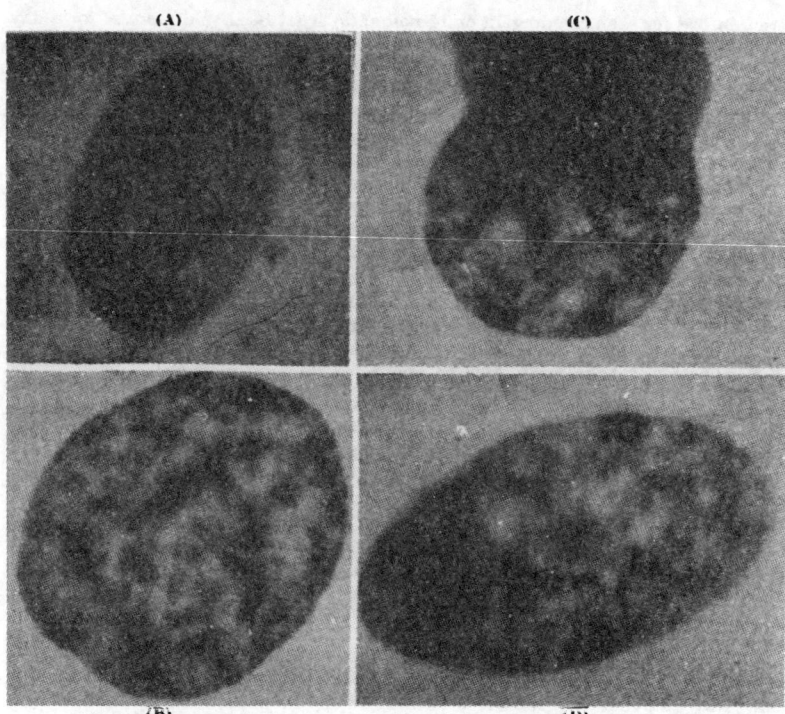

(B)   (D)

FIG. 273.—A chromatin-negative cell (A) from an oral mucosa smear and three chromatin-positive cells with one (B), two (C) and three (D) sex-chromatin masses. (Only the nuclei are shown.)
The negative cell (A) could be from a normal male or an XO female; the positive cell with one mass (B) from a normal female or an XXY male; the positive cell with two masses (C) from a triplo-X female—XXX—or an XXXY male; and the positive cell with three masses (D) from an XXXX female or an XXXXY male.
(Magnification approximately × 7,000.)

individually or to assign them to certain groups on morphological grounds. Having obtained a photograph of the cell, the individual chromosomes can be cut out from enlargements, arranged into matching pairs according (*a*) to a standard order of decreasing size, and (*b*) the position of the centromere. The latter is clearly seen at metaphase when each chromosome has made a replica and consists of two chromatids held together by the centromere. The orderly array of chromosomes is called a karyotype. The pairs are numbered but, whereas the morphological identification of some individual pairs of normal chromosomes is unequivocal, that of others is doubtful, and assignment is only possible to one of the groups of chromosomes with similar characters (Fig. 274).

Anomalies of development in about 1 in 200–300 liveborn babies may be caused by chromosome errors, mostly (A) extra sex chromosomes, or (B) extra autosomes (trisomic conditions); sometimes there is absence of one sex chromosome, and occasionally a visible structural change of either the autosomes or the sex chromosomes.

(A) ERRORS OF THE SEX CHROMOSOMES:
(i) OF NUMBER: XXY males, with a chromosome number of 47, present with Klinefelter's syndrome of small testes, azoospermia and at times endocrine changes after puberty (eunuchoidism, gynæcomastia) and some intellectual retardation. These males are chromatin positive. (Incidence about 1 in 400 males.)

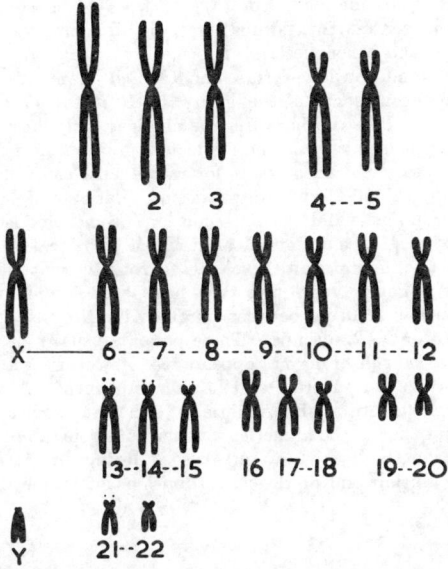

FIG. 274.—A diagrammatic representation of the 24 chromosomes of man (idiogram), numbered according to the Denve jsystem.

   Only one of each pair of autosomes is represented. Each chromosome is made up of two chromatids held together by the centromere. The uncertainty of individual classification is expressed by tracts between numbers, and by a solid line when difficulty of positive identification is even greater.

XXX (triple-X) females sometimes show intellectual impairment, usually without obvious error of sex or somatic development. The oral mucosa cells show two sex-chromatin masses and the chromosome number is 47. (Incidence about 1 in 700 females.)

XO females, with 45 chromosomes and chromatin negative on nuclear sexing, have short stature and often other associated anomalies (webbed neck, coarctation of the aorta, renal abnormalities, slight intellectual impairment) and, after puberty, lack of secondary sex characters (primary amenorrhœa, scanty axillary and pubic hair and no breast development) due to ovarian dysgenesis (Turner's syndrome). (Incidence about 1 in 3,000 females.)

Sex-chromosome mosaics: the name refers to men or women who are thought to have in their bodies cells with a different sex-chromosome complement and consequently different chromosome number. Clinically, they may have ovarian dysgenesis or features of Klinefelter's syndrome. Some true hermaphrodites have shown sex-chromosome mosaicism. More complex sex-chromosome anomalies are rarely found in males (with 48 chromosomes and XXXY or 49 chromosomes and XXXXY) or females (with 48 chromosomes and XXXX).

   (ii) OF STRUCTURE: Abnormal X chromosomes have been seen in women with variants of ovarian dysgenesis. These can be smaller than the normal X (and are thought to represent deletions), or they can be larger (probably isochromosomes made up of two long arms of the X chromosome).

   (B) ERRORS OF THE AUTOSOMES: The most common are those that cause mongolism (Down's syndrome), the incidence of which is one in 650 liveborn babies.

   (i) OF NUMBER: Trisomy for chromosome No. 21. The chromosome number is 47 because there are three instead of two chromosomes No. 21. (The clinical features are those of Down's syndrome.)

Trisòmy for chromosome No. 17 or 18, *i.e.*, three chromosomes 17 or 18, with a total of 47.   This presents with a peculiar face, digital anomalies, club feet, congenital heart disease, renal and other visceral abnormalities, spasticity and developmental retardation.   The condition is very rare and affected infants die within a few weeks.

Trisòmy for a chromosome of the group 13–15 (total 47): this rare anomaly manifests with cleft palate and hare lip, eye changes, polydactyly, congenital heart disease and developmental retardation ; affected children die in early infancy.

Chromosome mosaicism can account for rare examples of children with Down's syndrome, usually with odd features, for instance, relatively high intelligence.   There is a mixture of normal cells and cells trisomic for chromosome No. 21.

(ii) OF STRUCTURE: These are often the result of translocation: two chromosomes, usually belonging to different pairs, exchange chromatin material after a break has occurred in each.   Though very rare, they have been found in Down's syndrome when translocation has occurred between chromosome No. 21 and another autosome either of the 13–15 or 21–22 groups.   These patients usually have 46 chromosomes. One of the parents, though of normal appearance, often carries a translocation which can be transmitted to the offspring and has a complement of 45 chromosomes.

The origin of the structural abnormalities of either autosomes or sex chromosomes can be complex, but that of the numerical anomalies is generally the result of chromosome non-disjunction (faulty separation) or loss during one of the cell divisions of gametogenesis, or during one of the early divisions of the fertilised ovum.

INDEX

The principal references are in black type

Deer-fly fever, 740
Defæcation, disorders of, neurological, 1117
— painful, in women, 647
Defective feeding, causing emaciation, 845
— — — — in children, 845, 853
— vision, 1336
" Deficiency disease," 830, 924, 948
Degeneration, amyloid of liver, 495
— cerebro-macular, 1228, 1414
— fatty of liver, 38, 495
— hepato-lenticular, 1198
— myocardial, 89, 112, 119, 249
— of the cerebellum, 1209, 1210
— of the spinal cord, 1211, 1212, 1228
— reaction of, 1123, 1238
— subacute combined, 1212, 1228
Deglutition pneumonia, 202
Dehydration, 437, 440, 447
Deiter's nucleus, 1045, 1058, 1059, 1062
Delirious mania, acute, 1386
Delirium, 659, 1371, 1399
— causes of, 659, 1400
— cordis, 85
— drugs causing, 661, 1400
— è potu, 660
— febrile, 659, 660
— ferox, 659
— in heart failure, 45
— in specific fevers, 660
— in typhoid, 659, 662
— in uræmia, 529, 530, 660
— investigation of, 1399
— muttering, 529, 530, 660, 662
— non-febrile, 530, 660, 1399
— post-febrile, 660, 662, 1400
— reflex, 661
— treatment of, 661, 1400
— tremens, 660, 1395
— — treatment of, 1397
Delusion, definition of, 1371
Delusional insanity, 1391, 1401
Dementia, 1150, 1400
— alcoholic, 1395
— arteriosclerotic, 1401
— epileptic, 1145, 1402
— paralytica, 725, 1150, 1177, 1190, 1403
— post-traumatic, 1403
— præcox (Schizophrenia), 1391, 1401
— presenile, 1150, 1158, 1402
— senile, 1401
Demyelinating diseases, 1221
Dengue, 695
Dental caries, 308, 309
— causalgia, 1086
— infection, 310
Dentition, 308
Depilatory methods, 1029
Depression, in G.P.I., 1403
— in liver disorder, 472
— morbid, causes of, 1371, 1387
Depressor nerve, of heart, 32
Dercum's disease, 28

Dermacentor ticks, 698
Dermatitis artefacta, 939
— atopic, 972
— chemical, 969
— contact, 969
— dye, 1030
— exfoliative, 948, 966
— herpetiformis, 671, 979
— medicamentosa, 941
— occupational, 969
— repens, 987
— seborrhœic, 963
— streptococcal, 989
Dermatomyositis, 920, 948, 1019
Dermographism, 959
Desensitisation, 216, 959
Desert sore, 1004
Detachment of retina, 1349
Deviation of nasal septum, 292
— conjugate, of head and eyes, 1041, 1058, 1130, 1132, 1316
Devic's disease, 1219, 1342
" Devil's grip," 743
Dextrocardia, 177
Dhobie-itch (tinea cruris), 965, 1037
di Guglielmo's disease, 826
Diabetes, 586
— bronzed, 495, 516, 862
— coma in, 587, 588, 1137, 1190
— — pain in, 336, 354
— — treatment of, 590, 593
— diet in, 415, 590
— innocens, 585
— insipidus, 585, 596, 1063
— mellitus, 584, 586, 1137, 1190
— — arthritis in, 914
— — nephritis in, 566
— — polyneuritis in, 914, 1243
— — retinopathy in, 1350
— renal, 585, 586
Diacetic acid, 379, 538, 588
Diagnosis, method of, 9
Diaphragm, eventration of, 177
— hernia of, 177, 333, 375
Diaphragmatic pleurisy causing abdominal pain, 162, 355
Diarrhœa, 386, 433
— acute, 433
— chronic, 441
— — tetany in, 1288
— chyious, 796
— dysenteric, 447
— epidemic, 434
— — infantile, 437
— false, 446, 460
— gastrogenous, 453
— in amyloid disease, 453
— in portal obstruction, 446
— in typhoid fever, 438, 709
— infantile, 436
— lienteric, 446
— nervous, 446
— pancreatic, 453
— senile, 453

IDEAL WEIGHTS FOR MEN AND WOMEN

AGED 25 YEARS AND OVER

Weight in pounds according to frame (in indoor clothing)

Men

HEIGHT (with shoes on) 1-inch heels		Small frame	Medium frame	Large frame
Feet	Inches			
5	2	112-120	118-129	126-141
5	4	118-126	124-136	132-148
5	6	124-133	130-143	138-156
5	8	132-141	138-152	147-166
5	10	140-150	146-160	155-174
6	0	148-158	154-170	164-184
6	2	156-167	162-180	173-194
6	4	164-175	172-190	182-204

Women

HEIGHT (with shoes on) 2-inch heels				
Feet	Inches			
4	10	92- 98	96-107	104-119
5	0	96-104	101-113	109-125
5	2	102-110	107-119	115-131
5	4	108-116	113-126	121-138
5	6	114-123	120-135	129-146
5	8	122-131	128-143	137-154
5	10	130-140	136-151	145-163
6	0	138-148	144-159	153-173

For girls between 18 and 25, subtract 1 pound for each year under 25

(By Courtesy of Metropolitan Life Insurance Company)

Normal Blood Chemistry

(Values are those in the serum unless otherwise stated)

	m.Eq. per litre	content per 100 ml.
Amylase (Wohlegemuth units)		3–10 units per ml.
Bicarbonate (Alkali reserve)	22–34	53–77 ml.CO_2
Bilirubin, total		0·1–1·0 mg.
,, direct		0·1–0·2 mg.
,, indirect		0·1–0·8 mg.
Calcium	4·5–5·5	9–11 mg.
Chloride (as Cl)	95–110	350–375 mg.
,, (as NaCl)	95–110	560–620 mg.
Cholesterol (total in plasma)		150–260 mg.
,, (as esters in plasma)		100–180 mg.
,, ester fraction of total		60–75 per cent.
Copper		90–120 μg.
Creatinine		1–2 mg.
Glucose		80–160 mg.
Iron (Men)		80–150 μg.
,, (Women)		60–120 μg.
,, binding capacity		300–350 μg.
Phosphatase, acid		1–3 K.A. units
,, alkaline		3–13 K.A. units
Phosphate (adult as P)		2–4 mg.
,, (children as P)		4–6 mg.
Potassium	3·9–5·5	15–22 mg.
pH		7·36–7·44
Proteins, Total		5·6–8·5 G.
Albumen		4·0–6·7 G.
Fibrinogen (in plasma)		0·2–0·4 G.
Total globulin		1·2–2·9 G.
α_1 ,,		0·1–0·5 G.
α_2 ,,		0·4–1·4 G.
β ,,		0·4–1·2 G.
γ ,,		0·7–1·5 G.
Pyruvate (Whole blood, fasting)		0·6–1·4 mg.
Sodium	135–150	315–350 mg.
Sugar (fasting)		80–120 mg.
Transaminase, S.G.O.T.		up to 40 Sigma-Frankel
S.G.P.T.		units per ml.
Urea		15–40 mg.
Uric acid (colorimetric method)		1·5–6 mg.
Vitamin B_{12} (microbiological assay)		above 150 $\mu\mu$g.

Normal Cerebro-spinal Fluid

Cells (lymphocytes)	0–5 per c.mm.
Colloidal Gold (Lange)	not above 1 in any tube
Chloride (as NaCl)	720–750 mg. per cent.
Pressure (Recumbent)	60–150 mm.
Protein	20–50 mg. per cent.
Sugar	50–70 mg. per cent.
Total volume	60–150 ml.